a LANGE medical book

Basic &
Clinical
Pharmacology

Seventh Edition

Edited By
Bertram G. Katzung, MD, PhD
Professor of Pharmacology
Department of Cellular and Molecular Pharmacology
University of California, San Francisco

Lange Medical Books/McGraw-Hill
Health Professions Division

New York St. Louis San Francisco Auckland Bogotá Caracas Lisbon London
Madrid Mexico City Milan Montreal New Delhi San Juan
Singapore Sydney Tokyo Toronto

McGraw-Hill

*A Division of The **McGraw·Hill** Companies*

99 00 01 02 / 10 9 8 7 6 5 4

ISBN: 0-8385-0565-1
ISSN: 0891-2033

Acquisitions Editor: John P. Butler
Development Editor: Jim Ransom
Production Editor: Christine Langan
Associate Art Manager: Maggie Belis Darrow
Illustrators: Teshin Associates

PRINTED IN THE UNITED STATES OF AMERICA

ISBN 0-8385-0565-1

9 780838 505656

90000

Contents

Preface vii

The Authors ix

I. BASIC PRINCIPLES

1. Introduction 1
   Bertram G. Katzung, MD, PhD

2. Drug Receptors & Pharmacodynamics 9
   Henry R. Bourne, MD

3. Pharmacokinetics & Pharmacodynamics: Dose Selection
   & the Time Course of Drug Action 34
   Nicholas H.G. Holford, MB, ChB, FRACP, & Leslie Z. Benet, PhD

4. Drug Biotransformation 50
   Maria Almira Correia, PhD

5. Basic & Clinical Evaluation of New Drugs. 62
   Barry A. Berkowitz, PhD, & Bertram G. Katzung, MD, PhD

II. AUTONOMIC DRUGS

6. Introduction to Autonomic Pharmacology. 73
   Bertram G. Katzung, MD, PhD

7. Cholinoceptor-Activating & Cholinesterase-Inhibiting Drugs. 90
   Achilles J. Pappano, PhD

8. Cholinoceptor-Blocking Drugs. 105
   Bertram G. Katzung, MD, PhD

9. Adrenoceptor-Activating & Other Sympathomimetic Drugs. 118
   Brian B. Hoffman, MD

10. Adrenoceptor Antagonist Drugs 136
    Brian B. Hoffman, MD

III. CARDIOVASCULAR-RENAL DRUGS

11. Antihypertensive Agents 153
    Neal L. Benowitz, MD

12. Vasodilators & the Treatment of Angina Pectoris 179
    Bertram G. Katzung, MD, PhD, & Kanu Chatterjee, MB, FRCP

13. Cardiac Glycosides & Other Drugs Used in Congestive Heart Failure 197
    Bertram G. Katzung, MD, PhD, & William W. Parmley, MD

14. **Agents Used in Cardiac Arrhythmias** **216**
Luc M. Hondeghem, MD, PhD, & Dan M. Roden, MD

15. **Diuretic Agents**. **242**
Harlan E. Ives, MD, PhD

IV. DRUGS WITH IMPORTANT ACTIONS ON SMOOTH MUSCLE

16. **Histamine, Serotonin, & the Ergot Alkaloids**. **261**
Alan Burkhalter, PhD, David J. Julius, PhD, & Bertram G. Katzung, MD, PhD

17. **Vasoactive Peptides**. **287**
Ian A. Reid, PhD

18. **The Eicosanoids: Prostaglandins, Thromboxanes, Leukotrienes,
& Related Compounds**. **304**
Marie L. Foegh, MD, Markus Hecker, PhD, & Peter W. Ramwell, PhD

19. **Nitric Oxide, Donors, & Inhibitors** **319**
George Thomas, PhD, & Peter W. Ramwell, PhD

20. **Bronchodilators & Other Agents Used in Asthma** **325**
Homer A. Boushey, MD

V. DRUGS THAT ACT IN THE CENTRAL NERVOUS SYSTEM

21. **Introduction to the Pharmacology of CNS Drugs** **343**
Roger A. Nicoll, MD

22. **Sedative-Hypnotic Drugs** **354**
Anthony J. Trevor, PhD, & Walter L. Way, MD

23. **The Alcohols** **372**
Susan B. Masters, PhD, & Nancy M. Lee, PhD

24. **Antiepileptic Drugs**. **386**
Roger J. Porter, MD, & Brian S. Meldrum, MB, PhD

25. **General Anesthetics**. **409**
Anthony J. Trevor, PhD, & Ronald D. Miller, MD

26. **Local Anesthetics**. **425**
Ronald D. Miller, MD

27. **Skeletal Muscle Relaxants** **434**
Ronald D. Miller, MD

28. **Pharmacologic Management of Parkinsonism & Other Movement Disorders** **450**
Michael J. Aminoff, MD, FRCP

29. **Antipsychotic Agents & Lithium** **464**
William Z. Potter, MD, PhD, & Leo E. Hollister, MD

30. **Antidepressant Agents** **483**
William Z. Potter, MD, PhD, & Leo E. Hollister, MD

31. **Opioid Analgesics & Antagonists** **496**
Walter L. Way, MD, Howard L. Fields, MD, PhD, & E. Leong Way, PhD

32. **Drugs of Abuse** **516**
Thomas R. Kosten, MD, & Leo E. Hollister, MD

VI. DRUGS USED TO TREAT DISEASES OF THE BLOOD, INFLAMMATION, & GOUT

33. Agents Used in Anemias; Hematopoietic Growth Factors **533**
Daniel V. Santi, MD, PhD, & Curt A. Ries, MD

34. Drugs Used in Disorders of Coagulation **547**
Robert A. O'Reilly, MD

35. Agents Used in Hyperlipidemia **563**
Mary J. Malloy, MD, & John P. Kane, MD, PhD

36. Nonsteroidal Anti-inflammatory Drugs; Disease-Modifying Antirheumatic Drugs; Nonopioid Analgesics; Drugs Used in Gout **578**
Bertram G. Katzung, MD, PhD, & Daniel E. Furst, MD

VII. ENDOCRINE DRUGS

37. Hypothalamic & Pituitary Hormones **603**
Paul A. Fitzgerald, MD, & David C. Klonoff, MD

38. Thyroid & Antithyroid Drugs **619**
Francis S. Greenspan, MD, & Betty J. Dong, PharmD

39. Adrenocorticosteroids & Adrenocortical Antagonists **635**
Alan Goldfien, MD

40. The Gonadal Hormones & Inhibitors **653**
Alan Goldfien, MD

41. Pancreatic Hormones & Antidiabetic Drugs **684**
John H. Karam, MD

42. Agents That Affect Bone Mineral Homeostasis **706**
Daniel D. Bikle, MD, PhD

VIII. CHEMOTHERAPEUTIC DRUGS

43. Beta-Lactam Antibiotics & Other Inhibitors of Cell Wall Synthesis **724**
Henry F. Chambers, MD, W. Keith Hadley, MD, PhD, & Ernest Jawetz, MD, PhD

44. Chloramphenicol, Tetracyclines, Macrolides, Clindamycin, & Streptogramins **743**
Henry F. Chambers, MD

45. Aminoglycosides & Spectinomycin **752**
Henry F. Chambers, MD, W. Keith Hadley, MD, PhD, & Ernest Jawetz, MD, PhD

46. Sulfonamides, Trimethoprim, & Quinolones **761**
Henry F. Chambers, MD, & Ernest Jawetz, MD, PhD

47. Antimycobacterial Drugs **770**
Henry F. Chambers, MD, & Ernest Jawetz, MD, PhD

48. Antifungal Agents **780**
Don Sheppard, MD, & Harry W. Lampiris, MD

49. Antiviral Agents **788**
Sharon Safrin, MD, & Henry F. Chambers, MD

50. Miscellaneous Antimicrobial Agents; Disinfectants, Antiseptics, & Sterilants **803**
Henry F. Chambers, MD, & W. Keith Hadley, MD, PhD

51. Clinical Use of Antimicrobial Agents 812
Harry W. Lampiris, MD, & Daniel S. Maddix, PharmD

52. Basic Principles of Antiparasitic Chemotherapy 827
Ching Chung Wang, PhD

53. Antiprotozoal Drugs 838
Robert S. Goldsmith, MD, DTM&H

54. Clinical Pharmacology of the Anthelmintic Drugs 862
Robert S. Goldsmith, MD, DTM&H

55. Cancer Chemotherapy 881
Sydney E. Salmon, MD, & Alan C. Sartorelli, PhD

56. Immunopharmacology 916
Jose Alexandre M. Barbuto, MD, PhD, Emmanuel T. Akporiaye, PhD, & Evan M. Hersh, MD

IX. TOXICOLOGY

57. Introduction to Toxicology: Occupational & Environmental 945
Gabriel L. Plaa, PhD

58. Chelators & Heavy Metal Intoxication 956
Michael J. Kosnett, MD, MPH, & Charles E. Becker, MD

59. Management of the Poisoned Patient 968
Kent R. Olson, MD, & Charles E. Becker, MD

X. SPECIAL TOPICS

60. Special Aspects of Perinatal & Pediatric Pharmacology 979
Gideon Koren, MD

61. Special Aspects of Geriatric Pharmacology 989
Bertram G. Katzung, MD, PhD

62. Dermatologic Pharmacology 999
Dirk B. Robertson, MD, & Howard I. Maibach, MD

63. Drugs Used in Gastrointestinal Diseases 1017
David F. Altman, MD

64. Therapeutic & Toxic Potential of Over-the-Counter Agents 1030
Mary Anne Koda-Kimble, PharmD

65. Rational Prescribing & Prescription Writing 1041
Paul W. Lofholm, PharmD, & Bertram G. Katzung, MD, PhD

Appendix I. Vaccines, Immune Globulins, & Other Complex Biologic Products 1051
Harry W. Lampiris, MD, Daniel S. Maddix, PharmD, & Steven L. Barriere, PharmD

Appendix II. Important Drug Interactions & Their Mechanisms 1059
Philip D. Hansten, PharmD

Index 1071

Preface

This book is designed to provide a complete, authoritative, current, and readable pharmacology text for medical, pharmacy, and other health science students. It also offers special features that make it useful to house officers and practicing clinicians.

Information is organized according to the sequence used in many pharmacology courses: basic principles; autonomic drugs; cardiovascular-renal drugs; drugs with important actions on smooth muscle; central nervous system drugs; drugs used to treat inflammation, gout, and diseases of the blood; endocrine drugs; chemotherapeutic drugs; toxicology; and special topics. This sequence builds new information on a foundation of information already assimilated. For example, early presentation of autonomic pharmacology allows students to integrate the physiology and neuroscience they know with the pharmacology they are learning and prepares them to understand the autonomic effects of other drugs. This is especially important for the cardiovascular and central nervous system groups. However, chapters can be used equally well in courses that present these topics in a different sequence.

Within each chapter, emphasis is placed on drug groups and prototypes rather than repetitive detail about individual drugs. The selection and order of presentation of material are drawn from the accumulated experience of teaching this material to several thousand medical, pharmacy, dental, podiatry, nursing, and other health science students.

Major features that make this book especially useful to professional students include sections that specifically address the clinical choice and use of drugs in patients and the monitoring of their effects; *clinical pharmacology* is an integral part of this text. In addition, lists of the preparations available, including trade and generic names and dosage formulations, are provided at the end of each chapter for easy reference by the house officer or practitioner who is writing a chart order or prescription.

Because of the explosive increase in the number of recognized receptors, receptor nomenclature is unstable at present. In order to minimize discrepancies, we have in most cases chosen to use the receptor names given in the 1996 issue of *Receptor Nomenclature Supplement* (special annual issue of *Trends in Pharmacological Sciences*). Enzymes are named according to the contributor's judgment of the best current usage, usually that of *1992 Enzyme Nomenclature,* Academic Press, 1992.

Significant revisions in this edition include the following:

- Many new figures, most in color, that help to clarify important concepts in pharmacology
- Additional special interest text boxes that provide working examples of the text material or serve to point out items of special interest such as the cardiac toxicity of second generation antihistamines
- Continuing expansion of the coverage of general concepts relating to receptors and listings of newly discovered receptors
- A new chapter on nitric oxide, an important endogenous substance and potential therapeutic agent
- Major revision of the entire section on antimicrobial chemotherapy
- Major revisions of chapters on CNS drugs, including antipsychotic and antidepressant agents, and the coverage of substance abuse
- Recent changes in the clinical management of asthma, congestive heart failure, hypertension, AIDS, and Alzheimer's disease
- A new section on prescribing by health professionals other than physicians
- Descriptions of important new drugs released through December 1996
- Revised bibliographies with many new references through 1996

Two related sources of information are:

Pharmacology: Examination & Board Review, 4th ed. (Katzung BG, Trevor AJ; Appleton & Lange, 1995) provides a succinct review of pharmacology with one of the largest available collections of sample examination questions and answers. It is especially helpful to students preparing for board-type examinations.

Drug Therapy, 2nd ed. (Katzung BG [editor]; Appleton & Lange, 1991), is a pocket-size reference to the properties, prescribing, and use of drugs on hospital wards and in outpatient practice. This clinical manual is designed for students in clinical training, house staff, and practicing physicians.

The widespread acceptance of the first six editions of *Basic & Clinical Pharmacology* over more than a decade suggests that this book fills an important need. We believe that the seventh edition will satisfy this need even more effectively. Spanish, Portuguese, Italian, Czech, and Indonesian translations are available. Translations into other languages are under way; the publisher may be contacted for additional information.

I wish to acknowledge the ongoing efforts of my contributing authors and the major contributions of the staff at Appleton & Lange and of our editor, James Ransom. I also wish to thank my wife, Alice, for her expert proofreading contributions since the first edition.

Suggestions and comments about *Basic & Clinical Pharmacology* are always welcome. They may be sent to me at the Department of Cellular & Molecular Pharmacology, Box 0450, S-1210, University of California, San Francisco, CA 94143-0450.

Bertram G. Katzung, MD, PhD

San Francisco
September, 1997

The Authors

Emmanuel T. Akporiaye, PhD
Associate Professor, College of Medicine, Department of Microbiology and Immunology, University of Arizona, Tucson

David F. Altman, MD
The Lewin Group, Sausalito, California

Michael J. Aminoff, MD, FRCP
Professor of Neurology and Attending Physician, Department of Neurology, University of California, San Francisco

Jose Alexandre M. Barbuto, MD, PhD
Assistant Professor, Institute of Biomedical Science, Department of Immunology, University of São Paulo, São Paulo, Brazil

Steven L. Barriere, PharmD
Consultant, New Product Development, Smith-Kline Beecham Pharmaceuticals, Longmont, Colorado

Charles E. Becker, MD
Clinical Professor of Medicine, University of Colorado, Denver

Leslie Z. Benet, PhD
Professor and Chairman, Department of Pharmacy, School of Pharmacy, University of California, San Francisco

Neal L. Benowitz, MD
Professor of Medicine and Chief, Division of Clinical Pharmacology and Experimental Therapeutics, Department of Medicine, University of California, San Francisco

Barry A. Berkowitz, PhD
President and CEO, ChemGenics Pharmaceuticals, Inc, Cambridge, Massachusetts

Daniel D. Bikle, MD, PhD
Professor of Medicine, Department of Medicine, and Co-director, Special Diagnostic and Treatment Unit, University of California, San Francisco, and Veterans Administration Medical Center, San Francisco

Henry R. Bourne, MD
Professor, Departments of Cellular and Molecular Pharmacology and Medicine, University of California, San Francisco

Homer A. Boushey, MD
Professor of Medicine, Department of Medicine, University of California, San Francisco

Alan Burkhalter, PhD
Professor of Pharmacology, Department of Cellular and Molecular Pharmacology, University of California, San Francisco

Henry F. Chambers, MD
Associate Professor of Medicine in Residence, University of California, San Francisco General Hospital

Kanu Chatterjee, MB, FRCP
Lucie Stern Professor of Cardiology and Professor of Medicine, Cardiology Division, Department of Medicine, University of California, San Francisco

Maria Almira Correia, PhD
Professor of Pharmacology, Department of Cellular and Molecular Pharmacology, University of California, San Francisco

Betty J. Dong, PharmD
Clinical Professor of Pharmacy and Family and Community Medicine, Schools of Pharmacy and Medicine, University of California, San Francisco

Howard L. Fields, MD, PhD
Professor of Neurology and Physiology, Departments of Neurology and Physiology, University of California, San Francisco

Paul A. Fitzgerald, MD
Associate Clinical Professor of Medicine, Department of Medicine, University of California, San Francisco

Marie L. Foegh, MD, DSc
Research Professor, Department of Surgery, Georgetown University Medical Center, Washington, DC

ix

Daniel E. Furst MD
Clinical Professor of Medicine and Rheumatology, University of Washington and Director, Arthritis Clinical Research Unit, Virginia Mason Research Center, Seattle

Alan Goldfien, MD
Professor of Medicine, Departments of Medicine, Obstetrics, Gynecology and Reproductive Sciences, and Senior Staff Member, Cardiovascular Research Institute, University of California, San Francisco

Robert S. Goldsmith, MD, DTM&H
Professor of Tropical Medicine and Epidemiology, Department of Epidemiology and International Health, University of California, San Francisco

Francis S. Greenspan, MD
Clinical Professor of Medicine and Radiology, Department of Medicine, and Chief, Thyroid Clinic, University of California, San Francisco

W. Keith Hadley, MD
Professor of Clinical Laboratory Medicine, University of California, San Francisco General Hospital

Philip D. Hansten, PharmD
Professor of Pharmacy, School of Pharmacy, University of Washington, Seattle, Washington

Markus Hecker, PhD
Associate Professor of Physiology, Johann Wolfgang Goethe-University Clinic, Frankfurt am Main, Germany

Evan M. Hersh, MD
Professor of Medicine, Department of Medicine, University of Arizona, and Chief, Hematology/Oncology, Arizona Cancer Center, Tucson

Brian B. Hoffman, MD
Professor of Medicine and Pharmacology, Stanford University School of Medicine, Stanford, California, and Veterans Administration Medical Center, Palo Alto, California

Nicholas H.G. Holford, MB, ChB, MSc, MRCP(UK), FRACP
Senior Lecturer, Department of Pharmacology and Clinical Pharmacology, University of Auckland Medical School, Auckland, New Zealand

Leo E. Hollister, MD
Professor of Psychiatry and Pharmacology, University of Texas Medical School, Houston, and Medical Director, Harris County Psychiatric Center, Houston

Luc M. Hondeghem, MD, PhD
President and CEO, Hondeghem Pharmaceutical Consulting NV, Oostende, Belgium

Harlan E. Ives, MD, PhD
Professor of Medicine, Department of Medicine, University of California, San Francisco

Ernest Jawetz, MD, PhD
Professor of Microbiology and Medicine, Emeritus, Department of Microbiology, University of California, San Francisco

David J. Julius, PhD
Associate Professor of Pharmacology, Department of Cellular and Molecular Pharmacology, University of California, San Francisco

John P. Kane MD, PhD
Professor of Medicine, Department of Medicine, University of California, San Francisco

John H. Karam, MD
Professor of Medicine, University of California, San Francisco

Bertram G. Katzung, MD, PhD
Professor of Pharmacology, Department of Cellular and Molecular Pharmacology, University of California, San Francisco

David C. Klonoff, MD
Associate Clinical Professor of Medicine, Department of Medicine, University of California, San Francisco

Mary Anne Koda-Kimble, PharmD
Long Professor of Clinical Pharmacy and Vice Chairman, Division of Clinical Pharmacy, School of Pharmacy, University of California, San Francisco

Gideon Koren, MD
Associate Professor of Pediatrics, Pharmacology, and Pharmacy, Departments of Pediatrics, Pharmacology, and Pharmacy, University of Toronto, Canada

Michael J. Kosnett, MD, MPH
Assistant Clinical Professor, Division of Clinical Pharmacology and Toxicology, University of Colorado Health Sciences Center, Denver

Thomas R. Kosten, MD
Professor of Psychiatry, Department of Psychiatry and Director, Substance Abuse Center, Yale University School of Medicine, New Haven

Harry W. Lampiris, MD
Assistant Professor of Medicine, Department of Medicine, University of California, Veterans Administration Hospital, San Francisco

Nancy M. Lee, PhD
Professor of Pharmacology, Department of Pharmacology, University of Minnesota, Minneapolis

Paul W. Lofholm, PharmD
Clinical Professor of Pharmacy, School of Pharmacy, University of California, San Francisco

Daniel S. Maddix, PharmD
Assistant Clinical Professor of Pharmacy, University of California, Veterans Administration Medical Center, San Francisco

Howard I. Maibach, MD
Professor of Dermatology, Department of Dermatology, University of California, San Francisco

Mary J. Malloy, MD
Clinical Professor of Pediatrics and Medicine, Departments of Pediatrics and Medicine, University of California, San Francisco

Susan B. Masters, PhD
Adjunct Assistant Professor of Pharmacology, Department of Cellular and Molecular Pharmacology, University of California, San Francisco

Brian S. Meldrum, MB, PhD
Professor of Experimental Neurology, Department of Neurology, Institute of Psychiatry, London

Ronald D. Miller, MD
Professor and Chairman of Anesthesia and Professor of Pharmacology, Department of Anesthesia, University of California, San Francisco

Roger A. Nicoll, MD
Professor of Pharmacology and Physiology, Departments of Cellular and Molecular Pharmacology and Physiology, University of California, San Francisco

Kent R. Olson, MD
Associate Clinical Professor of Medicine and Adjunct Lecturer in Pharmacy, University of California, San Francisco, and Director, San Francisco Bay Area Regional Poison Control Center

Robert A. O'Reilly, MD
Chairman, Department of Medicine, Santa Clara Valley Medical Center, Professor of Medicine, Stanford University School of Medicine, Stanford, California, and Clinical Professor of Medicine, Department of Medicine, University of California, San Francisco

Achilles J. Pappano, PhD
Professor and Chairman, Department of Pharmacology, University of Connecticut, Farmington

William W. Parmley, MD
Professor of Medicine, Department of Medicine, Cardiology Division, University of California, San Francisco, and Chief of Cardiology, Herbert C. Moffitt Hospital, San Francisco

Gabriel L. Plaa, PhD
Professeur Emerité de Pharmacologie, Départment de Pharmacologie, Faculté de Médecine, Université de Montréal

Roger J. Porter, MD
Adjunct Professor of Neurology, University of Pennsylvania, Philadelphia, Adjunct Professor of Pharmacology, Uniformed Services University of the Health Sciences, Bethesda, and Vice President, Clinical Pharmacology, Wyeth-Ayerst Research, Radnor, Pennsylvania

William Z. Potter, MD, PhD
Vice President, Eli Lilly Research, Indianapolis

Peter W. Ramwell, PhD
Professor, Department of Physiology and Biophysics, Georgetown University Medical Center, Washington, DC

Ian A. Reid, PhD
Professor of Physiology, Department of Physiology, University of California, San Francisco

Curt A. Ries, MD
Clinical Professor of Medicine and Hematology-Oncology, Department of Medicine, University of California, San Francisco

Dirk B. Robertson, MD
Associate Professor of Dermatology, Department of Dermatology, Emory University School of Medicine, Atlanta

Dan M. Roden, MD
Professor of Medicine and Pharmacology, Departments of Medicine and Pharmacology, Vanderbilt University, Nashville

Sharon Safrin, MD
Associate Professor, Departments of Medicine and Epidemiology and Statistics, University of California, San Francisco and Director, Clinical Research, Gilead Sciences, Inc

Sydney E. Salmon, MD
Professor of Internal Medicine and of Hematology and Oncology, University of Arizona College of Medicine, Tucson, and Director, Arizona Cancer Center, Tucson

Daniel V. Santi, MD, PhD
Professor of Biochemistry and Pharmaceutical Chemistry, Departments of Biochemistry and Biophysics and Pharmaceutical Chemistry, University of California, San Francisco

Alan C. Sartorelli, PhD
Alfred Gilman Professor of Pharmacology and Epidemiology, Yale University School of Medicine, New Haven

Don Sheppard, MD
Fellow, Infectious Diseases, Department of Medicine, University of California, San Francisco

George Thomas, PhD
Senior Scientist, Liposomes, Inc., Princeton, New Jersey

Anthony J. Trevor, PhD
Professor of Pharmacology and Toxicology, Department of Cellular and Molecular Pharmacology, University of California, San Francisco

Ching Chung Wang, PhD
Professor of Chemistry and Pharmaceutical Chemistry, Department of Pharmaceutical Chemistry, University of California, San Francisco

E. Leong Way, PhD
Professor Emeritus of Pharmacology, Toxicology, and Pharmaceutical Chemistry, Department of Cellular and Molecular Pharmacology, University of California, San Francisco

Walter L. Way, MD
Professor of Anesthesia and Pharmacology, Department of Anesthesia, University of California, San Francisco

Section I.
Basic Principles

Introduction

1

Bertram G. Katzung, MD, PhD

Pharmacology can be defined as the study of substances that interact with living systems through chemical processes, especially by binding to regulatory molecules and activating or inhibiting normal body processes. These substances may be chemicals administered to achieve a beneficial therapeutic effect on some process within the patient or for their toxic effects on regulatory processes in parasites infecting the patient. Such deliberate therapeutic applications may be considered the proper role of **medical pharmacology**, which is often defined as the science of substances used to prevent, diagnose, and treat disease. **Toxicology** is that branch of pharmacology that deals with the undesirable effects of chemicals on living systems, from individual cells to complex ecosystems.

History

Prehistoric people undoubtedly recognized the beneficial or toxic effects of many plant and animal materials. The earliest written records from China and from Egypt list remedies of many types, including a few still recognized today as useful drugs. Most, however, were worthless or actually harmful. In the 2500 years or so preceding the modern era there were sporadic attempts to introduce rational methods into medicine, but none were successful owing to the dominance of systems of thought that purported to explain all of biology and disease without the need for experimentation and observation. These schools promulgated bizarre notions such as the idea that disease was caused by excesses of bile or blood in the body, that wounds could be healed by applying a salve to the weapon that caused the wound, and so on.

Around the end of the 17th century, reliance on observation and experimentation began to replace theorizing in medicine, following the example of the physical sciences. As the value of these methods in the study of disease became clear, physicians in Great Britain and elsewhere in Europe began to apply them to the effects of traditional drugs used in their own practices. Thus, materia medica, the science of drug preparation and the medical use of drugs, began to develop as the precursor to pharmacology. However, any understanding of the mechanisms of action of drugs was prevented by the absence of methods for purifying active agents from the crude materials that were available and—even more—by the lack of methods for testing hypotheses about the nature of drug actions. However, in the late 18th and early 19th centuries, François Magendie and later his student Claude Bernard began to develop the methods of experimental animal physiology and pharmacology. Advances in chemistry and the further development of physiology in the 18th, 19th, and early 20th centuries laid the foundation needed for understanding how drugs work at the organ and tissue levels. Paradoxically, real advances in basic pharmacology during the 19th century were accompanied by an outburst of unscientific promotion by manufacturers and marketers of worthless "patent medicines." It was not until the concepts of rational therapeutics, especially that of the controlled clinical trial, were reintroduced into medicine—about 50 years ago—that it became possible to accurately evaluate therapeutic claims.

About 50 years ago, there also began a major expansion of research efforts in all areas of biology. As new concepts and new techniques were introduced, information accumulated about drug action and the biologic substrate of that action, the receptor. During this half-century, many fundamentally new drug groups and new members of old groups have been introduced. The last 3 decades have seen an even more rapid growth of information and understanding of the molecular basis for drug action. The molecular mechanisms of action of many drugs have now been identified, and numerous receptors have been isolated, structurally characterized, and cloned. Much of that progress is summarized in this book.

The extension of scientific principles into everyday therapeutics is still going on, though the medication-consuming public, unfortunately, is still exposed to vast amounts of inaccurate, incomplete, or unscientific information regarding the pharmacologic effects of chemicals. This has resulted in the faddish use of innumerable expensive, ineffective, and sometimes harmful remedies and the growth of a huge "alternative health care" industry. Conversely, lack of understanding of basic scientific principles in biology and statistics and the absence of critical thinking about public health issues has led to rejection of medical science by a segment of the public and a tendency to assume that all adverse drug effects are the result of malpractice.

The Nature of Drugs

In the most general sense, a drug may be defined as any substance that brings about a change in biologic function through its chemical actions. In the great majority of cases, the drug molecule interacts with a specific molecule in the biologic system that plays a regulatory role, ie, a **receptor** molecule. The nature of receptors is discussed more fully in Chapter 2. In a very small number of cases, drugs known as chemical antagonists may interact directly with other drugs, while a few drugs (eg, osmotic agents) interact almost exclusively with water molecules. Drugs may be synthesized within the body (eg, hormones) or may be chemicals *not* synthesized in the body, ie, xenobiotics (from Gr *xenos* "stranger"). Poisons are drugs. Toxins are usually defined as poisons of biologic origin, ie, synthesized by plants or animals, in contrast to inorganic poisons such as lead and arsenic.

In order to interact chemically with its receptor, a drug molecule must have the appropriate size, electrical charge, shape, and atomic composition. Furthermore, a drug is often administered at a location distant from its intended site of action, eg, a pill given orally to relieve a headache. Therefore, a useful drug must have the necessary properties to be transported from its site of administration to its site of action. Finally, a practical drug should be inactivated or excreted from the body at a reasonable rate so that its actions will be of appropriate duration.

A. The Physical Nature of Drugs: Drugs may be solid at room temperature (eg, aspirin, atropine), liquid (eg, nicotine, ethanol), or gaseous (eg, nitrous oxide). These factors often determine the best route of administration. For example, some liquid drugs are easily vaporized and can be inhaled in that form, eg, halothane, amyl nitrite. The common routes of administration are listed in Table 3–3. The various classes of organic compounds—carbohydrates, proteins, lipids, and their constituents—are all represented in pharmacology. Many drugs are weak acids or bases. This fact has important implications for the way they are handled by the body, because pH differences in the various compartments of the body may alter the degree of ionization of such drugs (see below).

B. Drug Size: The molecular size of drugs varies from very small (lithium ion, MW 7) to very large (eg, alteplase [t-PA], a protein of MW 59,050). However, the vast majority of drugs have molecular weights between 100 and 1000. The lower limit of this narrow range is probably set by the requirements for specificity of action. In order to have a good "fit" to only one type of receptor, a drug molecule must be sufficiently unique in shape, charge, etc, to prevent its binding to other receptors. To achieve such selective binding, it appears that a molecule should in most cases be at least 100 MW units in size. The upper limit in molecular weight is determined primarily by the requirement that drugs be able to move within the body (eg, from site of administration to site of action). Drugs much larger than MW 1000 will not diffuse readily between compartments of the body (see Permeation, below). Therefore, very large drugs (usually proteins) must be administered directly into the compartment where they have their effect. In the case of alteplase, a clot-dissolving enzyme, the drug is administered directly into the vascular compartment by intravenous infusion.

C. Drug Reactivity and Drug-Receptor Bonds: Drugs interact with receptors by means of chemical forces or bonds. These are of three major types: covalent, electrostatic, and hydrophobic. Covalent bonds are very strong and in many cases not reversible under biologic conditions. Thus, the covalent bond formed between the activated form of phenoxybenzamine and the alpha receptor for norepinephrine (which results in blockade of the receptor) is not readily broken. The blocking effect of phenoxybenzamine lasts long after the free drug has disappeared from the bloodstream and is reversed only by the synthesis of new alpha receptors, a process that takes about 48 hours. Other examples of highly reactive, covalent bond-forming drugs are the DNA-alkylating agents used in cancer chemotherapy to disrupt cell division in the neoplastic tissue.

Electrostatic bonding is much more common than covalent bonding in drug-receptor interactions. Electrostatic bonds vary from relatively strong linkages between permanently charged ionic molecules to weaker hydrogen bonds and very weak induced dipole interactions such as van der Waals forces and similar phenomena. Electrostatic bonds are weaker than covalent bonds.

Hydrophobic bonds are usually quite weak and are probably important in the interactions of highly lipid-soluble drugs with the lipids of cell membranes and perhaps in the interaction of drugs with the internal walls of receptor "pockets."

The specific nature of a particular drug-receptor bond is of less practical importance than the fact that drugs which bind through weak bonds to their receptors are generally more selective than drugs which bind through very strong bonds. This is because weak bonds require a very precise fit of the drug to its receptor if an interaction is to occur. Only a few receptor types are likely to provide such a precise fit for a particular drug structure. Thus, if we wished to design a highly selective short-acting drug for a particular receptor, we would avoid highly reactive molecules that form covalent bonds and instead choose molecules that form weaker bonds.

A few substances that are almost completely inert in the chemical sense nevertheless have significant pharmacologic effects. For example, xenon, an "inert gas," has anesthetic effects at elevated pressures.

D. Drug Shape: The shape of a drug molecule must be such as to permit binding to its receptor site. Optimally, the drug's shape is complementary to that of the receptor site in the same way that a key is complementary to a lock. Furthermore, the phenomenon of **chirality** (stereoisomerism) is so common in biology that more than half of all useful drugs are chiral molecules, ie, they exist as enantiomeric pairs. Drugs with two asymmetric centers have four diastereomers, eg, labetalol, an alpha- and beta-receptor-blocking drug. In the great majority of cases, one of these enantiomers will be much more effective than its mirror image enantiomer, reflecting a better fit to the receptor molecule. For example, the $S(+)$ enantiomer of methacholine, a parasympathomimetic drug, is over 250 times more potent than the $R(-)$ enantiomer. If one imagines the receptor site to be like a glove into which the drug molecule must fit to bring about its effect, it is clear why a "left-oriented" drug will be more effective in binding to a left-hand receptor than will its "right-oriented" enantiomer.

The more active enantiomer at one type of receptor site may not be more active at another type, eg, a receptor type that may be responsible for some unwanted effect. For example, carvedilol, a drug that interacts with adrenoceptors, has a single chiral center and thus two enantiomers (Table 1–1). One of these enantiomers, the $S(-)$ isomer, is a potent beta receptor blocker. The $R(+)$ isomer is 100-fold weaker at the beta receptor. However, the isomers are approximately equipotent as alpha receptor blockers. Ketamine is an intravenous anesthetic. The $(+)$ enantiomer is a more potent anesthetic and is less toxic than the $(-)$ enantiomer. Unfortunately, the drug is still used as the racemic mixture.

Finally, because enzymes are usually stereoselective, one drug enantiomer is often more susceptible than the other to drug-metabolizing enzymes. As a result, the duration of action of one enantiomer may be quite different from that of the other.

Unfortunately, most studies of clinical efficacy and drug elimination in humans have been carried out with racemic mixtures of drugs rather than with the separate enantiomers. At present, only about 45% of the chiral drugs used clinically are marketed as the active isomer—the rest are available only as racemic mixtures. As a result, many patients are receiving drug doses of which 50% or more is either inactive or actively toxic. However, there is increasing interest—at both the scientific and the regulatory levels—in making more chiral drugs available as their active enantiomers.

E. Rational Drug Design: Rational design of drugs implies the ability to predict the appropriate molecular structure of a drug on the basis of information about its biologic receptor. Until recently, no receptor was known in sufficient detail to permit such drug design. Instead, drugs were developed through random testing of chemicals or modification of drugs already known to have some effect (Chapter 5). However, during the past 2 decades, many receptors have been isolated and characterized. A few drugs now in use were developed through molecular design based on a knowledge of the three-dimensional structure of the receptor site. Computer programs are now available that can iteratively optimize drug structures to fit known receptors. As more becomes known about receptor structure, rational drug design will become more feasible.

F. Receptor Nomenclature: The spectacular success of the newer, more efficient ways to identify and characterize receptors (see Chapter 2, box: How Are Receptors Discovered?) has resulted in a variety of differing systems for naming them. This in turn has led to a number of suggestions regarding more rational methods of naming them. The interested reader is referred for details to the efforts of the International Union of Pharmacology (IUPHAR) *Committee on Receptor Nomenclature and Drug Classification* report (Pharmacol Rev 1994;46:111–229) and to the annual *Receptor and Ion Channel Nomenclature Supplements* published as special issues by the journal *Trends in Pharmacological Sciences* (TIPS). The chapters in this book mainly use these sources for naming receptors.

Table 1–1. Dissociation constants (K_d) of the enantiomers and racemate of carvedilol. The K_d is the concentration for 50% saturation of the receptors and is inversely proportionate to the affinity of the drug for the receptors.[1]

Form of Carvedilol	Inverse of Affinity for Alpha Receptors (K_d, nmol/L)	Inverse of Affinity for Beta Receptors (K_d, nmol/L)
$R(+)$ enantiomer	14	45
$S(-)$ enantiomer	16	0.4
$R,S(+/-)$ enantiomer	11	0.9

[1]Data from Ruffolo RR et al: The pharmacology of carvedilol. Eur J Pharmacol 1990;38:S82.

Drug-Body Interactions

The interactions between a drug and the body are conveniently divided into two classes. The actions o the drug on the body are termed **pharmacodynamic** processes and are presented in greater detail in Chapter 2. These properties determine the group in which the drug is classified and often play the major role in deciding whether that group is appropriate therapy for a particular symptom or disease. The actions of the body on the drug are called **pharmacokinetic** processes and are described in Chapters 3 and 4. Pharmacokinetic processes govern the absorption, distribution, and elimination of drugs and are of great practical importance in the choice and administration of a particular drug for a particular patient, eg, one with impaired renal function. The following paragraphs provide a brief introduction to pharmacodynamics and pharmacokinetics.

Pharmacodynamic Principles

As noted above, most drugs must bind to a receptor to bring about an effect. However, at the molecular level, drug binding is only the first in what is often a complex sequence of steps.

A. Types of Drug-Receptor Interactions: **Agonist** drugs bind to and *activate* the receptor in some fashion, which directly or indirectly brings about the effect. Some receptors incorporate effector machinery in the same molecule, so that drug binding brings about the effect directly, eg, opening of an ion channel or activation of enzyme activity. Other receptors are linked through one or more intervening **coupling molecules** to a separate **effector molecule.** The several types of drug-receptor-effector coupling systems are discussed in Chapter 2. Pharmacologic **antagonist** drugs, by binding to a receptor, *prevent* binding by other molecules. For example, acetylcholine receptor blockers such as atropine are antagonists because they prevent access of acetylcholine and similar agonist drugs to the acetylcholine receptor. These agents reduce the effects of acetylcholine and similar drugs in the body.

B. Agonists That Inhibit Their Binding Molecules and Partial Agonists: Some drugs mimic agonist drugs by inhibiting the molecules responsible for terminating the action of an endogenous agonist. For example, acetylcholinesterase inhibitors, by slowing the destruction of endogenous acetylcholine, cause cholinomimetic effects that closely resemble the actions of cholinoceptor agonist molecules even though cholinesterase inhibitors do not—or only incidentally do—bind to cholinoceptors (see Chapter 7: Cholinoceptor-Activating & Cholinesterase-Inhibiting Drugs). Other drugs bind to receptors and activate them but do not evoke as great a response as so-called full agonists. Thus, pindolol, a β adrenoceptor "partial agonist," may act as either an agonist (if no full agonist is present) or as an antagonist (if a full agonist such as isoproterenol is present). (See Chapter 2.)

C. Duration of Drug Action: Termination of drug action at the receptor level results from one of several processes. In some cases, the effect lasts only

as long as the drug occupies the receptor, so that dissociation of drug from the receptor automatically terminates the effect. In many cases, however, the action may persist after the drug has dissociated, because, for example, some coupling molecule is still present in activated form. In the case of drugs that bind covalently to the receptor, the effect may persist until the drug-receptor complex is destroyed and new receptors are synthesized, as described previously for phenoxybenzamine. Finally, some receptor-effector systems incorporate **desensitization** mechanisms for preventing excessive activation when drug molecules continue to be present for long periods. See Chapter 2 for additional details.

D. Receptors and Inert Binding Sites: To function as a receptor, an endogenous molecule must first be selective in choosing ligands (drug molecules) to bind; and second, it must change its function upon binding in such a way that the function of the biologic system (cell, tissue, etc) is altered. The first characteristic is required to avoid constant activation of the receptor by promiscuous binding of large numbers of ligands. The second characteristic is clearly necessary if the ligand is to cause a pharmacologic effect. The body contains many molecules that are capable of binding drugs, however, and not all of these endogenous molecules are regulatory molecules. Binding of a drug to a nonregulatory molecule such as plasma albumin will result in no detectable change in the function of the biologic system, so the endogenous molecule can be called an inert binding site. Such binding is not completely without significance, however, since it affects the distribution of drug within the body and will determine the amount of free drug in the circulation. Both of these factors are of pharmacokinetic importance (see below and Chapter 3).

Pharmacokinetic Principles

In practical therapeutics, a drug should be able to reach its intended site of action after administration by some convenient route. In only a few situations is it possible to directly apply a drug to its target tissue, eg, by topical application of an anti-inflammatory agent to inflamed skin or mucous membrane. In other cases, drugs may be given intravenously and circulate in the blood directly to target blood vessels in another part of the body where they bring about useful effects. Much more commonly, a drug is given into one body compartment, eg, the gut, and must move to its site of action in another compartment, eg, the brain. This requires that the drug be **absorbed** into the blood from its site of administration and **distributed** to its site of action, **permeating** through the various barriers that separate these compartments. For a drug given orally to produce an effect in the central nervous system, these barriers include the tissues that comprise the wall of the intestine, the walls of the capillaries that perfuse the gut, and the "blood-brain barrier," the walls of the capillaries that perfuse the brain. Finally, after bringing about its effect, a drug should be **eliminated** at a reasonable rate by metabolic inactivation, by excretion from the body, or by a combination of these processes.

A. Permeation: Drug permeation proceeds by four primary mechanisms. Passive diffusion in an aqueous or lipid medium is most common, but active processes play a role in the movement of some drugs, especially those whose molecules are too large to diffuse readily.

1. Aqueous diffusion–Aqueous diffusion occurs within the larger aqueous compartments of the body (interstitial space, cytosol, etc) and across epithelial membrane tight junctions and the endothelial lining of blood vessels through aqueous pores that permit the passage of molecules as large as MW 20,000–30,000.* Aqueous diffusion of drug molecules is usually driven by the concentration gradient of the permeating drug, a downhill movement described by Fick's law (see below). Drug molecules that are bound to large plasma proteins (eg, albumin) will not permeate these aqueous pores. If the drug is charged, its flux is also influenced by electrical fields (eg, the membrane potential and—in parts of the nephron—the transtubular potential).

2. Lipid diffusion–Lipid diffusion is the most important limiting factor for drug permeation because of the large number of lipid barriers that separate the compartments of the body. Because these lipid barriers separate aqueous compartments, the lipid:aqueous partition coefficient of a drug determines how readily the molecule moves between aqueous and lipid media. In the case of weak acids and weak bases (which gain or lose electrical charge-bearing protons, depending on the pH), the ability to move from aqueous to lipid or vice versa varies with the pH of the medium, because charged molecules attract water molecules. The ratio of lipid-soluble form to aqueous-soluble form for a weak acid or weak base is expressed by the **Henderson-Hasselbalch equation** (see below).

3. Special carriers–Special carrier molecules exist for certain substances that are important for cell function and too large or too insoluble in lipid to diffuse passively through membranes, eg, peptides, amino acids, glucose. These carriers bring about movement by active transport or facilitated diffusion and, unlike passive diffusion, are saturable and inhibitable. Because many drugs are or resemble such naturally occurring peptides, amino acids, or sugars, they can use these carriers to cross membranes.

4. Endocytosis and exocytosis–A few substances are so large that they can enter cells only by endocytosis, the process by which the substance is engulfed by the cell membrane and carried into the cell by pinching off of the newly formed vesicle inside the membrane. The substance can then be released inside the cytosol by breakdown of the vesicle membrane. This process is responsible for the transport of iron and vitamin B_{12}, each complexed with appropriate binding proteins, across the wall of the gut into the blood. The reverse process (exocytosis) is responsible for the secretion of many substances from cells. For example, many neurotransmitter substances are stored in membrane-bound vesicles in nerve endings to protect them from metabolic destruction in the cytoplasm. Appropriate activation of the nerve ending causes fusion of the storage vesicle with the cell membrane and expulsion of its contents into the extracellular space.

B. Fick's Law of Diffusion: The passive flux of molecules down a concentration gradient is given by Fick's law:

Flux (molecules per unit time) =

$$(C_1 - C_2) \times \frac{\text{Area} \times \text{Permeability coefficient}}{\text{Thickness}}$$

where C_1 is the higher concentration, C_2 is the lower concentration, area is the area across which diffusion is occurring, permeability coefficient is a measure of the mobility of the drug molecules in the medium of the diffusion path, and thickness is the thickness (length) of the diffusion path. In the case of lipid diffusion, the lipid:aqueous partition coefficient is a major determinant of mobility of the drug, since it determines how readily the drug enters the lipid membrane from the aqueous medium.

C. Ionization of Weak Acids and Weak Bases; the Henderson-Hasselbalch Equation: The electrostatic charge of an ionized molecule attracts water dipoles and results in a polar, relatively water-soluble and lipid-insoluble complex. Since lipid diffusion depends on relatively high lipid solubility, ionization of drugs may markedly reduce their ability to permeate membranes. A very large fraction of the drugs in use are weak acids or weak bases (Table 1–2). For drugs, a weak acid is best defined as a neutral molecule that can reversibly dissociate into an anion (a negatively charged molecule) and a proton (a hydrogen ion). For example, aspirin dissociates as follows:

$$C_8H_7O_2COOH \rightleftharpoons C_8H_7O_2COO^- + H^+$$

| **Neutral aspirin** | **Aspirin anion** | **Proton** |

A drug that is a weak base can be defined as a neutral molecule that can form a cation (a positively charged molecule) by combining with a proton. For example, pyrimethamine, an antimalarial drug, undergoes the following association-dissociation process:

---

*The capillaries of the brain and the testes are characterized by an absence of the pores that permit aqueous diffusion of many drug molecules into the tissue. These tissues are therefore "protected" or "sanctuary" sites from many circulating drugs.

Table 1–2. Ionization constants of some common drugs.

Drug	pKa[1]	Drug	pKa[1]	Drug	pKa[1]
Weak acids		**Weak bases (cont'd)**		**Weak bases (cont'd)**	
Acetaminophen	9.5	Amiloride	8.7	Methamphetamine	10.0
Acetazolamide	7.2	Amiodarone	6.56	Methyldopa	10.6
Ampicillin	2.5	Amphetamine	9.8	Methysergide	6.6
Aspirin	3.5	Atropine	9.7	Metoprolol	9.8
Chlorothiazide	6.8, 9.4[2]	Bupivacaine	8.1	Morphine	7.9
Chlorpropamide	5.0	Chlordiazepoxide	4.6	Nicotine	7.9, 3.1[2]
Ciprofloxacin	6.09, 8.74[2]	Chloroquine	10.8, 8.4[2]	Norepinephrine	8.6
Cromolyn	2.0	Chlorpheniramie	9.2	Pentazocine	9.7
Ethacrynic acid	3.5	Chlorpromazine	9.3	Phenylephrine	9.8
Furosemide	3.9	Clonidine	8.3	Physostigmine	7.9, 1.8[2]
Ibuprofen	4.4, 5.2[2]	Cocaine	8.5	Pilocarpine	6.9, 1.4[2]
Levodopa	2.3	Codeine	8.2	Pindolol	8.8
Methotrexate	4.8	Cyclizine	8.2	Procainamide	9.2
Methyldopa	2.2, 9.2[2]	Desipramine	10.2	Procaine	9.0
Penicillamine	1.8	Diazepam	3.3	Promazine	9.4
Pentobarbital	8.1	Dihydrocodeine	8.8	Promethazine	9.1
Phenobarbital	7.4	Diphenhydramine	9.0	Propranolol	9.4
Phenytoin	8.3	Diphenoxylate	7.1	Pseudoephedrine	9.8
Propylthiouracil	8.3	Ephedrine	9.6	Pyrimethamine	7.0
Salicylic acid	3.0	Epinephrine	8.7	Quinidine	8.5, 4.4[2]
Sulfadiazine	6.5	Ergotamine	6.3	Scopolamine	8.1
Sulfapyridine	8.4	Fluphenazine	8.0, 3.9[2]	Strychnine	8.0, 2.3[2]
Theophylline	8.8[2]	Guanethidine	11.4, 8.3[2]	Terbutaline	10.1
Tolbutamide	5.3	Hydralazine	7.1	Thioridazine	9.5
Warfarin	5.0	Imipramine	9.5	Tolazoline	10.6
Weak bases		Isoproterenol	8.6		
Albuterol	9.3	Kanamycin	7.2		
(salbutamol)		Lidocaine	7.9		
Allopurinol	9.4, 12.3[2]	Metaraminol	8.6		
Alprenolol	9.6	Methadone	8.4		

[1]The pKa is that pH which the concentrations of the ionized and un-ionized forms are equal.
[2]More than one ionizable group.

$$C_{12}H_{11}ClN_3NH_3^+ \rightleftharpoons C_{12}H_{11}ClN_3NH_2 + H^+$$

Pyrimethamine cation	Neutral pyrimethamine	Proton

Note that the protonated form of a weak acid is the neutral, more lipid-soluble form, whereas the unprotonated form of a weak base is the neutral form. The law of mass action requires that these reactions move to the left in an acid environment (low pH, excess protons available) and to the right in an alkaline environment. The Henderson-Hasselbalch equation relates the ratio of protonated to unprotonated weak acid or weak base to the molecule's pKa and the pH of the medium as follows:

$$\log \frac{(Protonated)}{(Unprotonated)} = pK_a - pH$$

This equation applies to both acidic and basic drugs. Inspection confirms that the lower the pH relative to the pKa, the greater will be the fraction of drug in the protonated form. Because the uncharged form is the more lipid-soluble, more of a weak acid will be in the lipid-soluble form at acid pH, while more of a basic drug will be in the lipid-soluble form at alkaline pH.

The most important application of this principle is in the manipulation of drug excretion by the kidney. Almost all drugs are filtered at the glomerulus. If a drug is in a lipid-soluble form during its passage down the renal tubule, a significant fraction will be reabsorbed by simple passive diffusion. If the goal is to accelerate excretion of the drug, it is important to prevent its reabsorption from the tubule. This can often be accomplished by adjusting urine pH to make certain that most of the drug is in the ionized state, as shown in Figure 1–1. As a result of this pH partitioning effect, the drug will be "trapped" in the urine. Thus, weak acids are usually excreted faster in alkaline urine; weak bases are usually excreted faster in acidic urine. Other body fluids in which pH differences from blood pH may cause trapping or reabsorption are the contents of the stomach and small intestine; breast milk; aqueous humor; and vaginal and prostatic secretions (Table 1–3).

As suggested by Table 1–2, a large number of drugs are weak bases. Most of these bases are amine-containing molecules. The nitrogen of a neutral amine has three atoms associated with it plus a pair of unshared electrons—see the display below. The three atoms may consist of one carbon (designated "R") and two hydrogens (a *primary* amine), two carbons and one hydrogen (a *secondary* amine), or three car-

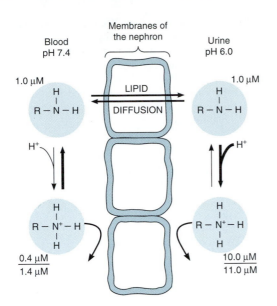

	Primary	Secondary	Tertiary	Quaternary
	H	R	R	R
	R:N̈:	R:N̈:	R:N̈:	R:N̈:+ R
	H	H	R	R

Figure 1–1. Trapping of a weak base (pyrimethamine) in the urine when the urine is more acidic than the blood. In the hypothetical case illustrated, the diffusible uncharged form of the drug has equilibrated across the membrane but the total concentration (charged plus uncharged) in the urine is almost eight times higher than in the blood.

Drug Groups

To learn each pertinent fact about each of the many hundreds of drugs mentioned in this book would be an impractical goal and, fortunately, is in any case unnecessary. Almost all of the several thousand drugs currently available can be arranged in about 70 groups. Many of the drugs within each group are very similar in pharmacodynamic actions and often in their pharmacokinetic properties as well. For most groups, one or more **prototype drugs** can be identified that typify the most important characteristics of the group. This permits classification of other important drugs in the group as variants of the prototype, so that only the prototype must be learned in detail and, for the remaining drugs, only the differences from the prototype.

Sources of Information

Students who wish to review the field of pharmacology in preparation for an examination are referred to *Pharmacology: Examination and Board Review*, by Katzung and Trevor (Appleton & Lange, 1995). *Drug Therapy*, edited by the present author (Appleton & Lange, 1991), is intended for use by house officers and practitioners who need ready access to a compendium of available drugs and drug doses.

The references at the end of each chapter in this book were selected to provide information specific to those chapters. Three textbooks (listed alphabetically on page eight) provide more general discussions and more extensive reference lists.

bon atoms (a *tertiary* amine). Each of these three forms may reversibly bind a proton with the unshared electrons. A fourth carbon-nitrogen bond may be formed, resulting in a *quaternary* amine. However, the quaternary amine is permanently charged and has no unshared electrons with which to reversibly bind a proton. Therefore, primary, secondary, and tertiary amines may undergo reversible protonation and vary their lipid solubility with pH, but quaternary amines are always in the poorly lipid-soluble charged form.

Table 1–3. Body fluids with potential for drug "trapping" through the pH-partitioning phenomenon.

Body Fluid	Range of pH	Total Fluid: Blood Concentration Ratios for Sulfadiazine (acid, pK$_a$ 6.5)[1]	Total Fluid: Blood Concentration Ratios for Pyrimethamine (base, pK$_a$ 7.0)[1]
Urine	5.0–8.0	0.12–4.65	72.24–0.79
Breast milk	6.4–7.6[2]	0.2–1.77	3.56–0.89
Jejunum, ileum contents	7.5–8.0[3]	1.23–3.54	0.94–0.79
Stomach contents	1.92–2.59[2]	0.11[4]	85,993–18,386
Prostatic secretions	6.45–7.4[2]	0.21	3.25–1.0
Vaginal secretions	3.4–4.2[3]	0.11[4]	2,848–452

[1]Body fluid protonated-to-unprotonated drug ratios were calculated using each of the pH extremes cited; a blood pH of 7.4 was used for blood drug ratio. For example, the urine:blood ratio for sulfadiazine is 0.12 at a urine pH of 5.0; this ratio is 4.65 at a urine pH of 8.0. Thus, sulfadiazine is much more effectively trapped and excreted in alkaline urine.
[2]Lentner C (editor): *Geigy Scientific Tables*, vol 1, 8th ed. Ciba Geigy, 1981.
[3]Bowman WC, Rand MJ: *Textbook of Pharmacology*, 2nd ed. Blackwell, 1980.
[4]Insignificant change in ratios over the physiologic pH range.

Bowman WC, Rand MJ: *Textbook of Pharmacology,* 2nd ed. Blackwell Scientific, 1980. (A large textbook with a chemical and comparative pharmacology orientation.)

Hardman JG et al (editors): *Goodman and Gilman's The Pharmacological Basis of Therapeutics,* 9th ed. Mc-Graw-Hill, 1996. (A large textbook with a medical orientation.)

Pratt WB, Taylor P: *Principles of Drug Action. The Basis of Therapeutics,* 3rd ed. Churchill Livingstone, 1990. (A specialized text emphasizing general principles: receptor concepts, dose-response principles, pharmacokinetics, and biochemical toxicology.)

Specific questions relating to basic or clinical research are best answered by resort to the general pharmacology and clinical specialty serials. For the student and the physician, three periodicals can be recommended as especially useful sources of current information about drugs: *The New England Journal of Medicine,* which publishes much original drug-related clinical research as well as frequent reviews of topics in pharmacology; *The Medical Letter on Drugs and Therapeutics,* which publishes brief critical reviews of new and old therapies, mostly pharmacologic; and *Drugs,* which publishes extensive reviews of drugs and drug groups.

Other sources of information pertinent to the USA should be mentioned as well. The "package insert" is a summary of information the manufacturer is required to place in the prescription sales package; *Physicians' Desk Reference (PDR)* is a compendium of package inserts published annually with supplements twice a year; *Facts and Comparisons* is a more complete loose-leaf drug information service with monthly updates; and the *USP DI* (vol 1, *Drug Information for the Health Care Professional*) is a large drug compendium with monthly updates. The package insert consists of a brief description of the pharmacology of the product. While this brochure contains much practical information, it is also used as a means of shifting liability for untoward drug reactions from the manufacturer onto the practitioner. Therefore, the manufacturer typically lists every toxic effect ever reported, no matter how rare. A useful and objective handbook that presents information on drug toxicity and interactions is *Drug Interactions.* Finally, the FDA has an Internet World Wide Web site that carries news regarding recent drug approvals, withdrawals, warnings, etc. It can be reached using a personal computer equipped with Internet browser software at http://www.fda.gov/fdahomepage.html.

The following addresses are provided for the convenience of readers wishing to obtain any of the publications mentioned above:

Drug Interactions
Lea & Febiger
600 Washington Square
Philadelphia, PA 19106

Facts and Comparisons
J.B. Lippincott Co.
111 West Port Plaza, Suite 423
St. Louis, MO 63146

Drug Therapy, 2nd ed
Appleton & Lange
Four Stamford Plaza
POB 120041
Stamford, CT 06912

Pharmacology: Examination & Board Review, 3rd ed
Appleton & Lange
Four Stamford Plaza
POB 120041
Stamford, CT 06912

The Medical Letter on Drugs and Therapeutics
56 Harrison St
New Rochelle, NY 10801

The New England Journal of Medicine
10 Shattuck Street
Boston, MA 02115

Physicians' Desk Reference
Box 2017
Mahopac, NY 10541

United States Pharmacopeia Dispensing Information
12601 Twinbrook Parkway
Rockville, MD 20852

Drug Receptors & Pharmacodynamics

Henry R. Bourne, MD

The therapeutic and toxic effects of drugs result from their interactions with molecules in the patient. Most drugs act by associating with specific macromolecules in ways that alter the macromolecules' biochemical or biophysical activities. This idea, now almost a century old, is embodied in the terms **receptive substance** and **receptor:** the component of a cell or organism that interacts with a drug and initiates the chain of biochemical events leading to the drug's observed effects.

Initially, the existence of receptors was inferred from observations of the chemical and physiologic specificity of drug effects. Thus, Ehrlich noted that certain synthetic organic agents had characteristic antiparasitic effects while other agents did not, though their chemical structures differed only slightly. Langley noted that curare did not prevent electrical stimulation of muscle contraction but did block contraction triggered by nicotine. From these simple beginnings, receptors have now become the central focus of investigation of drug effects and their mechanisms of action (pharmacodynamics). The receptor concept, extended to endocrinology, immunology, and molecular biology, has proved essential for explaining many aspects of biologic regulation. Drug receptors are now being isolated and characterized as macromolecules, thus opening the way to precise understanding of the molecular basis of drug action.

In addition to its usefulness for explaining biology, the receptor concept has important practical consequences for the development of drugs and for arriving at therapeutic decisions in clinical practice. These consequences—explained more fully in later sections of this chapter—form the basis for understanding the actions and clinical uses of drugs described in every chapter of this book. They may be briefly summarized as follows:

(1) Receptors largely determine the quantitative relations between dose or concentration of drug and pharmacologic effects: The receptor's affinity for binding a drug determines the concentration of drug required to form a significant number of drug-receptor complexes, and the total number of receptors often limits the maximal effect a drug may produce.

(2) Receptors are responsible for selectivity of drug action: The molecular size, shape, and electrical charge of a drug determine whether—and with what avidity—it will bind to a particular receptor among the vast array of chemically different binding sites available in a cell, animal, or patient. Accordingly, changes in the chemical structure of a drug can dramatically increase or decrease a new drug's affinities for different classes of receptors, with resulting alterations in therapeutic and toxic effects.

(3) Receptors mediate the actions of pharmacologic antagonists: Many drugs and endogenous chemical signals, such as hormones, regulate the function of receptor macromolecules as **agonists;** ie, they change the function of a macromolecule as a more or less direct result of binding to it. Pure pharmacologic **antagonists,** however, bind to receptors without directly altering their function. Thus, the effect of a pure antagonist on a cell or in a patient depends entirely upon its preventing the binding of agonist molecules and blocking their biologic actions. Some of the most useful drugs in clinical medicine are pharmacologic antagonists.

MACROMOLECULAR NATURE OF DRUG RECEPTORS

Until recently, the chemical structures and even the existence of receptors for most drugs could only be inferred from the chemical structures of the drugs themselves. Now, however, receptors for many drugs have been biochemically purified and characterized. The accompanying box describes some of the methods by which receptors are discovered and defined. Most receptors are proteins, presumably because the structures of polypeptides provide both the necessary diversity and the necessary specificity of shape and electrical charge.

The best-characterized drug receptors are **regulatory proteins,** which mediate the actions of endogenous chemical signals such as neurotransmitters, autacoids, and hormones. This class of receptors mediates the effects of many of the most useful therapeutic agents. The molecular structures and bio-

HOW ARE NEW RECEPTORS DISCOVERED?

Because today's new receptor sets the stage for tomorrow's new drug, it is important to know how new receptors are discovered. The discovery process follows a few key steps, summarized in Figure 2–1. As presented in greater detail elsewhere in this chapter, the process of defining a new receptor begins by studying the relations between structures and activities of a group of drugs on some conveniently measured response (stage 1 in Figure 2–1). Binding of radioactive ligands defines the molar abundance and binding affinities of the putative receptor and provides an assay to aid in its biochemical purification. Analysis of the pure receptor protein tells us the number of its subunits, its size, and (sometimes) provides a clue to how it works (eg, agonist-stimulated autophosphorylation on tyrosine residues, seen with receptors for insulin and many growth factors).

These "classic" steps in receptor identification serve as a warming-up exercise for a powerful new experimental strategy aimed at molecular cloning of the segment of DNA that encodes the receptor (stages 2–5 in Figure 2–1). The core of this strategy is the ability to identify a putative receptor DNA sequence in a representative population of cDNAs (DNA sequences complementary to their RNAs expressed in an appropriate cell or tissue, obtained by using reverse transcriptase). To do so (stage 2), investigators use biochemical and functional features of the receptor protein as handles for picking out the corresponding DNA. Thus, an antibody raised against the pure receptor protein or nucleic acid sequences based on the receptor's amino acid sequence may distinguish a bacterial colony containing putative receptor cDNA from colonies containing irrelevant DNA, by binding to receptor antigen expressed in the bacterium (2A), or by hybridizing to receptor DNA (2B), respectively. Alternatively, the population of cDNAs may be expressed as proteins in frog oocytes or vertebrate cells, and the putative receptor cDNA can then be detected by virtue of the protein's signaling function (2C) or its ability to bind a specific ligand (2D). Once the putative receptor cDNA has been identified, it is "validated" by carefully com-

paring the function and biochemical properties of the recombinant protein with those of the endogenous receptor that originally triggered the search (3A). The base sequence of the receptor DNA is also determined (3B), so that the amino acid sequence of the complete receptor protein can be deduced and compared with sequences of known receptors. Based on these criteria, it may then be possible to announce the identification of a new receptor (step 4).

A much greater quantity and quality of information flows from molecular cloning of the cDNA encoding a new receptor than from identifying a receptor in the "classic" way. The deduced amino acid sequence almost always resembles those of previously known receptors. Investigators can immediately place the new receptor into a specific class of known receptors, and the structural class tells us how the receptor works—whether it is a receptor tyrosine kinase, a seven-transmembrane region receptor coupled to G proteins, etc. The DNA sequence provides a probe to identify cells and tissues that express messenger RNA encoding the new receptor. Expression of the cDNA in cultured cells gives the pharmaceutical chemist an unlimited supply of recombinant receptor protein for precise biochemical analysis, tests of agonist and antagonist binding, and development of new drugs.

Finally (step 5), the receptor DNA itself provides a tool for identifying yet more receptors. Receptors within a specific class or subclass contain highly conserved regions of similar or identical amino acid (and therefore DNA) sequence. The DNA sequences corresponding to these conserved regions can be used as probes to find sequences of related but potentially novel receptors, either by DNA–DNA hybridization (2B) or as primers in a polymerase chain reaction (PCR) designed to amplify receptor DNA sequences (2E). These probes may lead to cloning DNA encoding a receptor whose ligand is unknown (an "orphan" receptor); the appropriate ligand is then sought by testing for functional and binding interactions with the recombinant receptor.

---

chemical mechanisms of these regulatory receptors are described in a later section entitled Signaling Mechanisms and Drug Action.

Other classes of proteins that have been clearly identified as drug receptors include **enzymes,** which may be inhibited (or, less commonly, activated) by binding a drug (eg, dihydrofolate reductase, the receptor for the antineoplastic drug methotrexate);

transport proteins (eg, Na^+/K^+ ATPase, the membrane receptor for cardioactive digitalis glycosides); and **structural proteins** (eg, tubulin, the receptor for colchicine, an anti-inflammatory agent).

This chapter deals with three aspects of drug receptor function, presented in increasing order of complexity: (1) The first aspect is their function as determinants of the quantitative relation between the

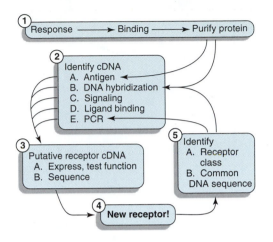

Figure 2–1. Methods used in the discovery and description of receptors.

concentration of a drug and the pharmacologic response. From this point of view, receptors are simple entities, principally characterized by their affinity for binding drug ligands and their abundance in target cells or tissues. (2) The second aspect is their function as regulatory proteins and components of chemical signaling mechanisms that provide targets for important drugs. Here receptors are considered as complex molecules whose structures and biochemical functions help to explain key features of concentration-effect relations, as well as pharmacologic selectivity. (3) The third aspect is their function as key elements of the therapeutic and toxic effects of drugs in patients. At this highest level of complexity, we discuss the crucial roles receptors play in determining selectivity of drug action, the relation between the dose of a drug and its effects, and the therapeutic usefulness of a drug (ie, therapeutic effectiveness versus toxicity).

RELATION BETWEEN DRUG CONCENTRATION & RESPONSE

The relation between dose of a drug and the clinically observed response may be quite complex. In carefully controlled in vitro systems, however, the relation between concentration of a drug and its effect is often simple and can be described with mathematical precision. This idealized relation underlies the more complex relations between dose and effect that occur when drugs are given to patients.

Concentration-Effect Curves & Receptor Binding of Agonists

Even in intact animals or patients, responses to low doses of a drug usually increase in direct proportion to dose. As doses increase, however, the response increment diminishes; finally, doses may be reached at

which no further increase in response can be achieved. In idealized or in vitro systems, the relation between drug concentration and effect is described by a hyperbolic curve (Figure 2–2A) according to the following equation:

$$E = \frac{E_{max} \times C}{C + EC50}$$

where E is the effect observed at concentration C, E_{max} is the maximal response that can be produced by the drug, and EC50 is the concentration of drug that produces 50% of maximal effect.

This hyperbolic relation resembles the mass action law, which predicts association between two molecules of a given affinity. This resemblance suggests that drug agonists act by binding to ("occupying") a distinct class of biologic molecules with a characteristic affinity for the drug receptor. With the advent of radioactive receptor ligands, including both agonists and antagonists, this occupancy assumption has been amply confirmed for a number of drug-receptor systems. In these systems, the relation between drug bound to receptors (B) and the concentration of free (unbound) drug (C) depicted in Figure 2–2B is described by an analogous equation:

$$B = \frac{B_{max} \times C}{C + K_D}$$

in which B_{max} indicates the total concentration of receptor sites (ie, sites bound to the drug at infinitely high concentrations of free drug). K_D (the equilibrium dissociation constant) represents the concentration of free drug at which half-maximal binding is observed. This constant characterizes the receptor's affinity for binding the drug in a reciprocal fashion: If the K_D is low, binding affinity is high, and vice versa.

Note also that the EC50 and K_D may be identical but need not be, as discussed below.

Graphic representation of dose-response data is frequently improved by plotting the drug effect (ordinate) against the *logarithm* of the dose or concentration (abscissa). The effect of this mathematical maneuver is to transform the hyperbolic curve of Figure 2–2 into a sigmoid curve with a linear midportion (eg, Figure 2–3). This transformation makes it easier to compare dose-response curves graphically because it expands the scale of the concentration axis at low concentrations (where the effect is changing rapidly) and compresses it at high concentrations (where the effect is changing slowly). This transformation has no special biologic or pharmacologic significance.

Receptor-Effector Coupling & Spare Receptors

When a receptor is occupied by an agonist, the resulting conformational change is only the first of

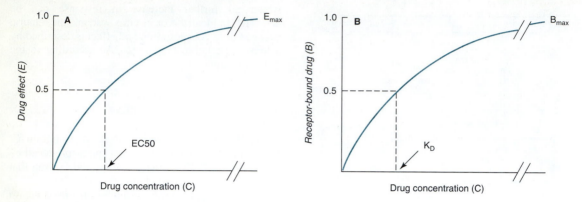

Figure 2–2. Relations between drug concentration and drug effect *(panel A)* or receptor-bound drug *(panel B)*. The drug concentrations at which effect or receptor occupancy is half-maximal are denoted EC50 and K_D, respectively.

many steps usually required to produce a pharmacologic response. The transduction process between occupancy of receptors and drug response is often termed coupling. The relative efficiency of occupancy-response coupling is partially determined by the initial conformational change in the receptor—thus, the effects of full agonists can be considered more efficiently coupled to receptor occupancy than can the effects of partial agonists, as described below.

Coupling efficiency is also determined by the biochemical events that transduce receptor occupancy into cellular response.

High efficiency of receptor-effector interaction may also be envisioned as the result of spare receptors. Receptors are said to be "spare" for a given pharmacologic response when the maximal response can be elicited by an agonist at a concentration that does not result in occupancy of the full complement of

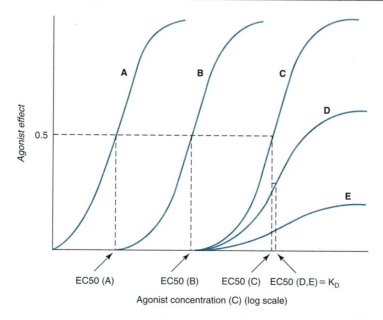

Figure 2–3. Experimental demonstration of spare receptors, using different concentrations of an irreversible antagonist. Curve **A** shows agonist response in the absence of antagonist. After treatment with a low concentration of antagonist (curve **B**), the curve is shifted to the right; maximal responsiveness is preserved, however, because the remaining available receptors are still in excess of the number required. In curve **C,** produced after treatment with a larger concentration of antagonist, the available receptors are no longer "spare"; instead, they are just sufficient to mediate an undiminished maximal response. Still higher concentrations of antagonist (curves **D** and **E**) reduce the number of available receptors to the point that maximal response is diminished. The apparent EC50 of the agonist in curves **D** and **E** may approximate the K_D that characterizes the binding affinity of the agonist for the receptor.

available receptors. Spare receptors are not qualitatively different from nonspare receptors. They are not hidden or unavailable, and when they are occupied they can be coupled to response. Experimentally, spare receptors may be demonstrated by using irreversible antagonists to prevent binding of agonist to a proportion of available receptors and showing that high concentrations of agonist can still produce an undiminished maximal response (Figure 2–3). Thus, a maximal inotropic response of heart muscle to catecholamines can be elicited even under conditions where 90% of the beta receptors are occupied by a quasi-irreversible antagonist. Accordingly, myocardium is said to contain a large proportion of spare beta receptors.

How can we account for the phenomenon of spare receptors? In a few cases, the biochemical mechanism is understood, such as for drugs that act on some regulatory receptors. In this situation, the effect of receptor activation—eg, binding of GTP by an intermediate—may greatly outlast the agonist-receptor interaction (see the following section on G Proteins and Second Messengers). In such a case, the "spareness" of receptors is *temporal* in that the response initiated by an individual ligand-receptor binding event persists longer than the binding event itself.

In other cases, where the biochemical mechanism is not understood, we imagine that the receptors are *spare in number*. If the concentration or amount of a cellular component other than the receptor limits the coupling of receptor occupancy to response, then a maximal response can occur without occupancy of all receptors. Figure 2–4 illustrates the notion of receptors that are spare in this sense and helps to explain how the sensitivity of a cell or tissue to a particular concentration of agonist may depend not only on the affinity of the receptor for binding an agonist (characterized by the K_D but also on the total concentration of receptors. Sensitivity may be expressed in terms of EC50, the concentration of agonist that results in half-maximal response. The K_D of the agonist-receptor interaction determines what fraction (B/B_{max}) of total receptors will be occupied at a given free concentration (C) of agonist regardless of the receptor concentration:

$$\frac{B}{B_{max}} = \frac{C}{C + K_D}$$

Imagine a responding cell with four receptors and four effectors (as in Figure 2–4). Here the number of effectors does not limit the maximal response, and the

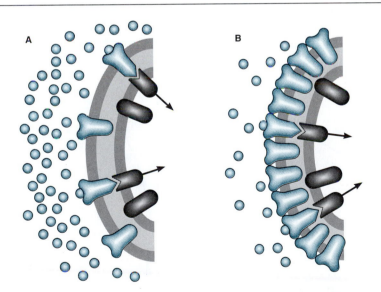

Figure 2–4. Spare receptors increase sensitivity to drug. In panel **A,** the free concentration of agonist is equal to the K_D concentration; this is sufficient to bind 50% of the four receptors present, resulting in the formation of two agonist-receptor complexes. (**Note:** When the agonist concentration is equal to the K_D, half the receptors will be occupied. Remember that $B/B_{max} = C/[C + K_D]$.) Agonist occupancy of these two receptors changes their conformation so that they bind to and activate two effector molecules, resulting in a response. Because two of four effectors are stimulated by agonist-receptor complexes, the response is 50% of maximum. In panel **B,** the receptor concentration has been increased tenfold (not all receptors are shown), and the K_D for binding of agonist to receptors remains unchanged. Now a very much smaller concentration of free agonist (= 0.05 × K_D) suffices to occupy two receptors and consequently to activate two effector molecules. Thus, the response is 50% of maximum (just as in panel **A**), even though the agonist concentration is very much lower than the K_D.

receptors are *not* spare in number. Consequently, an agonist present at a concentration equal to the K_D will occupy 50% of the receptors, and half of the effectors will be activated, producing a half-maximal response (ie, two receptors stimulate two effectors). Now imagine that the number of receptors increases tenfold to 40 receptors but that the total number of effectors remains constant. Most of the receptors are now spare in number. As a result, a much lower concentration of agonist suffices to occupy two of the 40 receptors (5% of the receptors), and this same low concentration of agonist is able to elicit a half-maximal response (two of four effectors activated). Thus, it is possible to change the sensitivity of tissues with spare receptors by changing the receptor concentration. (*Note:* Changing the number of receptors does not usually change the free concentration of drug achieved by administering a given dose. This is because the concentration of receptors in a tissue is usually very small relative to effective concentrations of drugs.)

An important biologic consequence of spare receptors is that they allow agonists with low affinity for receptors to produce full responses at low concentrations, to the extent that EC50 is lower than K_D. This is important because ligands with low affinity (high K_D) dissociate rapidly from receptors, allowing rapid termination of biologic responses. High binding affinity (low K_D), on the other hand, would result in slow dissociation of agonist from receptor and correspondingly slower reversal of a biologic response.

Competitive & Irreversible Antagonists

Receptor antagonists bind to the receptor but do not activate it. The effects of these antagonists result from preventing agonists (other drugs or endogenous regulatory molecules) from binding to and activating receptors. Such antagonists are divided into two classes depending on whether or not they reversibly compete with agonists for binding to receptors. The two classes of receptor antagonism produce quite different concentration-effect and concentration-binding curves in vitro and exhibit important practical differences in therapy of disease.

In the presence of a fixed concentration of agonist, increasing concentrations of a **competitive antagonist** progressively inhibit the agonist response; high antagonist concentrations prevent response completely. Conversely, sufficiently high concentrations of agonist can completely surmount the effect of a given concentration of the antagonist; ie, the E_{max} for the agonist remains the same for any fixed concentration of antagonist (Figure 2–5A). Because the antagonism is competitive, the presence of antagonist increases the agonist concentration required for a given degree of response, and so the agonist concentration-effect curve shifts to the right.

The concentration (C′) of an agonist required to produce a given effect in the presence of a fixed concentration ([I]) of competitive antagonist is greater than the agonist concentration (C) required to produce the same effect in the absence of the antagonist. The

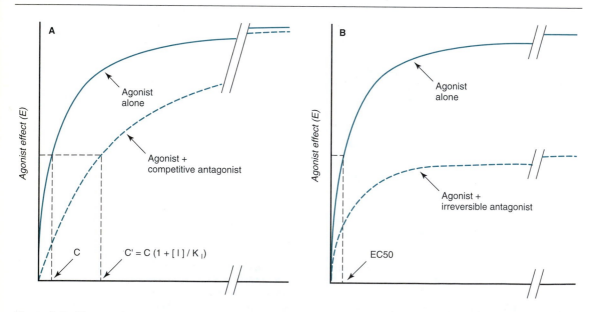

Figure 2–5. Changes in agonist concentration-effect curves produced by a competitive antagonist *(panel A)* or by an irreversible antagonist *(panel B)*. In the presence of a competitive antagonist, higher concentrations of agonist are required to produce a given effect; thus the agonist concentration (C′) required for a given effect in the presence of concentration [I] of an antagonist is shifted to the right, as shown. High agonist concentrations can overcome inhibition by a competitive antagonist. This is not the case with an irreversible antagonist, which reduces the maximal effect the agonist can achieve, though it may not change its EC50.

ratio of these two agonist concentrations (the "dose ratio") is related to the dissociation constant (K_I) of the antagonist by the Schild equation:

$$\frac{C'}{C} = 1 + \frac{[I]}{K_I}$$

Pharmacologists often use this relation to determine the K_I of a competitive antagonist. Even without knowledge of the relationship between agonist occupancy of the receptor and response, the K_I can be determined simply and accurately. As shown in Figure 2–5, concentration response curves are obtained in the presence and in the absence of a fixed concentration of competitive antagonist; comparison of the agonist concentrations required to produce identical degrees of pharmacologic effect in the two situations reveals the antagonist's K_I. If C′ is twice C, for example, then [I] = K_I. K_I values derived from such experiments agree with those determined by direct measurements of binding of radiolabeled competitive antagonists to receptors.

For the clinician, this mathematical relation has two important therapeutic implications:

(1) The degree of inhibition produced by a competitive antagonist depends upon the concentration of antagonist. Thus, the extent and duration of action of such a drug will depend upon its concentration in plasma and will be critically influenced by the rate of its metabolic clearance or excretion. Different patients receiving a fixed dose of propranolol, for example, exhibit a wide range of plasma concentrations, owing to differences in clearance of the drug. As a result, the effects of a fixed dose of this competitive antagonist of norepinephrine may vary widely in patients, and the dose must be adjusted accordingly.

(2) The equation defines another important source of variability in clinical response to a competitive antagonist, ie, the concentration of agonist that is competing for binding to receptors. Here also propranolol provides a useful example: When this competitive beta-adrenoceptor antagonist is administered in doses sufficient to block the effect of basal levels of the neurotransmitter norepinephrine, resting heart rate is decreased. However, the increase in release of norepinephrine and epinephrine that occurs with exercise, postural changes, or emotional stress may suffice to overcome competitive antagonism by propranolol and increase heart rate. Consequently, the prescriber who devises a dosage regimen for a competitive antagonist must always consider possible changes in endogenous agonist concentration that could influence therapeutic response.

Some receptor antagonists bind to the receptor in an **irreversible** or nearly irreversible fashion, ie, not competitive. The antagonist's affinity for the receptor may be so high that for practical purposes, the receptor is unavailable for binding of agonist. Other antagonists in this class produce irreversible effects because after binding to the receptor they form covalent bonds with it. After occupancy of some proportion of receptors by such an antagonist, the number of remaining unoccupied receptors may be too low to permit the previous maximal agonist response to be obtained (Figure 2–5B). However, if spare receptors are present, a lower dose of an irreversible antagonist may leave enough receptors unoccupied to allow achievement of maximum response to agonist, though a higher agonist concentration will be required (Figures 2–3B and 2–3C; see Receptor-Effector Coupling and Spare Receptors, above).

Therapeutically, irreversible antagonists present distinctive advantages and disadvantages. Once the irreversible antagonist has occupied the receptor, it need not be present in unbound form to inhibit agonist responses. Consequently, the duration of action of such an irreversible antagonist is relatively independent of its own rate of elimination and more dependent upon the rate of turnover of receptor molecules.

Phenoxybenzamine, an irreversible alpha-adrenoceptor antagonist, is used to control the hypertension caused by catecholamines released from pheochromocytoma, a tumor of the adrenal medulla. If administration of phenoxybenzamine lowers blood pressure, blockade will be maintained even when the tumor episodically releases very large amounts of catecholamine. In this case, the ability to prevent responses to varying and high concentrations of agonist is a therapeutic advantage. If overdose occurs, however, a real problem may arise. If the alpha-adrenoceptor blockade cannot be overcome, excess effects of the drug must be antagonized "physiologically," eg, by using a pressor agent that does not act via alpha receptors.

Partial Agonists

Based on the maximal pharmacologic response that occurs when all receptors are occupied, agonists can be divided into two classes: **Partial agonists** produce a lower response, at full receptor occupancy, than do **full agonists.** As compared with full agonists, partial agonists produce concentration-effect curves that resemble those observed with full agonists in the presence of an antagonist that irreversibly blocks receptor sites (compare Figures 2–3D and 2–6B). Nonetheless, radioligand-binding experiments have demonstrated that partial agonists may occupy all receptor sites (Figure 2–6A) at concentrations that will fail to produce a maximal response comparable to that seen with full agonists (Figure 2–4B). In addition, the failure of partial agonists to produce a "full" maximal response is not due to decreased affinity for binding to receptors. Such drugs compete, frequently with high affinity, for the full complement of receptors. Indeed, the partial agonists' ability to occupy the total receptor population is indicated by the fact that they competitively inhibit the responses produced by full agonists (Figure 2–6C).

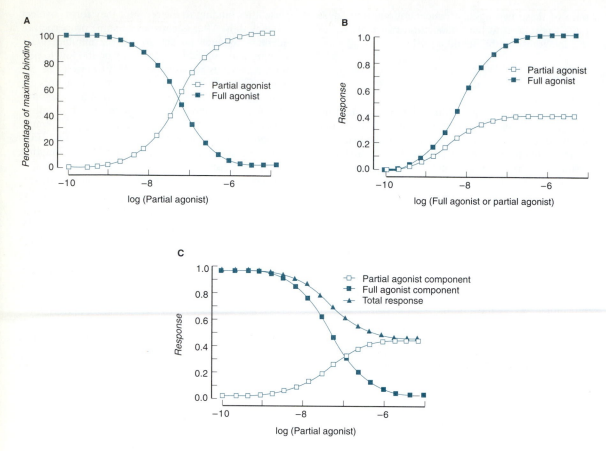

Figure 2–6. ***Panel A:*** The percentage of receptor occupancy resulting from full agonist (present at a single concentration) binding to receptors in the presence of increasing concentrations of a partial agonist. Because the full agonist (filled squares) and the partial agonist (open squares) compete to bind to the same receptor sites, when occupancy by the partial agonist increases, binding of the full agonist decreases. ***Panel B:*** When each of the two drugs is used alone and response is measured, occupancy of all the receptors by the partial agonist produces a lower maximal response than does similar occupancy by the full agonist. ***Panel C:*** Simultaneous treatment with a single concentration of full agonist and increasing concentrations of the partial agonist produces the response patterns shown in the bottom panel. The fractional response caused by a single concentration of the full agonist (filled squares) decreases as increasing concentrations of the partial agonist compete to bind to the receptor with increasing success; at the same time the portion of the response caused by the partial agonist (open squares) increases, while the total response—ie, the sum of responses to the two drugs (filled triangles)—gradually decreases, eventually reaching the value produced by partial agonist alone (compare panel B).

The reader will see that many drugs used as competitive antagonists are in fact weak partial agonists. The precise molecular mechanism that accounts for blunted maximal responses to partial agonists is not known, however. (See box: How Can an Agonist Be "Partial"?)

Other Mechanisms of Drug Antagonism

Not all of the mechanisms of antagonism involve interactions of drugs or endogenous ligands at a single type of receptor. Indeed, **chemical antagonists** need not involve a receptor at all. Thus, one drug may antagonize the actions of a second drug by binding to and inactivating the second drug. For example, prota-

mine, a protein that is positively charged at physiologic pH, can be used clinically to counteract the effects of heparin, an anticoagulant that is negatively charged; in this case, one drug antagonizes the other simply by binding it and making it unavailable for interactions with proteins involved in formation of a blood clot.

The clinician often uses drugs that take advantage of **physiologic antagonism** between endogenous regulatory pathways. Many physiologic functions are controlled by opposing regulatory pathways. For example, several catabolic actions of the glucocorticoid hormones lead to increased blood sugar, an effect that is physiologically opposed by insulin. Although gluco-

HOW CAN AN AGONIST BE "PARTIAL"?

We cannot precisely explain any individual partial agonist in molecular terms. Partial agonists are easier to understand, however, by envisioning the receptor as capable of taking on either of two shapes (see the top half of Figure 2–7): R, the inactive form, and R′, the active form, *in the absence as well as the presence of bound ligand (L)*. This implies that the receptor oscillates in an equilibrium between the two conformations (although the concentration of R′ is low) even in the absence of any ligand whatever. Considerable evidence confirms this surprising notion—eg, when an excessive number of normal recombinant receptors for thyroid-stimulating hormone are present in a cultured cell, the pharmacologic effect that is ordinarily produced by an agonist can be detected even in the absence of any agonist (Van Sande et al, 1995).

Now imagine that a receptor ligand L is added to the system. As depicted in the diagram, an equilibrium will now exist between four states of the receptor—free (unbound) R and R′, as well as LR and LR′. If L is a full agonist, it will bind to the active form, R′, very much more tightly than to R, for which its affinity is negligible. This will result in a shift of the equilibrium, strongly favoring formation of LR′. Conversely, a pure antagonist will bind well to R, but with negligible affinity to R′, resulting in formation of a preponderance of the inactive LR form. In this context it is easy to imagine a partial agonist as a ligand that can bind reasonably well to both R and R′. Thus, at any concentration of such a ligand some of the receptor will be in the LR′ form—and therefore capable of promoting (to some degree) the pharmacologic effect characteristic of the active receptor. As the concentration of partial agonist rises to the point that all receptors are occupied, however, some receptors will be in the LR form, so that the effect will be less than the maximum that might be achieved if all receptors were in the LR′ form. Thus, the relative efficacy of a partial agonist depends upon its relative affinities for R and R′.

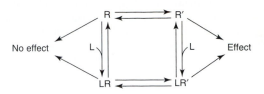

Figure 2–7. Possible mechanism for the partial agonist phenomenon. (R, receptor; L, ligand; R′, activated receptor.)

In general, use of a drug as a physiologic antagonist produces effects that are less specific and less easy to control than are the effects of a receptor-specific antagonist. Thus, for example, to treat bradycardia caused by increased release of acetylcholine from vagus nerve endings, which may be caused by the pain of myocardial infarction, the physician could use isoproterenol, a beta-adrenoceptor agonist that increases heart rate by mimicking sympathetic stimulation of the heart. However, use of this physiologic antagonist would be less rational—and potentially more dangerous—than would use of a receptor-specific antagonist such as atropine (a competitive antagonist at the receptors at which acetylcholine slows heart rate).

SIGNALING MECHANISMS & DRUG ACTION

Until now we have considered receptor interactions and drug effects in terms of equations and concentration-effect curves. This abstract analysis explains some quantitative aspects of drug action. For a more complete explanation, we must also understand the molecular mechanisms by which a drug acts. This understanding is particularly important for drugs that mimic or block intercellular signaling by hormones and neurotransmitters.

The research of the past 10 years has revealed in considerable detail the molecular processes that transduce extracellular signals into intracellular messages that control cell function. Understanding these remarkable signaling mechanisms allows us to ask basic questions with important clinical implications: Why do some drugs produce effects that persist for minutes, hours, or even days after the drug is no longer present? How do cellular mechanisms for amplifying external chemical signals explain the phenomenon of spare receptors? Why do chemically similar drugs often exhibit extraordinary selectivity in their actions? Can the signaling mechanisms explain actions of drugs that do not interact with receptors? Do these mechanisms provide targets for developing new drugs? Our new understanding allows us not only to ask these questions but also—in many cases—to answer them.

corticoids and insulin act on quite distinct receptor-effector systems, the clinician must sometimes administer insulin to oppose the hyperglycemic effects of glucocorticoid hormone, whether the latter is elevated by endogenous synthesis (eg, a tumor of the adrenal cortex) or as a result of glucocorticoid therapy.

Most transmembrane signaling is accomplished by only a few different molecular mechanisms. Each type of mechanism has been adapted, through the evolution of distinctive protein families, to transduce many different signals. These protein families include receptors on the cell surface and within the cell, as well as enzymes and other components that generate, amplify, coordinate, and terminate postreceptor signaling by chemical second messengers in the cytoplasm. This section first discusses the mechanisms for carrying chemical information across the plasma membrane and then outlines key features of cytoplasmic second messengers.

Five basic mechanisms of transmembrane signaling are well understood (Figure 2–8). Each uses a different strategy to circumvent the barrier posed by the lipid bilayer of the plasma membrane. These strategies use (1) a lipid-soluble ligand that crosses the membrane and acts on an intracellular receptor; (2) a transmembrane receptor protein whose intracellular enzymatic activity is allosterically regulated by a ligand that binds to a site on the protein's extracellular domain; (3) a transmembrane receptor that binds and stimulates a protein tyrosine kinase; (4) a ligand-gated transmembrane ion channel that can be induced to open or close by the binding of a ligand; or (5) a transmembrane receptor protein that stimulates a GTP-binding signal transducer protein (G protein), which in turn generates an intracellular second messenger.

While the five established mechanisms do not account for all the chemical signals conveyed across cell membranes, they do transduce many of the most important signals exploited in pharmacotherapy.

Intracellular Receptors for Lipid-Soluble Agents

Several biologic signals are sufficiently lipid-soluble to cross the plasma membrane and act on intracellular receptors. One of these is a gas, nitric oxide (NO), that acts by stimulating an intracellular enzyme, guanylyl cyclase, which produces cGMP. Signaling via cGMP is described in more detail later in this chapter. Receptors for another class of ligands—including **corticosteroids, mineralocorticoids, sex steroids, vitamin D,** and **thyroid hormone**—stimulate the transcription of genes in the nucleus by binding to specific DNA sequences near the gene whose expression is to be regulated. Many of the target DNA sequences (called **response elements**) have been identified.

The detailed molecular mechanisms used by these "gene-active" receptors are well understood. Structural features common to these receptors suggest that they belong to a protein family that evolved from a common precursor. Dissection of the receptors by recombinant DNA techniques has provided insights into their molecular mechanisms. For example, removal of a carboxyl terminal segment of the glucocorticoid receptor results in a protein that binds to the DNA response element and stimulates transcription of the target gene, even in the absence of glucocorticoids. Like this experimental truncation, binding of glucocorticoid hormone to the normal receptor relieves an inhibitory constraint on the transcription-stimulating activity of the protein. Figure 2–9 schematically depicts the molecular mechanism of glucocorticoid action: In the absence of hormone, the receptor is bound to hsp90, a protein that appears to prevent normal folding of several structural domains of the receptor.

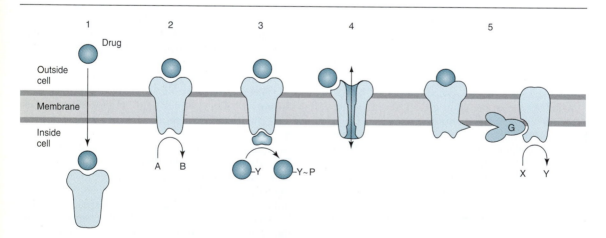

Figure 2–8. Known transmembrane signaling mechanisms: **1:** A lipid-soluble chemical signal crosses the plasma membrane and acts on an intracellular receptor (which may be an enzyme or a regulator of gene transcription); **2:** the signal binds to the extracellular domain of a transmembrane protein, thereby activating an enzymatic activity of its cytoplasmic domain; **3:** the signal binds to the extracellular domain of a transmembrane receptor bound to a protein tyrosine kinase, which it activates; **4:** the signal binds to and directly regulates the opening of an ion channel; **5:** the signal binds to a cell-surface receptor linked to an effector enzyme by a G protein.

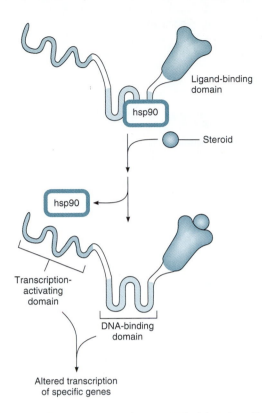

Figure 2–9. Mechanism of glucocorticoid action. The glucocorticoid receptor polypeptide is schematically depicted as a protein with three distinct domains. A heat-shock protein, hsp90, binds to the receptor in the absence of hormone and prevents folding into the active conformation of the receptor. Binding of a hormone ligand causes dissociation of the hsp90 stabilizer and permits conversion to the active configuration.

Binding of hormone to the ligand-binding domain triggers release of hsp90. This allows the DNA-binding and transcription-activating domains of the receptor to fold into their functionally active conformations, so that the activated receptor can initiate transcription of target genes.

The mechanism used by hormones that act by regulating gene expression has two therapeutically important consequences: (1) All of these hormones produce their effects after a characteristic lag period of 30 minutes to several hours—the time required for the synthesis of new proteins. This means that the gene-active hormones cannot be expected to alter a pathologic state within minutes—eg, glucocorticoids will not immediately relieve the symptoms of acute bronchial asthma. (2) The effects of these agents can persist for hours or days after the agonist concentration has been reduced to zero. The persistence of effect is primarily due to the relatively slow turnover of most enzymes and proteins, which can remain active in cells for hours or days after they have been synthe-

sized. (The persistence may also be partially due to the high affinity of receptors for the hormone, which results in slow dissociation of the hormone.) Therapeutically, it means that the beneficial (or toxic) effects of a gene-active hormone will usually decrease slowly when administration of the hormone is stopped and that there will be no simple temporal correlation between plasma concentration of the hormone and its effects.

Ligand-Regulated Transmembrane Enzymes Including Receptor Tyrosine Kinases

This class of receptor molecules mediates the first steps in signaling by **insulin, epidermal growth factor (EGF), platelet-derived growth factor (PDGF), atrial natriuretic factor (ANF), transforming growth factor-beta (TGFβ),** and several other trophic hormones. These receptors are polypeptides consisting of an extracellular hormone-binding domain and a cytoplasmic enzyme domain, which may be a protein tyrosine kinase, a serine kinase, or a guanylyl cyclase (Figure 2–10). In all these receptors, the two domains are connected by a hydrophobic segment of the polypeptide that crosses the lipid bilayer of the plasma membrane.

The receptor tyrosine kinase signaling pathway begins with hormone binding to the receptor's extracellular domain. The resulting change in receptor conformation causes receptor molecules to bind to one another, which in turn brings together the protein tyrosine kinase domains, which become enzymatically active. Tyrosine residues in both cytoplasmic domains become phosphorylated (each is probably phosphorylated by the other). This cross-phosphorylation can intensify or prolong the duration of allosteric regulation by the hormonal ligand. For example, the tyrosine kinase activity of the autophosphorylated insulin receptor persists after insulin is removed from the binding site. Different receptors catalyze phosphorylation of tyrosine residues on different downstream signaling proteins, but only a few of these substrate proteins have been identified. Insulin, for example, uses a single class of receptors to trigger increased uptake of glucose and amino acids and to regulate metabolism of glycogen and triglycerides in the cell. Similarly, each of the growth factors initiates in its specific target cells a complex program of cellular events ranging from altered membrane transport of protons, other ions, and metabolites to characteristic changes in the expression of many genes. Some of these responses involve phosphorylation by serine and threonine kinases, while others work via transcription factors that may themselves be kinase substrates. The tyrosine kinase receptors provide attractive targets for drug development. At present, a few compounds have been found to produce effects that may be due to inhibition of tyrosine kinase activities. It is easy to imagine therapeutic uses for specific inhibitors of growth factor receptors, especially in neoplastic disorders.

Figure 2–10. Mechanism of activation of the EGF receptor, a representative receptor tyrosine kinase. The receptor polypeptide has extracellular and cytoplasmic domains, depicted above and below the plasma membrane. Upon binding of EGF (circle), the receptor converts from its inactive monomeric state *(left)* to an active dimeric state *(right)*, in which two receptor polypeptides bind noncovalently in the plane of the membrane. The cytoplasmic domains become phosphorylated *(P)* on specific tyrosine residues *(Y)* and their enzymatic activities are activated, catalyzing phosphorylation of substrate proteins *(S)*.

The intensity and duration of action of EGF, PDGF, and other agents that act via this class of receptors are limited by receptor down-regulation. Ligand binding induces accelerated endocytosis of receptors from the cell surface, followed by the degradation of those receptors (and their bound ligands). When this process occurs at a rate faster than de novo synthesis of receptors, the total number of cell-surface receptors is reduced (down-regulated) and the cell's responsiveness to ligand is correspondingly diminished.

A growing number of regulators of growth and differentiation, including TGFβ, act on receptor serine kinases, another class of transmembrane receptor enzymes. ANF, an important regulator of blood volume and vascular tone, acts on a transmembrane receptor whose intracellular domain, a guanylyl cyclase, generates cGMP (see below). Receptors in both groups, like the protein tyrosine kinases, are active in their dimeric forms.

Cytokine Receptors

Cytokine receptors respond to a heterogeneous group of peptide ligands that includes growth hormone, erythropoietin, several kinds of interferon, and other regulators of growth and differentiation. These receptors use a recently discovered mechanism (Figure 2–11) that closely resembles that of receptor tyrosine kinases, but with a difference. In this case, the protein tyrosine kinase activity is not intrinsic to the receptor molecule; instead, a separate protein tyrosine kinase, from the Janus-kinase (JAK) family, binds noncovalently to the receptor. As in the case of the EGF-receptor, cytokine receptors dimerize after they bind the activating ligand, allowing the bound JAKs to become activated and to phosphorylate tyrosine residues on the receptor. Tyrosine phosphates on the receptor then set in motion a complex signaling dance by binding another set of proteins, called STATs (signal transducers and activators of transcription). Then the bound STATs are themselves phosphorylated by the JAKs, and two STAT molecules dimerize (attaching to one another's tyrosine phosphates). Finally, the STAT/STAT dimer dissociates from the receptor and travels to the nucleus, where it regulates transcription of specific genes. This multistep signaling process furnishes several attractive targets for potential drugs presently undergoing active investigation.

Ligand-Gated Channels

Many of the most useful drugs in clinical medicine act by mimicking or blocking the actions of endogenous ligands that regulate the flow of ions through plasma membrane channels. The natural ligands include **acetylcholine, gamma-aminobutyric acid,** and the **excitatory amino acids** (glycine, aspartate, glutamate, etc). All of these agents are synaptic transmitters.

Each of these receptors transmits its signal across the plasma membrane by increasing transmembrane conductance of the relevant ion and thereby altering the electrical potential across the membrane. For example, acetylcholine causes the opening of the ion channel in the nicotinic acetylcholine receptor (AchR), which allows Na^+ to flow down its concentration gradient into cells, producing a localized excitatory postsynaptic potential—a depolarization.

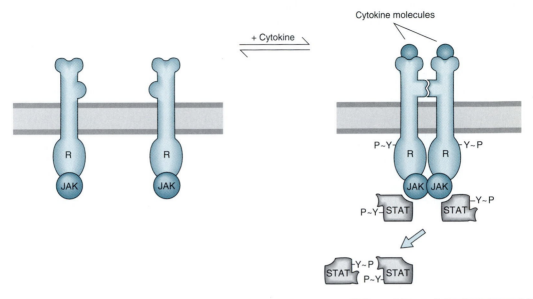

Figure 2–11. Cytokine receptors, like receptor tyrosine kinases, have extracellular and intracellular domains and form dimers. However, after activation by an appropriate ligand, separate mobile protein tyrosine kinase molecules (JAK) are activated, resulting in phosphorylation of STAT molecules. STAT dimers then travel to the nucleus, where they regulate transcription.

The nicotinic Ach receptor (Figure 2–12) is one of the best characterized of all cell-surface receptors for hormones or neurotransmitters. This receptor is a pentamer made up of five polypeptide subunits (eg, two alpha chains plus one beta, one gamma, and one delta chain, all with molecular weights ranging from 43,000 to 50,000). These polypeptides, each of which crosses the lipid bilayer four times, form a cylindric structure 8 nm in diameter. When acetylcholine binds to sites on the alpha subunits, a conformational change occurs that results in the transient opening of a central aqueous channel through which sodium ions penetrate from the extracellular fluid into the cell.

The time elapsed between the binding of the agonist to a ligand-gated channel and the cellular response can often be measured in milliseconds. The rapidity of this signaling mechanism is crucially important for moment-to-moment transfer of information across synapses. It contrasts sharply with other molecular signaling mechanisms, which may require seconds, minutes, or even hours, as is the case with gene-active hormones.

G Proteins & Second Messengers

Many extracellular ligands act by increasing the intracellular concentrations of second messengers such as cyclic adenosine-3′,5′-monophosphate (cAMP), calcium ion, or the phosphoinositides (described below). In most cases they use a transmembrane signaling system with three separate components. First, the extracellular ligand is specifically detected by a cell-surface receptor. The receptor in turn triggers the ac-

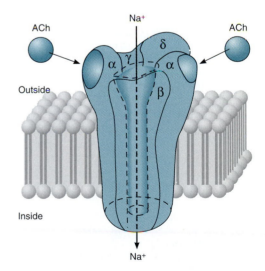

Figure 2–12. The nicotinic acetylcholine receptor, a ligand-gated ion channel. The receptor molecule is depicted as embedded in a rectangular piece of plasma membrane, with extracellular fluid above and cytoplasm below. Composed of five subunits (two α, one β, one γ, and one δ), the receptor opens a central transmembrane ion channel when acetylcholine (ACh) binds to sites on the extracellular domain of its α subunits.

tivation of a G protein located on the cytoplasmic face of the plasma membrane. The activated G protein then changes the activity of an effector element, usually an enzyme or ion channel. This element then changes the concentration of the intracellular second messenger. For cAMP, the effector enzyme is adenylyl cyclase, a transmembrane protein that converts intracellular ATP to cAMP. The corresponding G protein, called G_s, stimulates adenylyl cyclase after being activated by a host of hormones and neurotransmitters, each of which acts via a specific receptor (see Table 2–1).

G_s and other G proteins use a molecular mechanism that involves binding and hydrolysis of GTP (Figure 2–13). Significantly, this mechanism separates ligand excitation of the receptor from G protein-mediated activation of the effector, thereby allowing the transduced signal to be amplified. For example, a neurotransmitter such as norepinephrine may encounter its membrane receptor for a very short time—only a few milliseconds. When the encounter generates a GTP-bound G_s molecule, however, the duration of activation of adenylyl cyclase depends upon the longevity of GTP binding to G_s rather than upon the receptor's affinity for norepinephrine. Indeed, like other G proteins, GTP-bound G_s characteristically remains active for tens of seconds, which enormously amplifies the original signal. This mechanism explains how signaling by G proteins produces the phenomenon of spare receptors (described above). Even though one ligand-activated receptor molecule is required to initiate GTP binding by one G protein, the slow hydrolysis of GTP

causes the active G protein to persist long after the receptor has dissociated from its agonist molecule. So at low concentrations of agonist the proportion of agonist-bound receptors may be much less than the proportion of G proteins in the active (GTP-bound) state; if the proportion of active G proteins correlates with pharmacologic response, receptors will appear to be spare—ie, a small fraction of receptors occupied by agonist at any given time will appear to produce a proportionately larger response.

The family of G proteins is quite diverse (Table 2–2); in addition to G_s, the stimulator of adenylyl cyclase, it includes other subfamilies. Members of the G_i ("i" for inhibitory) subfamily couple receptors to inhibition of adenylyl cyclase; G_i proteins also mediate receptor stimulation of the phosphoinositide second messenger system in some cells (see below) and regulation of K^+ and Ca^{2+} channels. The G_i subfamily includes two G proteins (G_{t1} and G_{t2}, also called "transducins"), that mediate phototransduction in retinal rods and cones.

Not surprisingly, receptors coupled to G proteins are structurally related to one another, comprising a family of "serpentine receptors," so called because the receptor polypeptide chain crosses the plasma membrane seven times (Figure 2–14). Receptors for adrenergic amines, serotonin, acetylcholine (muscarinic but not nicotinic), many peptide hormones, odorants, and even visual receptors (in retinal rod and cone cells) all belong to the serpentine family. The amino and carboxyl terminals of each of these receptors are located on the extracellular and cytoplasmic sides of the membrane, respectively. Different serpentine receptors resemble one another rather closely in amino

Table 2–1. A partial list of endogenous ligands and their associated second messengers.

Ligand	Second Messenger
Adrenocorticotropic hormone	cAMP
Acetylcholine (muscarinic receptors)	Ca^{2+}, phosphoinositides
Angiotensin	Ca^{2+}, phosphoinositides
Catecholamines (α_1-adrenoceptors)	Ca^{2+}, phosphoinositides
Catecholamines (β-adrenoceptors)	cAMP
Chorionic gonadotropin	cAMP
Follicle-stimulating hormone	cAMP
Glucagon	cAMP
Histamine (H_2 receptors)	cAMP
Luteinizing hormone	cAMP
Melanocyte-stimulating hormone	cAMP
Parathyroid hormone	cAMP
Platelet-activating factor	Ca^{2+}, phosphoinositides
Prostacyclin, prostaglandin E_2	cAMP
Serotonin (5-HT_4 receptors)	cAMP
Serotonin (5-HT_{1C} and 5-HT_2 receptors)	Ca^{2+}, phosphoinositides
Thyrotropin	cAMP
Thyrotropin-releasing hormone	Ca^{2+}, phosphoinositides
Vasopressin (V_1 receptors)	Ca^{2+}, phosphoinositides
Vasopressin (V_2 receptors)	cAMP

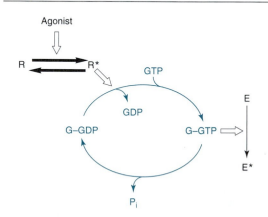

Figure 2–13. The guanine nucleotide-dependent activation-inactivation cycle of G proteins. The agonist activates the receptor *(R)*, which promotes release of GDP from the G protein *(G)*, allowing entry of GTP into the nucleotide binding site. In its GTP-bound state *(G-GTP)*, the G protein regulates activity of an effector enzyme or ion channel *(E)*. The signal is terminated by hydrolysis of GTP, followed by return of the system to the basal unstimulated state. Open arrows denote regulatory effects. (P_i, inorganic phosphate.)

Table 2–2. G proteins and their receptors and effectors.

G Protein	Receptors for:	Effector/Signaling Pathway
G_s	β-Adrenergic amines, glucagon, histamine, serotonin, and many other hormones	↑ Adenylyl cyclase → ↑ cAMP
G_{i1}, G_{i2}, G_{i3}	α_2-Adrenergic amines, acetylcholine (muscarinic), opioids, serotonin, and many others	Several, including: ↓Adenylyl cyclase → ↓ cAMP Open cardiac K^+ channels → ↓heart rate
G_{olf}	Odorants (olfactory epithelium)	↑Adenylyl cyclase → ↑ cAMP
G_o	Neurotransmitters in brain (not yet specifically identified)	Not yet clear
G_q	Acetylcholine (eg, muscarinic), bombesin, serotonin (5-HT_{1C}), and many others	↑Phospholipase C → ↑ IP_3, diacylglycerol, cytoplasmic Ca^{2+}
G_{t1}, G_{t2}	Photons (rhodopsin and color opsins in retinal rod and cone cells)	↑cGMP phosphodiesterase → ↓ cGMP (phototransduction)

acid sequences and in the locations of their hydrophobic transmembrane regions and hydrophilic extra- and intracellular loops, suggesting that all were derived from a common evolutionary precursor.

In parallel with these structural similarities, it appears that serpentine receptors transduce signals across the plasma membrane in essentially the same way. Often the agonist ligand—eg, a catecholamine, acetylcholine, or the photon-activated chromophore of retinal photoreceptors—is bound in a pocket enclosed by the transmembrane regions of the receptor (as in Figure 2–14). The resulting change in conformation of these regions is transmitted to cytoplasmic loops of the receptor, which in turn activate the appropriate G protein by promoting replacement of GDP by GTP, as described above. Considerable biochemical evidence indicates that the G proteins interact with amino acids in the third cytoplasmic loop of the receptor polypeptide (shown by arrows in Figure 2–14). The carboxyl terminal tails of these receptors, also located in the cytoplasm, can regulate the receptors' ability to interact with G proteins, as described below.

Receptor Desensitization

Receptor-mediated responses to drugs and hormonal agonists often "desensitize" with time (Figure 2–15, top). After reaching an initial high level, the response (eg, cellular cAMP accumulation, Na^+ influx, contractility, etc) gradually diminishes over seconds or minutes, even in the continued presence of the agonist. This desensitization is usually reversible. Thus, 15 minutes after removal of the agonist, a second exposure to agonist results in a response similar to the initial response. (Note that this ready reversibility distinguishes desensitization from down-regulation of the *number* of receptors, as described above for receptor tyrosine kinases.)

Although many kinds of receptors undergo desensitization, the mechanism is in most cases obscure (eg, agonist-induced desensitization of the nicotinic acetylcholine receptor). The molecular mechanism of agonist desensitization has been worked out in some

detail, however, in the case of the beta adrenoceptor (Figure 2–15, bottom): Binding of agonist induces a change in conformation of the receptor's carboxyl terminal tail, causing it to bind, activate, and serve as a substrate for a specific serine or threonine kinase, β-adrenoceptor kinase (also termed βARK). The presence of phosphoserines increases the receptor's affinity for binding a third protein, β-arrestin. Binding of β-arrestin to cytoplasmic loops of the receptor diminishes the receptor's ability to interact with G_s, thereby reducing the agonist response (ie, stimulation of adenylyl cyclase). Upon removal of agonist, however, cellular phosphatases remove phosphates from the receptor and βARK stops putting them back on, so that the receptor—and consequently the agonist response—return to normal.

Well-Established Second Messengers

A. cAMP: Acting as an intracellular second messenger, cAMP mediates such hormonal responses as the mobilization of stored energy (the breakdown of carbohydrates in liver or triglycerides in fat cells stimulated by beta-adrenomimetic catecholamines), conservation of water by the kidney (mediated by vasopressin), Ca^{2+} homeostasis (regulated by parathyroid hormone), and increased rate and contraction force of the heart muscle (beta-adrenomimetic catecholamines). It also regulates the production of adrenal and sex steroids (in response to corticotropin or follicle-stimulating hormone), the relaxation of smooth muscle, and many other endocrine and neural processes.

cAMP exerts most of its effects by stimulating cAMP-dependent protein kinases (Figure 2–16). These tetrameric kinases are composed of a cAMP-binding regulatory (R) dimer and two catalytic (C) chains. When cAMP binds to the R dimer, active C chains are released which then diffuse through the cytoplasm and nucleus, where they transfer phosphate from ATP to appropriate substrate proteins, often enzymes.

The specificity of cAMP's regulatory effects resides in the distinct protein substrates of the kinase that are expressed in different cells. For example, liver

Figure 2–14. Transmembrane topology of a typical serpentine receptor. The receptor's amino *(N)* terminal is extracellular (above the plane of the membrane), and its carboxyl *(C)* terminal intracellular. The terminals are connected by a polypeptide chain that traverses the plane of the membrane seven times. The hydrophobic transmembrane segments (speckled) are designated by roman numerals *(I–VII)*. The agonist *(Ag)* approaches the receptor from the extracellular fluid and binds to a site surrounded by the transmembrane regions of the receptor protein. G proteins *(G)* interact with cytoplasmic regions of the receptor, especially with portions of the third cytoplasmic loop between transmembrane regions *V* and *VI*. The receptor's cytoplasmic terminal tail contains numerous serine and threonine residues whose hydroxyl (–OH) groups can be phosphorylated. This phosphorylation may be associated with diminished receptor-G protein interaction.

is rich in phosphorylase kinase and glycogen synthase, enzymes whose reciprocal regulation by cAMP-dependent phosphorylation governs carbohydrate storage and release; adipocytes are rich in a lipase whose cAMP-dependent phosphorylation mediates free fatty acid release from fat cells. Similarly, phosphorylation of a kinase specific for the light chains of myosin (called myosin light chain kinase, or MLCK) is involved in relaxation of smooth muscle by beta-adrenomimetic amines. Other cell-specific responses to cAMP as a second messenger similarly depend upon the many enzymes available for regulation by phosphorylation.

When the hormonal stimulus stops, the intracellular actions of cAMP are terminated by an elaborate series of enzymes. cAMP-stimulated phosphorylation of enzyme substrates is rapidly reversed by a diverse group of specific and nonspecific phosphatases. cAMP itself is degraded to 5′-AMP by several distinct cyclic nucleotide phosphodiesterases (PDE, Figure 2–16). Competitive inhibition of cAMP degradation is one way caffeine, theophylline, and other methylxanthines produce their effects (see Chapter 20).

B. Calcium and Phosphoinositides: A second well-studied second messenger system involves hormonal stimulation of phosphoinositide hydrolysis (Figure 2–17). Some of the hormones, neurotransmitters, and growth factors that trigger this pathway (Table 2–1) bind to receptors linked to G proteins, while others bind to receptor tyrosine kinases. In all cases, however, the crucial step is stimulation of a membrane enzyme, phospholipase C (PLC), which specifically hydrolyzes a minor phospholipid component of the plasma membrane called phosphatidylinositol-4,5-bisphosphate (PIP_2). PIP_2 is split into two second messengers, diacylglycerol and inositol-1,4,5-trisphosphate (IP_3 or $InsP_3$). The first of these messengers is confined to the membrane, where it activates a phospholipid- and calcium-sensitive protein kinase called protein kinase C. The other messenger, IP_3, is water-soluble and diffuses through the cytoplasm, where it triggers the release of Ca^{2+} from internal storage vesicles. Elevated cytoplasmic Ca^{2+} concentration promotes the binding of Ca^{2+} to the calcium-binding protein calmodulin, which regulates activities of other enzymes, including calcium-dependent protein kinases.

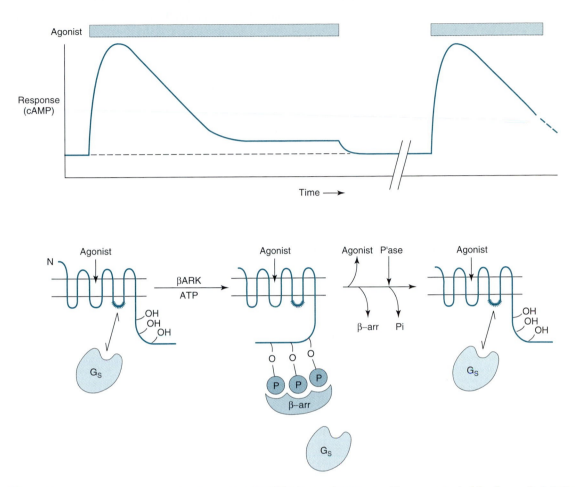

Figure 2–15. Possible mechanism for desensitization of the beta adrenoceptor. The upper part of the figure depicts the response to a β-adrenoceptor agonist (ordinate) versus time (abscissa). The break in the time axis indicates passage of time in the absence of agonist. Temporal duration of exposure to agonist is indicated by the hatched bar. The lower part of the figure schematically depicts agonist-induced phosphorylation (P) by β-adrenoceptor kinase (beta-adrenergic receptor kinase, βARK) of carboxyl terminal hydroxyl groups (–OH) of the beta adrenoceptor. This phosphorylation induces binding of a protein, β-arrestin *(β-arr)*, which prevents the receptor from interacting with G_s. Removal of agonist for a short period of time allows dissociation of β-arr, removal of phosphate *(Pi)* from the receptor by phosphatases *(P'ase)*, and restoration of the receptor's normal responsiveness to agonist.

With its multiple second messengers and protein kinases, the phosphoinositide signaling pathway is much more complex than the cAMP pathway. For example, different cell types may contain one or more specialized calcium- and calmodulin-dependent kinases with limited substrate specificity (eg, myosin light chain kinase) in addition to a general calcium- and calmodulin-dependent kinase that can phosphorylate a wide variety of protein substrates. Furthermore, at least nine structurally distinct types of protein kinase C have been identified.

Much of our understanding of the biologic roles of phosphoinositide second messengers comes from the use of pharmacologic agents that activate either the Ca^{2+} or the protein kinase C pathways. The concentration of cytoplasmic Ca^{2+} can be elevated by calcium ionophores, while protein kinase C is directly stimulated by binding phorbol esters or synthetic diacylglycerols. One or both of these classes of agents may reproduce the biologic response triggered by a physiologic signal using the phosphoinositide pathway.

As in the cAMP system, multiple mechanisms exist to damp or terminate signaling by this pathway. IP_3 is rapidly inactivated by dephosphorylation; diacylglycerol is either phosphorylated to yield phosphatidic acid, which is then converted back into phospholipids, or it is deacylated to yield arachidonic acid; Ca^{2+} is actively removed from the cytoplasm by Ca^{2+} pumps.

These and other nonreceptor elements of the calcium-phosphoinositide signaling pathway are now becoming targets for drug development. For example, the therapeutic effects of lithium ion, an established

Figure 2–16. The cAMP second messenger pathway. Key proteins include hormone receptors *(Rec)*, a stimulatory G protein *(G$_s$)*, catalytic adenylyl cyclase *(AC)*, phosphodiesterases *(PDE)* that hydrolyze cAMP, cAMP-dependent kinases, with regulatory *(R)* and catalytic *(C)* subunits, protein substrates *(S)* of the kinases, and phosphatases *(P'ase)*, which remove phosphates from substrate proteins. Open arrows denote regulatory effects.

ing) domain; this binding event triggers activation of the guanylyl cyclase activity that resides in the receptor's intracellular domain. The other mechanism takes advantage of the fact that cell membranes are permeable to the stimulating ligand, nitric oxide (NO, a gas; Chapter 19). The nitric oxide is generated in vascular endothelial cells in response to natural vasodilator agents such as acetylcholine and histamine (nitric oxide is also called endothelium-derived relaxing factor [EDRF]). After entering the cell, nitric oxide binds to and activates a cytoplasmic guanylyl cyclase. A number of useful vasodilating drugs act by generating or mimicking nitric oxide (see Chapters 11 and 12).

Interplay Among Signaling Mechanisms

The calcium-phosphoinositide and cAMP signaling pathways oppose one another in some cells and are complementary in others. For example, vasopressor agents that contract smooth muscle act by IP$_3$-mediated mobilization of Ca^{2+}, whereas agents that relax smooth muscle often act by elevation of cAMP. In contrast, cAMP and phosphoinositide second messengers act together to stimulate glucose release from the liver.

Phosphorylation: A Common Theme

Almost all second messenger signaling involves reversible phosphorylation. It plays a key role at every step, from regulation of receptors (autophosphorylation of tyrosine kinases and desensitization of recep-

agent for treating manic-depressive illness, may be mediated by effects on the metabolism of phosphoinositides (see Chapter 29).

C. cGMP: Unlike cAMP, the ubiquitous and versatile carrier of diverse messages, cGMP (cyclic guanosine-3′,5′-monophosphate) has established signaling roles in only a few cell types. In intestinal mucosa and vascular smooth muscle, the cGMP-based signal transduction mechanism closely parallels the cAMP-mediated signaling mechanism. Ligands detected by cell surface receptors stimulate membrane-bound guanylyl cyclase to produce cGMP, and cGMP acts by stimulating a cGMP-dependent protein kinase. The actions of cGMP in these cells are terminated by enzymatic degradation of the cyclic nucleotide and by dephosphorylation of kinase substrates.

Increased cGMP concentration causes relaxation of vascular smooth muscle by a kinase-mediated mechanism that results in dephosphorylation of myosin light chains. In these smooth muscle cells, cGMP synthesis can be elevated by two different transmembrane signaling mechanisms utilizing two different guanylyl cyclases. Atrial natriuretic factor (ANF), a blood-borne peptide hormone, stimulates a transmembrane receptor by binding to its extracellular (ligand-bind-

Figure 2–17. The Ca^{2+}-phosphoinositide signaling pathway. Key proteins include hormone receptors *(R)*, a G protein *(G)*, a phosphoinositide-specific phospholipase C *(PLC)*, protein kinase C *(PK-C)*, substrates of the kinase *(S)*, calmodulin *(CaM)*, and calmodulin-binding enzymes *(E)*, including kinases, phosphodiesterases, etc. (PIP$_2$, phosphatidylinositol-4,5-bisphosphate; DAG, diacylglycerol. Asterisk denotes activated state. Open arrows denote regulatory effects.)

tors linked to G proteins) to kinases regulated by second messengers and finally to substrates of these kinases that may themselves be kinases. These covalent modifications perform two principal functions in signaling, amplification and flexible regulation. In **amplification,** rather like GTP bound to a G protein, the attachment of a phosphoryl group to a serine, threonine, or tyrosine residue powerfully amplifies the initial regulatory signal by recording a molecular memory that the pathway has been activated; dephosphorylation erases the memory, taking a longer time to do so than is required for dissociation of an allosteric ligand. In **flexible regulation,** differing substrate specificities of the multiple protein kinases regulated by second messengers provide branch points in signaling pathways that may be independently regulated. In this way, cAMP, Ca^{2+}, or other second messengers can use the presence or absence of particular kinases or kinase substrates to produce quite different effects in different cell types.

RECEPTOR CLASSES & DRUG DEVELOPMENT

As we have seen, the existence of a specific drug receptor is usually inferred from studying the **structure-activity relationship** of a group of structurally similar congeners of the drug that mimic or antagonize its effects. Thus, if a series of related agonists exhibits identical relative potencies in producing two distinct effects, it is likely that the two effects are mediated by similar or identical receptor molecules. In addition, if identical receptors mediate both effects, a competitive antagonist will inhibit both responses with the same K_I; a second competitive antagonist will inhibit both responses with its own characteristic K_I. Thus, studies of the relation between structure and activity of a series of agonists and antagonists can identify a species of receptor that mediates a set of pharmacologic responses.

Exactly the same experimental procedure can show that observed effects of a drug are mediated by *different* receptors. In this case, effects mediated by different receptors may exhibit different orders of potency among agonists and different K_I values for each competitive antagonist.

Wherever we look, more than one class of receptor seems to have evolved for every chemical signal. For example, structure-activity studies with chemical congeners of acetylcholine, histamine, and catecholamines have identified multiple receptors for each of these endogenous ligands. Ligand-binding and molecular cloning techniques continue to reveal additional receptors, eg, two classes of vasopressin receptors, five molecular species of muscarinic receptors (only three of which are distinguishable by ligand-binding techniques), and multiple classes of receptors for dopamine, opioid peptides, serotonin, and others.

Why do multiple receptors for a single ligand exist? The answer is quite straightforward: Cells use more than one signaling pathway to respond to each endogenous ligand and therefore need more than one receptor for the same ligand. Thus, acetylcholine uses a nicotinic Ach receptor to initiate a fast excitatory postsynaptic potential (EPSP) in the postganglionic cells of autonomic ganglia and muscarinic receptors to evoke a slow EPSP, which modulates responsiveness to the fast EPSP in the same cells.

The existence of multiple receptors for each endogenous signaling ligand creates many important opportunities for drug development. Although each endogenous ligand produces multiple clinical effects, it is often therapeutically advantageous to block or mimic one set of effects without affecting the others. Subtle structural differences in the binding sites of two receptors for a ligand can make them bind congeners of the ligand with different affinities. If the affinities are sufficiently different, it may be possible to develop a drug that acts selectively, producing its effects through one receptor and not the other. Thus, β-adrenoceptor antagonists can block cardioacceleration produced by norepinephrine without preventing norepinephrine from constricting blood vessels via α_1 adrenoceptors. Clinical uses of receptor-selective drugs are described in almost every chapter of this book.

New drug development is not confined to agents that act on receptors for extracellular chemical signals. Pharmaceutical chemists are now determining whether elements of signaling pathways distal to the receptors may also serve as targets of selective and useful drugs. For example, clinically useful agents might be developed that act selectively on specific G proteins, kinases, phosphatases, or the enzymes that degrade second messengers.

RELATION BETWEEN DRUG DOSE & CLINICAL RESPONSE

We have dealt with receptors as molecules and shown how receptors can quantitatively account for the relation between dose or concentration of a drug and pharmacologic responses, at least in an idealized system. When faced with a patient who needs treatment, the prescriber must make a choice among a variety of possible drugs and devise a dosage regimen that is likely to produce maximal benefit and minimal toxicity. Because the patient is never an idealized system, the prescriber will not have precise information about the physicochemical nature of the receptors involved, the number of receptors, or their affinity for drugs. Nonetheless, in order to make rational therapeutic decisions, the prescriber must understand how drug-receptor interactions underlie the relations between dose and response in patients, the nature and causes of variation in pharmacologic responsiveness, and the clinical implications of selectivity of drug action.

Dose & Response in Patients

A. Graded Dose-Response Relations: To choose among drugs and to determine appropriate doses of a drug, the prescriber must know the relative **pharmacologic potency** and **maximal efficacy** of the drugs in relation to the desired therapeutic effect. These two important terms, often confusing to students and clinicians, can be explained by reference to Figure 2–18, which depicts graded dose-response curves that relate dose of four different drugs to the magnitude of a particular therapeutic effect, eg, lowering of blood pressure in a hypertensive patient or increasing urinary excretion of sodium in a patient with congestive heart failure.

1. Potency–Drugs A and B are said to be more potent than drugs C and D because of the relative positions of their dose-response curves along the dose axis of Figure 2–18. Potency refers to the concentration (EC50) or dose (ED50) of a drug required to produce 50% of that drug's maximal effect. Thus, the pharmacologic potency of drug A in Figure 2–18 is less than that of drug B, a partial agonist, because the EC50 of A is greater than the EC50 of B. Note that some doses of drug A can produce larger effects than any dose of drug B, despite the fact that we term drug B pharmacologically more potent. The reason for this is that drug A has a larger **maximal efficacy,** as described below.

Potency of a drug depends in part on the affinity (K_D) of receptors for binding the drug and in part on the efficiency with which drug-receptor interaction is coupled to response. As described above, both affinity and coupling efficiency contribute to the EC50 of a particular concentration-response relation in vitro.

For clinical use, it is helpful to distinguish between a drug's **potency** and its **efficacy.** The clinical effectiveness of a drug depends not on its potency (EC50),

but on its maximal efficacy (see below) and its ability to reach the relevant receptors. This ability can depend on its route of administration, absorption, distribution through the body, and clearance from the blood or site of action. In deciding which of two drugs to administer to a patient, the prescriber must usually consider their relative effectiveness rather than their relative potency. However, pharmacologic potency can largely determine the administered dose of the chosen drug. In general, low potency is important only if the drug has to be administered in inconveniently large amounts.

For therapeutic purposes, the potency of a drug should be stated in dosage units, usually in terms of a particular therapeutic end point (eg, 50 mg for mild sedation, 1 µg/kg/min for an increase in heart rate of 25 beats/min). Relative potency, the ratio of equi-effective doses (0.2, 10, etc), may be used in comparing one drug with another.

2. Maximal efficacy–This parameter reflects the limit of the dose-response relation on the **response axis.** Drugs A, C, and D in Figure 2–18 have equal maximal efficacy, while all have greater maximal efficacy than does drug B. The maximal efficacy (sometimes referred to simply as efficacy) of a drug is obviously crucial for making clinical decisions when a large response is needed. It may be determined by the drug's mode of interactions with receptors (as with partial agonists, described above)* or by characteristics of the receptor-effector system involved. Thus, diuretics that act on one portion of the nephron may produce much greater excretion of fluid and electrolytes than diuretics that act elsewhere. In addition, the efficacy of a drug for achieving a therapeutic end point (eg, increased cardiac contractility) may be limited by the drug's propensity to cause a toxic effect (eg, fatal cardiac arrhythmia) even if the drug could otherwise produce a greater therapeutic effect.

B. Shape of Dose-Response Curves: While the responses depicted in curves A, B, and C of Figure 2–18 approximate the shape of a simple Michaelis-Menten relation (transformed to a logarithmic plot), some clinical responses do not. Extremely steep dose-response curves (eg, curve D) may have important clinical consequences if the upper portion of the curve represents an undesirable extent of response (eg, coma caused by a sedative-hypnotic). Steep dose-response curves in patients could result

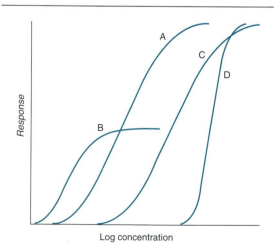

Figure 2–18. Graded dose-response curves for four drugs, illustrating different pharmacologic potencies and different maximal efficacies.

---

*Note that "maximal efficacy," used in a therapeutic context, does not have exactly the meaning the term denotes in the more specialized context of drug-receptor interactions described earlier in this chapter. In an idealized in vitro system, efficacy denotes the relative maximal efficacy of agonists and partial agonists that act via the same receptor. In therapeutics, efficacy denotes the extent or degree of an effect that can be achieved in the intact patient. Thus, therapeutic efficacy may be affected by the characteristics of a particular drug-receptor interaction, but it also depends upon a host of other factors as noted in the text.

from cooperative interactions of several different actions of a drug (eg, effects on brain, heart, and peripheral vessels, all contributing to lowering of blood pressure). Such steep dose-response curves could also be produced by a receptor-effector system in which most receptors must be occupied before any effect is seen.

C. Quantal Dose-Effect Curves: Despite their usefulness for characterizing the actions of drugs, graded dose-response curves of the sort described above have certain limitations in their application to clinical decision making. For example, such curves may be impossible to construct if the pharmacologic response is an either-or (quantal) event, such as prevention of convulsions, arrhythmia, or death. Furthermore, the clinical relevance of a quantitative dose-response relationship in a single patient, no matter how precisely defined, may be limited in application to other patients, owing to the great potential variability among patients in severity of disease and responsiveness to drugs.

Some of these difficulties may be avoided by determining the dose of drug required to produce a specified magnitude of effect in a large number of individual patients or experimental animals and plotting the cumulative frequency distribution of responders versus the log dose (Figure 2–19). The specified quantal effect may be chosen on the basis of clinical relevance (eg, relief of headache) or for preservation of safety of experimental subjects (eg, using low doses of a car-

diac stimulant and specifying an increase in heart rate of 20 beats/min as the quantal effect), or it may be an inherently quantal event (eg, death of an experimental animal). For most drugs, the doses required to produce a specified quantal effect in individuals are lognormally distributed; ie, a frequency distribution of such responses plotted against the log of the dose produces a gaussian normal curve of variation (Figure 2–19). When these responses are summated, the resulting cumulative frequency distribution constitutes a quantal dose-effect curve (or dose-percent curve) of the proportion or percentage of individuals who exhibit the effect plotted as a function of log dose (Figure 2–19).

The quantal dose-effect curve is often characterized by stating the **median effective dose (ED50)**, the dose at which 50% of individuals exhibit the specified quantal effect. (Note that the abbreviation ED50 has a different meaning in this context from its meaning in relation to graded dose-effect curves, described above.) Similarly, the dose required to produce a particular toxic effect in 50% of animals is called the **median toxic dose (TD50)**. If the toxic effect is death of the animal, a **median lethal dose (LD50)** may be experimentally defined. Such values provide a convenient way of comparing the potencies of drugs in experimental and clinical settings: Thus, if the ED50s of two drugs for producing a specified quantal effect are 5 and 500 mg, respectively, then the first drug can be said to be 100 times more potent than the second for that particular effect. Similarly, one can obtain a valuable index of the selectivity of a drug's action by comparing its ED50s for two different quantal effects in a population (eg, cough suppression versus sedation for opiate drugs; increase in heart rate versus increased vasoconstriction for sympathomimetic amines; antiinflammatory effects versus sodium retention for corticosteroids; etc).

Quantal dose-effect curves may also be used to generate information regarding the margin of safety to be expected from a particular drug used to produce a specified effect. One measure, which relates the dose of a drug required to produce a desired effect to that which produces an undesired effect, is the **therapeutic index.** In animal studies, the therapeutic index is usually defined as the ratio of the TD50 to the ED50 for some therapeutically relevant effect. The precision possible in animal experiments may make it useful to use such a therapeutic index to estimate the potential benefit of a drug in humans. Of course, the therapeutic index of a drug in humans is almost never known with real precision; instead, drug trials and accumulated clinical experience often reveal a range of usually effective doses and a different (but sometimes overlapping) range of possibly toxic doses. The clinically acceptable risk of toxicity depends critically on the severity of the disease being treated. For example, the dose range that provides relief from an ordinary headache in the great majority of patients should be

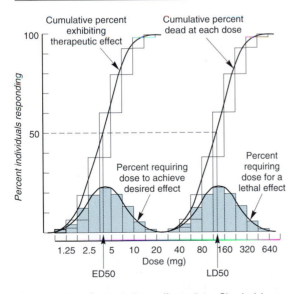

Figure 2–19. Quantal dose-effect plots. Shaded boxes (and the accompanying curves) indicate the frequency distribution of doses of drug required to produce a specified effect; ie, the percentage of animals that required a particular dose to exhibit the effect. The open boxes (and the corresponding curves) indicate the cumulative frequency distribution of responses, which are lognormally distributed.

very much lower than the dose range that produces serious toxicity, even if the toxicity occurs in a small minority of patients. However, for treatment of a lethal disease such as Hodgkin's lymphoma, the acceptable difference between therapeutic and toxic doses may be smaller.

Finally, note that the quantal dose-effect curve and the graded dose-response curve summarize somewhat different sets of information, although both appear sigmoid in shape on a semilogarithmic plot (compare Figures 2–18 and 2–19). Critical information required for making rational therapeutic decisions can be obtained from each type of curve: Both curves provide information regarding the **potency** and **selectivity** of drugs; the graded dose-response curve indicates the **maximal efficacy** of a drug; and the quantal dose-effect curve indicates the potential **variability** of responsiveness among individuals.

Variation in Drug Responsiveness

Individuals may vary considerably in their responsiveness to a drug; indeed, a single individual may respond differently to the same drug at different times during the course of treatment. Occasionally, individuals exhibit an unusual or **idiosyncratic** drug response, one that is infrequently observed in most patients. The idiosyncratic responses are usually caused by genetic differences in metabolism of the drug or by immunologic mechanisms, including allergic reactions.

Quantitative variations in drug response are in general more common and more clinically important: An individual patient is **hyporeactive** or **hyperreactive** to a drug in that the intensity of effect of a given dose of drug is diminished or increased in comparison to the effect seen in most individuals. (*Note:* The term **hypersensitivity** usually refers to allergic or other immunologic responses to drugs.) With some drugs, the intensity of response to a given dose may change during the course of therapy; in these cases, responsiveness usually decreases as a consequence of continued drug administration, producing a state of relative **tolerance** to the drug's effects. When responsiveness diminishes rapidly after administration of a drug, the response is said to be subject to **tachyphylaxis.**

The general clinical implications of individual variability in drug responsiveness are clear: The prescriber must be prepared to change either the dose of drug or the choice of drug, depending upon the response observed in the patient. Even before administering the first dose of a drug, the prescriber should consider factors that may help in predicting the direction and extent of possible variations in responsiveness. These include the propensity of a particular drug to produce tolerance or tachyphylaxis as well as the effects of age, sex, body size, disease state, and simultaneous administration of other drugs.

Four general mechanisms may contribute to variation in drug responsiveness among patients or within an individual patient at different times. The classification described below is necessarily artificial in that most variation in clinical responsiveness is caused by more than one mechanism. Nonetheless, the classification may be useful because certain mechanisms of variation are best dealt with according to different therapeutic strategies.

A. Alteration in Concentration of Drug That Reaches the Receptor: Patients may differ in the rate of absorption of a drug, in distributing it through body compartments, or in clearing the drug from the blood (see Chapter 3). Any of these pharmacokinetic differences may alter the concentration of drug that reaches relevant receptors and thus alter clinical response. Some differences can be predicted on the basis of age, weight, sex, disease state, or liver and kidney function of the patient, and such predictions may be used to guide quantitative decisions regarding an initial dosing regimen. Repeated measurements of drug concentrations in blood during the course of treatment are often helpful in dealing with the variability of clinical response caused by pharmacokinetic differences among individuals.

B. Variation in Concentration of an Endogenous Receptor Ligand: This mechanism contributes greatly to variability in responses to pharmacologic antagonists. Thus, propranolol, a β-adrenoceptor antagonist, will markedly slow the heart rate of a patient whose endogenous catecholamines are elevated (as in pheochromocytoma) but will not affect the resting heart rate of a well-trained marathon runner. A partial agonist may exhibit even more dramatically different responses: Saralasin, a weak partial agonist at angiotensin II receptors, lowers blood pressure in patients with hypertension caused by increased angiotensin II production and raises blood pressure in patients who produce low amounts of angiotensin.

C. Alterations in Number or Function of Receptors: Experimental studies have documented changes in drug responsiveness caused by increases or decreases in the number of receptor sites or by alterations in the efficiency of coupling of receptors to distal effector mechanisms. Although such changes have not been rigorously documented in human beings, it is likely that they account for much of the individual variability in response to some drugs, particularly those that act at receptors for hormones, biogenic amines, and neurotransmitters. In some cases, the change in receptor number is caused by other hormones; for example, thyroid hormones increase both the number of beta receptors in rat heart muscle and cardiac sensitivity to catecholamines. Similar changes probably contribute to the tachycardia of thyrotoxicosis in patients and may account for the usefulness of propranolol, a β-adrenoceptor antagonist, in ameliorating symptoms of this disease.

In other cases, the agonist ligand itself induces a decrease in the number ("down-regulation") or coupling efficiency of its receptors. Receptor-specific desensitization mechanisms presumably act physiologically to allow cells to adapt to changes in rates of stimulation by hormones and neurotransmitters in their environment. These mechanisms (discussed above, under Signaling Mechanisms and Drug Actions) may contribute to two clinically important phenomena: first, tachyphylaxis or tolerance to the effects of some drugs (eg, biogenic amines and their congeners), and second, the "overshoot" phenomena that follow withdrawal of certain drugs. These phenomena can occur with either agonists or antagonists. An antagonist may increase the number of receptors in a critical cell or tissue by preventing down regulation caused by an endogenous agonist. When the antagonist is withdrawn, the elevated number of receptors can produce an exaggerated response to physiologic concentrations of agonist. Potentially disastrous withdrawal symptoms can result for the opposite reason when administration of an agonist drug is discontinued. In this situation the number of receptors, which has been decreased by drug-induced down regulation, is too low for endogenous agonist to produce effective stimulation. For example, the withdrawal of clonidine (a drug whose α_2-adrenoceptor agonist activity reduces blood pressure) can produce hypertensive crisis, probably because the drug down-regulates α_2 adrenoceptors (see Chapter 11).

Various therapeutic strategies can be used to deal with receptor-specific changes in drug responsiveness, depending on the clinical situation. Tolerance to the action of a drug may require raising the dose or substituting a different drug. The down- (or up-) regulation of receptors may make it dangerous to discontinue certain drugs. The patient may have to be weaned slowly from the drug and watched carefully for signs of a withdrawal reaction.

D. Changes in Components of Response Distal to Receptor: Although a drug initiates its actions by binding to receptors, the response observed in a patient depends on the functional integrity of biochemical processes in the responding cell and physiologic regulation by interacting organ systems. Clinically, changes in these postreceptor processes represent the largest and most important class of mechanisms that cause variation in responsiveness to drug therapy.

Before initiating therapy with a drug, the prescriber should be aware of patient characteristics that may limit the clinical response. These characteristics include the age and general health of the patient and—most importantly—the severity and pathophysiologic mechanism of the disease. Once treatment is begun, the most important potential cause of failure to achieve a satisfactory response is that the diagnosis is wrong or physiologically incomplete. Thus, congestive heart failure will not respond satisfactorily to agents that increase myocardial contractility if the underlying pathologic mechanism is unrecognized stenosis of the mitral valve rather than myocardial insufficiency. Conversely, drug therapy will always be most successful when it is accurately directed at the pathophysiologic mechanism responsible for the disease.

When the diagnosis is correct and the drug is appropriate, treatment may still not produce an optimal result. An unsatisfactory therapeutic response can often be traced to compensatory mechanisms in the patient that respond to and oppose the beneficial effects of the drug. Compensatory increases in sympathetic nervous tone and fluid retention by the kidney, for example, can contribute to tolerance to antihypertensive effects of a vasodilator drug. In such cases, additional drugs may be required to achieve a useful therapeutic response.

Clinical Selectivity: Beneficial Versus Toxic Effects of Drugs

Although we classify drugs according to their principal actions, it is clear that *no drug causes only a single, specific effect.* Why is this so? It is exceedingly unlikely that any kind of drug molecule will bind to only a single type of receptor molecule, if only because the number of potential receptors in every patient is astronomically large. (Consider that the human genome encodes more than 10^5 different peptide gene products and that the chemical complexity of each of these peptides is sufficient to provide many different potential binding sites.) Even if the chemical structure of a drug allowed it to bind to only one kind of receptor, the biochemical processes controlled by such receptors would take place in multiple cell types and would be coupled to many other biochemical functions; as a result, the patient and the prescriber would probably perceive more than one drug effect.

Accordingly, drugs are only *selective*—rather than specific—in their actions, because they bind to one or a few types of receptor more tightly than to others and because these receptors control discrete processes that result in distinct effects. As we have seen, selectivity can be measured by comparing binding affinities of a drug to different receptors or by comparing ED50s for different effects of a drug in vivo. In drug development and in clinical medicine, selectivity is usually considered by separating effects into two categories: **beneficial** or **therapeutic effects** versus **toxic effects.** Pharmaceutical advertisements and prescribers occasionally use the term **side effect,** implying that the effect in question is insignificant or occurs via a pathway that is to one side of the principal action of the drug; such implications are frequently erroneous.

It is important to recognize that the designation of a particular drug effect as either therapeutic or toxic is a value judgment and not a statement about the pharmacologic mechanism underlying the effect. As a value judgment, such a designation depends on the clinical context in which the drug is used.

It is only because of their selectivity that drugs are useful in clinical medicine. Thus, it is important, both in the management of patients and in the development and evaluation of new drugs, to analyze ways in which beneficial and toxic effects of drugs may be related, in order to increase selectivity and usefulness of drug therapy. Figure 2–20 depicts three possible relations between the therapeutic and toxic effects of a drug based on analysis of the receptor-effector mechanisms involved.

A. Beneficial and Toxic Effects Mediated by the Same Receptor-Effector Mechanism: Much of the serious drug toxicity in clinical practice represents a **direct pharmacologic extension** of the therapeutic actions of the drug. In some of these cases (bleeding caused by anticoagulant therapy; hypoglycemic coma due to insulin), toxicity may be avoided by judicious management of the dose of drug administered, guided by careful monitoring of effect (measurements of blood coagulation or serum glucose) and aided by ancillary measures (avoiding tissue trauma that may lead to hemorrhage; regulation of carbohydrate intake). In still other cases, the toxicity may be avoided by not administering the drug at all, if the therapeutic indication is weak or if other therapy is available (eg, sedative-hypnotics ordinarily should not be used to treat patients whose complaints of insomnia are due to underlying psychiatric depression).

In certain situations, a drug is clearly necessary and beneficial but produces unacceptable toxicity when given in doses that produce optimal benefit. In such situations, it may be necessary to add another drug to the treatment regimen. For example, prazosin (Chapter 11) lowers blood pressure in essential hypertension by acting as an alpha$_1$-selective antagonist on receptors in vascular smooth muscle; as an inevitable consequence, patients will suffer from symptoms of postural hypotension if the dose of drug is large enough. (Note that postural hypotension has been called a "side effect" of prazosin, though in fact it is a direct effect, closely related to the drug's principal therapeutic action.) Appropriate management of such a problem takes advantage of the fact that blood pressure is regulated by changes in blood volume and tone of arterial smooth muscle in addition to the sympathetic nerves. Thus, concomitant administration of diuretics and vasodilators may allow the dose of prazosin to be lowered, with relief of postural hypotension and continued control of blood pressure.

B. Beneficial and Toxic Effects Mediated by Identical Receptors but in Different Tissues or by Different Effector Pathways: Examples of drugs in this category include digitalis glycosides, which may be used to augment cardiac contractility but also produce cardiac arrhythmias, gastrointestinal effects, and changes in vision (all probably mediated by inhibition of Na^+/K^+ ATPase in cell membranes); methotrexate, used to treat leukemia and other neoplastic diseases, which also kills normal cells in bone marrow and gastrointestinal mucosa (all mediated by inhibition of the enzyme dihydrofolate reductase); and congeners of glucocorticoid hormones, used to treat asthma or inflammatory disorders, which also can produce protein catabolism, psychosis, and other toxicities (all thought to be mediated by similar or identical glucocorticoid receptors). In addition to these and other well-documented examples, it is likely that adverse effects of many drugs are mediated by receptors identical to those which produce the recognized beneficial effect.

Three therapeutic strategies are used to avoid or mitigate this sort of toxicity. First, the drug should always be administered at the lowest dose that produces acceptable benefit, recognizing that complete abolition of signs or symptoms of the disease may not be achieved. Second (as described above for prazosin), adjunctive drugs that act through different receptor mechanisms and produce different toxicities may allow lowering the dose of the first drug, thus limiting its toxicity (eg, use of other immunosuppressive agents added to glucocorticoids in treating inflammatory disorders). Third, selectivity of the drug's actions may be increased by manipulating the concentrations of drug available to receptors in different parts of the body. Such "anatomic" selectivity may be achieved, for example, by aerosol administration of a glucocorticoid to bronchi or by selective arterial infusion of an antimetabolite into an organ containing tumor cells.

C. Beneficial and Toxic Effects Mediated by Different Types of Receptors: Therapeutic advantages resulting from new chemical entities with improved receptor selectivity were mentioned earlier in this chapter and are described in detail in later chapters. Such drugs include the alpha- and beta-selective adrenoceptor agonists and antagonists, the H$_1$ and H$_2$ antihistamines, nicotinic and muscarinic blocking agents, and receptor-selective steroid hor-

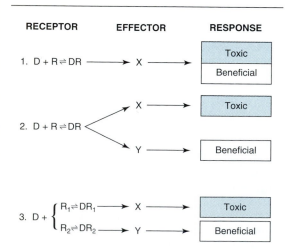

Figure 2–20. Possible relations between the therapeutic and toxic effects of a drug, based on different receptor-effector mechanisms. Therapeutic implications of these different relations are discussed in the text.

mones. All of these receptors are grouped in functional families, each responsive to a small class of endogenous agonists. The receptors and their associated therapeutic uses were discovered by analyzing effects of the physiologic chemical signals—catecholamines, histamine, acetylcholine, and corticosteroids.

A number of other drugs were discovered in a similar way, although they may not act at receptors for known hormones or neurotransmitters. These drugs were discovered by exploiting toxic effects of other agents, observed in a different clinical context. Examples include quinidine, the sulfonylureas, thiazide diuretics, tricyclic antidepressants, monoamine oxidase inhibitors, and phenothiazine antipsychotics among many others.

It is likely that some of these drugs will eventually be shown to act via receptors for endogenous agonists, as is the case with morphine, a potent analgesic agent. Morphine has been shown to act on receptors physiologically stimulated by the opioid peptides. Pharmacologists have now defined several subclasses of opioid receptors in a fashion reminiscent of earlier studies of autonomic receptors.

Thus, the propensity of drugs to bind to different classes of receptor sites is not only a potentially vexing problem in treating patients—it also presents a continuing challenge to pharmacology and an opportunity for developing new and more useful drugs.

REFERENCES

Becker AB, Roth RA: Insulin receptor structure and function in normal and pathological conditions. Annu Rev Med 1990;41:99.

Bell RM, Burns DJ: Lipid activation of protein kinase C. J Biol Chem 1990;266:4661

Berridge MJ: The biology and medicine of calcium signaling. Mol Cell Endocrinol 1994;98:119.

Bourne HR, DeFranco AL: Signal transduction and intracellular messengers. In: *Oncogenes and the Molecular Origins of Cancer.* Weinberg R (editor). Cold Spring Harbor Press, 1989.

Changeux JP: Thudicum Medal Lecture: The acetylcholine receptor: a model for allosteric membrane proteins. Biochem Soc Trans 1995;23:195.

Edelman AM, Blumenthal DK, Krebs EG: Protein serine/threonine kinases. Annu Rev Biochem 1987;56:567.

Goldstein A, Aronow L, Kalman SM: *Principles of Drug Action: The Basis of Pharmacology,* 2nd ed. Wiley, 1974.

Ihle JN, Kerr IM: Jaks and Stats in signaling by the cytokine receptor superfamily. Trends Genet 1995;11:69.

Kenakin T: The classification of seven transmembrane receptors in recombinant expression systems. Pharmacol Rev 1996;48:413.

Kenakin TP: *Pharmacologic Analysis of Drug-Receptor Interaction.* Raven Press, 1987.

Kobilka B: Adrenergic receptors as models for G protein-coupled receptors. Annu Rev Neurosci 1992;15:87.

Lowenstein CJ, Snyder SH: Nitric oxide, a novel biologic messenger. Cell 1992;70:705.

Neer EJ: Heterotrimeric G proteins: organizers of transmembrane signals. Cell 1995;80:249.

Schlessinger J: Cellular signaling by receptor tyrosine kinases. Harvey Lect 1993;89;105.

Van Sande J et al: In Chinese hamster ovary K1 cells dog and human thyrotropin receptors activate both the cyclic AMP and the phosphatidylinositol 4,5-bisphosphate cascades in the presence of thyrotropin and the cyclic AMP cascade in its absence. Eur J Biochem 1995;229:338.

Wong SK, Garbers DL: Receptor guanylyl cyclases. J Clin Invest 1992; 90:299.

3

Pharmacokinetics & Pharmacodynamics: Dose Selection & the Time Course of Drug Action

Nicholas H.G. Holford, MB, ChB, FRACP, & Leslie Z. Benet, PhD

The goal of therapeutics is to achieve a desired beneficial effect with minimal adverse effects. When a medicine has been selected for a patient, the clinician must determine the dose that most closely achieves this goal. A rational approach to this objective combines the principles of pharmacokinetics with pharmacodynamics to clarify the dose-effect relationship (Figure 3–1). Pharmacodynamics governs the concentration-effect part of the interaction, whereas pharmacokinetics deals with the dose-concentration part (Holford et al, 1981). The pharmacokinetic processes of absorption, distribution, and elimination determine how rapidly and in what concentration and for how long the drug will appear at the target organ. The pharmacodynamic concepts of maximum response and sensitivity determine the magnitude of the effect at a particular concentration (see E_{max} and EC50, Chapter 2).

Figure 3–1 illustrates a fundamental hypothesis of pharmacology, namely, that a relationship exists between a beneficial or toxic effect of a drug and the concentration of the drug in a readily accessible site of the body (eg, blood). This hypothesis has been documented for many drugs, as indicated by the Effective Concentrations and Toxic Concentrations columns in Table 3–1. The apparent lack of such a relationship for some drugs does not weaken the basic hypothesis but points to the need to consider the time course of concentration at the actual site of pharmacologic effect (see below).

Knowing the relationship between drug concentrations and effects allows the clinician to take into account the various pathologic and physiologic features of a particular patient that make him or her different from the average individual in responding to a drug. The importance of pharmacokinetics and pharmacodynamics in patient care thus rests upon the improvement in therapeutic efficacy and reduction in toxicity that can be achieved by application of their principles.

PHARMACOKINETICS

The "standard" dose of a drug is based on trials in healthy volunteers and patients with average ability to absorb, distribute, and eliminate the drug (see Clinical Trials: The IND & NDA in Chapter 5). This dose will not be suitable for every patient. Several physiologic (eg, maturation of organ function in infants) and pathologic processes (eg, heart failure, renal failure) dictate dosage adjustment in individual patients. These processes modify specific pharmacokinetic parameters. The two basic parameters are **clearance,** the measure of the ability of the body to eliminate the drug; and **volume of distribution,** the measure of the apparent space in the body available to contain the drug. These parameters are illustrated schematically in Figure 3–2, where the volume of the compartments into which the drugs diffuse represents the volume of distribution and the size of the outflow "drain" in Figures 3–2B and 3–2D represents the clearance.

Volume of Distribution

Volume of distribution (V_d) relates the amount of drug in the body to the concentration of drug (C) in blood or plasma:

$$V_d = \frac{\text{Amount of drug in body}}{C} \tag{1}$$

The volume of distribution may be defined with respect to blood, plasma, or water (unbound drug), depending on the concentration used in equation (1) (C = C_b, C_p, or C_u).

That the V_d calculated from equation (1) is an *apparent* volume may be appreciated by comparing the volumes of distribution of drugs such as digoxin or chloroquine (Table 3–1) with some of the physical volumes of the body (Table 3–2). V_d can vastly exceed

Figure 3–1. The relationship between dose and effect can be separated into pharmacokinetic (dose-concentration) and pharmacodynamic (concentration-effect) components. Concentration provides the link between pharmacokinetics and pharmacodynamics and is the focus of the target concentration approach to rational dosing. The three primary processes of pharmacokinetics are absorption, distribution, and elimination.

any physical volume in the body because the V_d is the volume necessary to contain the amount of drug *homogeneously* at the concentration found in the blood, plasma, or plasma water. Drugs with very high volumes of distribution have much higher concentrations in extravascular tissue than in the vascular compartment, ie, they are *not* homogeneously distributed. Drugs that are completely retained within the vascular compartment, on the other hand, have a minimum possible V_d equal to the blood component in which they are distributed, eg, 0.04 L/kg body weight (Table 3–2) or 2.8 L/70 kg for a drug that is restricted to the plasma compartment.

Clearance

Drug clearance principles are similar to the clearance concepts of renal physiology, in which creatinine clearance is defined as the rate of elimination of creatinine in the urine relative to its serum concentration (UV/P). At the simplest level, clearance of a drug is the ratio of the rate of elimination by all routes to the concentration of drug in a biologic fluid:

$$CL = \frac{\textbf{Rate of elimination}}{C} \qquad (2)$$

Clearance, like volume of distribution, may be defined with respect to blood (CL_b), plasma (CL_p), or unbound in the plasma water (CL_u), depending on the concentration measured.

It is important to note the additive character of clearance. Elimination of drug from the body may involve processes occurring in the kidney, the lung, the liver, and other organs. Dividing the rate of elimina-

tion at each organ by the concentration of drug presented to it yields the respective clearance at that organ. Added together, these separate clearances equal total systemic clearance:

$$CL_{renal} = \frac{\textbf{Rate of elimination}_{kidney}}{C} \qquad (3a)$$

$$CL_{liver} = \frac{\textbf{Rate of elimination}_{liver}}{C} \qquad (3b)$$

$$CL_{other} = \frac{\textbf{Rate of elimination}_{other}}{C} \qquad (3c)$$

$$CL_{systemic} = CL_{renal} + CL_{liver} + CL_{other} \qquad (3d)$$

"Other" tissues of elimination could include the lungs and additional sites of metabolism, eg, blood or muscle. The example provided in equations (3a–3d) indicates that the drug is eliminated by liver, kidney, and other tissues and that these routes of elimination account for all the pathways by which the drug leaves the body.

The two major sites of drug elimination are the kidneys and the liver. Clearance of unchanged drug in the urine represents renal clearance. Within the liver, drug elimination occurs via biotransformation of parent drug to one or more metabolites, or excretion of unchanged drug into the bile, or both. The pathways of biotransformation are discussed in Chapter 4. For most drugs, clearance is constant over the plasma or blood concentration range encountered in clinical settings, ie, elimination is not saturable, and the rate of

Table 3–1. Pharmacokinetic and pharmacodynamic parameters for selected drugs.

Drug	Oral Availability (F) (%)	Urinary Excretion (%)	Bound in Plasma (%)	Clearance (L/h/70 kg)[1]	Volume of Distribution (L/70 kg)	Half-Life (h)	Effective Concentrations	Toxic Concentrations
Acetaminophen	88	3	0	21	67	2	10–20 mg/L	>300 mg/L
Acyclovir	23	75	15	19.8	48	2.4	. . .	. . .
Amikacin	. . .	98	4	5.46	19	2.3	. . .	. . .
Amoxicillin	93	86	18	10.8	15	1.7	. . .	. . .
Amphotericin	. . .	4	90	1.92	53	18	. . .	. . .
Ampicillin	62	82	18	16.2	20	1.3	. . .	. . .
Aspirin	68	1	49	39	11	0.25	. . .	. . .
Atenolol	56	94	5	10.2	67	6.1	1 mg/L	. . .
Atropine	50	57	18	24.6	120	4.3	. . .	. . .
Captopril	65	38	30	50.4	57	2.2	50 ng/mL	. . .
Carbamazepine	70	1	74	5.34	98	15	6.5 mg/L	>9 mg/L
Cephalexin	90	91	14	18	18	0.9	. . .	. . .
Cephalothin	. . .	52	71	28.2	18	0.57	. . .	. . .
Chloramphenicol	80	25	53	10.2	66	2.7	. . .	. . .
Chlordiazepoxide	100	1	97	2.28	21	10	>0.7 mg/L	. . .
Chloroquine	89	61	61	45	13000	214	15–30 ng/mL	250 ng/mL
Chlorpropamide	90	20	96	0.126	6.8	33	. . .	. . .
Cimetidine	62	62	19	32.4	70	1.9	0.8 mg/L	. . .
Ciprofloxacin	60	65	40	25.2	130	4.1	. . .	. . .
Clonidine	95	62	20	12.6	150	12	0.2–2 ng/mL	. . .
Cyclosporine	23	1	93	24.6	85	5.6	100–400 ng/mL	>400 ng/mL
Diazepam	100	1	99	1.62	77	43	300–400 ng/mL	. . .
Digitoxin	90	32	97	0.234	38	161	>10 ng/mL	>35 ng/mL
Digoxin	70	60	25	7.8	440	39	>0.8 ng/mL	>2 ng/mL
Diltiazem	44	4	78	50.4	220	3.7	. . .	. . .
Disopyramide	83	55	2	5.04	41	6	3 mg/L	>8 mg/L
Enalapril	95	90	55	9	40	3	>0.5 ng/mL	. . .
Erythromycin	35	12	84	38.4	55	1.6	. . .	. . .
Ethambutol	77	79	5	36	110	3.1	. . .	>10 mg/L
Fluoxetine	60	3	94	40.2	2500	53	. . .	. . .
Furosemide	61	66	99	8.4	7.7	1.5	. . .	25 mg/L
Gentamicin	. . .	90	10	5.4	18	2.5	. . .	. . .
Hydralazine	40	10	87	234	105	1	100 ng/mL	. . .
Imipramine	40	2	90	63	1600	18	100–300 ng/mL	>1 mg/L
Indomethacin	98	15	90	8.4	18	2.4	0.3–3 mg/L	>5 mg/L
Labetalol	18	5	50	105	660	4.9	0.13 mg/L	. . .
Lidocaine	35	2	70	38.4	77	1.8	1.5–6 mg/L	>6 mg/L
Lithium	100	95	0	1.5	55	22	0.5–1.25 meq/L	>2 meq/L

Table 3–1. Pharmacokinetic and pharmacodynamic parameters for selected drugs (cont'd).

Drug	Oral Availability (F) (%)	Urinary Excretion (%)	Bound in Plasma (%)	Clearance (L/h/70 kg)[1]	Volume of Distribution (L/70 kg)	Half-Life (h)	Effective Concentrations	Toxic Concentrations[2]
Meperidine	52	12	58	72	310	3.2	0.4–0.7 mg/L	...
Methotrexate	70	48	34	9	39	7.2	...	10 µmol/L
Metoprolol	38	10	11	63	290	3.2	25 ng/mL	...
Metronidazole	99	10	10	5.4	52	8.5	3–6 mg/L	...
Midazolam	44	56	95	27.6	77	1.9	...	...
Morphine	24	8	35	60	230	1.9	65 ng/mL	...
Nifedipine	50	0	96	29.4	55	1.8	47 ng/mL	...
Nortriptyline	51	2	92	30	1300	31	50–140 ng/mL	>500 ng/mL
Phenobarbital	100	24	51	0.258	38	98	10–25 mg/L	>30 mg/L
Phenytoin	90	2	89	Conc-dependent[3]	45	Conc-dependent[4]	10 mg/L	>20 mg/L
Prazosin	68	1	95	12.6	42	2.9	...	...
Procainamide	83	67	16	36	130	3	3–14 mg/L	>14 mg/L
Propranolol	26	1	87	50.4	270	3.9	20 ng/mL	...
Pyridostigmine	14	85	...	36	77	1.9	50–100 ng/mL	...
Quinidine	80	18	87	19.8	190	6.2	2–6 mg/L	>8 mg/L
Ranitidine	52	69	15	43.8	91	2.1	100 ng/mL	...
Rifampin	?	7	89	14.4	68	3.5	...	...
Salicylic acid	100	15	85	0.84	12	13	150–300 mg/L	>200 mg/L
Sulfamethoxazole	100	14	62	1.32	15	10	...	...
Terbutaline	14	56	20	14.4	125	14	2.3 ng/mL	...
Tetracycline	77	58	65	7.2	105	11	...	...
Theophylline	96	18	56	2.88	35	8.1	10–20 mg/L	>20 mg/L
Tobramycin	...	90	10	4.62	18	2.2	...	...
Tocainide	89	38	10	10.8	210	14	6–15 mg/L	...
Tolbutamide	93	0	96	1.02	7	5.9	80–240 mg/L	...
Trimethoprim	100	69	44	9	130	11	...	...
Tubocurarine	...	63	50	8.1	27	2	0.6 mg/L	...
Valproic acid	100	2	93	0.462	9.1	14	30–100 mg/L	>150 mg/L
Vancomycin	...	79	30	5.88	27	5.6	...	...
Verapamil	22	3	90	63	350	4	...	...
Warfarin	93	3	99	0.192	9.8	37	...	...
Zidovudine	63	18	25	61.8	98	1.1	...	...

[1]Convert to mL/min by multiplying the number given by 16.6.
[2]Varies with concentration.
[3]Can be estimated from measured C_p using $CL = V_{max}/(K_m + C_p)$; V_{max} = 415 mg/d, K_m = 5 mg/L. See text.
[4]Varies because of concentration-dependent clearance.

Figure 3–2. Models of drug distribution and elimination. The effect of adding drug to the blood by rapid intravenous injection is represented by expelling a known amount of the agent into a beaker. The time course of the amount of drug in the beaker is shown in the graphs at the right. In the first example **(A)**, there is no movement of drug out of the beaker, so the graph shows only a steep rise to maximum followed by a plateau. In the second example **(B)**, a route of elimination is present, and the graph shows a slow decay after a sharp rise to a maximum. Because the level of material in the beaker falls, the "pressure" driving the elimination process also falls, and the slope of the curve decreases, approaching the steady state asymptotically. This is an exponential decay curve. In the third model **(C)**, drug placed in the first compartment (blood) equilibrates rapidly with the second compartment (extravascular volume) and the amount of drug in "blood" declines exponentially to a new steady state. The fourth model **(D)** illustrates a more realistic combination of elimination mechanism and extravascular equilibration. The resulting graph shows an early distribution phase followed by the slower elimination phase. These curves can be linearized by plotting the logarithm of the amount of drug against time.

Table 3–2. Physical volumes (in L/kg body weight) of some body compartments into which drugs may be distributed.

Compartment and Volume	Examples of Drugs
Water	
Total body water (0.6 L/kg[1])	Small water-soluble molecules: eg, ethanol
Extracellular water (0.2 L/kg)	Larger water-soluble molecules: eg, mannitol
Blood (0.08 L/kg); plasma (0.04 L/kg)	Strongly plasma protein-bound molecules and very large molecules: eg, heparin
Fat (0.2–0.35 L/kg)	Highly lipid-soluble molecules: eg, DDT
Bone (0.07 L/kg)	Certain ions: eg, lead, fluoride

[1]An average figure. Total body water in a young lean man might be 0.7 L/kg; in an obese woman, 0.5 L/kg.

drug elimination is directly proportionate to concentration (rearranging equation [2]):

$$\text{Rate of elimination} = CL \times C \qquad (4)$$

This is sometimes referred to as "first-order" elimination. When clearance is first-order, it can be measured by calculating the area under the curve (AUC) of the time-concentration curve after a dose. Clearance is proportionate to the dose divided by AUC.

A. Capacity-Limited Elimination: For drugs that exhibit capacity-limited elimination (eg, phenytoin, ethanol), clearance will vary depending on the concentration of drug that is achieved (Table 3–1). Capacity-limited elimination is also known as saturable, dose- or concentration-dependent, nonlinear, and Michaelis-Menten elimination.

Most drug elimination pathways will become saturated if the dose is high enough. When blood flow to an organ does not limit elimination (see below), the relation between elimination rate and concentration (C) is expressed mathematically in equation (5):

$$\text{Rate of elimination} = \frac{V_{max} \times C}{K_m + C} \qquad (5)$$

This equation is similar to the Michaelis-Menten statement of enzyme kinetics. The maximum elimination capacity corresponds to V_{max} of the Michaelis-Menten equation, and K_m is the drug concentration at which the rate of elimination is 50% of V_{max}. It is important to note that in the nonlinear region, the increment in elimination rate becomes less as concentration increases. At concentrations that are high relative to the K_m, the elimination rate is almost independent of concentration—a state of "pseudo-zero order"

elimination. If dosing rate exceeds elimination capacity, steady state cannot be achieved: The concentration will keep on rising as long as dosing continues. This pattern of capacity-limited elimination is important for three drugs in common use: ethanol, phenytoin, and aspirin. It is also the mechanism of elimination for ethanol and is important when assessing the forensic significance of ethanol blood concentrations.

B. Flow-Dependent Elimination: In contrast to capacity-limited drug elimination, some drugs are cleared very readily by the organ of elimination, so that at any clinically realistic concentration of the drug, most of the drug in the blood perfusing the organ is eliminated on the first pass of the drug through it. The elimination of these drugs will thus depend primarily on the blood flow through the organ of elimination. Such drugs (listed in Table 4–7) can be called "high-extraction" drugs, since they are almost completely extracted from the blood by the organ.

Half-Life

Half-life $(t_{1/2})$ is the time required to change the amount of drug in the body by one-half during elimination (or during a constant infusion). In the simplest case—and the most useful in designing drug dosage regimens—the body may be considered as a single compartment (as illustrated in Figure 3–2B) of a size equal to the volume of distribution (V_d). While the organs of elimination can only clear drug from the blood or plasma in direct contact with the organ, this blood or plasma is in equilibrium with the total volume of distribution. Thus, the time course of drug in the body will depend on both the volume of distribution and the clearance:

$$t_{1/2} = \frac{0.7^* \times V_d}{CL} \qquad (6)$$

However, many drugs will exhibit multicompartment pharmacokinetics (as illustrated in Figures 3–2C and 2D). Under these conditions, where more than one half-life term may apply to a single drug, the "true" terminal half-life as given in Table 3–1 will be greater than that calculated from equation (6). Nevertheless, half-life is a useful kinetic parameter in that it indicates the time required to attain 50% of steady state, or to decay 50% from steady-state conditions, after a change (ie, starting or stopping) in a particular rate of drug administration (the dosing regimen). Figure 3–3 shows the time course of drug accumulation during a constant-rate drug infusion and the time

*The constant 0.7 in equation (6) is an approximation to 0.693, the natural logarithm of 2. Because drug elimination can be described by an exponential process, the time taken for a twofold decrease can be shown to be proportionate to ln(2).

Figure 3–3. The time course of drug accumulation and elimination. *Solid line:* Plasma concentrations reflecting drug accumulation during a constant rate infusion of a drug. 50% of the steady state concentration is reached after one half-life, 75% after two half-lives, and over 90% after four half-lives. *Dashed line:* Plasma concentrations reflecting drug elimination after a constant rate infusion of a drug had reached steady state. Fifty percent of the drug is lost after one half-life, 75% after two half-lives, etc. The "rule of thumb" that 3.3–4 half-lives must elapse after starting a drug dosing regimen before full effects will be seen is based on the approach of the accumulation curve to over 90% of the final steady state concentration.

course of drug elimination after stopping an infusion that has reached steady state.

As an indicator of either drug elimination or distribution, half-life alone can be misleading. Disease states can affect both of the physiologically related parameters, volume of distribution, and clearance; thus, the derived parameter, $t_{1/2}$, will not necessarily reflect the expected change in drug elimination. For example, patients with chronic renal failure have a decreased renal clearance of digoxin and also a decreased volume of distribution; the increase in digoxin half-life is not as great as might be expected based on the change in renal function. The decrease in V_d is due to the decreased renal and skeletal muscle mass and consequent decreased tissue binding of digoxin.

Drug Accumulation

Whenever drug doses are repeated, the drug will accumulate in the body until dosing stops. This is because it takes an infinite time (in theory) to eliminate all of a given dose. In practical terms, this means that if the dosing interval is shorter than four half-lives, accumulation will be detectable.

Accumulation is inversely proportionate to the fraction of the dose lost in each dosing interval. The fraction lost is 1 minus the fraction remaining just before the next dose. The fraction remaining can be predicted from the dosing interval and the half-life. A convenient index of accumulation is the **accumulation factor.**

$$\text{Accumulation factor} = \frac{1}{\text{Fraction lost in one dosing interval}}$$

$$= \frac{1}{1 - \text{Fraction remaining}}$$

(7)

For a drug given once every half-life, the accumulation factor is 1/0.5, or 2. The accumulation factor predicts the ratio of the steady state concentration to that following the first dose. Thus, the peak concentrations after intermittent doses at steady state will be equal to the peak concentration after the first dose multiplied by the accumulation factor.

Bioavailability

Bioavailability is defined as the fraction of unchanged drug reaching the systemic circulation following administration by any route (Table 3–3). For an intravenous dose of the drug, bioavailability is equal to unity. Data on bioavailability following oral drug administration are set forth in Table 3–1 as percentages of dose available to the systemic circulation. For a drug administered orally, bioavailability may be less than 100% for two main reasons—incomplete extent of absorption and first-pass elimination.

A. Extent of Absorption: After oral administration, a drug may be incompletely absorbed, eg, only

Table 3–3. Routes of administration, bioavailability, and general characteristics.

Route	Bioavailability (%)	Characteristics
Intravenous	100 (by definition)	Most rapid onset
Intramuscular	≤100	Large volumes often feasible; may be painful
Subcutaneous	≤100	Smaller volumes than IM; may be painful
Oral	<100	Most convenient; first-pass effect may be significant
Rectal	<100	Less first-pass effect than oral
Inhalation	<100	Often very rapid onset
Transdermal	≤100	Usually very slow absorption; used for lack of first-pass effect; prolonged duration of action

70% of a dose of digoxin reaches the systemic circulation. This is mainly due to lack of absorption from the gut and is in part explained by bacterial metabolism of digoxin within the intestine. Other drugs are either too hydrophilic (eg, atenolol) or too lipophilic (eg, acyclovir) to be absorbed easily, and their low bioavailability is also due to incomplete absorption. If too hydrophilic, the drug cannot cross the lipid cell membrane; if too lipophilic, the drug is not soluble enough to cross the water layer adjacent to the cell.

B. First-Pass Elimination: Following absorption across the gut wall, the portal blood delivers the drug to the liver prior to entry into the systemic circulation. A drug can be metabolized in the gut wall or even in the portal blood, but most commonly it is the liver that is responsible for metabolism before the drug reaches the systemic circulation. In addition, the liver can excrete the drug into the bile. Any of these sites can contribute to this reduction in bioavailability, and the overall process is known as first-pass loss or elimination. The effect of first-pass hepatic elimination on bioavailability is expressed as the **extraction ratio** (ER):

$$ER = \frac{CL_{liver}}{Q} \qquad (8a)$$

where Q is hepatic blood flow, normally about 90 L/h in a person weighing 70 kg.

The systemic bioavailability of the drug (F) can be predicted from the extent of absorption (f) and the extraction ratio (ER):

$$F = f \times (1 - ER) \qquad (8b)$$

This process is shown schematically in Figure 3–4. A drug like morphine is almost completely absorbed (f = 1), so that loss in the gut is negligible. However, the hepatic extraction ratio for morphine is 0.67, so (1 − ER) is 0.33. The bioavailability of morphine is therefore expected to be about 33%, which is close to the observed value (Table 3–1).

C. Rate of Absorption: In addition to the definition given above, bioavailability is sometimes used (confusingly) to indicate both the extent *and* the rate at which an administered dose reaches the general circulation.

The distinction between rate and extent of absorption is clarified in Figure 3–5. The rate of absorption is determined by the site of administration and the drug formulation. Both the rate of absorption and the extent of input can influence the clinical effectiveness of a drug. For the three different dosage forms depicted in Figure 3–5, there would be significant differences in the intensity of clinical effect. Dosage form B would require twice the dose to attain blood concentrations equivalent to those of dosage form A. Differences in rate of availability may become important for drugs given as a single dose, such as a hypnotic used to induce sleep. In this case, drug from dosage form A would reach its minimum effective concentration earlier than drug from dosage form C; concentrations from A would also reach a higher level and remain above the minimum effective concentration for a longer period. In a multiple dosing regimen, dosage forms A and C would yield the same average blood level concentrations, though dosage form A would show somewhat greater maximum and lower minimum concentrations.

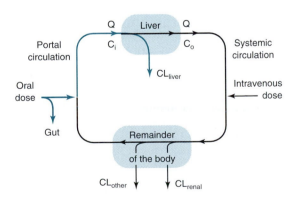

Figure 3–4. The clearance of drug by the liver is separated from the remaining systemic clearance to illustrate the effects of blood flow *(Q)* and extraction ratio ([C_i − C_o]/C_i) on organ clearance. The processes involved in first-pass metabolism are shown in color.

A: Drug rapidly and completely available

B: Only half of availability of A but rate equal to A

C: Drug completely available but rate only half of A

Figure 3–5. Blood concentration-time curves, illustrating how changes in the rate of absorption and extent of bioavailability can influence both the duration of action and the efficacy of the same total dose of a drug administered in three different formulations. The dashed line indicates the minimum effective concentration (MEC) of the drug in the blood.

The mechanism of drug absorption is said to be zero-order when the rate is independent of the amount of drug remaining in the gut, eg, when it is determined by the rate of gastric emptying or by a controlled-release drug formulation. In contrast, when the full dose is dissolved in gastrointestinal fluids, the rate of absorption is usually proportionate to the concentration and is said to be first-order.

Extraction Ratio & the First-Pass Effect

Disposition—systemic clearance, loss from the biologic system—is not affected by bioavailability. However, disposition can markedly affect the extent of availability because it determines the extraction ratio (equation [8a]). Of course, therapeutic blood levels may still be reached by the oral route of administration if larger doses are given. However, in this case, the levels of the drug *metabolites* will be increased significantly over those that would occur following intravenous administration. Lidocaine and verapamil are both used to treat cardiac arrhythmias and have similar bioavailability (20%), but lidocaine is never given orally because its metabolites are believed to contribute to central nervous system toxicity. Other drugs that are highly extracted by the liver include isoniazid, morphine, propranolol, verapamil, and several tricyclic antidepressants (Table 4–7).

Drugs with high extraction ratios will show marked intersubject variations in bioavailability because of differences in hepatic function and blood flow. These differences can explain the marked variation in drug concentrations that occurs among individuals given similar doses of highly extracted drugs. These considerations are also pertinent for hepatic diseases that are accompanied by significant intrahepatic or extrahepatic circulatory shunting and in the presence of surgically created anastomoses between the portal system and the systemic venous circulation. For drugs that are highly extracted by the liver, shunting of blood past hepatic sites of elimination will result in substantial increases in drug availability, whereas for drugs that are poorly extracted by the liver (for which the difference between entering and exiting drug concentration is small), shunting of blood past the liver will cause little change in availability. Drugs in Table 3–1 that are poorly extracted by the liver include chlorpropamide, diazepam, digitoxin, phenytoin, theophylline, tolbutamide, and warfarin.

Alternative Routes of Administration & the First-Pass Effect

Many routes of administration are used in clinical medicine (Table 3–3)—for convenience (eg, oral), to maximize concentration at the site of action and minimize it elsewhere (eg, topical), to prolong the duration of drug absorption (eg, transdermal), or to avoid the first-pass effect.

The hepatic first-pass effect can be avoided to a great extent by use of sublingual tablets and transdermal preparations and to a lesser extent by use of rectal suppositories. Sublingual absorption provides direct access to systemic—not portal—veins. The transdermal route offers the same advantage. Drugs absorbed from suppositories in the lower rectum enter vessels that drain into the inferior vena cava, thus bypassing the liver. However, suppositories tend to move upward in the rectum into a region where veins that lead to the liver, such as the superior hemorrhoidal vein, predominate. In addition, there are extensive anastomoses between the superior and middle hemorrhoidal veins; thus, only about 50% of a rectal dose can be assumed to bypass the liver.

Although drugs administered by inhalation bypass the hepatic first-pass effect, the lung may also serve as a site of first-pass loss by excretion and possibly metabolism for drugs administered by nongastrointestinal ("parenteral") routes. The lungs also provide a filtering function for particulate matter that may be given by intravenous injection.

THE TIME COURSE OF DRUG EFFECT

The principles of pharmacokinetics (discussed in this chapter) and those of pharmacodynamics (discussed in Chapter 2) provide a framework for understanding the time course of drug effect.

Immediate Effects

In the simplest case, drug effects are directly related to plasma concentrations, but this does not necessarily mean that effects simply parallel the time course of concentrations. Because the relationship between drug concentration and effect is not linear (recall the E_{max} model described in Chapter 2), the effect will not be always be directly proportionate to the concentration.

Consider the effect of an angiotensin-converting enzyme inhibitor, such as enalapril, on plasma angiotensin-converting enzyme (ACE). The half-life of enalapril is about 3 hours. After an oral dose of 10 mg, the peak plasma concentration at 3 hours is about 64 ng/mL. Enalapril is usually given once a day, so seven half-lives will elapse from the time of peak concentration to the end of the dosing interval. The concentration of enalapril after each half-life and the corresponding extent of ACE inhibition are shown in Figure 3–6. The extent of inhibition of ACE is calculated using the E_{max} model, where E_{max}, the maximum extent of inhibition, is 100% and the EC50 is about 1 ng/mL.

Note that plasma concentrations of enalapril change by a factor of 16 over the first 12 hours (four half-lives) after the peak, but ACE inhibition has only decreased by 20%. Because the concentrations over this time are so high in relation to the EC50, the effect on ACE is almost constant. After 24 hours, ACE is

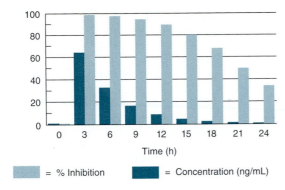

= % Inhibition   = Concentration (ng/mL)

Figure 3–6. Time course of ACE inhibitor concentrations and effects. The darker bars show the plasma enalapril concentrations in nanograms per milliliter after a single oral dose. The lighter bars indicate the percentage inhibition of its target, angiotensin-converting enzyme. Note the different shapes of the concentration-time course (exponentially decreasing) and the effect-time course (linearly decreasing in its central portion).

still 33% inhibited. This explains why a drug with a short half-life can be given once a day and still maintain its effect throughout the day. The key factor is a high initial concentration in relation to the EC50. Even though the plasma concentration at 24 hours is less than 1% of its peak, this low concentration is still half the EC50. This is very common for drugs that act on enzymes, eg, ACE inhibitors, or compete at receptors, eg, propranolol.

When concentrations are in the range between one-fourth and four times the EC50, the time course of effect is essentially a linear function of time—13% of the effect is lost every half-life over this concentration range. At concentrations below one-fourth the EC50, the effect becomes almost directly proportionate to concentration and the time course of drug effect will follow the exponential decline of concentration. It is only when the concentration is low in relation to the EC50 that the concept of a "half-life of drug effect" has any meaning.

Delayed Effects

Changes in the intensity of drug effects are often delayed in relation to changes in plasma concentration. This delay may reflect the time required for the drug to distribute from plasma to the site of action. This will be the case for almost all drugs. The delay due to distribution is a pharmacokinetic phenomenon that can account for delays of a few minutes up to a few hours. The distributional delay can account for the lag of effects after rapid intravenous injection of CNS-active agents such as thiopental.

A common reason for more delayed drug effects—especially those that take many hours or even days to occur—is the slow turnover of a physiologic sub-

stance that is involved in the expression of the drug effect. For example, warfarin works as an anticoagulant by inhibiting vitamin K epoxidase in the liver. This action of warfarin occurs rapidly, and inhibition of the enzyme is probably closely related to plasma concentrations of warfarin. The clinical effect of warfarin, eg, on the prothrombin time, reflects a decrease in the concentration of the prothrombin complex of clotting factors (Figure 34–7). Inhibition of vitamin K epoxidase decreases the synthesis of these clotting factors, but the complex has a long half-life (about 14 hours), and it is this half-life that determines how long it takes for the concentration of clotting factors to reach a new steady state and for a drug effect to become manifest reflecting the warfarin plasma concentration.

Cumulative Effects

Some drug effects are more obviously related to a cumulative action than to a rapidly reversible one. The renal toxicity of aminoglycoside antibiotics (eg, gentamicin) is greater when administered as a constant infusion as compared with intermittent dosing. It is the accumulation of aminoglycoside in the renal cortex that is thought to cause renal damage. Even though both dosing schemes produce the same average steady state concentration, the intermittent dosing scheme produces much higher peak concentrations, which saturate an uptake mechanism into the cortex; thus, total aminoglycoside accumulation is less. The difference in toxicity is a predictable consequence of the different patterns of concentration and the saturable uptake mechanism.

The effect of many drugs used to treat cancer also reflects a cumulative action, eg, the extent of binding of a drug to DNA is proportionate to drug concentration and is usually irreversible. The effect on tumor growth is therefore a consequence of cumulative exposure to the drug. Measures of cumulative exposure, such as area under the concentration time curve of the drug (AUC), have shown promise as predictors of response and—as a target AUC—provide a means to individualize treatment.

THE TARGET CONCENTRATION APPROACH TO DESIGNING A RATIONAL DOSAGE REGIMEN

A rational dosage regimen is based on the assumption that there is a *target concentration* that will produce the desired therapeutic effect. By considering the pharmacokinetic factors that determine the dose-concentration relationship, it is possible to individualize the dose regimen to achieve the target concentration. The effective concentration ranges shown in Table 3–1 are a guide to the concentrations measured when patients are being effectively treated. The initial target concentration should usually be chosen from the lower end of this range. In some cases, the target concentration will also depend on the specific therapeutic objective—eg, the control of atrial fibrillation by digoxin often requires a target concentration of 2 ng/mL, while heart failure is usually adequately managed with a target concentration of 1 ng/mL.

Maintenance Dose

In most clinical situations, drugs are administered in such a way as to maintain a steady state of drug in the body, ie, just enough drug is given in each dose to replace the drug eliminated since the preceding dose. Thus, calculation of the appropriate maintenance dose is a primary goal. Clearance is the most important pharmacokinetic term to be considered in defining a rational steady state drug dosage regimen. At steady state (SS), the dosing rate ("rate in") must equal the rate of elimination ("rate out"). Substitution of the target concentration (TC) for concentration (C) in equation (4) predicts the maintenance dosing rate:

$$\text{Dosing rate}_{ss} = \text{Rate of elimination}_{ss}$$

$$= CL \times TC \qquad (9)$$

Thus, if the desired target concentration is known, the clearance in that patient will determine the dosing rate. If the drug is given by a route that has a bioavailability less than 100%, then the dosing rate predicted by equation (9) must be modified. For oral dosing:

$$\text{Dosing rate}_{oral} = \frac{\text{Dosing rate}}{F_{oral}} \qquad (10)$$

If intermittent doses are given, the maintenance dose is calculated from:

Maintenance dose =

$$\text{Dosing rate} \times \text{Dosing interval} \qquad (11)$$

(See box: Example: Maintenance Dose Calculation.)

Note that the steady state concentration achieved by continuous infusion or the *average* concentration following intermittent dosing depends only on clearance. The volume of distribution and the half-life need not be known in order to determine the average plasma concentration expected from a given dosing rate or to predict the dosing rate for a desired target concentration. Figure 3–7 shows that at different dosing intervals, the concentration time curves will have different maximum and minimum values even though the average level will always be 10 mg/L.

Estimates of dosing rate and average steady state concentrations, which may be calculated using clearance, are independent of any specific pharmacokinetic model. In contrast, the determination of maximum and minimum steady state concentrations requires assumptions about the pharmacokinetic model. The accumulation factor (equation [7]) assumes that the drug follows a one-compartment body model (Figure 3–2B), and the peak concentration prediction assumes that the absorption rate is much faster than the elimination rate. For the calculation of estimated maximum and minimum concentrations in a clinical situation, these assumptions are usually reasonable.

Figure 3–7. Relationship between frequency of dosing and maximum and minimum plasma concentrations when a steady-state theophylline plasma level of 10 mg/L is desired. The smoothly rising line (solid black) shows the plasma concentration achieved with an intravenous infusion of 28 mg/h. The doses for 8-hourly administration (light color) are 224 mg; for 24-hourly administration (dark color), 672 mg. In each of the three cases, the mean steady state plasma concentration is 10 mg/L.

EXAMPLE: MAINTENANCE DOSE CALCULATION

A target plasma theophylline concentration of 10 mg/L is desired to relieve acute bronchial asthma in a patient (Holford et al, 1993). If the patient is a nonsmoker and otherwise normal except for asthma, we may use the mean clearance given in Table 3–1, ie, 2.8 L/h/70 kg. Since the drug will be given as an intravenous infusion, F = 1.

$$\text{Dosing rate} = CL \times TC$$
$$= 2.8 \text{ L/h/70kg} \times 10\text{mg/L}$$
$$= 28 \text{ mg/h/70kg}$$

Therefore, in this patient, the proper infusion rate would be 28 mg/h/70 kg.

If the asthma attack is relieved, the clinician might want to maintain this plasma level using oral theophylline, which might be given every 12 hours using an extended release formulation to approximate a continuous intravenous infusion. According to Table 3–1, F_{oral} is 0.96. When the dosing interval is 12 hours, the size of each maintenance dose would be:

$$\text{Maintenance dose} = \frac{\text{Dosing rate}}{F} \times \text{Dosing interval}$$
$$= \frac{28 \text{ mg/h}}{0.96} \times 12 \text{ hours}$$
$$= 350 \text{ mg}$$

A tablet or capsule size close to the ideal dose of 350 mg would then be prescribed at 12-hourly intervals. If an 8-hour dosing interval was used, the ideal dose would be 233 mg; and if the drug was given once a day, the dose would be 700 mg. In practice, F could be omitted from the calculation since it is so close to 1.

Loading Dose

When the time to reach steady state is appreciable, as it is for drugs with long half-lives, it may be desirable to administer a loading dose that promptly raises the concentration of drug in plasma to the target concentration. In theory, only the amount of the loading dose need be computed—not the rate of its administration—and, to a first approximation, this is so. The volume of distribution is the proportionality factor that relates the total amount of drug in the body to the concentration in the plasma (C_p); if a loading dose is to achieve the target concentration, then from equation (1):

$$\text{Loading dose} = \text{Amount in the body immediately following the loading dose}$$
$$= V_d \times TC \qquad (12)$$

For the theophylline example in the box above, the loading dose would be 350 mg (35 L × 10 mg/L) for a 70 kg person. For most drugs, the loading dose can be given as a single dose by the chosen route of administration.

Up to this point, we have ignored the fact that some drugs follow more complex multicompartment pharmacokinetics, eg, the distribution process illustrated by the two-compartment model in Figure 3–2. This is justified in the great majority of cases. However, in some cases the distribution phase may not be ignored, particularly in connection with the calculation of loading doses. If the rate of absorption is rapid relative to distribution (this is always true for intravenous bolus administration), the concentration of drug in plasma that results from an appropriate loading dose—calculated using the apparent V_d—can initially be considerably higher than desired. Severe toxicity may occur, albeit transiently. This may be particularly important, for example, in the administration of antiarrhythmic drugs such as lidocaine, where an almost immediate toxic response may occur. Thus, while the estimation of the *amount* of a loading dose may be quite correct, the *rate of administration* can sometimes be crucial in preventing excessive drug concentrations, and slow administration of an intravenous drug (over minutes rather than seconds) is almost always prudent practice. For intravenous doses of theophylline, initial injections should be given over a 20-minute period to avoid the possibility of high plasma concentrations during the distribution phase.

When intermittent doses are given, the loading dose calculated from equation (12) will only reach the average steady state concentration and will not match the peak steady state concentration (see Figure 3–7). To match the peak steady state concentration, the loading dose can be calculated from equation (13):

$$\text{Loading dose} = \text{Maintenance dose} \times \text{Accumulation factor} \qquad (13)$$

THERAPEUTIC DRUG MONITORING: RELATING PHARMACOKINETICS & PHARMACODYNAMICS

The basic principles outlined above can be applied to the interpretation of clinical drug concentration measurements on the basis of three major pharmacokinetic variables: absorption, clearance, and volume of distribution (and the derived variable, half-life); and two pharmacodynamic variables: maximum effect attainable in the target tissue and the sensitivity of the tissue to the drug. Diseases may modify all of these parameters, and the ability to predict the effect of disease states on pharmacokinetic parameters is important in properly adjusting dosage in such cases. (See box: The Target Concentration Strategy.)

Pharmacokinetic Variables

A. Absorption: The amount of drug that enters the body depends on the patient's compliance with the prescribed regimen and on the rate and extent of transfer from the site of administration to the blood.

Overdosage and underdosage relative to the prescribed dosage—both aspects of failure of compliance—can frequently be detected by concentration measurements when gross deviations from expected values are obtained. If compliance is found to be adequate, absorption abnormalities in the small bowel may be the cause of abnormally low concentrations. Variations in the extent of bioavailability are rarely caused by irregularities in the manufacture of the particular drug formulation. More commonly, variations in bioavailability are due to metabolism during absorption.

THE TARGET CONCENTRATION STRATEGY

Recognition of the essential role of concentration in linking pharmacokinetics and pharmacodynamics leads naturally to the target concentration strategy. Pharmacodynamic principles can be used to predict the concentration required to achieve a particular degree of therapeutic effect. This target concentration can then be achieved by using pharmacokinetic principles to arrive at a suitable dosing regimen. The target concentration strategy is a process for optimizing the dose in an individual on the basis of a measured surrogate response such as drug concentration:

1. Choose the target concentration.
2. Predict V_d and CL based on typical population values (eg, Table 3–1) and adjustments for factors such as weight and renal function.
3. Give a loading dose or maintenance dose calculated from TC, V_d, and CL.
4. Measure the patient's response and drug concentration.
5. Revise V_d and CL based on the measured concentration.
6. Repeat steps 3–6, adjusting the maintenance dose as needed to optimize the response.

B. Clearance: Abnormal clearance may be anticipated when there is major impairment of the function of the kidney, liver, or heart. Creatinine clearance is a useful quantitative indicator of renal function. Conversely, drug clearance may be a useful indicator of the functional consequences of heart, kidney, or liver failure, often with greater precision than clinical findings or other laboratory tests. For example, when renal function is changing rapidly, estimation of the clearance of aminoglycoside antibiotics may be a more accurate indicator of glomerular filtration than serum creatinine.

Hepatic disease has been shown to reduce the clearance and prolong the half-life of many drugs. However, for many other drugs known to be eliminated by hepatic processes, no changes in clearance or half-life have been noted with similar hepatic disease. This reflects the fact that hepatic disease does not always affect the hepatic intrinsic clearance. At present, there is no reliable marker of hepatic drug-metabolizing function that can be used to predict changes in liver clearance in a manner analogous to the use of creatinine clearance as a marker of renal drug clearance.

C. Volume of Distribution: The apparent volume of distribution reflects a balance between binding to tissues, which decreases plasma concentration and makes the apparent volume larger, and binding to plasma proteins, which increases plasma concentration and makes the apparent volume smaller. Changes in either tissue or plasma binding can change the apparent volume of distribution determined from plasma concentration measurements. Older people have a relative decrease in skeletal muscle mass and tend to have a smaller apparent volume of distribution of digoxin. The volume of distribution may be overestimated in obese patients if based on body weight and the drug does not enter fatty tissues well, as is the case with digoxin. In contrast, theophylline has a volume of distribution similar to that of total body water. Adipose tissue has almost as much water in it as other tissues, so that the apparent total volume of distribution of theophylline is proportionate to body weight even in obese patients.

Abnormal accumulation of fluid—edema, ascites, pleural effusion—can markedly increase the volume of distribution of drugs such as tobramycin that are hydrophilic and—in the absence of such accumulation—have small volumes of distribution.

D. Half-Life: The differences between clearance and half-life are important in defining the underlying mechanisms for the effect of a disease state on drug disposition. For example, the half-life of diazepam increases with age. When clearance is related to age, it is found that clearance of this drug does not change with age. The increasing half-life for diazepam actually results from changes in the volume of distribution with age; the metabolic processes responsible for eliminating the drug are fairly constant.

Pharmacodynamic Variables

A. Maximum Effect: All pharmacologic responses must have a maximum effect (E_{max}). No matter how high the drug concentration goes, a point will be reached beyond which no further increment in response is achieved.

If increasing the dose in a particular patient does not lead to a further clinical response, it is possible that the maximum effect has been reached. This can be verified by demonstrating that an increase in dose results in increased drug concentration without increased drug effect. Recognition of maximum effect is helpful in avoiding ineffectual increases of dose with the attendant risk of toxicity.

B. Sensitivity: The sensitivity of the target organ to drug concentration is reflected by the concentration required to produce 50% of maximum effect, the EC50. Failure of response due to diminished sensitivity to the drug can be detected by measuring—in a patient who is not getting better—drug concentrations that are usually associated with therapeutic response. This may be a result of abnormal physiology—eg, hyperkalemia diminishes responsiveness to digoxin—or drug antagonism—eg, calcium channel blockers impair the inotropic response to digoxin.

Increased sensitivity to a drug is usually signaled by exaggerated responses to small or moderate doses. The pharmacodynamic nature of this sensitivity can be confirmed by drug concentrations that are low in relation to the observed effect.

INTERPRETATION OF DRUG CONCENTRATION MEASUREMENTS

Clearance

Clearance is the single most important factor determining drug concentrations. The interpretation of measurements of drug concentrations depends upon a clear understanding of three factors that may influence clearance. These are the dose, the blood flow, and the intrinsic function of the liver or kidneys. Each of these factors should be considered when interpreting clearance estimated from a drug concentration measurement. It must also be recognized that changes in protein binding may lead the unwary to believe there is a change in clearance when in fact drug elimination is not altered (see box: Plasma Protein Binding: Is It Important?). Factors affecting protein binding include the following:

A. Albumin Concentration: Drugs such as phenytoin, salicylates, and disopyramide are extensively bound to plasma albumin. Albumin levels are low in many disease states, resulting in lower total drug concentrations.

B. α_1-Acid Glycoprotein Concentration: α_1-Acid glycoprotein is an important binding protein with binding sites for drugs such as quinidine, lido-

caine, and propranolol. It is increased in acute inflammatory disorders and causes major changes in total plasma concentration of these drugs even though drug elimination is unchanged.

C. Capacity-Limited Protein Binding: The binding of drugs to plasma proteins is capacity-limited. Therapeutic concentrations of salicylates, disopyramide, and prednisolone show concentration-dependent protein binding. Because unbound drug concentration is determined by dosing rate and clearance—which is not altered, in the case of these low-extraction-ratio drugs, by protein binding—increases in dosing rate will cause corresponding changes in the pharmacodynamically important unbound concentration. Total drug concentration will increase less rapidly than the dosing rate would suggest as protein binding approaches saturation at higher concentrations.

Dosing History

An accurate dosing history is essential if one is to obtain maximum value from a drug concentration measurement. In fact, if the dosing history is unknown or incomplete, a drug concentration measurement loses all predictive value.

Timing of Samples for Concentration Measurement

Information about the rate and extent of drug absorption in a particular patient is rarely of great clinical importance. However, absorption usually occurs during the first 2 hours after a drug dose and varies according to food intake, posture, and activity. Therefore, it is important to avoid drawing blood until absorption is complete (about 2 hours after an oral dose). Attempts to measure peak concentrations early after oral dosing are usually unsuccessful and compromise the validity of the measurement, because one cannot be certain that absorption is complete.

Some drugs such as digoxin and lithium take several hours to distribute to tissues. Digoxin samples should be taken at least 6 hours after the last dose and lithium just before the next dose (usually 24 hours after the last dose). Aminoglycosides distribute quite rapidly, but it is still prudent to wait 1 hour after giving the dose before taking a sample.

Clearance is readily estimated from the dosing rate and mean steady state concentration. Blood samples should be appropriately timed to estimate steady state concentration. Provided steady state has been reached (at least three half-lives of constant dosing), a sample obtained near the midpoint of the dosing interval will usually be close to the mean steady state concentration.

Initial Predictions of Volume of Distribution & Clearance

A. Volume of Distribution: Volume of distribution is commonly calculated for a particular patient using body weight (70 kg body weight is assumed for

PLASMA PROTEIN BINDING: IS IT IMPORTANT?

Plasma protein binding is often mentioned as a factor playing a role in pharmacokinetics, pharmacodynamics, and drug interactions. However, there are no clinically relevant examples of changes in drug disposition or effects that can be clearly ascribed to changes in plasma protein binding. The idea that if a drug is displaced from plasma proteins it would increase the unbound drug concentration and increase the drug effect and, perhaps, produce toxicity seems a simple and obvious mechanism. Unfortunately, this simple theory, which is appropriate for a test tube, does not work in the body, which is an open system capable of eliminating unbound drug.

First, a seemingly dramatic change in the unbound fraction from 1% to 10% releases less than 5% of the total amount of drug in the body into the unbound pool because less than one-third of the drug in the body is bound to plasma proteins even in the most extreme cases, eg, warfarin. Drug displaced from plasma protein will of course distribute throughout the volume of distribution, so that a 5% increase in the amount of unbound drug in the body produces at most a 5% increase in pharmacologically active unbound drug at the site of action.

Second, when the amount of unbound drug in plasma increases, the rate of elimination will increase (if clearance is unchanged), and after four half-lives the unbound concentration will return to its previous steady state value. When drug interactions associated with protein binding displacement and clinically important effects have been studied, it has been found that the displacing drug is also an inhibitor of clearance, and it is the change in *clearance* of the unbound drug that is the relevant mechanism explaining the interaction.

the values in Table 3–1. If a patient is obese, drugs that do not readily penetrate fat (eg, tobramycin and digoxin) should have their volumes calculated from ideal body weight as shown below:

$$\text{Ideal body wt (kg)} = 52 + 1.9 \text{ kg/in height over 5 ft (men)} \quad (14)$$
$$= 49 + 1.7 \text{ kg/in height over 5 ft (women)}$$

Patients with edema, ascites, or pleural effusions offer a larger volume of distribution to the aminoglycoside antibiotics (eg, tobramycin) than is predicted by body weight. In such patients, the weight should be corrected as follows: Subtract an estimate of the weight of the excess fluid accumulation. Use the resultant "normal" body weight to calculate the normal volume of distribution. Finally, this normal volume should be increased by 1 L for each estimated kilogram of excess fluid. This correction is important because of the relatively small volumes of distribution of these water-soluble drugs.

B. Clearance: Drugs cleared by the renal route often require adjustment of clearance in proportion to renal function. This can be conveniently estimated from the creatinine clearance, determined from a single blood sample (Bjornsson, 1979).*

$$\text{Creatinine clearance (L/h)} = \frac{160 - \text{Age (years)}}{22 \times \text{Serum creatinine (mg/dL)}} \quad (15)$$
$$\times \frac{\text{Weight (kg)}}{70} \quad (\times\, 0.9 \text{ if female})$$

Note: If serum creatinine is measured in mmol/L, the 22 in the denominator should be replaced by 250.

The predicted clearance in women is 90% of the calculated value, because they have a smaller muscle mass per kilogram and it is muscle mass that determines creatinine production. Because of the difficulty of obtaining complete urine collections, creatinine clearance calculated in this way is at least as reliable as estimates based on urine collections. Ideal body weight should be used for obese patients, and correction should be made for muscle wasting in severely ill patients.

Revising Individual Estimates of Volume of Distribution & Clearance

The commonsense approach to the interpretation of drug concentrations compares predictions of pharmacokinetic parameters and expected concentrations to measured values. If measured concentrations differ by more than 20% from predicted values, revised estimates of V_d or CL for that patient should be calculated using equation (1) or equation (2). If the change calculated is more than a 100% increase or 50% decrease in either V_d or CL, the assumptions made about the timing of the sample and the dosing history should be critically examined.

For example, if a patient is taking 0.25 mg of digoxin a day, a clinician may expect the digoxin concentration to be about 1 ng/mL. This is based on typical values for bioavailability of 70% and total clearance of about 7 L/h (CL_{renal} 4 L/h, $CL_{nonrenal}$ 3 L/h). If the patient has heart failure, the nonrenal (hepatic) clearance might be halved because of hepatic congestion and hypoxia, so the expected clearance would be-

---

*A similar equation, the Cockcroft-Gault equation, is given in Chapter 61.

come 5.5 L/h. The concentration is then expected to be about 1.3 ng/mL. Suppose that the concentration actually measured is 2 ng/mL. Common sense would suggest halving the daily dose to achieve a target concentration of 1 ng/mL. This approach implies a revised clearance of 3.5 L/h. The smaller clearance compared with the expected value of 5.5 L/h may reflect additional renal functional impairment due to heart failure.

This technique will often be misleading if steady state has not been reached. At least a week of regular dosing (three to four half-lives) must elapse before the implicit method will be reliable.

Failure to compare the expected concentration with the measured value in patients taking digoxin and quinidine explains why the major pharmacokinetic interaction between these two drugs went unnoticed for over 10 years, yet the doubling of steady state concentrations by the action of quinidine on digoxin clearance can be detected in almost every patient taking this drug combination.

REFERENCES

Benet LZ, Kroetz DL, Sheiner LB: Pharmacokinetics: The dynamics of drug absorption, distribution, and elimination. In: *Goodman and Gilman's The Pharmacological Basis of Therapeutics,* 9th ed. Hardman JG et al (editors). McGraw-Hill, 1996.

Benet LZ, Oie S, Schwartz JB: Appendix II. Design and optimization of dosage regimens: Pharmacokinetic data. In: *Goodman and Gilman's The Pharmacological Basis of Therapeutics,* 9th ed. Hardman JG et al (editors). McGraw-Hill, 1996.

Bjornsson TD: Use of serum creatinine concentrations to determine renal function. Clin Pharmacokinet 1979;4: 200.

Burton ME, Vasko MR, Brater DC: Comparison of drug dosing methods. Clin Pharmacokinet 1985;10:1.

Holford NHG et al: Theophylline target concentration in severe airways obstruction—10 or 20 mg/L? A randomised concentration-controlled trial. Clin Pharmacokinet 1993;25:495.

Holford NHG, Sheiner LB: Understanding the dose-effect relationship. Clin Pharmacokinet 1981;6:429.

Morgan DJ, Mclean AJ: Clinical pharmacokinetics and pharmacodynamic considerations in patients with liver disease: An update. Clin Pharmacokinet 1995;29:370.

Drug Biotransformation

Maria Almira Correia, PhD

Humans are exposed daily to a wide variety of foreign compounds called **xenobiotics**—substances absorbed across the lungs or skin or, more commonly, ingested either unintentionally as compounds present in food and drink or deliberately as drugs for therapeutic or "recreational" purposes. Exposure to environmental xenobiotics may be inadvertent and accidental or—when they are present as components of air, water, and food—inescapable. Some xenobiotics are innocuous, but many can provoke biologic responses. Some of the toxic effects of these substances are discussed in Chapters 57–59. Such biologic responses often depend on conversion of the absorbed substance into an active metabolite. The discussion that follows is applicable to xenobiotics in general (including drugs) and to some extent to endogenous compounds.

WHY IS DRUG BIOTRANSFORMATION NECESSARY?

Renal excretion plays a pivotal role in terminating the biologic activity of a few drugs, particularly those that have small molecular volumes or possess polar characteristics such as functional groups that are fully ionized at physiologic pH. Most drugs do not possess such physicochemical properties. Pharmacologically active organic molecules tend to be lipophilic and remain un-ionized or only partially ionized at physiologic pH. They are often strongly bound to plasma proteins. Such substances are not readily filtered at the glomerulus. The lipophilic nature of renal tubular membranes also facilitates the reabsorption of hydrophobic compounds following their glomerular filtration. Consequently, most drugs would have a prolonged duration of action if termination of their action depended solely on renal excretion. An alternative process that may lead to the termination or alteration of biologic activity is metabolism. In general, lipophilic xenobiotics are transformed to more polar and hence more readily excretable products. The role metabolism may play in the inactivation of lipid-soluble drugs can be quite dramatic. For example, lipophilic barbiturates such as thiopental and pentobarbital would have extremely long half-lives if it were not for their metabolic conversion to more water-soluble compounds. On the other hand, lipophilic substances such as DDT that are stored in fat and protected from the major organs of drug metabolism may persist in body fat years after exposure has ceased.

Metabolic products are often less pharmacodynamically active than the parent drug and may even be inactive. However, some biotransformation products have *enhanced* activity or toxic properties, including mutagenicity, teratogenicity, and carcinogenicity. It is noteworthy that the synthesis of endogenous substrates such as steroid hormones, cholesterol, and bile acids involves many enzyme-catalyzed pathways associated with the metabolism of xenobiotics. The same is true of the formation and excretion of endogenous metabolic products such as bilirubin, the end catabolite of heme. Finally, drug-metabolizing enzymes have been exploited through the design of pharmacologically inactive prodrugs that are converted in vivo to pharmacologically active molecules.

THE ROLE OF BIOTRANSFORMATION IN DRUG DISPOSITION

Most metabolic biotransformations occur at some point between absorption of the drug into the general circulation and its renal elimination. A few transformations occur in the intestinal lumen or intestinal wall. In general, all of these reactions can be assigned to one of two major categories called phase I and phase II reactions (Figure 4–1).

Figure 4–1. Phase I and phase II reactions in drug biodisposition. Phase II reactions may also precede phase I reactions.

Phase I reactions usually convert the parent drug to a more polar metabolite by introducing or unmasking a functional group (–OH, –NH$_2$, –SH). Often these metabolites are inactive, though in some instances activity is only modified.

If phase I metabolites are sufficiently polar, they may be readily excreted. However, many phase I products are not eliminated rapidly and undergo a subsequent reaction in which an endogenous substrate such as glucuronic acid, sulfuric acid, acetic acid, or an amino acid combines with the newly established functional group to form a highly polar conjugate. Such conjugation or synthetic reactions are the hallmarks of phase II metabolism. A great variety of drugs undergo these sequential biotransformation reactions, although in some instances the parent drug may already possess a functional group that may form a conjugate directly. For example, the hydrazide moiety of isoniazid is known to form an *N*-acetyl conjugate in a phase II reaction. This conjugate is then a substrate for a phase I type reaction, namely, hydrolysis to isonicotinic acid (Figure 4–2). Thus, phase II reactions may actually precede phase I reactions.

WHERE DO DRUG BIOTRANSFORMATIONS OCCUR?

Although every tissue has some ability to metabolize drugs, the liver is the principal organ of drug metabolism. Other tissues that display considerable activity include the gastrointestinal tract, the lungs, the skin, and the kidneys. Following oral administration, many drugs (eg, isoproterenol, meperidine, pentazocine, morphine) are absorbed intact from the small intestine and transported first via the portal system to the liver, where they undergo extensive metabolism. This process has been called a **first-pass effect.** Some orally administered drugs (eg, clonazepam, chlorpro-

mazine) are more extensively metabolized in the intestine than in the liver. Thus, intestinal metabolism may contribute to the overall first-pass effect. First-pass effects may so greatly limit the bioavailability of orally administered drugs that alternative routes of administration must be employed to achieve therapeutically effective blood levels. The lower gut harbors intestinal microorganisms that are capable of many biotransformation reactions. In addition, drugs may be metabolized by gastric acid (eg, penicillin), by digestive enzymes (eg, polypeptides such as insulin), or by enzymes in the wall of the intestine (eg, sympathomimetic catecholamines).

Although drug biotransformation in vivo can occur by spontaneous, noncatalyzed chemical reactions, the vast majority of transformations are catalyzed by specific cellular enzymes. At the subcellular level, these

Figure 4–2. Phase II activation of isoniazid (INH) to a hepatotoxic metabolite.

enzymes may be located in the endoplasmic reticulum, mitochondria, cytosol, lysosomes, or even the nuclear envelope or plasma membrane.

MICROSOMAL MIXED FUNCTION OXIDASE SYSTEM & PHASE I REACTIONS

Many drug-metabolizing enzymes are located in the lipophilic membranes of the endoplasmic reticulum of the liver and other tissues. When these lamellar membranes are isolated by homogenization and fractionation of the cell, they re-form into vesicles called **microsomes.** Microsomes retain most of the morphologic and functional characteristics of the intact membranes, including the rough and smooth surface features of the rough (ribosome-studded) and smooth (no ribosomes) endoplasmic reticulum. Whereas the rough microsomes tend to be dedicated to protein synthesis, the smooth microsomes are relatively rich in enzymes responsible for oxidative drug metabolism. In particular, they contain the important class of enzymes known as the mixed function oxidases (MFOs), or monooxygenases. The activity of these enzymes requires both a reducing agent (NADPH) and molecular oxygen; in a typical reaction, one molecule of oxygen is consumed (reduced) per substrate molecule, with one oxygen atom appearing in the product and the other in the form of water.

In this oxidation-reduction process, two microsomal enzymes play a key role. The first of these is a flavoprotein, NADPH-cytochrome P450 reductase. One mole of this enzyme contains 1 mol each of flavin mononucleotide (FMN) and flavin adenine dinucleotide (FAD). Because cytochrome c can serve as an electron acceptor, the enzyme is often referred to as NADPH-cytochrome c reductase. The second microsomal enzyme is a hemoprotein called cytochrome P450 that serves as the terminal oxidase. In fact, the microsomal membrane harbors multiple forms of this hemoprotein, and this multiplicity is increased by repeated administration of exogenous chemicals (see below). The name cytochrome P450 is derived from the spectral properties of this hemoprotein. In its reduced (ferrous) form, it binds carbon monoxide to give a complex that absorbs light maximally at 450 nm. The relative abundance of cytochrome P450, as compared with that of the reductase in the liver, contributes to making cytochrome P450 heme reduction a rate-limiting step in hepatic drug oxidations.

Microsomal drug oxidations require cytochrome P450, cytochrome P450 reductase, NADPH, and molecular oxygen. A simplified scheme of the oxidative cycle is presented in Figure 4–3. Briefly, oxidized (Fe^{3+}) cytochrome P450 combines with a drug substrate to form a binary complex (step ①). NADPH donates an electron to the flavoprotein reductase, which in turn reduces the oxidized cytochrome P450-drug

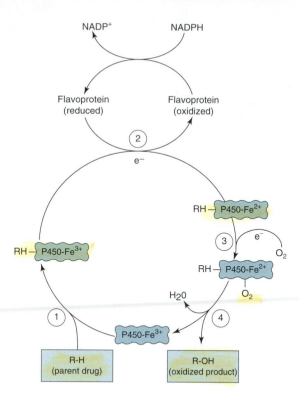

Figure 4–3. Cytochrome P450 cycle in drug oxidations. (RH, parent drug; ROH, oxidized metabolite; e^-, electron.)

complex (step ②). A second electron is introduced from NADPH via the same flavoprotein reductase, which serves to reduce molecular oxygen and to form an "activated oxygen-cytochrome P450-substrate" complex (step ③). This complex in turn transfers "activated" oxygen to the drug substrate to form the oxidized product (step ④).

The potent oxidizing properties of this activated oxygen permit oxidation of a large number of substrates. Substrate specificity is very low for this enzyme complex. High solubility in lipids is the only common structural feature of the wide variety of structurally unrelated drugs and chemicals that serve as substrates in this system (Table 4–1).

Enzyme Induction

An interesting feature of some of these chemically dissimilar drug substrates is their ability, on repeated administration, to "induce" cytochrome P450 by enhancing the rate of its synthesis or reducing its rate of degradation. Induction results in an acceleration of metabolism and usually in a decrease in the pharmacologic action of the inducer and also of coadministered drugs. However, in the case of drugs metabolically transformed to reactive metabolites, enzyme induction may exacerbate metabolite-mediated tissue toxicity.

Various substrates appear to induce forms of cytochrome P450 having different molecular masses

Table 4–1. Phase I reactions.

Reaction Class	Structural Change	Drug Substrates
Oxidations		
Cytochrome P450-dependent oxidations: Aromatic hydroxylations		Acetanilide, propranolol, phenobarbital, phenytoin, phenylbutazone, amphetamine, warfarin, 17α-ethinyl estradiol, naphthalene, benzpyrene
Aliphatic hydroxylations	$RCH_2CH_3 \rightarrow RCH_2CH_2OH$ $RCH_2CH_3 \rightarrow RCHCH_3$ $\quad\quad\quad\quad\quad\quad OH$	Amobarbital, pentobarbital, secobarbital, chlorpropamide, ibuprofen, meprobamate, glutethimide, phenylbutazone, digitoxin
Epoxidation	$RCH = CHR \rightarrow R - \overset{H}{\underset{}{C}} - \overset{O}{\underset{}{C}} - R$ (with H)	Aldrin
Oxidative dealkylation *N*-Dealkylation	$RNHCH_3 \rightarrow RNH_2 + CH_2O$	Morphine, ethylmorphine, benzphetamine, aminopyrine, caffeine, theophylline
O-Dealkylation	$ROCH_3 \rightarrow ROH + CH_2O$	Codeine, *p*-nitroanisole
S-Dealkylation	$RSCH_3 \rightarrow RSH + CH_2O$	6-Methylthiopurine, methitural
N-Oxidation Primary amines	$RNH_2 \rightarrow RNHOH$	Aniline, chlorphentermine
Secondary amines	$\underset{R_2}{\overset{R_1}{>}} NH \rightarrow \underset{R_2}{\overset{R_1}{>}} N - OH$	2-Acetylaminofluorene, acetaminophen
Tertiary amines	$\underset{R_3}{\overset{R_1}{\underset{}{}}} R_2 - N \rightarrow R_2 - N \rightarrow O$	Nicotine, methaqualone
S-Oxidation	$\underset{R_2}{\overset{R_1}{>}} S \rightarrow \underset{R_2}{\overset{R_1}{>}} S = O$	Thioridazine, cimetidine, chlorpromazine
Deamination	$\underset{NH_2}{\overset{}{RCHCH_3}} \rightarrow R - \overset{OH}{\underset{NH_2}{C}} - CH_3 \rightarrow R - CCH_3 + NH_3 \;(\overset{\|}{O})$	Amphetamine, diazepam
Desulfuration	$\underset{R_2}{\overset{R_1}{>}} C = S \rightarrow \underset{R_2}{\overset{R_1}{>}} C = O$	Thiopental

Table 4–1. Phase I reactions (cont'd).

Reaction Class	Structural Change	Drug Substrates
Cytochrome P450-dependent oxidations: (cont'd)	$\begin{array}{c} R_1 \\ \backslash \\ P=S \\ / \\ R_2 \end{array} \rightarrow \begin{array}{c} R_1 \\ \backslash \\ P=O \\ / \\ R_2 \end{array}$	Parathion
Dechlorination	$CCl_4 \rightarrow [CCl_3^{\cdot}] \rightarrow CHCl_3$	Carbon tetrachloride
Cytochrome P450-independent oxidations:		
Flavin monooxygenase (Ziegler's enzyme)	$R_3N \longrightarrow R_3N^+{\rightarrow}O^- \xrightarrow{H^+} R_3N^+OH$	Chlorpromazine, amitriptyline, benzphetamine
	$RCH_2N-CH_2R \rightarrow RCH_2-\underset{\underset{OH}{\mid}}{N}-CH_2R \rightarrow$ $\quad\quad\; \overset{\mid}{H}$ $RCH=N-CH_2R$ $\quad\quad\;\; \overset{\mid}{O^-}$	Desipramine, nortriptyline
	$\begin{array}{c} -N \\ \diagdown \\ \diagup \; -SH \rightarrow \\ -N \end{array} \begin{array}{c} -N \\ \diagdown \\ \diagup \; -SOH \rightarrow \\ -N \end{array} \begin{array}{c} -N \\ \diagdown \\ \diagup \; -SO_2H \\ -N \end{array}$	Methimazole, propylthiouracil
Amine oxidases	$RCH_2NH_2 \rightarrow RCHO + NH_3$	Phenylethylamine, epinephrine
Dehydrogenations	$RCH_2OH \rightarrow RCHO$	Ethanol
Reductions Azo reductions	$RN=NR_1 \rightarrow RNH-NHR_1 \rightarrow RNH_2 + R_1NH_2$	Prontosil, tartrazine
Nitro reductions	$RNO_2 \rightarrow RNO \rightarrow RNHOH \rightarrow RNH_2$	Nitrobenzene, chloramphenicol, clonazepam, dantrolene
Carbonyl reductions	$\underset{O}{RC}R' \rightarrow \underset{OH}{RCHR'}$	Metyrapone, methadone, naloxone
Hydrolyses Esters	$R_1COOR_2 \rightarrow R_1COOH + R_2OH$	Procaine, succinylcholine, aspirin, clofibrate, methylphenidate
Amides	$RCONHR_1 \rightarrow RCOOH + R_1NH_2$	Procainamide, lidocaine, indomethacin

and exhibiting different substrate specificities and immunochemical and spectral characteristics. The two forms that have been most extensively studied are CYP2B1 (cytochrome P450 2B1, formerly P450b), which is induced by treatment with phenobarbital; and CYP1A1 (cytochrome P450 1A1, cytochrome P_1450, or P448), which is induced by polycyclic aromatic hydrocarbons (PAHs), of which benzo[a]pyrene and 3-methylcholanthrene are prototypes. In addition, glucocorticoids, macrolide antibiotics, anticonvulsants, and some steroids induce specific forms called CYP3A. Isoniazid or chronic ethanol administration induces a different form, CYP2E1, that oxidizes ethanol and activates carcinogenic nitrosamines. The VLDL-lowering drug clofibrate induces other distinct enzymes of the CYP4A class that are responsible for ω-hydroxylation of several fatty acids, leukotrienes, and prostaglandins.

Environmental pollutants are capable of inducing cytochrome P450 enzymes. For example, exposure to benzo[a]pyrene and other polycyclic aromatic hydrocarbons, which are present in tobacco smoke, charcoal-broiled meat, and other organic pyrolysis products, is known to induce CYP1A enzymes and to alter the rates of drug metabolism in both experimental animals and in humans. Other environmental chemicals known to induce specific cytochromes P450 include the polychlorinated biphenyls (PCBs), which are used widely in industry as insulating materials and plasticizers, and 2,3,7,8-tetrachlorodibenzo-p-dioxin (dioxin, TCDD), a trace by-product of the chemical synthesis of the defoliant 2,4,5-T (Chapter 57).

Increased P450 synthesis requires enhanced transcription and translation. A cytoplasmic receptor for polycyclic aromatic hydrocarbons (eg, benzo[a]pyrene, dioxin) has been identified, and the translocation of the inducer-receptor complex into the nucleus and subsequent activation of regulatory elements of genes have been documented. A similar receptor for the other class of inducing chemicals (eg, phenobarbital) has not yet been identified (Gonzalez, 1989).

P450 enzymes may also be induced by "stabilization," ie, decreased degradation, as is the case with troleandomycin-mediated induction of CYP3A enzymes.

Enzyme Inhibition

Certain drug substrates may inhibit cytochrome P450 enzyme activity. A well-known inhibitor is proadifen (SK&F 525-A). This compound binds avidly to the cytochrome molecule and thereby competitively inhibits the metabolism of potential substrates. Imidazole-containing drugs such as cimetidine and ketoconazole bind tightly to the heme iron of cytochrome P450 and effectively reduce the metabolism of endogenous substrates (testosterone) or other coadministered drugs through competitive inhibition. However, macrolide antibiotics such as troleandomycin, erythromycin, and other erythromycin derivatives are metabolized, apparently by CYP3A, to metabolites that complex the cytochrome heme-iron and render it catalytically inactive. Some substrates irreversibly inhibit cytochrome P450 via covalent interaction of a metabolically generated reactive intermediate that may react with either the apoprotein or the heme moiety of the cytochrome. The antibiotic chloramphenicol is metabolized by cytochrome P450 to a species that alkylates its protein and thus also inactivates the enzyme. A growing list of inactivators that attack the heme moiety includes the steroids ethinyl estradiol, norethindrone, and spironolactone; the anesthetic agent fluroxene; the barbiturate allobarbital; the analgesic sedatives allylisopropylacetylurea, diethylpentenamide, and ethchlorvynol; the solvent carbon disulfide; and propylthiouracil. On the other hand, the barbiturate secobarbital is found to inactivate CYP2B1 by alkylation of both its heme and protein moieties.

Human Liver P450 Enzymes

Immunoblotting analyses—coupled with the use of relatively selective functional markers and selective P450 inhibitors—have identified numerous P450 isoforms (CYP1A2, 2A6, 2C9, 2C19, 2D6, 2E1, 3A4, 3A5, 4A11 and 7) in human liver microsomal preparations. Of these, CYP1A2, 2A6, 2C9, 2D6, 2E1, and 3A4 appear to be the major forms, accounting for approximately, 12, 4, 20, 4, 6, and 28 percent, respectively, of the total human liver P450 content. Together they are responsible for catalyzing the bulk of the hepatic drug and xenobiotic metabolism (Table 4–2). It is noteworthy that CYP3A4 alone is responsible for more than 60% of the clinically prescribed drugs metabolized by the liver. The involvement of individual P450s in the metabolism of a given drug may be screened in vitro by means of selective functional markers, selective chemical P450 inhibitors, and anti-P450 antibodies. In vivo, such screening may be accomplished by means of relatively selective noninvasive markers, which include breath tests or urinary analyses of specific metabolites after administration of a P450-selective substrate probe.

PHASE II REACTIONS

Parent drugs or their phase I metabolites that contain suitable chemical groups often undergo coupling or conjugation reactions with an endogenous substance to yield drug conjugates (Table 4–3). In general, conjugates are polar molecules that are readily excreted and often inactive. Conjugate formation involves high-energy intermediates and specific transfer enzymes. Such enzymes (transferases) may be located in microsomes or in the cytosol. They catalyze the coupling of an activated endogenous substance (such as the uridine 5′-diphosphate [UDP] derivative of glucuronic acid) with a drug (or endogenous compound), or of an activated drug (such as the S-CoA derivative of benzoic acid) with an endogenous substrate. Because the endogenous substrates originate in the diet, nutrition plays a critical role in the regulation of drug conjugations.

Drug conjugations were once believed to represent terminal inactivation events and as such have been viewed as "true detoxification" reactions. However, this concept must be modified, since it is now known that certain conjugation reactions (acyl glucuronidation of nonsteroidal anti-inflammatory drugs, O-sulfation of N-hydroxyacetylaminofluorene, and N-acetylation of isoniazid) may lead to the formation of reactive species responsible for the hepatotoxicity of the drug.

METABOLISM OF DRUGS TO TOXIC PRODUCTS

It is becoming increasingly evident that metabolism of drugs and other foreign chemicals may not always be an innocuous biochemical event leading to detoxification and elimination of the compound. Indeed, several compounds have been shown to be metabolically transformed to reactive intermediates that are toxic to various organs. Such toxic reactions may not be apparent at low levels of exposure to parent compounds when alternative detoxification mechanisms are not yet overwhelmed or compromised and the availability of endogenous detoxifying cosubstrates (glutathione, glucuronic acid, sulfate) is not limited. However, when these resources are exhausted, the toxic pathway may prevail, resulting in overt organ toxicity or carcinogenesis. The number of specific ex-

Table 4–2. Human liver P450s (CYPs), the drugs metabolized (substrates), inducers, and some drugs used for screening (noninvasive markers).

CYP	Substrates			Inducers	Noninvasive Markers
1A2	Acetaminophen Antipyrine Caffeine	Clomipramine Phenacetin Tamoxifen	Theophylline Warfarin	Smoking Charcoal-broiled foods Cruciferous vegetables	Caffeine
2A6	Coumarin			None	Coumarin
2C9	Hexobarbital Ibuprofen	Phenytoin Tolbutamide	Trimethadione S-Warfarin	Barbiturates Rifampin	Tolbutamide Warfarin
2C19	Diazepam S-Mephenytoin	Naproxen Omeprazole	Propranolol	None	S-Mephenytoin
2D6	Amitriptyline Clomipramine Clozapine Codeine Debrisoquin Desipramine Dextromethorphan Encainide Flecainide Fluoxetine	Guanoxan Haloperidol Hydrocodone Imipramine 4-Methoxyamphet- amine Metoprolol Mexiletine Nortriptyline Oxycodone	Paroxetine Phenformin Propafenone Propoxyphene Selegilene Sparteine Thioridazine Timolol	None	Debrisoquin Dextromethorphan
2E1	Acetaminophen Chlorzoxazone	Enflurane Halothane	Ethanol (a minor pathway)	Ethanol Isoniazid	Chlorzoxazone
3A4	Acetaminophen Alfentanil Amiodarone Astemizole Cocaine Cortisol Cyclosporine Dapsone Diazepam Dihydroergotamine Diltiazem Erythromycin	Ethinyl estradiol Felodipine Gestodene Lidocaine Lovastatin Miconazole Midazolam Nifedipine Niludipine Nitrendipine Paclitaxel Progesterone	Quinidine Rapamycin Sulfamethoxazole Sufentanil Tacrolimus Tamoxifen Terfenadine Testosterone Triazolam Troleandomycin Verapamil	Barbiturates Glucocorticoids Macrolide antibiotics Rifampin	Erythromycin 6β-Hydroxycortisol

amples of such drug-induced toxicity is expanding rapidly. An example is acetaminophen (paracetamol)-induced hepatotoxicity (Figure 4–4). This analgesic antipyretic drug is quite safe in therapeutic doses (1.2 g/d for an adult). It normally undergoes glucuronidation and sulfation to the corresponding conjugates, which together comprise 95% of the total excreted metabolites. The alternative cytochrome P450-dependent glutathione (GSH) conjugation pathway accounts for the remaining 5%. When acetaminophen intake far exceeds therapeutic doses, the glucuronidation and sulfation pathways are saturated, and the cytochrome P450-dependent pathway becomes increasingly important. Little or no hepatotoxicity results as long as glutathione is available for conjugation. However, with time, hepatic glutathione is depleted faster than it can be regenerated, and accumulation of a reactive and toxic metabolite occurs. In the absence of intracellular nucleophiles such as glutathione, this reactive metabolite (thought to be an *N*-hydroxylated product or an *N*-acetylbenzoiminoquinone) reacts with nucleophilic groups present on cellular macromolecules such as protein, resulting in hepatotoxicity (Figure 4–4).

The chemical and toxicologic characterization of the electrophilic nature of the reactive acetaminophen metabolite has led to the development of effective antidotes—cysteamine and *N*-acetylcysteine. Administration of *N*-acetylcysteine (the safer of the two) within 8–16 hours following acetaminophen overdosage has been shown to protect victims from fulminant hepatotoxicity and death.

Similar mechanistic interpretations can be invoked to explain the nephrotoxicity of phenacetin and the hepatotoxicity of aflatoxin and of benzo[*a*]pyrene.

CLINICAL RELEVANCE OF DRUG METABOLISM

The dose and the frequency of administration required to achieve effective therapeutic blood and tissue levels vary in different patients because of individual differences in drug distribution and rates of drug metabolism and elimination. These differences are determined by genetic factors and nongenetic variables such as age, sex, liver size, liver function, circadian rhythm, body temperature, and nutritional

Table 4–3. Phase II reactions.

Type of Conjugation	Endogenous Reactant	Transferase (Location)	Types of Substrates	Examples
Glucuronidation	UDP glucuronic acid	UDP glucuronosyl transferase (microsomes)	Phenols, alcohols, carboxylic acids, hydroxylamines, sulfonamides	Nitrophenol, morphine, acetaminophen, diazepam, N-hydroxydapsone, sulfathiazole, meprobamate, digitoxin, digoxin
Acetylation	Acetyl-CoA	N-Acetyl transferase (cytosol)	Amines	Sulfonamides, isoniazid, clonazepam, dapsone, mescaline
Glutathione conjugation	Glutathione	GSH-S-transferase (cytosol, microsomes)	Epoxides, arene oxides, nitro groups, hydroxylamines	Ethacrynic acid, bromobenzene
Glycine conjugation	Glycine	Acyl-CoA glycine transferase (mitochondria)	Acyl-CoA derivatives of carboxylic acids	Salicylic acid, benzoic acid, nicotinic acid, cinnamic acid, cholic acid, deoxycholic acid
Sulfate conjugation	Phosphoadenosyl phosphosulfate	Sulfotransferase (cytosol)	Phenols, alcohols, aromatic amines	Estrone, aniline, phenol, 3-hydroxycoumarin, acetaminophen, methyldopa
Methylation	S-Adenosyl-methionine	Transmethylases (cytosol)	Catecholamines, phenols, amines, histamine	Dopamine, epinephrine, pyridine, histamine, thiouracil
Water conjugation	Water	Epoxide hydrolase (microsomes)	Arene oxides, cis-disubstituted and monosubstituted oxiranes	Benzopyrene 7,8-epoxide, styrene 1,2-oxide, carbamazepine epoxide
		(cytosol)	Alkene oxides, fatty acid epoxides	Leukotriene A_4

and environmental factors such as concomitant exposure to inducers or inhibitors of drug metabolism. The discussion that follows will summarize the most important variables relating to drug metabolism that are of clinical relevance.

Individual Differences

Individual differences in metabolic rate depend on the nature of the drug itself. Thus, within the same population, steady state plasma levels may reflect a 30-fold variation in the metabolism of one drug and only a twofold variation in the metabolism of another.

Genetic Factors

Genetic factors that influence enzyme levels account for some of these differences. Succinylcholine, for example, is metabolized only half as rapidly in persons with genetically determined defects in pseudocholinesterase as in persons with normally functioning pseudocholinesterase. Analogous pharmacogenetic differences are seen in the acetylation of isoniazid (Figure 4–5) and the hydroxylation of war-

Figure 4–4. Metabolism of acetaminophen (Ac) to hepatotoxic metabolites. (GSH, glutathione; GS, glutathione moiety; Ac*, reactive intermediate.)

Figure 4–5. Genetic polymorphism in drug metabolism. The graph shows the distribution of plasma concentrations of isoniazid in 267 individuals 6 hours after an oral dose of 9.8 mg\kg. This distribution is clearly bimodal. Individuals with a plasma concentration greater than 2.5 mg\mL at 6 hours are considered slow acetylators. (Redrawn, with permission, from Evans DAP, Manley KA, McKusick VA: Genetic control of isoniazid metabolism in man. Br Med J 1960;2:485.)

farin. The defect in slow acetylators (of isoniazid and similar amines) appears to be caused by the synthesis of less of the enzyme rather than of an abnormal form of it. Inherited as an autosomal recessive trait, the slow acetylator phenotype occurs in about 50% of blacks and whites in the USA, more frequently in Europeans living in high northern latitudes, and much less commonly in Asians and Inuits (Eskimos). Similarly, genetically determined defects in the oxidative metabolism of debrisoquin, phenacetin, guanoxan, sparteine, phenformin, and others have been reported (Table 4–4). The defects are apparently transmitted as autosomal recessive traits and may be expressed at any one of the multiple metabolic transformations that a chemical might undergo in vivo.

Two genetic variations of these drug metabolism polymorphisms have been particularly well investi-gated and so afford some insight into possible under-lying mechanisms. First is the debrisoquin-sparteine oxidation type of polymorphism, which apparently occurs in 3–10% of whites and is inherited as an autosomal recessive trait. In affected individuals, the CYP2D6-dependent oxidations of debrisoquin and other drugs (Table 4–3) are impaired. These defects in oxidative drug metabolism are probably co-inherited. The precise molecular basis for the defect appears to be faulty expression of the cytochrome P450 protein, resulting in the absence of the necessary isozyme.

A second well-studied genetic drug polymorphism involves the stereoselective aromatic (4)-hydroxyla-tion of the anticonvulsant mephenytoin, catalyzed by CYP2C19. This polymorphism, which is also inher-ited as an autosomal recessive trait, occurs in 3–5% of Caucasians and 18–23% of Japanese populations. It is genetically independent of the debrisoquin-sparteine polymorphism. In normal "extensive metabolizers," S-mephenytoin is extensively hydroxylated by CYP2C19 at the 4 position of the phenyl ring before its glucuronidation and rapid excretion in the urine, whereas R-mephenytoin is slowly N-demethylated to nirvanol. "Poor metabolizers," however, appear to to-tally lack the stereospecific S-mephenytoin hydrox-ylase activity, so both S- and R-mephenytoin enan-tiomers are N-demethylated to nirvanol before excretion. The molecular basis for this defect is a sin-gle base pair mutation (G→A) in exon 5 of the CYP2C19 gene that creates an aberrant splice site, a correspondingly altered reading frame of the mRNA, and, finally, a truncated nonfunctional protein. It is clinically important to recognize that the safety of a drug may be severely reduced in individuals who are poor metabolizers. For example, poor metabolizers of mephenytoin show signs of profound sedation and ataxia after doses of the drug that are well tolerated by normal metabolizers.

Additional genetic polymorphisms in drug metabo-lism that are inherited independently from those al-ready described are being discovered. Studies of theo-phylline metabolism in monozygotic and dizygotic twins that included pedigree analysis of various fami-lies have revealed that a distinct polymorphism may exist for this drug and may be inherited as a recessive genetic trait. Genetic drug metabolism polymor-

Table 4–4. Some examples of genetic polymorphisms in drug metabolism.

Defect	Drug & Therapeutic Use	Clinical Consequences[1]
Oxidation	Bufuralol (β-adrenoceptor blocker)	Exacerbation of β-blockade, nausea
Oxidation	Debrisoquin (antihypertensive)	Orthostatic hypotension
Oxidation	Ethanol	Facial flushing, cardiovascular symptoms
N-Acetylation	Hydralazine (antihypertensive)	Lupus erythematosus-like syndrome
N-Acetylation	Isoniazid (antitubercular)	Peripheral neuropathy
Oxidation	Mephenytoin (antiepileptic)	Overdose toxicity
Oxidation	Sparteine	Oxytocic symptoms
Ester hydrolysis	Succinylcholine (neuromuscular blocker)	Prolonged apnea
Oxidation	Tolbutamide (hypoglycemic)	Cardiotoxicity

[1]Observed or predictable.

phisms also appear to occur for aminopyrine, tolbutamide, and carbocysteine oxidations.

Although genetic polymorphisms in drug oxidations often involve specific cytochrome P450 enzymes, such genetic variations can occur at other sites. The recent descriptions of a polymorphism in the oxidation of trimethylamine, believed to be metabolized largely by the flavin monooxygenase (Ziegler's enzyme), suggest that genetic variants of other non-P450-dependent oxidative enzymes may also contribute to such polymorphisms.

Diet & Environmental Factors

Diet and environmental factors also contribute to individual variations in drug metabolism. Charcoal-broiled foods and cruciferous vegetables are known to induce CYP1A enzymes, whereas grapefruit juice is known to inhibit the CYP3A metabolism of coadministered drug substrates. Cigarette smokers metabolize some drugs more rapidly than nonsmokers because of enzyme induction (see above). Industrial workers exposed to some pesticides metabolize certain drugs more rapidly than nonexposed individuals. Such differences make it difficult to determine effective and safe doses of drugs that have narrow therapeutic indices.

Age & Sex

Increased susceptibility to the pharmacologic or toxic activity of drugs has been reported in very young and old patients as compared with young adults (Chapters 60 and 61). Although this may reflect differences in absorption, distribution, and elimination, differences in drug metabolism cannot be ruled out—a possibility supported by studies in other mammalian species indicating that drugs are metabolized at reduced rates during the prepubertal period and senescence. Slower metabolism could be due to reduced activity of metabolic enzymes or reduced availability of essential endogenous cofactors. Similar trends have been observed in humans, but incontrovertible evidence is yet to be obtained.

Sex-dependent variations in drug metabolism have been well documented in rats but not in other rodents. Young adult male rats metabolize drugs much faster than mature female rats or prepubertal male rats. These differences in drug metabolism have been clearly associated with androgenic hormones. A few clinical reports suggest that similar sex-dependent differences in drug metabolism also exist in humans for ethanol, propranolol, benzodiazepines, estrogens, and salicylates.

Drug-Drug Interactions During Metabolism

Many substrates, by virtue of their relatively high lipophilicity, are retained not only at the active site of the enzyme but remain nonspecifically bound to the lipid membrane of the endoplasmic reticulum. In this state, they may induce microsomal enzymes; depending on the residual drug levels at the active site, they also may competitively inhibit metabolism of a simultaneously administered drug.

Enzyme-inducing drugs include various sedative-hypnotics, tranquilizers, anticonvulsants, and insecticides (Table 4–5). Patients who routinely ingest barbiturates, other sedative-hypnotics, or tranquilizers may require considerably higher doses of warfarin, when being treated with this oral anticoagulant, to maintain a prolonged prothrombin time. On the other hand, discontinuance of the sedative may result in reduced metabolism of the anticoagulant and bleeding—a toxic effect of the enhanced plasma levels of the anticoagulant. Similar interactions have been observed in individuals receiving various combination drug regimens such as antipsychotics or sedatives with contraceptive agents, sedatives with anticonvulsant drugs, and even alcohol with hypoglycemic drugs (tolbutamide).

It must also be noted that an inducer may enhance not only the metabolism of other drugs but also its own metabolism. Thus, continued use of some drugs may result in a pharmacokinetic type of tolerance—progressively reduced effectiveness due to enhancement of their own metabolism.

Conversely, simultaneous administration of two or more drugs may result in impaired elimination of the more slowly metabolized drug and prolongation or potentiation of its pharmacologic effects (Table 4–6). Both competitive substrate inhibition and irreversible substrate-mediated enzyme inactivation may augment

Table 4–5. Partial list of drugs that enhance drug metabolism in humans.

Inducer	Drug Whose Metabolism Is Enhanced
Benzo[a]pyrene	Theophylline
Chlorcyclizine	Steroid hormones
Ethchlorvynol	Warfarin
Glutethimide	Antipyrine, glutethimide, warfarin
Griseofulvin	Warfarin
Phenobarbital and other barbiturates[1]	Barbiturates, chloramphenicol, chlorpromazine, cortisol, coumarin anticoagulants, desmethylimipramine, digitoxin, doxorubicin, estradiol, phenylbutazone, phenytoin, quinine, testosterone
Phenylbutazone	Aminopyrine, cortisol, digitoxin
Phenytoin	Cortisol, dexamethasone, digitoxin, theophylline
Rifampin	Coumarin anticoagulants, digitoxin, glucocorticoids, methadone, metoprolol, oral contraceptives, prednisone, propranolol, quinidine

[1]Secobarbital is an exception. See Table 4–6 and text.

Table 4–6. Partial list of drugs that inhibit drug metabolism in humans.

Inhibitor	Drug Whose Metabolism Is Inhibited
Allopurinol, chloramphenicol, isoniazid	Antipyrine, dicumarol, probenecid, tolbutamide
Cimetidine	Chlordiazepoxide, diazepam, warfarin, others
Dicumarol	Phenytoin
Diethylpentenamide	Diethylpentenamide
Disulfiram	Antipyrine, ethanol, phenytoin, warfarin
Ethanol	Chlordiazepoxide (?), diazepam (?), methanol
Ketoconazole	Cyclosporine, astemizole, terfenadine
Nortriptyline	Antipyrine
Oral contraceptives	Antipyrine
Phenylbutazone	Phenytoin, tolbutamide
Secobarbital	Secobarbital
Troleandomycin	Theophylline, methylprednisolone

plasma drug levels and lead to toxic effects from drugs with narrow therapeutic indices. For example, it has been shown that erythromycin inhibits the metabolism of the antihistamine terfenadine and leads to the expression of adverse effects such as cardiac arrhythmias. Similarly, allopurinol both prolongs the duration and enhances the chemotherapeutic action of mercaptopurine by competitive inhibition of xanthine oxidase. Consequently, to avoid bone marrow toxicity, the dose of mercaptopurine is usually reduced in patients receiving allopurinol. Cimetidine, a drug used in the treatment of peptic ulcer, has been shown to potentiate the pharmacologic actions of anticoagulants and sedatives. The metabolism of chlordiazepoxide has been shown to be inhibited by 63% after a single dose of cimetidine; such effects are reversed within 48 hours after withdrawal of cimetidine.

Impairment of metabolism may also result if a simultaneously administered drug irreversibly inactivates a common metabolizing enzyme, as is the case with secobarbital or diethylpentenamide overdoses. These compounds, in the course of their metabolism by cytochrome P450, inactivate the enzyme and result in impairment of their own metabolism and that of other cosubstrates.

Interactions Between Drugs & Endogenous Compounds

Various drugs require conjugation with endogenous substrates such as glutathione, glucuronic acid, and sulfate for their inactivation. Consequently, different drugs may compete for the same endogenous substrates, and the faster-reacting drug may effectively deplete endogenous substrate levels and impair the metabolism of the slower-reacting drug. If the latter has a steep dose-response curve or a narrow margin of safety, potentiation of its pharmacologic and toxic effects may result.

Diseases Affecting Drug Metabolism

Acute or chronic diseases that affect liver architecture or function markedly affect hepatic metabolism of some drugs. Such conditions include fat accumulation, alcoholic hepatitis, active or inactive alcoholic cirrhosis, hemochromatosis, chronic active hepatitis, biliary cirrhosis, and acute viral or drug-induced hepatitis. Depending on their severity, these conditions impair hepatic drug-metabolizing enzymes, particularly microsomal oxidases, and thereby markedly affect drug elimination. For example, the half-lives of chlordiazepoxide and diazepam in patients with liver cirrhosis or acute viral hepatitis are greatly increased, with a corresponding prolongation of their effects. Consequently, these drugs may cause coma in patients with liver disease when given in ordinary doses.

Liver cancer has been reported to impair hepatic drug metabolism in humans. For example, aminopyrine metabolism is slower in patients with malignant hepatic tumors than in normal controls. These patients also exhibit markedly diminished aminopyrine clearance rates. Studies of liver biopsy specimens from patients with hepatocellular carcinoma also indicate impaired ability to oxidatively metabolize drugs in vitro. This is associated with a correspondingly reduced cytochrome P450 content.

Cardiac disease, by limiting blood flow to the liver, may impair disposition of those drugs whose metabolism is flow-limited (Table 4–7). These drugs are so readily metabolized by the liver that hepatic clearance is essentially equal to liver blood flow. Pulmonary disease may also affect drug metabolism as indicated by the impaired hydrolysis of procainamide and procaine in patients with chronic respiratory insufficiency and the increased half-life of antipyrine in patients with lung cancer. Impairment of enzyme activity or defective formation of enzymes associated with heavy metal poisoning or porphyria also results in reduction of hepatic drug metabolism. For example, lead poisoning has been shown to increase the half-life of antipyrine in humans.

Table 4–7. Rapidly metabolized drugs whose hepatic clearance is blood flow-limited.

Alprenolol	Lidocaine
Amitriptyline	Meperidine
Clomethiazole	Morphine
Desipramine	Pentazocine
Imipramine	Propoxyphene
Isoniazid	Propranolol
Labetalol	Verapamil

Although the effects of endocrine dysfunction on drug metabolism have been well explored in experimental animal models, corresponding data for humans with endocrine disorders are scanty. Thyroid dysfunction has been associated with altered metabolism of some drugs and of some endogenous compounds as well. Hypothyroidism increases the half-life of antipyrine, digoxin, methimazole, and practolol, whereas hyperthyroidism has the opposite effect. A few clinical studies in diabetic patients indicate no apparent impairment of drug metabolism, as reflected by the half-lives of antipyrine, tolbutamide, and phenylbutazone. In contrast, the metabolism of several drugs is impaired in male rats treated with diabetogenic agents such as alloxan or streptozocin. These alterations are abolished by administration of insulin, which has no direct influence on hepatic drug-metabolizing enzymes. Malfunctions of the pituitary, adrenal cortex, and gonads markedly impair hepatic drug metabolism in rats. On the basis of these findings, it may be supposed that such disorders could significantly affect drug metabolism in humans. However, until sufficient evidence is obtained from clinical studies in patients, such extrapolations must be considered tentative.

REFERENCES

Correia MA, Ortiz de Montellano P: Inhibitors of cytochrome P-450 and possibilities for their therapeutic application. In: *Frontiers in Biotransformation,* vol 8. Ruckpaul K (editor). Taylor & Francis, 1993.

Correia MA: Rat and human liver cytochromes P450: Substrate and inhibitor specificities and functional markers. In: *Cytochrome P450: Structure, Mechanism and Biochemistry,* 2nd ed. Ortiz de Montellano P (editor). Plenum Press, 1995.

Dayer P et al: Contribution of the genetic status of oxidative metabolism to variability in the plasma concentrations of beta-adrenoceptor blocking agents. Eur J Clin Pharmacol 1983;24:797.

Desmond PV et al: Cimetidine impairs elimination of chlordiazepoxide (Librium) in man. Ann Intern Med 1980;93:266.

Gilmore DA et al: Age and gender influence the stereoselective pharmacokinetics of propranolol. J Pharmacol Exp Ther 1992;261:1181.

Gonzalez F: The molecular biology of cytochrome P450s. Pharmacol Rev 1989;40:243.

Gonzalez FJ et al: Characterization of the common genetic defect in humans deficient in debrisoquine metabolism. Nature 1988;331:442.

Gonzalez FJ: Human cytochromes P450: Problems and prospects. Trends Pharmacol Sci 1992;13:346.

Guengerich FP: Reactions and significance of cytochrome P-450 enzymes. J Biol Chem 1991:266:10019.

Guengerich FP: Human cytochrome P450 enzymes. In: *Cytochrome P450: Structure, Mechanism and Biochemistry,* 2nd ed. Ortiz de Montellano P (editor). Plenum Press, 1995.

Jenner P, Testa B (editors): *Concepts in Drug Metabolism.* Part B of: *Drugs and the Pharmaceutical Science Series,* vol 10. Marcel Dekker, 1981.

Kroemer HK, Klotz U: Glucuronidation of drugs: A reevaluation of the pharmacological significance of the conjugates and modulating factors. Clin Pharmacokinet 1992;23:292.

Miller LG: Recent developments in the study of the effects of cigarette smoking on clinical pharmacokinetics and clinical pharmacodynamics. Clin Pharmacokinet 1989; 17:90.

Minchin RF, Boyd MR: Localization of metabolic activation and deactivation systems in the lung: Significance to the pulmonary toxicity of xenobiotics. Annu Rev Pharmacol Toxicol 1983;23:217.

Murray M: P450 enzymes: Inhibition mechanisms, genetic regulation, and effects of liver disease. Clin Pharmacokinet 1992;23:132.

Nelson DR et al: The P450 superfamily; update on new sequences, gene mapping, accession numbers, and nomenclature. Pharmacogenetics 1996;6:1.

Ortiz de Montellano PR, Correia MA: Inhibition of cytochrome P450 enzymes. In: *Cytochrome P450: Structure, Mechanism and Biochemistry,* 2nd ed. Ortiz de Montellano (editor). Plenum Press, 1995.

Testa B, Jenner P (editors): *Drug Metabolism: Chemical and Biological Aspects.* Marcel Dekker, 1976.

Vessell ES: Genetic and environmental factors causing variation in drug response. Mutat Res 1991;247:241.

Waxman DJ, Azaroff L: Phenobarbital induction of cytochrome P-450 gene expression. Biochem J 1992; 281:577.

Wood AJJ, Zhou H-H: Ethnic differences in drug disposition and responsiveness. Clin Pharmacokinet 1991;20:350.

Zanger UM et al: Absence of hepatic cytochrome P450bufI causes genetically deficient debrisoquin oxidation in man. Biochemistry 1988;27:5447.

Zhou H-H et al: Racial differences in drug response: Altered sensitivity to and clearance of propranolol in men of Chinese descent as compared with American males. N Engl J Med 1989;320:565.

5

Basic & Clinical Evaluation of New Drugs

Barry A. Berkowitz, PhD, & Bertram G. Katzung, MD, PhD

During the past 60 years, new drug developments have revolutionized the practice of medicine, converting many once fatal diseases into almost routine therapeutic exercises. One cause of this medical advance has been a fundamental improvement in the means of developing and testing new drugs. This process has been greatly accelerated by new technology, by financial motivation, and by governmental support of medical research. In most countries, the testing of drugs is now regulated by legislation and closely monitored by governmental agencies. This chapter summarizes the process by which new therapeutic agents are discovered, developed, and regulated. While the examples used reflect the USA experience, the pathway of new drug development generally is the same worldwide.

The first step in the development of a new drug is the discovery or synthesis of a potential new drug molecule (Figure 5–1). By law, the safety and efficacy of drugs must be defined before they can be marketed. In addition to in vitro studies, most of the biologic effects of the molecule must be characterized in animals before human drug trials can be started. Human testing must then go forward in three conventional phases before the drug can be considered for approval for general use. A fourth phase of data gathering follows after approval for general use.

Enormous costs, from $100 million to over $500 million, are involved in the development of a single successful new drug. These costs include the labor invested in searching for useful new molecules—5000–10,000 may be synthesized for each successful new drug introduced—and the costs of detailed basic and clinical studies and promotion of the ultimate candidate molecule. It is primarily because of the economic investment and risks involved that most new drugs are now developed in the laboratories of pharmaceutical companies. At the same time, the incentives to succeed in drug development are equally enormous. The worldwide market for ethical (prescription) pharmaceuticals in 1991 was estimated to be $284 billion. Moreover, it has been estimated that

over the past 50 years medications produced by the pharmaceutical industry have saved more than 1.5 million lives and $140 billion in the treatment of tuberculosis, poliomyelitis, coronary artery disease, and cerebrovascular disease alone (Billstein 1994).

DRUG DISCOVERY

Most new drug candidates are identified through one or more of four approaches: (1) chemical modification of a known molecule; (2) random screening for biologic activity of large numbers of natural products, banks of previously discovered chemical entities, or large libraries of peptides, nucleic acids, or other organic molecules; (3) rational drug design based on an understanding of biologic mechanisms and chemical structure; and, increasingly, (4) biotechnology and cloning using genes to produce larger peptides and proteins. Moreover, automation permits millions of assays per month. In addition to these efforts, major attention is now being given to the discovery of entirely new targets for drug therapy, eg, the intracellular receptors for second messengers.

The development of the thiazide diuretics from the much less useful carbonic anhydrase inhibitors (Chapter 15) is an example of the first approach. The discovery of many antibiotics and cyclosporine, an immunosuppressant drug, illustrates the second approach. An early example of the third approach was the development of H_2 histamine antagonists. Based on the suspected existence of different types of histamine receptors, rational molecular modification led to the gradual improvement of antagonist selectivity and potency, culminating in the introduction of cimetidine (Table 5–1). Rational drug design has made major strides recently, as illustrated by the development of angiotensin-converting enzyme inhibitors from a study of the structure-activity relationships of enzyme active site inhibitors and by the current development of hypothetical drug structures with computer assis-

Figure 5–1. The development and testing process required to bring a drug to market in the USA. Some of the requirements may be different for drugs used in life-threatening diseases.

Table 5–1. A history of the development of H_2 receptor blockers.

Compound and Characteristics	Structure	Antagonist Activity (in vivo ID_{50} μmol/kg)[1]
Histamine The starting point.	$CH_2-CH_2-NH_2$	Agonist
N-Guanylhistamine The first lead compound. A weak partial agonist.	$CH_2-CH_2-NHC-NH_2$ $+NH_2$	800
Burimamide Thiourea compound with a longer side chain. Weakly active in humans.	$CH_2-CH_2-CH_2-CH_2-NHCNH-CH_3$ S	6.1
Metiamide Active in humans but toxic.	$CH_3-CH_2-S-CH_2-CH_2-NHCNH-CH_3$ S	1.6
Cimetidine Replaces the thiourea with an N–CN substituent. Retains high potency with decreased toxicity. Launched the major series of drugs for the treatment of acid-peptic disorders.	$CH_3-CH_2-S-CH_2-CH_2-NHCNH-CH_3$ $N-C\equiv N$	1.4

[1]Activity in the anesthetized rat against histamine stimulation of acid secretion. The ID_{50} is the intravenous dose required to produce 50% inhibition. From Brimblecombe RW et al, 1978; and Black J, 1989.

tance. The fourth approach is illustrated by the development of recombinant tissue plasminogen activator (rt-PA) as described in the case study on the next page (see box: Case Study: The Discovery and Development of Recombinant Tissue Plasminogen Activator).

Regardless of the source of the candidate molecule, testing it involves a sequence of experimentation and characterization called **drug screening.** A variety of biologic assays at the molecular, cellular, organ, and whole animal levels are used to define the activity and selectivity of the drug. The type and number of initial screening tests depend on the pharmacologic goal. Anti-infective drugs will generally be tested first against a variety of infectious organisms, hypoglycemic drugs for their ability to lower blood sugar, etc. However, the molecule is usually studied for a broad array of actions to establish the selectivity of the drug. This has the advantage of demonstrating unsuspected toxic effects and occasionally discloses a previously unsuspected therapeutic action. The selection of molecules for further study is most efficiently conducted in animal models of human disease. Where good models exist (eg, hypertension or thrombotic disease), we generally have adequate drugs. Good drugs are conspicuously lacking for diseases for which models are not yet available, eg, Alzheimer's disease.

Some of the studies performed during drug screening are listed in Table 5–2 and define the **pharmacologic profile** of the drug. For example, a broad range of tests would be performed on a drug designed to act as an antagonist at vascular alpha adrenoceptors for the treatment of hypertension. At the molecular level, the compound would be screened for receptor binding affinity to cell membranes containing alpha receptors, other receptors, and binding sites on enzymes. Early studies would be done on liver cytochrome P450 to determine whether the molecule of interest is likely to be a substrate or inhibitor of these enzymes.

Effects on cell function would be studied to determine the efficacy of the compound. Evidence would be obtained about whether the drug is an agonist, partial agonist, or antagonist at alpha receptors. Isolated tissues would be utilized to further determine the pharmacologic activity and selectivity of the new compound in comparison with reference compounds. Comparison with other drugs would also be undertaken in other vitro preparations such as gastrointestinal and bronchial smooth muscle. At each step in this pathway, the compound would have to meet specific performance criteria to be carried further.

Whole animal studies are generally necessary to determine the effect of the drug on organ systems and disease models. Cardiovascular and renal function studies would be first performed in normal animals. For the hypothetical antihypertensive drug, animals with hypertension would then be treated to see if blood pressure was lowered and to characterize other effects of the compound. Evidence would be collected on duration of action and efficacy following oral and parenteral administration. If the agent possessed useful activity, it would be further studied for possible adverse effects on other major organ systems, including the respiratory, gastrointestinal, endocrine, and central nervous systems.

These studies might suggest the need for further chemical modification to achieve more desirable pharmacokinetic or pharmacodynamic properties. For example, oral administration studies might show that the drug was poorly absorbed or rapidly metabolized in the liver; modification to improve bioavailability might be indicated. If the drug is to be administered chronically, an assessment of tolerance development would be made. For drugs related to those known to cause physical dependency, abuse potential would also be studied. An explanation of pharmacologic mechanism would be sought.

The result of this procedure (which may have to be repeated several times with variants of the original molecules to produce a promising molecule) is a **lead compound,** ie, a leading candidate for a successful new drug. A patent application may then be filed for a novel compound that is efficacious or for a previously known chemical entity that has been discovered to have a new therapeutic use.

Advances in molecular biology and biotechnology have introduced new approaches and new problems to the drug discovery and development process. New information about the structure of receptors is making possible more rational drug design. A better understanding of second messenger processes is revealing second messenger receptors as a new class of drug targets. Insertion of the genes for active peptides or proteins into bacteria, yeast, or mammalian cells makes it possible to synthesize, isolate, and purify large quantities of the desired molecule. Human insulin, human growth hormone, interferon, hepatitis vaccines, tissue plasminogen activator, erythropoietin, antihemophilic factor, and bone marrow growth factors produced by these biotechnology approaches are now available for general clinical use.

PRECLINICAL SAFETY & TOXICITY TESTING

Candidate drugs that survive the initial screening and profiling procedures must be carefully evaluated for potential risks before clinical testing is begun. Depending on the proposed use of the drug, preclinical toxicity testing includes most or all of the procedures shown in Table 5–3. While no chemical can be certified as completely "safe" (*free* of risk), since every chemical is toxic at some level of dosage, it is usually possible to estimate the risk associated with exposure to the chemical under specified conditions if appropriate tests are performed.

The major kinds of information needed from the preclinical toxicity study are (1) acute toxicity—ef-

Table 5–2. Pharmacologic profile tests.

Experimental Method or Target Organ	Species or Tissue	Route of Administration	Measurement
Molecular			
Receptor binding (example: β-adrenoceptors)	Cell membrane fractions from organs or cultured cells; cloned receptors	In vitro	Receptor affinity and selectivity
Enzyme activity (examples: tyrosine hydroxylase, dopamine-β-hydroxylase, monoamine oxidase)	Sympathetic nerves adrenal glands; purified enzymes	In vitro	Enzyme inhibition and selectivity
Cytochrome P-450	Liver	In vitro	Enzyme inhibition; effects on drug metabolism
Cellular			
Cell function	Cultured cells	In vitro	Evidence for receptor activity—agonism or antagonism (example: effects on cyclic nucleotides)
Isolated tissue	Blood vessels, heart, lung, ileum (rat or guinea pig)	In vitro	Effects on vascular contraction and relaxation; selectivity for vascular receptors; effects on other smooth muscles
Systems/disease models			
Blood pressure	Dog, cat (anesthetized)	Parenteral	Systolic-diastolic changes
	Rat, hypertensive (conscious)	Oral	Antihypertensive effects
Cardiac effects	Dog (conscious)	Oral	Electrocardiography
	Dog (anesthetized)	Parenteral	Inotropic, chronotropic effects, cardiac output, total peripheral resistance
Peripheral autonomic nervous system	Dog (anesthetized)	Parenteral	Effects on response to known drugs and electrical stimulation of central and peripheral autonomic nerves
Respiratory effects	Dog, guinea pig	Parenteral	Effects on respiratory rate and amplitude, bronchial tone
Diuretic activity	Dog	Oral, parenteral	Natriuresis, kaliuresis, water diuresis, renal blood flow, glomerular filtration rate
Gastrointestinal effects	Rat	Oral	Gastrointestinal motility and secretions
Circulating hormones, cholesterol, blood sugar	Rat, dog	Parenteral, oral	Serum concentration
Blood coagulation	Rabbit	Oral	Coagulation time, clot retraction, prothrombin time
Central nervous system	Mouse, rat	Parenteral, oral	Degree of sedation, muscle relaxation, locomotor activity, stimulation

fects of large single doses up to the lethal level; (2) subacute and chronic toxicity—effects of multiple doses, which are especially important if the drug is intended for chronic use in humans; (3) effects on reproductive functions, including teratogenicity; (4) carcinogenicity; (5) mutagenicity; and (6) investigative toxicology. In addition to the studies shown in Table 5–3, several quantitative estimates are desirable. These include the "no-effect" dose—the maximum dose at which the specified toxic effect is not seen; the mini-mum lethal dose—the smallest dose that is observed to kill any animal; and, if necessary, the median lethal dose (LD50)—the dose that kills approximately 50% of the animals (see Chapter 2). Historically, the LD50 was determined with a high degree or precision and was used to compare toxicities of compounds relative to their therapeutic doses. It is now realized that high precision may not be necessary to compare toxicities (Malmfors et al, 1983). Therefore, the median lethal dose is now estimated from the smallest number of an-

Table 5–3. Safety tests.

Type of Test	Approach	Comment
Acute toxicity	Acute dose that is lethal in approximately 50% of animals. Determine maximum tolerated dose. Usually two species, two routes, single dose.	Compare with therapeutic dose
Subacute toxicity	Three doses, two species. Up to 6 months may be necessary prior to clinical trial. The longer the duration of expected clinical use, the longer the subacute test.	Clinical chemistry, physiologic signs, autopsy studies, hematology, histology, electron microscopy studies. Identify target organs of toxicity.
Chronic toxicity	One to 2 years. Required when drug is intended to be used in humans for prolonged periods. Usually run concurrently with clinical trial.	Goals of subacute and chronic tests are to show which organs are susceptible to drug toxicity. Tests as noted above for subacute.
Effect on reproductive performance	Effects on animal mating behavior, reproduction, parturition, progeny, birth defects	Examines fertility, teratology, perinatal and postnatal effects, lactation.
Carcinogenic potential	Two years, two species. Required when drug is intended to be used in humans for prolonged periods.	Hematology, histology, autopsy studies
Mutagenic potential	Effects on genetic stability of bacteria (Ames test) or mammalian cells in culture; dominant lethal test in mice	Increasing interest in this problem
Investigative toxicology	Determine sequence and mechanisms of toxic action. Develop new methods for assessing toxicity.	May allow rational and earlier design of safer drugs

imals possible. These doses are used to calculate the initial dose to be tried in humans, usually taken as 1\100–1\10 of the no-effect dose in animals.

It is important to recognize the limitations of preclinical testing. These include the following:

(1) Toxicity testing is time-consuming and expensive. During the last decade, the total cost of preclinical pharmacology and toxicology studies was estimated to be at least $41 million per successful drug. Two to 5 years may be required to collect and analyze data.

(2) Large numbers of animals are used to obtain preclinical data. Scientists are properly concerned about this situation, and progress is being made toward reducing the numbers required while still obtaining valid data (Malmfors et al, 1983; Zbinden et al, 1981). Cell and tissue culture in vitro methods are increasingly being used, but their predictive value is still severely limited. Nevertheless, some segments of the public attempt to bring to a halt all animal testing in the unfounded belief that it has become unnecessary.

(3) Extrapolation of toxicity data from animals to humans is not completely reliable (Jelovsek et al, 1989; Dixon, 1980). For any given compound, the total toxicity data from all species have a very high predictive value for its toxicity in humans. However, there are limitations on the amount of information it is practical to obtain.

(4) For statistical reasons, rare adverse effects are unlikely to be detected, just as in clinical trials (see below).

EVALUATION IN HUMANS

Less than one-third of the drugs tested in clinical trials reach the marketplace (DiMasi 1995). Federal law in the USA requires that the study of new drugs in humans be conducted in accordance with stringent guidelines. Scientifically valid results are not guaranteed simply by conforming to government regulations, however, and the design and execution of a good clinical trial requires the efforts of a clinician-scientist or clinical pharmacologist, a statistician, and frequently other professionals as well. The need for careful design and execution is based upon three major factors inherent in the study of any therapeutic measure—pharmacologic or nonpharmacologic—in humans.

Confounding Factors in Clinical Trials

A. The Variable Natural History of Most Diseases: Many diseases tend to wax and wane in severity; some disappear spontaneously with time; even malignant neoplasms may on occasion undergo spontaneous remissions. A good experimental design must take into account the natural history of the disease under study by evaluating a large enough population of subjects over a sufficient period of time. Further protection against errors of interpretation caused by fluctuations in severity of the manifestations of disease is provided by utilizing a **crossover design,** which consists of alternating periods of administration of test drug, placebo preparation (the control), and the standard treatment (positive control), if any, in each subject. These sequences are systematically varied, so that different subsets of patients receive each of the possible sequences of treatment. An example of such a design is shown in Table 5–4.

B. The Presence of Other Diseases and Risk Factors: Known or unknown diseases and risk factors (including life-styles of subjects) may influence the results of a clinical study. For example, some diseases alter the pharmacokinetics of drugs (Chapters 3 and 4). Concentrations of a blood component being monitored as a measure of the effect of the new agent may be influenced by other diseases or other drugs. Attempts to avoid this hazard usually involve the crossover technique (when feasible) and proper selection and assignment of patients to each of the study groups. This requires that careful medical and pharmacologic histories (including use of recreational drugs) be obtained and that statistically valid methods of randomization be used in assigning subjects to particular study groups.

C. Subject and Observer Bias: Most patients tend to respond in a positive way to any therapeutic intervention by interested, caring, and enthusiastic medical personnel. The manifestation of this phenomenon in the subject is the **placebo response** (Latin "I shall please") and may involve objective physiologic and biochemical changes as well as changes in subjective complaints associated with the disease. The placebo response is usually quantitated by administration of an inert material, with exactly the same physical appearance, odor, consistency, etc, as the active dosage form. The magnitude of the response varies considerably from patient to patient. However, the incidence of the placebo response is fairly constant, being observed in 20–40% of patients in almost all studies. Placebo "toxicity" also occurs but usually involves subjective effects: stomach upset, insomnia, sedation, etc.

Subject bias effects can be quantitated—and discounted from the response measured during active therapy—by the **single-blind design.** This involves use of a placebo or dummy medication, as described above, which is administered to the same subjects in a crossover design, if possible, or to a separate control group of subjects. Observer bias can be taken into account by disguising the identity of the medication being used–placebo or active form–from both the subjects and the personnel evaluating the subjects'

responses **(double-blind design).** In this design, a third party holds the code identifying each medication packet, and the code is not broken until all of the clinical data have been collected.

The Food and Drug Administration

The Food and Drug Administration (FDA) is the administrative body that oversees the drug evaluation process in the United States and grants approval for marketing of new drug products. The FDA's authority to regulate drug marketing derives from several pieces of legislation (Table 5–5). If a drug has not been shown through adequately controlled testing to be "safe and effective" for a specific use, it cannot be marketed in interstate commerce for this use.* Unfortunately, "safe" means different things to the patient, the physician, and society. As noted above, complete absence of risk is impossible to demonstrate (and probably never occurs), but this fact is not understood by the average member of the public, who assumes that any medication sold with the approval of the FDA must indeed be free of serious, if not minor, "side effects." This confusion continues to be a major cause of litigation and dissatisfaction with medical care (Feinstein, 1988; Shulman, 1989).

The history of drug regulation reflects several medical and public health events that precipitated major shifts in public opinion. The Pure Food and Drug Act of 1906 (Table 5–5) became law mostly in response to revelations of unsanitary and unethical practices in the meat-packing industry. The Federal Food, Drug, and Cosmetic Act of 1938 was largely a reaction to a series of deaths associated with the use of a preparation of sulfanilamide that was marketed before it and its vehicle were adequately tested. Thalidomide is another example of a drug that altered drug testing methods and stimulated drug-regulating legislation. This agent was introduced in Europe in 1957 and 1958 and, based on animal tests then commonly used, was promoted as a "nontoxic" hypnotic. In 1961, the first reports were published suggesting that thalidomide was responsible for a dramatic increase in the incidence of a rare birth defect called **phocomelia,** a condition involving shortening or complete absence of the limbs. Epidemiologic studies soon provided strong evidence for the association of this defect with thalidomide use by women during the first trimester of pregnancy, and the drug was withdrawn from sale worldwide. An estimated 10,000 children were born with birth defects because of maternal exposure to this one agent. The tragedy led to the requirement for more extensive testing of new drugs for teratogenic effects and played an important role in stimulating passage of the Kefauver-Harris Amendments of 1962,

Table 5–4. Typical crossover design for comparing a mythical new analgesic, "Novent," with placebo and a known active drug, aspirin, in the management of chronic pain. Each therapeutic period lasts 7 days, with 1 week between each treatment period for washout of the preceding medication.

Patient Group	Medication Given		
	Week 1	Week 3	Week 5
I	Aspirin	Placebo	"Novent"
II	Placebo	"Novent"	Aspirin
III	"Novent"	Aspirin	Placebo

---

*Although the FDA does not directly control drug commerce within states, a variety of state and federal laws control intrastate production and marketing of drugs.

Table 5–5. Major legislation pertaining to drugs in the USA.

Law	Purpose and Effect
Pure Food and Drug Act of 1906	Prohibited mislabeling and adulteration of drugs
Opium Exclusion Act of 1909	Prohibited importation of opium
Amendment (1912) to the Pure Food and Drug Act	Prohibited false or fraudulent advertising claims
Harrison Narcotic Act of 1914	Established regulations for use of opium, opiates, and cocaine (marijuana added in 1937)
Food, Drug, and Cosmetic Act of 1938	Required that new drugs be safe as well as pure (but did not require proof of efficacy). Enforcement by FDA
Durham-Humphrey Act of 1952	Vested in the FDA the power to determine which products could be sold without prescription
Kefauver-Harris Amendments (1962) to the Food, Drug, and Cosmetic Act	Required proof of efficacy as well as safety for new drugs and for drugs released since 1938; established guidelines for reporting of information about adverse reactions, clinical testing, and advertising of new drugs
Comprehensive Drug Abuse Prevention and Control Act (1970)	Outlined strict controls in the manufacture, distribution, and prescribing of habit-forming drugs; established programs to prevent and treat drug addiction
Orphan Drug Amendments of 1983	Amends Food, Drug, and Cosmetic Act of 1938, providing incentives for development of drugs that treat diseases with less than 200,000 patients in USA
Drug Price Competition and Patent Restoration Act of 1984	Abbreviated new drug applications for generic drugs. Required bioequivalence data. Patent life extended by amount of time drug delayed by FDA review process. Cannot exceed 5 extra years or extend to more than 14 years post-NDA approval.
Expedited Drug Approval Act (1992)	Allowed accelerated FDA approval for drugs of high medical need. Required detailed postmarketing patient surveillance.
Prescription Drug User Fee Act (1992)	Manufacturers pay user fees for certain new drug applications. FDA claims review time for new chemical entities dropped from 30 months in 1992 to 20 months in 1994.

even though the drug was never approved for use in the USA. Unfortunately, this episode also generated widespread fear of all drugs used in pregnancy, caused much unnecessary litigation, and resulted in the withdrawal from the market of drugs that are probably not teratogenic. In spite of its disastrous fetal toxicity, thalidomide is a relatively safe drug for humans after birth. Even the most serious risk of toxicities may be avoided or managed if understood, and despite its toxicity thalidomide is currently undergoing clinical trials as a potent immunoregulatory agent.

Of course it is impossible, as noted above, to certify that a drug is absolutely safe, ie, free of all risk. It is possible, however, to identify most of the hazards likely to be associated with use of a new drug and to place some statistical limits on frequency of occurrence of such events in the population under study. As a result, an operational and pragmatic definition of "safety" can usually be reached that is based upon the nature and incidence of drug-associated hazards as compared to the hazard of nontherapy of the target disease.

Clinical Trials: The IND & NDA

Once a drug is judged ready to be studied in humans, a Notice of Claimed Investigational Exemption for a

New Drug (IND) must be filed with the FDA (Figure 5–1). The IND includes (1) information on the composition and source of the drug, (2) manufacturing information, (3) all data from animal studies, (4) clinical plans and protocols, and (5) the names and credentials of physicians who will conduct the clinical trials.

It often requires 4–6 years of clinical testing to accumulate all required data. Testing in humans is begun after sufficient acute and subacute animal toxicity studies have been completed. Chronic safety testing in animals is usually done concurrently with clinical trials. In each of the three formal phases of clinical trials, volunteers or patients must be informed of the investigational status of the drug as well as possible risks and must be allowed to decline or to consent to participate and receive the drug. These regulations are based on the ethical principles set forth in the Declaration of Helsinki (Editor's Page, 1966). In addition to the approval of the sponsoring organization and the FDA, an interdisciplinary institutional review board at the facility where the clinical drug trial will be conducted critically reviews the plans for testing in humans.

In **phase 1,** the effects of the drug as a function of dosage are established in a small number (25–50) of healthy volunteers. (If the drug is expected to have significant toxicity, as is usually the case in cancer and AIDS therapy, volunteer patients with the disease are used in phase 1 rather than normal volunteers.) Phase 1 trials are done to determine whether humans and animals show significantly different responses to the drug and to establish the probable limits of the safe clinical dosage range. These trials are nonblind or "open," ie, both the investigators and the subjects know what is being given. Many predictable toxicities are detected in this phase. Pharmacokinetic measurements of absorption, half-life, and metabolism are often done in phase 1. Phase 1 studies are usually performed in research centers by specially trained clinical pharmacologists.

In **phase 2,** the drug is studied for the first time in patients with the target disease to determine its efficacy. A small number of patients (10–200) are studied in great detail. A single-blind design is often used, with an inert placebo medication and an older active drug (positive control) in addition to the investigational agent. Phase 2 trials also are usually done in special clinical centers (eg, university hospitals). A broader range of toxicities may be detected in this phase.

In **phase 3,** the drug is evaluated in much larger numbers of patients—sometimes thousands—to further establish safety and efficacy. Using information gathered in phases 1 and 2, trials are designed to minimize errors caused by placebo effects, variable course of the disease, etc. Therefore, double-blind and crossover techniques (like that set out in Table 5–4) are frequently employed. Phase 3 trials are usually performed in settings similar to those anticipated for the ultimate use of the drug. Phase 3 studies can be difficult to design and execute and are usually expensive because of the large numbers of patients involved and the masses of data that must be collected and analyzed. The investigators are usually specialists in the disease being treated. Certain toxic effects—especially those caused by immunologic processes—may first become apparent in phase 3.

If phase 3 results meet expectations, application will be made for permission to market the new agent. The process of applying for marketing approval requires submission of a **New Drug Application (NDA)** to the FDA. The application contains, often in hundreds of volumes, full reports of all preclinical and clinical data pertaining to the drug under review. A decision on approval by the FDA may take 3 years or longer. In cases where an urgent need is perceived (eg, cancer chemotherapy), the process of preclinical and clinical testing and FDA review may be accelerated. For serious diseases, the FDA may permit extensive but controlled marketing of a new drug before phase 3 studies are completed; for life-threatening diseases, it may permit controlled marketing even before phase 2 studies are finished (Young et al, 1988).

Once approval to market a drug has been obtained, **phase 4** begins. This constitutes monitoring the safety of the new drug under actual conditions of use in large numbers of patients. Final release of a drug for general prescription use should be accompanied by a vigilant postmarketing surveillance program. The importance of careful and complete reporting of toxicity after marketing approval by the FDA can be appreciated by noting that many important drug-induced effects have an incidence of 1:10,000 or less. Table 5–6 shows the sample size required to disclose drug-induced increases of events that occur with different frequencies in the untreated population (and some examples of such events). Because of the small numbers of subjects in phases 1–3, such low-incidence drug effects will not generally be detected before phase 4 no matter how carefully the studies are executed. Phase 4 has no fixed duration.

The time from the filing of a patent application to approval for marketing of a new drug may be 5 years or even longer. Since the lifetime of a patent is 20 years in the USA, the owner of the patent (usually a pharmaceutical company) has exclusive rights for marketing the product for only a limited time after approval of the NDA. Because the FDA review process can be lengthy, the time consumed by the review process is sometimes added to the patent life. However, the extension (up to 5 years) cannot increase the total life of the patent to more than 14 years post NDA approval. After expiration of the patent, any company may produce and market the drug as a **generic** product without paying license fees to the original patent owner. However, a trademark (the drug's proprietary

Table 5–6. Study size as a function of effect frequency.[1]

Number of exposed people required to detect a twofold increase in incidence of a rare effect with a 20% probability of missing a real effect and a 5% probability of concluding that an effect exists when one does not. One nonexposed control is required per exposed subject. If the drug increases the risk more than twofold, the number of subjects required is decreased.

Frequency of Effect in Nonexposed Controls	Example	Number of Exposed Subjects Required
1/100	Any congenital cardiac defect[2]	1800
1/1000	Facial clefts[3]	18,000
1/10,000	Tricuspid atresia[4]	180,000
1/100,000	Myocardial infarction[5]	1,800,000

[1]Modified and reproduced with permission, from Finkle W: Sample size requirements for detection of drug-induced disease. Report of Joint Commission on Prescription Drug Use, Appendix V, 1980.
[2]Frequency of all forms of congenital cardiac malformations is about one in 111 live births.
[3]Frequency of facial cleft malformations is about one in 700 live births.
[4]Frequency of tricuspid valve atresia is about one in 8500 live births.
[5]Frequency of myocardial infarction in women nonsmokers 30–39 years of age is about 4 in 100,000.

trade name) may be legally protected indefinitely. Therefore, pharmaceutical companies are strongly motivated to give their new drugs easily remembered trade names. For example, "Librium" is the trade name for the antianxiety drug "chlordiazepoxide." For the same reason, the company's advertising material will emphasize the trade name. (See section on generic prescribing in Chapter 65.)

Orphan Drugs

Drugs for rare diseases—so-called orphan drugs—can be difficult to research, develop, and market. Proof of drug safety and efficacy in small populations must be established, but doing so effectively is a complex process. For example, clinical testing of drugs in children is severely restricted, even for common diseases, and a number of rare diseases affect the very young. Furthermore, because basic research in the pathophysiology and mechanisms of rare diseases tends to receive little attention or funding in both academic and industrial settings, rational targets for drug action may be relatively few. In addition, the cost of developing a drug can greatly influence decisions and priorities when the target population is relatively small.

The Orphan Drug Act of 1983, which amended the 1938 Federal Food, Drug, and Cosmetic Act, provides incentives for the development of drugs for treatment of diseases affecting fewer than 200,000 patients in the United States. The FDA maintains an office of Orphan Product Development (301-827-3666) to provide special assistance and grants to scientists with an interest in these products. Information on orphan drugs is also available from The National Organization for Rare Disorders (800-447-6673).

As of 1996, over 630 biologic or drug products were registered with the FDA as orphan drugs, of which most were for products currently in development. The FDA has approved marketing applications for 120 orphan drugs to treat more than 82 rare diseases.

Adverse Reactions to Drugs

Severe adverse reactions to marketed drugs are uncommon, though less dangerous toxic effects, as noted elsewhere in this book, are frequent for some drug groups. Life-threatening reactions probably occur in less than 2% of patients admitted to medical wards (Adverse drug reactions, 1981). The mechanisms of these reactions fall into two main categories. Those in the first group are often extensions of known pharmacologic effects and thus are predictable. These toxicities are generally discovered by pharmacologists, toxicologists, and clinicians involved in phase 1–3 testing. Those in the second group, which may be immunologic or of unknown mechanism (Rawlins, 1981), are generally unexpected and may not be recognized until a drug has been marketed for many years. These toxicities are therefore usually discov-

ered by clinicians. It is thus important that practitioners be aware of the various types of allergic reactions to drugs. These include IgE-mediated reactions such as anaphylaxis, urticaria, and angioedema; IgG- or IgM-mediated reactions of the lupus erythematosus type; IgG-mediated responses of the serum sickness type, which involve vasculitis; and cell-mediated allergies involved in contact dermatitis. They are discussed in Chapter 56.

Evaluating a Clinical Drug Study

The periodical literature is the chief source of clinical information about new drugs, especially those very recently released for general use. Such information may include new indications or major new toxicities and contraindications. Therefore, health practitioners should be familiar with the sources of such information (noted in Chapter 1) and should be prepared to evaluate it. Certain general principles can be applied to such evaluations and are discussed in detail in the Cohen (1994), Nowak (1994), and Riegelman (1981) references listed below. These principles are conveniently stated in the form of questions every reader should ask while examining the paper.

A. Ethical Considerations: Were appropriate ethical and procedural safeguards available to the patients? Was informed consent obtained?

B. Statement of Objectives: What were the objectives of the study? Are the goals clearly defined and stated? A poorly defined goal such as "to study the effects of minoxidil" (an antihypertensive drug) is much less likely to lead to useful results than a clearly defined objective such as, "to measure the effect of minoxidil on renal function in severely hypertensive adults."

C. Experimental Methods: Were the experimental methods appropriate to the study goals? Does the author state the accuracy (precision) and reliability (reproducibility) of the methods? Are the methods sensitive enough so that small but biologically important changes could be detected?

D. Statistical Methods: How were the patients selected? Were there enough subjects? Are the subjects representative of the population most likely to receive the drug or of the population for which the reader would like to use the drug? If the project was a long-term or outpatient study, were any patients lost to follow-up? How was this accounted for? Were placebo and positive control treatments included? How were patients assigned to the various groups or subgroups, and were patients properly randomized between treatment groups? Was a crossover design feasible, and was one used? Were patients receiving any other therapy during the trial? How was this controlled or accounted for? Were appropriate statistical tests applied?

E. Conclusions: Do the data, even if sound, justify the conclusions? Does the drug offer significant advantages of cost, efficacy, or safety over existing

CASE STUDY: THE DISCOVERY & DEVELOPMENT OF RECOMBINANT TISSUE PLASMINOGEN ACTIVATOR (rt-PA)

The idea: The thrombotic complications of cardiovascular disease are a major cause of death and disability. Use of drugs to dissolve blood clots, however, is relatively recent, emerging only over the last decade. Central to current thrombolytic therapy and a clear example of progress in the use of biotechnology for drug discovery was the research, development, and marketing of rt-PA.

In 1980 Désiré Collen, a Belgian physician and scientist long interested in blood clotting, had begun using a human cell line as a source of a little-studied naturally occurring fibrin-selective thrombolytic substance. Only traces of it were detectable in the body. While the data were of considerable interest, there appeared to be no practical way to produce enough of this large molecule to effectively characterize or use it. Diane Pennica, a newly hired molecular biologist at the then young California biotechnology company Genentech, heard Collen present his preliminary data at a scientific meeting. Pennica, also new to the field, had just started working on approaches to produce—by biotechnology methods—another naturally occurring blood clot dissolving protein, urokinase. As the two scientists discussed how they could collaborate, an idea was born that was to lead to the first successful clot-busting drug, establish the value of thrombolysis, and jump-start the biotechnology industry.

The clinical need: The only available thrombolytic drugs during the early 1980s were the naturally occurring substances streptokinase (from streptococci) and urokinase (from cultured human renal cells). Uncertainty about their efficacy, the great risk of hemorrhage due to a generalized proteolytic effect of these drugs on key proteins involved in blood clotting, and the lack of clot and fibrin selectivity restricted their use to a few academic centers. Moreover, streptokinase was associated with the significant additional risk of antigenicity and occasionally anaphylaxis. However, it was increasingly believed that a more selective or effective thrombolytic agent could have a dramatic clinical impact.

The biologic hypothesis: Collen was searching for thrombolytic drugs that would have improved efficacy and safety and could be manufactured efficiently. The hypothesis was that t-PA, one of the body's endogenous thrombolytic substances, might have an enhanced affinity for fibrin in blood clots compared with its affinity for circulating fibrinogen. The local conversion of plasminogen to the active proteolytic plasmin thus might result in selective lytic activity in preformed clots as the insoluble fibrin was degraded to soluble forms. At the same time, t-PA should have less effect on other clotting-related proteins and therefore fewer adverse effects, especially less risk of bleeding.

The chemical hypothesis: Pennica and the Genentech team believed that once they had a reliable source of t-PA for chemical sequencing and a source of the human gene, they could clone the gene and transfer it to a microbial or animal cell line for large-scale rt-PA production. No one had ever successfully cloned and expressed a protein as large and complex as t-PA. On the other hand, a successful approach would probably be proprietary and patentable. The project became a priority at Genentech.

Research and development: It took Pennica and colleagues 2 years to determine the genetic code, transfect and express the gene, and complete the initial in vitro studies. Collen, who was now a consultant to Genentech, had meanwhile demonstrated for the first time—in two patients—the clinical thrombolytic efficacy of t-PA from the Bowes cell line.

It took 5 more years for clinical trials and regulatory approval of the recombinant material. In November of 1987, rt-PA received NDA approval, and the utility of rt-PA has been confirmed and extended in numerous large-scale clinical trials (TIMI, GUSTO). The time from the birth of the idea to drug approval for rt-PA was 7 years—one of the fastest times on record for drug discovery and development. In 1994, rt-PA sales were $280 million.

Postscript: Serendipity frequently plays a role in drug discovery. Pennica met Collen only by accident. She had arrived at the meeting early but was told in error that the meeting had already started and in fact was misdirected to Collen's pre-conference satellite meeting.

Thrombolysis is now an essential feature of therapeutics. Désiré Collen continues in Belgium doing cutting-edge basic and clinical research in thrombolysis. His university receives a royalty from Genentech. Diane Pennica continues as a research scientist at Genentech. Several years ago in the halls of Genentech, a colleague asked Pennica if she had a few minutes to see someone who wanted to meet her. It was the first patient who had received rt-PA for treatment of myocardial infarction.

agents, or is it merely new? Extrapolation from the study population to other groups must be very carefully scrutinized.

A well-written report in a journal subject to peer review usually provides explicit answers to all of the above questions. Absence of clear answers to these questions justifies skepticism about the investigation and the authors' conclusions.

REFERENCES

Adverse drug reactions. (Editorial.) Br Med J 1981; 282:1819.

Beyer KH: *Discovery, Development, and Delivery of New Drugs.* SP Medical & Scientific Books, 1978.

Billstein SA: How the pharmaceutical industry brings an antibiotic drug to market in the United Sates. Antimicrob Agents Chemother 1994;38:2679.

Black J: Drugs from emasculated hormones: The principle of syntopic antagonism. Science 1989;245:486.

Brimblecombe RW et al: Characterization and development of cimetidine as histamine H_2-receptor antagonist. Gastroenterology 1978;74:339.

Chappell WR, Mordenti J: Extrapolation of toxicological and pharmacological data from animals to humans. Adv Drug Res 1991 ;20:1.

Cohen J: Clinical trial monitoring: Hit or miss? Science 1994;264:1534.

Collins JM, Grieshaber CK, Chabner BA: Pharmacologically guided phase I clinical trials based upon preclinical drug development. J Natl Cancer Inst 1990;82:1321.

Dixon RL (editor): Extrapolation of laboratory toxicity data to man: Factors influencing the dose-toxic response relationship. (Symposium.) Fed Proc 1980;39:53.

DiMasi JA: Success rates for new drugs entering clinical testing in the United States. Clin Pharmacol Ther 1995;58:1.

Editor's Page: Code of ethics of the World Medical Association: Declaration of Helsinki. Clin Res 1966;14:193.

Feinstein AR: Scientific standards in epidemiologic studies of the menace of daily life. Science 1988;242:1257.

Fredd S: The FDA and the physician. Am J Gastroenterol 1988:83:1088.

Jelovsek FR, Mattison DR, Chen JJ: Prediction of risk for human developmental toxicity: How important are animal studies? Obstet Gynecol 1989;74:624.

Jick H: Drugs: Remarkably nontoxic. N Engl J Med 1974;291:824.

Kessler DA: The regulation of investigational drugs. N Engl J Med 1989;320:281.

Laughren TP: The review of clinical safety data in a new drug application. Psychopharmacol Bull 1989;25:5.

Malmfors T, Teiling A: LD50: Its value for the pharmaceutical industry in safety evaluation of drugs. Acta Pharmacol Toxicol 1983;52(Suppl 2):229.

Mattison N, Trimble AG, Lasagna L: New drug development in the United States, 1963 through 1984. Clin Pharmacol 1988;43:290.

McKhann GM: The trials of clinical trials. Arch Neurol 1989;46:611.

Moscucci M et al: Blinding, unblinding, and the placebo effect: An analysis of patients' guesses of treatment assignment in a double-blind clinical trial. Clin Pharmacol Ther 1987;41:259.

Nolan PE Jr: Generic substitution of antiarrhythmic drugs. Am J Cardiol 1989:64:1371.

Nowak R: Problems in clinical trials go far beyond misconduct. Science 1994;264:1538.

Pennica D et al: Cloning and expression of human tissue-type plasminogen activator cDNA in *E. coli.* Nature 1983:301:214.

Rawlins MD: Clinical pharmacology: Adverse reactions to drugs. Br Med J 1981:282:974.

Riegelman RK: *Studying a Study and Testing a Test: How to Read the Medical Literature.* Little, Brown, 1981.

Schwartzman D: *Innovation in the Pharmaceutical Industry.* Johns Hopkins Univ Press, 1976.

Sheiner LB: The intellectual health of clinical drug evaluation. Clin Pharmacol Ther 1991;50:4.

Shulman SR: The broader message of Accutane. Am J Public Health 1989;79:1565.

Sibille M et al: Adverse events in phase one studies: A study in 430 healthy volunteers. Eur J Clin Pharmacol 1992;42:389.

Spilker B: *Guide to Clinical Interpretation of Data.* Raven Press, 1986.

Spilker B: The development of orphan drugs: An industry perspective. In: *Orphan Diseases and Orphan Drugs.* Scheinberg JH, Walshe JM (editors). Manchester Univ Press, 1986.

Venning GR: Identification of adverse reactions to new drugs. (Five parts.) Br Med J 1983;286:199, 289, 365, 458, 544.

Waller PC: Measuring the frequency of adverse drug reactions. Br J Clin Pharmacol 1992:33:249.

Young FE, Nightingale SL: FDA's newly designated treatment INDs. JAMA 1988:260:224.

Zbinden G, Flury-Reversi M: Significance of LD50-test for the toxicological evaluation of chemical substances. Arch Toxicol 1981;47:77.

Section II.
Autonomic Drugs

Introduction to Autonomic Pharmacology

6

Bertram G. Katzung, MD, PhD

The motor (efferent) portion of the nervous system can be divided into two major subdivisions: **autonomic** and **somatic.** The autonomic nervous system (ANS) is largely autonomous (independent) in that its activities are not under direct conscious control. It is concerned primarily with visceral functions—cardiac output, blood flow to various organs, digestion, etc—that are necessary for life. The somatic division is largely nonautomatic and is concerned with consciously controlled functions such as movement, respiration, and posture. Both systems have important afferent (sensory) inputs that provide sensation and modify motor output through reflex arcs of varying size and complexity.

The nervous system has several properties in common with the endocrine system, which is the other major system for control of body function. These include high-level integration in the brain, the ability to influence processes in distant regions of the body, and extensive use of negative feedback. Both systems use chemicals for the transmission of information. In the nervous system, chemical transmission occurs between nerve cells and between nerve cells and their effector cells. Chemical transmission takes place through the release of small amounts of transmitter substances from the nerve terminals into the synaptic cleft. The transmitter crosses the cleft by diffusion and activates or inhibits the postsynaptic cell by binding to a specialized receptor molecule.

By using drugs that mimic or block the actions of chemical transmitters, we can selectively modify many autonomic functions. These functions involve a variety of effector tissues, including cardiac muscle, smooth muscle, vascular endothelium, exocrine glands, and presynaptic nerve terminals. Autonomic drugs are useful in many clinical conditions. Conversely, a very large number of drugs used for other purposes have unwanted effects on autonomic function.

ANATOMY OF THE AUTONOMIC NERVOUS SYSTEM

The autonomic nervous system lends itself to division on anatomic grounds into two major portions: the **sympathetic (thoracolumbar)** division and the **parasympathetic (craniosacral)** division (Figure 6–1). Both divisions originate in nuclei within the central nervous system and give rise to preganglionic efferent fibers that exit from the brain stem or spinal cord and terminate in motor ganglia. The sympathetic preganglionic fibers leave the central nervous system through the thoracic and lumbar spinal nerves, giving rise to the alternative name "thoracolumbar system." The parasympathetic preganglionic fibers leave the central nervous system through the cranial nerves (especially the third, seventh, ninth, and tenth) and the third and fourth sacral spinal roots.

Most of the sympathetic preganglionic fibers terminate in ganglia located in the paravertebral chains that lie on either side of the spinal column. The remaining sympathetic preganglionic fibers terminate in prevertebral ganglia, which lie in front of the vertebrae. From the ganglia, postganglionic sympathetic fibers run to the tissues innervated. Some preganglionic parasympathetic fibers terminate in parasympathetic ganglia located outside the organs innervated: the ciliary, pterygopalatine, submandibular, otic, and several pelvic ganglia. The majority of parasympathetic preganglionic fibers terminate on ganglion cells distributed diffusely or in networks in the walls of the innervated organs. It is important to remember that the terms "sympathetic" and "parasympathetic" are anatomic ones and do not depend on the type of transmitter chemical released from the nerve endings nor on the kind of effect—excitatory or inhibitory—evoked by nerve activity.

In addition to these clearly defined peripheral motor portions of the autonomic nervous system, there

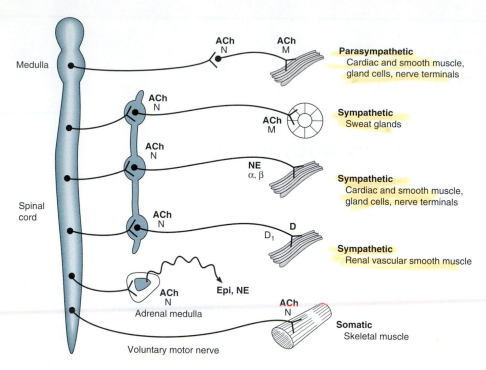

Figure 6–1. Schematic diagram comparing some anatomic and neurotransmitter features of autonomic and somatic motor nerves. Only the primary transmitter substances are shown. Parasympathetic ganglia are not shown because most are in or near the wall of the organ innervated. Note that some sympathetic postganglionic fibers release acetylcholine or dopamine rather than norepinephrine. The adrenal medulla, a modified sympathetic ganglion, receives sympathetic preganglionic fibers and releases epinephrine and norepinephrine into the blood. (ACh, acetylcholine; D, dopamine; Epi, epinephrine; NE, norepinephrine; N, nicotinic receptors; M, muscarinic receptors.)

are large numbers of afferent fibers that run from the periphery to integrating centers, including the enteric plexuses in the gut, the autonomic ganglia, and the central nervous system. Many of the sensory neurons that end in the central nervous system terminate in the integrating centers of the hypothalamus and medulla and evoke reflex motor activity that is carried to the effector cells by the efferent fibers described above. There is increasing evidence that some of these sensory fibers also have important peripheral motor functions (see Nonadrenergic, Noncholinergic Systems, below).

The **enteric nervous system (ENS)** is a very large and highly organized collection of neurons located in the walls of the gastrointestinal system (Figure 6–2). It is sometimes considered a third division of the ANS. The enteric nervous system includes the myenteric plexus (the plexus of Auerbach) and the submucous plexus (the plexus of Meissner) (see Furness et al, 1987; Goyal et al, 1996). These neuronal networks receive preganglionic fibers from the parasympathetic system as well as postganglionic sympathetic axons. They also receive sensory input from within the wall of the gut. Fibers from the cell bodies in these plexuses travel to the smooth muscle of the gut to control motility. Other motor fibers go to the se-

cretory cells. Sensory fibers transmit information from the mucosa and from stretch receptors to motor neurons in the plexuses and to postganglionic neurons in the sympathetic ganglia. The parasympathetic and sympathetic fibers that synapse on enteric plexus neurons appear to play a modulatory role, as indicated by the observation that deprivation of input from both ANS divisions does not halt activity in the plexuses nor in the smooth muscle and glands innervated by them.

NEUROTRANSMITTER CHEMISTRY OF THE AUTONOMIC NERVOUS SYSTEM

An important traditional classification of autonomic nerves is based on the primary transmitter molecules—acetylcholine or norepinephrine—released from their terminal boutons and varicosities. A large number of peripheral autonomic nervous system fibers synthesize and release acetylcholine; they are **cholinergic** fibers, ie, they act by releasing acetylcholine. As shown in Figure 6–1, these include all preganglionic efferent autonomic fibers and the somatic (nonautonomic) motor fibers to skeletal muscle

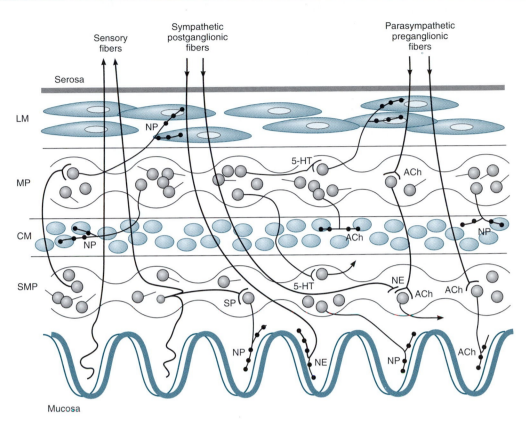

Figure 6–2. A highly simplified diagram of some of the circuitry of the enteric nervous system (ENS). The ENS receives input from both the sympathetic and the parasympathetic systems and sends afferent impulses to sympathetic ganglia and to the central nervous system. Many transmitter or neuromodulator substances have been identified in the ENS; see Table 6–1. (LM, longitudinal muscle layer; MP, myenteric plexus; CM, circular muscle layer; SMP, submucosal plexus; ACh, acetylcholine; NE, norepinephrine; NP, neuropeptides; SP, substance P; 5-HT, serotonin.)

as well. Thus, almost all efferent fibers leaving the central nervous system are cholinergic. In addition, all parasympathetic postganglionic and a few sympathetic postganglionic fibers are cholinergic. Most postganglionic sympathetic fibers release norepinephrine (noradrenaline); they are **noradrenergic** (often called simply "adrenergic") fibers—ie, they act by releasing norepinephrine. These transmitter characteristics are presented schematically in Figure 6–1. As noted above, a few sympathetic fibers release acetylcholine. There is considerable evidence that dopamine is released by some peripheral sympathetic fibers. Adrenal medullary cells, which are embryologically analogous to postganglionic sympathetic neurons, release a mixture of epinephrine and norepinephrine. In recent years it has been recognized that most autonomic nerves also release several transmitter substances, or *cotransmitters*, in addition to the primary transmitter.

Four key features of neurotransmitter function represent potential targets of pharmacologic therapy: synthesis, storage, release, and termination of action. These processes are discussed in detail below.

Cholinergic Transmission

The terminals of cholinergic neurons contain large numbers of small membrane-bound vesicles concentrated near the synaptic portion of the cell membrane (Figure 6–3) as well as a smaller number of large dense-cored vesicles located farther from the synaptic membrane. The large vesicles contain a high concentration of peptides, while the smaller clear vesicles contain most of the acetylcholine. Vesicles are initially synthesized in the neuron soma and transported to the terminal. They may also be recycled several times within the terminal. These vesicles contain acetylcholine in high concentration and other molecules (eg, peptides) that may act as cotransmitters. Acetylcholine is synthesized in the cytoplasm from acetyl-CoA and choline through the catalytic action of the enzyme choline acetyltransferase (ChAT). Acetyl-CoA is synthesized in mitochondria, which are present in large numbers in the nerve ending. Choline is transported from the extracellular fluid into the neuron terminal by a sodium-dependent membrane carrier (Figure 6–3, carrier A). This carrier can be blocked by a group of drugs called **hemi-**

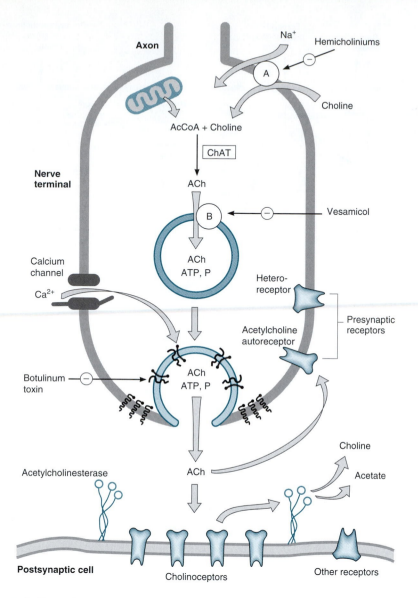

Figure 6–3. Schematic illustration of a generalized cholinergic junction (not to scale). Choline is transported into the presynaptic nerve terminal by a sodium-dependent carrier *(A)*. This transport can be inhibited by hemicholinium drugs. ACh is transported into the storage vesicle by a second carrier *(B)* that can be inhibited by vesamicol. Peptides *(P)*, ATP, and proteoglycan are also stored in the vesicle. Release of transmitter occurs when voltage-sensitive calcium channels in the terminal membrane are opened, allowing an influx of calcium. The resulting increase in intracellular calcium causes fusion of vesicles with the surface membrane and exocytotic expulsion of ACh and cotransmitters into the junctional cleft. This step is blocked by botulinum toxin. Acetylcholine's action is terminated by metabolism by the enzyme acetylcholinesterase. Receptors on the presynaptic nerve ending regulate transmitter release.

choliniums. Once synthesized, acetylcholine is transported from the cytoplasm into the vesicles by an antiporter that removes protons (Figure 6–3, carrier B). This transporter can be blocked by **vesamicol** (Usdin et al, 1995). Acetylcholine synthesis is a rapid process capable of supporting a very high rate of transmitter release. Storage of acetylcholine is accomplished by the packaging of "quanta" of acetyl-

choline molecules (usually 1000–50,000 molecules in each vesicle).

Release of transmitter is dependent on extracellular calcium and occurs when an action potential reaches the terminal and triggers sufficient influx of calcium ions. It has recently been shown that the increased Ca^{2+} concentration "destabilizes" the storage vesicles by interacting with a special protein associated with the vesicular membrane (probably synaptotagmin; Brose et al, 1992). Fusion of the vesicular membranes with the terminal membrane occurs through the interaction of another vesicular protein, synaptobrevin, with several proteins of the terminal membrane, eg, SNAP-25 and syntaxin. Fusion of the membranes results in exocytotic expulsion of—in the case of somatic motor nerves—several hundred quanta of acetylcholine into the synaptic cleft. The amount of transmitter released by one depolarization of an autonomic postganglionic nerve terminal is probably smaller. In addition to acetylcholine, one or more cotransmitters may be released at the same time (Table 6–1). The ACh vesicle release process is blocked by botulinum toxin through the enzymatic removal of two amino acids from synaptobrevin (Schiavo et al, 1992).

After release from the presynaptic terminal, acetylcholine molecules may bind to and activate an acetylcholine receptor **(cholinoceptor).** Eventually (and usually very rapidly), all of the acetylcholine released will diffuse within range of an **acetylcholinesterase** (AChE) molecule. AChE very efficiently splits acetylcholine into choline and acetate, neither of which has significant transmitter effect, and thereby terminates the action of the transmitter (Figure 6–3). Most cholinergic synapses are richly supplied with acetylcholinesterase; the half-life of acetylcholine in the synapse is therefore very short. Acetylcholinesterase is also found in other tissues, eg, red blood cells. (Another cholinesterase with a lower specificity for acetylcholine, butyrylcholinesterase [pseudocholinesterase], is found in blood plasma, liver, glia, and many other tissues.)

Adrenergic Transmission

Adrenergic neurons (Figure 6–4) also transport a precursor molecule into the nerve ending, then synthesize the transmitter, and finally store it in membrane-bound vesicles, but—as indicated in Figure

Table 6–1. Some of the transmitter substances found in autonomic nervous system (ANS), enteric nervous system (ENS), and nonadrenergic, noncholinergic neurons.

Substance	Probable Roles
Acetylcholine (ACh)	The primary transmitter at ANS ganglia, at the somatic neuromuscular junction, and at parasympathetic postganglionic nerve endings. A primary excitatory transmitter to smooth muscle and secretory cells in the ENS. Probably also the major neuron-to-neuron ("ganglionic") transmitter in the ENS.
Adenosine triphosphate (ATP)	May act as a cotransmitter at inhibitory ENS neuromuscular junctions. Inhibits release of ACh and norepinephrine from ANS nerve endings. An excitatory transmitter in the nerves of the vas deferens.
Calcitonin gene-related peptide (CGRP)	Found with substance P in cardiovascular sensory nerve fibers. Present in some secretomotor ENS neurons and interneurons. A cardiac stimulant.
Cholecystokinin (CCK)	May act as a cotransmitter in some excitatory neuromuscular ENS neurons
Dopamine	An important postganglionic sympathetic transmitter in renal blood vessels. Probably a modulatory transmitter in some ganglia and the ENS.
Enkephalin and related opioid peptides	Present in some secretomotor and interneurons in the ENS. Appear to inhibit ACh release and thereby inhibit peristalsis. May *stimulate* secretion.
Galanin	Present in secretomotor neurons; may play a role in appetite-satiety mechanisms
GABA (γ-aminobutyric acid)	May have presynaptic effects on excitatory ENS nerve terminals. Has some relaxant effect on the gut. Probably not a major transmitter in the ENS.
Gastrin-releasing peptide (GRP)	Extremely potent excitatory transmitter to gastrin cells. Also known as mammalian bombesin.
Neuropeptide Y (NPY)	Present in some secretomotor neurons in the ENS and may inhibit secretion of water and electrolytes by the gut. Causes long-lasting vasoconstriction. It is also a cotransmitter in many parasympathetic postganglionic neurons and sympathetic postganglionic norarenergic vascular neurons.
Nitric oxide (NO)	A cotransmitter at inhibitory ENS neuromuscular junctions
Norepinephrine (NE)	The primary transmitter at most sympathetic postganglionic nerve endings
Serotonin (5-HT)	A cotransmitter at excitatory neuron-to-neuron junctions in the ENS
Substance P (and related "tachykinins")	Substance P is an important sensory neuron transmitter in the ENS and elsewhere. Tachykinins appear to be excitatory cotransmitters with ACh at ENS neuromuscular junctions. Found with CGRP in cardiovascular sensory neurons. Substance P is a vasodilator (probably via release of nitric oxide).
Vasoactive intestinal peptide (VIP)	Excitatory secretomotor transmitter in the ENS; may also be an inhibitory ENS neuromuscular cotransmitter. A probable cotransmitter in many cholinergic neurons. A vasodilator (found in many perivascular neurons) and cardiac stimulant.

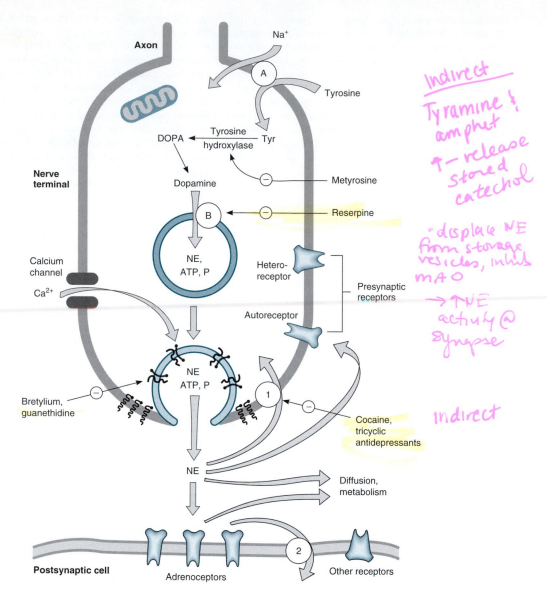

Handwritten annotations:

Indirect

Tyramine & amphet ↑-release stored catechol

°displace NE from storage vesicles, inhib mAO

→ ↑NE activity @ synapse

Indirect

Figure 6–4. Schematic diagram of a generalized noradrenergic junction (not to scale). Tyrosine is transported into the noradrenergic ending or varicosity by a sodium-dependent carrier *(A)*. Tyrosine is converted to dopamine (see Figure 6–5 for details), which is transported into the vesicle by a carrier *(B)* that can be blocked by reserpine. The same carrier transports norepinephrine *(NE)* and several other amines into these granules. Dopamine is converted to NE in the vesicle by dopamine-β-hydroxylase. Release of transmitter occurs when an action potential opens voltage-sensitive calcium channels and increases intracellular calcium. Fusion of vesicles with the surface membrane results in expulsion of norepinephrine, cotransmitters, and dopamine-β-hydroxylase. Release can be blocked by drugs such as guanethidine and bretylium. After release, norepinephrine diffuses out of the cleft or is transported into the cytoplasm of the terminal (uptake 1 *[1]*, blocked by cocaine, tricyclic antidepressants) or into the postjunctional cell (uptake 2 *[2]*). Regulatory receptors are present on the presynaptic terminal.

6–5—the synthesis of the adrenergic transmitters is more complex than that of acetylcholine. In the adrenal medulla and certain areas of the brain, norepinephrine is further converted to epinephrine. Several important processes in the noradrenergic nerve terminal are potential sites of drug action. One of these, the conversion of tyrosine to dopa, is the rate-limiting step in norepinephrine synthesis. It can be inhibited by the tyrosine analog metyrosine (Figure 6–4). A high-affinity carrier for catecholamines located in the wall of the storage vesicle can be inhibited by the reserpine alkaloids (Figure 6–4, carrier B).

Figure 6–5. Biosynthesis of catecholamines. The rate-limiting step, conversion of tyrosine to Dopa, can be inhibited by metyrosine (α-methyltyrosine) The alternative pathways shown by the dashed arrows have not been found to be of physiologic significance in humans. However, tyramine and octopamine may accumulate in patients treated with monoamine oxidase inhibitors. (Reproduced, with permission, from Greenspan FS, Strewler GJ: *Basic and Clinical Endocrinology,* 5th ed. Appleton & Lange, 1996.)

Depletion of transmitter stores results. Another carrier transports norepinephrine and similar molecules into the cell cytoplasm (Figure 6–4, carrier 1, commonly called uptake 1). It can be inhibited by cocaine and tricyclic antidepressant drugs, resulting in an increase of transmitter activity in the synaptic cleft.

Release of the vesicular transmitter store from noradrenergic nerve endings is similar to the calcium-dependent process described above for cholinergic terminals. In addition to the primary transmitter (norepinephrine), ATP, dopamine-β-hydroxylase, and certain peptide cotransmitters are also released into the synaptic cleft. Indirectly acting sympathomimetics—eg, tyramine and amphetamines—are capable of releasing stored transmitter from noradrenergic nerve endings. These drugs are poor agonists (some are inactive) at adrenoceptors but are taken up into noradrenergic nerve endings by uptake 1. In the nerve ending, they may displace norepinephrine from storage vesicles, inhibit monoamine oxidase, and have other effects that result in increased norepinephrine activity in the synapse. Their action does not require vesicle exocytosis and is not calcium-dependent.

Norepinephrine and epinephrine can be metabolized by several enzymes, as shown in Figure 6–6. Because of the high activity of monoamine oxidase in

Figure 6–6. Metabolism of catecholamines by catechol-*O*-methyltransferase *(COMT)* and monoamine oxidase *(MAO)*. (Modified and reproduced, with permission, from Greenspan FS, Strewler GJ: *Basic and Clinical Endocrinology,* 5th ed. Appleton & Lange, 1996.)

the mitochondria of the nerve terminal, there is a significant turnover of norepinephrine even in the resting terminal. Since the metabolic products are excreted in the urine, an estimate of catecholamine turnover can be obtained from laboratory analysis of total metabolites (sometimes referred to as "VMA and metanephrines") in a 24-hour urine sample. However, metabolism is not the primary mechanism for termination of action of norepinephrine physiologically released from noradrenergic nerves. Termination of noradrenergic transmission results from several processes, including simple diffusion away from the receptor site (with eventual metabolism in the plasma or liver) and reuptake into the nerve terminal **(uptake 1)** or into perisynaptic glia or smooth muscle cells **(uptake 2)** (Figure 6–4).

Cotransmitters in Cholinergic & Adrenergic Nerves

As previously noted, the vesicles of both cholinergic and adrenergic nerves contain other substances in addition to the primary transmitter (Burnstock, 1995). Furthermore, the large vesicles found in nerve endings release transmitter peptides, especially at high rates of nerve firing. Some of the substances identified to date are listed in Table 6–1. Many of these substances are also *primary* transmitters in the nonadrenergic, noncholinergic nerves described below. Their roles in the function of nerves that release acetylcholine or norepinephrine are not fully understood. They may provide a slow, long-lasting action to supplement or modulate the more transient effects of the primary transmitter. They may also participate in feedback inhibition of the same or nearby nerve terminals.

AUTONOMIC RECEPTORS

A great deal has been learned about the chemical nature of autonomic receptors during the past 2 decades, and this field is one of the most active research areas in pharmacology. Historically, structure-activity analyses, with careful comparisons of the potency of series of autonomic analogs, led to the definition of different autonomic receptor subtypes, including muscarinic and nicotinic cholinoceptors, and alpha, beta, and dopamine adrenoceptors (Table 6–2). Molecular biology has provided a new approach by making possible the discovery and expression of genes that code for related receptors within these groups. (See Chapter 2 box: How Are New Receptors Discovered?)

The primary acetylcholine receptor subtypes were named after the alkaloids originally used in their iden-

tification: muscarine and nicotine. These nouns are readily converted into adjectives—thus, muscarinic and nicotinic receptors. In the case of receptors associated with noradrenergic nerves, the coining of simple adjectives from the names of the agonists (noradrenaline, phenylephrine, isoproterenol, etc) was not practicable. Therefore, the term **adrenoceptor** is widely used to describe receptors that respond to catecholamines such as norepinephrine. By analogy, the term **cholinoceptor** denotes receptors (both muscarinic and nicotinic) that respond to acetylcholine. In North America, receptors were colloquially named after the nerves that usually innervate them; thus, **adrenergic** (or noradrenergic) **receptors** and **cholinergic receptors.** The adrenoceptors can be subdivided into alpha-adrenoceptor and beta-adrenoceptor types on the basis of both agonist and antagonist selectivity. Development of more selective blocking drugs has led to the naming of subclasses within these major types; eg, within the alpha-adrenoceptor class, α_1 and α_2 receptors differ in both agonist and antagonist selectiv-

Table 6–2. Autonomic receptor types with documented or probable effects on peripheral autonomic effector tissues.

Receptor Name	Typical Locations	Result of Ligand Binding
Cholinoceptors		
Muscarinic M_1	CNS neurons, sympathetic postganglionic neurons, some presynaptic sites	Formation of IP_3 and DAG, increased intracellular calcium
Muscarinic M_2	Myocardium, smooth muscle, some presynaptic sites	Opening of potassium channels, inhibition of adenylyl cyclase
Muscarinic M_3	Exocrine glands, vessels (smooth muscle and endothelium)	Formation of IP_3 and DAG, increased intracellular calcium
Nicotinic N_N	Postganglionic neurons, some presynaptic cholinergic terminals	Opening of Na^+, K^+ channels, depolarization
Nicotinic N_M	Skeletal muscle neuromuscular endplates	Opening of Na^+, K^+ channels, depolarization
Adrenoceptors		
Alpha$_1$	Postsynaptic effector cells, especially smooth muscle	Formation of IP_3 and DAG, increased intracellular calcium
Alpha$_2$	Presynaptic adrenergic nerve terminals, platelets, lipocytes, smooth muscle	Inhibition of adenylyl cyclase, decreased cAMP
Beta$_1$	Postsynaptic effector cells, especially heart, lipocytes, brain, presynaptic adrenergic and cholinergic nerve terminals	Stimulation of adenylyl cyclase, increased cAMP
Beta$_2$	Postsynaptic effector cells, especially smooth muscle and cardiac muscle	Stimulation of adenylyl cyclase and increased cAMP
Beta$_3$	Postsynaptic effector cells, especially lipocytes	Stimulation of adenylyl cyclase and increased cAMP
Dopamine receptors		
D_1 (DA_1), D_5	Brain; effector tissues, especially smooth muscle of the renal vascular bed	Stimulation of adenylyl cyclase and increased cAMP
D_2 (DA_2)	Brain; effector tissues especially smooth muscle; presynaptic nerve terminals	Inhibition of adenylyl cyclase; increased potassium conductance
D_3	Brain	Inhibition of adenylyl cyclase
D_4	Brain, cardiovascular system	Inhibition of adenylyl cyclase

ity. Specific examples of such selective drugs are given in the chapters that follow.

Much progress has been made in isolating and purifying receptor proteins, and in many cases this has permitted the determination of the peptide sequences of these proteins and their three-dimensional conformations. Independent studies based on cDNA libraries have confirmed and extended the numbers of subtypes of cholinoceptors and adrenoceptors. For example, genes have been discovered for five different muscarinic cholinoceptors (Buckley et al, 1989).

NONADRENERGIC, NONCHOLINERGIC NEURONS

It has been known for many years that autonomic effector tissues (eg, gut, airways, bladder) contain nerve fibers that do not show the histochemical characteristics of either cholinergic or adrenergic fibers. Both motor and sensory nonadrenergic, noncholinergic fibers are present. Although peptides are the most common transmitter substances found in these nerve endings, other substances, especially purines, are also present in many nerve terminals (Table 6–1). Improved immunologic assay methods now permit accurate identification and quantitation of peptides stored in and released from the fiber terminals. In addition, it has been found that capsaicin, a neurotoxin derived from chili peppers, can cause the release of transmitter from such neurons and, if given in high doses, destruction of the neuron. Use of these research tools has led to the accumulation of a large amount of information, much of which is still incompletely understood.

The enteric system in the gut wall (Figure 6–2) is the most extensively studied system containing nonadrenergic, noncholinergic neurons in addition to cholinergic and adrenergic fibers. In the guinea pig small intestine, for example, these neurons respond to immunofluorescent probes for one or more of the following: calcitonin gene-related peptide, cholecystokinin, dynorphin, enkephalins, gastrin-releasing peptide, 5-hydroxytryptamine (serotonin), neuropeptide Y, somatostatin, substance P, and vasoactive intestinal peptide. Some neurons contain as many as five different possible transmitters. This system functions in a semiautonomous manner, utilizing input from the motor outflow of the ANS for modulation of gastrointestinal activity and sending sensory information back to the central nervous system. The ENS provides the necessary synchronization of impulses that, for example, ensures forward, not backward, propulsion of gut contents and relaxation of sphincters when the gut wall contracts.

The sensory fibers in the nonadrenergic, noncholinergic systems are probably better termed "sensory-efferent" or "sensory-local effector" fibers because, when activated by a sensory input, they are capable of releasing transmitter peptides from the sensory ending itself, from local axon branches, and from collaterals that terminate in the autonomic ganglia. These peptides are potent agonists at many autonomic effector tissues.

FUNCTIONAL ORGANIZATION OF AUTONOMIC ACTIVITY

A basic understanding of the interactions of autonomic nerves with each other and with their effector organs is essential for an appreciation of the actions of autonomic drugs, especially because of the significant "reflex" effects that may be evoked by these agents.

Central Integration

At the highest level—midbrain and medulla—the two divisions of the autonomic nervous system and the endocrine system are integrated with each other, with sensory input, and with information from higher central nervous system centers. These interactions are such that early investigators called the parasympathetic system a **trophotropic** one (ie, leading to growth) and the sympathetic system an **ergotropic** one (ie, leading to energy expenditure) that was activated for "fight or flight." While such terms offer little insight into the mechanisms involved, they do provide simple descriptions applicable to many of the actions of the systems (Table 6–3). For example, slowing of the heart and stimulation of digestive activity are typical energy-conserving "rest and digest" actions of the parasympathetic system. In contrast, cardiac stimulation, increased blood sugar, and cutaneous vasoconstriction are responses produced by sympathetic discharge that are suited to fighting or surviving attack.

At a more subtle level of interactions in the brain stem, medulla, and spinal cord, there are important cooperative interactions between the parasympathetic and sympathetic systems. For some organs, sensory fibers associated with the parasympathetic system exert reflex control over motor outflow in the sympathetic system. Thus, the sensory carotid sinus baroreceptor fibers in the glossopharyngeal nerve have a major influence on sympathetic outflow from the vasomotor center. This example is described in greater detail below. Similarly, parasympathetic sensory fibers in the wall of the urinary bladder significantly influence sympathetic inhibitory outflow to that organ. Within the enteric nervous system, sensory fibers from the wall of the gut synapse on both preganglionic and postganglionic motor cells that control intestinal smooth muscle and secretory cells (Figure 6–2).

Integration of Cardiovascular Function

Autonomic reflexes are particularly important in understanding cardiovascular responses to autonomic

Table 6–3. Direct effects of autonomic nerve activity on some organ systems.

Organ	Effect of			
	Sympathetic		Parasympathetic	
	Action[1]	Receptor[2]	Action	Receptor[2]
Eye				
Iris				
Radial muscle	Contracts	α_1	. . .	. . .
Circular muscle	. . .	. . .	Contracts	M_3
Ciliary muscle	[Relaxes]	β	Contracts	M_3
Heart				
Sinoatrial node	Accelerates	β_1,β_2	Decelerates	M_2
Ectopic pacemakers	Accelerates	β_1,β_2	. . .	. . .
Contractility	Increases	β_1,β_2	Decreases (atria)	M_2
Blood vessels				
Skin, splanchnic vessels	Contracts	α	. . .	
Skeletal muscle vessels	Relaxes	β_2	. . .	. . .
	[Contracts]	α	. . .	. . .
	Relaxes	M^3	. . .	. . .
Endothelium			Releases EDRF	$M_3{}^4$
Bronchiolar smooth muscle	Relaxes	β_2	Contracts	M_3
Gastrointestinal tract				
Smooth muscle				
Walls	Relaxes	$\alpha_2{}^5, \beta_2$	Contracts	M_3
Sphincters	Contracts	α_1	Relaxes	M_3
Secretion	. . .		Increases	M_3
Myenteric plexus			Activates	M_1
Genitourinary smooth muscle				
Bladder wall	Relaxes	β_2	Contracts	M_3
Sphincter	Contracts	α_1	Relaxes	M_3
Uterus, pregnant	Relaxes	β_2	. . .	. . .
	Contracts	α	Contracts	M_3
Penis, seminal vesicles	Ejaculation	α	Erection	M
Skin				
Pilomotor smooth muscle	Contracts	α	. . .	. . .
Sweat glands			. . .	. . .
Thermoregulatory	Increases	M	. . .	. . .
Apocrine (stress)	Increases	α	. . .	. . .
Metabolic functions				
Liver	Gluconeogenesis	β_2,α	. . .	. . .
Liver	Glycogenolysis	β_2,α	. . .	. . .
Fat cells	Lipolysis	β_3	. . . . . .	
Kidney	Renin release	β_1	. . .	. . .
Autonomic nerve endings				
Sympathetic	. . .	. . .	Decreases NE release	M^6
Parasympathetic	Decreases ACh release	α	. . .	. . .

[1]Less important actions are shown in brackets.
[2]Specific receptor type: α = alpha, β = beta, M = muscarinic.
[3]Vascular smooth muscle in skeletal muscle has sympathetic cholinergic dilator fibers.
[4]The endothelium of most blood vessels releases EDRF (endothelium-derived relaxing factor), which causes marked vasodilation, in response to muscarinic stimuli. However, unlike the receptors innervated by sympathetic cholinergic fibers in skeletal muscle blood vessels, these muscarinic receptors are not innervated and respond only to circulating muscarinic agonists.
[5]Probably through presynaptic inhibition of parasympathetic activity.
[6]Probably M_1 but M_2 may participate in some locations.

drugs. As indicated in Figure 6–7, the primary controlled variable in cardiovascular function is **mean arterial pressure.** Changes in any variable contributing to mean arterial pressure (eg, peripheral vascular resistance) will evoke powerful **homeostatic** secondary responses that tend to compensate for the directly evoked change. The homeostatic response may sometimes be sufficient to prevent any change in mean arterial pressure and to reverse the drug's effects on heart rate. A slow infusion of norepinephrine provides a useful example. This agent produces direct effects on both vascular and cardiac muscle. It is a powerful

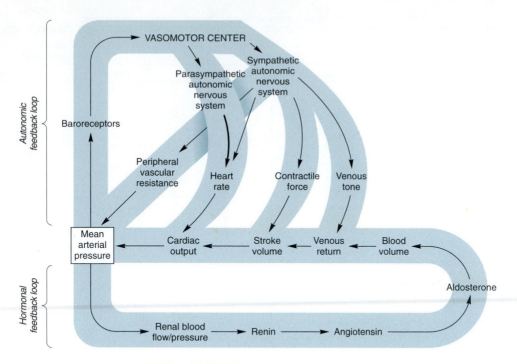

Figure 6–7. Autonomic and hormonal control of cardiovascular function. Note that two feedback loops are present: the autonomic nervous system loop and the hormonal loop. The sympathetic nervous system directly influences four major variables: peripheral vascular resistance, heart rate, force, and venous tone. It also directly modulates renin production (not shown). The parasympathetic nervous system directly influences heart rate. Angiotensin II directly increases peripheral vascular resistance (not shown). The net feedback effect of each loop is to compensate for changes in arterial blood pressure. Thus, decreased blood pressure due to blood loss would evoke increased sympathetic outflow and renin release. Conversely, elevated pressure due to the administration of a vasoconstrictor drug would cause reduced sympathetic outflow and renin release and increased parasympathetic (vagal) outflow.

vasoconstrictor and, by increasing peripheral vascular resistance, increases mean arterial pressure. In the absence of reflex control—in a patient who has had a heart transplant, for example—the drug's effect on the heart is also stimulatory; ie, it increases heart rate and contractile force. However, in a subject with intact reflexes, the negative feedback baroreceptor response to increased mean arterial pressure causes decreased sympathetic outflow to the heart and a powerful increase in parasympathetic (vagus nerve) discharge at the cardiac pacemaker. As a result, the *net* effect of ordinary pressor doses of norepinephrine is to produce a marked increase in peripheral vascular resistance, a moderate increase in mean arterial pressure, and a consistent *slowing* of heart rate. Bradycardia, the reflex compensatory response elicited by this agent, is *the exact opposite of the drug's direct action;* yet it is completely predictable if the integration of cardiovascular function by the autonomic nervous system is understood.

Presynaptic Regulation

The principle of negative feedback control is also found at the presynaptic level of autonomic function.

While not yet as well understood as the baroreceptor reflex, important presynaptic feedback inhibitory control mechanisms have been shown to exist in noradrenergic fibers. The best-documented mechanism involves an α_2 receptor located on the nerve terminals. This receptor is activated by norepinephrine and similar molecules; activation diminishes further release of norepinephrine from these nerve endings (Table 6–4). Conversely, a presynaptic beta receptor may facilitate the release of norepinephrine. Presynaptic receptors that respond to the transmitter substances released by the nerve ending have been called **autoreceptors.** Autoreceptors are usually inhibitory, but some cholinergic fibers, especially somatic motor fibers, may have excitatory autoreceptors for acetylcholine.

Control of transmitter release is not limited to modulation by the transmitter itself. Nerve terminals also carry regulatory receptors that respond to many other substances (heteroreceptors). Heteroreceptors may be activated by substances released from nerve terminals that synapse with the nerve ending. Alternatively, the ligands for these receptors may diffuse to the receptors from the blood or from nearby tissues. Some of the transmitters and receptors identified to date are

Table 6–4. Autoreceptor, heteroreceptor, and modulatory effects in peripheral synapses.[1]

Transmitter/Modulator	Receptor Type	Neuron Terminals Where Found
Inhibitory effects		
Acetylcholine	M_2	Adrenergic, enteric nervous system
Norepinephrine	Alpha$_2$	Adrenergic
Dopamine	D_2; less evidence for D_1	Adrenergic
Serotonin (5-HT)	5-HT$_1$, 5-HT$_2$, 5-HT$_3$	Cholinergic preganglionic
ATP and adenosine	P_1	Adrenergic, autonomic presynaptic, and ENS cholinergic neurons
Histamine	H_3, possibly H_2	H_3 type identified on CNS adrenergic and serotonergic neurons
Enkephalin	Delta (also mu, kappa)	Adrenergic, ENS cholinergic
Neuropeptide Y	NPY	Adrenergic, some cholinergic
Prostaglandin E$_1$, E$_2$	EP$_3$	Adrenergic
Excitatory effects		
Epinephrine	Beta$_2$	Adrenergic, somatic motor cholinergic
Acetylcholine	N_M	Somatic motor cholinergic
Angiotensin II	AII-1	Adrenergic

[1]A provisional list. The number of transmitters and locations will undoubtedly increase with additional research.

listed in Table 6–4. Presynaptic regulation by a variety of endogenous chemicals probably occurs in all nerve fibers.

Postsynaptic Regulation

Postsynaptic regulation can be considered from two perspectives: modulation by the prior history of activity at the primary receptor (which may up- or downregulate receptor number or desensitize receptors; see Chapter 2) and modulation by other temporally associated events.

The first mechanism has been well documented in several receptor-effector systems. Up- and down-regulation are known to occur in response to decreased or increased activation, respectively, of the receptors. An extreme form of up-regulation occurs after denervation of some tissues, resulting in "denervation supersensitivity" of the tissue to activators of that receptor type. In skeletal muscle, for example, nicotinic receptors are normally restricted to the endplate regions underlying somatic motor nerve terminals. Surgical denervation results in marked proliferation of nicotinic cholinoceptors over all parts of the fiber, including areas not previously associated with any motor nerve junctions. A related pharmacologic denervation supersensitivity phenomenon occurs in autonomic effector tissues after administration of drugs that deplete transmitter stores and prevent activation of the postsynaptic receptors for a sufficient period of time. For example, administration of large doses of reserpine, a norepinephrine depleter, can cause increased sensitivity of the smooth muscle and cardiac muscle effector cells served by the depleted sympathetic fibers.

The second mechanism involves modulation of the primary transmitter-receptor event by events evoked by the same or other transmitters acting on different postsynaptic receptors. Ganglionic transmission is a good example of this phenomenon (Figure 6–8). The postganglionic cells are activated (depolarized) as a result of binding of an appropriate ligand to a nicotinic (N_N) acetylcholine receptor. The resulting fast excitatory postsynaptic potential (EPSP) evokes a propagated action potential if threshold is reached. This event is often followed by a small and slowly developing but longer-lasting hyperpolarizing afterpotential—a slow inhibitory postsynaptic potential (IPSP). The hyperpolarization involves opening of potassium channels by M_2 cholinoceptors. The IPSP is followed by a small, slow excitatory postsynaptic potential apparently caused by closure of potassium channels linked to M_1 cholinoceptors. Finally, a late, very slow EPSP may be evoked by peptides released from other fibers. These slow potentials serve to modulate the responsiveness of the postsynaptic cell to subsequent primary excitatory presynaptic nerve activity. (See Chapter 21 for additional examples.)

PHARMACOLOGIC MODIFICATION OF AUTONOMIC FUNCTION

Because transmission involves different mechanisms in different segments of the autonomic nervous system, some drugs produce highly specific effects while others are much less selective in their actions. A summary of the steps in transmission of impulses, from the central nervous system to the autonomic effector cells, is presented in Table 6–5. Drugs that block action potential propagation (local anesthetics)

Table 6–5. Steps in autonomic transmission: Effects of drugs.

Process	Drug Example	Site	Action
Action potential propagation	Local anesthetics, tetrodotoxin,[1] saxitoxin[2]	Nerve axons	Block sodium channels; block conduction
Transmitter synthesis	Hemicholinium	Cholinergic nerve terminals: membrane	Blocks uptake of choline and slows synthesis
	α-Methyltyrosine (metyrosine)	Adrenergic nerve terminals and adrenal medulla: cytoplasm	Blocks synthesis
Transmitter storage	Vesamicol	Cholinergic terminals: vesicles	Prevents storage, depletes
	Reserpine	Adrenergic terminals: vesicles	Prevents storage, depletes
Transmitter release	Many[3]	Nerve terminal membrane receptors	Modulate release
	ω-Conotoxin GVIA[4]	Nerve terminal calcium channels	Reduces transmitter release
	Botulinus toxin	Cholinergic vesicles	Prevents release
	Alpha-latrotoxin[5]	Cholinergic and adrenergic vesicles	Causes explosive release
	Tyramine, amphetamine	Adrenergic nerve terminals	Promote transmitter release
Transmitter uptake after release	Cocaine, tricyclic antidepressants	Adrenergic nerve terminals	Inhibit uptake; increase transmitter effect on postsynaptic receptors
	6-Hydroxydopamine	Adrenergic nerve terminals	Destroys the terminals
Receptor activation or blockade	Norepinephrine	Receptors at adrenergic junctions	Binds α receptors; causes activation
	Phentolamine	Receptors at adrenergic junctions	Binds α receptors; prevents activation
	Isoproterenol	Receptors at adrenergic junctions	Binds β receptors; activates adenylyl cyclase
	Propranolol	Receptors at adrenergic junctions	Binds β receptors; prevents activation
	Nicotine	Receptors at nicotinic cholinergic junctions (autonomic ganglia, neuromuscular end-plates)	Binds nicotinic receptors; opens ion channel in postsynaptic membrane
	Tubocurarine	Neuromuscular end-plates	Prevents activation
	Bethanechol	Receptors, parasympathetic effector cells (smooth muscle, glands)	Binds and activates muscarinic receptors
	Atropine	Receptors, parasympathetic effector cells	Binds muscarinic receptors; prevents activation
Enzymatic inactivation of transmitter	Neostigmine	Cholinergic synapses (acetylcholinesterase)	Inhibits enzyme; prolongs and intensifies transmitter action
	Tranylcypromine	Adrenergic nerve terminals (monoamine oxidase)	Inhibits enzyme; increases stored transmitter pool

[1]Toxin of puffer fish, California newt.
[2]Toxin of *Gonyaulax* (red tide organism).
[3]Norepinephrine, dopamine, acetylcholine, angiotensin II, various prostaglandins, etc.
[4]Toxin of marine snails of the genus *Conus*.
[5]Black widow spider venom.

Figure 6–8. Excitatory and inhibitory postsynaptic potentials *(EPSP and IPSP)* in an autonomic ganglion cell. The postganglionic neuron shown at the left with a recording electrode might undergo the membrane potential changes shown schematically in the recording. The response begins with two EPSP responses to nicotinic *(N)* receptor activation, the first not achieving threshold. The action potential is followed by an IPSP, probably evoked by M_2 receptor activation (with possible participation from dopamine receptor activation). The IPSP is, in turn, followed by a slower M_1-dependent EPSP, and this is sometimes followed by a still slower peptide-induced excitatory postsynaptic potential.

are very nonselective in their action, since they act on a process that is common to all neurons. On the other hand, drugs that act on the biochemical processes involved in transmitter synthesis and storage are more selective, since the biochemistry of adrenergic transmission is very different from that of cholinergic transmission. Activation or blockade of effector cell receptors offers maximum flexibility and selectivity

of effect: adrenoceptors are easily distinguished from cholinoceptors. Furthermore, individual subgroups can often be selectively activated or blocked within each major type. Some examples are given in the box: Pharmacology of the Eye.

The next four chapters provide many more examples of this useful diversity of autonomic control processes.

PHARMACOLOGY OF THE EYE

The eye is a good example of an organ with multiple ANS functions, controlled by several different autonomic receptors. As shown in Figure 6–9, the anterior chamber is the site of several tissues controlled by the ANS. These tissues include three different muscles (pupillary dilator and constrictor muscles in the iris and the ciliary muscle) and the secretory epithelium of the ciliary body.

Muscarinic cholinomimetics cause contraction of the circular pupillary constrictor muscle and of the ciliary muscle. Contraction of the pupillary constrictor muscle causes miosis, a reduction in pupil size. Miosis is usually present in patients exposed to large systemic or small topical doses of cholinomimetics, especially organophosphate cholinesterase inhibitors. Ciliary muscle contraction causes accommodation of focus for near vision. Marked contraction of the ciliary muscle, which often occurs with cholinesterase inhibitor

intoxication, is called *cyclospasm*. Ciliary muscle contraction also puts tension on the trabecular meshwork, opening its pores and facilitating outflow of the aqueous humor into the canal of Schlemm. Increased outflow reduces intraocular pressure, a very useful result in patients with glaucoma. All of these effects are prevented or reversed by muscarinic blocking drugs such as atropine.

Alpha adrenoceptors cause contraction of the radially oriented pupillary dilator muscle fibers in the iris and result in mydriasis. This occurs during sympathetic discharge and when alpha agonist drugs such as phenylephrine are placed in the conjunctival sac. Beta adrenoceptors on the ciliary epithelium facilitate the secretion of aqueous humor. Blocking these receptors (with beta-blocking drugs) reduces the secretory activity and reduces intraocular pressure, providing another therapy for glaucoma.

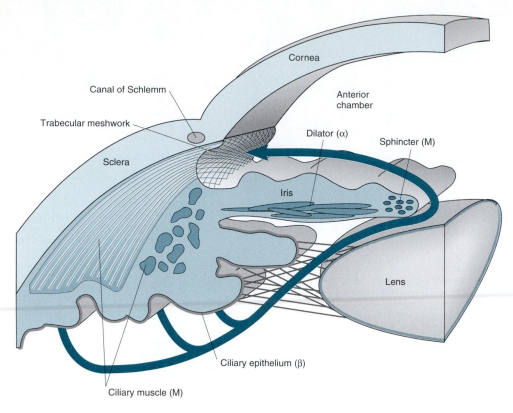

Figure 6–9. Structures of the anterior chamber of the eye. Tissues with significant autonomic functions and the associated ANS receptors are shown in this schematic diagram. Blockade of the beta adrenoceptors associated with the ciliary epithelium causes decreased secretion of aqueous humor (arrow). Blood vessels (not shown) in the sclera are also under autonomic control and influence aqueous drainage.

REFERENCES

Allen TGJ, Burnstock G: M_1 and M_2 muscarinic receptors mediate excitation and inhibition of guinea-pig intracardiac neurones in culture. J Physiol 1990;422:463.

Anderson K-E: Pharmacology of lower urinary tract smooth muscles and penile erectile tissues. Pharmacol Rev 1993; 45:253.

Bernardi L et al: Demonstrable cardiac reinnervation after human heart transplantation by carotid baroreflex modulation of RR interval. Circulation 1995;92:2895.

Bevan JA, Brayden JE: Nonadrenergic neural vasodilator mechanisms. Circ Res 1987;60:309.

Brose N et al: Synaptotagmin: A calcium sensor on the synaptic vesicle surface. Science 1992;256:1021.

Buckley NJ et al: Antagonist binding properties of five cloned muscarinic receptors expressed in CHO-K1 cells. Mol Pharmacol 1989;35:469.

Burnstock G: Noradrenaline and ATP: Cotransmitters and neuromodulators. J Physiol Pharmacol 1995;46:365.

Burnstock G, Hoyle CHV: *Autonomic Neuroeffector Mechanisms.* Harwood Academic Publishers, 1992.

Cassis LA, Dwoskin LP: Presynaptic modulation of transmitter release by endogenous angiotensin II in brown adipose tissue. J Neural Transm 1991;34(Suppl):129.

DiFrancesco D: The onset and autonomic regulation of cardiac pacemaker activity: relevance of f current. Cardiovasc Res 1995;29:449.

Duckles SP, Garcia-Villalon L: Characterization of vascular muscarinic receptors: Rabbit ear artery and bovine coronary artery. J Pharmacol Exp Ther 1990;253:608.

Eglen RM et al: Muscarinic acetylcholine receptor subtypes in smooth muscle. Trends Pharmacol Sci 1994;15:114.

Eglen RM, Hegde SS, Watson N: Muscarinic receptor subtypers and smooth muscle function. Pharmacol Rev 1996;48:531.

Furchgott RF: Role of endothelium in responses of vascular smooth muscle to drugs. Annu Rev Pharmacol Toxicol 1984;24:175.

Furness JB et al: Roles of peptides in transmission in the enteric nervous system. Trends Neurosci 1992;15:66.

Furness JB, Costa M: *The Enteric Nervous System.* Churchill Livingstone, 1987.

Gershon MD, Kirchgessner AL, Wade PR: Functional anatomy of the enteric nervous system. In: *Physiology of the Gastrointestinal Tract,* 3rd ed. Johnson LR (editor). Raven Press, 1994.

Goyal RK, Hirano I: The enteric nervous system. N Engl J Med 1996;334:1106.

Goyal RK: Muscarinic receptor subtypes. Physiology and clinical implications. N Engl J Med 1989;321:1022.

Holzer P: Local effector functions of capsaicin-sensitive sensory nerve endings: Involvement of tachykinins, calcitonin gene-related peptide and other neuropeptides. Neuroscience 1988;24:739.

Hökfelt T et al: Coexistence of peptides with classical neurotransmitters. Experientia 1989;56(Suppl):154.

Jankovic J, Brin MF: Therapeutic uses of botulinum toxin. N Engl J Med 1991;324:1186.

Kellogg DL Jr et al: Cutaneous active vasodilation in humans is mediated by cholinergic nerve cotransmission. Circ Res 1995;77:1222.

Kromer W: Endogenous opioids, the enteric nervous system and gut motility. Dig Dis 1990;8:361.

Kumada M, Terui N, Kuwaki T: Arterial baroreceptor reflex: Its central and peripheral neural mechanisms. Prog Neurobiol 1990;35:331.

Langer SZ: Presynaptic regulation of monoaminergic neurons. In: *Psychopharmacology: The Third Generation of Progress.* Meltzer HY (editor). Raven Press, 1987.

Lefkowitz RJ, Hausdorff WP, Caron MG: Role of phosphorylation in desensitization of the β-adrenoceptor. Trends Pharmacol Sci 1990;11:190.

Limberger N, Spädth L, Starke K: Presynaptic α_2-adrenoceptor, opioid k-receptor and adenosine A_1-receptor interactions on noradrenalin release in rabbit brain cortex. Naunyn Schmiedebergs Arch Pharmacol 1988;338:53.

Lundberg JM: Pharmacology of cotransmission in the autonomic nervous system: Integrative aspects on amines, neuropeptides, adenosine triphosphate, amino acids and nitric oxide. Pharmacol Rev 1996;48:113.

Lundgren O, Svanvik J, Jivegård L: Enteric nervous system. I. Physiology and pathophysiology of the intestinal tract. Dig Dis Sci 1989;34:264.

MacDonald A et al: Contributions of α_1-adrenoceptors, α_2-adrenoceptors, and P_{2x}-purinoceptors to neurotransmission in several rabbit isolated blood vessels: Role of neuronal uptake and autofeedback. Br J Pharmacol 1992;105:347.

Maggi CA, Meli A: The sensory-efferent function of capsaicin-sensitive sensory neurons. Gen Pharmacol 1988; 19:1.

Makhlouf GM: Neuromuscular function of the small intestine. In: *Physiology of the Gastrointestinal Tract,* 3rd ed. Johnson LR (editor). Raven 1994.

1996 Receptor and ion channel nomenclature supplement. Trends Pharmacol Sci 1996(suppl):1.

Ohia SE, Jumblatt JE: Prejunctional inhibitory effects of prostanoids on sympathetic neurotransmission in the rabbit iris-ciliary body. J Pharmacol Exp Ther 1990;255:11.

Palmer RM, Ferrige AG, Moncada S: Nitric oxide release accounts for the biological activity of endothelium-derived relaxing factor. Nature 1987;327:524.

Pappano AJ, Mubagwa K: Actions of muscarinic agents and adenosine on the heart. In: *The Heart and Cardiovascular System.* Fozzard HA (editor). Raven Press, 1992.

Parsons SM et al: Transport in the cholinergic synaptic vesicle. Fed Proc 1982;41:2765.

Pfeiffer A et al: Muscarinic receptors mediating acid secretion in isolated rat parietal cells are of M_3 type. Gastroenterology 1990;98:218.

Polinsky RJ: Central nervous system control of blood pressure. In: *Mild Hypertension.* Weber MA, Mathias CJ (editors). Steinkopff, 1984.

Rubanyi GM, Vanhoutte PM: Nature of endothelium-derived relaxing factor: Are there two relaxing factors? Circ Res 1987;61(Suppl 2):II–61.

Ruffolo RR Jr et al: Drug receptors and control of the cardiovascular system: Recent advances. Prog Drug Res 1991;36:117.

Schiavo G et al: Tetanus and botulinum-B neurotoxins block neurotransmitter release by proteolytic cleavage of synaptobrevin. Nature 1992;359:832.

Schwartz J-C et al: The dopamine receptor family: Molecular biology and pharmacology. Semin Neurosci 1992; 4:99.

Seeman P, Grigoriades D: Dopamine receptors in brain and periphery. Neurochem Int 1987;10:1.

Starke K, Göthert M, Kilbinger H: Modulation of neurotransmitter release by presynaptic autoreceptors. Physiol Rev 1989;69:864.

Südhof TC: The synaptic vesicle cycle: A cascade of protein-protein interactions. Nature 1995;375:645.

Takiyyudidin MA et al: Sympatho-adrenal secretion in humans: Factors governing catecholamine and storage vesicle peptide co-release. J Auton Pharmacol 1994;14:187.

Taylor P, Radić Z: The cholinesterases: from genes to proteins. Annu Rev Pharmacol Toxicol 1994;34:281.

Taylor SJ, Kilpatrick GJ: Characterization of histamine-H_3 receptors controlling non-adrenergic non-cholinergic contractions of the guinea-pig isolated ileum. Br J Pharmacol 1992;105:667.

Tetrodotoxin poisoning associated with eating puffer fish transported from Japan—California, 1996. MMWR Morbid Mortal Wkly Rep 1996;45:389.

Thiel G: Recent breakthroughs in neurotransmitter release: Paradigm for regulated exocytosis. News Physiol Sci 1995;10:42.

Usdin TB et al: Molecular biology of the vesicular ACh transporter. Trends Neurosci 1995;18:218.

Valtorta F et al: Neurotransmitter release and synaptic vesicle recycling. Neuroscience 1990;35:477.

Wagner G, Sjöstrand NO: Autonomic pharmacology and sexual function. In: *Handbook of Sexology.* Vol 6: *The Pharmacology and Endocrinology of Sexual Function.* Sitsen JMA (editor). Elsevier, 1988.

Wharton J, Gulbenkian S: Peptides in the mammalian cardiovascular system. Experientia 1989;56(Suppl):292.

Wilson RF et al: Regional differences in sympathetic reinnervation after human orthotopic cardiac transplantation. Circulation 1993;88:165.

Wood JD: Physiology of the enteric nervous system. In: *Physiology of the Gastrointestinal Tract,* 3rd ed. Johnson LR (editor). Raven Press, 1994.

7

Cholinoceptor-Activating & Cholinesterase-Inhibiting Drugs

Achilles J. Pappano, PhD

The acetylcholine receptor stimulants and cholinesterase inhibitors together comprise a large group of drugs that mimic acetylcholine (cholinomimetic agents) (Figure 7–1). Cholinoceptor stimulants are classified pharmacologically by their spectrum of action depending upon the receptor type—muscarinic or nicotinic—that is activated. They are also classified by their mechanism of action, because some cholinomimetic drugs bind directly to (and activate) cholinoceptors while others act indirectly by inhibiting the hydrolysis of endogenous acetylcholine.

SPECTRUM OF ACTION OF CHOLINOMIMETIC DRUGS

In some of the first studies of the parasympathetic nervous system, Sir Henry Dale found that the alkaloid **muscarine** mimicked the effects of parasympathetic nerve discharge, ie, the effects were **parasympathomimetic.** Direct application of muscarine to ganglia and to autonomic effector tissues (smooth muscle, heart, exocrine glands) showed that the parasympathomimetic action of the alkaloid was mediated by receptors at the effector cells, not those in the ganglia. Therefore, by convention, the effects of acetylcholine itself and of other cholinomimetic drugs at autonomic neuroeffector junctions are referred to as parasympathomimetic effects, mediated by muscarinic receptors.

In contrast, the alkaloid **nicotine** was found to stimulate autonomic ganglia and skeletal muscle neuromuscular junctions but to have little effect on autonomic effector cells when applied in low concentrations. The ganglion and skeletal muscle receptors were therefore labeled nicotinic. When acetylcholine was later identified as the physiologic transmitter at both muscarinic and nicotinic receptors, it was recognized that both receptors are subtypes of cholinoceptors.

Cholinoceptors are members of either G protein-linked (muscarinic) or ion channel (nicotinic) families on the basis of their transmembrane signaling mechanisms. Muscarinic receptors contain seven transmembrane domains whose third cytoplasmic loop is coupled to G proteins that function as intramembrane transducers (Figure 2–14). In general, these receptors regulate the production of intracellular second messengers. Agonist selectivity is determined by the subtypes of muscarinic receptors and G proteins that are present in a given cell (Table 7–1). Muscarinic receptors are located on plasma membranes of cells of organs innervated by parasympathetic nerves as well as on some tissues that are not innervated by these nerves, eg, endothelial cells (Table 7–1), and on those tissues innervated by cholinergic postganglionic sympathetic nerves.

Nicotinic receptors are part of a transmembrane polypeptide whose subunits form cation-selective ion channels (Figure 2–12). These receptors are located on plasma membranes of parasympathetic and sympathetic postganglionic cells in autonomic ganglia and also on membranes of muscles innervated by somatic motor fibers (Figure 6–1).

Unselective cholinoceptor stimulants in sufficient dosage can produce very diffuse and marked alterations in organ system function because acetylcholine has multiple sites of action where it initiates both excitatory and inhibitory effects. Fortunately, drugs are available that have a degree of selectivity, so that desired effects can often be achieved while avoiding or minimizing adverse effects. This selectivity of action is based on several factors. Some drugs stimulate muscarinic receptors selectively, whereas others activate nicotinic receptors selectively. Some agents stimulate nicotinic receptors in ganglia preferentially and have less effect on nicotinic receptors at neuromuscular junctions. Organ selectivity can also be achieved by utilizing appropriate routes of administration ("pharmacokinetic selectivity"). For example, muscarinic stimulants can be administered topically to the

Figure 7–1. The major groups of cholinoceptor-activating drugs, receptors, and target tissues.

external surface of the eye to modify ocular function while minimizing systemic effects.

MODE OF ACTION OF CHOLINOMIMETIC DRUGS

Cholinomimetic agents can be either direct-or indirect-acting (Figure 7–1). The direct-acting agents directly bind to and activate muscarinic or nicotinic receptors. The indirect-acting agents produce their primary effects by inhibiting the action of acetylcholinesterase, which hydrolyzes acetylcholine to choline and acetic acid (Figure 6–3). By inhibiting acetylcholinesterase, the indirect-acting drugs increase the concentration of endogenous acetylcholine in the synaptic clefts and neuroeffector junctions, and the excess acetylcholine in turn stimulates cholinoceptors to evoke increased responses. These drugs are, in effect, *amplifiers* of endogenous acetylcholine and act primarily where acetylcholine is physiologically released.

Table 7–1. Subtypes and characteristics of cholinoceptors.

Receptor Type	Other Names	Location	Structural Features	Postreceptor Mechanism
M_1	M_{1a}	Nerves	Seven-transmembrane segments, G protein-linked	IP_3, DAG cascade
M_2	M_{2a}, cardiac M_2	Heart, nerves, smooth muscle	Seven-transmembrane segments, G protein-linked	Inhibition of cAMP production, activation of K^+ channels
M_3	M_{2b}, glandular M_2	Glands, smooth muscle, endothelium	Seven-transmembrane segments, G protein-linked	IP_3, DAG cascade
m_4[1]		?CNS	Seven-transmembrane segments, G protein-linked	Inhibition of cAMP production
m_5[1]		?CNS	Seven-transmembrane segments, G protein-linked	IP_3, DAG cascade
N_M	Muscle type, end plate receptor	Skeletal muscle neuromuscular junction	Pentamer $(\alpha_2\beta\delta\gamma)$[2]	Na^+, K^+ depolarizing ion channel
N_N	Neuronal type, ganglion receptor	Postganglionic cell body, dendrites	α and β subunits only as $\alpha_2\beta_2$ or $\alpha_3\beta_3$	Na^+, K^+ depolarizing ion channel

[1]Genes have been cloned, but functional receptors have not been incontrovertibly identified.
[2]Structure in *Torpedo* electric organ and fetal muscle. In adult muscle, the γ subunit is replaced by an ε subunit. Several different α and β subunits have been identified in different mammalian tissues (Lindstrom et al, 1990).

Figure 7–2. Molecular structures of four choline esters and carbamic acid. Acetylcholine and methacholine are acetic acid esters of choline and β-methylcholine, respectively. Carbachol and bethanechol are carbamic acid esters of the same alcohols.

Some cholinesterase inhibitors, even in low concentration, also inhibit butyrylcholinesterase (pseudocholinesterase), and most inhibit this enzyme when they are present in high concentrations. However, since butyrylcholinesterase is not important in the physiologic termination of action of synaptic acetylcholine, inhibition of its action plays little role in the action of indirect-acting cholinomimetic drugs. Some cholinesterase inhibitors also have a modest direct action as well; this is especially true of some quaternary carbamates, eg, neostigmine, which activate neuromuscular nicotinic cholinoceptors directly in addition to blocking cholinesterase.

I. BASIC PHARMACOLOGY OF THE DIRECT-ACTING-CHOLINOCEPTOR STIMULANTS

The direct-acting cholinomimetic drugs can be divided on the basis of chemical structure into esters of choline (including acetylcholine) and alkaloids (such as muscarine and nicotine). A few of these drugs are highly selective for the muscarinic or for the nicotinic receptor. Many have effects on both receptors; acetylcholine is typical.

Chemistry & Pharmacokinetics

A. Structure: Four important esters of choline that have been studied extensively are shown in Figure 7–2. They are permanently charged and relatively insoluble in lipids because they contain the quaternary ammonium group. Many naturally occurring and synthetic cholinomimetic drugs that are not choline esters have been identified; a few of these are shown in Figure 7–3. The muscarinic receptor is strongly stereoselective: *(S)*-bethanechol is almost 1000 times more potent than *(R)*-bethanechol.

B. Absorption, Distribution, and Metabolism: The choline esters are poorly absorbed and poorly distributed into the central nervous system because they are hydrophilic. Although they are all hydrolyzed in the gastrointestinal tract (and less active by the oral route), they differ markedly in their susceptibility to hydrolysis by cholinesterase in the body. Acetylcholine is very rapidly hydrolyzed, as described in Chapter 6; large amounts must be infused intravenously to achieve levels high enough to produce detectable effects. A large intravenous bolus injection has a brief effect, typically 5–20 seconds, whereas intramuscular and subcutaneous injections produce only local effects. Methacholine is at least three times more resistant to hydrolysis and produces systemic effects even when given subcutaneously. The carbamic acid esters, carbachol and bethanechol, are extremely resistant to hydrolysis by cholinesterase and have correspondingly longer durations of action. Presence of the β-methyl group (methacholine, bethanechol) reduces the potency of these drugs at the nicotinic receptor (Table 7–2).

The tertiary cholinomimetic alkaloids (pilocarpine, nicotine, lobeline; Figure 7–3) are well absorbed from most sites of administration. Nicotine, a liquid, is sufficiently lipid-soluble to be absorbed across the skin. Muscarine, a quaternary amine, is less completely absorbed from the gastrointestinal tract than the tertiary amines but is nevertheless toxic when ingested, eg, in certain mushrooms. Excretion of these amines is chiefly by the kidneys. Clearance of the tertiary amines can be accelerated by acidification of the urine. Oxotremorine is an extremely potent synthetic mus-

Figure 7–3. Structures of some cholinomimetic alkaloids and synthetic analogs.

carinic agonist that has been used as a research tool. It is well distributed into the central nervous system. Lobeline is a plant derivative with lower potency than nicotine but with a similar spectrum of action. Dimethylphenylpiperazinium (DMPP) is a potent synthetic nicotinic stimulant with little access to the central nervous system. It is a research tool used for selective stimulation of ganglionic nicotinic receptors.

Pharmacodynamics

A. Mechanism of Action: Activation of the parasympathetic nervous system modifies organ function by two major mechanisms. First, acetylcholine released from parasympathetic nerves can activate muscarinic receptors on effector organs to alter organ function directly. Second, acetylcholine released from parasympathetic nerves can interact with muscarinic receptors on nerve terminals to inhibit the release of their neurotransmitter. By this mechanism, acetylcholine release—and, possibly, circulating muscarinic agonists—indirectly alter organ function by modulating the effects of the parasympathetic and sympathetic nervous systems and perhaps noncholinergic, nonadrenergic systems.

The subcellular mechanism by which muscarinic stimulants alter cellular function continues to be investigated. As indicated in Chapter 6, multiple muscarinic receptor types have been cloned and several have been characterized by binding studies. Several cellular events occur when muscarinic receptors are activated, one or more of which might serve as "second messengers" for muscarinic activation. All muscarinic receptors appear to be of the G-protein coupled type (Chapter 2) with seven segments (Table 7–1) arranged in serpentine fashion across the membrane. An important result of muscarinic agonist binding is activation of the IP_3, DAG cascade. Some evidence implicates diacylglycerol in the opening of smooth muscle calcium channels; IP_3 evokes release of calcium from endoplasmic and sarcoplasmic reticulum. Muscarinic agonists also increase cellular concentrations of cGMP. The activation of muscarinic re-

Table 7–2. Properties of choline esters.

Choline Ester	Susceptibility to Cholinesterase	Muscarinic Action	Nicotinic Action
Acetylcholine chloride	++++	+++	+++
Methacholine chloride	+	++++	None
Carbachol chloride	Negligible	++	+++
Bethanechol chloride	Negligible	++	None

ceptors also increases potassium flux across cell membranes. This effect is mediated by the binding of an activated G protein directly to the channel. Finally, it has been shown that activation of muscarinic receptors in some tissues (eg, heart) results in inhibition of adenylyl cyclase activity. Moreover, muscarinic agonists can attenuate the activation of adenylyl cyclase and modulate the increase in cAMP levels induced by hormones such as catecholamines. These muscarinic effects on cAMP generation are paralleled by attenuation of the physiologic response of the organ to stimulatory hormones.

The mechanism of nicotinic receptor activation has been studied in great detail, taking advantage of three factors: The receptor is present in extremely high concentration in the membranes of the electric organs of electric fish; α-bungarotoxin, a component of certain snake venoms, is tightly bound to the receptors and readily labeled as a marker for isolation procedures; and activation of the receptor results in easily measured electrical and ionic changes in the cells involved. The nicotinic receptor in muscle tissues appears to be a pentamer of four types of glycoprotein subunits (one monomer occurs twice) with a total molecular weight of about 250,000 (see Figure 2–12). The nicotinic receptor in neurons consists of alpha and beta subunits only (Table 7–1). Each subunit appears to have four membrane-crossing segments. Each alpha subunit has a receptor site that, when occupied by a nicotinic agonist, causes a conformational change in the protein (channel opening) that allows sodium and potassium ions to diffuse rapidly down their concentration gradients. While binding of an agonist molecule by one of the two alpha subunit receptor sites only modestly increases the probability of channel opening, simultaneous binding of agonist by both of the receptor sites greatly enhances opening probability. Thus, the primary effect of nicotinic receptor activation is depolarization of the nerve cell or neuromuscular endplate bearing the receptor.

If agonist occupancy of the nicotinic receptor is prolonged, the effector response is abolished; ie, the postganglionic neuron stops firing (ganglionic effect), and the skeletal muscle cell relaxes (neuromuscular endplate effect). Furthermore, the continued presence of the nicotinic agonist prevents electrical recovery of the postjunctional membrane. In this way, a state of "depolarizing blockade" is induced that is refractory to reversal by other agonists. As noted below, this effect can be exploited for producing muscle paralysis.

B. Organ System Effects: Most of the direct organ system effects of muscarinic cholinoceptor stimulants are readily predicted from a knowledge of the effects of parasympathetic nerve stimulation (Table 6–3) and the distribution of muscarinic receptors. Effects of a typical agent such as acetylcholine are listed in Table 7–3. The effects of nicotinic agonists are similarly predictable from a knowledge of the physiology of the autonomic ganglia and skeletal muscle motor endplate.

Table 7–3. Effects of direct-acting cholinoceptor stimulants. Only the direct effects are indicated; homeostatic responses to these direct actions may be important (see text).

Organ	Response
Eye	
Sphincter muscle of iris	Contraction (miosis)
Ciliary muscle	Contraction for near vision
Heart	
Sinoatrial node	Decrease in rate (negative chronotropy)
Atria	Decrease in contractile strength (negative inotropy). Decrease in refractory period.
Atrioventricular node	Decrease in conduction velocity (negative dromotropy). Increase in refractory period.
Ventricles	Small decrease in contractile strength
Blood vessels	
Arteries	Dilation (via EDRF). Constriction (high-dose direct effect).
Veins	Dilation (via EDRF). Constriction (high-dose direct effect).
Lung	
Bronchial muscle	Contraction (bronchoconstrictor)
Bronchial glands	Stimulation
Gastrointestinal tract	
Motility	Increase
Sphincters	Relaxation
Secretion	Stimulation
Urinary bladder	
Detrusor	Contraction
Trigone and sphincter	Relaxation
Glands	
Sweat, salivary, lacrimal, nasopharyngeal	Secretion

1. Eye–Muscarinic agonists instilled into the conjunctival sac cause contraction of the smooth muscle of the iris sphincter (resulting in miosis) and of the ciliary muscle (resulting in accommodation). As a result, the iris is pulled away from the angle of the anterior chamber, and the trabecular meshwork at the base of the ciliary muscle is opened up. Both effects facilitate the outflow of aqueous humor into the canal of Schlemm, which drains the anterior chamber.

2. Cardiovascular system–The primary cardiovascular effects of muscarinic agonists are reduction in peripheral vascular resistance and changes in heart rate. The direct effects listed in Table 7–3 are modified by important homeostatic reflexes, as described in Chapter 6 and depicted in Figure 6–7. Intravenous infusions of minimal effective doses of acetylcholine in humans (eg, 20–50 µg/min) cause vasodilation, resulting in a reduction in blood pressure, often accompanied by a reflex increase in heart rate. Larger doses of acetylcholine produce bradycardia and decrease conduction velocity through the atrioventricular node in addition to the hypotensive effect.

The direct cardiac actions of muscarinic stimulants include the following: (1) an increase in a potassium current ($I_{K(ACh)}$) in atrial muscle cells and in the cells of the sinoatrial and atrioventricular nodes as well; (2) a decrease in the slow inward calcium current (I_{Ca}) in heart cells; and (3) a reduction in the hyperpolarization-activated current (I_f) that underlies diastolic depolarization. All of these actions contribute to the observed slowing of pacemaker rate. Effects (1) and (2) cause hyperpolarization and decreased contractility of atrial cells. As noted above, the direct slowing of sinoatrial rate and atrioventricular conduction that is produced by muscarinic agonists is often opposed by reflex sympathetic discharge, elicited by the decrease in blood pressure. The resultant interaction between sympathetic and parasympathetic effects is complex because of the previously described muscarinic modulation of sympathetic influences that occurs by inhibition of norepinephrine release and by postjunctional cellular effects. Muscarinic receptors are also present on postganglionic parasympathetic nerves and allow neurally released acetylcholine to inhibit its own secretion. The neuronal muscarinic receptors need not be the same subtype as found on effector cells. Therefore, the net effect on heart rate depends on local concentrations of the agonist in the heart and in the vessels and on the level of reflex responsiveness.

Parasympathetic innervation of the ventricles is much less extensive than that of the atria. Also, activation of muscarinic receptors in ventricles results in much less physiologic effect than that seen following activation of these receptors in atria. However, during sympathetic stimulation, the effects of muscarinic agonists on ventricular function are clearly evident because of muscarinic modulation of sympathetic ef-

fects ("accentuated antagonism"; Levy et al, 1994) as described above.

In the intact organism, muscarinic agonists produce marked vasodilation. However, in earlier studies, isolated vascular smooth muscle preparations often showed a contractile response to these agents. It is now known (Furchgott et al, 1980) that acetylcholine-induced vasodilation requires the presence of intact endothelium (Figure 7–4). Muscarinic agonists release a relaxing substance (endothelium-derived relaxing factor, or EDRF) from the endothelial cells that causes smooth muscle relaxation. Isolated vessels prepared with the endothelium preserved consistently reproduce the vasodilation seen in the intact organism. EDRF appears to be largely nitric oxide (NO) (reviewed in Moncada et al, 1991). This substance activates guanylyl cyclase and increases cGMP in smooth muscle, resulting in relaxation (see Figure 12–2). Nitric oxide may also participate in muscarinic regulation of I_{Ca} in pacemaker and contracting cardiac tissues.

The cardiovascular effects of all of the choline esters are similar to those of acetylcholine, the main difference being in their potency and duration of action. Because of the resistance of methacholine, carbachol, and bethanechol to acetylcholinesterase, lower doses given intravenously are sufficient to produce effects similar to those of acetylcholine, and the duration of action of these synthetic choline esters is longer. The cardiovascular effects of most of the cholinomimetic natural alkaloids and synthetic analogs are also generally similar to those of acetylcholine.

Pilocarpine is an interesting exception to the above statement. If given intravenously (an experimental exercise), it may produce hypertension after a brief initial hypotensive response. The longer-lasting hypertensive effect can be traced to sympathetic ganglionic discharge caused by activation of M_1 receptors in the postganglionic cell membrane, which close K^+ channels and elicit slow excitatory (depolarizing) postsynaptic potentials. This effect, like the hypotensive effect, can be blocked by atropine, an antimuscarinic drug.

Figure 7–4. Activation of endothelial cell muscarinic receptors by acetylcholine releases EDRF (NO), which causes relaxation of vascular smooth muscle precontracted with norepinephrine. Removal of the endothelium by rubbing eliminates the relaxant effect and reveals contraction caused by direct action of acetylcholine on vascular smooth muscle. (Modified and reproduced, with permission, from Furchgott RF, Zawadzki JV: The obligatory role of endothelial cells in the relaxation of arterial smooth muscle by acetylcholine. Nature 1980;288:373.)

3. Respiratory system–The smooth muscle of the bronchial tree is contracted by muscarinic stimulants. In addition, the glands of the tracheobronchial mucosa are stimulated to secrete. This combination of effects can occasionally cause symptoms, especially in individuals with asthma.

4. Gastrointestinal tract–Administration of muscarinic agonists, like stimulation of the parasympathetic nervous system, causes an increase in secretory and motor activity of the gut. The salivary and gastric glands are strongly stimulated; the pancreas and small intestinal glands less so. Peristaltic activity is increased throughout the gut, and most sphincters are relaxed. Stimulation of contraction in this organ system has been shown to involve depolarization of the smooth muscle cell membrane and increased calcium influx.

5. Genitourinary tract–Muscarinic agonists stimulate the detrusor muscle and relax the trigone and sphincter muscles of the bladder, thus promoting voiding. The human uterus is not notably sensitive to muscarinic agonists.

6. Miscellaneous secretory glands–Muscarinic agonists stimulate the secretory activity of sweat, lacrimal, and nasopharyngeal glands.

7. Central nervous system–The central nervous system contains both muscarinic and nicotinic receptors, the brain being relatively richer in muscarinic sites and the spinal cord containing a preponderance of nicotinic sites. The physiologic role of these receptors is discussed in Chapter 21. In spite of the smaller ratio of nicotinic to muscarinic receptors in the brain, nicotine and lobeline (Figure 7–3) have important effects on the brain stem and cortex. The mild alerting action of nicotine absorbed from inhaled tobacco smoke is the best-known of these effects. In larger concentrations, nicotine induces tremor, emesis, and stimulation of the respiratory center. At still higher levels, nicotine causes convulsions, which may terminate in fatal coma. The lethal effects on the central nervous system and the fact that nicotine is readily absorbed form the basis for the use of nicotine as an insecticide. Dimethylphenylpiperazinium (DMPP), a synthetic nicotinic stimulant (Figure 7–3), is relatively free of these central effects because it does not cross the blood-brain barrier.

8. Peripheral nervous system–The autonomic ganglia are important sites of nicotinic synaptic action. All of the nicotinic agents shown in Figure 7–3 are capable of causing marked activation of the nicotinic receptors, resulting in firing of action potentials in the postganglionic neurons. Nicotine itself has a somewhat greater affinity for neuronal than for skeletal muscle nicotinic receptors. The action is the same on both parasympathetic and sympathetic ganglia. The initial response therefore often resembles simultaneous discharge of both the parasympathetic and the sympathetic nervous systems. In the case of the cardiovascular system, the effects of nicotine are chiefly

sympathomimetic. Dramatic hypertension is produced by parenteral injection of nicotine; sympathetic tachycardia may alternate with a vagally mediated bradycardia. In the gastrointestinal and urinary tracts, the effects are largely parasympathomimetic: nausea, vomiting, diarrhea, and voiding of urine are commonly observed. Prolonged exposure may result in depolarizing blockade.

A second class of nicotinic sites consists of chemoreceptors on sensory nerve endings—especially certain chemosensitive nerve endings in the coronary arteries and the carotid and aortic bodies. Activation of these endings elicits complex medullary responses, including respiratory alterations and vagal discharge.

9. Neuromuscular junction–The nicotinic receptors on the neuromuscular endplate apparatus are similar but not identical to the receptors in the autonomic ganglia (Table 7–1). Both types respond to acetylcholine and nicotine. (However, as discussed in Chapter 8, the receptors differ in their structural requirements for nicotinic blocking drugs.) When a nicotinic agonist is applied directly (by iontophoresis or by intra-arterial injection), an immediate depolarization of the endplate results, caused by an increase in permeability to sodium and potassium ions. Depending on the synchronization of depolarization of endplates throughout the muscle, the contractile response will vary from disorganized fasciculations of independent motor units to a strong contraction of the entire muscle. Depolarizing nicotinic agents that are not rapidly hydrolyzed (like nicotine itself) cause rapid development of depolarization blockade; transmission blockade persists even when the membrane has repolarized (discussed further in Chapters 8 and 27). In the case of skeletal muscle, this block is manifested as flaccid paralysis.

II. BASIC PHARMACOLOGY OF THE INDIRECT-ACTING CHOLINOMIMETICS

The actions of acetylcholine released from autonomic and somatic motor nerves are terminated by enzymatic destruction of the molecule. Hydrolysis is accomplished by the action of acetylcholinesterase, a protein with a molecular weight of about 320,000, which is present in high concentrations in cholinergic synapses. The indirect-acting cholinomimetics have their primary effect at the active site of this enzyme, though some also have direct actions at nicotinic receptors. By far the most important use (in terms of amount manufactured) of these chemicals is as insecticides; a few have therapeutic applications. The chief differences between members of the group are chemical and pharmacokinetic—their pharmacodynamic properties are almost identical.

Chemistry & Pharmacokinetics

A. Structure: The commonly used cholinesterase inhibitors fall into three chemical groups: (1) simple alcohols bearing a quaternary ammonium group, eg, edrophonium; (2) carbamic acid esters of alcohols bearing quaternary or tertiary ammonium groups (carbamates, eg, neostigmine); and (3) organic derivatives of phosphoric acid (organophosphates, eg, isoflurophate). Examples of the first two groups are shown in Figure 7–5. Edrophonium, neostigmine, and ambenonium are synthetic quaternary ammonium agents used in medicine. Physostigmine (eserine) is a naturally occurring tertiary amine of greater lipid solubility that is also used in therapeutics. Carbaryl (carbaril) is typical of a large group of carbamate insecticides designed for very high lipid solubility, so that absorption into the insect and distribution to its central nervous system are very rapid.

A few of the estimated 50,000 organophosphates are shown in Figure 7–6. Many of the organophosphates (echothiophate is an exception) are highly lipid-soluble liquids. Isoflurophate (diisopropylfluorophosphate, DFP) was one of the first organophosphates synthesized and is one of the best-studied. It is still available for clinical use but has been largely superseded by drugs like echothiophate. Echothiophate, a thiocholine derivative, is of clinical interest because it retains the very long duration of action of other organophosphates but is more stable in aqueous solution. Soman is an extremely potent "nerve gas." Parathion and malathion are thiophosphate insecticides that are inactive as such; they are converted to the phosphate derivatives in animals and plants. They are somewhat more stable than compounds like isoflurophate and soman, making them more suitable for use as insecticides.

B. Absorption, Distribution, and Metabolism: Absorption of the quaternary carbamates from the conjunctiva, skin, and lungs is predictably poor, since their permanent charge renders them relatively insoluble in lipids. Similarly, much larger doses are required for oral administration than for parenteral injection. Distribution into the central nervous system is negligible. Physostigmine, in contrast, is well absorbed from all sites and can be used topically in the eye (Table 7–4). It is distributed into the central nervous system and is more toxic than the more polar quaternary carbamates. However, even the nonpolar carbamates used as insecticides are poorly absorbed across the skin—the ratio of dermal:oral lethal doses for this group is much higher than the ratios for the organophosphate pesticides. The carbamates are rela-

Figure 7–5. Cholinesterase inhibitors. Neostigmine exemplifies the typical compound that is an ester of carbamic acid ([1]) and a phenol bearing a quaternary ammonium group ([2]). Physostigmine, a naturally occurring carbamate, is a tertiary amine. Acetylcholine is shown in the same orientation (acid left, alcohol right) for reference. Edrophonium is not an ester but binds to the active site of the enzyme.

Figure 7–6. Structures of some organophosphate cholinesterase inhibitors. The dashed lines indicate the bond that is hydrolyzed in binding to the enzyme. The shaded ester bonds in malathion represent the points of detoxification of the molecule in mammals and birds.

tively stable in aqueous solution but can be metabolized by nonspecific esterases in the body, as well as by cholinesterase. However, the duration of their effect is determined chiefly by the stability of the inhibitor-enzyme complex (see Mechanism of Action, below), not by metabolism or excretion.

The organophosphate cholinesterase inhibitors (except for echothiophate) are well absorbed from the skin, lung, gut, and conjunctiva—thereby making them dangerous to humans and highly effective as insecticides. They are relatively less stable than the carbamates when dissolved in water and thus have a limited half-life in the environment (as compared to the other major class of insecticides, the halogenated hydrocarbons, eg, DDT). Echothiophate is highly polar and more stable than most other organophosphates. It can be made up in aqueous solution for ophthalmic use and retains its activity for weeks.

The thiophosphate insecticides (parathion, malathion, and related compounds) are quite lipid-soluble and are rapidly absorbed by all routes. They must be activated in the body by conversion to the oxygen analogs (Figure 7–6), a process that occurs rapidly in both insects and vertebrates. Malathion and certain other organophosphate insecticides are also rapidly metabolized by other pathways to inactive products in birds and mammals, but not in insects; these agents are therefore considered safe enough for sale to the general public. Unfortunately, fish are not able to

Table 7–4. Therapeutic uses and durations of action of cholinesterase inhibitors.

	Uses	Approximate Duration of Action
Alcohols		
Edrophonium	Myasthenia gravis, ileus, arrhythmias	5–15 minutes
Carbamates and related agents		
Neostigmine	Myasthenia gravis, ileus	0.5–2 hours
Pyridostigmine	Myasthenia gravis	3–6 hours
Physostigmine	Glaucoma	0.5–2 hours
Ambenonium	Myasthenia gravis	4–8 hours
Demecarium	Glaucoma	4–6 hours
Organophosphates		
Echothiophate	Glaucoma	100 hours

detoxify malathion, and significant numbers of fish have died from the heavy use of this agent on and near waterways. Parathion is not detoxified effectively in vertebrates; thus, it is considerably more dangerous than malathion to humans and livestock and is not available for general public use.

All of the organophosphates except echothiophate are fully distributed to all parts of the body, including the central nervous system. Poisoning with these agents therefore includes an important component of central nervous system toxicity.

Pharmacodynamics

A. Mechanism of Action: Acetylcholinesterase is the primary target of these drugs, but butyrylcholinesterase is also inhibited. Acetylcholinesterase is an extremely active enzyme. In the initial step, acetylcholine binds to the enzyme's active site and is hydrolyzed, yielding free choline and the *acetylated* enzyme. In the second step, the covalent acetylenzyme bond is split, with the addition of water (hydration). The entire process takes place in approximately 150 microseconds.

All of the cholinesterase inhibitors exert their effects by inhibiting acetylcholinesterase and thereby increasing the concentration of endogenous acetylcholine in the vicinity of cholinoceptors. However, the molecular details of their interaction with the enzyme vary according to the three chemical subgroups mentioned above.

The first group, of which edrophonium is the major example, consists of quaternary alcohols. These agents bind reversibly to the active site, thus preventing access of acetylcholine. The enzyme-inhibitor complex does not involve a covalent bond and is correspondingly short-lived (on the order of 2–10 minutes). The second group consists of carbamate esters, eg, neostigmine and physostigmine. These agents undergo a two-step hydrolysis sequence analogous to that described for acetylcholine. However, the covalent bond of the *carbamoylated* enzyme is considerably more resistant to the second (hydration) process, and this step is correspondingly prolonged (on the order of 30 minutes to 6 hours). The third group consists of the organophosphates. These agents also undergo initial binding and hydrolysis by the enzyme, resulting in a *phosphorylated* active site. The covalent phosphorus-enzyme bond is extremely stable and hydrolyzes in water at a very slow rate (hundreds of hours). After the initial binding-hydrolysis step, the phosphorylated enzyme complex may undergo a process called **aging.** This process apparently involves the breaking of one of the oxygen-phosphorus bonds of the inhibitor and results in further strengthening of the phosphorus-enzyme bond. The rate of aging varies with the particular organophosphate compound. If given before aging has occurred, strong nucleophiles like pralidoxime are able to split the phosphorus-enzyme bond and can be used as "cholinesterase regenerator" drugs for organophosphate insecticide poisoning (Chapter 8). Once aging has occurred, the enzyme-inhibitor complex is even more stable and is more difficult to split, even with oxime regenerator compounds.

Because of the marked differences in duration of action, the organophosphate inhibitors are sometimes referred to as "irreversible" cholinesterase inhibitors, and edrophonium and the carbamates are considered "reversible" inhibitors. In fact, the molecular mechanisms of action of the three groups do not support this simplistic description, but the terms are frequently used.

B. Organ System Effects: The most prominent pharmacologic effects of cholinesterase inhibitors are on the cardiovascular and gastrointestinal systems, the eye, and the skeletal muscle neuromuscular junction. Because the primary action is to amplify the action of endogenous acetylcholine, the effects are similar (but not always identical) to the effects of the direct-acting cholinomimetic agonists.

1. Central nervous system–In low concentrations, the lipid-soluble cholinesterase inhibitors cause diffuse activation of the EEG and a subjective alerting response. In higher concentrations, they cause generalized convulsions, which may be followed by coma and respiratory arrest.

2. Eye, respiratory tract, gastrointestinal tract, urinary tract–The effects of the cholinesterase inhibitors on these organ systems, all of which are well innervated by the parasympathetic nervous system, are qualitatively quite similar to the effects of the direct-acting cholinomimetics.

3. Cardiovascular system–The cholinesterase inhibitors can increase activation in both sympathetic and parasympathetic ganglia supplying the heart and at the acetylcholine receptors on neuroeffector cells (cardiac and vascular smooth muscles) that receive cholinergic innervation.

In the heart, the effects on the parasympathetic limb predominate. Thus, administration of cholinesterase inhibitors such as edrophonium, physostigmine, or neostigmine leads to effects on the heart that mimic the effects of vagal nerve activation. Negative chronotropic, dromotropic, and inotropic effects are produced, and cardiac output falls. The fall in cardiac output is attributable to bradycardia, decreased atrial contractility, and some reduction in ventricular contractility. The latter effect occurs as a result of prejunctional modulation of sympathetic activity (inhibition of norepinephrine release) as well as inhibition of postjunctional cellular sympathetic effects.

The effects of cholinesterase inhibitors on vascular smooth muscle and on blood pressure are less marked than the effects of direct-acting muscarinic agonists. This is because indirect-acting drugs can modify the tone of only those vessels that are innervated by cholinergic nerves and because the net effects on vascular tone may reflect activation of both the parasympathetic and sympathetic nervous systems. Since few vascular beds receive cholinergic innervation, the cholinomimetic effect at the smooth muscle effector tissue is minimal. Activation of sympathetic ganglia would tend to increase vascular resistance.

The *net* cardiovascular effects of moderate doses of cholinesterase inhibitors therefore consist of modest bradycardia, a fall in cardiac output, and no change or a modest fall in blood pressure. Large (toxic) doses of these drugs cause more marked bradycardia and hypotension.

4. Neuromuscular junction–The cholinesterase inhibitors have important therapeutic and toxic effects at the skeletal muscle neuromuscular junction. Low (therapeutic) concentrations moderately prolong and intensify the actions of physiologically released acetylcholine. This results in increased strength of contraction, especially in muscles weakened by curare-like neuromuscular blocking agents or by myasthenia gravis. At higher concentrations, the accumulation of acetylcholine may result in fibrillation of muscle fibers. Antidromic firing of the motor neuron may also occur, resulting in fasciculations that involve an entire motor unit. With marked inhibition of acetylcholinesterase, the initial phase of depolarizing neuromuscular blockade may be followed by a phase of nondepolarizing blockade as seen with succinylcholine (see Table 27–2 and Table 27–6).

Some quaternary carbamate cholinesterase inhibitors, eg, neostigmine, have an additional *direct* nicotinic agonist effect at the neuromuscular junction. This may contribute to the effectiveness of these agents in the therapy of myasthenia.

III. CLINICAL PHARMACOLOGY OF THE CHOLINOMIMETICS

The major therapeutic uses of the cholinomimetics are for diseases of the eye (glaucoma, accommodative esotropia), the gastrointestinal and urinary tracts (postoperative atony, neurogenic bladder), the neuromuscular junction (myasthenia gravis, curare-induced neuromuscular paralysis), and the heart (certain atrial arrhythmias). Cholinesterase inhibitors are occasionally used in the treatment of atropine overdosage. **Tacrine** is a drug with anticholinesterase and other cholinomimetic actions that has been approved for the treatment of mild to moderate Alzheimer's disease. It is discussed in Chapter 61.

Clinical Uses

A. The Eye: Glaucoma is a disease characterized by increased intraocular pressure. There are two types of acquired glaucoma: primary, which can be subdivided into angle-closure and open-angle types; and secondary, eg, caused by trauma, inflammation, or surgical procedures. Muscarinic stimulants and cholinesterase inhibitors can reduce intraocular pressure by causing contraction of the ciliary body so as to facilitate outflow of aqueous humor and perhaps also by diminishing the rate of its secretion (see Figure 6–9). Glaucoma can be treated with either direct agonists (pilocarpine, methacholine, carbachol) or cholinesterase inhibitors (physostigmine, demecarium, echothiophate, isoflurophate). Pilocarpine is by far the most commonly used.

Acute angle-closure glaucoma is a medical emergency that is usually treated initially with drugs but frequently requires surgery for permanent correction. Initial therapy often consists of a combination of a direct muscarinic agonist and a cholinesterase inhibitor (eg, pilocarpine plus physostigmine). Once the intraocular pressure is controlled and the danger of loss of vision is diminished, the patient can be prepared for corrective surgery (iridectomy). Open-angle glaucoma and some cases of secondary glaucoma are chronic diseases that are not amenable to surgical correction (although newer laser techniques may prove useful). Consequently, therapy is based on long-term pharmacologic management that relies greatly on the use of parasympathomimetics as well as epinephrine, the β-adrenoceptor-blocking drugs, and acetazolamide. Of the parasympathomimetics, the ones in current favor include pilocarpine (as drops, or a long-acting plastic film reservoir of drug placed in the conjunctival sac) and carbachol (drops). Longer-acting agents (demecarium, echothiophate) are reserved for cases in which control of the intraocular pressure cannot be achieved with other drugs. Other treatments for glaucoma are described in the box: The Treatment of Glaucoma, Chapter 10.

Accommodative esotropia (strabismus caused by hypermetropic accommodative error) in young children is sometimes diagnosed and treated with cholinomimetic agonists. Dosage is similar to or higher than that used for glaucoma.

B. Gastrointestinal and Urinary Tracts: In clinical disorders that involve depression of smooth muscle activity *without obstruction,* cholinomimetic drugs with direct or indirect muscarinic effects may be helpful. These disorders include postoperative ileus (atony or paralysis of the stomach or bowel following surgical manipulation) and congenital megacolon. Urinary retention may occur postoperatively or postpartum or may be secondary to spinal cord injury or disease (neurogenic bladder). Cholinomimetics are also sometimes used to increase the tone of the lower esophageal sphincter in patients with reflux esophagitis. Of the choline esters, bethanechol is the most widely used for these disorders. For gastrointestinal problems, it is usually administered orally in a dose of 10–25 mg three or four times daily. In patients with urinary retention, bethanechol can be given subcutaneously in a dose of 5 mg and repeated in 30 minutes if necessary. Of the cholinesterase inhibitors, neostigmine is the most widely used for these applications. For paralytic ileus or atony of the urinary bladder, neostigmine can be given subcutaneously in a dose of 0.5–1 mg. If patients are able to take the drug by mouth, neostigmine can be given orally in a dose of 15 mg. In all of these situations, the clinician must be certain that there is no mechanical obstruction to outflow prior to using the cholinomimetic. Otherwise, the drug may exacerbate the problem and may even cause perforation as a result of increased pressure.

C. Neuromuscular Junction: Myasthenia gravis is a disease affecting skeletal muscle neuromuscular junctions. An autoimmune process causes production of antibodies that decrease the number of functional nicotinic receptors on the postjunctional endplates. The characteristic symptoms of weakness and fatigability that remit with rest and worsen with exercise may affect any skeletal muscle but most often involve the small muscles of the head, neck, and extremities. Frequent findings are ptosis, diplopia, difficulty in speaking and swallowing, and extremity weakness. Severe disease may affect all the muscles, including those necessary for respiration. The disease resembles the neuromuscular paralysis produced by *d*-tubocurarine and similar nondepolarizing neuromuscular blocking drugs (Chapter 27). Patients with myasthenia are exquisitely sensitive to the action of curariform drugs and other drugs that interfere with neuromuscular transmission, eg, aminoglycoside antibiotics.

Cholinesterase inhibitors—but not direct-acting acetylcholine receptor agonists—are extremely valuable in the therapy of myasthenia. (Some patients also respond to thymectomy or immunosuppressant therapy with adrenocorticosteroids and cyclosporine.)

Edrophonium is sometimes used as a diagnostic test for myasthenia. A dose of 2 mg is injected intravenously after baseline measurements of muscle strength have been obtained. If no reaction occurs after 45 seconds, an additional 8 mg may be injected. Some clinicians divide the 8 mg dose into two doses of 3 and 5 mg given at 45-second intervals. If the patient has myasthenia gravis, an improvement in muscle strength that lasts about 5 minutes will usually be observed.

Edrophonium is also used to assess the adequacy of treatment with the longer-acting cholinesterase inhibitors in patients with documented myasthenia gravis. If excessive amounts of cholinesterase inhibitor have been used, patients may become paradoxically weak because of nicotinic depolarizing blockade of the motor endplate. These patients may also exhibit symptoms of excessive stimulation of muscarinic receptors (abdominal cramps, diarrhea, increased salivation, excessive bronchial secretions, miosis, bradycardia). Small doses of edrophonium (1–2 mg intravenously) will produce no relief or even worsen weakness if the patient is receiving excessive cholinesterase inhibitor therapy. On the other hand, if the patient improves with edrophonium, an increase in cholinesterase inhibitor dosage may be indicated.

Clinical situations in which severe myasthenia (myasthenic crisis) must be distinguished from excessive drug therapy (cholinergic crisis) usually occur in very ill myasthenic patients and must be managed in a hospital with adequate emergency and support systems (eg, mechanical ventilators) available.

Chronic long-term therapy of myasthenia gravis is usually accomplished with neostigmine, pyridostigmine, or ambenonium. The doses are titrated to optimum levels based on changes in muscle strength. These agents are relatively short-acting and therefore require frequent dosing (every 2–4 hours for neostigmine and every 3–6 hours for pyridostigmine and ambenonium; Table 7–4). Sustained-release preparations are available but should be used only at night and if needed. Longer-acting cholinesterase inhibitors such as the organophosphate agents are not used, because the dose requirement in this disease changes too rapidly to permit smooth control with long-acting drugs.

If muscarinic effects of such therapy are prominent, they can be controlled by the administration of antimuscarinic drugs such as atropine. Frequently, tolerance to the muscarinic effects of the cholinesterase inhibitors develops, so atropine treatment is not required.

Neuromuscular blockade is frequently produced as an adjunct to surgical anesthesia, using nondepolarizing neuromuscular relaxants such as curare, pancuronium, and newer agents. Following the surgical procedure, it is usually desirable to reverse this pharmacologic paralysis promptly. This can be easily accomplished with cholinesterase inhibitors; neostigmine and edrophonium are the drugs of choice. They are given intravenously or intramuscularly for prompt effect.

D. Heart: The short-acting cholinesterase inhibitor edrophonium was often used in the past for treatment of supraventricular tachyarrhythmias, particularly paroxysmal supraventricular tachycardia. In this application, edrophonium has been replaced by newer drugs (adenosine and the calcium channel blockers verapamil and diltiazem).

E. Antimuscarinic Drug Intoxication: Atropine intoxication is potentially lethal in children (Chapter 8) and may cause prolonged severe behavioral disturbances and arrhythmias in adults. The tricyclic antidepressants, when taken in overdosage (often with suicidal intent), also cause severe muscarinic blockade (Chapter 30). Because the muscarinic receptor blockade produced by all these agents is competitive in nature, it can be overcome by increasing the amount of endogenous acetylcholine present at the neuroeffector junctions. Theoretically, a cholinesterase inhibitor could be used to reverse these effects. Physostigmine has been used for this application, because it enters the central nervous system and reverses the central as well as the peripheral signs of muscarinic blockade. However, as explained in the next chapter, physostigmine itself can produce dangerous central nervous system effects, and such therapy is therefore used only in patients with dangerous elevation of body temperature or very rapid supraventricular tachycardia.

Toxicity

The toxic potential of the cholinoceptor stimulants varies markedly depending on their absorption, access to the central nervous system, and metabolism.

A. Direct-Acting Muscarinic Stimulants: Drugs such as pilocarpine and the choline esters cause predictable signs of muscarinic excess when given in overdosage. These effects include nausea, vomiting, diarrhea, salivation, sweating, cutaneous vasodilation, and bronchial constriction. The effects are all blocked competitively by atropine and its congeners.

Certain mushrooms, especially those of the genus *Inocybe,* contain muscarinic alkaloids. Ingestion of these mushrooms causes typical signs of muscarinic excess within 15–30 minutes. Treatment is with atropine, 1–2 mg parenterally. (*Amanita muscaria,* the first source of muscarine, contains very low concentrations of the alkaloid.)

B. Direct-Acting Nicotinic Stimulants: Nicotine itself is the only common cause of this type of poisoning. The acute toxicity of the alkaloid is well-defined but much less important than the chronic effects associated with smoking. In addition to tobacco products, nicotine is also used in a number of insecticides.

1. Acute toxicity–The fatal dose of nicotine is approximately 40 mg, or 1 drop of the pure liquid. This is the amount of nicotine in two regular cigarettes. Fortunately, most of the nicotine in cigarettes is destroyed by burning or escapes via the "sidestream" smoke. Ingestion of nicotine insecticides or of tobacco by infants and children is usually followed by vomiting, limiting the amount of the alkaloid absorbed.

The toxic effects of a large dose of nicotine are simple extensions of the effects described previously. The most dangerous are (1) central stimulant actions, which cause convulsions and may progress to coma and respiratory arrest; (2) skeletal muscle endplate depolarization, which may lead to depolarization blockade and respiratory paralysis; and (3) hypertension and cardiac arrhythmias.

Treatment of acute nicotine poisoning is largely symptom-directed. Muscarinic excess resulting from parasympathetic ganglion stimulation can be controlled with atropine. Central stimulation is usually treated with parenteral anticonvulsants such as diazepam. Neuromuscular blockade is not responsive to pharmacologic treatment and may require mechanical respiration.

Fortunately, nicotine is metabolized and excreted relatively rapidly. Patients who survive the first 4 hours usually recover completely if hypoxia and brain damage have not occurred.

2. Chronic nicotine toxicity–The health costs of tobacco smoking to the smoker and its socioeconomic costs to the general public are still incompletely understood. However, the 1979 *Surgeon General's Report on Health Promotion and Disease Prevention* stated that "cigarette smoking is clearly the largest single preventable cause of illness and premature death in the United States." This statement was underscored by the 1983 and 1985 reports of the US Department of Health and Human Services, which estimated that up to 30% of the over 500,000 coronary heart disease deaths and 30% of the over 400,000 cancer deaths in the USA each year were attributable to smoking. Unfortunately, the fact that the most important of the tobacco-associated diseases are delayed in onset reduces the health incentive to stop smoking.

It is not known to what extent nicotine per se contributes to the well-documented adverse effects of chronic tobacco use. It appears highly probable that nicotine contributes to the increased risk of vascular disease and sudden coronary death associated with smoking. It is also probable that nicotine contributes to the high incidence of ulcer recurrences in smokers with peptic ulcer.

C. Cholinesterase Inhibitors: The acute toxic effects of the cholinesterase inhibitors, like those of the direct-acting agents, are direct extensions of their pharmacologic actions. The major source of such intoxications is pesticide use in agriculture and in the home. Approximately 100 organophosphate and 20 carbamate cholinesterase inhibitors are available in pesticides and veterinary vermifuges used in the USA.

Acute intoxication must be recognized and treated promptly in patients with heavy exposure. The dominant initial signs are those of muscarinic excess: miosis, salivation, sweating, bronchial constriction, vomiting, and diarrhea. Central nervous system involvement usually follows rapidly, accompanied by peripheral nicotinic effects, especially depolarizing neuromuscular blockade. Therapy always includes (1) maintenance of vital signs—respiration in particular may be impaired; (2) decontamination to prevent further absorption—this may require removal of all clothing and washing of the skin in cases of exposure to dusts and sprays; and (3) atropine parenterally in large doses, given as often as required to control signs of muscarinic excess. Therapy often also includes treatment with pralidoxime as described in Chapter 8.

Chronic exposure to certain organophosphate compounds, including some organophosphate cholinesterase inhibitors, causes neuropathy associated with demyelination of axons. **Triorthocresylphosphate,** an additive in lubricating oils, is the prototype agent of this class. The effects are not caused by cholinesterase inhibition.

PREPARATIONS AVAILABLE

Direct-Acting Cholinomimetics
  Acetylcholine (Miochol)
    Ophthalmic: 1:100 (10 mg/mL) intraocular solution
  Bethanechol (generic, Urecholine)
    Oral: 5, 10, 25, 50 mg tablets
    Parenteral: 5 mg/mL for SC injection
  Carbachol
    Ophthalmic (topical, Isopto Carbachol): 0.75, 1.5, 2.25, 3% drops
    Ophthalmic (intraocular, Miostat): 0.01% solution
  Pilocarpine (generic, Isopto Carpine)
    Ophthalmic (topical): 0.25, 0.5, 1, 2, 3, 4, 6, 8, 10% solutions, 4% gel
    Ophthalmic sustained-release inserts (Ocusert Pilo-20, Ocusert Pilo-40): release 20 and 40 μg pilocarpine per hour for 1 week, respectively

Cholinesterase Inhibitors
  Ambenonium (Mytelase)

Oral: 10 mg tablets
  Demecarium (Humorsol)
    Ophthalmic: 0.125, 0.25% drops
  Echothiophate (Phospholine)
    Ophthalmic: powder to reconstitute for 0.03, 0.06, 0.125, 0.25% drops
  Edrophonium (generic, Tensilon)
    Parenteral: 10 mg/mL for IM or IV injection
  Isoflurophate (Floropryl)
    Ophthalmic: 0.025% ointment
  Neostigmine (generic, Prostigmin)
    Oral: 15 mg tablets
    Parenteral: 1:1000 in 10 mL; 1:2000, 1:4000 in 1 mL
  Physostigmine, eserine (generic)
    Ophthalmic: 0.25% ointment
    Parenteral: 1 mg/mL for IM or slow IV injection
  Pyridostigmine (Mestinon)
    Oral: 60 mg tablets; 180 mg sustained-release tablets; 15 mg/mL syrup
    Parenteral: 5 mg/mL for IM or slow IV injection

REFERENCES

Abou-Donia MB, Lapadula DM: Mechanisms of organophosphorus ester-induced delayed neurotoxicity: Type I and type II. Annu Rev Pharmacol 1990;30:405.

Aquilonius S-M, Hartvig P: Clinical pharmacology of cholinesterase inhibitors. Clin Pharmacokinet 1986;11:236.

Barnes PJ, Minette P, Maclagan J: Muscarinic receptor subtypes in airways. Trends Pharmacol Sci 1988;9:412.

Berridge MJ, Irvine RF: Inositol phosphates and cell signalling. Nature 1989;341:197.

Bognar IT, Wesner MT, Fuder H: Muscarine receptor types mediating autoinhibition of acetylcholine release and sphincter contraction in the guinea-pig iris. Naunyn Schmiedebergs Arch Pharmacol 1990;341:22.

Bonner TI et al: Identification of a family of muscarinic acetylcholine receptor genes. Science 1987;237:527.

Brown JH (editor): *The Muscarinic Receptors.* Humana Press, 1989.

Buckley NJ et al: Antagonist binding properties of five cloned muscarinic receptors expressed in CHO-K1 cells. Mol Pharmacol 1989;35:469.

Cady B: Cost of smoking. (Letter.) N Engl J Med 1983;308:1105.

Cerbai E, Klockner U, Isenberg G: The α subunit of the GTP binding protein activates muscarinic potassium channels of the atrium. Science 1988;240:1782.

Deighton NM et al: Muscarinic cholinoceptors in the human heart: Demonstration, subclassification, and distribution. Naunyn Schmiedebergs Arch Pharmacol 1990;341:14.

DiFrancesco D, Tromba C: Muscarinic control of the hyperpolarization-activated current (i_f) in rabbit sino-atrial node myocytes. J Physiol 1988;405:493.

Drachman DH: Myasthenia gravis. N Engl J Med 1994;330:1797.

Eglen RM, Whiting RL: Heterogeneity of vascular muscarinic receptors. J Auton Pharmacol 1990;19:233.

Fielding JE: Smoking: Health effects and control. (Two parts.) N Engl J Med 1985;313:491, 555.

Freedman SB, Beer MS, Harley EA: Muscarinic M_1, M_2 receptor binding: Relationship with functional efficacy. Eur J Pharmacol 1988;156:133.

Furchgott RF, Zawadzki JV: The obligatory role of endothelial cells in the relaxation of arterial smooth muscle by acetylcholine. Nature 1980;288:373.

Goyal RK: Muscarinic receptor subtypes: Physiology and clinical implications. N Engl J Med 1989;321:1022.

Grana E et al: Determination of dissociation constants and relative efficacies of some potent muscarinic agonists at postjunctional muscarinic receptors. Naunyn Schmiedebergs Arch Pharmacol 1987;335:8.

Han X et al: An obligatory role for nitric oxide in autonomic control of mammalian heart rate. J Physiol 1994;476:309.

Hobbiger F: Pharmacology of anticholinesterase drugs. In: Neuromuscular Junction—Vol 42 of Handbook of Experimental Pharmacology. Zaimis E (editor). Springer Verlag, 1976.

Honkanen RE, Howard EF, Abdel-Latif AA: M3-muscarinic receptor subtype predominates in the bovine sphincter smooth muscle and ciliary processes. Invest Ophthalmol Vis Sci 1990;31:590.

Levy MN, Schwartz PJ (editors): *Vagal Control of the Heart.* Futura, 1994.

Lindstrom J et al: Structural and functional heterogeneity of nicotinic receptors. In: *The Biology of Nicotine Depen-*

dence. Ciba Symposium 152. Bock G, Marsh J (editors). Wiley, 1990.

Marrion NV et al: Muscarinic suppression of the M-current in the rat sympathetic ganglion is mediated by receptors of the M_1-subtype. Br J Pharmacol 1989;98:557.

Molitor H: A comparative study of the effects of five choline compounds used in therapeutics: Acetylcholine chloride, acetyl-beta-methylcholine chloride, carbaminoyl choline, ethyl ether beta-methylcholine chloride, carbaminoyl beta-methylcholine chloride. J Pharmacol Exp Ther 1936;58:337.

Moncada S et al: Nitric oxide: Physiology, pathophysiology, and pharmacology. Pharmacol Rev 1991;43:109.

Nathanson NM: Molecular properties of the muscarinic acetylcholine receptor. Annu Rev Neurosci 1987;10:195.

Noronha-Blob L et al: Muscarinic receptors: Relationships among phosphoinositide breakdown, adenylate cyclase inhibition, in vitro detrusor muscle contraction, and in vivo cystometrogram studies in guinea pig bladder. J Pharmacol Exp Therap 1989;249:843.

Pappano AJ: Modulation of the heartbeat by the vagus nerve. In: *Cardiac Electrophysiology: From Cell to Bedside.* Zipes DP, Jalife J (editors). Saunders, 1995.

Pfeiffer A et al: Muscarinic receptors mediating acid secretion in isolated rat gastric mucosa cells are of M3 type. Gastroenterology 1990;98:218.

Raftery MA et al: Acetylcholine receptor: Complex of homologous subunits. Science 1980;208:1454.

Rand MJ: Neuropharmacological effects of nicotine in relation to cholinergic mechanisms. Prog Brain Res 1989;79:3.

Rockwood EJ: The pharmacology of medical management: Practical aspects. In: *Management of Difficult Glaucoma.* Higginbotham EJ, Lee DA (editors). Blackwell, 1994.

Smoking and cardiovascular disease. MMWR Morb Mortal Wkly Rep 1984;32:677.

Starke K et al: Modulation of neurotransmitter release by presynaptic autoreceptors. Physiol Rev 1989;69:864.

Watanabe AM et al: Cardiac autonomic receptors: Recent concepts from radiolabeled ligand-binding studies. Circ Res 1982;50:161.

Cholinoceptor-Blocking Drugs

8

Bertram G. Katzung, MD, PhD

Just as cholinoceptor agonists are divided into muscarinic and nicotinic subgroups on the basis of their specific receptor affinities, so the antagonists acting on these receptors fall into two major families: the **antimuscarinic** and **antinicotinic** agents. The nicotinic receptor-blocking drugs consist of ganglion-blockers and neuromuscular junction blockers. The ganglion-blocking drugs have very limited use and are discussed at the end of this chapter. The neuromuscular blockers are discussed in Chapter 27. The major emphasis in this chapter is on drugs that block muscarinic cholinoceptors.

As noted in Chapters 6 and 7, five subtypes of muscarinic receptors have been described, primarily on the basis of data from ligand-binding and cDNA-cloning experiments. A standard terminology (M_1 through M_5) for these subtypes is now in common use, and good evidence, based mostly on selective agonists and antagonists, suggests that functional differences do exist between several of these subtypes.

As suggested in Chapter 6, the M_1 receptor subtype appears to be located on central nervous system neurons, sympathetic postganglionic cell bodies, and many presynaptic sites. M_3 receptors are most common on effector cell membranes, especially glandular and smooth muscle cells. M_2 receptors are located in the myocardium, smooth muscle organs, and some neuronal sites.

I. BASIC PHARMACOLOGY OF THE MUSCARINIC RECEPTOR-BLOCKING DRUGS

Because the effects of parasympathetic autonomic discharge can be blocked by muscarinic antagonists, they are often called parasympatholytic drugs. However, they do not "lyse" parasympathetic nerves, and they have some effects that are not predictable from block of the parasympathetic nervous system. For these reasons, the term "antimuscarinic" is preferable.

Naturally occurring compounds with antimuscarinic effects have been known and used for millennia as medicines, poisons, and cosmetics. The prototype of these drugs is atropine. Many similar plant alkaloids are known, and hundreds of synthetic antimuscarinic compounds have been prepared.

Chemistry & Pharmacokinetics

A. Source and Chemistry: Atropine and its naturally occurring congeners are tertiary ammonium alkaloid esters of tropic acid (Figure 8–1).

Atropine (hyoscyamine) is found in the plant *Atropa belladonna,* or deadly nightshade, and in *Datura stramonium,* also known as jimsonweed (Jamestown weed) or thorn apple. **Scopolamine** (hyoscine) occurs in *Hyoscyamus niger,* or henbane. Scopolamine occurs as the *l*(–) stereoisomer in the plant. Naturally occurring atropine is *l*(–)-hyoscyamine, but the compound readily racemizes, so the commercial material is racemic *d,l*-hyoscyamine. The *l*(–) isomers of both alkaloids are at least 100 times more potent than the *d*(+) isomers.

Semisynthetic tertiary ammonium analogs can be produced by esterifying a natural base, eg, tropine, the base in atropine, with different acids. Thus, homatropine is the mandelic acid ester of tropine. A variety of fully synthetic molecules have antimuscarinic effects.

The tertiary members of these classes (Figure 8–2) are often used for their effects on the eye or the central nervous system. Many antihistaminic (Chapter 16), antipsychotic (Chapter 29), and antidepressant (Chapter 30) drugs have similar structures and, predictably, significant antimuscarinic effects.

Quaternary ammonium antimuscarinic agents have been developed to produce more peripheral effects with reduced central nervous system effects. These drugs include both semisynthetic and synthetic molecules (Figure 8–2).

B. Absorption: The natural alkaloids and most tertiary antimuscarinic drugs are well absorbed from the gut and across the conjunctival membrane. When applied in a suitable vehicle, some, eg, scopolamine,

Figure 8–1. The structure of atropine (oxygen at *[1]* is missing) or scopolamine (oxygen present). In homatropine, the hydroxymethyl at *[2]* is replaced by a hydroxyl group, and the oxygen at *[1]* is absent.

are even absorbed across the skin (transdermal route). In contrast, only 10–30% of a dose of a quaternary antimuscarinic drug is absorbed after oral administration, reflecting the decreased lipid solubility of the charged molecule.

C. Distribution: Atropine and the other tertiary agents are widely distributed after absorption. Significant levels are achieved in the central nervous system within 30 minutes to 1 hour, and this may limit the dose tolerated when the drug is taken for its peripheral effects. Scopolamine is rapidly and fully distributed into the central nervous system and has greater effects there than most other antimuscarinic drugs. In contrast, the quaternary derivatives are poorly taken up by the brain and therefore are relatively free—at low doses—of these central nervous system effects.

D. Metabolism and Excretion: Atropine disappears rapidly from the blood after administration, with a half-life of 2 hours. About 60% of the dose is excreted unchanged in the urine. Most of the rest appears in the urine as hydrolysis and conjugation products. The effect of the drug on parasympathetic function declines rapidly in all organs except the eye. Effects on the iris and ciliary muscle persist for 72 hours or longer.

Certain species, notably rabbits, have a specific enzyme—atropine esterase—that confers almost complete protection against the toxic effects of atropine by rapidly metabolizing the drug.

Pharmacodynamics

A. Mechanism of Action: Atropine causes reversible (surmountable) blockade of the actions of cholinomimetics at muscarinic receptors—ie, blockade by a small dose of atropine can be overcome by a larger concentration of acetylcholine or equivalent muscarinic agonist. This suggests competition for a common binding site on the receptor protein. Mutation experiments suggest that a specific amino acid is required in the receptor to form the characteristic bond with the nitrogen atom of acetylcholine; this amino acid is also required for binding of antimuscarinic drugs. When atropine binds to the muscarinic

receptor, it prevents the actions described in Chapter 7 such as the release of inositol trisphosphate (IP_3) and the inhibition of adenylyl cyclase that are brought about by muscarinic agonists.

The effectiveness of antimuscarinic drugs varies with the tissue under study and with the source of agonist. The tissues most sensitive to atropine are the salivary, bronchial, and sweat glands. Secretion of acid by the gastric parietal cells is the least sensitive. Smooth muscle autonomic effectors and the heart are intermediate in responsiveness. In most tissues, antimuscarinic agents are more effective in blocking exogenously administered cholinoceptor agonists than endogenously released acetylcholine.

Atropine is highly selective for muscarinic receptors. Its potency at nicotinic receptors is much lower than at muscarinic receptors; in clinical use, actions at nonmuscarinic receptors are generally undetectable.

Atropine does not distinguish between the M_1, M_2, and M_3 subgroups of muscarinic receptors. In contrast, other antimuscarinic drugs have been found that do have moderate selectively for one or another of these subgroups (Table 8–1). Most synthetic antimuscarinic drugs are considerably less specific than atropine in interactions with nonmuscarinic receptors. For example, some quaternary ammonium antimuscarinic agents have significant ganglion-blocking actions, and others are potent histamine receptor blockers. The antimuscarinic effects of other groups, eg, antihistaminic and antidepressant drugs, have been mentioned. Their relative selectivity for muscarinic receptor subtypes has not been defined.

B. Organ System Effects:

1. Central nervous system–In the doses usually used clinically, atropine has minimal stimulant effects on the central nervous system, especially the parasympathetic medullary centers, and a slower, longer-lasting sedative effect on the brain. A central vagal stimulant effect has been inferred from the fact that low doses of atropine can cause bradycardia, which is later supplanted by tachycardia as the drug's antimuscarinic effects at the sinoatrial node become manifest (see below). Scopolamine has more marked central effects, producing drowsiness when given in recommended dosages and amnesia in sensitive individuals. In toxic doses, scopolamine and to a lesser degree atropine can cause excitement, agitation, hallucinations, and coma.

The tremor of Parkinson's disease is reduced by centrally acting antimuscarinic drugs, and atropine—in the form of belladonna extract—was one of the first drugs used in the therapy of this disease. As discussed in Chapter 28, parkinsonian tremor and rigidity seem to result from a *relative* excess of cholinergic activity because of a deficiency of dopaminergic activity in the basal ganglia-striatum system. Thus, the combination of an antimuscarinic agent with a dopamine precursor drug (levodopa) may provide a more effective therapeutic approach than either drug alone.

Quaternary amines for gastrointestinal applications (peptic disease, hypermotility):

Propantheline

Glycopyrrolate

Tertiary amines for peripheral applications:

Pirenzepine
(peptic disease)

Dicyclomine
(peptic disease, hypermotility)

Tropicamide
(mydriatric, cycloplegic)

Quaternary amine for use in asthma:

Tertiary amine for Parkinson's disease:

Ipratropium

Benztropine

Figure 8–2. Structures of some semisynthetic and synthetic antimuscarinic drugs.

Vestibular disturbances, especially motion sickness, appear to involve muscarinic cholinergic transmission. Scopolamine is often effective in preventing or reversing these disturbances.

2. Eye—The pupillary constrictor muscle (Figure 6–9) is dependent on muscarinic cholinoceptor activation. This activation is effectively blocked by topical atropine and other tertiary antimuscarinic drugs

Table 8–1. Three muscarinic receptor subgroups and their antagonists. (Acronyms identify selective antagonists used in research studies only.)

Property	Subgroup		
	M_1	M_2	M_3
Primary locations	Nerves	Heart, nerves, smooth muscle	Glands, smooth muscle, endothelium
Dominant effector system	↑ IP_3, ↑ DAG	↓ cAMP, ↑ K+ channel current	↑ IP_3, ↑ DAG
Antagonists	Pirenzepine, telenzepine dicyclomine,[2] trihexyphenidyl[3]	Gallamine,[1] 1-methoctramine, AF-DX 116	4-DAMP, HHSD
Approximate dissociation constant[4]			
Atropine	1	1	1
Pirenzepine	10	50	200
AF-DX 116	800	100	3000
HHSD	40	200	2

[1]In clinical use as a neuromuscular blocking agent.
[2]In clinical use as an intestinal antispasmodic agent.
[3]In clinical use in the treatment of Parkinson's disease.
[4]Relative to atropine. Smaller numbers indicate higher affinity.
Key:

AF-DX 116	= 11-({2-[(Diethylamino)methyl]-1-piperidinyl}acetyl)-5,11-dihydro-6H-pyrido-[2,3-b](1,4)benzodiaz-epin-6-one
DAG	= Diacylglycerol
IP_3	= Inositol trisphosphate
4-DAMP	= 4-Diphenylacetoxy-N-methylpiperidine
HHSD	= Hexahydrosiladifenidol

and results in unopposed sympathetic dilator activity and **mydriasis** (Figure 8–3). Dilated pupils were apparently considered cosmetically desirable during the Renaissance and account for the name belladonna (Italian, "beautiful lady") applied to the plant and its active extract because of the use of the extract as eye drops during that time.

The second important ocular effect of antimuscarinic drugs is weakening of contraction of the ciliary muscle, or **cycloplegia.** The result of cycloplegia is loss of the ability to accommodate; the fully atropinized eye cannot focus for near vision (Figure 8–3).

Both mydriasis and cycloplegia are useful in ophthalmology. They are also potentially hazardous, since acute glaucoma may be precipitated in patients with a narrow anterior chamber angle.

A third ocular effect of antimuscarinic drugs is reduction of lacrimal secretion. Patients occasionally complain of dry or "sandy" eyes when receiving large doses of antimuscarinic drugs.

3. Cardiovascular system–The atria of the heart are richly innervated by parasympathetic (vagal) nerve fibers, and the sinoatrial node is therefore sensitive to muscarinic receptor blockade. The effect of moderate to high therapeutic doses of atropine in the innervated and spontaneously beating heart is a clear blockade of vagal slowing and a relative tachycardia.

However, as noted above, lower doses cause parasympathetic *stimulation* and often result in initial bradycardia before the effects of peripheral vagal block become manifest (Figure 8–4). Although this effect has been ascribed to central stimulation of the vagal nucleus, other evidence suggests that it may be due to block of presynaptic muscarinic receptors on vagal postganglionic fibers that normally limit acetylcholine release in the sinus node. The same mechanisms operate in the control of atrioventricular node function; in the presence of high vagal tone, administration of atropine can significantly reduce the PR interval of the ECG by blocking muscarinic receptors in the AV node. Muscarinic effects on atrial muscle are similarly blocked, but except in atrial flutter and fibrillation these effects are of no clinical significance. The ventricles, because of a lesser degree of muscarinic control, are less affected by antimuscarinic drugs at therapeutic levels. In toxic concentrations, the drugs can cause intraventricular conduction block by an unknown mechanism.

The blood vessels receive little or no direct innervation from the parasympathetic nervous system. However, as noted in Chapter 6, sympathetic cholinergic nerves cause vasodilation in the skeletal muscle vascular bed. This vasodilation can be blocked by atropine. Furthermore, almost all vessels contain uninnervated muscarinic receptors that mediate vasodila-

Figure 8–3. Effects of topical scopolamine drops on pupil diameter (mm) and accommodation (diopters) in the normal human eye. One drop of 0.5% solution of drug was applied at zero time, and a second drop was administered at 30 minutes (arrows). The responses of 42 eyes were averaged. Note the extremely slow recovery. (Redrawn from Marron J: Cycloplegia and mydriasis by use of atropine, scopolamine, and homatropine-paredrine. Arch Ophthal 1940;23:340.)

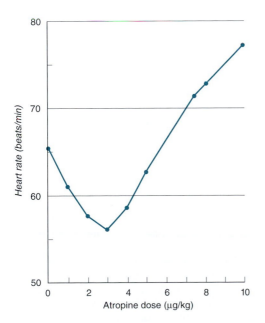

Figure 8–4. Dose-response curve for the effects of atropine on heart rate in eight healthy human subjects. Intravenous doses were given cumulatively. Lower doses slow the rate (see text). (Data from Porter TR et al: J Clin Invest 1990;85:1362.)

tion (Chapter 7). These receptors, which are located on endothelial cells, cause the release of endothelium-derived relaxing factor (EDRF) in response to circulating direct-acting muscarinic agonists, and are readily blocked by antimuscarinic drugs. At toxic doses, and in some individuals at normal doses, antimuscarinic agents cause cutaneous vasodilation, especially in the upper portion of the body. The mechanism is unknown.

The net cardiovascular effects of atropine in patients with normal hemodynamics are not dramatic: tachycardia may occur, but there is little effect on blood pressure. However, the effects of administered direct-acting muscarinic stimulants are easily prevented.

4. Respiratory system–Both smooth muscle and secretory glands of the airway receive vagal innervation and contain muscarinic receptors. Even in normal individuals, some bronchodilation and reduction of secretion can be measured after administration of atropine. The effect is much more dramatic in patients with airway disease, though the antimuscarinic drugs are not as useful as the beta-adrenoceptor stimulants in the treatment of asthma (Chapter 20). Nevertheless, the antimuscarinic agents are valuable in some patients with asthma or chronic obstructive pulmonary disease (COPD). In addition, they are frequently used prior to administration of inhalant anesthetics to reduce the accumulation of secretions in the trachea and the possibility of laryngospasm.

5. Gastrointestinal tract–Blockade of muscarinic receptors has dramatic effects on motility and some of the secretory functions of the gut. However, since local hormones and noncholinergic neurons in the enteric nervous system (see Chapter 6) also modulate gastrointestinal function, even complete muscarinic block cannot totally abolish activity in this organ system. As in other tissues, exogenously administered muscarinic stimulants are more effectively blocked than the effects of parasympathetic (vagal) nerve activity.

The effects of antimuscarinic drugs on salivary secretion are marked; dry mouth is a frequent symptom in patients taking antimuscarinic drugs for Parkinson's disease or peptic ulcer (Figure 8–5). Gastric secretion is blocked less effectively: the volume and amount of acid, pepsin, and mucin are all reduced, but large doses of atropine may be required. Basal secretion is blocked more effectively than that stimulated by food, nicotine, or alcohol. Pirenzepine and a more potent analog, telenzepine, appear to reduce gastric acid secretion with fewer adverse effects than atropine and other less selective agents. This may result from a selective blockade of presynaptic excitatory muscarinic receptors on vagal nerve endings as suggested by their high ratio of M_1 to M_3 affinity (Table 8–1), but this hypothesis is not universally accepted. Pirenzepine and telenzepine are investigational in the USA. Pancreatic and intestinal secretion are little affected by atropine; these processes are primarily under hormonal rather than vagal control.

Motility of gastrointestinal smooth muscle is affected from the stomach to the colon. In general, the walls of the viscera are relaxed, and both tone and propulsive movements are diminished. Therefore, gastric emptying time is prolonged, and intestinal transit time is lengthened. Diarrhea due to overdosage with parasympathomimetic agents is readily eliminated, and even that caused by nonautonomic agents can usually be temporarily controlled. However, intestinal "paralysis" induced by antimuscarinic drugs is temporary; local mechanisms within the enteric nervous system will usually reestablish at least some peristalsis after 1–3 days of antimuscarinic drug therapy.

Several of the synthetic antimuscarinic agents are said to have "spasmolytic" activity in excess of their antimuscarinic effects. This is the result of selection of agents, through screening tests in isolated tissue, that relax the gut in the absence as well as the presence of cholinoceptor stimulants.

6. Genitourinary tract–Smooth muscle of the ureters and bladder wall is relaxed and voiding is slowed (Figure 8–5) by the antimuscarinic action of atropine and its analogs. This action is useful in the treatment of spasm induced by mild inflammatory conditions and certain neurologic conditions, but it also poses a hazard of precipitating urinary retention in elderly men, who may have prostatic hyperplasia (see Clinical Pharmacology). The antimuscarinic drugs have no significant effect on the uterus.

7. Sweat glands–Thermoregulatory sweating is suppressed by atropine. The muscarinic receptors on eccrine sweat glands are innervated by sympathetic cholinergic fibers and are readily accessible to antimuscarinic drugs. In adults, body temperature is elevated by this effect only if large doses are administered, but in infants and children even ordinary doses may cause "atropine fever."

II. CLINICAL PHARMACOLOGY OF THE MUSCARINIC RECEPTOR-BLOCKING DRUGS

Therapeutic Applications
A. Central Nervous System Disorders:
1. Parkinson's disease–As described in Chapter 28, the treatment of Parkinson's disease is often an exercise in polypharmacy, since no single agent is fully effective over the course of the disease. Most of the antimuscarinic drugs promoted for this application (Table 28–1) were developed before levodopa became available. Their use is accompanied by all of the adverse effects described below, but the drugs remain useful as adjunctive therapy in some patients.

2. Motion sickness–Certain vestibular disorders respond to antimuscarinic drugs (and to antihistaminic agents with antimuscarinic effects). Scopolamine is one of the oldest remedies for seasickness and is as effective as any more recently introduced agent. It can be given by injection or by mouth. It was available as a transdermal patch, which produced significant blood levels over 24–48 hours. Unfortunately, useful doses by any route usually cause significant sedation and dry mouth. The patch form has been tem-

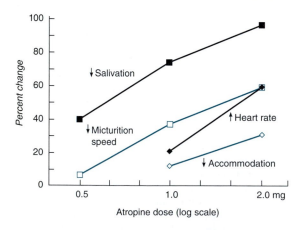

Figure 8–5. Effects of subcutaneous injection of atropine on salivation, speed of micturition (voiding), heart rate, and accommodation in normal adults. Note that salivation is the most sensitive of these variables, accommodation the least. (Data from Herxheimer A: Br J Pharmacol 1958;13:184.)

porarily withdrawn in the USA because of manufacturing problems.

B. Ophthalmologic Disorders: Accurate measurement of refractive error in uncooperative patients, eg, young children, requires ciliary paralysis. In addition, ophthalmoscopic examination of the retina is greatly facilitated by mydriasis. Therefore, antimuscarinic agents, administered topically as eye drops or ointment, are extremely helpful in doing a complete examination. For adults and older children, the shorter-acting drugs are preferred (Table 8–2). For younger children, the greater efficacy of atropine is sometimes necessary, but the possibility of antimuscarinic poisoning is correspondingly increased. Loss of drug from the conjunctival sac via the nasolacrimal duct into the nasopharynx can be diminished by the use of the ointment form in preference to drops. In the past, ophthalmic antimuscarinic drugs have been selected from the tertiary ammonium subgroup to ensure good penetration after conjunctival application. Recent experiments in animals, however, suggest that glycopyrrolate, a quaternary agent, is as rapid in onset and as long-lasting as atropine.

Antimuscarinic drugs should never be used for mydriasis unless cycloplegia or prolonged action is required. Alpha-adrenoceptor stimulant drugs, eg, phenylephrine, produce a short-lasting mydriasis that is usually sufficient for funduscopic examination (Chapter 9).

A second ophthalmologic use is to prevent synechia (adhesion) formation in uveitis and iritis. The longer-lasting preparations, especially homatropine, are valuable for this indication.

C. Respiratory Disorders: The use of atropine became part of routine preoperative medication when anesthetics such as ether were used, because these irritant anesthetics caused a marked increase in airway secretions and were associated with frequent episodes of laryngospasm. These hazardous effects could be prevented by preanesthetic injection of atropine or scopolamine. The latter drug also produced significant amnesia for the events associated with surgery and obstetric delivery, a side effect that was considered desirable. On the other hand, urinary retention and intestinal hypomotility following surgery could be significantly exacerbated by the use of the antimuscarinic drug. With the advent of effective and nonirritant inhalational anesthetics such as halothane and enflurane, one reason for the routine use of antimuscarinic drugs as preanesthetic medication has been eliminated.

Inhalation of smoke from burning leaves of *Datura stramonium* has been used for centuries as a remedy for bronchial asthma. "Asthmador" cigarettes containing *D stramonium* were available without prescription for this application until recently. As described in Chapter 20, the hyperactive neural bronchoconstrictor reflex present in most individuals with asthma is mediated by the vagus, acting on muscarinic receptors on bronchial smooth muscle cells. **Ipratropium** (Figure 8–2), a synthetic analog of atropine, is used as an inhalational drug in asthma. The aerosol route of administration provides the advantages of maximal concentration at the bronchial target tissue with reduced systemic effects. This application is discussed in greater detail in Chapter 20. Ipratropium has also proved useful in chronic obstructive pulmonary disease, a condition that occurs with higher frequency in older patients, particularly chronic smokers. Patients with COPD benefit from bronchodilators, especially antimuscarinic agents such as ipratropium. Investigational agents in this category include **tiotropium,** a long-acting quaternary aerosol antimuscarinic drug.

D. Cardiovascular Disorders: Marked vagal discharge sometimes accompanies the pain of myocardial infarction and may result in sufficient depression of sinoatrial or atrioventricular node function to impair cardiac output. Parenteral atropine or a similar antimuscarinic drug is appropriate therapy in this situation. Rare individuals without other detectable cardiac disease have hyperactive carotid sinus reflexes and may experience faintness or even syncope as a result of vagal discharge in response to pressure on the neck, eg, from a tight collar. Such individuals may benefit from the judicious use of atropine or a related antimuscarinic agent.

E. Gastrointestinal Disorders: The antimuscarinic drugs were mainly used to treat peptic ulcer until the introduction of the H_2 histamine receptor-blocking agents (see Chapter 63). Antimuscarinic agents are now rarely used for this indication, though the development of selective M_1 blockers such as pirenzepine may reverse the trend. When the older agents are used for this application, quaternary antimuscarinic drugs such as glycopyrrolate are preferred; large doses (Table 8–3) are required to significantly reduce gastric acid secretion. Patients who receive this treatment will have blurred vision, dry mouth, and urinary hesitancy. In the case of *gastric* peptic ulcer, antimuscarinic drugs may be contraindicated because they can slow gastric emptying and prolong the exposure of the ulcer bed to acid.

In the treatment of common traveler's diarrhea and other mild or self-limited conditions of hypermotility, the antimuscarinic agents can provide some relief. They are often combined with an opioid antidiarrheal

Table 8–2. Antimuscarinic drugs used in ophthalmology.

Drug	Duration of Effect (days)	Usual Concentration (%)
Atropine	7–10	0.5–1
Scopolamine	3–7	0.25
Homatropine	1–3	2–5
Cyclopentolate	1	0.5–2
Tropicamide	0.25	0.5–1

Table 8–3. Antimuscarinic drugs used in gastrointestinal and genitourinary conditions.

Drug	Usual Dosage
Quaternary amines	
Anisotropine	50 mg tid
Clidinium	2.5 mg tid–qid
Glycopyrrolate	1 mg bid–tid
Isopropamide	5 mg bid
Mepenzolate	25–50 mg qid
Methantheline	50–100 mg qid
Methscopolamine	2.5 mg qid
Oxyphenonium	5–10 mg qid
Propantheline	15 mg qid
Tertiary amines	
Atropine	0.4 mg tid–qid
Dicyclomine	10–20 mg qid
Oxybutynin	5 mg tid
Oxyphencyclimine	10 mg bid
Scopolamine	0.4 mg tid
Tridihexethyl	25–50 mg tid–qid

drug, an extremely effective therapy. In this combination, however, the very low dosage of the antimuscarinic drug functions primarily to discourage abuse of the opioid agent. The classic combination of atropine with diphenoxylate, a nonanalgesic congener of meperidine, is available under many names (eg, Lomotil) in both tablet and liquid form (Chapter 63).

F. Urinary Disorders: Atropine and other antimuscarinic drugs have been used in the treatment of urinary urgency caused by minor inflammatory bladder disorders (Table 8–3). This approach does provide some symptomatic relief, though it is no substitute for specific antimicrobial therapy in bacterial cystitis.

Oxybutynin is often used to relieve bladder spasm after urologic surgery, eg, prostatectomy. It is also valuable in reducing involuntary voiding in patients with neurologic disease, eg, children with meningomyelocele. Oral oxybutynin or instillation of the drug by catheter into the bladder in such patients appears to improve bladder capacity and continence and to reduce infection and renal damage. **Tolterodine** is investigational for this purpose.

Imipramine, a tricyclic antidepressant drug with strong antimuscarinic actions, has long been used to reduce incontinence in the institutionalized elderly. It is moderately effective but at the cost of significant central nervous system toxicity. **Propiverine** is a newer antimuscarinic agent that is investigational for this purpose.

The antimuscarinic agents have also been used in urolithiasis to relieve the ureteral smooth muscle spasm caused by passage of the stone. However, their usefulness in this condition is debatable.

G. Cholinergic Poisoning: Severe cholinergic excess is an important medical emergency, especially in rural communities where the use of cholinesterase inhibitor insecticides is common and in cultures where wild mushrooms are commonly eaten. The potential use of these agents as chemical warfare "nerve gases" also requires an awareness of the methods for treating acute poisoning.

1. Antimuscarinic therapy–As noted in Chapter 7, both the nicotinic and the muscarinic effects of the cholinesterase inhibitors can be life-threatening. Unfortunately, there is no effective method for directly blocking the nicotinic effects of cholinesterase inhibition, because nicotinic agonists *and* blockers cause blockade of transmission (Chapter 27). To reverse the muscarinic effects, a tertiary (not quaternary) amine drug must be used (preferably atropine), since the central nervous system effects as well as the peripheral effects of the organophosphate inhibitors must be treated. Large doses of atropine may be needed to combat the muscarinic effects of extremely potent agents like parathion and chemical warfare nerve gases: 1–2 mg of atropine sulfate may be given intravenously every 5–15 minutes until signs of effect (dry mouth, reversal of miosis) appear. The drug may have to be repeated many times, since the acute effects of the anticholinesterase agent may last for 24–48 hours or longer. There is no theoretical limit to the use of atropine in this life-threatening situation, and as much as 1 g per day may be required for as long as 1 month for full control of muscarinic excess (LeBlanc et al, 1986).

2. Cholinesterase regenerator compounds–A second class of compounds, capable of regenerating active enzyme from the organophosphorus-cholinesterase complex, is also available for the treatment of organophosphorus inhibitor poisoning. These **oxime** agents include **pralidoxime (PAM),** diacetylmonoxime (DAM), and others.

Pralidoxime

Diacetylmonoxime

HLö7

The oxime group (=NOH) has a very high affinity for the phosphorus atom, and these drugs are able to hydrolyze the phosphorylated enzyme if the complex has not "aged" (Chapter 7). HLö7 is the most effective of these oximes in experimental animals (Eyer et al, 1992). Pralidoxime is the most extensively studied—in humans—of the three agents shown and the only one available for clinical use in the USA. It is most effective in regenerating the cholinesterase associated with skeletal muscle neuromuscular junctions. Because of its positive charge, it does not enter the central nervous system and is ineffective in reversing the central effects of organophosphate poisoning. Diacetylmonoxime, on the other hand, does cross the blood-brain barrier and, in experimental animals, can regenerate some of the central nervous system cholinesterase.

Pralidoxime is administered by intravenous infusion, 1–2 g given over 15–30 minutes. In spite of the likelihood of aging of the phosphate-enzyme complex, recent reports suggest that administration of multiple doses of pralidoxime over several days may be useful in severe poisoning. In excessive doses, pralidoxime can induce neuromuscular weakness and other adverse effects. Pralidoxime is *not* recommended for the reversal of inhibition of acetylcholinesterase by carbamate inhibitors. Further details of treatment of anticholinesterase toxicity are given in Chapter 59.

A third approach to protection against excessive AChE inhibition lies in *pretreatment* with reversible inhibitors of the enzyme to prevent binding of the irreversible organophosphate inhibitor. This prophylaxis can be achieved with pyridostigmine or physostigmine but is reserved for situations in which possibly lethal poisoning is anticipated, eg, chemical warfare. An experimental cholinesterase ligand derived from hemicholinium-3 is particularly effective in animal tests (Cannon et al, 1991). Simultaneous use of atropine is required to control muscarinic excess.

Mushroom poisoning has traditionally been divided into rapid-onset and delayed-onset types. The rapid-onset type is usually apparent within 15–30 minutes following ingestion of the mushrooms. It is often characterized entirely by signs of muscarinic excess: nausea, vomiting, diarrhea, vasodilation, reflex tachycardia (occasionally bradycardia), sweating, salivation, and sometimes bronchoconstriction. Although *Amanita muscaria* contains muscarine (the alkaloid was named after the mushroom), numerous other alkaloids, including antimuscarinic agents, are found in this fungus. In fact, ingestion of *A muscaria* may produce signs of atropine poisoning, not muscarine excess. Other mushrooms, especially those of the *Inocybe* genus, cause rapid-onset poisoning of the muscarinic excess type. Parenteral atropine, 1–2 mg, is effective treatment in such intoxications.

Delayed-onset mushroom poisoning, usually caused by *Amanita phalloides, A virosa, Galerina au-*tumnalis, or *G marginata*, manifests its first symptoms 6–12 hours after ingestion. Although the initial symptoms usually include nausea and vomiting, the major toxicity involves hepatic and renal cellular injury by amatoxins that inhibit RNA polymerase. Atropine is of no value in this form of mushroom poisoning (see Chapter 59).

H. Other Applications: Hyperhidrosis is sometimes reduced by antimuscarinic agents. However, relief is incomplete at best, probably because apocrine rather than eccrine glands are usually involved.

Adverse Effects

Because of the broad range of antimuscarinic effects, treatment with atropine or its congeners directed at one organ system almost always induces undesirable effects in other organ systems. Thus, mydriasis and cycloplegia are "adverse" effects when an antimuscarinic agent is being used to reduce gastrointestinal secretion or motility, even though they are "therapeutic" effects when the drug is used in ophthalmology.

At higher concentrations, atropine causes block of all parasympathetic functions; these are predictable from the organ system effects described above. However, even in gram quantities, atropine is a remarkably safe drug *in adults*. Atropine poisoning has occurred as a result of attempted suicide, but most cases are due to attempts to induce hallucinations. Poisoned individuals manifest dry mouth, mydriasis, tachycardia, hot and flushed skin, agitation, and delirium for as long as a week. Body temperature is frequently elevated. These effects are memorialized in the adage, "dry as a bone, blind as a bat, red as a beet, mad as a hatter."

Unfortunately, children, especially infants, are very sensitive to the hyperthermic effects of atropine. Although accidental administration of over 400 mg has been followed by recovery, deaths have followed doses as small as 2 mg. Therefore, atropine should be considered a highly dangerous drug when overdose occurs in infants or children.

Overdoses of atropine or its congeners are generally treated symptomatically (see Chapter 59). In the past, physostigmine or another cholinesterase inhibitor was recommended, but most poison control experts now consider physostigmine more dangerous and no more effective in most patients than symptomatic management. When physostigmine is deemed necessary, *small* doses are given *slowly* intravenously (1–4 mg in adults, 0.5–1 mg in children). Symptomatic treatment may require temperature control with cooling blankets and seizure control with diazepam.

Poisoning caused by high doses of the quaternary antimuscarinic drugs is associated with all of the peripheral signs of parasympathetic blockade but few or none of the central nervous system effects of atropine. These more polar drugs may cause significant ganglionic blockade, however, with marked orthostatic hypotension (see below). Treatment of the antimuscarinic effects, if required, can be carried out with a quaternary cholinesterase inhibitor such as neostigmine. Control of hypotension may require the administration of a sympathomimetic drug such as phenylephrine or methoxamine.

Contraindications

Contraindications to the use of antimuscarinic drugs are relative, not absolute. *Obvious muscarinic excess, especially that caused by cholinesterase inhibitors, can always be treated with atropine.*

Antimuscarinic drugs are contraindicated in patients with glaucoma, especially angle-closure glaucoma. Even systemic use of moderate doses may precipitate angle closure (and acute glaucoma) in patients with shallow anterior chambers.

In elderly men, antimuscarinic drugs should always be used with caution and should be avoided in those with a history of prostatic hyperplasia.

Because the antimuscarinic drugs slow gastric emptying, they may *increase* symptoms in patients with gastric ulcer. If a stomach ulcer is to be treated pharmacologically, H_2 histamine antagonists and other agents are preferred (see Chapter 63).

III. BASIC & CLINICAL PHARMACOLOGY OF THE GANGLION-BLOCKING DRUGS

These agents block the action of acetylcholine and similar agonists at the nicotinic receptors of both parasympathetic and sympathetic autonomic ganglia. Some members of the group also block the ionic channel that is gated by the nicotinic cholinoceptor. Because of their ability to block all autonomic outflow, the ganglion-blocking drugs are still important and useful in pharmacologic and physiologic research. However, their lack of selectivity confers such a broad range of undesirable effects that they have been abandoned for clinical use.

Chemistry & Pharmacokinetics

All of the ganglion-blocking drugs of interest are synthetic amines. The first to be recognized as having this action was **tetraethylammonium (TEA).** Because of the very short duration of action of TEA, **hexamethonium ("C6")** was developed and was soon introduced into clinical medicine as the first effective drug for management of hypertension. As shown in Figure 8–6, there is an obvious relationship between the structures of the normal agonist acetylcholine and the nicotinic antagonists tetraethylammonium and hexamethonium. It is interesting that decamethonium, the "C10" analog of hexamethonium, is an effective neuromuscular depolarizing blocking agent.

Figure 8–6. Some ganglion-blocking drugs. Acetylcholine is shown for reference.

Because the quaternary ammonium ganglion-blocking compounds were poorly and erratically absorbed after oral administration, **mecamylamine,** a secondary ammonium compound, was developed to improve the degree and extent of absorption from the gastrointestinal tract. Mecamylamine is the only ganglion-blocking drug still available in the USA. **Trimethaphan,** a short-acting ganglion blocker, is inactive by the oral route and was given by intravenous infusion for the emergency treatment of malignant hypertension (Chapter 11).

Pharmacodynamics

A. Mechanism of Action: The nicotinic receptors of the ganglia, like those of the skeletal muscle neuromuscular junction, are subject to both depolarizing and nondepolarizing blockade (Chapters 7 and 27). Nicotine itself, carbamoylcholine, and even acetylcholine (if amplified with a cholinesterase inhibitor) can produce depolarizing ganglion block.

All of the drugs presently used as ganglion-blockers are classified as nondepolarizing competitive antagonists. However, evidence from many studies suggests that hexamethonium actually produces most of its blockade by occupying sites in or on the ion channel that is controlled by the acetylcholine receptor, not by occupying the cholinoceptor itself. In contrast, trimethaphan appears to block the nicotinic receptor, not the channel. According to older studies, blockade can be at least partially overcome by increasing the concentration of normal agonists, eg, acetylcholine.

As noted in Chapter 6, other receptors on the postganglionic cell modulate the ganglionic transmission process. However, their effects are not sufficient to overcome large doses of the hexamethonium-trimethaphan group.

B. Organ System Effects:

1. Central nervous system–The quaternary ammonium agents and trimethaphan are devoid of central effects because they do not cross the blood-brain barrier. Mecamylamine, however, readily enters the central nervous system. Sedation, tremor, choreiform movements, and mental aberrations have all been reported as effects of the latter drug.

2. Eye–Because the ciliary muscle receives innervation primarily from the parasympathetic nervous system, the ganglion-blocking drugs cause a predictable cycloplegia with loss of accommodation. The effect on the pupil is not so easily predicted, since the iris receives both sympathetic innervation (mediating pupillary dilation) and parasympathetic innervation (mediating pupillary constriction). Because parasympathetic tone is usually dominant in this tissue, ganglionic blockade usually causes moderate dilation of the pupil.

3. Cardiovascular system–The blood vessels receive chiefly vasoconstrictor fibers from the sympathetic nervous system; therefore, ganglionic blockade causes a very important decrease in arteriolar and venomotor tone. The blood pressure may drop precipitously, because both peripheral vascular resistance and venous return are decreased (see Figure 6–7). Hypotension is especially marked in the upright position (orthostatic or postural hypotension), because postural reflexes that normally prevent venous pooling are blocked.

Cardiac effects include diminished contractility and, because the sinoatrial node is usually dominated by the parasympathetic nervous system, a moderate tachycardia.

4. Gastrointestinal tract–Secretion is reduced, though not enough to effectively treat peptic disease. Motility is profoundly inhibited, and constipation may be marked.

5. Other systems–Genitourinary smooth muscle is partially dependent on autonomic innervation for normal function. Ganglionic blockade therefore causes hesitancy in urination and may precipitate urinary retention in men with prostatic hyperplasia. Sexual function is impaired in that both erection and ejaculation may be prevented by moderate doses.

Thermoregulatory sweating is blocked by the ganglion-blocking drugs. However, hyperthermia is not a problem except in very warm environments, because cutaneous vasodilation is usually sufficient to maintain a normal body temperature.

6. Response to autonomic drugs–Because the effector cell receptors (muscarinic, alpha, and beta) are not blocked, patients receiving ganglion-blocking drugs are fully responsive to autonomic drugs acting on these receptors. In fact, responses may be exaggerated or even reversed (eg, norepinephrine may cause tachycardia rather than bradycardia), because homeostatic reflexes, which normally moderate autonomic responses, are absent.

Clinical Applications & Toxicity

Because of the availability of more selective autonomic blocking agents, the applications of the ganglion blockers have disappeared. These drugs were used in the treatment of hypertensive emergencies and to produce controlled hypotension, which can be of value in neurosurgery to reduce bleeding in the operative field. However, other rapid-onset, short-acting agents are available (eg, nitroprusside), and most physicians have more experience with these alternative agents.

The toxicity of the ganglion-blocking drugs is limited to the autonomic effects already described. For most patients, these effects are intolerable except for acute use.

PREPARATIONS AVAILABLE

Antimuscarinic Anticholinergic Drugs*

Anisotropine (generic, Valpin)
  Oral: 50 mg tablets
Atropine (generic)
  Oral: 0.4, 0.6 mg tablets
  Parenteral: 0.05, 0.1, 0.3, 0.4, 0.5, 0.8, 1, mg/mL for injection
  Ophthalmic (generic, Isopto Atropine): 0.5, 1, 2, 3% drops; 0.5, 1% ointments
Belladonna alkaloids, extract or tincture
    (generic)

*Antimuscarinic drugs used in parkinsonism are listed in Chapter 29.

  Oral: 0.27–0.33 mg/mL liquid
Clidinium (Quarzan)
  Oral: 2.5, 5 mg capsules
Cyclopentolate (generic, Cyclogyl, others)
  Ophthalmic: 0.5, 1, 2% drops
Dicyclomine (generic, Bentyl, others)
  Oral: 10, 20 mg capsules; 20 mg tablets; 10 mg/5mL syrup
  Parenteral: 10 mg/mL for injection
Flavoxate (Urispas)
  Oral: 100 mg tablets
Glycopyrrolate (generic, Robinul)
  Oral: 1, 2 mg tablets Parenteral: 0.2 mg/mL for injection

Homatropine (generic, Isopto Homatropine)
Ophthalmic: 2, 5% drops
Isopropamide (Darbid)
Oral: 5 mg tablets
l-**Hyoscyamine** (Anaspaz, Cystospaz-M, Levsinex)
Oral: 0.125, 0.15 mg tablets; 0.375 mg timed-release capsules; 0.125 mg/5 mL oral elixir and solution
Parenteral: 0.5 mg/mL for injection
Ipratropium (Atrovent)
Aerosol: 200 dose metered dose inhaler
Mepenzolate (Cantil)
Oral: 25 mg tablets
Methantheline (Banthine)
Oral: 50 mg tablets
Methscopolamine (Pamine)
Oral: 2.5 mg tablets
Oxybutynin (generic, Ditropan)
Oral: 5 mg tablets, 5 mg/5 mL syrup
Oxyphencyclimine (Daricon)
Oral: 10 mg tablets

Propantheline (generic, Pro-Banthine)
Oral: 7.5, 15 mg tablets
Scopolamine (generic)
Oral: 0.25 mg capsules
Parenteral: 0.3, 0.4, 0.65, 0.86, 1 mg/mL for injection
Ophthalmic (generic, Isopto Hyoscine): 0.25% solution
Tridihexethyl (Pathilon)
Oral: 25 mg tablets
Tropicamide (generic, Mydriacyl Ophthalmic, others)
Ophthalmic: 0.5, 1% drops

Ganglion Blockers
Mecamylamine (Inversine)
Oral: 2.5 mg tablets

Cholinesterase Regenerator
Pralidoxime (generic, Protopam)
Parenteral: 1 g vial with 20 mL diluent for IV administration; 600 mg in 2 mL autoinjector)

REFERENCES

Antimuscarinic Drugs

Amitai Y et al: Atropine poisoning in children during the Persian Gulf crisis. JAMA 1992;268:630.

Berdie GJ et al: Angle closure glaucoma precipitated by aerosolized atropine. Arch Intern Med 1991;151:1658.

Brown JH (editor): *The Muscarinic Receptors* Humana Press, 1989.

Christofi FL, Palmer JM, Wood JD: Neuropharmacology of the muscarinic antagonist telenzepine in myenteric ganglia of the guinea-pig small intestine. Eur J Pharmacol 1991;195:333.

Crowell EB, Ketchum JS: The treatment of scopolamine-induced delirium with physostigmine. Clin Pharmacol Ther 1967;8:409.

Doods HN et al: Selectivity of muscarinic antagonists in radioligand and *in vivo* experiments for the putative M_1, M_2, and M_3 receptors. J Pharmacol Exp Therap 1987;242:257.

Feldman M: Inhibition of gastric acid secretion by selective and nonselective anticholinergics. Gastroenterology 1984;86:361.

Higgins ST, Lamb RJ, Henningfield JE: Dose-dependent effects of atropine on behavioral and physiologic responses in humans. Pharmacol Biochem Behav 1989; 34:303.

Holtmann G, Küppers U, Singer MV: Telenzepine, a new M_1-receptor antagonist, is a more potent inhibitor of pentagastrin-stimulated gastric acid output than pirenzepine in dogs. Scand J Gastroenterol 1990; 25:293.

Hsu CK et al: Anticholinergic poisoning associated with herbal tea. Arch Intern Med 1995;155:2245.

Jimson weed poisoning—Texas, New York, and California, 1994. MMWR Morbid Mortal Wkly Rep 1995;44:41.

Kaplinsky R et al: Expanded followup of intravesical oxybutynin chloride use in children with neurogenic bladder. J Urol 1996;156:753.

Maesen FP et al: Tiotropium bromide, a new long-acting antimuscarinic bronchodilator: A pharmacodynamic study in patients with chronic obstructive pulmonary disease (COPD). Eur Respir J 1995;8:1506.

Mazur D et al: Clinical and urodynamic effects of propiverine in patients suffering from urgency and urge incontinence: A multicentre dose-optimizing study. Scand J Urol Nephrol 1995;29:289.

Melchiorre C et al: Antimuscarinic action of methoctramine, a new cardioselective M-2 muscarinic receptor antagonist, alone and in combination with atropine and gallamine. Europ J Pharmacol 1987; 144:117.

Mikolich JR, Paulson GW, Cross CJ: Acute anticholinergic syndrome due to Jimson seed ingestion: Clinical and laboratory observation in six cases. Ann Intern Med 1975;83:321.

Olson K: Mushrooms. In: *Poisoning & Drug Overdose*, 2nd ed. Olson K (editor). Appleton & Lange, 1994.

O'Rourke ST, Vanhoutte PM: Subtypes of muscarinic receptors on adrenergic nerves and vascular smooth muscle of the canine saphenous vein. J Pharmacol Exp Ther 1987;241:64.

Peters NL: Snipping the thread of life: Antimuscarinic side effects of medications in the elderly. Arch Intern Med 1989;149:2414.

Rascol O et al: Antivertigo medications and drug-induced vertigo: A pharmacological review. Drugs 1995; 50:777.

Ren J, Harty RF: Presynaptic muscarinic receptors modulate acetylcholine release from rat antral mucosal/submucosal nerves. Dig Dis Sci 1994;39: 1099.

Rusted JM, Warburton DM: The effects of scopolamine on working memory in healthy young volunteers. Psychopharmacology 1988;96:145.

Schneider F et al: Plasma and urine concentrations of atropine after the ingestion of cooked deadly nightshade berries. J Toxicol 1996;34:113.

Sigman HH, Poleski MH, Gillich A: Effects of pirenzepine on acute mucosal erosions, gastric acid, and mucosal blood flow in the spinal rat stomach. Digestion 1991;49:185.

Skorodin MS: Pharmacotherapy for asthma and chronic obstructive pulmonary disease. Current thinking, practices, and controversies. Arch Int Med 1993;153:814.

Smellie JM et al: Nocturnal enuresis: A placebo-controlled trial of two antidepressant drugs. Arch Dis Child 1996;75:62.

Teramoto S, Fukuchi Y: Improvements in exercise capacity and dyspnoea by inhaled anticholinergic drug in elderly patients with chronic obstructive pulmonary disease. Age Aging 1995;24:278.

Varssano D et al: The mydriatic effect of topical glycopyr-rolate. Graefes Arch Clin Exp Ophthalmol 1996;234:205.

Vybiral T et al: Effects of transdermal scopolamine on heart rate variability in normal subjects. Am J Cardiol 1990;65:604.

Wada Y et al: Comparison of the effects of various anticholinergic drugs on human isolated urinary bladder. Arch Int Pharmacodyn Ther 1995;330:76.

Wellstein A, Pitschner HF: Complex dose-response curves of atropine in man explained by different functions of M_1- and M_2-cholinoceptors. Naunyn Schmiedebergs Arch Pharmacol 1988;338:19.

Ganglion-Blocking Drugs

Fahmy NR: Nitroprusside vs. a nitroprusside-trimethaphan mixture for induced hypotension: Hemodynamic effects and cyanide release. Clin Pharmacol Ther 1985;70:264.

Gurney AM, Rang HP: The channel-blocking action of methonium compounds on rat submandibular ganglion cells. Br J Pharmacol 1984;82:623.

Rang HP: The action of ganglionic blocking drugs on the synaptic responses of rat submandibular ganglion cells. Br J Pharmacol 1982;75:151.

Treatment of Anticholinesterase Poisoning

Cannon JG et al: Structure-activity studies on a potent antagonist to organophosphate-induced toxicity. J Med Chem 1991;34:1582.

deKort WLAM, Kiestra SH, Sangster B: The use of atropine and oximes in organophosphate intoxications: A modified approach. Clin Toxicol 1988;26:199.

DeSilva HJ, Wijewickrema R, Senanayake N: Does pralidoxime affect outcome of management in acute organophosphorus poisoning? Lancet 1992;339:1136.

Eyer P et al: HLx 7 dimethanesulfonate, a potent bispyridinium-dioxime against anticholinesterases. Arch Toxicol 1992;66:603.

Farrar HC, Wells TG, Kearns GL: Use of continuous infusion of pralidoxime for treatment of organophosphate poisoning in children. J Pediatr 1990;116:658.

Leadbeater L, Inns RH, Rylands JM: Treatment of poisoning by soman. Fundam Appl Toxicol 1985;5:S225.

LeBlanc FN, Benson BE, Gilg AD: A severe organophosphate poisoning requiring the use of an atropine drip. Clin Toxicol 1986;24:69.

Sharabi Y et al: Survey of symptoms following intake of pyridostigmine during the Persian Gulf war. Israel J Med Sci 1991;27:656.

Solana RP et al: Evaluation of a two-drug combination pretreatment against organophosphorus exposure. Toxicol Appl Pharmacol 1990;102:421.

Adrenoceptor-Activating & Other Sympathomimetic Drugs

Brian B. Hoffman, MD

The sympathetic nervous system is an important regulator of the activities of organs such as the heart and peripheral vasculature, especially in responses to stress (see Chapter 6). The ultimate effects of sympathetic stimulation are mediated by release of norepinephrine from nerve terminals that serve to activate the adrenoceptors on postsynaptic sites. Also, in response to stress, the adrenal medulla releases epinephrine, which is transported in the blood to target tissues. Drugs that mimic the actions of epinephrine or norepinephrine—**sympathomimetic drugs**—would be expected to have a wide range of effects. An understanding of the pharmacology of these agents is thus a logical extension of what we know about the physiologic role of the catecholamines.

The Mode & Spectrum of Action of Sympathomimetic Drugs

Like the cholinomimetic drugs, the sympathomimetics can be grouped by mode of action and by the spectrum of receptors that they affect. Some of these drugs (eg, norepinephrine, epinephrine) act by a *direct* mode, ie, they directly interact with and activate adrenoceptors. Others act *indirectly;* their actions are dependent on the release of endogenous catecholamines. These indirect agents may have either of two different mechanisms: (1) displacement of stored catecholamines from the adrenergic nerve ending (eg, amphetamine and tyramine) or (2) inhibition of reuptake of catecholamines already released (eg, cocaine and tricyclic antidepressants). Both types of sympathomimetics, direct and indirect, ultimately cause activation of adrenoceptors, leading to some or all of the characteristic effects of catecholamines. The selectivity of different sympathomimetics for various types of adrenoceptors is discussed below.

I. BASIC PHARMACOLOGY OF SYMPATHOMIMETIC DRUGS

IDENTIFICATION OF ADRENOCEPTORS

The effort to understand the molecular mechanisms by which catecholamines act has a long and rich history. A great conceptual debt is owed to the work done by Langley and Ehrlich 75–100 years ago in putting forth the hypothesis that drugs have their effects by interacting with specific "receptive" substances. Ahlquist in 1948 rationalized a large body of observations by his conjecture that catecholamines acted via two principal receptors. He termed these receptors alpha and beta. Alpha receptors are those that exhibit the potency series epinephrine ≥ norepinephrine >> isoproterenol. Beta receptors have the potency series isoproterenol > epinephrine ≥ norepinephrine. Ahlquist's hypothesis was dramatically confirmed by the development of drugs that selectively antagonize beta receptors but not alpha receptors (see Chapter 10). More recent evidence suggests that alpha receptors comprise two major families. At present, therefore, it appears appropriate to classify adrenoceptors into three major groups, namely β, α_1, and α_2 receptors.

A. Beta Adrenoceptors: Soon after the demonstration of separate alpha and beta receptors, it was found that there are at least two *subtypes* of beta receptors, designated β_1 and β_2. Beta$_1$ and β_2 receptors are operationally defined by their affinities for epinephrine and norepinephrine: β_1 receptors have approximately equal affinity for epinephrine and norepinephrine, whereas β_2 receptors have a higher affinity for epinephrine than for norepinephrine. More recently, β_3 receptors have been identified as a novel and distinct third β adrenoceptor. Some of the properties of each of these receptor types are listed in Table 9–1.

B. Alpha Adrenoceptors: Following the demonstration of the beta subtypes, it was found that there are two major groups of alpha receptors, α_1 and α_2. These receptors were originally identified with antagonist drugs that distinguished between α_1 and α_2 receptors. For example, alpha adrenoceptors were identified in a variety of tissues by measuring the binding of radiolabeled antagonist compounds that are considered to have a high affinity for these receptors, eg, dihydroergocryptine (α_1 and α_2), prazosin (α_1), and yohimbine (α_2). These radioligands were used to measure the number of receptors in tissues and to determine the affinity (by displacement of the radiolabeled ligand) of other drugs that interact with the receptors.

The concept of subtypes *within* the α_1 group emerged out of pharmacologic experiments that indicated complex shapes of agonist dose-response curves of smooth muscle contraction in some tissues as well as differences in antagonist affinities in certain contractile responses. These experiments demonstrated the existence of two subtypes of α_1 receptor that could be distinguished on the basis of their reversible affinities for a variety of drugs and experimental compounds. A third α_1 receptor subtype has been identified by molecular cloning techniques. These α_1 receptors are termed α_{1A}, α_{1B}, and α_{1D} receptors. There is evidence that the α_{1A} receptor has splice vari-

ants. In addition, there is pharmacologic evidence suggesting that there may be a novel subtype of α_1 receptor with relatively low affinity for prazosin (the so-called α_{1L} receptor). A major current area of investigation is determining the importance of each of these various subtypes for mediating α_1 receptor responses in a variety of organs.

The hypothesis that there are subtypes of α_2 receptors similarly emerged from pharmacologic experiments and radioligand-binding assays. Human platelets appear to contain only the α_{2A} subtype. Clinically used drugs such as prazosin, chlorpromazine, yohimbine, and oxymetazoline have different affinities for α_{2A} and α_{2B} receptors. There is additional pharmacologic evidence supporting the existence of an α_{2C} receptor. Molecular cloning has identified three α_2 receptor proteins that are products of distinct genes.

C. Dopamine Receptors: The endogenous catecholamine dopamine produces a variety of biologic effects that are mediated by interactions with specific dopamine receptors (Table 9–1). These receptors are distinct from alpha and beta receptors and are particularly important in the brain (see Chapters 21 and 29) and in the splanchnic and renal vasculature. As with alpha and beta adrenoceptors, there is now considerable evidence for the existence of multiple forms of dopamine receptors. Pharmacologically distinct dopamine receptor subtypes, termed D_1 and D_2, have been known for some time. More recently, molecular cloning has identified several distinct genes encoding

Table 9–1. Adrenoceptor types and subtypes.

Receptor	Agonist	Antagonist	Effects	Gene on Chromosome
Alpha$_1$ type Alpha$_{1A}$ Alpha$_{1B}$ Alpha$_{1D}$	Phenylephrine, methoxamine	Prazosin, corynanthine WB4101, prazosin CEC (irreversible) WB4101	↑ IP$_3$, DAG common to all	 C5 C8 C20
Alpha$_2$ type Alpha$_{2A}$ Alpha$_{2B}$ Alpha$_{2C}$	Clonidine, BHT920 Oxymetazoline	Rauwolscine, yohimbine Prazosin Prazosin	↓ cAMP common to all ↓ cAMP; ↑ K$^+$ channels; ↓ Ca^{2+} channels ↓ cAMP; ↓ Ca^{2+} channels ↓ cAMP	 C10 C2 C4
Beta type Beta$_1$ Beta$_2$ Beta$_3$	Isoproterenol Dobutamine Procaterol, terbutaline BRL37344	Propranolol Betaxolol Butoxamine	↑ cAMP common to all ↑ cAMP ↑ cAMP ↑ cAMP	
Dopamine type D$_1$ D$_2$ D$_4$ D$_5$	Dopamine Fenoldopam Bromocriptine	 Clozapine	 ↑ cAMP ↓ cAMP; ↑ K$^+$ channels; ↑ Ca^{2+} channels ↓ cAMP ↑ cAMP	 C5 C11 C4

Key:	BRL37344	=	Sodium-4-(2-[2-hydroxy-{3-chlorophenyl}ethylamino]propyl)phenoxyacetate
	BHT920	=	6-Allyl-2-amino-5,6,7,8-tetrahydro-4H-thiazolo-[4,5-d]-azepine
	CEC	=	Chloroethylclonidine
	DAG	=	Diacylglycerol
	IP$_3$	=	Inositol trisphophate
	WB4101	=	N-[2-(2,6-dimethoxyphenoxy)ethyl]-2,3-dihydro-1,4-benzodioxan-2-methanamine

each of these subtypes. Further complexity occurs because of the presence of introns within the coding region of the D_2-like receptors, which allows for alternative splicing of the exons in this major subtype. In addition, a restriction length polymorphism has been associated with a human D_2-like receptor (Gingrich et al, 1993). The terminology of the various subtypes is particularly unsettled, with the alternative series names D_1, D_2, D_3, D_4, D_5 or D_{1A}, D_{2A}, D_{2C}, D_{1B} being used. (See 1996 Receptor Nomenclature Supplement.)

Receptor Selectivity

Examples of clinically useful sympathomimetic agonists that are relatively selective for α_1-, α_2-, and β-adrenoceptor subgroups are compared with some nonselective agents in Table 9–2. Selectivity means that a drug may preferentially bind to one subgroup of receptors at concentrations too low to interact with another subgroup. For example, norepinephrine preferentially activates β_1 receptors as compared to β_2 receptors. However, selectivity is not usually absolute, and at higher concentrations related classes of receptor may also interact with the drug. As a result, the "numeric" subclassification of adrenoceptors is clinically important only for drugs that have relatively marked selectivity.

Nomenclature

The nomenclature for adrenoceptor subtypes is confusing because there is no generally agreed upon formal system; different authors may use similar names for talking about what appear to be quite different receptors. Consequently, caution is advised in reading research reports.

The exact number of adrenoceptor subtypes that are actually expressed in human tissues is uncertain, but expression of subtypes has been demonstrated in tissues where the physiologic or pharmacologic importance of the subtype is not yet known. These results

Table 9–2. Relative selectivity of adrenoceptor agonists.

	Relative Receptor Affinities
Alpha agonists	
Phenylephrine, methoxamine	$\alpha_1 > \alpha_2 >>>>> \beta$
Clonidine, methylnorepinephrine	$\alpha_2 > \alpha_1 >>>>> \beta$
Mixed alpha and beta agonists	
Norepinephrine	$\alpha_1 = \alpha_2; \beta_1 >>\beta_2$
Epinephrine	$\alpha_1 = \alpha_2; \beta_1 = \beta_2$
Beta agonists	
Dobutamine[1]	$\beta_1 > \beta_2 >>>> \alpha$
Isoproterenol	$\beta_1 = \beta_2 >>>> \alpha$
Terbutaline, metaproterenol,	$\beta_2 >> \beta_1 >>>> \alpha$
albuterol, ritodrine	
Dopamine agonists	
Dopamine	$D_1 = D_2 >> \beta >> \alpha$

[1]See text.

suggest the possibility of designing novel drugs to exploit the expression of a particular receptor subtype in a single target tissue. For example, determining which blood vessels express which subtypes of α_1 and α_2 receptors could lead to design of drugs having selectivity for certain vascular beds such as the splanchnic or coronary vessels. Similarly, there is enormous interest in the α_1 receptor subtypes that mediate pharmacologic responses in the human prostate.

MOLECULAR MECHANISMS OF SYMPATHOMIMETIC ACTION

The effects of catecholamines are mediated by cell surface receptors. As described in Chapter 2, these receptors are coupled by G proteins to the various effector proteins whose activities are regulated by those receptors. Each G protein is a heterotrimer consisting of alpha, beta, and gamma subunits. G proteins are classified on the basis of their distinctive alpha subunits. G proteins of particular importance for adrenoceptor function include G_s, the stimulatory G protein of adenylyl cyclase; G_i, the inhibitory G protein of adenylyl cyclase; and G_q, the protein coupling alpha receptors to phospholipase C. The activation of G protein-coupled receptors by catecholamines promotes the dissociation of GDP from the alpha subunit of the appropriate G protein. GTP then binds to this G protein, and the alpha subunit dissociates from the beta-gamma unit. The activated GTP-bound alpha subunit then regulates the activity of its effector. Some effectors of adrenoceptor-activated alpha subunits include adenylyl cyclase, cGMP phosphodiesterase, phospholipase C, and ion channels. The alpha subunit is inactivated by hydrolysis of the bound GTP to GDP and P_i, and the subsequent reassociation of the alpha subunit with the beta-gamma subunit. The beta-gamma subunit may have additional independent effects, acting on a variety of effectors such as ion channels and enzymes.

Receptor Types

A. Alpha Receptors: The mechanism of activation of alpha receptors by catecholamines is not as well understood as that of beta receptors. Typically, α_1 receptors can be shown to stimulate polyphosphoinositide hydrolysis, leading to the formation of inositol 1,4,5-trisphosphate and diacylglycerol.

In certain smooth muscle cells, α_1-receptor activation leads to an influx of calcium across the membrane. Alpha$_1$-receptor activation in many cells leads to the breakdown of polyphosphoinositides into inositol trisphosphate and diacylglycerol (Figure 9–1). G proteins in the G_q family couple α_1 receptors to phospholipase C. Inositol 1,4,5-trisphosphate (IP_3) promotes the release of sequestered Ca^{2+} from intracellular stores, which increases the cytoplasmic

[handwritten annotations on figure:]
$\alpha_1 \rightarrow \uparrow Ca^{+2}$ via $IP_3 + DAG$

$\alpha_2 \dashv\!\!\dashv AC, \downarrow cAMP$ via G_i also $\uparrow K^+$ chan

Figure 9–1. Activation of α_1 responses. Stimulation of α_1 receptors by catecholamines leads to the activation of a G_q coupling protein. The α subunit of this G protein activates the effector, phospholipase C, which leads to the release of IP_3 (inositol 1,4,5-trisphosphate) and DAG (diacylglycerol) from phosphatidylinositol 4,5-bisphosphate (PtdIns 4, 5-P_2). IP_3 stimulates the release of sequestered stores of calcium, leading to an increased concentration of cytoplasmic Ca^{2+}. Ca^{2+} may then activate Ca^{2+}-dependent protein kinases, which in turn phosphorylate their substrates. DAG activates protein kinase C. See text for additional effects of α_1 receptor activation.

concentration of free Ca^{2+} and the activation of various calcium-dependent protein kinases. Inositol 1,4,5-trisphosphate is sequentially dephosphorylated, which ultimately leads to the formation of free inositol. However, several other phosphorylated isomers of inositol may be produced and accumulate owing to the metabolism of 1,4,5-trisphosphate; the biologic significance of these other molecules is unclear. Diacylglycerol activates protein kinase C. In addition, recent evidence indicates that α_1 receptors activate signal transduction pathways that have traditionally been associated with peptide growth factors. For example, α_1 receptors have been found to activate mitogen-activated kinases (MAP kinases) and polyphosphoinositol-3-kinase (PI-3-kinase). These pathways may have importance for the α_1 receptor-mediated stimulation of cell growth. The physiologic significance of this "cross talk" between major signaling pathways remains to be determined.

Alpha$_2$ receptors inhibit adenylyl cyclase activity and cause intracellular cAMP levels to decrease. While this effect has been well documented, it is not clear whether this action is the exclusive or major expression of α_2-receptor activation. Thus, α_2-receptor agonists cause platelet aggregation and a decrease in platelet cAMP levels, but it is not clear that aggregation is the result of the decrease in cAMP. Alpha$_2$ inhibition of adenylyl cyclase occurs through the mediation of the inhibitory regulatory protein, G_i, that couples the α_2 receptor to the inhibition of adenylyl cyclase (Figure 9–2). How the activation of G_i leads

to the inhibition of adenylyl cyclase is unclear. Two major possibilities are (1) that the free beta-gamma units of G_i combine with the free alpha subunits of G_s, rendering them inactive; and (2) that the alpha subunit of G_i directly inhibits adenylyl cyclase activity. Some evidence favors both of these possible mechanisms. In addition, some of the effects of α_2 adrenoceptors are independent of their ability to inhibit adenylyl cyclase; mechanisms include activation of potassium channels and closing of calcium channels. These actions may be mediated by G proteins of the G_i/G_o class.

B. Beta Receptors: The mechanism of action of beta agonists has been studied in considerable detail. Activation of all three receptor subtypes (β_1, β_2, and β_3) results in activation of adenylyl cyclase and increased conversion of ATP to cAMP (Figure 9–2). Activation of the cyclase enzyme is mediated by the stimulatory coupling protein G_s. cAMP is the major second messenger of β-receptor activation. For example, in the liver of many species, β-receptor activation increases cAMP synthesis, which leads to a cascade of events culminating in the activation of glycogen phosphorylase. In the heart, β-receptor activation increases the influx of calcium across the cell membrane and its sequestration inside the cell. Beta-receptor activation also promotes the relaxation of smooth muscle. While the mechanism is uncertain, it may involve the phosphorylation of myosin light chain kinase to an inactive form (see Figure 12–1). Beta adrenoceptors may activate voltage-sensitive calcium

[handwritten annotation at bottom:]
$\beta \rightarrow G_s \rightarrow \uparrow cAMP$

Handwritten annotations:

$B \rightarrow \uparrow cAMP$ via Gs

$\alpha_2 \dashv\dashv cAMP$ via G_i

Figure 9–2. Activation and inhibition of adenylyl cyclase by agonists that bind to catecholamine receptors. Binding to beta adrenoceptors stimulates adenylyl cyclase by activating the stimulatory G protein, G_s, which leads to the dissociation of its alpha subunit charged with GTP. This α_s subunit directly activates adenylyl cyclase, resulting in an increased rate of synthesis of cAMP. Alpha$_2$ adrenoceptor ligands inhibit adenylyl cyclase by causing dissociation of the inhibitory G protein, G_i, into its subunits; ie, an α_i subunit charged with GTP and a beta-gamma unit. The mechanism by which these subunits inhibit adenylyl cyclase is uncertain. cAMP binds to the regulatory subunit (R) of cAMP-dependent protein kinase, leading to the liberation of active catalytic subunits (C) that phosphorylate specific protein substrates and modify their activity. These catalytic units also phosphorylate the cAMP response element binding protein (CREB), which modifies gene expression.

channels in the heart independently of changes in cAMP concentration via G_s-mediated enhancement.

C. Dopamine Receptors: The D_1 receptor is typically associated with the stimulation of adenylyl cyclase (Table 9–1); for example, D_1-receptor-induced smooth muscle relaxation is presumably due to cAMP accumulation in the smooth muscle of those vascular beds where dopamine is a vasodilator. D_2 receptors have been found to inhibit adenylyl cyclase activity, open potassium channels, and decrease calcium influx.

Handwritten: $D_1 \rightarrow \uparrow cAMP$ ($\rightarrow$ vasodil) ; $D_2 \rightarrow \downarrow cAMP$

Receptor Regulation

Responses mediated by adrenoceptors are not fixed and static. The number and function of adrenoceptors on the cell surface and their responses may be regulated by catecholamines themselves, other hormones and drugs, age, and a number of disease states. These changes may modify the magnitude of a tissue's physiologic response to catecholamines. One of the best-studied examples of receptor regulation is the **desensitization** of adrenoceptors that may occur after exposure to catecholamines and other sympatho-

mimetic drugs. After a cell or tissue has been exposed for a period of time to an agonist, that tissue often becomes less responsive to further stimulation by that agent. Other terms such as tolerance, refractoriness, and tachyphylaxis have also been used to denote desensitization. This process has considerable clinical significance because it may limit the therapeutic response to sympathomimetic agents.

The mechanisms involved in desensitization of cells to responses mediated by beta adrenoceptors have been extensively studied. There appear to be at least three distinct mechanisms. In some cells, desensitization is caused by receptor sequestration (a rapid and transient event wherein the receptors are made temporarily unavailable for activation by agonists). A second process, down-regulation (ie, disappearance of the receptors from the cell), may take place by the action of enzymes on the receptor or by decreased synthesis. Third, phosphorylation of the receptor on the cytoplasmic side by protein kinase A or β-adrenergic receptor kinase (βARK) may impair coupling of beta adrenoceptors with G_s. βARK is a specific example of a large class of related proteins that phosphorylate G protein-coupled receptors. The phosphorylation induced by βARK may disrupt coupling to G_s, in part by facilitating association of β-arrestin, a 48 kDa protein, with phosphorylated beta adrenoceptors (Figure 2–15).

CHEMISTRY & PHARMACOKINETICS OF SYMPATHOMIMETIC DRUGS

Phenylethylamine may be considered the parent compound from which sympathomimetic drugs are derived (Figure 9–3). This compound consists of a benzene ring with an ethylamine side chain. Substitutions may be made (1) on the terminal amino group, (2) on the benzene ring, and (3) on the alpha or beta carbons. Substitution by –OH groups at the 3 and 4 positions yields sympathomimetic drugs collectively known as catecholamines. The effects of modification of phenylethylamine are to change the affinity of the drugs for alpha and beta receptors as well as to influence the intrinsic ability to activate the receptors. In addition, chemical structure determines the pharmacokinetic properties of these molecules. Sympathomimetic drugs may activate both alpha and beta receptors; however, the relative alpha-receptor versus beta-receptor activity spans the range from almost pure alpha activity (methoxamine) to almost pure beta activity (isoproterenol).

A. Substitution on the Amino Group: Increasing the size of alkyl substituents on the amino group tends to increase beta-receptor activity. For example, methyl substitution on norepinephrine, yielding epinephrine, enhances activity at β_2 receptors. Beta activity is further enhanced with isopropyl substitution at the amino nitrogen (isoproterenol). Beta$_2$-selective agonists generally require a large amino substituent group. The larger the substituent on the amino group, the lower the activity at alpha receptors; eg, isoproterenol is very weak at alpha receptors.

B. Substitution on the Benzene Ring: Maximal alpha and beta activity are found with catecholamines (drugs having –OH groups at the 3 and 4 positions). The absence of one or the other of these groups, particularly the hydroxyl at C_3, without other substitutions on the ring may dramatically reduce the potency of the drugs. For example, phenylephrine (Figure 9–4) is much less potent than epinephrine; indeed, alpha activity is decreased about 100-fold and beta activity is almost negligible except at very high concentrations. However, catecholamines are subject to inactivation by catechol-O-methyltransferase (COMT), an enzyme found in gut and liver (see Chapter 6). Therefore, absence of one or both –OH groups on the phenyl ring increases the bioavailability after oral administration and prolongs the duration of action. Furthermore, absence of ring –OH groups increases the distribution of the molecule to the central nervous system. For example, ephedrine and amphetamine (Figure 9–4) are orally active, have a prolonged duration of action, and produce central nervous system effects not observed with the catecholamines.

C. Substitution on the Alpha Carbon: Substitutions at the alpha carbon block oxidation by

Figure 9–3. Phenylethylamine and some important catecholamines. Catechol is shown for reference.

[handwritten margin note: substit @ α c block oxid by MAO → α methyl compounds displace catechol from storage sites → indirect sympathomim]

Figure 9–4. Some examples of noncatecholamine sympathomimetic drugs.

[handwritten note next to Ephedrine: orally active, into CNS]

monoamine oxidase (MAO) and prolong the action of such drugs, particularly the noncatecholamines. Ephedrine and amphetamine are examples of alpha-substituted compounds (Figure 9–4). Alpha-methyl compounds are also called phenylisopropylamines. In addition to their resistance to oxidation by MAO, phenylisopropylamines have an enhanced ability to displace catecholamines from storage sites in noradrenergic nerves. Therefore, at least a portion of their activity is dependent upon the presence of normal norepinephrine stores in the body; they are indirectly acting sympathomimetics.

D. Substitution on the Beta Carbon: Direct-acting agonists typically have a beta-hydroxyl group, though dopamine does not. In addition to activating adrenoceptors, this hydroxyl group may be important for storage of sympathomimetic amines in neural vesicles.

ORGAN SYSTEM EFFECTS OF SYMPATHOMIMETIC DRUGS

General outlines of the cellular actions of sympathomimetics are presented in Tables 6–3 and 9–3. The net effect of a given drug in the intact organism depends on its relative receptor affinity (alpha or beta), intrinsic activity, and the compensatory reflexes evoked by its direct actions.

Cardiovascular System

A. Blood Vessels: Vascular smooth muscle tone is regulated by adrenoceptors; consequently, catecholamines are important in controlling peripheral vascular resistance and venous capacitance. Alpha receptors increase arterial resistance, whereas β_2 receptors promote smooth muscle relaxation. There are major differences in receptor types in the various vascular beds (Table 9–4). The skin vessels have predominantly alpha receptors and constrict in the presence of epinephrine and norepinephrine, as do the splanchnic vessels. Vessels in skeletal muscle may

Table 9–3. Distribution of adrenoceptor subtypes.

Type	Tissue	Actions
Alpha$_1$	Most vascular smooth muscle (innervated)	Contraction
	Pupillary dilator muscle	Contraction (dilates pupil)
	Pilomotor smooth muscle	Erects hair
	Rat liver	Glycogenolysis
	Heart	Increases force of contraction
Alpha$_2$	Postsynaptic CNS adrenoceptors	Probably multiple
	Platelets	Aggregation
	Adrenergic and cholinergic nerve terminals	Inhibition of transmitter release
	Some vascular smooth muscle	Contraction
	Fat cells	Inhibition of lipolysis
Beta$_1$	Heart	Increases force and rate of contraction
Beta$_2$	Respiratory, uterine, and vascular smooth muscle	Promotes smooth muscle relaxation
	Skeletal muscle	Promotes potassium uptake
	Human liver	Activates glycogenolysis
Beta$_3$	Fat cells	Activates lipolysis
D$_1$	Smooth muscle	Dilates renal blood vessels
D$_2$	Nerve endings	Modulates transmitter release

Table 9–4. Cardiovascular response to sympathomimetic amines.[1]

	Phenyl-ephrine	Epi-nephrine	Isopro-terenol
Vascular resistance (tone)			
Cutaneous, mucous membranes (α)	↑↑	↑↑	0
Skeletal muscle (β_2, α)	↑	↓ or ↑	↓↓
Renal (α, D_1)	↑	↑	↓
Splanchnic (α)	↑↑	↓ or ↑[2]	↓
Total peripheral resistance	↑↑↑	↓ or ↑[2]	↓↓
Venous tone	↑	↑	↓
Cardiac			
Contractility (β_1)	0 or ↑	↑↑↑	↑↑↑
Heart rate (predominantly β_1)	↓↓ (vagal reflex)	↑ or ↓	↑↑↑
Stroke volume	0, ↓, ↑	↑	↑
Cardiac output	↓	↑	↑↑
Blood pressure			
Mean	↑↑	↑	↓
Diastolic	↑↑	↓ or ↑[2]	↓↓
Systolic	↑↑	↑↑	0 or ↓
Pulse pressure	0	↑↑	↑↑

[1]↑ = increase; ↓ = decrease; 0 = no change.
[2]Small doses decrease, large doses increase.

constrict or dilate depending on whether alpha or beta receptors are activated. Thus, the overall effects of a sympathomimetic drug on blood vessels depend on the relative activities of that drug at alpha and beta receptors and the anatomic sites of the vessels affected. In addition, D_1 receptors promote vasodilation of renal, splanchnic, coronary, and cerebral arteries. Activation of the D_1 receptors in the renal vasculature may play a major role in the natriuresis induced by pharmacologic administration of dopamine.

B. Heart: Direct effects on the heart are determined largely by β_1 receptors, though β_2 and to a lesser extent alpha receptors are also involved. Beta-receptor activation results in increased calcium influx in cardiac cells. This has both electrical (Figure 9–5) and mechanical consequences. Pacemaker activity, both normal (sinoatrial node) and abnormal (eg, Purkinje fibers), is increased (positive chronotropic effect). Conduction velocity in the atrioventricular node is increased, and the refractory period is decreased. Intrinsic contractility is increased (positive inotropic effect), and relaxation is accelerated. As a result, the twitch response of isolated cardiac muscle is increased in tension but abbreviated in duration. In the intact heart, intraventricular pressure rises and falls more rapidly, and ejection time is decreased. These direct effects are easily demonstrated in the absence of reflexes evoked by changes in blood pressure, eg, in isolated myocardial preparations and in patients with ganglionic blockade. In the presence of normal reflex activity, the direct effects on heart rate may be

dominated by a reflex response to blood pressure changes.

C. Blood Pressure: The effects of sympathomimetic drugs on blood pressure can be explained on the basis of their effects on the heart, the peripheral vascular resistance, and the venous return (see Figure 6–7 and Table 9–4). A relatively pure alpha agonist such as phenylephrine increases peripheral arterial resistance and decreases venous capacitance. The enhanced arterial resistance usually leads to a marked rise in blood pressure (Figure 9–6). In the presence of normal cardiovascular reflexes, the rise in blood pressure elicits a baroreceptor-mediated increase in vagal tone with slowing of heart rate, which may be dramatic. However, cardiac output may not diminish in proportion to this reduction in rate, since increased venous return may increase stroke volume; furthermore, direct alpha-adrenoceptor stimulation of the heart may have a modest positive inotropic action. While these are the expected effects of pure alpha agonists in normal subjects, their use in hypotensive patients usually does not lead to brisk reflex responses because in this situation blood pressure is returning to normal, not exceeding normal.

The blood pressure response to a pure beta-adrenoceptor agonist is quite different. Stimulation of beta receptors in the heart increases cardiac output. A relatively pure beta agonist such as isoproterenol also decreases peripheral resistance by dilating certain vascular beds (Table 9–4). The net effect is to maintain or slightly increase systolic pressure while permitting a fall in diastolic pressure owing to enhanced diastolic runoff (Figure 9–6). The actions of drugs

Figure 9–5. Effect of epinephrine on the transmembrane potential of a pacemaker cell in the frog heart. The arrowed trace was recorded after the addition of epinephrine. Note the increased slope of diastolic depolarization and decreased interval between action potentials. This pacemaker acceleration is typical of β_1-stimulant drugs. (Modified and reproduced, with permission, from Brown H, Giles W, Noble S: Membrane currents underlying rhythmic activity in frog sinus venosus. In: *The Sinus Node: Structure, Function, and Clinical Relevance.* Bonke FIM [editor]. Martinus Nijhoff, 1978.)

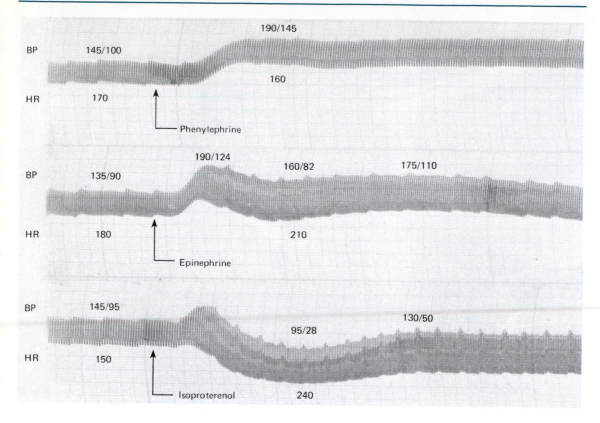

Figure 9–6. Effects of an alpha-selective (phenylephrine), beta-selective (isoproterenol), and nonselective (epinephrine) sympathomimetic, given as an intravenous bolus injection to a dog. (BP, blood pressure; HR, heart rate.) Reflexes are blunted but not eliminated in this anesthetized animal.

with both alpha and beta effects (eg, epinephrine and norepinephrine) are discussed below.

Eye

The radial pupillary dilator muscle of the iris contains alpha receptors; activation by drugs such as phenylephrine causes mydriasis (Figure 6–9). Alpha and beta stimulants also have important effects on intraocular pressure. Present evidence suggests that alpha agonists increase the outflow of aqueous humor from the eye, while beta antagonists decrease the production of aqueous humor. These effects are important in the treatment of glaucoma (Chapter 10), a leading cause of blindness. Beta stimulants relax the ciliary muscle to a minor degree, causing an insignificant decrease in accommodation.

Respiratory Tract

Bronchial smooth muscle contains β_2 receptors that cause relaxation. Activation of these receptors thus results in bronchodilation (see Chapter 19 and Table 9–3). The blood vessels of the upper respiratory tract mucosa contain α_1 receptors; the decongestant action of adrenoceptor stimulants is clinically useful (see Clinical Pharmacology).

Gastrointestinal Tract

Relaxation of gastrointestinal smooth muscle can be brought about by both alpha- and beta-stimulant agents. Beta receptors appear to be located directly on the smooth muscle cells and mediate relaxation via hyperpolarization and decreased spike activity in these cells. Alpha stimulants, especially α_2-selective agonists, decrease muscle activity *indirectly* by pre-synaptically reducing the release of acetylcholine and possibly other stimulants within the enteric nervous system (Chapter 6). The alpha-receptor-mediated response is probably of greater pharmacologic significance than the beta-stimulant response. Alpha$_2$ receptors may also decrease salt and water flux into the lumen of the intestine.

Genitourinary Tract

The human uterus contains alpha and β_2 receptors. The fact that the beta receptors mediate relaxation can be clinically useful in pregnancy (see Clinical Pharmacology). The bladder base, urethral sphincter, and prostate contain alpha receptors that mediate contraction and therefore promote urinary continence. The specific subtype of α_1 receptor involved in mediating constriction of the bladder base and prostate is uncertain and the subject of active investigation. The β_2 receptors of the bladder wall mediate relaxation. Ejaculation depends upon normal alpha-receptor (and possibly purinergic receptor) activation in the ductus deferens, seminal vesicles, and prostate. The detumescence of erectile tissue that normally follows ejaculation is also brought about by norepinephrine (and possibly neuropeptide Y) released from sympathetic nerves (deGroat et al, 1990). Alpha activation appears to have a similar detumescent effect on erectile tissue in female animals.

Exocrine Glands

The salivary glands contain adrenoceptors that regulate the secretion of amylase and water. However, certain sympathomimetic drugs, eg, clonidine, produce symptoms of dry mouth. The mechanism of this effect is uncertain; it is likely that central nervous system effects are responsible, though other (peripheral) effects may contribute.

The apocrine sweat glands, located on the palms of the hands and a few other areas, respond to adrenoceptor stimulants with increased sweat production. These are the apocrine nonthermoregulatory glands usually associated with psychologic stress. (The diffusely distributed thermoregulatory eccrine sweat glands are regulated by *sympathetic cholinergic* postganglionic nerves that activate muscarinic cholinoceptors; see Chapter 6.)

Metabolic Effects

Sympathomimetic drugs have important effects on intermediary metabolism. Activation of beta adrenoceptors in fat cells leads to increased lipolysis. The beta receptors mediating this effect have characteristics of β_3 adrenoceptors. There is considerable interest in developing β_3 receptor-selective agonists, which could be useful in some metabolic disorders. Human lipocytes also contain α_2 receptors that inhibit lipolysis by decreasing intracellular cAMP. Sympathomimetic drugs enhance glycogenolysis in the liver, which leads to increased glucose release into the circulation. In the human liver, the effects of catecholamines are probably mediated mainly by beta receptors, though α_1 receptors may also play a role. Catecholamines in high concentrations may also cause metabolic acidosis. Activation of β_2 adrenoceptors by endogenous epinephrine or by sympathomimetic drugs promotes the uptake of potassium into cells, leading to a fall in extracellular potassium. This may lead to a fall in the plasma potassium concentration during stress or protect against a rise in plasma potassium during exercise. Blockade of these receptors may accentuate the rise in plasma potassium that occurs during exercise.

Effects on Endocrine & Other Function

Catecholamines are important endogenous regulators of hormone secretion from a number of glands. Insulin secretion is stimulated by beta receptors and inhibited by α_2 receptors. Similarly, renin secretion is stimulated by β_1 and inhibited by α_2 receptors; indeed, beta-receptor antagonist drugs may lower plasma renin at least in part by this mechanism. Adrenoceptors also modulate the secretion of parathyroid hormone, calcitonin, thyroxine, and gastrin; however, the physiologic significance of these control mechanisms is unclear. In high concentrations, epinephrine and related agents cause leukocytosis, in part by promoting demargination of white blood cells sequestered away from the general circulation.

Effects on the Central Nervous System

The action of sympathomimetics on the central nervous system varies dramatically, depending on their ability to cross the blood-brain barrier. The catecholamines are almost completely excluded by this barrier, and subjective central nervous system effects are noted only at the highest rates of infusion. These effects have been described as ranging from "nervousness" to a "feeling of impending disaster," sensations that are universally regarded as undesirable. Furthermore, peripheral effects of β adrenoceptor agonists such as tachycardia and tremor are similar to the somatic manifestations of anxiety. In contrast, noncatecholamines with indirect actions, such as the amphetamine agents, which easily enter the central nervous system from the circulation, produce qualitatively very different central nervous system effects. These actions vary from mild alerting, with improved attention to boring tasks; through elevation of mood, insomnia, euphoria, and anorexia; to psychotic behavior at the very highest levels. These effects are not readily assigned to either alpha- or beta-mediated actions and probably represent enhancement of dopamine-mediated processes in the central nervous system.

SPECIFIC SYMPATHOMIMETIC DRUGS

Catecholamines

Epinephrine (adrenaline) is a very potent vasoconstrictor and cardiac stimulant. The rise in systolic blood pressure that occurs after epinephrine release or administration is caused by its positive inotropic and chronotropic actions on the heart (predominantly β_1 receptors) and the vasoconstriction induced in many vascular beds (alpha receptors). Epinephrine also activates β_2 receptors in some vessels (eg, skeletal muscle blood vessels), leading to their dilation. Consequently, total peripheral resistance may actually fall, explaining the fall in diastolic pressure that is sometimes seen with epinephrine injection (Figure 9–6).

Norepinephrine (levarterenol, noradrenaline) and epinephrine have similar effects on β_1 receptors in the

NE→ ↑ periph resist + bp

heart and similar potency at alpha receptors. Norepinephrine has relatively little effect on β_2 receptors. Consequently, norepinephrine increases peripheral resistance and both diastolic and systolic blood pressure. Compensatory vagal reflexes tend to overcome the direct positive chronotropic effects of norepinephrine; however, the positive inotropic effects on the heart are maintained.

Isoproterenol (isoprenaline) is an extremely potent beta-receptor agonist, having little effect on alpha receptors. The drug has positive chronotropic and inotropic actions; because isoproterenol activates beta receptors almost exclusively, it is a potent vasodilator. These actions lead to a marked increase in cardiac output associated with a fall in diastolic and mean arterial pressure and a lesser decrease or a slight increase in systolic pressure (Table 9–4 and Figure 9–6).

Dopamine, the immediate metabolic precursor of norepinephrine, activates D_1 receptors in several vascular beds, which leads to vasodilation. The effect this has on renal blood flow may be of considerable clinical value. The activation of presynaptic D_2 receptors, which suppress norepinephrine release, contributes to these effects to an unknown extent. In addition, dopamine activates β_1 receptors in the heart. At low doses it has relatively little effect on overall peripheral resistance. However, at higher rates of infusion, dopamine activates vascular alpha receptors, leading to vasoconstriction. Thus, high concentrations may mimic the actions of epinephrine.

Ibopamine is an orally active butyric acid ester of methyldopamine (also called epinine). The ester linkage is hydrolyzed by nonspecific esterases in the blood to yield epinine, which has pharmacologic effects similar to those of dopamine. This compound is presently in clinical trial; its usefulness is not yet clear, and the long-term effects are unknown.

Dobutamine is a relatively β_1-selective synthetic catecholamine. As discussed below, dobutamine also activates α_1 receptors.

Other Sympathomimetics

These agents are of interest because of pharmacokinetic features (oral activity, distribution to the central nervous system) or because of relative selectivity for specific receptor subclasses.

Phenylephrine was previously described as an example of a relatively pure alpha agonist (Table 9–2). It acts directly on the receptors. Because it is not a catechol derivative (Figure 9–4), it is not inactivated by COMT and has a much longer duration of action than the catecholamines. It is an effective mydriatic and decongestant and can be used to raise the blood pressure (Figure 9–6).

Methoxamine acts pharmacologically like phenylephrine, since it is predominantly a direct-acting $alpha_1$-receptor agonist. It may cause a prolonged

increase in blood pressure due to vasoconstriction; it also causes a vagally mediated bradycardia. Methoxamine is available for parenteral use, but clinical applications are rare and limited to hypotensive states. **Midodrine,** the *N*-acetamide derivative of methoxamine, has recently been introduced and approved for use in patients with disabling chronic orthostatic hypotension. It is active by the oral route.

Ephedrine occurs in various plants and has been used in China for over 2000 years; it was introduced into Western medicine approximately 70 years ago as the first orally active sympathomimetic drug. Because it is a noncatechol phenylisopropylamine (Figure 9–4), it has high bioavailability and a long duration of action. As is the case with many other phenylisopropylamines, a significant fraction of the drug is excreted unchanged in the urine. Since it is a weak base, its excretion can be accelerated by acidification of the urine.

Ephedrine acts primarily through the release of stored catecholamines; in addition, it has some direct actions on adrenoceptors. It is nonselective and mimics epinephrine in its spectrum of effects. Because it gains access to the central nervous system, it is a mild stimulant.

Clinically, ephedrine is utilized when a prolonged duration of effect is desired, particularly after oral administration. The main applications are as a nasal decongestant and as a pressor agent. Pseudoephedrine, one of the four ephedrine enantiomers, is available over-the-counter as a component of many decongestant mixtures. It was recently recommended for use in stress incontinence in women.

Xylometazoline and **oxymetazoline** are direct-acting alpha agonists. These drugs have been used as topical decongestants because of their ability to promote constriction of the nasal mucosa. When taken in large doses, oxymetazoline may cause hypotension, presumably because of a central clonidine-like effect (Chapter 11). (As noted in Table 9–1, oxymetazoline has significant affinity for alpha$_{2A}$ receptors.)

Amphetamine is a phenylisopropylamine (Figure 9–4) that is important chiefly because of its use and misuse as a central nervous system stimulant (see Chapter 32). Its pharmacokinetics are similar to those of ephedrine, but amphetamine enters the central nervous system even more readily and has a much more marked stimulant effect on mood and alertness and a depressant effect on appetite. Its peripheral actions are mediated primarily through the release of catecholamines. **Methamphetamine** (*N*-methylamphetamine) is very similar to amphetamine with an even higher ratio of central to peripheral actions. **Phenmetrazine** (see Figure 31–1) is a variant phenylisopropylamine with amphetamine-like effects. It has been promoted as an anorexiant and is also a popular drug of abuse. **Methylphenidate** and **pemoline** are amphetamine variants whose major pharmacologic effects and abuse potential are similar to those of amphetamine. Amphetamine-like drugs appear to have efficacy in some children with attention deficit hyper-activity disorder (see Clinical Pharmacology). **Phenylpropanolamine** is a sympathomimetic drug with weak effects on mood that is available over-the-counter in numerous weight reduction medications. Though apparently safe in recommended dosage, it has been associated with significant rises in blood pressure and target organ damage in case reports of persons ingesting large doses. There is no evidence that treatment of obesity with these drugs leads to weight loss that extends beyond the course of treatment (Bray, 1993).

Receptor-Selective Sympathomimetic Drugs

Alpha$_2$-selective agonists have an important ability to decrease blood pressure through actions in the central nervous system even though local application may cause vasoconstriction. Such drugs (eg, clonidine, methyldopa, guanfacine, guanabenz) are useful in the treatment of hypertension (and some other conditions) and are discussed in Chapter 11.

Beta-selective agonists are very important because of the separation of β_1 and β_2 effects that has been achieved (Table 9–2). Although this separation is incomplete, it is sufficient to reduce adverse effects in several clinical applications.

Beta$_1$-selective agents include dobutamine and a partial agonist, prenalterol (Figure 9–7). Because they are less effective in activating vasodilator β_2 receptors, they may increase cardiac output with less reflex tachycardia than occurs with nonselective beta agonists such as isoproterenol. Dobutamine consists of two isomers, administered as a racemic mixture. The (+) isomer is a potent beta$_1$ agonist and an α_1 receptor antagonist. The (–) isomer is a potent α_1 agonist, capable of causing significant vasoconstriction when given alone. This action tends to reduce vasodilation and may also contribute to the positive inotropic action caused by the isomer with predominantly beta-receptor activity. A major limitation with these drugs—as with other direct-acting sympathomimetic agents—is that tolerance to their effects may develop with prolonged use.

Beta$_2$-selective agents have achieved an important place in the treatment of asthma and are discussed in Chapter 19. An additional application is as uterine relaxants in premature labor (ritodrine; see below). Some examples of drugs currently in use are shown in Figures 9–7 and 20–6; many more are available or under investigation.

Special Sympathomimetics

Cocaine is a local anesthetic with a peripheral sympathomimetic action that results from inhibition of transmitter reuptake at noradrenergic synapses (see Chapter 6). It readily enters the central nervous system and produces an amphetamine-like effect that is shorter lasting and more intense. The major action of cocaine in the central nervous system is to inhibit dopamine reuptake into neurons in the "pleasure centers" of the brain. These properties and the fact that it can be smoked, "snorted," or injected for rapid onset of effect have made it a very heavily abused drug (see Chapter 32).

Tyramine (see Figure 6–5) is a normal by-product of tyrosine metabolism in the body and is also found in high concentrations in fermented foods such as cheese (Table 9–5). It is readily metabolized by MAO

Figure 9–7. Examples of β_1- and β_2-selective agonists.

Table 9–5. Foods reputed to have a high content of tyramine or other sympathomimetic agents. In a patient taking an irreversible MAO inhibitor drug, 6 mg of tyramine in a meal may increase the blood pressure significantly (see also Chapter 30). Note that only cheese, sausage, pickled fish, and yeast supplements contain sufficient tyramine to be consistently dangerous. This does not rule out the possibility that some preparations of other foods might contain significantly greater than average amounts of tyramine. Spoiled food may have greatly increased tyramine content.

Food	Tyramine Content of an Average Serving
Beer	Nil to 100 mg
Broad beans, fava beans	Negligible (but contains dopamine: avoid)
Cheese, natural or aged	Nil to 130 mg (Cheddar, Gruyère, and Stilton especially high)
Chicken liver	Nil to 9 mg
Chocolate	Negligible (but contains phenylethylamine: caution)
Sausage, fermented (eg, salami, pepperoni, summer sausage)	Nil to 74 mg
Smoked or pickled fish (eg, pickled herring)	Nil to 198 mg
Wine (red)	Nil to 3 mg/dL
Yeast (eg, dietary brewer's yeast supplements)	2–68 mg

in the liver and is normally inactive if ingested because of a very high first-pass effect. If administered parenterally, it has an indirect sympathomimetic action caused by the release of stored catecholamines. Thus, its spectrum of action is similar to that of norepinephrine. In patients treated with MAO inhibitors—particularly inhibitors of the MAO-A isoform—this effect of tyramine may be greatly intensified, leading to marked increases in blood pressure. Such individuals must be very careful to avoid tyramine-containing foods.

II. CLINICAL PHARMACOLOGY OF SYMPATHOMIMETIC DRUGS

The rationale for the use of sympathomimetic drugs in therapy rests on a knowledge of the physiologic effects of catecholamines on tissues. Selection of a particular sympathomimetic drug from the host of compounds available depends upon such factors as whether activation of alpha, β_1, or β_2 receptors is desired; the duration of action desired; and the preferred route of administration. Sympathomimetic drugs are very potent and can have profound effects on a variety of organ systems, particularly the heart and pe-

ripheral circulation. Therefore, great caution is indicated when these agents are used parenterally. In most cases, rather than using fixed doses of the drugs, careful monitoring of pharmacologic response is required to determine the appropriate dosage, especially if the drug is being infused. Generally, it is desirable to use the minimum dose required to achieve the desired response. The adverse effects of these drugs are generally understandable in terms of their known physiologic effects.

Cardiovascular Applications

A. Conditions in Which Blood Flow or Pressure Is to Be Enhanced: Hypotension may occur in a variety of settings such as decreased blood volume, cardiac arrhythmias, neurologic disease, adverse reactions to medications such as antihypertensive drugs, and infection. If cerebral, renal, and cardiac perfusion is maintained, hypotension itself does not usually require vigorous direct treatment. Rather, placing the patient in the recumbent position and ensuring adequate fluid volume—while the primary problem is determined and treated—is usually the correct course of action. The use of sympathomimetic drugs merely to elevate a blood pressure that is not an immediate threat to the patient may increase morbidity (see Toxicity of Sympathomimetic Drugs, below). Sympathomimetic drugs may be used in a hypotensive emergency to preserve cerebral and coronary blood flow. Such situations might arise in severe hemorrhage, spinal cord injury, or overdoses of antihypertensive or central nervous system depressant medications. The treatment is usually of short duration while the appropriate intravenous fluid or blood is being administered. Direct-acting alpha agonists such as norepinephrine, phenylephrine, or methoxamine can be utilized in this setting if vasoconstriction is desired. For the treatment of **chronic orthostatic hypotension,** oral ephedrine has been the traditional therapy. Midodrine, a newer orally active alpha agonist, may be considered as a replacement for ephedrine in this application if further studies confirm its long-term safety and efficacy (Fouad-Tarazi et al, 1995).

Shock is a complex acute cardiovascular syndrome that results in a critical reduction in perfusion of vital tissues and a wide range of systemic effects. Shock is usually associated with hypotension, an altered mental state, oliguria, and metabolic acidosis. If untreated, shock usually progresses to a refractory deteriorating state and death. The three major mechanisms responsible for shock are hypovolemia, cardiac insufficiency, and altered vascular resistance. Volume replacement and treatment of the underlying disease are the mainstays of the treatment of shock. While sympathomimetic drugs have been used in the treatment of virtually all forms of shock, their efficacy is unclear. In most forms of shock, vasoconstriction mediated by the sympathetic nervous system is already intense. Indeed, efforts aimed at reducing rather than increasing peripheral resistance may be more fruitful if cerebral, coronary, and renal perfusion are improved. A decision to use vasoconstrictors or vasodilators is best made on the basis of information about the underlying cause, which may require invasive monitoring.

Cardiogenic shock, usually due to massive myocardial infarction, has a poor prognosis. Mechanically assisted perfusion and emergency cardiac surgery have been utilized in some settings. Optimal fluid replacement requires monitoring of pulmonary capillary wedge pressure. Positive inotropic agents such as dopamine or dobutamine may have a role in this situation. In low to moderate doses, these drugs may increase cardiac output and, compared with norepinephrine, cause relatively little peripheral vasoconstriction. Isoproterenol increases heart rate and work more than either dopamine or dobutamine. See Chapter 13 and Table 13–6 for a discussion of shock associated with myocardial infarction.

Unfortunately, the patient with shock may not respond to any of the above therapeutic maneuvers; the temptation is then great to use vasoconstrictors to maintain adequate blood pressure. While coronary perfusion may be improved, this gain may be offset by increased myocardial oxygen demands as well as more severe vasoconstriction in blood vessels to the abdominal viscera. Therefore, the goal of therapy in shock should be to optimize tissue perfusion, not blood pressure.

B. Conditions in Which Blood Flow Is to Be Reduced: Reduction of regional blood flow is desirable for achieving hemostasis in surgery, for reducing diffusion of local anesthetics away from the site of administration, and for reducing mucous membrane congestion. In each instance, alpha-receptor activation is desired, and the choice of agent depends upon the maximal efficacy required, the desired duration of action, and the route of administration.

Effective pharmacologic hemostasis, often necessary for facial, oral, and nasopharyngeal surgery, requires drugs of high efficacy that can be administered in high concentration by local application. Epinephrine is usually applied topically in nasal packs (for epistaxis) or in a gingival string (gingivectomy). **Cocaine** is still sometimes used for nasopharyngeal surgery, because it combines a hemostatic effect with local anesthesia. Occasionally, cocaine is mixed with epinephrine for maximum hemostasis and local anesthesia.

Combining alpha agonists with local anesthetics greatly prolongs the duration of infiltration nerve block; the total dose of local anesthetic (and the probability of toxicity) can therefore be reduced. **Epinephrine,** 1:200,000, is the favored agent for this application, but norepinephrine, phenylephrine, and other alpha agonists have also been used. Systemic effects on the heart and peripheral vasculature may occur even with local drug administration.

Mucous membrane decongestants are alpha agonists that reduce the discomfort of hay fever and, to a lesser extent, the common cold by decreasing the volume of the nasal mucosa, probably mediated by α_1 receptors. Unfortunately, rebound hyperemia may follow the use of these agents, and repeated topical use of high concentrations may result in ischemic changes in the mucous membranes, probably as a result of vasoconstriction of nutrient arteries. Constriction of these vessels may involve activation of α_2 receptors. Favored short-acting topical agents include phenylephrine and phenylpropanolamine in nasal sprays and ophthalmic drops. A longer duration of action, at the cost of much lower local concentrations and greater cardiac and central nervous system effects, can be achieved by the oral administration of agents such as ephedrine or one of its isomers, pseudoephedrine. Long-acting topical decongestants include xylometazoline and oxymetazoline. All of these mucous membrane decongestants are available as over-the-counter products.

C. Cardiac Applications: Episodes of **paroxysmal atrial tachycardia** were treated in the past with α agonist drugs such as phenylephrine or methoxamine. Because these drugs cause marked vasoconstriction and lead to a rise in blood pressure, a reflex vagal discharge is evoked that may convert the arrhythmia to sinus rhythm. If used for this indication, the drugs should be given by slow intravenous infusion; caution must be exercized to prevent a rise in systolic blood pressure to greater than about 160 mm Hg. While these drugs have been effective in the past in terminating this rhythm disturbance in patients who were hypotensive, safer alternatives such as verapamil, adenosine, and electrical cardioversion are currently preferred and have replaced the alpha agonists (Chapter 14).

Catecholamines such as isoproterenol and epinephrine have also been utilized in the temporary emergency management of **complete heart block** and **cardiac arrest.** Epinephrine may be useful in cardiac arrest in part by redistributing blood flow during cardiopulmonary resuscitation to coronaries and to the brain. However, electronic pacemakers are both safer and more effective in heart block and should be inserted as soon as possible if there is any indication of continued high-degree block.

Congestive heart failure may respond to the positive inotropic effects of drugs such as dobutamine and prenalterol. These applications are discussed in Chapter 13. The development of tolerance or desensitization is a major limitation to the use of catecholamines in congestive heart failure.

Respiratory Applications

One of the most important uses of sympathomimetic drugs is in the therapy of bronchial asthma. This use is discussed in Chapter 20. Nonselective drugs (epinephrine), beta-selective agents (isoproterenol), and beta$_2$-selective agents (metaproterenol, terbutaline, albuterol) are all available for this indication. For most patients, the beta$_2$-selective drugs are as effective as and less toxic than the less selective agents. In certain epidemiologic studies, the intensive use of beta-adrenoceptor agonists in asthma was associated with an increased mortality rate. However, the basis for this association is uncertain. It may represent inadequate treatment with other drugs, especially glucocorticoids, rather than direct adverse effects of sympathomimetics.

Anaphylaxis

Anaphylactic shock and related immediate (type I) IgE-mediated reactions affect both the respiratory and the cardiovascular systems. The syndrome of bronchospasm, mucous membrane congestion, angioedema, and cardiovascular collapse usually responds rapidly to subcutaneous administration of **epinephrine,** 0.3–0.5 mg (0.3–0.5 mL of 1:1000 epinephrine solution). This drug is the agent of choice because of its great efficacy at alpha, β$_1$, and β$_2$ receptors; stimulation of all three is helpful in reversing the pathophysiologic process. Glucocorticoids and antihistamines (both H$_1$ and H$_2$ receptor antagonists) may be useful as secondary therapy in anaphylaxis; however, epinephrine is the initial treatment.

Ophthalmic Applications

Phenylephrine is an effective mydriatic agent frequently used to facilitate examination of the retina. It is also a useful decongestant for minor allergic hyperemia of the conjunctival membranes. Sympathomimetics administered as ophthalmic drops are also useful in localizing the lesion in Horner's syndrome. (See box: An Application of Basic Pharmacology to a Clinical Problem.)

Glaucoma responds to a variety of sympathomimetic and sympathoplegic drugs. (See box in Chapter 10: The Treatment of Glaucoma.) **Epinephrine** and beta-blocking agents are among the most important therapies. Used chronically, topical epinephrine (1–2% solution) lowers intraocular pressure primarily by increasing aqueous outflow. The efficacy of epinephrine may be related in part to desensitization of β-adrenoceptor-mediated responses. **Dipivefrin** is a prodrug of epinephrine formed by esterification of epinephrine with pivalic acid. The ester enjoys enhanced penetration into the anterior chamber of the eye, where it is converted back into epinephrine by enzymatic hydrolysis. **Apraclonidine** and **brimonidine** are α$_2$-selective agonists that also lower intraocular pressure and are approved for use in glaucoma.

Genitourinary Applications

As noted above, β$_2$-selective agents relax the pregnant uterus. **Ritodrine, terbutaline,** and similar drugs have been used to suppress premature labor. The goal is to defer labor long enough to ensure adequate mat-

AN APPLICATION OF BASIC PHARMACOLOGY TO A CLINICAL PROBLEM

Horner's syndrome is a condition—usually unilateral—that results from interruption of the sympathetic nerves to the face. The effects include vasodilation, ptosis, miosis, and loss of sweating on the side affected. The syndrome can be caused by either a preganglionic or a postganglionic lesion, such as a tumor. Knowledge of the location of the lesion (preganglionic or postganglionic) helps determine the optimal therapy.

An understanding of the effects of denervation on neurotransmitter metabolism permits the clinician to use drugs to localize the lesion. In most situations, a localized lesion in a nerve will cause degeneration of the distal portion of that fiber and loss of transmitter contents from the degenerated nerve ending, without affecting neurons innervated by the fiber. Therefore, a preganglionic lesion will leave the postganglionic adrenergic neuron intact, whereas a postganglionic lesion results in degeneration of the adrenergic nerve endings and loss of stored catecholamines from them. Because indirectly acting sympathomimetics require normal stores of catecholamines, such drugs can be used to test for the presence of normal adrenergic nerve endings. The iris, because it is easily visible and responsive to topical sympathomimetics, is a convenient assay tissue in the patient.

If the lesion of Horner's syndrome is postganglionic, indirectly acting sympathomimetics (eg, cocaine, hydroxyamphetamine) will not dilate the abnormally constricted pupil—because catecholamines have been lost from the nerve endings in the iris. In contrast, the pupil will dilate in response to phenylephrine, which acts directly on the alpha receptors on the smooth muscle of the iris. A patient with a preganglionic lesion, on the other hand, will show a normal response to both drugs, since the postganglionic fibers and their catecholamine stores remain intact in this situation.

uration of the fetus. Several trials indicated that these drugs could defer delivery for days or even weeks (eg, Merkatz et al, 1980). However, meta-analysis of older trials and a recent randomized study suggest that beta-agonist therapy may have no significant benefit on perinatal infant mortality and may increase maternal morbidity (Canada Preterm Labor Investigators Group, 1992).

Oral sympathomimetic therapy is occasionally useful in the treatment of stress incontinence. Ephedrine or pseudoephedrine may be tried.

Central Nervous System Applications

As noted above, the amphetamine-like sympathomimetics have a mood-elevating (euphoriant) effect; this effect is the basis for the widespread abuse of this subgroup (see Chapter 32). The amphetamines also have an alerting, sleep-deferring action that is manifested by improved attention to repetitive tasks and by acceleration and desynchronization of the EEG. A therapeutic application of this effect is in the treatment of narcolepsy. The appetite-suppressing effect of these agents is easily demonstrated in experimental animals. In obese humans, an encouraging initial response may be observed, but there is no evidence that long-term improvement in weight control can be achieved with amphetamines alone. A final application of the CNS-active sympathomimetics is in the attention-deficit hyperkinetic syndrome of children, a poorly defined and overdiagnosed behavioral syndrome consisting of short attention span, hyperkinetic physical behavior, and learning problems. Some patients with this syndrome respond well to low doses of the amphetamine-like drugs or to clonidine.

Additional Therapeutic Uses

While the primary use of the α_2-agonist clonidine is in the treatment of hypertension (Chapter 11), the drug has been found to have efficacy in the treatment of diarrhea in diabetics with autonomic neuropathy, perhaps due to its ability to enhance salt and water absorption from the intestines. In addition, clonidine has efficacy in diminishing craving for narcotics and alcohol during withdrawal and may facilitate cessation of cigarette smoking. Clonidine has also been used to diminish menopausal hot flushes and is being used experimentally to reduce hemodynamic instability during general anesthesia.

TOXICITY OF SYMPATHOMIMETIC DRUGS

The adverse effects of adrenoceptor agonists are primarily extensions of their receptor effects in the cardiovascular and central nervous systems.

Adverse cardiovascular effects seen with pressor agents include marked elevations in blood pressure, which may cause cerebral hemorrhage or pulmonary edema. Increased cardiac work may precipitate severe angina or myocardial infarction. Beta-stimulant drugs frequently cause sinus tachycardia and may provoke serious ventricular arrhythmias. Sympathomimetic drugs may lead to myocardial damage, particularly after prolonged infusion. Special caution is indicated in elderly patients or those with hypertension or coronary artery disease.

If an adverse sympathomimetic effect requires urgent reversal, a specific adrenoceptor antagonist should be used (see Chapter 10). For example, extravasation into subcutaneous tissues of norepinephrine being given by the intravenous route may lead to marked ischemia that can be reversed by alpha-adrenoceptor antagonists.

Central nervous system toxicity is rarely observed with catecholamines or drugs such as phenylephrine. Amphetamines commonly cause restlessness, tremor, insomnia, and anxiety. In very high doses, a paranoid state may be induced. Cocaine may precipitate convulsions, cerebral hemorrhage, arrhythmias, or myocardial infarction. The last three of these effects represent sympathomimetic toxicity. Therapy is discussed in Chapter 59.

PREPARATIONS AVAILABLE*

Amphetamine, racemic mixture (generic)
  Oral: 5, 10 mg tablets
Apraclonidine (Iopidine)
  Topical: 0.5, 1% solutions
Brimonidine (Alphagan)
  Topical: 0.2% solution
Dextroamphetamine (generic, Dexedrine)
  Oral: 5, 10 mg tablets; 5 mg/5 mL elixir
  Oral sustained-release: 5, 10, 15 mg capsules
Dipivefrin (generic, Propine)
  Topical: 0.1% ophthalmic solution

Dobutamine (Dobutrex)
  Parenteral: 250 mg/20 mL for injection
Dopamine (generic, Intropin)
  Parenteral: 40, 80, 160 mg/mL for injection; 80, 160, 320 mg/100 mL in 5% D/W for injection
Ephedrine (generic, Vatronol Nose Drops, Efedron Nasal)
  Oral: 25, 50 mg capsules; 11, 20 mg/5 mL syrups
  Parenteral: 50 mg/mL for injection
  Nasal: 0.25% spray, 0.5% drops, 1% jelly
Epinephrine (generic, Adrenalin Chloride, others)
  Parenteral: 1:200 (5 mg/mL), 1:1000 (1 mg/mL), 1:10,000 (0.1 mg/mL), 1:100,000 (0.01 mg/mL) for injection

---

*Alpha$_2$ agonists used in hypertension are listed in Chapter 11. Beta$_2$ agonists used in asthma are listed in Chapter 20.

Parenteral autoinjector (Epipen): 1:2000 (0.5 mg/mL)

Ophthalmic: 0.1, 0.5, 1, 2% drops

Nasal: 0.1% drops and spray

Aerosol for bronchospasm (Primatene Mist, Bronkaid Mist): 0.16, 0.2, 0.25 mg/spray

Solution for aerosol: 1:100

Isoproterenol (generic, Isuprel)

Parenteral: 1:5000 (0.2 mg/mL), 1:50,000 (0.02 mg/mL) for injection

Mephentermine (Wyamine Sulfate)

Parenteral: 15, 30 mg/mL for injection

Metaraminol (generic, Aramine)

Parenteral: 10 mg/mL for injection

Methamphetamine (generic, Desoxyn)

Oral: 5 mg tablets

Oral sustained-release: 5, 10, 15 mg tablets

Methoxamine (Vasoxyl)

Parenteral: 20 mg/mL for injection

Methylphenidate (generic, Ritalin, Ritalin-SR)

Oral: 5, 10, 20 mg tablets

Oral sustained-release: 20 mg tablets

Midodrine (ProAmatine)

Oral: 2.5, 5 mg tablets

Naphazoline (Privine)

Nasal: 0.05% drops and spray

Norepinephrine (Levophed)

Parenteral: 1 mg/mL for injection

Oxymetazoline (generic, Afrin, Neo-Synephrine 12 Hour, others)

Nasal: 0.025, 0.05% sprays

Pemoline (Cylert)

Oral: 18.75, 37.5, 75 mg tables; 37.5 mg chewable tablets

Phendimetrazine (generic)

Oral: 35 mg tablets, capsules; 105 mg sustained-release capsules

Phenylephrine (generic, Neo-Synephrine)

Parenteral: 10 mg/mL for injection

Nasal: 0.125, 0.16, 0.25, 0.5, 1% drops and spray; 0.5% jelly

Phenylpropanolamine (generic)

Oral: 25 mg tablets; 37.5 mg capsules

Oral sustained-release: 75 mg tablets; 25, 75 mg capsules

Pseudoephedrine (generic, Sudafed, others)

Oral: 30, 60 mg tablets; 15, 30 mg/5 mL syrups; 7.5 mg/0.8 mL drops

Oral sustained-release: 120 mg tablets, capsules

Tetrahydrozoline (generic, Tyzine)

Nasal: 0.05 drops, 0.1% drops, spray

Xylometazoline (generic, Otrivin, Neo-Synephrine Long-Acting, Chlorohist LA)

Nasal: 0.05 drops, 0.1% drops and spray

REFERENCES

Aantaa R, Marjamaki A, Scheinin M: Molecular pharmacology of alpha 2-adrenoceptor subtypes. Ann Med 1995;27:439.

Arch JR, Wilson S: Prospects for beta$_3$-adrenoceptor agonists in the treatment of obesity and diabetes. Int J Obes Relat Metab Disord 1996;20:191.

Barach EM et al: Epinephrine for treatment of anaphylactic shock. JAMA 1984;251:2118.

Brown CG et al: A comparison of standard dose and high dose epinephrine in cardiac arrest outside the hospital. N Engl J Med 1992;327:1051.

Bylund DB et al: International Union of Pharmacology nomenclature of adrenoceptors. Pharmacol Rev 1994;46:121.

Bylund DB et al: Vascular alpha-adrenoceptors: from the gene to the human. Can J Physiol Pharmacol 1995; 73:533.

The Canada Preterm Labor Investigators Group: Treatment of preterm labor with the beta-adrenergic agonist ritodrine. N Engl J Med 1992;327:308.

Caron MG, Lefkowitz RJ: Catecholamine receptors: Structure, function, and regulation. Recent Prog Horm Res 1993;48:277.

Cobb MH, Goldsmith EJ: How MAP kinases are regulated. J Biol Chem 1995;270:14843.

Conklin BR, Bourne HR: Structural elements of G alpha subunits that interact with G beta gamma, receptors, and effectors. Cell 1993;73:631.

deGroat WC, Steers WD: Autonomic regulation of the urinary bladder and sexual organs. In: *Central Regulation of Autonomic Functions.* Loewy AD, Spyer KM (editors). Oxford Univ Press, 1990.

Fouad-Tarazi FM, Okabe M, Goren H: Alpha sympathomimetic treatment of autonomic insufficiency with orthostatic hypotension. Am J Med 1995;99:604.

Gingrich JA, Caron MG: Recent advances in the molecular biology of dopamine receptors. Annu Rev Neurosci 1993;16:299.

Glassman AH et al: Heavy smokers, smoking cessation, and clonidine: Results of a double-blind, randomized trial. JAMA 1988;259,2863.

Graham RM et al: Alpha$_1$-adrenergic receptor subtypes. Molecular structure, function, and signaling. Circ Res 1996;78:737.

Hepler JR, Gilman AG: G proteins. Trends Biochem Sci 1992;17:383.

Hieble JP et al: International Union of Pharmacology. X. Recommendation for nomenclature of alpha 1-adrenoceptors: consensus update. Pharmacol Rev 1995;47:267.

Hurvitz LM et al: New developments in the drug treatment of glaucoma. Drugs 1991;41:514.

Insel PA: Seminars in medicine of the Beth Israel Hospital, Boston. Adrenergic receptors: Evolving concepts and clinical implications. N Engl J Med 1996;334:580.

Kobilka B: Adrenergic receptors as models for G protein-coupled receptors. Annu Rev Neurosci 1992;15:87.

Koch WJ, Milano CA, Lefkowitz RJ: Transgenic manipulation of myocardial G protein-coupled receptors and receptor kinases. Circ Res 1996;78:511.

LaMorte VJ et al: G_q- and ras-dependent pathways mediate hypertrophy of neonatal rat ventricular myocytes following alpha$_1$-adrenergic stimulation. J Biol Chem 1994; 269:13490.

McCabe BJ: Dietary tyranine and other pressor amines in MAOI regimens: A review. J Am Diet Assoc 1986;86:1059.

Merkatz IR, Peter JB, Barden TP: Ritodrine hydrochloride: A betamimetic agent for use in preterm labor. II. Evidence of efficacy. Obstet Gynecol 1980;56:7.

1996 Receptor and Ion Channel Nomenclature Supplement. Trends Pharmacol Sci 1996.

Raymond JR: Multiple mechanisms of receptor-G protein signaling specificity. (Editorial.) Am J Physiol 1995;269:F141.

Ruffolo RR Jr et al: Pharmacologic and therapeutic applications of α_2-adrenoceptor subtypes. Annu Rev Pharmacol Toxicol 1993;32:243.

Ruffolo RR Jr et al: Structure and function of alpha-adrenoceptors. Pharmacol Rev 1991;43:475

Ruffolo RR Jr: Fundamentals of receptor theory: Basics for shock research. Circ Shock 1992;37:176.

Spiegel AM: Mutations in G proteins and G protein-coupled receptors in endocrine disease. J Clin Endocrinol Metab 1996;81:2434.

Spitzer WO et al: The use of β-agonists and the risk of death and near death from asthma. N Engl J Med 1992; 326:501.

Tang WJ, Gilman AG: Adenylyl cyclases. Cell 1992;70:869.

10

Adrenoceptor Antagonist Drugs

Brian B. Hoffman, MD

Since catecholamines play a role in a variety of physiologic and pathophysiologic responses, drugs that block adrenoceptors have important effects, some of which are of great clinical value. These effects vary dramatically according to the drug's selectivity for alpha and beta receptors. The classification of adrenoceptors into alpha$_1$, alpha$_2$, and beta subtypes and the effects of activating these receptors are discussed in Chapters 6 and 9. Blockade of peripheral dopamine receptors is of no recognized clinical importance at present. In contrast, blockade of central nervous system dopamine receptors is very important; drugs that act on these receptors are discussed in Chapters 21 and 29. This chapter deals with pharmacologic antagonist drugs whose major effect is to occupy either alpha$_1$, alpha$_2$, or beta receptors outside the central nervous system and prevent their activation by catecholamines and related agonists.

In basic pharmacology, alpha$_1$ and alpha$_2$ adrenoceptor antagonist drugs have been very useful in the experimental exploration of autonomic nervous system function. In clinical therapeutics, they have had only limited application (in pheochromocytoma and essential hypertension). Although alpha$_1$ receptor antagonists effectively block the vasoconstricting effect of catecholamines and are capable of lowering blood pressure, they have not been as popular as many other classes of drugs in treatment of essential hypertension (Chapter 11). Recently, however, interest in these antagonists has surged as their efficacy in treating symptoms of prostatic hyperplasia has become more firmly established. Beta-receptor antagonist drugs have been found useful in a wide variety of clinical conditions and are firmly established in the treatment of hypertension, ischemic heart disease, arrhythmias, endocrinologic and neurologic disorders, and other conditions.

I. BASIC PHARMACOLOGY OF THE ALPHA-RECEPTOR-ANTAGONIST DRUGS

Mechanism of Action

Alpha-receptor antagonists may be reversible or irreversible in their interaction with these receptors. Reversible antagonists dissociate from receptors; irreversible drugs do not. Phentolamine and tolazoline are examples of reversible antagonists (Figure 10–1). Prazosin (and analogs) and labetalol—drugs used primarily for their antihypertensive effects—as well as several ergot derivatives (see Chapter 16) are also reversible alpha-adrenoceptor blockers. Phenoxybenzamine, an agent related to the nitrogen mustards, forms a reactive ethyleneimonium intermediate (Figure 10–1) that covalently binds to alpha receptors, resulting in irreversible blockade. Figure 10–2 illustrates the effects of a reversible drug in comparison with those of an irreversible agent.

The duration of action of a reversible antagonist is largely dependent on the half-life of the drug in the body and the rate at which it dissociates from its receptor: The shorter the half-life of the drug in the body or of binding to its receptor, the less time it takes for the effects of the drug to disappear. However, the effects of an irreversible antagonist may persist long after the drug has been cleared from the plasma. In the case of phenoxybenzamine, the restoration of tissue responsiveness after extensive alpha-receptor blockade is dependent on synthesis of new receptors, which may take several days.

Pharmacologic Effects

A. Cardiovascular Effects: Because arteriolar and venous tone are determined to a large extent by alpha receptors on vascular smooth muscle, alpha-receptor antagonist drugs cause a lowering of peripheral vascular resistance and blood pressure (Figure 10–3). They can prevent the pressor effects of usual doses of alpha agonists; indeed, in the case of agonists with both alpha and beta$_2$ effects (eg, epinephrine), they convert a pressor to a depressor response (Figure 10–3). This change in response is called **epinephrine reversal.** Alpha receptor antagonists may cause postural hypotension and reflex tachycardia. Postural hypotension is due to antagonism of sympathetic nervous system stimulation of alpha$_1$ receptors in venous smooth muscle; contraction of veins is an important component of the capacity to stand up. Tachycardia may be more marked with agents that block alpha$_2$ presynaptic receptors in the heart (Table 10–1), since the augmented release of norepinephrine will further stimulate beta receptors in the heart. Chronic use of

Phentolamine

Tolazoline

Phenoxybenzamine

Active (ethyleneimonium) intermediate

Prazosin

Figure 10–1. Structure of several alpha-receptor-blocking drugs.

Figure 10–2. Dose-response curves to norepinephrine in the presence of two different alpha adrenoceptor-blocking drugs. The tension produced in isolated strips of cat spleen, a tissue rich in alpha receptors, was measured in response to graded doses of norepinephrine. **Left:** Tolazoline, a reversible blocker, shifted the curve to the right without decreasing the maximum response when present at concentrations of 10 and 20 μmol/L. **Right:** Dibenamine, an analog of phenoxybenzamine and irreversible in its action, reduced the maximum response attainable at both concentrations tested. (Modified and reproduced, with permission, from Bickerton RK: The response of isolated strips of cat spleen to sympathomimetic drugs and their antagonists. J Pharmacol Exp Ther 1963;142:99.)

Figure 10–3. Top: Effects of phentolamine, an alpha receptor-blocking drug, on blood pressure in an anesthetized dog. Epinephrine reversal is demonstrated by tracings showing the response to epinephrine before **(middle)** and after **(bottom)** phentolamine. All drugs given intravenously. (BP, blood pressure; HR, heart rate.)

alpha antagonists may result in a compensatory increase in blood volume.

B. Other Effects: Minor effects that signal the blockade of alpha receptors in other tissues include miosis and nasal stuffiness. Alpha-receptor blockade of the base of the bladder and the prostate is associ-

Table 10–1. Relative selectivity of antagonists for adrenoceptors.

	Receptor Affinity
Alpha antagonists	
Prazosin, terazosin, doxazosin	$\alpha_1 >>>> \alpha_2$
Phenoxybenzamine	$\alpha_1 > \alpha_2$
Phentolamine	$\alpha_1 = \alpha_2$
Rauwolscine, yohimbine, tolazoline	$\alpha_2 >> \alpha_1$
Mixed antagonists	
Labetalol, carvedilol	$\beta_1 = \beta_2 \geq \alpha_1 > \alpha_2$
Beta antagonists	
Metoprololol, acebutolol, alprenolol, atenolol, betaxolol, celiprolol, esmolol	$\beta_1 >>> \beta_2$
Propranolol, carteolol, nadolol, penbutolol, pindolol, timolol	$\beta_1 = \beta_2$
Butoxamine	$\beta_2 >>> \beta_1$

ated with decreased resistance to the flow of urine. Individual agents may have other important effects in addition to alpha blockade (see below).

SPECIFIC AGENTS

Phentolamine, an imidazoline derivative, is a potent competitive antagonist at both alpha$_1$ and alpha$_2$ receptors. Phentolamine causes a reduction in peripheral resistance through blockade of alpha$_1$ receptors and possibly alpha$_2$ receptors on vascular smooth muscle. The cardiac stimulation induced by phentolamine may be due to activation of sympathetic stimulation of the heart in response to baroreflex mechanisms. Since phentolamine potently blocks both alpha$_1$ and alpha$_2$ receptors, antagonism of presynaptic alpha$_2$ receptors may lead to enhanced release of norepinephrine from sympathetic nerves. Enhanced norepinephrine release may contribute to marked cardiac stimulation via unblocked beta adrenoceptors. In addition to being an alpha$_1$ and alpha$_2$ receptor antagonist, phentolamine also inhibits responses to serotonin. Phentolamine is an agonist at muscarinic and H$_1$ and H$_2$ histamine receptors. Thus, phentolamine is a relatively "dirty" drug with multiple potential actions.

Phentolamine is poorly absorbed after oral administration. Its pharmacokinetics are not well known. The principal adverse effects are related to cardiac stimulation, which may cause severe tachycardia, arrhythmias, and myocardial ischemia. Gastrointestinal stimulation may cause diarrhea and increased gastric acid production.

Phentolamine has been used in the treatment of pheochromocytoma (see below). **Tolazoline** is similar to phentolamine. It is somewhat less potent but is better absorbed from the gastrointestinal tract. It is rapidly excreted in the urine. Tolazoline has very limited clinical applications in peripheral vasospastic disease and in the treatment of pulmonary hypertension in newborn infants with respiratory distress syndrome. Its efficacy in these conditions is doubtful and it is rarely used.

Ergot derivatives—eg, ergotamine, dihydroergotamine—cause reversible alpha-receptor blockade. However, most of the clinically significant effects of these drugs are the result of other actions; eg, ergotamine probably acts at serotonin receptors in the treatment of migraine (Chapter 16).

Phenoxybenzamine binds covalently to alpha receptors, causing irreversible blockade of long duration (14–48 hours or longer). It is somewhat selective for alpha$_1$ receptors but less so than prazosin (Table 10–1). The drug also inhibits reuptake of released norepinephrine by presynaptic adrenergic nerve terminals. Phenoxybenzamine blocks histamine (H$_1$), acetylcholine, and serotonin receptors as well as alpha receptors. The role (if any) of these secondary actions in human pharmacology is not well defined.

The pharmacologic actions of phenoxybenzamine are primarily related to antagonism of alpha receptor-mediated events. Most importantly, phenoxybenzamine blocks catecholamine-induced vasoconstriction. While phenoxybenzamine causes relatively little fall in blood pressure in supine individuals, it reduces blood pressure when sympathetic tone is high, eg, as a result of upright posture or because of reduced blood volume. Cardiac output may be increased because of reflex effects and because of some blockade of presynaptic alpha$_2$ receptors in cardiac sympathetic nerves.

Phenoxybenzamine is absorbed after oral administration, though bioavailability is low and its kinetics are not well known. The drug is usually given orally, starting with low doses of 10–20 mg/d and progressively increasing the dose until the desired effect is achieved. Less than 100 mg/d is usually sufficient to achieve adequate alpha-receptor blockade. The major use of phenoxybenzamine is in the treatment of pheochromocytoma (see below).

The adverse effects of phenoxybenzamine derive from its alpha receptor-blocking action; the most important are postural hypotension and tachycardia.

Nasal stuffiness and inhibition of ejaculation also occur. Since phenoxybenzamine enters the central nervous system, it may cause less specific effects, including fatigue, sedation, and nausea. Since phenoxybenzamine is an alkylating agent, it may have other adverse effects that have not yet been characterized. Phenoxybenzamine causes tumors in animals, but the clinical implications of this observation are unknown.

Prazosin is a piperazinyl quinazoline effective in the management of hypertension (Chapter 11). It was originally thought to be a direct-acting vasodilator, but it is now clear that the major pharmacologic action of prazosin is that of an extremely potent alpha-receptor antagonist. It is highly selective for alpha$_1$ receptors, having relatively low affinity for alpha$_2$ receptors (typically 1000-fold less potent). This may partially explain the relative absence of tachycardia seen with prazosin as compared to what is reported with phentolamine and phenoxybenzamine. Prazosin leads to relaxation of both arterial and venous smooth muscle due to blockade of alpha$_1$ receptors.

Prazosin is extensively metabolized in humans; because of metabolic degradation by the liver, only about 50% of the drug is available after oral administration. The half-life is normally about 3 hours.

Terazosin is another reversible alpha$_1$-selective antagonist that is effective in hypertension (Chapter 11); it has also been approved for use in men with urinary symptoms due to prostatic hyperplasia. Terazosin has high bioavailability yet is extensively metabolized in the liver, with only a small fraction of parent drug excreted in the urine. The half-life of terazosin is about 9–12 hours.

Doxazosin is the third alpha$_1$-selective antagonist approved for use in hypertension in the United States. It has moderate bioavailability and is extensively metabolized, with very little parent drug excreted in urine or feces. Doxazosin has active metabolites, though their contribution to the drug's effects is probably small. The parent compound has a half-life of about 22 hours. Doxazosin is also effective in the symptomatic treatment of prostatic hyperplasia.

Several newer alpha antagonists are under investigation for possible use in the treatment of benign prostatic hyperplasia. **Alfuzosin**, an alpha$_1$-selective quinazoline derivative, has a bioavailability of about 60%, is extensively metabolized, and has an elimination half-life of about 5 hours. Alfuzosin has been shown to be efficacious in blocking alpha$_1$ receptors in prostate smooth muscle. **Tamsulosin** is a methoxybenzene sulfonamide competitive alpha$_1$ receptor antagonist with a structure quite different from that of most other alpha$_1$ receptor blockers. It has very high bioavailability and a long half-life. Tamsulosin has some selectivity for the alpha$_{1A}$ subtype and also appears be efficacious in preventing contraction of prostate smooth muscle.

OTHER ALPHA-ADRENOCEPTOR ANTAGONISTS

Indoramin is another alpha$_1$-selective antagonist that also has efficacy as an antihypertensive. **Urapidil** is an alpha$_1$ antagonist (its primary effect) that also has weak alpha$_2$-agonist and 5-HT$_{1A}$-agonist actions and weak antagonist action at beta$_1$ receptors. It is used in Europe as an antihypertensive agent. **Labetalol** has both alpha$_1$-selective and beta-blocking effects; it is discussed below. Neuroleptic drugs such as chlorpromazine and haloperidol are potent alpha-receptor and dopamine-receptor antagonists. Although these drugs are not used clinically to block alpha receptors, this action may contribute to their adverse effects (eg, hypotension).

Yohimbine, an indole alkaloid, is an alpha$_2$-selective antagonist. It has no established clinical role. Theoretically, it could be useful in autonomic insufficiency by promoting neurotransmitter release through blockade of presynaptic alpha$_2$ receptors. Yohimbine may improve symptoms in some patients with painful diabetic neuropathies. It has been suggested that yohimbine improves male sexual function; however, evidence for this effect in humans is limited.

II. CLINICAL PHARMACOLOGY OF THE ALPHA-RECEPTOR-BLOCKING DRUGS

Pheochromocytoma

The major clinical use of both phenoxybenzamine and phentolamine is in the management of pheochromocytoma. Pheochromocytoma is a tumor usually found in the adrenal medulla that releases a mixture of epinephrine and norepinephrine. Patients have many signs of catecholamine excess, including hypertension, tachycardia, and arrhythmias.

The diagnosis of pheochromocytoma is usually made on the basis of chemical assay of circulating catecholamines and urinary excretion of catecholamine metabolites, especially 3-hydroxy-4-methoxymandelic acid, metanephrine, and normetanephrine. Infusion of phentolamine has been advocated as a diagnostic test when pheochromocytoma is suspected, since patients with this tumor often manifest a greater-than-average drop in blood pressure in response to alpha-blocking drugs. However, measurement of circulating catecholamines and urinary catecholamines and their metabolites is a more reliable and safer diagnostic approach. Injection of a bolus dose of phentolamine may lead to a dangerous fall in blood pressure in a patient with a pheochromocytoma. Provocative testing for pheochromocytoma by infusion of drugs such as histamine may cause dangerous blood pressure elevation. Unavoidable release of stored catecholamines

sometimes occurs during operative manipulation of pheochromocytoma; the resulting hypertension may be controlled with phentolamine or nitroprusside. Nitroprusside has many advantages, particularly since its effects can be more readily titrated and it has a shorter duration of action.

Alpha-receptor antagonists are most useful in the preoperative management of patients with pheochromocytoma (Figure 10–4). Administration of phenoxybenzamine in the preoperative period will prevent precipitation of acute hypertensive episodes during studies undertaken to localize the tumor and will tend to reverse chronic changes resulting from excessive catecholamine secretion such as plasma volume contraction, if present. Furthermore, the patient's opera-

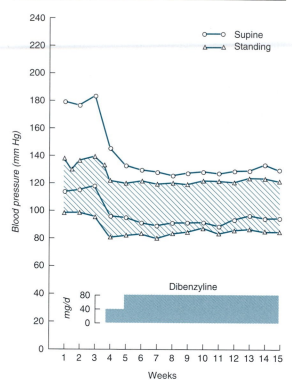

Figure 10–4. Effects of phenoxybenzamine (Dibenzyline) on blood pressure in a patient with pheochromocytoma. Dosage of the drug was begun in the third week as shown by the shaded bar. Supine systolic and diastolic pressures are indicated by the circles, the standing pressures by triangles and the hatched area. Note that the alpha-blocking drug dramatically reduced blood pressure. The reduction in orthostatic hypotension, which was marked before treatment, is probably due to normalization of blood volume, a variable that is sometimes markedly reduced in patients with long-standing pheochromocytoma-induced hypertension. (Redrawn and reproduced, with permission, from Engelman E, Sjoerdsma A: Chronic medical therapy for pheochromocytoma. Ann Intern Med 1961;61:229.)

tive course may be simplified. Oral doses of 10–20 mg/d may be increased at intervals of several days until hypertension is controlled. Some physicians give phenoxybenzamine to patients with pheochromocytoma for 1–3 weeks before surgery. Other surgeons prefer to operate on patients in the absence of treatment with phenoxybenzamine, counting on modern anesthetic techniques to control blood pressure and heart rate during surgery. Phenoxybenzamine may be very useful in the chronic treatment of inoperable or metastatic pheochromocytoma. Although there is less experience with alternative drugs, hypertension in patients with pheochromocytoma may also respond to reversible alpha$_1$-selective antagonists or to conventional calcium channel antagonists. Beta-blocking drugs may be required after alpha-receptor blockade has been instituted to reverse the cardiac effects of excessive catecholamines. Beta antagonists should not be employed prior to establishing effective alpha-receptor blockade, since unopposed beta-receptor blockade could theoretically cause blood pressure elevation from increased vasoconstriction.

Pheochromocytoma is rarely treated with **metyrosine,** the alpha-methyl analog of tyrosine (alpha-methyltyrosine). This agent is a competitive inhibitor of tyrosine hydroxylase and, in oral doses of 1–4 g/d, interferes with synthesis of dopamine (see Figure 6–5), thereby decreasing the amounts of norepinephrine and epinephrine secreted by the tumor. Metyrosine has no alpha-blocking effects but may act synergistically with phenoxybenzamine in the treatment of pheochromocytoma. Metyrosine is especially useful in symptomatic patients with inoperable or metastatic pheochromocytoma.

Hypertensive Emergencies

The alpha adrenoceptor-blocking drugs have limited application in the management of hypertensive emergencies, though labetalol has been increasingly used. In theory, alpha-adrenoceptor antagonists are most useful when increased blood pressure reflects excess circulating concentrations of alpha agonists. In this circumstance, which may result from pheochromocytoma, overdosage of sympathomimetic drugs, or clonidine withdrawal, phentolamine can be used to control high blood pressure. However, other drugs are generally preferable (Chapter 11), since considerable experience is necessary to use phentolamine safely in these settings and few physicians have such experience.

Chronic Hypertension

Members of the prazosin family of alpha$_1$-selective antagonists are efficacious drugs in the treatment of mild to moderate systemic hypertension. They are generally well tolerated by most patients. Their major adverse effect is postural hypotension, which may be severe after the first dose (Chapter 11). Nonselective alpha antagonists are not used in primary systemic hypertension.

Peripheral Vascular Disease

Although alpha receptor-blocking drugs have been tried in the treatment of peripheral vascular occlusive disease, there is no evidence that the effects are significant when morphologic changes limit flow in the vessels. Occasionally, individuals with Raynaud's phenomenon and other conditions involving excessive reversible vasospasm in the peripheral circulation do benefit from phentolamine, tolazoline, or phenoxybenzamine, though calcium channel blockers may be preferable for many patients.

Local Vasoconstrictor Excess

Phentolamine is also useful to reverse the intense local vasoconstriction caused by inadvertent infiltration of alpha agonists (eg, norepinephrine) into subcutaneous tissue during intravenous administration. The alpha antagonist is administered by local infiltration into the ischemic tissue.

Urinary Obstruction

Benign prostatic hyperplasia (BPH) is a prevalent disorder, especially in elderly men. A variety of surgical treatments are effective in relieving the urinary symptoms of BPH, but there is growing interest in drug therapy for it. Alpha-receptor blockade was first found to be helpful in BPH using phenoxybenzamine in selected patients who were poor operative risks. The mechanism of action presumably involves partial reversal of smooth muscle contraction in the enlarged prostate and in the bladder base.

A number of well-controlled studies have demonstrated reproducible efficacy of several alpha$_1$ receptor antagonists in patients with BPH. Prazosin, doxazosin, and terazosin have been used successfully. Considerable interest has focused on which alpha$_1$ receptor subtype is most important for smooth muscle contraction in the prostate: *subtype-selective* alpha$_1$-receptor antagonists might lead to improved efficacy and safety in treating this disease. Some evidence (Lepor et al, 1996) suggests that the efficacy of alpha$_1$ receptor antagonists exceeds that of finasteride, the 5α-reductase inhibitor (see Chapter 40 and Lepor et al, 1996).

Male Sexual Dysfunction

A combination of the alpha-adrenoceptor antagonist phentolamine with the nonspecific vasodilator papaverine, when injected directly into the penis, may cause erections in men with sexual dysfunction. The long-term efficacy of this form of therapy is not known; there is a risk of fibrotic reactions with long-term administration. Systemic absorption may lead to orthostatic hypotension; priapism may require direct treatment with an alpha-adrenoceptor agonist such as phenylephrine. Alternative therapies include prostaglandins (approved; Chapter 18) and alpha$_1$ receptor antagonists and nitric oxide-releasing agents (under investigation).

Applications of Alpha$_2$ Antagonists

It is surprising that alpha$_2$ antagonists have so little clinical usefulness. There is experimental interest in the development of highly selective antagonists for use in Raynaud's phenomenon to inhibit smooth muscle contraction and for use in type II diabetes (alpha$_2$ receptors inhibit insulin secretion) and psychiatric depression (Ruffolo et al, 1993). It is not known to what extent the recognition of multiple subtypes of alpha$_2$ receptors will lead to development of clinically useful subtype-selective new drugs.

III. BASIC PHARMACOLOGY OF THE BETA RECEPTOR ANTAGONIST DRUGS

Drugs in this category share the common feature of antagonizing the effects of catecholamines at beta adrenoceptors. Beta-blocking drugs occupy beta receptors and competitively reduce receptor occupancy by catecholamines and other beta agonists. (A few members of this group, used only for experimental purposes, bind irreversibly to beta receptors.) Most beta-blocking drugs in clinical use are pure antagonists; ie, the occupancy of a beta receptor by such a drug causes no activation of the receptor. However, a few beta receptor-blocking drugs are partial agonists; ie, they cause partial activation of the receptor, albeit less than that caused by the full agonists epinephrine and isoproterenol. Another major difference among the many beta receptor-blocking drugs concerns their relative affinities for beta$_1$ and beta$_2$ receptors (Table 10–1). Some of these antagonists have a higher affinity for beta$_1$ than for beta$_2$ receptors, and this selectivity may have important clinical implications. Other major differences among beta antagonists relate to their pharmacokinetic characteristics and local anesthetic membrane-stabilizing effects.

Chemically, the beta receptor-antagonist drugs (Figure 10–5) resemble isoproterenol (see Figure 9–3), a potent beta receptor agonist.

Pharmacokinetic Properties of the Beta Receptor Antagonists

A. Absorption: Most of the drugs in this class are well absorbed after oral administration; peak concentrations occur 1–3 hours after ingestion. Sustained-release preparations of propranolol and metoprolol are available.

B. Bioavailability: Propranolol undergoes extensive hepatic (first-pass) metabolism; its bioavailability is relatively low (Table 10–2). The proportion of drug reaching the systemic circulation increases as the dose is increased, suggesting that hepatic extraction mechanisms may become saturated. A major consequence of the low bioavailability of propranolol is that oral administration of the drug leads to much lower drug concentrations than are achieved after intravenous injection of the same dose. Because the first-pass effect varies among individuals, there is great individual variability in the plasma concentrations achieved after oral propranolol. Bioavailability is limited to varying degrees for most beta antagonists with the exception of betaxolol, penbutolol, pindolol, and sotalol.

C. Distribution and Clearance: The beta antagonists are rapidly distributed and have large volumes of distribution. Propranolol and penbutolol are quite lipophilic and readily cross the blood-brain barrier (Table 10–2). Most beta antagonists have half-lives in the range of 2–5 hours. A major exception is esmolol, which is rapidly hydrolyzed and has a half-life of approximately 10 minutes. Propranolol and metoprolol are extensively metabolized in the liver, with little unchanged drug appearing in the urine. Atenolol, celiprolol, and pindolol are less completely metabolized. Nadolol is excreted unchanged in the urine and has the longest half-life of any available beta antagonist (up to 24 hours). The half-life of nadolol is prolonged in renal failure. The elimination of drugs such as propranolol may be prolonged in the presence of liver disease, diminished hepatic blood flow, or hepatic enzyme inhibition. It is notable that the clinical effects of these drugs are often prolonged well beyond the time predicted from half-life data.

Pharmacodynamics of the Beta Receptor Antagonist Drugs

Most of the effects of these drugs are due to occupancy and blockade of beta receptors. However, some actions may be due to other effects, including partial agonist activity at beta receptors and local anesthetic action, which differ among the beta-blockers (Table 10–2).

A. Effects on the Cardiovascular System: Beta-blocking drugs given chronically lower blood pressure in patients with hypertension. The factors involved may include effects on the heart and blood vessels, the renin-angiotensin system, and perhaps the central nervous system. Beta adrenoceptor-blocking drugs are of major clinical importance in the treatment of hypertension (Chapter 11). In conventional doses, these drugs do not usually cause hypotension in healthy individuals with normal blood pressure.

Beta receptor antagonists have prominent effects on the heart (Figure 10–6). The negative inotropic and chronotropic effects are predictable from the role of adrenoceptors in regulating these functions. Slowed atrioventricular conduction with an increased PR interval is a related result of adrenoceptor blockade in the atrioventricular node. These effects may be clinically valuable in some patients but are potentially hazardous in others. In the vascular system, beta receptor blockade opposes beta$_2$-mediated vasodilation. This may result initially in a rise in peripheral resistance from unopposed alpha receptor-mediated effects. Beta-blocking drugs antagonize the release of

Figure 10–5. Structures of some beta receptor antagonists.

renin caused by the sympathetic nervous system. As noted in Chapter 11, the relation between the effects on renin release and those on blood pressure is still being debated. In any event, while the acute effects of these drugs may include a rise in peripheral resistance, chronic drug administration leads to a fall in peripheral resistance.

B. Effects on the Respiratory Tract: Blockade of the beta$_2$ receptors in bronchial smooth muscle may lead to an increase in airway resistance, particularly in patients with asthma. Beta$_1$ receptor antagonists such as metoprolol or atenolol may have some advantage over nonselective beta antagonists when blockade of beta$_1$ receptors in the heart is desired and beta$_2$ receptor blockade is undesirable. However, no currently available beta$_1$-selective antagonist is sufficiently specific to *completely* avoid interactions with beta$_2$ adrenoceptors. Consequently, these drugs should generally be avoided in patients with asthma.

C. Effects on the Eye: Several beta-blocking agents reduce intraocular pressure, especially in glaucomatous eyes. The mechanism usually reported is decreased aqueous humor production. (See Clinical Pharmacology and box: The Treatment of Glaucoma.)

D. Metabolic and Endocrine Effects: Beta antagonists such as propranolol inhibit sympathetic nervous system stimulation of lipolysis. The effects on carbohydrate metabolism are less clear, though glycogenolysis in the human liver is at least partially inhibited after beta$_2$ receptor blockade. However, glucagon is the primary hormone employed to combat hypoglycemia. It is unclear to what extent beta antagonists impair recovery from hypoglycemia, but they should be used with great caution in insulin-dependent diabetic patients. This may be particularly important in diabetic patients with inadequate glucagon reserve and in pancreatectomized patients since catecholamines may be the major factors in stimulating

Table 10–2. Properties of several beta-receptor-blocking drugs.

	Selectivity	Partial Agonist Activity	Local Anesthetic Action	Lipid Solubility	Elimination Half-Life (Hours)	Approximate Bioavailability
Acebutolol	β_1	Yes	Yes	Low	3–4	50
Atenolol	β_1	No	No	Low	6–9	40
Betaxolol	β_1	No	Slight	Low	14–22	90
Bisoprolol	β_1	No	No	Low	9–12	80
Carteolol	None	Yes	No	Low	6	85
Carvedilol[1]	None	No	No	No data	7–10	25–35
Celiprolol	β_1	Yes[2]	No	No data	4–5	70
Esmolol	β_1	No	No	Low	10	~0
Labetalol[1]	None	Yes[1]	Yes	Moderate	5	30
Metoprolol	β_1	No	Yes	Moderate	3–4	50
Nadolol	None	No	No	Low	14–24	33
Penbutolol	None	Yes	No	High	5	>90
Pindolol	None	Yes	Yes	Moderate	3–4	90
Propranolol	None	No	Yes	High	3.5–6	30[3]
Sotalol	None	No	No	Low	12	90
Timolol	None	No	No	Moderate	4–5	50

[1]Carvedilol and labetalol also cause α_1 adrenoceptor blockade.
[2]Partial agonist effects at β_2 receptors.
[3]Bioavailability is dose-dependent.

glucose release from the liver in response to hypoglycemia. However, beta receptor antagonists are much safer in those non-insulin-dependent diabetic patients who do not have hypoglycemia reactions.

The chronic use of beta adrenoceptor antagonists has been associated with increased plasma concentrations of VLDL and decreased concentrations of HDL cholesterol. Both of these changes are potentially unfavorable in terms of risk of cardiovascular disease. Although LDL concentrations generally do not change, there is a variable decline in the HDL cholesterol/LDL cholesterol ratio that may increase the risk of coronary artery disease. These changes tend to occur with both selective and nonselective beta-

Figure 10–6. The effect in an anesthetized dog of the injection of epinephrine before and after propranolol. In the presence of a beta receptor-blocking agent, epinephrine no longer augments the force of contraction (measured by a strain gauge attached to the ventricular wall) nor increases cardiac rate. Blood pressure is still elevated by epinephrine because vasoconstriction is not blocked. (Reproduced, with permission, from Shanks RG: The pharmacology of beta sympathetic blockade. Am J Cardiol 1966;18:312.)

blockers, though they are less likely to occur with beta-blockers possessing intrinsic sympathomimetic activity (partial agonists). Interestingly, the use of *alpha*-adrenoceptor antagonists such as prazosin has been found to be associated with either no changes in plasma lipids or increased concentrations of HDL, which could be a favorable alteration. The mechanisms by which alpha- and beta-receptor antagonists cause these changes are not understood.

E. Effects Not Related to Beta Blockade:
Partial beta-agonist activity was significant in the first beta-blocking drug synthesized, dichloroisoproterenol. It has been suggested that retention of some intrinsic sympathomimetic activity is desirable to prevent untoward effects such as precipitation of asthma. Pindolol and other partial agonists are noted in Table 10–2. It is not yet clear to what extent partial agonism is clinically valuable. However, these drugs may be useful in patients who develop symptomatic bradycardia or bronchoconstriction with nonselective beta-adrenoceptor antagonists. Nonetheless, a beta-blocker should be used with great caution in these settings and only if the drug is strongly indicated for a particular clinical indication. Furthermore, the possibly smaller adverse effects of partial agonist drugs on plasma lipids warrant continuing study.

Local anesthetic action, also known as "membrane-stabilizing" action, is a prominent effect of several beta-blockers (Table 10–2). This action is the result of typical local anesthetic blockade of sodium channels and can be demonstrated in neurons, heart muscle, and skeletal muscle membrane. However, it is unlikely that this effect is important after systemic administration, since the concentration usually achieved by that route is too low for the anesthetic effects to be evident. These drugs are not used topically on the eye, where local anesthesia of the cornea would be highly undesirable. Sotalol is a nonselective beta receptor antagonist that lacks local anesthetic action but has marked class III antiarrhythmic effects, reflecting potassium channel blockade (see Chapter 14).

SPECIFIC AGENTS
(See Table 10–2.)

Propranolol is the prototype beta-blocking drug. It has low and dose-dependent bioavailability, the result of extensive first-pass metabolism in the liver. A long-acting form of propranolol is available; prolonged absorption of the drug may occur over a 24-hour period. The drug has negligible effects at alpha and muscarinic receptors; however, it may block some serotonin receptors in the brain, though the clinical significance is unclear. It has no detectable partial agonist action at beta receptors.

Metoprolol, atenolol, and several other drugs (see Table 10–2) are members of the beta$_1$-selective group. These agents may be safer in patients who experience

bronchoconstriction responses to propranolol. However, since their beta$_1$ selectivity is rather modest, they should be used with great caution, if at all, in patients with a history of bronchospasm. Beta$_1$-selective antagonists may be preferable in patients with diabetes or peripheral vascular disease when therapy with a beta-blocker is required since beta$_2$ receptors are probably important in liver (recovery from hypoglycemia) and blood vessels (vasodilation).

Nadolol is noteworthy for its very long duration of action; its spectrum of action is similar to that of timolol. **Timolol** is a nonselective agent with no local anesthetic activity. It has excellent ocular hypotensive effects. **Levobunolol** (nonselective) and **betaxolol** (beta$_1$-selective) are used for direct ophthalmic application in glaucoma; the latter drug may be less likely to induce bronchoconstriction than nonselective antagonists. **Carteolol** is a nonselective beta receptor antagonist.

Pindolol, acebutolol, carteolol, bopindolol,* **oxprenolol,*** **celiprolol,** and **penbutolol** are of interest because they have partial beta-agonist activity. They are effective in the major cardiovascular applications of the beta-blocking group (hypertension and angina). Although these partial agonists may be less likely to cause bradycardia and abnormalities in plasma lipids than are antagonists, the overall clinical significance of intrinsic sympathomimetic activity remains uncertain.

Celiprolol is a beta$_1$-selective antagonist with a modest capacity to activate beta$_2$ receptors. The drug is efficacious in hypertension and in treating angina. There is limited evidence suggesting that celiprolol may have less adverse bronchoconstrictor effects in asthma and may even promote bronchodilation (van Zyl et al, 1989). If absence of unfavorable effects in asthmatics is confirmed in longer and more extensive clinical trials, celiprolol would have significant advantages for some patients requiring a beta receptor antagonist (see Clinical Pharmacology, Hypertension, below). Acebutolol is also a beta$_1$-selective antagonist.

Labetalol is a reversible adrenoceptor antagonist available as a racemic mixture of two pairs of chiral isomers (the molecule has two centers of asymmetry). The *SS* and *RS* isomers are inactive, *SR* is a potent alpha-blocker, and the *RR* isomer is a potent beta-blocker. Labetalol's affinity for alpha receptors is less than that of phentolamine, but labetalol is alpha$_1$-selective. Its beta-blocking potency is somewhat lower than that of propranolol. Hypotension induced by labetalol is accompanied by less tachycardia than occurs with phentolamine and similar alpha-blockers.

Carvedilol, medroxalol,* and **bucindolol*** are nonselective beta receptor antagonists with some capacity to block alpha$_1$-adrenergic receptors.

---

*Not available in the USA.

Esmolol is an ultra-short-acting beta$_1$-selective adrenoceptor antagonist. The structure of esmolol contains an ester linkage; esterases in red blood cells rapidly metabolize esmolol to a metabolite that has a low affinity for beta receptors. Consequently, esmolol has a short half-life (about 10 minutes). Therefore, during continuous infusions of esmolol, steady state concentrations are achieved quickly, and the therapeutic actions of the drug are terminated rapidly when its infusion is discontinued. Esmolol is potentially much safer to use than longer-acting antagonists in critically ill patients who require a beta-adrenoceptor antagonist. Esmolol may be useful in controlling supraventricular arrhythmias, perioperative hypertension, and myocardial ischemia in acutely ill patients.

Butoxamine is selective for beta$_2$ receptors. Selective beta$_2$-blocking drugs have not been actively sought because there is no obvious clinical application for them.

IV. CLINICAL PHARMACOLOGY OF THE BETA RECEPTOR BLOCKING DRUGS

Hypertension

Many of the beta adrenoceptor-blocking drugs have proved to be effective and well tolerated in hypertension. While many hypertensive patients will respond to a beta-blocker used alone, the drug is often used with either a diuretic or a vasodilator. In spite of the short half-life of many beta antagonists, these drugs may be administered once or twice daily and still have an adequate therapeutic effect. Labetalol, a competitive alpha and beta antagonist, is effective in hypertension, though its ultimate role is yet to be determined. Use of these agents is discussed in detail in Chapter 11. There is some evidence that drugs in this class may be less effective in blacks and the elderly. However, these differences are relatively small and may not apply to an individual patient. Indeed, since effects on blood pressure are easily measured, the therapeutic outcome for this indication can be readily detected in any patient.

Considerable attention has been paid during the last decade to claims that partial agonists (eg, pindolol) have increased safety in patients with airway disease. In theory, there is much to recommend this idea, since the partial agonist beta-blockers are better agonists at beta$_2$ than at beta$_1$ receptors. This should result in useful bronchodilation and even added hypotensive action from the smooth muscle-relaxing action of beta$_2$ agonism while the beta$_1$ antagonist action reduces blood pressure. Unfortunately, there is little evidence of practical clinical differences to support this hypothesis at present. One potential advantage of partial agonist beta-blockers that has not yet been disproved is a relative lack of deleterious effect on plasma lipids.

Ischemic Heart Disease

Beta adrenoceptor blockers reduce the frequency of anginal episodes and improve exercise tolerance in many patients with angina (see Chapter 12). These actions relate to the blockade of cardiac beta receptors, resulting in decreased cardiac work and reduction in oxygen demand. Slowing and regularization of the heart rate may contribute to clinical benefits (Figure 10–7). Large-scale prospective studies indicate that the long-term use of timolol, propranolol, oxprenolol, or metoprolol in patients who have had a myocardial infarction prolongs survival (Figure 10–8). Studies in experimental animals suggest that use of beta receptor antagonists during the acute phase of a myocardial infarction may limit infarct size. However, this use is still controversial.

Cardiac Arrhythmias

Beta antagonists are effective in the treatment of both supraventricular and ventricular arrhythmias (see Chapter 14). In cases of sinus tachycardia and supraventricular ectopic beats, treatment should not be limited to the use of a beta antagonist; attention should be given to the underlying disease. By increasing the atrioventricular nodal refractory period, beta antagonists will slow ventricular response rates in atrial flutter and fibrillation. These drugs can also reduce ventricular ectopic beats, particularly if the ectopic activity has been precipitated by catecholamines. Sotalol has additional antiarrhythmic effects in addition to its beta-blocking action; these are discussed in Chapter 14.

Other Cardiovascular Disorders

Beta receptor antagonists have been found to increase stroke volume in some patients with obstructive cardiomyopathy. This beneficial effect is thought to result from the slowing of ventricular ejection and decreased outflow resistance. Beta antagonists are useful in dissecting aortic aneurysm to decrease the rate of development of systolic pressure. Recent experimental evidence suggests that—paradoxically—beta antagonists may be effective in treating congestive heart failure in certain carefully selected patients, though this possibility requires more extensive studies. Carvedilol, a beta receptor antagonist with antioxidant activity, has recently been found to prolong life in some patients with congestive failure, though the mechanism is uncertain. Beta receptor antagonists may be useful in the treatment of heart failure when used by skilled and experienced physicians in carefully selected patients. However, these drugs are generally contraindicated in patients with congestive heart failure, who depend on sympathetic drive to maintain cardiac output except under special conditions.

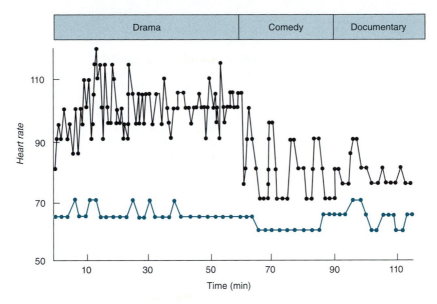

Figure 10–7. Heart rate in a patient with ischemic heart disease measured by telemetry while watching television. Measurements were begun 1 hour after receiving placebo (solid circles, black) or 40 mg of oxprenolol (color), a nonselective beta-antagonist with partial agonist activity. Not only was the heart rate decreased by the drug under the conditions of this experiment; it also varied much less in response to stimuli. (Modified and reproduced, with permission, from Taylor SH: Oxprenolol in clinical practice. Am J Cardiol 1983;52:34D.)

Glaucoma
(See box: The Treatment of Glaucoma)

Systemic administration of beta-blocking drugs for other indications was found serendipitously to reduce intraocular pressure in patients with glaucoma. Subsequently, it was found that topical administration also reduces intraocular pressure. The mechanism ap-

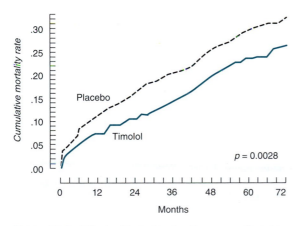

Figure 10–8. Effects of beta-blocker therapy on life-table cumulated rates of mortality from all causes over 6 years among 1884 patients surviving myocardial infarctions. Patients were randomly assigned to treatment with placebo (dashed line) or timolol (color). (Reproduced, with permission, from Pederson TR: Six-year follow-up of the Norwegian multicenter study on timolol after acute myocardial infarction. N Engl J Med 1985;313:1055.)

pears to involve reduced production of aqueous humor by the ciliary body, which is physiologically activated by cAMP. Timolol has been favored for local use in the eye because it lacks local anesthetic properties and is a pure antagonist. Timolol appears to have an efficacy comparable to that of epinephrine or pilocarpine in open-angle glaucoma. While the maximal daily dose applied locally (1 mg) is small compared with the systemic doses commonly used in the treatment of hypertension or angina (10–60 mg), sufficient timolol may be absorbed from the eye to cause serious adverse effects on the heart and airways in susceptible individuals. Topical timolol may interact with orally administered verapamil and increase risk of heart block.

Betaxolol, carteolol, levobunolol, and metipranolol are newer beta-receptor antagonists approved for the treatment of glaucoma. Betaxolol has the potential advantage of being beta$_1$-selective; to what extent this potential advantage might diminish systemic adverse effects remains to be determined. The drug apparently has caused worsening of pulmonary symptoms in some patients.

Hyperthyroidism

Excessive catecholamine action is an important aspect of the pathophysiology of hyperthyroidism, especially in relation to the heart (see Chapter 38). The beta antagonists have salutary effects in this condition. These beneficial effects presumably relate to blockade of adrenoceptors and perhaps to the inhibi-

THE TREATMENT OF GLAUCOMA

Glaucoma is a major cause of blindness and of great pharmacologic interest because the chronic form often responds to drug therapy. The primary manifestation is increased intraocular pressure not initially associated with symptoms. Without treatment, increased intraocular pressure results in damage to the retina and optic nerve, with restriction of visual fields and, eventually, blindness. Intraocular pressure is easily measured as part of the routine ophthalmologic examination. Two major types of glaucoma are recognized: open-angle and closed-angle (or narrow-angle). The closed-angle form is associated with a shallow anterior chamber, in which a dilated iris can occlude the outflow drainage pathway at the angle between the cornea and the ciliary body (Figure 6–9). This form is associated with acute and painful increases of pressure, which must be controlled on an emergency basis with drugs or prevented by surgical removal of part of the iris (iridectomy). The open-angle form of glaucoma is a chronic condition, and treatment is largely pharmacologic. Because intraocu-

lar pressure is a function of the balance between fluid input and drainage out of the globe, the strategies for the treatment of closed-angle glaucoma fall into two classes: reduction of aqueous humor secretion and enhancement of aqueous outflow. Four general groups of drugs—cholinomimetics, alpha agonists, beta-blockers, and diuretics—have been found to be useful in reducing intraocular pressure and can be related to these strategies as shown in Table 10–3. Of the four drug groups listed in Table 10–3, the beta-blockers are by far the most popular. This popularity results from convenience (once- or twice-daily dosing) and relative lack of adverse effects (except in patients with asthma or cardiac pacemaker or conduction pathway disease). Other drugs that have been reported to reduce intraocular pressure include alpha$_2$ agonists, prostaglandin E$_2$, and marijuana. The use of drugs in acute closed-angle glaucoma is limited to cholinomimetics and osmotic agents preceding surgery. The onset of action of the other agents is too slow in this situation.

---

tion of peripheral conversion of thyroxine to triiodothyronine. The latter action may vary from one beta antagonist to another. Propranolol is particularly efficacious in thyroid storm; it has been used cautiously in patients with this condition to control supraventricular tachycardias that often precipitate congestive heart failure.

Neurologic Diseases

Several studies show a beneficial effect of propranolol in reducing the frequency and intensity of migraine headache. The mechanism is not known. Since sympathetic activity may enhance skeletal muscle tremor, it is not surprising that beta antagonists have been found to reduce certain tremors (Chapter 28). The somatic manifestations of anxiety may respond dramatically to low doses of propranolol, particularly when taken prophylactically. For example, benefit has been found in musicians with performance anxiety ("stage fright"). Propranolol is also of benefit in treating alcohol withdrawal.

Miscellaneous

Beta receptor antagonists have been found to diminish portal vein pressure in patients with cirrhosis. There is evidence that both propranolol and nadolol decrease the incidence of the first episode of bleeding from esophageal varices and decrease the mortality rate associated with bleeding in patients with cirrhosis. Recently, nadolol in combination with isosorbide mononitrate was found to be more efficacious than

sclerotherapy in preventing re-bleeding in patients who have previously bled from esophageal varices.

CHOICE OF A BETA-BLOCKING DRUG

Propranolol is the standard against which newer beta antagonists developed for systemic use should be compared. In many years of very wide use, it has been found to be a safe and effective drug for many indications. Since it is possible that some actions of a beta receptor antagonist may relate to some other effect of the drug, these drugs should not be considered interchangeable for all applications. For example, only beta antagonists known to be effective in hyperthyroidism or in prophylactic therapy after myocardial infarction should be used for those indications. It is possible that the beneficial effects of one drug in these settings might not be shared by another drug in the same class. The possible advantages and disadvantages of beta-blockers that are partial agonists have not been clearly defined in clinical settings.

CLINICAL TOXICITY OF THE BETA RECEPTOR ANTAGONIST DRUGS

A variety of minor toxic effects have been reported for propranolol. Rash, fever, and other manifestations of drug allergy are rare. Central nervous system effects include sedation, sleep disturbances, and depres-

Table 10–3. Drugs used in open-angle glaucoma.

	Mechanism	Methods of Administration
Cholinomimetics Pilocarpine, carbachol, physostigmine, echothiophate	Ciliary muscle contraction, opening of trabecular meshwork; increased outflow	Topical drops or gel; plastic film slow-release insert
Alpha agonists Unselective Epinephrine, dipivefrin	Increased outflow	Topical drops
Alpha$_2$-selective Apraclonidine Brimonidine	Decreased aqueous secretion	Topical, postlaser only Topical
Beta-blockers Timolol, betaxolol, carteolol, levobunolol, metipranolol	Decreased aqueous secretion from the ciliary epithelium	Topical drops
Diuretics Dorzolamide	Decreased secretion due to lack of HCO$_3^-$	Topical
Acetazolamide		Oral
Ethacrynic acid (investigational)	Decreased secretion	Intraocular injection at long intervals, eg, annually

sion. Rarely, psychotic reactions may occur. Discontinuing the use of beta-blockers in any patient who develops a depression should be seriously considered if clinically feasible. It has been claimed that beta receptor antagonist drugs with low lipid solubility will be associated with a lower incidence of central nervous system adverse effects than compounds with higher lipid solubility (Table 10–2). Further studies designed to compare the central nervous system adverse effects of various drugs are required before specific recommendations can be made, though it seems reasonable to try nadolol or atenolol in a patient who experiences unpleasant central nervous system effects with other beta-blockers. Experience with the newer members of this group is too limited to permit comparison of the incidence of toxic effects.

The major adverse effects of beta receptor antagonist drugs relate to the predictable consequences of beta blockade. Beta$_2$ receptor blockade associated with the use of nonselective agents commonly causes worsening of preexisting asthma and other forms of airway obstruction without having these consequences in normal individuals. Indeed, relatively trivial asthma may become severe after beta blockade. While beta$_1$-selective drugs may have less effect on airways than nonselective beta antagonists, they must be used very cautiously, if at all, in patients with reactive airways. While beta$_1$-selective antagonists are generally well tolerated in patients with mild to moderate peripheral vascular disease, caution is required in patients with severe peripheral vascular disease or vasospastic disorders.

Beta receptor blockade depresses myocardial contractility and excitability. In patients with abnormal myocardial function, cardiac output may be dependent on sympathetic drive. If this stimulus is removed by beta blockade, cardiac decompensation may ensue. Great caution must be exercised in using beta receptor antagonists in patients with myocardial infarction or compensated congestive heart failure. In a life-threatening situation, an adverse cardiac effect of a beta antagonist may be overcome directly with isoproterenol or with glucagon (glucagon stimulates the heart via glucagon receptors, which are not blocked by beta antagonists), but neither of these methods is without hazard. A very small dose of a beta antagonist (eg, 10 mg of propranolol) may provoke severe cardiac failure in a susceptible individual. Beta-blockers may interact with the calcium antagonist verapamil; severe hypotension, bradycardia, congestive heart failure, and cardiac conduction abnormalities have all been described. These adverse effects may also arise in susceptible patients taking a topical (ophthalmic) beta-blocker and oral verapamil.

There are hazards associated with abruptly discontinuing beta antagonist therapy after chronic use. Evidence suggests that patients with ischemic heart disease may be at increased risk if beta blockade is suddenly interrupted. The mechanism of this effect is uncertain but might involve "up-regulation" of the number of beta receptors. Until better evidence is available regarding the magnitude of the risk, prudence dictates the gradual tapering rather than abrupt cessation of dosage when these drugs are discontinued.

The incidence of hypoglycemic episodes in diabetics that are exacerbated by beta-blocking agents is unknown. Nevertheless, it is inadvisable to use beta antagonists in insulin-dependent diabetic patients who are subject to frequent hypoglycemic reactions if alternative therapies are available. Beta$_1$-selective antagonists offer some advantage in these patients, since the rate of recovery from hypoglycemia may be faster compared with diabetics receiving nonselective beta adrenoceptor antagonists.

Beta blockade may mask clinical signs of developing hyperthyroidism. With the growing number of patients taking beta antagonists for prolonged periods, this effect may become increasingly important.

PREPARATIONS AVAILABLE

Alpha-Blockers
Doxazosin (Cardura)
Oral: 1, 2, 4, 8 mg tablets
Phenoxybenzamine (Dibenzyline)
Oral: 10 mg capsules
Phentolamine (Regitine)
Parenteral: 5 mg/mL for injection
Prazosin (generic, Minipress)
Oral: 1, 2, 5 mg capsules
Terazosin (Hytrin)
Oral: 1, 2, 5, 10 mg tablets, capsules
Tolazoline (Priscoline)
Parenteral: 25 mg/mL for injection

Beta-Blockers
Acebutolol (Sectral)
Oral: 200, 400 mg capsules
Atenolol (generic, Tenormin)
Oral: 25, 50, 100 mg tablets
Parenteral: 0.5 mg/mL for IV injection
Betaxolol
Oral: 10, 20 mg tablets (Kerlone)
Ophthalmic: 0.5% drops (Betoptic)
Bisoprolol (Zebeta)
Oral: 5, 10 mg tablets
Carteolol
Oral: 2.5, 5 mg tablets (Cartrol)
Ophthalmic: 1% drops (Ocupress)
Carvedilol (Coreg)
Oral: 6.25, 12.5, 25 mg tablets
Esmolol (Brevibloc)
Parenteral: 10 mg/mL for IV injection; 250 mg/mL for IV infusion

Labetalol (Normodyne, Trandate)
Oral: 100, 200, 300 mg tablets
Parenteral: 5 mg/mL for injection
Levobunolol (Betagan Liquifilm, others)
Ophthalmic: 0.25, 0.5% drops
Metipranolol (Optipranolol)
Ophthalmic: 0.3% drops
Metoprolol (Lopressor, Toprol)
Oral: 50, 100 mg tablets
Oral sustained-release: 50, 100, 200 mg tablets
Parenteral: 1 mg/mL for injection
Nadolol (Corgard)
Oral: 20, 40, 80, 120, 160 mg tablets
Penbutolol (Levatol)
Oral: 20 mg tablets
Pindolol (Visken)
Oral: 5, 10 mg tablets
Propranolol (generic, Inderal)
Oral: 10, 20, 40, 60, 80, 90 mg tablets; 4, 8, 80 mg/mL solutions
Oral sustained release: 60, 80, 120, 160 mg capsules
Parenteral: 1 mg/mL for injection
Sotalol (Betapace)
Oral: 80, 160, 240 mg tablets
Timolol
Oral: 5, 10, 20 mg tablets (generic, Blocadren)
Ophthalmic: 0.25, 0.5% drops, gel (Timoptic)

Synthesis Inhibitor
Metyrosine (Demser)
Oral: 250 mg capsules

REFERENCES

Abrams P et al: Tamsulosin, a selective alpha$_{1C}$- adrenoceptor antagonist: A randomized, controlled trial in patients with benign prostatic obstruction (symptomatic BPH). Br J Urol 1995;76:325.

Adams KF Jr: Current perspectives on beta-receptor antagonists in the treatment of symptomatic ventricular dysfunction. Pharmacotherapy 1996;16:69S.

Ariens EJ: Chirality in bioactive agents and its pitfalls. Trends Pharmacol Sci 1986;7:200.

Babamoto K, Hirokawa WT: Doxazosin: A new alpha$_1$-adrenergic antagonist. Clin Pharm 1992;11:415.

Benfield P, Clissold SP, Brogden RN: Metoprolol. Drugs 1986;31:376.

Beta blockers and lipophilicity. (Editorial.) Lancet 1987;1:900.

Blaufarb I, Pfeifer TM, Frishman WH: Beta-blockers: Drug interactions of clinical significance. Drug Saf 1995; 13:359.

Brantigan CO, Brantigan TA, Joseph N: Effect of beta blockade and beta stimulation on stage fright. Am J Med 1982;72:88.

Doughty RN, MacMahon S, Sharpe N: Beta-blockers in heart failure: Promising or proved? J Am Coll Cardiol 1994;23:814.

Fallon B: Intracavernous injection therapy for male erectile dysfunction. Urol Clin North Am 1995;22:833.

Fitzgerald JD: Do partial agonist beta-blockers have improved clinical utility? Cardiovasc Drugs Ther 1993;7:303.

Frishman WH, Fuksbrumer MS, Tannenbaum M: Topical ophthalmic beta-adrenergic blockade for the treatment of glaucoma and ocular hypertension. J Clin Pharmacol 1994;34:795.

Frishman WH, Lazar EJ, Gorodokin G: Pharmacokinetic optimisation of therapy with beta-adrenergic blocking agents. Clin Pharmacokinet 1991;20:311.

Gengo FM, Huntoon L, McHugh WB: Lipid-soluble and water-soluble beta blockers: Comparison of the central nervous system depressant effect. Arch Intern Med 1987;147:39.

Gold EH et al: Synthesis and comparison of some cardiovascular properties of the stereoisomers of labetalol. J Med Chem 1982;25:1363.

Goldberg MR, Robertson D: Yohimbine: A pharmacological probe of the alpha$_2$ adrenoceptor. Pharmacol Rev 1983;35:143.

Goldstein S: Beta-blockers in hypertensive and coronary heart disease. Arch Intern Med 1996;156:1267.

Hampton JR: Choosing the right beta-blocker: A guide to selection. Drugs 1994;48:549.

Heintzen MP, Strauer BE: Peripheral vascular effects of beta-blockers. Eur Heart J 1994;15(Suppl C):2.

Hjalmarson A et al: The Göteborg metoprolol trial: Effects on mortality and morbidity in acute myocardial infarction. Circulation 1983;67(Suppl I):I-26.

Janknegt RA et al: Efficacy and safety of the alpha$_1$ blocker doxazosin in the treatment of benign prostatic hyperplasia. Eur Urol 1993;24:319.

Jonler M, Riehmann M, Bruskewitz RC: Benign prostatic hyperplasia: Current pharmacological treatment. Drugs 1994;47:66.

Lepor H et al: The efficacy of terazosin, finasteride, or both in benign prostate hyperplasia. N Engl J Med 1996;335:533.

Lepor H: Prostate selectivity of alpha-blockers: From receptor biology to clinical medicine. Eur Urol 1996;29(Suppl 1):12.

Leren P: Comparison of effects on lipid metabolism of antihypertensive drugs with alpha- and beta-adrenergic antagonist properties. Am J Med 1987;82(Suppl 1A):31.

Lesar TS: Comparison of ophthalmic beta-blocking agents. Clin Pharm 1987;6:451.

Montorsi F et al: Pharmacological management of erectile dysfunction. Drugs 1995;50:465.

Morgan T: Clinical pharmacokinetics and pharmacodynamics of carvedilol. Clin Pharmacokinet 1994;26:335.

Nickerson M: The pharmacology of adrenergic blockade. Pharmacol Rev 1949;1:27.

Poynard T et al: Beta-adrenergic-antagonist drugs in the prevention of gastrointestinal bleeding in patients with cirrhosis and esophageal varices: An analysis of data and prognostic factors in 589 patients from four randomized clinical trials. N Engl J Med 1991;324:1532.

Reid D et al: Double-blind trial of yohimbine in treatment of psychogenic impotence. Lancet 1987;2:421.

Rosenthal J: Lipid metabolism: Implications of alpha 1-blockade. J Clin Pharmacol 1993;33:883.

Ruffolo RR Jr et al: Pharmacologic and therapeutic applications of alpha$_2$-adrenoceptor subtypes. Annu Rev Pharmacol Toxicol 1993;32:243.

Ruffolo RR Jr, Hieble JP: Alpha-adrenoceptors. Pharmacol Ther 1994;61:1.

Sidi AA: Vasoactive intracavernous pharmacotherapy. Urol Clin North Am 1988;15:95.

van Zwieten PA: An overview of the pharmacodynamic properties and therapeutic potential of combined alpha- and beta-adrenoceptor antagonists. Drugs 1993;45:509.

van Zyl AI et al: Comparison of respiratory effects of two cardioselective beta-blockers, celiprolol and atenolol, in asthmatics with mild to moderate hypertension. Chest 1989;95:209.

Villanueva C et al: Nadolol plus isosorbide mononitrate compared with sclerotherapy for prevention of variceal bleeding. N Engl J Med 1996;334:1624.

Wilde MI et al: Alfusosin: A review of its pharmacodynamic and pharmacokinetic properties, and therapeutic potential in benign prostatic hyperplasia. Drugs 1993;45:410.

Wilde MI, Fitton A, Sorkin EM: Terazosin. A review of its pharmacodynamic and pharmacokinetic properties, and therapeutic potential in benign prostatic hyperplasia. Drugs Aging 1993;3:258.

Yamada Y et al: Risk assessment of adverse pulmonary effects induced by adrenaline beta-receptor antagonists and rational drug dosage regimen based on receptor occupancy. J Pharmacokinet Biopharm 1995;5:463.

Yedinak KC: Formulary considerations in selection of beta-blockers. Pharmacoeconomics 1993;4:104.

Section III.
Cardiovascular-Renal Drugs

Antihypertensive Agents

11

Neal L. Benowitz, MD

Hypertension is the most common cardiovascular disease. Thus, the third National Health and Nutrition Examination Survey (NHANES III), conducted from 1988 through 1991, found that 24% of the United States adult population had hypertension. The prevalence varies with age, race, education, and many other variables. Sustained arterial hypertension damages blood vessels in kidney, heart, and brain and leads to an increased incidence of renal failure, coronary disease, cardiac failure, and stroke. Effective pharmacologic lowering of blood pressure has been shown to prevent damage to blood vessels and to substantially reduce morbidity and mortality rates. Many effective drugs are available. Knowledge of their antihypertensive mechanisms and sites of action allows accurate prediction of efficacy and toxicity. As a result, rational use of these agents, alone or in combination, can lower blood pressure with minimal risk of serious toxicity in most patients.

HYPERTENSION & REGULATION OF BLOOD PRESSURE

Diagnosis

The diagnosis of hypertension is based on repeated, reproducible measurements of elevated blood pressure. The diagnosis serves primarily as a prediction of consequences for the patient; it seldom includes a statement about the cause of hypertension.

Epidemiologic studies indicate that the risks of damage to kidney, heart, and brain are directly related to the extent of blood pressure elevation. Even mild hypertension (blood pressure ≥ 140/90 mm Hg) in young or middle-aged adults increases the risk of eventual end organ damage. The risks—and therefore the urgency of

instituting therapy—increase in proportion to the magnitude of blood pressure elevation. The risk of end organ damage at any level of blood pressure or age is greater in black people and relatively less in premenopausal women than in men. Other positive risk factors include smoking, hyperlipidemia, diabetes, manifestations of end organ damage at the time of diagnosis, and a family history of cardiovascular disease.

It should be noted that the diagnosis of hypertension depends on measurement of blood pressure and not upon symptoms reported by the patient. In fact, hypertension is usually asymptomatic until overt end organ damage is imminent or has already occurred.

Etiology of Hypertension

A specific cause of hypertension can be established in only 10–15% of patients. It is important to consider specific causes in each case, however, because some of them are amenable to definitive surgical treatment: renal artery constriction, coarctation of the aorta, pheochromocytoma, Cushing's disease, and primary aldosteronism.

Patients in whom no specific cause of hypertension can be found are said to have **essential hypertension.*** In most cases, elevated blood pressure is associated with an overall increase in resistance to flow of blood through arterioles, while cardiac output is usually normal. Meticulous investigation of autonomic nervous system function, baroreceptor reflexes, the renin-angiotensin-aldosterone system, and the kidney has failed to identify a primary abnormality as the cause of increased peripheral vascular resistance in essential hypertension.

---

*The adjective originally was intended to convey the now abandoned idea that blood pressure elevation was essential for adequate perfusion of diseased tissues.

Elevated blood pressure is usually caused by a combination of several abnormalities (multifactorial). Epidemiologic evidence points to genetic inheritance, psychologic stress, and environmental and dietary factors (increased salt and perhaps decreased potassium or calcium intake) as perhaps contributing to the development of hypertension. Increase in blood pressure with aging does not occur in populations with low daily sodium intake. Patients with labile hypertension appear more likely than normal controls to have blood pressure elevations after salt loading.

Normal Regulation of Blood Pressure

According to the hydraulic equation, arterial blood pressure (BP) is directly proportionate to the product of the blood flow (cardiac output, CO) and the resistance to passage of blood through precapillary arterioles (peripheral vascular resistance, PVR):

$$BP = CO \times PVR$$

Physiologically, in both normal and hypertensive individuals, blood pressure is maintained by moment-to-moment regulation of cardiac output and peripheral vascular resistance, exerted at three anatomic sites (Figure 11–1): arterioles, postcapillary venules (capacitance vessels), and heart. A fourth anatomic control site, the kidney, contributes to maintenance of blood pressure by regulating the volume of intravascular fluid. Baroreflexes, mediated by autonomic nerves, act in combination with humoral mechanisms, including the renin-angiotensin-aldosterone system, to coordinate function at these four control sites and to maintain normal blood pressure.

Blood pressure in a hypertensive patient is controlled by the same mechanisms that are operative in normotensive subjects. Regulation of blood pressure in hypertensives differs from normal in that the baroreceptors and the renal blood volume-pressure control systems appear to be "set" at a higher level of blood pressure. All antihypertensive drugs act by interfering with these normal mechanisms, which are reviewed below.

A. Postural Baroreflex: (Figure 11–2.) Baroreflexes are responsible for rapid, moment-to-moment adjustments in blood pressure, such as in transition from a reclining to an upright posture. Central sympathetic neurons arising from the vasomotor area of the medulla are tonically active. Carotid baroreceptors are stimulated by the stretch of the vessel walls brought about by the internal pressure (blood pressure). Baroreceptor activation inhibits central sympathetic discharge. Conversely, reduction in stretch results in a reduction in baroreceptor activity. Thus, in the case of a transition to upright posture, baroreceptors sense the reduction in arterial pressure that results from pooling of blood in the veins below the level of the heart as reduced wall stretch, and sympathetic discharge is disinhibited. The reflex increase in sympathetic outflow acts through nerve endings to increase peripheral vascular resistance (constriction of arterioles) and cardiac output (direct stimulation of the heart and constriction of capacitance vessels, which increases venous return to the heart), thereby restoring normal blood pressure. The same baroreflex acts in response to any event that lowers arterial pressure, including a primary reduction in peripheral vascular resistance (eg, caused by a vasodilating agent) or a reduction in intravascular volume (eg, due to hemorrhage or to loss of salt and water via the kidney).

B. Renal Response to Decreased Blood Pressure: By controlling blood volume, the kidney is primarily responsible for long-term blood pressure control. A reduction in renal perfusion pressure causes intrarenal redistribution of blood flow and increased reabsorption of salt and water. In addition, decreased pressure in renal arterioles as well as sympathetic neural activity (via beta adrenoceptors) stimulates production of renin, which increases production of angiotensin II (see Figure 11–1 and Chapter 17). Angiotensin II causes (1) direct constriction of resistance vessels and (2) stimulation of aldosterone synthesis in the adrenal cortex, which increases renal sodium absorption and intravascular blood volume.

Therapeutic Implications

Because antihypertensive therapy is not usually directed at a specific cause, it necessarily depends upon interfering with normal physiologic mechanisms that regulate blood pressure. Antihypertensive therapy is administered to an asymptomatic patient, for whom it provides no direct relief from discomfort; instead, the benefit of lowering blood pressure lies in preventing disease and death at some future time. The natural human tendency to weigh present inconvenience and discomfort more heavily than future benefit means

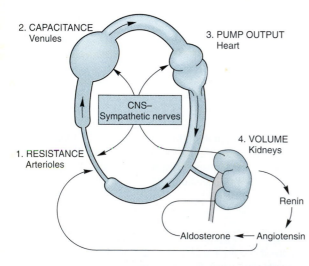

2. CAPACITANCE
   Venules

3. PUMP OUTPUT
   Heart

CNS–
Sympathetic nerves

4. VOLUME
   Kidneys

1. RESISTANCE
   Arterioles

Renin

Aldosterone ← Angiotensin

Figure 11–1. Anatomic sites of blood pressure control.

Figure 11–2. Baroreceptor reflex arc.

that a major problem—perhaps *the* major problem—in antihypertensive therapy is that of providing consistent, effective drug therapy over many years in a regimen the patient will adhere to ("patient compliance").

It is essential to balance the risks of toxicity from drug treatment against the risks of not treating, which are proportionate to the extent of blood pressure elevation before treatment and vary according to the characteristics of individual patients. Accordingly, no single mode of treatment will be suitable for more than a small proportion of hypertensive patients.

I. BASIC PHARMACOLOGY OF ANTIHYPERTENSIVE AGENTS

All antihypertensive agents act at one or more of the four anatomic control sites depicted in Figure 11–1 and produce their effects by interfering with normal mechanisms of blood pressure regulation. A useful classification of these agents categorizes them according to the principal regulatory site or mechanism on which they act (Figure 11–3). Because of their common mechanisms of action, drugs within each category tend to produce a similar spectrum of toxicities. The categories include the following:

(1) **Diuretics,** which lower blood pressure by depleting the body of sodium and reducing blood volume and perhaps by other mechanisms.

(2) **Sympathoplegic agents,** which lower blood pressure by reducing peripheral vascular resistance, inhibiting cardiac function, and increasing venous pooling in capacitance vessels. (The latter two effects reduce cardiac output.) These agents are further sub-

divided according to their putative sites of action in the sympathetic reflex arc (see below).

(3) **Direct vasodilators,** which reduce pressure by relaxing vascular smooth muscle, thus dilating resistance vessels and—to varying degrees—increasing capacitance as well.

(4) **Agents that block production or action of angiotensin** and thereby reduce peripheral vascular resistance and (potentially) blood volume.

The fact that these drug groups act by different mechanisms permits the combination of drugs from two or more groups with increased efficacy and, in some cases, decreased toxicity. (See box: Monotherapy Versus Polypharmacy in Hypertension.)

DRUGS THAT ALTER SODIUM & WATER BALANCE

Dietary sodium restriction has been known for many years to decrease blood pressure in hypertensive patients. With the advent of diuretics, sodium restriction was thought to be less important. However, there is now general agreement that dietary control of blood pressure is a relatively nontoxic therapeutic measure and may even be preventive. Several studies have shown that even modest dietary sodium restriction lowers blood pressure (though to varying extents) in many hypertensive individuals.

Mechanisms of Action & Hemodynamic Effects of Diuretics

Diuretics lower blood pressure primarily by depleting body sodium stores. Initially, diuretics reduce

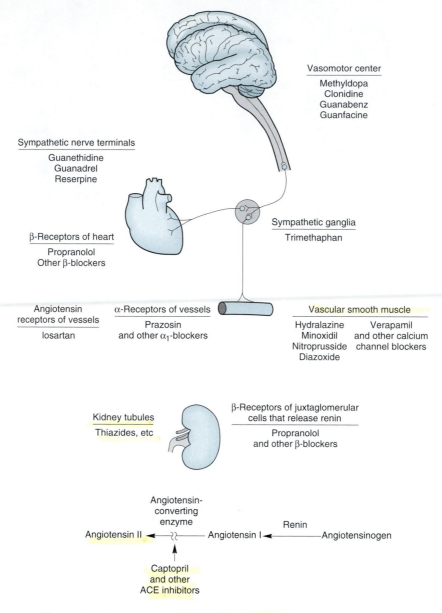

Vasomotor center
Methyldopa
Clonidine
Guanabenz
Guanfacine

Sympathetic nerve terminals
Guanethidine
Guanadrel
Reserpine

β-Receptors of heart
Propranolol
Other β-blockers

Sympathetic ganglia
Trimethaphan

Angiotensin receptors of vessels
losartan

α-Receptors of vessels
Prazosin
and other α₁-blockers

Vascular smooth muscle
Hydralazine   Verapamil
Minoxidil   and other calcium
Nitroprusside   channel blockers
Diazoxide

Kidney tubules
Thiazides, etc

β-Receptors of juxtaglomerular cells that release renin
Propranolol
and other β-blockers

Angiotensin-converting enzyme

Renin

Angiotensin II ◄——⟨⟩—— Angiotensin I ◄—————— Angiotensinogen

Captopril
and other
ACE inhibitors

Figure 11–3. Sites of action of the major classes of antihypertensive drugs.

blood pressure by reducing blood volume and cardiac output; peripheral vascular resistance may increase. After 6–8 weeks, cardiac output returns toward normal while peripheral vascular resistance declines. Sodium is believed to contribute to vascular resistance by increasing vessel stiffness and neural reactivity, possibly related to increased sodium-calcium exchange with a resultant increase in intracellular calcium. These effects are reversed by diuretics or sodium restriction.

Some diuretics have direct vasodilating effects in addition to their diuretic action. Indapamide is a nonthiazide sulfonamide diuretic with both diuretic and vasodilator activity. As a consequence of vasodilation, cardiac output remains unchanged or increases slightly. Amiloride inhibits smooth muscle responses to contractile stimuli, probably through effects on transmembrane and intracellular calcium movement that are independent of its action on sodium excretion.

Diuretics are effective in lowering blood pressure by 10–15 mm Hg in most patients, and diuretics alone often provide adequate treatment for mild or moderate essential hypertension. In more severe hypertension, diuretics are used in combination with sympathoplegic and vasodilator drugs to control the tendency toward sodium retention caused by these agents. Vascular responsiveness—ie, the ability to either constrict or dilate—is diminished by symphatoplegic and vasodilator drugs, so that the vasculature behaves like an inflexible tube. As a consequence, blood pressure becomes exquisitely sensitive to blood volume. Thus, in severe hypertension, when multiple drugs are used, blood pressure may be well controlled when blood volume is 95% of normal but much too high when blood volume is 105% of normal.

Selection of Diuretics

The sites of action within the kidney and the pharmacokinetics of various diuretic drugs are discussed in Chapter 15. Thiazide diuretics are appropriate for most patients with mild or moderate hypertension and normal renal and cardiac function. More powerful diuretics (eg, those acting on the loop of Henle) are necessary in severe hypertension, when multiple drugs with sodium-retaining properties are used; in renal insufficiency, when glomerular filtration rate is less than 30 or 40 mL/min; and in cardiac failure or cirrhosis, where sodium retention is marked.

Potassium-sparing diuretics are useful both to avoid excessive potassium depletion, particularly in patients taking digitalis, and to enhance the natriuretic effects of other diuretics.

Dosing Considerations

Although the pharmacokinetics and pharmacodynamics of the various diuretics differ, their common therapeutic end point in treating hypertension is daily natriuresis. However, it must be recognized that in steady-state conditions (as in long-term management of hypertension), daily sodium excretion is equal to dietary sodium intake. Diuretics are necessary to oppose the tendency toward sodium retention in a relatively sodium-depleted patient. Although thiazide diuretics are more natriuretic at higher doses (up to 100–200 mg of hydrochlorothiazide), when used as a single agent, lower doses (25–50 mg) exert as much antihypertensive effect as do higher doses. Thus, a threshold amount of body sodium depletion may be sufficient for antihypertensive efficacy. In contrast to thiazides, the blood pressure response to loop diuretics continues to increase at doses many times greater than the usual therapeutic dose.

Toxicity of Diuretics

In the treatment of hypertension, the most common adverse effect of diuretics (except for potassium-sparing diuretics) is potassium depletion. Although mild degrees of hypokalemia are tolerated well by many patients, hypokalemia may be hazardous in persons taking digitalis, those who have chronic arrhythmias, or those with acute myocardial infarction. Potassium loss is coupled to reabsorption of sodium, and restriction of dietary sodium intake will therefore minimize potassium loss. Diuretics may also cause magnesium depletion, impair glucose tolerance, and increase serum lipid concentrations. Diuretics may increase uric acid concentrations and precipitate gout. The possibility of an increased risk of coronary artery disease associated with the metabolic effects of diuretics is still under study. However, it has been found that the use of low doses minimizes these adverse metabolic effects without impairing the antihypertensive action.

DRUGS THAT ALTER SYMPATHETIC NERVOUS SYSTEM FUNCTION

In patients with moderate to severe hypertension, most effective drug regimens include an agent that inhibits function of the sympathetic nervous system. Drugs in this group are classified according to the site at which they impair the sympathetic reflex arc (Figure 11–2). This neuroanatomic classification explains prominent differences in cardiovascular effects of drugs and allows the clinician to predict interactions of these drugs with one another and with other drugs.

Most importantly, the subclasses of drugs exhibit different patterns of potential toxicity. Drugs that lower blood pressure by actions on the central nervous system tend to cause sedation and mental depression and may produce disturbances of sleep, including nightmares. Drugs that act by inhibiting transmission through autonomic ganglia produce toxicity from inhibition of parasympathetic regulation, in addition to profound sympathetic blockade. Drugs that act chiefly by reducing release of norepinephrine from sympathetic nerve endings cause effects that are similar to those of surgical sympathectomy, including inhibition of ejaculation, and hypotension that is increased by upright posture and after exercise. Drugs that block postsynaptic adrenoceptors produce a more selective spectrum of effects depending on the class of receptor to which they bind.

A few of the drugs to be discussed appear to act at more than one anatomic site, although each probably works by a single biochemical mechanism. No clinically useful drug acts primarily on baroreceptors. The **veratrum alkaloids** lower blood pressure by increasing sensitivity of baroreceptors, but they are of only academic interest because they produce erratic therapeutic effects and cause unacceptable toxicity in patients.

Finally, we should note that *all* of the agents that lower blood pressure by altering sympathetic function can elicit compensatory effects through mechanisms that are not dependent on adrenergic nerves. Thus, the antihypertensive effect of any of these agents used alone may be limited by retention of sodium by the kidney and expansion of blood volume. For these reasons, sympathoplegic antihypertensive drugs are most effective when used concomitantly with a diuretic.

CENTRALLY ACTING SYMPATHOPLEGIC DRUGS

Mechanism & Sites of Action

Methyldopa and clonidine reduce sympathetic outflow from vasopressor centers in the brain stem but allow these centers to retain or even increase their sensitivity to baroreceptor control. Accordingly, the antihypertensive and toxic actions of these drugs are generally less dependent on posture than are the effects of drugs such as guanethidine that act directly on peripheral sympathetic neurons.

Methyldopa (L-α-methyl-3,4-dihydroxyphenylalanine) is an analog of L-dopa and is converted to α-methyldopamine and α-methylnorepinephrine; this pathway directly parallels the synthesis of norepinephrine from dopa illustrated in Figure 6–5. Alpha-methylnorepinephrine is stored in adrenergic nerve vesicles, where it stoichiometrically replaces norepinephrine, and is released by nerve stimulation to interact with postsynaptic adrenoceptors. However, this replacement of norepinephrine by a false transmitter in peripheral neurons is *not* responsible for methyldopa's antihypertensive effect, because the α-methylnorepinephrine released is an effective agonist at the alpha adrenoceptors that mediate peripheral sympathetic constriction of arterioles and venules. Direct electrical stimulation of sympathetic nerves in methyldopa-treated animals produces sympathetic responses similar to those observed in untreated animals.

Indeed, methyldopa's antihypertensive action appears to be due to stimulation of central alpha adrenoceptors by α-methylnorepinephrine or α-methyldopamine, based on the following evidence: (1) Much lower doses of methyldopa are required to lower blood pressure in animals when the drug is administered centrally by cerebral intraventricular injection rather than intravenously. (2) Alpha-receptor antagonists, especially α_2-selective antagonists, administered centrally, block the antihypertensive effect of methyldopa, whether the latter is given centrally or intravenously. (3) Potent inhibitors of dopa decarboxylase, administered centrally, block methyldopa's antihypertensive effect, thus showing that metabolism of the parent drug is necessary for its action.

The antihypertensive action of **clonidine,** a 2-imidazoline derivative, was discovered in the course of testing the drug for use as a topically applied nasal decongestant. After intravenous injection, clonidine produces a brief rise in blood pressure followed by more prolonged hypotension. The pressor response is due to direct stimulation of alpha adrenoceptors in arterioles. The drug is classified as a partial agonist at alpha receptors because it also inhibits pressor effects of other alpha agonists.

Considerable evidence indicates that the hypoten-

sive effect of clonidine is exerted at alpha adrenoceptors in the medulla of the brain. In animals, the hypotensive effect of clonidine is prevented by central administration of alpha antagonists. Clonidine reduces sympathetic and increases parasympathetic tone, resulting in blood pressure lowering and bradycardia. The reduction in pressure is accompanied by a decrease in circulating catecholamine levels. These observations suggest that clonidine sensitizes brain stem pressor centers to inhibition by baroreflexes.

Thus, studies of clonidine and methyldopa suggest that normal regulation of blood pressure involves central adrenergic neurons that modulate baroreceptor reflexes. Both drugs bind more tightly to α_2 than to α_1 adrenoceptors. As noted in Chapter 6, α_2 receptors are located on presynaptic adrenergic neurons as well as some postsynaptic sites. It is possible that clonidine and α-methylnorepinephrine act in the brain to reduce norepinephrine release onto relevant receptor sites. Alternatively, these drugs may act on postsynaptic α_2 adrenoceptors to inhibit activity of appropriate neurons. Finally, clonidine also binds to a nonadrenoceptor site, the **imidazoline receptor,** which may also mediate antihypertensive effects (see text box: Clonidine: A Pointer to New Receptors and Clinical Applications).

Methyldopa and clonidine produce slightly different hemodynamic effects: clonidine lowers heart rate and cardiac output more than does methyldopa. This difference suggests that these two drugs do not have identical sites of action. They may act primarily on different populations of neurons in vasomotor centers of the brain stem.

Guanabenz and **guanfacine** are centrally active antihypertensive drugs that share the central alpha-adrenoceptor-stimulating effects of clonidine. They do not appear to offer any advantages over clonidine.

METHYLDOPA

Methyldopa is useful in the treatment of mild to moderately severe hypertension. It lowers blood pressure chiefly by reducing peripheral vascular resistance, with a variable reduction in heart rate and cardiac output.

Most cardiovascular reflexes remain intact after administration of methyldopa, and blood pressure reduction is not markedly dependent upon mainte-

α-Methyldopa
(α-methyl group in color)

CLONIDINE: A POINTER TO NEW RECEPTORS & CLINICAL APPLICATIONS

As noted in the text, the precise mechanism of the centrally acting sympathoplegic drugs is still not understood. Furthermore, clonidine has several actions unrelated to blood pressure control, including sedation, dry mouth, and analgesia, that are of interest. Studies of these questions have led to several new antihypertensive drugs and to potential therapies for glaucoma, preanesthetic medication, and other applications.

Blood Pressure Regulation

Many studies have been carried out with congeners of clonidine to resolve the question of how this drug exerts its sympathoplegic action. More than a decade ago, it was pointed out that there were differences between the central actions of catecholamine (eg, methyldopa metabolites) and imidazoline (eg, clonidine) drugs (Bousquet et al, 1984). It was found that clonidine and several congeners have significant affinity for a *non*adrenergic class of binding sites in addition to α_2 adrenoceptors. In contrast, methylnorepinephrine, the active metabolite of methyldopa, has high affinity for the α_2 receptors and only low affinity for the nonadrenergic binding site (Ernsberger, 1994). It was then discovered that the highest density of α-methylnorepinephrine binding sites is found in the nucleus tractus solitarius (NTS) of the medulla, whereas clonidine and its imidazole derivatives also bind strongly in the rostral ventrolateral medulla (RVLM), which is considered to be the final common pathway for sympathetic vasomotor outflow. One of the newest imidazole derivatives, moxonidine, binds almost exclusively in the RVLM but retains strong antihypertensive activity. The new group of binding sites in the RVLM was initially referred to as the imidazoline-preferring receptor group and later named the imidazoline receptor group after the distinctive ring structure found in clonidine but not in catecholamines.

Subgroups of imidazoline receptors have been identified and named I_1 and I_2. The I_1 subgroup seems to be the primary binding site for imidazoline drugs that have useful antihypertensive effects. These drugs include **moxonidine** and **rilmenidine,** both of which are currently available overseas. They are claimed to have much less sedative action than clonidine and a somewhat reduced tendency to cause dry mouth (Pritchard, 1994). It has been proposed that the I_1 receptor is a G protein-coupled receptor that utilizes the IP_3, DAG second messenger system (Separovic et al, 1996).

Other Actions of α_2 & I_1 Agonist Drugs

Clonidine and its derivatives have several intriguing noncardiovascular actions. It has long been recognized that clonidine has analgesic effects (Filos et al, 1992), can reduce the symptoms of withdrawal from addictive drugs (Gourlay et al, 1995), and may decrease intraocular pressure. The latter effect is already recognized by the availability of **apraclonidine** for the prevention of postoperative glaucoma.

The ability of α_2 agonists to alter neuronal activity in the spinal cord has resulted in the development of **tizanidine** for the treatment of spasticity (see Chapter 27), withdrawal syndromes (Koyuncuoglu, 1995), and chronic pain syndromes (Leiphart et al, 1995). These effects are believed to reflect α_2—not imidazoline—receptor agonist effects. **Dexmedetomidine** is another imidazoline congener of clonidine (see structures) and has been shown to have hypnotic effects and ocular hypotensive effects when given systemically and significant analgesic effects when given by the intrathecal route. These effects are probably mediated primarily by α_2 agonist action. Dexmedetomidine retains some sympathoplegic and hypotensive effect, which may limit its usefulness in surgery (Scheinin et al, 1993).

Clonidine

Moxonidine

Dexmedetomidine

Tizanidine

nance of upright posture. Postural (orthostatic) hypotension sometimes occurs, particularly in volume-depleted patients. One potential advantage of methyldopa is that it causes reduction in renal vascular resistance.

Pharmacokinetics & Dosage

Owing to extensive first-pass metabolism (primarily *O*-sulfate conjugation by the gastrointestinal mucosa), the bioavailability of methyldopa is low, averaging 25%, and varies among individuals. About two-thirds of the drug that reaches the systemic circulation is cleared by renal excretion, with a terminal elimination half-life of 2 hours. Impaired renal function results in reduced drug clearance.

Methyldopa enters the brain via a pump that actively transports aromatic amino acids. An oral dose of methyldopa produces its maximal antihypertensive effect in 4–6 hours, and the effect can persist for up to 24 hours. Because the effect depends upon accumulation of a metabolite, α-methylnorepinephrine, the action persists after the parent drug has disappeared from the circulation.

The maximal efficacy of methyldopa in lowering blood pressure is limited. In most patients, a dose of 2 g or less will produce maximal reduction in hypertension; if this result is not satisfactory, higher doses will usually not result in greater effects. The usual therapeutic dosage is about 1–2 g/d orally in divided doses. In many patients, once-daily therapy is effective.

Toxicity

Most of the undesirable effects of methyldopa are referable to the central nervous system. Of these, the most frequent is overt sedation, particularly at the onset of treatment. With long-term therapy, patients may complain of persistent mental lassitude and impaired mental concentration. Nightmares, mental depression, vertigo, and extrapyramidal signs may occur but are relatively infrequent. Lactation, associated with increased prolactin secretion, can occur both in men and in women treated with methyldopa. This toxicity is probably mediated by an inhibiting action on dopaminergic mechanisms in the hypothalamus.

Other important adverse effects of methyldopa are development of a positive Coombs test (occurring in 10–20% of patients undergoing therapy for longer than 12 months), which sometimes makes cross-matching blood for transfusion difficult and rarely is associated with hemolytic anemia, as well as hepatitis and drug fever. Discontinuation of the drug usually results in prompt reversal of these abnormalities.

CLONIDINE

Hemodynamic studies indicate that blood pressure lowering by clonidine results from reduction of cardiac output due to decreased heart rate and relaxation of capacitance vessels, with a reduction in peripheral vascular resistance, particularly when patients are upright (when sympathetic tone is normally increased).

Reduction in arterial blood pressure by clonidine is accompanied by decreased renal vascular resistance and maintenance of renal blood flow. As with methyldopa, clonidine reduces blood pressure in the supine position and only rarely causes postural hypotension. Pressor effects of clonidine are not observed after ingestion of therapeutic doses of clonidine, but severe hypertension can complicate overdosage.

Pharmacokinetics & Dosage

In healthy individuals, the bioavailability of clonidine averages 75% and the half-life is 8–12 hours. About half of the drug is eliminated unchanged in the urine, suggesting that lower than usual doses may be effective in patients with renal insufficiency.

Clonidine is lipid-soluble and rapidly enters the brain from the circulation. Because of its relatively short half-life and the fact that its antihypertensive effect is directly related to blood concentration, oral clonidine must be given twice a day to maintain smooth blood pressure control. Therapeutic dosages are commonly between 0.2 and 1.2 mg/d. However, as is not the case with methyldopa, the dose-response curve of clonidine is such that increasing doses are more effective (but also more toxic). The maximal recommended dosage is 1.2 mg/d.

A transdermal preparation of clonidine that reduces blood pressure for 7 days after a single application is also available. This preparation appears to produce less sedation than clonidine tablets but is often associated with local skin reactions.

Toxicity

Dry mouth and sedation are frequent and may be severe. Both effects are centrally mediated and dose-dependent and coincide temporally with the drug's antihypertensive effect.

The drug should not be given to patients who are at risk of mental depression and should be withdrawn if depression occurs during therapy. Concomitant treatment with tricyclic antidepressants may block the antihypertensive effect of clonidine. The interaction is believed to be due to alpha-adrenoceptor-blocking actions of the tricyclics.

Withdrawal of clonidine after protracted use, particularly with high dosages (greater than 1 mg/d), can result in life-threatening hypertensive crisis mediated by increased sympathetic nervous activity. Patients exhibit nervousness, tachycardia, headache, and sweating after omitting one or two doses of the drug. Although the incidence of severe hypertensive crisis is unknown, it is high enough to require that all patients who take clonidine be carefully warned of the possibility. If the drug must be stopped, this should be done gradually while other antihypertensive agents are being substituted. Treatment of the hypertensive crisis consists of reinstitution of clonidine therapy or administration of alpha- and beta-adrenoceptor-blocking agents.

GANGLION-BLOCKING AGENTS

Historically, drugs that block stimulation of postganglionic autonomic neurons by acetylcholine were among the first agents used in the treatment of hypertension. Most such drugs are no longer available clinically because of intolerable toxicities related to their primary action (see below). Until recently, one drug in this class (trimethaphan) was still used to treat hypertension. However, in 1996 trimethaphan was withdrawn from the market. It is described here because of its importance as a prototype drug. Mecamylamine, though still available, is almost never used for hypertension.

Ganglion blockers competitively block nicotinic cholinoceptors on postganglionic neurons in both sympathetic and parasympathetic ganglia. In addition, these drugs may directly block the nicotinic acetylcholine channel, in the same fashion as neuromuscular nicotinic blockers (see Figure 27–5).

TRIMETHAPHAN

Trimethaphan camsylate was administered intravenously to take advantage of its rapid action in treating hypertensive crisis, acute aortic dissection, and to induce controlled hypotension for neurosurgery. The dependence of ganglionic blockade on blood level and the short half-life of the drug allow precise titration of blood pressure while other drugs are taking effect.

The antihypertensive effect of trimethaphan is to a large extent dependent upon pooling of blood in capacitance vessels. The patient's bed must be tilted head up for effective blood pressure lowering. Conversely, excessive hypotension can be rapidly treated by reverse tilting.

The adverse effects of ganglion blockers are direct extensions of their pharmacologic effects. These effects include both sympathoplegia (excessive orthostatic hypotension and sexual dysfunction) and parasympathoplegia (constipation, urinary retention, precipitation of glaucoma, blurred vision, dry mouth, etc). These severe toxicities are the major reason for the abandonment of ganglion blockers for the therapy of hypertension.

ADRENERGIC NEURON-BLOCKING AGENTS

These drugs lower blood pressure by preventing normal physiologic release of norepinephrine from postganglionic sympathetic neurons.

GUANETHIDINE

In high enough doses, guanethidine can produce profound sympathoplegia. The resulting high maximal efficacy of this agent made it the mainstay of outpatient therapy of severe hypertension for many years. For the same reason, guanethidine can produce all of the toxicities expected from "pharmacologic sympathectomy," including marked postural hypotension, diarrhea, and impaired ejaculation. Because of these adverse effects, guanethidine is now rarely used.

The structure of guanethidine includes a highly basic nitrogen that makes the drug too polar to enter the central nervous system. As a result, this drug has none of the central effects seen with many of the other antihypertensive agents described in this chapter.

$$N-CH_2-CH_2-\underset{H}{N}-\underset{|}{\overset{NH}{\overset{||}{C}}}-NH_2$$

Guanethidine

Guanadrel is a guanethidine-like drug that is also available in the USA. **Bethanidine** and **debrisoquin,** antihypertensive agents not available for clinical use in the USA, are similar to guanethidine in mechanism of antihypertensive action.

Mechanism & Sites of Action

Guanethidine inhibits the release of norepinephrine from sympathetic nerve endings (Figure 11–4). This effect is probably responsible for most of the sympathoplegia that occurs in patients. Guanethidine is transported across the sympathetic nerve membrane by the same mechanism that transports norepinephrine itself (uptake 1), and uptake is essential for the drug's action. Once guanethidine has entered the nerve, it is concentrated in transmitter vesicles, where it replaces norepinephrine. Because it replaces norepinephrine, the drug causes a gradual depletion of norepinephrine stores in the nerve ending.

Inhibition of norepinephrine release is probably caused by guanethidine's local anesthetic properties on sympathetic nerve terminals. Although the drug does not impair axonal conduction in sympathetic fibers, local blockade of membrane electrical activity may occur in nerve endings because the nerve endings specifically take up and concentrate the drug.

Because neuronal uptake is necessary for the hypotensive activity of guanethidine, drugs that block the catecholamine uptake process or displace amines from the nerve terminal (see Chapter 6) block its effects. These include cocaine, amphetamine, tricyclic antidepressants, phenothiazines, and phenoxybenzamine.

Guanethidine increases sensitivity to the hypertensive effects of exogenously administered sympathomimetic amines. This results from inhibition of neu-

Figure 11–4. Guanethidine actions and drug interactions involving the adrenergic neuron. (G, guanethidine; NE, norepinephrine; TCA, tricyclic antidepressants.)

ronal uptake of such amines and, after long-term therapy with guanethidine, supersensitivity of effector smooth muscle cells, in a fashion analogous to the process that follows surgical sympathectomy (see Chapter 6).

The hypotensive action of guanethidine early in the course of therapy is associated with reduced cardiac output, due to bradycardia and relaxation of capacitance vessels, without consistent change in peripheral vascular resistance. With chronic therapy, peripheral vascular resistance decreases. Sodium and water retention may be marked during guanethidine therapy.

Pharmacokinetics & Dosage

The bioavailability of guanethidine is variable (3–50%). It is 50% cleared by the kidney. Retention of drug in nerve endings and uptake into other sites account for the very large volume of distribution and long half-life (5 days) of guanethidine. Thus, with constant daily dosing, the onset of sympathoplegia is gradual (maximal effect in 1–2 weeks), and sympathoplegia persists for a comparable period after cessation of therapy.

The daily dose required for a satisfactory antihypertensive response varies greatly among individual patients. For this reason, therapy is usually initiated at a low dose, eg, 10 mg/d. The dose should not ordinarily be increased at intervals shorter than 2 weeks. Be-

cause of the drug's long duration of action, maintenance doses need not be taken more than once a day.

Toxicity

Therapeutic use of guanethidine is often associated with symptomatic postural hypotension and hypotension following exercise, particularly when the drug is given in high doses. Injudicious treatment (excessive doses or too rapid escalation in dosage) may produce dangerously decreased blood flow to heart and brain or even overt shock. Guanethidine-induced sympathoplegia in men may be associated with delayed or retrograde ejaculation (into the bladder). Guanethidine commonly causes diarrhea, which results from increased gastrointestinal motility due to parasympathetic predominance in controlling the activity of intestinal smooth muscle.

Interactions with other drugs may complicate guanethidine therapy. Sympathomimetic agents such as phenylpropanolamine, at doses available in over-the-counter cold preparations, can produce hypertension in patients taking guanethidine. Similarly, guanethidine can produce hypertensive crisis by releasing catecholamines in patients with pheochromocytoma. When tricyclic antidepressants are administered to patients taking guanethidine, the drug's antihypertensive effect is attenuated, and severe hypertension may follow. A physician who is ignorant of this interaction may raise the dose of guanethidine; if the tricyclic antidepressant is then stopped, the patient may suffer severe hypotension or cardiovascular collapse from the unopposed action of guanethidine.

RESERPINE

Reserpine, an alkaloid extracted from the roots of an Indian plant, *Rauwolfia serpentina,* was one of the first effective drugs used on a large scale in the treatment of hypertension. At present, it is considered an effective and relatively safe drug for treating mild to moderate hypertension.

Mechanism & Sites of Action

Reserpine blocks the ability of aminergic transmitter vesicles to take up and store biogenic amines, probably by interfering with an uptake mechanism that depends on Mg^{2+} and ATP (Figure 6–4, carrier *B*). This effect occurs throughout the body, resulting in depletion of norepinephrine, dopamine, and serotonin in both central and peripheral neurons. Chromaffin granules of the adrenal medulla are also depleted of catecholamines, although to a lesser extent than are neurons elsewhere. Reserpine's effects on adrenergic vesicles appear irreversible; trace amounts of the drug remain bound to vesicular membranes for many days. Although sufficiently high doses of reserpine in animals can reduce catecholamine stores to zero, lower doses cause inhibition of neurotransmission that is roughly proportionate to the degree of amine depletion.

Depletion of peripheral amines probably accounts for much of the beneficial antihypertensive effect of reserpine, but a central component cannot be ruled out. The effects of low but clinically effective doses resemble those of centrally acting agents (eg, methyldopa) in that sympathetic reflexes remain largely intact, blood pressure is reduced in supine as well as in standing patients, and postural hypotension is mild.

Reserpine readily enters the brain, and depletion of cerebral amine stores causes sedation, mental depression, and parkinsonism symptoms.

At lower doses used for treatment of mild hypertension, reserpine lowers blood pressure by a combination of decreased cardiac output and decreased peripheral vascular resistance.

Pharmacokinetics & Dosage

Absorption, clearance, and metabolism have not been well defined. The drug disappears rapidly from the circulation, but its effects persist much longer, owing to irreversible inactivation of the carriers in catecholamine storage granules, as described above.

The usual daily dose is less than 1 mg (typically, 0.25 mg), administered orally as a single dose. Although reserpine is available in injectable form, parenteral administration is rarely indicated.

Toxicity

At the low doses usually administered, reserpine produces little postural hypotension. Most of the unwanted effects of reserpine result from actions on the brain or gastrointestinal tract.

High doses of reserpine characteristically produce sedation, lassitude, nightmares, and severe mental depression; occasionally, these occur even in patients receiving low doses (0.25 mg/d). Much less frequently, ordinary low doses of reserpine produce extrapyramidal effects resembling Parkinson's disease, probably as a result of dopamine depletion in the corpus striatum. Although these central effects are uncommon, it should be stressed that they may occur at any time, even after months of uneventful treatment. Patients with a history of mental depression should not receive reserpine, and the drug should be stopped if depression appears.

Reserpine rather often produces mild diarrhea and gastrointestinal cramps and increases gastric acid secretion. The drug should probably not be given to patients with a history of peptic ulcer.

Reserpine

PARGYLINE

Although pargyline and other inhibitors of monoamine oxidase lower blood pressure, they have no place in the modern treatment of hypertension. Pargyline is thought to lower blood pressure by increasing the concentration of an ineffective false transmitter in peripheral adrenergic nerve endings. Pargyline inhibits monoamine oxidase in gastrointestinal mucosa and the liver and thus allows unimpeded access of dietary tyramine to the systemic circulation. Tyramine is taken up into nerve endings and converted to octopamine (Figure 6–5), which partially replaces norepinephrine in catecholamine storage granules. Because octopamine is ineffective as a pressor agonist at postsynaptic alpha receptors, sympathoplegia results even though total stores of norepinephrine may be increased.

ADRENOCEPTOR ANTAGONISTS

The pharmacology of drugs that antagonize catecholamines at alpha and beta adrenoceptors is presented in Chapter 10. Here we will concentrate on two prototypical drugs, propranolol and prazosin, primarily in relation to their use in treatment of hypertension. Other adrenoceptor antagonists will be considered only briefly.

PROPRANOLOL

Propranolol, a beta-adrenoceptor-blocking agent, is very useful for lowering blood pressure in mild to moderate hypertension. In severe hypertension, propranolol is especially useful in preventing the reflex tachycardia that often results from treatment with direct vasodilators.

Mechanism & Sites of Action

Propranolol antagonizes catecholamines at both β_1 and β_2 adrenoceptors. Both its efficacy in treating hypertension as well as most of its toxic effects result from beta blockade. Propranolol decreases blood pressure primarily as a result of a decrease in cardiac output. Other beta-blockers may decrease cardiac output or decrease peripheral vascular resistance to various degrees, depending on cardioselectivity and partial agonist activities (van den Meiracker et al, 1989).

Beta blockade in brain, kidney, and peripheral adrenergic neurons has been proposed as contributing to the antihypertensive effect observed with beta-receptor blockers. In spite of conflicting evidence (Pearson, 1989), the brain appears unlikely to be the primary site of the hypotensive action of these drugs, because some beta-blockers that do not readily cross the blood-brain barrier (eg, nadolol, described below) are nonetheless effective antihypertensive agents.

Propranolol inhibits the stimulation of renin production by catecholamines (mediated by β_1 receptors). It is likely that propranolol's effect is due in part to depression of the renin-angiotensin-aldosterone system (Man in't Veld et al, 1983). Although most effective in patients with high plasma renin activity, propranolol also reduces blood pressure in hypertensive patients with normal or even low renin activity. Beta-blockers might also act on peripheral prejunctional β adrenoceptors to reduce sympathetic vasoconstrictor nerve activity.

In mild to moderate hypertension, propranolol produces a significant reduction in blood pressure without prominent postural hypotension.

Pharmacokinetics & Dosage

As described in Chapter 10, effective oral doses of propranolol are greater than effective intravenous doses, owing to first-pass hepatic inactivation. The prominent first-pass effect partially accounts for the variability in doses required for clinically useful effects. The half-life is 3–6 hours.

Treatment of hypertension is usually started with 80 mg/d in divided doses. Effective antihypertensive dosage ranges from 80 to 480 mg/d. Resting bradycardia and a reduction in the heart rate during exercise are indicators of propranolol's beta-blocking effect. Measures of these responses may be used as guides in regulating dosage. Propranolol can be administered once or twice daily.

Toxicity

The principal toxicities of propranolol result from blockade of cardiac, vascular, or bronchial beta receptors and are described in more detail in Chapter 10. The most important of these predictable extensions of the beta-blocking action occur in patients with reduced myocardial reserve, asthma, peripheral vascular insufficiency, and diabetes.

When propranolol is discontinued after prolonged regular use, some patients experience a withdrawal syndrome, manifested by nervousness, tachycardia, increased intensity of angina, or increase of blood pressure. Myocardial infarction has been reported in a few patients. Although the incidence of these complications is probably low, propranolol should not be discontinued abruptly. The withdrawal syndrome may involve "up-regulation" or supersensitivity of beta adrenoceptors.

Propranolol also produces a low incidence of effects not clearly attributable to beta blockade, including diarrhea, constipation, nausea, and vomiting. Not infrequently, patients receiving propranolol complain of central nervous system effects reminiscent of those caused by methyldopa and clonidine, including nightmares, lassitude, mental depression, and insomnia.

Finally, propranolol may increase plasma triglycerides and decrease HDL-cholesterol, which theoretically could contribute to atherogenesis.

OTHER BETA-ADRENOCEPTOR-BLOCKING AGENTS

Of the large number of beta-blockers tested, most have been shown to be effective in lowering blood pressure. The pharmacologic properties of several of these agents differ from those of propranolol in ways that may confer therapeutic benefits in certain clinical situations.

1. METOPROLOL

Metoprolol is approximately equipotent to propranolol in inhibiting stimulation of β_1 adrenoceptors such as those in the heart but 50- to 100-fold less potent than propranolol in blocking β_2 receptors. Although metoprolol is in other respects very similar to propranolol, its relative cardioselectivity may be advantageous in treating hypertensive patients who also suffer from asthma, diabetes, or peripheral vascular disease. Studies of small numbers of asthmatic patients have shown that metoprolol causes less bronchial constriction than propranolol at doses that produce equal inhibition of β_1-adrenoceptor responses. The cardioselectivity is not complete, however, and asthmatic symptoms have been exacerbated by metoprolol. Usual antihypertensive doses of metoprolol range from 100 to 450 mg/d.

2. NADOLOL, CARTEOLOL, ATENOLOL, BETAXOLOL, & BISOPROLOL

Nadolol and carteolol, nonselective beta-receptor antagonists, and atenolol, a β_1-selective blocker, are not appreciably metabolized and are excreted to a considerable extent in the urine. Betaxolol and bisoprolol are β_1-selective blockers that are primarily metabolized in the liver but have long half-lives. These drugs can be administered once daily because of their relatively long half-lives in plasma. Nadolol is usually begun at a dosage of 40 mg/d, atenolol at a dosage of 50 mg/d, carteolol at a dosage of 2.5 mg/d, betaxolol at a dosage of 10 mg/d, and bisoprolol at a dosage of 5 mg/d. Increases in dosage to obtain a satisfactory therapeutic effect should take place no oftener than every 4 or 5 days. Patients with reduced renal function should receive correspondingly reduced doses of nadolol, carteolol, and atenolol. It is claimed that atenolol produces fewer central nervous system-related effects than other more lipid-soluble beta antagonists.

3. PINDOLOL, ACEBUTOLOL, & PENBUTOLOL

Pindolol, acebutolol, and penbutolol are partial agonists, ie, beta-blockers with intrinsic sympathomimetic activity. They lower blood pressure by decreasing vascular resistance and appear to depress cardiac output or heart rate less than other beta-blockers, perhaps because of significantly greater agonist than antagonist effects at β_2 receptors. This may be particularly beneficial for patients with cardiac failure, bradyarrhythmias, or peripheral vascular disease. Daily doses of pindolol start at 10 mg; of acebutolol, at 400 mg; and of penbutolol, at 20 mg.

4. LABETALOL & CARVEDILOL

Labetalol is given clinically as a racemic mixture of four isomeric compounds (it has two centers of asymmetry). Two of these isomers (the *SS* and *RS* isomers) are inactive, a third *(SR)* is a potent alpha-blocker, and the last *(RR)* is a potent beta-blocker. The beta-blocking isomer is thought to have selective β_2 agonist and nonselective beta antagonist action. Labetalol has a 3:1 ratio of beta:alpha antagonism after oral dosing. Blood pressure is lowered by reduction of systemic vascular resistance without significant alteration in heart rate or cardiac output. Because of its combined alpha- and beta-blocking activity, labetalol is useful in treating the hypertension of pheochromocytoma and hypertensive emergencies. Oral daily doses of labetalol range from 200 to 2400 mg/d. Labetalol is given as repeated intravenous bolus injections of 20–80 mg to treat hypertensive emergencies.

Carvedilol, like labetalol, is administered as a racemic mixture. The $S(-)$ isomer is a nonselective β adrenoceptor blocker, but both $S(-)$ and $R(+)$ isomers have approximately equal α-blocking potency. The isomers are stereoselectively metabolized in the liver, which means that their elimination half-lives may differ. The average half-life is 7–10 hours. The usual starting dosage of carvedilol for ordinary hypertension is 6.25 mg twice daily. Preliminary studies suggest that carvedilol (like certain other beta-blockers) may be useful in some cases of congestive heart failure (see Chapter 13).

PRAZOSIN & OTHER α_1-BLOCKERS

Mechanism & Sites of Action

Prazosin, terazosin, and doxazosin produce most of their antihypertensive effect by blocking α_1 receptors in arterioles and venules. Selectivity for α_1 receptors may explain why these agents produce less reflex tachycardia than do nonselective alpha antagonists such as phentolamine. This receptor selectivity allows norepinephrine to exert unopposed negative feedback (mediated by presynaptic α_2 receptors) on its own release (see Chapter 6); in contrast, phentolamine blocks both pre- and postsynaptic alpha receptors, with the result that reflex stimulation of sympathetic neurons produces greater release of transmitter onto beta receptors and correspondingly greater cardioacceleration.

Alpha-blockers reduce arterial pressure by dilating both resistance and capacitance vessels. As expected, blood pressure is reduced more in the upright than in the supine position. Retention of salt and fluid occurs when these drugs are administered without a diuretic. The drugs are more effective when used in combination with other agents, such as a beta-blocker and a diuretic, than when used alone.

Pharmacokinetics & Dosage

Prazosin is well absorbed but undergoes substantial first-pass metabolism in the liver. It is eliminated almost entirely by metabolism, with a plasma half-life of 3–4 hours, although the duration of the antihypertensive effect is longer. Plasma concentrations are increased in patients with congestive heart failure, owing primarily to reduced first-pass metabolism. Terazosin is also extensively metabolized but undergoes very little first-pass metabolism and has a half-life of 12 hours. Doxazosin has an intermediate bioavailability and a half-life of 22 hours.

Treatment with prazosin should be initiated with a low dose (1 mg 3 times daily) to prevent postural hypotension and syncope. Doses may be increased to 20 or 30 mg/d. Terazosin can often be given once daily, with doses of 5–20 mg/d. Doxazosin is usually given once daily starting at 1 mg/d and progressing to 4 mg/d or more as needed. Although long-term treatment with these alpha-blockers causes relatively little postural hypotension, a number of patients develop a precipitous drop in standing blood pressure shortly after the first dose is absorbed. For this reason, the first dose should be small and should be administered at bedtime. While the mechanism of this first-dose phenomenon is not clear, it occurs more commonly in patients who are salt- and volume-depleted.

Aside from the first-dose phenomenon, the reported toxicities of the α_1 blockers are relatively infrequent and mild. These include dizziness, palpitations, headache, and lassitude. Some patients develop a positive test for antinuclear factor in serum while on prazosin therapy, but this has not been associated with rheumatic symptoms. Unlike diuretics and beta-blockers, the α_1-blockers do not adversely and may even beneficially affect plasma lipid profiles.

OTHER ALPHA-ADRENOCEPTOR-BLOCKING AGENTS

Investigational α_1-selective blockers include pinacidil, urapidil, and cromakalim. The nonselective agents, **phentolamine** and **phenoxybenzamine,** are useful in diagnosis and treatment of pheochromocytoma and in other clinical situations associated with exaggerated release of catecholamines (eg, phentolamine may be combined with propranolol to treat the clonidine withdrawal syndrome, described above). Their pharmacology is described in Chapter 10.

VASODILATORS

Mechanism & Sites of Action

Within this class of drugs are the oral vasodilators, hydralazine and minoxidil, which are used for long-term outpatient therapy of hypertension; the parenteral vasodilators, nitroprusside and diazoxide, which are used to treat hypertensive emergencies; and the calcium channel blockers, which are used in both circumstances.

Chapter 12 contains a general discussion of vasodilators. All of the vasodilators useful in hypertension relax smooth muscle of arterioles, thereby decreasing systemic vascular resistance. Sodium nitroprusside also relaxes veins. Decreased arterial resistance and decreased mean arterial blood pressure elicit compensatory responses, mediated by baroreceptors and the sympathetic nervous system (Figure 11–5), as well as renin, angiotensin, and aldosterone. These compensating responses oppose the antihypertensive effect of the vasodilator. Because sympathetic reflexes are intact, vasodilator therapy does not cause orthostatic hypotension or sexual dysfunction.

Vasodilators work best in combination with other antihypertensive drugs that oppose the compensatory cardiovascular responses (Figure 11–5). (See box: Monotherapy Versus Polypharmacy in Hypertension.)

HYDRALAZINE

Hydralazine, a hydrazine derivative, dilates arterioles but not veins. It has been available for many years, though it was initially thought not to be particularly effective because tachyphylaxis to hypertensive effects developed rapidly. Now the benefits of combination therapy are recognized, and hydralazine may be used more effectively, particularly in severe hypertension.

Hydralazine

Pharmacokinetics, Metabolism, & Dosage

Hydralazine is well absorbed and rapidly metabolized by the liver during the first pass, so that bioavail-

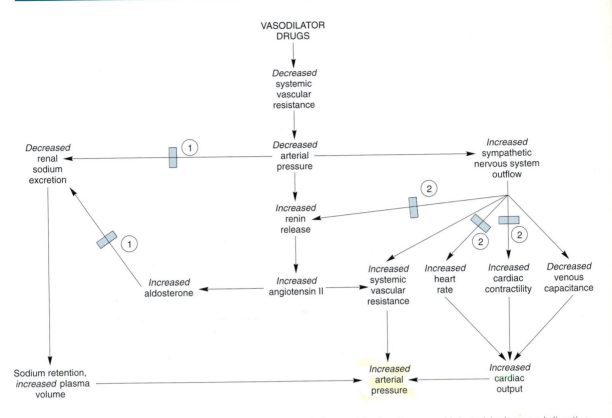

Figure 11–5. Compensatory responses to vasodilators; basis for combination therapy with beta-blockers and diuretics. ① Effect blocked by diuretics. ② Effect blocked by beta-blockers.

ability is low (averaging 25%) and variable among individuals. It is metabolized in part by acetylation at a rate that appears to be bimodally distributed in the population (see Chapter 4). As a consequence, rapid acetylators have greater first-pass metabolism, lower bioavailability, and less antihypertensive benefit from a given dose than do slow acetylators. The half-life of hydralazine ranges from 2 to 4 hours, but vascular effects appear to persist longer than do blood concentrations—an observation that is consistent with experimental evidence of avid binding to vascular tissue.

Usual dosage ranges from 40 to 200 mg/d. The higher dosage was selected as the dose at which there is a small possibility of developing the lupus erythematosus-like syndrome described in the next section. However, higher dosages result in greater vasodilation and may be used if necessary. Dosing 2 or 3 times daily provides smooth control of blood pressure.

Toxicity

The most common adverse effects of hydralazine are headache, nausea, anorexia, palpitations, sweating, and flushing. In patients with ischemic heart disease, reflex tachycardia and sympathetic stimulation may provoke angina or ischemic arrhythmias. With dosages of 400 mg/d or more, there is a 10–20% incidence—chiefly in persons who slowly acetylate the drug—of a syndrome characterized by arthralgia, myalgia, skin rashes, and fever that resembles lupus erythematosus. The syndrome is not associated with renal damage and is reversed by discontinuance of hydralazine. Peripheral neuropathy and drug fever are other serious but uncommon adverse effects.

MINOXIDIL

Minoxidil is a very efficacious orally active vasodilator. The effect appears to result from the opening of potassium channels in smooth muscle membranes by minoxidil sulfate, the active metabolite. This action stabilizes the membrane at its resting potential and makes contraction less likely. Like hydralazine, minoxidil dilates arterioles but not veins. Because of its greater potential antihypertensive effect, minoxidil should replace hydralazine when maximal doses of the latter are not effective or in patients with renal failure and severe hypertension, who do not respond well to hydralazine.

Minoxidil

Pharmacokinetics, Metabolism, & Dosage

Minoxidil is well absorbed from the gastrointestinal tract and is metabolized, primarily by conjugation, in the liver. Minoxidil is not protein-bound. Its half-life averages 4 hours, but its hypotensive effect after a single dose may persist for over 24 hours, probably reflecting the persistence of its active metabolite, minoxidil sulfate.

Minoxidil is available for hypertension only as an oral preparation. Generally, patients are started on 5 or 10 mg/d in two doses, and the daily dosage is then gradually increased to 40 mg/d. Higher dosages—up to 80 mg/d—have been used in treating severe hypertension.

Even more than with hydralazine, the use of minoxidil is associated with reflex sympathetic stimulation and sodium and fluid retention. Minoxidil must be used in combination with a beta-blocker and a loop diuretic.

Toxicity

Tachycardia, palpitations, angina, and edema are observed when doses of beta-blockers and diuretics are inadequate. Headache, sweating, and hypertrichosis, which is particularly bothersome in women, are relatively common. Minoxidil illustrates how one person's toxicity may become another person's therapy. Topical minoxidil (as Rogaine) is now used as a stimulant to hair growth for correction of baldness.

SODIUM NITROPRUSSIDE

Sodium nitroprusside is a powerful parenterally administered vasodilator that is used in treating hypertensive emergencies as well as severe cardiac failure. Nitroprusside dilates both arterial and venous vessels, resulting in reduced peripheral vascular resistance and venous return. The action occurs as a result of activation of guanylyl cyclase, either via release of nitric oxide or by direct stimulation of the enzyme. The result is increased intracellular cGMP, which relaxes vascular smooth muscle.

In the absence of cardiac failure, blood pressure decreases, owing to decreased vascular resistance, while cardiac output does not change or decreases slightly. In patients with cardiac failure and low cardiac output, output increases owing to afterload reduction.

Nitroprusside

Pharmacokinetics, Metabolism, & Dosage

Nitroprusside is a complex of iron, cyanide groups, and a nitroso moiety. It is rapidly metabolized by uptake into red blood cells with liberation of cyanide. Cyanide in turn is metabolized by the mitochondrial enzyme rhodanase, in the presence of a sulfur donor, to thiocyanate. Thiocyanate is distributed in extracellular fluid and slowly eliminated by the kidney.

Nitroprusside rapidly lowers blood pressure, and its effects disappear within 1–10 minutes after discontinuation. The drug is given by intravenous infusion. Sodium nitroprusside in aqueous solution is sensitive to light and must therefore be made up fresh before each administration and covered with opaque foil. Infusion solutions should be changed after several hours. Dosage typically begins at 0.5 µg/kg/min and may be increased up to 10 µg/kg/min as necessary to control blood pressure. Higher rates of infusion, if continued for more than an hour, may result in toxicity. Because of its efficacy and rapid onset of effect, the drug should be administered by infusion pump and arterial blood pressure continuously monitored via intra-arterial recording.

Toxicity

The most serious toxicity is related to accumulation of cyanide; metabolic acidosis, arrhythmias, excessive hypotension, and death have resulted. In a few cases, toxicity after relatively low doses of nitroprusside suggested a defect in cyanide metabolism. Administration of sodium thiosulfate as a sulfur donor facilitates metabolism of cyanide. Hydroxocobalamin combines with cyanide to form the nontoxic cyanocobalamin. Both have been advocated for prophylaxis or treatment of cyanide poisoning during nitroprusside infusion. Thiocyanate may accumulate over the course of prolonged administration, usually a week or more, particularly in patients with renal insufficiency who do not excrete thiocyanate at a normal rate. Thiocyanate toxicity is manifested as weakness, disorientation, psychosis, muscle spasms, and convulsions, and the diagnosis is confirmed by finding serum concentrations greater than 10 mg/dL. Rarely, delayed hypothyroidism occurs, owing to thiocyanate inhibition of iodide uptake by the thyroid. Methemoglobinemia during infusion of nitroprusside has also been reported.

DIAZOXIDE

Diazoxide is an effective and relatively long-acting parenterally administered arteriolar dilator that is used to treat hypertensive emergencies. Injection of diazoxide results in a rapid fall in systemic vascular resistance and mean arterial blood pressure associated with substantial tachycardia and increase in cardiac output. Studies of its mechanism suggest that it prevents vascular smooth muscle contraction by opening potassium channels and stabilizing the membrane potential at the resting level.

Diazoxide

Pharmacokinetics & Dosage

Diazoxide is similar chemically to the thiazide diuretics but has no diuretic activity. It is bound extensively to serum albumin and to vascular tissue. Diazoxide is both metabolized and excreted unchanged; its metabolic pathways are not well characterized. Its half-life is approximately 24 hours, but the relationship between blood concentration and hypotensive action is not well established. The blood pressure-lowering effect after a rapid injection is established within 5 minutes and lasts for 4–12 hours. It was initially thought that rapid injection was mandatory to saturate plasma protein binding so that free drug could reach vascular tissue, but this idea is no longer generally accepted. Blood pressure is in fact lowered by constant infusion, although the extent of lowering for a given total dose is greater after rapid administration.

When diazoxide was first marketed, a dose of 300 mg by rapid injection was recommended. It appears, however, that excessive hypotension can be avoided by beginning with smaller doses (50–150 mg). If necessary, doses of 150 mg may be repeated every 5 minutes until blood pressure is lowered satisfactorily. Nearly all patients respond to a maximum of three or four doses. Alternatively, diazoxide may be administered by intravenous infusion at rates of 15–30 mg/min. Because of reduced protein binding, hypotension occurs after smaller doses in persons with chronic renal failure, and smaller doses should be administered to these patients. The hypotensive effects of diazoxide are also greater if patients are pretreated with beta-blockers to prevent the reflex tachycardia and associated increase in cardiac output.

Toxicity

The most significant toxicity from diazoxide has been excessive hypotension, resulting from the recommendation to use a fixed dose of 300 mg in all patients. Such hypotension has resulted in stroke and myocardial infarction. The reflex sympathetic response can provoke angina, electrocardiographic evidence of ischemia, and cardiac failure in patients with ischemic heart disease, and diazoxide should be avoided in this situation.

Diazoxide inhibits insulin release from the pancreas (probably by opening potassium channels in the beta cell membrane) and is used to treat hypoglycemia secondary to insulinoma. Occasionally, hyperglycemia complicates diazoxide use, particularly in persons with renal insufficiency.

In contrast to the thiazide diuretics, diazoxide causes renal salt and water *retention*. However, because the drug is used for short periods only, this is rarely a problem.

CALCIUM CHANNEL BLOCKERS

In addition to their antianginal (Chapter 12) and antiarrhythmic effects (Chapter 14), calcium channel blockers also dilate peripheral arterioles and reduce blood pressure. The mechanism of action in hypertension (and, in part, in angina) is inhibition of calcium influx into arterial smooth muscle cells.

Verapamil, diltiazem, and the **dihydropyridine** family (**amlodipine, felodipine, isradipine, nicardipine, nifedipine, and nisoldipine**) are all equally effective in lowering blood pressure, and various formulations are currently approved for this use in the USA. Several others are under study. Hemodynamic differences among calcium channel blockers may influence the choice of a particular agent. Nifedipine and the other dihydropyridine agents are more selective as vasodilators and have less cardiac depressant effect than verapamil and diltiazem. Reflex sympathetic activation with slight tachycardia maintains or increases cardiac output in most patients given dihydropyridines. Verapamil has the greatest effect on the heart and may decrease heart rate and cardiac output. Diltiazem has intermediate actions. The pharmacology and toxicity of these drugs is discussed in more detail in Chapter 12. Doses of calcium channel blockers used in treating hypertension are similar to those used in treating angina or coronary spasm. Some recent epidemiologic studies reported an increased risk of myocardial infarction or mortality in patients receiving short-acting nifedipine for hypertension (Psaty et al, 1995; Pahor et al, 1995). While there is still debate about causation, it is recommended that short-acting nifedipine not be used for hypertension. In any case, sustained-release calcium blockers or calcium blockers with long half-lives provide smoother blood pressure control and are more appropriate for treatment of chronic hypertension. Intravenous nicardipine has recently been released for the treatment of hypertension when oral therapy is not feasible, though parenteral verapamil and diltiazem could be used for the same indication. Nicardipine is typically infused at rates of 2–15 mg/h. Oral short-acting nifedipine has gained some popularity in emergency management of severe hypertension.

INHIBITORS OF ANGIOTENSIN

Although the causative roles of renin, angiotensin, and aldosterone in essential hypertension are still controversial, there do appear to be differences in the activity of this system among individuals. When controlled for daily sodium intake (assessed as 24-hour urinary sodium excretion) and serum potassium concentration, approximately 20% of patients with essential hypertension have inappropriately low and 20% have inappropriately high plasma renin activity. Blood pressure of patients with high-renin hypertension responds well to beta-adrenoceptor blockers, which lower plasma renin activity, and to angiotensin inhibitors—supporting a role for excess renin and angiotensin in this population.

Mechanism & Sites of Action

Renin release from the kidney cortex is stimulated by reduced renal arterial pressure, sympathetic neural stimulation, and reduced sodium delivery or increased sodium concentration at the distal renal tubule. Renin acts upon renin substrate, an α_2-globulin, to split off the inactive decapeptide angiotensin I. Angiotensin I is then converted, primarily by endothelial angiotensin-converting enzyme (ACE) in the lung, to the arterial vasoconstrictor octapeptide angiotensin II (Figure 11–6), which is in turn converted in the adrenal gland to angiotensin III. Angiotensin II has vasoconstrictor and sodium-retaining activity. Angiotensin II and III both stimulate aldosterone release. Angiotensin may contribute to maintaining high vascular resistance in hypertensive states associated with high plasma renin activity, such as renal arterial stenosis, some types of intrinsic renal disease, and malignant hypertension, as well as in essential hypertension after treatment with sodium restriction, diuretics, or vasodilators.

New evidence suggests that a parallel system for angiotensin generation exists in several other tissues (eg, heart) and may be responsible for trophic changes such as cardiac hypertrophy. The converting enzyme involved in tissue angiotensin II synthesis is also inhibited by the ACE inhibitors.

Two classes of drugs act specifically on the renin-angiotensin system: the ACE inhibitors and the competitive inhibitors of angiotensin at its receptors, including losartan, valsartan, and saralasin (saralasin is no longer in clinical use).

ANGIOTENSIN-CONVERTING ENZYME (ACE) INHIBITORS

Captopril (Figure 17–3) and other drugs in this class inhibit the converting enzyme peptidyl dipeptidase that hydrolyzes angiotensin I to angiotensin II and (under the name plasma kininase) inactivates bradykinin, a potent vasodilator, which works at least in part by stimulating release of nitric oxide and prostacyclin. The hypotensive activity of captopril probably results both from an inhibitory action on the renin-angiotensin system and a stimulating action on the kallikrein-kinin system (Figure 11–6).

Enalapril (Figure 17–3) is a prodrug that is converted by deesterification to a converting enzyme inhibitor, enalaprilat, with effects similar to those of captopril. Enalaprilat itself is available only for intravenous use, primarily for hypertensive emergencies. **Lisinopril** is a lysine derivative of enalaprilat. **Benazepril, fosinopril, moexipril, quinapril,** and **ramipril** are more recently introduced long-acting members of the class. All are prodrugs, like enalapril, and are converted to the active agents by hydrolysis, primarily in the liver.

Angiotensin II inhibitors lower blood pressure principally by decreasing peripheral vascular resistance. Cardiac output and heart rate are not significantly changed. Unlike direct vasodilators, these agents do not result in reflex sympathetic activation and can be used safely in persons with ischemic heart disease. The absence of reflex tachycardia may be due to downward resetting of the baroreceptors or to enhanced parasympathetic activity.

Although converting enzyme inhibitors are most effective in conditions associated with high plasma renin activity, there is no good correlation among subjects between plasma renin activity and antihypertensive response. Accordingly, renin profiling is unnecessary.

ACE inhibitors have a particularly useful role in treating patients with diabetic nephropathy, diminishing proteinuria and stabilizing renal function (even in the absence of lowering of blood pressure). These benefits probably result from improved intrarenal hemodynamics, with decreased glomerular efferent arteriolar resistance and a resulting reduction of intraglomerular capillary pressure. ACE inhibitors have also proved to be extremely useful in the treatment of congestive heart failure, and after myocardial infarction. In the latter case, ACE inhibitors result in better preservation of left ventricular function in the years following infarction, acting by reducing postinfarction myocardial remodeling. These applications are discussed in Chapter 13.

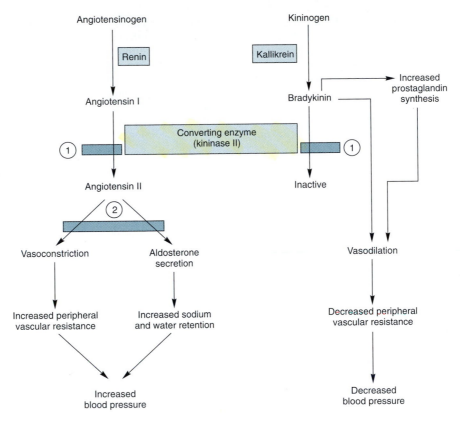

Figure 11–6. Sites of action of ACE inhibitors and receptor blockers. ① Site of ACE blockade. ② Site of receptor blockade.

Pharmacokinetics & Dosage

Captopril is rapidly absorbed, with a bioavailability of about 70% after fasting. Bioavailability is decreased by 30–40% if the drug is taken with food; however, the antihypertensive action of captopril is unaffected. It is metabolized chiefly to disulfide conjugates with other sulfhydryl-containing molecules. Less than half of an oral dose of captopril is excreted unchanged in the urine. Captopril is distributed to most body tissues, with the notable exception of the central nervous system. The half-life of captopril is less than 3 hours. Blood levels correlate poorly with clinical response (see Figure 3–6).

Captopril is initially administered in doses of 25 mg 2 or 3 times each day, 1–2 hours before meals. Maximal blood pressure response is seen 2–4 hours after the dose. At 1- to 2-week intervals, doses can be increased until blood pressure is controlled.

Peak concentrations of enalaprilat occur 3–4 hours after dosing with enalapril. The half-life of enalaprilat is about 11 hours. Typical doses of enalapril are 10–20 mg once or twice daily.

Lisinopril is slowly absorbed, with peak blood levels at about 7 hours after a dose. It has a half-life of 12 hours. Doses of 10–80 mg once daily are effective in most patients.

All of the ACE inhibitors except fosinopril and moexipril are eliminated primarily by the kidneys; doses of these drugs should be reduced in patients with renal insufficiency.

Toxicity

Severe hypotension can occur after initial doses of any ACE inhibitor in patients who are hypovolemic due to diuretics, salt restriction, or gastrointestinal fluid loss. Other adverse effects common to all ACE inhibitors include acute renal failure (particularly in patients with bilateral renal artery stenosis or stenosis of the renal artery of a solitary kidney), hyperkalemia, dry cough sometimes accompanied by wheezing, and angioedema. Hyperkalemia is more likely to occur in patients with renal insufficiency or diabetes. Bradykinin seems to be responsible for the cough and angioedema seen with ACE inhibition.

The use of ACE inhibitors is contraindicated during the second and third trimesters of pregnancy because of the risk of fetal hypotension, anuria, and renal failure, sometimes associated with fetal malformations or death. Captopril, particularly when given in high doses to patients with renal insufficiency, may cause neutropenia or proteinuria. Minor toxic effects seen more typically include altered sense of taste, allergic skin rashes, and drug fever, which may occur in as many as 10% of patients. The incidence of these adverse effects may be lower with the long-acting ACE inhibitors.

Important drug interactions include those with potassium supplements or potassium-sparing diuretics, which can result in hyperkalemia. Nonsteroidal anti-inflammatory drugs may impair the hypotensive effects of ACE inhibitors by blocking bradykinin-mediated vasodilation, which is at least in part, prostaglandin mediated.

ANGIOTENSIN RECEPTOR-BLOCKING AGENTS

Losartan and **valsartan** are recently released blockers of the angiotensin type 1 (AT_1) receptor. They have no effect on bradykinin metabolism and are therefore more selective blockers of angiotensin effects than ACE inhibitors. They also have the potential for more complete inhibition of angiotensin action compared with ACE inhibitors because there are enzymes other than ACE that are capable of generating angiotensin II. Losartan is orally active and extensively metabolized; its principal 5-carboxylic acid metabolite is active. The half-life of losartan is about 2 hours; the half-life of the metabolite is 6–9 hours. The typical starting dosage is 50 mg/d, with a usual dose range of 25–100 mg/d. The side effects are similar to those described for ACE inhibitors, including the hazard of use during pregnancy, with the exception of cough and angioedema, which are thought to be mediated by bradykinin.

Saralasin (1-sar-8-ala-angiotensin II) is an analog and competitive inhibitor of angiotensin II at its receptors (Figure 11–6). Saralasin blocks the pressor and aldosterone-releasing effects of infused angiotensin II and lowers blood pressure in high-renin states such as renal artery stenosis. Saralasin also has weak agonist activity, however, so that rapid injection or administration to persons without high circulating angiotensin II may increase rather than decrease blood pressure. Because it had to be administered by continuous intravenous infusion and because its vascular effects were unpredictable, saralasin was withdrawn from the market. However, this partial agonist drug has proved to be a valuable research tool in determining the role of angiotensin II in hypertension.

II. CLINICAL PHARMACOLOGY OF ANTIHYPERTENSIVE AGENTS

Hypertension presents a unique problem in therapeutics. It is usually a lifelong disease that causes few symptoms until the advanced stage. For effective treatment, medicines that are expensive and often produce adverse effects must be consumed daily. Thus, the physician must establish with certainty that hypertension is persistent and requires treatment and must exclude secondary causes of hypertension that might be treated by definitive surgical procedures. Persistence of hypertension, particularly in persons with mild elevation of blood pressure, should be established by finding an elevated blood pressure on at least three different office visits. Ambulatory blood pressure monitoring may be the best predictor of risk and therefore of need for therapy in mild hypertension. Recent evidence indicates that isolated systolic hypertension and hypertension in the elderly also benefit from therapy.

Once the presence of hypertension is established, the question of whether or not to treat and which drugs to use must be considered. The level of blood pressure, the age and sex of the patient, the severity of organ damage (if any) due to high blood pressure, and the presence of cardiovascular risk factors must all be considered.

Once the decision is made to treat, a therapeutic regimen must be developed and the patient must be educated about the nature of hypertension and the importance of treatment. Selection of drugs is dictated by the level of blood pressure, the presence and severity of end-organ damage, and the presence of other diseases. Severe high blood pressure with life-threatening complications requires more rapid treatment with more potent drugs. Most patients with essential hypertension, however, have had elevated blood pressure for months or years, and therapy is best initiated in a gradual fashion.

Successful treatment of hypertension requires that dietary instructions be followed and medications be taken as directed. Education about the natural history of hypertension and the importance of treatment as well as potential side effects of drugs is essential. Follow-up visits should be frequent enough to convince the patient that the physician thinks the illness is serious. With each follow-up visit, the importance of treatment should be reinforced and questions particularly concerning dosing or side effects of medication encouraged. Other factors that may improve compliance are simplifying dosing regimens and having the patient monitor blood pressure at home.

OUTPATIENT THERAPY OF HYPERTENSION

The initial step in treating hypertension may be nonpharmacologic. As discussed previously, sodium restriction may be effective treatment for as many as half of patients with mild hypertension. The average American diet contains about 200 meq of sodium per day. A reasonable dietary goal in treating hypertension is 70–100 meq of sodium per day, which can be achieved by not salting food during or after cooking and by avoiding processed foods that contain large amounts of sodium. Compliance with sodium restriction can be assessed by measuring 24-hour urinary excretion of sodium, which approximates sodium intake, before and after dietary instruction.

Weight reduction even without sodium restriction has been shown to normalize blood pressure in up to 75% of overweight patients with mild to moderate hypertension. Regular exercise has been shown in some but not all studies to lower blood pressure in hypertensive patients.

For pharmacologic management of mild hypertension, blood pressure can be normalized in most patients with a single drug. Such "monotherapy" is also sufficient for some patients with moderate hypertension. Thiazide diuretics and beta-blockers are the only drugs that have been shown to reduce morbidity and mortality and are recommended for initial drug therapy in such patients. There has been concern that diuretics and beta-blockers, by adversely affecting the serum lipid profile or impairing glucose tolerance, may add to the risk of coronary disease, thereby offsetting the benefit of blood pressure reduction. Alternative choices for initial monotherapy include ACE inhibitors, calcium channel blockers, selective α_1 blockers (eg, prazosin), $\alpha + \beta$ blockers (labetalol or

carvedilol), and central sympathoplegic agents (eg, clonidine), though none of these have yet been shown to affect long-term outcome. The presence of concomitant disease should influence selection of antihypertensive drugs because two diseases may benefit from a single drug. For example, beta-blockers or calcium channel blockers are particularly useful in patients who also have angina, diuretics or ACE inhibitors in patients who also have congestive heart failure. Race also affects drug selection: blacks respond well to diuretics and calcium channel blockers and less well to beta-blockers and ACE inhibitors.

If a single drug does not adequately control blood pressure, drugs with different sites of action can be combined to effectively lower blood pressure while minimizing toxicity ("stepped care"). If a diuretic is not used initially, it is often selected as the second drug. If three drugs are required, combining a diuretic, a sympathoplegic agent or an ACE inhibitor, and a direct vasodilator (eg, hydralazine or a calcium channel blocker) is often effective.

Assessment of blood pressure during office visits should include measurement of recumbent, sitting, and standing pressures. An attempt should be made to normalize blood pressure (mean blood pressure ≤ 100 mm Hg) in the posture or activity level that is customary for the patient. The extent of orthostatic hy-

---

MONOTHERAPY VERSUS POLYPHARMACY IN HYPERTENSION

Monotherapy of hypertension (treatment with a single drug) has become more popular since the introduction of ACE inhibitors and α_1-selective alpha-blockers because compliance is likely to be better and because in some cases adverse effects are fewer. However, moderate to severe hypertension is still commonly treated by a combination of two or more drugs, each acting by a different mechanism (polypharmacy). The rationale for polypharmacy is that each of the drugs acts on one of a set of interacting, mutually compensatory regulatory mechanisms for maintaining blood pressure (Figures 6–7 and 11–1).

For example, because an adequate dose of hydralazine causes a significant decrease in peripheral vascular resistance, there will initially be a drop in mean arterial blood pressure, evoking a strong response in the form of compensatory tachycardia and salt and water retention (Figure 11–5). The result is an increase in cardiac output that is capable of almost completely reversing the effect of hydralazine. The addition of a sympathoplegic drug (eg, propranolol) prevents the tachycardia; addition of a diuretic (eg, hydrochlorothiazide) prevents the salt and water retention. In effect, all three drugs increase the sensitivity of

the cardiovascular system to each other's actions. Thus, partial impairment of one regulatory mechanism (sympathetic discharge to the heart) increases the antihypertensive effect of impairing regulation by another mechanism (peripheral vascular resistance). Finally, in some circumstances, a normal compensatory response accounts for the toxicity of an antihypertensive agent, and the toxic effect can be prevented by administering a second type of drug. In the case of hydralazine, compensatory tachycardia and increased cardiac output may precipitate angina in patients with coronary atherosclerosis. Addition of the beta-blocker and diuretic can prevent this toxicity in many patients.

In practice, when hypertension does not respond adequately to a regimen of one drug, a second drug from a different class with a different mechanism of action and different pattern of toxicity is added. If the response is still inadequate and compliance is known to be good, a third drug may be added. The drugs least likely to be successful as monotherapy are hydralazine and minoxidil. It is not completely clear why other drugs such as α_1-blockers and calcium channel blockers cause less marked compensatory responses for the same amount of blood pressure lowering.

potension and inhibition of reflex or exercise tachycardia are useful indicators of the effectiveness of or compliance with sympathoplegic therapy. In addition to noncompliance with medication, causes of failure to respond to drug therapy include excessive sodium intake and inadequate diuretic therapy with excessive blood volume (this can be measured directly), and drugs such as antidepressants, nonsteroidal anti-inflammatory drugs, over-the-counter sympathomimetics, and oral contraceptives that can interfere with actions of some antihypertensive drugs or directly raise blood pressure.

MANAGEMENT OF HYPERTENSIVE EMERGENCIES

Despite the large number of patients with chronic hypertension, hypertensive emergencies are relatively rare. Marked or sudden elevation of blood pressure may be a serious threat to life, however, and prompt reduction of blood pressure is indicated. Most commonly, hypertensive emergencies occur in patients whose hypertension is severe and poorly controlled and in those who suddenly discontinue antihypertensive medications.

Clinical Presentation & Pathophysiology

Hypertensive emergencies include hypertension associated with vascular damage (termed malignant hypertension) and hypertension associated with hemodynamic complications such as cardiac failure, stroke, or dissecting aneurysm. The underlying pathologic process in malignant hypertension is a progressive arteriopathy with inflammation and necrosis of arterioles. Vascular lesions occur in the kidney, which releases renin, which in turn stimulates production of angiotensin and aldosterone, which further increase blood pressure.

Hypertensive encephalopathy is a classic feature of malignant hypertension. Its clinical presentation consists of severe headache, mental confusion, and apprehension. Blurred vision, nausea and vomiting, and focal neurologic deficits are common. If untreated, the syndrome may progress over a period of 12–48 hours to convulsions, stupor, coma, and even death.

Treatment of Hypertensive Emergencies

The general management of hypertensive emergencies requires monitoring the patient in an intensive care unit with continuous recording of arterial blood pressure. Fluid intake and output must be monitored carefully and body weight measured daily as an indicator of total body fluid volume during the course of therapy.

Parenteral antihypertensive medications are used to lower blood pressure rapidly (within a few hours); as soon as reasonable blood pressure control is achieved, oral antihypertensive therapy should be substituted, because this allows smoother long-term management of hypertension. The goal of treatment in the first few hours or days is not normalization of blood pressure because chronic hypertension is associated with autoregulatory changes in cerebral blood flow. Thus, rapid normalization of blood pressure may lead to cerebral hypoperfusion and brain injury. Rather, blood pressure should be lowered by about 25%, maintaining diastolic blood pressure at no less than 100–110 mm Hg. Subsequently, blood pressure can be reduced to normal levels using oral medications over several weeks. The drugs most commonly used to treat hypertensive emergencies are the vasodilators sodium nitroprusside and diazoxide. Other parenteral drugs that may be effective include nitroglycerin, labetalol, calcium channel blockers, hydralazine, reserpine, and methyldopa. Nonparenteral therapy with oral nifedipine, captopril, prazosin, or clonidine has also been shown to be useful in the therapy of severe hypertension.

Most patients with severe hypertension have a normal or contracted blood volume, although some, eg, those with renal failure, may be hypervolemic. Diuretics are administered to prevent the volume expansion that typically occurs during administration of powerful vasodilators. Because it is likely that the patient will have compromised renal function, a drug that works in the presence of renal insufficiency, such as furosemide, should be selected.

Dialysis may be a necessary alternative to the loop diuretics, particularly in patients with oliguric renal failure. Dialysis can remove excess fluid, correct electrolyte disturbances, and control symptoms of uremia. Uremic symptoms may be confusing in evaluating patients with hypertensive encephalopathy.

PREPARATIONS AVAILABLE

Beta-Adrenoceptor Blockers
  Acebutolol (Sectral)
    Oral: 200, 400 mg capsules
  Atenolol (generic, Tenormin)
    Oral: 25, 50, 100 mg tablets
    Parenteral: 0.5 mg/mL for injection

  Betaxolol (Kerlone)
    Oral: 10, 20 mg tablets
  Bisoprolol (Zelate)
    Oral: 5, 10 mg tablets
  Carteolol (Cartrol)
    Oral: 2.5, 5 mg tablets

Carvedilol (Coreg)
Oral: 6.25, 12.5, 25 mg tablets
Labetalol (Normodyne, Trandate)
Oral: 100, 200, 300 mg tablets
Parenteral: 5 mg/mL for injection
Metoprolol (Lopressor)
Oral: 50, 100 mg tablets
Oral extended release (Toprol-XL): 50, 100,
200 mg tablets
Parenteral: 1 mg/mL for injection
Nadolol (Corgard)
Oral: 20, 40, 80, 120, 160 mg tablets
Penbutolol (Levatol)
Oral: 20 mg tablets
Pindolol (generic, Visken)
Oral: 5, 10 mg tablets
Propranolol (generic, Inderal)
Oral: 10, 20, 40, 60, 80, 90 mg tablets; Intensol,
80 mg/mL solution
Oral sustained-release (generic, Inderal LA): 60,
80, 120, 160 mg capsules
Parenteral: 1 mg/mL for injection
Timolol (generic, Blocadren)
Oral: 5, 10, 20 mg tablets

Centrally Acting Sympathoplegic Drugs
Clonidine (generic, Catapres)
Oral: 0.1, 0.2, 0.3 mg tablets
Transdermal (Catapres-TTS): patches that re-
lease 0.1, 0.2, 0.3 mg/24 hr
Guanabenz (Wytensin)
Oral: 4, 8 mg tablets
Guanfacine (Tenex)
Oral: 1, 2 mg tablets
Methyldopa (generic, Aldomet)
Oral: 125, 250, 500 mg tablets; 250 mg/5 mL
suspension
Parenteral: 250 mg/5 mL for injection

Postganglionic Sympathetic Nerve Terminal Blockers
Guanadrel (Hylorel)
Oral: 10, 25 mg tablets
Guanethidine (generic, Ismelin Sulfate)
Oral: 10, 25 mg tablets
Reserpine (generic, Serpasil)
Oral: 0.1, 0.25 mg tablets

Alpha₁-Selective Adrenoceptor Blockers
Doxazosin (Cardura)
Oral 1, 2, 4, 8 mg tablets
Prazosin (Minipress)
Oral: 1, 2, 5 mg capsules
Terazosin (Hytrin)
Oral: 1, 2, 5, 10 mg tablets; 1, 2, 5, 10 mg
capsules

Ganglion Blocking Agents
Mecamylamine (Inversine)
Oral: 2.5 mg tablets

Vasodilators Used in Hypertension
Diazoxide (generic, Hyperstat IV)
Oral (Proglycem): 50 mg capsule; 50 mg/mL
oral suspension
Parenteral: 15 mg/mL, 300 mg/20 mL amp
Hydralazine (generic, Apresoline)
Oral: 10, 25, 50, 100 mg tablets
Parenteral: 20 mg/mL for injection
Minoxidil (generic, Loniten)
Oral: 2.5, 10 mg tablets
Topical (Rogaine, etc): 1.8 g/60 mL lotion
Nitroprusside (generic, Nipride)
Parenteral: 50 mg/vial

Calcium Channel Blockers
Amlodipine (Norvasc)
Oral 2.5, 5, 10 mg tablets
Diltiazem (generic, Cardizem)
Oral: 30, 60, 90, 120 mg tablets (unlabeled in
hypertension)
Oral sustained-release (Cardizem CD,
Cardizem SR, Dilacor XL): 60, 90, 120, 180,
240, 300 mg capsules
Parenteral: 5 mg/mL for injection
Felodipine (Plendil)
Oral extended release: 2.5, 5, 10 mg tablets
Isradipine (DynaCirc)
Oral: 2.5, 5 mg capsules
Nicardipine (Cardene)
Oral: 20, 30 mg capsules
Oral sustained release (Cardene SR): 30, 45,
60 mg capsules
Parenteral (Cardene IV): 25 mg/mL for
injection
Nisoldipine (Sular)
Oral: 10, 20, 30, 40 mg tablets
Nifedipine (generic, Adalat, Procardia)
Oral: 10, 20 mg capsules (unlabeled in hyper-
tension)
Oral extended-release (Adalat CC, Procardia-
XL): 30, 60, 90 mg tablets
Verapamil (generic, Calan, Isoptin)
Oral: 40, 80, 120 mg tablets
Oral sustained-release (generic, Calan SR, Vere-
lan): 120, 180, 240 mg tablets; 120, 180, 240
mg capsules
Parenteral: 5 mg/2 mL for injection

Angiotensin-Converting Enzyme Inhibitors
Benazepril (Lotensin)
Oral: 5, 10, 20, 40, mg tablets
Captopril (Capoten)
Oral: 12.5, 25, 50, 100 mg tablets

Enalapril (Vasotec)
Oral: 2.5, 5, 10, 20 mg tablets
Parenteral (Enalaprilat): 1.25 mg/mL for injection
Fosinopril (Monopril)
Oral: 10, 20 mg tablets
Lisinopril (Prinivil, Zestril)
Oral: 2.5, 5, 10, 20, 40 mg tablets
Moexipril (Univase)
Oral: 7.5, 15 mg tablets
Quinapril (Accupril)
Oral: 5, 10, 20, 40 mg tablets

Perindopril (Aceon)
Oral: 2, 4, 8 mg tablets
Ramipril (Altace)
Oral: 1.25, 2.5, 5, 10 mg capsules

Angiotensin Receptor Blockers
Losartan (Cozaar)
Oral: 25, 50 mg tablets
Valsartan (Diovan)
Oral: 80, 160 mg tablets

REFERENCES

Atlas D, Diamant S, Zonnenschein R: Is the imidazoline site a unique receptor? A correlation with clonidine-displacing substance activity. Am J Hypertens 1992;5:83S.

Bauer JH, Ream GP, Wu Z: Effects of losartan on the renin-angiotensin-aldosterone axis in essential hypertension. Am J Hypertens 1995;9:237.

Bousquet P, Feldman J, Schwartz J: Central cardiovascular effects of alpha adrenergic drugs: Differences between catecholamines and imidazolines. J Pharmacol Exp Ther 1984;230:232.

Buccafusco JJ et al: Role of medullary I_1 imidazoline and α_2-adrenergic receptors in the antihypertensive responses evoked by central administration of clonidine analogs in conscious spontaneously hypertensive rats. J Pharmacol Exp Ther 1995;273:1162.

Burt VL et al: Prevalence of hypertension in the US adult population. Hypertension 1995;25:305.

Calhoun DA, Oparil S: Treatment of hypertensive crisis. N Engl J Med 1990;323:1177.

Campese VM: Salt sensitivity in hypertension: Renal and cardiovascular implications. Hypertension 1994;23:531.

Cohn JN, Burke LP: Nitroprusside. Ann Intern Med 1979;91:752.

Croog SH et al: The effects of antihypertensive therapy on the quality of life. N Engl J Med 1986;314:1657.

Dahlof B et al: Morbidity and mortality in the Swedish trial in old patients with hypertension (STOP-Hypertension). Lancet 1991;338:1281.

Dominiak P: Historic aspects in the identification of the I_1 receptor and the pharmacology of the imidazolines. Cardiovasc Drugs Ther 1994;8:21.

Edelson JT et al: Long-term cost-effectiveness of various initial monotherapies for mild to moderate hypertension. JAMA 1990;263:407.

Eisenberg DM et al: Cognitive behavioral techniques for hypertension: Are they effective? Ann Intern Med 1993;118:964.

Ernsberger P et al: A novel mechanism of action for hypertension control: Moxonidine as a selective I_1-imidazoline agonist. Cardiovasc Drugs Ther 1994;27:49.

Ernsberger P et al: Moxonidine, a centrally acting antihypertensive agent, is a selective ligand for I_1-imidazoline sites. J Pharmacol Exp Ther 1993;264:172.

Filos KS et al: Intrathecal clonidine as a sole analgesic for pain relief after cesarean section. Anesthesiology 1992;77:267.

Fletcher AE, Bulpitt CJ: How far should blood pressure be lowered?: N Engl J Med 1992;326:251.

Frohlich ED: Methyldopa: Mechanisms and treatment 25 years later. Arch Intern Med 1980;140:954.

Gifford RW et al: Office evaluation of hypertension. Hypertension 1989;13:283.

Gifford RW: An algorithm for the management of resistant hypertension. Hypertension 1988;11(Suppl 2):II–101.

Gilford RW Jr: Management of hypertensive crises. JAMA 1991;266:829.

Goldberg AI, Dunlay MC, Sweet CS: Safety and tolerability of losartan potassium, an angiotensin I_1 receptor antagonist, compared with hydrochlorothiazide, atenolol, felodipine ER and angiotensin-converting enzyme inhibitors for the treatment of systemic hypertension. Am J Cardiol 1995;75:793.

Gourlay SG, Benowitz NL: Is clonidine an effective smoking cessation therapy? Drugs 1995;50:197.

Gurwitz JH et al: Initiation of antihypertensive treatment during nonsteroidal anti-inflammatory drug therapy. JAMA 1994;272:781.

Hanssens M et al: Fetal and neonatal effects of treatment with angiotensin-converting-enzyme inhibitors in pregnancy. Obstet Gynecol 1991;78:128.

Hypertension Detection and Follow-Up Program Cooperative Group: Five-year findings of the Hypertension Detection and Follow-Up Program. 1. Reduction in mortality of persons with high blood pressure, including mild hypertension. JAMA 1979;242:2562.

Hypertension Detection and Follow-Up Program Cooperative Group: Persistence of reduction in blood pressure and mortality of participants in the hypertension detection and follow-up program. JAMA 1988;259:2113.

Hypertension Detection and Follow-Up Program Cooperative Group: The effect of treatment on mortality in "mild" hypertension. N Engl J Med 1982;307:976.

Insua JT et al: Drug treatment of hypertension in the elderly: A meta-analysis. Ann Intern Med 1994;121:355.

Johnson AG, Nguyen TV, Day RO: Do nonsteroidal anti-inflammatory drugs affect blood pressure? A meta-analysis. Ann Intern Med 1994;121:289.

Joint National Committee on Detection, Evaluation, and Treatment of High Blood Pressure: The fifth report of the Joint National Committee on Detection, Evaluation, and Treatment of High Blood Pressure (JNC V). Arch Intern Med 1993;153:154.

Joint-National-Committee on Detection, Evaluation, and Treatment of High Blood Pressure: Nonpharmacological approaches to the control of high blood pressure. Hypertension 1986;8:444.

Kang PM et al: Angiotensin II receptor antagonists: A new approach to blockade of the renin-angiotensin-system. Am Heart J 1994;127:1388.

Kaplan NM: The appropriate goals of antihypertensive therapy: Neither too much nor too little. Ann Intern Med 1992;116:686.

Kasiske BL et al: Effect of antihypertensive therapy on the kidney in patients with diabetes: A meta-regression analysis. Ann Intern Med 1993;118:129.

Kasiske BL et al: Effects of antihypertensive therapy on serum lipids. Ann Intern Med 1995;122:133.

Khoury AF, Kaplan NM: Alpha-blocker therapy of hypertension: An unfulfilled promise. JAMA 1991;266:394.

Kokkinos PF et al: Effects of regular exercise on blood pressure and left ventricular hypertrophy in African-American men with severe hypertension. N Engl J Med 1995;333:1462.

Koyuncuoglu H: The combination of tizanidine markedly improves the treatment with dextromethorphan of heroin addicted outpatients. Int J Clin Pharmacol Ther 1995;33:13.

Kroin JS et al: Intrathecal clonidine and tizanidine in conscious dogs: Comparison of analgesic and hemodynamic effects. Anesth Analg 1996;82:627.

Lam YWF, Shepherd MM: Drug interactions in hypertensive patients: Pharmacokinetic, pharmacodynamic and genetic considerations. Clin Pharmacokinet 1990;18:295.

Langford HG et al: Dietary therapy slows the return of hypertension after stopping prolonged medication. JAMA 1985;253:657.

Law MR, Frost CD, Wald NJ: Analysis of data from trials of salt reduction. Br Med J 1991;302:819.

Leiphart JW et al: A comparison of intrathecally administered narcotic and nonnarcotic analgesics for experimental neuropathic pain. J Neurosurg 1995;82:595.

Lewis EJ et al: The effect of angiotensin-converting-enzyme inhibition on diabetic nephropathy. N Engl J Med 1993;329:1456.

Li G et al: Agmatine: An endogenous clonidine-displacing substance in the brain. Science 1994;263:966.

Linas SL, Nies AS: Minoxidil. Ann Intern Med 1981;94:61.

Linas SL: The role of potassium in the pathogenesis and treatment of hypertension. Kidney Int 1991;39:771.

Lowenstein J: Clonidine. Ann Intern Med 1980;92:74.

Luke RG: Essential hypertension: A renal disease? A review and update of the evidence. Hypertension 1993;21:380.

Maheswaran R et al: High blood pressure due to alcohol: A rapidly reversible effect. Hypertension 1991;17:787.

Makino N et al: Effect of angiotensin converting enzyme inhibitor on regression in cardiac hypertrophy. Mol Cell Biochem 1993;119:23.

Man in't Veld AJ, Schalekamp MADH: Effects of 10 different β-adrenoceptor antagonists on hemodynamics, plasma renin activity, and plasma norepinephrine in hypertension: The key role of vascular resistance changes in relation to partial agonist activity. J Cardiovasc Pharmacol 1983;5:S30.

Materson BJ et al: Single-drug therapy for hypertension in men: A comparison of six antihypertensive agents with placebo. N Engl J Med 1993;328:914.

McKaigue JP, Harron DWG: The effects of rilmenidine on tests of autonomic function in humans. Clin Pharmacol Ther 1992;52:511.

Michelson EL, Frishman WH: Labetalol: An alpha- and beta-adrenoceptor blocking drug. Ann Intern Med 1983;99:553.

Multiple Risk Factor Intervention Trial Research Group: Multiple risk factor intervention trial. JAMA 1982; 248:1465.

National High Blood Pressure Education Program Working Group on High Blood Pressure in Pregnancy: Working Group report on high blood pressure in pregnancy. Am J Obstet Gynecol 1990;163:1689.

National High Blood Pressure Education Program Working Group: Working Group report on hypertension and chronic renal failure. Arch Intern Med 1991;151:1280.

National High Blood Pressure Education Program Working Group: National High Blood Pressure Education Program Working Group report on hypertension in diabetes. Hypertension 1994;23:145.

Pahor M et al: Long-term survival and use of antihypertensive medications in older persons. J Am Geriatr Soc 1995;43:1191.

Pearson AA et al: A stereoselective central hypotensive action of atenolol. J Pharmacol Exp Ther 1989;250:759.

Perloff D et al: Human blood pressure determination by sphygmomanometry. Circulation 1993;88:2460.

Peterson JC et al: Blood pressure control, proteinuria, and the progression of renal disease. The Modification of Diet in Renal Disease study. Ann Intern Med 1995;123:754.

Pollare T, Lithell H, Berne C: A comparison of hydrochlorothiazide and captopril on glucose and lipid metabolism in patients with hypertension. N Engl J Med 1989;321:868.

Pritchard BNC: Clinical experience with moxonidine. Cardiovasc Drugs Ther 1994;8:49.

Psaty BM et al: The risk of myocardial infarction associated with antihypertensive drug therapies. JAMA 1995; 274:620.

Ragunathan S, Reis DJ: Imidazoline receptors and their endogenous ligands. Annu Rev Pharmacol Toxicol 1996; 36:511.

Report by the Management Committee: The Australian therapeutic trial in mild hypertension. Lancet 1980;1:1261.

Sanguinetti MC: Modulation of potassium channels by antiarrhythmic and antihypertensive drugs. Hypertension 1992;19:228.

Scheinin H et al: Intramuscular dexmedetomidine as premedication for general anesthesia: A comparative multicenter study. Anesthesiology 1993;78:1065.

Separovic D, Kester M, Ernsberger P: Coupling of I_1-imidazoline receptors to diacylglyceride accumulation in PC12 rat pheochromocytoma cells. Mol Pharmacol 1996; 49:668.

Setaro JF, Black HR: Refractory hypertension. N Engl J Med 1992;327:543.

SHEP Cooperative Research Group: Implications of the Systolic Hypertension in the Elderly Program. Hypertension 1993;21:335.

SHEP Cooperative Research Group: Prevention of stroke by antihypertensive drug treatment in older persons with isolated systolic hypertension. JAMA 1991;265:3255.

Siani A et al: Increasing the dietary potassium intake reduces the need for antihypertensive medication. Ann Intern Med 1991;115:753.

Stamler J et al: INTERSALT study findings: Public health and medical care implications. Hypertension 1989; 14:570.

Symposium: The imidazoline receptor: Pharmacology, functions, ligands, and relevance to biology and medicine. Ann N Y Acad Sci 1995;763:1.

Tädschner K-L: A controlled comparison of clonidine and doxepin in the treatment of the opiate withdrawal syndrome. Pharmacopsychiatry 1986;19:91.

Task Force on Blood Pressure Control in Children: Report of the Second Task Force on Blood Pressure Control in Children—1987. Pediatrics 1987;79:1.

Toto RD et al: Reversible renal insufficiency due to angiotensin converting enzyme inhibitors in hypertensive nephrosclerosis. Ann Intern Med 1991;115:513.

Treatment of Mild Hypertension Research Group: The Treatment of Mild Hypertension Study: A randomized, placebo-controlled trial of a nutritional-hygienic regimen along with various drug monotherapies. Arch Intern Med 1991;151:1413.

van den Meiracker AH et al: Hemodynamic and β-adrenergic receptor adaptations during long-term β adrenoceptor blockade. Studies with acebutolol, atenolol, pindolol, and propranolol in hypertensive patients. Circulation 1989;80:903.

van den Meiracker AH et al: Hemodynamic and hormonal adaptation to beta-adrenoceptor blockade: A 24-hour study of acebutolol, atenolol, pindolol, and propranolol in hypertensive patients. Circulation 1988;78:957.

Veterans Administration Cooperative Study Group on Antihypertensive Agents: Effects of treatment on morbidity in hypertension: 1. Results in patients with diastolic blood pressure averaging 115 through 129 mm Hg. JAMA 1967;202:1028.

Veterans Administration Cooperative Study Group on Antihypertensive Agents: Effects of treatment on morbidity in hypertension: 2. Results in patients with diastolic blood pressure averaging 90 through 114 mm Hg. JAMA 1970;213:1143.

Weber MA et al: Characterization of antihypertensive therapy by whole-day blood pressure monitoring. JAMA 1988;259:3281.

Weber MA: Clinical pharmacology of centrally acting antihypertensive agents. J Clin Pharmacol 1989;29:598.

Weber MA: Hypertension: Steps forward and steps backward—The Joint National Committee Fifth Report. Arch Intern Med 1993;153:149.

Williams GH: Converting enzyme inhibitors in the treatment of hypertension. N Engl J Med 1988;319:1517.

Woosley RL, Nies AS: Guanethidine. N Engl J Med 1976;295:1053.

Working Group on Ambulatory Blood Pressure Monitoring, National High Blood Pressure Education Program Coordinating Committee: National High Blood Pressure Education Program Working Group Report on ambulatory blood pressure monitoring. Arch Intern Med 1990; 150:2270.

Working Group on Management of Patients With Hypertension and High Blood Cholesterol: National Education Programs Working Group report on the management of patients with hypertension and high blood cholesterol. Ann Intern Med 1991;114:224.

World Health Organization: The 1993 guidelines for the treatment of mild hypertension. Hypertension 1993; 22:392.

World Hypertension League: Physical exercise in the management of hypertension: A consensus statement by the World Hypertension League. J Hypertens 1991;9:283.

Vasodilators & the Treatment of Angina Pectoris

12

Bertram G. Katzung, MD, PhD, & Kanu Chatterjee, MB, FRCP

Angina pectoris is the most common condition involving tissue ischemia in which vasodilator drugs are used. Angina (pain) is caused by the accumulation of metabolites in striated muscle; angina pectoris is the severe chest pain that occurs when coronary blood flow is inadequate to supply the oxygen required by the heart. The organic nitrates, eg, **nitroglycerin,** are the mainstay of therapy in angina. Another group of vasodilators, the **calcium channel blockers,** is also important, especially for prophylaxis, and the **beta-blockers,** which are *not* vasodilators, are also useful in prophylaxis.

Ischemic heart disease is the most common serious health problem in many Western societies. By far the most frequent cause of angina is atheromatous obstruction of the large coronary vessels (**atherosclerotic** or **classic** angina). However, transient spasm of localized portions of these vessels, which is usually associated with underlying atheromas, can also cause significant myocardial ischemia and pain (**angiospastic** or **variant** angina).

The primary cause of angina pectoris is an imbalance between the oxygen requirement of the heart and the oxygen supplied to it via the coronary vessels. In classic angina, the imbalance occurs when the myocardial oxygen requirement increases, as during exercise, and coronary blood flow does not increase proportionately. The resulting ischemia usually leads to pain. Classic angina is therefore "angina of effort." (In some individuals, the ischemia may not always be accompanied by pain, resulting in "silent" or "ambulatory" ischemia.) In variant angina, oxygen delivery decreases as a result of reversible coronary vasospasm (usually superimposed on chronic obstruction).

In theory, the imbalance between oxygen delivery and myocardial oxygen demand can be corrected by **increasing delivery** (by increasing coronary flow) or **decreasing oxygen demand** (by decreasing cardiac work). Both measures are used in clinical practice. In atherosclerotic angina, reduction of demand is the easier of these goals to achieve by pharmacologic means.

Traditional medical therapy achieves this goal through the use of organic nitrates—potent vasodilators—and several other classes of drugs, which decrease cardiac work. Increased delivery via increased coronary flow is difficult to achieve by pharmacologic means when flow is limited by fixed atheromatous plaques. In this situation, invasive measures (coronary bypass grafts or angioplasty) may be needed if reduction of oxygen demand does not control symptoms. In variant angina, on the other hand, spasm of coronary vessels can be reversed by nitrates or calcium channel blockers. It should be emphasized that not all vasodilators are effective in angina and, conversely, that some agents useful in angina (eg, propranolol) are not vasodilators.

When there is a change in the character, frequency, duration, and precipitating factors in patients with stable angina and when there are episodes of angina at rest, **unstable angina** is said to be present. This condition is caused by episodes of increased epicardial coronary artery tone or small platelet clots occurring in the vicinity of an atherosclerotic plaque. In most cases, formation of labile thrombi at the site of a fissured plaque is the mechanism for reduction in flow. It signals the imminent occurrence of a myocardial infarction and requires vigorous therapy.

History

Angina pectoris was first described as a distinct clinical entity by William Heberden in the latter half of the 18th century. In the second half of the 19th century, it was found that amyl nitrite could provide transient relief. However, it was not until the introduction of nitroglycerin in 1879 that effective relief of acute episodes of angina became possible. Subsequently, many other vasodilators (eg, theophylline, papaverine) were introduced for the treatment of angina. However, when careful double-blind clinical trials were done, these nonnitrate agents were found to be no better than placebo. In fact, several of the classic studies of the placebo effect were carried out in patients with angina. With the introduction of beta-adrenoceptor-blocking drugs, useful prophylactic therapy of angina became possible. More recently, the calcium channel blockers have been shown to be useful for prevention of anginal attacks, especially in variant angina.

PATHOPHYSIOLOGY OF ANGINA

Determinants of Myocardial Oxygen Demand

The major and minor determinants of myocardial oxygen requirement are set forth in Table 12–1. Unlike skeletal muscle, human cardiac muscle cannot develop an appreciable oxygen debt during stress and repay it later. As a consequence of its continuous activity, the heart's oxygen needs are relatively high, and it extracts approximately 75% of the available oxygen even under conditions of no stress. The myocardial oxygen requirement increases when there is an increase in heart rate, contractility, arterial pressure, or ventricular volume. These hemodynamic alterations frequently occur during physical exercise and sympathetic discharge, which often precipitate angina in patients with obstructive coronary artery disease. The relative contributions of basal metabolism and activation of contraction to the overall myocardial oxygen consumption appear to be small, but under pathologic conditions these apparently minor determinants of myocardial oxygen consumption may become relevant.

It is not possible to measure all of the determinants listed in Table 12–1 in the clinical setting. Therefore, indirect measures are often used to assess changes in myocardial oxygen demand and consumption. One commonly used index is the "double product" (heart rate × systolic blood pressure), a measure closely related to the tension-time index. The tension-time index is a more invasive measure of myocardial work and therefore of oxygen demand.

Determinants of Coronary Blood Flow & Myocardial Oxygen Supply

Oxygen supply is a function of myocardial oxygen delivery and extraction. Since myocardial oxygen ex-

Table 12–1. Determinants of myocardial oxygen consumption.

Major
  Wall stress
    Intraventricular pressure
    Ventricular radius (volume)
    Wall thickness
  Heart rate
  Contractility
Minor
  Activation energy
  Resting metabolism

traction is nearly maximal at rest, there is little reserve to meet increased demands; furthermore, the oxygen content of the blood cannot be significantly increased under normal atmospheric conditions. Thus, increased myocardial demands for oxygen in the normal heart are met by augmenting coronary blood flow.

Coronary blood flow is directly related to the perfusion pressure (aortic diastolic pressure) and the duration of diastole. Because coronary flow drops to negligible values during systole, the duration of diastole becomes a limiting factor for myocardial perfusion during tachycardia. Coronary blood flow is inversely proportionate to coronary vascular bed resistance. Resistance is determined by intrinsic factors, including metabolic products and autonomic activity; by various pharmacologic agents; and by the extravascular mechanical compression of the coronary arteries. The site of autoregulation appears to be the arteriolar resistance vessels. Damage to the endothelium of coronary vessels has been shown to alter their ability to dilate in response to normal stimuli.

Determinants of Vascular Tone

Arteriolar and venous tone both play a role in determining myocardial wall stress (Table 12–1). Arteriolar tone directly controls peripheral vascular resistance and thus arterial blood pressure. In systole, intraventricular pressure must exceed arterial pressure to eject blood; arterial blood pressure thus determines the *systolic* wall stress in an important way. Venous tone determines the capacity of the venous circulation and controls the amount of blood sequestered in the venules versus the amount returned to the heart. Venous tone thereby determines the *diastolic* wall stress.

The regulation of smooth muscle contraction and relaxation is shown schematically in Figure 12–1. As shown in Figures 12–1 and 12–2, drugs may relax vascular smooth muscle in several ways:

A. Increasing cGMP: As indicated in Figure 12–2, cGMP facilitates the dephosphorylation of myosin light chains, preventing the interaction of myosin with actin. Nitric oxide is an effective activator of soluble guanylyl cyclase and probably acts mainly through this mechanism. Important therapeutic donors of nitric oxide include nitroprusside (Chapter 11) and the **organic nitrates** used in angina.

B. Decreasing Intracellular Ca^{2+}: Calcium channel blockers predictably cause vasodilation because they reduce intracellular Ca^{2+}, a major modulator of the activation of myosin light chain kinase. (Beta-blockers and some calcium channel blockers reduce Ca^{2+} influx in cardiac muscle, thereby reducing rate and contractility—and oxygen requirement—by a direct myocardial mechanism.)

C. Stabilizing or Preventing Depolarization of the Vascular Smooth Muscle Cell Membrane: The membrane potential of excitable cells is stabilized near the resting potential by increasing potassium permeability (see Chapter 14, box: Effects

Figure 12–1. Control of smooth muscle contraction and site of action of calcium channel-blocking drugs. Contraction is triggered by influx of calcium (which can be blocked by calcium channel blockers) through transmembrane calcium channels. The calcium combines with calmodulin to form a complex that converts the enzyme myosin light chain kinase to its active form (MLCK*). The latter phosphorylates the myosin light chains, thereby initiating the interaction of myosin with actin. Beta$_2$ agonists (and other substances that increase cAMP) may cause relaxation in smooth muscle by accelerating the inactivation of MLCK (heavy arrows) and by facilitating the expulsion of calcium from the cell (not shown).

of Potassium). Potassium channel openers (Chapter 11; eg, minoxidil sulfate) increase the permeability of K$^+$ channels, probably ATP-dependent K$^+$ channels. Certain newer agents under investigation for use in angina, eg, **nicorandil,** may act, in part, by this mechanism.

D. Increasing cAMP in the Vascular Cells: As shown in Figure 12–1, an increase in cAMP appears to increase the rate of inactivation of myosin light chain kinase, the enzyme responsible for triggering the interaction of actin with myosin in these cells. This appears to be the mechanism of vasodilation caused by β$_2$ agonists, drugs that are *not* used in angina.

I. BASIC PHARMACOLOGY OF DRUGS USED TO TREAT ANGINA

Drug Action in Angina

All three of the drug groups useful in angina *decrease myocardial oxygen requirement* by decreasing peripheral vascular resistance, by decreasing cardiac output, or in both ways. In some patients, a redistri-

bution of coronary flow may increase oxygen delivery to ischemic tissue. In variant angina, the nitrates and the calcium channel blockers may also *increase myocardial oxygen delivery* by reversing coronary arterial spasm.

NITRATES & NITRITES

Chemistry

These agents are simple nitric and nitrous acid esters of polyalcohols (Figure 12–3). They vary from extremely volatile liquids (amyl nitrite) through moderately volatile liquids (nitroglycerin) to solids (isosorbide dinitrate). Nitroglycerin may be considered the prototype of the group. Although it is used in the manufacture of dynamite, the formulations of nitroglycerin used in medicine are not explosive. The conventional sublingual tablet form of nitroglycerin may lose potency when stored as a result of volatilization and adsorption to plastic surfaces. Therefore, it should be kept in tightly closed glass containers. It is not sensitive to light.

Structure-activity studies indicate that all therapeutically active agents in this group are capable of releasing nitric oxide (NO) in vascular smooth muscle target tissues (Harrison et al, 1993). Unfortunately, they all are capable of inducing cross-tolerance when given in large doses. Therefore, pharmacokinetic factors govern the choice of agent and mode of therapy when using the nitrates.

Figure 12–2. Mechanism of action of nitrates, nitrites, and other substances that increase the concentration of nitric oxide (NO) in smooth muscle cells. (MLCK*, activated myosin light chain kinase [see Figure 12–1]; guanylyl cyclase*, activated guanylyl cyclase; ?, unknown intermediate steps. Steps leading to relaxation are shown with heavy arrows.)

Figure 12–3. Chemical structures of three nitrates and amyl nitrite.

Pharmacokinetics

The use of organic nitrates is strongly influenced by the existence of a high-capacity hepatic organic nitrate reductase that removes nitrate groups in a stepwise fashion from the parent molecule and ultimately inactivates the drug. Therefore, bioavailability of the traditional oral organic nitrates (nitroglycerin and isosorbide dinitrate) is very low (typically < 10–20%). The sublingual route, which avoids the first-pass effect, is therefore preferred for achieving a therapeutic blood level rapidly. Nitroglycerin and isosorbide dinitrate are both absorbed efficiently by this route and reach therapeutic blood levels within a few minutes. However, the total dose administered by this route must be limited to avoid excessive effects; therefore, the total duration of effect is brief (15–30 minutes). When much longer duration of action is needed, oral preparations can be given that contain an amount of drug sufficient to result in sustained systemic blood levels of the parent drug or active metabolites. Other routes of administration available for nitroglycerin include transdermal and buccal absorption from slow-release preparations; these are described below.

Amyl nitrite and related nitrites are highly volatile liquids. Amyl nitrite is available in fragile glass ampules packaged in a protective cloth covering. The ampule can be crushed with the fingers, resulting in rapid release of inhalable vapors through the cloth covering. The inhalation route provides for very rapid absorption and, like the sublingual route, avoids the hepatic first-pass effect.

Once absorbed, the unchanged nitrate compounds have half-lives of only 2–8 minutes. The partially denitrated metabolites have much longer half-lives (up to 3 hours). Of the nitroglycerin metabolites (two dinitroglycerins and two mononitro forms), the dinitro derivatives have significant vasodilator efficacy; they probably provide most of the therapeutic effect of orally administered nitroglycerin. The 5-mononitrate metabolite of isosorbide dinitrate is an active metabolite of the latter drug and is available for clinical use as isosorbide mononitrate. It has a bioavailability of 100%.

Excretion, primarily in the form of glucuronide derivatives of the denitrated metabolites, is largely by way of the kidney.

Pharmacodynamics

Nitroglycerin and its analogs are unusually selective drugs: in therapeutic doses, their action is largely on smooth muscle cells. Another action of possible clinical significance is on platelet aggregation.

A. Mechanism of Action in Smooth Muscle: Nitroglycerin appears to be denitrated, releasing free nitrite ion, in the smooth muscle cell as it is in other tissues, by glutathione *S*-transferase. A different unknown enzymatic reaction releases nitric oxide (NO; Chapter 19) from the parent drug molecule (Harrison et al, 1993). Nitric oxide is a much more potent vasodilator than nitrite, which itself can release nitric oxide. As shown in Figure 12–2, nitric oxide (or an *S*-nitrosothiol derivative) causes activation of guanylyl cyclase and an increase in cGMP, which are the first steps toward smooth muscle relaxation. The production of prostaglandin E or prostacyclin (PGI$_2$) and membrane hyperpolarization may also be involved. There is no evidence that autonomic receptors are involved in the primary nitrate response (though autonomic *reflex* responses are evoked when hypotensive doses are given). As described below, tolerance is an important consideration in the use of nitrates. While tolerance may be caused in part by a decrease in tissue sulfhydryl groups, it can be only partially prevented or reversed with a sulfhydryl-regenerating agent. The site of this cellular tolerance may be in the unknown reaction responsible for the release of nitric oxide from the nitrate, since other agents, eg, acetylcholine, that cause vasodilation via release of nitric oxide from *endogenous* substrates, do not show cross tolerance with the nitrates. (See box: The Coronary Steal Phenomenon.)

Nicorandil and several other investigational antianginal agents appear to combine the activity of NO release with potassium channel-opening action, thus providing an additional mechanism for causing vasodilation.

B. Organ System Effects: Nitroglycerin relaxes all types of smooth muscle irrespective of the cause of the preexisting muscle tone (Figure 12–4). It has practically no direct effect on cardiac or skeletal muscle.

1. Vascular smooth muscle–All segments of the vascular system from large arteries through large veins relax in response to nitroglycerin. Veins respond at the lowest concentrations, arteries at slightly higher ones. Arterioles and precapillary sphincters are dilated less than the large arteries and the veins, partly because of reflex responses (Bassenge et al, 1986, 1992) and partly because different vessels vary in their ability to release nitric oxide (see box). The primary direct result of an effective blood concentration is marked relaxation of veins with increased venous capacitance and decreased ventricular preload. Pulmonary vascular pressures and heart size are significantly reduced. In the absence of heart failure, cardiac output is reduced. Because venous capacitance is increased, orthostatic hypotension may be marked and syncope can result. Dilation of some large arteries (including the aorta) may be significant because of their large compliance. Temporal artery pulsations and a throbbing headache associated with meningeal artery pulsations are frequent effects of nitroglycerin and amyl nitrite. In the presence of heart failure, preload is often abnormally high; the nitrates and other vasodilators, by reducing preload, may have a beneficial effect on cardiac output in this condition (see Chapter 13). However, in patients with chronic left ventricular heart failure, afterload reduction—by enhancing arterial compliance and ventriculo-aortic coupling—may also be an important mechanism for improved ventricular function.

The indirect effects of nitroglycerin consist of those compensatory responses evoked by baroreceptors and hormonal mechanisms responding to decreased arterial pressure (see Figure 6–7). The primary mechanism of the response is sympathetic discharge; this consistently results in tachycardia and increased cardiac contractility. In the case of very rapidly acting agents (eg, inhaled amyl nitrite), arterial dilation may be so marked as to cause a reflex venoconstriction. Retention of salt and water may also be significant, especially with intermediate- and long-acting nitrates. These compensatory responses contribute to the development of tolerance.

In the isolated coronary-perfused heart (Langendorff preparation) and in normal subjects without coronary disease, nitroglycerin can induce a significant, if transient, increase in total coronary blood flow. In contrast, there is no evidence that total coronary flow is increased in patients with angina due to

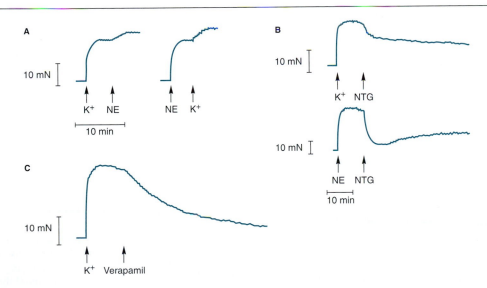

Figure 12–4. Effects of vasodilators on contractions of human vein segments studied in vitro. **Panel A** shows contractions induced by two vasoconstrictor agents, norepinephrine *(NE)* and potassium *(K+)*. **Panel B** shows the relaxation induced by nitroglycerin *(NTG)*, 4 μmol/L. The relaxation is prompt. **Panel C** shows the relaxation induced by verapamil, 2.2 μmol/L. The relaxation is slower but more sustained. (Modified and reproduced, with permission, from Mikkelsen E, Andersson KE, Bengtsson B: Effects of verapamil and nitroglycerin on contractile responses to potassium and noradrenaline in isolated human peripheral veins. Acta Pharmacol Toxicol 1978;42:14.)

THE CORONARY STEAL PHENOMENON

The development of useful vasodilators for management of angina has been marked by frustrating episodes when pharmacologists found that new drugs that were extremely effective vasodilators in normal animals were ineffective or even caused increased anginal symptoms in patients. It is now clear that potent arteriolar dilators (eg, hydralazine, dipyridamole) are generally ineffective in angina and may reduce perfusion of ischemic areas. In fact, dipyridamole is often used in imaging studies of the coronary circulation to demonstrate regions of poor perfusion. On the other hand, drugs that are more effective dilators of veins and large arteries and relatively ineffective dilators of resistance vessels (eg, nitrates) are very useful in angina. The reason for this apparent anomaly has been called the "coronary steal phenomenon."

Coronary steal occurs when two branches from a main coronary vessel have differing degrees of obstruction. For example, one branch may be relatively normal and capable of dilating and constricting in response to changes in oxygen demand, while the other branch is significantly obstructed and has significant arteriolar dilation even when cardiac oxygen demand is low, because of the accumulation of metabolites in the ischemic tissue. Perfusion in the obstructed region may be adequate at rest, because perfusion pressure is well maintained in the main coronary artery. (Recall that perfusion in a regional vascular bed is directly proportionate to perfusion pressure in the large supply vessels and inversely proportionate to the resistance to flow in the arterioles.) If a powerful arteriolar dilator drug is administered, the arterioles in the unobstructed vessel will be forced to dilate, reducing the resistance in this area and greatly increasing flow through the already adequately perfused tissue. As a result of the reduction in resistance in the normal branch, perfusion pressure in the main coronary will diminish, flow through the obstructed branch will *decrease,* and angina may worsen.

It has been suggested that the lesser potency of the nitrates in dilating arterioles is the result of a reduced ability of these vessels to release nitric oxide from the parent nitrate molecule. There is some evidence that supplementation with thiol-containing compounds such as cysteine can increase the ability of arterioles to release nitric oxide from nitroglycerin (Harrison and Bates, 1993). If this is true, administration of acetylcysteine to prevent tolerance might cause nitroglycerin to produce effects like those of the *ineffective* arteriolar vasodilators!

---

atherosclerotic obstructive coronary artery disease. While some studies suggest that *redistribution* of coronary flow from normal to ischemic regions may play a role, most evidence suggests that relief of effort angina by nitroglycerin is the result of decreased myocardial oxygen requirement secondary to decreased preload and arterial pressure (see Clinical Pharmacology, below).

2. Other smooth muscle organs–Relaxation of smooth muscle of the bronchi, gastrointestinal tract (including biliary system), and genitourinary tract has been demonstrated experimentally. Because of their brief duration, these actions of the nitrates are rarely of any clinical value. During recent years, the use of amyl nitrite and isobutyl nitrite by inhalation as purported recreational (sex-enhancing) drugs has become popular with some segments of the population. The basis for this use is described in Chapter 19. Isobutyl nitrite is not licensed or advertised as a drug but is sold over the counter under such names as Rush, Bolt, Locker Room, and Dr. Bananas.

3. Action on platelets–Nitric oxide released from nitroglycerin stimulates guanylyl cyclase in platelets as in smooth muscle. The increase in cGMP that results is responsible for a decrease in platelet aggregation (Karlberg et al, 1992). Unfortunately, recent prospective trials have established no survival benefit when nitroglycerin is used in acute myocardial infarction.

4. Other effects–*Nitrite* ion reacts with hemoglobin (which contains ferrous iron) to produce **methemoglobin** (which contains ferric iron). Because methemoglobin has a very low affinity for oxygen, large doses of nitrites can result in pseudocyanosis, tissue hypoxia, and death. The plasma level of *nitrite* resulting from even large doses of organic and inorganic *nitrates* is too low to cause significant methemoglobinemia in adults. However, sodium nitrite is used as a curing agent for meats. In nursing infants, the intestinal flora is capable of converting significant amounts of inorganic nitrate, eg, from well water, to nitrite ion. Thus, inadvertent exposure to large amounts of nitrite ion can occur and may produce serious toxicity. One therapeutic application of this otherwise toxic effect of nitrite has been discovered. **Cyanide poisoning** results from complexing of cytochrome iron by the CN^- ion. Methemoglobin iron has a very high affinity for CN^-; thus, administration of sodium nitrite ($NaNO_2$) soon after cyanide exposure will regenerate active cytochrome. The cyanmethemoglobin produced can be further detoxified by the intravenous administration of sodium thiosulfate ($Na_2S_2O_3$); this results in formation of thiocyanate ion

(SCN⁻), a less toxic ion that is readily excreted. Methemoglobinemia, if excessive, can be treated by giving methylene blue intravenously.

Toxicity & Tolerance

A. Acute Adverse Effects: The major acute toxicity of organic nitrates is a direct extension of therapeutic vasodilation: orthostatic hypotension, tachycardia, and throbbing headache. Glaucoma, once thought to be a contraindication, does not worsen, and nitrates can be used safely in the presence of increased intraocular pressure. Nitrates are contraindicated, however, if intracranial pressure is elevated.

B. Tolerance: With continuous exposure to nitrates, isolated smooth muscle may develop complete tolerance (tachyphylaxis), and the intact human becomes progressively more tolerant when long-acting preparations (oral, transdermal) or continuous intravenous infusions are used for more than a few hours without interruption (Steering Committee, 1991).

Continuous exposure to high levels of nitrates can occur in the chemical industry, especially where explosives are manufactured. When contamination of the workplace with volatile organic nitrate compounds is severe, workers find that upon starting their work week (Monday), they suffer headache and transient dizziness. After a day or so, these symptoms disappear owing to the development of tolerance. Over the weekend, when exposure to the chemicals is reduced, tolerance disappears, so symptoms recur each Monday. A more serious hazard of industrial exposure is the development of dependence. This may affect workers after months or years of exposure and manifests itself as variant angina occurring after 1–2 days away from the source of nitrates. In the most seriously affected individuals, coronary vasospasm may cause myocardial infarction. There is no evidence that physical dependence develops as a result of the therapeutic use of short-acting nitrates for angina, even in large doses.

The mechanisms by which tolerance develops are not completely understood. As noted above, cellular tolerance appears to play a role in that activation of guanylyl cyclase in cellular homogenates is decreased by preincubation with organic nitrates. Partial reversal of this loss of responsiveness by thiol-containing compounds (eg, acetylcysteine) and the absence of cross tolerance to other nitric oxide-dependent vasodilators (acetylcholine, nicorandil) suggests that diminished release of nitric oxide may be partly responsible for tolerance to nitroglycerin. Systemic compensation also plays a role in tolerance in the intact human. Initially, significant sympathetic discharge occurs; this increases vascular tone. After one or more days of therapy with long-acting nitrates, retention of salt and water may reverse the favorable hemodynamic changes normally caused by nitroglycerin (Parker, 1993).

C. Carcinogenicity of Nitrate and Nitrate Derivatives: Nitrosamines are small molecules with the structure R_2—N—NO formed from the combination of nitrates and nitrites with amines. Some nitrosamines are powerful carcinogens in animals, apparently through conversion to very reactive derivatives. While there is no direct proof that these agents cause cancer in humans, there is a strong epidemiologic correlation between the incidence of esophageal and gastric carcinoma and the nitrate content of food in different cultures. Nitrosamines are also found in tobacco and in cigarette smoke. There is no evidence that the small doses of nitrates used in the treatment of angina result in significant body levels of nitrosamines.

Mechanisms of Clinical Effect

The beneficial and deleterious effects of nitrate-induced vasodilation are summarized in Table 12–2.

A. Nitrate Effects in Angina of Effort: Decreased venous return to the heart and the resulting reduction of intracardiac volume are the principal hemodynamic effects. Arterial pressure decreases. Decreased intraventricular pressure and left ventricular volume are associated with decreased wall tension (Laplace relation) and decreased myocardial oxygen requirement. In rare instances, a paradoxical increase in myocardial oxygen demand may occur as a result of excessive reflex tachycardia and increased contractility.

Intracoronary, intravenous, and sublingual nitrate administration consistently increases the caliber of the epicardial coronary arteries. Coronary arteriolar resistance tends to decrease, though to a lesser extent. However, nitrates administered by the usual systemic routes also consistently *decrease* overall coronary blood flow and myocardial oxygen consumption. In-

Table 12–2. Beneficial and deleterious effects of nitrates in the treatment of angina.

Effect	Result
Potential beneficial effects	
Decreased ventricular volume	Decreased myocardial oxygen requirement
Decreased arterial pressure	
Decreased ejection time	
Vasodilation of epicardial coronary arteries	Relief of coronary artery spasm
Increased collateral flow	Improved perfusion to ischemic myocardium
Decreased left ventricular diastolic pressure	Improved subendocardial perfusion
Potential deleterious effects	
Reflex tachycardia	Increased myocardial oxygen requirement
Reflex increase in contractility	
Decreased diastolic perfusion time due to tachycardia	Decreased myocardial perfusion

tracoronary injection of small doses of nitroglycerin, which increases total coronary blood flow but does not produce systemic hemodynamic effects, does not relieve pacing-induced angina. Yet systemic administration of nitroglycerin, which decreases arterial pressure and left ventricular volume, does relieve angina despite decreased coronary blood flow. These findings indicate that the relief of effort angina with nitrates is due primarily to decreased myocardial oxygen demand, not to increased coronary blood flow.

B. Nitrate Effects in Variant Angina: Nitrates benefit patients with variant angina by relaxing the smooth muscle of the epicardial coronary arteries and relieving coronary artery spasm. Although intracoronary nitroglycerin injection appears to be the most effective method for relieving coronary artery spasm, this method of administration has little clinical relevance, and other routes of administration are also effective.

C. Nitrate Effects in Unstable Angina: Nitrates are also useful in the treatment of unstable angina, but the precise mechanism for their beneficial effects is not clear. Because both increased coronary vascular tone and increased myocardial oxygen demand can precipitate rest angina in these patients, nitrates may exert their beneficial effects both by dilating the epicardial coronary arteries and by simultaneously reducing myocardial oxygen demand.

The major mechanism for prolonged episodes of rest angina is now known to be recurrent thrombotic occlusion (presumably initiated by platelet aggregation) at the site of atherosclerotic plaques. As noted above, nitroglycerin decreases platelet aggregation, and this effect may be of importance in unstable angina.

Clinical Use of Nitrates

Some of the forms of nitroglycerin and its congeners are listed in Table 12–3. Because of its rapid onset of action (1–3 minutes), sublingual nitroglycerin is the most frequently used agent for the immediate treatment of angina. Because its duration of action is short (not exceeding 20–30 minutes), it is not suitable for maintenance therapy. The onset of action of

intravenous nitroglycerin is also rapid (minutes), but its hemodynamic effects are quickly reversed by stopping its infusion. Clinical application of intravenous nitroglycerin, therefore, is restricted to the treatment of severe, recurrent rest angina. Slowly absorbed preparations of nitroglycerin include a buccal form, an oral preparation, and several transdermal forms. These formulations have been shown to provide blood concentrations for long periods, but, as noted above, this leads to the development of tolerance.

The hemodynamic effects of sublingual or chewable isosorbide dinitrate and other organic nitrates are similar to those of nitroglycerin. The recommended dosage schedules for commonly used long-acting nitrate preparations, along with their duration of action, are listed in Table 12–3. Although transdermal administration may provide blood levels of nitroglycerin for 24 hours or longer, the full hemodynamic effects usually do not persist for more than 6–8 hours. The clinical efficacy of slow-release forms of nitroglycerin in maintenance therapy of angina is thus limited by the development of significant tolerance. It has been suggested that a nitrate-free period of at least 8 hours between doses should be observed to reduce or prevent tolerance.

CALCIUM CHANNEL-BLOCKING DRUGS

It has been known since the late 1800s that calcium influx was necessary for the contraction of muscle. However, the mechanism by which calcium entered the cell was unknown until much more recently. The discovery of a calcium channel in cardiac muscle (summarized in Reuter, 1983) was followed by the finding of several different types of calcium channels in different tissues (Table 12–4). These discoveries provided the necessary mechanisms for the triggering of cardiac and smooth muscle contraction and for excitation-secretion coupling in nerve and secretory tissues as well. The discovery of these channels also made possible the development of clinically useful blocking drugs. Although the therapeutic blockers de-

Table 12–3. Nitrate and nitrite drugs used in the treatment of angina.

Drug	Dose	Duration of Action
"Short-acting"		
Nitroglycerin, sublingual	0.15–1.2 mg	10–30 minutes
Isosorbide dinitrate, sublingual	2.5–5 mg	10–60 minutes
Amyl nitrite, inhalant	0.18–0.3 mL	3–5 minutes
"Long-acting"		
Nitroglycerin, oral sustained-action	6.5–13 mg per 6–8 hours	6–8 hours
Nitroglycerin, 2% ointment	1–1.5 inches per 4 hours	3–6 hours
Nitroglycerin, slow-release, buccal	1–2 mg per 4 hours	3–6 hours
Nitroglycerin, slow-release, transdermal	10–25 mg per 24 hours (one patch per day)	8–10 hours
Isosorbide dinitrate, oral	10–60 mg per 4–6 hours	4–6 hours
Isosorbide dinitrate, chewable	5–10 mg per 2–4 hours	2–3 hours
Isosorbide mononitrate, oral	20 mg per 12 hours	6–10 hours

Table 12–4. Properties of several recognized voltage-activated calcium channels.

Type	Where Found	Properties of the Calcium Current	Blocked By
L	Muscle, neurons	Long, large, high threshold	Verapamil, DHPs, Cd^{2+}
T	Heart, neurons	Short, small, low threshold	sFTX, flunarizine, Ni^{2+}
N	Neurons	Short, high threshold	ω-CTX-GVIA, Cd^{2+}
P	Cerebellar Purkinje neurons	Long, high threshold	ω-CTX-MVIIC, ω-Aga-IVA

Key:

Aga-IVA	= a toxin of the funnel web spider, *Agelenopsis aperta*
ω-CTX	= conotoxins extracted from several marine snails of the genus *Conus*
DHPs	= dihydropyridines, eg, nifedipine
Flunarizine	= an organic calcium channel blocker
sFTX	= synthetic funnel web spider toxin

veloped to date have been almost exclusively L-type channel blockers (because of the screening methods used), intensive studies are now under way for selective blockers of neuronal calcium channels in the hope that more effective drugs may be developed for the prevention of brain injury following stroke, etc.

Chemistry

Verapamil, the first clinically useful member of this group, was the result of attempts to synthesize more active analogs of papaverine, a vasodilator alkaloid found in the opium poppy. Since then, dozens of agents of varying structure have been found to have the same fundamental pharmacologic action. Four chemically dissimilar calcium channel blockers are shown in Figure 12–5. Nifedipine is the prototype of the dihydropyridine family of calcium channel blockers; dozens of molecules in this family have been investigated, and seven are currently approved in the USA for angina and other indications. Nifedipine is the most extensively studied of this group, but the properties of the other dihydropyridines can be assumed to be similar to it unless otherwise noted.

Pharmacokinetics (Table 12–5)

The calcium channel blockers are orally active agents. Verapamil and diltiazem are used by the intravenous route as well. They are characterized by high first-pass effect, high plasma protein binding, and extensive metabolism.

Pharmacodynamics

A. Mechanism of Action: The L-type calcium channel is the dominant type in cardiac and smooth muscle and is known to contain several drug receptors. It has been demonstrated that nifedipine and other dihydropyridines bind to one site, while verapamil and diltiazem appear to bind to closely related but not identical receptors in another region. Binding of a drug to the verapamil or diltiazem receptors also affects dihydropyridine binding. These receptor regions are stereoselective, since marked differences in both stereoisomer-binding affinity and pharmacologic potency are observed for enantiomers of verapamil,

diltiazem, and optically active nifedipine congeners.

Blockade by these drugs resembles that of sodium channel blockade by local anesthetics: the drugs act from the inner side of the membrane and bind more effectively to channels in depolarized membranes. Binding of the drug appears to convert the mode of operation of the channel from one in which openings occur consistently after depolarization to one in which such openings are rare. The result is a marked decrease in transmembrane calcium current (Figure 12–1) associated in smooth muscle with a long-lasting relaxation (Figure 12–4) and in cardiac muscle with a reduction in contractility throughout the heart and decreases in sinus node pacemaker rate and in atrioventricular node conduction velocity.* Smooth muscle responses to calcium influx through *receptor*-operated calcium channels are also reduced by these drugs but not as markedly. The block is partially reversed by elevating the concentration of calcium, though the levels of calcium required are not easily attainable. Block can also be partially reversed by the use of drugs that increase the transmembrane flux of calcium, such as sympathomimetics.

Other types of calcium channels are less sensitive to blockade by these calcium channel blockers (Table 12–4). Therefore, tissues in which these channel types play a major role—neurons and most secretory glands—are much less affected by these drugs than are cardiac and smooth muscle.

B. Organ System Effects:

1. Smooth muscle–Most types of smooth muscle are dependent on transmembrane calcium influx for normal resting tone and contractile responses. These cells are relaxed by the calcium channel blockers (Figure 12–4). Vascular smooth muscle appears to be the most sensitive, but similar relaxation can be shown for bronchiolar, gastrointestinal, and uterine smooth muscle. In the vascular system, arterioles appear to be more sensitive than veins; orthostatic hy-

---

*At very low doses and under certain circumstances, some dihydropyridines *increase* calcium influx. Some special dihydropyridines, eg, Bay K 8644, appear to increase calcium influx over most of their dose range.

Figure 12–5. Chemical structures of several calcium channel-blocking drugs.

potension is not a common adverse effect. Blood pressure can be reduced, especially with nifedipine. Women may be more sensitive than men to the hypotensive action of diltiazem. The reduction in peripheral vascular resistance is one mechanism by which these agents may benefit the patient with angina of effort. Reduction of coronary arterial tone has been demonstrated in patients with variant angina.

Important differences in "vascular selectivity" exist among the calcium channel blockers. In general, the dihydropyridines have a greater ratio of vascular smooth muscle effects relative to cardiac effects than do bepridil, diltiazem, and verapamil (Table 12–6). Furthermore, the dihydropyridines may differ in their potency in different vascular beds. For example, nimodipine is claimed to be particularly selective for cerebral blood vessels.

2. Cardiac muscle—Cardiac muscle is highly dependent upon calcium influx for normal function. Impulse generation in the sinoatrial node and conduction in the atrioventricular node—so-called "slow response," or calcium-dependent, action potentials—may be reduced or blocked by all of the calcium channel blockers. Excitation-contraction coupling in all cardiac cells requires calcium influx, so these drugs reduce cardiac contractility in a dose-dependent fashion. In some cases, cardiac output may also decrease. This reduction in mechanical function is another mechanism by which the calcium channel blockers may reduce the oxygen requirement in patients with angina.

An additional benefit of calcium influx inhibition has been demonstrated in experimental myocardial infarction. Because ischemia causes membrane depolarization, calcium influx in ischemic cells is increased. Elevated intracellular calcium accelerates the activity of several ATP-consuming enzymes, which further depletes already marginal cellular energy stores, making the heart even more susceptible to ischemic damage. The calcium channel blockers have been demonstrated to protect against the damaging effects of calcium by reducing the incidence of arrhythmias and the ultimate size of developing infarctions in experimental animals. Unfortunately, clinical studies have not consistently supported the notion of protection and in some instances have suggested an *increased* incidence of myocardial infarction.

Important differences between the available calcium channel blockers arise from the details of their

Table 12–5. Pharmacokinetics of some calcium channel blocking drugs.

Drug	Oral Bioavailability	Onset of Action (route)	Plasma Half-Life (hours)	Disposition
Dihydropyridines Amlodipine	65–90%	No data available	30–50	> 90% bound to plasma proteins; extensively metabolized.
Felodipine	15–20%	2–5 hours (oral)	11–16	> 99% bound to plasma proteins; extensively metabolized.
Isradipine	15–25%	2 hours (oral)	8	95% bound to plasma protein; extensively metabolized.
Nicardipine	35%	20 minutes (oral)	2–4	95% bound; extensively metabolized in the liver.
Nifedipine	45–70%	< 1 minute (IV); 5–20 minutes (sublingual or oral)	4	About 90% bound to plasma protein; metabolized to an acid lactate. 80% of the drug and metabolites excreted in urine.
Nimodipine	13%	No data available	1–2	Extensively metabolized.
Nisoldipine	< 10%	No data available	2–6	Extensively metabolized.
Nitrendipine	10–30%	4 hours (oral)	5–12	98% bound; extensively metabolized.
Miscellaneous Bepridil	60%	60 minutes (oral)	24–40	> 99% bound to plasma proteins; extensively metabolized.
Diltiazem	40–65%	< 3 minutes (IV), > 30 minutes (oral)	3–4	70–80% bound to plasma protein; extensively deacylated. Drug and metabolites excreted in feces.
Verapamil	20–35%	< 1.5 minutes (IV), 30 minutes (oral)	6	About 90% bound to plasma protein. 70% eliminated by kidney; 15% by gastrointestinal tract.

interactions with cardiac ion channels and, as noted above, differences in their relative smooth muscle versus cardiac effects. Cardiac *sodium* channels are blocked by bepridil but somewhat less effectively than are calcium channels. Sodium channel block is modest with verapamil and still less marked with diltiazem. It is negligible with nifedipine and other dihydropyridines. Verapamil and diltiazem interact kinetically with the calcium channel receptor in a different manner than the dihydropyridines; they block tachycardias in calcium-dependent cells, eg, the atrioventricular node, more selectively than do the dihydropyridines. (See Chapter 14 for additional details.) On the other hand, the dihydropyridines appear to block smooth muscle calcium channels at concentrations below those required for significant cardiac effects; they are therefore less depressant on the heart than verapamil or diltiazem. Bepridil also has a significant potassium channel blocking effect in the heart. This results in prolongation of cardiac repolarization (see Chapter 14) and a distinct risk of induction of arrhythmias.

3. Skeletal muscle–Skeletal muscle is not depressed by the calcium channel blockers because it utilizes intracellular pools of calcium to support excitation-contraction coupling and does not require as much transmembrane calcium influx.

4. Cerebral vasospasm and infarct following subarachnoid hemorrhage–Nimodipine, a member of the dihydropyridine group of calcium channel blockers, has a high affinity for cerebral blood vessels and appears to reduce morbidity following a subarachnoid hemorrhage—morbidity that is probably caused by vasospasm evoked by the extravasation of blood into the tissue. Nimodipine is therefore labeled for use in patients who have had a subarachnoid hemorrhage. Although evidence suggests that calcium channel blockers may also reduce cerebral damage following thromboembolic stroke in experimental animals, there is no evidence that this occurs in humans.

5. Other effects–Calcium channel blockers minimally interfere with stimulus-secretion coupling in glands and nerve endings because of differences be-

Table 12–6. Vascular selectivity and clinical properties of some calcium channel-blocking drugs. (Unlabeled indications are noted in parentheses.)

Drug	Vascular Selectivity[1]	Indications	Usual Dosage	Toxicity
Dihydropyridines				
Amlodipine	++	Angina, hypertension	5–10 mg once daily	Headache, edema
Felodipine	5.4	Hypertension (Raynaud's phenomenon, congestive heart failure)	5–10 mg once daily	Dizziness, headache
Isradipine	7.4	Hypertension	2.5–10 mg every 12 hours	Headache, fatigue
Nicardipine	17.0	Angina, hypertension (Congestive heart failure)	20–40 mg every 8 hours orally	Edema, dizziness, headache, flushing
Nifedipine	3.1	Angina (Hypertension, migraine, cardio-myopathy, Raynaud's phenomenon)	3–10 μg/kg IV; 20–40 mg every 8 hours orally	Hypotension, dizziness, flushing, nausea, constipation, dependent edema
Nimodipine	++	Subarachnoid hemorrhage (Migraine)	60 mg every 4 hours orally	Headache, diarrhea
Nisoldipine	++	Hypertension	20–40 mg once daily	Probably similar to nifedipine
Nitrendipine	14.4	Investigational for angina, hypertension	20 mg once or twice daily	Probably similar to nifedipine
Miscellaneous				
Bepridil	–	Angina	200–400 mg orally once a day	Arrhythmias, dizziness, nausea
Diltiazem	0.3	Angina, hypertension (Raynaud's phenomenon)	75–150 μg/kg IV; 30–80 mg every 6 hours orally	Hypotension, dizziness, flushing, bradycardia
Verapamil	1.3	Angina, hypertension, arrhythmias (Migraine, cardiomyopathy)	75–150 μg/kg IV; 80–160 mg every 8 hours orally	Hypotension, myocardial depression, constipation, dependent edema

[1]Numerical data (Spedding, 1990) give the ratio of vascular potency to cardiac potency; higher numbers mean greater vascular, less cardiac potency. Plus and minus signs reflect estimated ratio of vascular to cardiac potency: – = myocardial depression greater than vasodilation; ++ = significant degree of vasodilation greater than myocardial depression.

tween calcium channels in different tissues, as noted above. Verapamil has been shown to inhibit insulin release in humans, but the dosages required are greater than those used in management of angina.

A significant body of evidence suggests that the calcium channel blockers may interfere with platelet aggregation in vitro and prevent or attenuate the development of atheromatous lesions in animals. Clinical studies have not yet firmly established their role in human blood clotting and atherosclerosis.

Verapamil has been shown to block the P170 glycoprotein responsible for the transport of many foreign drugs out of cancer (and other) cells; other calcium channel blockers appear to have a similar effect. Unlike calcium channel blockade, this action is not stereospecific. Increased expression of the P170 multidrug transporter protein is associated with the development of resistance to chemotherapy in cancer cells. Verapamil has been shown to partially reverse the re-

sistance of cancer cells to many chemotherapeutic drugs in vitro. Early clinical results suggest similar effects in patients (see Chapter 55).

Toxicity

The most important toxic effects reported for the calcium channel blockers are direct extensions of their therapeutic action. Excessive inhibition of calcium influx can cause serious cardiac depression, including cardiac arrest, bradycardia, atrioventricular block, and congestive heart failure. These effects have been rare in clinical use. Recent reports suggest that prompt-acting nifedipine may increase the incidence of myocardial infarction. (See Psaty et al, 1995, and Pahor et al, 1995, references in Chapter 11.) If true, this effect might be due to the rapid onset of blood pressure lowering with this formulation of nifedipine and the resulting sympathetic response. While these findings have not been confirmed, caution is recommended in the use of prompt-release nifedipine. Bepridil consistently prolongs the cardiac action potential and in susceptible patients may cause a dangerous **torsade de pointes** arrhythmia. It is contraindicated in patients with a history of serious arrhythmias or prolonged QT syndrome. Patients receiving beta-adrenoceptor-blocking drugs are more sensitive to the cardiodepressant effects of calcium channel blockers. Minor toxicity (not usually requiring discontinuance of therapy) includes flushing, edema, dizziness, nausea, and constipation (Table 12–6).

Mechanisms of Clinical Effects

As mentioned previously, calcium channel blockers decrease myocardial contractile force, which in turn reduces myocardial oxygen requirements. Inhibition of calcium entry into arterial smooth muscle is associated with decreased arteriolar tone and systemic vascular resistance, resulting in decreased arterial and intraventricular pressure. Some of these drugs (eg, verapamil) also possess a nonspecific antiadrenergic effect, which may contribute to peripheral vasodilation. As a result of all of these effects, left ventricular wall stress declines, which reduces myocardial oxygen requirements. Decreased heart rate with the use of verapamil, diltiazem, or bepridil causes a further decrease in myocardial oxygen demand. Calcium channel-blocking agents also relieve and prevent focal coronary artery spasm—the primary mechanism of variant angina. Use of these agents has thus emerged as the most effective treatment for this form of angina pectoris.

As noted above, the calcium channel-blocking agents differ in their clinical cardiovascular effects. Sinoatrial and atrioventricular nodal tissues, which are mainly composed of slow response cells, are affected markedly by verapamil, moderately by diltiazem, and much less by nifedipine. Thus, verapamil and diltiazem decrease atrioventricular nodal conduction and are effective in the management of supraventricular reentry tachycardia and in decreasing ventricular responses in atrial fibrillation or flutter. Nifedipine does not affect atrioventricular conduction. Nonspecific sympathetic antagonism is most marked with diltiazem and much less with verapamil. Nifedipine does not appear to have this effect. Thus, significant reflex tachycardia in response to hypotension occurs most frequently with nifedipine and less so with verapamil. These differences in pharmacologic effects should be considered in selecting calcium channel-blocking agents for the management of angina.

Clinical Uses of Calcium Channel-Blocking Drugs

In addition to angina, calcium channel blockers have well-documented efficacy in hypertension (see Chapter 11) and supraventricular tachyarrhythmias

(see Chapter 14). They also show promise in a wide variety of other conditions, including hypertrophic cardiomyopathy, migraine, Raynaud's phenomenon, and atherosclerosis.

Approved and unlabeled indications and dosages for these drugs are set forth in Table 12–6. The choice of a particular calcium channel-blocking agent should be made with knowledge of its specific potential adverse effects as well as its pharmacologic properties. Nifedipine does not decrease atrioventricular conduction and therefore can be used more safely in the presence of atrioventricular conduction abnormalities. A combination of verapamil or diltiazem with beta-blockers may produce atrioventricular block and depression of ventricular function. In the presence of overt heart failure, all calcium channel blockers can cause further worsening of heart failure as a result of their negative inotropic effect. Controlled studies have reported a higher mortality rate in patients with congestive failure when treated with calcium channel blockers; they are therefore contraindicated in the vasodilator treatment of heart failure. In the presence of relatively low blood pressure, nifedipine can cause further deleterious lowering of blood pressure. Verapamil and diltiazem appear to produce less hypotension and may be better tolerated in these circumstances. In patients with a history of atrial tachycardia, flutter, and fibrillation, verapamil and diltiazem provide a distinct advantage because of their antiarrhythmic effects. In the digitalized patient, verapamil should be used with caution, because it may increase digoxin blood levels through a pharmacokinetic interaction. Although increases in digoxin blood level have also been demonstrated with diltiazem and nifedipine, such interactions are less consistent than with verapamil.

In patients with unstable angina, immediate-release short-acting calcium channel blockers can increase the risk of adverse cardiac events and therefore are contraindicated (see Toxicity, above). However, in patients with non-Q wave myocardial infarction, diltiazem can decrease the frequency of postinfarction angina and may be used. Slow-release and long-acting calcium channel blockers are effective in controlling angina, particularly in combination with nitrates and beta-blockers, and they are therefore not contraindicated in the long-term management of patients with angina or hypertension.

BETA-ADRENOCEPTOR-BLOCKING DRUGS

Although they are not vasodilators, beta-blocking drugs (see Chapter 10) are extremely useful in the management of angina pectoris. The beneficial effects of beta-blocking agents are related primarily to their hemodynamic effects—decreased heart rate, blood pressure, and contractility—which decrease myocardial oxygen requirements at rest and during exercise. Lower heart rate is also associated with an increase in diastolic perfusion time that may increase myocardial perfusion. It has been suggested that the beta-blocking agents can cause a favorable redistribution of coronary blood flow to the ischemic myocardium based on differential effects on the coronary vascular resistance in the relatively ischemic and nonischemic myocardial segments. However, reduction of heart rate and blood pressure and consequently decreased myocardial oxygen consumption appear to be the most important mechanisms for relief of angina and improved exercise tolerance. Beta-blockers may also be valuable in treating silent or ambulatory ischemia. Because this condition causes no pain, it is usually detected by the appearance of typical electrocardiographic signs of ischemia. As shown in Figure 12–6, the total amount of "ischemic time" is reduced by chronic therapy with a beta-blocker. This improvement may account, in part, for the reduction in reinfarction and mortality in patients who are placed on beta-blocker therapy after a myocardial infarct.

Undesirable effects of beta-blocking agents include an increase in end-diastolic volume that accompanies slowing of the heart rate and an increase in ejection time. Increased myocardial oxygen requirements associated with increased left ventricular diastolic volume partially offset the beneficial effects of beta-

blocking agents. These potentially deleterious effects of beta-blocking agents can be balanced by the concomitant use of nitrates as described below.

II. CLINICAL PHARMACOLOGY OF DRUGS USED TO TREAT ANGINA

Principles of Therapy of Angina

In addition to modification of the risk factors for coronary atherosclerosis (smoking, hypertension, hyperlipidemia), the treatment of angina and other manifestations of myocardial ischemia is based on reduction of myocardial oxygen demand and increase of coronary blood flow to the potentially ischemic myocardium to restore the balance between myocardial oxygen supply and demand.

Angina of Effort

Many studies have demonstrated that nitrates, calcium channel blockers, and beta-blockers increase time to onset of angina and ST depression during treadmill tests in patients with angina of effort (Figure 12–7). The double product remains consistently lower during exercise. However, although exercise tolerance increases, there is usually no change in the angina

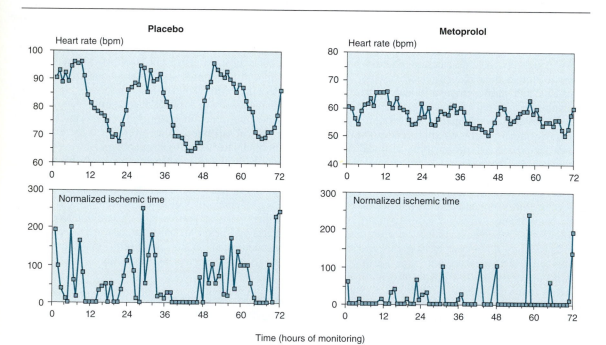

Figure 12–6. Effects of metoprolol on the heart rate and normalized ischemic time (measured by ambulatory electrocardiographic monitoring) in nine men with severe coronary artery disease over 72-hour periods. The drug reduced the mean heart rate, magnitude of diurnal heart rate changes, and the total time during which the ECG showed evidence of ischemia. (Reproduced, with permission, from Lambert CR et al: Influence of beta-adrenergic blockade defined by time series analysis on circadian variation of heart rate and ambulatory myocardial ischemia. Am J Cardiol 1989;64:835.)

Figure 12–7. Effects of diltiazem on the "double product" in a group of 20 patients with angina of effort. In a double-blind study using a standard protocol, patients were tested on a treadmill during treatment with placebo and three doses of the drug. Heart rate *(HR)* and systolic blood pressure *(BP)* were recorded at 180 seconds of exercise (midpoints of lines) and at the time of onset of anginal symptoms (rightmost points). Note that the drug treatment decreased the double product at all times during exercise and prolonged the time to appearance of symptoms. (Data from Lindenberg BS et al: Efficacy and safety of incremental doses of diltiazem for the treatment of angina. J Am Coll Cardiol 1983;2:1129. Used with permission of the American College of Cardiology.)

threshold, ie, the rate-pressure product at which symptoms occur.

For maintenance therapy of chronic stable angina, long-acting nitrates, calcium channel-blocking agents, or beta-blockers may be chosen; the best choice of drug will depend on the individual patient's response. In hypertensive patients, monotherapy with either slow-release or long-acting calcium channel blockers or beta-blockers may be adequate. In normotensive patients, long-acting nitrates may be suitable. The combination of a beta-blocker with a calcium channel blocker (eg, propranolol with nifedipine) or two different calcium channel blockers (eg, nifedipine and verapamil) has been shown to be more effective than individual drugs used alone. If response to a single drug is inadequate, a drug from a different class should be added to maximize the beneficial reduction of cardiac work while minimizing undesirable effects (Table 12–7). Some patients may require therapy with all three drug groups.

For patients with persistent hypertension, sinus bradycardia, or atrioventricular node dysfunction, slow-release nifedipine or a longer-acting dihydropyridine is the drug of choice.

In the case of beta-blocking drugs, there is no evidence that any one agent is significantly more effective or better tolerated than the others.

Surgical revascularization and catheter-based revascularization are the primary methods available that restore coronary blood flow and increase oxygen supply to the myocardium. Patients refractory to medical therapy or unable to adapt their life-style should be considered for this mode of therapy.

Vasospastic Angina

Nitrates and the calcium channel blockers are considerably more effective than the beta-adrenoceptor-blocking drugs in relieving and preventing ischemic episodes in patients with variant angina. In approximately 70% of patients treated with nitrates plus calcium channel blockers, angina attacks are completely abolished; in another 20%, marked reduction of frequency of anginal episodes is observed. Prevention of coronary artery spasm (in the presence or absence of fixed atherosclerotic coronary artery lesions) is the principal mechanism for this beneficial response. All presently available calcium channel blockers appear to be equally effective, and the choice of a particular drug should depend on the patient, as indicated above. Surgical revascularization and angioplasty are not indicated in patients with variant angina.

Unstable Angina

In patients with unstable angina with recurrent ischemic episodes at rest, recurrent thrombotic occlusions of the offending coronary artery occur as the result of fissuring of atherosclerotic plaques and platelet aggregation. Aspirin has been shown to reduce the in-

Table 12–7. Effects of nitrates alone and with beta-blockers or calcium blockers in angina pectoris. Undesirable effects are shown in italics.

	Nitrates Alone	β-Blockers or Calcium Channel Blockers	Combined Nitrates With β-Blockers or Calcium Channel Blockers
Heart rate	*Reflex increase*	Decrease[1]	Decrease
Arterial pressure	Decrease	Decrease	Decrease
End-diastolic volume	Decrease	*Increase*	None or decrease
Contractility	*Reflex increase*	Decrease[1]	None
Ejection time	Decrease	*Increase*	None

[1]Nifedipine may cause a reflex *increase* in heart rate and cardiac contractility.

cidence of cardiac events in such patients. Intravenous heparin is indicated in most patients. In addition to aspirin and heparin therapy, anti-ischemic therapy with nitroglycerin and beta-blockers should be considered; calcium channel blockers should be added in refractory patients. Catheter-based or surgical myocardial revascularization is often necessary in refractory patients.

PREPARATIONS AVAILABLE

Nitrates & Nitrites

Amyl nitrite (generic, Aspirols, Vaporole)
Inhalant: 0.3 mL capsules

Isosorbide dinitrate (generic, Isordil, Sorbitrate)
Oral: 5, 10, 20, 30, 40 mg tablets; 5, 10 mg chewable tablets
Oral sustained-release (generic, Sorbitrate SA, Iso-Bid): 40 mg tablets and capsules
Sublingual: 2.5, 5, 10 mg sublingual tablets

Isosorbide mononitrate (Ismo, others)
Oral: 10, 20 mg tablets; extended-release 60 mg tablets

Nitroglycerin
Sublingual: 0.15, 0.3, 0.4, 0.6 mg tablets; 0.4 mg/metered dose aerosol
Oral sustained-release (generic, Nitrong): 2.6, 6.5, 9 mg tablets; 2.5, 6.5, 9, 13 mg capsules
Buccal (Nitrogard): 1, 2, 3 mg buccal tablets
Parenteral (Nitro-Bid IV, Tridil, generic): 0.5, 5 mg/mL for IV administration
Transdermal patches (Minitran, Nitro-Dur, Transderm-Nitro): to release a total of 9, 12.5, 16, 18, 20, 24, 25, 32, 40, 60 mg at 0.1, 0.2, 0.3, 0.4, 0.6, or 0.8 mg/h.
Topical ointment (generic, Nitrol): 20 mg/mL ointment (1 inch, or 25 mm, of ointment contains about 15 mg nitroglycerin)

Calcium Channel Blockers

Amlodipine (Norvasc)
Oral: 2.5, 5, 10 mg tablets

Bepridil (Vascor)
Oral: 200, 300, 400 mg tablets

Diltiazem (Cardizem, generic) 432
Oral: 30, 60, 90, 120 mg tablets 432
Oral sustained-release (Cardizem SR, Dilacor XL): 60, 90, 120, 180, 240, 300 mg capsules
Parenteral: 5 mg/mL for injection

Felodipine (Plendil)
Oral extended-release: 2.5, 5, 10 mg tablets

Isradipine (DynaCirc)
Oral: 2.5, 5 mg capsules

Nicardipine (Cardene)
Oral: 20, 30 mg capsules
Oral sustained-release (Cardene SR): 30, 45, 60 mg capsules)
Parenteral (Cardene IV): 2.5 mg/mL

Nifedipine (Adalat, Procardia, others)
Oral: 10, 20 mg capsules
Oral sustained-release (Procardia XL, Adalat CC): 30, 60, 90 mg tablets

Nimodipine (Nimotop)
Oral: 30 mg capsules. (Labeled for use in subarachnoid hemorrhage, not angina.)

Nisoldipine (Sular)
Oral: 10, 20, 30, 40 mg extended-release tablets

Verapamil (generic, Calan, Isoptin)
Oral: 40, 80, 120 mg tablets
Oral sustained-release: 120, 180, 240 mg tablets, capsules
Parenteral: 5 mg/2 mL for injection

Beta-Blockers Labeled for Use in Angina

Atenolol (Tenormin)
Oral: 25, 50, 100 mg tablets

Metoprolol (Lopressor)
Oral: 50, 100 mg tablets; 50, 100, 200 mg extended-release tablets

Propranolol (generic, Inderal)
Oral: 10, 20, 40, 60, 80, 90 mg tablets; solution, 4 and 8 mg/mL; solution, concentrated, 80 mg/mL
Oral sustained-release (Inderal LA): 60, 80, 120, 160 mg capsules;

Nadolol (Corgard)
Oral: 20, 40, 80, 120, 160 mg tablets

REFERENCES

Abrams J: Nitrates. Med Clin North Am 1988;72:1.

Allen GS et al: Cerebral arterial spasm: A controlled trial of nimodipine in patients with subarachnoid hemorrhage. N Engl J Med 1983;308:619.

Andersson K-E, Vinge E: β-Adrenoceptor blockers and calcium antagonists in the prophylaxis and treatment of migraine. Drugs 1990;39:355.

Bassenge E, Stewart DJ: Effects of nitrates in various vascular sections and regions. Z Kardiol 1986;75(Suppl 3):1.

Bassenge E, Zanzinger J: Nitrates in different vascular beds, nitrate tolerance, and interactions with endothelial function. Am J Cardiol 1992;70(Suppl B):23B.

Beller GA: Calcium antagonists in the treatment of Prinzmetal's angina and unstable angina pectoris. Circulation 1989;80(Suppl IV):IV–78.

Boesgaard S et al: Nitrate tolerance in vivo is not associated with depletion of arterial or venous thiol levels. Circ Res 1994;74:115.

Bright GE: The effects of nitroglycerin on those engaged in its manufacture. JAMA 1914;62:201.

Carmichael P, Lieben J: Sudden death in explosives workers. Arch Environ Health 1963;7:50.

Chatterjee K: Ischemic heart disease. In: *Internal Medicine.* Stein JH (editor). Little, Brown, 1990.

Chobanian A: Effects of calcium channel antagonists and other antihypertensive drugs on atherogenesis. J Hypertens 1987;5(Suppl 4):S43.

Coffman JD: Raynaud's phenomenon. An update. Hypertension 1991;17:593.

Cohen RA, Vanhoutte PM: Endothelium-dependent hyperpolarization: Beyond nitric oxide and cyclic GMP. Circulation 1995;92:3337.

Cohn PF: Total ischemic burden: Definition, mechanisms, and therapeutic implications. Am J Med 1986;81(Suppl 4A):2.

Danish Study Group on Verapamil in Myocardial Infarction: Effect of verapamil on mortality and major events after acute myocardial infarction (The Danish Verapamil Infarction Trial II—DAVIT II). Am J Cardiol 1990;66:779.

Dickson RB, Gottesmann MM: Understanding of the molecular basis of drug resistance in cancer reveals new targets for chemotherapy. Trends Pharmacol Sci 1990; 11:305.

Freedman DD, Waters DD: "Second generation" dihydropyridine calcium antagonists. Greater vascular selectivity and some unique applications. Drugs 1987;34:578.

Fung H-L, Bauer JA: Mechanisms of nitrate tolerance. Cardiovasc Drugs Ther 1994;8:489.

Fuster V et al: The pathogenesis of coronary artery disease and the acute coronary syndromes. (Two parts.) N Engl J Med 1992;326:242, 310.

Ganz W, Marcus HS: Failure of intracoronary nitroglycerin to alleviate pacing-induced angina. Circulation 1972; 46:880.

Godfraind T, Miller R, Wibo M: Calcium antagonism and calcium entry blockade. Pharmacol Rev 1986;38:321.

Gollasch M et al: Pinacidil relaxes porcine and human coronary arteries by activating ATP-dependent potassium channels in smooth muscle cells. J Pharmacol Exp Ther 1995;275:681.

Harrison DG, Bates JN: The nitrovasodilators. New ideas about old drugs. Circulation 1993;87:1461.

Hartman PE: Review: Putative mutagens and carcinogens in foods. 1. Nitrate/nitrite ingestion and gastric cancer mortality. Environ Mutagen 1983;5:111.

Higginbotham MB et al: Comparison of nifedipine alone with propranolol alone for stable angina pectoris including hemodynamics at rest and during exercise. Am J Cardiol 1986;57:1022.

Ignarro LJ et al: Mechanism of vascular smooth muscle relaxation by organic nitrates, nitrites, nitroprusside, and nitric oxide: Evidence for the involvement of S-nitrosothiols as active intermediates. J Pharmacol Exp Ther 1981;218:739.

Jackson CL, Bush RC, Bowyer DE: Mechanism of antiatherogenic action of calcium antagonists. Atherosclerosis 1989;80:17.

Jugdutt BI, Warnica JW: Intravenous nitroglycerin therapy to limit myocardial infarct size, expansion, and complications. Circulation 1988;78:906.

Kar S, Waikada Y, Nordlander R: The high-risk unstable angina patient. An approach to treatment. Drugs 1992; 43:837.

Karlberg K-E et al: Dose-dependent effect of intravenous nitroglycerin on platelet aggregation, and correlation with plasma glyceryl dinitrate concentration in healthy men. Am J Cardiol 1992;69:802.

Kawanishi DT et al: Response of angina and ischemia to long-term treatment in patients with chronic stable angina: A double blind randomized individualized dosing trial of nifedipine, propranolol, and their combination. J Am Coll Cardiol 1992;19:409.

Klemsdal TO, Gjesdal K: Intermittent or continuous transdermal nitroglycerin: Still an issue, or is the case closed? Cardiovasc Drugs Ther 1996;10:5.

Kokubun S et al: Studies on Ca channels in intact cardiac cells: Voltage-dependent effects and cooperative interactions of dihydropyridine enantiomers. Mol Pharmacol 1987;30:571.

Kukovetz WR, Holzmann S: Mechanisms of nitrate-induced vasodilation and tolerance. Eur J Clin Pharm 1990;38 (Suppl 1):S–9.

Lambert CR et al: Influence of beta-adrenergic blockade defined by time series analysis on circadian variation of heart rate and ambulatory myocardial ischemia. Am J Cardiol 1989;64:835.

Lindenberg BS et al: Efficacy and safety of incremental doses of diltiazem for the treatment of stable angina pectoris. J Am Coll Cardiol 1983;2:1129.

McDonald KM et al: Long-term oral nitrate therapy prevents chronic ventricular remodeling in the dog. J Am Coll Cardiol 1993;21:514.

Miljanich GP, Ramachandran J: Antagonists of neuronal calcium channels: Structure, function, and therapeutic implications. Annu Rev Pharmacol Toxicol 1995;35:707.

Mohanty N et al: Prevention of nitrate tolerance with diuretics. Am Heart J 1995;130:522.

Multicenter Diltiazem Postinfarction Trial Research Group: The effect of diltiazem on mortality and reinfarction after myocardial infarction. N Engl J Med 1988;319:385.

Nesto RW et al: Comparison of nifedipine and isosorbide dinitrate when added to maximal propranolol therapy in stable angina pectoris. Am J Cardiol 1987;60:256.

Opie LH: Calcium channel antagonists in the management of anginal syndromes: Changing concepts in relation to the role of coronary vasospasm. Prog Cardiovasc Dis 1996;38:291.

Packer M: Combined beta-adrenergic and calcium-entry blockade in angina pectoris. N Engl J Med 1989;320:709.

Parker JD, Parker JO: Effect of therapy with an angiotensin-converting enzyme inhibitor on hemodynamic and counter-regulatory responses during continuous therapy with nitroglycerin. J Am Coll Cardiol 1993; 21:1445.

Parker JO et al: Effect of intervals between doses on the development of tolerance of isosorbide dinitrate. N Engl J Med 1987;316:1440.

Prida XE et al: Comparison of selective (β_1) and nonselective (β_1 and β_2) beta-adrenergic blockade on systemic and coronary hemodynamic findings in angina pectoris. Am J Cardiol 1987;60:244.

Quast U, Guillon J-M, Cavero I: Cellular pharmacology of potassium channel openers in vascular smooth muscle. Cardiovasc Res 1994;28:805.

Rankin JS et al: Clinical characteristics and current management of medically refractory unstable angina. Ann Surg 1984;200:457.

Rapoport RM et al: Effects of glyceryl trinitrate on endothelium-dependent and -independent relaxation and cyclic GMP levels in rat aorta and human coronary artery. J Cardiovasc Pharmacol 1987;10:82.

Reuter H: Calcium channel modulation by neurotransmitters, enzymes, and drugs. Nature 1983;301:569.

Roth A et al: Early tolerance to hemodynamic effects of high-dose transdermal nitroglycerin in responders with severe chronic heart failure. J Am Coll Cardiol 1987; 9:858.

Rouleau JL et al: Mechanism of relief of pacing-induced angina with oral verapamil: Reduced oxygen demand. Circulation 1983;67:94.

Schmidt HHHW et al: The nitric oxide and cGMP signal transduction system: Regulation and mechanism of action. Biochim Biophys Acta 1993;1178:153.

Spedding M et al: Factors modifying the tissue selectivity of calcium-antagonists. J Neural Transm 1990;31(Suppl):5.

Spedding M, Kenny B, Chatelain P: New drug binding sites in Ca^{2+} channels. Trends Pharmacol Sci 1995;16:139.

Steering Committee, Transdermal Nitroglycerin Cooperative Study: Acute and chronic antianginal efficacy of continuous twenty-four hour application of transdermal nitroglycerin. Am J Cardiol 1991;68:1263.

Stengele E et al: Short-term hemodynamic, anti-ischemic, and antianginal effects of pirsidomine, a new sydnonimine. Am J Cardiol 1996;77:937.

Strauss WE, Parisi AF: Combined use of calcium-channel and beta-adrenergic blockers for the treatment of chronic stable angina: Rationale, efficacy, and adverse effects. Ann Intern Med 19 1988;109:570.

Taira N: Differences in cardiovascular profile among calcium antagonists. Am J Cardiol 1987;59:24B.

Taira N: Nicorandil as a hybrid between nitrates and potassium channel activators. Am J Cardiol 1989;63(Suppl J):18–J.

Thadani U, Bittar N: Effects of 8:00 A.M. and 2:00 P.M. doses of isosorbide-5-mononitrate during twice-daily therapy in stable angina pectoris. Am J Cardiol 1992; 70:286.

Trost BN, Weidmann P: Effects of calcium antagonists on glucose homeostasis and serum lipids in non-diabetic and diabetic subjects: A review. J Hypertens 1987;5(Suppl 4):S81.

Uydeş-Doğan BS et al: The comparison of vascular reactivities of arterial and venous grafts to vasodilators: Management of graft spasm. Int J Cardiol 1996;53:137.

Vaghy PL, Williams JS, Schwartz A: Receptor pharmacology of calcium entry blocking agents. Am J Cardiol 1987;59(Suppl A):9–A.

Weinstein DB, Heider JG: Antiatherogenic properties of calcium antagonists. State of the art. Am J Med 1989; 86(Suppl 4A):27.

Wong MCW, Haley EC Jr: Calcium antagonists: Stroke therapy coming of age. Stroke 1990;21:494.

Cardiac Glycosides & Other Drugs Used in Congestive Heart Failure

13

Bertram G Katzung, MD, PhD, & William W. Parmley, MD

Congestive heart failure occurs when the cardiac output is inadequate to provide the oxygen needed by the body. It is a highly lethal condition, with a 5-year mortality rate of approximately 50%. Although many new drugs have been introduced for the treatment of heart failure, this unsatisfactory statistic has been remarkably resistant to change. However, recent developments suggest the possibility of improvement (Stevenson et al, 1995). Although it is believed that the primary defect in early heart failure resides in the excitation-contraction coupling machinery of the heart, the clinical condition also involves many other processes and organs, including the baroreceptor reflex, the sympathetic nervous system, the kidneys, the renin-angiotensin-aldosterone system, vasopressin, and death of cardiac cells.

Clinical research has shown that therapy directed at noncardiac targets may be more valuable in the long-term treatment of congestive failure than traditional positive inotropic agents (cardiac glycosides [digitalis]). Thus, drugs acting on the kidneys (diuretics) have long been considered at least as valuable as digitalis for this condition. More recently, ACE inhibitors and vasodilators have come into common use. Now even beta-adrenoceptor-blocking drugs are in clinical trials as potential treatment for congestive heart failure.

The cardiac glycosides (**digitalis derivatives and similar agents**) comprise a group of steroid compounds that can increase cardiac output and alter the electrical functions of the heart. They also have effects on smooth muscle and other tissues. The principal therapeutic effect in congestive heart failure is an increase in cardiac contractility (a positive inotropic action), which corrects the imbalance associated with failure. Nevertheless, there is some doubt regarding the long-term efficacy of cardiac glycosides in some patients with heart failure (see Clinical Pharmacology). There is general agreement that the glycosides have a narrow margin of safety and that less toxic compounds with positive inotropic actions are needed. Several agents have been candidates for this role in acute failure, including **phosphodiesterase in-**hibitors and certain **beta-adrenoceptor stimulants,** but they are not useful in chronic therapy.

Although traditional therapy of congestive failure has placed most emphasis on correcting the failure of cardiac contractility and reversing the retention of salt and water, clinical research has shown that unloading the stressed myocardium—by reduction of vascular tone—gives effective relief. Thus, certain vasodilators have been used with considerable success. Such agents include **nitroprusside, hydralazine, nitroglycerin,** and **angiotensin-converting enzyme inhibitors.**

Control of Normal Cardiac Contractility

The vigor of contraction of heart muscle is determined by several processes that lead to the movement of actin and myosin filaments in the cardiac sarcomere (Figure 13–1). Ultimately, contraction results from the interaction of calcium (during systole) with the actin-troponin-tropomyosin system, thereby releasing the actin-myosin interaction. This "activator" calcium is released from the sarcoplasmic reticulum (SR). The amount released depends upon the amount stored in the SR and upon the amount of "trigger" calcium that enters the cell during the plateau of the action potential. In theory, each of these processes could be a target of drug therapy, but only a few have proved useful thus far.

A. Sensitivity of the Contractile Proteins to Calcium: The determinants of calcium sensitivity, ie, the curve relating the shortening of cardiac myofibrils to the cytoplasmic calcium concentration, are poorly understood, but several types of drugs can be shown to affect it in vitro. For example, certain phosphodiesterase inhibitors (theophylline, etc) and some newer agents (Solaro, 1993; Zimmermann et al, 1996) appear to shift this curve to lower calcium concentrations.

B. The Amount of Calcium Released From the Sarcoplasmic Reticulum: A sudden small rise in free cytoplasmic calcium, brought about by calcium influx during the action potential, triggers the opening of specialized calcium channels in the mem-

Figure 13–1. Schematic diagram of a cardiac muscle sarcomere, with sites of action of several drugs that alter contractility (numbered structures). Site *1* is Na⁺/K⁺ ATPase, the sodium pump. Site *2* is the sodium/calcium exchanger. Site *3* is the voltage-gated calcium channel. Site *4* is a calcium transporter that pumps calcium into the sarcoplasmic reticulum (SR). Site *5* is a calcium channel in the membrane of the SR that is triggered to release stored calcium by activator calcium. Site *6* is the actin-troponin-tropomyosin complex at which activator calcium brings about the contractile interaction of actin and myosin.

brane of the SR and the rapid release of a large amount of the ion into the cytoplasm in the vicinity of the actin-troponin-tropomyosin complex. The amount released is proportionate to the amount stored in the SR and the amount of trigger calcium that enters the cell through the cell membrane. Ryanodine is a potent *negative* inotropic plant alkaloid that interferes with the release of calcium through the SR channels. No drugs are available that have been shown to increase the release of calcium through these channels.

C. The Amount of Calcium Stored in the Sarcoplasmic Reticulum: The SR membrane contains a very efficient calcium uptake transporter, which maintains free cytoplasmic calcium at very low levels during diastole by pumping calcium into the membrane-limited tubules of the SR. The amount of calcium sequestered in the SR is thus determined, in part, by the amount accessible to this transporter. This in turn is dependent on the balance of calcium influx (primarily through the voltage-gated membrane calcium channels) and calcium efflux, the amount removed from the cell (primarily via the sodium-calcium exchanger, a transporter in the cell membrane).

D. The Amount of Trigger Calcium: The amount of trigger calcium that enters the cell depends upon the availability of calcium channels and the du-

ration of their opening. As described in Chapters 6 and 9, sympathomimetics cause an increase in calcium influx through an action on these channels. Conversely, the calcium channel blockers (Chapter 12) reduce this influx and depress contractility. Some investigators have proposed that reverse sodium-calcium exchange (which occurs normally during sufficiently positive action potential plateaus) also contributes to the trigger calcium.

E. Activity of the Sodium-Calcium Exchanger: This antiporter uses the sodium gradient to move calcium against its concentration gradient from the cytoplasm to the extracellular space. Extracellular concentrations of these ions are much less labile than intracellular concentrations under physiologic conditions. The sodium-calcium exchanger's ability to carry out this transport is thus dependent primarily on the intracellular concentrations of both ions, especially sodium.

F. Intracellular Sodium Concentration and Activity of Na⁺/K⁺ ATPase: Na⁺/K⁺ ATPase, by removing intracellular sodium, is the major determinant of sodium concentration in the cell. The sodium influx through voltage-gated channels, which occurs as a normal part of almost all cardiac action potentials, is another determinant. As described below, Na⁺/K⁺ ATPase appears to be the primary target of cardiac glycosides. Several experimental drugs markedly increase sodium influx during action potentials by interfering with sodium channel inactivation (Hoey et al, 1993). They have been shown to have dramatic positive inotropic effects in vitro, but their role in clinical therapy has yet to be defined.

PATHOPHYSIOLOGY OF HEART FAILURE

Congestive heart failure is a syndrome with multiple causes that may involve the right ventricle, the left ventricle, or both. Cardiac output in congestive heart failure is usually below the normal range. This ventricular dysfunction may be primarily systolic (ie, inadequate force generation to eject blood normally) or diastolic (ie, inadequate relaxation to permit normal filling). Systolic dysfunction, with reduced cardiac output and significantly reduced ejection fraction (less than 45%), is typical of acute failure, especially that resulting from myocardial infarction. It is usually responsive to positive inotropic drugs, at least initially. Diastolic dysfunction often occurs as a result of hypertrophy and stiffening of the myocardium, and although cardiac output is reduced, ejection fraction may be normal. Congestive failure due to diastolic dysfunction does not usually respond optimally to positive inotropic drugs.

Rarely, "high-output" failure may occur. In this condition, the demands of the body are so great that even increased cardiac output is insufficient. High-output failure can result from hyperthyroidism, beriberi, anemia, and arteriovenous shunts. This form of failure responds poorly to positive inotropic agents and should be treated by correcting the underlying cause.

The primary signs and symptoms of all types of congestive heart failure include tachycardia, decreased exercise tolerance and shortness of breath, peripheral and pulmonary edema, and cardiomegaly. Decreased exercise tolerance with rapid muscular fatigue is the major direct consequence of diminished cardiac output. The other manifestations result from the attempts by the body to compensate for the intrinsic cardiac defect.

Neurohumoral reflex (extrinsic) compensation involves two major mechanisms previously presented in Figure 6–7: the sympathetic nervous system and the renin-angiotensin-aldosterone hormonal response. Some of the pathologic as well as beneficial features of these compensatory responses are illustrated in Figure 13–2. The baroreceptor reflex appears to be "reset," with a lower sensitivity to arterial pressure, in patients with heart failure. As a result, baroreceptor sensory input to the vasomotor center is reduced even at normal pressures; sympathetic outflow is increased; and parasympathetic outflow is decreased (Ferguson, 1992). Increased sympathetic outflow causes tachy-

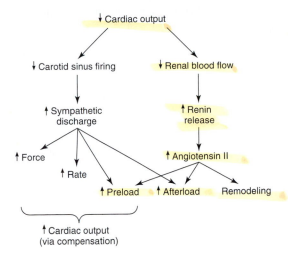

Figure 13–2. Some compensatory responses that occur during congestive heart failure. In addition to the effects shown, angiotensin II increases sympathetic effects by facilitating norepinephrine release.

cardia, increased cardiac contractility, and increased vascular tone. While the increased preload, force, and heart rate initially increase cardiac output, increased arterial tone results in increased afterload and decreased ejection fraction, cardiac output, and renal perfusion. Increased angiotensin II production leads to increased aldosterone secretion (with sodium and water retention), to increased afterload, and to remodeling of both heart and vessels (discussed below). Other hormones may also be released.

The most important intrinsic compensatory mechanism is **myocardial hypertrophy.** This increase in muscle mass helps to maintain cardiac performance in the face of adverse effects such as pressure or volume overload, loss of functional tissue (myocardial infarction), or decrease in cardiac contractility. However, after an initial beneficial effect, hypertrophy can lead to ischemic changes, impairment of diastolic filling, and alterations in ventricular geometry. **Remodeling** is a newer term now applied to slow structural changes that occur in the stressed myocardium. It may include proliferation of connective tissue cells as well as abnormal myocardial cells with some biochemical characteristics of fetal myocytes. Ultimately, myocytes may die at an accelerated rate, leaving the remaining myocytes subject to even greater overload (Katz, 1994).

Pathophysiology of Cardiac Performance

Cardiac performance is a function of four primary factors.

A. Preload: The effect of altered preload (atrial pressure) on cardiovascular performance is of considerable importance. When some measure of left ventricular performance such as stroke volume or stroke work is plotted as a function of left ventricular filling pressure, the resulting curve is termed the **left ventricular function curve** (Figure 13–3). The ascending limb (< 15 mm Hg filling pressure) represents the classic Frank-Starling relation. Beyond approximately 15 mm Hg, there is a plateau of performance. Preloads greater than 20–25 mm Hg result in pulmonary congestion. As noted above, preload is usually increased in heart failure because of increased blood volume and venous tone. Reduction of high filling pressure is the goal of salt restriction and diuretic therapy in congestive heart failure. Venodilator drugs (eg, nitroglycerin) also reduce preload by redistributing blood away from the chest into peripheral veins.

B. Afterload: Afterload is the resistance against which the heart must pump blood and is represented by aortic impedance and systemic vascular resistance. Systemic vascular resistance is frequently increased in patients with congestive heart failure. As cardiac output falls in chronic failure, there is a reflex increase in systemic vascular resistance, mediated in part by increased sympathetic outflow and circulating catecholamines and in part by activation of the renin-angiotensin system. However, elevated vascular resistance may further reduce cardiac output by increasing

resistance to ejection. This sets the stage for the use of drugs that reduce arteriolar tone in congestive heart failure.

C. Contractility: In patients with chronic low-output failure, the primary defect appears to be a reduction in the intrinsic contractility of the myocardium. As contractility decreases, there is a reduction in the velocity of muscle shortening and the rate of intraventricular pressure development (dP/dt). This results in the reduction in pump performance of the heart that accompanies heart failure, eg, after acute myocardial infarction (Figure 13–3). However, the heart is still capable of an increase in contractility in response to inotropic drugs.

D. Heart Rate: The heart rate is a major determinant of cardiac output. As the intrinsic function of the heart decreases in failure and stroke volume diminishes, an increase in heart rate—through sympathetic activation of beta adrenoceptors—is the first compensatory mechanism that comes into play to maintain cardiac output.

I. BASIC PHARMACOLOGY OF DRUGS USED IN CONGESTIVE HEART FAILURE

DIGITALIS

Medicinal plants containing cardiac glycosides were known to the ancient Egyptians 3000 years ago, but these agents were used erratically and with variable success until the 18th century, when William Withering, an English physician and botanist, published a monograph describing the clinical effects of an extract of the foxglove plant (*Digitalis purpurea*, a major source of these agents). His book, *An Account of the Foxglove and Some of Its Medical Uses: With Practical Remarks on Dropsy and Other Diseases*, published in 1785, described in detail the indications for the use of cardiac glycosides and offered cautionary remarks about their toxicity.

Chemistry

All of the commonly used cardiac glycosides, or cardenolides—of which **digoxin** (Figure 13–4) may be considered the prototype—combine a steroid nucleus with an unsaturated five-membered lactone ring at the 17 position and a series of sugars linked to carbon 3 of the nucleus. Because they lack an easily ionizable group, their solubility is not pH-dependent.

Sources of these drugs include white and purple foxglove (*Digitalis lanata* and *D purpurea*), Mediterranean sea onion (squill), *Strophanthus gratus*, oleander, lily of the valley, milkweed, and numerous other tropical and temperate zone plants. Certain toads have

Figure 13–3. Relation of left ventricular performance to filling pressure in patients with acute myocardial infarction. The cross-hatched area is the range for normal, healthy individuals. Following infarction, there is a wide range of performance characteristics. In some patients, performance is in the normal or hypernormal range (hyperreactor). As the size of the infarct increases, however, function is shifted down and to the right. Similar depression is observed in patients with chronic congestive heart failure. (Reproduced with permission, from Swan HJC, Parmley WW: Congestive heart failure. In: *Pathologic Physiology.* Sodeman WA Jr, Sodeman TM [editors]. Saunders, 1979.)

Figure 13–4. Structure of digoxin, a typical cardiac glycoside.

skin glands capable of elaborating **bufadienolides,** which differ from the cardenolides mainly in having a six-membered (rather than a five-membered) lactone ring at the 17 position.

Structure-activity studies indicate that the lactone ring and the steroid nucleus are essential for activity. The other substituents—especially the sugar molecules in the 3 position—influence pharmacokinetic variables, including absorption, half-life, and metabolism. There is no clinical evidence that any of the natural cardenolides differs from the others in therapeutic index or maximal efficacy.

Pharmacokinetics

A. Absorption and Distribution: Cardenolides have both lipophilic (steroid nucleus) and hydrophilic (lactone ring, hydroxyl, sugar) groups. The balance of these two factors has an important effect on absorption, distribution, metabolism, and excretion, as shown by comparison of three representative agents: **digoxin, digitoxin,** and **ouabain** (Table 13–1). Of these three, digoxin is by far the most widely used preparation.

As noted in the table, digoxin is fairly well absorbed after oral administration. However, about 10% of individuals harbor enteric bacteria that inactivate digoxin in the gut, greatly reducing bioavailability and requiring higher than average maintenance dosage. Treatment of such patients with antibiotics can result in a sudden increase in bioavailability and digitalis toxicity. Because the safety margin of cardiac glycosides is very narrow, even minor variations in bioavailability could cause serious toxicity or loss of effect. In fact, product formulation (factors in manufacture of the tablets) can modify the bioavailability of digoxin. As a result, digoxin preparations must pass dissolution tests before they can be marketed in the USA. Digitoxin, because it is well absorbed under almost all circumstances, is not subject to this restriction. Beta-methyldigoxin, a semisynthetic derivative of digoxin often used outside the USA, is almost completely absorbed from the gut and is metabolized to digoxin in the body.

Once absorbed into the blood, all cardiac glycosides are widely distributed to tissues, including the central nervous system. Their volumes of distribution differ, however, depending on their tendency to bind to plasma proteins versus tissue proteins. The highest tissue concentrations—for digoxin, 10–50 times higher than in plasma—are found in heart, kidney, and liver.

B. Metabolism and Excretion: Digoxin is not extensively metabolized in humans; almost two-thirds is excreted unchanged by the kidneys. Its renal clearance is proportionate to creatinine clearance and is significantly slowed in patients with renal disease. Equations and nomograms are available for adjusting digoxin dosage.

Digitoxin is metabolized in the liver and excreted into the gut via the bile. Cardioactive metabolites (which include digoxin) as well as unchanged digitoxin can then be reabsorbed from the intestine, thus establishing an **enterohepatic circulation** that con-

Table 13–1. Properties of three typical cardiac glycosides.

	Ouabain[1]	Digoxin	Digitoxin
Lipid solubility (oil/water coefficient)	Low	Medium	High
Oral availability (percentage absorbed)	0	75	> 90
Half-life in body (hours)	21	40	168
Plasma protein binding (percentage bound)	0	20–40	> 90
Percentage metabolized	0	< 20	> 80
Volume of distribution (L/kg)	18	6.3	0.6

[1]Ouabain is no longer in use as a drug in the USA, but see box: Endogenous Cardiac Glycosides.

ENDOGENOUS CARDIAC GLYCOSIDES

Do all receptors on regulatory enzymes and transporters have endogenous ligands as well as an affinity for the exogenous chemicals we use as drugs? Some biologists would answer this question affirmatively, reasoning that these regulators of important processes themselves require endogenous regulators. Others argue that proteins have sufficient complexity of structure so that there is a great likelihood they will bind some completely foreign ligand molecules. Furthermore, if the binding occurs in a critical region of the protein, it is highly probable that some alteration of function of that enzyme or transporter will result, thereby causing a pharmacologic response.

The receptor for the cardiac glycosides is a case in point. The very high affinity of the Na^+/K^+ ATPase for cardiac glycosides suggests that there might be an endogenous ligand of similar structure. Like the adrenocortical hormones, the cardiac glycosides have a steroid nucleus, but the stereochemistry of the rings is quite different from that of typical cholesterol derivatives. While many plants synthesize these glycosides, in the animal kingdom only a few amphibians (poisonous toads) had been thought to have this capability.

A significant new body of evidence (reviewed by Blaustein, 1993) based on extremely sensitive immunochemical techniques now suggests that ouabain is synthesized by the adrenal and perhaps by the brain in humans and other mammals. It is claimed that ouabain is released as an endocrine and paracrine agent under certain circumstances, such as high salt intake and heart failure. It has been postulated for almost 20 years that some forms of hypertension are caused by vasoconstriction evoked by an endogenous inhibitor of the sodium pump. Elevated endogenous ouabain secretion evoked by high salt intake would provide an important link in this hypothesis. In congestive heart failure, plasma ouabain levels are said to be positively correlated with the severity of failure.

There are chemical and physiologic reasons to question these proposals (Kelly et al: Circulation, 1992). Even if the controversial evidence is replicated, much remains to be explained about the role of endogenous ouabain. From the observation that serum ouabain is increased in patients with heart failure, we can probably conclude that failure—at least in some patients—is not caused by primary ouabain deficiency. If ouabain is indeed synthesized in the patient with heart failure, does the continued progression of the disease to the point of requiring exogenous glycoside therapy represent an inadequate endogenous supply, development of tolerance, or some other alteration?

In the meantime, it appears that one more receptor may have a surprising endogenous ligand, and if this is the case, convergent evolution in plants, toads, and mammals may have been demonstrated.

---

tributes to the very long half-life of this agent. Renal impairment does not significantly prolong the half-life of digitoxin, so this drug might rarely be useful in patients with erratic or rapidly failing renal function. On the other hand, a variety of hepatic enzyme-inducing drugs (see Chapter 4) can reduce the blood level of digitoxin by accelerating its metabolism.

Ouabain must be given parenterally and was therefore used only for acute therapy and rarely for more than a few doses. It is metabolized very little and excreted primarily by the kidney.

Pharmacodynamics

Digitalis has multiple direct and indirect cardiovascular effects, with both therapeutic and toxic (arrhythmogenic) consequences. In addition, it has undesirable effects on the central nervous system and gut. A small direct renal (diuretic) effect has been demonstrated.

At the molecular level, all therapeutically useful cardiac glycosides inhibit Na^+/K^+ ATPase, the membrane-bound transporter often called the "sodium pump." Several different forms of this enzyme, which consists of α and β subunits, have been identified. The binding sites for Na^+, K^+, ATP, and digitalis all appear to reside on the α subunit. Different isoforms of the subunits have been identified (3 α and 2 β), thus providing for different isoforms of the complete enzyme with differing affinities for cardiac glycosides in various tissues. Very low concentrations of these drugs have occasionally been reported to *stimulate* the enzyme. In contrast, inhibition over most of the dose range has been extensively documented in all tissues studied. It is probable that this action is largely responsible for the therapeutic effect (positive inotropy) in the heart. Since the sodium pump is necessary for maintenance of normal resting potential in most excitable cells, it is likely that a portion of the toxicity of digitalis is also caused by this enzyme-inhibiting action. Other molecular-level effects of digitalis have been studied in the heart and are discussed below. The fact that the receptor for cardiac glycosides exists on the sodium pump has prompted investigators to propose that an endogenous "digitalis-like" agent must exist. (See box: Endogenous Cardiac Glycosides.)

A. Cardiac Effects: For clarity, the effects of digitalis on mechanical and electrical function are discussed separately, but it should be realized that these changes occur simultaneously.

1. Mechanical effects–The therapeutic action of cardiac glycosides on mechanical function is to increase the intensity of the interaction of the actin and myosin filaments of the cardiac sarcomere (Figure 13–1). This increased intensity is caused by an increase in the free calcium concentration in the vicinity of the contractile proteins during systole. The increase in calcium concentration is the result of a two-step process: first, an increase of intracellular sodium concentration because of Na^+/K^+ ATPase inhibition (*1* in Figure 13–1); and second, a relative reduction of calcium expulsion from the cell by the sodium-calcium exchanger (*2* in Figure 13–1) caused by the increase in intracellular sodium. Two other mechanisms have been proposed (but never widely accepted) that might complement this well-documented action: facilitation of calcium entry through the voltage-gated calcium channels of the membrane (*3* in Figure 13–1); and an independent effect on sarcoplasmic reticulum that results in increased release of calcium from this intracellular storage site (*5* in Figure 13–1).

The net result of the action of therapeutic concentrations of a cardiac glycoside is a distinctive increase in cardiac contractility (Figure 13–5, bottom trace). In isolated myocardial preparations, the rate of development of tension and of relaxation are both increased, with little or no change in time to peak tension. The duration of the contractile response is neither shortened (as in the case of beta-adrenoceptor stimulation) nor prolonged (as in the case of methylxanthines such as theophylline). These effects occur in both normal and failing myocardium, but in the intact animal or patient the responses are modified by cardiovascular reflexes and the pathophysiology of congestive heart failure.

2. Electrical effects–The effects of digitalis on the electrical properties of the heart in the intact subject are a mixture of direct and autonomic actions. Direct actions on the membranes of cardiac cells follow a well-defined progression: an early, brief prolongation of the action potential, followed by a protracted period of shortening (especially the plateau phase). This decrease in action potential duration is probably the result of increased potassium conductance that is caused by increased intracellular calcium. (See Chapter 14 for a discussion of the effects of ionic conductances on the action potential.) All of these effects can be observed in the absence of overt toxicity. Shortening of the action potential contributes to the shortening of atrial and ventricular refractoriness (Table 13–2).

With more toxic concentrations, resting membrane potential is reduced (made less negative) as a result of inhibition of the sodium pump and reduced intracellular potassium. As toxicity progresses, oscillatory depolarizing afterpotentials appear following normally evoked action potentials (Figure 13–5, panel B). The afterpotentials (also known as "delayed afterdepolarizations") are associated with overloading of the intracellular calcium stores and oscillations in the free intracellular calcium ion concentration. When below threshold, these afterpotentials may interfere with normal conduction because of the further

Figure 13–5. Effects of a cardiac glycoside, ouabain, on isolated cardiac tissue. The top tracing shows action potentials evoked during the control period, early in the "therapeutic" phase, and later, when toxicity is present. The middle tracing shows the light (L) emitted by the calcium-detecting protein aequorin (relative to the maximum possible, L_{max}) and is roughly proportionate to the free intracellular calcium concentration. The bottom tracing records the tension elicited by the action potentials. The early phase of ouabain action (**A**) shows a slight shortening of action potential and a marked increase in free intracellular calcium concentration and contractile tension. The toxic phase (**B**) is associated with depolarization of the resting potential, a marked shortening of the action potential, and the appearance of an oscillatory depolarization, calcium increment, and contraction (*arrows*). (Unpublished data kindly provided by P Hess and H Gil Wier.)

Table 13–2. Major actions of digitalis on cardiac electrical functions.
(PANS) = parasympathetic actions
(Direct) = direct membrane actions

	Tissue		
Variable	**Atrial Muscle**	**AV Node**	**Purkinje System, Ventricles**
Effective refractory period	↓ (PANS)	↑ (PANS)	↓ (Direct)
Conduction velocity	↑ (PANS)	↓ (PANS)	Negligible
Automaticity	↑ (Direct)	↑ (Direct)	↑(Direct)
Electrocardiogram Before arrhythmias	Negligible	↑ PR interval	↓ QT interval; T wave inversion; ST segment depression
During arrhythmias	Atrial tachycardia, atrial fibrillation	AV nodal tachycardia, AV blockade	Premature ventricular contractions, bigeminy, ventricular tachycardia, ventricular fibrillation

reduction of resting potential. Eventually, an afterpotential may reach threshold, eliciting an action potential (premature ventricular depolarization or "ectopic beat") that is coupled to the preceding normal one. If afterpotentials in the Purkinje conducting system regularly reach threshold in this way, bigeminy will be recorded on the ECG (Figure 13–6). With further toxic deterioration, each afterpotential-evoked action potential will itself elicit a suprathreshold afterpotential, and a self-sustaining arrhythmia (ventricular tachycardia) will be established. If allowed to progress, such a tachycardia may deteriorate into ventricular fibrillation.

Autonomic actions of cardiac glycosides on the heart involve both the parasympathetic and the sympathetic systems and occur throughout the therapeutic and toxic dose ranges. In the lower portion of the dose range, cardioselective **parasympathomimetic** effects predominate. In fact, these atropine-blockable effects

are responsible for a significant portion of the early electrical effects of digitalis (Table 13–2). This action involves sensitization of the baroreceptors, central vagal stimulation, and facilitation of muscarinic transmission at the cardiac muscle cell. Because cholinergic innervation is much richer in the atria, these actions affect atrial and atrioventricular nodal function more than Purkinje or ventricular function. Some of the cholinomimetic effects are useful in the treatment of certain arrhythmias. At toxic levels, sympathetic outflow is increased by digitalis. This effect is not essential for typical cardenolide toxicity but sensitizes the myocardium and exaggerates all the toxic effects of the drug.

The most common cardiac manifestations of glycoside toxicity include atrioventricular junctional rhythm, premature ventricular depolarizations, bigeminal rhythm, and second-degree atrioventricular blockade. However, it is claimed that digitalis can cause virtually every variety of arrhythmia. The membrane cardiotoxicity of digitalis was described above as involving resting depolarization (due to sodium pump inhibition) and oscillatory afterdepolarizations (caused by overload of intracellular calcium). Resting depolarization may be responsible for a portion of the conduction abnormalities such as atrioventricular block. Afterdepolarizations are probably responsible for most glycoside arrhythmias involving abnormal automaticity, including premature ventricular depolarizations, bigeminy, and ventricular tachycardia.

B. Effects on Other Organs: Cardiac glycosides affect all excitable tissues, including smooth muscle and the central nervous system. The mechanism of these effects has not been fully explored but probably involves the inhibition of Na+/K+ ATPase in these tissues. The lower sensitivity of noncardiac tissues presumably depends upon the different enzyme isoforms found in these tissues. The depolarization resulting from depression of the sodium pump would

Figure 13–6. ECG record showing digitalis-induced bigeminy. The complexes marked NSR are normal sinus rhythm beats; an inverted T wave and depressed ST segment are present. The complexes marked PVB are premature ventricular beats and are the electrocardiographic manifestations of depolarizations evoked by delayed oscillatory afterpotentials as shown in Figure 13–5. (Modified and reproduced, with permission, from Goldman MJ: *Principles of Clinical Electrocardiography,* 12th ed. Lange, 1986.)

be expected to increase spontaneous activity both in neurons and in smooth muscle cells. In addition, an increase in intracellular calcium could increase smooth muscle tone. This may occur when an intravenous dose of digoxin is given rapidly. However, it should be remembered that in most cases of congestive heart failure successfully treated with digitalis, a *decrease* in vascular tone is the net effect, resulting from a beneficial reduction of sympathetic tone (see below).

The gastrointestinal tract is the most common site of digitalis toxicity outside the heart. These actions include anorexia, nausea, vomiting, and diarrhea. This toxicity may be partially caused by direct effects on the gastrointestinal tract but is also the result of central nervous system actions, including chemoreceptor trigger zone stimulation.

Central nervous system effects commonly include vagal and chemoreceptor zone stimulation, as noted above. Much less often, disorientation and hallucinations—especially in the elderly—and visual disturbances are noted. The latter effect may include aberrations of color perception. Agitation and even convulsions are occasionally reported in patients taking digitalis.

Gynecomastia is a rare effect reported in men taking digitalis; it is not certain whether this effect represents a peripheral estrogenic action of these steroid drugs or a manifestation of hypothalamic stimulation.

ATPase-dependent transport processes such as production of aqueous humor and cerebrospinal fluid, as well as sodium reabsorption in the kidney, can be shown experimentally to be inhibited by cardiac glycosides. These effects are of no clinical significance.

C. Interactions With Potassium, Calcium, and Magnesium: The concentrations of potassium and calcium in the extracellular compartment (usually measured as serum K^+ and Ca^{2+}) have important effects on sensitivity to digitalis. Potassium and digitalis interact in two ways. First, they inhibit each other's binding to Na^+/K^+ ATPase; therefore, hyperkalemia reduces the enzyme-inhibiting actions of cardiac glycosides, whereas hypokalemia facilitates these actions. Second, abnormal cardiac automaticity is inhibited by hyperkalemia (see Chapter 14); thus, moderately increased extracellular K^+ reduces the effects of digitalis, especially the toxic effects. Calcium ion facilitates the toxic actions of cardiac glycosides by accelerating the overloading of intracellular calcium stores that appears to be responsible for digitalis-induced abnormal automaticity. Hypercalcemia therefore increases the risk of a digitalis-induced arrhythmia. The effects of magnesium ion appear to be directly opposite to those of calcium. Hypomagnesemia is therefore a risk factor for arrhythmias. These interactions mandate careful evaluation of serum electrolytes in patients with digitalis-induced arrhythmias.

OTHER POSITIVE INOTROPIC DRUGS USED IN HEART FAILURE

Drugs that inhibit **phosphodiesterases,** the family of enzymes that inactivate cAMP and cGMP, have long been used in therapy of heart failure. Although they have positive inotropic effects, most of their benefits appear to derive from vasodilation, as discussed below. Aminophylline, a traditional methylxanthine compound with some phosphodiesterase-inhibiting effects, was often used in the treatment of acute pulmonary edema. It is of no value in the treatment of chronic congestive heart failure and is rarely used for acute therapy now. Newer phosphodiesterase inhibitors have been intensively studied for several decades with mixed results. The bipyridines amrinone and milrinone are the most successful of these agents found to date, but their utility is quite limited. Clinical trials first suggested that vesnarinone, a drug with a mixed mechanism of action, may significantly lower the risk of death in patients with heart failure. However, the recent VEST trial was stopped because of an apparent increase in mortality with vesnarinone. (See box: Vesnarinone.) A group of beta-adrenoceptor stimulants have also been used as digitalis substitutes, but they may increase mortality (Xamoterol, 1990).

BIPYRIDINES

Amrinone and **milrinone** are bipyridine compounds that can be given orally or parenterally but are only available in parenteral forms. They have elimination half-lives of 2–3 hours, with 10–40% being excreted in the urine.

Pharmacodynamics

The bipyridines increase myocardial contractility without inhibiting Na^+/K^+ ATPase or activating adrenoceptors. They appear to increase inward calcium flux in the heart during the action potential and alter the intracellular movements of calcium by influencing the sarcoplasmic reticulum. They also have a significant vasodilating effect that undoubtedly contributes to their therapeutic benefits in heart failure. Biochemical studies suggest that most of their action results from inhibition of phosphodiesterase, an action similar to that of the methylxanthines. These drugs and several investigational phosphodiesterase inhibitors appear to be relatively selective for phosphodiesterase isozyme III, a form found in cardiac and smooth muscle. Inhibition of this isozyme results in an increase in cAMP and the increase in contractility and vasodilation noted above.

When given to patients in acute heart failure, the bipyridines increase cardiac output and reduce pulmonary capillary wedge pressure and peripheral vas-

VESNARINONE

The difficulty of developing effective new drugs for congestive heart failure is well illustrated by a newer agent.

Vesnarinone is an orally active quinolinone agent that has been shown to have several effects on isolated cardiac muscle, including inhibition of phosphodiesterase, increase in calcium current, and prolongation of the action potential duration. Each of these effects could, in theory, produce a significant inotropic effect (see Control of Cardiac Contractility, above), and phosphodiesterase inhibition may also cause vasodilation with useful unloading of the overworked ventricles. Several clinical trials with this agent (eg, Feldman et al, 1993) have suggested that it may significantly decrease morbidity and mortality for at least 25 weeks. The latter study also showed, however, that the therapeutic margin of safety is narrow, with 60 mg daily causing a *decrease* in mortality and 120 mg daily causing a significant *increase* in deaths. It is uncertain that any of the proposed mechanisms of therapeutic effect are produced at the lower dose. Unfortunately, the clinical benefits were not reproduced in the larger VEST trial.

These results reinforce the facts that once congestive failure has occurred, the heart is extremely vulnerable to excessive stimulation and that drugs which produce clinically useful increases in cardiac contractility are operating near the absolute limits of clinical safety. Positive inotropic drugs appear to be especially hazardous.

Vesnarinone is not available for general clinical use in the USA at present.

cular resistance. There is little change in the heart rate or arterial pressure. Although the acute effects are clearly beneficial in some patients, their toxicity prevents their long-term use.

The toxicity of amrinone includes a relatively high incidence of nausea and vomiting; thrombocytopenia and liver enzyme changes have been reported in a smaller but significant number of patients. This agent is used only for short-term parenteral treatment. It may be less likely to cause cardiac arrhythmias than is digitalis. Milrinone appears less likely to cause bone marrow and liver toxicity than amrinone, but it does cause arrhythmias. In a placebo-controlled trial in patients with severe congestive heart failure, oral milrinone increased mortality (Packer et al, 1991). Therefore, like amrinone, it is now used only intravenously and only for acute heart failure.

BETA-ADRENOCEPTOR STIMULANTS

The general pharmacology of these agents is discussed in Chapter 9. The search for positive inotropic drugs with less arrhythmogenic potential than digitalis and less tendency to increase heart rate than isoproterenol has led to the development of β_1-selective agents. At the same time, the successful use of vasodilators in congestive heart failure has resulted in an interest in selective β_2 agents for this condition.

The selective β_1 agonist that has been most widely used in patients with heart failure is **dobutamine.** This drug produces an increase in cardiac output together with a decrease in ventricular filling pressure. Some tachycardia and an increase in myocardial oxygen consumption have been reported. Thus, although dobutamine clearly increases cardiac contractility, it is unclear what net benefit it may have in patients with ischemic heart disease. The potential for producing angina or arrhythmias in such patients must be considered, as well as the tachyphylaxis that accompanies the use of any beta stimulant. Intermittent dobutamine infusion may benefit some patients with chronic heart failure.

A variety of other agents with effects at beta and dopamine adrenoceptors have been studied. Most of these, like dopamine and dobutamine, are not active orally, so they are reserved for management of acute failure or failure refractory to oral agents. At the present time, only dobutamine and dopamine are used in significant quantities.

DRUGS WITHOUT POSITIVE INOTROPIC EFFECTS USED IN HEART FAILURE

The drugs most commonly used in chronic heart failure are diuretics, cardiac glycosides, and angiotensin-converting enzyme inhibitors. In acute failure, diuretics and vasodilators play important roles. Thus, drugs without positive inotropic actions on the heart play a major role in therapy.

Diuretics

The diuretics are discussed in detail in Chapter 15. Their mechanism of action in heart failure is to reduce salt and water retention, thereby reducing ventricular preload. The reduction in venous pressure has two useful effects: reduction of edema and its symptoms and reduction of cardiac size, which leads to improved efficiency of pump function.

Angiotensin-Converting Enzyme Inhibitors

The ACE inhibitors are introduced in Chapter 11 and discussed again in Chapter 17. Because of the per-

---

REDUCED SURVIVAL WITH POTENT POSITIVE INOTROPIC DRUGS

A number of potent inotropic agents have been shown to improve myocardial contractility when given acutely. Their effects include an increase in cardiac output, a reduction in left atrial pressure, a reduction in symptoms, and an improvement in exercise tolerance. When given chronically, however, several potent inotropic agents have been shown to reduce survival in placebo-controlled trials. The list includes milrinone (Packer et al, 1991), xamoterol (Xamoterol, 1990), enoximone (Uretsky et al, 1990), imazodan (Goldberg et al, 1990), flosequinan, and vesnarinone (see box: Vesnarinone). This adverse experience with potent inotropic agents seems to involve drugs that increase cAMP. It is now known that a drug which works by a different mechanism (digitalis) has a neutral effect on mortality (DIG Trial). We do not yet know what effects pimobendan (a calcium sensitizer) will have.

---

vasive involvement of angiotensin II in the undesirable compensatory responses to failure (Figure 13–2), reduction of this peptide has several positive effects on the course of the disease. These versatile drugs reduce peripheral resistance and thereby reduce afterload; they also reduce salt and water retention (by reducing aldosterone secretion) and in that way reduce preload. The reduction in tissue angiotensin levels also reduces sympathetic activity, probably through diminution of angiotensin's presynaptic effects on norepinephrine release. Finally, these drugs reduce the long-term remodeling of the heart and vessels, an effect that may be responsible for the observed reduction in mortality and morbidity. These agents are now usually considered ahead of digitalis in the treatment of chronic failure (see Clinical Pharmacology). Losartan and similar angiotensin receptor blockers (see Chapter 11) might be expected to have similar beneficial effects, but this remains to be documented.

Vasodilators

The vasodilators are effective in acute heart failure because they provide a reduction in preload (through venodilation), or reduction in afterload (through arteriolar dilation), or both. Some evidence suggests that long-term use of hydralazine and isosorbide dinitrate can also reduce damaging remodeling of the heart.

Beta-Adrenoceptor Blockers

Beta blockers are correctly considered dangerous in patients with congestive heart failure because they may precipitate acute decompensation of cardiac function. Therefore, it may come as a surprise that some patients respond favorably to these drugs. Evidence for this paradoxic effect began to appear many years ago but was initially considered to be limited to patients with diastolic dysfunction or cardiomyopathies, in whom slowing of cardiac rate and contraction velocity could improve cardiac output. More recent studies suggest a wider role for these drugs (Packer et al, 1996). A full understanding of the beneficial action of beta blockade is lacking, but suggested mechanisms include up-regulation of beta receptors, decreased heart rate, and reduced remodeling through inhibition of the mitogenic activity of catecholamines.

II. CLINICAL PHARMACOLOGY OF DRUGS USED IN CONGESTIVE HEART FAILURE

As the result of a remarkable number of large and sophisticated clinical trials in the last decade, the treatment of chronic congestive heart failure has undergone a radical reevaluation and considerable revision. Before these trials, prescription of a diuretic plus digitalis was almost automatic in every case of chronic congestive heart failure, and other drugs were rarely considered. At present, diuretics are still considered as first-line therapy, but other drugs (especially ACE inhibitors) are often considered before digitalis.

DIGITALIS IN CONGESTIVE HEART FAILURE

Because it has a moderate but persistent positive inotropic effect, digitalis can, in theory, reverse the signs and symptoms of congestive heart failure. In an appropriate patient, digitalis increases stroke work and cardiac output. The increased output (and possibly a direct action resetting the sensitivity of the baroreceptors) eliminates the stimuli evoking increased sympathetic outflow, and both heart rate and vascular tone diminish. With decreased end-diastolic fiber tension (the result of increased systolic ejection and decreased filling pressure), heart size and oxygen demand decrease. Finally, increased renal blood flow improves glomerular filtration and reduces aldosterone-driven sodium reabsorption. Thus, edema fluid can be excreted, further reducing ventricular preload and the danger of pulmonary edema. However, the apparent lack of ability to alter long-term mortality (Digitalis Investigation Group, 1997) suggests that digitalis is unable to maintain these effects over long periods and that other aspects of heart failure, eg, remodeling, are extremely important in the progression of the disease.

Administration & Dosage

Chronic treatment with digitalis agents requires careful attention to pharmacokinetics because of their long half-lives (Table 13–3). According to the rules set forth in Chapter 3, it will take three to four half-lives to approach steady-state total body load when given at a constant dosing rate, ie, approximately 1 week for digoxin and 1 month for digitoxin. Since it is very important not to exceed the therapeutic range of plasma digitalis concentration, such a slow approach to "digitalization" is the safest dosing technique. If a more rapid effect is required, digitalization can be achieved quickly with a large loading dose (divided into three or four portions and given over 24–36 hours) followed by maintenance doses. Typical doses used in adults are given in Table 13–3. A parenteral preparation of digoxin is available but is not used to achieve a faster onset of effect because the time to peak effect is determined mainly by time-dependent ion changes in the tissue. Thus, the parenteral preparation is only suitable for patients who cannot take drugs by mouth. It is essential that the patient be examined before each dose when using the rapid (three-dose) method of digitalization. Sensitive plasma digoxin assays are available at most medical centers and should be used when patient response is not as predicted from the dosing schedule.

Interactions

Important drug interactions must be considered in patients taking cardiac glycosides. All such patients are at risk of developing serious cardiac arrhythmias if hypokalemia develops, as in diuretic therapy or diarrhea. Furthermore, patients taking digoxin are at risk if given quinidine, which displaces digoxin from tissue binding sites (a minor effect) and depresses renal digoxin clearance (a major effect). The plasma level of the glycoside may double within a few days after beginning quinidine therapy, and toxic effects may become manifest. A similar interaction with other drugs, including nonsteroidal anti-inflammatory

agents and calcium channel-blocking agents, has been reported, but clinically significant effects have not been demonstrated in humans. Quinidine does not alter volume of distribution or protein binding of digitoxin. However, it may prolong the half-life of this glycoside. As noted above, antibiotics that alter gastrointestinal flora may increase digoxin bioavailability in about 10% of patients. Finally, agents that release catecholamines may sensitize the myocardium to digitalis-induced arrhythmias.

Reduced responsiveness to cardiac glycosides may be due to intractably severe disease or patient non-compliance. In patients concurrently taking cholestyramine (see Chapter 35), digitalis absorption is reduced. The digitalis dose required for therapeutic effect must be increased in most hyperthyroid patients because of reduction in elimination half-life.

Other Clinical Uses of Digitalis

Digitalis is useful in the management of atrial arrhythmias because of its cardioselective parasympathomimetic effects. In atrial flutter, the depressant effect of the drug on atrioventricular conduction will help control an excessively high ventricular rate. The effects of the drug on the atrial musculature may convert flutter to fibrillation, with a further decrease in ventricular rate. In atrial fibrillation, the same vagomimetic action helps control ventricular rate, thereby improving ventricular filling and increasing cardiac output. Digitalis has also been used in the control of paroxysmal atrial and atrioventricular nodal tachycardia. Oral or, if necessary, cautious intravenous administration of digoxin may abruptly terminate such attacks, probably as the result of its vagomimetic action. The availability of calcium channel blockers and adenosine has reduced the popularity of digoxin in this application.

Although it has been recommended in the past, digitalis is not the drug of choice in the therapy of arrhythmias associated with Wolff-Parkinson-White syndrome, because it increases the probability of conduction of arrhythmic atrial impulses through the alternative rapidly conducting atrioventricular pathway. It is explicitly contraindicated in patients with Wolff-Parkinson-White syndrome and atrial fibrillation (see Chapter 14).

Toxicity

In spite of its recognized hazards, digitalis toxicity is common. In a large multicenter study, 17–27% of patients admitted for all medical conditions were taking digitalis on admission, and 5–25% of the identified group showed evidence of toxicity requiring at least temporary cessation of digitalis therapy.

Therapy of digitalis toxicity manifested as visual changes or gastrointestinal disturbances generally requires no more than reducing the dose of the drug. If cardiac arrhythmia is present and can definitely be ascribed to digitalis, more vigorous therapy may be nec-

Table 13–3. Clinical use of cardiac glycosides.[1]

	Digoxin	Digitoxin
Half-life	40 hours	168 hours
Therapeutic plasma concentration	0.5–1.5 ng/mL	10–25 ng/mL
Toxic plasma concentration	> 2 ng/mL	> 35 ng/mL
Daily dose (slow loading or maintenance)	0.125–0.5 mg	0.05–0.2 mg
Rapid digitalizing dose	0.5–0.75 mg every 8 hours for three doses	0.2–0.4 mg every 12 hours for three doses

[1]These values are appropriate for adults with normal renal and hepatic function.

essary. Serum digitalis and potassium levels and the ECG should always be monitored during therapy of significant digitalis toxicity. Electrolyte status should be corrected if abnormal (see above). For patients who do not respond promptly (within one to two half-lives), calcium and magnesium as well as potassium levels should be checked. For occasional premature ventricular depolarizations or brief runs of bigeminy, oral potassium supplementation and withdrawal of the glycoside may be sufficient. If the arrhythmia is more serious, parenteral potassium and antiarrhythmic drugs may be required. Of the available antiarrhythmic agents, lidocaine is favored.

In very severe digitalis intoxication (which usually involves suicidal overdose), serum potassium will already be elevated at the time of diagnosis (because of potassium loss from the intracellular compartment of skeletal muscle and other tissues). Furthermore, automaticity is usually depressed, and antiarrhythmic agents administered in this setting may lead to cardiac arrest. Such patients are best treated with insertion of a temporary cardiac pacemaker catheter and administration of digitalis antibodies. These antibodies are produced in sheep, and although they are raised to digoxin they also recognize digitoxin and other cardiac glycosides. They are extremely useful in reversing severe intoxication with most glycosides.

Digitalis-induced arrhythmias are frequently made worse by cardioversion; this therapy should be reserved for ventricular fibrillation if the arrhythmia is glycoside-induced.

MANAGEMENT OF CHRONIC HEART FAILURE

The major steps in the management of patients with chronic heart failure are outlined in Table 13–4. Reduction of cardiac work is a traditional form of therapy that is extremely helpful in most cases. It can be accomplished by reducing activity levels, weight reduction, and—especially important—control of hypertension. Sodium restriction is the next important step. Despite the availability of efficacious diuretics, one should advise patients about the necessity for salt restriction and encourage them to avoid excess salt through dietary restraint.

If edema is present, a diuretic is usually required. It is reasonable to start with a thiazide diuretic, switching to more powerful agents as required. The loop diuretics are very efficacious agents that should be reserved for patients with resistant edema. Sodium loss causes secondary loss of potassium, which is particularly hazardous if the patient is to be given digitalis. Therefore, serum electrolytes should be checked periodically in patients so treated. Hypokalemia can be treated with potassium supplementation or through the addition of a potassium-sparing diuretic (see Chapter 15).

If reduction of cardiac work and diuresis are inadequate, either an ACE inhibitor or digoxin (or both) will be added. It should be emphasized that only about 50% of patients with normal sinus rhythm (usually those with documented *systolic* dysfunction) will have documentable relief of congestive failure. Better results are obtained in patients with atrial fibrillation. If the decision is made to use a cardiac glycoside, digoxin is the one chosen in the great majority of cases. When symptoms are mild, slow digitalization (Table 13–3) is safer and just as effective as the rapid method. If symptoms are moderately severe, the rapid oral method may be used, but the patient should be examined before each dose with particular attention to the cardiac rhythm. An ECG should be recorded if there is any doubt about the nature of the pretherapy rhythm or changes during digitalization. Intravenous digitalization is rarely required in chronic heart failure; it should be used only in hospitalized patients with careful monitoring.

A recent large mortality trial with digoxin (DIG Study; Digitalis Investigation Group, 1997) showed no increase or decrease in mortality compared with placebo. Digoxin did reduce the hospitalization rate and the number of deaths from progressive heart failure.

Determining the optimal level of digitalis effect may be difficult. In patients with atrial fibrillation, reduction of ventricular rate is the best measure of glycoside effect. In patients in normal sinus rhythm, symptomatic improvement and reductions in heart size, heart rate during exercise, venous pressure, or edema may signify optimum drug levels in the myocardium. Unfortunately, toxic effects may occur before the therapeutic end point is detected. If slow digitalization is being employed, simple omission of one dose and halving the maintenance dose will often bring the patient to the narrow range between suboptimal and toxic concentrations. Measurement of plasma digoxin levels is useful in patients who appear unusually resistant or sensitive; a level of 1.1 ng/mL or less is appropriate.

Vasodilator drugs (including ACE inhibitors) are very useful agents in chronic congestive heart failure. A useful classification divides the drugs into selective

---

Table 13–4. Steps in the treatment of chronic heart failure.

1. Reduce workload of the heart
   a. Limit activity level
   b. Reduce weight
   c. Control hypertension
2. Restrict sodium
3. Restrict water (rarely required)
4. Give diuretics
5. Give ACE inhibitor and digitalis[1]
6. Give vasodilators

[1]Many clinicians use angiotensin-converting enzyme inhibitors before digitalis.

arteriolar dilators, venous dilators, and drugs with nonselective vasodilatory effects (Table 13–5). The choice of agent should be based on the patient's signs and symptoms and hemodynamic measurements. Thus, in patients with high filling pressures in whom the principal symptom is dyspnea, the venous dilators will be most helpful in reducing filling pressures and the symptoms of pulmonary congestion. In patients in whom fatigue due to low left ventricular output is a primary symptom, an arteriolar dilator may be helpful in increasing forward cardiac output. In most patients with severe chronic failure that responds poorly to other therapy, the problem usually involves both elevated filling pressures and reduced cardiac output. In these circumstances, dilation of both arterioles and veins is required. In the V-HEFT trial, combined therapy with hydralazine (arteriolar dilation) and isosorbide dinitrate (venous dilation) prolonged life more than placebo in patients already receiving digitalis and diuretics (Cohn et al, 1986).

In a study comparing digoxin and captopril as first-line therapy for chronic heart failure, both agents produced similar effects (Captopril-Digoxin Multicenter Research Group, 1988). Several large studies have compared enalapril with placebo or with other vasodilators (CONSENSUS, 1987; SOLVD Investigators, 1991; Cohn et al, 1991). These studies suggest that angiotensin-converting enzyme inhibitors are superior to both placebo and other vasodilators and must be considered as first-line agents, together with diuretics and digitalis, for the treatment of chronic congestive heart failure. However, patients who are stable while receiving diuretics, digoxin, and angiotensin-converting enzyme inhibitors may deteriorate if digoxin is withdrawn, suggesting that the angiotensin-converting enzyme inhibitors cannot completely replace digitalis in these individuals (Packer et al, 1993).

Two recent studies suggest that angiotensin-converting enzyme inhibitors are also valuable in asymptomatic patients with ventricular dysfunction (Pfeffer et al, 1992; SOLVD Investigators, 1992). By reducing preload and afterload, these drugs appear to slow the rate of ventricular dilation and thus delay the onset of clinical congestive heart failure. Angiotensin-converting enzyme inhibitors thus are beneficial in all subsets of patients, from those who are asymptomatic to those in severe chronic failure.

It appears that all ACE inhibitors tested to date have beneficial effects in patients with chronic heart failure.

Recent studies have documented these beneficial effects with lisinopril, quinapril, and ramipril (Garg et al, 1995). Thus, this benefit appears to be a class effect.

The angiotensin II receptor antagonists (eg, losartan) produce beneficial hemodynamic effects similar to those of the ACE inhibitors. In a recent trial (Pitt et al, 1997), losartan even reduced mortality more than captopril in elderly patients with heart failure.

Many trials have evaluated beta-blocker therapy in patients with heart failure. The rationale is based on the hypothesis that excessive tachycardia and adverse effects of high catecholamine levels on the heart contribute to the downward course of heart failure patients. However, such therapy must be initiated very cautiously at low doses, since acutely blocking the supportive effects of catecholamines can worsen heart failure. Potential improvement is only seen after several months of therapy and consists of a slight rise in ejection fraction, slower heart rate, and reduction in symptoms (Waagstein et al, 1993). The beta-blockers with associated vasodilator activity such as bucindolol, carvedilol (Packer, 1996), nebirolol, celiprolol, and labetalol appear to be especially promising.

The calcium blocking drugs appear in general to have no role in the treatment of patients with heart failure. Their depressive effects on the heart may worsen heart failure. However, in the PRAISE Trial (O'Connor et al, 1995), amlodipine decreased mortality in patients with dilated cardiomyopathy who were on standard therapy consisting of digoxin, diuretics, and an ACE inhibitor. There was no benefit or harm to patients whose heart failure was due to coronary artery disease. Amlodipine is representative of several new vasoselective dihydropyridine calcium blockers, which primarily vasodilate but have minimal effects on the myocardium (Chapter 12). Additional studies are required to put this class of drugs in perspective.

MANAGEMENT OF ACUTE HEART FAILURE

Acute heart failure occurs frequently in patients with chronic failure. Such episodes are usually associated with increased exertion, emotion, salt in the diet, noncompliance with medical therapy, or increased metabolic demand occasioned by fever, anemia, etc. A particularly common and important cause of acute failure—with or without chronic failure—is acute myocardial infarction. Many of the signs and symptoms of acute and chronic failure are identical, but their therapies diverge because of the need for more rapid response and the relatively greater frequency and severity of pulmonary vascular congestion in the acute form.

Because of the need for rapid recognition and evaluation of changing hemodynamic status, it is much more important to obtain quantitative measurements in acute failure than in chronic failure. These measurements should include left ventricular filling pressure (pulmonary wedge pressure) and cardiac output in addition

Table 13–5. Vasodilators for use in congestive heart failure.

Drugs	Site of Dilating Action
Hydralazine, minoxidil	Arterioles
Nitrates	Veins and venules
Captopril and other ACE inhibitors	Both arterioles and veins

to heart rate and blood pressure. The stroke work index (approximately stroke volume index times arterial pressure) is a useful derived variable that estimates the external work performed by the left ventricle.

Measurements of stroke work index and pulmonary capillary wedge pressure from a large group of patients with acute myocardial infarction are illustrated in Figure 13–3. When filling pressure is greater than 15 mm Hg and stroke work index is less than 20 g-m/m², the mortality rate is high. Intermediate levels of these two variables imply a much better prognosis. It is apparent, therefore, that the effects of myocardial infarction on ventricular function are not uniform and that there can be no single standard therapy for the management of congestive failure in this condition.

Subsets of Patients Following Myocardial Infarction

Patients with acute congestive failure following myocardial infarction can be usefully characterized on the basis of three hemodynamic measurements: arterial pressure, left ventricular filling pressure, and cardiac index. One such classification is illustrated in Table 13–6.

(1) Hypovolemia: Subset 1 includes patients who are relatively hypovolemic following myocardial infarction as a result of diuretics or inadequate fluid intake. The primary hemodynamic abnormality is a low left ventricular filling pressure, which can be corrected by giving fluids. With an increase of filling pressure up to the optimal range of 15 mm Hg (Figure 13–7), hypotension often disappears and cardiac output increases.

(2) Pulmonary congestion: The second subset—patients with severe pulmonary congestion and dyspnea—is a very large one and is also representative

Figure 13–7. Effects of vasodilator therapy on left ventricular function. The dose is chosen to reduce filling pressure by 5 mm Hg. With the administration of a combined arteriolar dilator and venous dilator such as nitroprusside, function is shifted to a higher curve, reflecting the decreased impedance to ventricular ejection. However, the effect on stroke volume will depend on the initial filling pressure. A patient in heart failure with an initial filling pressure of 20 mm Hg will experience an increase in stroke volume along line *A*, up and to the left. If the patient was initially at a filling pressure of 10 mm Hg, nitroprusside would still shift performance to the upper curve, but this would result in a decrease of performance, along line *B*. (Reproduced, with permission, from Chatterjee K, Parmley WW: The role of vasodilator therapy in heart failure. Prog Cardiovasc Dis 1977;19:305.)

of other causes of acute heart failure. Diuretics are helpful in such patients because they reduce intravascular volume. In addition, when given intravenously, powerful diuretics such as furosemide produce an immediate increase in compliance of systemic veins. This leads to peripheral pooling of blood, which re-

Table 13–6. Therapeutic classification of subsets in acute myocardial infarction.[1]

Subset	Systolic Arterial Pressure (mm Hg)	Left Ventricular Filling Pressure (mm Hg)	Cardiac Index (L/min/m²)	Therapy
1. Hypovolemia	< 100	< 10	< 2.5	Volume replacement
2. Pulmonary congestion	100–150	> 20	> 2.5	Diuretics
3. Peripheral vasodilation	< 100	10–20	> 2.5	None, or vasoactive drugs
4. Power failure	< 100	> 20	< 2.5	Vasodilators, inotropic drugs
5. Severe shock	< 90	> 20	< 2.0	Vasoactive drugs, inotropic drugs, vasodilators, circulatory assist
6. Right ventricular infarct	< 100	RVFP > 10 LVFP < 15	< 2.5	Provide volume replacement for LVFP, inotropic drugs. Avoid diuretics.
7. Mitral regurgitation, ventricular septal defect	< 100	> 20	< 2.5	Vasodilators, inotropic drugs, circulatory assist, surgery

[1]The numerical values are intended to serve as general guidelines and not as absolute cutoff points. Arterial pressures apply to patients who were previously normotensive and should be adjusted upward for patients who were previously hypertensive. (RVFP and LVFP = right and left ventricular filling pressure.)

duces central blood volume and decreases right and left ventricular filling pressures. Morphine sulfate also is clinically effective in the management of acute pulmonary edema. Apart from its ability to relieve the pain of infarction, the mechanisms by which it reduces pulmonary congestion are uncertain. If bronchospasm is a prominent component of the pulmonary signs, aminophylline may also be helpful, since it combines bronchodilator, vasodilator, and positive inotropic actions (Chapter 20).

(3) Peripheral vasodilation: The third subset of patients are hypotensive and yet have warm extremities because of peripheral vasodilation. These patients may not need any therapy, since pulmonary wedge pressure is usually normal and cardiac output satisfactory. If blood pressure is extremely low, however, a vasoactive drug such as dopamine should be considered to maintain arterial perfusion pressure at the desired level.

(4) "Power failure": The fourth subset represents those patients who have a reduction in arterial pressure, though not to shock levels, together with an elevation of left ventricular filling pressure and a reduction of cardiac index. The goal of therapy in these patients is to increase cardiac output and reduce ventricular filling pressure without a further decrease in arterial pressure. Diuretics or nitrates are helpful in lowering filling pressures but will not increase cardiac output. A combined venous and arteriolar dilator such as nitroprusside is extremely beneficial in such patients. Its venodilating effects reduce right and left atrial pressures by redistributing more blood into the periphery. Its arteriolar dilating properties increase forward cardiac output by reducing systemic vascular resistance. The main limiting factor in the use of nitroprusside is the reduction in arterial pressure. If the dose is titrated carefully, however, this reduction in blood pressure may be minimized. A good rule of thumb is to consider giving nitroprusside if the systolic pressure is 90 mm Hg or higher. The effects of nitroprusside depend on the level of left ventricular filling pressure. This is illustrated diagrammatically in Figure 13–7. The middle curve in the figure represents a patient with moderately severe heart failure. If the patient has a high left ventricular filling pressure (20 mm Hg), the administration of sodium nitroprusside will shift ventricular function up and to the left, as illustrated by line A. If, however, the patient has been given large doses of diuretics and filling pressure has thereby been reduced to 10 mm Hg, nitroprusside will produce a different result. Although the patient moves to the upper curve with nitroprusside (line B), there is a reduction of stroke volume because the heart is on the steep ascending limb of the curve. This will worsen hypotension and tachycardia. If the patient is now volume-loaded to the optimal filling pressure of 15 mm Hg, the beneficial effect of nitroprusside will become evident. This example illustrates the importance of filling pressure: pul-

monary wedge pressure should be maintained at about 15 mm Hg by either diuresis or volume administration, as required.

(5) Severe shock: Subset 5 represents a group of patients with cardiogenic shock following myocardial infarction. These patients have very low arterial pressures, very high filling pressures, and low cardiac indices. Although diuretics may be helpful in lowering the elevated filling pressures, they will not increase cardiac output. Furthermore, the use of vasodilators in these patients is difficult, since the accompanying hypotension may be severe and may impair perfusion of vital organs. Since the mortality rate under these circumstances is high, it is often difficult to know whether any therapy is beneficial. Nevertheless, certain approaches may be helpful. If the arterial pressure is extremely low, it is useful to consider use of a catecholamine such as dopamine. By titrating the dose of this drug, one can produce an increase in arterial pressure that is adequate for peripheral tissue perfusion. At this point, one can cautiously add nitroprusside to lower pulmonary wedge pressure. The combined effects of these two agents on the heart tend to be additive, since they work through different mechanisms. Dopamine directly increases cardiac contractility, while nitroprusside produces venous and arteriolar dilation. The addition of inotropic agents such as amrinone or dobutamine may also be useful. This therapy should be combined with an attempt to optimize left ventricular filling pressure. These patients are also candidates for circulatory assist measures (intra-aortic balloon) and consideration of cardiac catheterization and possible revascularization.

(6) Right ventricular infarction: Group 6 comprises a subset of patients who have an inferior myocardial infarction that predominantly involves the right ventricle. Their hypotension is due to the fact that the right ventricle is unable to deliver sufficient blood to the left side of the heart to optimize left ventricular filling pressure and cardiac output. Therefore, the primary therapeutic goal is to optimize left ventricular filling pressure. This may require volume infusion despite elevated central venous pressure. One should avoid using diuretics, since reduction of volume may lead to further reduction of filling pressure with associated hypotension and tachycardia. Inotropic agents may be useful.

(7) Mitral regurgitation and ventricular septal defect: A seventh subset is mentioned for completeness, though these patients are also found in other subsets, particularly those with shock. These are patients with mechanical abnormalities such as acute severe mitral regurgitation or a ruptured interventricular septum. Depending on the severity of the defect, cardiac surgery must be considered urgently as the most definitive form of therapy. However, vasodilator therapy such as nitroprusside may be necessary to stabilize the patient before surgery is possible.

PREPARATIONS AVAILABLE
(Diuretics: See Chapter 15.)

Digitalis
  Digitoxin (Crystodigin)
    Oral: 0.05, 0.1 mg tablets
  Digoxin (generic, Lanoxicaps, Lanoxin)
    Oral: 0.125, 0.25, 0.5 mg tablets; 0.05, 0.1, 0.2 mg capsules; 0.05 mg/mL elixir
    Parenteral: 0.1, 0.25 mg/mL for injection

Digitalis Antibody
  Digoxin immune fab (ovine) (Digibind)
    Parenteral: 38 mg per vial with 75 mg sorbitol lyophilized powder to reconstitute for IV injection. Each vial will bind approximately 0.5 mg digoxin or digitoxin.

Sympathomimetics Most Commonly Used in Congestive Heart Failure
  Dobutamine (generic, Dobutrex)
    Parenteral: 250 mg/20 mL for IV infusion
  Dopamine (generic, Intropin)
    Parenteral: 40, 80, 160 mg/mL for IV injection; 80, 160, 320 mg/dL for IV infusion

Angiotensin-Converting Enzyme Inhibitors Labeled for Use in Congestive Heart Failure
  Captopril (Capoten)
    Oral: 12.5, 25, 50, 100 mg tablets
  Enalapril (Vasotec)
    Oral: 2.5, 5, 10, 20 mg tablets
  Fosinopril (Monopril)
    Oral: 10, 20 mg tablets
  Lisinopril (Prinivil, Zestril)
    Oral: 5, 10, 20, 40 mg tablets
  Quinipril (Accupril)
    Oral: 5, 10, 20, 40 mg tablets
  Ramipril (Altace)
    Oral: 1.25, 2.5, 5, 10 mg capsules

Other Drugs Labeled Only for Use in Congestive Heart Failure
  Amrinone (Inocor)
    Parenteral: 5 mg/mL for IV injection
  Milrinone (Primacor)
    Parenteral: 1 mg/mL for IV injection; 200 μg/mL premixed for IV infusion

REFERENCES

Basic Pharmacology

Blaustein MP: Physiological effects of endogenous ouabain: Control of intracellular Ca^{2+} stores and cell responsiveness. Am J Physiol 1993;264:C1367.

Doherty JE: Clinical use of digitalis glycosides. Cardiology 1985;72:225.

Hickey AR et al: Digoxin immune Fab therapy in the management of digitalis intoxication: Safety and efficacy results of an observational surveillance study. J Am Coll Cardiol 1991;17:590.

Hoey A et al: Inotropic actions of BDF 9148 and DPI 201-106 and their enantiomers in guinea-pig, rat and human atria. Eur J Pharmacol 1993;231:477.

Katz AM: Effects of digitalis on cell biochemistry: Sodium pump inhibition. J Am Coll Cardiol 1985;5(Suppl A):16A.

Kelly RA, Smith TW: Is ouabain the endogenous digitalis? (Editorial comment.) Circulation 1992;86:694.

Kelly RA, Smith TW: Recognition and management of digitalis toxicity. Am J Cardiol 1992;69:108G.

Lee JA, Allen DG: EMD 53998 sensitizes the contractile proteins to calcium in intact ferret ventricular muscle. Circ Res 1991;69:927.

LeGrand B, et al: Stimulatory effect of ouabain on T- and L-type calcium currents in guinea pig cardiac myocytes. Am J Physiol 1990;258:H1620.

Lindenbaum J et al: Inactivation of digoxin by the gut flora: Reversal by antibiotic therapy. N Engl J Med 1981; 305:789.

Perrault CL et al: Differential inotropic effects of flosequinan in ventricular muscle from normal ferrets versus patients with end-stage heart failure. Br J Pharmacol 1992;106:511.

Rodin SM, Johnson BF: Pharmacokinetic interactions with digoxin. Clin Pharmacokinet 1988;15:227.

Smith TW: Digitalis: Mechanisms of action and clinical use. N Engl J Med 1988;318:358.

Solaro RJ et al: Stereoselective actions of thiadiazinones on canine cardiac myocytes and myofilaments. Circ Res 1993;73:481.

Sonnenblick EH (editor): A symposium: The role of phosphodiesterase III inhibitors in contemporary cardiovascular medicine. Am J Cardiol 1989;63(2). (Entire issue.)

Sweadner KJ: Multiple digitalis receptors. A molecular perspective. Trends Cardiovasc Med 1993;3:2.

Vemuri R, Longoni S, Philipson KD: Ouabain treatment of cardiac cells induces enhanced Na^+-Ca^{2+} exchange activity. Am J Physiol 1989;256:C1273.

Wenger TL et al: Treatment of 63 severely digitalis-toxic patients with digoxin-specific antibody fragments. J Am Coll Cardiol 1985;5(Suppl A):118A.

Zimmermann N et al: Positive inotropic effects of the calcium sensitizer CGP 48506 in guinea pig myocardium. J Pharmacol Exp Ther 1996;277:1572.

Pathophysiology of Heart Failure

Ferguson DW: Digitalis and neurohormonal abnormalities in heart failure and implications for therapy. Am J Cardiol 1992;69:24G.

Francis GS, Cohn JN: Heart failure: Mechanisms of cardiac and vascular dysfunction and the rationale for pharmacologic intervention. FASEB J 1990;4:3068.

Goto A, Yamada K, Sugimoto T: Endogenous digitalis: Reality or myth? Life Sci 1991;48:2109.

Grossmann W: Diastolic dysfunction and congestive heart failure. Circulation 1990;81(Suppl III):III–1.

Katz AM: The cardiomyopathy of overload: An unnatural growth response in the hypertrophied heart. Ann Intern Med 1994;121:363.

Parmley WW: Pathophysiology and therapy of congestive heart failure. J Am Coll Cardiol 1989;13:771.

Rahimtoola SH: The pharmacologic treatment of chronic congestive heart failure. Circulation 1989;80:693.

Swan HJ, Parmley WW: Congestive heart failure. In: *Pathologic Physiology,* 7th ed. Sodeman WA Jr, Sodeman TM (editors). Saunders, 1985.

van Zwieten PA: Compensatory mechanisms associated with congestive heart failure as targets for drug treatment. Prog Pharmacol Clinical Pharmacol 1990;7:49.

Acute Myocardial Infarction

Califf RM, Bengtson JR: Cardiogenic shock. N Engl J Med 1994;330:1724.

Hennekens CH et al: Adjunctive drug therapy of acute myocardial infarction: Evidence from clinical trials. N Engl J Med 1996;335:1660.

Parmley W, Chatterjee K: Evaluation of cardiac function in the coronary care unit. In: *Acute Myocardial Infarction.* Donoso E, Lipski J (editors). Stratton Intercontinental, 1978.

Pasternak RC, Braunwald E, Sobel BE: Acute myocardial infarction. In: *Heart Disease,* 3rd ed. Braunwald E (editor). Saunders, 1987.

Shah PK, Swan HJC: Complications of acute myocardial infarction. In: *Cardiology.* Parmley WW, Chatterjee K (editors). Lippincott, 1988.

Verma SP et al: Modulation of inotropic therapy by venodilation in acute heart failure: A randomised comparison of four inotropic agents, alone and combined with isosorbide dinitrate. J Cardiovasc Pharmacol 1992;19:24.

Chronic Heart Failure

Brodde O-E: β_1- and β_2-adrenoceptors in the human heart: Properties, function, and alterations in chronic heart failure. Pharmacol Rev 1991;43:203.

Captopril-Digoxin Multicenter Research Group: Comparative effects of therapy with captopril and digoxin of patients with mild to moderate heart failure. JAMA 1988;259:539.

Cavero PG et al: Flosequinan, a new vasodilator: Systemic and coronary hemodynamics and neuroendocrine effects in congestive heart failure. J Am Coll Cardiol 1992; 20:1542.

Chatterjee K: Digitalis, catecholamines, and other positive inotropic agents. In: *Cardiology.* Parmley WW, Chatterjee K (editors). Lippincott, 1988.

Cheitlin MD: Digitalis: Is it useful in congestive heart failure in patients in normal sinus rhythm? Cardiology 1987;74:376.

Cohn JN et al: A comparison of enalapril with hydralazine-isosorbide dinitrate in the treatment of chronic congestive heart failure. N Engl J Med 1991;325:303.

Cohn JN: The management of chronic heart failure. N Engl J Med 1996;335:490.

CONSENSUS Trial Study Group: Effects of enalapril on mortality in severe congestive heart failure. N Engl J Med 1987;316:1429.

DiBianco R et al: A comparison of oral milrinone, digoxin, and their combination in the treatment of patients with chronic heart failure. N Engl J Med 1989;320:677.

Digitalis Investigation Group: The effect of digoxin on mortality and morbidity in patients with heart failure. N Engl J Med 1997;336:525

Feldman AM et al: Effects of vesnarinone on morbidity and mortality in patients with heart failure. N Engl J Med 1993;329:149.

Fonarow GC et al: Effect of direct vasodilation with hydralazine versus angiotensin-converting enzyme inhibition with captopril on mortality in advanced heart failure: The Hy-C Trial. J Am Coll Cardiol 1992;19:842.

Francis GS, McDonald KM, Cohn JN: Neurohumoral activation in preclinical heart failure: Remodeling and the potential for intervention. Circulation 1993;87(Suppl IV):IV–90.

Garg R, Yusuf S: Overview of randomized trials of angiotensin-converting enzyme inhibitors on mortality and morbidity in patients with heart failure. JAMA 1995;273:1450.

Goldberg AD, Goldstein S, Nichlas J: Multicenter trial of imazodan in patients with chronic congestive heart failure. Circulation 1990;(Suppl III):III-673.

Hall D, Zeitler H, Rudolph W: Counteraction of the vasodilator effects of enalapril by aspirin in severe heart failure. J Am Coll Cardiol 1992;20:1549.

Horn PT, Murphy MB: New dopamine receptor agonists in heart failure and hypertension: Implications for therapy. Drugs 1990;40:487.

Konstam MA et al: Effects of the angiotensin converting enzyme inhibitor enalapril on the long-term progression of left ventricular dysfunction in patients with heart failure. Circulation 1992;86:431.

Krum H et al: Effect of long-term digoxin therapy on autonomic function in patients with chronic heart failure. J Am Coll Cardiol 1995;25:289.

Newton GE, Parker JD: Acute effects of β_1-selective and nonselective β-adrenergic receptor blockade on cardiac sympathetic activity in congestive heart failure. Circulation 1996;94:353.

O'Connor CM et al: Effect of amlodipine on mode of death in severe chronic heart failure: The PRAISE Trial. Circulation 1995;(Suppl I)92:I-143.

Packer M et al, for the PROMISE Study Research Group: Effect of milrinone on mortality in severe chronic heart failure. N Engl J Med 1991;325:1468.

Packer M et al: The effect of carvedilol on morbidity and mortality in patients with chronic heart failure. N Engl J Med 1996;334:334.

Packer M et al: Withdrawal of digoxin from patients with chronic heart failure treated with angiotensin-converting-enzyme inhibitors. N Engl J Med 1993;329:1.

Papadakis MA, Massie BM: Appropriateness of digoxin use in medical outpatients. Am J Med 1988;85:365.

Parmley WW: Principles in the management of congestive heart failure. In: *Cardiology.* Parmley WW, Chatterjee K (editors). Lippincott, 1988.

Pfeffer MA et al, on behalf of the SAVE investigators: Effect of captopril on mortality and morbidity in patients with left ventricular dysfunction after myocardial infarction. N Engl J Med 1992;327:669.

Pitt B et al: Randomized trial of losartan versus captopril in patients over 65 with heart failure (Evaluation of Losartan in the Elderly Study, ELITE.) Lancet 1997; 349:747.

Smith TW, Braunwald E: The management of heart failure. In: *Heart Disease,* 3rd ed. Braunwald E (editor). Saunders, 1987.

The SOLVD Investigators: Effect of enalapril on mortality and the development of heart failure in asymptomatic patients with reduced left ventricular ejection fractions. N Engl J Med 1992;327:685

The SOLVD Investigators: Effect of enalapril on survival in patients with reduced left ventricular ejection fractions and congestive heart failure. N Engl J Med 1991; 325:293.

Stevenson WG et al: Improving survival for patients with advanced heart failure: A study of 737 consecutive patients. J Am Coll Cardiol 1995;26:1417.

Uretsky BF et al: Multicenter trial of oral enoximone in patients with moderate to moderately severe congestive heart failure: Lack of benefit compared with placebo. Circulation 1990;82:774.

Uretsky BF: Digoxin in the treatment of patients with chronic heart failure: Its place in therapy. Drugs Aging 1995;7:1.

Waagstein F et al: Beneficial effects of metoprolol in idiopathic dilated cardiomyopathy. Lancet 1993;342: 1441.

The Xamoterol in Severe Heart Failure Study Group: Xamoterol in severe heart failure. Lancet 1990;336:1.

14 Agents Used in Cardiac Arrhythmias

Luc M Hondeghem, MD, PhD, & Dan M Roden, MD

Cardiac arrhythmias are a frequent problem in clinical practice, occurring in up to 25% of patients treated with digitalis, 50% of anesthetized patients, and over 80% of patients with acute myocardial infarction. Arrhythmias may require treatment because rhythms that are too rapid, too slow, or asynchronous can reduce cardiac output. Some arrhythmias can precipitate more serious or even lethal rhythm disturbances—eg, early premature ventricular depolarizations can precipitate ventricular fibrillation. In such patients, antiarrhythmic drugs may be lifesaving. On the other hand, the hazards of antiarrhythmic drugs—and in particular the fact that they can (paradoxically) *precipitate* lethal arrhythmias in some patients—has led to a reevaluation of their relative risks and benefits. In general, treatment of asymptomatic or minimally symptomatic arrhythmias should be avoided for this reason.

Arrhythmias can be treated with the drugs discussed in this chapter and with nonpharmacologic therapies such as pacemakers, cardioversion, catheter ablation, and surgery. This chapter describes the pharmacology of agents that suppress arrhythmias by a direct action on the cardiac cell membrane. Other modes of therapy are discussed briefly.

ELECTROPHYSIOLOGY OF NORMAL CARDIAC RHYTHM

The electrical impulse that triggers a normal cardiac contraction originates at regular intervals in the sinoatrial node (Figure 14–1), usually at a frequency of 60–100 beats per minute. This impulse spreads rapidly through the atria and enters the atrioventricular node, which is normally the only conduction pathway between the atria and ventricles. Conduction through the atrioventricular node is slow, requiring about 0.15 s. (This delay provides time for atrial contraction to propel blood into the ventricles.) The impulse then propagates over the His-Purkinje system and invades all parts of the ventricles. Ventricular activation is complete in less than 0.1 s; therefore, contraction of all of the ventricular muscle is synchronous and hemodynamically effective.

Arrhythmias consist of cardiac depolarizations that deviate from the above description in one or more aspects—ie, there is an abnormality in the site of origin of the impulse, its rate or regularity, or its conduction.

Ionic Basis of Membrane Electrical Activity

The transmembrane potential of cardiac cells is determined by the concentrations of several ions—chiefly sodium (Na^+), potassium (K^+), and calcium (Ca^{2+})—on either side of the membrane and the permeability of the membrane to each ion. These water-soluble ions are unable to freely diffuse across the lipid cell membrane in response to their electrical and concentration gradients; they require aqueous channels (specific pore-forming proteins) for such diffusion. Thus, ions move across cell membranes in response to their gradients only at specific times during the cardiac cycle when these ion channels are open. The movements of these charged ions produce currents that form the basis of the cardiac action potential. Individual channels are relatively ion-specific, and the flux of ions through them is thought to be controlled by "gates" (probably flexible peptide chains or energy barriers). Each type of channel has its own type of gate (sodium, calcium, and some potassium channels are each thought to have two types of gates), and each type of gate is opened and closed by specific transmembrane voltage, ionic, or metabolic conditions.

At rest, most cells are not significantly permeable to sodium, but at the start of each action potential, they become quite permeable (see below). Similarly, calcium enters and potassium leaves the cell with each action potential. Therefore, the cell must have a mechanism to maintain stable transmembrane ionic conditions by establishing and maintaining ion gradients. The most important of these active mechanisms is the sodium pump, Na^+/K^+ ATPase, described in Chapter 13. This pump and other active ion carriers contribute indirectly to the transmembrane potential by maintaining the gradients necessary for diffusion

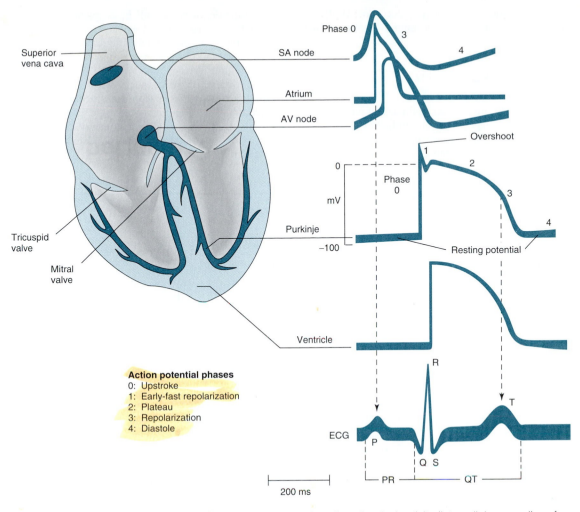

Action potential phases
0: Upstroke
1: Early-fast repolarization
2: Plateau
3: Repolarization
4: Diastole

Figure 14–1. Schematic representation of the heart and normal cardiac electrical activity (intracellular recordings from areas indicated and ECG). SA node, AV node, and Purkinje cells display pacemaker activity (phase 4 depolarization). The ECG is the body surface manifestation of the depolarization and repolarization waves of the heart. The P wave is generated by atrial depolarization, the QRS by ventricular muscle depolarization, and the T wave by ventricular repolarization. Thus, the PR interval is a measure of conduction time from atrium to ventricle, and the QRS duration indicates the time required for all of the ventricular cells to be activated (ie, the intraventricular conduction time). The QT interval reflects the duration of the ventricular action potential.

through channels. In addition, some pumps and exchangers produce net current flow (eg, by exchanging three Na^+ for two K^+ ions) and hence are termed "electrogenic."

When the cardiac cell membrane becomes permeable to a specific ion (ie, when the channels selective for that ion are open), movement of that ion across the cell membrane is determined by Ohm's law: current = voltage ÷ resistance, or voltage × conductance. Conductance is determined by the properties of the individual ion channel protein. The voltage term is the difference between the actual membrane potential and the membrane potential at which no ion current would flow even if channels were open. For example, in the case of sodium in a cardiac cell at rest, there is a sub-

stantial concentration gradient (140 mmol/L Na^+ outside; 10–15 mmol/L Na^+ inside) and electrical gradient (0 mV outside; –90 mV inside) which would drive Na^+ into cells. Sodium does not enter the cell at rest because sodium channels are closed; when sodium channels open, the very large influx of Na^+ ions accounts for phase 0 depolarization. The situation for K^+ ions in the resting cardiac cell is quite different. Here, the concentration gradient (140 mmol/L inside; 4 mmol/L outside) would drive the ion out of the cell, but the electrical gradient would drive it in, ie, the inward gradient is in equilibrium with the outward gradient. In fact, certain potassium channels ("inward rectifier" channels) are open in the resting cell, but little current flows through them because of this balance. The equilibrium, or **reversal potential,** for sodium or potassium is determined by the **Nernst equation:**

$$E_{ion} = 61 \times \log\left(\frac{C_e}{C_i}\right)$$

where C_e and C_i are the extracellular and intracellular concentrations, respectively, multiplied by their activity coefficients. Note that raising extracellular potassium makes E_K less negative. When this occurs, the membrane depolarizes until E_K is reached. Thus, extracellular potassium and inward rectifier channel function are the major factors determining the membrane potential of the resting cardiac cell. The conditions required for application of the Nernst equation are approximated at the peak of the overshoot and during rest in most nonpacemaker cardiac cells. If the permeability is significant for both potassium and sodium, the Nernst equation is not a good predictor of membrane potential, but the **Goldman-Hodgkin-Katz equation** may be used.

EFFECTS OF POTASSIUM

Just as drugs may act on two or more receptors, potassium affects several different membrane properties. As described in the text, the potassium concentration gradient (outside versus inside concentrations) determines the *potassium equilibrium potential* (E_K) as given by the Nernst equation. This is true of all cells and of artificial systems containing semipermeable membranes as well. Therefore, an increase in extracellular potassium concentration reduces (makes less negative) E_K. A second important effect of potassium is the ability of the extracellular potassium concentration to alter the membrane permeability to potassium (P_K). The consequences of the resulting changes in P_K are best appreciated by examining the resting potential (E_{mem}) predicted by the Goldman-Hodgkin-Katz equation. As the equation indicates, it is the *ratio of potassium permeability to sodium permeability* that determines how the concentration gradients for these two ions will influence the membrane potential. Anything that increases the potassium permeability will increase the influence of the potassium gradient and force the membrane potential closer to E_K. Since experimental evidence shows that an increase in extracellular potassium concentration increases P_K, it is not surprising that hyperkalemia shifts the membrane potential closer to E_K.

If we combine these two effects of potassium, we find that hyperkalemia will depolarize E_K and simultaneously shift E_{mem} closer to E_K. In a nonpacemaker cell, P_K is very high during diastole even at low and normal extracellular potassium concentrations, and E_{mem} lies relatively close to E_K at all times. On the other hand, in pacemaker cells, P_K is relatively low at normal potassium concentrations, and an increase in P_K, caused by hyperkalemia, can shift E_{mem} significantly closer to E_K. The following table shows some hypothetical examples of these effects, with Na_e, Na_i, and P_{Na} taken as 140, 10, and 1, respectively, in each condition.

Extracellular K (K_e)	K_i	P_K	E_K	E_{mem}
Nonpacemaker cell				
Low: 2.5	150	75	−108	−94
Normal: 4.0	150	100	−96	−88
High: 10.0	150	300	−72	−71
Pacemaker cell				
Low: 2.5	150	15	−108	−67
Normal: 4.0	150	20	−96	−69
High: 10.0	150	60	−72	−66

As the table shows, both the potassium equilibrium potential (E_K) and the resting potential (E_{mem}) become significantly less negative in a nonpacemaker as extracellular potassium increases. The pacemaker cell shows the same alterations in E_K, but E_{mem} is changed much less because the changes in potassium permeability are more important than changes in K_e in this cell type and have the opposite effect on resting potential. The result of increasing extracellular potassium will be to stabilize the membrane potential closer to the potassium equilibrium potential.

With the identification of the individual currents that make up the action potential has come the description of yet another important effect of changing K_e. The amplitude of one important repolarizing current, I_{Kr} (see box: Molecular Basis of Cardiac Excitability), paradoxically increases when K_e is increased despite the fact that the electrochemical driving forces decrease. The mechanism underlying this effect is not yet known. The fact that cardiac action potentials are longer at low K_e than at high K_e may be determined in part by this effect. In addition, changing K_e may alter the potencies of blocking drugs; at low K_e, I_{Kr} is much smaller and more sensitive to drug block. This effect, in turn, may contribute to the tendency for I_{Kr} blockers (such as quinidine or sotalol) to prolong action potentials and to cause torsade de pointes to a much greater extent when K_e is low.

$$E_{mem} = 61 \times \log \left(\frac{P_k \times K_e + P_{Na} \times Na_e}{P_k \times K_i + P_{Na} \times Na_i} \right)$$

In pacemaker cells (whether normal or ectopic), spontaneous depolarization (the pacemaker potential) occurs during diastole (phase 4, Figure 14–1). This depolarization results from a gradual increase of depolarizing current (caused by increasing permeability to sodium or calcium), a decrease in repolarizing potassium current (caused by a decrease in potassium permeability), or both. The effect of changing extracellular potassium is more complex in a pacemaker cell than it is in a nonpacemaker cell because the effect on permeability to potassium is much more important in a pacemaker (see box: Effects of Potassium). In a pacemaker—especially an ectopic one—the end result of an increase in extracellular potassium will usually be to slow or stop the pacemaker. Conversely, hypokalemia will often facilitate ectopic pacemakers.

The Active Cell Membrane

In normal atrial, Purkinje, and ventricular cells, the action potential upstroke (phase 0) is dependent on sodium current. From a functional point of view, it is convenient to describe the behavior of the sodium current in terms of three channel states (Figure 14–2). The cardiac sodium channel protein has been cloned, and it is now recognized that these channel states actually represent different protein conformations. In addition, regions of the protein that confer specific behaviors, such as voltage sensing, pore formation, or inactivation, are now being identified. The gates described below and in Figure 14–2 represent such regions.

Depolarization to the threshold voltage results in opening of the activation (m) gates of sodium channels (Figure 14–2, panel A, middle). If the inactivation (h) gates of these channels have not already closed, the channels are now open or activated, and sodium permeability is markedly increased, greatly exceeding the permeability for any other ion. Extracellular sodium therefore diffuses down its electrochemical gradient into the cell, and the membrane potential very rapidly approaches the sodium equilibrium potential, E_{Na} (about +70 mV when $Na_e = 140$ mmol/L and $Na_i = 10$ mmol/L). This intense sodium current is very brief, because opening of the m gates upon depolarization is promptly followed by closure of the h gates and inactivation of the sodium channels (Figure 14–2, panel A, right).

Most calcium channels become activated and inactivated in what appears to be the same way as sodium channels, but in the case of the most common type of cardiac calcium channel (the "L" type), the transitions occur more slowly and at more positive potentials. The action potential plateau (phases 1 and 2) reflects the turning off of most of the sodium current, the waxing and waning of calcium current, and the slow development of a repolarizing potassium current.

Final repolarization (phase 3) of the action potential results from completion of sodium and calcium channel inactivation and the growth of potassium permeability, so that the membrane potential once again approaches the potassium equilibrium potential. These processes are diagrammed in Figure 14–3.

The Effect of Resting Potential on Action Potentials

A key factor in the pathophysiology of arrhythmias and the actions of antiarrhythmic drugs is the relationship between the resting potential of a cell and the action potentials that can be evoked in it (Figure 14–4, left panel). Because the inactivation gates of sodium channels in the resting membrane close over the potential range –75 to –55 mV, fewer sodium channels are "available" for diffusion of sodium ions when an action potential is evoked from a resting potential of –60 mV than when it is evoked from a resting potential of –80 mV. Important consequences of the reduction in peak sodium permeability include reduced upstroke velocity (called V_{max}, for maximum rate of change of membrane voltage), reduced action potential amplitude, reduced excitability, and reduced conduction velocity.

During the plateau of the action potential, most sodium channels are inactivated. Upon repolarization, recovery from inactivation takes place (in the terminology of Figure 14–2, the h gates reopen), making the channels again available for excitation. The time between phase 0 and sufficient recovery of sodium channels in phase 3 to permit a propagated response to external stimulus is the "refractory period." Changes in refractoriness (determined by either altered recovery from inactivation or altered action potential duration) can be important in the genesis or suppression of certain arrhythmias. Another important effect of less negative resting potential is prolongation of this recovery time, as shown in Figure 14–4 (right panel). The prolongation of recovery time is reflected in an increase in the effective refractory period.

A brief depolarizing stimulus, whether caused by a propagating action potential or by an external electrode arrangement, causes the opening of large numbers of activation gates before a significant number of inactivation gates can close. In contrast, slow reduction (depolarization) of the resting potential, whether brought about by hyperkalemia, sodium pump blockade, or ischemic cell damage, results in depressed sodium currents during the upstrokes of action potentials. Depolarization of the resting potential to levels positive to –55 mV abolishes sodium currents, since all sodium channels are inactivated. However, such severely depolarized cells have been found to support special action potentials under circumstances that increase calcium permeability or decrease potassium permeability. These "slow responses"—slow upstroke velocity and slow conduction—depend on a calcium

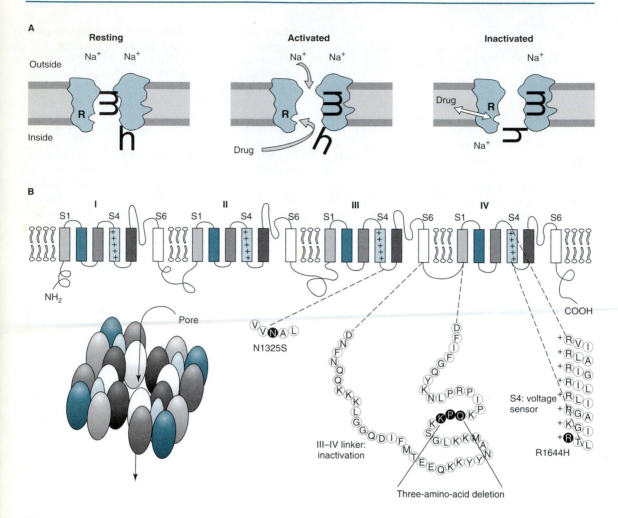

Figure 14–2. Schematic diagrams of a cardiac sodium channel. **Panel A:** A functional representation. The shapes shown for the channel and its gates are purely symbolic (compare with panel B). The channel protein (color) spans the membrane. In the resting, fully polarized membrane (left), the *h* gate is open and the *m* gate is closed, preventing any movement of sodium through the channel. With an appropriate activating stimulus, the *m* gate opens, allowing a rapid influx of sodium ions (middle). About a millisecond later, the *h* gate closes, inactivating the channel and shutting off the sodium current (right). Additional stimuli applied to the inactivated channel cannot open it (the *h* gate is closed); therefore it is "unavailable." The area designated R in the channel is a putative local anesthetic-antiarrhythmic drug receptor. Drugs can access the receptor via the aqueous pathway from the inside of the cell (arrow, middle) or from the membrane phase (arrow, right). **Panel B:** A protein structure representation. Cloning of the human sodium channel reveals a large protein whose inferred orientation in the membrane is indicated in the upper part of panel B. The protein consists of four roughly homologous domains (labeled *I–IV,*) each consisting of six membrane spanning segments *(S).* It is thought that the protein folds upon itself, forming a pore, as shown in the lower left. The S5 and S6 segments (black, white) in each domain are thought to line the pore, while the S4 segments (light color) may form the voltage-sensing elements needed to open the *m* gates and close the *h* gate (refer to panel A). The *h* gate is thought to consist of the peptide chain linking domains III and IV *(III–IV linker: inactivation).* Mutations in the sodium channel that result in incomplete inactivation can cause the congenital long QT syndrome. The sites of three such mutations are indicated in the figure (black amino acids). (Panel B redrawn, with permission, from Roden DM, George AL Jr, Bennett PB: Recent advances in understanding the molecular mechanisms of the long QT syndrome. J Cardiovasc Electrophysiol 1995;6:1023.)

inward current and constitute the normal electrical activity in the sinoatrial and atrioventricular nodes, since these tissues have a normal resting potential in the range of –50 to –70 mV. Slow responses may also be important for certain arrhythmias. Modern techniques of molecular biology and electrophysiology can identify multiple subtypes of calcium and potassium channels. One way in which such subtypes may differ is in sensitivity to drug therapy, so drugs targeting specific channel subtypes may be developed in the future.

Figure 14–3. Schematic diagram of the ion permeability changes and transport processes that occur during an action potential and the diastolic period following it. The size and weight of the arrows indicate approximate magnitudes of the ion channel currents. Multiple subtypes of potassium and calcium currents, with different sensitivities to blocking drugs, have been identified.

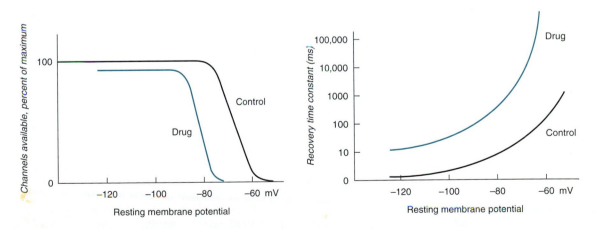

Figure 14–4. Dependence of sodium channel function on the membrane potential preceding the stimulus. *Left:* The fraction of sodium channels available for opening in response to a stimulus is determined by the membrane potential immediately preceding the stimulus. The decrease in the fraction available when the resting potential is depolarized in the absence of a drug (control curve) results from the voltage-dependent closure of h gates in the channels. The curve labeled "Drug" illustrates the effect of a typical "local anesthetic" antiarrhythmic drug. Most sodium channels are inactivated during the plateau of the action potential. *Right:* The time constant for recovery from inactivation after repolarization also depends on the resting potential. In the absence of drug, recovery occurs in less than 10 ms at normal resting potentials (–85 to –95 mV). Depolarized cells recover more slowly (note logarithmic scale). In the presence of a sodium channel-blocking drug, the time constant of recovery is increased, but the increase is far greater at depolarized potentials than at more negative ones.

MECHANISMS OF ARRHYTHMIAS

Many factors can precipitate or exacerbate arrhythmias: ischemia, hypoxia, acidosis or alkalosis, electrolyte abnormalities, excessive catecholamine exposure, autonomic influences, drug toxicity (eg, digitalis or antiarrhythmic drugs), overstretching of cardiac fibers, and the presence of scarred or otherwise diseased tissue. However, all arrhythmias result from (1) disturbances in impulse formation, (2) disturbances in impulse conduction, or (3) both.

Disturbances of Impulse Formation

The interval between depolarizations of a pacemaker cell is the sum of the duration of the action potential and the duration of the diastolic interval. Shortening of either duration results in an increase in pacemaker rate. The more important of the two, diastolic interval, is determined by three factors: maximum diastolic potential, slope of phase 4 depolarization, and threshold potential (Figure 14–5). Thus, vagal discharge slows normal pacemaker rate by making the maximum diastolic potential more negative and reducing the phase 4 slope; beta receptor-blocking drugs also reduce phase 4 slope. Acceleration of pacemaker discharge is often brought about by increased phase 4 depolarization slope, caused by hypokalemia, beta adrenoceptor stimulation, fiber stretch, acidosis, and partial depolarization by currents of injury.

Latent pacemakers (cells that show slow phase 4 depolarization even under normal conditions, eg, some Purkinje fibers) are particularly prone to acceleration by the above mechanisms. However, all car-

Figure 14–6. Two forms of abnormal activity, early *(top)* and delayed afterdepolarizations *(bottom)*. In both cases, abnormal depolarizations arise during or after a normally evoked action potential. They are therefore often referred to as "triggered" automaticity, ie, they require a normal action potential for their initiation.

diac cells, including normally quiescent atrial and ventricular cells, may show repetitive pacemaker activity when depolarized under appropriate conditions, especially if hypokalemia is also present.

Afterdepolarizations (Figure 14–6) are depolarizations that interrupt phase 3 (early afterdepolarizations, EADs) or phase 4 (delayed afterdepolarizations, DADs). Delayed afterdepolarizations, discussed in Chapter 13, often occur when intracellular calcium is increased. They are exacerbated by fast heart rates and are thought to be responsible for some arrhythmias related to digitalis excess, to catecholamines, and to myocardial ischemia. EADs, on the other hand, are exacerbated at slow heart rates and thought to be contribute to the development of long QT-related arrhythmias.

All pacemakers, normal and abnormal, are dependent upon phase 4 diastolic depolarization. Hyperkalemia, as described above, will *stabilize* the membrane potential and thus will reduce the rate of firing.* In hypokalemia, the membrane is less permeable to potassium and consequently more easily displaced from the potassium equilibrium potential (see box: Effects of Potassium), ie, spontaneous firing is facilitated.

Figure 14–5. Determinants of pacemaker rate. Transmembrane potential in a Purkinje fiber pacemaker cell is shown. The rate of a pacemaker can be slowed by four mechanisms. *1,* more negative maximum diastolic potential, shown as a change from –80 to –100 mV; *2,* reduction of the slope of diastolic depolarization; *3,* more positive threshold potential, shown as a change from –65 to –45 mV; and *4,* (not shown because not a common mechanism), prolongation of the action potential duration. Note that each of the changes shown results in prolongation of the interval between the first action potential and the second from the short interval (solid line) to a longer one (dashed line).

---

*Even though potassium depolarizes the membrane and depolarization can promote pacemaker activity, the effect of membrane stabilization is more important than that of the depolarization, so that increased potassium normally reduces pacemaker rate.

Figure 14–7. Electrocardiogram from a patient with the long QT syndrome during two episodes of torsade de pointes. The polymorphic ventricular tachycardia is seen at the start of this tracing and spontaneously halts at the middle of the panel. A single normal sinus beat *(NSB)* with an extremely prolonged QT interval follows, succeeded immediately by another episode of ventricular tachycardia of the torsade type. The usual symptoms would be dizziness or transient loss of consciousness.

THE MOLECULAR BASIS OF CARDIAC EXCITABILITY: LESSONS FROM THE CONGENITAL LONG QT SYNDROME

The polymorphic ventricular tachycardia torsade de pointes (Figure 14–7) can occur both during therapy with QT-prolonging drugs such as quinidine or sotalol and also as a familial condition. The electrocardiographic hallmark of both the acquired and congenital syndromes is prolongation of the QT interval, especially at the onset of the tachycardia (above). As can be inferred from Figure 14–1, this must represent prolongation of the action potential of at least some ventricular cells. This effect can, in theory, be attributed either to increased inward current or decreased outward current during the plateau of the action potential. In fact, recent molecular genetic studies have identified mutations in ion channel genes that produce the long QT syndrome by either mechanism. In some families, there are mutations in the region of the sodium channel gene that is important for normal inactivation (Figure 14–2, panel B); the result is a maintained inward current through sodium channels during the plateau. In other families, there is a mutation in a gene termed *HERG*. Interestingly, *HERG* encodes a potassium channel, the rapid component of the delayed rectifier current (termed I_{Kr}), that is blocked by many drugs, such as quinidine or sotalol, that also produce torsade de pointes. Thus, these molecular genetic studies have identified the reason why congenital and acquired cases of torsade de pointes can be so strikingly similar. The identification of

the precise molecular mechanisms underlying various forms of the long QT syndromes now raises the possibility that specific therapies may be developed for individuals with defined molecular abnormalities. Indeed, preliminary reports do suggest that the sodium channel blocker mexiletine can correct the clinical manifestations of the long QT syndrome in patients with abnormal sodium channel inactivation as the underlying problem.

Hypokalemia and bradycardia have been identified as important risk factors for torsade de pointes. The role of hypokalemia is discussed further in the box: Effects of Potassium. In vitro and clinical data demonstrate that most available action potential-prolonging drugs exert greater effects at slow rates (where torsade de pointes is a risk) than at fast rates (where arrhythmia suppression would occur). This "reverse use-dependent" action potential prolongation seems to be absent with amiodarone, which may help explain that drug's apparently greater clinical efficacy with its low rate of torsade de pointes. It is likely that torsade de pointes originates from triggered upstrokes arising from early afterdepolarizations (Figure 14–6). Thus, therapy is directed at correcting hypokalemia, eliminating triggered upstrokes (eg, by using beta-blockers or magnesium), or shortening the action potential (eg, by increasing heart rate with isoproterenol or pacing)—or all of these.

Disturbances of Impulse Conduction

Severely depressed conduction may result in simple block, eg, atrioventricular nodal block or bundle branch block. Because parasympathetic control of atrioventricular conduction is significant, partial atrioventricular block is sometimes relieved by atropine. A more common abnormality of conduction is **reentry** (also known as "circus movement"), in which one impulse reenters and excites areas of the heart more than once (Figure 14–8). The path of the reentering impulse may be confined to very small areas, eg, within or near the atrioventricular node, or it may involve large portions of the atrial or ventricular walls. Some forms of reentry are strictly anatomically determined; for example, in the Wolff-Parkinson-White syndrome, the reentry circuit consists of atrial tissue, the AV node, ventricular tissue, and an accessory atrioventricular connection (a "bypass tract"). In other cases (eg, atrial or ventricular fibrillation), multiple reentry circuits, determined by the properties of the cardiac tissue, may meander through the heart. Furthermore, the circulating impulse often gives off "daughter impulses" that can spread to the rest of the heart. Depending on how many round trips through the pathway the impulse makes before dying out, the arrhythmia may be manifest as one or a few extra beats or as a sustained tachycardia.

In order for reentry to occur, three conditions must coexist, as indicated in Figure 14–8: (1) There must be an obstacle (anatomic or physiologic) to homogeneous conduction, thus establishing a circuit around which the reentrant wavefront can propagate; (2) there must be unidirectional block at some point in the circuit, ie, conduction must die out in one direction but continue in the opposite direction (as shown in Figure 14–8, the impulse can gradually decrease as it invades progressively more depolarized tissue until it finally blocks—a process known as decremental conduction); and (3) conduction time around the circuit must be long enough so that the retrograde impulse does not enter refractory tissue as it travels around the obstacle, ie, the conduction time must exceed the effective refractory period. Importantly, reentry depends upon conduction that has been depressed by some critical amount, usually as a result of injury or ischemia. If conduction velocity is too *slow,* bidirectional block rather than unidirectional block occurs; if the reentering impulse is too weak, conduction may fail, or the impulse may arrive so late that it collides with the next regular impulse. On the other hand, if conduction is too *rapid,* ie, almost normal, bidirectional conduction rather than unidirectional block will occur. Even in the presence of unidirectional block, if the impulse travels around the obstacle too rapidly, it will reach tissue that is still refractory.

Slowing of conduction may be due to depression of sodium current, depression of calcium current (the latter especially in the atrioventricular node), or both. Drugs that abolish reentry usually work by further slowing depressed conduction (by blocking the sodium or calcium current) or, less commonly, by accelerating it (by increasing the sodium or calcium current).

Lengthening (or shortening) of the refractory period may also make reentry less likely. The longer the refractory period in tissue near the site of block, the greater the chance that the tissue will still be refractory when reentry is attempted. (Alternatively, the shorter the refractory period in the depressed region, the less likely it is that unidirectional block will occur.) Thus, increased "dispersion" of refractoriness is one contributor to reentry, and drugs may suppress arrhythmias by reducing such dispersion.

I. BASIC PHARMACOLOGY OF THE ANTIARRHYTHMIC AGENTS

Mechanisms of Action

Arrhythmias are caused by abnormal pacemaker activity or abnormal impulse propagation. Thus, the aim of therapy of the arrhythmias is to reduce ectopic pacemaker activity and modify conduction or refractoriness in reentry circuits to disable circus movement. The major mechanisms currently available for accomplishing these goals are (1) sodium channel blockade, (2) blockade of sympathetic autonomic effects in the heart, (3) prolongation of the effective refractory period, and (4) calcium channel blockade.

Antiarrhythmic drugs decrease the automaticity of ectopic pacemakers more than that of the sinoatrial node. They also reduce conduction and excitability and increase the refractory period to a greater extent in depolarized tissue than in normally polarized tissue. This is accomplished chiefly by selectively blocking the sodium or calcium channels of depolarized cells (Figure 14–9). Therapeutically useful channel-blocking drugs have a high affinity for activated channels (ie, during phase 0) or inactivated channels (ie, during phase 2) but very low affinity for rested channels. Therefore, these drugs block electrical activity when there is a fast tachycardia (many channel activations and inactivations per unit time) or when there is significant loss of resting potential (many inactivated channels during rest). This type of drug action is often described as **use-dependent** or **state-dependent,** ie, channels that are being used frequently, or in an inactivated state, are more susceptible to block. Channels in normal cells that become blocked by a drug during normal activation-inactivation cycles will rapidly lose the drug from the receptors during the resting portion of the cycle (Figure 14–9). Channels in myocardium that is chronically depolarized (ie, has a resting potential more positive than –75 mV) will recover from block very slowly if at all (see also right panel, Figure 14–4).

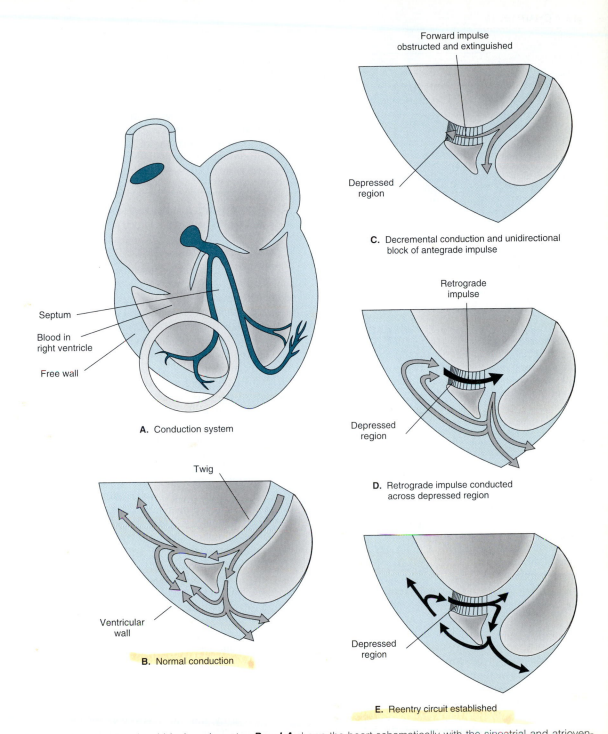

Forward impulse
obstructed and extinguished

Depressed
region

C. Decremental conduction and unidirectional
block of antegrade impulse

Retrograde
impulse

Depressed
region

D. Retrograde impulse conducted
across depressed region

Depressed
region

E. Reentry circuit established

Septum

Blood in
right ventricle

Free wall

A. Conduction system

Twig

Ventricular
wall

B. Normal conduction

Figure 14–8. Unidirectional block and reentry. *Panel A* shows the heart schematically with the sinoatrial and atrioventricular nodes and the conducting system in color. A small bifurcating twig of the Purkinje system is circled where it enters the ventricular wall. *Panel B* shows the normal passage and fate of an impulse that is conducted down the twig. It splits into two impulses at the bifurcation, and these collide (and extinguish each other) after exciting the ventricular muscle. *Panels C–E* show the sequence of events when the normal impulse finds an area of unidirectional block (blocked depressed region) in one of the branches. As shown by the path of the impulse in the depressed region (panel C), this weak stimulus is unable to conduct through or to "jump over" the area of block. In contrast, the wave in the undepressed branch is able to excite the entire ventricular wall (panel D). Because the ventricular wall constitutes a large mass of cells, the strong ventricular depolarization is able to jump the depressed region and results in a retrograde impulse (shown by the black arrow, panels D and E). The retrograde impulse may be propagated if the impulse finds excitable tissue, ie, the refractory period is shorter than the conduction time. This impulse will then reexcite tissue it had previously passed through, and a reentry arrhythmia will be established in the circuit indicated by the black arrows in panel E.

225

Figure 14–9. Diagram of a mechanism for the selective depressant action of antiarrhythmic drugs on sodium channels. The upper portion of the figure shows the population of channels moving through a cycle of activity during an action potential in the absence of drugs: R (rested) → A (activated) → I (inactivated). Recovery takes place via the I → R pathway. Antiarrhythmic drugs (D) that act by blocking sodium channels can bind to their receptors in the channels, as shown by the vertical arrows, to form drug-channel complexes, indicated as R-D, A-D, and I-D. Affinity of the drugs for the receptor varies with the state of the channel, as indicated by the separate rate constants (k and l) for the R ⇌ R-D, A ⇌ A-D, and I ⇌ I-D steps. The data available for a variety of sodium channel blockers indicate that the affinity of the drugs for the active and inactivated channel receptor is much higher than the affinity for the rested channel. Furthermore, recovery from the I-D state to the R-D state is much slower than from I to R. As a result, rapid activity (more activations and inactivations) and depolarization of the resting potential (more channels in the I state) will favor blockade of the channels and selectively suppress arrhythmic cells.

In cells with abnormal automaticity, most of these drugs reduce the phase 4 slope (Figure 14–5) by blocking either sodium or calcium channels and thereby reducing the ratio of sodium (or calcium) permeability to potassium permeability. As a result, the membrane potential during phase 4 stabilizes closer to the potassium equilibrium potential. In addition, some agents may increase the threshold (make it more positive). Beta adrenoceptor-blocking drugs indirectly reduce the phase 4 slope by blocking the positive chronotropic action of norepinephrine in the heart.

In reentry arrhythmias, which depend upon critically depressed conduction, most antiarrhythmic agents slow conduction further by one or both of two mechanisms: (1) steady-state reduction in the number of available unblocked channels, which reduces the excitatory currents to a level below that required for propagation (Figure 14–4, left); and (2) prolongation of recovery time of the channels still able to reach the rested and available state, which increases the effective refractory period (Figure 14–4, right). As a result, early extrasystoles are unable to propagate at all; later impulses propagate more slowly and are subject to bidirectional conduction block.

By these mechanisms, antiarrhythmic drugs can suppress ectopic automaticity and abnormal conduction occurring in depolarized cells—rendering them electrically silent—while minimally affecting the elec-

trical activity in normally polarized parts of the heart. However, as dosage is increased, these agents also depress conduction in normal tissue, eventually resulting in *drug-induced* arrhythmias. Furthermore, a drug concentration that is therapeutic (antiarrhythmic) under the initial circumstances of treatment may become "proarrhythmic" (arrhythmogenic) during fast heart rates (more development of block), acidosis (slower recovery from block for most drugs), or hyperkalemia.

II. SPECIFIC ANTIARRHYTHMIC AGENTS

The antiarrhythmic agents have traditionally been divided into four distinct classes on the basis of their dominant mechanism of action. **Class I action** is sodium channel block, ie, a local anesthetic action. In fact, a widely used parenteral antiarrhythmic drug, lidocaine, is also a popular local anesthetic. Class I agents are frequently subdivided according to their effects on action potential duration or on the kinetics of their interactions with cardiac sodium channels: Class IA drugs (quinidine, procainamide, disopyramide) lengthen the duration, IB agents (lidocaine, mexiletine, tocainide, phenytoin) shorten it, and IC drugs (flecainide) have no effect or may minimally increase action potential duration. As a group, IB agents interact (bind and unbind) rapidly with sodium channels, IC drugs interact slowly, and IA drugs are intermediate. This classification is somewhat arbitrary, and some drugs (moricizine, propafenone) do not readily fit these simplified definitions. **Class II action** is sympathoplegic; drugs include those that reduce adrenergic activity in the heart, especially beta-blockers. The **class III** action is prolongation of the action potential duration—by block of outward or augmentation of inward currents. This, in turn, prolongs the effective refractory period, which provides the antiarrhythmic action. The **class IV** action is block of cardiac calcium currents, which may slow conduction and increase refractory period in calcium-dependent tissues such as the AV node.

While drugs of a similar class or subclass tend to produce similar electrophysiologic effects, their clinical actions may differ substantially. Moreover, other compounds (eg, adenosine, digitalis, magnesium) exerting antiarrhythmic actions do so by unclassified mechanisms. Thus, certain *actions* of the drugs can be conveniently separated (block of sodium channels, prolongation of action potential duration, etc), but classifying drug action does not mean that drugs from the same class will produce the same overall effects. This is because a given drug with (for example) class I effects may also have significant class III effects, while a different drug with class I action may also have class IV effects.

In recognition of the inadequacies of the traditional classification, a new approach to classification that recognizes the multiplicity of actions of most of the drugs and the variable mechanisms of arrhythmogenesis has been proposed (Task Force, 1991). However, this system is not yet widely used.

SODIUM CHANNEL-BLOCKING DRUGS (CLASS I)

QUINIDINE

Although quinine was used sporadically as an antiarrhythmic drug during the 18th and 19th centuries, it was not until the early years of the 20th century that quinidine, a diastereomer of quinine, came into wide use. Quinidine remains among the most commonly used oral antiarrhythmic agents in the USA, although its use is declining.

Quinidine

Cardiac Effects

Quinidine depresses pacemaker rate (especially that of ectopic pacemakers) and depresses conduction and excitability (especially in depolarized tissue) (Table 14–1). To a large extent, these actions result from quinidine's ability to bind to and block activated sodium channels. Recovery from block is slower and less complete in depolarized than in fully polarized tissue. Thus, quinidine lengthens the refractory period and depresses excitability and conduction in depolarized tissue more than in normal tissue.

Quinidine also lengthens the action potential duration, which is reflected in the ECG as a lengthening of the QT interval. Block of potassium channels with a reduction in repolarizing outward current is responsible for this effect. This lengthening of the action potential duration reduces the time spent at more negative diastolic membrane potentials and therefore—at least theoretically—enhances the sodium channel-blocking efficacy of quinidine. Lengthening of the action potential duration and effective refractory period reduces the maximum reentry frequency and can slow tachycardias. As discussed below, this effect may be associated with torsade de pointes. Torsade de pointes is estimated to occur in 2–8% of patients receiving quinidine. In contrast to torsade de pointes with many

other drugs, plasma concentrations of quinidine are often normal or even subtherapeutic in patients with this toxic effect.

Extracardiac Effects

Quinidine possesses alpha adrenoceptor-blocking properties that can cause vasodilation and a reflex increase in sinoatrial nodal rate. These effects are most prominent after intravenous administration (see below).

Toxicity

A. Cardiac: Quinidine has antimuscarinic actions in the heart that inhibit vagal effects. This can overcome some of its direct membrane effect and lead to increased sinus rate and increased atrioventricular conduction. In atrial fibrillation or flutter, this antimuscarinic action on the AV node may result in an excessively high ventricular rate. For example, in atrial flutter, the ratio of the frequency of impulses in the atria to that in the ventricle can decrease from 2:1 or 4:1 to 1:1, with a resultant (often dramatic) increase in ventricular rate, a highly undesirable effect. This can be prevented by prior administration of a drug that slows atrioventricular conduction, eg, verapamil, a beta-blocker, or digitalis.

A small percentage (1–5%) of patients given quinidine develop a syndrome called **quinidine syncope,** characterized by recurrent lightheadedness and episodes of fainting. These symptoms are a result of torsade de pointes, which usually terminates spontaneously but may recur frequently or even occasionally be fatal by degenerating into ventricular fibrillation.

In patients with sick sinus syndrome, quinidine may depress the pacemaker activity of the sinoatrial node. In toxic concentrations, this drug can depress cardiac electrical activity in any part of the heart to the point of precipitating arrhythmias or asystole. These toxic effects are more likely to occur when the serum concentrations exceed 5 µg/mL and in the presence of high serum potassium levels (> 5 mmol/L). Widening of the QRS duration by 30% by quinidine administration is usually considered premonitory of serious toxicity. Toxic concentrations may depress contractility and lower blood pressure.

B. Extracardiac: The most common adverse effects are gastrointestinal: diarrhea, nausea, and vomiting. These may occur in one-third to one-half of patients. The drug can also cause cinchonism (headache, dizziness, tinnitus). Rarely, quinidine can cause rashes, angioneurotic edema, fever, hepatitis, and thrombocytopenia. Quinidine increases digoxin plasma levels and may precipitate digitalis toxicity in patients taking digoxin or digitoxin (see Chapter 13).

Pharmacokinetics & Dosage

Quinidine is usually administered orally and is rapidly absorbed from the gastrointestinal tract. It is

Table 14–1. Membrane actions of antiarrhythmic drugs.

Drug	Block of Sodium Channels		Refractory Period		Calcium Channel Blockade	Effect on Pacemaker Activity	Sympatholytic Action
	Normal Cells	Depolarized Cells	Normal Cells	Depolarized Cells			
Adenosine	0	0	0	0	0	0	+
Amiodarone	+	+++	↑↑	↑↑↑	+	↓↓	+
Bretylium	0	0	↑↑↑	↑↑↑	0	↑↓[1]	++
Diltiazem	0	0	0	0	+++	↓↓	0
Disopyramide	+	+++	↑	↑↑	+	↓↓	0
Esmolol	0	+	0	NA[2]	0	↓↓	+++
Flecainide	+	+++	0	↑	0	↓↓	0
Ibutilide	0	0	↑	?	0	0	0
Lidocaine	0	+++	↓	↑↑	0	↓↓	0
Mexiletine	0	+++	0	↑↑	0	↓↓	0
Moricizine	+	++	↓	↓	0	↓↓	0
Procainamide	+	+++	↑	↑↑↑	0	↓	+
Propafenone	+	++	↑	↑↑	+	↓↓	+
Propranolol	0	+	↓	↑↑	0	↓↓	+++
Quinidine	+	++	↑	↑↑	0	↓↓	+
Sotalol	0	0	↑↑	↑↑↑	0	↓↓	++
Tocainide	0	+++	0	↑↑	0	↓↓	0
Verapamil	0	+	0	↑	+++	↓↓	+

[1]Bretylium may transiently increase pacemaker rate by causing catecholamine release.
[2]Data not available.

80% bound to plasma proteins. Quinidine is metabolized in the liver, but 20% is excreted unchanged in the urine. Its half-life is about 6 hours (Table 14–2) and may be longer in patients with congestive heart failure or hepatic or renal disease. Urinary excretion is enhanced in acid urine. The drug is usually administered orally as the sulfate, gluconate, or polygalacturonate salt. The usual dose of 0.2–0.6 g of quinidine sulfate is given two to four times daily. The therapeutic concentration in plasma is 3–5 μg/mL. Although quinidine can be given parenterally, this is very rarely done because of the risk of hypotension.

Therapeutic Use

Quinidine has been used in nearly every form of arrhythmia. Its most common indications are atrial fibrillation and flutter and, occasionally, ventricular tachycardia. Quinidine is also occasionally used for the intravenous treatment of malaria.

PROCAINAMIDE

Cardiac Effects

The electrophysiologic effects of procainamide are similar to those of quinidine. The drug may be somewhat less effective in suppressing abnormal ectopic pacemaker activity but more effective in blocking sodium channels in depolarized cells.

Perhaps the most important difference between quinidine and procainamide is the less prominent antimuscarinic action of procainamide. Therefore, the directly depressant actions of procainamide on sinoatrial and atrioventricular nodes are not as effectively counterbalanced by drug-induced vagal block as in the case of quinidine.

Procainamide

Extracardiac Effects

Procainamide has ganglion-blocking properties. This action reduces peripheral vascular resistance and can cause hypotension, particularly with intravenous use. However, in therapeutic concentrations, its peripheral vascular effects are less prominent than those of quinidine. Hypotension is usually associated with excessively rapid procainamide infusion or the presence of severe underlying left ventricular dysfunction.

Table 14–2. Clinical pharmacologic properties of antiarrhythmic drugs.

Drug	Effect on SA Nodal Rate	Effect on AV Nodal Refractory Period	PR Interval	QRS Duration	QT Interval	Usefulness in Arrhythmias		Half-Life
						Supraventricular	Ventricular	
Adenosine	Little	↑↑↑	↑↑↑	0	0	++++	?	< 10 s
Amiodarone	↓↓[1]	↑↑	↑↑	↑	↑↑↑↑	+++	+++	(weeks)
Bretylium	↑↓[2]	↑↓[2]	0	0	0	0	+	4 h
Diltiazem	↑↓	↑↑	↑	0	0	+++	−	4–8 h
Disopyramide	↑↓[1,3]	↑↓[3]	↑↓[3]	↑↑	↑↑	+	+++	6–8 h
Esmolol	↓↓	↑↑	↑↑	0	0	+	+	10 min
Flecainide	None	↑	↑	↑↑↑	0	+[4]	++++	20 h
Ibutilide	↓(?)	0	0	0	↑↑	++	?	6 h
Lidocaine	None[1]	None	0	0	0	None[5]	+++	1 h
Mexiletine	None[1]	None	0	0	0	None[6]	+++	12 h
Moricizine	None	None	↑	↑↑	0	None	+++	2–6 h[6]
Procainamide	↓[1]	↑↓[3]	↑↓[3]	↑↑	↑↑	+	+++	3–4 h
Propafenone	0	↑	↑	↑↑↑	0	+	+++	7 h
Propranolol	↓↓	↑↑	↑↑	0	0	+	+	8 h
Quinidine	↑↓[1,3]	↑↓[3]	↑↓[3]	↑↑	↑↑	+	+++	6 h
Sotalol	↓↓	↑↑	↑↑	0	↑↑↑	+++	+++	7 h
Tocainide	None[1]	None	0	0	0	None[5]	+++	12 h
Verapamil	↓↓	↑↑	↑↑	0	0	+++	−	7 h

[1]May suppress diseased sinus nodes.
[2]Initial stimulation by release of endogenous norepinephrine followed by depression.
[3]Anticholinergic effect and direct depressant action.
[4]Especially in Wolff-Parkinson-White syndrome.
[5]May be effective in atrial arrhythmias caused by digitalis.
[6]Half-life of active metabolites much longer.

Toxicity

A. Cardiac: Procainamide's cardiotoxic effects are similar to those of quinidine. Antimuscarinic and direct depressant effects may occur. New arrhythmias may be precipitated.

B. Extracardiac: The most troublesome adverse effect of long-term procainamide therapy is a syndrome resembling lupus erythematosus and usually consisting of arthralgia and arthritis. In some patients, pleuritis, pericarditis, or parenchymal pulmonary disease also occurs. Renal lupus is rarely induced by procainamide. During long-term therapy, serologic abnormalities (eg, increased antinuclear antibody titer) occur in nearly all patients, and in the absence of symptoms these are not an indication to stop drug therapy. Approximately one-third of patients receiving long-term procainamide therapy develop these reversible lupus-related symptoms.

Other adverse effects include nausea and diarrhea (about 10% of cases), rash, fever, hepatitis (< 5%), and agranulocytosis (approximately 0.2%).

Pharmacokinetics & Dosage

Procainamide can be administered safely by the intravenous and intramuscular routes and is well absorbed orally, with 75% systemic bioavailability. The major metabolite is *N*-acetylprocainamide (NAPA), which has class III activity. Excessive accumulation of NAPA has been implicated in torsade de pointes during procainamide therapy, especially in patients with renal failure. Some individuals rapidly acetylate procainamide and develop high levels of NAPA. The lupus syndrome appears to be less common in these patients.

Procainamide is eliminated by hepatic metabolism to NAPA and by renal elimination. Its half-life is only 3–4 hours, which necessitates frequent dosing. NAPA is eliminated by the kidneys. Thus, procainamide dosage must be reduced in patients with renal failure. The reduced volume of distribution and renal clearance associated with congestive heart failure also require reduction in dosage. The half-life of NAPA is considerably longer than that of procainamide, and it therefore accumulates more slowly. Thus, it is important to measure plasma levels of both procainamide and NAPA, especially in patients with circulatory or renal impairment.

If a rapid procainamide effect is needed, an intravenous loading dose of up to 12 mg/kg can be given at a rate of 0.3 mg/kg/min or less rapidly. This dose is followed by a maintenance dosage of 2–5 mg/min, with careful monitoring of plasma levels. The risk of gastrointestinal or cardiac toxicity rises at plasma concentrations greater than 8 µg/mL or NAPA concentrations greater than 20 µg/mL.

Oral procainamide is frequently used improperly. If around-the-clock antiarrhythmic activity is required, a sustained-release preparation must be administered every 6 hours in most cases. In order to control ventricular arrhythmias, a total dosage of 2–5 g/d is usually required. In an occasional patient who accumulates high levels of NAPA, less frequent dosing may be possible. This is also possible in renal disease, where procainamide elimination is also slowed.

Therapeutic Use

Like quinidine, procainamide is effective against most atrial and ventricular arrhythmias. However, many clinicians attempt to avoid long-term therapy because of the frequent dosing requirement and the common occurrence of lupus-related effects. Procainamide is the drug of second choice (after lidocaine) in most coronary care units for the treatment of sustained ventricular arrhythmias associated with acute myocardial infarction.

DISOPYRAMIDE

Disopyramide

Cardiac Effects

The effects of disopyramide are very similar to those of quinidine. Its cardiac antimuscarinic effects are even more marked than those of quinidine. Therefore, a drug that slows atrioventricular conduction should be administered with disopyramide when treating atrial flutter or fibrillation.

Toxicity

A. Cardiac: Toxic concentrations of disopyramide can precipitate all of the electrophysiologic disturbances described under quinidine. In addition, disopyramide's negative inotropic actions are frequently troublesome in patients with preexisting left ventricular dysfunction. Moreover, in rare instances, it may produce heart failure in subjects without prior

myocardial dysfunction. Because of this effect, disopyramide is not used as a first-line antiarrhythmic agent in the USA. It must be used with great caution in patients with congestive heart failure.

B. Extracardiac: Disopyramide's atropine-like activity accounts for most of its symptomatic adverse effects: urinary retention (most often, but not exclusively, in male patients with prostatic hyperplasia), dry mouth, blurred vision, constipation, and worsening of preexisting glaucoma. These effects may require discontinuation of the drug.

Pharmacokinetics & Dosage

In the USA, disopyramide is only available for oral use. Bioavailability is about 50%. The drug is extensively protein-bound, but binding sites become saturated with increasing dosage, which results in a nonlinear rise in free (active) drug levels when doses are increased. As a result, measurements of total plasma concentration may be misleading. The drug is excreted by the kidneys and has a half-life of approximately 6–8 hours. The usual oral dosage of disopyramide is 150 mg three times a day, but as much as 1 g/d has been used. In patients with renal impairment, dosage must be reduced. Because of the danger of precipitating congestive heart failure, the use of loading doses is not recommended.

Therapeutic Use

Although disopyramide has been shown to be effective in a variety of supraventricular arrhythmias, in the USA it is approved only for the treatment of ventricular arrhythmias.

AMIODARONE

Amiodarone has been widely used as an antiarrhythmic and antianginal agent in Europe and South America. In the USA, it is only approved for use in serious ventricular arrhythmias. It is very effective against a wide variety of arrhythmias. It has prominent adverse effects and unusual pharmacokinetic properties that have limited its use in the USA. However, it is being increasingly used, possibly because of the recognition that other drugs may be more dangerous than heretofore appreciated (see boxes: The Molecular Basis of Cardiac Excitability and The Cardiac Arrhythmia Suppression Trial).

Amiodarone

Cardiac Effects

Amiodarone has a broad spectrum of actions on the heart. It is a very effective blocker of sodium channels, but unlike quinidine it has a low affinity for activated channels, combining instead almost exclusively with channels in the inactivated state. Thus, the sodium-blocking action of amiodarone is most pronounced in tissues that have long action potentials, frequent action potentials, or less negative diastolic potentials. In therapeutic concentrations, amiodarone also markedly lengthens action potential duration, probably by blocking potassium channels. Amiodarone sustains its lengthening of action potential duration quite well at fast heart rates, ie, it lacks the undesirable reverse use-dependent effects of other action potential-prolonging drugs (see box: The Molecular Basis of Cardiac Excitability). This is probably an important reason for its efficacy against tachycardias. Amiodarone is a weak calcium channel blocker as well as a noncompetitive inhibitor of beta adrenoceptors. The drug has also been shown to be a powerful inhibitor of abnormal automaticity. These latter actions may explain the rarity of torsade de pointes during amiodarone therapy, despite the QT interval prolongation the drug produces.

Amiodarone slows the sinus rate and atrioventricular conduction, markedly prolongs the QT interval, and prolongs QRS duration. It increases atrial, atrioventricular nodal, and ventricular refractory periods. Induction of new ventricular arrhythmias or worsening of preexisting ones occurs rarely during therapy with amiodarone.

Amiodarone also has antianginal effects. This may result from its noncompetitive alpha and beta adrenoceptor-blocking properties as well as from its apparent ability to block calcium influx in vascular smooth muscle.

Extracardiac Effects

Amiodarone causes peripheral vascular dilation, presumably through its alpha adrenoceptor-blocking and calcium channel-inhibiting effects. In some patients, this may be beneficial; rarely, it may require discontinuation of the drug.

Toxicity

A. Cardiac: In patients with sinus or atrioventricular nodal disease, amiodarone may produce symptomatic bradycardia or heart block. It may also precipitate heart failure in susceptible patients.

B. Extracardiac: Amiodarone causes a remarkable variety of extracardiac adverse effects, including potentially fatal pulmonary fibrosis. The number of amiodarone's toxic effects increases with the cumulative dose and can limit the utility of this drug (especially at higher dosage, eg, 400 mg/d or more) in long-term therapy.

Amiodarone is concentrated in tissue and can be found in virtually every organ. The most readily detected deposits are those in the cornea, which appear as yellowish-brown microcrystals in a few weeks after initiation of therapy. These corneal deposits rarely cause visual symptoms except for occasional halos in the peripheral visual fields, most prominent at night. Only infrequently does reduction of visual acuity occur, requiring discontinuation or reduction of amiodarone dosage. Skin deposits result in photodermatitis in about 25% of patients, and patients receiving the drug must avoid exposure to the sun. In less than 5% of patients, a grayish-blue skin discoloration develops.

Adverse neurologic effects are common and include paresthesias, tremor, ataxia, and headaches.

Thyroid dysfunction—both hypo- and hyperthyroidism—occurs in about 5% of patients. Thyroid function should be assessed prior to and throughout the duration of amiodarone therapy.

Amiodarone may affect the gastrointestinal tract (eg, constipation, 20%), liver (eg, hepatocellular necrosis), or lung (eg, inflammation and fibrosis). Pulmonary fibrosis has been reported in 5–15% of patients; in a fraction of these, it may be fatal.

Drug interactions are very common. Amiodarone reduces clearance of warfarin, theophylline, quinidine, procainamide, flecainide, and other drugs.

An intravenous formulation of amiodarone was marketed in the USA in 1995. Therapy with the intravenous form usually lasts only a few days, so the side effects seen with the oral drug (which reflect cumulative dose) are rare during intravenous administration. Rather, hypotension and bradycardia are the common adverse effects.

Pharmacokinetics & Dosage

Amiodarone has an extremely long half-life (13–103 days). The effective plasma concentration is approximately 1–2 μg/mL, while the cardiac tissue concentration is about 30 times higher. Even with large loading doses, 15–30 days or more are required to load the body stores with sufficient amiodarone to estimate the drug's efficacy. Loading doses of 0.8–1.2 g daily for about 2 weeks are used, after which the patient is maintained on 200–400 mg daily. Because of the drug's long half-life, once-daily dosage is adequate. If toxicity occurs, it may persist long after drug administration is discontinued.

Therapeutic Use

Amiodarone is very effective against both supraventricular and ventricular arrhythmias. In general, relatively low maintenance dosages (100–200 mg/d) can be used against paroxysmal atrial fibrillation. Amiodarone appears to be quite effective against supraventricular arrhythmias in children, in whom it appears to be relatively safe. However, long-term experience is not yet available. Large-scale clinical trials suggest that amiodarome, unlike many other drugs, does not increase mortality in patients with advanced heart disease (see box: The Cardiac Arrhythmia Suppression Trial).

Intravenous amiodarone is used in patients with recurrent ventricular tachycardia or fibrillation. With initial doses of 150 mg over 30 minutes (and 1 g over the first day), arrhythmias are often promptly suppressed. The mechanisms underlying this antiarrhythmic action are unknown but may reflect the drug's antiadrenergic properties. Phlebitis and physical compatibility with other intravenous fluids or drugs can be problems during intravenous treatment.

LIDOCAINE

Lidocaine is an antiarrhythmic drug that is used only by the intravenous route. It has a low incidence of toxicity and a high degree of effectiveness in arrhythmias associated with acute myocardial infarction.

Lidocaine

Cardiac Effects

Lidocaine is a potent suppressor of abnormal cardiac activity, and it appears to act exclusively on the sodium channel. Its interaction with this channel differs substantially from that of quinidine. Whereas quinidine mostly blocks sodium channels in the activated state, lidocaine rapidly blocks both activated and inactivated sodium channels (Figure 14–10). As a result, a large fraction (>50%) of the unblocked sodium channels become blocked during each action potential in Purkinje fibers and ventricular cells, which have long plateaus (and correspondingly long periods of inactivation). During diastole, most of the sodium channels in normally polarized cells rapidly become drug-free. Since lidocaine may shorten the action potential duration, diastole may be prolonged, thereby extending the time available for recovery. As a result, lidocaine has few electrophysiologic effects in normal cardiac tissue. In contrast, depolarized (inactivated) sodium channels remain largely blocked during diastole, and more may become blocked. Thus, lidocaine suppresses the electrical activity of the depolarized, arrhythmogenic tissues while minimally interfering with the electrical activity of normal tissues. These factors appear to be responsible for the fact that lidocaine is a very effective agent for suppressing arrhythmias associated with depolarization (eg, ischemia, digitalis toxicity), but it is relatively ineffective against arrhythmias occurring in normally polarized tissues (eg, atrial flutter and fibrillation).

Figure 14–10. Effect of membrane potential on the blocking and unblocking of sodium channels by lidocaine. **Upper tracing:** Action potentials in a ventricular muscle cell; **lower trace:** percentage of channels blocked by the drug. As the membrane depolarizes through –80, –75, –70 and –65 mV, an 800 ms time segment is shown. Extra passage of time is indicated by breaks in the traces. **Left side:** At the normal resting potential of –85 mV, the drug combines with open (activated) and inactivated channels during each action potential, but block is rapidly reversed during diastole because the affinity of the drug for its receptor is so low when the channel recovers to the resting state at –85 mV. **Middle:** Metabolic injury has occurred, eg, ischemia due to coronary occlusion, that causes gradual depolarization over time. With subsequent action potentials arising from more depolarized potentials, the fraction of channels blocked increases because more channels remain in the inactivated state at less negative potentials (Figure 14–4, left), and the time constant for unblocking during diastole rapidly increases at less negative resting potentials (Figure 14–4, right). **Right:** Because of marked drug binding, conduction block and loss of excitability in this tissue result, ie, the "sick" (depolarized) tissue is selectively suppressed.

Toxicity

A. Cardiac: Lidocaine is one of the least cardiotoxic of the currently used sodium channel blockers. The drug exacerbates ventricular arrhythmias in fewer than 10% of patients (a good record). However, in about 1% of patients with acute myocardial infarction, lidocaine precipitates sinoatrial nodal standstill or worsens impaired conduction.

In large doses, especially in patients with preexisting heart failure, lidocaine may cause hypotension—partly by depressing myocardial contractility.

B. Extracardiac: Lidocaine's most common adverse effects—like those of other local anesthetics—are neurologic: paresthesias, tremor, nausea of central origin, lightheadedness, hearing disturbances, slurred speech, and convulsions. These occur most commonly in elderly or otherwise vulnerable patients or when a bolus of the drug is given too rapidly. The ef-

GABA
valium

fects are dose-related and usually short-lived; seizures respond to intravenous diazepam. In general, if plasma levels above 9 μg/mL are avoided, lidocaine is well tolerated.

Pharmacokinetics & Dosage

Because of its very extensive first-pass hepatic metabolism, only 3% of orally administered lidocaine appears in the plasma. Thus, lidocaine must be given parenterally. Lidocaine has a half-life of about 2 hours. In adults, a loading dose of 150–200 mg administered over about 15 minutes (as a single infusion or as a series of slow boluses) should be followed by a maintenance infusion of 2–4 mg/min to achieve a therapeutic plasma level of 2–6 μg/mL. Determination of lidocaine plasma levels is of great value in adjusting the infusion rate. Occasional patients with myocardial infarction or other acute illness require (and tolerate) higher concentrations. This may be due to increased plasma α$_1$-acid glycoprotein, an acute phase reactant protein that binds lidocaine, making less free drug available to exert its pharmacologic effects.

In patients with congestive heart failure, lidocaine's volume of distribution and total body clearance may both be decreased. Thus, both loading and maintenance doses should be decreased. Since these effects counterbalance each other, the half-life may not be increased as much as predicted from clearance changes alone. In patients with liver disease, plasma clearance is markedly reduced and the volume of distribution is often increased; the elimination half-life in such cases may be increased threefold or more. In liver disease, the maintenance dose should be decreased, but usual loading doses can be given. Elimination half-life determines the time to steady state. Thus, while steady state concentrations may be achieved in 8–10 hours in normal patients and patients with heart failure, 24–36 hours may be required in those with liver disease. Drugs that decrease liver blood flow (eg, propranolol, cimetidine) reduce lidocaine clearance and so increase the risk of toxicity unless infusion rates are decreased. With infusions lasting more then 24 hours, clearance falls and plasma concentrations rise. Renal disease has no major effect on lidocaine disposition.

Therapeutic Use

Lidocaine is the agent of choice for suppression of ventricular tachycardia and fibrillation after cardioversion. Most evidence also suggests that lidocaine reduces the incidence of ventricular fibrillation in the first few days after acute myocardial infarction. However, some analyses suggest that routine prophylactic use of lidocaine in this setting may actually increase total mortality, possibly by increasing the incidence of asystole. Thus, most physicians administer lidocaine only to patients with arrhythmias and do not use the drug prophylactically in myocardial infarction.

TOCAINIDE & MEXILETINE

Tocainide and mexiletine are congeners of lidocaine that are resistant to first-pass hepatic metabolism. Therefore, they can be used by the oral route. Their electrophysiologic and antiarrhythmic actions are similar to those of lidocaine. (The anticonvulsant phenytoin [see Chapter 24] exerts similar electrophysiologic effects and has been used as an antiarrhythmic.) Tocainide and mexiletine are used in the treatment of ventricular arrhythmias. The elimination half-life of both drugs is 8–20 hours, and they are administered two or three times a day. The usual daily dosage of mexiletine is 600–1200 mg/d; of tocainide, 800–2400 mg/d. Both drugs cause dose-related adverse effects that are seen frequently at therapeutic dosage. These are predominantly neurologic, including tremor, blurred vision, and lethargy. Nausea is also a common effect. Rash, fever, and agranulocytosis occur in about 0.5% of patients receiving tocainide.

Mexiletine has also shown significant efficacy in relieving chronic pain, especially pain due to diabetic neuropathy and nerve injury. The usual dosage is 450–750 mg/d orally. This application is unlabeled.

Tocainide

Mexiletine

FLECAINIDE

Flecainide is a potent blocker of sodium and potassium channels. It is currently used for patients with otherwise normal hearts who have supraventricular arrhythmias. It has no antimuscarinic effects. It is very effective in suppressing premature ventricular contractions. However, it may cause severe exacerbation of arrhythmia even when normal doses are administered to patients with preexisting ventricular tachyarrhythmias and those with a previous myocardial infarction and ventricular ectopy (see box: The Cardiac Arrhythmia Suppression Trial). The drug is well absorbed and has a half-life of approximately 20 hours. Elimination is both by hepatic metabolism and by the kidney. The usual dosage of flecainide is 100–200 mg twice a day.

PROPAFENONE

Propafenone has some structural similarities to propranolol and possesses weak beta-blocking activity. Its spectrum of action is very similar to that of quinidine.

THE CARDIAC ARRHYTHMIA SUPPRESSION TRIAL

Premature ventricular contractions (PVCs) are commonly recorded in patients convalescing from myocardial infarction. Since such arrhythmias have been associated with an increased risk of sudden cardiac death, it had been the empiric practice of many physicians to treat PVCs, even if asymptomatic, in such patients. In CAST (Cardiac Arrhythmia Suppression Trial [CAST] Investigators, 1989; Echt et al, 1991), an attempt was made to document the efficacy of such therapy in a controlled clinical trial. The effects of several antiarrhythmic drugs on arrhythmia frequency were first evaluated in an open-label fashion. Then, patients in whom antiarrhythmic therapy suppressed PVCs were randomly assigned, in a double-blind fashion, to continue that therapy or its corresponding placebo.

The results showed that mortality among patients treated with the drugs flecainide and encainide (which is now available only under special circumstances) was *increased* more than twofold compared with those treated with placebo. The mechanism underlying this effect is not known, though an interaction between conduction depression by sodium channel block and chronic or acute myocardial ischemia seems likely. Indirect evidence suggests that other sodium channel blockers may produce a similar effect. Whatever the mechanism, the important lesson reinforced by CAST was that the decision to initiate any form of drug therapy (antiarrhythmic or otherwise) should be predicated on the knowledge (or at least a reasonable assumption) that any risk is outweighed by real or potential benefit. Large trials suggest that amiodarone (unlike flecainide) has little effect on survival of patients with advanced heart disease, while many studies indicate a beneficial effect of β-blockade.

Its potency as a sodium channel blocker is similar to that of flecainide. Its average elimination half-life is 5 hours except in poor metabolizers (7% of whites), in whom it is as much as 17 hours. The usual daily dosage of propafenone is 450–900 mg in three doses. The drug is used primarily for supraventricular arrhythmias. The most common adverse effects are a metallic taste and constipation; arrhythmia exacerbation can occur.

MORICIZINE

Moricizine is an antiarrhythmic phenothiazine derivative that is used for treatment of ventricular arrhythmias. It is a relatively potent sodium channel blocker that does not prolong action potential duration.

Moricizine produces in humans multiple metabolites, some of which are probably active and have long half-lives. Its most common adverse effects are dizziness and nausea. Like other potent sodium channel blockers, it can exacerbate arrhythmias.

The usual dosage of moricizine is 200–300 mg by mouth three times a day.

BETA ADRENOCEPTOR-BLOCKING DRUGS (CLASS II)

Cardiac Effects

Propranolol and similar drugs have antiarrhythmic properties by virtue of their beta receptor-blocking action and direct membrane effects. As described in Chapter 10, some of these drugs have selectivity for cardiac β_1 receptors; some have intrinsic sympathomimetic activity; some have marked direct membrane effects; and some prolong the cardiac action potential. The relative contributions of the beta-blocking and direct membrane effects to the antiarrhythmic effects of these drugs are not fully known. Although beta-blockers are fairly well tolerated, their efficacy for suppression of ventricular ectopic depolarizations is lower than that of sodium channel blockers. However, there is good evidence that these agents can prevent recurrent infarction and sudden death in patients recovering from acute myocardial infarction (Chapter 10).

Esmolol is a short-acting beta-blocker used primarily as an antiarrhythmic drug for intraoperative and other acute arrhythmias. See Chapter 10 for more information. Sotalol is a nonselective beta-blocking drug that prolongs the action potential (class III action).

DRUGS THAT PROLONG EFFECTIVE REFRACTORY PERIOD BY PROLONGING ACTION POTENTIAL (CLASS III)

These drugs prolong action potentials, usually by blocking potassium channels in cardiac muscle or by enhancing inward current, eg, through sodium or calcium channels. Many agents in this category exert additional effects that also place them in one of the other subgroups. Quinidine and amiodarone prolong action potential duration. However, as noted above, their actions on sodium channels also contribute to the measured increase in effective refractory period. Bretylium and sotalol have prominent autonomic effects and also prolong action potential duration and refractory period and are discussed below. A new action potential-prolonging drug, ibutilide, was approved in 1996. Ibutilide, unlike other drugs discussed here, is a "pure" class III agent in that it appears to be devoid of other significant pharmacologic effects. Action potential prolongation by these drugs often exhibits the undesirable property of "reverse use-dependence": Action potential prolongation is least marked at fast rates (where it is desirable) and most marked at slow rates, where it can contribute to the risk of torsade de pointes. Amiodarone may be an exception, prolonging action potential duration equally at all rates.

BRETYLIUM

Bretylium was first introduced as an antihypertensive agent. It interferes with the neuronal release of catecholamines but also has direct antiarrhythmic properties.

Bretylium

Cardiac Effects

Bretylium lengthens the ventricular (but not the atrial) action potential duration and effective refractory period. This effect is most pronounced in ischemic cells, which have shortened action potential durations. Thus, bretylium may reverse the shortening of action potential duration caused by ischemia. Experimentally, it has been shown that bretylium markedly increases the strength of electrical stimulation needed to induce ventricular fibrillation (ventricular fibrillation threshold) and delays the onset of fib-

rillation after acute coronary ligation. This antifibrillatory action appears to be independent of its sympatholytic properties.

Since bretylium causes an initial release of catecholamines, it has some positive inotropic actions when first administered. This action may also *precipitate* ventricular arrhythmias and must be watched for at the onset of therapy with the drug.

Extracardiac Effects

These result from the drug's sympathoplegic actions. The major adverse effect is postural hypotension. This effect can be almost totally prevented by concomitant administration of a tricyclic antidepressant agent such as protriptyline. Nausea and vomiting may occur after the intravenous administration of a bolus of bretylium.

Pharmacokinetics & Dosage

Bretylium is available only for intravenous use in the USA. In adults, an intravenous bolus of bretylium tosylate, 5 mg/kg, is administered over a 10-minute period. This dosage may be repeated after 30 minutes. Maintenance therapy is achieved by a similar bolus every 4–6 hours or by a constant infusion of 0.5–2 mg/min.

Therapeutic Use

Bretylium is usually used in an emergency setting, often during attempted resuscitation from ventricular fibrillation when lidocaine and cardioversion have failed. Only rarely does bretylium suppress premature ventricular contractions.

SOTALOL

Sotalol is a nonselective beta-blocker that also prolongs action potential duration and is an effective antiarrhythmic agent. Sotalol can be used in both supraventricular and ventricular arrhythmias. The usual effective dosage is 80–320 mg twice daily. Its major toxicities are associated with beta blockade (see Chapter 10) and with prolongation of repolarization, including torsade de pointes. Unlike quinidine, the risk of torsade de pointes is greater at higher dosages and plasma concentrations of sotalol. Thus, only lower dosages (80–160 mg twice daily) are usually used in atrial fibrillation. Sotalol is excreted unchanged by the kidneys, so dosage should be lowered in patients with renal failure to avoid the risk of torsade de pointes.

Sotalol

IBUTILIDE

Ibutilide prolongs cardiac action potentials but does not produce other significant pharmacologic effects. In vitro data suggest that it acts by enhancing an inward sodium current, by blocking I_{Kr}, or by both mechanisms. With oral administration, it is rapidly converted to inactive metabolites. Intravenous ibutilide (1 mg over 10 minutes) restores sinus rhythm in about 50% of patients with atrial flutter and about 30% of those with atrial fibrillation. There is a 4–8% incidence of torsade de pointes.

CALCIUM CHANNEL-BLOCKING DRUGS (CLASS IV)

These drugs, of which verapamil is the prototype, were first introduced as antianginal agents and are discussed in greater detail in Chapter 12. Verapamil, diltiazem, and bepridil also have antiarrhythmic effects. Nifedipine and other dihydropyridine calcium channel-blocking drugs have little antiarrhythmic activity.

VERAPAMIL

Cardiac Effects

Verapamil blocks both activated and inactivated calcium channels. Thus, its effect is more marked in tissues that fire frequently, those that are less completely polarized at rest, and those in which activation depends exclusively on the calcium current, such as the sinoatrial and atrioventricular nodes. It is therefore not surprising that verapamil has marked effects on these tissues. Atrioventricular nodal conduction and effective refractory period are invariably prolonged by therapeutic concentrations. Verapamil usually slows the sinoatrial node by its direct action, but its hypotensive action may occasionally result in a small reflex increase of sinoatrial nodal rate.

Verapamil can suppress both early and delayed afterdepolarizations and may antagonize slow responses arising in severely depolarized tissue.

Extracardiac Effects

Verapamil causes peripheral vasodilation, which may be beneficial in hypertension and peripheral vasospastic disorders. Its effects upon smooth muscle produce a number of extracardiac effects (see Chapter 12).

Toxicity

A. Cardiac: Verapamil's cardiotoxic effects are dose-related and usually avoidable. A common error has been to administer intravenous verapamil to a patient with ventricular tachycardia misdiagnosed as supraventricular tachycardia. In this setting, hypotension and ventricular fibrillation can occur. Verapamil's negative inotropic effects may limit its clinical usefulness in damaged hearts (see Chapter 12). Verapamil can lead to atrioventricular block when used in large doses or in patients with partial atrioventricular block. This block can be treated with atropine, beta receptor stimulants, or calcium. In patients with sinus node disease, verapamil can precipitate sinus arrest.

B. Extracardiac: Adverse effects include constipation, lassitude, nervousness, and peripheral edema.

Pharmacokinetics & Dosage

The half-life of verapamil is approximately 7 hours. It is extensively metabolized by the liver; after oral administration, its bioavailability is only about 20%. Therefore, verapamil must be administered with caution in patients with hepatic dysfunction.

In adult patients without heart failure or sinoatrial or atrioventricular nodal disease, parenteral treatment of supraventricular tachycardia consists of an initial bolus of 5 mg administered over 2–5 minutes, followed a few minutes later by a second 5 mg bolus if needed. Thereafter, doses of 5–10 mg can be administered every 4–6 hours, or a constant infusion of 0.4 µg/kg/min may be used.

Effective oral dosages are higher than with intravenous drug because of first pass metabolism and range from 120 to 640 mg daily, divided into three or four doses.

Therapeutic Use

Reentrant supraventricular tachycardia is the major indication for verapamil, and adenosine or verapamil are preferred over older treatments (propranolol, digoxin, edrophonium, vasoconstrictor agents, and cardioversion). Verapamil can also reduce the ventricular rate in atrial fibrillation and flutter. It only rarely converts atrial flutter and fibrillation to sinus rhythm. Verapamil is very rarely useful in ventricular arrhythmias. In fact, the use of intravenous verapamil in a patient with sustained ventricular tachycardia can cause hemodynamic collapse.

DILTIAZEM & BEPRIDIL

These agents appear to be similar in efficacy to verapamil in the management of supraventricular arrhythmias, including rate control in atrial fibrillation. An intravenous form of diltiazem is available for the latter indication and seems to cause hypotension or bradyarrhythmias relatively infrequently. Bepridil also has action potential- and QT-prolonging actions that theoretically may make it more useful in some ventricular arrhythmias but also create the risk of torsade de pointes. Bepridil is only rarely used, primarily to control refractory angina.

MISCELLANEOUS ANTIARRHYTHMIC AGENTS

Certain agents used for the treatment of arrhythmias do not fit the conventional class I–IV organization. These include digitalis (already discussed in Chapter 13), adenosine, magnesium, and potassium.

ADENOSINE

Mechanism & Clinical Use

Adenosine is a nucleoside that occurs naturally throughout the body. Its half-life in the blood is estimated to be less than 10 seconds. Its mechanism of action involves enhanced potassium conductance and inhibition of cAMP-induced calcium influx. The results of these actions are marked hyperpolarization and suppression of calcium-dependent action potentials. When given as a bolus dose, adenosine directly inhibits atrioventricular nodal conduction and increases the atrioventricular nodal refractory period but has only mild effects on sinoatrial nodal function. Adenosine is currently the drug of choice for prompt conversion of paroxysmal supraventricular tachycardia to sinus rhythm because of its high efficacy (90–95%) and very short duration of action. It is usually given in a bolus dose of 6 mg followed, if necessary, by a dose of 12 mg. The drug may also be effective in rare patients with ventricular tachycardia. It is less effective in the presence of adenosine receptor blockers such as theophylline or caffeine, and its effects are potentiated by adenosine uptake inhibitors such as dipyridamole.

Toxicity

Adenosine causes flushing in about 20% of patients and shortness of breath or chest burning (perhaps related to bronchospasm) in over 10%. Induction of high-grade atrioventricular block may occur but is very short-lived. Atrial fibrillation may occur. Less common toxicities include headache, hypotension, nausea, and paresthesias.

MAGNESIUM

Originally used for patients with digitalis-induced arrhythmias who were hypomagnesemic, magnesium infusion has been found to have antiarrhythmic effects in some patients with normal serum magnesium levels. The mechanisms of these effects are not known, but magnesium is recognized to influence Na^+/K^+ ATPase, sodium channels, certain potassium channels, and calcium channels. Magnesium therapy appears to be indicated in patients with digitalis-induced arrhythmias if hypomagnesemia is present; it is also indicated in some patients with torsade de pointes and in some with acute myocardial infarction even if serum magnesium is normal. The usual dosage is 1 g (as sulfate) given intravenously over 20 minutes and repeated once if necessary. The full details of the action and indications of magnesium as an antiarrhythmic drug await further investigation.

POTASSIUM

The significance of the potassium ion concentrations inside and outside the cardiac cell membrane has been discussed earlier in this chapter. The effects of increasing serum K^+ can be summarized as (1) a resting potential depolarizing action and (2) a membrane potential stabilizing action, caused by increased potassium permeability. Hypokalemia results in an increased risk of early and delayed afterdepolarizations, and ectopic pacemaker activity, especially in the presence of digitalis; hyperkalemia is characterized by depression of ectopic pacemakers (severe hyperkalemia is required to suppress the sinoatrial node) and slowing of conduction. Because both insufficient and excess potassium are potentially arrhythmogenic, potassium therapy is directed toward normalizing potassium gradients and pools in the body.

III. PRINCIPLES IN THE CLINICAL USE OF ANTIARRHYTHMIC AGENTS

The likelihood that therapy with any drug will be effective depends in part on the relationship between drug doses required to produce a desired therapeutic effect and drug doses associated with toxicity. This margin between efficacy and toxicity is particularly narrow for antiarrhythmic drugs. Therefore, individuals prescribing antiarrhythmic drugs must be thoroughly familiar with the indications, contraindications, risks, and clinical pharmacologic characteristics of each compound they use.

Pretreatment Evaluation

Several important determinations must be made prior to initiation of any antiarrhythmic therapy:

(1) Any factor that might precipitate arrhythmias must be recognized and eliminated if possible. These include not only abnormalities of internal homeostasis, such as hypoxia or electrolyte abnormalities (especially hypokalemia or hypomagnesemia), but also drug therapy. Drugs that can precipitate arrhythmias include digitalis, all antiarrhythmic drugs, and many compounds generally not thought to have primary cardiovascular actions. For example, high doses of erythromycin, pentamidine, tricyclic antidepressants, antipsychotics (notably thioridazine), and the nonsedating antihistamines terfenadine and astemizole have

all been associated with torsade de pointes. Other important reversible causes of arrhythmias include underlying disease states. For example, antiarrhythmic drug therapy for atrial fibrillation is not likely to be effective in hyperthyroidism; rather, the underlying pathophysiology should be addressed with antithyroid maneuvers. Most patients who have arrhythmias have some form of underlying cardiac disease. It is important to separate this abnormal substrate from triggering factors, such as myocardial ischemia or acute cardiac dilation, which may be treatable and reversible.

(2) A firm arrhythmia diagnosis should be established. For example, the misuse of verapamil in patients with ventricular tachycardia mistakenly diagnosed as supraventricular tachycardia can lead to catastrophic hypotension and cardiac arrest. As increasingly sophisticated methods to characterize underlying arrhythmia mechanisms become available and are validated, it may be possible to direct certain drugs (or other therapies—see box: The Nonpharmacologic Therapy of Cardiac Arrhythmias) toward specific arrhythmia mechanisms.

(3) It is important to establish a reliable baseline upon which to judge the efficacy of any subsequent antiarrhythmic intervention. A number of methods are now available for such baseline quantitation. These include prolonged ambulatory monitoring, electrophysiologic studies that reproduce a target arrhythmia, reproduction of a target arrhythmia by treadmill exercise, or the use of transtelephonic monitoring for recording of sporadic but symptomatic arrhythmias. Whatever the baseline modality chosen, the prescriber should also recognize the phenomenon of "ascertainment" bias: Arrhythmia frequency may fluctuate over months, and patients are most likely to present to a physician when they are symptomatic. Therefore, even a completely ineffective drug intervention may appear to have antiarrhythmic properties.

(4) The mere identification of an abnormality of cardiac rhythm does not necessarily require that the arrhythmia be treated. An excellent justification for conservative treatment was provided by the Cardiac Arrhythmia Suppression Trial (CAST) (see box: The Cardiac Arrhythmia Suppression Trial).

Benefits & Risks

The benefits of antiarrhythmic therapy are actually relatively difficult to establish. Two types of benefits can be envisioned: reduction of arrhythmia-related symptoms, such as palpitations, syncope, or cardiac arrest; or reduction in long-term mortality in asymptomatic patients. Among drugs discussed here, only beta-blockers have been definitely associated with reduction of mortality in relatively asymptomatic patients, and the mechanism underlying this effect is not established (see Chapter 10).

Antiarrhythmic therapy carries with it a number of risks. In some cases, the risk of an adverse reaction is clearly related to high dosages or plasma concen-

---

THE NONPHARMACOLOGIC THERAPY OF CARDIAC ARRHYTHMIAS

It was recognized at the start of the 20th century that reentry in simple in vitro models (eg, rings of conducting tissues) was permanently interrupted by transecting the reentry circuit. This concept has now been applied to treat clinical arrhythmias that occur as a result of reentry in anatomically delineated pathways. For example, interruption of accessory atrioventricular connections can permanently cure arrhythmias in patients with the Wolff-Parkinson-White syndrome. Such interruption was originally performed at open heart surgery but is now readily accomplished by delivery of radiofrequency energy through an appropriately positioned intracardiac catheter. Since the procedure carries only minimal morbidity, it is being increasingly applied to other reentry arrhythmias with defined pathways, such as AV nodal reentry, atrial flutter, and some forms of ventricular tachycardia.

Another form of nonpharmacologic therapy is the implantable cardioverter-defibrillator (ICD), a device that can automatically detect and treat potentially fatal arrhythmias such as ventricular fibrillation. ICDs are now widely used in patients who have been resuscitated from such arrhythmias, and trials are under way to determine if they should be used in patients with advanced heart disease who have not yet had such arrhythmias but are judged to be at high risk. The increasing use of nonpharmacologic antiarrhythmic therapies reflects both advances in the relevant technologies and an increasing appreciation of the dangers of long-term therapy with currently available drugs.

---

trations. Examples include lidocaine-induced tremor or quinidine-induced cinchonism. In other cases, adverse reactions are unrelated to high plasma concentrations (eg, procainamide- or tocainide-induced agranulocytosis). For many serious adverse reactions to antiarrhythmic drugs, the *combination* of drug therapy and the underlying heart disease appears important. For example, patients with advanced conduction system disease are at increased risk for complete heart block during treatment with drugs such as quinidine or flecainide, whereas this risk is very small in patients without conduction system disease. Similarly, the development of congestive heart failure is more common during drug treatment in patients with underlying left ventricular dysfunction. Beta-blockers, verapamil, disopyramide, and flecainide are particularly prone to produce heart failure in this setting.

Several specific syndromes of arrhythmia provocation by antiarrhythmic drugs have also been identified, each with its underlying pathophysiologic mechanism and risk factors. Drugs such as quinidine or sotalol, which act—at least in part—by prolonging cardiac action potentials can result in marked QT prolongation and torsade de pointes. Treatment of torsade de pointes requires recognition of the arrhythmia, withdrawal of any offending agent, correction of hypokalemia, and treatment with maneuvers to increase heart rate (pacing or isoproterenol); intravenous magnesium also appears effective, even in patients with normal magnesium levels. Drugs that markedly slow conduction, such as flecainide, or high concentrations of quinidine, can result in an increased frequency of reentry arrhythmias, notably reentry ventricular tachycardia in patients with prior myocardial infarction in whom a potential reentry circuit may be present. Treatment here consists of recognition, withdrawal of the offending agent, and intravenous sodium. Some patients with this form of arrhythmia aggravation cannot be resuscitated, and deaths have been reported. Thus, the prescriber is faced with the paradox that the patient most likely to benefit from antiarrhythmic therapy, such as one with advanced coronary artery disease, conduction system disease, left ventricular dysfunction, and recurrent ventricular tachycardia, is exactly that patient who is at greatest risk for adverse reactions to antiarrhythmic drugs.

In practice, the choice of drug therapies is frequently dictated not so much by expected efficacy but by toxicity profiles. The presence of certain disease states may lead the prescribing clinician away from drugs with certain toxicities and toward other drugs. In addition to left ventricular dysfunction and underlying conduction system disturbances mentioned above, noncardiovascular diseases may also influence the choice of drug therapy. For example, prostatism is a relative contraindication to disopyramide, since the drug commonly causes urinary retention even in normal individuals. It may be difficult in patients with chronic arthritis to detect the development of the procainamide-induced lupus syndrome, and this drug is therefore relatively contraindicated as well. Similarly, it may be difficult to detect amiodarone-induced pulmonary injury in patients with advanced lung disease, so the drug is relatively contraindicated. Moreover, some data suggest that such patients may actually be at increased risk for amiodarone-induced pulmonary injury.

Conduct of Antiarrhythmic Therapy

Once a decision has been made to initiate drug therapy, the next step is to decide whether the arrhythmia is immediately life-threatening. If it is, then the use of loading doses is appropriate. If it is not, loading doses may expose patients to a greater risk of toxicity and do not alter the ultimate steady state achieved. Therefore, unless the clinical situation demands it, loading doses should be avoided.

Drug therapy can be considered effective when the target arrhythmia is suppressed (according to the measure used to quantify at baseline) and toxicities are absent. Conversely, drug therapy should not be considered ineffective unless toxicities occur at a time when arrhythmias are not suppressed. Occasionally, arrhythmias may recur at a time when plasma drug concentrations are relatively high but toxicities have not recurred. Under these conditions, the prescriber must decide whether a judicious increase in dose might suppress the arrhythmia and still leave the patient free of toxicity.

Monitoring plasma drug concentrations can be a useful adjunct to managing antiarrhythmic therapy. Widely quoted therapeutic ranges are actually derived from two concentration-response curves. The lower limit of the therapeutic range is defined as a concentration below which clinically beneficial drug actions do not usually occur. The upper limit of the therapeutic range is a concentration beyond which additional drug efficacy is unlikely or toxicities become increasingly frequent. For a specific patient, drug efficacy or adverse effects may occur below the usual lower limit of the therapeutic range; conversely, occasional patients can be effectively treated at plasma concentrations above the upper limit and without adverse effects. Thus, the use of a concentration monitoring strategy mandates that the prescriber be aware of the potential toxicity associated with high concentrations. Plasma drug concentrations are also important in establishing compliance during long-term therapy as well as in detecting drug interactions that may result in very high concentrations at low drug dosages or very low concentrations at high dosages. For some drugs, active metabolites (which may exert pharmacologic actions similar to or different from the parent drug) contribute to a variable extent to drug actions in patients. The presence of such active drug metabolites makes interpretation of data obtained during plasma concentration monitoring particularly difficult and, in some cases, makes routine plasma concentration drug monitoring impractical.

PREPARATIONS AVAILABLE

Sodium Channel Blockers

Amiodarone (Cordarone)
Oral: 200 mg tablets
Parenteral: 150 mg/3 mL for intravenous infusion

Disopyramide (generic, Norpace)
Oral: 100, 150 mg capsules;
Oral controlled-release (generic, Norpace CR): 100, 150 capsules

Flecainide (Tambocor)
Oral: 50, 100, 150 mg tablets

Lidocaine (generic, Xylocaine)
Parenteral: 100 mg/mL for IM injection; 10, 20 mg/mL for IV injection; 40, 100, 200 mg/mL for IV admixtures; premixed IV (5% D/W) solution

Mexiletine (Mexitil)
Oral: 150, 200, 250 mg capsules

Moricizine (Ethmozine)
Oral: 200, 250, 300 mg tablets

Procainamide (generic, Pronestyl, others)
Oral: 250, 375, 500 mg tablets and capsules
Oral sustained-release (generic, Procan-SR): 250, 500, 750, 1000 mg tablets
Parenteral: 100, 500 mg/mL for injection

Propafenone (Rythmol)
Oral: 150, 300 mg tablets

Quinidine sulfate [83% quinidine base] (generic)
Oral: 200, 300 mg tablets; 300 mg capsules
Oral sustained-release (Quinidex Extentabs): 300 mg tablets

Quinidine gluconate [62% quinidine base] (generic)
Oral sustained-release: 324 mg tablets
Parenteral: 80 mg/mL for injection

Quinidine polygalacturonate [60% quinidine base] (Cardioquin)
Oral: 275 mg tablets

Tocainide (Tonocard)
Oral: 400, 600 mg tablets

Beta-Blockers Labeled for Use as Antiarrhythmics

Acebutolol (Sectral)
Oral: 200, 400 mg capsules

Esmolol (Brevibloc)
Parenteral: 10 mg/mL, 250 mg/mL for IV injection

Propranolol (generic, Inderal)
Oral: 10, 20, 40, 60, 80, 90 mg tablets; 4 mg/mL, 8 mg/mL solutions; Intensol, 80 mg/mL
Oral sustained-release: 60, 80, 120, 160 mg capsules
Parenteral: 1 mg/mL for injection

Action Potential-Prolonging Agents

Bretylium (generic, Bretylol)
Parenteral: 50 mg/mL for injection

Sotalol (Betapace) Oral: 80, 160, 240 mg capsules

Ibutilide (Corvert)
Parenteral: 0.1 g/mL solution for IV infusion

Calcium Channel Blockers

Bepridil (generic, Vascor; *not labeled for use in arrhythmias*)
Oral: 200, 300, 400 mg tablets

Diltiazem (generic, Cardizem, Dilacor)
Oral: 30, 60, 90, 120 mg tablets; 60, 90, 120, 180, 240, 300 mg sustained-release capsules *(not labeled for use in arrhythmias)*
Parenteral: 5 mg/mL for intravenous injection

Verapamil (generic, Calan, Isoptin)
Oral: 40, 80, 120 mg tablets;
Oral sustained-release (Calan SR, Isoptin SR): 120, 180, 240 mg tablets and capsules
Parenteral: 5 mg/2 mL for injection

Miscellaneous

Adenosine (Adenocard)
Parenteral: 6 mg/2 mL for injection

Magnesium chloride
Parenteral: 0.2 g/mL for intravenous infusion

REFERENCES

Akhtar M et al: CAST and beyond: Implications of the cardiac arrhythmia suppression trial. Circulation 1990; 81:1123.

Akhtar M, Tchou P, Jazayeri M: Use of calcium entry blockers in the treatment of cardiac arrhythmias. Circulation 1989;80(Suppl IV):IV-31.

Balser JR et al: Suppression of time-dependent outward current in guinea pig ventricular myocytes: Actions of quinidine and amiodarone. Circ Res 1991;69:519.

Cairns JA et al: Randomized trial of outcome after myocardial infarction in patients with frequent or repetitive ventricular premature depolarizations. Canadian Amiodarone Myocardial Infarction Arrhythmia Trial. Lancet 1997;349:675.

Coplen SE et al: Efficacy and safety of quinidine therapy for maintenance of sinus rhythm after cardioversion. Circulation 1990;82:1106.

Curran ME et al: A molecular basis for cardiac arrhythmia: *HERG* mutations cause long QT syndrome. Cell 1995;80:795.

Dusman RE et al: Clinical features of amiodarone-induced pulmonary toxicity. Circulation 1990;82:51.

Echt DS et al for the CAST Investigators: Mortality and morbidity in patients receiving encainide, flecainide, or placebo. N Eng J Med 1991;324:781.

Funck-Brentano C et al: Propafenone. N Engl J Med 1990;322:518.

Greene HL, The CASCADE Investigators: The CASCADE Study: Randomized antiarrhythmic drug therapy in survivors of cardiac arrest in Seattle. Am J Cardiol 1993;72:70F.

Greene HL: Antiarrhythmic drugs versus implantable defibrillators: The need for a randomized controlled study. Am Heart J 1994;127:1171.

Greene HL: The efficacy of amiodarone in the treatment of ventricular tachycardia or ventricular fibrillation. Prog Cardiovasc Dis 1989;31:319.

Hennekens CH et al: Adjunctive drug therapy of acute myocardial infarction: Evidence from clinical trials. N Engl J Med 1996;335:1660.

Hohnloser SH, Woosley RL: Sotalol. N Engl J Med 1994;331:31.

Hondeghem LM, Katzung BG: Antiarrhythmic agents: Modulated receptor mechanism of action of sodium and calcium channel-blocking drugs. Annu Rev Pharmacol Toxicol 1984;24:387.

Hondeghem LM: Ideal antiarrhythmic agents: Chemical defibrillators. J Cardiovasc Electrophysiol 1991;2:169.

Julian DG et al: Randomized trial of effect of amiodarone on mortality in patients with left-ventricular dysfunction after recent myocardial infarction. Lancet 1997;349:667.

Kopelman HA, Horowitz LN: Efficacy and toxicity of amiodarone for the treatment of supraventricular arrhythmias. Prog Cardiovasc Dis 1989;31:355.

Kowey PR et al and Intravenous Amiodarone Multicenter Investigators Group: Randomized, double-blind comparison of intravenous amiodarone and bretylium in the treatment of patients with recurrent, hemodynamically destabilising ventricular tachycardia or fibrillation. Circulation 1995;92:3255.

Lerman BB, Belardinelli L: Cardiac electrophysiology of adenosine: Basic and clinical concepts. Circulation 1991;83:1499.

Levine JH, Morganroth J, Kadish AH: Mechanisms and risk factors for proarrhythmia with type Ia compared with Ic antiarrhythmic drug therapy. Circulation 1989;80:1063.

Manolis AS, Wang PJ, Estes NA: Radiofrequency catheter ablation for cardiac tachyarrhythmias. Ann Intern Med 1994;121:452.

Mason JW, Hondeghem LM, Katzung BG: Block of inactivated sodium channels and of depolarization-induced automaticity in guinea pig papillary muscles by amiodarone. Circ Res 1984;55:278.

Mason JW: A comparison of seven antiarrhythmic drugs in patients with ventricular tachyarrhythmias: Electrophysiologic study versus electrocardiographic monitoring investigators. N Engl J Med 1993;329:452.

Mason JW: Amiodarone. N Engl J Med 1987;316:455.

Mitchell LB, Schroeder JS, Mason JW: Comparative clinical electrophysiologic effects of diltiazem, verapamil and nifedipine: A review. Am J Cardiol 1982;49:629.

Myers M et al: Benefits and risks of long-term amiodarone therapy for sustained ventricular tachycardia/fibrillation: Minimum of three-year follow-up in 145 patients. Am Heart J 1990;119:8.

Roden DM, George AL Jr, Bennett PB: Recent advances in understanding the molecular mechanisms of the long QT syndrome. J Cardiovasc Electrophysiol 1995;6:1023.

Roden DM, George AL Jr: The cardiac ion channels: Relevance to management of arrhythmias. Annu Rev Med 1996;47:135.

Roden DM, Woosley RL: Flecainide. N Engl J Med 1986; 315:361.

Roden DM: Early after-depolarizations and torsade de pointes: Implications for the control of cardiac arrhythmias by prolonging repolarization. Eur Heart J 1993; 14(Suppl H):56.

Roden DM: Risks and benefits of antiarrhythmic therapy. N Engl J Med 1994;331:785.

Stanton MS et al: Arrhythmogenic effects of antiarrhythmic drugs: A study of 506 patients treated for ventricular tachycardia or fibrillation. J Am Coll Cardiol 1989; 14:209.

Stewart RB, Bardy GH, Greene HL: Wide complex tachycardia: Misdiagnosis and outcome after emergent therapy. Ann Intern Med 1986;104:766.

Task Force of the Working Group on Arrhythmias of the European Society of Cardiology: The Sicilian gambit: A new approach to the classification of antiarrhythmic drugs based on their actions on arrhythmic mechanisms. Circulation 1991;84:1831.

Tzivoni D et al: Treatment of torsade de pointes with magnesium sulfate. Circulation 1988;77:392.

Wang Q et al: Cardiac sodium channel mutations in patients with long QT syndrome, an inherited cardiac arrhythmia. Hum Mol Gen 1995;4:1603.

Wang Q et al: Positional cloning of a novel potassium channel gene: *KVLQT1* mutations cause cardiac arrhythmias. Nat Genet 1996;12:17.

Woods KL et al: Intravenous magnesium sulphate in suspected acute myocardial infarction: Results of the second Leicester Intravenous Magnesium Intervention Trial (LIMIT-2). Lancet 1992;339:1553.

Yang T, Roden DM: Extracellular potassium modulation of drug block of I_{Kr}: Implications for torsades de pointes and reverse use-dependence. Circulation 1996;93:407.

15

Diuretic Agents

Harlan E. Ives, MD, PhD

Abnormalities in fluid volume and electrolyte composition are common and important clinical problems that can become life-threatening if untreated. Drugs that block the transport functions of the renal tubules are important clinical tools in the treatment of these disorders.

Although various agents that increase urine flow have been described since antiquity, it was not until 1957, with the synthesis of chlorothiazide, that a practical and powerful diuretic agent became available for widespread use. Thus, the science of diuretics is relatively new. Technically, the term "diuresis" signifies an increase in urine volume, while "natriuresis" denotes an increase in renal sodium excretion. Because the important natriuretic drugs almost always also increase water excretion, they are usually called diuretics, and the increase in sodium excretion is assumed.

Many diuretic agents (loop diuretics, thiazides, amiloride, and triamterene) exert their effects on specific membrane transport proteins at the luminal surface of renal tubular epithelial cells. Others exert osmotic effects that prevent water reabsorption in the water-permeable segments of the nephron (mannitol), inhibit enzymes (acetazolamide), or interfere with hormone receptors in renal epithelial cells (spironolactone).

For the most part, each diuretic agent acts upon a single anatomic segment of the nephron (Figure 15–1). Because these segments have distinctive transport functions, the actions of each diuretic agent can be best understood in relation to its site of action in the nephron and the normal physiology of that segment. Therefore, the first section of this chapter is devoted to a review of those features of renal tubule physiology that are relevant to diuretic action. The second section is devoted to the basic pharmacology of diuretics, and the third section discusses the clinical applications of these drugs.

I. RENAL TUBULE TRANSPORT MECHANISMS

PROXIMAL TUBULE

Sodium bicarbonate, sodium chloride, glucose, amino acids, and other organic solutes are preferentially reabsorbed via specific transport systems in the early proximal tubule. Water is reabsorbed passively so as to maintain constant osmolality of proximal tubular fluid. As tubule fluid is processed along the length of the proximal tubule, the luminal concentrations of the solutes decrease relative to the concentration of inulin, an experimental marker that is neither secreted nor absorbed by renal tubules (Figure 15–2). The inulin concentration itself rises owing to water reabsorption by the proximal tubule. Approximately 85% of the filtered sodium bicarbonate, 40% of the sodium chloride, 60% of the water, and virtually all of the filtered organic solutes are reabsorbed in the proximal tubule.

Of the various solutes reabsorbed in the proximal tubule, the most relevant to diuretic action are sodium bicarbonate and sodium chloride. Of the currently available diuretic agents, only one (acetazolamide) acts predominantly in the proximal tubule, and that agent blocks only sodium bicarbonate reabsorption. However, proximal tubule sodium chloride reabsorption is of great theoretical interest. In view of the large quantity of sodium chloride absorbed at this site, a drug that specifically blocked proximal tubule sodium chloride transport might be a particularly powerful diuretic agent.

Sodium bicarbonate reabsorption by the proximal tubule is initiated by the action of a Na^+-H^+ exchanger located in the apical (luminal) membrane of the proximal tubule epithelial cell (Figure 15–3). This transport system allows sodium to enter the cell from the tubular lumen in one-for-one exchange with a proton from inside the cell. As in all portions of the nephron, Na^+/K^+ ATPase in the basolateral membrane pumps

Figure 15–1. Tubule transport systems and sites of action of diuretics.

the reabsorbed Na+ out of the cells into the interstitium and keeps the intracellular concentration of sodium low. Protons secreted into the lumen combine with bicarbonate to form carbonic acid, H_2CO_3. Carbonic acid, like bicarbonate, is not directly transported by proximal tubule cells. Instead, carbonic acid is dehydrated to CO_2 and H_2O, which readily move across the membranes. This dehydration reaction requires enzymatic catalysis, which is provided by carbonic anhydrase. Carbon dioxide produced by dehydration of carbonic acid enters the proximal tubule cell by simple diffusion and is then rehydrated back to carbonic acid. After dissociation, the H+ is again available for transport by the Na+/H+ exchanger, and the bicarbonate is transported across the basolateral membrane and into the blood by a specific transporter (Figure 15–3). Thus, bicarbonate reabsorption by the proximal tubule is critically dependent upon carbonic anhydrase activity. Carbonic anhydrase is inhibited by an important diuretic: acetazolamide.

In the late proximal tubule, as bicarbonate and organic solutes have been largely removed from the tubular fluid, the residual luminal fluid contains predominantly NaCl. Under these conditions, Na+ reabsorption continues, but the proton secreted by the Na+/H+ exchanger is no longer titrated by bicarbonate. This causes luminal pH to fall, activating a still poorly defined Cl−/base exchanger (Figure 15–3). The net effect of parallel Na+/H+ exchange and Cl−/base exchange is NaCl reabsorption. As yet, there are no diuretic agents that are known to act on this process. Thus, diuretic action in the proximal tubule is currently limited to inhibition of sodium bicarbonate reabsorption by carbonic anhydrase inhibitors.

Because of the high water permeability of the proximal tubule, the luminal fluid osmolality and sodium concentration remain relatively constant along the length of the proximal tubule (Figure 15–2). Thus, water is reabsorbed in direct proportion to salt reabsorption in this segment. An experimental impermeant solute like inulin will therefore rise in concentration as water is reabsorbed (Figure 15–2). If large amounts of impermeant solutes, eg, glucose or mannitol, are present in the tubular fluid, water reabsorption would cause the concentration of these solutes to rise to the point where osmolality of the tubular fluid is increased and further water reabsorption is prevented. This is the mechanism by which osmotic diuretics act (see below).

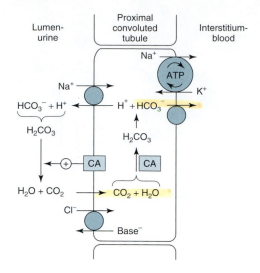

Figure 15–3. Apical membrane Na⁺/H⁺ exchanger and bicarbonate reabsorption in the proximal convoluted tubule cell. Na⁺/K⁺ ATPase is present in the basolateral membrane to maintain intracellular sodium and potassium levels within the normal range. Because of rapid equilibration, concentrations of the solutes shown are approximately equal in the interstitial fluid and the blood. Carbonic anhydrase (CA) is found in other locations in addition to the brush border of the luminal membrane.

Figure 15–2. Reabsorption of various solutes in the proximal tubule in relation to tubule length. (TF/P, tubular fluid to plasma concentration ratio; PD, potential difference across the tubule.) (Reproduced, with permission, from Ganong WF: *Review of Medical Physiology*, 17th ed. Lange, 1993.)

Organic acid secretory systems are located in the middle third of the proximal tubule (S_2 segment). These systems secrete a variety of organic acids (uric acid, *p*-aminohippuric acid, diuretics, antibiotics, etc) into the luminal fluid from the blood. Organic base secretory systems (creatinine, procainamide, choline, etc) are localized in the early (S_1) and middle (S_2) segments of the proximal tubule. These systems are important determinants in delivery of diuretics to their active sites at the luminal aspects of tubule segments along the entire nephron. In addition, these sites account for several interactions between diuretics and uric acid or other exogenous organic compounds (eg, interactions between diuretics and probenecid).

LOOP OF HENLE

The thin limb of Henle's loop does not participate in active salt reabsorption, but it does contribute to water reabsorption. Water is extracted from the thin descending limb of the loop of Henle by osmotic forces generated in the hypertonic medullary interstitium. As in the proximal tubule, impermeant solutes like mannitol or glucose in the lumen will oppose water extraction and increase the delivery of water to more distal sites. Thus, the thin limb is an additional site of action for osmotic diuretics. The thick ascending limb of the loop of Henle actively reabsorbs NaCl from the lumen (about 35% of the filtered sodium), but unlike the proximal tubule and thin limb, it is extremely impermeable to water. Salt reabsorption in the thick ascending limb therefore dilutes the tubular fluid, leading to its designation as a "diluting segment." Medullary portions of the thick ascending limb contribute to medullary hypertonicity and thereby also play an important role in concentration of urine.

The NaCl transport system in the luminal membrane of the thick ascending limb is a Na⁺/K⁺/2Cl⁻ cotransporter (Figure 15–4). This transporter is selectively blocked by diuretic agents known as "loop" diuretics (see below). Although the Na⁺/K⁺/2Cl⁻ transporter is itself electrically neutral (two cations and two anions are cotransported), the action of the transporter leads to excess K⁺ accumulation within the cell since the Na⁺/K⁺ ATPase is also pumping potassium into the cell (from the basolateral side). This results in back diffusion of K⁺ into the tubular lumen, which leads to the development of a lumen-positive electrical potential. This electrical potential

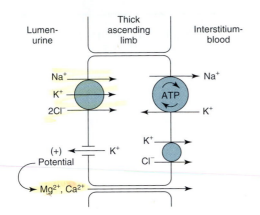

Figure 15–4. Ion transport pathways across the luminal and basolateral membranes of the thick ascending limb cell. The lumen positive electrical potential created by K+ back diffusion drives divalent cation reabsorption via the paracellular pathway.

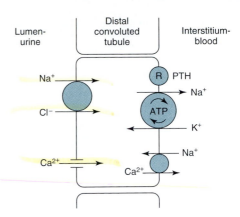

Figure 15–5. Ion transport pathways across the luminal and basolateral membranes of the distal convoluted tubule cell. As in all tubular cells, Na+/K+ ATPase is present in the basolateral membrane. (R, PTH receptor.)

provides the driving force for reabsorption of the divalent cations—Mg^{2+} and Ca^{2+}—via the paracellular pathway (between the cells). Thus, inhibition of salt transport in the thick ascending limb by loop diuretics causes an increase in urinary excretion of these divalent cations in addition to NaCl.

DISTAL CONVOLUTED TUBULE

Less NaCl is reabsorbed in the distal convoluted tubule (only about 10% of the filtered NaCl) than in the thick ascending limb. Like the thick ascending limb, this segment is relatively impermeable to water, and the NaCl reabsorption therefore further dilutes the tubular fluid. The mechanism of NaCl transport in the distal convoluted tubule is electrically neutral Na^+ and Cl^- cotransport (Figure 15–5), which is pharmacologically distinct from the $Na^+/K^+/2Cl^-$ cotransporter in the thick ascending limb. The NaCl transporter is blocked by diuretics of the thiazide class. Because K^+ does not recycle across the apical membrane of the distal convoluted tubule as it does in the loop of Henle, there is no lumen-positive potential in this segment, and Ca^{2+} and Mg^{2+} are not driven out of the tubular lumen by electrical forces.

However, Ca^{2+} is actively reabsorbed by the distal convoluted tubule epithelial cell via an apical Ca^{2+} channel and basolateral Na^+/Ca^{2+} exchanger (Figure 15–5). This process is regulated by parathyroid hormone. As will be seen below, the differences in the mechanism of Ca^{2+} transport in the distal convoluted tubule and in the loop of Henle have important implications for the effects of various diuretics on Ca^{2+} transport.

COLLECTING TUBULE

The collecting tubule is responsible for only 2–5% of NaCl reabsorption by the kidney. Despite this seemingly small contribution, the collecting tubule plays a vital role in renal physiology and in diuretic action. As the final site of NaCl reabsorption, the collecting tubule is responsible for determining the final Na^+ concentration of the urine. Furthermore, the collecting tubule (and the late distal tubule) is the site at which mineralocorticoids exert a significant influence, and this segment therefore plays an important role in volume regulation. Lastly, the collecting tubule is the major site of potassium secretion by the kidney and is thus the site at which virtually all diuretic-induced changes in potassium metabolism occur.

The mechanism of NaCl reabsorption in the collecting tubule is again distinct from the mechanisms described for the other tubule segments. The **principal cells** are the major sites of Na^+, K^+, and H_2O transport (Figure 15–6), and the **intercalated cells** are the primary sites of proton secretion. Unlike the epithelial cells in the earlier nephron segments, the apical membrane of the collecting tubule principal cells does not contain cotransport systems for Na^+ and other ions. Rather, these membranes exhibit separate ion channels for Na^+ and K^+. Since these channels exclude anions, transport of Na^+ or K^+ leads to a net movement of charge across the membrane. Because the driving force for Na^+ entry into the principal cell greatly exceeds that for K^+ exit, Na^+ reabsorption predominates, and a significant (10–50 mV) lumen-negative electrical potential develops. Na^+ that enters the principal cell by this mechanism is then transported into the blood via the basolateral Na^+/K^+ ATPase as in the other nephron segments (Figure 15–6). The lumen-negative electrical potential drives the

Figure 15–6. Ion and H$_2$O transport pathways across the luminal and basolateral membranes of collecting tubule and collecting duct cells. Inward diffusion of Na$^+$ leaves a lumen-negative potential, which drives reabsorption of Cl$^-$ and efflux of K$^+$. (R, aldosterone or ADH receptor.)

with the apical membranes of the principal cells and thus increases the membrane permeability to water (Figure 15–6). ADH secretion is regulated by serum osmolality and by volume status. Thus, practical ADH antagonists would theoretically be very useful drugs for inducing water diuresis. Such agents are not yet available for clinical application.

II. BASIC PHARMACOLOGY OF DIURETIC AGENTS

CARBONIC ANHYDRASE INHIBITORS

Carbonic anhydrase is present in many nephron sites, including the luminal and basolateral membranes, the cytoplasm of the epithelial cells, and the red blood cells in the renal circulation. However, the predominant location of this enzyme is the luminal membrane of the proximal tubule (Figure 15–3), where it catalyzes the dehydration of H$_2$CO$_3$, a critical step in the proximal reabsorption of bicarbonate. Inhibitors of carbonic anhydrase thus block sodium bicarbonate reabsorption, causing sodium bicarbonate diuresis and a reduction in total body bicarbonate stores.

The carbonic anhydrase inhibitors were the forerunners of modern diuretics (see box: Development of Modern Diuretics). They are unsubstituted sulfonamide derivatives and were developed when it was noted that bacteriostatic sulfonamides caused an alkaline diuresis and hyperchloremic metabolic acidosis.

transport of Cl$^-$ back to the blood via the paracellular pathway and also drives K$^+$ out of the cell through the apical membrane K$^+$ channel. Thus, there is an important relation between Na$^+$ delivery to the collecting tubule and the resulting secretion of K$^+$. Diuretics that act upstream of the collecting tubule will increase Na$^+$ delivery to this site and will enhance K$^+$ secretion. Furthermore, if the Na$^+$ is delivered with an anion such as bicarbonate, which cannot be reabsorbed as readily as Cl$^-$, the lumen-negative potential is increased, and K$^+$ secretion will be even further enhanced. This mechanism, combined with enhanced aldosterone secretion due to volume depletion, is the basis for most diuretic-induced K$^+$ wasting.

Reabsorption of Na$^+$ and its coupled secretion of K$^+$ is regulated by aldosterone. This steroid hormone, through its actions on gene transcription, increases the activity of both apical membrane channels and the basolateral Na$^+$/K$^+$ ATPase. This leads to an increase in the transepithelial electrical potential and a dramatic increase in both Na$^+$ reabsorption and K$^+$ secretion (see box: Electrical Potential & Potassium Secretion and Figure 15–7).

In the absence of antidiuretic hormone (ADH), the collecting tubule (and duct) is impermeable to water, and dilute urine is produced. However, this is the only site in the nephron at which membrane water permeability can be regulated. ADH causes intracellular vesicles containing preformed water channels to fuse

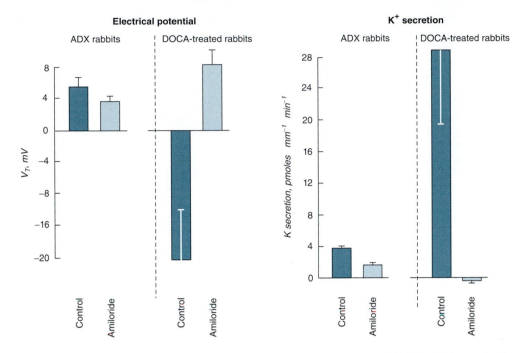

Figure 15–7. Electrical potential and potassium secretion. In adrenalectomized (ADX) rabbits, collecting tubule transepithelial voltage (left, dark color bar) is positive and K⁺ secretion (right, solid bar) is negligible. When rabbits are treated with a mineralocorticoid (DOCA-treated), voltage changes to –20 mV and K⁺ secretion is increased more than sevenfold. The effects of DOCA are completely reversed by amiloride (light color bars). ADX, adrenalectomized; DOCA, desoxycorticosterone acetate. (Modified and reproduced, with permission, from Wingo CS: Cortical collecting tubule potassium secretion: Effect of amiloride, ouabain, and luminal sodium concentration. Kidney Int 1985;27:886.)

With the development of newer agents, the carbonic anhydrase inhibitors are now rarely used, but there are still several specific applications that will be discussed below. The prototypical carbonic anhydrase inhibitor is **acetazolamide.**

Chemistry

The structure of acetazolamide is shown in the accompanying box. The $-SO_2NH_2$ (sulfonamide) group is essential for activity. Alkyl substitutions at this point completely block the effects on carbonic anhydrase activity.

Pharmacokinetics

The carbonic anhydrase inhibitors are well absorbed after oral administration. An increase in urine pH from the bicarbonate diuresis is apparent within 30 minutes, maximal at 2 hours, and persists for 12 hours after a single dose. Excretion of the drug is by tubular secretion in the S_2 segment of the proximal tubule, and for that reason dosing must be reduced in renal insufficiency.

Pharmacodynamics

Inhibition of carbonic anhydrase activity profoundly depresses bicarbonate reabsorption in the proximal tubule. At its maximal safely administered dosage, 85% of the bicarbonate reabsorptive capacity of the superficial proximal tubule is inhibited by acetazolamide, with an apparent IC_{50} (concentration for 50% inhibition) of 4 μmol/L. However, some bicarbonate can still be absorbed at other nephron sites by carbonic anhydrase-independent mechanisms. The overall effect of maximal acetazolamide administration is about 45% inhibition of whole kidney bicarbonate reabsorption. Nevertheless, carbonic anhydrase inhibition causes significant bicarbonate losses, resulting in hyperchloremic metabolic acidosis. Because of the toxicity of this acidosis and the fact that HCO_3^- depletion leads to enhanced NaCl reabsorption by the remaining tubule segments in the nephron, the diuretic effectiveness of acetazolamide decreases significantly with use over several days.

The major clinical applications of acetazolamide involve carbonic anhydrase-dependent bicarbonate transport at sites other than the kidney. The ciliary body of the eye secretes bicarbonate into the aqueous humor by a process similar to the reabsorption of bicarbonate from proximal tubular fluid. The only difference is that the process is reversed—bicarbonate is removed from the blood by the ciliary body and returned to the blood in the proximal tubule. Likewise, formation of cerebrospinal fluid by the choroid plexus involves bicarbonate secretion into the cerebrospinal fluid. Although these processes are in the opposite di-

DEVELOPMENT OF MODERN DIURETICS

Development of the thiazides and other modern diuretics began when a perceptive physician noticed that patients receiving sulfanilamide, an early antimicrobial drug, developed metabolic acidosis and a very alkaline urine. Careful study revealed that the drug was causing sodium bicarbonate diuresis. The realization that this could be a useful diuretic effect led first to the development of acetazolamide and then, by the steps shown below, to the thiazides.

The arrows in the figure indicate historical steps, not chemical reactions. When dichlorphenamide was synthesized as a competitor to acetazolamide, it was found to cause an increased ratio of sodium chloride excretion relative to sodium bicarbonate excretion—a desirable change indicating an action different from (or in addition to) carbonic anhydrase inhibition. Further molecular manipulation led to disulfamoylchloraniline, a weak diuretic but one that was cyclized to chlorothiazide, the first thiazide. This molecule has little effect on carbonic anhydrase and selectively inhibits NaCl reabsorption in the distal tubule. The loop diuretics were subsequently derived from the thiazides.

Sulfanilamide   Acetazolamide   Dichlorphenamide   Disulfamoylchloraniline   Chlorothiazide

rection from that in the proximal tubule, they are equally well inhibited by carbonic anhydrase inhibitors, which in both cases dramatically alter the pH and quantity of fluid produced.

Clinical Indications & Dosage (Table 15–1)

A. Glaucoma: Inhibition of carbonic anhydrase decreases the rate of aqueous humor formation, causing a decrease in intraocular pressure. This effect is of value in the management of several forms of glaucoma, making it the most common indication for use of carbonic anhydrase inhibitors.

A topically active carbonic anhydrase inhibitor **(dorzolamide)** has recently become available. This new compound achieves reductions in intraocular pressure comparable to oral agents. Although the drug is taken up by red blood cells, plasma levels of dorzolamide are undetectable. Thus, diuretic and systemic metabolic effects are eliminated.

Table 15–1. Carbonic anhydrase inhibitors used orally in treatment of glaucoma.

	Usual Oral Dose (1–4 Times Daily)
Acetazolamide	250 mg
Dichlorphenamide	50 mg

B. Urinary Alkalinization: Uric acid and cystine are relatively insoluble in acidic urine, and enhanced renal excretion can be achieved by increasing urinary pH with carbonic anhydrase inhibitors. Similarly, renal excretion of weak acids (eg, aspirin) is enhanced by acetazolamide. In the absence of continuous bicarbonate administration, these effects of acetazolamide are of relatively short duration and are only useful in the initiation of a response. Prolonged therapy requires concomitant bicarbonate administration.

C. Metabolic Alkalosis: In most cases, sustained metabolic alkalosis is a consequence either of decreased total body K^+ and intravascular volume or of high levels of mineralocorticoids. It is therefore generally treated by correction of these underlying conditions and not with acetazolamide. However, when the alkalosis is due to excessive use of diuretics in patients with severe heart failure, saline administration may be contraindicated because of elevated cardiac filling pressures. In these cases, acetazolamide can be useful in correcting the alkalosis as well as producing a small additional diuresis for the correction of heart failure. Acetazolamide has also been used to rapidly correct the metabolic alkalosis that may develop in the setting of respiratory acidosis.

D. Acute Mountain Sickness: Weakness, dizziness, insomnia, headache, and nausea can occur in mountain travelers who rapidly ascend above 3000 m. The symptoms are usually mild and last for a few days. In more serious cases, rapidly progressing pulmonary or cerebral edema can be life-threatening. By decreasing cerebrospinal fluid formation and by decreasing the pH of the cerebrospinal fluid and brain, acetazolamide can enhance performance status and diminish symptoms of mountain sickness. Prophylaxis can be achieved by starting oral acetazolamide 24 hours before the ascent. One study (Zell et al, 1988) recommended against routine prophylaxis for recreational hikers because the symptoms are usually mild.

E. Other Uses: Carbonic anhydrase inhibitors have been used as adjuvants for the treatment of epilepsy, in some forms of hypokalemic periodic paralysis, and to increase urinary phosphate excretion during severe hyperphosphatemia.

Toxicity

A. Hyperchloremic Metabolic Acidosis: Acidosis predictably results from chronic reduction of body bicarbonate stores by carbonic anhydrase inhibitors. Bicarbonate wasting limits the diuretic efficacy of these drugs to 2 or 3 days.

B. Renal Stones: Phosphaturia and hypercalciuria occur during the bicarbonaturic response to carbonic anhydrase inhibition. Renal excretion of solubilizing factors (eg, citrate) may also decline with chronic use. Calcium salts are relatively insoluble at alkaline pH, which means that the potential for renal stone formation from these salts is enhanced.

C. Renal Potassium Wasting: Potassium wasting can occur because $NaHCO_3$ presented to the collecting tubule causes an increase in the lumen-negative electrical potential in that segment and enhances K^+ excretion. This effect can be counteracted by simultaneous administration of KCl.

D. Other Toxicities: Drowsiness and paresthesias are common following large doses. These agents accumulate in patients with renal failure, and central nervous system toxicity can be marked in this setting. Hypersensitivity reactions (fever, rashes, bone marrow suppression, interstitial nephritis) can also occur.

Contraindications

Carbonic anhydrase inhibitors should be avoided in hepatic cirrhosis. Alkalinization of the urine will decrease urinary trapping—and thus excretion—of NH_4^+ and may contribute to the development of hepatic encephalopathy.

LOOP DIURETICS

Loop diuretics selectively inhibit NaCl reabsorption in the thick ascending limb of the loop of Henle. Owing to the large NaCl absorptive capacity of this segment and the fact that diuresis is not limited by development of acidosis, as it is with the carbonic anhy-

drase inhibitors, these drugs are the most efficacious diuretic agents available.

Chemistry

The two prototypical drugs of this group are **furosemide** and **ethacrynic acid.** The structures of several loop diuretics are shown in Figure 15–8. Like the carbonic anhydrase inhibitors, furosemide and bumetanide are sulfonamide derivatives. These agents have a carboxyl group with a sulfamoyl moiety in the meta position (carbon number 5). A halide or phenoxy substitution is present at carbon 4, and a substituted amino group is present at carbon 2 or 3. Torsemide, a newer loop diuretic, is another sulfonamide compound derived from 4-amino-3-pyridine-sulfonylurea.

Ethacrynic acid—not a sulfonamide derivative—is chemically distinct from furosemide. It is a phenoxyacetic acid derivative containing an adjacent ketone and methylene group (Figure 15–8). The methylene group (shaded) forms an adduct with the free sulfhydryl group of cysteine. The cysteine adduct appears to be the active form of the drug.

Organic **mercurial diuretics** inhibit salt transport in the thick ascending limb. They are no longer used

Figure 15–8. Loop diuretics. The shaded methylene group on ethacrynic acid is reactive and may combine with free sulfhydryl groups.

because of their high toxicity and are of only historical interest.

Pharmacokinetics

The loop agents are rapidly absorbed. They are eliminated by renal secretion as well as by glomerular filtration. Absorption of oral torsemide is more rapid (1 hour) than that of furosemide (2–3 hours) and is nearly comparable with intravenous administration. Diuretic response is extremely rapid following intravenous injection. The duration of effect for furosemide is usually 2–3 hours and for torsemide 4–6 hours. Half-life is dependent on renal function. Since loop agents act on the luminal side of the tubule, the diuretic response correlates positively with their excretion in the urine. Defects in the secretory component of its clearance may result from simultaneous administration of agents such as indomethacin and probenecid, which inhibit weak acid secretion in the proximal tubule. Metabolites of ethacrynic acid and furosemide have been identified, but it is not known if they have any diuretic activity. Torsemide has at least one active metabolite with a half-life considerably longer than that of the parent compound.

Pharmacodynamics

These drugs inhibit the coupled $Na^+/K^+/2Cl^-$ transport system in the luminal membrane of the thick ascending limb of Henle's loop. By inhibiting this transporter, the loop diuretics reduce the reabsorption of NaCl and also diminish the normal lumen-positive potential that derives from K^+ recycling (Figure 15–4). This electrical potential normally drives divalent cation reabsorption in the loop. Loop diuretics, by abolishing the lumen-positive potential, cause an increase in Mg^{2+} and Ca^{2+} excretion. Prolonged use can cause significant hypomagnesemia in some patients. Since Ca^{2+} is actively reabsorbed in the distal convoluted tubule, loop diuretics do not generally cause hypocalcemia. However, in disorders that cause hypercalcemia, Ca^{2+} excretion can be greatly enhanced by combining loop agents with saline infusions. This effect is of great value in the acute management of hypercalcemia.

In addition to their diuretic activity, loop agents appear to have direct effects on blood flow through several vascular beds. The mechanisms for this action are not well defined. Furosemide increases renal blood flow and causes redistribution of blood flow within the renal cortex. Furosemide and ethacrynic acid have also been shown to relieve pulmonary congestion and reduce left ventricular filling pressures in congestive heart failure before a measurable increase in urinary output occurs, and in anephric patients.

Clinical Indications & Dosage (Table 15–2)

The most important indications for the use of the loop diuretics include acute pulmonary edema, other edematous conditions, and acute hypercalcemia. The

Table 15–2. Loop diuretics: Dosages.[1]

Drug	Daily Oral Dose
Bumetanide	0.5–2 mg
Ethacrynic acid	50–200 mg
Furosemide	20–80 mg
Torsemide	2.5–20 mg

[1]As single dose or in two divided doses.

use of loop diuretics in these conditions is discussed in Section III, Clinical Pharmacology. Other indications for loop diuretics include the following.

A. Hyperkalemia: In mild hyperkalemia—or after acute management of severe hyperkalemia by other measures—loop diuretics can significantly enhance urinary excretion of K^+ as a means of reducing total body K^+ stores. This response is enhanced by simultaneous NaCl and water administration.

B. Acute Renal Failure: Loop agents can increase the rate of urine flow and enhance K^+ excretion in acute renal failure. These drugs may convert oliguric renal failure to nonoliguric failure, which facilitates management of the patient. However, they do not seem to shorten the duration of renal failure. If a large pigment load has precipitated acute renal failure or threatens to do so, loop agents may help flush out intratubular casts and ameliorate intratubular obstruction. On the other hand, loop agents can theoretically worsen cast formation in myeloma and light chain nephropathy.

C. Anion Overdose: Bromide, fluoride, and iodide are all reabsorbed in the thick ascending limb; loop diuretics are therefore useful in treating toxic ingestions of these ions. Saline solution must be administered to replace urinary losses of Na^+ and to provide Cl^-, so as to avoid extracellular fluid volume depletion.

Toxicity

A. Hypokalemic Metabolic Alkalosis: Loop diuretics increase delivery of salt and water to the collecting duct and thus enhance the renal secretion of K^+ and H^+, causing hypokalemic metabolic alkalosis. This toxicity is a function of the magnitude of the diuretic effect and can be reversed by K^+ replacement and correction of hypovolemia.

B. Ototoxicity: The loop diuretics can cause dose-related hearing loss that is usually reversible. It is most common in patients who have diminished renal function or who are also receiving other ototoxic agents such as aminoglycoside antibiotics.

C. Hyperuricemia: Loop diuretics can cause hyperuricemia and precipitate attacks of gout. This is caused by hypovolemia-associated enhancement of uric acid reabsorption in the proximal tubule. It may be avoided by using lower doses of the diuretic.

D. Hypomagnesemia: Magnesium depletion is a predictable consequence of the chronic use of loop agents and occurs most often in patients with dietary deficiency of magnesium. It can be readily reversed by administration of oral magnesium preparations.

E. Allergic Reactions: Skin rash, eosinophilia, and, less often, interstitial nephritis are occasional side effects of furosemide therapy. These usually resolve rapidly after drug withdrawal. Experience with torsemide is limited, but similar allergic reactions are likely in view of its chemical structure. Allergic reactions are probably related to the sulfonamide moiety; they are much less common with ethacrynic acid.

F. Other Toxicities: Even more than other diuretics, loop agents can cause severe dehydration. Hyponatremia is less common than with the thiazides (see below) because loop agents diminish maximal concentrating ability. Nevertheless, patients who increase water intake in response to hypovolemia-induced thirst can become severely hyponatremic with loop agents. Loop agents are known for their calciuric effect, but hypercalcemia can occur, generally in patients who become severely dehydrated and who have another, previously occult, cause for hypercalcemia, such as an oat cell carcinoma of the lung.

Contraindications

Furosemide, bumetanide, and torsemide may demonstrate cross-reactivity in patients who are sensitive to other sulfonamides. Overzealous use of any diuretic is dangerous in hepatic cirrhosis, borderline renal failure, or congestive heart failure (see below).

THIAZIDES

The thiazide diuretics emerged during efforts to synthesize more potent carbonic anhydrase inhibitors (see box: Development of Modern Diuretics). It subsequently became clear that the thiazides inhibit NaCl transport independently of their effect on carbonic anhydrase activity and that they act on salt transport in the distal convoluted tubule. Some members of this group retain significant carbonic anhydrase inhibitory activity, but this effect is not related to the primary mode of action. The prototypical thiazide is **hydrochlorothiazide.**

Chemistry

The drugs in this group are formally called benzothiadiazides, usually shortened to thiazides. The nature of the heterocyclic rings and the substitutions on these rings may vary among the congeners, but all of them retain, in common with the carbonic anhydrase inhibitors, an unsubstituted sulfonamide group (Figure 15–9).

Pharmacokinetics

All of the thiazides are absorbed when given orally, but there are differences in their metabolism. Chlorothiazide, the parent of the group, is less lipid-soluble and must be given in relatively large doses. Chlorthalidone is slowly absorbed and has a longer duration of action. Although indapamide is excreted primarily by the biliary system, enough of the active form is cleared by the kidney to exert its diuretic effect in the distal convoluted tubule.

All of the thiazides are secreted by the organic acid secretory system and compete to some extent with the secretion of uric acid by that system. As a result, the uric acid secretory rate may be reduced, with a concomitant elevation in serum uric acid level. In the steady state, uric acid production and therefore renal excretion are not affected by the thiazides.

Pharmacodynamics

Thiazides inhibit NaCl reabsorption from the luminal side of epithelial cells in the distal convoluted tubule. There may also be a small effect on NaCl reabsorption in the late proximal tubule, but this is not observed in the usual clinical setting.

Relatively little is known about the NaCl transport system that is inhibited by thiazides. As described above (under Distal Convoluted Tubule), the mode of transport appears to be an electrically neutral NaCl cotransporter that is distinct from the transporter in the loop of Henle. There is also an active reabsorptive process for Ca^{2+} in the distal convoluted tubule, which is modulated by parathyroid hormone (PTH) (Figure 15–5). In contrast to the situation in the loop of Henle, where loop diuretics inhibit Ca^{2+} reabsorption, thiazides actually enhance Ca^{2+} reabsorption in the distal convoluted tubule. The mechanism for this enhancement is not known, but it has been postulated to result from a lowering of cell Na^+ upon blockade of Na^+ entry by thiazides. The lower cell Na^+ might then enhance Na^+/Ca^{2+} exchange in the basolateral membrane (Figure 15–5), increasing overall reabsorption of Ca^{2+}. While thiazides rarely cause hypercalcemia as the result of this enhanced reabsorption, they can unmask hypercalcemia due to other causes (eg, hyperparathyroidism, carcinoma, sarcoidosis). Thiazides have proved useful in the treatment of kidney stones caused by hypercalciuria.

Clinical Indications & Dosage (Table 15–3)

The major indications for thiazide diuretics are (1) hypertension, (2) congestive heart failure, (3) nephrolithiasis due to idiopathic hypercalciuria, and (4) nephrogenic diabetes insipidus. Use of the thiazides in each of these conditions is described below in the section on clinical pharmacology.

Toxicity

A. Hypokalemic Metabolic Alkalosis and Hyperuricemia: These toxicities are similar to those observed with loop diuretics (see above).

B. Impaired Carbohydrate Tolerance: Hyperglycemia may occur in patients who are overtly diabetic or who have even mildly abnormal glucose tol-

Figure 15–9. Hydrochlorothiazide and related agents.

Table 15–3. Thiazides and related diuretics: Dosages.

	Daily Oral Dose	Frequency of Dosage
Bendroflumethazide	2.5–10 mg	As single dose
Benzthiazide	25–100 mg	In two divided doses
Chlorothiazide	0.5–1 g	In two divided doses
Chlorthalidone[1]	50–100 mg	As single dose
Hydrochlorothiazide	25–100 mg	As single dose
Hydroflumethiazide	25–100 mg	In two divided doses
Indapamide[1]	2.5–10 mg	As single dose
Methyclothiazide	2.5–10 mg	As single dose
Metolazone[1]	2.5–10 mg	As single dose
Polythiazide	1–4 mg	As single dose
Quinethazone[1]	50–100 mg	As single dose
Trichlormethiazide	2–8 mg	As single dose

[1]Not a thiazide but a sulfonamide qualitatively similar to the thiazides.

erance tests. The effect is due both to impaired pancreatic release of insulin and to diminished tissue utilization of glucose. Hyperglycemia may be partially reversible with correction of hypokalemia.

C. Hyperlipidemia: Thiazides cause a 5–15% increase in serum cholesterol and increased low-density lipoproteins (LDL). These levels may return toward baseline after prolonged use.

D. Hyponatremia: Hyponatremia is an important adverse effect of thiazide diuretics and can on rare occasions be life-threatening. It is due to a combination of hypovolemia-induced elevation of ADH, reduction in the diluting capacity of the kidney, and increased thirst. It can be prevented by reducing the dose of the drug or limiting water intake.

E. Allergic Reactions: The thiazides are sulfonamides and share cross-reactivity with other members of this chemical group. Photosensitivity or generalized dermatitis occurs rarely. Serious allergic reactions are extremely rare but do include hemolytic anemia, thrombocytopenia, and acute necrotizing pancreatitis.

F. Other Toxicities: Weakness, fatigability, and paresthesias may be similar to those of carbonic anhydrase inhibitors. Impotence has been reported but is probably related to volume depletion.

Contraindications

Overzealous use of any diuretic is dangerous in hepatic cirrhosis, borderline renal failure, or congestive heart failure (see below).

POTASSIUM-SPARING DIURETICS

The members of this group antagonize the effects of aldosterone at the cortical collecting tubule and late distal tubule. Inhibition may occur by direct pharmacologic antagonism of mineralocorticoid receptors (**spironolactone**) or by inhibition of Na⁺ transport through ion channels in the luminal membrane (**triamterene, amiloride**). Lesser potassium-sparing effects are occasionally seen with drugs that suppress renin or angiotensin II action (nonsteroidal anti-inflammatory agents, beta-blockers, converting enzyme inhibitors, angiotensin receptor inhibitors).

Chemistry & Pharmacokinetics

Spironolactone is a synthetic steroid that acts as a competitive antagonist to aldosterone. Its onset and duration of action are therefore determined by the kinetics of aldosterone response in the target tissue. Substantial inactivation of spironolactone occurs in the liver. The overall result is a rather slow onset of action, requiring several days before full therapeutic effect is achieved.

Triamterene is metabolized in the liver, but renal excretion is a major route of elimination for the active form and the metabolites. Very little is known about the diuretic effects of the metabolites. Amiloride is excreted unchanged in the urine. Because triamterene is extensively metabolized, it has a shorter half-life and must be given more frequently than amiloride. The structures of spironolactone, triamterene, and amiloride are shown in Figure 15–10.

Pharmacodynamics

The potassium-sparing diuretics reduce Na⁺ absorption in the collecting tubules and ducts. Na⁺ absorption (and K⁺ secretion) at this site is regulated by aldosterone. At any given rate of Na⁺ delivery, the rate of distal K⁺ secretion is positively correlated with the aldosterone level. As described above, aldosterone enhances K⁺ secretion by increasing Na⁺/K⁺ ATPase activity and Na⁺ and K⁺ channel activities. Na⁺ absorption in the collecting tubule generates a lumen-negative electrical potential, which enhances K⁺ secretion. Aldosterone antagonists interfere with this process. Similar effects are observed with respect to H⁺ handling by the collecting tubule, in part explaining the metabolic acidosis seen with aldosterone antagonists.

Spironolactone is a synthetic steroid that binds to cytoplasmic mineralocorticoid receptors and prevents translocation of the receptor complex to the nucleus in the target cell. The drug may also reduce the

Figure 15–10. Aldosterone antagonists.

intracellular formation of active metabolites of aldosterone by inhibition of 5α-reductase activity. Triamterene and amiloride do not block the aldosterone receptor but instead directly interfere with Na⁺ entry through the sodium-selective ion channels in the apical membrane of the collecting tubule. Since K⁺ secretion is coupled with Na⁺ entry in this segment, these agents are also effective K⁺-sparing diuretics.

Other Potassium-Sparing Agents

Converting enzyme inhibitors and angiotensin receptor antagonists are discussed in Chapters 11 and 17. Although not used therapeutically as potassium-sparing diuretics, these agents do antagonize the effects of aldosterone by interfering with its secretion and are often associated with hyperkalemia.

Clinical Indications & Dosage (Table 15–4)

These agents are most useful in states of mineralocorticoid excess, due either to primary hypersecretion (Conn's syndrome, ectopic ACTH production) or to secondary aldosteronism. Secondary aldosteronism results from congestive heart failure, hepatic cirrhosis, nephrotic syndrome, and other conditions associated with renal salt retention and diminished effective intravascular volume. Use of other diuretics, like thiazides or loop agents, can cause or exacerbate volume contraction and thus intensify secondary aldostero-

Table 15–4. Potassium-sparing diuretics and combination preparations.

Trade Name	Potassium-Sparing Agent	Hydrochlorothiazide	Frequency of Dosage
Aldactazide	Spironolactone 25 mg	25 mg	1–4 times daily
Aldactone	Spironolactone 25 mg	. . .	1–4 times daily
Dyazide	Triamterene 50 mg	25 mg	1–4 times daily
Dyrenium	Triamterene 50 mg	. . .	1–3 times daily
Maxzide	Triamterene 75 mg	50 mg	Once daily
Maxzide-25 mg	Triamterene 37.5 mg	25 mg	Once daily
Midamor	Amiloride 5 mg	. . .	Once daily
Moduretic	Amiloride 5 mg	50 mg	Once or twice daily

nism. In the setting of enhanced mineralocorticoid secretion and continuing delivery of Na^+ to distal nephron sites, renal K^+ wasting occurs. This is due to K^+ secretion by the collecting tubule. K^+-sparing diuretics of either type are used in this setting to blunt the K^+ secretory response and prevent depletion of the intracellular K^+ stores.

Toxicity

A. Hyperkalemia: Unlike other diuretics, these agents can cause mild, moderate, or even life-threatening hyperkalemia. The risk of this complication is greatly increased in the presence of renal disease or of other drugs that reduce renin (beta-blockers, NSAIDs) or angiotensin II activity (ACE inhibitors, angiotensin receptor inhibitors). Since most other diuretic agents lead to K^+ losses, hyperkalemia is more common when aldosterone antagonists are used as the sole diuretic agent, especially in patients with renal insufficiency. With fixed-dosage combinations of potassium-sparing and thiazide diuretics, there may be a fairly even balance, so that both the hypokalemia and the metabolic alkalosis due to the thiazide are ameliorated by the aldosterone antagonist. However, owing to variations in the bioavailability of the components of some of the fixed-dosage forms, the thiazide-associated adverse effects may predominate (eg, metabolic alkalosis, hyponatremia). For these reasons, it is generally preferable to adjust the doses of the two drugs separately.

B. Hyperchloremic Metabolic Acidosis: By inhibiting H^+ secretion in parallel with K^+ secretion, the potassium-sparing diuretics can cause acidosis similar to that seen with type IV renal tubular acidosis.

C. Gynecomastia: Synthetic steroids may cause endocrine abnormalities by effects on other steroid receptors. Gynecomastia and other adverse effects (impotence, benign prostatic hyperplasia) have been reported with spironolactone.

D. Acute Renal Failure: The combination of triamterene with indomethacin has been reported to cause acute renal failure. This has not yet been reported with other potassium-sparing agents.

E. Kidney Stones: Triamterene is poorly soluble and may precipitate in the urine, causing kidney stones.

Contraindications

These agents can cause severe, even fatal hyperkalemia in susceptible patients. Oral K^+ administration should be discontinued if aldosterone antagonists are administered. Patients with chronic renal insufficiency are especially vulnerable and should rarely be treated with aldosterone antagonists. Concomitant use of other agents that blunt the renin-angiotensin system (beta-blockers or ACE inhibitors) increases the likelihood of hyperkalemia. Patients with liver disease may have impaired metabolism of triamterene and spironolactone, and dosing must be carefully adjusted.

AGENTS THAT ENHANCE WATER EXCRETION

1. OSMOTIC DIURETICS

The proximal tubule and descending limb of Henle's loop are freely permeable to water. An osmotic agent that is not transported causes water to be retained in these segments and promotes a water diuresis. One such agent, mannitol, is used mainly to reduce increased intracranial pressure, but it is occasionally used to promote prompt removal of renal toxins, which may be required in acute hemolysis or after use of radiocontrast agents.

Pharmacokinetics

Mannitol is not metabolized and is handled primarily by glomerular filtration, without any important tubular reabsorption or secretion. By definition, osmotic diuretics are poorly absorbed, which means that they must be given parenterally. Mannitol is excreted by glomerular filtration within 30–60 minutes. If administered orally, mannitol causes osmotic diarrhea. This effect can be used to potentiate the effects of potassium-binding resins or eliminate toxic substances from the gastrointestinal tract in conjunction with activated charcoal (see Chapter 59).

Pharmacodynamics

Osmotic diuretics limit water reabsorption primarily in those segments of the nephron that are freely permeable to water: the proximal tubule and the descending limb of the loop of Henle. The presence of a nonreabsorbable solute such as mannitol prevents the normal absorption of water by interposing a countervailing osmotic force. As a result, urine volume increases in conjunction with mannitol excretion. The concomitant increase in urine flow rates decreases the contact time between fluid and the tubular epithelium, thus reducing Na^+ reabsorption. However, the resulting natriuresis is of lesser magnitude than the water diuresis, leading eventually to hypernatremia.

Clinical Indications & Dosage

A. To Increase Urine Volume: Osmotic diuretics are used to increase water excretion in preference to sodium excretion. This effect can be useful when renal hemodynamics are compromised or when avid Na^+ retention limits the response to conventional agents. It can be used to maintain urine volume and to prevent anuria that might otherwise result from presentation of large pigment loads to the kidney (eg, hemolysis or rhabdomyolysis). Some oliguric patients do not respond to an osmotic diuretic. Therefore, a test dose of mannitol (12.5 g intravenously) should be given prior to starting a continuous infusion. Mannitol should not be continued unless there is an increase in urine flow rate to more than 50 mL/h during the 3 hours following the test dose. If there is a response, mannitol administration (12.5–25 g) can be repeated in 1–2 hours to maintain urine flow rate greater than 100 mL/h. Prolonged use of mannitol is not advised.

B. Reduction of Intracranial and Intraocular Pressure: Osmotic diuretics reduce total body water more than total body cation content and thus reduce intracellular volume. This effect is used to reduce intracranial pressure in neurologic conditions and to reduce intraocular pressure before ophthalmologic procedures. A dose of 1–2 g/kg mannitol is administered intravenously. Intracranial pressure, which must be monitored, should fall in 60–90 minutes.

Toxicity

A. Extracellular Volume Expansion: Mannitol is rapidly distributed in the extracellular compartment and extracts water from the intracellular compartment. Initially, this leads to expansion of the extracellular fluid volume and hyponatremia. This effect can complicate congestive heart failure and may produce florid pulmonary edema. Headache, nausea, and vomiting are commonly observed in patients treated with osmotic diuretics.

B. Dehydration and Hypernatremia: Excessive use of mannitol without adequate water replacement can ultimately lead to severe dehydration, free water losses, and hypernatremia. This complication can be avoided by careful attention to serum ion composition and fluid balance.

2. ADH ANTAGONISTS

A variety of medical conditions, eg, tumors that secrete ADH-like peptides, cause water retention as the result of ADH excess. Unfortunately, specific ADH antagonists are available only for investigational purposes. Two nonselective agents, Li^+ and demeclocycline, are of limited use in a few specific situations.

Pharmacokinetics

ADH antagonists currently available include Li^+ salts and tetracycline derivatives (demeclocycline). Both are orally active. Lithium is reabsorbed to some extent in the proximal tubule and thereafter is neither secreted nor absorbed. Demeclocycline is metabolized in the liver.

Pharmacodynamics

ADH antagonists inhibit the effects of ADH at the collecting tubule. While the mechanisms by which Li^+ and demeclocycline exert this action have never been conclusively demonstrated, it appears that both agents act to reduce the formation of cAMP in response to ADH and also to interfere with the actions of cAMP in the collecting tubule cells.

Clinical Indications & Dosage

A. Syndrome of Inappropriate ADH Secretion (SIADH): ADH antagonists are clinically used to manage SIADH when water restriction has failed to correct the abnormality. This generally occurs in the outpatient setting, where water restriction cannot be enforced, or in the hospital when large quantities of intravenous fluid are administered with drugs. Lithium carbonate has been used to treat this syndrome, but the response is unpredictable. Serum levels of Li^+ must be monitored closely, as serum concentrations greater than 1 mmol/L are toxic. Demeclocycline, in dosages of 600–1200 mg/d, yields a more predictable result and is less toxic. Appropriate plasma levels (2 μg/mL) can be approximated by using standard determinations of plasma tetracyclines.

B. Other Causes of Elevated ADH: ADH is also elevated in response to diminished effective circulating blood volume. When treatment by volume replacement is not possible, as in heart failure or liver disease, hyponatremia may result. As for SIADH, water restriction is the treatment of choice, but if it is not successful, demeclocycline may be considered.

Toxicity

A. Nephrogenic Diabetes Insipidus: If serum Na^+ is not monitored closely, SIADH can be replaced with nephrogenic diabetes insipidus, and severe hypernatremia can result. If Li^+ is being used for an affective disorder, nephrogenic diabetes insipidus can be treated with a thiazide diuretic or amiloride (see below).

B. Renal Failure: Both Li^+ and demeclocycline have been reported to cause acute renal failure. Long-term Li^+ therapy may also cause chronic interstitial nephritis.

C. Other: Adverse effects associated with Li^+ therapy include tremulousness, mental obtundation, cardiotoxicity, thyroid dysfunction, and leukocytosis (see Chapter 29). Demeclocycline should be avoided in patients with liver disease (see Chapter 44).

DIURETIC COMBINATIONS

LOOP AGENTS & THIAZIDES

Some patients are refractory to the usual doses of loop agents or become refractory after an initial response. Since these agents have a short half-life, refractoriness may be due to an excessively long interval between doses. Renal Na^+ retention is enhanced during the time period when the drug is no longer active. After the dosing interval for loop agents is minimized or the dose is maximized, the use of two drugs acting at different nephron sites may exhibit synergy. Loop agents and thiazides in combination will often produce diuresis when neither agent acting alone is even minimally effective. There are several reasons for this phenomenon. First, salt and water reabsorption in either the thick ascending limb or the distal convoluted tubule can increase when the other is blocked. Inhibition of both will therefore produce more than an additive diuretic response. Secondly, thiazide diuretics may produce a mild natriuresis in the proximal tubule which is usually masked by increased reabsorption in the thick ascending limb. The combination of loop diuretics and thiazides will therefore blunt Na^+ reabsorption, at least to some extent, from all three segments.

Metolazone is the usual choice of thiazide-like drug in patients refractory to loop agents alone. It has been reported that metolazone may be more effective than other thiazides in renal failure, but this point is controversial, and it is likely that other members of the thiazide group are as effective as metolazone. Moreover, metolazone is available only in an oral preparation, while chlorothiazide can be given parenterally.

The combination of loop diuretics and thiazides can mobilize large amounts of fluid, even in patients who have been refractory to single agents. Therefore, close hemodynamic monitoring of these patients is essential. Routine outpatient use cannot be recommended. Furthermore, potassium wasting is extremely common and may require parenteral K^+ administration with careful monitoring of the fluid and electrolyte status.

POTASSIUM-SPARING DIURETICS & LOOP AGENTS OR THIAZIDES

Many patients who are placed on loop diuretics or thiazides develop hypokalemia at some point in their therapy. This can often be managed with dietary salt restriction, which will limit sodium delivery to the collecting tubule. When hypokalemia cannot be managed in this way, or with KCl supplements, the addition of a potassium-sparing diuretic can significantly lower potassium excretion. While this approach is generally safe, it should probably be avoided in patients with renal insufficiency, who can develop life-threatening hyperkalemia in response to potassium-sparing diuretics.

III. CLINICAL PHARMACOLOGY OF DIURETIC AGENTS

This section discusses the clinical use of diuretic agents in edematous and nonedematous states. The effects of these agents on urinary electrolyte excretion are shown in Table 15–5.

EDEMATOUS STATES

The most common reason for diuretic use is for reduction of peripheral or pulmonary edema that has accumulated as a result of diseases of the heart, kidney, or vasculature, or abnormalities in the blood oncotic pressure. Salt and water retention with edema formation often occurs when diminished blood delivery to the kidney is sensed as insufficient "effective" arterial blood volume. Judicious use of diuretics can mobilize interstitial edema fluid without significant reductions in plasma volume. However, excessive diuretic therapy in this setting may lead to further compromise of the effective arterial blood volume with reduction in perfusion of vital organs. Therefore, the use of diuretics to mobilize edema requires careful monitoring of the patient's hemodynamic status and an understanding of the pathophysiology of the underlying condition.

CONGESTIVE HEART FAILURE

When cardiac function is decreased by disease, the resultant changes in blood pressure and blood flow to the kidney are sensed as hypovolemia and thus induce renal retention of salt and water. This physiologic response initially expands the intravascular volume and venous return to the heart and may partially restore the cardiac output towards normal.

Table 15–5. Changes in urinary electrolyte patterns in response to diuretic drugs.

Agent	Urinary Electrolyte Patterns		
	NaCl	NaHCO$_3$	K$^+$
Carbonic anhydrase inhibitors	+	+++	+
Loop agents	++++	−	+
Thiazides	++	±	+
Loop agents plus thiazides	+++++	+	++
K$^+$-sparing agents	+	−	−

+, increase; −, decrease.

If the underlying disease causes cardiac function to deteriorate despite expansion of plasma volume, the kidney continues to retain salt and water, which then leaks from the vasculature and becomes interstitial or pulmonary edema. At this point, diuretic use becomes necessary to reduce the accumulation of edema, particularly that which is in the lungs. Reduction of pulmonary vascular congestion with diuretics may actually improve oxygenation and thereby improve myocardial function. Edema associated with congestive heart failure is generally managed with loop diuretics. In some instances, salt and water retention may become so severe that a combination of thiazides and loop diuretics is necessary.

In treating the heart failure patient with diuretics, it must always be remembered that cardiac output in these patients is being maintained in part by high filling pressures and that excessive use of diuretics may diminish venous return and thereby impair cardiac output. This issue is especially critical in right ventricular failure. Systemic rather than pulmonary vascular congestion is the hallmark of this disorder. Diuretic-induced volume contraction will predictably reduce venous return and can severely compromise cardiac output if left ventricular filling pressure is reduced below 15 mm Hg.

Diuretic-induced metabolic alkalosis is another adverse effect that may further compromise cardiac function. While this effect is generally treated with replacement of potassium and restoration of intravascular volume with saline, severe heart failure may preclude the use of saline even in patients who have received too much diuretic. In these cases, adjunctive use of acetazolamide can help correct the alkalosis.

Another serious toxicity of diuretic use, particularly in the cardiac patient, is hypokalemia. Hypokalemia can exacerbate underlying cardiac arrhythmias and contribute to digitalis toxicity. This can often be avoided by having the patient reduce sodium intake, thus decreasing sodium delivery to the K$^+$-secreting collecting tubule. Patients who are noncompliant with a low Na$^+$ diet must take oral KCl supplements or a K$^+$-sparing diuretic or must stop using the thiazide diuretic.

Finally, it should be kept in mind that diuretics can never correct the underlying cardiac disease. Drugs that improve myocardial contractility or reduce peripheral vascular resistance are more direct approaches to the basic problem. Diuretics are at best adjunctive therapy.

KIDNEY DISEASE

A variety of renal diseases may interfere with the kidney's normally critical role in volume homeostasis. Although kidney disease will occasionally cause salt wasting, most kidney diseases cause retention of salt and water. When loss of renal function is severe, diuretic agents are of little benefit, because there is insufficient glomerular filtration to sustain a natriuretic response. However, a large number of patients with milder degrees of renal insufficiency can be treated with diuretics when they retain sodium.

Many primary and secondary glomerular diseases, such as those associated with diabetes mellitus, systemic lupus erythematosus, and other disorders involving vascular damage exhibit primary retention of salt and water by the kidney. The cause of this sodium retention is not precisely known, but it probably involves disordered regulation of the renal microcirculation and tubular function through release of vasoconstrictors, prostaglandins, cytokines, and other inflammatory mediators. When these patients develop edema or hypertension, diuretic therapy can be very effective. If heart failure is present simultaneously, the warnings mentioned above should apply.

Certain forms of renal disease, particularly diabetic nephropathy, are frequently associated with development of hyperkalemia at a relatively early stage in the progression of chronic renal failure. In these cases, a thiazide or loop diuretic will enhance K$^+$ excretion by increasing delivery of salt to the K$^+$-secreting collecting tubule.

Patients with renal diseases leading to the nephrotic syndrome often present complex problems in volume management. It was taught traditionally that these patients have reduced plasma volume in conjunction with reduced plasma oncotic pressures. This explanation is probably correct in many patients with "minimal change" nephropathy. In these patients, diuretic use may cause further reductions in plasma volume that can impair glomerular filtration rate and may lead to orthostatic hypotension. However, most other causes of nephrotic syndrome are associated with an unexplained primary retention of salt and water by the kidney, leading to expanded plasma volume and hypertension despite the low plasma oncotic pressure. In these cases, diuretic therapy may be beneficial in controlling the volume-dependent component of hypertension and reducing the contribution hypertension may make to the underlying renal disease.

In choosing a diuretic for the patient with kidney disease, a number of important limitations must be kept in mind. Acetazolamide and K^+-sparing diuretics must usually be avoided because of their tendency to exacerbate acidosis and hyperkalemia, respectively. Thiazide diuretics are generally ineffective when GFR falls below 30 mL/min. Thus, loop diuretics are often the best choice in treating edema associated with kidney failure. Lastly, overzealous use of diuretics will cause renal function to decline in all patients, but in those with underlying renal disease, the consequences are all the more serious.

HEPATIC CIRRHOSIS

Liver disease is often associated with edema and with ascites in conjunction with elevated portal hydrostatic pressures and reduced plasma oncotic pressures. The mechanisms for the sodium retention are complex. They probably involve a combination of factors, including diminished renal perfusion resulting from systemic vascular alterations, diminished plasma volume as the result of ascites formation, and diminished oncotic pressure from hypoalbuminemia. In addition, there may be primary sodium retention by the kidney. Plasma aldosterone levels are usually high in response to the reduction in effective circulating volume.

When ascites and edema become severe, diuretic therapy can be useful in initiating and maintaining diuresis. Cirrhotic patients are often resistant to loop diuretics, in part because of an unexplained decrease in secretion of the drug into the tubular fluid and in part because of high aldosterone levels leading to enhanced collecting duct salt reabsorption. On the other hand, cirrhotic edema is unusual in its high degree of responsiveness to spironolactone. The combination of loop diuretics and spironolactone may be useful in some patients. However, even more than in heart failure, overly aggressive use of diuretics in this setting can be disastrous. Vigorous diuretic therapy can cause marked depletion of intravascular volume, hypokalemia, and metabolic alkalosis. Hepatorenal syndrome and hepatic encephalopathy are the unfortunate consequences of overzealous diuretic use in the cirrhotic patient.

IDIOPATHIC EDEMA

This syndrome, which occurs almost exclusively in women, consists of fluctuating salt retention and edema. Despite intensive study, the pathophysiology of this disorder remains obscure. Some studies suggest that intermittent diuretic use may actually contribute to the syndrome. Therefore, idiopathic edema should be managed with mild salt restriction alone if possible.

NONEDEMATOUS STATES

HYPERTENSION

It has long been known that the diuretic and mild vasodilator actions of the thiazides are useful in the treatment of virtually all patients with essential hypertension and may be sufficient therapy in nearly two-thirds. Moderate restriction of dietary Na^+ intake (60–100 meq/d) has been shown to potentiate the effects of diuretics in essential hypertension and to lessen renal K^+ wasting.

Until recently, a thiazide diuretic was usually the first drug to be tried in treating patients with mild essential hypertension. With increasing recognition of the adverse effects of thiazides (see above) and the development of newer antihypertensives (see Chapter 11), the use of thiazides as first-line treatment has declined somewhat. Diuretics still play an important role in patients who require multiple drugs to control blood pressure. Diuretics enhance the efficacy of many agents, particularly the angiotensin-converting enzyme inhibitors. Patients being treated with powerful vasodilators such as hydralazine or minoxidil usually require diuretics simultaneously, because the vasodilators cause significant volume retention and, sometimes, edema.

Despite their adverse effects, diuretics are likely to continue as important tools in the management of hypertension. This is particularly true in light of their low cost and effectiveness.

NEPHROLITHIASIS

Approximately two-thirds of all renal stones contain calcium phosphate or calcium oxalate. Many patients with such stones exhibit a renal "leak" of calcium that causes hypercalciuria. This can be treated with thiazide diuretics, which enhance calcium reabsorption in the distal convoluted tubule and thus reduce the urinary calcium concentration. Salt intake must be reduced in this setting, as excess dietary NaCl will overwhelm the hypocalciuric effect of thiazides. Calcium stones may also be caused by increased intestinal absorption of calcium, or they may be idiopathic. In these situations, thiazides are also effective, but should be used as adjunctive therapy with decreased calcium intake and other measures.

HYPERCALCEMIA

Hypercalcemia can be a medical emergency. Since the loop of Henle is an important site of calcium reabsorption, loop diuretics can be quite effective in promoting calcium diuresis. However, loop diuretics alone can cause marked volume contraction. If this occurs, loop diuretics are ineffective (and potentially counterproductive) because calcium reabsorption in the proximal tubule is enhanced. Thus, saline must be administered simultaneously with loop diuretics if an effective calcium diuresis is to be achieved. The usual approach is to infuse normal saline and give furosemide (80–120 mg) intravenously. Once the diuresis begins, the rate of saline infusion can be matched with the urine flow rate to avoid volume depletion. Potassium may be added to the saline infusion as needed.

DIABETES INSIPIDUS

Thiazide diuretics can reduce polyuria and polydipsia in patients who are not responsive to ADH. The beneficial effect is mediated through plasma volume reduction, with an attendant fall in glomerular filtration rate, enhanced proximal reabsorption of NaCl and water, and decreased delivery of fluid to the diluting segments. Thus, the maximum volume of dilute urine that can be produced is lowered. This seemingly paradoxical effect of thiazides can significantly reduce urine flow in the polyuric patient. Dietary sodium restriction can potentiate the beneficial effects of thiazides on urine volume in this setting. Lithium, used in the treatment of manic-depressive disorder, is a common cause of drug-induced diabetes insipidus, and thiazide diuretics have been found to be helpful in treating it. Serum Li^+ levels must be carefully monitored in this situation, since diuretics may *reduce* renal clearance of Li^+ and raise Li^+ levels into the toxic range (Chapter 28). Lithium polyuria can also be partially reversed by amiloride, which appears to block lithium entry into collecting duct cells, much as it blocks Na^+ entry.

PREPARATIONS AVAILABLE

Acetazolamide (generic, Diamox)
    Oral: 125, 250 mg tablets
    Oral sustained-release: 500 mg capsules
    Parenteral: 500 mg powder for injection
Amiloride (generic, Midamor)
    Oral: 5 mg tablets
Bendroflumethiazide (Naturetin)
    Oral: 5, 10 mg tablets
Benzthiazide (Exna)
    Oral: 50 mg tablets
Bumetanide (Bumex)
    Oral: 0.5, 1, 2 mg tablets
    Parenteral: 0.5 mg/2 mL ampule for IV or IM injection
Chlorothiazide (generic, Diuril, others)
    Oral: 250, 500 mg tablets; 250 mg/5 mL suspension
    Parenteral: 500 mg for injection
Chlorthalidone (generic, Hygroton, others)
    Oral: 15, 25, 50, 100 mg tablets
Demeclocycline (Declomycin)
    Oral: 150 mg tablets and capsules; 300 mg tablets
Dichlorphenamide (Daranide)
    Oral: 50 mg tablets
Dorzolamide (Trusopt)
    Ophthalmic: 2% solution
Ethacrynic acid (Edecrin)
    Oral: 25, 50 mg tablets
    Parenteral: 50 mg for IV injection
Furosemide (generic, Lasix, others)
    Oral: 20, 40, 80 mg tablets; 8, 10 mg/mL solutions
    Parenteral: 10 mg/mL for IM or IV injection

Hydrochlorothiazide (generic, Esidrix, Hydro-DIURIL, others)
    Oral: 25, 50, 100 mg tablets; 10, 100 mg/mL solution
Hydroflumethiazide (generic, Diucardin, Saluron)
    Oral: 50 mg tablets
Indapamide (Lozol)
    Oral: 1.25, 2.5 mg tablets
Mannitol (generic, Osmitrol)
    Parenteral: 5, 10, 15, 20, 25% for injection
Methyclothiazide (generic, Enduron, others)
    Oral: 2.5, 5 mg tablets
Metolazone (Mykrox, Zaroxolyn) (**Note:** Bioavailability of Mykrox is greater than that of Zaroxolyn.)
    Oral: 0.5 (Mykrox); 2.5, 5, 10 mg (Zaroxolyn) tablets
Polythiazide (Renese)
    Oral: 1, 2, 4 mg tablets
Quinethazone (Hydromox)
    Oral: 50 mg tablets
Spironolactone (generic, Aldactone)
    Oral: 25, 50, 100 mg tablets
Torsemide (Demadex)
    Oral: 5, 10, 20, 100 mg tablets
    Parenteral: 10 mg/mL for injection
Triamterene (Dyrenium)
    Oral: 50, 100 mg tablets
Trichlormethiazide (generic, Naqua)
    Oral: 2, 4 mg tablets

REFERENCES

General

Brenner BM (editor): *The Kidney,* 5th ed. Saunders, 1996.

Ellison DH: Diuretic drugs and the treatment of edema: From clinic to bench and back again. Am J Kidney Dis 1994;23:623.

Rose BD: Diuretics. Kidney Int 1991;39:336.

Specific Agents

Aiza I, Perez GO, Schiff ER: Management of ascites in patients with chronic liver disease. Am J Gastroenterol 1994;89:1949.

Ashraf N, Locksley R, Arieff AI: Thiazide-induced hyponatremia associated with death or neurologic damage in outpatients. Am J Med 1981;70:1163.

Baglin A et al: Metabolic adverse reactions to diuretics: Clinical relevance to elderly patients. Drug Saf 1995; 12:161.

Barr WH et al: Comparison of bioavailability, pharmacokinetics, and pharmacodynamics of torasemide in young and elderly healthy volunteers. Prog Pharm Clinical Pharmacol 1990;8:1.

Battle DC et al: Amelioration of polyuria by amiloride in patients receiving long-term lithium therapy. N Engl J Med 1985;312:408.

Biollaz J et al: Whole-blood pharmacokinetics and metabolic effects of the topical carbonic anhydrase inhibitor dorzolamide. Eur J Clin Pharmacol 1995;47:453.

Blose JS, Adams KF Jr, Patterson JH: Torsemide: A pyridine-sulfonylurea loop diuretic. Ann Pharmacother 1995;29:396.

Brater DC: Pharmacokinetics and pharmacodynamics of torasemide in health and disease. J Cardiovasc Pharmacol 1993;22(Suppl 3):S24.

Brater DC: Diuretic resistance: Mechanisms and therapeutic strategies. Cardiology 1994;84(Suppl 2):57.

Brown CB et al: High dose frusemide in acute renal failure: A controlled trial. Clin Nephrol 1981;15:90.

De Marchi S, Ceddhin E: Severe metabolic acidosis and disturbances of calcium metabolism induced by acetazol-amide in patients on haemodialysis. Clin Sci 1990; 78:295.

DeTroyer A: Demeclocycline: Treatment for syndrome of inappropriate antidiuretic hormone secretion. JAMA 1977;237:2723.

Ellison DH et al: Adaptation of the distal convoluted tubule of the rat: Structural and functional effects of dietary salt intake and chronic diuretic infusion. J Clin Invest 1989;83:113.

Forns X et al: Management of ascites and renal failure in cirrhosis. Semin Liver Dis 1994;14:82.

Giebisch G et al: Renal and extrarenal sites of action of diuretics. Cardiovasc Drugs Ther 1993;7:11.

Goldberg H et al: Mechanism of Li inhibition of vasopressin-sensitive adenylate cyclase in cultured renal epi-thelial cells. Am J Physiol 1988;255:F995.

Greene MK et al: Acetazolamide in prevention of acute mountain sickness: A double-blind controlled crossover study. Br Med J 1981;283:811.

Hollifield JW, Slaton PE: Thiazide diuretics, hypokalemia, and cardiac arrhythmias. Acta Med Scand 1981; 647(Suppl):67.

Horisberger J-D, Giebisch G: Potassium-sparing diuretics. Renal Physiol 1987;10:198.

Indapamide: A new indoline diuretic agent. (Symposium.) Am Heart J 1983;106:183.

Koechel DA: Ethacrynic acid and related diuretics: Relationship of structure to beneficial and detrimental actions. Annu Rev Pharmacol Toxicol 1981;21:265.

Levy ST, Forrest JM, Heninger GR: Lithium-induced diabetes insipidus: Manic symptoms, brain and electrolyte correlates, and chlorothiazide treatment. Am J Psychiatry 1973;130:1014.

Loon NR et al: Mechanism of impaired natriuretic response to furosemide during prolonged therapy. Kidney Int 1989;36:682.

Nakahama H et al: Pharmacokinetic and pharmacodynamic interactions between furosemide and hydrochlorothiazide in nephrotic patients. Nephron 1988;49:223.

Pollare T et al: A comparison of the effects of hydrochlorothiazide and captopril on glucose and lipid metabolism in patients with hypertension. N Engl J Med 1989;321:868.

Preisig PA, Rector FC Jr: Role of the Na^+/H^+ antiporter in rat proximal tubule NaCl absorption. Am J Physiol 1988;255:F461.

Puschett JB: Pharmacological classification and renal actions of diuretics. Cardiology 1994;84(Suppl 2):4.

Shimuzu T et al: Effects of PTH, calcitonin, and cAMP on calcium transport in rabbit distal nephron. Am J Physiol 1990;259:F408.

Stanton BA: Cellular actions of thiazide diuretics in the distal tubule. J Am Soc Nephrol 1990;1:832.

Stokes JB: Electroneutral NaCl transport in the distal tubule. Kidney Int 1989;36:427.

Strahlman E, Tiping R, Vogel R: A double-masked randomized 1-year study comparing dorzolamide (Trusopt), timolol, and betaxolol. Arch Ophthalmol 1995;113:1009.

Townsend RR, Holland B: Combination of converting enzyme inhibitor with diuretic for the treatment of hypertension. Arch Intern Med 1990;150:1175.

Van Brummelen P, Woerlee M, Schalekamp MA: Long-term versus short-term effects of hydrochlorothiazide on renal haemodynamics in essential hypertension. Clin Sci 1979;56:463.

Vargo DL et al: Bioavailability, pharmacokinetics, and pharmacodynamics of torsemide and furosemide in patients with congestive heart failure. Clin Pharmacol Ther 1995;57:601.

Ward ME, Musa MN, Bailey L: Clinical pharmacokinetics of lithium. J Clin Pharmacol 1994;34:280.

Warren SE, Blantz RC: Mannitol. Arch Intern Med 1981; 141:493.

Weinberg MS et al: Anuric renal failure precipitated by indomethacin and triamterene. Nephron 1985;40:216.

Wingo CS: Cortical collecting tubule potassium secretion: Effect of amiloride, ouabain, and luminal sodium concentration. Kidney Int 1985;27:886.

Wollam GL et al: Diuretic potency of combined hydrochlorothiazide and furosemide therapy in patients with azotemia. Am J Med 1982;72:929.

Zell SC, Goodman PH: Acetazolamide and dexamethasone in the prevention of acute mountain sickness. West J Med 1988;148:541.

Section IV.
Drugs With Important Actions on Smooth Muscle

Histamine, Serotonin, & the Ergot Alkaloids

16

Alan Burkhalter, PhD, David J. Julius, PhD, & Bertram G. Katzung, MD, PhD

Histamine and serotonin (5-hydroxytryptamine) are biologically active amines that are found in many tissues, have complex physiologic and pathologic effects through multiple receptor subtypes, and are often released locally. Together with endogenous peptides (Chapter 17) and prostaglandins and leukotrienes (Chapter 18), they are sometimes called *autacoids* (Gk "self-remedy") or *local hormones* in recognition of these properties.

The roles of histamine and serotonin in normal physiology are not completely understood, and because of their broad and largely undesirable effects, these compounds have no clinical application in the treatment of disease. However, compounds that selectively activate certain receptor subtypes or selectively antagonize the actions of these amines are of considerable clinical usefulness. This chapter therefore emphasizes the basic pharmacology of the agonist amines and the clinical pharmacology of the more selective agonist and antagonist drugs. The ergot alkaloids, compounds with partial agonist activity at serotonin and several other receptors, are discussed at the end of the chapter.

HISTAMINE

Histamine was synthesized in 1907 and later isolated from mammalian tissues. Early hypotheses concerning the possible physiologic roles of tissue histamine were based on similarities between histamine's actions and the symptoms of anaphylactic shock and tissue injury. Marked species variation has been observed, but in humans histamine is an important medi-

ator of immediate allergic and inflammatory reactions; has an important role in gastric acid secretion; and functions as a neurotransmitter and neuromodulator.

I. Basic Pharmacology of Histamine

Chemistry & Pharmacokinetics

Histamine is 2-(4-imidazoyl)ethylamine. It occurs in plants as well as in animal tissues and is a component of some venoms and stinging secretions.

Histamine is formed by decarboxylation of the amino acid L-histidine, a reaction catalyzed in mammalian tissues by the enzyme histidine decarboxylase (E.C.4.1.1.22). Pyridoxal phosphate is required as cofactor. Once formed, histamine is either stored or rapidly inactivated. The major inactivation pathway involves, first, conversion to methylhistamine, catalyzed by imidazole-*N*-methyltransferase, and then oxidation to methylimidazoleacetic acid, catalyzed by diamine oxidase. A second important pathway of metabolism involves direct conversion of histamine to imidazoleacetic acid by diamine oxidase. Very little histamine is excreted unchanged. Certain neoplasms (systemic mastocytosis, urticaria pigmentosa, gastric carcinoid, and occasionally myelogenous leukemia) are associated with increased numbers of mast cells or basophils and with increased excretion of histamine and its metabolites.

Although histamine is found in most tissues, it is very unevenly distributed. Most tissue histamine exists in bound form in granules in mast cells or basophils; the histamine content of many tissues is directly related to their mast cell content. The bound form of histamine is biologically inactive, but many stimuli, as noted below, can trigger the release of mast cell histamine, allowing the free amine to exert its actions on surrounding tissues.

Mast cells are especially rich at sites of potential tissue injury—nose, mouth, and feet; internal body surfaces; and blood vessels, particularly at pressure points and bifurcations. Mast cells in different tissues also differ. Some mast cells found in the gastrointestinal mucosa are similar to those found in connective tissue, but others exhibit different properties. Such mucosal or atypical mast cells contain—in addition to histamine—chondroitin sulfate instead of heparin sulfate in the storage granules and exhibit different sensitivities to chemicals that cause histamine release.

Non-mast cell histamine is found in several tissues, including the brain, where it functions as a neurotransmitter (Chapter 21). Cell bodies of histaminergic neurons are found in the tuberomamillary nucleus and other sites. Endogenous neurotransmitter histamine may play a role in many brain functions such as neuroendocrine control, cardiovascular regulation, thermoregulation, and arousal.

A second important nonneuronal site of histamine storage and release is the enterochromaffin-like cell of the fundus of the stomach. These cells release histamine, one of the primary acid secretagogues, to activate the acid-producing parietal cells of the mucosa (Chapter 63).

Storage & Release of Histamine

In human mast cells and basophils, storage granules contain histamine complexed with a sulfated polysaccharide, heparin or chondroitin sulfate, and an acidic protein. The bound form of histamine can be released through several mechanisms.

A. Immunologic Release: The important pathophysiologic mechanism of mast cell and basophil histamine release is immunologic. These cells, if sensitized by IgE antibodies attached to their surface membranes, degranulate when exposed to the appropriate antigen (see Figure 56–5). This type of release also requires energy and calcium. Degranulation leads to the simultaneous release of histamine, ATP, and other mediators that are stored together in secretory granules. Some of these compounds, most notably ATP, serve to further potentiate mast cell degranulation via a paracrine or autocrine mechanism. Degranulated mast cells will reaccumulate histamine over a period of days to weeks. Histamine released by this mechanism is a mediator in immediate (type I) allergic reactions. Substances released during IgG- or IgM-mediated immune reactions that activate the complement cascade also release histamine from mast cells and basophils.

By a negative feedback control mechanism mediated by H_2 receptors, histamine appears to modulate its own release and that of other mediators from sensitized mast cells in some tissues. In humans, mast cells in skin and basophils show this negative feedback mechanism; lung mast cells do not. Thus, histamine may act to limit the intensity of the allergic reaction in the skin and blood.

Endogenous histamine may also have a modulating role in a variety of inflammatory and immune responses. Histamine probably plays a part in acute inflammatory responses. Upon injury to a tissue, released histamine causes local vasodilation and leakage of plasma containing mediators of acute inflammation (complement, C-reactive protein), antibodies, and inflammatory cells (neutrophils, eosinophils, basophils, monocytes, and lymphocytes). Histamine inhibits the release of lysosome contents and several T and B lymphocyte functions. Most of these actions are mediated by H_2 receptors acting through increased intracellular cAMP. Release of peptides from nerves in response to inflammation is also probably modulated by histamine, in this case acting through presynaptic H_3 receptors.

B. Chemical and Mechanical Release: Certain amines, including drugs such as morphine and tubocurarine, can displace histamine from the heparin-protein complex within cells. This type of release does not require energy and is not associated with mast cell injury or degranulation. Loss of granules from the mast cell will also release histamine, since sodium ions in the extracellular fluid rapidly displace the amine from the complex. Chemical and mechanical mast cell injury causes degranulation and histamine release. Compound 48/80, an experimental diamine polymer, specifically releases histamine from tissue mast cells by an exocytotic degranulation process requiring energy and calcium.

Pharmacodynamics

A. Mechanism of Action: Histamine exerts its biologic actions by combining with specific cellular receptors located on the surface membrane. The three different histamine receptors thus far characterized are designated H_1, H_2, and H_3 and are described in Table 16–1. All three receptor subtypes belong to the large superfamily of receptors having seven membrane-spanning regions and intracellular association with G proteins. The structures of the H_1 and H_2 receptors have been determined. In the brain, H_1 and H_2 receptors are located on postsynaptic membranes, while H_3 receptors are predominantly presynaptic. Activation of these presynaptic receptors is associated with a reduction of transmitter release, including histamine itself, norepinephrine, serotonin, and acetylcholine. Activation of H_1 receptors, which are present in endothelial and smooth muscle cells, usually elicits an increase in phosphoinositol hydrolysis and an increase in intracellular calcium. Activation of H_2 receptors, present in gastric mucosa, cardiac muscle cells, and some immune cells, increases intracellular cAMP. Activation of H_3 receptors, which are found in several areas of the

Table 16–1. Histamine receptor subtypes.

Receptor Subtype	Distribution	Postreceptor Mechanism	Partially Selective Agonists	Partially Selective Antagonists
H_1	Smooth muscle, endothelium, brain	↑ IP_3, DAG	2-(m-fluorophenyl)-histamine[1]	Mepyramine, triprolidine
H_2	Gastric mucosa, cardiac muscle, mast cells, brain	↑ cAMP	Dimaprit, impromidine, amthamine	Ranitidine, tiotidine
H_3	Presynaptic: brain, myenteric plexus, other neurons	G protein-coupled	R-α-Methylhistamine, imetit, immepip	Thioperamide, iodophenpropit, clobenpropit

[1]Partial agonist.

central nervous system, decreases transmitter release from histaminergic and other neurons, possibly mediated by a decrease in calcium influx through N-type calcium channels in nerve endings.

B. Tissue and Organ System Effects of Histamine: Histamine exerts powerful effects on smooth and cardiac muscle, on certain endothelial and nerve cells, and on the secretory cells of the stomach. However, sensitivity to histamine varies greatly among species. Humans, guinea pigs, dogs, and cats are quite sensitive, while mice and rats are much less so.

1. Cardiovascular system–In humans, injection or infusion of histamine causes a decrease in systolic and diastolic blood pressure and an increase in heart rate (Figure 16–1). The acute blood pressure changes are caused by the direct vasodilator action of histamine on arterioles and precapillary sphincters; the increase in

heart rate involves both stimulatory actions of histamine on the heart and a reflex tachycardia. Flushing, a sense of warmth, and headache may also occur during histamine administration, consistent with the vasodilation. Histamine-induced vasodilation is mediated, at least in part, by release of endothelium-derived relaxing factor (EDRF; see Chapter 6). Studies with histamine receptor antagonists show that both H_1 and H_2 receptors are involved in these cardiovascular responses to high doses, since a combination of H_1 and H_2 receptor-blocking agents is more effective in preventing the actions of histamine than either blocking agent alone (Figure 16–1). However, in humans, the cardiovascular effects of small doses of histamine can usually be antagonized by H_1 receptor antagonists alone.

Histamine-induced edema results from the action of the amine on H_1 receptors in the vessels of the

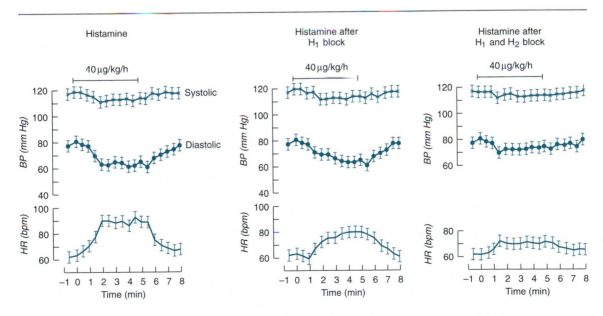

Figure 16–1. Effects of histamine and histamine antagonists on blood pressure and heart rate in humans. Histamine was infused at 40 µg/kg/h for 5 minutes as shown at the top of each panel. The H_1 antagonist was chlorpheniramine (10 mg intravenously). The H_2 antagonist was cimetidine (2 mg intravenously). (Modified and reproduced, with permission, from Torsoli A, Lucchelli PE, Brimblecombe RW [editors]: *H_2Antagonists: H_2Receptor Antagonists in Peptic Ulcer Disease and Progress in Histamine Research.* Excerpta Medica, 1980.)

microcirculation, especially the postcapillary vessels. The effect is associated with an increase in permeability of the vessel wall that has been ascribed to the separation of the endothelial cells, thus permitting the transudation of fluid and molecules as large as small proteins into the perivascular tissue. This effect is responsible for the urticaria (hives) that signals the release of histamine in the skin. New studies of endothelial cells suggest that actin and myosin within these *nonmuscle* cells contract in response to calcium influx evoked by drugs such as histamine. This contraction results in separation of the endothelial cells and increased permeability (Curry, 1992).

Direct cardiac effects of histamine include both increased contractility and increased pacemaker rate. These effects are mediated chiefly by H_2 receptors. In human atrial muscle, histamine can also decrease contractility; this effect is mediated by H_1 receptors. The physiologic significance of these cardiac actions is not clear. The cardiovascular effects may also be produced by the release of endogenous histamine from mast cells. Many of the cardiovascular signs and symptoms of anaphylaxis are due to released histamine, though other mediators are also involved.

2. Gastrointestinal tract smooth muscle– Histamine causes contraction of intestinal smooth muscle, and histamine-induced contraction of guinea pig ileum is a standard bioassay for histamine. The human gut is not as sensitive as that of the guinea pig, but large doses of histamine may cause diarrhea, partly as a result of this effect. This action of histamine is mediated by H_1 receptors.

3. Bronchiolar smooth muscle–In both humans and guinea pigs, histamine causes bronchoconstriction mediated by H_1 receptors. In the guinea pig, this effect is the cause of death from histamine toxicity, but in normal humans, bronchoconstriction following the usual doses of histamine is not marked. However, patients with asthma are very sensitive to histamine. The bronchoconstriction induced in these patients probably represents a hyperactive neural response, since such patients also respond excessively to many other stimuli, and the response to histamine can be blocked by autonomic blocking drugs such as ganglionic blocking agents as well as by H_1 receptor antagonists (see Chapter 20). Provocative tests using increasing doses of inhaled histamine are of diagnostic value for bronchial hyperreactivity in patients with suspected asthma or cystic fibrosis. Such individuals may be 100- to 1000-fold more sensitive to histamine than are normal subjects.

4. Other smooth muscle organs–In humans, histamine generally has insignificant effects on the smooth muscle of the eye and genitourinary tract. However, pregnant women suffering anaphylactic reactions may abort as a result of histamine-induced contractions, and in some species the sensitivity of the uterus is sufficient to form the basis for a bioassay.

5. Nerve endings–Histamine is a powerful stimulant of sensory nerve endings, especially those mediating pain and itching. This H_1-mediated effect is an important component of the urticarial response and reactions to insect and nettle stings. Some evidence suggests that local high concentrations can also depolarize efferent (axonal) nerve endings (see ¶ 7, below).

6. Secretory tissue–Histamine has long been recognized as a powerful stimulant of gastric acid secretion and, to a lesser extent, of gastric pepsin and intrinsic factor production. The effect is caused by activation of H_2 receptors on gastric parietal cells and is associated with increased adenylyl cyclase activity, cAMP concentration, and intracellular Ca^{2+} concentration. Other stimulants of gastric acid secretion such as acetylcholine and gastrin do not increase cAMP even though their maximal effects on acid output can be reduced—but not abolished—by H_2 receptor antagonists. Histamine also stimulates secretion in the small and large intestine.

Histamine has insignificant effects on the activity of other glandular tissue at ordinary concentrations. Very high concentrations can cause adrenal medullary discharge.

7. The "triple response"–Intradermal injection of histamine causes a characteristic wheal-and-flare response that was first described over 60 years ago. The effect involves three separate cell types: smooth muscle in the microcirculation, capillary or venular endothelium, and sensory nerve endings. At the site of injection, a reddening appears owing to dilation of small vessels, followed soon by an edematous wheal at the injection site and a red irregular flare surrounding the wheal. The flare is said to be caused by an axon reflex. As noted above, histamine stimulates nerve endings; the resulting impulses are thought to travel through other branches of the same axon, causing vasodilation through the release of a vasodilatory neuromediator. The sensation of itch may also accompany the appearance of these effects. The wheal is due to local edema.

Similar local effects may be produced by injecting histamine liberators (compound 48/80, morphine, etc) intradermally or by applying the appropriate antigens to the skin of a sensitized person. Although most of these local effects can be blocked by prior administration of an H_1 receptor-blocking agent, H_2 receptors may also be involved.

Other Histamine Agonists

Small substitutions on the imidazole ring of histamine significantly modify the selectivity of the compounds for the histamine receptor subtypes. For example, 2-methylhistamine is relatively more selective for H_1 receptors, while 4-methylhistamine is a relatively specific H_2 agonist. **Betazole**—a drug that was used in testing gastric acid-secreting ability—and **impromidine** are agonists at H_2 receptors and antagonists at H_3 receptors. R-α-Methylhistamine is a potent and selective H_3 receptor agonist that crosses the blood-brain barrier. It is also a potent inhibitor of histamine synthesis and release and can reduce the release of other transmitters from peripheral nerves through activation of presynaptic H_3 receptors.

II. Clinical Pharmacology of Histamine

Clinical Uses

A. Testing Gastric Acid Secretion: Histamine was used in the past as a diagnostic agent in testing for gastric acid secreting ability. However, pentagastrin is currently used for this purpose with a much lower incidence of adverse effects.

B. Diagnosis of Pheochromocytoma: Histamine can cause release of catecholamines from adrenal medullary cells. Although this effect is not prominent in normal humans, massive release can occur in patients with pheochromocytoma. This hazardous provocative test is now obsolete, since chemical assays are available for determination of the catecholamines and their metabolites in patients suspected of having this tumor.

C. Pulmonary Function Testing: In pulmonary function laboratories, histamine aerosol (in addition to other agents) is sometimes used as a provocative test of bronchial hyperreactivity.

Toxicity & Contraindications

Adverse effects following administration of histamine, like those of histamine release, are dose-related. Flushing, hypotension, tachycardia, headache, wheals, bronchoconstriction, and gastrointestinal upset are noted. These effects are also observed after the ingestion of spoiled fish (scombroid fish poisoning), and there is evidence that histamine produced by bacterial action in the flesh of the fish is the major causative agent.

Histamine should not be given to asthmatics (except as part of a carefully monitored test of pulmonary function) or to patients with active ulcer disease or gastrointestinal bleeding.

HISTAMINE ANTAGONISTS

The effects of histamine released in the body can be reduced in several ways. **Physiologic antagonists,** especially epinephrine, have smooth muscle actions opposite to those of histamine, but they act at different receptors. This is important clinically because injection of epinephrine can be lifesaving in systemic anaphylaxis and in other conditions in which massive release of histamine—and other mediators—occurs.

Release inhibitors reduce the degranulation of mast cells that results from immunologic triggering by antigen-IgE interaction. Cromolyn and nedocromil appear to have this effect (see Chapter 20) and are used in the treatment of asthma, though the molecular mechanism underlying their action is presently unknown. Beta$_2$-adrenoceptor agonists also appear capable of reducing histamine release.

Histamine **receptor antagonists** represent a third approach to the reduction of histamine-mediated responses. For over 45 years, compounds have been available that competitively antagonize many of the actions of histamine on smooth muscle. However, not until the H_2 receptor antagonist burimamide was described in 1972 was it possible to antagonize the gastric acid-stimulating activity of histamine. The development of selective H_2 receptor antagonists has led not only to more precise definition of histamine's actions in terms of receptors involved but also to more effective therapy for peptic ulcer. Selective H_3 antagonists are not yet available for clinical use. However, a potent and selective H_3 receptor antagonist, thioperamide, has been introduced that competes for the binding of radiolabeled R-α-methylhistamine to this site at nanomolar concentration. Like R-α-methylhistamine, thioperamide crosses the blood-brain barrier. The availability of this agonist and antagonist will help to define the physiologic role of H_3 receptors.

H$_1$-RECEPTOR ANTAGONISTS

Compounds that competitively block histamine at H_1 receptors have been used clinically for many years, and many H_1 antagonists are currently marketed in the USA. Several are available without prescription, both alone and in combination formulations such as "cold pills" and sleep aids (see Chapter 64).

I. Basic Pharmacology of H$_1$-Receptor Antagonists

Chemistry & Pharmacokinetics

The H_1 antagonists are conveniently divided into first-generation and second-generation agents. These groups are distinguished by the relatively strong sedative effects of most of the first-generation drugs. The first-generation agents are also more likely to block autonomic receptors. The relatively less sedating characteristic of the second-generation H_1 blockers is due mainly to their less complete distribution into the central nervous system. All of the H_1 antagonists are stable amines with the general structure illustrated in Figure 16–2. There are several chemical subgroups, and the structures of compounds representing different sub-

$$X - Y - C - C - N$$

X is: C or N
Y is: C, O, or omitted

GENERAL STRUCTURE

ETHERS OR ETHANOLAMINE DERIVATIVE

$$CH - O - CH_2 - CH_2 - N \begin{array}{c} CH_3 \\ CH_3 \end{array}$$

Diphenhydramine or dimenhydrinate

ETHYLENEDIAMINE DERIVATIVE

$$CH_2 \quad N - CH_2 - CH_2 - N \begin{array}{c} CH_3 \\ CH_3 \end{array}$$

Tripelennamine

PIPERAZINE DERIVATIVE

$$CH - N \bigcirc N - CH_3$$

Cyclizine

ALKYLAMINE DERIVATIVE

$$Cl \qquad CH - CH_2 - CH_2 - N \begin{array}{c} CH_3 \\ CH_3 \end{array}$$

Chlorpheniramine

PHENOTHIAZINE DERIVATIVE

$$N - CH_2 - CH - N \begin{array}{c} CH_3 \\ CH_3 \end{array}$$
$$\quad\quad CH_3$$

Promethazine

PIPERIDINE DERIVATIVES

$$CH_2 - CH_2 - CH_2 - CH - R$$

R: $\quad\quad C - CH_3$ (with CH_3, CH_3)

Terfenadine

R: $\quad\quad C - COOH$ (with CH_3, CH_3, OH)

Fexofenadine

Figure 16–2. General structure of H$_1$ antagonist drugs and examples of the major subgroups.

groups are shown in the figure. Doses of some of these drugs are given in Table 16–2. During the last decade, chemists have learned to use the active metabolites of several antihistamines as active drugs (see box: Antihistamines & Their Active Metabolites).

These agents are rapidly absorbed following oral administration, with peak blood concentrations occurring in 1–2 hours. They are widely distributed throughout the body, and the first-generation drugs enter the central nervous system readily. They are extensively metabolized, primarily by microsomal systems in the liver. Several of the second-genera-

tion agents are metabolized by the CYP3A4 system and thus are subject to important interactions when other drugs (such as ketoconazole) inhibit this subtype of P450 enzymes. Most of the drugs have an effective duration of action of 4–6 hours following a single dose, but meclizine and several second-generation agents are longer-acting, with a duration of action of 12–24 hours. The newer agents also are considerably less lipid-soluble and enter the central nervous system with difficulty or not at all. Astemizole, ebastine (investigational), hydroxyzine, loratadine, and terfenadine have active metabolites. The

Table 16–2. Some H₁ antihistaminic drugs in clinical use.

Drugs	Usual Adult Dose	Anti-cholinergic Activity	Comments
FIRST-GENERATION ANTIHISTAMINES			
Ethanolamines			
Carbinoxamine (Clistin)	4–8 mg	+++	Slight to moderate sedation.
Dimenhydrinate (salt of diphenhydramine) (Dramamine)	50 mg	+++	Marked sedation; anti-motion sickness activity.
Diphenhydramine (Benadryl, etc)	25–50 mg	+++	Marked sedation; anti-motion sickness activity.
Doxylamine (Decapryn)	1.25–25 mg	nd	Marked sedation; now available only in OTC "sleep aids."
Ethylenediamines			
Pyrilamine (Neo-Antergan)	25–50 mg	+	Moderate sedation; component of OTC "sleep aids."
Tripelennamine (PBZ, etc)	25–50 mg	+	Moderate sedation.
Piperazine derivatives			
Hydroxyzine (Atarax, etc)	25–100 mg	nd	Marked sedation.
Cyclizine (Marezine)	25–50 mg	—	Slight sedation; anti-motion sickness activity.
Meclizine (Bonine, etc)	25–50 mg	—	Slight sedation; anti-motion sickness activity.
Alkylamines			
Brompheniramine (Dimetane, etc)	4–8 mg	+	Slight sedation.
Chlorpheniramine (Chlor-Trimeton, etc)	4–8 mg	+	Slight sedation; common component of OTC "cold" medication.
Phenothiazine derivatives			
Promethazine (Phenergan, etc)	10–25 mg	+++	Marked sedation; antiemetic.
Miscellaneous			
Cyproheptadine (Periactin, etc)	4 mg	+	Moderate sedation; also has antiserotonin activity.
SECOND-GENERATION ANTIHISTAMINES			
Piperidines			
Astemizole (Hismanal)	10 mg	—	Slow onset of action.
Fexofenadine (Allegra)	60 mg	—	Lower risk of arrhythmia.
Terfenadine (Seldane)	60 mg	—	Prompt onset of action.
Miscellaneous			
Loratadine (Claritin)	10 mg	—	Longer action.
Cetirizine (Zyrtec)	5–10 mg	—	

active metabolites of hydroxyzine and terfenadine are available as drugs (cetirizine and fexofenadine, respectively).

Pharmacodynamics

A. Histamine Receptor Blockade: H₁-receptor antagonists block the actions of histamine by reversible competitive antagonism at the H₁ receptor. They have negligible potency at the H₂ receptor and little at the H₃ receptor. For example, histamine-induced contraction of bronchiolar or gastrointestinal smooth muscle can be completely blocked by these agents, but the effects of histamine on the cardiovascular system are only partly blocked because of H₂ receptor-mediated actions (Figure 16–1). H₂ receptor-mediated actions such as increase in gastric acid secretion and inhibition of histamine release from mast cells are unaffected.

B. Actions Not Caused by Histamine Receptor Blockade: The first-generation H₁-receptor antagonists have many actions not ascribable to blockade of the actions of histamine. The large number of these actions probably results from the similarity of the general structure (Figure 16–2) to the structure of drugs that have effects at muscarinic cholinoceptor, alpha-adrenoceptor, serotonin, and local anesthetic receptor sites. Some of these actions are of therapeutic value and some are undesirable.

1. Sedation—A common effect of first-generation H₁ antagonists is sedation, but the intensity of this ef-

---

ANTIHISTAMINES & THEIR ACTIVE METABOLITES

The pharmacokinetics of the H_1 antihistamines have proved to be of immense importance since the introduction of the second-generation agents. The first significant pharmacokinetic contribution was the demonstration that their lack of sedative effect was largely the result of poor distribution to the central nervous system. The popularity of these nonsedating agents then came under attack when it was found that the metabolism of terfenadine was easily inhibited by a variety of hepatic microsomal enzyme inhibitors, even including grapefruit juice, and that the resulting high concentrations could cause a lethal arrhythmia, torsades de pointes. The fact that the parent compound was the toxic agent in this interaction and lacked useful antihistaminic effect logically led to the development of the active metabolite, fexofenadine, as a drug in its own right. Fexofenadine is carboxylated terfenadine (Figure 16–2) and lacks cardiac toxicity.

Synthetic art has imitated nature in the development of several other antihistamines with second-generation characteristics. As shown in the following table, four compounds that contain the carboxylated structure can now be prescribed. In addition, ebastine, an investigational long-acting second-generation drug, is known to be a prodrug and is rapidly converted to its carboxylated derivative, cerebastine, in the body.

Carboxylated Drug	$t_{1/2}$	Prodrug
Fexofenadine	25 h	Terfenadine
Cetirizine	7–9 h	Hydroxyzine
Acrivastine[1]	2–3 h	. . .
Levocabastine	35–40 h	. . .

[1]Not available in the USA.

These drugs (or their active metabolites) are highly selective for H_1 receptors.

2. Antinausea and antiemetic actions–Several first-generation H_1 antagonists have significant activity in preventing motion sickness (Table 16–2). They are less effective against an episode of motion sickness already present. Certain H_1 antagonists, notably doxylamine (in Bendectin), were used widely in the past in the treatment of nausea and vomiting of pregnancy (see below).

3. Antiparkinsonism effects–Perhaps because of their anticholinergic effects (cf benztropine, Chapter 28), some of the H_1 antagonists have significant acute suppressant effects on the parkinsonism symptoms associated with certain antipsychotic drugs.

4. Anticholinoceptor actions–Many of the first-generation agents, especially those of the ethanolamine and ethylenediamine subgroups, have significant atropine-like effects on peripheral muscarinic receptors. This action may be responsible for some of the (uncertain) benefits reported for nonallergic rhinorrhea but may also cause urinary retention and blurred vision.

5. Adrenoceptor-blocking actions–Alpha receptor-blocking effects can be demonstrated for many H_1 antagonists, especially those in the phenothiazine subgroup. This action may cause orthostatic hypotension in susceptible individuals. Beta receptor blockade is not observed.

6. Serotonin-blocking action–Strong blocking effects at serotonin receptors have been demonstrated for some first-generation H_1 antagonists, notably cyproheptadine. This drug is promoted as an antiserotonin agent and is discussed with that drug group. Nevertheless, it has a chemical structure that resembles that of the phenothiazine antihistamines and is a potent H_1 blocking agent.

7. Local anesthesia–Many first-generation H_1 antagonists are effective local anesthetics. They block sodium channels in excitable membranes in the same fashion as procaine and lidocaine. Diphenhydramine and promethazine are actually more potent than procaine as local anesthetics. They are occasionally used to produce local anesthesia in patients allergic to the conventional local anesthetic drugs.

---

fect varies among chemical subgroups (Table 16–2) and among patients as well. The effect is sufficiently prominent with some agents to make them useful as "sleep aids" (see Chapter 64) and unsuitable for daytime use. The effect resembles that of some antimuscarinic drugs and is considered very unlike the disinhibited sedation produced by sedative-hypnotic drugs. At ordinary dosages, children occasionally (and adults rarely) manifest excitation rather than sedation. At very high toxic dose levels, marked stimulation, agitation, and even convulsions may precede coma. Newer H_1 antagonists have little or no sedative action.

II. Clinical Pharmacology of H_1-Receptor Antagonists

Clinical Uses

A. Allergic Reactions: The H_1 antihistaminic agents are often the first drugs used to prevent or treat the symptoms of allergic reactions. In allergic rhinitis and urticaria, in which histamine is the primary mediator, the H_1 antagonists are the drugs of choice and are often quite effective. However, in bronchial asthma, which involves several mediators, the H_1 antagonists are largely ineffective.

Angioedema may be precipitated by histamine release but appears to be maintained by bradykinins that are not affected by antihistaminic agents. For atopic dermatitis, antihistaminic drugs such as diphenhydramine are used mostly for their sedative side effects and for some control of the itching.

The H_1 antihistamines used for treating allergic conditions such as hay fever are usually selected with the goal of minimizing sedative effects; in the USA, the drugs in widest use are the alkylamines and the newer piperidines. However, the sedative effect and the therapeutic efficacy of different agents vary widely among individuals, so it is common practice to give a patient samples from each major group to determine which is the most effective with the least adverse effects in that individual. In addition, the clinical effectiveness of one group may diminish with continued use, and switching to another group may restore drug effectiveness for as yet unexplained reasons.

The second-generation H_1 antagonists are used mainly for the treatment of allergic rhinitis and chronic urticaria. Several double-blind comparisons with older agents (such as chlorpheniramine) indicated about equal therapeutic efficacy. However, sedation and interference with safe operation of machinery, which occur in about 50% of subjects taking conventional antihistamines, occurred in only about 7% of subjects taking terfenadine or astemizole. The newer drugs are much more expensive.

B. Motion Sickness and Vestibular Disturbances: Scopolamine and certain first-generation H_1 antagonists are the most effective agents available for the prevention of motion sickness. The antihistaminic drugs with the greatest effectiveness in this application are diphenhydramine and promethazine. The piperazines (cyclizine and meclizine) also have significant activity in preventing motion sickness and are less sedative in most patients. Dosage is the same as that recommended for allergic disorders (Table 16–2). Both scopolamine and the H_1 antagonists are more effective in preventing motion sickness when combined with ephedrine or amphetamine.

It has been claimed that the antihistaminic agents effective in prophylaxis of motion sickness are also useful in Meniere's syndrome, but efficacy in the latter application is not well established.

C. Nausea and Vomiting of Pregnancy: Several H_1 antagonist drugs have been studied for possible use in treating "morning sickness." The piperazine derivatives were withdrawn from such use when it was demonstrated that they have teratogenic effects in rodents. Doxylamine, an ethanolamine H_1 antagonist, was promoted for this application as a component of Bendectin, a prescription medication that also contained pyridoxine. The question of fetal malforma-

tions resulting from this use of Bendectin is discussed below.

Toxicity

The wide spectrum of adverse effects of the H_1 antihistamines is described above. Several of these effects (sedation, antimuscarinic action) have been used for therapeutic purposes, especially in OTC remedies (see Chapter 64). Nevertheless, these two effects constitute the most common undesirable actions when these drugs are used to block histamine receptors. Appropriate selection of drugs with a lower incidence of these effects (Table 16–2) and trial of several drugs by the patient are the most effective methods for minimizing both toxicities.

Less common toxic effects of systemic use include excitation and convulsions in children, postural hypotension, and allergic responses. Drug allergy is relatively common, especially after topical use of H_1 antagonists. The effects of severe systemic overdosage of the older agents resemble those of atropine overdosage and are treated in the same way (see Chapters 8 and 59). Overdosage of the newer H_1-blockers, especially astemizole, may induce cardiac arrhythmias (Woosley, 1996; Saviuc et al, 1993), and the same effect may be caused by interaction with enzyme inhibitors (see Drug Interactions, below).

Possible teratogenic effects of doxylamine were widely publicized in the lay press after 1978 as a result of case reports of fetal malformation associated with maternal ingestion of Bendectin. However, several large prospective studies involving over 60,000 pregnancies, of which more than 3000 involved maternal **Bendectin** ingestion, disclosed no increase in the incidence of birth defects. In contrast, a few case-control studies of infants with malformations suggested a weak correlation between Bendectin use and certain abnormalities. Because of the continuing controversy, adverse publicity, and lawsuits, the manufacturer of Bendectin withdrew the product from the market. Our inability to define the existence and extent of risk in this situation illustrates the difficulties involved in detecting small changes in the incidence of rare pathologic events (see Chapter 5).

Drug Interactions

Significant cardiac toxicity, including QT prolongation and potentially lethal ventricular arrhythmias, has occurred in patients taking either terfenadine or astemizole combined with ketoconazole, itraconazole, or macrolide antibiotics such as erythromycin. These antimicrobial drugs inhibit the metabolism of many drugs by CYP3A4 and cause significant increases in blood concentrations of the antihistamines. The seriousness of this interaction is such that terfenadine and astemizole are contraindicated in patients taking ketoconazole, itraconazole, or macrolides and in patients with liver disease. Grapefruit juice also inhibits CYP3A4 and has been shown to increase terfenadine's blood levels significantly. The FDA has indicated that it may try to have terfenadine withdrawn from the market since its safer active metabolite, fexofenadine, is now available.

For those H_1 antagonists that cause significant sedation, addition of other drugs that cause central nervous system depression produces additive effects and is contraindicated while driving or operating machinery.

H_2-RECEPTOR ANTAGONISTS (Table 16–3)

The development of H_2-receptor antagonists was based on the observation that H_1 antagonists had no effect on histamine-induced acid secretion in the stomach. Molecular manipulation of the histamine molecule resulted in a series of drugs with progressive increases in the acid secretion-blocking action and reduction in irrelevant effects. This development led to renewed interest in possible physiologic roles for histamine and to a classification of effects of both agonists and antagonists based upon histamine receptor subtypes. The high incidence of peptic ulcer disease and related gastrointestinal complaints created great interest in the therapeutic potential of H_2-receptor antagonists. Because of the ability of this class of drugs to reduce gastric acid secretion, they are now among the most frequently prescribed drugs in the USA and have recently become OTC items.

I. Basic Pharmacology of H_2-Receptor Antagonists

Chemistry & Pharmacokinetics

The first two H_2 receptor antagonists discovered, burimamide and metiamide, are imidazole compounds with long side chains containing a thiourea group. Because of their toxic effects, these agents are no longer used. Four H_2 antagonists are currently available in the USA: cimetidine, ranitidine, famotidine, and nizatidine. Their structures and some of their pharmacokinetic properties are set out in Table 16–3.

Pharmacodynamics

A. Mechanisms of Action: Presently available H_2-receptor antagonists reversibly compete with histamine at H_2-receptor sites. This action is quite selective in that the H_2 antagonists do not affect H_1 receptor-mediated actions.

B. Organ System Effects:

1. Acid secretion and gastric motility–The most important action of H_2 receptor antagonists is to reduce the secretion of gastric acid (Figure 16–3). These drugs block the acid secretion stimulated by histamine, gastrin, cholinomimetic drugs, and vagal stimulation. The volume of gastric secretion and the concentration of pepsin are also reduced. While the ability of H_2 receptor antagonists to inhibit all phases

Table 16–3. H_2-receptor-blocking drugs.

Drug	Bioavailability (Oral)	V_d	$t_{1/2\beta}$	Elimination
Cimetidine	30–80%	0.8–1.2 L/kg	1.5–2.3 hours, increased in severe renal failure	Mostly renal. Major metabolite, S-oxide.
Ranitidine	30–88%	1.2–1.9 L/kg	1.6–2.4 hours, increased in severe renal failure	Mostly renal. Small amounts of S-oxide, N-oxide, and N-desmethyl metabolites.
Famotidine	37–45%	1.1–1.4 L/kg	2.5–4 hours, increased in severe renal failure	Mostly renal. Major metabolite, S-oxide.
Nizatidine	75–100%	1.2–1.6 L/kg	1.1–1.6 hours, increased in severe renal failure	Mostly renal. Small amounts of S-oxide, N-oxide, and N-desmethyl metabolites.

Figure 16–3. Effects of ranitidine on hypersecretion of pepsin and acid secretion in a patient. Gastric contents were collected by gastric tube for two 6-hour periods. Pepsin is quantitated as thousands of units and acid as millimoles per 30 minutes. During the first period, intravenous saline (placebo) injections were made at 40-minute intervals. During the second period, increasing intravenous ranitidine doses were given at 40-minute intervals as shown by the arrows. Ranitidine had a marked and long-lasting effect on acid secretion and a shorter but significant effect on pepsin production. (Modified and reproduced, with permission, from Danilewith M et al: Ranitidine suppression of gastric hypersecretion resistant to cimetidine. N Engl J Med 1982;306:20.)

of acid secretion has been interpreted as implicating histamine as a final common mediator of acid secretion, a more plausible hypothesis suggests that the full expression of stimuli such as gastrin and parasympathetic impulses requires the participation of histamine in some manner. See Chapter 63 for further details.

Cimetidine, ranitidine, and famotidine have little effect on gastric smooth muscle function and on lower esophageal sphincter pressure. Other gastrointestinal secretions are not significantly reduced. While there are marked potency differences among the members of this class, no agent appears to be more efficacious than the others in reducing acid secretion. Nizatidine stimulates contractile activity in the stomach, leading to decreased emptying time. This effect may be related to the ability of nizatidine to inhibit acetylcholinesterase.

2. Other effects related to H$_2$-receptor blockade—In doses that suppress gastric acid secretion, cimetidine and ranitidine have little effect on the heart or blood pressure. Early reports that famotidine reduces cardiac output have not been confirmed in more recent studies. Nizatidine has been reported to reduce heart rate and cardiac output in healthy subjects. These observations are consistent with the idea that endogenous histamine has a negligible role in the normal regulation of cardiovascular function and in patients with congestive heart failure (Solomon et al, 1993). As shown in Figure 16–1, cimetidine is effective in reducing some of the actions of administered histamine on the heart and vessels.

It has been predicted that H$_2$ receptor antagonists may enhance certain immune responses by blocking histamine's ability to decrease mediator release from mast cells and basophils; experimentally, increases in delayed hypersensitivity reactions can be shown in some patients receiving cimetidine. However, there is no evidence that clinical hypersensitivity reactions are increased in such patients.

3. Effects not related to H$_2$-receptor blockade—Cimetidine and, to a much lesser extent, ranitidine can inhibit the cytochrome P450 oxidative drug-metabolizing system. Famotidine and nizatidine do not inhibit the P450 system. There is evidence that cimetidine, ranitidine, and nizatidine—but not famotidine—inhibit the first-pass gastric metabolism of ethanol. Ranitidine has been shown to inhibit the glucuronidation of acetaminophen in animals. Both cimetidine and ranitidine can inhibit the renal clearance of basic drugs that are secreted by the renal tubule. Cimetidine binds to androgen receptors and causes antiandrogen effects. Ranitidine, famotidine, and nizatidine do not bind to androgen receptors.

II. Clinical Pharmacology of H$_2$-Receptor Antagonists

Clinical Uses

A. Peptic Duodenal Ulcer: An estimated 10% of adults in the Western world will suffer an episode of peptic ulcer disease during their lifetime. Although the mortality rate of this condition is low, the recurrence rate is high and the socioeconomic cost is great.

Because it was known that "no acid = no ulcer," medical therapy—before the era of H_2-blockers—focused on reducing acidity with antimuscarinic drugs and antacids. However, antimuscarinic drugs must be used in high doses that cause significant adverse effects. Antacids relieve symptoms and, in high doses, can promote healing. However, frequent doses are required, and patient compliance is poor except during the acute symptomatic phase of the disease. The effectiveness of H_2-receptor antagonists in reducing gastric acidity coupled with their low toxicity represents a significant advance in the treatment of this disease. Results of many clinical trials show that these drugs effectively control symptoms during acute episodes and promote healing of duodenal ulcers. Prophylactic use at reduced dosage helps to prevent recurrence in many patients. Omeprazole, a very efficacious blocker of gastric acid secretion (by proton pump blockade), and sucralfate, a drug that promotes healing by coating the ulcer bed, are also available. Surgery for peptic ulcer has markedly declined as a result of drug therapy since the introduction of H_2 blockers. See Chapter 63 for further details.

For short-term management of active duodenal ulcer, once-daily doses of an H_2-blocker given at bedtime appear to be effective. Healing is promoted by cimetidine 800 mg, ranitidine 300 mg, famotidine 40 mg, or nizatidine 300 mg given once daily for up to 8 weeks. Because these drugs are eliminated by the kidney, doses should be reduced in patients with poor renal function. Maintenance therapy for patients with a healed duodenal ulcer can also be accomplished by once-daily doses; cimetidine 400 mg, ranitidine 150 mg, famotidine 20 mg, or nizatidine 150 mg is effective in reducing recurrence. Most patients respond adequately, but some may become refractory to these agents for unknown reasons. These drugs are usually administered orally; cimetidine, ranitidine, and famotidine are also available for intravenous use. Hypotension and cardiac arrhythmias have been reported (rarely) following intravenous administration.

B. Gastric Ulcer: For patients with active benign gastric ulcers, administration of H_2-receptor antagonists relieves symptoms and promotes healing. Dosages are the same as for duodenal disease.

C. Erosive Esophagitis (Gastroesophageal Reflux Disorder): Erosive esophagitis is much more difficult to treat than peptic ulcer and often requires more frequent dosing than peptic ulcer. All four of the H_2 blockers are approved for this indication in the same or slightly higher total daily dosage, but divided into at least two daily doses. Many patients require significantly higher doses than those listed or do not respond adequately at any dosage. Such patients usually require proton pump inhibitors for relief (Chapter 63).

D. Hypersecretory Conditions: Zollinger-Ellison syndrome is a usually fatal disorder in which hypersecretion of acid is caused by a gastrin-secreting tumor. Systemic mastocytosis and multiple endocrine adenomas often result in hypersecretion. In many patients, H_2 receptor-blocking drugs effectively control symptoms related to excess acid secretion. The drugs can be used before surgery or as primary treatment when surgery is not indicated. The dosages of H_2 antagonists required to reduce secretion and control symptoms are usually much larger than in ulcer patients. Multiple daily doses adjusted for each patient are usually required.

E. Other Conditions: In patients with hiatal hernia, stress-induced ulcers, and iatrogenic ulcers, the benefit of these drugs is not clearly documented.

Toxicity

H_2-blocking drugs are well tolerated, and adverse effects are reported in only 1–2% of cases. The most commonly reported effects are diarrhea, dizziness, somnolence, headache, and rash. Others include constipation, vomiting, and arthralgia. Cimetidine is associated with the most adverse effects, while nizatidine seems to produce the fewest. Other less common but more serious effects are discussed below.

A. Central Nervous System Dysfunction: Slurred speech, delirium, and confusional states are most common in elderly patients. These effects are most often associated with cimetidine, rare for ranitidine, and of unknown prevalence for famotidine and nizatidine.

B. Endocrine Effects: Cimetidine binds to androgen receptors, and antiandrogenic effects such as gynecomastia (in men) and galactorrhea (in women) have been reported. In addition, a reduction in sperm count and reversible impotence have been reported in male patients receiving high doses for hypersecretory states such as Zollinger-Ellison syndrome. These effects are rarely observed with therapy that continues for no longer than 8 weeks. Ranitidine, famotidine, and nizatidine appear to be free of endocrine effects.

C. Blood Dyscrasias: Cimetidine therapy has been associated with granulocytopenia, thrombocytopenia, neutropenia, and even aplastic anemia in a very few instances. There are also rare reports of similar effects associated with ranitidine. There is less information about these effects for famotidine or nizatidine.

D. Liver Toxicity: Reversible cholestatic effects have been reported for cimetidine. Reversible hepatitis, with or without jaundice, has been reported for ranitidine. Reversible abnormalities in liver enzyme tests have been reported for famotidine and nizatidine.

E. Pregnancy and Nursing Mothers: Studies have not shown any harmful effects on the fetus when H_2-blockers are administered to pregnant women. However, they cross the placenta, so these drugs should be given in this context only when absolutely necessary. All four agents are secreted into breast milk and therefore may affect the nursing infant.

Drug Interactions

Cimetidine inhibits the cytochrome P450-catalyzed oxidative drug metabolism pathway. The drug also reduces hepatic blood flow, which may further reduce clearance of other drugs. Coadministration of cimetidine with any of the following drugs may result in increased pharmacologic effects or toxicity: warfarin, phenytoin, propranolol, metoprolol, labetalol, quinidine, caffeine, lidocaine, theophylline, alprazolam, diazepam, flurazepam, triazolam, chlordiazepoxide, carbamazepine, ethanol, tricyclic antidepressants, metronidazole, calcium channel blockers, and sulfonylureas. Dosage adjustments may be necessary, especially in patients with reduced kidney function. Ranitidine in ordinary therapeutic doses does not appear to inhibit the oxidative metabolism of most other drugs. As noted above, however, all of the H_2 blockers except famotidine significantly increase the bioavailability of ethanol by inhibiting its gastric first-pass metabolism.

SEROTONIN (5-HYDROXYTRYPTAMINE)

Before the identification of 5-hydroxytryptamine (5-HT), it was known that when blood is allowed to clot, a vasoconstrictor substance is released from the clot; this substance was called serotonin. Independent studies established the existence of a smooth muscle stimulant in intestinal mucosa; this was called enteramine. The synthesis of 5-hydroxytryptamine in 1951 permitted the identification of serotonin and enteramine as the same metabolite of 5-hydroxytryptophan.

Serotonin is known to play a role in several diseases and is probably involved in many more. One of the more dramatic of these conditions is called **"serotonin syndrome"** and is evoked by an interaction between serotonergic agents, especially 5-HT reuptake blockers, and MAO inhibitors. This condition is described in Chapter 30. Serotonin is also one of the mediators of the signs and symptoms of carcinoid syndrome, an unusual manifestation of carcinoid tumor, a neoplasm of enterochromaffin cells. In patients whose tumor is not operable, serotonin antagonists may constitute the best treatment.

I. Basic Pharmacology of Serotonin

Chemistry & Pharmacokinetics

Like histamine, serotonin is widely distributed in nature, being found in plant and animal tissues, ven-

oms, and stings. It is an indoleethylamine formed in biologic systems from the amino acid L-tryptophan by hydroxylation of the indole ring followed by the decarboxylation of the amino acid. Hydroxylation at C5 is the rate-limiting step and can be blocked by p-chlorophenylalanine (PCPA, fenclonine) and by p-chloroamphetamine. These agents have been used experimentally to reduce serotonin synthesis in carcinoid syndrome.

Serotonin

After synthesis, the free amine is stored or is rapidly inactivated, usually by oxidation catalyzed by the enzyme monoamine oxidase. In the pineal gland, serotonin serves as a precursor of melatonin, a melanocyte-stimulating hormone. In mammals (including humans), over 90% of the serotonin in the body is found in enterochromaffin cells in the gastrointestinal tract. In the blood, serotonin is found in platelets, which are able to concentrate the amine by means of an active carrier mechanism similar to that in the vesicles of noradrenergic and serotonergic nerve endings. Serotonin is also found in the raphe nuclei of the brain stem, which contain cell bodies of tryptaminergic (serotonergic) neurons that synthesize, store, and release serotonin as a transmitter. Brain serotonergic neurons are involved in various functions such as mood, sleep, appetite, temperature regulation, the perception of pain, the regulation of blood pressure, and vomiting (see Chapter 21). Serotonin may also be involved in conditions such as depression, anxiety, and migraine. Serotonergic neurons are also found in the enteric nervous system of the gastrointestinal tract and around blood vessels. In rodents (but not in humans), serotonin is found in mast cells.

The function of serotonin in enterochromaffin cells is not clear. These cells synthesize serotonin, store the amine in a complex with ATP and with other substances in granules, and can release serotonin in response to mechanical and neuronal stimuli. Some of the released serotonin diffuses into blood vessels and is taken up and stored in platelets.

Stored serotonin can be depleted by reserpine in much the same manner as this drug depletes catecholamines from vesicles in adrenergic nerves (see Chapter 6).

Serotonin is metabolized by monoamine oxidase, and the intermediate product, 5-hydroxyindole-acetaldehyde, is further oxidized by aldehyde dehydrogenase. When the latter enzyme is saturated, eg, by large amounts of acetaldehyde from ethanol metabolism, a significant fraction of the 5-hydroxyindole-acetaldehyde may be *reduced* in the liver to the alcohol 5-hydroxytryptophol. In humans consuming a normal diet, the excretion of 5-hydroxyindoleacetic acid (5-HIAA) is a measure of serotonin synthesis. Therefore, the 24-hour excretion of 5-HIAA can be used as a diagnostic test for tumors that synthesize excessive quantities of serotonin, especially carcinoid tumor. A few foods (eg, bananas) contain large amounts of serotonin or its precursors and must be prohibited during such diagnostic tests.

Pharmacodynamics

A. Mechanisms of Action: Serotonin exerts many actions and, like histamine, has many species differences, making generalizations difficult. The actions of serotonin are mediated through a variety of cell membrane receptors. The serotonin receptors that have been characterized thus far are described in Table 16–4. Seven major 5-HT-receptor subtypes have been identified, six involving G protein-coupled receptors and one a ligand-gated ion channel. Among these receptor subtypes, several lack any recognized physiologic function. Discovery of these functions awaits the development of subtype-selective drugs or the use of genetic methods to mutate or delete genes encoding these receptors from the mouse genome.

B. Tissue and Organ System Effects:

1. Cardiovascular system–Serotonin directly causes the contraction of smooth muscle, mainly through $5-HT_2$ receptors. In humans, serotonin is a powerful vasoconstrictor except in skeletal muscle and heart, where it dilates blood vessels. At least part of this 5-HT-induced vasodilation requires the presence of vascular endothelial cells. When the endothelium is damaged, coronary vessels constrict (Golino et al, 1991). Serotonin can also elicit reflex bradycardia by activation of $5-HT_3$ receptors on chemoreceptor nerve endings. A triphasic blood pressure response is often seen following injection of serotonin. Initially, there is a decrease in heart rate, cardiac output, and blood pressure caused by the chemoreceptor response. Following this decrease, blood pressure increases as a result of vasoconstriction. The third phase is again a decrease in blood pressure attributed to vasodilation in vessels supplying skeletal muscle. Pulmonary and renal vessels seem especially sensitive to the vasoconstrictor action of serotonin.

Serotonin also constricts veins, and venoconstriction with a resulting increased capillary filling appears responsible for the flush that is observed following serotonin administration. Serotonin has small

Table 16–4. Serotonin receptor subtypes.

Receptor Subtype	Distribution	Postreceptor Mechanism	Partially Selective Agonists	Partially Selective Antagonists
$5-HT_{1A}$	Raphe nuclei, hippocampus	↓ cAMP, K^+ channels	8-OH-DPAT	WAY100635
$5-HT_{1B}$	Substantia nigra, globus pallidus, basal ganglia	↓ cAMP	CP 93129	
$5-HT_{1Da,b}$	Brain	↓ cAMP	Sumatriptan	
$5-HT_{1E}$	Cortex, putamen	↓ cAMP		
$5-HT_{1F}$	Cortex, hippocampus	↓ cAMP		
$5-HT_{2A}$	Platelets, smooth muscle, cerebral cortex	↑ IP_3	α-Methyl-5-HT	Ketanserin
$5-HT_{2B}$	Stomach fundus	↑ IP_3	α-Methyl-5-HT	SB204741
$5-HT_{2C}$	Choroid, hippocampus, substantia nigra	↑ IP_3	α-Methyl-5-HT	Mesulergine
$5-HT_3$	Area postrema, sensory and enteric nerves	Receptor is a Na^+-K^+ ion channel	2-Methyl-5-HT, m-chlorophenyl-biguanide	Tropisetron, ondansetron, granisetron
$5-HT_4$	CNS and myenteric neurons, smooth muscle	↑ cAMP	5-Methoxytryp-tamine, renzapride, metoclopramide	See Bockaert, 1992, reference.
$5-HT_{5A,B}$	Brain	Unknown		
$5-HT_{6,7}$	Brain	↑ cAMP		Clozapine ($5-HT_7$)

Key: 8-OH-DPAT = 8-Hydroxy-2-(di-*n*-propylamine)tetralin
CP93129 = 5-Hydroxy-3(4-1,2,5,6-tetrahydropyridyl)-4-azaindole
SB204741 = *N*-(1-methyl-5-indolyl)-*N*′-(3-methyl-5-isothiazolyl)urea
WAY100635 = *N*-*tert*-butyl 3-4-(2-methoxyphenyl)piperazin-1-yl-2-phenylpropanamide

MELATONIN PHARMACOLOGY

Melatonin is N-acetyl-5-methoxytryptamine, a simple methylated and N-acetylated product of serotonin found in the pineal gland. It is produced and released primarily at night and has long been suspected of playing a role in diurnal cycles of animals and the sleep-wake behavior of humans (Brzezinski, 1997; Dubocovich, 1995; Hagan et al, 1995).

Melatonin receptors have now been characterized in several central nervous system and peripheral tissues. In the brain, the MEL_1 receptor is found in membranes of neurons in the suprachiasmatic nucleus of the hypothalamus, an area associated—from lesioning experiments—with circadian rhythm. MEL_1 is a seven-transmembrane (7TM) receptor that is coupled to its effector via a G_i protein. The result of receptor binding is inhibition of adenylyl cyclase. Most species studied have three variants of the receptor (1a, 1b, and 1c) but thus far only 1a and 1b have been found in humans.[*] The MEL_1 family shows little homology with any other family of 7TM receptors and may represent a new subfamily of the group. Activation of this receptor with pharmacologic doses of

melatonin appears to entrain the circadian clock and reset the sleep-wake behavior and temperature cycles of experimental animals and probably humans as well.

Melatonin is relatively lipid-soluble and appears to interact with intracellular receptors as well as those in the cell membrane. Candidates for such intracellular sites include a novel receptor related to the retinoid receptor and currently called $RZR\beta$. This protein has very high affinity for melatonin and modulates expression of genes. The mRNA associated with $RZR\beta$ is found in the visual system and the suprachiasmatic nucleus. Melatonin can also act as a Ca^{2+}-calmodulin antagonist.

Though very little is known about this potent neurohormone, the drug is freely available in health food stores in the USA and elsewhere because its commercial purveyors have labeled it a food and not a drug. In the few clinical studies done to date, melatonin does appear to be able to regularize sleep patterns—even though it has no observable direct hypnotic actions—in both young adults and in elderly patients with severely disturbed sleep. These encouraging findings suggest that melatonin, in addition to being the latest health-food fad, may find actual clinical utility.

[*]An alternative naming system uses ML_{1A}, ML_{1B}, etc.

---

direct positive chronotropic and inotropic effects on the heart that are probably of no clinical significance. However, prolonged elevation of the blood level of serotonin (which occurs in carcinoid syndrome) is associated with pathologic alterations in the endocardium (subendocardial fibroplasia) that may result in valvular or electrical malfunction.

Serotonin causes blood platelets to aggregate by activating surface $5-HT_2$ receptors. This response, in contrast to aggregation induced during clot formation, is not accompanied by the release of serotonin stored in the platelets. The physiologic role of this effect is unclear.

2. Gastrointestinal tract—Serotonin causes contraction of gastrointestinal smooth muscle, increasing tone and facilitating peristalsis. This action is caused by the direct action of serotonin on $5-HT_2$ smooth muscle receptors plus a stimulating action on ganglion cells located in the enteric nervous system (Chapter 6). Activation of $5-HT_4$ receptors in this system causes increased acetylcholine release and thereby mediates a motility-enhancing or "prokinetic" effect of selective serotonin agonists such as cisapride (Craig et al, 1990). These agents are useful in several gastrointestinal disorders. Overproduction of serotonin (and other substances) in carcinoid tumor is associated with severe diarrhea. Serotonin has little ef-

fect on secretions, and what effects it has are generally inhibitory.

3. Respiration—Serotonin has a small direct stimulant effect on bronchiolar smooth muscle in normal humans. In patients with carcinoid syndrome, episodes of bronchoconstriction occur in response to elevated levels of the amine. Serotonin may also cause hyperventilation as a result of the chemoreceptor reflex or bronchial sensory nerve ending stimulation.

4. Nervous system—Like histamine, serotonin is a potent stimulant of pain and itch sensory nerve endings and is responsible for some of the symptoms caused by insect and plant stings. In addition, serotonin is a powerful activator of chemosensitive endings located in the coronary vascular bed. Activation of $5-HT_3$ receptors on these afferent vagal nerve endings is associated with the chemoreceptor reflex (also known as the Bezold-Jarisch reflex). The reflex response consists of marked bradycardia and hypotension. The bradycardia is mediated by vagal outflow to the heart and can be blocked by atropine. The hypotension is a consequence of the decrease in cardiac output that results from bradycardia. A variety of other agents can activate the chemoreceptor reflex. These include nicotinic cholinoceptor agonists and some cardiac glycosides, eg, ouabain.

5-HT_3 receptors in the gastrointestinal tract and in the vomiting center of the medulla participate in the vomiting reflex. They are particularly important in vomiting caused by chemical triggers such as cancer chemotherapy drugs.

Serotonin is present in a variety of sites in the brain. Its role as a neurotransmitter and its relation to the actions of drugs acting in the central nervous system are discussed in Chapters 21 and 30. Serotonin is also a precursor of melatonin (see box: Melatonin Pharmacology).

II. Clinical Pharmacology of Serotonin

SEROTONIN AGONISTS

Serotonin has no clinical applications as a drug. However, several receptor subtype-selective agonists have proved to be of value. **Buspirone,** a 5-HT_{1a} agonist, has received wide attention for its utility as an effective nonbenzodiazepine anxiolytic (see Chapter 22). **Dexfenfluramine,** another selective 5-HT agonist, is widely used as an appetite suppressant (see box: Appetite Control Through Serotonin). **Sumatriptan** is a 5-HT_{1d} agonist effective in the treatment of acute migraine and cluster headache attacks.

Sumatriptan

Following the administration of 6 mg of sumatriptan succinate subcutaneously or 25 mg orally, a majority of patients suffering migraine attacks will experience relief of symptoms. This degree of efficacy is equal to or greater than that of other drug treatments, eg, parenteral or oral ergot alkaloids. Most adverse effects are mild and include altered sensations (tingling, warmth, etc), dizziness, muscle weakness, neck pain, and injection site reactions. Chest discomfort occurs in 5% of patients, and chest pain has been reported. Sumatriptan is contraindicated in patients with ischemic coronary artery disease and in patients with Prinzmetal's angina. Other disadvantages of this drug include the fact that its duration of effect is often shorter than the duration of the headache. As a result, several doses may be required during a prolonged migraine attack, though the drug is approved for only two doses per 24 hours. In addition, the drug is extremely expensive at present.

Other Agonists in Clinical Use

Dexfenfluramine, used in weight control, is described in the box: Appetite Control Through Serotonin. Cisapride, a 5-HT_4 agonist, is used in the treatment of gastroesophageal reflux and is described in Chapter 63.

In addition to agonists and antagonists, compounds such as fluoxetine and other serotonin-selective reuptake inhibitors, which modulate serotonergic transmission by blocking reuptake of the transmitter, are among the most widely prescribed drugs for the management of depression and other behavioral disorders. These drugs are discussed in Chapter 30.

APPETITE CONTROL THROUGH SEROTONIN

As noted above, serotonin appears to be related to several general behaviors such as sleep, emotion, sex, and appetite, and early studies with the amine suggested that it could reduce food intake in animals, an anorexigenic effect.

Fenfluramine, a racemic chemical more closely related to amphetamine than to serotonin, affects brain levels of serotonin and its metabolites at relatively low doses. It was introduced as an anorexigenic drug more than a decade ago in Europe. Its *d-* isomer, *d-*fenfluramine **(dexfenfluramine, Redux)** is about twice as potent an anorexigenic drug as fenfluramine, suggesting that all of fenfluramine's activity resides in the *d-* form. Several controlled clinical trials have demonstrated that the drug can help patients maintain caloric restriction and a lower body weight for at least a year, a better record than that of other anorexigenic drugs. Unlike amphetamine, dexfenfluramine appears to reduce appetite more in obese than in nonobese individuals. Dexfenfluramine has become a widely used weight control medication at a dosage of 30 mg/d.

Dexfenfluramine causes serotonin release and inhibits reuptake at moderately low concentrations. It also stimulates 5-HT receptors at relatively low concentrations. Metergoline, an ergot derivative with high affinity for 5-HT receptors, completely blocks the anorexic effect of dexfenfluramine, further suggesting a serotonergic action.

Most of the adverse effects of dexfenfluramine are mild and reversible, eg, headache or insomnia. However, since the introduction of the drug, several cases of fatal and nonfatal pulmonary hypertension have been reported in individuals with no known risk factor for this devastating condition other than consumption of dexfenfluramine. Other anorexigenic drugs have been similarly associated with cases of pulmonary hypertension. Therefore, patients taking this medication should be carefully monitored.

SEROTONIN ANTAGONISTS

The actions of serotonin, like those of histamine, can be antagonized in several different ways. Such antagonism is clearly desirable in those rare patients who have carcinoid tumor and may also be valuable in certain other conditions.

As noted above, serotonin synthesis can be inhibited by *p*-chlorophenylalanine and *p*-chloroamphetamine. However, these agents are too toxic for general use. Storage of serotonin can be inhibited by the use of reserpine, but the sympatholytic effects of this drug (see Chapter 11) and the high levels of circulating serotonin that result from release prevent its use in carcinoid. Therefore, receptor blockade is the major approach to therapeutic limitation of serotonin effects.

SEROTONIN RECEPTOR ANTAGONISTS

A wide variety of drugs with actions at other receptors (alpha adrenoceptors, H_1 histamine receptors, etc) are also serotonin receptor-blocking agents. In addition, the ergot alkaloids discussed in the last portion of the chapter are partial agonists at serotonin receptors.

Cyproheptadine resembles the phenothiazine antihistaminic agents in chemical structure and has potent H_1 receptor-blocking actions. The actions of cyproheptadine are predictable from its H_1 histamine and serotonin receptor affinities. It prevents the smooth muscle effects of both amines but has no effect on the gastric secretion stimulated by histamine. It has significant antimuscarinic effects and causes sedation.

The major clinical applications of cyproheptadine are in the treatment of the smooth muscle manifestations of carcinoid tumor and in the postgastrectomy dumping syndrome. The usual dosage in adults is 12–16 mg/d in three or four divided doses. It is also the preferred drug in cold-induced urticaria.

Ketanserin blocks 5-HT_{1c} and 5-HT_2 receptors and has little or no reported antagonist activity at other 5-HT or H_1 receptors. This drug also blocks vascular α_1 adrenoceptors. The drug blocks 5-HT_2 receptors on platelets and antagonizes platelet aggregation promoted by serotonin. Interest in this compound is generated by observations that it lowers blood pressure both in hypertensive animals and in hypertensive human patients. The mechanism involved in this hypotensive action is not clear but probably involves α_1 adrenoceptors more than 5-HT_2 receptors. Ketanserin is available in Europe for the treatment of hypertension and vasospastic conditions but has not been approved in the USA.

Ritanserin, another 5-HT_2 antagonist, has little or no alpha-blocking action. It has been reported to alter bleeding time and to reduce thromboxane formation, presumably by altering platelet function.

Ondansetron, a 5-HT_3 antagonist, is approved for use in the prevention of nausea and vomiting associated with surgery and with cancer chemotherapy. It is effective at a dose level of 0.1–0.2 mg/kg intravenously. **Granisetron**, a drug with similar properties, is also available. Other congeners are in clinical trials. These drugs have become extremely important in cancer chemotherapy because of their powerful ability to prevent or reduce the severe nausea and vomiting associated with anticancer drugs.

Considering the diverse effects attributed to serotonin and the heterogeneous nature of 5-HT receptors, other selective 5-HT antagonists may prove to be useful clinically.

THE ERGOT ALKALOIDS

Ergot alkaloids are produced by *Claviceps purpurea*, a fungus that infects grain—especially rye—under damp growing or storage conditions. This fungus synthesizes histamine, acetylcholine, tyramine, and other biologically active products in addition to a score or more of unique ergot alkaloids. These alkaloids affect alpha adrenoceptors, dopamine receptors, 5-HT receptors, and perhaps other receptor types.

The accidental ingestion of ergot alkaloids in contaminated grain can be traced back more than 2000 years from descriptions of epidemics of ergot poisoning (**ergotism**). The most dramatic effects of poisoning are dementia with florid hallucinations; prolonged vasospasm, which may result in gangrene; and stimulation of uterine smooth muscle, which in pregnancy may result in abortion. The severity of each effect varies among reported epidemics and may represent a different mix of individual alkaloids in different crops of the fungus. In medieval times, ergot poisoning was called **St. Anthony's fire** after the saint whose help was sought in relieving the burning pain of vasospastic ischemia. Identifiable epidemics have occurred sporadically up to modern times (see box: Ergot Poisoning: Not Just an Ancient Disease) and mandate continuous surveillance of all grains used for food. Poisoning of grazing animals is common in many areas because the same and related fungi may grow on pasture grasses (Porter et al, 1992).

In addition to the effects noted above, the ergot alkaloids produce a variety of other central nervous system and peripheral effects. Detailed structure-activity analysis and appropriate semisynthetic modifications have yielded a large number of agents with documented or potential clinical value.

ERGOT POISONING: NOT JUST AN ANCIENT DISEASE

As noted in the text, epidemics of ergotism, or poisoning by ergot-contaminated grain, are known to have occurred sporadically in ancient times and through the Middle Ages. It is easy to imagine the social chaos that might occur if fiery pain, gangrene, hallucinations, convulsions, and abortions appeared simultaneously throughout a community in which all or most of the people believed in witchcraft, demonic possession, and the visitation of supernatural punishments upon humans for their misdeeds. Such beliefs are uncommon in most cultures today. However, ergotism has not disappeared in modern times. A most convincing demonstration of ergotism occurred in the small French village of Pont-Saint-Esprit in 1951. It was described in the British Medical Journal in 1951 (Gabbai et al, 1951) and in a later book-length narrative account (Fuller, 1968). Several hundred individuals suffered symptoms of hallucinations, convulsions, and ischemia—and several died—after eating bread made from contaminated flour. Similar events have occurred even more recently when poverty, famine, or incompetence resulted in the consumption of contaminated grain.

Iatrogenic ergot toxicity caused by excessive use of medical ergot preparations is still fre-quently reported. The following case history is typical (Andersen et al, 1977).

A 58-year-old woman with a history of moderate ergotamine use for migraine was admitted to the hospital after 3 days of increasing symptoms of ischemia in the legs (pain, tenderness, cyanosis, and low skin temperature). No pulses could be palpated below the femoral vessels. The initial aortogram is shown in Figure 16–4 *(left)*. An epidural local anesthetic was administered to block sympathetic vasoconstrictor impulses to the vessels in the pelvis and legs, but no improvement was observed. After 3 hours, an infusion of nitroprusside was started. The temperature of the skin of the large toe rose rapidly from 22 °C (71.6 °F) to 31 °C (87.8 °F). Cyanosis disappeared, and popliteal and tibial pulses became palpable. An attempt to discontinue the nitroprusside infusion after 11 hours was followed by immediate vasoconstriction and cyanosis in the legs, so nitroprusside was restarted and continued for another 25 hours with good maintenance of circulation. Thirty-six hours after the start of the infusion, nitroprusside was discontinued with no signs of recurrent vasoconstriction. A repeat aortogram 1 week after the event appeared normal (Figure 16–4 [*right*]).

I. Basic Pharmacology of Ergot Alkaloids

Chemistry & Pharmacokinetics

Two major families of compounds that incorporate the tetracyclic **ergoline** nucleus may be identified; the amine alkaloids and the peptide alkaloids (Table 16–5). Drugs of therapeutic and toxicologic importance are found in both groups.

The ergot alkaloids are variably absorbed from the gastrointestinal tract. The oral dose of ergotamine is about ten times larger than the intramuscular dose, but the speed of absorption and peak blood levels after oral administration can be improved by administration with caffeine (see below). The amine alkaloids are also absorbed from the rectum and the buccal cavity and after administration by aerosol inhaler. Absorption after intramuscular injection is slow but usually reliable. Bromocriptine is well absorbed from the gastrointestinal tract.

The ergot alkaloids are extensively metabolized in the body. The primary metabolites are hydroxylated in the A ring, and peptide alkaloids are also modified in the peptide moiety. Most of the excretory products of methysergide are demethylated at the N_1 position.

Pharmacodynamics

A. Mechanism of Action: As suggested above, the ergot alkaloids act on several types of receptors. Their effects include agonist, partial agonist, and antagonist actions at alpha adrenoceptors and serotonin receptors and agonist actions at central nervous system dopamine receptors (Table 16–6). In addition, as yet undefined receptors may be activated. Furthermore, some members of the ergot family have a high affinity for presynaptic receptors, while others are more selective for postjunctional receptors. There is a powerful stimulant effect on the uterus that seems to be most closely associated with agonist (or partial agonist) effects at 5-HT_2 receptors. Structural variations increase the selectivity of certain members of the family for specific receptor types.

B. Organ System Effects:

1. Central nervous system–As indicated by

Table 16–5. Major ergoline derivatives (ergot alkaloids).

Amine alkaloids	Peptide alkaloids

	R_1	R_8
6-Methylergoline	—H	—H
Lysergic acid	—H	—COOH
Lysergic acid diethylamide (LSD)	—H	$-\overset{\overset{\text{O}}{\|\|}}{C}-N(CH_2-CH_3)_2$
Ergonovine (ergometrine)	—H	$-\overset{\overset{\text{O}}{\|\|}}{C}-NHCHCH_3$ with CH_2OH
Methysergide	—CH$_3$	$-\overset{\overset{\text{O}}{\|\|}}{C}-NH-CH-CH_2-CH_3$ with CH_2OH

	R_2	R_2'	R_5'
Ergotamine[1]	—H	—CH$_3$	—CH$_2$— (phenyl)
α-Ergocryptine	—H	—CH(CH$_3$)$_2$	—CH$_2$—CH(CH$_3$)$_2$
Bromocriptine	—Br	—CH(CH$_3$)$_2$	—CH$_2$—CH(CH$_3$)$_2$

[1]Dihydroergotamine lacks the double bond between carbons 9 and 10.

traditional descriptions of ergotism, certain of the naturally occurring alkaloids are powerful hallucinogens. Lysergic acid diethylamide (LSD, "acid") is the ergot compound that most clearly demonstrates this action. The drug has been used in the laboratory as a potent peripheral 5-HT$_2$ antagonist, but current evidence suggests that its behavioral effects are mediated by *agonist* effects at prejunctional (Sadzot et al, 1989) or postjunctional (Buckholtz et al, 1990) 5-HT$_2$ receptors in the central nervous system. In spite of extensive research, no clinical value has been discovered for LSD's dramatic effects. Abuse of this drug was widespread for several decades and is discussed in Chapter 32.

Table 16–6. Effects of ergot alkaloids at several receptors.[1]

Ergot Alkaloid	Alpha-Adrenoceptor	Dopamine Receptor	Serotonin Receptor (5-HT$_2$)	Uterine Smooth Muscle Stimulation
Bromocriptine	–	+++	–	0
Ergonovine	+	+	– (PA)	+++
Ergotamine	– – (PA)	0	+ (PA)	+++
Lysergic acid diethylamide (LSD)	0	+++	– –	+
Methysergide	+/0	+/0	– – – (PA)	+/0

[1]Agonist effects are indicated by +, antagonist by –, no effect by 0. Relative affinity for the receptor is indicated by the number of + or – signs. PA means partial agonist (both agonist and antagonist effects can be detected).

Dopamine receptors in the central nervous system play important roles in extrapyramidal motor control and the regulation of prolactin release. The actions of bromocriptine on the extrapyramidal system are discussed in Chapter 28. Of all the currently available ergot derivatives, bromocriptine and pergolide have the highest selectivity for the pituitary dopamine receptors. These drugs directly suppress prolactin secretion from pituitary cells by activating regulatory dopamine receptors (Chapter 37). They compete for binding to these sites with dopamine itself and with other dopamine agonists such as apomorphine.

2. Vascular smooth muscle—The action of ergot alkaloids on vascular smooth muscle is drug-, species-, and vessel-dependent, so few generalizations are possible. Ergotamine and related compounds constrict most human blood vessels in a predictable, prolonged, and potent manner (Figure 16–5). This response is partially blocked by conventional alpha-blocking agents. However, ergotamine's effect is also associated with "epinephrine reversal" (see Chapter 10) and with *blockade* of the response to other alpha agonists. This dual action represents partial agonist action (Table 16–5). Because ergotamine dissociates very slowly from the alpha receptor, it produces very long-lasting agonist and antagonist effects at this receptor. There is little or no effect at beta adrenoceptors.

While much of the vasoconstriction elicited by ergot alkaloids can be ascribed to partial agonist effects at alpha adrenoceptors, some may be the result of effects at 5-HT receptors. Ergotamine, ergonovine, and methysergide all have partial agonist effects at 5-HT$_2$ vascular receptors. Furthermore, different vascular beds have different sensitivities, and it is claimed that cerebral vessels, especially cerebral arteriovenous anastomotic vessels, are most sensitive to drugs such as ergotamine, dihydroergotamine, and sumatriptan (den Boer et al, 1992). The remarkably specific antimigraine action of the ergot derivatives is thought to be related to their actions on neuronal or vascular serotonin receptors. Ergotamine, ergonovine, and methysergide are the ergot drugs most commonly used for the treatment of migraine.

After overdosage with ergotamine and similar agents, vasospasm is severe and prolonged (see Toxicity, below). This vasospasm is not reversed by alpha antagonists, serotonin antagonists, or combinations of both.

Ergotamine is typical of the ergot alkaloids that have a strong vasoconstrictor spectrum of action. The hydrogenation of ergot alkaloids at the 9 and 10 positions (Table 16–5) yields dihydro derivatives that have much lower direct smooth muscle and serotonin effects and more selective alpha receptor-blocking actions.

3. Uterine smooth muscle—The stimulant ac-

Figure 16–4. Vasospasm induced by ergotamine. Aortic angiograms taken at the time of maximum vasospasm (left panel) and 1 week after (right panel) infusion of nitroprusside. The major vessels distal to the common iliac arteries *(arrows)* are thread-like and occluded in the left panel; in the right panel, normal flow has been restored. (Modified and reproduced, with permission, from Andersen PK et al: Sodium nitroprusside and epidural blockade in the treatment of ergotism. N Engl J Med 1977;296:1271.)

Figure 16–5. Effects of ergot derivatives on contraction of isolated segments of human basilar artery strips removed at surgery. All of the ergot derivatives are partial agonists, and all are more potent than the full agonists, norepinephrine and serotonin. (NE, norepinephrine; 5-HT, serotonin; ERG, ergotamine; MT, methylergometrine; DHE, dihydroergotamine; MS, methysergide.) (Modified and reproduced, with permission, from Müller-Schweinitzer E in: *5-Hydroxytryptamine Mechanisms in Primary Headaches.* Oleson J, Saxena PR [editors]. Raven Press, 1992.)

tion of ergot alkaloids on the uterus, as on vascular smooth muscle, appears to combine alpha agonist, serotonin, and other effects. Furthermore, the sensitivity of the uterus to the stimulant effects of ergot changes dramatically during pregnancy, perhaps because of increasing dominance of alpha₁ receptors as pregnancy progresses. As a result, the uterus at term is more sensitive than earlier in pregnancy and far more sensitive than the nonpregnant organ.

In very small doses, ergot preparations can evoke rhythmic contraction and relaxation of the uterus. At higher concentrations, these drugs induce powerful and prolonged contracture. Ergonovine is more selective than other ergot alkaloids in affecting the uterus and is the agent of choice in obstetric applications of these drugs.

4. Other smooth muscle organs–In most patients, the ergot alkaloids have no significant effect on bronchiolar smooth muscle. The gastrointestinal tract, on the other hand, varies dramatically in sensitivity among patients. Nausea, vomiting, and diarrhea may be induced by low doses in some patients but only by high doses in others. The effect is consistent with action on the central nervous system emetic center and on gastrointestinal serotonin receptors.

II. Clinical Pharmacology of Ergot Alkaloids

Clinical Uses

A. Migraine: Migraine headache in its classic form is characterized by a brief "aura" that may involve vi-

sual scotomas or even hemianopia and speech abnormalities, followed by a severe throbbing unilateral headache that lasts for a few hours to 1–2 days. The disease is familial in 60–80% of patients, more common in women, and usually has its onset in early adolescence through young adulthood, waning with advancing years. Attacks are frequently precipitated by stress but often occur after rather than during the stressful episode. They vary in frequency from one attack a year to two or more a week. Excellent written descriptions by patients are available (eg, Creditor, 1982).

Although the symptom pattern varies among patients, the severity of migraine headache justifies vigorous therapy in the great majority of cases.

The pathophysiology of migraine clearly includes some vasomotor mechanism, because the onset of headache is associated with a marked increase in amplitude of temporal artery pulsations, and relief of pain by administration of ergotamine is accompanied by diminution of arterial pulsations. On the other hand, these vasomotor changes may be the result of more basic processes underlying migraine, since a number of drugs with very different vascular actions are effective in migraine. For example, even though many vasoconstrictors are able to reduce or abort a migraine attack, drug-induced dilation of the cranial vessels does not provoke a typical migraine attack. Histologic study of cranial vessels from migraine patients shows that migraine attacks are associated with a sterile neurogenic perivascular edema and inflammation. Since these tissues are well supplied with sensory nerves, such pathologic changes could indeed be associated with prolonged headache. Finally, it is claimed that many of the drugs known to be effective in clinical migraine (ergot, nonsteroidal anti-inflammatory agents) are capable of preventing or reducing the perivascular tissue inflammation (Moskowitz et al, 1989; Buzzi et al, 1990).

Evidence suggests that the onset of a migrainous aura is associated with an abnormal release of serotonin from platelets, while the throbbing headache is associated with decrease of platelet and serum serotonin below normal concentrations. Other evidence implicating serotonin in migraine includes the facts that numerous serotonergic nerve fiber endings are found in and around meningeal blood vessels and that many of the drugs useful in migraine directly or indirectly influence serotonergic nerve transmission. Other chemical triggers (which may operate through serotonin) include falling levels of estrogen in women whose headache is linked to the menstrual cycle and elevated levels of prostaglandin E_1.

The efficacy of ergot derivatives in the therapy of migraine is so specific as to constitute a diagnostic test. Traditional therapy (**ergotamine**) is most effective when given during the prodrome of an attack and becomes progressively less effective if delayed. Ergotamine tartrate is available for oral, sublingual, rectal suppository, and inhaler use. It is often combined with caffeine (100 mg caffeine for each 1 mg ergotamine tartrate) to facilitate absorption of the ergot alkaloid.

The vasoconstriction induced by ergotamine is long-lasting and cumulative when the drug is taken repeatedly, as in a severe attack. Therefore, patients must be carefully informed that no more than 6 mg of the oral preparation may be taken for each attack and no more than 10 mg per week. For very severe attacks, ergotamine tartrate, 0.25–0.5 mg, may be given intravenously or intramuscularly. **Dihydroergotamine,** 0.5–1 mg intravenously, is favored by some clinicians for treatment of intractable migraine. Intranasal or oral dihydroergotamine, currently investigational, may also be effective.

Because of the cumulative toxicity of ergotamine, safer agents useful for the prophylaxis of migraine have been sought. When available, **ergonovine,** 0.2–0.4 mg three times daily, has been used. **Methysergide,** a derivative of the amine subgroup (Table 16–5), has been shown to be effective in this application in about 60% of patients. Unfortunately, significant toxicity (discussed below) occurs in almost 40% of patients. As suggested in Table 16–6, there is some evidence of a difference in the agonist:antagonist ratios of methysergide and ergotamine when assayed on serotonin receptors. Regardless of the cause, methysergide is relatively *ineffective* in treatment of impending or active episodes of migraine. The dosage of methysergide maleate for prophylaxis of migraine is 4–8 mg/d.

Although relatively free of the rapidly cumulative vasospastic toxicity of ergotamine, chronic use of methysergide may induce retroperitoneal fibroplasia and subendocardial fibrosis, possibly through its vascular effects. Therefore, it is important that patients taking methysergide have drug holidays of 3–4 weeks every 6 months (see Toxicity).

Propranolol and **amitriptyline** have also been found to be effective for the prophylaxis of migraine in some patients. Like methysergide, they are of no value in the treatment of acute migraine. **Flunarizine,** an investigational calcium channel blocker, has been reported in preliminary trials to effectively reduce the severity of the acute attack and prevent recurrences.

Sumatriptan, discussed above, is an effective alternative to ergotamine for the treatment of acute migraine attacks in many patients. However, it should not be used in patients at risk for coronary artery disease.

B. Hyperprolactinemia: Increased serum levels of the anterior pituitary hormone prolactin are associated with secreting tumors of the gland and also with the use of centrally acting dopamine antagonists, especially the antipsychotic drugs. Because of negative feedback effects, hyperprolactinemia is associated with amenorrhea and infertility in women as well as galactorrhea in both sexes.

Bromocriptine is extremely effective in reducing the high levels of prolactin that result from pituitary tumors and has even been associated with regression of the tumor in some cases. The usual dosage of bromocriptine is 2.5 mg two or three times daily. Bromocriptine has also been used in the same dosage to suppress physiologic lactation. A few cases of serious postpartum cardiovascular toxicity have been reported in association with the latter use of bromocriptine (Ruch et al, 1989). **Pergolide** is also used to suppress lactation (Chapter 37).

C. Postpartum Hemorrhage: The uterus at term is extremely sensitive to the stimulant action of ergot, and even moderate doses produce a prolonged and powerful spasm of the muscle quite unlike natural labor. This was not appreciated when the drugs were introduced into obstetrics in the 18th century. Their use at that time to accelerate delivery caused a dramatic *increase* in fetal and maternal mortality rates. Therefore, ergot derivatives are useful only for control of late uterine bleeding and should never be given before delivery. Ergonovine maleate, 0.2 mg usually given intramuscularly, is effective within 1–5 minutes and is less toxic than other ergot derivatives for this application. It is given at the time of delivery of the placenta or immediately afterward if bleeding is significant.

D. Diagnosis of Variant Angina: Ergonovine produces prompt vasoconstriction during coronary angiography to diagnose variant angina.

E. Senile Cerebral Insufficiency: Dihydroergotoxine, a mixture of dihydro-α-ergocryptine and three similar dihydrogenated peptide ergot alkaloids (ergoloid mesylates), has been promoted for many years for the relief of senility and more recently for the treatment of Alzheimer's dementia. There is no evidence of significant benefit.

Toxicity & Contraindications

The most common toxic effects of the ergot derivatives are gastrointestinal disturbances, including diarrhea, nausea, and vomiting. Activation of the medullary vomiting center and of the gastrointestinal serotonin receptors is involved. Since migraine attacks are often associated with these symptoms before therapy is begun, these adverse effects are rarely contraindications to the use of ergot. However, in prophylactic management with methysergide, nausea, vomiting, and diarrhea are important factors limiting use of the drug.

A more dangerous toxic effect of overdosage with agents like ergotamine and ergonovine is prolonged vasospasm. As described above, this sign of vascular smooth muscle stimulation may result in gangrene and require amputation. Most cases involve the circulation to the arms and legs. However, bowel infarction resulting from mesenteric artery vasospasm has also been reported. Peripheral vascular vasospasm caused by ergot is refractory to most vasodilators, but infusions of large doses of nitroprusside (Dierckx et al, 1986) or nitroglycerin (Tfelt-Hansen, 1982), have been successful in some cases. (See box: Ergot Poisoning: Not Just an Ancient Disease.)

Chronic therapy with methysergide is associated with development of fibroplastic changes in the retroperitoneal space, the pleural cavity, and the endocardial tissue of the heart. These changes occur insidiously over months and may present as hydronephrosis (from obstruction of the ureters) or a cardiac murmur (from distortion of the valves of the heart). In some cases, valve damage may require surgical replacement (Redfield et al, 1992). Fortunately, in most patients, signs of toxicity regress when administration of the drug is halted. However, the potential for injury is such that all patients taking methysergide should have periodic drug holidays and should be carefully studied if signs or symptoms of fibroplasia occur.

Other toxic effects of the ergot alkaloids include drowsiness and, in the case of methysergide, occasional instances of central stimulation and hallucinations. In fact, methysergide has been used as a substitute for LSD by members of the "drug culture."

Contraindications to the use of ergot derivatives consist of the obstructive vascular diseases and collagen diseases.

There is no evidence that ordinary use of ergotamine or methysergide for migraine is hazardous in pregnancy. However, most clinicians counsel restraint in the use of these agents by pregnant patients.

PREPARATIONS AVAILABLE

Antihistamines (H₁ Blockers)

Astemizole (Hismanal)
Oral: 10 mg tablets
Azatadine (Optimine)
Oral: 1 mg tablets
Brompheniramine (generic, Dimetane, Bromphen, others)
Oral: 4, 8, 12 mg tablets; 2 mg/5 mL elixir
Oral sustained-release: 8, 12 mg tablets
Parenteral: 10 mg/mL for injection
Buclizine (Bucladin-S Softabs)
Oral: 50 mg tablets
Carbinoxamine (Clistin)
Oral: 4 mg tablets
Cetirizine (Zyrtec)
Oral: 5, 10 mg tablets.
Chlorpheniramine (generic, Chlor-Trimeton, Teldrin, others)
Oral: 2 mg chewable tablets; 4, 12 mg tablets; 2 mg/5 mL syrup
Oral sustained-release: 8, 12 mg tablets and capsules
Parenteral: 10, 100 mg/mL for injection
Clemastine (Tavist)
Oral: 1.34, 2.68 mg tablets; 0.67 mg/5 mL syrup
Cyclizine (Marezine)
Oral: 50 mg tablets

Parenteral: 50 mg/mL for injection
Cyproheptadine (generic, Periactin)
Oral: 4 mg tablets; 2 mg/5 mL syrup
Dexchlorpheniramine (generic, Polamine, others)
Oral: 2 mg tablets; 2 mg/5 mL syrup
Oral sustained release: 4, 6 mg tablets
Dimenhydrinate* (generic, Dramamine)
Oral: 50 mg tablets and capsules; 50 mg chewable tablets; 12.5 mg/4 mL; 15.62 mg/5 mL
Diphenhydramine (generic, Benadryl)
Oral: 25, 50 mg capsules; 25, 50 mg tablets; 12.5 mg/5 mL elixir and syrup
Parenteral: 10, 50 mg/mL for injection
Fexofenadine (Allegra)
Oral: 60 mg tablets
Hydroxyzine (generic, Atarax, Vistaril)
Oral: 10, 25, 50, 100 mg tablets; 25, 50, 100 mg capsules; 10 mg/5 mL syrup; 25 mg/5 mL suspension
Parenteral: 25, 50 mg/mL for injection
Loratidine (Claritin)
Oral: 10 mg tablets

---

*Dimenhydrinate is the chlorotheophylline salt of diphenhydramine.

Meclizine (generic, Antivert, others)
Oral: 12.5, 25, 50 mg tablets; 25 mg capsules; 25 mg chewable tablets
Methdilazine (Tacaryl)
Oral: 4 mg chewable tablets; 8 mg tablets; 4 mg/5 mL syrup
Phenindamine (Nolahist)
Oral: 25 mg tablets
Promethazine (generic, Phenergan, others)
Oral: 12.5, 25, 50 mg tablets; 6.25, 25 mg/5 mL syrups
Parenteral: 25 mg/mL for injection; 50 mg/mL for IM injection
Rectal: 12.5, 25, 50 mg suppositories
Pyrilamine (generic)
Oral: 25 mg tablets
Terfenadine (generic, Seldane)
Oral: 60 mg tablets
Trimeprazine (Temaril)
Oral: 2.5 mg tablets; 2.5 mg/5 mL syrup
Oral sustained-release: 5 mg capsules
Tripelennamine (generic, Pelamine, PBZ)
Oral: 25, 50 mg tablets; 37.5 mg/5 mL elixir
Oral sustained-release: 100 mg tablets
Triprolidine (generic, Actidil, Myidil)
Oral: 2.5 mg tablets; 1.25 mg/5 mL syrup

H$_2$ Blockers
Cimetidine (Tagamet)
Oral: 75, 100, 200, 300, 400, 800 mg tablets; 300 mg/5 mL liquid
Parenteral: 300 mg/2 mL, 300 mg/50 mL for injection
Famotidine (Pepcid)
Oral: 10,* 20, 40 mg tablets; powder to reconstitute for 40 mg/5 mL suspension
Parenteral: 10 mg/mL for injection
Nizatidine (Axid)
Oral: 75,* 150, 300 mg tablets
Ranitidine (Zantac)
Oral: 75,* 150, 300 mg tablets; 150 mg effervescent tablets; 150, 300 mg capsules; 15 mg/mL syrup
Parenteral: 0.5, 25 mg/mL for injection

5-HT Agonists
Dexfenfluramine (Redux)
Oral: 15 mg capsules
Sumatriptan (Imitrex)
Oral: 25, 50 mg tablets
Parenteral: 6 mg/0.5 mL in *SELFdose* autoinjection units for subcutaneous injection
Cisapride (Propulsid)
Oral: 10, 20 mg tablets; 1 mg/mL suspension

5-HT Antagonists
Granisetron (Kytril)
Oral: 1 mg tablets
Parenteral: 1 mg/mL for IV administration
Ondansetron (Zofran)
Oral: 4, 8 mg tablets
Parenteral: 2 mg/mL for IV administration

Ergot Alkaloids
Dihydroergotamine (D.H.E. 45)
Parenteral: 1 mg/mL for injection
Ergonovine (generic, Ergotrate maleate)
Oral: 0.2 mg tablets†
Parenteral: 0.2 mg/mL for injection
Ergotamine [mixtures] (generic, Cafergot, others)
Oral: 1 mg ergotamine/100 mg caffeine tablets
Rectal: 2 mg ergotamine/100 mg caffeine suppositories
Ergotamine tartrate (Ergomar, Ergostat, others)
Sublingual: 2 mg sublingual tablets; 9 mg/mL metered-dose aerosol, 0.36 mg/dose
Methylergonovine (Methergine)
Oral: 0.2 mg tablets
Parenteral: 0.2 mg/mL for injection
Methysergide (Sansert)
Oral: 2 mg tablets

REFERENCES

Histamine

Black JW et al: Definition and antagonism of histamine H$_2$ receptors. Nature 1972;236:385.

Bochner BS, Lichtenstein LM: Anaphylaxis. N Engl J Med 1991;324:1785.

Curry FE: Modulation of venular microvessel permeability by calcium influx into endothelial cells. FASEB J 1992;6:2456.

DiPadova C et al: Effects of ranitidine on blood alcohol levels after ethanol ingestion: Comparison with other H$_2$-receptor antagonists. JAMA 1992;267:83.

Desager J-P, Horsmans Y: Pharmacokinetic-pharmacodynamic relationships of H$_1$-antihistamines. Clin Pharmacokinet 1995;28:418.

Feldman M, Burton ME: Drug therapy: Histamine$_2$ receptor antagonists: Standard therapy for acid-peptic disease. (Two parts.) N Engl J Med 1990;323:1672,1749.

Gugler R: H$_2$-antagonists and alcohol: Do they interact? Drug Saf 1994;10:271.

Haaksma EEJ, Leurs R, Timmerman H: Histamine receptors: Subclasses and specific ligands. Pharmacol Ther 1990;47:73.

*OTC preparation.

†Not always available.

Hill SJ: Distribution, properties, and functional characteristics of three classes of histamine receptors. Pharmacol Rev 1990;42:45.

Hinrichsen H, Halabi A, Kirsh W: Hemodynamic effect of H_2 receptor antagonists. Eur J Clin Invest 1992;22:9.

Hinrichsen H et al: Dose-dependent heart rate reducing effect of nizatidine, a histamine H_2-receptor antagonist. Br J Clin Pharmacol 1993;35:461.

Holmes LB: Teratogen update: Bendectin. Teratology 1983;27:277.

Honig PK et al: Terfenadine-ketoconazole interaction. Pharmacokinetic and electrocardiographic consequences. JAMA 1993;269:1513.

Lin JH: Pharmacokinetic and pharmacodynamic properties of histamine H_2-receptor antagonists. Relationship between intrinsic potency and effective plasma concentrations. Clin Pharmacokinet 1991;20:218.

Mezey E, Palkovits M: Localization of targets for anti-ulcer drugs in cells of the immune system. Science 1992; 258:1662.

Naclerio RM: Allergic rhinitis. N Engl J Med 1991; 325:860.

Nielsen HJ: Histamine-2 receptor antagonists as immunomodulators: New therapeutic views? Ann Med 1996;28:107.

Pelikan Z, Knottnerus I: Inhibition of the late asthmatic response by nedocromil sodium administered more than two hours after allergen challenge. J Allergy Clin Immunol 1993;92:19.

Poli E et al: Signal transducing mechanisms coupled to histamine H_3 receptors and alpha-2 adrenoceptors in the guinea pig duodenum: possible involvement of N-type Ca^{++} channels. J Pharmacol Exp Ther 1994;270:788.

Pollard H et al: A detailed autoradiographic mapping of histamine H_3 receptors in rat brain areas. Neuroscience 1993;52:169.

Rangachari PK: Histamine: mercurial messenger in the gut. (Editorial.) Am J Physiol 1992;262(1 Part 1):G1.

Rascol O et al: Antivertigo medications and drug-induced vertigo: A pharmacological review. Drugs 1995;50:777.

Sachs G, Prinz C: Gastric enterochromaffin-like cells and the regulation of acid secretion. News Physiol Sci 1996;11:57.

Saviuc P, Danel V, Dixmerias F: Prolonged QT interval and torsade de pointes following astemizole overdose. Clin Toxicol 1993;31:121.

Schwartz J-C et al: Histamine. In: *Psychopharmacology: The Fourth Generation of Progress.* Bloom FE, Kupfer DJ (editors). Raven Press, 1995

Schwartz J-C et al: Histaminergic transmission in the mammalian brain. Physiol Rev 1991;71:1.

Simons FE, Simons KJ: The pharmacology and use of H_1-receptor-antagonist drugs. N Engl J Med 1994;330:1663.

Solomon SD et al: Effects of histamine type 2-receptor antagonists *cimetidine* and *famotidine* on left ventricular systolic function in chronic congestive heart failure. Am J Cardiol 1993;72:1163.

Torsoli A, Lucchelli PE, Brimblecombe RW (editors): H_2 Antagonists: H_2 Receptor Antagonists in Peptic Ulcer Disease and Progress in Histamine Research. (Symposium.) International Congress Series 521. Excerpta Medica, 1980.

Ueki S et al: Gastroprokinetic activity of nizatidine, a new H_2-receptor antagonist, and its possible mechanism of action in dogs and rats. J Pharmacol Exper Ther 1993;264:152.

Wiley JF II et al: Cardiotoxic effects of astemizole overdose in children. J Pediatr 1992;120:799.

Woosley RL: Cardiac actions of antihistamines. Annu Rev Pharmacol Toxicol 1996;36:233.

Serotonin

Abenheim L et al: Appetite-suppressant drugs and the risk of primary pulmonary hypertension. N Engl J Med 1996;335:609.

Bateman DN: Sumatriptan. Lancet 1993;341:221.

Baxter G et al: 5-HT_2 receptors: a family reunited? Trends Pharmacol Sci 1995;16:105.

Bockaert J et al: The 5-HT_4 receptor: A place in the sun. Trends Pharmacol Sci 1992;13:141.

Brzezinski A: Melatonin in humans. N Engl J Med 1997;336:186.

Buckholtz NS et al: Lysergic acid diethylamide (LSD) selectively downregulates serotonin$_2$ receptors in rat brain. Neuropsychopharmacology 1990;3:137.

Cacoub P et al: Pulmonary hypertension and dexfenfluramine. Eur J Clin Pharmacol 1995;48:81.

Craig DA, Clarke DE: Pharmacological characterization of a neuronal receptor for 5-hydroxytryptamine in guinea pig ileum with properties similar to the 5-hydroxytryptamine$_4$ receptor. J Pharmacol Exp Ther 1990;252:1378.

Derkach V, Surprenant A, North RA: 5-HT_3 receptors are membrane ion channels. Nature 1989;339:706.

Dubocovich ML: Melatonin receptors: Are there multiple subtypes? Trends Pharmacol Sci 1995;16:50.

Ferrari MD: Sumatriptan in the treatment of migraine. Neurology 1993;43(Suppl 3):S43.

Fozard JR, Kalkman HO: 5-Hydroxtryptamine (5-HT) and the initiation of migraine: New perspectives. Naunyn-Schmiedeberg's Arch Pharmacol 1994; 350:225.

Freeman AJ et al: The vomiting reflex and the role of 5-HT_3 receptors. Anticancer Drugs 1993;4(Suppl 2):9.

Glennon RA, Dukat M: Serotonin receptor subtypes. In: *Psychopharmacology: The Fourth Generation of Progress.* Bloom FE, Kupfer DJ (editors). Raven Press, 1995.

Golino P et al: Divergent effects of serotonin on coronary-artery dimensions and blood flow in patients with coronary atherosclerosis and control patients. N Engl J Med 1991;324:641.

Guy-Grand B et al: International trial of long-term dexfenfluramine in obesity. Lancet 1989;2:1142.

Gyermek L: 5-HT3 receptors: Pharmacologic and therapeutic aspects. J Clin Pharmacol 1995;35:845.

Hagan RM, Oakley NR: Melatonin comes of age? Trends Pharmacol Sci 1995;16:81.

Hartig P et al: Alignment of receptor nomenclature with the human genome: Classification of 5-HT_{1B} and 5-HT_{1D} receptor subtypes. Trends Pharmacol Sci 1996;17:103.

Hesketh PJ, Gandara DR: Serotonin antagonists: A new class of antiemetic agents. J Natl Cancer Inst 1991; 83:613.

Humphrey PP et al: Serotonin and migraine. Ann NY Acad Sci 1990;600:587.

Julius D: Molecular biology of serotonin receptors. Annu Rev Neurosci 1991;14:335.

Kenny GNC et al: Efficacy of orally administered ondansetron in the prevention of postoperative nausea and vomiting: A dose ranging study. Br J Anaesth 1992; 68:466.

Lejoyeux M, Adés J, Rouillon F: Serotonin Syndrome: Incidence, symptoms, and treatment. CNS Drugs 1994; 2:132.

Matthes H et al: Mouse 5-hydroxytryptamine$_{5CA}$ and 5-hydroxytryptamine$_{5CB}$ receptors define a new family of serotonin receptors: Cloning, functional expression, and chromosomal localization. Mol Pharmacol 1993;43:313.

Ottervanger JP, Stricker BHCh: Cardiovascular adverse reactions to sumatriptan. Cause for concern? CNS Drugs 1995;3:90.

Peroutka SJ: Serotonin receptor subtypes. Their evolution and clinical relevance. CNS Drugs 1995;4:19.

Reppert SM, Weaver DR, Godson C: Melatonin receptors step into the light: Cloning and classification of subtypes. Trends Pharmacol Sci 1996;17:100.

Saxena PR: Serotonin receptors: Subtypes, functional responses and therapeutic relevance. Pharmacol Ther 1995;66:339.

Spring B et al: Efficacies of dexfenfluramine and fluoxetine in preventing weight gain after smoking cessation. Am J Clin Nutr 1995;62:1181.

Sternbach H: The serotonin syndrome. Am J Psychiatry 1991;148:705.

Tecott LH, Julius D: A new wave of serotonin receptors. Curr Opin Neurobiol 1993;3:310.

The Subcutaneous Sumatriptan International Study Group: Treatment of migraine attacks with sumatriptan. N Engl J Med 1991;325:322.

Wagner B et al: Effect of ritanserin, a 5-hydroxytryptamine antagonist, on platelet function and thrombin generation at the site of plug formation in vivo. Clin Pharmacol Therap 1990;48:419.

Watcha MF et al: The dose-response relationship of ondansetron in preventing postoperative emesis in pediatric patients undergoing ambulatory surgery. Anesthesiology 1995;82:47.

Ergot Alkaloids: Historical

Fuller JG: *The Day of St. Anthony's Fire*. Macmillan, 1968; Signet, 1969.

Gabbai Dr, Lisbonne Dr, Pourquier Dr: Ergot poisoning at Pont St. Esprit. Br Med J (Sept 15) 1951;650.

Ergot Alkaloids: Basic Pharmacology

Berde B: Ergot compounds: A synopsis. Adv Biochem Psychopharmacol 1980;23:3.

MacLennan SJ, Martin GR: Actions of non-peptide ergot alkaloids at 5-HT$_1$-like and 5-HT$_2$ receptors mediating vascular smooth muscle contraction. Naunyn Schmiedebergs Arch Pharmacol 1990;342:120.

Müller-Schweinitzer E: Responsiveness of isolated canine cerebral and peripheral arteries to ergotamine. Naunyn Schmiedebergs Arch Pharmacol 1976;292:113.

Müller-Schweinitzer E, Weidman H: Basic pharmacological properties. In: *Ergot Alkaloids and Related Compounds*—Vol 49 of *Handbook of Experimental Pharmacology*. Berde B, Schild HO (editors). Springer Verlag, 1978.

Sadzot B et al: Hallucinogenic drug interactions at human brain 5-HT$_2$ receptors: implications for treating LSD-induced hallucinogenesis. Psychopharmacology 1989; 98:495.

Saxena PR, Ferrari MD: 5-HT$_1$-like receptor agonists and the pathophysiology of migraine. Trends Pharmacol Sci 1989;10:200.

Ergot Alkaloids: Clinical Pharmacology

Andersen PK et al: Sodium nitroprusside and epidural blockade in the treatment of ergotism. N Engl J Med 1977;296:1271.

Buzzi MG, Moskowitz MA: The antimigraine drug, sumatriptan (GR43175) selectively blocks neurogenic plasma extravasation from blood vessels in dura mater. Br J Pharmacol 1990;99:202.

Creditor MC: Occasional notes: Me and migraine. N Engl J Med 1982;307:1029.

den Boer MO, Somers JAE, Saxena PR: Lack of effect of the antimigraine drugs, sumatriptan, ergotamine, and dihydroergotamine on arteriovenous shunting in the dura mater of the pig. Br J Pharmacol 1992;107:577.

Dierckx RA et al: Intraarterial sodium nitroprusside infusion in the treatment of severe ergotism. Clin Neuropharmacol 1986;9:542.

Ferrari MD et al: Serotonin metabolism in migraine. Neurology 1989;39:1239.

Lewis PJ et al: Rapid reversal of ergotamine-induced vasospasm. Can J Neurol Sci 1986;13:72.

Malaquin F et al: Pleural and retroperitoneal fibrosis from dihydroergotamine. (Letter.) N Engl J Med 1989; 321:1760.

Moskowitz MA et al: Pain mechanisms underlying vascular headaches. Rev Neurol 1989;145:181.

Moskowitz MA, Macfarlane R: Neurovascular and molecular mechanisms in migraine headaches. Cerebrovasc Brain Metab Rev 1993;5:159.

Olesen J, Saxena PR (editors): *5-Hydroxytryptamine Mechanisms in Primary Headaches*. Raven Press, 1992.

Nappi G, Micieli G: Sumatriptan in the treatment of migraine attacks. Curr Therap Res 1993;53:599.

Porter JK, Thompson FN Jr: Effects of fescue toxicosis on reproduction in livestock. J Animal Sci 1992;70:1594.

Raskin NH: Acute and prophylactic treatment of migraine: Practical approaches and pharmacologic rationale. Neurology 1993;43(Suppl 3):S39.

Redfield MM et al: Valve disease associated with ergot alkaloid use: Echocardiographic and pathologic correlations. Ann Intern Med 1992;117:50.

Ruch A, Duhring JL: Postpartum myocardial infarction in a patient receiving bromocriptine. Obstet Gynecol 1989; 74:448.

Saxena PR, Villalon CM: Cardiovascular effects of serotonin agonists and antagonists. J Cardiovasc Pharmacol 1990;15(Suppl 7):S17.

Tfelt-Hansen P: Nitroglycerin for ergotism: Experimental studies in vitro and in migraine patients and treatment of an overt case. Eur J Clin Pharmacol 1982;22:105.

Titeler M, Lyon RA, Glennon RA: Radioligand binding evidence implicates the brain 5-HT$_2$ receptor as a site of action for LSD and phenylisopropylamine hallucinogens. Psychopharmacology 1988;94:213.

Welch KMA: Drug therapy of migraine. N Engl J Med 1993;329:1476.

Vasoactive Peptides

17

Ian A. Reid, PhD

Peptides are used by most tissues for cell-to-cell communication. As noted in Chapters 6 and 21, they play important roles in the autonomic and central nervous systems. Several peptides exert important direct effects on vascular and other smooth muscles. These peptides include vasoconstrictors (angiotensin II, vasopressin, endothelins, and neuropeptide Y) and vasodilators (bradykinin and related kinins, natriuretic peptides, vasoactive intestinal peptide, substance P, neurotensin, and calcitonin gene-related peptide). This chapter focuses on the smooth muscle actions of the peptides.

ANGIOTENSIN

BIOSYNTHESIS OF ANGIOTENSIN

The pathway for the formation and metabolism of angiotensin II is summarized in Figure 17–1. The principal steps include enzymatic cleavage of angiotensin I from angiotensinogen by renin, conversion of angiotensin I to angiotensin II by converting enzyme, and degradation of angiotensin II by several peptidases.

Renin & Factors Controlling Renin Secretion

Renin is an aspartyl protease that specifically catalyzes the hydrolytic release of the decapeptide angiotensin I from angiotensinogen. It is synthesized as a preprohormone that is processed to prorenin, which is inactive, and then to active renin, a glycoprotein consisting of 340 amino acids.

Most (probably all) of the renin in the circulation originates in the kidneys. Enzymes with renin-like activity are present in several extrarenal tissues, including blood vessels, uterus, salivary glands, and adrenal cortex, but no physiologic role for these enzymes has been established. Within the kidney, renin is synthesized and stored in a specialized area of the nephron, the juxtaglomerular apparatus, which is composed of the afferent and efferent arterioles and the macula densa. The afferent arteriole and, to a lesser extent, the efferent arteriole contain specialized granular cells called juxtaglomerular cells that are the site of synthesis, storage, and release of renin. The macula densa is a specialized tubular segment closely associated with the vascular components of the juxtaglomerular apparatus. The vascular and tubular components of the juxtaglomerular apparatus, including the juxtaglomerular cells, are innervated by adrenergic neurons.

The rate at which renin is secreted by the kidney is the primary determinant of activity of the renin-angiotensin system. Renin secretion is controlled by a variety of factors, including a renal vascular receptor, the macula densa, the sympathetic nervous system, and angiotensin II.

A. Renal Vascular Receptor: The renal vascular receptor functions as a stretch receptor, decreased stretch leading to increased renin release and vice versa. The receptor is apparently located in the afferent arteriole, and it is possible that the juxtaglomerular cells themselves are sensitive to changes in stretch.

B. Macula Densa: The macula densa contains a different type of receptor, sensitive to changes in the rate of delivery of sodium or chloride to the distal tubule. Decreases in distal delivery result in stimulation of renin secretion and vice versa. These changes are apparently mediated by a luminal $Na^+/K^+/2Cl^-$ cotransporter sensitive to changes in luminal Cl^- concentration (Lorenz et al, 1991).

C. Sympathetic Nervous System: The sympathetic innervation of the juxtaglomerular apparatus plays an important role in the control of renin secretion. Maneuvers that increase renal nerve activity cause stimulation of renin secretion, while renal denervation results in suppression of renin secretion. Norepinephrine stimulates renin secretion by a direct

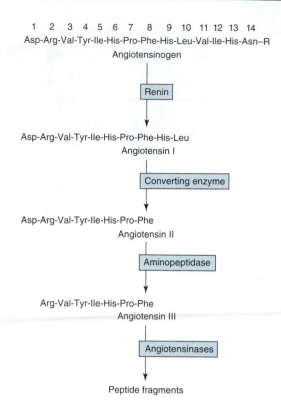

1 2 3 4 5 6 7 8 9 10 11 12 13 14
Asp-Arg-Val-Tyr-Ile-His-Pro-Phe-His-Leu-Val-Ile-His-Asn–R

Angiotensinogen

Renin

Asp-Arg-Val-Tyr-Ile-His-Pro-Phe-His-Leu

Angiotensin I

Converting enzyme

Asp-Arg-Val-Tyr-Ile-His-Pro-Phe

Angiotensin II

Aminopeptidase

Arg-Val-Tyr-Ile-His-Pro-Phe

Angiotensin III

Angiotensinases

Peptide fragments

Figure 17–1. Chemistry of the renin-angiotensin system. The amino acid sequence of the amino terminal of human angiotensinogen is shown. R denotes the remainder of the protein molecule.

action on the juxtaglomerular cells. This effect is mediated by beta adrenoceptors, activation of adenylyl cyclase and formation of cAMP. In humans, these beta receptors are of the β_1 subtype. In some situations, norepinephrine stimulates renin secretion indirectly by means of alpha receptors. This stimulation apparently results from constriction of the afferent arteriole, with resultant activation of the renal vascular receptor and decreased delivery of sodium chloride to the macula densa. In other situations, alpha adrenoceptor stimulation may inhibit renin secretion.

The rate of renin secretion is also influenced by circulating epinephrine and norepinephrine. These catecholamines may act via the same mechanisms as the norepinephrine released locally from the renal sympathetic nerves, but there is evidence that a major component of the renin secretory response to circulating catecholamines is mediated by extrarenal beta receptors.

D. Angiotensin: Angiotensin II inhibits renin secretion. The inhibition, which results from a direct action of the peptide on the juxtaglomerular cells, forms the basis of a short-loop negative feedback mechanism controlling renin secretion. Interruption of this feedback with inhibitors of the renin-angiotensin system (see below) results in stimulation of renin secretion.

E. Pharmacologic Alteration of Renin Release: The release of renin is altered by a wide variety of pharmacologic agents. Renin release is stimulated by vasodilators (hydralazine, minoxidil, nitroprusside), beta-adrenoceptor agonists (isoproterenol), alpha-adrenoceptor antagonists, and most diuretics and anesthetics. This stimulation can be accounted for by the control mechanisms just described. Drugs that inhibit renin release are discussed below in the section on inhibition of the renin-angiotensin system.

Angiotensinogen

Angiotensinogen is the circulating protein substrate from which renin cleaves angiotensin I. It is synthesized in the liver. Human angiotensinogen is a glycoprotein with a molecular weight of approximately 57,000. The 14 amino acids at the amino terminal of the molecule are shown in Figure 17–1. In humans, the concentration of angiotensinogen in the circulation is less than the K_m of the renin-angiotensinogen reaction and is therefore an important determinant of the rate of formation of angiotensin.

The production of angiotensinogen is increased by corticosteroids, estrogens, thyroid hormones, and angiotensin II. Plasma angiotensinogen concentration increases in patients with Cushing's syndrome and in patients being treated with glucocorticoids. It is also elevated during pregnancy and in women taking estrogen-containing oral contraceptives. The increased plasma angiotensinogen concentration is thought to contribute to the hypertension that may occur in these situations. Evidence for a genetic linkage between the angiotensinogen gene and essential hypertension has been presented (Hata et al, 1994).

Angiotensin I

Although angiotensin I contains the peptide sequences necessary for all of the actions of the renin-angiotensin system, it has little or no biologic activity. Instead, it must be converted to angiotensin II by converting enzyme (Figure 17–1). Angiotensin I may also be acted on by plasma or tissue aminopeptidases to form [des-Asp[1]]angiotensin I; this in turn is converted to [des-Asp[1]]angiotensin II (commonly known as angiotensin III) by converting enzyme.

Converting Enzyme (Peptidyl Dipeptidase [PDP], Kininase II)

Converting enzyme is a dipeptidyl carboxypeptidase that catalyzes the cleavage of dipeptides from the carboxyl terminal of certain peptides. Its most important substrates are angiotensin I, which it converts to angiotensin II, and bradykinin, which it inactivates (see below). It also cleaves enkephalins and substance P, but the physiologic significance of these effects has not been established. The action of converting enzyme is prevented by a penultimate prolyl residue, and angiotensin II is therefore not hydrolyzed by converting enzyme. Converting enzyme is distributed widely in the body. In most tissues, converting enzyme is located on the luminal surface of vascular endothelial cells and is thus in close contact with the circulation.

Angiotensinase

Angiotensin II is removed rapidly from the circulation, with a half-life of 15–60 seconds. It is metabolized during passage through most vascular beds (a notable exception being the lung) by a variety of peptidases collectively referred to as angiotensinase. Most metabolites of angiotensin II are biologically inactive, but the initial product of aminopeptidase action—[des-Asp^1]angiotensin II—retains considerable biologic activity.

ACTIONS OF ANGIOTENSIN II

Angiotensin II exerts important actions at several sites in the body, including vascular smooth muscle, adrenal cortex, kidney, and brain. Through these actions, the renin-angiotensin system plays a key role in the regulation of fluid and electrolyte balance and arterial blood pressure. Excessive activity of the renin-angiotensin system can result in hypertension and disorders of fluid and electrolyte homeostasis.

Effects on Blood Pressure

Angiotensin II is a very potent pressor agent—on a molar basis, approximately 40 times more potent than norepinephrine. The pressor response to intravenous angiotensin II is rapid in onset (10–15 seconds) and sustained during long-term infusions of the peptide. A large component of the pressor response to intravenous angiotensin II is due to direct contraction of vascular—especially arteriolar—smooth muscle. In addition, however, angiotensin II can also increase blood pressure through actions on the brain and autonomic nervous system. The pressor response to angiotensin is usually accompanied by little or no reflex bradycardia because the peptide acts on the brain to reset the baroreceptor reflex control of heart rate to a higher pressure (Reid, 1992).

Angiotensin II also interacts with the autonomic nervous system. It stimulates autonomic ganglia, increases the release of epinephrine and norepinephrine from the adrenal medulla, and—what is most important—facilitates sympathetic transmission by an action at adrenergic nerve terminals. The latter effect results from both increased release and reduced reuptake of norepinephrine. Angiotensin II also has a less important direct positive inotropic action on the heart.

Effects on the Adrenal Cortex

Angiotensin II acts directly on the zona glomerulosa of the adrenal cortex to stimulate aldosterone biosynthesis. In higher doses, angiotensin II also stimulates glucocorticoid biosynthesis.

Effects on the Kidney

Angiotensin II acts on the kidney to cause renal vasoconstriction, increase proximal tubular sodium reabsorption, and inhibit the secretion of renin.

Effects on the Central Nervous System

In addition to its central effects on blood pressure, angiotensin II acts on the central nervous system to stimulate drinking (dipsogenic effect) and increase the secretion of vasopressin and ACTH. The physiologic significance of the effects of angiotensin II on drinking and pituitary hormone secretion is not known.

Effects on Cell Growth

Angiotensin II is mitogenic for vascular and cardiac muscle cells and may contribute to the development of cardiovascular hypertrophy (Schelling et al, 1991). Considerable evidence now indicates that angiotensin-converting enzyme inhibitors will slow or prevent morphologic changes (remodeling) following myocardial infarction that would otherwise lead to congestive heart failure (Konstam et al, 1992).

ANGIOTENSIN RECEPTORS & MECHANISM OF ACTION

Angiotensin II receptors are widely distributed in the body. Like the receptors for other peptide hormones, angiotensin II receptors are located on the plasma membrane of target cells, and this permits rapid onset of the various actions of angiotensin II.

Two distinct subtypes of angiotensin II receptors termed AT$_1$ and AT$_2$ (Bumpus et al, 1991) have been identified on the basis of their differential affinity for peptide (CGP 42112A) and nonpeptide (losartan [DuP 753], PD 123177) antagonists (see below), and their sensitivity to sulfhydryl-reducing agents. AT$_1$ receptors have a high affinity for losartan and a low affinity for PD 123177 and CGP 42112A, while AT$_2$ receptors have a high affinity for PD 123177 and CGP 42112A and a low affinity for losartan. Angiotensin II and saralasin bind equally to both subtypes. Binding of angiotensin II to AT$_1$ but not AT$_2$ receptors is reduced by sulfhydryl-reducing agents such as dithiothreitol. The relative proportion of the two subtypes varies from tissue to tissue: AT$_1$ receptors predominate in vascular smooth muscle.

Most of the known actions of angiotensin II are mediated by the AT$_1$ receptor subtype. This receptor belongs to the G protein-coupled receptor super-family. Binding of angiotensin II to AT$_1$ receptors in vascular smooth muscle results in the phospholipase C-mediated generation of inositol trisphosphate and diacylglycerol; these two events result in smooth muscle contraction. In other tissues, AT$_1$ receptors are coupled to different signal transduction mechanisms, including inhibition of adenylyl cyclase. The function and signal transduction pathways for AT_2 receptors are still being investigated.

INHIBITION OF THE RENIN-ANGIOTENSIN SYSTEM

A wide variety of agents are now available that block the formation or actions of angiotensin II. These drugs may block renin secretion, the enzymatic action of renin, the conversion of angiotensin I to angiotensin II, or angiotensin II receptors.

Drugs That Block Renin Secretion

Several drugs that interfere with the sympathetic nervous system inhibit the secretion of renin. Examples are clonidine, methyldopa, and propranolol. Clonidine inhibits renin secretion by causing a centrally mediated reduction in neural activity to the kidney, and it may also exert a direct intrarenal action. The mechanism by which methyldopa inhibits renin secretion has not been established, but it may be similar to the central action of clonidine. Propranolol and other beta adrenoceptor-blocking drugs act by blocking the intrarenal and extrarenal beta receptors involved in the neural control of renin secretion.

Renin Inhibitors

The action of renin can be blocked by pepstatin, a pentapeptide that also inhibits the action of other proteases such as pepsin and cathepsin D. The use of pepstatin in vivo is restricted by its low solubility, but a more soluble form, N-acetylpepstatin, is available for research use. Competitive inhibitors of renin based on the amino acid sequence around the cleavage site of angiotensinogen have been synthesized. The problem with most of these is low solubility. However, one of these peptides, Pro-His-Pro-Phe-His-Phe-Phe-Val-Tyr-Lys, is reasonably soluble and is an effective inhibitor of renin in vivo.

Recently, orally active renin inhibitors have been developed. Two of the new renin inhibitors that have been tested in humans are shown in Figure 17–2. These peptidomimetic compounds are transition-state analogs of the cleavage site of human angiotensinogen. They have a high specificity for renin, cause marked suppression of plasma renin activity and plasma angiotensin II concentration, and lower blood pressure in hypertensive patients. However, the bioavailability of these inhibitors is generally poor, mainly because of poor absorption and a considerable first pass effect. They also increase plasma active renin levels because of interruption of the negative feedback effect of angiotensin II on renin secretion, and this further limits the reduction in plasma renin activity that can be achieved. Renin inhibitors have the potential to be as effective as converting enzyme

inhibitors in inhibiting the renin-angiotensin system, but further improvement of their bioavailability and efficacy is needed.

Converting Enzyme Inhibitors

A nonapeptide inhibitor of converting enzyme was originally isolated from the venom of the South American pit viper, *Bothrops jararaca*. The synthetic form of this peptide, teprotide, is an effective inhibitor of converting enzyme. However, it is active only when administered intravenously. An important class of orally active angiotensin-converting enzyme (ACE) inhibitors, directed against the active site of ACE, is now extensively used. Captopril and enalapril are typical (Figure 17–3). Many potent new ACE inhibitors have been synthesized. It should be noted that ACE inhibitors not only block the conversion of angiotensin I to angiotensin II but also inhibit the degradation of other substances, including bradykinin, substance P, and enkephalins. The action of ACE inhibitors to inhibit bradykinin metabolism contributes significantly to their hypotensive action (Panzenbeck et al, 1995) and is apparently responsible for adverse side effects, including cough and angioedema. As noted in Chapters 11 and 13, extensive studies document the value of the ACE inhibitors in hypertension and congestive heart failure. Evidence suggests that these drugs also protect against renal vascular injury in diabetes and possibly in other conditions (Björck et al, 1992).

Angiotensin Antagonists

Substitution of aliphatic residues such as glycine, alanine, leucine, isoleucine, or threonine for the phenylalanine in position 8 of angiotensin II results in the formation of potent antagonists of the action of angiotensin II. Substitution of sarcosine (N-methylglycine) for the amino terminal aspartic acid prolongs the half-life of the peptides and thereby enhances their potency. The best-known of these antagonists is [Sar^1,Val^5,Ala^8]angiotensin-(1–8)octapeptide, or **saralasin.**

Asp-Arg-Val-Tyr-Ile-His-Pro-Phe

Angiotensin II

Sar-Arg-Val-Tyr-Val-His-Pro-Ala

Saralasin

Saralasin exhibits some agonist activity and may elicit pressor responses, particularly when circulating angiotensin II levels are low. Saralasin must be administered intravenously, and this severely restricts its use as an antihypertensive agent. However, it has been used for the detection of renin-dependent hypertension and other hyperreninemic states. In general, angiotensin analogs are less effective in lowering blood pressure than are angiotensin-converting enzyme inhibitors. This difference reflects both the partial ago-

Figure 17–2. The cleavage site of angiotensinogen and two renin inhibitors that have been tested in humans. (Modified and redrawn, with permission, from Rongen GA et al: Clinical pharmacokinetics and efficacy of renin inhibitors. Clin Pharmacokinet 1995;29:6.)

nist activity of angiotensin analogs and the bradykinin-potentiating action of ACE inhibitors.

Recently, a new class of nonpeptide angiotensin II antagonists has been developed (Bauer et al, 1995). One of these, **losartan,** is a potent and specific competitive antagonist of angiotensin AT$_1$ receptors (Figure 17–4). Losartan is orally active and does not exhibit agonist activity. It lowers blood pressure in patients with essential hypertension and shows considerable promise for use in the treatment of hypertension and congestive heart failure (Chapter 11). The blood pressure-lowering efficacy of losartan is similar to that of the converting enzyme inhibitor enalapril, but treatment with losartan is associated with a lower incidence of adverse effects, especially cough, than is treatment with enalapril (Figure 17–5). **Valsartan** is a similar more recently released drug. AT$_2$ receptor antagonists, including PD 123177 (Figure 17–4), are also available but have no clinical use at this time.

Figure 17–3. Two orally active converting enzyme inhibitors: captopril and enalapril. Enalapril is a prodrug ethyl ester that is hydrolyzed in the body.

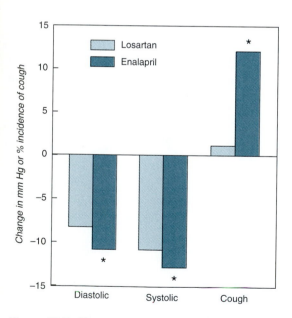

Figure 17–4. Structures of the angiotensin AT$_1$ receptor antagonist losartan and the AT$_2$ antagonist PD 123177.

KININS

BIOSYNTHESIS OF KININS

Kinins are a group of potent vasodilator peptides. They are formed enzymatically by the action of enzymes known as kallikreins or kininogenases acting on protein substrates called kininogens. From the biochemical point of view, the kallikrein-kinin system has several features in common with the renin-angiotensin system.

Kallikreins

Kallikreins are glycoprotein enzymes present in plasma and in several tissues, including the kidneys, pancreas, intestine, sweat glands, and salivary glands. They are serine proteases with active sites and catalytic properties similar to those of enzymes such as trypsin, chymotrypsin, elastase, thrombin, plasmin, and other serine proteases. Tissue kallikreins have molecular weights between 25,000 and 40,000; plasma kallikrein has a molecular weight of approximately 100,000.

Plasma kallikrein circulates in the blood as a precursor, prekallikrein, which is produced by the liver. Plasma kallikrein can be activated by trypsin, Hageman factor, and possibly kallikrein itself. Some glandular kallikreins exist as prekallikreins; others are present in active forms. In general, the biochemical properties of glandular kallikreins are quite different from those of plasma kallikreins. Kallikreins can convert prorenin to active renin, but the physiologic significance of this action has not been established.

Figure 17–5. Changes in diastolic and systolic pressure and incidence of dry cough in hypertensive patients treated for 12 weeks with enalapril (20 mg/d) or losartan (50 mg/d). *, P < 0.01 compared to losartan. (Data from Tikkanen I, Omvik P, Jensen HAE: Comparison of the angiotensin II antagonist losartan with the angiotensin converting enzyme inhibitor enalapril in patients with essential hypertension. J Hypertens 1995;13:1343.)

INHIBITION OF THE RENIN-ANGIOTENSIN SYSTEM

The involvement of the renin-angiotensin system in cardiovascular diseases such as hypertension and congestive heart failure prompted the development of several classes of drugs that inhibit the formation or actions of angiotensin II. The renin-angiotensin system can be inhibited by drugs that suppress renin secretion, slow the enzymatic action of renin or converting enzyme, or block angiotensin receptors. Renin secretion can be reduced by β-adrenoceptor-blocking drugs such as propranolol, and this may contribute to their antihypertensive action. However, these agents clearly also reduce blood pressure by actions unrelated to the renin-angiotensin system. Converting enzyme inhibitors such as captopril and enalapril are much more selective in their action and have proved to be very useful in the treatment of hypertension and heart failure. However, these drugs not only block the conversion of angiotensin I to angiotensin II but also inhibit the degradation of other peptides such as bradykinin. This latter action contributes to the hypotensive action of the drugs but is also responsible for adverse side effects such as cough and angioedema.

A new class of drugs that block angiotensin II receptors has been developed recently. Losartan, the first of these to be released, is a potent and selective antagonist of angiotensin AT_1 receptors. The angiotensin II receptor blockers are orally active and lower blood pressure almost as effectively as converting enzyme inhibitors but with fewer side effects such as cough.

Finally, drugs that block the enzymatic action of renin are now available. Examples are remikiren and enalkiren (Figure 17–2). These drugs cause marked suppression of plasma renin activity and plasma angiotensin II concentration and lower blood pressure in hypertensive patients. They have the potential to be as effective as converting enzyme inhibitors and angiotensin receptor antagonists, but significant improvement of their oral bioavailability is required.

Kininogens

Kininogens—the precursors of kinins and substrates of kallikreins—are present in plasma, lymph, and interstitial fluid. Two kininogens are known to be present in plasma: a low-molecular-weight form (LMW kininogen) and a high-molecular-weight form (HMW kininogen). Both are acidic glycoproteins consisting of a single polypeptide chain. About 15–20% of the total plasma kininogen is in the HMW form. It is thought that LMW kininogen crosses capillary walls and serves as the substrate for tissue kallikreins, while HMW kininogen is confined to the bloodstream and serves as the substrate for plasma kallikrein.

FORMATION OF KININS IN PLASMA & TISSUES

The pathway for the formation and metabolism of kinins is shown in Figure 17–6. Three kinins have been identified in mammals: bradykinin, lysylbradykinin (also known as kallidin), and methionyllysylbradykinin. Their structures are shown below:

Arg-Pro-Pro-Gly-Phe-Ser-Pro-Phe-Arg
  1   2   3   4   5   6   7   8   9

Bradykinin

Lys-Arg-Pro-Pro-Gly-Phe-Ser-Pro-Phe-Arg

Lysylbradykinin (kallidin; Lys-bradykinin)

Met-Lys-Arg-Pro-Pro-Gly-Phe-Ser-Pro-Phe-Arg

Methionyllysylbradykinin (Met-Lys-bradykinin)

Note that each kinin contains bradykinin in its structure. Each kinin is formed from a kininogen by the action of a different enzyme. Bradykinin is released by plasma kallikrein, lysylbradykinin by glandular kallikrein, and methionyllysylbradykinin by pepsin and pepsin-like enzymes. The preferred substrate for plasma kallikrein is HMW kininogen, and the preferred substrate for tissue kallikrein is LMW kininogen. Some lysylbradykinin is converted to

Figure 17–6. The kallikrein-kinin system. Kininase II is identical to converting enzyme peptidyl dipeptidase.

bradykinin by an aminopeptidase. The three kinins have been found in plasma, but bradykinin is the predominant one. All three kinins are also present in urine. Lysylbradykinin is the major urinary kinin and is probably formed by the action of renal kallikrein. Bradykinin is generated from lysylbradykinin by a renal aminopeptidase. Methionyllysylbradykinin occurs in acidified urine: acid activates uropepsinogen, which then catalyzes the release of methionyllysylbradykinin from urinary kininogens.

ACTIONS OF KININS

Effects on the Cardiovascular System

Kinins produce marked vasodilation in several vascular beds, including the heart, kidney, intestine, skeletal muscle, and liver. In this respect, kinins are approximately ten times more potent than histamine. The vasodilation may result from a direct inhibitory effect of kinins on arteriolar smooth muscle or may be mediated by the release of endothelium-derived relaxing factor (EDRF, nitric oxide) or vasodilator prostaglandins such as PGE_2 and PGI_2. In contrast, the predominant effect of kinins on veins is contraction; again, this may result from direct stimulation of venous smooth muscle or from the release of venoconstrictor prostaglandins such as $PGF_{2\alpha}$. Kinins also produce contraction of most visceral smooth muscle.

When injected intravenously, kinins produce a rapid fall in blood pressure that is due to their vasodilator action. The hypotensive response to bradykinin is of very brief duration. Intravenous infusions of the peptide fail to produce a sustained decrease in blood pressure; prolonged hypotension can only be produced by progressively increasing the rate of infusion. The rapid reversibility of the hypotensive response to kinins is due primarily to reflex increases in heart rate, myocardial contractility, and cardiac output. In some species, bradykinin produces a biphasic change in blood pressure—an initial hypotensive response followed by an increase above the preinjection level. The increase in blood pressure may be due to a reflex activation of the sympathetic nervous system, but under some conditions, bradykinin can directly release catecholamines from the adrenal medulla and stimulate sympathetic ganglia. Bradykinin also increases blood pressure when injected into the central nervous system, but the physiologic significance of this effect is not clear, since it is unlikely that kinins cross the blood-brain barrier. Kinins have no consistent effect on sympathetic or parasympathetic nerve endings.

The arteriolar dilation produced by kinins causes an increase in pressure and flow in the capillary bed, thus favoring efflux of fluid from blood to tissues. This effect may be facilitated by increased capillary permeability resulting from contraction of endothelial cells and widening of intercellular junctions, and by increased venous pressure secondary to constriction of veins. As a result of these changes, water and solutes pass from the blood to the extracellular fluid, lymph flow increases, and edema may result.

Effects on Endocrine & Exocrine Glands

As noted earlier, prekallikreins and kallikreins are present in several glands, including the pancreas, kidney, intestine, salivary glands, and sweat glands, and can be released into the secretory fluids of these glands. The function of the enzymes in these tissues is not known. The enzymes (or active kinins) may diffuse from the organs to the blood and act as local modulators of blood flow. Since kinins have such marked effects on smooth muscle, they may also modulate the tone of salivary and pancreatic ducts and help to regulate gastrointestinal motility. Kinins also influence the transepithelial transport of water, electrolytes, glucose, and amino acids and may regulate the transport of these substances in the gastrointestinal tract and kidney. Finally, kallikreins may play a role in the physiologic activation of various prohormones, including proinsulin and prorenin.

Role in Inflammation

Kinins play an important role in the inflammatory process. Kallikreins and kinins can produce all the symptoms of inflammation, and the production of kinins is increased in inflammatory lesions produced by a variety of methods.

Effects on Sensory Nerves

Kinins are potent pain-producing substances when applied to a blister base or injected intradermally. They elicit pain by stimulating nociceptive afferents in the skin and viscera.

KININ RECEPTORS & MECHANISMS OF ACTION

The biologic actions of kinins are mediated by specific receptors located on the membranes of the target tissues. Two types of kinin receptors, termed B_1 and B_2, have been defined based on the rank orders of agonist potencies: for B_1 receptors, [des-Arg⁹]bradykinin > [Tyr(Me)⁸] bradykinin > bradykinin. For B_2 receptors, [Tyr(Me)⁸] bradykinin > bradykinin > [des-Arg⁹]bradykinin. (Note that *B* here stands for bradykinin, not for beta adrenoceptor.) In B_1 receptor systems, Lys-bradykinin and Met-Lys-bradykinin are approximately 10 and 76 times (respectively) more potent than bradykinin. The octapeptide [des-Arg⁹] bradykinin is ten times more potent, while the heptapeptide [des-Phe⁸-des-Arg⁹]bradykinin is inactive. Bradykinin displays the highest affinity in most B_2 receptor systems, followed by Lys-bradykinin and then by Met-Lys-bradykinin. One exception is the B_2 receptor that mediates contraction of venous smooth muscle; this appears to be most sensitive to Lys-bradykinin. Recent evidence suggests the existence of two B_2 receptor subtypes which have been termed B_{2A} and B_{2B} (Regoli et al, 1994).

B_1 receptors appear to have a very limited distribution in mammalian tissues. Known functional roles for B_1 receptors are limited but may involve inflammation and long-lasting effects of kinins such as collagen synthesis and cell multiplication. By contrast, B_2 receptors have a widespread distribution which is consistent with the multitude of biologic effects that are mediated by this receptor type. B_2 receptors belong to the G protein-coupled family of receptors. Receptor binding sets in motion multiple signal transduction events, including calcium mobilization, chloride transport, formation of nitric oxide, and activation of phospholipase C, phospholipase A_2, and adenylyl cyclase.

METABOLISM OF KININS

Kinins are metabolized rapidly (half-life < 15 seconds) by nonspecific exo- or endopeptidases, commonly referred to as kininases. Two plasma kininases have been well characterized. Kininase I, apparently synthesized in the liver, is a carboxypeptidase that releases the carboxyl terminal arginine residue. Kininase II is present in plasma and vascular endothelial cells throughout the body. It is identical to angiotensin converting enzyme (peptidyl dipeptidase), discussed above. Kininase II inactivates kinins by cleaving the carboxyl terminal dipeptide phenylalanyl-arginine. Like angiotensin I, bradykinin is almost completely hydrolyzed during a single passage through the pulmonary vascular bed.

DRUGS AFFECTING THE KALLIKREIN-KININ SYSTEM

Drugs that modify the activity of the kallikrein-kinin system are available, though none is in wide clinical use. Kinin synthesis can be inhibited with the kallikrein inhibitor aprotinin. Considerable effort has been directed toward developing kinin receptor antagonists, since such drugs have considerable therapeutic potential as anti-inflammatory and antinociceptive agents. Competitive antagonists of both B_1 and B_2 receptors are available for research use. An example of a B_1 receptor antagonist is [Leu[8]-des-Arg[9]]bradykinin. B_2 receptor antagonists include DArg[Hyp[3], Thi[5], DTic[7], Oic[8]] bradykinin (HOE 140 or icatibant) and DArg[Hyp[3],DPhe[7],Leu[8]] bradykinin, which specifically and potently inhibit a wide variety of responses to bradykinin. WIN 64338 is a recently developed nonpeptide competitive bradykinin B_2 receptor antagonist. Actions of kinins mediated by prostaglandin generation can be blocked nonspecifically by inhibitors of prostaglandin synthesis. Finally, the actions of kinins can be enhanced by angiotensin-converting enzyme inhibitors, which block the degradation of these peptides. Indeed, as noted above, inhibition of bradykinin metabolism by ACE inhibitors contributes significantly to their hypotensive action.

VASOPRESSIN

Vasopressin (antidiuretic hormone, ADH) plays an important role in the long-term control of blood pressure through its action on the kidney to increase water reabsorption. This and other aspects of the physiology of vasopressin are discussed in Chapters 15 and 37 and will not be reviewed here.

Considerable evidence indicates that vasopressin also plays an important role in the short-term regulation of arterial pressure by its vasoconstrictor action. The peptide increases total peripheral resistance when infused in doses less than those required to produce maximum urine concentration. Such doses do not normally increase arterial pressure because the vasopressor activity of the peptide is buffered by a reflex decrease in cardiac output. When the influence of this reflex is removed, eg, in shock, pressor sensitivity to vasopressin is greatly increased. Pressor sensitivity to vasopressin is also enhanced in patients with idiopathic orthostatic hypotension. Higher doses of vasopressin increase blood pressure even when baroreceptor reflexes are intact. These doses are generally higher than those required to produce maximum urine concentration; however, pressor responses can be elicited when plasma vasopressin concentration is increased to levels reached during nonhypotensive hemorrhage.

VASOPRESSIN RECEPTORS & ANTAGONISTS

The actions of vasopressin are mediated by activation of specific membrane receptors. Two subtypes of vasopressin receptors have been identified: V_1 receptors that mediate the vasoconstrictor action of the peptide and V_2 receptors that mediate the antidiuretic action. V_1 effects are mediated by activation of phospholipase C, formation of inositol trisphosphate, and increased intracellular calcium concentration. V_2 effects are mediated by activation of adenylyl cyclase.

Vasopressin-like peptides selective for either vasoconstrictor or antidiuretic activity have been synthesized. The most specific V_1 vasoconstrictor agonist synthesized to date is [Phe[2], Ile[3], Orn[8]]vasotocin. Selective V_2 antidiuretic analogs include 1-deamino[D-

Arg[8]]arginine vasopressin (dDAVP) and 1-deamino [Val[4],D-Arg[8]]arginine vasopressin (dVDAVP). Specific antagonists of the vasoconstrictor action of vasopressin are also now undergoing clinical investigation. One of the most potent V₁ antagonists is [1-(β-mercapto-β,β-cyclopentamethylenepropionic acid)-2-(*O*-methyl)tyrosine] arginine vasopressin. This compound also has antioxytocic activity but does not antagonize the antidiuretic action of vasopressin. It does not interfere with the actions of other pressor agents such as angiotensin and norepinephrine. An orally active competitive vasopressin V₁ receptor antagonist is now investigational (Yamamura et al, 1991). Antagonists of the antidiuretic action of vasopressin are also investigational.

The vasopressor antagonists have been particularly useful for investigating the role of endogenous vasopressin in cardiovascular regulation. The antagonists have no cardiovascular effects when administered to animals in which circulating vasopressin levels are within or below the normal range. However, when they are administered to water-deprived rats or dogs in which circulating vasopressin levels are elevated, prompt decreases in arterial pressure or total peripheral resistance occur. Vasopressin blockade also decreases blood pressure in adrenal-insufficient animals and impairs blood pressure regulation during hemorrhage. Taken together, these and other observations demonstrate that, through its vasoconstrictor action, vasopressin plays an important role in cardiovascular regulation.

There is also some evidence that vasopressin plays a role in experimental hypertension in animals and may be involved in some forms of human hypertension. Vasopressin antagonists of the type described above will be of value in the investigation of this important question.

NATRIURETIC PEPTIDES

The atria and other tissues of mammals contain a family of peptides with natriuretic, diuretic, vasorelaxant and other properties. The family currently consists of atrial natriuretic peptide (ANP), brain natriuretic peptide (BNP) and C-type natriuretic peptide (CNP). The structures of the three peptides are similar (Figure 17–7), but there are differences in their biologic effects. ANP is derived from the carboxyl terminal end of a common precursor termed preproANP which, in humans, is a 151-amino-acid peptide. ANP is synthesized primarily in cardiac atriocytes, but small amounts are synthesized in ventriculocytes. It is also synthesized by neurons in the central and peripheral nervous systems and in the lungs. ANP circulates as a 28-amino-acid peptide with a single disulfide bridge that forms a 17-residue ring.

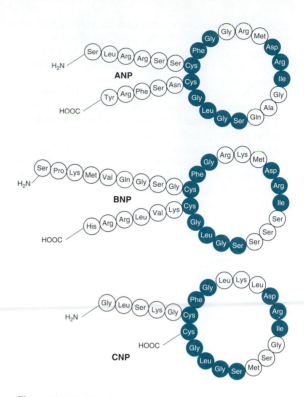

Figure 17–7. Structures of the atrial natriuretic peptides ANP, BNP, and CNP. Sequences *common* to the peptides are indicated in blue.

In healthy humans, plasma ANP concentration, as measured by radioimmunoassay, is 15–60 pg/mL. Several factors increase the release of ANP from the heart, but the most important one appears to be atrial distention. How distention increases ANP release is not known, but cardiac innervation is not required. ANP release is also increased by volume expansion, head-out water immersion, changing from the standing to the supine position, and exercise. In each case, the increase in ANP release is probably due to increased atrial stretch, but the cellular mechanisms that link ANP release to atrial stretch have not been elucidated. ANP release can also be increased by α-adrenoceptor agonists, glucocorticoids, endothelin (see below), and vasopressin. Finally, plasma ANP concentration increases in various pathologic states, including congestive heart failure, primary aldosteronism, chronic renal failure, and inappropriate ADH secretion syndrome.

Administration of ANP produces prompt and marked increases in sodium excretion and urine flow. Glomerular filtration rate increases, with little or no change in renal blood flow, so that the filtration fraction increases. The ANP-induced natriuresis is apparently due to both the increase in glomerular filtration rate and a decrease in proximal tubular sodium reabsorption. ANP also inhibits the secretion of renin, aldosterone, and vasopressin; these changes may also increase sodium and water excretion. Finally, ANP decreases arterial blood pressure. This hypotensive action is due to vasodilation, which results from stimulated particulate guanylyl cyclase activity, increased cGMP levels, and decreased cytosolic free calcium concentration. ANP also antagonizes the vasoconstrictor action of angiotensin II and other vasoconstrictors, and this action may also contribute to the hypotensive action of the peptide.

ANP apparently participates in the physiologic regulation of sodium excretion. For example, the natriuretic response to volume expansion is reduced, at least in some species, by ANP antibodies or by partial removal of the source of circulating ANP by atrial appendectomy.

BNP was originally isolated from porcine brain, but, like ANP, it is synthesized primarily in the heart. It consists of 26 amino acids (Figure 17–7). Like ANP, the release of BNP appears to be volume-related; indeed, the two peptides may be co-secreted. BNP exhibits natriuretic, diuretic, and hypotensive activities similar to those of ANP but circulates at a lower concentration.

CNP consists of 22 amino acids (Figure 17–7). It is located predominantly in the central nervous system but is also present in several tissues including the vascular endothelium, kidneys, and intestine. It has not been found in significant concentrations in the circulation. CNP has less natriuretic and diuretic activity than ANP and BNP but is a potent vasodilator. Its physiologic role remains unclear.

The biologic actions of the natriuretic peptides are mediated through association with specific high-affinity receptors located on the surface of the target cells. Three receptor subtypes termed ANP_A, ANP_B, and ANP_C have been identified. The ANP_A receptor consists of a 120 kDa protein; its primary ligands are ANP and BNP. The ANP_B receptor is similar in structure to the ANP_A receptor, but its primary ligand appears to be CNP. Both the ANP_A and ANP_B receptors are coupled to guanylyl cyclase. The ANP_C receptor is not coupled to guanylyl cyclase, binds all three peptides with equal affinity, and is thought to function in the clearance of the natriuretic peptides.

The natriuretic peptides have a short half-life in the circulation. They are metabolized in the kidneys, liver, and lungs by the neutral endopeptidase NEP 24.11. Inhibition of this endopeptidase results in increases in circulating levels of the natriuretic peptides, natriuresis, and diuresis. The peptides are also removed from the circulation by binding to ANP_C receptors in the vascular endothelium.

Because of their ability to reduce blood volume and arterial pressure, both ANP and BNP, as well as inhibitors of the endopeptidase NEP 24.11, are being evaluated as natriuretic-diuretic agents in the treatment of congestive heart failure, hypertension, renal failure, and states of fluid overload.

ENDOTHELINS

The endothelium is the source of a variety of substances with vasodilator (PGI_2 and nitric oxide) and vasoconstrictor activities. The latter include the endothelin family, potent vasoconstrictor peptides that were first isolated from aortic endothelial cells.

Three isoforms of endothelin have been identified: the originally described endothelin (ET-1) and two similar peptides, ET-2 and ET-3. Each isoform is a product of a different gene and is synthesized as a prepro form which is processed to a propeptide and then to the mature peptide. Each endothelin is a 21-amino-acid peptide containing two disulfide bridges. The structures of the endothelins are shown in Figure 17–8.

Endothelins are widely distributed in the body. ET-1 is produced in endothelial and vascular smooth muscle cells. It is also produced by neurons and astrocytes in the central nervous system and in endometrial, renal mesangial, Sertoli, breast epithelial, and other cells. ET-2 is produced predominantly in the kidneys and intestine, while ET-3 is found in highest concentration in the brain but is also present in the gastrointestinal tract, lungs, and kidneys. Endothelins are present in the blood but in low concentration; they probably act locally in a paracrine or autocrine fashion rather than as circulating hormones.

Endothelins exert widespread actions in the body. In particular, they cause dose-dependent vasoconstriction in most vascular beds. Intravenous administration of ET-1 causes a rapid and transient decrease in arterial blood pressure followed by a prolonged increase. The depressor response apparently results from release of PGI_2 or nitric oxide from the vascular endothelium, while the pressor response is due to direct constriction of vascular smooth muscle. Endothelins also exert direct positive inotropic and chronotropic actions on the heart and are potent coronary vasoconstrictors. They act on the kidneys to cause vasoconstriction and decrease glomerular filtration rate and sodium and water excretion. In the respiratory system, they cause potent constriction of tracheal and bronchial smooth muscle. Endothelins interact with several endocrine systems, increasing the secretion of renin, aldosterone, vasopressin and atrial natriuretic peptide. Finally, they exert a variety of actions on the central and peripheral nervous systems, the gastrointestinal system, the liver, the urinary tract, the male and female reproductive systems, the eye, the skeletal system, and the skin.

Endothelin receptors are present in many tissues and organs, including the blood vessel wall, cardiac muscle, central nervous system, lung, kidney, adrenal, spleen, and intestine. Two receptor subtypes, termed ET_A and ET_B, have been cloned and sequenced. ET_A receptors have a high affinity for ET-1 and a low affinity for ET-3 and are located on smooth muscle cells, where they mediate vasoconstriction. ET_B receptors have approximately equal affinities for ET-1 and

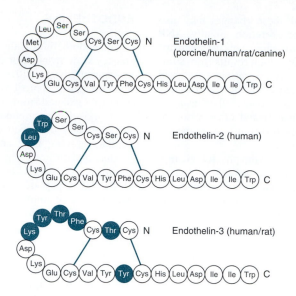

Figure 17–8. Structures of the endothelin peptides endothelin-1, endothelin-2, and endothelin-3. Sequences *different* in the three peptides are shown in blue.

ET-3 and are located on vascular endothelial cells, where they mediate release of PGI_2 and nitric oxide. Both receptor subtypes belong to the G protein-coupled seven-transmembrane domain family of receptors. There may be a third receptor selective for ET-3, but the existence of such an ET_C receptor has not been demonstrated in mammalian tissues.

The signal transduction mechanisms triggered by binding of ET-1 to ET_A receptors have been studied most extensively. As shown in Figure 17–9, these effects include an increase in intracellular calcium concentration resulting from increased influx of extracellular calcium via calcium channels and from stimulation of phospholipase C, formation of inositol trisphosphate, and release of calcium from the endoplasmic reticulum. In addition, there is activation of protein kinase C and phospholipase A_2 and stimulation of Na^+/H^+ exchange.

Antagonists of ET_A and ET_B receptors have recently been developed. Examples are shown in Figure 17–10. ET_A-selective antagonists include BQ-123, FR-139317, and 50-235. IRL 1038 is the only ET_B-selective antagonist currently available. Nonselective antagonists include [Thr[18],MeLeu[19]]ET-1, PD 145065, and Ro 46-2005.

The physiologic role of endothelins remains to be determined, but it seems likely that the peptides play important roles in cardiovascular regulation. They may also participate in hypertension and other cardiovascular diseases, but again their pathologic significance remains to be elucidated. The endothelin antagonists should help resolve these questions and also have considerable potential for the treatment of hypertension and vascular disease.

VASOACTIVE INTESTINAL PEPTIDE

Vasoactive intestinal peptide (VIP) is a 28-amino-acid peptide closely related structurally to secretin and glucagon. Its structure is shown below.

His-Ser-Asp-Ala-Val-Phe-Thr-Asp-Asn-Tyr-Thr-Arg-Leu-Arg-Lys-Gln-Met-Ala-Val-Lys-Lys-Tyr-Leu-Asn-Ser-Ile-Leu-Asn-NH₂

Vasoactive intestinal peptide (VIP)

VIP was originally extracted from porcine lung and was subsequently purified from porcine duodenum. It is now known that VIP is widely distributed in the central and peripheral nervous systems of humans and several animal species. It is also present in the circulation, but most evidence suggests that VIP functions as a neurotransmitter or neuromodulator rather than as a classic hormone.

VIP produces marked vasodilation in most vascular beds, including the splanchnic, pulmonary, coronary, renal, and cerebral vessels. The vasodilator action of VIP is independent of norepinephrine, acetylcholine, serotonin, and histamine receptors and apparently results from a direct action of the peptide on vascular smooth muscle. As a result of this action, arterial pres-

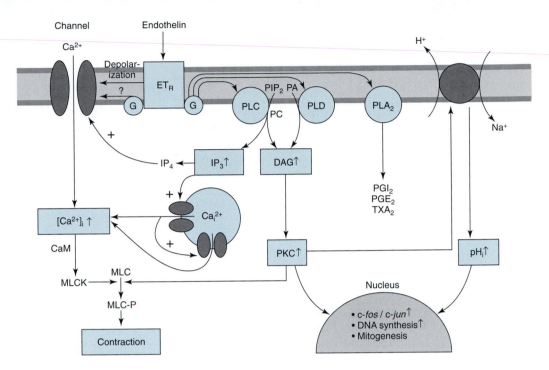

Figure 17–9. Signal transduction mechanisms involved in ET-1-induced short-term (eg, contraction of vascular smooth muscle) and long-term (eg, mitogenesis) modulation of cell function. See text for details. (Modified and redrawn, with permission, from Rubanyi GM, Polokoff MA: Endothelins: Molecular biology, biochemistry, pharmacology, physiology, and pathophysiology. Pharmacol Rev 1994;46:325.)

sure falls and cardiac output increases. The mechanism of the vasodilator action of VIP is not fully understood. However, it has been suggested that VIP binds to specific receptors in the blood vessels and stimulates cAMP production. This effect could be produced by VIP released from the nonadrenergic, noncholinergic VIP-containing nerve fibers that are associated with blood vessels or by VIP in the circulation.

In addition to dilating blood vessels, VIP relaxes tracheobronchial and gastrointestinal smooth muscle, stimulates intestinal water and electrolyte secretion, promotes hepatic glycogenolysis, causes neuronal excitation, and stimulates the release of several hormones including growth hormone, prolactin, and renin. The physiologic significance of these actions remains to be defined.

SUBSTANCE P

Substance P is an undecapeptide of the tachykinin family. It has the following structure:

Arg-Pro-Lys-Pro-Gln-Gln-Phe-Phe-Gly-Leu-Met

Substance P

Substance P is present in the central nervous system, where it is a neurotransmitter (Chapter 21), and in the gastrointestinal tract, where it may play a role as a transmitter in the enteric nervous system and as a local hormone (Chapter 6).

Substance P is a potent vasodilator and produces a marked hypotensive action in humans and in several animal species. The vasodilation apparently results from a direct inhibitory effect of the peptide on arteriolar smooth muscle. This action is mediated via specific receptors that differ from those mediating the actions of other vasodilators. In contrast to its effects on arteriolar smooth muscle, substance P stimulates contraction of venous, intestinal, and bronchial smooth muscle. It also causes secretion in the salivary glands, diuresis and natriuresis in the kidneys, and a variety of effects in the central and peripheral nervous systems. These diverse effects may result from the activation of more than one receptor type.

The amino terminal region of substance P is not essential for activity, and several carboxyl terminal fragments of the peptide, including the octa (4–11), hepta (5–11), and hexa (6–11) fragments, are also active. Indeed, depending on the preparation being studied, these peptides may be as potent as the intact undecapeptide or even more so. Analogs of substance P

Figure 17–10. Endothelin receptor antagonists. (Reproduced, with permission, from Huggins JP, Pelton JT, Miller RC: The structure and specificity of endothelin receptors: Their importance in physiology and medicine. Pharmacol Ther 1993;59:55.)

that are antagonists in vivo and in vitro are now available for experimental use (Regoli et al, 1994).

NEUROTENSIN

Neurotensin is a tridecapeptide that was first isolated from the central nervous system but subsequently was found to be present in the gastrointestinal tract and in the circulation. It has the following structure:

Glu-Leu-Tyr-Glu-Asn-Lys-Pro-Arg-Arg-Pro-Tyr-Ile-Leu

Neurotensin

When administered into the peripheral circulation, neurotensin produces a variety of effects, including vasodilation, hypotension, increased vascular permeability, increased secretion of several anterior pituitary hormones, hyperglycemia, inhibition of gastric acid and pepsin secretion, and inhibition of gastric motility. Following administration into the cerebrospinal fluid, it produces hypothermia and analgesia. Structure-activity studies indicate that the five or

six amino acid residues at the carboxyl terminal of the molecule are required for biologic activity. At present, the physiologic significance of the actions of neurotensin is not known.

CALCITONIN GENE-RELATED PEPTIDE

Calcitonin gene-related peptide (CGRP) is one of three products of the calcitonin gene. CGRP consists of 37 amino acids and displays approximately 30% structural homology with salmon calcitonin.

Like calcitonin, CGRP is present in large quantities in the C cells of the thyroid gland. It is also distributed widely in the central and peripheral nervous systems, in the cardiovascular system, the gastrointestinal tract, and the urogenital system. CGRP is found with substance P (see above) in some of these regions and with acetylcholine in others.

When CGRP is injected into the central nervous system, it produces a variety of effects, including suppression of feeding and hypertension. The peptide also produces several effects when injected into the systemic circulation, including hypotension and tachycardia. The hypotensive action of CGRP results from the potent vasodilator action of the peptide; indeed, CGRP is the most potent vasodilator yet discovered.

NEUROPEPTIDE Y

Neuropeptide Y is a 36-amino-acid peptide that was first isolated from porcine brain. Its structure is closely related to that of pancreatic polypeptide. Neuropeptide Y is present in high concentrations in the brain and peripheral nervous system and is one of the most abundant neuropeptides. In the sympathetic nervous system, neuropeptide Y is frequently localized in noradrenergic neurons and apparently functions both as a vasoconstrictor and as a cotransmitter with norepinephrine.

Neuropeptide Y produces a variety of central nervous system effects including increased feeding, hypotension, hypothermia, and respiratory depression. Peripheral effects include vasoconstriction of cerebral blood vessels, positive chronotropic and inotropic actions on the heart, and hypertension. These effects result from prejunctional actions, including inhibition of transmitter release from sympathetic and parasympathetic nerves, and from postjunctional actions, including direct vasoconstriction, potentiation of the action of vasoconstrictors, and inhibition of the action of vasodilators. These actions are apparently mediated by multiple receptor subtypes, including postjunctional Y_1 receptors and prejunctional Y_2 receptors. There also appear to be Y_3 and other receptor types. The Y_1 receptor is the best-characterized. Depending on the cell in which it is expressed, this receptor can couple either to phosphatidylinositol hydrolysis or inhibition of adenylyl cyclase. The vasoconstrictor action of neuropeptide Y can be antagonized by the inositol derivative D-myo-inositol-1,2,6-trisphosphate, but useful competitive antagonists of neuropeptide Y receptors are not yet available.

Preparations of angiotensin-converting enzyme inhibitors and losartan are found in Chapter 11; preparations of vasopressin in Chapter 15.

REFERENCES

General

Hedner T et al: Peptides as targets for antihypertensive drug development. J Hypertens 1992;10:S121.

Regoli D et al: Vasoactive peptides and characterization of their receptors. Regul Pept 1993;45:323.

Angiotensin

Bauer JH, Reams GP: The angiotensin II type 1 receptor antagonists: A new class of antihypertensive drugs. Arch Intern Med 1995;155:1361.

Bernstein KE, Alexander RW: Counterpoint: molecular analysis of the angiotensin II receptor. Endocr Rev 1992; 13:381.

Björck S et al: Renal protective effect of enalapril in diabetic nephropathy. Br Med J 1992;304:339.

Bumpus FM et al: Nomenclature for angiotensin receptors. Hypertension 1991;17:720.

Cody RJ: The clinical potential of renin inhibitors and angiotensin antagonists. Drugs 1994;47:586.

Corvol P et al: Human renin inhibitor peptides. Hypertension 1990;16:1.

Costerousse O et al: The angiotensin I converting enzyme (kininase II): Molecular organization and regulation of its expression in humans. J Cardiovasc Pharmacol 1992;20:S10.

Crozier I et al: Losartan in heart failure: Hemodynamic effects and tolerability. Circulation 1995;91:691.

Goldberg MR et al: Effects of losartan on blood pressure, plasma renin activity, and angiotensin II in volunteers. Hypertension 1993;21:704.

Greenlee WJ: Renin inhibitors. Med Res Rev 1990;10:173.

Griendling KK, Lassegue B, Alexander RW: Angiotensin receptors and their therapeutic implications. Ann Rev Pharmacol Toxicol 1996;36:281.

Hata A et al: Angiotensinogen as a risk factor for essential hypertension in Japan. J Clin Invest 1994;93:1285.

Inagami T, Harris RC: Molecular insights into angiotensin II receptor subtypes. News Physiol Sci 1993;8:215.

Kang PM et al: Angiotensin II receptor antagonists: A new approach to blockade of the renin-angiotensin system. Am Heart J 1994;127:1388.

Keeton TK, Campbell WB: The pharmacologic alteration of renin release. Pharmacol Rev 1980;32:81.

Konstam MA et al: Effects of the angiotensin converting enzyme inhibitor enalapril on the long-term progression of left ventricular dysfunction in patients with heart failure. Circulation 1992;86:431.

Lorenz JN et al: Renin release from isolated juxtaglomerular apparatus depends on macula densa chloride transport. Am J Physiol 1991;260:F486.

Menard J et al: Dose-dependent effects of the renin inhibitor zankiren HCl after a single oral dose in mildly sodium-depleted normotensive subjects. Circulation 1995; 91:330.

Panzenbeck MJ et al: Captopril-induced hypotension is inhibited by the bradykinin blocker HOE-140 in Na$^+$-depleted marmosets. Am J Physiol 1995;38:H1221.

Regitz-Zagrosek V et al: Molecular biology of angiotensin receptors and their role in human cardiovascular disease. J Mol Med 1996;74:233.

Reid IA: Actions of angiotensin II on the brain: Mechanisms and physiologic role. Am J Physiol 1984;246:F533.

Reid IA: Interactions between ANG II, sympathetic nervous system, and baroreceptor reflexes in regulation of blood pressure. Am J Physiol 1992;262:E763.

Rongen GA et al: Clinical pharmacokinetics and efficacy of renin inhibitors. Clin Pharmacokinet 1995;29:6.

Schelling P, Fischer H, Ganten D: Angiotensin and cell growth: A link to cardiovascular hypertrophy? J Hypertens 1991;9:3.

Tikkanen I, Omvik P, Jensen HAE: Comparison of the angiotensin II antagonist losartan with the angiotensin converting enzyme inhibitor enalapril in patients with essential hypertension. J Hypertens 1995;13:1343.

Timmermans PBMWM et al: Angiotensin II receptors and angiotensin II receptor antagonists. Pharmacol Rev 1993;45:205.

van Paassen P, de Zeeuw D, de Jong PE: Renal and systemic effects of the renin inhibitor remikiren in patients with essential hypertension. J Cardiovasc Pharmacol 1995;26:39.

Wexler RR et al: Nonpeptide angiotensin II receptor antagonists: The next generation in antihypertensive therapy. J Med Chem 1996;39:625.

Wyvratt MJ, Patchett AA: Recent developments in the design of angiotensin-converting enzyme inhibitors. Med Res Rev 1985;5:483.

Kinins

Bathon JM, Proud D: Bradykinin antagonists. Ann Rev Pharmacol Toxicol 1991;31:129.

Bhoola KD, Figueroa CD, Worthy K: Bioregulation of kinins: kallikreins, kininogens, and kininases. Pharmacol Rev 1992;44:1.

Dray A, Perkins M: Bradykinin and inflammatory pain. Trends Neurosci 1993;16:99.

Hall JM: Bradykinin receptors: Pharmacological properties and biological roles. Pharmacol Ther 1992;56:131.

Linz W et al: Contribution of kinins to the cardiovascular actions of angiotensin-converting enzyme inhibitors. Pharmacol Rev 1995;47:25.

Regoli D et al: Bradykinin receptor types and B_2 subtypes. Life Sci 1994;55:735.

Vasopressin

Laszlo FA, Laszlo F, De Wied D: Pharmacology and clinical perspectives of vasopressin antagonists. Pharmacol Rev 1991;43:73.

Manning M, Sawyer WH: Design, synthesis, and some uses of receptor specific agonists and antagonists of vasopressin and oxytocin. J Recept Res 1993;13:195.

Reid IA, Schwartz J: Role of vasopressin in the control of blood pressure. In: *Frontiers in Neuroendocrinology,* vol 8. Martini L, Ganong WF (editors). Raven Press, 1984.

Thibonnier M: Signal transduction of V_1-vascular vasopressin receptors. Regul Pept 1992;38:1.

Yamamura Y et al: OPC-21268, an orally effective, nonpeptide vasopressin V_1 receptor antagonist. Science 1991;252:572.

Natriuretic Peptides

Anand-Srivastava MB, Trachte GJ: Atrial natriuretic factor receptors and signal transduction mechanisms. Pharmacol Rev 1993;45:455.

Awazu M, Ichikawa I: Biological significance of atrial natriuretic peptide in the kidney. Nephron 1993;63:1.

McDowell G et al: The natriuretic peptide family. Eur J Clin Invest 1995;25:291.

Nakao K et al: Molecular biology and biochemistry of the natriuretic peptide system. I: Natriuretic peptides. J Hypertens 1992;10:907.

Nakao K et al: Molecular biology and biochemistry of the natriuretic peptide system. II: Natriuretic peptide receptors. J Hypertens 1992;10:1111.

Ruskoaho H: Atrial natriuretic peptide: Synthesis, release, and metabolism. Pharmacol Rev 1992;44:479.

Tan ACITL et al: Atrial natriuretic peptide. An overview of clinical pharmacology and pharmacokinetics. Clin Pharmacokinet 1993;24:28.

Wilkins MR, Unwin RJ, Kenny AJ: Endopeptidase 24.11 and its inhibitors: Potential therapeutic agents for edematous disorders and hypertension. Kidney Int 1993;43:273.

Endothelins

Clavell A et al: Physiologic significance of endothelin: Its role in congestive heart failure. Circulation 1993; 87(Suppl V):V–45.

Ferro CJ, Webb DJ: The clinical potential of endothelin receptor antagonists in cardiovascular medicine. Drugs 1996;51:12.

Haynes WG, Webb DJ: The endothelin family of peptides: Local hormones with diverse roles in health and disease? Clin Sci 1993;84:485.

Huggins JP, Pelton JT, Miller RC: The structure and specificity of endothelin receptors: Their importance in physiology and medicine. Pharmacol Ther 1993;59:55.

Levin ER: Endothelins. N Engl J Med 1995;333:356.

Masaki T, Vane JR, Vanhoutte PM: International union of pharmacology nomenclature of endothelin receptors. Pharmacol Rev 1994;46:137.

Masaki T, Yanagisawa M: Physiology and pharmacology of endothelins. Med Res Rev 1992;12:391.

Miller RC, Pelton JT, Huggins JP: Endothelins: from receptors to medicine. Trends Pharmacol Sci 1993;14:54.

Rubanyi GM, Polokoff MA: Endothelins: Molecular biology, biochemistry, pharmacology, physiology, and pathophysiology. Pharmacol Rev 1994;46:325.

Simonson MS: Endothelins: Multifunctional renal peptides. Physiol Rev 1993;73:375.

Thomas CP, Simonson MS, Dunn MJ: Endothelin: Receptors and transmembrane signals. News Physiol Sci 1992;7:207.

Vasoactive Intestinal Peptide

Said SI (editor): *Vasoactive Intestinal Peptide.* Raven Press, 1982.

Substance P

Maggio JE: Tachykinins. Ann Rev Neurosci 1988;11:13.

Nakanishi S: Substance P precursor and kininogen: Their structures, gene organizations, and regulation. Physiol Rev 1987;67:1117.

Regoli D, Boudon A, Fauchere J-L: Receptors and antagonists for substance P and related peptides. Pharmacol Rev 1994;46:551.

Neurotensin

Nemeroff CB, Prange AJ (editors): Neurotensin: A brain and gastrointestinal peptide. Ann NY Acad Sci 1982;400:1.

Vincent J-P: Neurotensin receptors: Binding properties, transduction pathways, and structure. Cell Mol Neurobiol 1995;15:501.

Calcitonin Gene-Related Peptide

Goodman EC, Iversen LL: Calcitonin gene-related peptide: Novel neuropeptide. Life Sci 1986;38:2169.

Zaidi M, Breimer LH, MacIntyre I: Biology of peptides from the calcitonin genes. Q J Exp Physiol 1987; 72:371.

Neuropeptide Y

Gehlert DR: Subtypes of receptors for neuropeptide Y: Implications for the targeting of therapeutics. Life Sci 1994;55:551.

Gray TS, Morley JE: Neuropeptide Y: Anatomical distribution and possible function in mammalian nervous system. Life Sci 1986;38:389.

McDermott BJ, Millar BC, Piper HM: Cardiovascular effects of neuropeptide Y: Receptor interactions and cellular mechanisms. Cardiovasc Res 1993;27:893.

Sundler F et al: Neuropeptide Y in the peripheral adrenergic and enteric nervous systems. Int Rev Cytol 1986; 102:243.

Walker P et al: The role of neuropeptide Y in cardiovascular regulation. Trends Pharmacol Sci 1991;12:111.

18

The Eicosanoids: Prostaglandins, Thromboxanes, Leukotrienes, & Related Compounds

Marie L. Foegh, MD, DSc, Markus Hecker, PhD, & Peter W. Ramwell, PhD

The eicosanoids are oxygenation products of polyunsaturated long chain fatty acids. They are ubiquitous in the animal kingdom and are also found—together with their precursor oils—in a variety of plants. They constitute a very large family of compounds that are not only highly potent but also display an extraordinarily wide spectrum of biologic activity. Because of their biologic activity, the eicosanoids, their specific receptor and enzyme inhibitors, and their plant and fish oil precursors have great therapeutic potential. Their short half-lives—seconds to minutes—make special delivery systems or synthesis of stable analogs mandatory for their clinical use.

ARACHIDONIC ACID & OTHER POLYUNSATURATED PRECURSORS

Arachidonic acid is the most abundant and probably the most important of the precursors of the eicosanoids. Arachidonic acid is a 20-carbon (C20) fatty acid that contains four double bonds beginning at the omega-6 position to yield a 5,8,11,14-eicosatetraenoic acid (denoted 20:4-6). For eicosanoid synthesis to occur, arachidonate must first be released or mobilized from membrane phospholipids by one or more lipases of the phospholipase A_2 (PLA_2) type (Figure 18–1). At least three phospholipases mediate arachidonate release from membrane lipids: cardiac PLA_2 ($cPLA_2$), cytosolic PLA_2, and secretory PLA_2. The first does not require calcium. The second and third enzymes are calcium-dependent and are more widely involved in arachidonate release. $cPLA_2$ is more involved in late phase stimulation by lipopolysaccharide (endotoxin), tumor necrosis factor, and mitogenic growth factors. $cPLA_2$ is thought to be activated by hormone stimulation of phospholipase C, which promotes Ca^{2+}-dependent membrane activation and MAP kinase-mediated phosphorylation. In addition, arachidonate can also be released by a combination of phospholipase C and diglyceride lipase. These lipase pathways are interdicted by steroidal anti-inflammatory drugs such as corticosteroids. The precise mechanisms are still conjectural.

ACRONYMS USED IN THIS CHAPTER	
ACTH	Adrenocorticotropic hormone
ADH	Antidiuretic hormone
EDRF	Endothelium-derived relaxing factor
EETE	Epoxyeicosatetraenoic (acid)
FSH	Follicle-stimulating hormone
HETE	Hydroxyeicosatetraenoic (acid)
HPETE	Hydroperoxyeicosatetraenoic (acid)
LH	Luteinizing hormone
LHRH	Luteinizing hormone-releasing hormone
LT	Leukotriene
LX	Lipoxin
NSAID	Nonsteroidal anti-inflammatory drugs
PAF	Platelet-activating factor
PG	Prostaglandin
PMN	Polymorphonuclear
PTH	Parathyroid hormone
SRS-A	Slow-reacting substance of anaphylaxis
TSH	Thyroid-stimulating hormone
TX	Thromboxane

Following mobilization, arachidonic acid is oxygenated by four separate routes: the cyclooxygenase, lipoxygenase, P450 epoxygenase, and isoprostane pathways. A number of factors determine the type of eicosanoid synthesized: (1) the species, (2) the type of cell, and (3) the cell's particular phenotype. The pattern of eicosanoids synthesized also frequently reflects (4) the manner in which the cell is stimulated. Finally, an important factor governing the pattern of eicosanoid release is (5) the nature of the precursor polyunsaturated

Figure 18–1. Pathways of arachidonic acid release and metabolism.

fatty acid that has been esterified in specific membrane phospholipids. For example, homo-γ-linoleic acid (C20:3–6), which is trienoic, yields products that differ from those derived from arachidonate (C20:4–6), which has four double bonds. Similarly, the products derived from eicosapentaenoic acid (C20:5–3), which has five double bonds, are also quantitatively different. This is the basis for using as nutritional supplements in humans the structurally different fatty acids obtained from cold water fish or from plants. An example of the significance of the polyunsaturated fatty acid precursors is evident when one considers thromboxane A (TXA) derived from the cyclooxygenase pathway. TXA_2 is synthesized from arachidonate, a *tetraenoic* acid and is a powerful vasoconstrictor and aggregator of platelets. However 5,8,11,14,17-eicosapentaenoic acid yields TXA_3, which is relatively inactive. In theory, dietary eicosapentaenoate substitution for arachidonate should minimize thrombotic events due to the displacement of tetraenoic arachidonate in the membrane by a pentaenoic acid.

SYNTHESIS OF EICOSANOIDS

Products of Prostaglandin Endoperoxide Synthases (Cyclooxygenases)

Two unique but related cyclooxygenase isozymes have been discovered that convert arachidonic acid into prostaglandin endoperoxide. PGH synthase-1 (COX-I) is constitutively expressed, ie, it is always present. In contrast, PGH synthase-2 (COX-II) is inducible, ie, its expression varies markedly depending on the stimulus. The two isozymes also differ in function in that COX-I is widely distributed and has housekeeping functions, eg, gastric cytoprotection. Two to fourfold increases occur following humoral stimulation. In contrast, COX-II is an immediate early response gene product in inflammatory and immune cells and is prominently expressed (tenfold to eighteenfold) by growth factors, tumor promoters, and cytokines. Lipopolysaccharide (endotoxin) is particularly potent in this respect.

The synthases are important because it is at this step that the nonsteroidal anti-inflammatory drugs exert their therapeutic effects. Indomethacin and sulindac act primarily on COX-I. Meclofenamate and ibuprofen are equipotent on COX-I and II, while the active metabolite of nabumetone preferentially inhibits COX-II. The steroidal anti-inflammatory drugs such as dexamethasone can inhibit COX-II gene expression. Specific COX-II inhibitors do not cause gastric erosion, as do COX-I inhibitors, and will become important drugs for treating chronic inflammation. Aspirin acetylates and inhibits both enzymes to different extents.

Both cyclooxygenases promote the uptake of two molecules of oxygen by cyclization of arachidonic acid to yield a C_9–C_{11} endoperoxide C_{15} hydroperoxide (Figure 18–2). This product is PGG_2, which is then rapidly modified by the peroxidase moiety of the cyclooxygenase enzyme to add a 15-hydroxyl group that is essential for biologic activity. This product is PGH_2. Both endoperoxides are highly unstable. Analogous families—PGH_1 and PGH_3 and all their subsequent products—are derived from homo-γ-linolenic acid and eicosapentaenoic acid, respectively.

PGH_2 then yields the prostaglandins, thromboxane, and prostacyclin by separate pathways. The prostaglandins differ from each other in two ways: (1) in the substituents of the pentane ring (indicated by the last letter, eg, E and F in PGE and PGF) and (2) in the number of double bonds in the side chains (indi-cated by the subscript, eg, PGE_1, PGE_2). Six products of the arachidonate series are of current clinical importance. **Alprostadil** (PGE_1) is used for its smooth muscle relaxing effects. **Misoprostol**, a PGE_1 derivative, is a cytoprotective prostaglandin used in preventing peptic ulcer. **PGE_2** and **$PGF_{2\alpha}$** are used in obstetrics. **Latanoprost**, a topically active $PGF_{2\alpha}$ derivative, is used in ophthalmology. **Prostacyclin** (PGI_2, epoprostenol) is synthesized mainly by the vascular endothelium and is a powerful vasodilator and inhibitor of platelet aggregation. In contrast, **thromboxane (TXA_2)** has undesirable properties (aggregation of platelets, vasoconstriction). Therefore

Figure 18–2. Prostagandin and thromboxane biosynthesis. Compound names are enclosed in boxes. The asterisks indicate that both cyclooxygenase and peroxidase steps are catalyzed by the single enzyme prostaglandin endoperoxide (PGH) synthase.

TXA$_2$ receptor *antagonists* and synthesis *inhibitors* have been synthesized for cardiovascular indications.

All the naturally occurring cyclooxygenase products rapidly undergo metabolism by β-oxidation, ω-oxidation, and oxidation of the key 15-hydroxyl group to the corresponding ketone. These inactive metabolites can then be determined in blood and urine by immunoassay or mass spectrometry as a measurement of the in vivo synthesis of their parent compound.

Products of Lipoxygenase

The metabolism of arachidonic acid by the 5-, 12-, and 15-lipoxygenases results in the production of hy-droperoxyeicosatetraenoic acids (HPETEs), which rapidly convert to hydroxy derivatives (HETEs) and leukotrienes (Figure 18–3). The most actively investigated leukotrienes are those produced by the 5-lipoxygenase present in inflammatory cells (PMNs, basophils, mast cells, eosinophils, macrophages). This pathway is of great interest since it is associated with asthma and anaphylactic shock. Stimulation of these cells elevates intracellular Ca^{2+}, releases arachidonate, and incorporates molecular oxygen by 5-lipoxygenase to yield the unstable epoxide leukotriene A$_4$ (LTA$_4$). This intermediate either converts to the dihydroxy leukotriene B$_4$ (LTB$_4$) or conjugates with glutathione to yield leukotriene C$_4$

Figure 18–3. Leukotriene biosynthesis. The asterisks indicate that both the lipoxygenase and dehydrase reactions are driven by the single enzyme 5-lipoxygenase. (GGTP, γ-glutamyltranspeptidase.)

(LTC$_4$), which can then undergo sequential degradation of the glutathione moiety by peptidases to yield LTD$_4$ and LTE$_4$. These three products are often called cysteinyl leukotrienes or peptidoleukotrienes.

LTC$_4$ and **LTD$_4$** are potent bronchoconstrictors and are now recognized as the primary components of the **slow-reacting substance of anaphylaxis (SRS-A)** that is secreted in asthma and anaphylaxis. There are four current approaches to anti-leukotriene drug development: 5-lipoxygenase enzyme inhibitors, leukotriene receptor antagonists, inhibitors of an important membrane-bound 5-lipoxygenase activating protein (FLAP), and phospholipase A$_2$ inhibitors.

Another group of 5-lipoxygenase products are the **lipoxins** LXA and LXB. Their biologic roles have not been elucidated.

Epoxygenase Products

Specific isozymes of microsomal P450 monooxygenases convert arachidonic acid to four epoxyeicosatrienoic acids (EETs) (Figure 18–1). These are the 5,6-, 6,9-, 11,12-, and 14,15-oxido products. Each EET has two stereoisomers. These epoxides are unstable and rapidly form the corresponding dihydroxyeicosatrienoic (DHET) acid, eg, 5,6-DHET. Unlike the prostaglandins, both the EETs and the DHETs can be incorporated into phospholipids that then act as storage sites. The epoxygenase products are active on smooth muscle cells and in cell signaling pathways and are thought to have important roles in renal function.

Isoprostanes

The generation of isoprostanes from arachidonic acid is another potentially important pathway. The isoprostanes are prostaglandin stereoisomers. Because prostaglandins have many asymmetric centers, they have a very large number of potential stereoisomers. Prostaglandin synthase (cyclooxygenase) is not needed for the formation of the isoprostanes, and aspirin and other nonsteroidal inhibitors of cyclooxygenase should not affect the isoprostane pathway. The primary epimerization mechanism is peroxidation of arachidonate by free radicals. Peroxidation occurs while arachidonic acid is still esterified to the membrane phospholipids. Thus, unlike prostaglandins, these stereoisomers are "stored" as part of the membrane. The importance of the isoprostane pathway lies in the relatively large amounts of these products (tenfold greater in blood and urine than the cyclooxygenase-derived prostaglandins) and their potent vasoconstrictor effects in the renal and other vascular beds. It has been proposed that isoprostanes play an important role in the hepatorenal syndrome.

I. BASIC PHARMACOLOGY OF EICOSANOIDS

MECHANISMS & EFFECTS OF EICOSANOIDS

Receptor Mechanisms

The eicosanoids act in an autocrine and paracrine fashion. These ligands bind to receptors on the cell surface, and pharmacologic specificity is determined by receptor density and type on different cells. A number of these receptors and their subtypes have been cloned. All of the receptors appear to be G protein-linked, and they contain sequences that predict seven membrane-spanning domains (see Chapter 2).

Binding of PGI$_2$, PGE$_1$, and PGD$_2$ to their platelet receptors inhibits platelet aggregation by activating adenylyl cyclase. This leads to increased intracellular cAMP levels, which in turn activates specific protein kinases. These kinases phosphorylate internal calcium pump proteins, an action that decreases free intracellular calcium concentration. In contrast, the binding of TXA$_2$ to its specific receptors activates phosphatidylinositol metabolism, leading to the formation of inositol-1,4,5-trisphosphate (IP$_3$). IP$_3$ causes mobilization of Ca^{2+} stores and an increase of free intracellular calcium. LTB$_4$ also generates IP$_3$ release and causes activation, degranulation, and superoxide anion generation in polymorphonuclear leukocytes.

Subtypes are described for PGE$_2$ receptors (EP$_1$, EP$_2$, and EP$_3$), each of which activates distinct signaling pathways. The EP$_1$ receptor is coupled to activation of phospholipase C, the EP$_2$ receptor to stimulation of adenylyl cyclase, and the EP$_3$ receptor to inhibition of adenylyl cyclase. The recent description of isoforms of receptor subtypes with coupling to different G proteins makes the issue of second messenger activation more complex. However this multiplicity of pathways may help clarify seemingly paradoxical experimental results.

The contractile effects of eicosanoids on smooth muscle are mediated by the release of calcium, while their relaxing effects are mediated by the generation of cAMP. The effects of eicosanoids on many target systems, including the immune system, can be similarly explained (see below). Many of the cicosanoids' contractile effects on smooth muscle can be inhibited by lowering extracellular calcium or by using calcium channel-blocking drugs.

Effects of Prostaglandins & Thromboxanes

The prostaglandins and thromboxanes have major effects on four types of smooth muscle: airway, gastrointestinal, reproductive, and vascular. Other important targets include platelets and monocytes, the central nervous system, autonomic presynaptic nerve terminals, sensory nerve endings, endocrine organs, adipose tissue, and the eye (the effects on the eye may involve smooth muscle).

A. Smooth Muscle:

1. Vascular—TXA_2 is a smooth muscle cell mitogen and is the only eicosanoid that has convincingly been shown to have this effect. The mitogenic effect is potentiated by exposure of smooth muscle cells to testosterone, which up-regulates smooth muscle cell TXA_2 receptors. In addition to its mitogenic effect, TXA_2 is a potent vasoconstrictor. $PGF_{2\alpha}$ is also a vasoconstrictor but is not a mitogen for smooth muscle cells. Another potent vasoconstrictor is 8-epi-$PGF_{2\alpha}$. In patients with cirrhosis, it is produced in large amounts in the liver and is thought to play a pathophysiologic role as an important vasoconstrictor substance in the hepatorenal syndrome.

Vasodilator prostaglandins promote vasodilation by decreasing smooth muscle intracellular calcium. Vascular prostacyclin is synthesized by both smooth muscle and endothelial cells, with the latter as the major contributor. PGI_2 undergoes rapid metabolism in a few seconds to more stable but inactive products. In the microcirculation, PGE_2 is another important endothelial vasodilator product.

2. Gastrointestinal tract—Most of the prostaglandins and thromboxanes activate gastrointestinal smooth muscle. Longitudinal muscle is contracted by PGE_2 and $PGF_{2\alpha}$, while circular muscle is contracted by PGI_2 and $PGF_{2\alpha}$ and relaxed by PGE_2. Administration of either PGE_2 or $PGF_{2\alpha}$ results in colicky cramps (see Clinical Pharmacology of Eicosanoids, below).

3. Airways—Respiratory smooth muscle is relaxed by PGE_1, PGE_2, and PGI_2 and contracted by TXA_2 and $PGF_{2\alpha}$.

B. Platelets and Blood Cells:

Platelet aggregation is markedly affected by eicosanoids. PGE_1 and especially PGI_2 effectively inhibit aggregation, while TXA_2 is a potent platelet aggregator. Platelets release TXA_2 during activation and aggregation, suggesting that thrombotic events such as myocardial infarction may result in the release of TXA_2. In fact, a measurable increase in urinary metabolites of TXA_2 following myocardial infarction has been reported. A more surprising finding was that urinary metabolites of TXA_2 also increased in patients experiencing a myocardial infarction while on low-dosage aspirin. At this aspirin dosage, thromboxane synthesis is significantly inhibited only in platelets. This suggests that other cells may contribute to the increase in TXA_2; these other cells may be monocytes, since monocytes have a high capacity for sustained release of TXA_2. Neutrophils and lymphocytes synthesize little if any prostaglandins, while monocytes have a substantial capacity for prostaglandin and thromboxane synthesis through both constitutive and inducible cyclooxygenases. Human eosinophils also seem to have a high capacity for prostaglandin and thromboxane synthesis.

C. Kidney:

Both the renal medulla and the renal cortex synthesize prostaglandins, the medulla substantially more than the cortex. Both parts of the kidney synthesize several hydroxyeicosatetraenoic acids, leukotrienes, cytochrome P450 products, and epoxides. These compounds play important autoregulatory roles in renal function by modifying renal hemodynamics and glomerular and tubular function. This regulatory role is especially important in marginally functioning kidneys, as shown by the decline in kidney function associated with the use of cyclooxygenase inhibitors in elderly patients and those with renal disease.

The major eicosanoid products of the renal cortex are PGE_2 and PGI_2. Both compounds increase renin release; normally, however, renin release is more directly under β_1 adrenoceptor control. The glomeruli also synthesize small amounts of TXA_2. This very potent vasoconstrictor does not appear to be responsible for regulating glomerular function in healthy humans.

PGE_1, PGE_2, and PGI_2 increase glomerular filtration through their vasodilating effects. These prostaglandins also increase water and sodium excretion. The increase in water clearance probably results from an attenuation of the action of antidiuretic hormone on adenylyl cyclase. It is uncertain whether the natriuretic effect is caused by the direct inhibition of sodium resorption in the distal tubule or by increased medullary blood flow. Loop diuretics, eg, furosemide, produce some of their effect by stimulating cyclooxygenase activity. In the normal kidney, this increases the synthesis of the vasodilator prostaglandins. Therefore, patient response to a loop diuretic will be diminished if a cyclooxygenase inhibitor is administered concurrently.

Like antidiuretic hormone, TXA_2 appears to increase water transport in the toad bladder. This and other findings have led to the suggestion that ADH may exert part of its effect by increasing TXA_2 synthesis. The normal kidney synthesizes only small amounts of TXA_2. However, in renal conditions involving inflammatory cell infiltration (such as glomerulonephritis and renal transplant rejection), the inflammatory cells (monocyte-macrophages) release substantial amounts of TXA_2. This increased concentration causes intrarenal vasoconstriction (and perhaps an ADH-like effect), resulting in a decline in renal function. Theoretically, TXA_2 synthase inhibitors or receptor antagonists should improve renal function in these patients, but no such drug is clinically available.

Hypertension is reportedly associated with increased TXA_2 and decreased PGE_2 and PGI_2 synthesis in some animal models. It is not known whether these changes are primary contributing factors or secondary responses. Similarly, increased TXA_2 formation has been reported in cyclosporine-induced nephrotoxicity, but no causal relationship has been established.

PGE_2 may also be involved in renal phosphate excretion, because exogenous PGE_2 antagonizes the inhibition of phosphate resorption by parathyroid hormone in the proximal tubule. However, the physiologic role of this eicosanoid may be limited because the proximal tubule, the major site for phosphate transport, produces few prostaglandins.

D. Reproductive Organs:

1. Female reproductive organs–The effects of prostaglandins on uterine function are of great clinical importance. They are discussed below. (See Clinical Pharmacology of Eicosanoids.)

2. Male reproductive organs–The role of prostaglandins in semen is still conjectural. The major source of these prostaglandins is the seminal vesicle; the prostate and the testes synthesize only small amounts. Thus, the term prostaglandin (referring to the prostate gland) is now known to be a misnomer. Semen from fertile men contains about 400 μg/mL of PGE and PGF and their 19-hydroxy metabolites. There is about 20 times more PGE than PGF in fertile semen, though this ratio varies greatly among individuals. However, within individuals, this ratio remains fairly constant as long as the sperm characteristics are unchanged. The factors that regulate the concentration of prostaglandins in human seminal plasma are not known in detail, but testosterone does promote prostaglandin production. Thromboxane and leukotrienes have not been found in seminal plasma. Men with a low seminal fluid concentration of prostaglandins are relatively infertile. Large doses of aspirin reduce the prostaglandin content of seminal plasma.

Smooth muscle-relaxing prostaglandins such as PGE_1 enhance penile erection by relaxing the smooth muscle of the corpora cavernosa. (See Clinical Pharmacology of the Eicosanoids.)

E. Central and Peripheral Nervous Systems:

1. Fever–PGE_1 and PGE_2 increase body temperature, especially when administered into the cerebral ventricles. Pyrogens release interleukin-1, which in turn promotes the synthesis and release of PGE_2. This synthesis is blocked by aspirin and other antipyretic compounds.

2. Sleep–When infused into the cerebral ventricles, PGD_2 induces natural sleep (as determined by electroencephalographic analysis) in a number of species, including primates.

3. Neurotransmission–PGE compounds inhibit the release of norepinephrine from postganglionic sympathetic nerve endings. Moreover, NSAIDs increase norepinephrine release in vivo, suggesting that the prostaglandins play a physiologic role in this process. Thus, vasoconstriction observed during treatment with cyclooxygenase inhibitors may be due to increased release of norepinephrine as well as to inhi-

bition of the endothelial synthesis of the vasodilators PGE_2 and PGI_2.

F. Neuroendocrine Organs: Both in vitro and in vivo tests have shown that some of the eicosanoids affect the secretion of neurohormones. PGE compounds promote the release of growth hormone, prolactin, TSH, ACTH, FSH, and LH. However, endocrine changes reflecting significant release of these hormones have not been reported in patients receiving PGE compounds. LTC_4 and LTD_4 stimulate LHRH and LH secretion (see below).

G. Bone Metabolism: Prostaglandins are abundant in skeletal tissue and are produced by the osteoblasts and the adjacent hematopoietic cells. The major effect of prostaglandins in vivo is to increase bone turnover, ie, stimulation of bone resorption and formation. Prostaglandins may mediate the effects of mechanical forces on bones and some of the changes that occur in bones with inflammation. Finally, prostaglandins may play a role in the bone loss that occurs at menopause.

H. Eye: PGE and PGF derivatives lower the intraocular pressure. The mechanism of this action is unclear but probably involves increased outflow of aqueous humor from the anterior chamber.

Effects of Lipoxygenase & Cytochrome P450-Derived Metabolites

The actions of lipoxygenases generate compounds that can regulate specific cellular responses important in inflammation and immunity. Other cytochrome P450-derived metabolites affect nephron transport functions either directly or via metabolism to active compounds (see below). The biologic functions of the various forms of hydroxy- and hydroperoxyeicosaenoic acids are largely unknown, but their pharmacologic potency is impressive.

A. Heart and Smooth Muscle:

1. Cardiovascular–12(S)-HETE is a potent chemoattractant for smooth muscle cells, causing migration at concentrations as low as 1 fmol/L; it may play a role in myointimal proliferation that occurs after vascular injury such as that caused by angioplasty. Its stereoisomer, 12(R)-HETE, is not a chemoattractant but is a potent inhibitor of the Na^+/K^+ ATPase in the cornea. LTC_4 and LTD_4 reduce myocardial contractility and coronary blood flow, leading to cardiac depression. Lipoxin A and lipoxin B seem to exert similar vasoconstrictor effects.

2. Gastrointestinal–Human colonic epithelial cells synthesize LTB_4, a chemoattractant for neutrophils. The colonic mucosa of patients with inflammatory bowel disease contains substantially increased amounts of LTB_4, as might be expected.

3. Airways–The peptidoleukotrienes, particularly LTC_4 and LTD_4, are potent bronchoconstrictors and cause increased microvascular permeability, plasma exudation, and mucus secretion in the airways. Controversies exist over whether the pattern and specificity of the leukotriene receptors differ in animal models and humans. LTC_4-specific receptors have not been found in human lung tissue, whereas both high- and low-affinity LTD_4 receptors are present.

B. Blood Cells: LTB_4 is a potent chemoattractant for neutrophils; LTC_4 and LTD_4 are potent chemoattractants for eosinophils. These leukotrienes also promote eosinophil adherence, degranulation, and oxygen radical formation. The leukotrienes have been implicated in the pathogenesis of inflammation, especially in chronic diseases. Lipoxin A seems to exert effects similar to those of LTB_4 on neutrophils. Lymphocyte proliferation and differentiation are modified by LTB_4. Both Lipoxin A and lipoxin B inhibit natural killer cell cytotoxicity.

C. Renal System: The roles of leukotrienes and cytochrome P450 products in the human kidney are currently speculative. Recently, the 5,6-epoxide has been shown to be a powerful vasodilator in animal experiments. Another recent discovery is that free radicals attack arachidonic acid-containing phospholipids to yield an 8-*epi*-$PGF_{2\alpha}$ that has powerful thromboxane-like properties. Synthesis is not blocked by cyclooxygenase inhibitors but can be blocked by antioxidants. This vasoconstrictor, which is present in humans, is thought to be an important mediator causing renal failure in the hepatorenal syndrome.

D. Miscellaneous: The effects of these products on the reproductive organs remain to be elucidated. Similarly, actions on the nervous system have been suggested (recent data indicate that 12-HPETE acts as a neurotransmitter in *Aplysia* neurons), but this has not been confirmed in higher organisms. Very low concentrations of LTC_4 increase and higher concentrations of arachidonate-derived epoxides augment LH and LHRH release from isolated rat anterior pituitary cells.

INHIBITION OF EICOSANOID SYNTHESIS

Corticosteroids block all the known pathways of eicosanoid synthesis, perhaps by stimulating the synthesis of several inhibitory proteins collectively called **annexins** or **lipocortins.** They inhibit phospholipase A_2 activity, probably by interfering with phospholipid binding and thus preventing the release of arachidonic acid.

The nonsteroidal anti-inflammatory drugs (eg, aspirin, indomethacin, ibuprofen) block both prostaglandin and thromboxane formation by inhibiting cyclooxygenase activity. For example, aspirin is a long-lasting inhibitor of platelet cyclooxygenase and of TXA_2 biosynthesis because it irreversibly acetylates the enzyme. Once acetylated, platelet cyclooxygenase cannot be restored via protein biosynthesis because platelets lack a nucleus.

The development of selective thromboxane synthase inhibitors and TXA_2 receptor antagonists has re-

quired considerable effort. The resulting compounds, eg, sulotroban, have been quite useful for characterizing TXA_2-related effects in vitro and in vivo. They are being tested in the treatment of unwanted clotting, pulmonary hypertension, and preeclampsia-eclampsia.

Selective inhibitors of the lipoxygenase pathway are also mainly investigational. With a few exceptions, NSAIDs do not inhibit lipoxygenase activity at concentrations that markedly inhibit cyclooxygenase activity. In fact, by preventing arachidonic acid conversion via the cyclooxygenase pathway, NSAIDs may cause more substrate to be metabolized through the lipoxygenase pathways, leading to an increased formation of the inflammatory leukotrienes. Even among the cyclooxygenase-dependent pathways, inhibiting the synthesis of one derivative may increase the synthesis of an enzymatically related product. Therefore, researchers are attempting to develop drugs that inhibit both cyclooxygenase and lipoxygenase.

II. CLINICAL PHARMACOLOGY OF EICOSANOIDS

Several approaches have been used in the clinical application of eicosanoids. First, stable oral or parenteral long-acting analogs of the naturally occurring prostaglandins have been developed. Several such compounds have been approved for clinical use overseas and are being introduced in the USA (Figure 18–4). Second, enzyme inhibitors and receptor antagonists have been developed to interfere with the synthesis or effects of the "pathologic" eicosanoids (ie, thromboxanes and leukotrienes). For example, knowledge of eicosanoid synthesis and metabolism has led to the development of new nonsteroidal anti-inflammatory drugs that inhibit cyclooxygenase, with improved pharmacokinetic and pharmacodynamic characteristics. One objective, described earlier, is to develop dual inhibitors that block both the cyclooxygenase (especially COX-II) and lipoxygenase pathways. Another goal is to decrease gastrointestinal and renal toxicity. Third, dietary manipulation—to change the polyunsaturated fatty acid precursors in the cell membrane phospholipids and so change eicosanoid synthesis—is used extensively in over-the-counter products and in diets emphasizing increased consumption of cold water fish.

Female Reproductive System

The physiologic role of prostaglandins in reproduction has been intensively studied since the discovery of prostaglandins in the seminal plasma of primates and sheep. It has been suggested that the prostaglandins in seminal plasma facilitate blastocyst implantation or egg transport and that uterine secretion of prostaglandins causes luteolysis. The latter is not true

Figure 18–4. Chemical structures of prostaglandins and prostaglandin analogs currently in clinical use.

in humans but appears to be true in cattle and pigs. This finding has led to the marketing of veterinary preparations of $PGF_{2\alpha}$ and its analogs for synchronizing ovulation in animals.

A. Abortion: PGE_2 and $PGF_{2\alpha}$ have potent oxytocic actions. The ability of the E and F prostaglandins and their analogs to terminate pregnancy at any stage by promoting uterine contractions has been adapted to routine clinical use. Many studies worldwide have established that prostaglandin administration efficiently terminates pregnancy. The drugs are used for first- and second-trimester abortion and for priming or ripening the cervix before abortion. These prostaglandins appear to soften the cervix by increasing proteoglycan content and changing the biophysical properties of collagen.

Early studies found that intravenous PGE_2 and $PGF_{2\alpha}$ produced abortion in about 80% of cases. The success rate is dependent on the dose, the duration of the infusion, and parity of the woman. Dose-limiting adverse effects include vomiting, diarrhea, fever, and bronchoconstriction. Hypotension, hypertension, syncope, dizziness, and flushing can occur and may be related to the vasomotor and vasovagal effects of PGE_2.

In current practice, dinoprostone, a synthetic preparation of naturally occurring PGE_2, is administered vaginally for oxytocic use. In the USA it is approved for inducing abortion in the second trimester of pregnancy, for missed abortion, for benign hydatidiform mole, and for ripening of the cervix for induction of labor in patients at or near term.

Dinoprostone stimulates the contraction of the uterus throughout pregnancy. As the pregnancy progresses, the uterus increases its contractile response, and the contractile effect of oxytocin is potentiated as well. Dinoprostone also directly affects the collagenase of the cervix and breaks down the collagen network with an increase in hydrophilic glycosaminoglycan and hyaluronic acid and a decrease in dermatan sulfate, resulting in softening of the cervix. The vaginal dose enters the maternal circulation, and a small amount is absorbed directly by the uterus via the cervix and the lymphatic system. Dinoprostone is metabolized in local tissues and on the first pass through the lungs (about 95%). The metabolites are mainly excreted in the urine. The plasma half-life is 2.5–5 minutes.

For the induction of labor, dinoprostone is available either as a gel (0.5 mg PGE_2) or as a controlled-release formulation (10 mg PGE_2) that releases PGE_2 in vivo at a rate of about 0.3 mg/h over 12 hours. An advantage of the controlled-release formulation is a lower incidence of gastrointestinal side effects

($< 1\%$). A further advantage of this delivery system is that the medication is contained within a vaginal insert that can be retrieved at any time.

For abortifacient purposes, the recommended dosage is a 20 mg dinoprostone vaginal suppository repeated at 3- to 5-hour intervals depending on the response of the uterus. For softening of the cervix at term, the preparations used are either a single vaginal insert containing 10 mg PGE_2 or a vaginal gel containing 0.5 mg PGE_2 administered every 6 hours. The mean time to abortion is 17 hours, but in more than 25% of cases the abortion is incomplete and requires additional intervention. The softening of the cervix for induction of labor substantially shortens the time to onset of labor and the delivery time.

The use of PGE analogs for "menstrual regulation" or very early abortions—within 1–2 weeks after the last menstrual period—has been explored extensively. There are two problems: prolonged vaginal bleeding and severe menstrual cramps.

Antiprogestins (eg, RU 486) have been combined with an oral oxytocic prostaglandin (eg, misoprostol) to produce early abortion. This regimen is available in Europe. The ease of use and the effectiveness of the combination have aroused considerable opposition in some quarters (see Chapter 39), but the drug has completed clinical testing in the United States and has been recommended for approval by the FDA committee. The major toxicities are cramping pain and diarrhea.

$PGF_{2\alpha}$ is no longer available for clinical use in the USA. The drug previously available for this route of administration, carboprost tromethamine (15-methyl-$PGF_{2\alpha}$—the C_{15} methyl group prolongs the duration of action) was withdrawn from the USA market. In other countries, the intra-amniotic, intramuscular, and intravaginal routes are commonly used for administration of $PGF_{2\alpha}$. Intra-amniotic administration has close to a 100% success rate, with fewer and less severe adverse effects than intravenous administration.

Where still available, carboprost is used to induce second-trimester abortions and is usually administered as a single 40 mg intra-amniotic injection. The abortion is normally completed within 20 hours. The most serious adverse effects of this route of administration involve cardiovascular collapse. Most of the reported cases have been diagnosed as anaphylactic shock, but others may have been due to the drug escaping into the circulation and causing severe pulmonary hypertension. In pregnant anesthetized women, $PGF_{2\alpha}$, 300 μg/min intravenously, doubles pulmonary resistance and increases the work of the right side of the heart threefold. Thus, only minimal amounts of the 40 mg intra-amniotic dose need to reach the circulation to cause cardiovascular effects. This problem may be avoided by instilling the drug under ultrasonic guidance.

Intramuscular injection of carboprost tromethamine can also be used to induce abortion. Unlike the one-time intrauterine instillation of dinoprost, carboprost is given repeatedly up to the total dose of 2.6 mg normally required to cause abortion.

B. Facilitation of Labor: Numerous studies have shown that PGE_2, $PGF_{2\alpha}$, and their analogs effectively initiate and stimulate labor. However, this is an unlabeled use. There appears to be no difference in the efficacy of the two drugs when they are administered intravenously, but $PGF_{2\alpha}$ is one-tenth as potent as PGE_2. These agents and oxytocin have similar success rates and comparable induction-to-delivery intervals. The adverse effects of the prostaglandins are moderate, with a slightly higher incidence of nausea, vomiting, and diarrhea than that produced by oxytocin. $PGF_{2\alpha}$ has more gastrointestinal toxicity than PGE_2. Neither drug has significant maternal cardiovascular toxicity in the recommended doses. In fact, PGE_2 must be infused at a rate about 20 times faster than that used for induction of labor to decrease blood pressure and increase heart rate. $PGF_{2\alpha}$ is a bronchoconstrictor and should be used with caution in asthmatics; however, neither asthmatic attacks nor bronchoconstriction have been observed during the induction of labor. Although both PGE_2 and $PGF_{2\alpha}$ pass the fetoplacental barrier, fetal toxicity is uncommon.

The effects of oral PGE_2 administration (0.5–1.5 mg/h) have been compared to those of intravenous oxytocin and oral demoxytocin, an oxytocin derivative, in the induction of labor. Oral PGE_2 is superior to the oral oxytocin derivative and in most studies is as efficient as intravenous oxytocin. However, the only available form of PGE_2 in the USA at present is dinoprostone for vaginal administration, and by this route of administration the drug is slightly less effective than oxytocin. Vaginal PGE_2 is also used to soften the cervix before inducing labor. Oral $PGF_{2\alpha}$ causes too much gastrointestinal toxicity to be useful by this route.

Theoretically, PGE_2 and $PGF_{2\alpha}$ should be superior to oxytocin for inducing labor in women with preeclampsia-eclampsia or cardiac and renal diseases because, unlike oxytocin, they have no antidiuretic effect. In addition, PGE_2 has natriuretic effects. However, the clinical benefits of these effects have not been documented. In cases of intrauterine fetal death, the prostaglandins alone or with oxytocin seem to cause delivery effectively. In some cases of postpartum bleeding, 15-methyl-$PGF_{2\alpha}$ will successfully control hemorrhage when oxytocin and methylergonovine fail to do so.

C. Dysmenorrhea: Primary dysmenorrhea is attributable to increased endometrial synthesis of PGE_2 and $PGF_{2\alpha}$ during menstruation, with contractions of the uterus that lead to ischemic pain. NSAIDs successfully inhibit the formation of these prostaglandins (see Chapter 36) and so relieve dysmenorrhea in 75–85% of cases. Some of these drugs are available over the counter. Aspirin is also effective in dysmenorrhea, but because it has low potency and is quickly hydrolyzed, large doses and frequent administration are necessary. In addition, the acetylation of platelet cyclooxygenase, causing permanent abolition of platelet TXA_2, may have an adverse effect on the amount of menstrual bleeding.

Male Reproductive System

Intracavernosal injection therapy with the vasodilator alprostadil (PGE_1) has become important in the treatment of impotence. Doses of 0.2–140 µg are used. Penile pain is a frequent side effect that may be related to the algesic effects of PGE derivatives; however, only a few patients discontinue the use due to pain. Prolonged erection and priapism are less frequent side effects that occur in fewer than 4% of patients and are minimized by careful titration to the minimal effective dose. Alprostadil may be used as monotherapy or in combination with either papaverine or phentolamine. A minisuppository preparation has recently been approved. This formulation is placed in the urethra and dissolves, releasing alprostadil into the cavernosa.

Cardiovascular System

The vasodilator effects of PGE compounds have been studied extensively in hypertensive patients. These compounds also promote sodium diuresis. Practical application will require derivatives with oral activity, longer half-lives, and fewer adverse effects.

A. Pulmonary Hypertension: Prostacyclin lowers peripheral, pulmonary, and coronary resistance. It has been used to treat both primary pulmonary hypertension and secondary pulmonary hypertension, which sometimes occurs after mitral valve surgery. However, its pulmonary vasodilator effects are not specific enough, so the patient's blood pressure must also be supported with pressor drugs. A commercial preparation of prostacyclin (epoprostenol) is approved for treatment of primary pulmonary hypertension, in which it appears to improve symptoms and prolong survival. The drug is administered as a continuous intravenous infusion through a central line. Because of its extremely short plasma half-life, the effects of PGI_2 cease within a few minutes of ending the infusion. PGI_2 is metabolized to two major metabolites and a series of minor metabolites. The most common adverse effects are nausea, vomiting, headache, hypotension, and flushing.

B. Peripheral Vascular Disease: A number of studies have investigated the use of PGE and PGI_2 compounds in Raynaud's phenomenon and peripheral atherosclerosis. In the latter case, prolonged infusions have been used to permit remodeling of the vessel wall and to enhance regression of ischemic ulcers.

C. Patent Ductus Arteriosus: Patency of the fetal ductus arteriosus is now generally believed to depend on local PGE_2 and PGI_2 synthesis. In certain types of congenital heart disease (eg, transposition of the great arteries, pulmonary atresia, pulmonary

artery stenosis), it is important to maintain the patency of the neonate's ductus arteriosus before surgery. This is done with alprostadil, PGE_1. Like PGE_2, PGE_1 is a vasodilator and an inhibitor of platelet aggregation, and it contracts uterine and intestinal smooth muscle. There are no absolute contraindications to the use of this drug, but in cases of respiratory distress syndrome it is not recommended. Adverse effects include apnea, bradycardia, hypotension, and hyperpyrexia. Because of rapid pulmonary clearance, the drug must be continuously infused at an initial rate of 0.05–0.1 µg/kg/min, which may be increased to 0.4 µg/kg/min. Prolonged treatment has been associated with ductal fragility and rupture.

In delayed closure of the ductus arteriosus, cyclooxygenase inhibitors are often used to inhibit synthesis of PGE_2 and PGI_2 and so close the ductus. Premature infants who develop respiratory distress due to failure of ductus closure can be treated with a high degree of success with indomethacin. This treatment often precludes the need for surgical closure of the ductus.

Blood

As noted above, eicosanoids are involved in thrombosis because TXA_2 promotes platelet aggregation and PGI_2 inhibits it. Aspirin inhibits platelet cyclooxygenase to produce a mild clotting defect. The mildness of this defect is supported by the fact that very modest hemostatic defects are noted in patients with diseases involving deficiencies of platelet cyclooxygenase and thromboxane synthase—eg, these patients have no history of increased or decreased bleeding. Blockade of either of these two enzymes inhibits secondary aggregation of platelets induced by ADP, by low concentrations of thrombin and collagen, or by epinephrine. Thus, these platelet enzymes are not necessary for platelet function but may amplify an aggregating stimulus.

Epidemiologic studies in the USA and United Kingdom indicate that low doses of aspirin reduce the risk of death due to infarction but may *increase* overall mortality rates because they may increase the incidence of stroke (see Chapter 34). It is now difficult to find patients at risk for thromboembolism—as in orthopedic surgery or angioplasty for coronary artery stenosis—who do not take aspirin. However, the beneficial effects of aspirin may relate to its other acetylating properties and not to acetylation of cyclooxygenase.

During the development of deep vein thrombosis, thromboxane and its metabolites are excreted in the urine, probably because the entire platelet pool is activated. This phenomenon is seen to a lesser extent in kidney transplant patients experiencing organ rejection. Elevated excretion of thromboxane metabolites is also seen in patients before infarction and during unstable angina.

Prostacyclin is not a circulating hormone, as originally claimed; it inhibits platelet aggregation but does not inhibit platelet adhesion to the endothelium, platelet spreading, or granule release. Finally, PGI_2 and PGE_2 analogs can inhibit the development of atherosclerosis in cholesterol-fed animals, but hypotension is an adverse effect in this setting.

Respiratory System

PGE_2 is a powerful bronchodilator when given in aerosol form. Unfortunately, it also promotes coughing, and an analog that possesses only the bronchodilator properties has been difficult to obtain.

$PGF_{2\alpha}$ and TXA_2 are both strong bronchoconstrictors and were once thought to be primary mediators in asthma. However, the identification of the peptidoleukotrienes— LTC_4, LTD_4, and LTE_4—expanded the role of eicosanoids as important mediators in asthma and other immune responses. Recent clinical trials indicate that a 5-lipoxygenase inhibitor, **zileuton,** does have a bronchodilator effect in humans. It remains unclear whether leukotrienes are partially responsible for the acute respiratory distress syndrome.

Corticosteroids and cromolyn are currently the major eicosanoid-related drugs used in asthma (see Chapter 20). Corticosteroids inhibit eicosanoid synthesis and thus limit the amounts of eicosanoid mediator available for release. Cromolyn probably inhibits the release of eicosanoids and other mediators such as histamine and platelet-activating factor. In the future, leukotriene antagonists and lipoxygenase inhibitors may become useful in treating acute asthmatic attacks and hypersensitivity reactions.

Gastrointestinal System

The word "cytoprotection" was coined to signify the remarkable protective effect of the E prostaglandins against gastric ulcers in animals at doses that do not reduce acid secretion. These prostaglandins were independently discovered also to inhibit gastric acid secretion (at higher doses). Since then, numerous experimental and clinical investigations have shown that the PGE compounds and their analogs protect against gastric ulcers produced by either steroids or NSAIDs. Misoprostol is an orally active synthetic analog of PGE_1 available in Europe and the USA for ulcer treatment. The FDA-approved indication is for prevention of NSAID-induced gastric ulcers only. The drug is administered at a dosage of 200 μg four times daily. This and other PGE analogs (eg, enprostil) are cytoprotective at low doses and inhibit gastric acid secretion at higher doses. The adverse effects are abdominal discomfort and occasional diarrhea; both effects are dose-related. More recently, dose dependent bone pain and hyperostosis have been described in patients with liver disease who were given long-term PGE treatment. This adverse effect can be explained by a PGE-induced acceleration of osteoclast and osteoblast activity. Recurrent calcium oxalate kidney stones were described in the same group of patients. This may be related to PGE-induced hypercalciuria.

Gastrointestinal side effects seen in many patients using NSAIDs may be reduced by the development of selective inhibitors of COX-II that spare the gastric COX-I so that the natural cytoprotection by locally synthesized PGE2 is undisturbed. Such agents are not yet available.

Increased leukotriene formation in colonic mucosa has been demonstrated in patients with inflammatory bowel diseases. Whether these products play a significant pathophysiologic role has not yet been established.

Immune System

Monocyte-macrophages are the only principal cells of the immune system that can synthesize all the eicosanoids. T and B lymphocytes are interesting exceptions to the general rule that all nucleated cells produce eicosanoids. However, in a B lymphoma cell line, there is non-receptor-mediated uptake of LTB_4 and 5-HETE. Interaction between lymphocytes and monocyte-macrophages may cause the lymphocytes to release arachidonic acid from their cell membranes. The arachidonic acid is then used by the monocyte-macrophages for eicosanoid synthesis. In addition to these cells, there is evidence for eicosanoid-mediated cell-cell interaction by platelets, erythrocytes, PMNs, and endothelial cells.

The eicosanoids modulate the effects of the immune system, as illustrated by the cell-mediated immune response. As shown in Figure 18–5, PGE_2 and PGI_2 affect T cell proliferation in vitro as corticosteroids do. T cell clonal expansion is attenuated though inhibition of interleukin-1 and interleukin-2 and class II antigen expression by macrophages or other antigen-presenting cells. The leukotrienes, TXA_2, and platelet-activating factor stimulate T cell clonal expansion. These compounds stimulate the formation of interleukin-1 and interleukin-2 as well as the expression of interleukin-2 receptors. The leukotrienes also promote interferon-γ release and can replace interleukin-2 as a stimulator of interferon-γ. These in vitro effects of the eicosanoids agree with in vivo findings in animals with acute organ transplant rejection, as described below. The association between the use of the anti-inflammatory steroids and increased risk of infection is well established; however, the nonsteroidal anti-inflammatory drugs do not seem to alter patient responses to infection.

A. Cell-Mediated Organ Transplant Rejection: Acute organ transplant rejection is a cell-mediated immune response. Administration of PGI_2 to renal transplant patients has reversed the rejection process in some cases. Experimental in vitro and in vivo data show that PGE_2 and PGI_2 can attenuate T cell proliferation and rejection, which can also be seen with drugs that inhibit TXA_2 and leukotriene for-

Figure 18–5. Modulation of macrophage and lymphocyte interactions by eicosanoids, platelet activating factor, and corticosteroids. Corticosteroids, PGE_2, and possibly PGI_2 inhibit the expression of interleukin-1 (IL-1) and its effect on T lymphocytes. Platelet-activating factor (PAF), LTB_4, and LTD_4 increase IL-1 expression. Similar inhibitory and stimulant effects are exerted on the action of interferon-gamma on the macrophage and on the action of interleukin-2 (IL-2). Agents marked with an asterisk are suspected, but not yet proved, to have the effects indicated. (DR, class II MHC [major histocompatibility complex] receptor; T, T lymphocytes.) (Modified and reproduced, with permission, from Foegh ML, Ramwell PW: PAF and transplant immunology. In: Braquet P [editor]: *The Role of Platelet Activating Factor in Immune Disorders.* Karger, 1988.)

mation. In organ transplant patients, urinary excretion of TXB_2, a metabolite of TXA_2, increases during acute rejection. Corticosteroids, the primary drugs used for treatment of acute rejection due to their effects on lymphocytes, inhibit both phospholipase and COX-II activity.

B. Inflammation: Aspirin has been used to treat arthritis for nearly a century, but its mechanism of action—inhibition of cyclooxygenase activity—was not discovered until 1971. Aspirin and other anti-inflammatory agents that inhibit cyclooxygenase are discussed in Chapter 36. Cox-II appears to be the form of the enzyme associated with cells involved in the inflammatory process. The prostaglandins are not chemoattractants, but the leukotrienes and some of the HETEs (eg, 12-HETE) are strong chemoattractants. Drugs that inhibit COX-II, 5-lipoxygenase, and 12-lipoxygenase are in clinical development. PGE_2 inhibits both antigen-driven and mitogen-induced B lymphocyte proliferation and differentiation to plasma cells, resulting in inhibition of IgM synthesis

(Figure 18–6). The concomitant elevation of serum IgE and monocyte PGE_2 synthesis, seen in patients with severe trauma and patients with Hodgkin's disease, is explained by PGE_2 ability to enhance immunoglobulin class switching to IgE.

C. Rheumatoid Arthritis: In rheumatoid arthritis, immune complexes are deposited in the affected joints, causing an inflammatory response that is amplified by eicosanoids. Lymphocytes and macrophages accumulate in the synovium, while PMNs localize mainly in the synovial fluid. The major eicosanoids produced by PMNs are leukotrienes, which facilitate T cell proliferation and act as chemoattractants. Human macrophages synthesize the cyclooxygenase products PGE_2 and TXA_2 and large amounts of leukotrienes.

Glaucoma

Latanoprost, a stable long-acting $PGF_{2\alpha}$ derivative, has been introduced as a drug for glaucoma. It is administered as drops into the conjunctival sac once or twice daily.

DIETARY MANIPULATION OF ARACHIDONIC ACID METABOLISM

Because arachidonic acid is derived from dietary linoleic and α-linolenic acids, which are essential fatty acids, the effects of dietary manipulation on arachidonic acid metabolism have been extensively

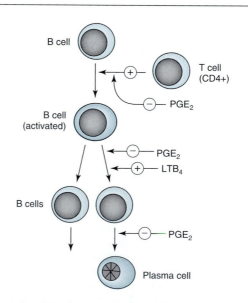

Figure 18–6. The activation and proliferation of B lymphocytes by T lymphocytes (CD4+) are inhibited by PGE_2. Both mitogen- and antigen-induced B cell proliferation is inhibited by PGE_2 and stimulated by LTB_4. PGE_2 inhibits the differentiation of B cells into plasma cells and thus indirectly inhibits IgM synthesis.

studied and are still under investigation. Two approaches have been used. The first adds corn, safflower, and sunflower oils, which contain linoleic acid (C18:2), to the diet. The second approach adds oils containing eicosapentaenoic (C20:5) and docosahexaenoic acids (C22:6) from cold water fish. These are so-called ω3 fatty acids. Both types of diet change the phospholipid composition of cell membranes by replacing arachidonic acid with the dietary fatty acids. It has been claimed that the synthesis of both TXA_2 and PGI_2 is reduced and that changes in platelet aggregation, vasomotor spasm, and cholesterol metabolism follow.

As indicated above, there are many possible oxidation products of the different polyenoic acids. It is probably naive to ascribe the effects of dietary intervention reported thus far to such metabolites. Carefully controlled clinical studies will be needed before these questions can be satisfactorily answered. However, subjects on diets containing highly saturated fatty acids clearly show increased platelet aggregation when compared with other study groups. Such diets (eg, in Finland and the USA) are associated with higher rates of myocardial infarction than are more polyunsaturated diets (eg, in Italy).

PREPARATIONS AVAILABLE

Alprostadil
Penile injection (Caverject): 10, 20 μg sterile powder for reconstitution
Penile pellet (Muse): 125, 250, 500, 1000 μg
Parenteral (Prostin VR Pediatric): 500 μg/mL ampules
Carboprost tromethamine*
Parenteral: 250 μg carboprost and 83 μg tromethamine per mL ampules
Dinoprostone [prostaglandin E_2] (Prostin E2, Prepidil, Cervidil)

Vaginal: 20 mg suppositories, 0.5 mg gel, 10 mg controlled release system
Epoprostenol [prostacyclin] (Flolan, Cyclo-prostin)
Intravenous: 3, 5, 10, 15 μg/mL
Latanoprost (Xalatan)
Topical: 50 μg/mL ophthalmic solution
Misoprostol (Cytotec)
Oral: 100 and 200 μg tablets
Zileuton (Zyflow)
Oral: 600 mg tablets

REFERENCES

Agrawal NM: Epidemiology and prevention of nonsteroidal anti-inflammatory drug effects in the gastrointestinal tract. Br J Rheumatol 1995;34(Suppl 1):5.

Baulieu EE: The combined use of prostaglandin and antiprogestin in human fertility control. Adv Prostaglandin Thromboxane Leukot Res 1995;23:55.

Borgida AF et al: Second-trimester abortion by intramuscular 15-methyl-prostaglandin $F_{2α}$ or intravaginal prostaglandin E_2 suppositories: A randomized trial. Obstet Gynecol 1995;85:697.

Christ GJ: The penis as a vascular organ: The importance of corporal smooth muscle tone in the control of erection. Urol Clin North Am 1995;22:727.

Claesson HE, Odlander B, Jakobsson PJ: Leukotriene B_4 in the immune system. Int J Immunopharmacol 1992; 14:441.

Dahlen S-E et al (editors): Leukotrienes as mediators of asthma and inflammation: Basic and applied research. Second International Symposium on Trends in Eicosanoid Biology, Interlaken, Switzerland. Vol 22 of: *Advances in Prostaglandin, Thromboxane, and Leukotriene Research.* Raven Press, 1994.

Eberhart CE, DuBois RN: Eicosanoids and the gastrointestinal tract. Gastroenterology 1995;109:285.

Foegh ML: Obstetrics and gynecology. In: *Prostaglandins in Clinical Practice.* Watkins WD et al (editors). Raven Press, 1989.

Foegh ML et al: Urinary thromboxane A_2 metabolites in patients presenting in the emergency room with acute chest pain. J Int Med 1994;235:153.

Goetzl EJ, An S, Smith WL: Specificity of expression and effects of eicosanoid mediators in normal physiology and human diseases. FASEB J 1995;9:1051.

Hayashi RH: Pharmacological application of prostaglandins, their analogues, and their inhibitors in obstetrics. In: *Uterine Function: Molecular and Cellular Aspects.* Carsten ME, Miller JD (editors). Plenum, 1990.

Holtzman MJ: Arachidonic acid metabolism in airway epithelial cells. Annu Rev Physiol 1992;54:303.

Lands WEM: Biochemistry and physiology of n-3 fatty acids. FASEB J 1992;6:2530.

Lewis RA, Austen KF, Soberman RJ: Leukotrienes and other products of the 5-lipoxygenase pathway: Biochemistry and relation to pathobiology in human diseases. N Engl J Med 1990;323:645.

McGiff JC: Cytochrome P-450 metabolism of arachidonic acid. Annu Rev Pharmacol Toxicol 1991;31:339.

Mitchell JA et al: Selectivity of nonsteroidal antiinflammatory drugs as inhibitors of constitutive and inducible cyclooxygenase. Proc Natl Acad Sci USA 1994;90:11693.

---

*Not available in the USA.

Olschewski H et al: Aerosolized prostacyclin and iloprost in severe pulmonary hypertension. Ann Intern Med 1996;124:820.

Phipps RP, Stein SH, Roper RL: A new view of prostaglandin E regulation of the immune response. Immunol Today 1991;12:349.

Porst H: The rationale for prostaglandin E_1 (alpha-alprostadil) in the management of male impotence. Adv Prostaglandin Thromboxane Leukot Res 1995;23:539.

Raisz LG: Physiologic and pathologic roles of prostaglandins and other eicosanoids in bone metabolism. J Nutr 1995;125(7 Suppl):2024S.

Rand JH et al: Reduction of annexin-V (placental anticoagulant protein-I) on placental villi of women with antiphospholipid antibodies and recurrent spontaneous abortion. Am J Obstet Gynecol 1994;171:1566.

Reichler A, Romem Y, Divon MY: Induction of labor. Curr Opin Obstet Gynecol 1995;7:432.

Resul B et al: Phenyl-substituted prostaglandins—potent and selective antiglaucoma agents. J Med Chem 1993;36:243.

Savage MP et al: Effect of thromboxane A_2 blockade on clinical outcome and restenosis after successful coronary angioplasty. Multi-Hospital Eastern Atlantic Restenosis Trial (M-Heart II). Circulation 1995;92:3194.

Silverstein FE et al: Misoprostol reduces serious gastrointestinal complications in patients with rheumatoid arthritis receiving nonsteroidal anti-inflammatory drugs. A randomized, double-blind, placebo-controlled trial. Ann Intern Med 1995;123:241.

Samuelsson B et al (editors): Prostaglandins and related compounds. Vols 21A and 21B of: *Advances in Prostaglandin, Thromboxane, and Leukotriene Research.* Raven Press, 1991.

Samuelsson B et al (editors): Ninth International Conference on Prostaglandins and Related Compounds. Vol 23 of: *Advances in Prostaglandin, Thromboxane, and Leukotriene Research.* Raven Press, 1995.

Smith SF et al: Lipocortin-1 distribution in bronchoalveolar lavage from healthy human lung: Effect of prednisolone. J Appl Physiol 1995;79:121.

Smith WL, DeWitt DL: Biochemistry of prostaglandin endoperoxide H synthase-1 and synthase-2 and their differential susceptibility to nonsteroidal anti-inflammatory drugs. Semin Nephrol 1995;15:179.

Williams CS, DuBois RN: Prostaglandin endoperoxide synthase: Why two isoforms? Am J Physiol 1996;270:G393.

Nitric Oxide, Donors, & Inhibitors 19

George Thomas, PhD, & Peter W. Ramwell, PhD

Until recently, endogenous production of oxides of nitrogen—in the form of nitrate ion—was known to occur only in macrophages as part of the defense system against parasitic and bacterial infection. Nitric oxide (NO) was considered a toxic smog pollutant. Recent findings, however, have shown that many cells synthesize nitric oxide and that this simple molecule plays major roles in the regulation of the cardiovascular, immune, and nervous systems.

DISCOVERY OF ENDOGENOUS NITRIC OXIDE

The first observations of the biologic role of NO were in rodent macrophages and neutrophils: In vitro exposure of these cells to endotoxin lipopolysaccharide released significant amounts of nitrite and nitrate into the cell culture medium. Furthermore, injection of endotoxin in vivo elevated urinary nitrite and nitrate, the two oxidation products of nitric oxide. This nitric oxide was found to originate from oxidation of the guanidino group of L-arginine.

The second observation was made by Furchgott and Zawadzki in 1980 using isolated vascular smooth muscle preparations. They discovered that following stimulation with acetylcholine or carbachol, the endothelium released a short-lived vasodilator, which—unlike endothelium-derived prostacyclin—was not blocked by cyclooxygenase inhibitors. They named this vasodilator **"endothelium-derived relaxing factor" (EDRF)** since it promoted relaxation of precontracted smooth muscle preparations as shown in Figure 19–1. Other workers confirmed and extended these findings. In 1987, by comparing the pharmacologic and biochemical properties of the suspect molecule, three independent groups reported that EDRF and nitric oxide are the same molecule. It was later reported that other vasodilator molecules may be a part of EDRF, but it appears clear that nitric oxide provides the major part of its activity. Subsequent studies revealed that nitric oxide was generated by many cells and was, like the eicosanoids (Chapter 18), found in almost all tissues.

BIOLOGIC SYNTHESIS & INACTIVATION OF NITRIC OXIDE

Synthesis

Although biologic investigation of nitric oxide is recent, the first synthesis of nitric oxide was reported by Joseph Priestly (the discoverer of oxygen) in 1790. Nitric oxide, written as NO· or simply NO, is a highly diffusible stable gas composed of one atom each of nitrogen and oxygen. It is synthesized by a family of enzymes that are collectively called nitric oxide synthase, NOS (EC 1.14.13.49). Three isoforms of NOS have been identified (Table 19–1). These three isoforms are heme-containing flavoproteins employing L-arginine as a substrate and requiring NADPH, flavin adenine dinucleotide, and tetrahydrobiopterin as cofactors. Phosphorylation may also have a regulatory effect on the activity of NO synthase. For example phosphorylation significantly reduces the activity of isoform I. However, very little is known about the effect of phosphorylation on the activities of isoform II and III.

Formation of nitric oxide from L-arginine and several nitric oxide donors is shown in Figure 19–2. Activation of NOS by the influx of extracellular calcium, as in the case of the constitutive enzyme, or following the activation of the inducible NOS (isoform II) by cytokines, results in the metabolism of L-arginine to L-citrulline and nitric oxide. The conversion of L-arginine to NO and L-citrulline is inhibited by several arginine competitors such as N^G-monomethyl-L-arginine (L-NMMA). Some NO donors, eg, nitro-

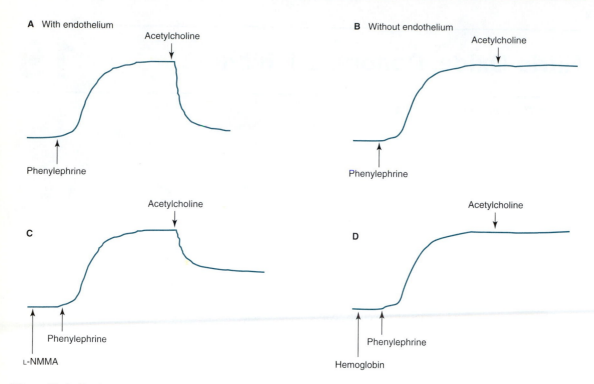

Figure 19–1. The isometric contractile response of the isolated rat aorta preparation to phenylephrine. **A:** Endothelium-dependent generation of EDRF (NO) from rat aorta by the vasodilator acetylcholine. **B:** Lack of generation of EDRF in the absence of endothelium. **C:** Inhibition of EDRF by the NO-synthase inhibitor L-NMMA. **D:** Inhibition of EDRF by hemoglobin, a scavenger of NO.

prusside, spontaneously generate NO in aqueous solutions whereas others, such as furoxans and organic nitrates and nitrites such as nitroglycerin, require the presence of a thiol compound such as cysteine. Once generated, NO interacts with the heme moiety of soluble guanylyl cyclase (Figure 19–2, right). This results in allosteric transformation and activation of the enzyme and leads to the formation of cGMP from GTP. Activation of the soluble guanylyl cyclase by NO can be inhibited by methylene blue. The affinity of nitric oxide for iron is also responsible for its inhibitory effect on several enzymes by interacting with the iron-sulfur centers of these enzymes. Interestingly, carbon monoxide, another gaseous compound produced endogenously from the catabolism of heme, also shares many of the properties of nitric oxide such as activation of soluble guanylyl cyclase. However, unlike nitric oxide, which has an extra electron, carbon monoxide is a stable molecule in the presence of oxygen. The affinity of nitric oxide for hemoglobin is several orders of magnitude greater than that of carbon monoxide. Nitric oxide undergoes both oxidative and reductive reactions, resulting in the formation of a variety of oxides of nitrogen (Table 19–2).

Inactivation

Nitric oxide is inactivated by heme and by the free radical, superoxide. Thus, scavengers of superoxide

Table 19–1. Properties of the three isoforms of nitric oxide synthase (NOS).

Property	Isoform I	Isoform II	Isoform III
Name	cNOS	iNOS	eNOS
Tissue	Neuronal, epithelial cells	Macrophages, smooth muscle cells	Endothelial cells
Expression	Constitutive	Transcriptional induction	Constitutive
Calcium requirement	Yes	No	Yes
Chromosome	12	17	7
Approximate mass of protein	150–160 kDa	125–135 kDa	133 kDa

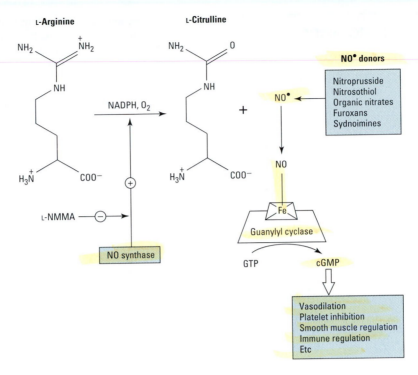

Figure 19–2. NO generation from L-arginine and NO donors and the formation of cGMP. L-NMMA inhibits NO-synthase. Some of the NO donors such as furoxans and organic nitrates and nitrites require a thiol cofactor such as cysteine or glutathione to form NO.

anion such as superoxide dismutase may protect nitric oxide, enhancing its potency and prolonging its duration of action. Conversely, interaction of nitric oxide with superoxide may generate the potent tissue-damaging moiety, peroxynitrite ($ONOO^-$), which has a high affinity for sulfhydryl groups and thus inactivates several key sulfhydryl-bearing enzymes. This effect of peroxynitrite is regulated by the cellular content of glutathione. Since glutathione is the major intracellular soluble sulfhydryl-containing compound, factors that regulate the biosynthesis and decomposition of glutathione may have important consequences.

Glutathione also interacts with nitric oxide under physiologic conditions to generate *S*-nitrosoglutathione, a more stable form of nitric oxide. Nitrosoglutathione may serve as an endogenous long-lived adduct or carrier of nitric oxide. Vascular glutathione is decreased in diabetes mellitus and atherosclerosis, and this may account for the increased incidence of cardiovascular complications in these conditions. Ischemia followed by reperfusion is another situation in which endothelial function is compromised owing to increased production of free radicals, resulting in reduced nitric oxide formation.

Table 19–2. Oxides of nitrogen.

Name	Symbol	Known Function
Nitric oxide	$NO^\bullet$	Vasodilator, platelet inhibitor, immune regulator, neurotransmitter
Nitroxyl anion	NO^-	Smooth muscle relaxant
Nitrogen dioxide	$NO_2^\bullet$	Free radical, nitrosating agent
Nitrous oxide	N_2O	Anesthetic
Dinitrogen trioxide	N_2O_3	Nitrosating agent
Dinitrogen tetraoxide	N_2O_4	Nitrosating agent
Nitrite	NO_2^-	Produce $NO^\bullet$ at acidic pH
Nitrate	NO_3^-	Stable oxidation product of $NO^\bullet$

EFFECTS OF NITRIC OXIDE

The field of nitric oxide research has exploded during the last decade. An extraordinary amount of data has been collected using a variety of experimental methods in systems ranging from isolated enzymes to small groups of patients. While final conclusions regarding the effects of this molecule will require much more research, the following paragraphs provide an introduction to some of the most interesting and provocative observations reported to date.

VASCULAR EFFECTS

Nitric oxide has a significant effect on vascular smooth muscle tone and blood pressure. As stated previously, it is released by acetylcholine and other endothelium-dependent vasodilators. It may play a role in the normal regulation of vascular tone as suggested by the fact that a reduction of nitric oxide synthesis (caused either by infusion of NOS inhibitors such as L-NMMA or by injury to the vascular endothelium) increases vascular tone and elevates mean arterial pressure. The effects of vasopressor drugs are increased by inhibition of NOS.

The vasodilator action of nitric oxide in vascular smooth muscle is mediated by its activation of soluble guanylyl cyclase. As described in Chapter 12 and shown in Figure 12–2, increased cGMP synthesis by guanylyl cyclase results in smooth muscle relaxation.

Apart from being a vasodilator, nitric oxide is also a potent inhibitor of neutrophil adhesion to the vascular endothelium. This is due to the inhibitory effect of nitric oxide on the expression of adhesion molecules on the endothelial surface. The role of nitric oxide in protecting the endothelium has been demonstrated by studies that showed that treatment with NO donors (see Figure 19–2 for examples) protects against ischemia- and reperfusion-mediated endothelial dysfunction.

HYPERTENSION ASSOCIATED WITH PREGNANCY

Preeclampsia is a major cause of maternal and perinatal mortality and morbidity throughout the world, and no satisfactory unifying theory of its causation has been advanced. The manifestations of preeclampsia appear to result from suppression of normal physiologic responses to pregnancy and resemble a combined deficiency of NO and prostacyclin. These manifestations include generalized vasoconstriction, increased blood pressure, increased capillary permeability, edema, a decrease in plasma volume, disseminated intravascular coagulation, decreased organ perfusion, decreased glomerular filtration rate, proteinuria, glomerular endotheliosis, liver dysfunction, and intrauterine growth retardation. Many investigators have reported maternal endothelial dysfunction in preeclampsia in that vascular prostacyclin and nitric oxide production is reduced and thromboxane and free radical formation enhanced. Attempts to decrease the incidence of preeclampsia with low-dose aspirin therapy have not been successful, and it has been proposed that enhancing nitric oxide levels through nutritional supplementation with L-arginine may be effective. This remains to be tested.

RESPIRATORY DISORDERS

Nitric oxide has been administered by inhalation to newborns with pulmonary hypertension and acute respiratory distress syndrome. The current treatment for severely defective gas exchange in the newborn is with extracorporeal membrane oxygenation (ECMO), which does not directly affect pulmonary vascular pressures. NO inhalation decreases pulmonary arterial pressure and improves blood oxygenation. Thus, when pulmonary resistance is elevated, it is possible to exploit the vasodilator properties of nitric oxide by administering NO via inhalation of a few parts per million. Adults with respiratory distress syndrome also appear—in open trials—to benefit from NO inhalation. Nitric oxide may have an additional role in relaxing airway smooth muscle and thus acting as a bronchodilator. For these reasons, NO inhalation therapy is being widely tested in both infants and adults with acute respiratory distress syndrome. The adverse effects of this use of NO are being assessed.

SEPTIC SHOCK

As mentioned previously, increased urinary excretion of nitrate, the oxidative product of nitric oxide, is reported in gram-negative bacterial infection. Lipopolysaccharide components from the bacterial wall activate the inducible NOS, resulting in exaggerated hypotension, shock, and possible death. This hypotension is reversed by NOS inhibitors and by compounds such as methylene blue, which prevent the action of nitric oxide. However, there has been no correlation between the hemodynamic effects of the nitric oxide inhibitors and survival rate in gram-negative sepsis thus far.

ATHEROSCLEROSIS

Vascular plaque formation in hypercholesterolemia leads to reduced NO formation and endothelium-dependent vasodilator responses. In vitro, NO carriers and donors and cGMP analogs inhibit smooth muscle cell proliferation. In animal models, myointimal proliferation following angioplasty can be blocked by feeding arginine, by using NO donors, by NOS gene transfer, and by NO inhalation. In addition, nitric oxide may act as an antioxidant, blocking the oxidation of low-density lipoproteins (LDL) and thus preventing the formation of foam cells in the vascular wall.

PLATELETS

Abnormal activation of platelets is associated with increased platelet adhesion and aggregation and therefore a higher incidence of thrombotic events. Platelet activation also leads to release of smooth muscle mitogens such as growth factors and thromboxane. Nitric oxide is a potent inhibitor of platelet adhesion and aggregation. Thus, endothelial dysfunction and the associated decrease in nitric oxide generation may result in abnormal platelet function. Platelets also contain both constitutive and inducible NOS, though to a much lesser extent than endothelial cells. As in vascular smooth muscle, cGMP mediates the protective effect of nitric oxide in platelets. Nitric oxide may have an additional beneficial effect on blood coagulation by enhancing fibrinolysis via an effect on plasminogen.

ORGAN TRANSPLANTATION

Accelerated graft atherosclerosis following organ transplantation is a chronic condition and is a major cause of transplant failure, leading to retransplantation or death. Continuous vascular smooth muscle proliferation occurs within the vasculature of most grafts and is a central event in luminal narrowing. Ischemic and reperfusion injuries at the time of organ harvesting, preservation, and revascularization initiate myointimal proliferation, which is also promoted by the continuous immune response to the allogeneic organ graft. By reducing free radical toxicity under these conditions, nitric oxide may act as a cytoprotective agent, inhibiting platelet and neutrophil aggregation and adhesion to the vascular wall. Dietary L-arginine supplementation increases plasma nitrite and nitrate formation and has been shown to attenuate accelerated graft atherosclerosis. However, excessively high concentrations of NO may be detrimental during *acute* organ rejection due to up-regulation of inducible NOS by cytokines; under these circumstances, *inhibition* of NO synthesis has been shown to prolong graft survival in experimental animals.

THE CENTRAL NERVOUS SYSTEM

Nitric oxide may have a major role in the central nervous system—as a neurotransmitter, as a modulator of ligand-gated receptors, or both. The likely cellular targets of nitric oxide in the central nervous system include pre- and postsynaptic nerve terminals. Nitric oxide modifies neurotransmitter release in different areas of the brain. Postsynaptic release of nitric oxide following activation of the NMDA receptor may initiate presynaptic transmitter release of glutamate, ie, NO may function as a *retrograde* messenger that is synthesized in postsynaptic sites following opening of the Ca^{2+} channels and activation of NOS. It is proposed that the NO thus produced rapidly diffuses to the presynaptic nerve terminal where guanylyl cyclase is activated to yield cGMP and thus facilitate transmitter release. In the cerebellum and in neuroblastoma cells, this effect is blocked by NOS inhibitors such as L-NMMA and is enhanced by L-arginine. It has been suggested that nitric oxide (like many other substances) may have a role in short- and long-term potentiating effects on excitatory amino acids in brain development and learning.

However, as in the case of acute rejection of organ transplants, not all the central nervous system effects of nitric oxide are physiologic or benign. It is well known that prolonged NMDA glutamate receptor activation results in degeneration of neurons (excitotoxicity). This has been attributed to a large increase in calcium influx, which activates the calmodulin-dependent NOS isoform I and leads to sustained elevation of nitric oxide concentrations. The increase in neurodegeneration caused by excitatory amino acids may be due to enhanced oxygen radical formation since superoxide dismutase has a beneficial effect in experimental models. The damage may also be mediated by the generation of secondary radicals such as peroxynitrite, which has a high affinity for sulfhydryl-containing enzymes such as calcium ATPase. Inhibition of calcium ATPases by peroxynitrite may in turn lead to enhanced Ca^{2+} accumulation and associated neurodegeneration.

High levels of nitric oxide have also been shown to cause destruction of photoreceptor cells in the retina. This is believed to be due to a prolonged increase in cGMP formation. Finally, nitric oxide and cGMP have been reported to have a role in epileptic seizures.

THE PERIPHERAL NERVOUS SYSTEM

There are extensive nonadrenergic, noncholinergic (NANC) neurons that are widely distributed in peripheral tissues, especially the gastrointestinal and reproductive tracts (see Chapter 6). Considerable evidence implicates nitric oxide as a mediator of certain NANC actions, and some NANC neurons appear to release NO. Penile erection is thought to be caused by the release of nitric oxide from NANC neurons; it is well documented that NO promotes relaxation of the smooth muscle in the corpus cavernosum—the initiating factor in penile erection—and inhibitors of NOS have been shown to prevent erection caused by pelvic nerve stimulation in the rat. Thus, impotence is a possible clinical indication for the use of a NO donor, and trials have been carried out with nitroglycerin ointment and the nitroglycerin patch. However, it appears that a better drug delivery system will be required for successful exploitation of this approach. At present, prostaglandin E_1 is employed, administered into the urethra or directly into the corpus cavernosum.

INFLAMMATION

Nitric oxide has a role in both acute and chronic inflammation. In experimental models of acute inflammation, inhibitors of NOS have a dose-dependent protective effect, suggesting that nitric oxide promotes edema and vascular permeability. Nitric oxide also has a detrimental effect in chronic models of arthritis; dietary L-arginine supplementation exacerbates arthritis whereas protection is seen with NOS inhibitors. Synovial fluid from patients with arthritis contains increased oxidation products of nitric oxide, particu-

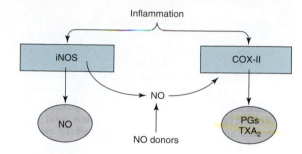

Figure 19–3. Model of the interaction between NO synthase and cyclooxygenase pathways in inflammation. (iNOS, i isoform of nitric oxide synthase; NO, nitric oxide; COX-II, isoform II of cyclooxygenase; PGs, prostaglandins; TXA_2, thromboxane A_2.)

larly peroxynitrite. Recent studies have shown that nitric oxide stimulates the synthesis of inflammatory prostaglandins by activating cyclooxygenase isoenzyme II (COX-2) (Figure 19–3 and Chapter 36). Thus, inhibition of the nitric oxide pathway may have a beneficial effect on inflammatory diseases, including joint diseases.

REFERENCES

Czapski G, Goldstein S: The role of the reactions of NO· with superoxide and oxygen in biological systems: A kinetic approach. Free Radic Biol Med 1995;19:785.

Furchgott RF, Khan MT, Jothianandan D: Comparison of endothelium-dependent relaxation and nitric oxide induced relaxation in rabbit aorta. Fed Proc 1987;46:385.

Furchgott RF, Zawadzki JV: The obligatory role of endothelial cells in the relaxation of arterial smooth muscle by acetylcholine. Nature 1980;288:373.

Hibbs JB Jr, Taintor RR, Vavrin Z: Macrophage cytotoxicity: Role of L-arginine deiminase activity and iminonitrogen oxidation to nitrite. Science 1987;235:473.

Ignarro LJ et al: Endothelium-derived relaxing factor from artery and vein is nitric oxide. Proc Natl Acad Sci USA 1987;84:92965.

Ignarro LJ: Physiology and pathophysiology of nitric oxide. Kidney Int 1996;(Suppl 55):S2.

Kelly RA, Balligand J-L, Smith TW: Nitric oxide and cardiac function. Circ Res 1996;79:363.

Lou H et al: L-Arginine prevents cardiac transplant arteriosclerosis by modulating the vascular cell proliferative response to insulin-like growth factor-I and interleukin-6. J Heart Lung Transplant. [In press.]

Lowe PN et al: Identification of the domains of neuronal nitric oxide synthase by limited proteolysis. Biochem Pharmacol 1996;314:55.

Moncada S, Higgs EA: Molecular mechanisms and therapeutic strategies related to nitric oxide. FASEB J 1995;9:1319.

Nakaki T, Nakayama M, Kato R: Inhibition by nitric oxide and nitric oxide-producing vasodilators of DNA synthesis in vascular smooth muscle cells. Eur J Pharmacol 1990;189:347.

Palmer RMJ, Ferrige AG, Moncada S: Nitric oxide release accounts for the biological activity of endothelium-derived relaxing factor. Nature 1987;327:524.

Ramwell PW, Thomas G: Nitric oxide and its role in transplantation. Transplant Proc 1995;27:2074.

Rossaint R et al: Inhaled nitric oxide for the adult respiratory distress syndrome. N Engl J Med 1993;328:399.

Salvemini D et al: Nitric oxide activates cyclooxygenase enzymes. Proc Natl Acad Sci USA 1993;90:7240.

Volk T et al: Endothelial damage induced by nitric oxide: Synergism with reactive oxygen species. Biochem Biophys Res Commun 1995;213:196.

Bronchodilators & Other Agents Used in Asthma

Homer A. Boushey, MD

The clinical hallmarks of asthma are recurrent, episodic bouts of coughing, shortness of breath, chest tightness, and wheezing. Most people with asthma have a mild form of the disease, with symptoms occurring only occasionally, eg, on exposure to allergens or certain pollutants, on exercise, or after a viral upper respiratory infection. More severe forms of asthma are associated with frequent attacks of wheezing dyspnea, especially at night, or even chronic limitation of activity. Indeed, asthma is the most common chronic disabling disease of childhood, but it affects all age groups. Asthma is physiologically characterized by increased responsiveness of the trachea and bronchi to various stimuli and by widespread narrowing of the airways that changes in severity either spontaneously or as a result of therapy. Its pathologic features are contraction of airway smooth muscle, mucosal thickening from edema and cellular infiltration, and inspissation in the airway lumen of abnormally thick, viscid plugs of mucus. Of these causes of airway obstruction, contraction of smooth muscle is most easily reversed by current therapy; reversal of the edema and cellular infiltration requires sustained treatment with anti-inflammatory agents. Asthma therapies are thus sometimes divided into two categories: "short-term relievers" and "long-term controllers."

Short-term relief is most effectively achieved with bronchodilators, agents that increase airway caliber by relaxing airway smooth muscle, and of these the β-adrenoceptor stimulants (Chapter 9) are the most widely used. Theophylline, a methylxanthine drug, and antimuscarinic agents (Chapter 8) are also used for reversal of airway constriction. Long-term control is most often achieved with an anti-inflammatory agent such as an inhaled corticosteroid or an inhibitor of mast cell degranulation, eg, cromolyn or nedocromil. The distinction between "short-term relievers" and "long-term controllers" has become blurred by the finding that theophylline inhibits some lymphocyte functions and modestly reduces airway mu-

cosal inflammation and that budesonide, an inhaled corticosteroid, produces modest immediate bronchodilation. Similarly, a recently released long-acting β-adrenoceptor stimulant, salmeterol, appears effective in improving asthma control when taken regularly. Finally, agents in the newly developed class of therapy, the leukotriene pathway inhibitors, also seem to produce benefit over both the short and long term.

This chapter presents the basic pharmacology of cromolyn, methylxanthines, and the leukotriene pathway inhibitors—agents whose medical use is almost exclusively for pulmonary disease. The other classes of drugs listed above are discussed in relation to the therapy of asthma.

PATHOGENESIS OF ASTHMA

A rational approach to the pharmacotherapy of asthma depends on an understanding of the disease's pathogenesis. In the classic immunologic model, asthma is a disease mediated by reaginic (IgE) antibodies bound to mast cells in the airway mucosa (Figure 20–1). On reexposure to an antigen, antigen-antibody interaction on the surface of the mast cells triggers both the release of mediators stored in the cells' granules and the synthesis and release of other mediators. The agents responsible for the early reaction—immediate bronchoconstriction—include histamine, tryptase and other neutral proteases, leukotrienes C_4 and D_4, and prostaglandins. These agents diffuse throughout the airway wall and cause muscle contraction and vascular leakage. Other mediators are responsible for the more sustained bronchoconstriction, cellular infiltration of the airway mucosa, and mucus hypersecretion of the late asthmatic reaction that occurs 2–8 hours later. These mediators are thought to be cytokines characteristically produced by TH2 lymphocytes, especially GM-CSF and interleukins 4 and 5, which attract and activate eosinophils and stimulate IgE production by B lymphocytes. It is

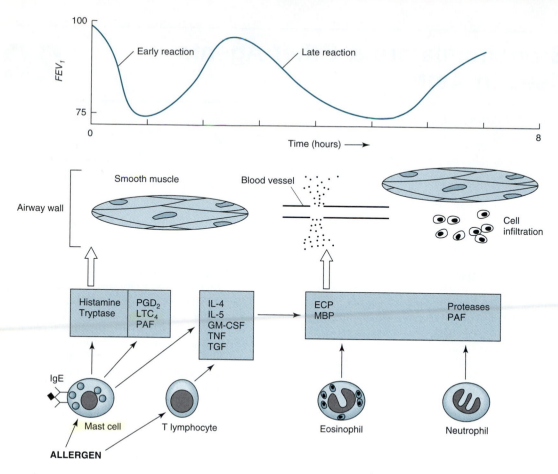

Figure 20–1. Conceptual model for the immunopathogenesis of asthma. Exposure to allergen causes synthesis of IgE, which binds to mast cells in the airway mucosa. On reexposure to allergen, antigen-antibody interaction on mast cell surfaces triggers release of mediators of anaphylaxis: histamine, tryptase, prostaglandin D_2 (PGD_2), leukotriene C_4, and platelet-activating factor (PAF). These agents provoke contraction of airway smooth muscle, causing the immediate fall in FEV_1. Reexposure to allergen also causes the synthesis and release of a variety of cytokines: interleukins 4 and 5, granulocyte-macrophage colony stimulating factor (GM-CSF), tumor necrosis factor (TNF), and tissue growth factor (TGF) from T cells and mast cells. These cytokines in turn attract and activate eosinophils and neutrophils, whose products include eosinophil cationic protein (ECP), major basic protein (MBP), proteases, and platelet-activating factor. These mediators cause the edema, mucus hypersecretion, smooth muscle contraction, and increase in bronchial reactivity associated with the late asthmatic response, indicated by a fall in FEV_1 2–8 hours after the exposure.

not clear whether lymphocytes or mast cells in the airway mucosa are the primary source of the cytokines and other mediators responsible for the late inflammatory response, but it is now thought that the benefits of corticosteroid therapy may result from their inhibition of cytokine production in the airways.

Not all of the features of asthma can be accounted for by the antigen challenge model. Some adults with asthma have no evidence of immediate hypersensitivity to antigens, and most severe exacerbations of asthma appear to be provoked by viral respiratory infection rather than by recent exposure to an unusual quantity of antigen. Even in patients with a history of asthma during the ragweed season and positive cutaneous and bronchial responses to ragweed antigen, the severity of symptoms correlates poorly with the quantity of antigen in the atmosphere. Furthermore, bronchospasm can be provoked by nonantigenic stimuli such as distilled water, exercise, cold air, sulfur dioxide, and rapid respiratory maneuvers.

This tendency to develop bronchospasm upon encountering stimuli that do not affect healthy nonasthmatic airways is characteristic of asthma and is sometimes called "nonspecific bronchial hyperreactivity" to distinguish it from bronchial responsiveness to specific antigens. Bronchial hyperreactivity is quantitated by measuring the fall in forced expiratory volume in 1 second (FEV_1) provoked by inhaling serially increasing concentrations of aerosolized histamine or methacholine. This exaggerated sensitivity of the airways appears to be fundamental to asthma's pathogenesis, for it is nearly ubiquitous in patients with asthma and its degree correlates with the symptomatic severity of the disease.

The mechanisms underlying bronchial hyperactivity are somehow related to inflammation of the airway mucosa. The agents that increase bronchial reactivity, such as ozone exposure, allergen inhalation, and infection with respiratory viruses, also cause airway inflammation. In both dogs and humans, the increase in bronchial reactivity induced by ozone is associated with an increase in the number of polymorphonuclear leukocytes found in fluid obtained by bronchial lavage or from bronchial mucosal biopsies. The increase in reactivity due to allergen inhalation is associated with an increase in both eosinophils and polymorphonuclear leukocytes in bronchial lavage fluid. The increase in reactivity that is associated with the

late asthmatic response to allergen inhalation (Figure 20–2) is sustained and, because it is prevented by treatment with inhaled corticosteroids immediately before antigen challenge, is thought to be caused by airway inflammation.

How the increase in airway reactivity is linked to inflammation is uncertain, but accumulating evidence points to the eosinophil. The most consistent difference in bronchial mucosal biopsies obtained from asthmatic and healthy subjects is an increase in the number of eosinophils found beneath the airway epithelium. Immunohistochemical staining shows increased levels of eosinophil cationic protein, indicating activation of the cells. The number of eosinophils in expectorated sputum or in fluid lavaged from the lungs correlates with the degree of bronchial hyperreactivity. Eosinophil products have in turn been shown to cause epithelial sloughing and an increase in contractile responsiveness of airway smooth muscle. However, the products of other cells in the airways,

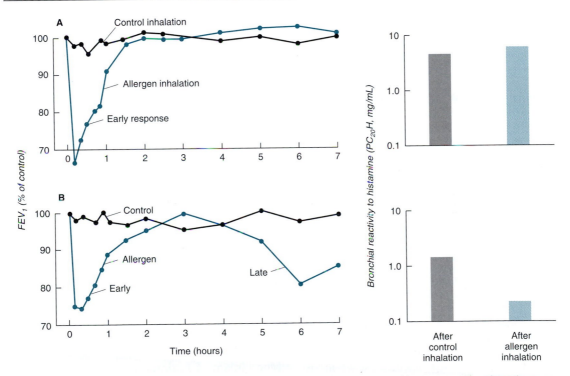

Figure 20–2. Comparison of responses to control and allergen inhalation in two subjects, one with only early responses (panel A) and one with both early and late bronchial responses (panel B). Forced expiratory volume in 1 second (FEV_1) is shown on the left as a percentage of the control value. Bronchoconstriction results in a fall in FEV_1. The doses (mg/mL) of inhaled histamine required to cause a 20% fall in FEV_1 ($PC_{20}H$) 8 hours after the control inhalation and 8 hours after the allergen inhalation are shown in the bar graphs on the right. An increase in responsiveness is shown by a decrease in the dose of histamine required. The subject shown in panel A had a transient drop in FEV_1 immediately after inhaling allergen but recovered rapidly and showed no later fall in this variable. He showed no increase in responsiveness to histamine 8 hours later (panel A). In contrast, the subject who showed a late bronchoconstriction response to the inhaled allergen (panel B, dip at 6 hours in the graph at left) also showed a marked reduction in the dose of histamine required to cause a further bronchoconstrictor response (bar graph, after allergen inhalation). (Redrawn from Cockcroft DW et al: Allergen-induced increase in non-allergic bronchial reactivity. Clin Allergy 1977;7:503.)

such as macrophages, mast cells, sensory nerves, and epithelial cells, have also been shown to alter airway smooth muscle function, so a specific antagonist to a single mediator or class of mediators might not prove wholly effective as asthma therapy. A possible example is zafirlukast, the leukotriene receptor antagonist recently approved for use. While clinical trials show it to improve asthma control, it is not curative and is not effective in all patients (see below).

Whatever the mechanisms responsible for bronchial hyperreactivity, bronchoconstriction itself seems to result not simply from the direct effect of the released mediators but also from their activation of neural or humoral pathways. Evidence for the importance of neural pathways stems largely from studies of laboratory animals. Thus, the bronchospasm provoked in dogs by histamine can be greatly reduced by pretreatment with an inhaled topical anesthetic agent, by transection of the vagus nerves, and by pretreatment with atropine, a competitive antagonist of acetylcholine. Studies of asthmatic humans, however, have shown that treatment with atropine causes only a reduction in—not abolition of—the bronchospastic responses to antigens and to nonantigenic stimuli, such as exercise or inhalation of cold air, sulfur dioxide, or distilled water. While it is possible that activity in some other neural pathway (eg, the nonadrenergic, noncholinergic system; Chapter 6) contributes to bronchomotor responses to nonspecific (ie, nonantigenic) stimuli, their inhibition by cromolyn, a drug that appears to inhibit mast cell degranulation, suggests that both antigenic and nonantigenic stimuli may provoke the release from mast cells of mediators that stimulate smooth muscle contraction by direct and indirect mechanisms (Figure 20–3).

The hypothesis suggested by these studies—that asthmatic bronchospasm results from a combination of release of mediators and an exaggeration of responsiveness to their effects—predicts that asthma may be effectively treated by drugs with different modes of action. Asthmatic bronchospasm might be reversed or prevented, for example, by drugs that prevent mast cell degranulation (cromolyn or nedocromil, sympathomimetic agents, calcium channel blockers), inhibit the effect of acetylcholine released from vagal motor nerves (muscarinic antagonists), or directly relax airway smooth muscle (sympathomimetic agents, theophylline).

Another approach to the treatment of asthma is aimed not just at preventing or reversing acute bronchospasm but at reducing the level of bronchial responsiveness. Because increased responsiveness appears to be linked to airway inflammation and because airway inflammation is a feature of late asthmatic responses, this strategy is implemented both by reducing exposure to the allergens that provoke inflammation and by prolonged therapy with anti-inflammatory agents, especially inhaled corticosteroids.

I. BASIC PHARMACOLOGY OF AGENTS USED IN THE TREATMENT OF ASTHMA

CROMOLYN & NEDOCROMIL

Cromolyn sodium (disodium cromoglycate) and nedocromil sodium differ from most antiasthmatic medications in that they are only of value when taken prophylactically. They are stable but extremely insoluble salts (see structures below). When used as aerosols (metered-dose inhalers), they effectively inhibit both antigen- and exercise-induced asthma, and chronic use (four times daily) may reduce the overall level of bronchial reactivity; however, these drugs have no effect on airway smooth muscle tone and are ineffective in reversing asthmatic bronchospasm.

Cromolyn sodium

Nedocromil sodium

Cromolyn is poorly absorbed from the gastrointestinal tract. For use in asthma, it must be applied topically by inhalation of a microfine powder or aerosolized solution as described below. When given by inhalation or orally, less than 10% is absorbed, and most is excreted unchanged. Nedocromil also has a very low bioavailability and is available only in metered-dose aerosol form.

Mechanism of Action

Cromolyn and nedocromil differ structurally but are thought to share a common mechanism of action. The fundamental action, best shown for nedocromil, appears to be alteration in the function of delayed chloride channels in the cell membrane, inhibiting cellular activation (Barnes et al, 1995). This action on airway nerves is thought to be responsible for nedocromil's inhibition of cough; on mast cells, for inhibition of the early response to antigen challenge; and on eosinophils, for the inhibition of the late re-

Figure 20–3. Mechanisms of response to inhaled irritants. The airway is represented microscopically by a cross-section of the wall with branching vagal sensory endings lying adjacent to the lumen. Afferent pathways in the vagus nerves travel to the central nervous system; efferent pathways from the central nervous system travel to efferent ganglia. Postganglionic fibers release acetylcholine (ACh), which binds to muscarinic receptors on airway smooth muscle. Inhaled materials may provoke bronchoconstriction by several possible mechanisms. First, they may trigger the release of chemical mediators from mast cells. Second, they may stimulate afferent receptors to initiate reflex bronchoconstriction or to release tachykinins (eg, substance P) that directly stimulate smooth muscle contraction.

sponse. The inhibitory effect on mast cells appears to be specific for cell type, since cromolyn has little inhibitory effect on mediator release from human basophils. It may also be specific for different organs, since cromolyn inhibits mast cell degranulation in human and primate lung but not in skin. This in turn may reflect differences in mast cells found in different sites. For example, mast cells from human lung and skin differ in their neutral protease content. Lung mast cells contain only tryptase, while skin mast cells contain both tryptase and chymase.

Until recently, the idea that cromolyn inhibits mast cell degranulation was so well accepted that the inhibition of a response by cromolyn was thought to indicate the involvement of mast cells in the response.

This simplistic idea has been overturned in part by the finding that cromolyn and nedocromil inhibit the function of cells other than mast cells and in part by the finding that nedocromil inhibits appearance of the late response even when given after the early response to antigen challenge, ie, after mast cell degranulation has occurred (Pelikan et al, 1993).

Clinical Use of Cromolyn & Nedocromil

The efficacy of cromolyn has been demonstrated in patients in several circumstances. Pretreatment with cromolyn blocks the bronchoconstriction caused by antigen inhalation, by exercise, by aspirin, and by a variety of causes of occupational asthma, including toluene diisocyanate, wood dusts, soldering fluxes, piperazine hydrochloride, and certain enzymes. This acute protective effect of a single treatment makes cromolyn useful for administration shortly before exercise or before unavoidable exposure to an allergen.

Cromolyn is also effective in reducing the symptomatic severity and the need for bronchodilator medications in patients with perennial asthma. Not all patients benefit from chronic therapy, and although young patients with extrinsic asthma are most likely to respond favorably, some older patients with intrinsic disease also improve. At present, the only way of determining whether a patient will respond is by a therapeutic trial for 4 weeks. In those who respond, the effectiveness of regular use of cromolyn in controlling asthmatic symptoms appears to be roughly equal to that of maintenance theophylline therapy.

It has been proposed that chronic treatment with cromolyn causes a decrease in bronchial hyperreactivity, perhaps by protecting the airway against the inflammatory effects of the chemical mediators of anaphylaxis. At present, cromolyn appears to effectively prevent seasonal increases in bronchial reactivity in patients with allergic asthma, but it seems to be less effective than inhaled corticosteroids in reducing bronchial reactivity.

Cromolyn is effective in asthma only when inhaled directly into the airways. Two methods of administration are currently used. In adults, the drug is given by metered-dose inhaler. The usual dose is 2–4 mg inhaled four times daily. In children, who may have difficulty coordinating the use of the inhaler device, cromolyn may be given by aerosol of a 1% solution.

Cromolyn solution is also useful in reducing symptoms of **allergic rhinitis.** Applying the solution by nasal spray or eye drops several times a day is effective in about 75% of patients with **hay fever,** even during the peak pollen season.

Because it is so poorly absorbed, adverse effects of cromolyn are minor and are localized to the sites of deposition. These include such symptoms as throat irritation, cough, mouth dryness, chest tightness, and wheezing. Some of these symptoms can be prevented by inhaling a β_2-adrenoceptor agonist before cromolyn treatment. Serious adverse effects are rare. Reversible dermatitis, myositis, or gastroenteritis occurs in about 2% of patients, and a very few cases of pulmonary infiltration with eosinophilia and anaphylaxis have been reported.

Nedocromil appears to have greater inhibitory action on primate lung mast cells in vitro and has given promising results in large clinical trials. Nedocromil may offer greater antiasthmatic potency than cromolyn.

Nedocromil appears to be roughly equipotent to standard doses of inhaled corticosteroids in patients with moderate asthma (Ruffin et al, 1987), and the addition of nedocromil to a standard dose of an inhaled corticosteroid appears to improve asthma control.

METHYLXANTHINE DRUGS

The three important methylxanthines are theophylline, theobromine, and caffeine. Their major source is, of course, beverages (tea, cocoa, and coffee, respectively). The importance of theophylline as a therapeutic agent in the treatment of asthma is waning as the greater effectiveness of inhaled adrenoceptor agents for acute asthma and of inhaled anti-inflammatory agents for chronic asthma has been established.

Chemistry

As shown below, theophylline is 1,3-dimethylxanthine; theobromine is 3,7-dimethylxanthine; and caffeine is 1,3,7-trimethylxanthine. The theophylline preparation most commonly used for therapeutic purposes is aminophylline, a theophylline-ethylenediamine complex. A synthetic analog of theophylline (dyphylline) is both less potent and shorter-acting than theophylline. The pharmacokinetics of theophylline are discussed below (see Clinical Use of Methylxanthines). The metabolic products, partially demethylated xanthines (not uric acid), are excreted in the urine.

Xanthine

Theobromine

Caffeine

Theophylline

Mechanism of Action

Several mechanisms have been proposed for the action of the methylxanthines, but none have been established as responsible for the bronchodilating effect. At high concentrations, the drugs can be shown in vitro to inhibit the enzyme phosphodiesterase (Figure 20–4). Since phosphodiesterase hydrolyzes cyclic nucleotides, this inhibition results in higher concentrations of intracellular cAMP. This effect could explain the cardiac stimulation and smooth muscle relaxation produced by these drugs, but it is not certain that sufficiently high concentrations are achieved in

Figure 20–4. Bronchodilation is promoted by cAMP. Intracellular levels of cAMP can be increased by beta-adrenoceptor agonists, which increase the rate of its synthesis by adenylyl cyclase (AC); or by phosphodiesterase (PDE) inhibitors such as theophylline, which slow the rate of its degradation. Bronchoconstriction can be inhibited by muscarinic antagonists and possibly by adenosine antagonists.

vivo to inhibit phosphodiesterase. Another proposed mechanism is the inhibition of cell surface receptors for adenosine. These receptors modulate adenylyl cyclase activity, and adenosine has been shown to cause contraction of isolated airway smooth muscle and to enhance histamine release from cells present in the lung. These effects are antagonized by theophylline, which blocks cell surface adenosine receptors. It has also been shown, however, that xanthine derivatives devoid of adenosine-antagonistic properties (eg, enprofylline) may be more potent than theophylline in inhibiting bronchoconstriction in asthmatic subjects.

An anti-inflammatory action of theophylline has recently been proposed (Ward et al, 1993). Low doses of theophylline—below those necessary for bronchodilation—inhibit the late response to antigenic challenge, and withdrawal of theophylline causes worsening of asthmatic symptoms, a fall in spirometry, and significant increases in CD4+ and CD8+ lymphocytes in bronchial biopsies (Kidney et al, 1995).

Pharmacodynamics of Methylxanthines

The methylxanthines have effects on the central nervous system, kidney, and cardiac and skeletal muscle as well as smooth muscle. Of the three agents, theophylline is most selective in its smooth muscle effects, while caffeine has the most marked central nervous system effects.

A. Central Nervous System Effects: In low and moderate doses, the methylxanthines—especially caffeine—cause mild cortical arousal with increased alertness and deferral of fatigue. In unusually sensitive individuals, the caffeine contained in beverages, eg, 100 mg in a cup of coffee, is sufficient to cause nervousness and insomnia. At very high doses, medullary stimulation and convulsions may occur. Nervousness and tremor are primary side effects in

patients taking large doses of aminophylline for asthma.

B. Cardiovascular Effects: The methylxanthines have direct positive chronotropic and inotropic effects on the heart. At low concentrations, these effects appear to result from increased catecholamine release that is caused by inhibition of presynaptic adenosine receptors. At higher concentrations (> 10 μmol/L), calcium influx may be increased directly through the increase in cAMP that results from inhibition of phosphodiesterase. At very high concentrations (> 100 μmol/L), sequestration of calcium by the sarcoplasmic reticulum is impaired. In unusually sensitive individuals, consumption of a few cups of coffee may result in arrhythmias; but in most people, parenteral administration of higher doses of the methylxanthines produces only sinus tachycardia and increased cardiac output. Methylxanthines were once commonly used in the treatment of pulmonary edema associated with heart failure (Chapter 13). In large doses, these agents also relax vascular smooth muscle except in cerebral blood vessels, where they cause contraction. Ordinary consumption of coffee and other methylxanthine-containing beverages, however, usually raises the peripheral vascular resistance and blood pressure slightly, probably through the release of catecholamines.

Methylxanthines decrease blood viscosity and may improve blood flow under certain conditions. The mechanism of this action is not well defined, but the effect is exploited in the treatment of intermittent claudication with pentoxifylline, a dimethylxanthine agent. However, no evidence suggests that this therapy is superior to other approaches.

C. Effects on Gastrointestinal Tract: The methylxanthines stimulate secretion of both gastric acid and digestive enzymes. However, even decaffeinated coffee has a potent stimulant effect on secretion, which means that the primary secretagogue in coffee is not caffeine.

D. Effects on Kidney: The methylxanthines—especially theophylline—are weak diuretics. This effect may involve both increased glomerular filtration and reduced tubular sodium reabsorption. The diuresis is not of sufficient magnitude to be therapeutically useful.

E. Effects on Smooth Muscle: The bronchodilation produced by the methylxanthines is the major therapeutic action. Tolerance does not develop, but adverse effects, especially in the central nervous system, may limit the dose (see below). In addition to this direct effect on the airway smooth muscle, these agents—in sufficient concentration—inhibit antigen-induced release of histamine from lung tissue; their effect on mucociliary transport is unknown.

F. Effects on Skeletal Muscle: The therapeutic actions of the methylxanthines may not be confined to the airways, for they also strengthen the contractions of isolated skeletal muscle in vitro and have potent effects in improving contractility and in reversing fatigue of the diaphragm in patients with chronic obstructive lung diseases. This effect on diaphragmatic performance, rather than an effect on the respiratory center, may account for theophylline's ability to improve the ventilatory response to hypoxia and to diminish dyspnea even in patients with irreversible airflow obstruction.

Clinical Use of Methylxanthines

Of the xanthines, theophylline is the most effective bronchodilator, and it has been shown repeatedly both to relieve airflow obstruction in acute asthma and to reduce the severity of symptoms and time lost from work or school in chronic asthma. Theophylline base is only slightly soluble in water, so it has been administered as several salts containing varying amounts of theophylline base. The two commonly used theophylline salts are aminophylline, which contains 86% theophylline by weight; and oxtriphylline, which contains 64% by weight. Corrections must be made to ensure equivalent doses of theophylline for different preparations. Most preparations are well absorbed from the gastrointestinal tract; their absorption is not affected significantly by food. The absorption of rectal suppositories is unreliable, and these preparations should be used only in special circumstances.

Improvements in theophylline preparations have come from alterations in the physical state of the drugs rather than from new chemical formulations. For example, several companies now provide anhydrous theophylline in a microcrystalline form in which the increased surface area facilitates solubilization for complete and rapid absorption after oral administration. In addition, several sustained-release preparations (eg, Slo-Phyllin, Theo-Dur) are available and can produce therapeutic blood levels of theophylline for 12 hours or more. These preparations offer the advantages of less frequent drug administration, less fluctuation of theophylline blood levels, and, in many cases, more effective treatment of nocturnal bronchospasm.

Theophylline should only be used where methods to measure theophylline blood levels are available, because its therapeutic and toxic effects are related to its plasma concentrations. Improvement in pulmonary function is correlated with plasma concentration in the range of 5–20 mg/L. Anorexia, nausea, vomiting, abdominal discomfort, headache, and anxiety begin to occur at concentrations of 15 mg/L in some patients and become common at concentrations greater than 20 mg/L. Higher levels (> 40 mg/L) may cause seizures or arrhythmias; these may not be preceded by gastrointestinal or neurologic warning symptoms. Rational administration of theophylline, therefore, requires knowledge of its pharmacokinetics.

As described in Chapter 3, the initial or loading dose of a drug is determined by its volume of distribution (V_d) and the subsequent or maintenance dose by the rate of plasma clearance. The V_d for theophylline is proportionate to lean body weight but otherwise varies only slightly among individuals. On the average, the V_d is 0.5 L/kg, so a plasma concentration of 10 mg/L will be achieved by a loading dose of 5 mg of theophylline per kilogram of body weight. Because aminophylline contains 86% theophylline by weight, this is approximately equivalent to 6 mg/kg of aminophylline. If administered intravenously, the loading dose should be given over 30 minutes, since rapid injection ("IV push") may result in transient toxic plasma levels with the risk of seizures or cardiac arrhythmias.

The plasma clearance of theophylline has been shown to vary widely. Because theophylline is metabolized by the liver, a decrease in hepatic function caused by cirrhosis or a decrease in hepatic blood flow caused by heart failure may result in toxic concentrations of the drug. Conversely, clearance may be increased through the induction of hepatic enzymes by cigarette smoking or by changes in diet. In normal adults, the mean plasma clearance is 0.69 mL/kg/min (0.041 L/kg/h). Children appear to clear theophylline faster than adults (1–1.5 mL/kg/min; 0.06–0.09 L/kg/h). Neonates and young infants have the slowest clearance (Chapter 60). Even when maintenance doses are altered to correct for the above factors, plasma concentrations vary widely.

Intravenous therapy is now given only in unusual circumstances, because theophylline has been shown to add insignificantly to the bronchodilation achieved with frequent administration of aerosolized sympathomimetics. When it is given, an infusion rate of 0.7 mg/kg/h may be used in stable patients; but it should be decreased to approximately 0.6 mg/kg/h in acutely ill patients—and further still (to 0.3 mg/kg/h) in the presence of liver disease or heart failure. Theophylline levels should be measured 24 hours after starting treatment.

Theophylline is effective when taken orally, but its once dominant place in maintenance therapy is now unsettled. It improves long-term control of asthma when taken as the sole maintenance treatment or when added to inhaled corticosteroids. It is inexpensive, and it can be taken orally. Its use, however, also requires occasional measurement of plasma levels; it often causes unpleasant minor side effects (especially insomnia); and accidental or intentional overdose can result in severe toxicity or death. For oral therapy, the usual dose is 3–4 mg/kg of theophylline every 6 hours. Changes in dosage will result in a new steady-state concentration of theophylline in 1–2 days, so the dose may be increased at intervals of 2–3 days until therapeutic plasma concentrations are achieved (10–20 mg/L) or until adverse effects develop.

SYMPATHOMIMETIC AGENTS

The adrenoceptor agonists, discussed in detail in Chapter 9, have several pharmacologic actions that are important in the treatment of asthma—ie, they relax airway smooth muscle and inhibit release of some bronchoconstricting substances from mast cells. They may also inhibit microvascular leakage and increase mucociliary transport by increasing ciliary activity or by affecting the composition of mucous secretions. As in other tissues, the beta agonists stimulate adenylyl cyclase and catalyze the formation of cAMP in the airway tissues (Figure 20–4).

The best-characterized action of the adrenoceptor agonists on airways is relaxation of airway smooth muscle that results in bronchodilation. Although there is no evidence for direct sympathetic innervation of human airway smooth muscle, there is ample evidence for the presence of adrenoceptors on airway smooth muscle. In general, stimulation of β_2 receptors relaxes airway smooth muscle, inhibits mediator release, and causes skeletal muscle tremor as a toxic effect.

The sympathomimetic agents that have been widely used in the treatment of asthma include epinephrine, ephedrine, isoproterenol, and a number of β_2-selective agents (Figure 20–5). Because epinephrine and isoproterenol cause more cardiac stimulation (mediated by β_1 receptors), they should probably be reserved for special situations (see below).

Epinephrine is an effective, rapidly acting bronchodilator when injected subcutaneously (0.4 mL of 1:1000 solution) or inhaled as a microaerosol from a pressurized canister (320 μg per puff). Maximal bronchodilation is achieved 15 minutes after inhalation and lasts 60–90 minutes. Because epinephrine stimulates β_1 as well as β_2 receptors, tachycardia, arrhythmias, and worsening of angina pectoris are troublesome adverse effects.

Ephedrine probably has the longest history of any drug used in treating asthma, for it was used in China for more than 2000 years before it was introduced into Western medicine in 1924. Compared with epinephrine, ephedrine has a longer duration, oral activity, more pronounced central effects, and much lower potency. Because of the development of more efficacious and β_2-selective agonists, ephedrine is now used infrequently in treating asthma. It was formerly prescribed in fixed-dose combination with theophylline and a sedative in commercial formulations. These fixed-dose combinations make adjustment of dosage of the individual agents impossible and should be avoided.

Isoproterenol is a potent bronchodilator; when inhaled as a microaerosol from a pressurized canister, 80–120 μg causes maximal bronchodilation within 5 minutes. When the drug is given as an aerosolized solution from a nebulizer, the larger particle size generated results in a smaller quantity being delivered to the tracheobronchial tree, so that larger doses must be given to achieve the same effect. Isoproterenol has a 60- to 90-minute duration of action. An increase in the asthma mortality rate that occurred in the United Kingdom in the mid 1960s was attributed to cardiac arrhythmias resulting from the use of high doses of inhaled isoproterenol, though this attribution remains a subject of controversy.

Beta$_2$-Selective Drugs

The β_2-selective adrenoceptor agonist drugs are the most widely used sympathomimetics for the treatment of asthma at the present time (Figure 20–5). These agents differ structurally from epinephrine in having a larger substitution on the amino group and in the position of the hydroxyl groups on the aromatic ring. They are effective after inhaled or oral administration and have a long duration of action and significant β_2 selectivity. **Albuterol, terbutaline, metaproterenol,** and **bitolterol** are available as metered-dose inhalers; 2.5–5 mg of albuterol and 15 mg of metaproterenol can be diluted in 1–2.5 mL of saline for delivery from a hand-held nebulizer. When given by inhalation, these agents cause bronchodilation equivalent to that produced by isoproterenol. Bronchodilation is maximal by 30 minutes and persists for 3–4 hours.

Albuterol, metaproterenol, and terbutaline are also prepared in tablet form. One tablet two or three times daily is the usual regimen; the principal adverse effects of skeletal muscle tremor, nervousness, and occasional weakness may be reduced by starting the patient on half-strength tablets for the first 2 weeks of therapy.

Of these agents, only terbutaline is available for subcutaneous injection (0.25 mg). The indications for this route are similar to those for subcutaneous epinephrine—severe asthma requiring emergency treatment when aerosolized therapy is not available or has

Figure 20–5. Structures of isoproterenol and several β₂-selective analogs.

been ineffective—but it should be remembered that terbutaline's longer duration of action means that cumulative effects may be seen after repeated injections.

A new generation of long-acting β₂-selective agonists has been under investigation. Of these agents, **salmeterol** has been approved and **formoterol** may be approved in the near future. These agents were developed for an increased duration of action (12 hours or more). Both drugs are potent selective β₂ agonists that appear to achieve their long duration of action as a result of high lipid solubility rather than resistance to metabolism. Their high lipid solubility permits them to dissolve in the smooth muscle cell membrane in high concentration. It is postulated that this dissolved drug functions as a "slow release depot" that provides drug to adjacent beta receptors over a long period (Anderson, 1993).

Although adrenoceptor agonists may be administered by inhalation or by the oral or parenteral routes, delivery by inhalation results in the greatest local effect on airway smooth muscle with the least systemic toxicity. Aerosol deposition depends on the particle size, the pattern of breathing (tidal volume and rate of airflow), and the geometry of the airways. Even with

particles in the optimal size range of 2–5 μm, 80–90% of the total dose of aerosol is deposited in the mouth or pharynx. Particles under 1–2 μm in size remain suspended and may be exhaled. Deposition can be increased by holding the breath in inspiration.

Toxicities

The use of sympathomimetic agents by inhalation at first raised fears about possible tachyphylaxis or tolerance to beta agonists and cardiac arrhythmias from β₁-adrenoceptor stimulation, hypoxemia, and fluorinated hydrocarbons in freon aerosol propellants. The concept that beta-agonist drugs cause worsening of clinical asthma by inducing tachyphylaxis to their own action remains unestablished. Most studies have shown only a small change in the bronchodilator response to beta stimulation after prolonged treatment with beta-agonist drugs, but other studies have shown a loss in the ability of beta-agonist treatment to inhibit the response to subsequent challenge with exercise, methacholine, or antigen challenge (referred to as a loss of "bronchoprotective" action).

A highly publicized epidemiologic study overseas reported an association between the risk of death or near-death from asthma and the use of two or more inhalers per month of **fenoterol,** a beta agonist not approved in the USA (Spitzer et al, 1992). Subsequent analysis of the data from this study suggested that increased beta-agonist use was a marker of disease severity, not an independent risk factor. A later meta-analysis of several published studies of the relationship found no association between risk of death from asthma and use of beta agonists by either oral or metered dose inhaler administration (Mullen et al, 1993).

Other experiments have demonstrated that arterial oxygen tension (PaO_2) may decrease after administration of beta agonists if ventilation/perfusion ratios in the lung worsen. This effect is usually small, however, and may occur with any bronchodilator drug; the significance of such an effect will depend on the initial PaO_2 of the patient. Supplemental oxygen may be necessary if the initial PaO_2 is decreased markedly or if there is a large decrease in PaO_2 during treatment with bronchodilators. Finally, there is concern over myocardial toxicity from freon propellants contained in all of the commercially available metered-dose canisters. While fluorocarbons may sensitize the heart to toxic effects of catecholamines, such an effect occurs only at very high myocardial concentrations, which are not achieved if inhalers are used as recommended. Under the terms of an international agreement, fluorocarbons will be removed from all inhalers before the end of this century. In general, β_2-adrenoceptor agonists are safe and effective bronchodilators when given in doses that avoid systemic adverse effects.

MUSCARINIC ANTAGONISTS

Leaves from *Datura stramonium* have been used in treating asthma for hundreds of years. Interest in the potential value of antimuscarinic agents has recently been increased by demonstration of the importance of the vagus in bronchospastic responses of laboratory animals and by the development of a potent antimuscarinic agent that is poorly absorbed after aerosol administration to the airways and is therefore not associated with systemic atropine effects.

Mechanism of Action

Muscarinic antagonists competitively inhibit the effect of acetylcholine at muscarinic receptors (Chapter 8). In the airways, acetylcholine is released from efferent endings of the vagus nerves, and muscarinic antagonists can effectively block the contraction of airway smooth muscle and the increase in secretion of mucus that occurs in response to vagal activity (Figure 20–4). Very high concentrations—well above those achieved even with maximal therapy—are required to inhibit the response of airway smooth muscle to nonmuscarinic stimulation. This selectivity of muscarinic antagonists accounts for their usefulness

as investigative tools in examining the role of parasympathetic pathways in bronchomotor responses but limits their usefulness in preventing bronchospasm. In the doses given, antimuscarinic agents inhibit only that portion of the response mediated by muscarinic receptors, and the involvement of parasympathetic pathways in bronchospastic responses appears to vary among individuals.

Clinical Use of Muscarinic Antagonists

Antimuscarinic agents are effective bronchodilators. When given intravenously, atropine, the prototypical muscarinic antagonist, causes bronchodilation at a lower dose than that needed to cause an increase in heart rate. The selectivity of atropine's effect can be increased further by administering the drug by inhalation. Studies of **atropine sulfate aerosol** have shown that it can cause an increase in baseline airway caliber—nearly equivalent to that achieved with beta-agonist agents—and that this effect persists for 5 hours. The dose required depends on the particle size of the aerosol used. Using a nebulizer producing particles with a diameter of 1–1.5 μm, systemic effects commonly occur when 2 mg is inhaled. The initial dose, then, should be 1 mg or less. Deposition of the aerosol in the mouth frequently causes a local drying effect. Adverse effects due to systemic absorption include urinary retention, tachycardia, loss of visual accommodation, and agitation.

The dose of an antimuscarinic drug causing maximal change in resting airway caliber is smaller than the dose needed to maximally inhibit bronchospastic responses (Figure 20–6), probably because the quan-

Figure 20–6. Inhibition of bronchomotor response to sulfur dioxide by two doses of atropine sulfate and by 10 mg of metaproterenol aerosol in one asthmatic subject. Specific airway resistance was measured after 5 minutes of eucapnic hyperpnea (40 L/min) of filtered air containing increasing amounts of SO_2. Note that all treatments caused equal changes in baseline-specific resistance but different degrees of inhibition of the response to SO_2.

tity of acetylcholine released under resting conditions is smaller than the quantity released in response to an inhaled irritant. This is an important consideration because asthma is characterized by episodic bouts of bronchospasm, often occurring in response to exercise or to inhalation of antigens or irritants.

Systemic adverse effects limit the quantity of atropine sulfate that can be given, but the development of a more selective quaternary ammonium derivative of atropine, **ipratropium bromide,** permits delivery of high doses to muscarinic receptors in the airways because the compound is poorly absorbed and does not readily enter the central nervous system. Studies with this agent have shown that the degree of involvement of parasympathetic pathways in bronchomotor responses varies among subjects. In some, bronchoconstriction is inhibited effectively; in others, only modestly. The failure of higher doses of the muscarinic antagonist to further inhibit the response in these individuals indicates that mechanisms other than parasympathetic reflex pathways must be involved.

Even in the subjects least protected by this antimuscarinic agent, however, the bronchodilation and partial inhibition of provoked bronchoconstriction are of potential clinical value, and antimuscarinic agents are valuable for patients intolerant of inhaled beta-agonist agents. While antimuscarinic agents generally appear to be slightly less effective than beta-agonist agents in reversing asthmatic bronchospasm, they appear to be at least as effective in patients with chronic obstructive pulmonary disease (COPD) that includes a partially reversible component. In acute severe asthma, the addition of ipratropium enhances the bronchodilation produced by nebulized albuterol.

CORTICOSTEROIDS

Mechanism of Action

Although corticosteroids have been used to treat asthma since 1950, their precise mechanism of action remains unknown. Like cromolyn, these drugs do not relax airway smooth muscle directly but reduce bronchial reactivity, increase airway caliber, and reduce the frequency of asthma exacerbations if administered for some time. Their effect on airway obstruction may be due in part to their potentiation of the effects of beta-receptor agonists, but their most important action is their inhibition of the eosinophilic airway mucosal inflammation in asthmatic airways. The principal anti-inflammatory action was once thought to be inhibition of the release of arachidonic acid from cell membranes and therefore reduction of the production of leukotrienes and prostaglandins, but the action now considered most important is their inhibition of the production of cytokines believed to be central in the initiation of the inflammatory cascade provoked by antigen inhalation and viral infection.

Clinical Use of Corticosteroids

Despite the consistency of clinical studies showing their efficacy, there is still controversy over the indications for initiating corticosteroid treatment of asthma and the appropriate dosage schedule. Because of severe adverse effects when given chronically, oral and parenteral corticosteroids are generally reserved for patients who require more urgent treatment, ie, those who have not improved adequately with bronchodilators or who experience worsening symptoms despite maintenance therapy. Patients with milder disease are treated with aerosol corticosteroids.

Urgent treatment is often begun with an oral dose of 30–60 mg of prednisone per day or an intravenous dose of 1 mg/kg of methylprednisolone every 6 hours; the daily dose is decreased gradually after airway obstruction has improved. In most patients, systemic cortico-steroid therapy can be discontinued in a week or 10 days, but in other patients symptoms may worsen as the dose is decreased to lower levels. Because adrenal suppression by corticosteroids is related to dose and because secretion of corticosteroids has a diurnal variation, it has become customary to administer corticosteroids early in the morning, after endogenous ACTH secretion has peaked. For prevention of nocturnal asthma, however, oral or inhaled corticosteroids are most effective when given in the late afternoon.

Aerosol treatment is the most effective way to decrease the systemic adverse effects of corticosteroid therapy. The introduction of lipid-soluble corticosteroids such as **beclomethasone, triamcinolone, flunisolide, fluticasone,** and **budesonide** makes it possible to deliver corticosteroids to the airways with minimal systemic absorption. An average daily dose of four puffs twice daily of beclomethasone is equivalent to about 10–15 mg/d of prednisone for the control of asthma, with far fewer systemic effects. Indeed, one of the cautions in switching patients from oral to inhaled corticosteroid therapy is to taper oral therapy slowly to avoid precipitation of adrenal insufficiency. In patients requiring continued prednisone treatment despite inhalation of standard doses of an inhaled corticosteroid, higher doses appear to be more effective; dosages up to 2000 µg/d of fluticasone have been used effectively to wean patients from chronic oral prednisone therapy. While these high doses of inhaled steroids may cause adrenal suppression, the risks of systemic toxicity from chronic use appear negligible compared with those of the oral corticosteroid therapy they replace. A special problem caused by inhaled topical corticosteroids is the occurrence of oropharyngeal candidiasis. The risk of this complication can be reduced by having patients gargle water and spit after each inhaled treatment. Hoarseness can also result from a direct local effect of inhaled corticosteroids on the vocal cords. These agents are remarkably free of other complications in adults, but not all concerns about the possible risks of osteoporosis or cataracts have been put to rest. In children, some concern persists over possible retardation of growth with inhaled corticosteroid therapy, but asthma itself delays puberty, and many studies have found no evidence of growth impairment.

Chronic use of inhaled corticosteroids effectively reduces symptoms and improves pulmonary function in patients with mild asthma. Such use also reduces or eliminates the need for oral corticosteroids in patients with more severe disease. In contrast to beta-stimulant agents and theophylline, chronic use of inhaled corticosteroids reduces bronchial reactivity. This important effect, which usually becomes apparent after 2–4 weeks, is both dose- and time-dependent. Bronchial reactivity is greatly reduced in some individuals, and the maximal reduction may not be achieved until the ninth to twelfth months of therapy. Because of the efficacy and safety of inhaled corticosteroids, they are now often prescribed for patients who require more than occasional inhalations of a beta agonist for relief of symptoms. Others give them as first-line therapy for mild asthma in combination with use of a beta agonist when needed. This therapy is continued for 10–12 weeks and then withdrawn to determine if more prolonged therapy is needed.

LEUKOTRIENE PATHWAY INHIBITORS

Because of the evidence of leukotriene involvement in many inflammatory diseases (Chapter 18) and in anaphylaxis, considerable effort has been expended on the development of drugs that block the synthesis of these arachidonic acid derivatives or their receptors. Leukotrienes result from the action of 5-lipoxygenase on arachidonic acid and are synthesized by a variety of inflammatory cells in the airways, including eosinophils, mast cells, macrophages, and basophils. Leukotriene B_4 is a potent neutrophil chemoattractant, and LTC_4 and LTD_4 exert many effects known to occur in asthma, including bronchoconstriction, increased bronchial reactivity, mucosal edema, and mucus hypersecretion. Early studies established that antigen challenge of sensitized human lung tissue results in the generation of leukotrienes, while other studies of human subjects have shown that inhalation of leukotrienes causes not only bronchoconstriction but also an increase in bronchial reactivity to histamine that persists for several days.

Two approaches to interrupting the leukotriene pathway have been pursued: inhibition of 5-lipoxygenase, thereby preventing leukotriene synthesis; and inhibition of the binding of leukotriene D_4 to its receptor on target tissues, thereby preventing its action. Efficacy in blocking airway responses to exercise and to antigen challenge has been shown for drugs in both categories: **zileuton**, a 5-lipoxygenase inhibitor, and **zafirlukast**, an LTD_4-receptor antagonist. Both have

the advantage of being effective when taken orally, and both have been shown to be effective (though apparently less so than inhaled cortico-steroids) when taken regularly in outpatient clinical trials (Holgate et al, 1996). Some patients appear to have particularly favorable responses, but no clinical features allow identification of "responders" before a trial of therapy. Zafirlukast has been approved for use in the USA in an oral dose of 20 mg twice daily. Zileuton has been approved for use in an oral dose of 600 mg given four times daily.

Zafirlukast

Zileuton

Trials with leukotriene inhibitors have demonstrated an important role for leukotrienes in aspirin-induced asthma. It has long been known that 5–10% of asthmatics are exquisitely sensitive to aspirin, so that ingestion of even a very small dose causes profound bronchoconstriction and symptoms of systemic release of histamine, such as flushing and abdominal cramping. Because this reaction to aspirin is not associated with any evidence of sensitization to aspirin or its metabolites, and because it is produced by any of the nonsteroidal anti-inflammatory agents, it is thought to result from inhibition of prostaglandin synthetase, shifting arachidonic acid metabolism from the prostaglandin to the leukotriene pathway. Support for this idea was provided by the demonstration that leukotriene pathway inhibitors impressively reduce the response to aspirin challenge.

OTHER DRUGS IN THE TREATMENT OF ASTHMA

Calcium Channel Blockers

Each of the cell functions that may become abnormal in patients with asthma—contraction of airway smooth muscle, secretion of mucus and of various mediators, and transmission along airway nerves—depends to some degree on the movement of calcium into cells. The calcium channel blockers have no effect on baseline airway diameter but do significantly inhibit the airway narrowing that is induced by various stimuli. In patients, both **nifedipine** and **verapamil** given by inhalation significantly inhibited the bronchoconstriction induced by exercise, hyperventilation, or inhalation of aerosolized histamine, methacholine, or antigen but were much less effective than inhaled albuterol. Indeed, in only one study was the protection against bronchoconstriction completely effective. Other studies showed only partial protection and considerable variability in drug effect between subjects. The reasons for the small effects of calcium channel blockers are uncertain.

Nitric Oxide Donors

Preliminary studies in animals suggest that airway smooth muscle, like that in the vasculature, is effectively relaxed by nitric oxide. This very lipophilic drug can be inhaled as a gas in acute asthma and dilates the pulmonary blood vessels as well as the airway smooth muscle. Although nitric oxide itself—or nitric oxide donors—may prove of value in acute severe asthma, it appears more likely that they will be used in pulmonary hypertension.

Potassium Channel Openers

Cromakalim is an investigational drug with vasodilating actions that are ascribed partly to alpha-adrenoceptor blockade and partly to direct hyperpolarization of smooth muscle cells by activation of potassium channels. A similar hyperpolarization may occur in the smooth muscle of the airways. Although relaxation of airway smooth muscle can be readily demonstrated in vitro, conflicting results have been obtained in asthma patients (Williams et al, 1990; Kidney et al, 1993).

Anti-IgE Monoclonal Antibodies

An entirely new approach to the treatment of asthma exploits the advances in molecular biology to target IgE antibody. From a collection of monoclonal antibodies raised in mice against IgE antibody itself, a monoclonal antibody was selected that appeared to be targeted against the portion of IgE that binds to its receptors (FCe-R1 and -R2 receptors) on mast cells and other inflammatory cells. This anti-IgE antibody inhibits the binding of IgE to mast cells but does not activate IgE already bound to these cells and thus does not provoke mast cell degranulation. In mice, it also appears to inhibit IgE synthesis by B lymphocytes. The murine antibody has been genetically "humanized" by replacing all but a small fraction of its amino acids with those found in human proteins, and it does not appear to cause sensitization when given to human subjects. A study aimed at examining the activity of the humanized monoclonal anti-IgE antibody in asthmatic volunteers showed that its administration over 10 weeks lowered plasma IgE to undetectable

levels and significantly reduced the magnitude of both the early and the late bronchospastic responses to antigen challenge (Fahy et al, 1996). Whether this innovative therapy will actually be effective in clinical treatment remains to be established.

II. CLINICAL PHARMACOLOGY OF DRUGS USED IN THE TREATMENT OF ASTHMA

BRONCHODILATORS

Patients with mild asthma and only occasional symptoms generally require no more than an inhaled beta-receptor agonist (eg, albuterol) on an "as-needed" basis. If symptoms require frequent aerosol inhalations (more often than twice a week), or if nocturnal symptoms occur, additional treatment is needed, preferably with an inhaled anti-inflammatory agent such as a corticosteroid or cromolyn. Theophylline is now largely reserved for patients in whom symptoms remain poorly controlled despite the combination of regular treatment with an inhaled anti-inflammatory agent and as-needed use of a β_2 agonist. If the addition of theophylline fails to improve symptoms or if adverse effects become bothersome, it is important to check the plasma level of theophylline to be sure it is in the therapeutic range (10–20 mg/L).

CORTICOSTEROIDS

If asthmatic symptoms occur frequently or if functionally limiting airflow obstruction persists despite bronchodilator therapy, inhaled corticosteroids should be started. For patients with severe symptoms or severe airflow obstruction (eg, $FEV_1 < 1.5$ L), initial treatment with oral corticosteroid (eg, 30 mg/d of prednisone for 3 weeks) is appropriate. Once clinical improvement is noted, inhaled corticosteroid treatment should be started and the oral dose reduced to the minimum necessary to control symptoms. For patients with milder symptoms but still inadequately controlled by as-needed use of an inhaled bronchodilator, corticosteroids may be initiated by the inhaled route.

Two recent studies in patients whose symptoms were inadequately controlled by a standard dose of an inhaled corticosteroid have compared the results from addition of salmeterol, a long-acting inhaled beta-receptor agonist, with doubling the dose of the inhaled corticosteroid. Both studies showed a prompt and sustained difference in favor of addition of the long-acting beta-receptor agonist. In patients on such a combined treatment regimen, it is important to provide explicit instructions that a standard, short-acting inhaled beta-agonist, like albuterol, be used for relief of acute symptoms.

CROMOLYN & NEDOCROMIL

Cromolyn or nedocromil may be considered as an alternative to inhaled corticosteroids in patients with symptoms occurring more than twice a week or who are wakened from sleep by asthma. They may also be useful in patients whose symptoms occur seasonally or after clear-cut inciting stimuli such as exercise or exposure to animal danders or irritants. In patients whose symptoms are continuous or occur without an obvious inciting stimulus, the value of these drugs can only be established with a therapeutic trial of inhaled drug four times a day for 4 weeks. If the patient responds to this therapy, the dose can be reduced. Maintenance therapy with cromolyn appears to be as effective as maintenance therapy with theophylline and, because of concerns over the possible long-term toxicity of systemic absorption of inhaled corticosteroids, has become widely used for treating children in the USA.

MUSCARINIC ANTAGONISTS

Inhaled muscarinic antagonists have so far earned a limited place in the treatment of asthma. When adequate doses are given, their effect on baseline airway resistance is nearly as great as that of the sympathomimetic drugs. The airway effects of antimuscarinic and sympathomimetic drugs given in full doses have been shown to have significant additive effects only in patients with severe airflow obstruction who present for emergency care. Antimuscarinic agents appear to be of significant value in chronic obstructive pulmonary disease—perhaps more so than in asthma. They are useful as alternative therapies for patients intolerant of beta-adrenoceptor agonists.

When muscarinic antagonists are used for long-term treatment, they appear to be effective bronchodilators. Although it was predicted that muscarinic antagonists might dry up airway secretions, direct measurements of fluid volume secretion from single airway submucosal glands in animals show that atropine decreases secretory rates only slightly; however, the drug does prevent excessive secretion caused by vagal reflex stimulation. No cases of inspissation of mucus have been reported following administration of these drugs.

OTHER ANTI-INFLAMMATORY THERAPIES

Some recent reports suggest that agents commonly used to treat rheumatoid arthritis might also be used to treat patients with chronic steroid-dependent asthma. The development of an alternative treatment is important, since chronic treatment with oral corticosteroids may cause osteoporosis, cataracts, glucose intolerance, worsening of hypertension, and cushingoid changes in appearance. Two double-blind prospective studies of prednisone-dependent asthmatic patients suggested that the use of methotrexate (15–50 mg/wk) permitted a reduction in prednisone dosage (Mullarkey et al, 1990; Shiner et al, 1990). However, subsequent studies have shown no such effect (Erzurum et al, 1991). Similarly, studies of prednisone-dependent asthmatics have reported benefit from treatment with oral gold (auranofin) and with cyclosporine. These promising results offer hope for the small proportion of patients whose asthma can be managed only with high doses of oral prednisone, but these results must be confirmed by larger studies before either treatment can be recommended.

MANAGEMENT OF ACUTE ASTHMA

The treatment of acute attacks of asthma in patients reporting to the hospital requires more continuous assessment and objective measurement of lung function than is necessary for chronic outpatient therapy. For patients with mild attacks, inhalation of a beta-receptor agonist is as effective as subcutaneous injection of epinephrine. Both of these treatments are more effective than intravenous administration of aminophylline. Severe attacks require treatment with oxygen, frequent or continuous administration of aerosolized albuterol, and systemic treatment with prednisone or methylprednisolone (0.5 mg/kg every 6 hours). Even this aggressive treatment is not invariably effective, and patients must be watched closely for signs of deterioration. Intubation and mechanical ventilation of asthmatic patients cannot be undertaken lightly but may be life-saving if respiratory failure supervenes.

PREPARATIONS AVAILABLE

Sympathomimetics Used in Asthma
Albuterol (Proventil, Ventolin, generic)
Inhalant: 90 μg/puff aerosol; 0.083, 0.5% solution for nebulization; 200 μg microfine capsules for inhalation
Oral: 2, 4 mg tablets; 2 mg/5 mL syrup
Oral sustained-release (Proventil Repetabs): 4 mg tablets
Bitolterol (Tornalate)
Inhalant: 0.37 mg/puff aerosol in 300 dose container
Ephedrine (generic)
Oral: 25, 50 mg capsules
Parenteral: 25, 50 mg/mL for injection
Epinephrine (generic, Adrenalin, others)
Inhalant: 1, 2.25% for nebulization; 0.16, 0.2, 0.25 mg epinephrine base aerosol in 233 and 350 dose containers
Parenteral: 1:1000 (1 mg/mL), 1:200 (5 mg/mL) for injection
Ethylnorepinephrine (Bronkephrine)
Parenteral: 2 mg/mL for injection
Isoetharine (generic, others)
Inhalant: 0.062, 0.08, 0.1, 0.125, 0.167, 0.17, 0.2, 0.25, 1% for nebulization; 340 μg/puff aerosol
Isoproterenol (generic, Isuprel, others)
Inhalant: 0.25, 0.5, 1% for nebulization; 80, 131 μg/puff aerosols
Oral: 10, 15 mg sublingual tablets
Parenteral: 0.2 mg/mL for injection
Metaproterenol (Alupent, Metaprel, generic)
Inhalant: 0.65 mg/puff aerosol in 75, 150 mg containers; 0.4, 0.6, 5% for nebulization
Oral: 10, 20 mg tablets; 10 mg/5 mL syrup
Pirbuterol (Maxair)
Inhalant: 0.2 mg/puff aerosol in 300 dose container
Salmeterol (Serevent)
Inhalant: 25μg salmeterol base/puff in 60 and 120 dose containers
Terbutaline (Brethine, Bricanyl)
Inhalant: 0.2 mg/puff aerosol
Oral: 2.5, 5 mg tablets
Parenteral: 1 mg/mL for injection

Antimuscarinic Drugs Used in Asthma
Ipratropium (Atrovent)
Aerosol: 18 μg/puff in 200 metered-dose inhaler; 0.02% (500 μg/vial) for nebulization
Nasal spray: 21 μg/spray

Cromolyn Sodium & Nedocromil Sodium
Cromolyn sodium
Pulmonary aerosol (Intal): 800 μg/puff in 200 dose container; 20 mg capsules for inhalation; 20 mg/2 mL for nebulization (for asthma)
Nasal aerosol (Nasalcrom)*: 5.2 mg/puff (for hay fever)
Oral (Gastrocrom): 100 mg capsules (for gastrointestinal allergy)

Nedocromil sodium (Tilade)
Pulmonary aerosol: 1.75 mg/puff in 112 metered-dose container

Aerosol Corticosteroids (See also Chapter 39.)
Beclomethasone (Beclovent, Vanceril)
Aerosol: 42 μg/puff in 200 dose container
Dexamethasone (Decadron Phosphate Respihaler)
Aerosol: 84 μg/puff in 170 dose container
Flunisolide (AeroBid)
Aerosol: 250 μg/puff in 100 dose container
Triamcinolone acetonide (Azmacort)
Aerosol: 100 μg/puff in 240 dose container
Fluticasone (Flovent)
Aerosol: 44, 110, and 220 μg/puff in 120 dose container

Methylxanthines: Theophylline & Derivatives
Aminophylline (theophylline ethylenediamine, 79% theophylline) (generic, others)
Oral: 105 mg/5 mL liquid; 100, 200 mg tablets,
Oral sustained-release: 225 mg tablets
Rectal: 250, 500 mg suppositories
Parenteral: 250 mg/10 mL for injection
Oxtriphylline, choline theophyllinate (64% theophylline) (generic, Choledyl)
Oral: 50 mg/5 mL mg syrup, 100 mg/5 mL elixir; 100, 200 mg tablets
Oral sustained-release: 400, 600 mg tablets
Theophylline (generic, Elixophyllin, Slo-Phyllin, Uniphyl, Theo-Dur, Theo-24, others)
Oral: 100, 125, 200, 250, 300 mg tablets; 100, 200 mg capsules; 26.7, 50 mg/5 mL elixirs, syrups, and solutions
Oral sustained-release: 8–12 hours: 50, 60, 65, 75, 100, 125, 130, 200, 250, 260, 300 mg capsules
Oral sustained-release: 8–24 hours: 100, 200, 300, 450 mg tablets
Oral sustained-release: 12 hours: 50, 75, 125, 130, 200, 250, 260 mg capsules
Oral sustained-release: 12–24 hours: 100, 200, 300 tablets
Oral sustained-release: 24 hours: 100, 200, 300, 400 mg tablets and capsules
Parenteral: 200, 400, 800 mg/container, theophylline and 5% dextrose for injection

Other Methylxanthines
Dyphylline (generic, other)
Oral: 200, 400 mg tablets; 33.3, 53.3 mg/5 mL elixir
Parenteral: 250 mg/mL for injection
Pentoxifylline (Trental)
Oral: 400 mg controlled-release tablets

Leukotriene Inhibitors
Zafirlukast (Accolate)
Oral: 20 mg tablets
Zileuton (Zyflo)
Oral: 600 mg tablets

*OTC preparation.

REFERENCES

Pathophysiology of Airway Disease

Barnes PJ, Chung KF, Page CP: Inflammatory mediators and asthma. Pharmacol Rev 1988;40:49.

Bousquet J et al: Eosinophilic inflammation in asthma. N Engl J Med 1990;323:1033.

Cockcroft DW: The bronchial late response in the pathogenesis of asthma and its modulation by therapy. Ann Allergy 1985;55:857.

Djukanović R et al: Mucosal inflammation in asthma. Am Rev Respir Dis 1990;142:434.

Gleich GJ, Loegering DA, Adolphson CR: Eosinophils and bronchial inflammation. Chest 1985;87(Suppl):10S.

Goldie RG: Receptors in asthmatic airways. Am Rev Respir Dis 1990;141(Suppl):S151.

Kay AB: Asthma and inflammation. J Allergy Clin Immunol 1991;87:893.

McFadden ER, Gilbert IA: Asthma. N Engl J Med 1992; 327:1928.

Weitzman M et al: Recent trends in the prevalence and severity of childhood asthma. JAMA 1992;268:2673.

Methylxanthines

Aubier M et al: Aminophylline improves diaphragmatic contractility. N Engl J Med 1981;305:249.

Becker AB et al: The bronchodilator effects and pharmacokinetics of caffeine in asthma. N Engl J Med 1984; 310:743.

Benowitz N: Clinical pharmacology of caffeine. Annu Rev Med 1990;41:277.

Brackett LE, Shamim MT, Daly JW: Activities of caffeine, theophylline, and enprofylline analogs as tracheal relaxants. Biochem Pharmacol 1990;39:1897.

Hirsh K: Central nervous system pharmacology of the dietary methylxanthines. In: *The Methylxanthine Beverages and Foods: Chemistry, Consumption, and Health Effects.* Spiller GA (editor). Alan Liss, 1984.

Kidney J et al: Immunomodulation by theophylline in asthma: Demonstration by withdrawal of therapy. Am J Respir Crit Care Med 1995;151:1907.

Murciano D et al: Effects of theophylline on diaphragmatic strength and fatigue in patients with chronic obstructive pulmonary disease. N Engl J Med 1984;311:349.

Murphy DG et al: Aminophylline in the treatment of acute asthma when β_2-adrenergics and steroids are provided. Arch Intern Med 1993;153:1784.

Persson CGA: The pharmacology of anti-asthmatic xanthines and the role of adenosine. Asthma Rev 1987;1:61.

Pincomb GA et al: Effects of caffeine on vascular resistance, cardiac output, and myocardial contractility in young men. Am J Cardiol 1985;56:119.

Thelle DS, Arnesen E, Frde OH: The Tromsø heart study: Does coffee raise serum cholesterol? N Engl J Med 1983;308:1454.

Ward AJ et al: Theophylline—an immunomodulating role in asthma? Am Rev Resp Dis 1993;147:518.

Cromolyn & Nedocromil

Aalbers R et al: The effect of nedocromil sodium on the early and late reaction and allergen-induced bronchial hyperresponsiveness. J Allergy Clin Immunol 1991; 87:993.

Barnes PJ et al: Asthma mechanisms, determinants of severity and treatment: the role of nedocromil sodium. Clin Exper Allergy 1995;25:771.

Bergmann K-Ch, Bauer CP, Overlack A: A placebo-controlled blinded comparison of nedocromil sodium and beclomethasone dipropionate in bronchial asthma. Lung 1990;168(Suppl):230.

Bruijnzeel PLB et al: Inhibition of neutrophil and eosinophil induced chemotaxis by nedocromil sodium and sodium cromoglycate. Br J Pharmacol 1990;99: 798.

Dahlen S-E et al: Dual inhibitory action of nedocromil sodium on antigen-induced inflammation. Drugs 1989;37(Suppl 1):63.

Neale MG et al: The pharmacokinetics of sodium cromoglycate in man after intravenous and inhalation administration. Br J Clin Pharm 1986;22:373.

Pelikan Z, Knotterus I: Inhibition of the late response asthmatic response by nedocromil sodium administered more than two hours after antigen challenge. J Allergy Clin Immunol 1993;92:19.

Rebuck AS et al: A 3-month evaluation of the efficacy of nedocromil sodium in asthma: A randomized, double-blind, placebo-controlled trial of nedocromil sodium conducted by a Canadian multicenter study group. J Allergy Clin Immunol 1990;85:612.

Ruffin RE et al: The efficacy of nedocromil sodium (Tilade) in asthma. Aust N Z J Med 1987;17:557.

Svendsen UG et al: A comparison of the effects of sodium cromoglycate and beclomethasone dipropionate on pulmonary function and bronchial hyperreactivity in subjects with asthma. J Allergy Clin Immunol 1987;80:68.

Corticosteroids

Harding SM: The human pharmacology of fluticasone propionate. Respir Med 1990;84:25.

Juniper EF et al: Effect of long-term treatment with an inhaled corticosteroid (budesonide) on airway hyperresponsiveness and clinical asthma in nonsteroid-dependent asthmatics. Am Rev Respir Dis 1990;142:832.

Noonan M et al: Fluticasone propionate reduces oral prednisone use while it improves asthma control and quality of life. Am J Respir Crit Care Med 1995;152:1467.

Robinson DS, Geddes DM: Inhaled corticosteroids: Benefits and risks. J Asthma 1996;33:5.

Stein LM, Cole RP: Early administration of corticosteroids in emergency room treatment of acute asthma. Ann Intern Med 1990;112:822.

Toogood JH: Bronchial asthma and glucocorticoids. In: *Anti-inflammatory Steroid Action: Basic And Clinical Aspects.* Schleimer RP, Claman HN, Oronsky AL (editors). Academic Press, 1989.

Woolcock AJ et al: Effect of therapy on bronchial hyperresponsiveness in the long-term management of asthma. Clin Allergy 1988;18:165.

Beta Agonists

Anderson GP: Formoterol: Pharmacology, molecular basis of agonism, and mechanism of long duration of a highly potent and selective β_2-adrenoceptor agonist bronchodilator. Life Sci 1993;52:2145.

Coleman JJ et al: Cardiac arrhythmias during the combined use of β-adrenergic agonist drugs and theophylline. Chest 1986;89:45.

Greening AP et al: Added salmeterol versus higher-dose corticosteroid in asthma patients with symptoms on existing inhaled corticosteroid. Lancet 1994;344:219.

Mullen M, Mullen B, Carey M: The association between β-agonist use and death from asthma. A meta-analytic integration of case-control studies. JAMA1993; 270:1842.

Schatz M et al: The safety of inhaled β-agonist bronchodilators during pregnancy. J Allergy Clin Immunol 1988; 82:686.

Spitzer WO et al: The use of β-agonists and the risk of death and near death from asthma. N Engl J Med 1992; 326:501.

Svedmyr N: The current place of β_2-agonists in the management of asthma. Lung 1990;168(Suppl):105.

Ullman A, Svedmyr N: Salmeterol, a new long acting inhaled β_2-adrenoceptor agonist: comparison with salbutamol in adult asthmatic patients. Thorax 1988;43:674.

Woolcock A et al: Comparison of addition of salmeterol to inhaled steroids with doubling of the dose of inhaled steroids. Am J Respir Crit Care Med 1996;153:1481.

Antimuscarinic Drugs

Gross NJ: Ipratropium bromide. N Engl J Med 1988; 319:486.

Gross NJ, Skorodin MS: Role of the parasympathetic system in airway obstruction due to emphysema. N Engl J Med 1984;311:421.

Karpel JP et al: A comparison of the effects of ipratropium bromide and metaproterenol sulfate in acute exacerbations of COPD. Chest 1990;98:835.

Schleuter DP: Ipratropium bromide in asthma: A review of the literature. Am J Med 1986;81(Suppl 5A):55.

Leukotriene Pathway Inhibitors

Cloud ML et al: A specific LTD4/LTE4-receptor antagonist improves pulmonary function in patients with mild, chronic asthma. Am Rev Respir Dis 1989;140:1336.

Friedman BS et al: Oral leukotriene inhibitor (MK-886) blocks allergen-induced airway responses. Am Rev Respir Dis 1993;147:839.

Holgate ST, Bradding P, Sampson AP: Leukotriene antagonists and synthesis inhibitors: New directions in asthma therapy. J Allergy Clin Immunol 1996;98:1.

Israel E et al: The effect of inhibition of 5-lipoxygenase by zileuton in mild-to-moderate asthma. Ann Intern Med 1993;119:1059.

Lewis RA, Austen KF, Soberman RJ: Leukotrienes and other products of the 5-lipoxygenase pathway: Biochemistry and relation to pathobiology in human diseases. N Engl J Med 1990;323:645.

Manning PJ et al: Inhibition of exercise-induced bronchoconstriction by MK-571, a potent leukotriene D4-receptor antagonist. N Engl J Med 1990;323:1736.

Other Drugs for Asthma

Bernstein DI et al: An open study of auranofin in the treatment of steroid-dependent asthma. J Allergy Clin Immunol 1988;81:6.

Dupuy PM et al: Bronchodilator action of inhaled nitric oxide in guinea pigs. J Clin Invest 1992;90:421.

Erzurum SC et al: Lack of effect of methotrexate in severe, steroid-dependent asthma: A double-blind, placebo-controlled study. Ann Intern Med 1991;114: 353.

Fahy JV et al: The effect of anti-IgE recombinant humanized monoclonal antibody-E25 on the early and late phase response to airway challenge with allergen in asthmatic subjects. Am J Respir Crit Care Med 1996. [Submitted.]

Garty M et al: Effect of nifedipine and theophylline in asthma. Clin Pharmacol Ther 1986;40:195.

Heusser CH et al: New concepts of IgE regulation. Int Arch Allergy Appl Immunol 1991;94:87.

Jardieu P: Anti-IgE therapy. Curr Opin Immunol 1995; 7:779.

Kidney JC et al: Effect of an oral potassium channel activator, BRL 38227, on airway function and responsiveness in asthmatic patients: comparison with oral salbutamol. Thorax 1993;48:130.

Mullarkey MF, Lammert JK, Blumenstein BA: Long-term methotrexate treatment in corticosteroid-dependent asthma. Ann Intern Med 1990;112:577.

Ozenne G et al: Nifedipine in chronic bronchial asthma: A randomized double-blind crossover trial against placebo. Eur J Respir Dis 1985;67:238.

Shiner RJ et al: Randomised, double-blind, placebo-controlled trial of methotrexate in steroid-dependent asthma. Lancet 1990;336:137.

Williams AJ et al: Attenuation of nocturnal asthma by cromakalim. Lancet 1990;336:334.

Clinical Management of Airway Disease

Barnes PJ: A new approach to the treatment of asthma. N Engl J Med 1989;321:1517.

Corbridge TC, Hall JB: The assessment and management of adults with status asthmaticus. Am J Respir Crit Care Med 1995;151:1296.

Guidelines for the diagnosis and management of asthma: National Heart, Lung, and Blood Institute National Asthma Education Program Expert Panel Report. J Allergy Clin Immunol 1991;88:425.

Haahtela T et al: Comparison of a β_2-agonist, terbutaline, with an inhaled corticosteroid, budesonide, in newly detected asthma. N Engl J Med 1991;325:388.

Juniper EF et al: Reduction of budesonide use after a year of increased use: A randomized controlled trial to evaluate whether improvements in airway responsiveness and clinical asthma are maintained. J Allergy Clin Immunol 1991;87:483.

Kesten S, Rebuck AS: Management of chronic obstructive pulmonary disease. Drugs 1989;38:160.

Szefler SJ: Anti-inflammatory drugs in the treatment of allergic disease. Med Clin North Am 1992;76:953.

Section V.
Drugs That Act in the Central Nervous System

Introduction to the Pharmacology of CNS Drugs

21

Roger A. Nicoll, MD

Drugs acting in the central nervous system (CNS) were among the first to be discovered by primitive humans and are still the most widely used group of pharmacologic agents. In addition to their use in therapy, drugs acting on the CNS are used without prescription to increase one's sense of well-being. Caffeine, alcohol, and nicotine are socially accepted drugs in many countries, and their consumption is practiced worldwide. Because some of the drugs in this group are addictive and cause severe personal, social, and economic dysfunction, societies have found it necessary to control their use and availability.

The mechanisms by which various drugs act in the CNS have not always been clearly understood. Since the causes of many of the conditions for which these drugs are used (schizophrenia, anxiety, etc) are themselves poorly understood, it is not surprising that in the past much of CNS pharmacology has been purely descriptive. In the last 2 decades, however, dramatic advances have been made in the methodology of CNS pharmacology. It is now possible to study the action of a drug on individual cells and even single ion channels within synapses. The information obtained from such studies is the basis for several major developments in studies of the CNS.

First, it is clear that nearly all drugs with CNS effects act on specific receptors that modulate synaptic transmission. A very few agents such as general anesthetics and alcohol may have nonspecific actions on membranes (although these exceptions are not fully accepted), but even these non-receptor-mediated actions result in demonstrable alterations in synaptic transmission.

Second, drugs are among the most important tools for studying all aspects of the physiology of CNS, from the mechanism of convulsions to the laying down of long-term memory. As will be described below, agonists that mimic natural transmitters (and in many cases are more selective than the endogenous substances) and antagonists are both extremely useful in such studies.

Third, unraveling the actions of drugs with known clinical efficacy has led to some of the most fruitful hypotheses regarding the mechanisms of disease. For example, information on the action of antipsychotic drugs on dopamine receptors has provided the basis for important hypotheses regarding the pathophysiology of schizophrenia. Studies of the effects of a variety of agonists and antagonists on γ-aminobutyric acid (GABA) receptors are resulting in new concepts pertaining to the pathophysiology of several diseases, including anxiety and epilepsy.

This chapter provides an introduction to the functional organization of the CNS and its synaptic transmitters as a basis for understanding the actions of the drugs described in the following chapters.

Methods for the Study of CNS Pharmacology

Although scientists (and the public) have always been interested in the action of drugs in the CNS, a detailed description of synaptic transmission was not possible until glass microelectrodes, which permit intracellular recording, were developed. Detailed electrophysiologic studies of the action of drugs on both voltage- and transmitter-operated channels were greatly facilitated by the introduction of the patch clamp technique, which permits the recording of current through single channels. Histochemical, immunologic, and radioisotopic methods are widely used to map the distribution of specific transmitters, their associated enzyme systems, and their receptors.

Molecular cloning is now having a major impact on our understanding of CNS receptors. These techniques make it possible to determine the precise molecular structure of the receptors and their associated channels.

ION CHANNELS

The membranes of nerve cells contain two types of channels defined on the basis of the mechanisms controlling their gating (opening and closing). The first mechanism is that of membrane *voltage-sensitive* gating; the second is that of *chemically activated* gating. The voltage-sensitive sodium channel described in Chapter 14 for the heart is an example of the first type and is very important in the CNS. In nerve cells, these channels are concentrated on the initial segment and the axon and are responsible for the fast action potential, which transmits the signal from cell body to nerve terminal. There are many types of voltage-sensitive calcium and potassium channels on the cell body, dendrites, and initial segment, which act on a much slower time scale and modulate the rate at which the neuron discharges. For example, some types of potassium channels opened by depolarization of the cell result in slowing of further depolarization and act as a brake to limit further action potential discharge.

Chemically activated channels, also called receptor-operated channels, are opened by the action of neurotransmitters and other chemical agents. The receptor is formed of subunits, and the channel is an integral part of the receptor complex. These channels are insensitive or only weakly sensitive to membrane potential. Neurotransmitter receptors are concentrated on subsynaptic membranes, eg, the nicotinic neuromuscular receptor of the skeletal muscle end plate.

It is now well-established that the traditional view of completely separate electrically gated and chemically gated channels requires modification. In particular, many neurotransmitter receptors are coupled to voltage-sensitive channels via second messenger systems.

THE SYNAPSE & SYNAPTIC POTENTIALS

The communication between neurons in the CNS occurs through chemical synapses in the vast majority of cases. (A few instances of electrical coupling between neurons have been documented, and such coupling may play a role in synchronizing neuronal discharge. However, it is unlikely that these electrical synapses are an important site of drug action.) The events involved in the release of transmitter from the presynaptic terminal have been studied most extensively at the vertebrate neuromuscular junction and at the giant synapse of the squid. An action potential in the presynaptic fiber propagates into the synaptic ter-

minal and activates voltage-sensitive calcium channels in the membrane of the terminal (Figure 6–3). The calcium channels responsible for the release of transmitter are generally resistant to the calcium channel-blocking agents discussed in Chapter 12 (verapamil, etc) but are sensitive to blockade by certain marine toxins and metal ions (Table 12–4). Calcium flows into the terminal, and the increase in intraterminal calcium concentration promotes the fusion of synaptic vesicles with the presynaptic membrane. The transmitter contained in the vesicles is released into the synaptic cleft and diffuses to the receptors on the postsynaptic membrane. Binding of the transmitter to its receptor causes a brief change in membrane conductance (permeability to ions) of the postsynaptic cell. The time delay from the arrival of the presynaptic action potential to the onset of the postsynaptic response is approximately 0.5 ms. Most of this delay is consumed by the release process, particularly the time required for calcium channels to open.

The first systematic analysis of synaptic potentials in the CNS was in the early 1950s by Eccles and associates, who recorded intracellularly from spinal motoneurons. When a microelectrode enters a cell, there is a sudden change in the potential recorded by the electrode, which is typically about –70 mV (Figure 21–1). This is the resting membrane potential of the neuron. Two types of pathways, excitatory and inhibitory, impinge on the motoneuron. When an excitatory pathway is stimulated, a small depolarization or excitatory postsynaptic potential (EPSP) is recorded. This potential is due to the excitatory transmitter activating a large increase in sodium and potassium permeability. The duration of these potentials is quite brief, usually less than 20 ms. Changing the stimulus intensity to the pathway and therefore the number of presynaptic fibers activated results in a graded change in the size of the depolarization. This indicates that

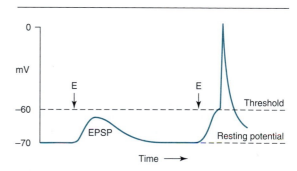

Figure 21–1. Excitatory synaptic potentials and spike generation. The figure shows a resting membrane potential of –70 mV in a postsynaptic cell. Stimulation of an excitatory pathway *(E)* generates transient depolarization. Increasing the stimulus strength (second *E*) increases the size of the depolarization, so that the threshold for spike generation is reached.

the contribution a single fiber makes to the EPSP is quite small. When a sufficient number of excitatory fibers are activated, the EPSP depolarizes the post-synaptic cell to threshold, and an all-or-none action potential is generated.

When an inhibitory pathway is stimulated, the post-synaptic membrane is hyperpolarized, producing an inhibitory postsynaptic potential (IPSP) (Figure 21–2). A number of inhibitory synapses must be activated simultaneously to appreciably alter the membrane potential. This hyperpolarization is due to a selective increase in membrane permeability to chloride ions that flow into the cell during the IPSP. If an EPSP that under resting conditions would evoke an action potential in the postsynaptic cell (Figure 21–2) is elicited during an IPSP, it no longer evokes an action potential, because the IPSP has moved the membrane potential farther away from the threshold for action potential generation. A second type of inhibition is termed presynaptic inhibition. In the CNS, this inhibition is mainly limited to the sensory fibers entering the brain stem and spinal cord. The excitatory synaptic terminals of these sensory fibers receive synapses called axoaxonic synapses (Figure 21–4B). When activated, the axoaxonic synapses reduce the amount of transmitter released from the synapses of sensory fibers. Synaptic inhibition in an unanesthetized subject lasts tens of milliseconds.

SITES OF DRUG ACTION

Virtually all of the drugs that act in the CNS produce their effects by modifying some step in chemical synaptic transmission. Figure 21–3 illustrates some

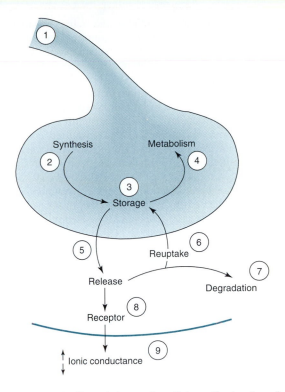

Figure 21–3. Sites of drug action. Schematic drawing of steps at which drugs can alter synaptic transmission. *(1)* Action potential in presynaptic fiber; *(2)* synthesis of transmitter; *(3)* storage; *(4)* metabolism; *(5)* release; *(6)* reuptake; *(7)* degradation; *(8)* receptor for the transmitter; *(9)* receptor-induced increase or decrease in ionic conductance.

of the steps that can be altered. These transmitter-dependent actions can be divided into presynaptic and postsynaptic categories.

Drugs acting on the synthesis, storage, metabolism, and release of neurotransmitters fall into the presynaptic category. Synaptic transmission can be depressed by blockade of transmitter synthesis or storage. For example, *p*-chlorophenylalanine blocks the synthesis of serotonin, and reserpine depletes the synapses of monoamines by interfering with intracellular storage. Blockade of transmitter catabolism can increase transmitter concentrations and has been reported to increase the amount of transmitter released per impulse. Drugs can also alter the release of transmitter. The stimulant amphetamine induces the release of catecholamines from adrenergic synapses. Capsaicin causes the release of the peptide substance P from sensory neurons, and tetanus toxin blocks the release of transmitters. After a transmitter has been released into the synaptic cleft, its action is terminated either by uptake or degradation. For most neurotransmitters, there are uptake mechanisms into the synaptic terminal and also into surrounding neuroglia. Cocaine, for example, blocks the uptake of catecholamines at adrenergic

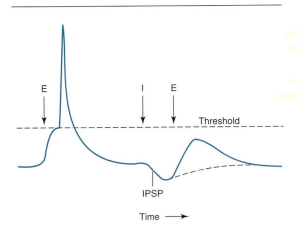

Figure 21–2. Interaction of excitatory and inhibitory synapses. On the left, a suprathreshold stimulus is given to an excitatory pathway *(E)*. On the right, this same stimulus is given shortly after stimulating an inhibitory pathway *(I)*, which prevents the excitatory potential from reaching threshold.

synapses and thus potentiates the action of these amines. However, acetylcholine is inactivated by enzymatic degradation. Anticholinesterases block the degradation of acetylcholine and thereby prolong its action. No uptake mechanism has been found for any of the numerous CNS peptides, and it has yet to be demonstrated whether specific enzymatic degradation terminates the action of peptide transmitters.

In the postsynaptic region, the transmitter receptor provides the primary site of drug action. Drugs can act either as neurotransmitter agonists, such as the opioids, which mimic the action of enkephalin, or they can block receptor function. Receptor antagonism is a common mechanism of action for CNS drugs. An example is strychnine's blockade of the receptor for the inhibitory transmitter glycine. This block, which underlies strychnine's convulsant action, illustrates how the blockade of inhibitory processes results in excitation. Receptors control membrane excitability in one of two ways. First, they can directly form an ion channel. The receptors at most synapses in the central nervous system are of this type, and receptor activation typically results in a brief (a few milliseconds to tens of milliseconds) opening of the channel. Drugs can act directly on the ion channel. For example, barbiturates enter and block the channel coupled to many excitatory neurotransmitter receptors. Second, receptors can act indirectly via G proteins (Chapter 2). The activated G protein can directly modulate voltage-gated ion channels, or it can act by generating a diffusible second messenger that then modulates voltage-gated ion channels. These effects can persist long after the transmitter has left the receptor, ie, tens of seconds to minutes. The methylxanthines are the best-known examples of drugs that can modify neurotransmitter responses mediated through the second messenger cAMP. At high concentrations, the methylxanthines elevate the level of cAMP by blocking its metabolism and thereby prolong its action in the postsynaptic cell.

General anesthetics and ethanol are not thought to produce their effects by binding to specific receptors. Their actions are closely correlated with their lipophilicity. These drugs are believed to alter transmitter release and postsynaptic responsiveness by interacting with membrane lipids as well as membrane proteins.

The selectivity of CNS drug action is based almost entirely on the fact that different transmitters are used by different groups of neurons. Furthermore, these transmitters are often segregated into neuronal systems that subserve broadly different CNS functions. Without such segregation, it would be impossible to selectively modify CNS function even if one had a drug that operated on a single neurotransmitter system. It is not entirely clear why the CNS has relied on so many neurotransmitters and segregated them into different neuronal systems, since the primary function of a transmitter is either excitation or inhibition; this could be accomplished with two transmitter sub-

stances or perhaps even one. That such segregation does occur has provided neuroscientists with a powerful pharmacologic approach for analyzing CNS function and treating pathologic conditions.

IDENTIFICATION OF CENTRAL NEUROTRANSMITTERS

Since drug selectivity is based on the fact that different pathways utilize different transmitters, it is a primary goal of neuropharmacologists to identify the transmitters in CNS pathways. Establishing that a chemical substance is a transmitter has been far more difficult for central synapses than for peripheral synapses. In theory, to identify a transmitter it is sufficient to show that stimulation of a pathway releases enough of the substance to produce the postsynaptic response. In practice, this experiment cannot be done satisfactorily for at least two reasons. First, the anatomic complexity of the CNS prevents the selective activation of a single set of synaptic terminals. Second, available techniques for measuring the released transmitter and applying the transmitter are not sufficiently precise to satisfy the quantitative requirements. Therefore, the following criteria have been established for transmitter identification.

Localization

A number of approaches have been used to prove that a suspected transmitter resides in the presynaptic terminal of the pathway under study. These include biochemical analysis of regional concentrations of suspected transmitters, often combined with interruption of specific pathways, and microcytochemical techniques. Immunocytochemical techniques have proved very useful in localizing peptides and enzymes that synthesize or degrade nonpeptide transmitters.

Release

To determine whether the substance can be released from a particular region, local collection (in vivo) of the extracellular fluid can sometimes be accomplished. In addition, slices of brain tissue can be electrically or chemically stimulated in vitro and the released substances measured. To determine if the release is relevant to synaptic transmission, it is important to establish that the release is calcium-dependent. As mentioned above, anatomic complexity often prevents identification of the synaptic terminals responsible for the release, and the amount collected in the perfusate is a small fraction of the amount actually released.

Synaptic Mimicry

Finally, application of the suspected substance should produce a response that mimics the action of the transmitter released by nerve stimulation. Microiontophoresis, which permits highly localized drug administration, has been a valuable technique in assessing the action of suspected transmitters. In practice, this criterion has two parts: physiologic and pharmacologic identity. To establish physiologic identity of action, the substance must be shown to initiate the same change in ionic conductance in the postsynaptic cell as synaptically released transmitter. This requires intracellular recording and determination of the reversal potential and ionic dependencies of the responses. However, since different transmitters can elicit identical ionic conductance changes, this finding is not sufficient. Thus, selective pharmacologic antagonism is used to further establish that the suspected transmitter is acting in a manner identical to synaptically released transmitter. Because of the complexity of the CNS, specific pharmacologic antagonism of a synaptic response provides a particularly powerful technique for transmitter identification.

CELLULAR ORGANIZATION OF THE BRAIN

Most of the neuronal systems in the CNS can be divided into two broad categories: hierarchical systems and nonspecific or diffuse neuronal systems.

Hierarchical Systems

These systems include all of the pathways directly involved in sensory perception and motor control. The pathways are generally clearly delineated, being composed of large myelinated fibers that can often conduct action potentials at a rate in excess of 50 m/s. The information is typically phasic, and in sensory systems the information is processed sequentially by successive integrations at each relay nucleus on its way to the cortex. A lesion at any link will incapacitate the system. Within each nucleus and in the cortex, there are two types of cells: relay or projection neurons and local circuit neurons (Figure 21–4A). The projection neurons that form the interconnecting pathways transmit signals over long distances. The cell bodies are relatively large, and their axons emit collaterals that arborize extensively in the vicinity of the neuron. These neurons are excitatory, and their synaptic influences are very short-lived. The excitatory transmitter released from these cells is, in most instances, glutamate. Local circuit neurons are typically smaller than projection neurons, and their axons arborize in the immediate vicinity of the cell body. The vast majority of these neurons are inhibitory, and they release either GABA or glycine. They synapse primarily on the cell body of the projection neurons but can also synapse on the dendrites of projection neurons as well as with each other. A special class of local circuit neurons in the spinal cord forms axoaxonic synapses on the terminals of sensory axons (Figure 21–4B). Two common types of pathways for these

neurons (Figure 21–4A) include recurrent feedback pathways and feed-forward pathways. In many sensory pathways, local circuit neurons may actually lack an axon and release neurotransmitter from dendritic synapses in a graded fashion in the absence of action potentials. Some pathways involving presynaptic dendrites of local circuit neurons are shown in Figure 21–4C.

Although there is a great variety of synaptic connections in these hierarchical systems, the fact that a limited number of transmitters are utilized by these neurons indicates that any major pharmacologic manipulation of this system will have a profound effect on the overall excitability of the CNS. For instance, selectively blocking GABA receptors with a drug such as picrotoxin results in generalized convulsions. Thus, while the mechanism of action of picrotoxin is quite specific in blocking the effects of GABA, the overall functional effect appears to be quite nonspecific, since GABA-mediated synaptic inhibition is so widely utilized in the brain.

Nonspecific or Diffuse Neuronal Systems

Neuronal systems that contain one of the monoamines—norepinephrine, dopamine, or 5-hydroxytryptamine (serotonin)—provide examples in this category. Certain other pathways emanating from the reticular formation and possibly some peptide-containing pathways also fall into this category. These systems differ in fundamental ways from the hierarchical systems, and the noradrenergic systems will serve to illustrate the differences.

Noradrenergic cell bodies are found primarily in a compact cell group called the locus ceruleus located in the caudal pontine central gray matter. The number of neurons in this cell group is quite small, approximately 1500 on each side of the brain in the rat. The axons of these neurons are very fine and unmyelinated. Indeed, they were entirely missed with classic anatomic techniques. It was not until the mid 1960s, when the formaldehyde fluorescence histochemical technique was applied to the study of CNS tissues, that the anatomy of the monoamine-containing systems was described. Because these axons are fine and unmyelinated, they conduct very slowly, at about 0.5 m/s. The axons branch repeatedly and are extraordinarily divergent. Branches from the same neuron can innervate several functionally different parts of the CNS. In the neocortex, these fibers have a tangential organization and therefore can monosynaptically influence large areas of cortex. The pattern of innervation in the cortex and nuclei of the hierarchical systems is diffuse, and the noradrenergic fibers form a very small percentage of the total number in the area. In addition, the axons are studded with periodic enlargements called varicosities that contain large numbers of vesicles. In some instances, these varicosities do not form synaptic contacts, suggesting that norepinephrine may be released in a

A Feed-forward and recurrent interaction

Feed-forward

Recurrent

B Axoaxonic interaction

C Dendrodendritic interaction

Triad

Axon

Reciprocal synapse

Electrotonic (gap) junction

Serial synapse

Inhibitory

Excitatory

Figure 21–4. Pathways in the central nervous system. **A** shows two relay neurons and two types of inhibitory pathways, recurrent and feed-forward. The inhibitory neurons are shown in black. **B** shows the pathway responsible for presynaptic inhibition in which the axon of an inhibitory neuron synapses on the axon terminal of an excitatory fiber. **C:** Diagram illustrating that dendrites may be both pre- and postsynaptic to each other, forming reciprocal synapses, two of which are shown between the same dendrite pair. In triads, an axon synapses on two dendrites, and one of these dendrites synapses on the second. In serial synapses, a dendrite may be postsynaptic to one dendrite and presynaptic to another, thus connecting a series of dendrites. Dendrites also interact through low-resistance electrotonic ("gap") junctions (two of which are shown). Except for one axon, all structures shown in *C* are dendrites. (Reproduced, with permission, from Schmitt FO, Dev P, Smith BH: Electrotonic processing of information by brain cells. Science 1976;193:114. Copyright © 1976 by the American Association for the Advancement of Science.)

rather diffuse manner, as occurs with the noradrenergic innervation of smooth muscle. This indicates that the cellular targets of these systems will be determined largely by the location of the receptors rather than the location of the release sites. Based on all of these observations, it is clear that the monoamine systems cannot be conveying specific topographic types of information—rather, vast areas of the CNS must be affected simultaneously and in a rather uniform way. It is not surprising, then, that these systems have been implicated in such global functions as sleeping and waking, attention, appetite, and emotional states.

CENTRAL NEUROTRANSMITTERS

A vast number of small molecules have been isolated from brain, and studies using a variety of approaches suggest that the agents listed in Table 21–1 are neurotransmitters. A brief summary of the evidence for some of these compounds follows.

Amino Acids

The amino acids of primary interest to the pharmacologist fall into two categories: the neutral amino acids **glycine** and **GABA** and the acidic amino acids **glutamate** and **aspartate.** All of these compounds are

Table 21–1. Summary of neurotransmitter pharmacology in the central nervous system.

Transmitter	Anatomy	Receptor Subtypes and Preferred Agonists	Receptor Antagonists	Mechanisms
Acetylcholine	Cell bodies at all levels; long and short connections	Muscarinic (M_1): muscarine, McN-A-343	Pirenzepine, atropine	Excitatory: $\downarrow$ in K^+ conductance; $\uparrow$ IP_3, DAG
		Muscarinic (M_2): muscarine, bethanechol	Atropine	Inhibitory: $\uparrow$ K^+ conductance; $\downarrow$ cAMP.
	Motoneuron-Renshaw cell synapse.	Nicotinic: nicotine	Dihydro-β-erythroidine	Excitatory: $\uparrow$ cation conductance.
Dopamine	Cell bodies at all levels; short, medium, and long connections.	D_1: SKF 38393	Phenothiazines, SCH 23390	Inhibitory (?): $\uparrow$ cAMP
		D_2: quinpirole	Phenothiazines, butyrophenones	Inhibitory (presynaptic): $\downarrow$ Ca^{2+} Inhibitory (postsynaptic): $\uparrow$ in K^+ conductance, $\downarrow$ cAMP.
GABA	Supraspinal interneurons; spinal interneurons involved in presynaptic inhibition.	$GABA_A$: muscimol	Bicuculline, picrotoxin	Inhibitory: $\uparrow$ Cl^- conductance.
		$GABA_B$: baclofen	2-OH saclofen, CGP35348 CGP55845	Inhibitory (presynaptic): $\downarrow$ Ca^{2+} conductance. Inhibitory (postsynaptic): $\uparrow$ K^+ conductance.
Glutamate; aspartate	Relay neurons at all levels.	N-Methyl-D-aspartate (NMDA): NMDA	2-Amino-5-phosphonovalerate, CPP	Excitatory: $\uparrow$ cation conductance, particularly Ca^{2+}.
		AMPA: AMPA	CNQX; GYKI52466	Excitatory: $\uparrow$ cation conductance
		Kainate: kainate, domoic acid	CQNX	
		Metabotropic: ACPD, quisqualate	MCPG	Inhibitory (presynaptic): $\downarrow$ Ca^{2+} conductance; $\downarrow$ cAMP. Excitatory: $\downarrow$ K^+ conductance, $\uparrow$ IP_3, DAG.
Glycine	Spinal interneurons and some brain stem interneurons.	Taurine, β-alanine	Strychnine	Inhibitory: $\uparrow$ Cl^- conductance
5-Hydroxytryptamine (serotonin)	Cell bodies in midbrain and pons project to all levels.	$5-HT_{1A}$: LSD, 8-OH-DPAT	Metergoline, spiperone	Inhibitory: $\uparrow$ K^+ conductance, $\downarrow$ cAMP
		$5-HT_{2A}$: LSD, DOB	Ketanserin	Excitatory: $\downarrow$ K^+ conductance; $\uparrow$ IP_3, DAG
		$5-HT_3$: 2-methyl-5-HT, phenylbiguanide	ICS 205930, ondansetron	Excitatory: $\uparrow$ cation conductance.
		$5HT_4$: BIMU8	GR113808	Excitatory: $\downarrow$ K^+ conductance

Table 21–1. Summary of neurotransmitter pharmacology in the central nervous system (cont'd).

Transmitter	Anatomy	Receptor Subtypes and Preferred Agonists	Receptor Antagonists	Mechanisms
Norepinephrine	Cell bodies in pons and brain stem project to all levels.	Alpha$_1$: phenylephrine	Prazosin	Excitatory: ↓ K$^+$ conductance; ↑ IP$_3$, DAG
		Alpha$_2$: Clonidine	Yohimbine	Inhibitory (presynaptic): ↓ Ca^{2+} conductance. Inhibitory: ↑ K$^+$ conductance; ↓ cAMP
		Beta$_1$: isoproterenol, dobutamine	Atenolol, practolol	Excitatory: ↓ K$^+$ conductance; ↑ cAMP
		Beta$_2$: salbutamol	Butoxamine	Inhibitory: may involve ↑ in electrogenic sodium pump; ↑ cAMP.
Histamine	Cells in ventral posterior hypothalamus	H$_1$: 2(m-F-phenyl) histamine	Mepyramine	Excitatory: ↓ K$^+$ conductance, ↑ IP$_3$, DAG
		H$_2$: Dimaprit	Ranitidine	Excitatory: ↓ K$^+$ conductance, ↑ cAMP
Opioid peptides	Cell bodies at all levels; long and short connections	Mu: Bendorphin, DAMGO	Naloxone	Inhibitory (presynaptic): ↓ Ca^{2+} conductance, ↓ cAMP
		Delta: enkephalin, DPDPE	Naloxone	Inhibitory (postsynaptic): ↑ K$^+$ conductance, ↓ cAMP
		Kappa: dynorphin, U69593	Naloxone, nor-BNI	
Tachykinins	Primary sensory neurons, cell bodies at all levels; long and short connections	NK1: Substance P methylester	CP99994	Excitatory: ↓ K$^+$ conductance, ↑ IP$_3$, DAG
		NK2: β-[Ala^8] NKA$_{4-10}$	SR48968	
		NK3: GR138676	[Pro^7]NKB	

Abbreviations:

8-OH DPAT, 8-hydroxy-2(di-n-propylamino)tetralin
ACPD, *trans*-1-amino-cyclopentyl-1,3-dicarboxylate
AMPA, DL-α-amino-3-hydroxy-5-methylisoxazole-4-propionate
BIMU8, (endo-N-8-methyl-8-azabicyclo[3.2.1]oct-3-yl)-2,3-dihydro-3-isopropyl-2-oxo-1H-benzimidazol-1-carboxamide hydrochloride
CGP 35348, 3-aminopropyl(diethoxymethyl)phosphinic acid
CNQX, 6-cyano-7-nitroquinoxaline-2,3-dione
CPP, 3-(2-carboxypiperazin-4-yl)propyl-1-phosphonic acid
DAG, diacylglycerol
DAMGO, D-ala-2,Me-Phe^4,Gly^1-enkephalin
DOB, 5-bromo-2,5-dimethoxyamphetamine
DPDPE, [D-pen^{2}D-pen^5]-enkephalin
GR 113808, [1-[2-[(methylsulfonyl)amino]ethyl]-4-piperidinyl]methyl-1-methyl-1H-indole-3-carboxylate
GYKI 52466, 1-(4-aminophenyl)-4-methyl-7,8-methylenedioxy-5H-2,3-benzodiazepine
IP3, inositol trisphosphate
MCPG, α-methyl-4-carboxyphenylglycine
NK, NK1,2,3,A,B, neurokinin and derivatives
nor-BNI, nor-binaltorphimine
U-69593, (+)-(5α,7α,8β)-N-methyl-N-[7-(1-pyrrolidinyl)]-1-oxaspiro[4,5]dec-8-yl-benzenacetamide

present in high concentrations in the CNS and are extremely potent modifiers of neuronal excitability.

A. Neutral Amino Acids: The neutral amino acids are inhibitory and increase membrane permeability to chloride ions, thus mimicking the IPSP. Glycine concentrations are particularly high in the gray matter of the spinal cord, and destruction of the neurons in this area results in a marked decrease in the concentration of glycine. In addition, strychnine, which is a potent spinal cord convulsant and has been used in some rat poisons, selectively antagonizes both the action of glycine and the IPSPs recorded in spinal cord neurons. Thus, it is generally agreed that glycine is released from spinal cord inhibitory local circuit neurons involved in postsynaptic inhibition.

GABA receptors are divided into two types: $GABA_A$ and $GABA_B$. $GABA_A$ receptors open chloride channels and are antagonized by picrotoxin and bicuculline, which both cause generalized convulsions. $GABA_B$ receptors, which can be selectively activated by the antispastic drug baclofen, are coupled to G proteins that either inhibit calcium channels or activate potassium channels. In most regions of the brain, IPSPs have a fast and slow component. Good evidence suggests that GABA is the inhibitory transmitter mediating both components. The fast IPSPs are blocked by $GABA_A$ antagonists, while the slow IPSPs are blocked by $GABA_B$ antagonists. Immunohistochemical studies indicate that a large majority of the local circuit neurons synthesize GABA. A special class of local circuit neuron localized in the dorsal horn of the spinal cord also synthesizes GABA. These neurons form axoaxonic synapses with primary sensory nerve terminals and are responsible for presynaptic inhibition (Figure 21–4B).

B. Acidic Amino Acids: Both glutamate and aspartate are present in very high concentrations in the CNS. Virtually all neurons that have been tested are strongly excited by these two amino acids. This excitation is caused by the activation of receptors that can be divided into two classes: *ionotropic* and *metabotropic*, which have been extensively characterized by molecular cloning. As their name suggests, the ionotropic receptors directly gate cation-selective channels and are further divided into three subtypes based on the action of the selective agonists: kainate (K), α-amino-3-hydroxy-5-methylisoxazole-4-propionate (AMPA), and N-methyl-D-aspartate (NMDA). The AMPA- and K-activated channels are permeable to sodium and potassium ions and, for certain subtypes, calcium as well. They are often grouped together and referred to as non-NMDA channels. The NMDA-activated channel is highly permeable to sodium, potassium, and calcium ions.

The metabotropic glutamate receptors act indirectly on ion channels via G proteins. They are selectively activated by *trans*-1-amino-cyclopentyl-1,3-dicarboxylate (ACPD). These G protein-coupled receptors are either positively coupled to (ie, stimulate) phospholipase C or negatively coupled to adenylyl cyclase. Although the role of metabotropic glutamate receptors in synaptic transmission remains unclear, pharmacologic studies indicate that both NMDA and non-NMDA receptors are present at most excitatory synapses in the brain.

The role of NMDA receptors has recently received considerable attention. These receptors play a critical role in synaptic plasticity, which is thought to underlie certain forms of learning and memory. They are selectively blocked by the dissociative anesthetic ketamine and the hallucinogenic drug phencyclidine.

These drugs exert their effects by entering and blocking the open channel. Some drugs that block this receptor channel have potent antiepileptic activity in animal models, though these drugs have yet to be tested clinically. Considerable evidence exists that the release of glutamate during neuronal injury can, by activating the NMDA receptor, cause further cell injury and death. Thus, a particularly exciting finding is that blocking the NMDA receptor can attenuate the neuronal damage caused by anoxia in experimental animals. The potential therapeutic benefits of this action are considerable.

Acetylcholine

Acetylcholine was the first compound to be identified pharmacologically as a transmitter in the CNS. Eccles showed in the early 1950s that excitation of Renshaw cells by motor axon collaterals was blocked by nicotinic antagonists. Furthermore, Renshaw cells were extremely sensitive to nicotinic agonists. These experiments were remarkable for two reasons. First, this early success at identifying a transmitter for a central synapse was followed by disappointment, because it remained the sole central synapse for which the transmitter was known until the late 1960s, when comparable data became available for the neutral amino acids. Second, the motor axon collateral synapse remains the only clearly documented example of a cholinergic nicotinic synapse in the mammalian CNS, despite the rather widespread distribution of nicotinic receptors as defined by in situ hybridization studies. Most CNS responses to acetylcholine are mediated by a large family of G protein-coupled muscarinic receptors. At a few sites, acetylcholine causes slow inhibition of the neuron by activating the M_2 subtype of receptor, which opens potassium channels. A far more widespread muscarinic action in response to acetylcholine is a slow excitation that in some cases may be mediated by M_1 receptors. These muscarinic effects are much slower than either nicotinic effects on Renshaw cells or the effect of amino acids. Furthermore, this muscarinic excitation is unusual in that acetylcholine produces it by *decreasing* the membrane permeability to potassium, ie, the opposite of conventional transmitter action.

A number of pathways contain acetylcholine, including neurons in the neostriatum, the medial septal nucleus, and the reticular formation. The introduction of monoclonal antibodies that bind to choline acetyltransferase has greatly improved the histochemical localization of this transmitter. Cholinergic pathways appear to play an important role in cognitive functions, especially memory. Presenile dementia of the Alzheimer type is reportedly associated with a profound loss of cholinergic neurons. However, the specificity of this loss has been questioned since the levels of other putative transmitters, eg, somatostatin, are also decreased.

Monoamines

Monoamines include the catecholamines (dopamine and norepinephrine) and 5-hydroxytryptamine. Although these compounds are present in very small amounts in the CNS, they can be localized using extremely sensitive histochemical methods. These include formaldehyde-induced fluorescence of the monoamines and immunohistochemical methods for localizing the individual synthetic enzymes. These pathways are the site of action of many drugs; for example, the CNS stimulants cocaine and amphetamine are believed to act primarily at catecholamine synapses. Cocaine blocks the reuptake of dopamine and norepinephrine, while amphetamines cause presynaptic terminals to release these transmitters.

A. Dopamine: The major pathways containing dopamine are the projection linking the substantia nigra to the neostriatum and the projection linking the ventral tegmental region to limbic structures, particularly the limbic cortex. The therapeutic action of the antiparkinsonism drug levodopa is associated with the former area, whereas the therapeutic action of the antipsychotic drugs is thought to be associated with the latter area. Dopamine-containing neurons in the tuberobasal ventral hypothalamus play an important role in regulating hypothalamohypophysial function. Dopamine generally exerts a slow inhibitory action on CNS neurons. This action has been best characterized on dopamine-containing substantia nigra neurons, where D_2 receptor activation opens potassium channels.

B. Norepinephrine: This system has already been discussed. Most noradrenergic neurons are located in the locus ceruleus or the lateral tegmental area of the reticular formation. Although the density of fibers innervating various sites differs considerably, most regions of the central nervous system receive diffuse noradrenergic input. When applied to neurons, norepinephrine can hyperpolarize them by increasing potassium conductance. This effect is mediated by alpha$_2$ receptors and has been characterized most thoroughly on locus ceruleus neurons. In many regions of the CNS, norepinephrine actually enhances excitatory inputs by both indirect and direct mechanisms. The indirect mechanism involves disinhibition, ie, inhibitory local circuit neurons are inhibited. The direct mechanism is blockade of potassium conductances that slow neuronal discharge. Depending on the type of neuron, this effect is mediated by either alpha$_1$ or beta receptors. Facilitation of excitatory synaptic transmission is in accordance with many of the behavioral processes thought to involve noradrenergic pathways—attention, arousal, and so on.

C. 5-Hydroxytryptamine: Most 5-hydroxytryptamine (5-HT, serotonin) pathways originate from neurons in the raphe or midline regions of the pons and upper brain stem. 5-HT is contained in unmyelinated fibers that diffusely innervate most regions of the CNS, but the density of the innervation varies. In most areas of the central nervous system, 5-HT has a strong inhibitory action. This action is mediated by 5-HT$_{1A}$ receptors and is associated with membrane hyperpolarization caused by an increase in potassium conductance. It has been found that 5-HT$_{1A}$ receptors and GABA$_B$ receptors share the same potassium channels. These receptors and the potassium channels are coupled using a GTP-binding protein. Some cell types are slowly excited by 5-HT owing to its blockade of potassium channels via 5-HT$_2$ or 5-HT$_4$ receptors. Both excitatory and inhibitory actions can occur on the same neurons. It has often been speculated that 5-HT pathways may be involved in the hallucinations induced by LSD, since this compound can antagonize the peripheral actions of 5-HT. However, LSD does not appear to be a 5-HT antagonist in the central nervous system, and typical LSD-induced behavior is still seen in animals after raphe nuclei are destroyed. Other proposed regulatory functions of 5-HT-containing neurons include sleep, temperature, appetite, and neuroendocrine control.

Peptides

A great many CNS peptides have been discovered that produce dramatic effects both on animal behavior and on the activity of individual neurons. Many of the peptides have been mapped with immunohistochemical techniques and include opioid peptides (enkephalins, endorphins, etc), neurotensin, substance P, somatostatin, cholecystokinin, vasoactive intestinal polypeptide, neuropeptide Y, and thyrotropin-releasing hormone. As in the peripheral autonomic nervous system, peptides often coexist with a conventional nonpeptide transmitter in the same neuron. A good example of the approaches used to define the role of these peptides in the central nervous system comes from studies on substance P and its association with sensory fibers. Immunohistochemical studies have found substance P to be present in some of the small unmyelinated primary sensory neurons of the spinal cord and brain stem. In addition, stimulation of the sensory neurons releases substance P from the spinal cord. Application of substance P to neurons in the spinal cord excites neurons that are activated by painful stimuli. Painful stimuli are known to selectively activate unmyelinated sensory fibers. Thus, it is believed that substance P may be an excitatory transmitter released from unmyelinated fibers that respond to painful stimulation. However, although substance P antagonists can modify the response to certain types of pain, they do not block the response. Thus, other transmitters, most likely glutamate, are co-released from unmyelinated sensory afferents. Substance P is certainly involved in many other functions, since it is found in many areas of the central nervous system that are unrelated to pain pathways.

Many of these peptides are also found in peripheral structures, including peripheral synapses. They are described in Chapters 6 and 17.

Nitric Oxide

The CNS contains a substantial amount of nitric oxide synthase (NOS), which is found within certain classes of neurons. This neuronal NOS is an enzyme activated by calcium-calmodulin, and activation of NMDA receptors, which increases intracellular calcium, results in the generation of nitric oxide. While a physiologic role for nitric oxide has been clearly established for vascular smooth muscle, its role in synaptic transmission and synaptic plasticity remains controversial.

REFERENCES

Amara SG, Arriza JL: Neurotransmitter transporters: Three distinct gene families. Curr Opin Neurobiol 1993;3:337.

Bettler B, Mulle C: Review: Neurotransmitter receptors 11. AMPA and kainate receptors. Neuropharmacology 1995;34:123.

Betz H: Structure and function of inhibitory glycine receptors. Q Rev Biophys 1992;25:381.

Bliss TVP, Collingridge GL: A synaptic model of memory: Long-term potentiation in the hippocampus. Nature 1993;361:31.

Bloom FE: Neurotransmitters: Past, present, and future directions. FASEB J 1988;2:32.

Bourne HR, Nicoll R: Molecular machines integrate coincident synaptic signals. Cell 1993;72(Suppl):65.

Bowery NG: GABA$_B$ receptor pharmacology. Annu Rev Pharmacol Toxicol 1993;33:109.

Brake AJ, Julius D: Signaling by extracellular nucleotides. Annu Rev Cell Dev Biol 1996;12:519.

Catterall WA: Structure and function of voltage-gated ion channels. Trends Neurosci 1993;16:500.

Cooper JR, Bloom FE, Roth RH: In: *The Biochemical Basis of Neuropharmacology,* 6th ed. Oxford Univ Press, 1991.

Eccles JC: In: *The Physiology of Synapses.* Springer, 1964.

Grandy DK, Civelli O: G-protein-coupled receptors: The new dopamine receptor subtypes. Curr Opin Neurobiol 1992;2:275.

Hall ZW: In: *An Introduction to Molecular Neurobiology.* Sinauer, 1992.

Hille B: *Ionic Channels of Excitable Membranes.* 2nd ed. Sinauer, 1992.

Hokfelt T: Neuropeptides in perspective: The last ten years. Neuron 1991;7:867.

Hollmann M, Heinemann S: Cloned glutamate receptors. Annu Rev Neurosci 1994;17:31.

Hyman SE, Nestler EJ: *The Molecular Foundations of Psychiatry.* American Psychiatric Press, 1993.

Linden DJ: Long-term synaptic depression in the mammalian brain. Neuron 1994;12:457.

Llinas RR: The intrinsic electrophysiological properties of mammalian neurons: Insights into central nervous system function. Science 1988;242:1654.

Martin GR, Humphrey PP: Receptors for 5-hydroxytryptamine: Current perspectives on classification and nomenclature. Neuropharmacology 1994;33:261.

Nakanishi S: Metabotropic glutamate receptors: Synaptic transmission, modulation, and plasticity. Neuron 1994;13:1031.

Nakanishi S: Molecular diversity of glutamate receptors and implications for brain function. Science 1992;258:597.

Nicoll RA: The coupling of neurotransmitter receptors to ion channels in the brain. Science 1988;241:545.

Nicoll RA, Malenka RC: Contrasting properties of two forms of long-term potentiation in the hippocampus. Nature 1995;377:115.

Pin J-P, Duvosin R: The metabotropic glutamate receptors: Structure and functions. Neuropharmacology 1995;34:1.

Seeburg PH: The TiNS/TiPS Lecture. The molecular biology of mammalian glutamate receptor channels. Trends Neurosci 1993;16:359.

Südhof TC: The synaptic vesicle cycle: A cascade of protein-protein interactions. Nature 1995;375:645.

Tecott LH, Julius D: A new wave of serotonin receptors. Curr Opin Neurobiol 1993;3:310.

Wagner JJ, Terman GW, Chavkin C: Endogenous dynorphins inhibit excitatory neurotransmission and block LTP induction in the hippocampus. Nature 1993;363:451.

Weisskopf MG, Zalutsky RA, Nicoll RA: The opioid peptide dynorphin mediates heterosynaptic depression of hippocampal mossy fiber synapses and modulates long-term potentiation. Nature 1993;362:423.

Wisden W, Seeburg PH: GABA$_A$ receptor channels: From subunits to functional entities. Curr Opin Neurobiol 1992;2:263.

22

Sedative-Hypnotic Drugs

Anthony J. Trevor, PhD, & Walter L. Way, MD

Assignment of a drug to the sedative-hypnotic class indicates that its major therapeutic use is to cause sedation (with concomitant relief of anxiety) or to encourage sleep. There is considerable chemical variation within this group, so this is an example of drug classification based on clinical uses rather than on similarities in chemical structures or mechanisms of action. Anxiety states and sleep disorders are common problems, and sedative-hypnotics are among the most widely prescribed drugs worldwide.

I. BASIC PHARMACOLOGY OF SEDATIVE-HYPNOTICS

An effective **sedative** (anxiolytic) agent should reduce anxiety and exert a calming effect with little or no effect on motor or mental functions. The degree of central nervous system depression caused by a sedative should be the minimum consistent with therapeutic efficacy. A **hypnotic** drug should produce drowsiness and encourage the onset and maintenance of a state of sleep* that as far as possible resembles the natural sleep state. Hypnotic effects involve more pronounced depression of the central nervous system than sedation, and this can be achieved with most sedative drugs simply by increasing the dose.

Graded dose-dependent depression of central nervous system function is a characteristic of sedative-hypnotics. However, individual drugs differ in the relationship between the dose and the degree of central nervous system depression. Two examples of such dose-response relationships are shown in Figure 22–1. The linear slope for drug A is typical of many of the older sedative-hypnotics, including the barbiturates and alcohols. With such drugs, an increase in dose above that needed for hypnosis may lead to a state of general anesthesia. At still higher doses, sedative-hypnotics may depress respiratory and vasomotor centers in the medulla, leading to coma and death. Deviations from a linear dose-response relationship, as shown for drug B, will require proportionately greater dosage increments in order to achieve central nervous system depression more profound than hypnosis. This appears to be the case for most drugs of the benzodiazepine class, and the greater margin of safety this offers is an important reason for their extensive clinical use to treat anxiety states and sleep disorders.

CHEMICAL CLASSIFICATION

The benzodiazepines (Figure 22–2) are the most important sedative-hypnotics. All of the structures shown are 1,4-benzodiazepines, and most contain a carboxamide group in the 7-membered heterocyclic ring structure. A substituent in the 7 position, such as a halogen or a nitro group, is required for sedative-hypnotic activity. The structures of triazolam and alprazolam include the addition of a triazole ring at the 1,2-position, and such drugs are sometimes referred to as triazolobenzodiazepines.

The chemical structures of some older and less commonly used sedative-hypnotics are shown in Figure 22–3. The motivation to develop the benzodiazepines and other newer sedative-hypnotics can be attributed to efforts to avoid undesirable features of the barbiturates, including their potential for inducing psychologic and physiologic dependence. Such efforts have not always been successful. For example, the piperidinediones (glutethimide, others), introduced as "nonbarbiturate sedative-hypnotics," are in fact chemically related to and virtually indistinguish-

---

*We use the word "hypnosis" in its original sense, ie, "sleep"— not a trancelike state.

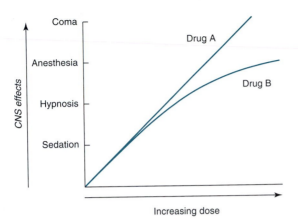

Figure 22–1. Dose-response curves for two hypothetical sedative-hypnotics.

able from barbiturates in their pharmacologic properties. The propanediol carbamates such as meprobamate are of distinctive chemical structure but are practically equivalent to barbiturates in their pharmacologic effects, and their clinical use is rapidly declining. The sedative-hypnotic class also includes compounds of simple chemical structure, including alcohols (ethanol, chloral hydrate) and the cyclic ethers. Chloral hydrate and its congeners, such as trichloroethanol, together with paraldehyde (not shown), continue to be used, particularly in institutionalized patients. Several drugs with novel chemical structures have been introduced recently. Buspirone, an azaspirodecanedione, is an anxiolytic agent that has actions different from those of conventional sedative-hypnotic drugs. Zolpidem is an imidazopyridine hypnotic, structurally unrelated to benzodiazepines.

Other classes of drugs not included in Figure 22–3 may exert sedative effects. For example, β-blocking drugs are effective in certain anxiety states and functional disorders, particularly those in which somatic and autonomic symptoms are prominent. Clonidine, a partial agonist at α_2 receptors, including presynaptic adrenoceptors in the brain, also has anxiolytic properties. Sedative effects can also be obtained with the antipsychotic tranquilizers, the tricyclic antidepressant drugs, and certain antihistaminic agents. As discussed in other chapters, these agents differ from conventional sedative-hypnotics in both their effects and their major therapeutic uses. Most importantly, they do not produce general anesthesia, and they have low abuse liability. Since they commonly exert marked effects on the peripheral autonomic nervous system, they are sometimes referred to as **"sedative-autonomic"** drugs. Compounds of the antihistaminic type are present in a number of over-the-counter sleep preparations, in which their autonomic properties as well as their long duration of action can result in adverse effects.

THE BENZODIAZEPINES & BARBITURATES

Pharmacokinetics

A. Absorption: When used to treat anxiety or sleep disorders, sedative-hypnotics are usually given orally. The rates of oral absorption of benzodiazepines differ depending on a number of factors, including lipophilicity. Oral absorption of triazolam is extremely rapid, and that of diazepam and the active metabolite of clorazepate is more rapid than other commonly used benzodiazepines. Clorazepate is converted to its active form, desmethyldiazepam (nordiazepam), by acid hydrolysis in the stomach. Oxazepam, lorazepam, and temazepam are absorbed at slower rates than other benzodiazepines. The bioavailability of several benzodiazepines, including chlordiazepoxide and diazepam, may be unreliable after intramuscular injection. The barbiturates are usually absorbed very rapidly into the blood following oral administration.

B. Distribution: Transport of a sedative-hypnotic in the blood is a dynamic process in which drug molecules enter and leave tissues at rates dependent upon blood flow, concentration gradients, and permeabilities. Lipid solubility plays a major role in determining the rate at which a particular sedative-hypnotic enters the central nervous system. For example, diazepam and triazolam are more lipid-soluble than chlordiazepoxide and lorazepam; thus, the central nervous system actions of the latter drugs are slower in onset. The thiobarbiturates (eg, thiopental), in which the oxygen on C_2 is replaced by sulfur, are very lipid-soluble, and a high rate of entry into the central nervous system contributes to the rapid onset of their central effects (see Chapter 25). In contrast, meprobamate has quite low solubility in lipids and penetrates the brain slowly even when given intravenously.

Redistribution of drug from the central nervous system to other tissues is an important feature of the biodisposition of sedative-hypnotics. Classic studies on the thiobarbiturates have shown that they are rapidly redistributed from the brain, first to highly perfused tissues such as skeletal muscle and subsequently to poorly perfused adipose tissue. These processes contribute to the termination of their major central nervous system effects. This may also be the case for other sedative-hypnotics, including the benzodiazepines, where the rate of metabolic transformation and elimination in humans is much too slow to account for the relatively short time required for dissipation of major pharmacologic effects.

All sedative-hypnotics cross the placental barrier during pregnancy. The rate at which maternal and fetal blood concentrations equilibrate is slower than that for the maternal blood and central nervous system, partly because of lower blood flow to the placenta. Nonetheless, if sedative-hypnotics are given in the predelivery period, they may contribute to the depres-

Figure 22–2. Chemical structures of benzodiazepines.

sion of neonatal vital functions. Sedative-hypnotics are detectable in breast milk and may exert depressant effects on central nervous system function in the nursing infant.

Benzodiazepines and most other sedative-hypnotics bind extensively to plasma proteins. For example, plasma protein binding of benzodiazepines ranges from 60% to over 95%. However, few clinically significant interactions involving sedative-hypnotic drugs appear to be based on competition for common binding sites on the plasma proteins. One exception is chloral hydrate, which transiently increases the anticoagulant effects of warfarin by displacement of the anticoagulant from such binding sites.

C. Biotransformation: Metabolic transformation to more water-soluble metabolites is necessary for clearance from the body of almost all drugs in this class. The microsomal drug-metabolizing enzyme systems of the liver are most important in this regard. Since few sedative-hypnotics are excreted from the body unchanged, the elimination half-life depends mainly on the rate of their metabolic transformation.

1. Benzodiazepines–Hepatic metabolism accounts for the clearance or elimination of all benzodiazepines. The patterns and rates of metabolism depend on the individual drugs. Most benzodiazepines undergo microsomal oxidation (phase I reactions), including N-dealkylation and aliphatic hydroxylation. The metabolites are subsequently conjugated (phase

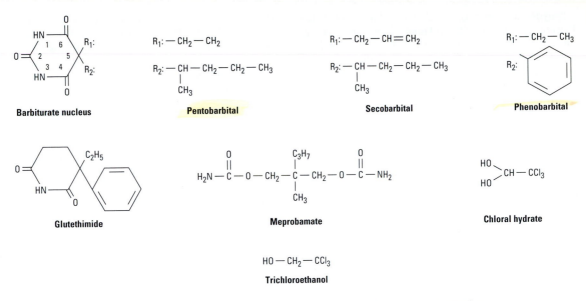

Figure 22–3. Chemical structures of barbiturates and other sedative-hypnotics.

II reactions) by glucuronosyltransferases to form glucuronides that are excreted in the urine. However, many phase I metabolites of benzodiazepines are active, with half-lives greater than the parent drugs.

As shown in Figure 22–4, desmethyldiazepam, which has an elimination half-life of more than 40 hours, is an active metabolite of chlordiazepoxide, diazepam, prazepam, and clorazepate. Desmethyldiazepam in turn is biotransformed to the active compound oxazepam. Other active metabolites of chlordiazepoxide include desmethylchlordiazepoxide and demoxepam. While diazepam is metabolized mainly to desmethyldiazepam, it is also converted to temazepam (not shown in Figure 22–4), which is further metabolized in part to oxazepam. Flurazepam, which is used mainly for hypnosis, is oxidized by hepatic enzymes to three active metabolites, desalkylflurazepam, hydroxyethylflurazepam, and flurazepam

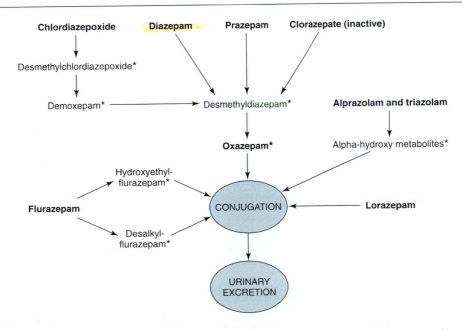

Figure 22–4. Biotransformation of benzodiazepines. (Boldface, drugs available for clinical use; *, active metabolite.)

aldehyde (not shown), which have elimination half-lives ranging from 30 to 100 hours. This may result in unwanted central nervous system depression, including daytime sedation. The triazolobenzodiazepines alprazolam and triazolam undergo alpha-hydroxylation, and the resulting metabolites appear to exert short-lived pharmacologic effects since they are rapidly conjugated to form inactive glucuronides.

The formation of active metabolites has complicated studies on the pharmacokinetics of the benzodiazepines in humans because the elimination half-life of the parent drug may have little relationship to the time course of pharmacologic effects. Those benzodiazepines for which the parent drug or active metabolites have long half-lives are more likely to cause cumulative effects with multiple doses. Cumulative and residual effects such as excessive drowsiness appear to be less of a problem with such drugs as estazolam, oxazepam, and lorazepam, which have shorter half-lives and are metabolized directly to inactive glucuronides. Some pharmacokinetic properties of selected benzodiazepines are listed in Table 22–1.

2. Barbiturates—With the exception of phenobarbital, only insignificant quantities of the barbiturates are excreted unchanged. The major metabolic pathways involve oxidation by hepatic enzymes of chemical groups attached to C_5, which are different for the individual barbiturates. The alcohols, acids, and ketones formed appear in the urine as glucuronide conjugates. With very few exceptions, the metabolites of the barbiturates lack pharmacologic activity. The overall rate of hepatic metabolism in humans depends on the individual drug but (with the exception of the thiobarbiturates) is usually slow. The elimination half-lives of secobarbital and pentobarbital range from 18 to 48 hours in different individuals. The elimination half-life of phenobarbital in humans is 4–5 days. Multiple dosing with these agents can lead to cumulative effects.

D. Excretion: The water-soluble metabolites of benzodiazepines and other sedative-hypnotics are excreted mainly via the kidney. In most cases, changes in renal function do not have a marked effect on the elimination of parent drugs. Phenobarbital is excreted unchanged in the urine to a certain extent (20–30% in humans), and its elimination rate can be increased significantly by alkalinization of the urine. This is partly due to increased ionization at alkaline pH, since phenobarbital is a weak acid with a pK_a of 7.4. Only trace amounts of the benzodiazepines and less than 10% of a hypnotic dose of meprobamate appear in the urine unchanged.

E. Factors Affecting Biodisposition: The biodisposition of sedative-hypnotics can be influenced by several factors, particularly alterations in hepatic function resulting from disease, old age, or drug-induced increases or decreases in microsomal enzyme activities.

As described in Chapter 4, decreased hepatic function may result in reduction of the clearance of drugs metabolized via oxidative pathways. Many of the benzodiazepines, almost all of the barbiturates, the piperidinediones, and meprobamate fall into this category. In very old patients and in patients with severe liver disease, the elimination half-lives of these drugs are usually increased significantly. In such cases, multiple normal doses of these sedative-hypnotics often result in excessive central nervous system effects. Thus, it is common practice to reduce the dosage of such

Table 22–1. Pharmacokinetic properties of benzodiazepines in humans.

Drug	Peak Blood Level (hours)	Elimination Half-Life[1] (hours)	Comments
Alprazolam	1–2	12–15	Rapid oral absorption
Chlordiazepoxide	2–4	15–40	Active metabolites; erratic bioavailability from IM injection
Clorazepate	1–2 (nordiazepam)	50–100	Prodrug; hydrolyzed to active form in stomach
Diazepam	1–2	20–80	Active metabolites; erratic bioavailability from IM injection
Estazolam	2	10–24	No active metabolites
Flurazepam	1–2	40–100	Active metabolites with long half-lives
Lorazepam	1–6	10–20	No active metabolites
Oxazepam	2–4	10–20	No active metabolites
Prazepam	1–2	50–100	Active metabolites with long half-lives
Quazepam	2	30–100	Active metabolites with long half-lives
Temazepam	2–3	10–40	Slow oral absorption
Triazolam	1	2–3	Rapid onset; short duration of action

[1]Includes half-lives of major metabolites.

sedative-hypnotics in patients who are elderly or who may have limited hepatic function. Metabolism involving glucuronide conjugation appears to be less affected by old age or liver disease than oxidative metabolism.

The activity of hepatic microsomal drug-metabolizing enzymes may be increased in patients exposed to certain older sedative-hypnotics on a chronic basis (enzyme induction; see Chapter 4). Drugs with long elimination half-lives such as phenobarbital and meprobamate are most likely to cause this effect and result in an increase in their own hepatic metabolism as well as that of certain other drugs. Self-induction of metabolism is a possible but poorly documented mechanism that contributes to the development of tolerance to sedative-hypnotics. Increased biotransformation of other pharmacologic agents as a result of enzyme induction by barbiturates is a potential mechanism underlying drug interactions (Appendix II). In contrast, the benzodiazepines do not change hepatic drug-metabolizing enzyme activity with continuous use.

Pharmacodynamics of Benzodiazepines & Barbiturates

A. Molecular Pharmacology of the GABA$_A$ Receptor: The benzodiazepines, the barbiturates, and the imidazopyridines bind to molecular components of the GABA$_A$ receptor present in neuronal membranes in the central nervous system. This ionotropic receptor, a transmembrane heteroligomeric protein that functions as a chloride ion channel, is activated by the inhibitory neurotransmitter GABA.

Molecular cloning techniques show the GABA$_A$ receptor to have a pentameric structure comprised of multiple subunits (alpha, beta, gamma, etc), each with four transmembrane spanning domains. Several different subunits of each type have been identified, ie, six different alpha, four beta, and three gamma. Although alpha subunits alone or beta units alone can form chloride channels with weak GABA responsiveness, combinations of the three major subunits—alpha, beta, and gamma—appear to be essential for normal physiologic and pharmacologic function of the macromolecule. GABA$_A$ receptors in different areas of the central nervous system contain different combinations of the essential subunits conferring different pharmacologic properties on GABA$_A$ subtypes. Analyses of mRNAs from various regions of the brain have shown that at least 16 genes are currently known to encode the five subunits that are assembled in GABA$_A$ receptors.

Reconstitution of channels with various combinations of the subunits indicates that GABA binds to receptor sites on the alpha or beta subunits and that this interaction initiates gating of the chloride channel current. Sensitivity of the complex to benzodiazepines requires a gamma$_2$ subunit, suggesting that the benzodiazepine (BDZ) receptor sites are probably located on or near this structure (see box: Benzodiazepine Receptor Heterogeneity). At least two benzodiazepine

receptor subtypes (BZ$_1$ and BZ$_2$) occur in the brain and differ in their affinities for specific drugs. A model of the hypothetical GABA-BDZ receptor-chloride ion channel macromolecular complex is shown in Figure 22–5.

B. Neuropharmacology: Gamma-aminobutyric acid (GABA) is the major inhibitory neurotransmitter in the central nervous system. Electrophysiologic studies have shown that benzodiazepines potentiate GABAergic inhibition at all levels of the neuraxis, including the spinal cord, hypothalamus, hippocampus, substantia nigra, cerebellar cortex, and cerebral cortex. Benzodiazepines appear to increase the efficiency of GABAergic synaptic inhibition (via membrane hyperpolarization), which leads to a decrease in the firing rate of critical neurons in many regions of the brain. The benzodiazepines do not substitute for GABA but appear to enhance GABA's effects without directly activating GABA receptors or opening the associated chloride channels. The enhancement in chloride ion conductance induced by

Figure 22–5. A model of the GABA$_A$ receptor-chloride ion channel macromolecular complex (many others could be proposed). A heteroligomeric glycoprotein, the complex consists of five or more membrane-spanning subunits. Multiple forms of alpha, beta, and gamma subunits are arranged in different pentameric combinations so that GABA$_A$ receptors exhibit molecular heterogeneity. GABA appears to interact with alpha or beta subunits triggering chloride channel opening with resultant membrane hyperpolarization. Binding of benzodiazepines to gamma subunits or to an area of the alpha unit influenced by the gamma unit facilitates the process of channel opening but does not directly initiate chloride current. (Modified and reproduced, with permission, from Zorumsky CF, Isenberg KE: Insights into the structure and function of GABA-benzodiazepine receptors: Ion channels and psychiatry. Am J Psychiatry 1991;148:162.)

BZ ↑ GABA chan freq *barbit ↑ GABA durat*

BENZODIAZEPINE RECEPTOR HETEROGENEITY

Benzodiazepine receptors in the central nervous system have been classified as BZ_1 (also called omega$_1$) and BZ_2 (omega$_2$) subtypes on the basis of their relative affinities for different benzodiazepines and for nonbenzodiazepine drugs that appear to act via benzodiazepine receptors. Differences in binding affinities of receptor ligands are due to heterogeneity in GABA$_A$ receptor subunit composition. Activators of BZ_1 receptors have a high affinity for GABA receptors containing the alpha$_1$ subunit and a very low affinity for receptors containing an alpha$_5$ subunit (corresponding to one type of BZ_2 receptor). Most benzodiazepines used clinically are able to interact with both BZ_1 and BZ_2 receptor subtypes, but the imidazopyridines (eg, zolpidem) are BZ_1-selective. As noted in the text, zolpidem exerts hypnotic actions with minimal muscle relaxing or anticonvulsant effects and produces little tolerance or dependence with continued use. Thus, the spectrum of pharmacologic actions elicited by drugs that modulate GABA actions is influenced by the composition of the subunits assembled to form the GABA$_A$ receptor. With further molecular characterization of these ligand-binding sites on the various GABA$_A$ receptors in different regions of the brain, it may be possible to design drugs that are even more selective than the currently available benzodiazepines and imidazopyridines in their central nervous system actions.

---

the interaction of benzodiazepines with GABA takes the form of an increase in the *frequency* of channel-opening events (Figure 22–6). This effect may be due in part to enhanced receptor affinity for GABA.

Barbiturates also facilitate the actions of GABA at multiple sites in the central nervous system, but—in contrast to benzodiazepines—they appear to increase the *duration* of the GABA-gated channel openings (Figure 22–6). At high concentrations, the barbiturates may also be GABA-mimetic, directly activating chloride channels. These effects involve a binding site or sites distinct from the benzodiazepine binding site. Barbiturates are less selective in their actions than benzodiazepines, since they also depress the actions of excitatory neurotransmitters and exert nonsynaptic membrane effects in parallel with their effects on GABA neurotransmission. This multiplicity of sites of action of barbiturates may be the basis for their ability to induce full surgical anesthesia (see Chapter 25) and for their more pronounced central depressant

effects (which result in their low margin of safety) compared to benzodiazepines.

C. Benzodiazepine Receptor Ligands: Three types of ligand-benzodiazepine receptor interactions have been reported: (1) **Agonists** facilitate GABA action and act as positive allosteric modulators of receptor function. These actions are typically produced by the clinically useful benzodiazepines, which exert anxiolytic and anticonvulsant effects. Zolpidem and related imidazopyridines are selective agonists at the BZ_1 (omega$_1$) receptor subtype. Endogenous agonist ligands for the BZ receptors have been proposed, since benzodiazepine-like chemicals have been isolated from brain tissue of animals never exposed to these drugs, and benzodiazepine-like immunoreactivity has been detected in human brains stored in paraffin 15 years before the first benzodiazepine drug was synthesized. Nonbenzodiazepine molecules that have affinity for benzodiazepine receptors have also been detected in human brain. Such "endozepines" facilitate GABA-mediated chloride channel gating in cultured neurons. (2) **Antagonists** are typified by the synthetic benzodiazepine derivative **flumazenil,** which blocks the actions of benzodiazepines and zolpidem but does not antagonize the actions of barbiturates, meprobamate, or ethanol. Certain endogenous compounds, eg, diazepam-binding inhibitor (DBI), are also capable of blocking the interaction of benzodiazepines with benzodiazepine receptors. (3) **Inverse agonists** act as negative allosteric modulators of GABA receptor function. Their interaction with benzodiazepine receptors can produce anxiety and seizures, an action that has been demonstrated for several compounds, especially the **β-carbolines,** eg, n-butyl-β-carboline-3-carboxylate (β-CCB). In addition to their direct actions, these molecules can block the effects of benzodiazepines.

The physiologic significance of endogenous modulators of the functions of GABA in the central nervous system remain unclear. To date it has not been established that these putative endogenous ligands of BZ receptors play a role in the control of states of anxiety, sleep patterns, or any other characteristic behavioral expression of central nervous system function.

D. Organ Level Effects:

1. Sedation—Sedation can be defined as a suppression of responsiveness to a constant level of stimulation, with decreased spontaneous activity and ideation. These behavioral changes occur at the lowest effective doses of the commonly used sedative-hypnotics, and it is not yet clear whether such antianxiety actions seen clinically are equivalent to or different from sedative effects. In experimental animal models, benzodiazepines and the older sedative-hypnotic drugs are able to release punishment-suppressed behavior, and this disinhibition has been equated with antianxiety effects. However, the release of previously suppressed behavior may be more relevant to behavioral disinhibitory effects of these drugs, including euphoria, impaired judgment, and loss of self-control, which can occur at dosages in the range of those used for management of anxiety. While most sedative-hypnotic drugs are capable of releasing punishment-suppressed behavior in animals, the benzodiazepines exert such effects at dosages that cause only minor central nervous system depression. Although they have sedative actions, antipsychotic drugs and tricyclic antidepressants are not effective in this experimental model. The benzodiazepines also exert anterograde amnesic effects (inability to remember events occurring during the drug's action) at sedative dosages. Buspirone is the most distinctive drug in terms of anti-anxiety actions, since these are achieved with minimal effects on psychomotor functions.

2. Hypnosis–By definition, all of the sedative-hypnotics will induce sleep if high enough doses are given. Normal sleep consists of distinct stages, based on three physiologic measures: the electroencephalogram, the electromyogram, and the electronystagmogram (a measure of lateral movements of the eye). Based on the latter, two major categories can be distinguished: non-rapid eye movement (NREM) sleep, which represents approximately 70–75% of total sleep; and rapid eye movement (REM) sleep. REM and NREM sleep occur cyclically over an interval of about 90 minutes. The REM sleep stage is that in which most

Figure 22–6. Patch-clamp recording of single-channel GABA-evoked currents in mouse spinal cord neurons. **A:** Control. **B:** Channel opening (downward deflections) elicited by GABA. **C:** Diazepam increases the frequency of channel opening without marked effects on duration of openings. **D:** Phenobarbital prolongs the duration of channel openings without marked effects on frequency. (Reproduced, with permission, from, Twyman RE et al: Differential regulation of GABA receptor channels by diazepam and phenobarbital. Ann Neurol 1989;25:213.)

recallable dreams occur. NREM sleep progresses through four stages (1–4), with the greatest proportion (50%) of sleep being spent in stage 2. This is followed by delta or slow-wave sleep (stages 3 and 4), in which somnambulism and night terrors occur. During slow wave sleep, the secretion of adrenal steroids is at its lowest and secretion of somatotropin is at its highest.

The effects of sedative-hypnotics on the sleep stages have been studied extensively, though often with normal volunteer subjects rather than patients with sleep disorders. The effects observed depend on several factors, including the specific drug, the dose, and the frequency of its administration. While some exceptions exist, the effects of sedative-hypnotics on patterns of normal sleep are as follows: (1) the latency of sleep onset is decreased (time to fall asleep); (2) the duration of stage 2 NREM sleep is increased; (3) the duration of REM sleep is decreased; and (4) the duration of slow-wave sleep is decreased.

More rapid onset of sleep and prolongation of stage 2 are presumably clinically useful effects. However, the significance of sedative-hypnotic drug effects on REM and slow-wave sleep is not clear. Deliberate interruption of REM sleep causes anxiety and irritability followed by a rebound increase in REM sleep at the end of the experiment. A similar pattern of "REM rebound" can be detected following cessation of drug treatment with most sedative-hypnotics. Despite possible reductions in slow wave sleep there are no reports of disturbances in the secretion of pituitary or adrenal hormones when either barbiturates or benzodiazepines are used as hypnotics. The use of sedative-hypnotics for more than 1–2 weeks leads to some tolerance to their effects on sleep patterns.

3. Anesthesia–As shown in Figure 22–1, certain sedative-hypnotics in high doses will depress the central nervous system to the point known as stage III of general anesthesia (see Chapter 25). However, the suitability of a particular agent as an adjunct in anesthesia depends mainly on the physicochemical properties that determine its rapidity of onset and duration of effect. Among the barbiturates, thiopental and methohexital are very lipid-soluble, penetrating brain tissue rapidly following intravenous administration. Rapid tissue redistribution accounts for the short duration of action of these drugs, which are therefore useful in anesthesia practice.

Certain benzodiazepines, including diazepam and midazolam, are used intravenously in anesthesia (see Chapter 24) but have not proved to be fully successful as induction agents capable of producing surgical anesthesia by themselves. This statement is supported by the fact that the MAC (minimum alveolar anesthetic concentration, Chapter 25) of another anesthetic cannot be reduced to zero by the substitution of a benzodiazepine. Not surprisingly, benzodiazepines given in large doses as adjuncts to general anesthetics may contribute to a persistent postanesthetic respiratory depression. This is probably related to their rela-

tively long half-lives and the formation of active metabolites.

4. Anticonvulsant effects–Most of the sedative-hypnotics are capable of inhibiting the development and spread of epileptiform activity in the central nervous system. Some selectivity exists in that certain drugs can exert anticonvulsant effects without marked central nervous system depression, so that mentation and physiologic activity are relatively unaffected. Several benzodiazepines, including clonazepam, nitrazepam, lorazepam, and diazepam, have selective actions that are clinically useful in the management of seizure states (see Chapter 24). Of the barbiturates, phenobarbital and metharbital (converted to phenobarbital in the body) are effective in the treatment of generalized tonic-clonic seizures.

5. Muscle relaxation–Some sedative-hypnotics, particularly members of the carbamate and benzodiazepine groups, exert inhibitory effects on polysynaptic reflexes and internuncial transmission and at high doses may also depress transmission at the skeletal neuromuscular junction. Somewhat selective actions of this type that lead to muscle relaxation can be readily demonstrated in animals and have led to claims of usefulness for relaxing contracted voluntary muscle in joint disease or muscle spasm (see Clinical Pharmacology).

6. Effects on respiration and cardiovascular function–At hypnotic doses in healthy patients, the effects of sedative-hypnotics on respiration are comparable to changes during natural sleep. However, sedative-hypnotics even at therapeutic doses can produce significant respiratory depression in patients with pulmonary disease. Effects on respiration are dose-related, and depression of the medullary respiratory center is the usual cause of death due to overdose of sedative-hypnotics.

At doses up to those causing hypnosis, no significant effects on the cardiovascular system are observed in healthy patients. However, in hypovolemic states, congestive heart failure, and other diseases that impair cardiovascular function, normal doses of sedative-hypnotics may cause cardiovascular depression, probably as a result of actions on the medullary vasomotor centers. At toxic doses, myocardial contractility and vascular tone may both be depressed by central and peripheral effects, leading to circulatory collapse. Respiratory and cardiovascular effects become more apparent when sedative-hypnotics are given intravenously.

Tolerance; Psychologic & Physiologic Dependence

Tolerance—decreased responsiveness to a drug following repeated exposure—is a common feature of sedative-hypnotic use. It may result in an increase in the dose needed to maintain symptomatic improvement or to promote sleep. It is important to recognize that partial cross-tolerance occurs between the sedative-hypnotics described here and also with ethanol (Chapter 23)—a feature of some clinical importance, as explained below. The mechanisms responsible for tolerance to sedative-hypnotics are not well understood. An alteration in the rate of metabolic inactivation with chronic administration may be partly responsible (metabolic tolerance) in the case of barbiturates, but changes in responsiveness of the central nervous system (pharmacodynamic tolerance) are of greater importance for most sedative-hypnotics. In the case of benzodiazepines, the development of tolerance in animals is associated with down-regulation of brain benzodiazepine receptors.

The perceived desirable properties of relief of anxiety, euphoria, disinhibition, and promotion of sleep have led to the compulsive misuse of virtually all sedative-hypnotics. (See Chapter 32 for a detailed discussion of drug abuse.) The consequences of abuse of these agents can be defined in both psychologic and physiologic terms. The psychologic component may initially parallel simple neurotic behavior patterns difficult to differentiate from those of the inveterate coffee drinker or cigarette smoker. When the pattern of sedative-hypnotic use becomes compulsive, more serious complications develop, including physiologic dependence and tolerance.

Physiologic dependence can be described as an altered physiologic state that requires continuous drug administration to prevent the appearance of an abstinence or withdrawal syndrome. As described more fully later, in the case of sedative-hypnotics this syndrome is characterized by states of increased anxiety, insomnia, and central nervous system excitability that may progress to convulsions. Most sedative-hypnotics—including benzodiazepines—are capable of causing physiologic dependence when used on a chronic basis. However, the severity of withdrawal symptoms differs between individual drugs and depends also on the magnitude of the dose used immediately prior to cessation of use. When higher doses of sedative-hypnotics are used, abrupt withdrawal leads to more serious withdrawal signs. Differences in the severity of withdrawal symptoms between individual sedative-hypnotics relate in part to half-life, since drugs with long half-lives are eliminated slowly enough to accomplish gradual withdrawal with few physical symptoms. The use of drugs with very short half-lives for hypnotic effects may lead to signs of withdrawal even between doses. For example, triazolam, a benzodiazepine with a half-life of about 4 hours, has been reported to cause daytime anxiety when used to treat sleep disorders.

BENZODIAZEPINE ANTAGONISTS: FLUMAZENIL

Flumazenil is one of several 1,4-benzodiazepine derivatives with high affinity for the benzodiazepine receptor that act as competitive antagonists. It is the only benzodiazepine receptor antagonist available for clinical use at present. It blocks many of the actions of benzodiazepines (and imidazopyridines) but does not antagonize the central nervous system effects of other sedative-hypnotics, ethanol, opioids, or general anesthetics. Flumazenil is approved for use in reversing the central nervous system depressant effects of benzodiazepine overdose and to hasten recovery following use of these drugs in anesthetic and diagnostic procedures. While the drug reverses the sedative effects of benzodiazepines, antagonism of benzodiazepine-induced respiratory depression is less predictable. When given intravenously, flumazenil acts rapidly but has a short half-life (0.7–1.3 hours) due to rapid hepatic clearance. Since all benzodiazepines have a longer duration of action than flumazenil, sedation commonly recurs, requiring repeated administration of the antagonist.

Adverse effects of flumazenil include agitation, confusion, dizziness, and nausea. Flumazenil may cause a severe precipitated abstinence syndrome in patients who have developed physiologic benzodiazepine dependence. In patients who have ingested benzodiazepines with tricyclic antidepressants, seizures and cardiac arrhythmias may occur following flumazenil administration. Transient improvement in mental status has been reported with flumazenil when used in patients with hepatic encephalopathy.

NEWER DRUGS FOR ANXIETY & SLEEP DISORDERS

Although the benzodiazepines continue to be the agents of choice in the treatment of most anxiety states and for insomnia, their pharmacologic effects include daytime sedation and drowsiness, synergistic depression of the central nervous system with other drugs (especially alcohol), and the possibility of psychologic and physiologic dependence with repeated use. Anxiolytic drugs that act through non-GABAergic systems might have a reduced propensity for such actions. Several new nonbenzodiazepines, including buspirone, have such characteristics. In addition, certain imidazopyridines, including zolpidem, may be more selective in their central actions even though they appear to act through benzodiazepine receptors.

Buspirone

Buspirone relieves anxiety without causing marked sedative or euphoric effects. Unlike benzodiazepines, the drug has no hypnotic, anticonvulsant, or muscle relaxant properties. Buspirone does not interact directly with GABAergic systems and may exert its anxiolytic effects by acting as a partial agonist at brain 5-HT$_{1A}$ receptors. Buspirone-treated patients show no rebound anxiety or withdrawal signs on abrupt discontinuance. The drug is not effective in blocking the acute withdrawal syndrome resulting from abrupt cessation of use of benzodiazepines or other sedative-hypnotics. Buspirone has minimal abuse liability. In contrast to the benzodiazepines, the anxiolytic effects of buspirone may take more than a week to become established, making this drug suitable mainly for generalized anxiety states. The drug is not very effective in panic disorders.

Buspirone is rapidly absorbed orally but undergoes extensive first-pass metabolism via hydroxylation and dealkylation reactions to form several active metabolites. The major metabolite is 1-(2-pyrimidyl)-piperazine (1-PP), which has α_2-adrenoceptor-blocking actions and which enters the central nervous system to reach higher levels than the parent drug. It is not known what role (if any) 1-PP plays in the central actions of buspirone. The elimination half-life of buspirone is 2–4 hours, and liver dysfunction may decrease its clearance.

Buspirone causes less psychomotor impairment than diazepam and does not affect driving skills. The drug does not potentiate the central nervous system depressant effects of conventional sedative-hypnotic drugs, ethanol, or tricyclic antidepressants, and elderly patients do not appear to be more sensitive to its actions. Tachycardia, palpitations, nervousness, gastrointestinal distress, and paresthesias may occur more frequently than with benzodiazepines. Buspirone also causes a dose-dependent pupillary constriction. Blood pressure may be elevated in patients receiving MAO inhibitors. A number of buspirone analogs have been developed (eg, **ipsapirone, gepirone, tandospirone**) and are under study.

Zolpidem

Zolpidem, an imidazopyridine derivative structurally unrelated to benzodiazepines, has hypnotic actions. The drug binds selectively to the BZ_1 (omega$_1$) subtype of benzodiazepine receptors and facilitates GABA-mediated neuronal inhibition. Like the benzodiazepines, the actions of zolpidem are antagonized by flumazenil. Unlike benzodiazepines, zolpidem has minimal muscle relaxing and anticonvulsant effects. When used for the short-term treatment of insomnia, zolpidem has an efficacy similar to that of hypnotic benzodiazepines. The drug has an onset of action similar to that of flurazepam, but its duration of action is closer to that of triazolam. Zolpidem causes minor effects on sleep patterns at the recommended hypnotic dose but can suppress REM sleep at higher doses. Respiratory depression may occur if large doses of zolpidem are ingested with other central nervous system depressants, including ethanol.

The risk of development of tolerance and dependence with extended use of zolpidem appears to be less than with the use of hypnotic benzodiazepines. Zolpidem is rapidly metabolized to inactive metabolites by the liver via oxidation and hydroxylation. The elimination half-life of the drug is 1.5–3.5 hours, with

clearance decreased in elderly patients. Dosage reductions are recommended in patients with hepatic dysfunction, in elderly patients, and in patients taking cimetidine. **Alpidem,** a related imidazopyridine used as an anxiolytic, is reported to cause acute hepatitis. Alpidem is not approved in the USA.

OLDER SEDATIVE-HYPNOTICS

These drugs include alcohols (**ethchlorvynol, chloral hydrate**), piperidinediones (**glutethimide, methyprylon**), and carbamates (**meprobamate**). They are rarely used in therapy, though the low cost of chloral hydrate makes it attractive for institutional use. Little is known about their molecular mechanisms of action. Most of these drugs are biotransformed to more water-soluble compounds by hepatic enzymes. Trichloroethanol is the pharmacologically active metabolite of chloral hydrate and has a half-life of 6–10 hours. However, its toxic metabolite, trichloroacetic acid, is cleared very slowly and can accumulate with the nightly administration of chloral hydrate. Furthermore, recurrent concerns regarding the possible carcinogenicity of chloral hydrate itself—or its metabolites—suggest that this drug should not be used until more data are available.

II. CLINICAL PHARMACOLOGY OF SEDATIVE-HYPNOTICS

TREATMENT OF ANXIETY STATES

The psychologic, behavioral, and physiologic responses that characterize anxiety can take many forms. Typically, the psychic awareness of anxiety is accompanied by enhanced vigilance, motor tension, and autonomic hyperactivity. Before prescribing sedative-hypnotics, one should analyze the patient's symptoms carefully. Anxiety is in many cases secondary to organic disease states—acute myocardial infarction, angina pectoris, gastrointestinal ulcers, etc—which themselves require specific therapy. Another class of secondary anxiety states (situational anxiety) results from circumstances that may have to be dealt with only once or only a few times, including anticipation of frightening medical or dental procedures and family illness or other tragedy. Even though situational anxiety tends to be self-limiting, the short-term use of sedative-hypnotics may be appropriate for the treatment of this and certain disease-associated anxiety states. Similarly, the use of a sedative-hypnotic as premedication prior to surgery or some unpleasant medical procedure is rational and proper (Table 22–2). If the patient presents with chronic anxiety as the primary complaint, it may be appropriate to

Table 22–2. Clinical uses of sedative-hypnotics.

For relief of anxiety
For insomnia
For sedation and amnesia before medical and surgical procedures
Treatment of epilepsy and seizure states
Intravenous administration, as a component of balanced anesthesia
For control of ethanol or other sedative-hypnotic withdrawal states
For muscle relaxation in specific neuromuscular disorders
As diagnostic aids or for treatment in psychiatry

review the diagnostic criteria set forth in the *Diagnostic & Statistical Manual of Mental Disorders (DSM IV)* to determine whether the diagnosis is correct and if treatment should include drug therapy. For example, excessive or unreasonable anxiety about life circumstances (generalized anxiety disorder), panic disorders, and agoraphobia are amenable to drug therapy, usually in conjunction with psychotherapy. In some cases, anxiety may be a symptom of other psychiatric problems that may warrant the use of pharmacologic agents such as antidepressant or antipsychotic drugs.

The benzodiazepines are the drugs most commonly used for treatment of anxiety states. Since anxiety symptoms may be relieved by many sedatives, it is not always easy to demonstrate superiority of one drug over another. Thus, a preference for a particular drug in a specific situation is often based on factors other than anxiolytic efficacy. An exception to this generalization is alprazolam, which is particularly effective in the treatment of panic disorders and agoraphobia and is more selective in this regard than other benzodiazepines. Alprazolam is also reported to have efficacy similar to that of tricyclic antidepressants in major depressive disorders. The choice of benzodiazepines for anxiety is based on several sound pharmacologic principles: (1) a relatively high therapeutic index (see drug B in Figure 22–1), plus availability of flumazenil for treatment of overdose; (2) a low risk of drug interactions based on liver enzyme induction; (3) slow elimination rates, which may favor persistence of useful central nervous system effects; and (4) a low risk of physiologic dependence, with minor withdrawal symptoms.

Disadvantages of the benzodiazepines include the tendency to develop psychologic dependence, the formation of active metabolites, amnesic effects, and their higher cost. In addition, the benzodiazepines exert additive central nervous system depression when administered with other drugs, including ethanol. The patient should be warned of this possibility to avoid impairment of performance of any task requiring mental alertness and motor coordination. Many of the disadvantages of benzodiazepines are not shared by buspirone, which appears to be the most selective anxiolytic of the currently available drugs. However, limitations of buspirone include the extremely slow onset of its anxiolytic actions—confining its use to generalized anxiety—and its limited efficacy in anxiety states that feature panic attacks and phobic characteristics.

Perhaps the most important guide to therapy is the recommendation to use the drug selected with appropriate restraint so as to minimize adverse effects. A dose should be prescribed that does not impair mentation or motor functions during working hours. Some patients may tolerate the drug better if most of the daily dose is given at bedtime, with smaller doses during the day. Prescriptions should be written for short periods, since there is little justification for long-term therapy. The physician should make an effort to assess the efficacy of therapy from the patient's subjective responses. Combinations of antianxiety agents should be avoided, and people taking sedatives should be cautioned about the consumption of alcohol and the concurrent use of over-the-counter medications containing antihistaminic or anticholinergic drugs (see Chapter 64).

Phenobarbital, meprobamate, and sedative-autonomic drugs are used occasionally as antianxiety agents. For example, the antihistaminics (diphenhydramine, hydroxyzine, promethazine) continue to be used presurgically for their sedative and muscarinic receptor blocking actions.

Beta-blocking drugs (eg, propranolol) may be used as antianxiety agents in a number of situations. The sympathetic nervous system overactivity associated with anxiety appears to be satisfactorily relieved by the β-blockers, and a slight improvement in the nonsomatic components of anxiety may also occur. Adverse central nervous system effects of propranolol include lethargy, vivid dreams, and hallucinations.

The antihypertensive drug clonidine has also been used in the treatment of anxiety states, including panic attacks. Clonidine also has usefulness in suppressing anxiety in the management of withdrawal from dependence on nicotine or opioid analgesics. Concomitant treatment with drugs that exert α-adrenoceptor-blocking actions (including tricyclic antidepressants) may decrease the effects of clonidine. Withdrawal from clonidine after protracted use, especially at high doses, has led to life-threatening hypertensive crisis (see Chapter 11).

TREATMENT OF SLEEP PROBLEMS

The complaint of insomnia embraces a wide variety of sleep problems that include difficulty in falling asleep, frequent awakenings, short duration of sleep, and "unrefreshing" sleep. Insomnia is a serious complaint calling for careful evaluation to uncover possible causes (organic, psychologic, situational, etc) that can perhaps be managed without hypnotic drugs. Nonpharmacologic therapies that are sometimes useful include proper diet and exercise, avoiding stimulants before retiring, ensuring a comfortable sleeping place, and retiring at a regular time each night. In some cases, however, the patient will need and should be given a sedative-hypnotic for a limited period. It should be noted that the discontinuance of most drugs in this class can lead to rebound insomnia.

Claims have sometimes been made for superiority of one sedative-hypnotic over another based on differential actions on sleep architecture. Benzodiazepines can cause a dose-dependent decrease in both REM and slow wave sleep, though to a lesser extent than the barbiturates. Zolpidem appears to be even less likely than the benzodiazepines to change sleep patterns. However, so little is known about the clinical impact of these effects that statements about the desirability of a particular drug based on its effects on sleep architecture have more theoretical than practical significance. Clinical criteria of efficacy in alleviating a particular sleeping problem are more useful. The drug selected should be one that provides sleep of fairly rapid onset (decreased sleep latency) and sufficient duration, with minimal "hangover" effects such as drowsiness, dysphoria, and mental or motor depression the following day. While older drugs such as chloral hydrate, secobarbital, and pentobarbital are still used, benzodiazepines are generally preferred. Daytime sedation is more common with benzodiazepines that have slow elimination rates (eg, lorazepam) and those that are biotransformed to active metabolites (eg, flurazepam, quazepam). Conversely, early morning awakening may occur with a short-acting drug such as triazolam, the most frequently prescribed hypnotic drug in the United States. If hypnotics are used every night, tolerance can occur, leading to dose increases by the patient to produce the desired effect. It should be recalled that if physiologic dependence develops, the shorter-acting drugs are associated with more intense withdrawal signs when discontinued. These can include rebound anxiety and insomnia, restlessness, tinnitus, increased reflex activity, and possibly seizures. Anterograde amnesia occurs to some degree with all hypnotic benzodiazepines. Zolpidem has efficacy similar to that of the hypnotic benzodiazepines in the management of sleep disorders and appears less likely to lead to tolerance or dependence. The drugs commonly used for sedation and hypnosis are listed in Table 22–3 together with recommended doses. *Note: Long-term use of hypnotics is irrational and dangerous medical practice.*

OTHER THERAPEUTIC USES

Table 22–2 summarizes several other important clinical uses of drugs in the sedative-hypnotic class. Drugs used in the management of seizure disorders and for intravenous anesthesia are discussed in Chapters 24 and 25.

For sedative and possible amnesic effects during medical or surgical procedures such as endoscopy and bronchoscopy—as well as for premedication prior to anesthesia—oral formulations of shorter-acting drugs are preferred. When drug administration is under close supervision, the danger of accidental or intentional overdosage is less than in the outpatient situation, and a barbiturate may be as appropriate as any other sedative-hypnotic.

Long-acting drugs such as chlordiazepoxide and diazepam and, to a lesser extent, phenobarbital are administered in progressively decreasing doses to patients during withdrawal from physiologic dependence on ethanol or other sedative-hypnotics.

Meprobamate and, more recently, the benzodiazepines have frequently been used as central muscle relaxants, though evidence for general efficacy without accompanying sedation is lacking. A possible exception is diazepam, which has useful relaxant effects in skeletal muscle spasticity of central origin (see Chapter 27).

Psychiatric uses of benzodiazepines other than treatment of anxiety states include the initial manage-

Table 22–3. Dosages of drugs used commonly for sedation and hypnosis.

Sedation		Hypnosis	
Drug	**Dosage**	**Drug**	**Dosage (at Bedtime)**
Alprazolam (Xanax)	0.25–0.5 mg 2–3 times daily	Chloral hydrate	500–1000 mg
Buspirone (Buspar)	5–10 mg 2–3 times daily	Estazolam (ProSom)	0.5–2 mg
Chlordiazepoxide (Librium)	10–20 mg 2–3 times daily	Flurazepam (Dalmane)	15–30 mg
Clorazepate (Tranxene)	5–7.5 mg twice daily	Lorazepam (Ativan)	2–4 mg
Diazepam (Valium)	5 mg twice daily	Pentobarbital	100–200 mg
Halazepam (Paxipam)	20–40 mg 3–4 times daily	Quazepam (Doral)	7.5–15 mg
Lorazepam (Ativan)	1–2 mg once or twice daily	Secobarbital	100–200 mg
Oxazepam (Serax)	15–30 mg 3–4 times daily	Temazepam (Restoril)	10–30 mg
Phenobarbital	15–30 mg 2–3 times daily	Triazolam (Halcion)	0.125–0.5 mg
Prazepam (Centrax)	10–20 mg 2–3 times daily	Zolpidem (Ambien)	5–10 mg

ment of mania, the control of drug-induced hyperexcitability states (eg, phencyclidine intoxication), and possibly the treatment of major depressive disorders with alprazolam. Sedative-hypnotics are also used occasionally as diagnostic aids in neurology and psychiatry.

CLINICAL TOXICOLOGY OF SEDATIVE-HYPNOTICS

Direct Toxic Actions

Many of the common adverse effects of drugs in this class are those resulting from dose-related depression of central nervous system functions. Relatively low doses may lead to drowsiness, impaired judgment, and diminished motor skills, sometimes with a significant impact on driving ability, job performance, and personal relationships. Benzodiazepines may cause a significant dose-related anterograde amnesia; they can significantly impair ability to learn new information, particularly that involving effortful cognitive processes, while leaving the retrieval of previously learned information intact. This effect is utilized to advantage in uncomfortable procedures, eg, endoscopy, since the appropriate dose leaves the patient able to cooperate during the procedure but amnesic regarding it afterward. Hangover effects are not uncommon following use of hypnotic drugs with long elimination half-lives. Because elderly patients are more sensitive to the effects of sedative-hypnotics, doses approximately half of those used in younger adults are safer and usually as effective. The most common reversible cause of confusional states in the elderly is overuse of sedative-hypnotics. At higher doses, toxicity may present as lethargy or a state of exhaustion or, alternatively, in the form of gross symptoms equivalent to those of ethanol intoxication. The titration of useful therapeutic effects against such unwanted effects is usually more difficult with sedative-hypnotics that exhibit steep dose-response relationships of the type shown in Figure 22–1 (drug A), including the barbiturates, chloral hydrate, and piperidinediones. The physician should be aware of variability among patients in terms of doses causing adverse effects. An increased sensitivity to sedative-hypnotics is more common in patients with cardiovascular disease, respiratory disease, or hepatic impairment and in older patients. Sedative-hypnotics can exacerbate breathing problems in patients with chronic pulmonary disease and in those with symptomatic sleep apnea.

Sedative-hypnotics are the drugs most frequently involved in deliberate overdoses, in part because of their general availability as very commonly prescribed pharmacologic agents. The benzodiazepines are considered to be "safer" drugs in this respect, since they have flatter dose-response curves. Epi-

demiologic studies on the incidence of drug-related deaths support this general assumption—eg, 0.3 deaths per million tablets of diazepam prescribed versus 11.6 deaths per million capsules of secobarbital in one study. Of course, many factors other than the specific sedative-hypnotic could influence such data—particularly the presence of other central nervous system depressants, including ethanol. In fact, most serious cases of drug overdosage, intentional or accidental, do involve polypharmacy; and when combinations of agents are taken, the practical safety of benzodiazepines may be less than the foregoing would imply.

The lethal dose of any sedative-hypnotic varies with the patient and the circumstances (Chapter 59). If discovery of the ingestion is made early and a conservative treatment regimen is started, the outcome is rarely fatal, even following very high doses. On the other hand, for most sedative-hypnotics—with the exception of benzodiazepines—a dose as low as ten times the hypnotic dose may be fatal if the patient is not discovered or does not seek help in time. With severe toxicity, the respiratory depression from central actions of the drug may be complicated by aspiration of gastric contents in the unattended patient—an even more likely occurrence if ethanol is present. Loss of brain stem vasomotor control, together with direct myocardial depression, further complicates successful resuscitation. In such patients, treatment consists of ensuring a patent airway, with mechanical ventilation if needed, and maintenance of plasma volume, renal output, and cardiac function. Use of a positive inotropic drug such as dopamine, which preserves renal blood flow, is sometimes indicated. Hemodialysis or hemoperfusion may be used to hasten elimination of some of these drugs (see Table 59–4).

Flumazenil reverses the sedative actions of benzodiazepines. However, its duration of action is short and its antagonism of respiratory depression unpredictable. Therefore, the use of flumazenil in benzodiazepine overdose *must* be accompanied by adequate monitoring and support of respiratory function.

The extensive clinical use of triazolam has led to reports of "serious" central nervous system effects including behavioral disinhibition, delirium, aggression, and violence. While behavioral disinhibition may occur with sedative-hypnotic drugs, it does not appear to be more prevalent with triazolam than with other benzodiazepines. Disinhibitory reactions during benzodiazepine treatment are more clearly associated with the use of very high doses and the pretreatment level of patient hostility.

Adverse effects of the sedative-hypnotics that are not referable to their CNS actions occur infrequently. Hypersensitivity reactions, including skin rashes, occur only occasionally with most drugs of this class. Reports of teratogenicity leading to fetal deformation following use of piperidinediones and certain benzodiazepines justify caution in the use of these drugs during pregnancy. Because barbiturates enhance porphyrin synthesis, they are absolutely contraindicated in patients with a history of acute intermittent porphyria, variegate porphyria, hereditary coproporphyria, or symptomatic porphyria.

Alterations in Drug Response

Depending on the dosage and the duration of use, tolerance occurs in varying degrees to many of the pharmacologic effects of sedative-hypnotics. This can be demonstrated experimentally during chronic use in humans by changes in the effects of these drugs on the electroencephalogram and other characteristics of the stages of sleep. Clearly, tolerance must occur with respect to other effects, since it is known that chronic abusers sometimes ingest quantities of sedative-hypnotics many times the conventional dosage without experiencing severe toxicity. However, it should not be assumed that the degree of tolerance achieved is identical for all pharmacologic effects: There is evidence that the lethal dose range is not altered significantly by the chronic use of sedative-hypnotics. Cross-tolerance between the different sedative-hypnotics, including ethanol, can lead to an unsatisfactory therapeutic response when standard doses of a drug are used in a patient with a recent history of excessive use of these agents.

With the chronic use of sedative-hypnotics, especially if doses are increased, a state of physiologic dependence can occur. This may develop to a degree unparalleled by any other drug group, *including the opioids*. Withdrawal from a sedative-hypnotic can have severe and life-threatening manifestations. Withdrawal symptoms range from restlessness, anxiety, weakness, and orthostatic hypotension to hyperactive reflexes and generalized seizures. The severity of withdrawal symptoms depends to a large extent on the dosage range used immediately prior to discontinuance but also on the particular drug. For example, barbiturates such as secobarbital or pentobarbital in a dosage of less than 400 mg/d, or diazepam in a dosage of less than 40 mg/d, may produce only mild symptoms of withdrawal when discontinued. On the other hand, the use of more than 800 mg/d of barbiturates or 50–60 mg/d of diazepam for 60–90 days is likely to result in seizures if abrupt withdrawal is attempted.

Symptoms of withdrawal are usually more severe following discontinuance of sedative-hypnotics with shorter half-lives. Symptoms are less pronounced with longer-acting drugs, which may partly accomplish their own "tapered" withdrawal by virtue of their slow elimination. Cross-dependence, defined as the ability of one drug to suppress abstinence symptoms from discontinuance of another drug, is quite marked among sedative-hypnotics. This provides the rationale for therapeutic regimens in the management of withdrawal states: Longer-acting drugs such as chlordiazepoxide, diazepam, and phenobarbital can be used to alleviate withdrawal symptoms of shorter-acting drugs, including ethanol.

Drug Interactions

The most frequent drug interactions involving sedative-hypnotics are interactions with other central nervous system depressant drugs, leading to additive effects. These interactions have some therapeutic utility with respect to the use of these drugs as premedicants or anesthetic adjuvants. However, if not anticipated, they can lead to serious consequences, including enhanced depression with concomitant use of many other drugs. Additive effects can be predicted with concomitant use of alcoholic beverages, opioid analgesics, anticonvulsants, and phenothiazines. Less obvious but just as important is enhanced central nervous system depression with a variety of antihistamines, antihypertensive agents, and antidepressant drugs of the tricyclic class.

Interactions involving changes in the activity of hepatic drug-metabolizing enzyme systems can occur, especially following continuous use of barbiturates or meprobamate. For example, in humans, barbiturates have been shown to increase the rate of metabolism of dicumarol, phenytoin, digitalis compounds, and griseofulvin—effects that could lead to decreased response to these agents. This type of drug interaction has not been reported following continuous use of benzodiazepines. Cimetidine, which is known to inhibit hepatic metabolism of many drugs, doubles the elimination half-life of diazepam, presumably via inhibition of its metabolism. As mentioned above, chloral hydrate may displace warfarin from plasma proteins to cause enhanced anticoagulant effects.

PREPARATIONS AVAILABLE

Benzodiazepines
Alprazolam (Xanax)
Oral: 0.25, 0.5, 1, 2 mg tablets
Chlordiazepoxide (generic, Librium, others)
Oral: 5, 10, 25 mg tablets, capsules
Parenteral: 100 mg powder for injection
Clorazepate (Tranxene)
Oral: 3.75, 7.5, 15 mg tablets and capsules
Oral sustained-release: 11.25, 22.5 mg tablets
Clonazepam (Klonopin)
Oral: 0.5, 1, 2 mg tablets
Diazepam (generic, Valium, others)
Oral: 2, 5, 10 mg tablets; 5 mg/5 mL, 5 mg/mL solutions
Oral sustained-release: 15 mg capsules
Parenteral: 5 mg/mL for injection
Estazolam (ProSom)
Oral: 1, 2 mg tablets
Flurazepam (generic, Dalmane)
Oral: 15, 30 mg capsules
Halazepam (Paxipam)
Oral: 20, 40 mg tablets
Lorazepam (generic, Ativan, Alzapam)
Oral: 0.5, 1, 2 mg tablets
Parenteral: 2, 4 mg/mL for injection
Midazolam (Versed)
Parenteral: 1, 5 mg/mL in 1, 2, 5, 10 mL vials for injection
Oxazepam (generic, Serax)
Oral: 10, 15, 30 mg capsules, 15 mg tablets
Prazepam (Centrax)
Oral: 5, 10, 20 mg capsules, 10 mg tablets
Quazepam (Doral)
Oral: 7.5, 15 mg tablets
Temazepam (generic, Restoril)
Oral: 15, 30 mg capsules
Triazolam (Halcion)
Oral: 0.125, 0.25 mg tablets

Benzodiazepine Antagonist
Flumazenil (Romazicon)
Parenteral: 0.1 mg/mL for IV injection

Barbiturates
Amobarbital (generic, Amytal)
Parenteral: powder in 250, 500 mg vials to reconstitute for injection

Aprobarbital (Alurate)
Oral: 40 mg/5 mL elixir
Butabarbital sodium (generic, Butisol, others)
Oral: 15, 30, 50, 100 mg tablets; 30 mg/5 mL elixirs
Mephobarbital (Mebaral)
Oral: 32, 50, 100 mg tablets
Pentobarbital (generic, Nembutal Sodium)
Oral: 50, 100 mg capsules
Rectal: 30, 60, 120, 200 mg suppositories
Parenteral: 50 mg/mL for injection
Phenobarbital (generic, Luminal Sodium, others)
Oral: 15, 30, 60, 100 mg tablets; 16 mg capsules; 15, 20 mg/5 mL elixirs
Parenteral: 30, 60, 65, 130 mg/mL for injection
Secobarbital (generic, Seconal)
Oral: 100 mg capsules
Parenteral: 50 mg/mL for injection

Miscellaneous Drugs
Buspirone (BuSpar)
Oral: 5, 10 mg tablets
Chloral hydrate (generic, Noctec, Aquachloral Supprettes)
Oral: 250, 500 mg capsules; 250, 500 mg/5 mL syrups
Rectal: 324, 500, 648 mg suppositories
Ethchlorvynol (Placidyl)
Oral: 200, 500, 750 mg capsules
Ethinamate (Valmid Pulvules)
Oral: 500 mg capsules
Hydroxyzine (generic, Atarax, Vistaril)
Oral: 10, 25, 50, 100 mg tablets; 25, 50, 100 mg capsules; 10 mg/5 mL syrup; 25 mg/5 mL suspension
Parenteral: 25, 50 mg/mL for injection
Meprobamate (generic, Miltown, Equanil, others)
Oral: 200, 400, 600 mg tablets
Oral sustained-release: 200, 400 mg capsules
Paraldehyde (generic)
Oral, rectal liquids
Zolpidem (Ambien)
Oral: 5, 10 mg tablets

REFERENCES

Barrett JE, Vanover KE: 5-HT receptors as targets for the development of novel anxiolytic drugs: Models, mechanisms, and future directions. Psychopharmacology 1993;112:1.

Basile AS et al: Elevated brain concentrations of 1,4-benzodiazepines in fulminant hepatic failure. N Engl J Med 1991;325:473.

Besset A et al: Effects of zolpidem on the architecture and cyclical structure of sleep in poor sleepers. Drugs Exp Clin Res 1995;21:161.

Cadronel JF et al: Flumazenil therapy for hepatic encephalopathy in cirrhotic patients: A double-blind, pragmatic randomized, placebo study. Eur J Gastroenterol Hepatol 1995;7:325.

Costa E, Guidotti A: Benzodiazepines on trial: A research strategy for their rehabilitation. Trends Pharmacol Sci 1996;17:192.

Delle Chiaie R et al: Assessment of the efficacy of buspirone in patients affected by generalized anxiety disorder, shifting to buspirone from lorazepam: A placebo-controlled, double-blind study. J Clin Psychopharmacol 1995;15:12.

Dubovsky SL: Generalized anxiety disorder: New concepts and psychopharmacologic therapies. J Clin Psychiatry 1990;51(Suppl):3.

Garnier R et al: Acute zolpidem poisoning: Analysis of 344 cases. J Toxicol Clin Toxicol 1994;32:391.

Garzone PD, Kroboth PD: Pharmacokinetics of the newer benzodiazepines. Clin Pharmacokinet 1989;16:337.

Ghonheim MM, Mewaldt SP: Benzodiazepines and human memory: A review. Anesthesiology 1990;72:926.

Gillin JC et al: Rebound insomnia: A critical review. J Clin Psychopharmacol 1989;9:161.

Gillin JC, Byerly WF: The diagnosis and management of sleep disorders. N Engl J Med 1990;322:239.

Gottlieb GL: Sleep disorders and their management: Special considerations in the elderly. Am J Med 1990;88(Suppl 3B):29S.

Greenblatt DJ, Harmatz JS, Shader RI: Clinical pharmacokinetics of anxiolytics and hypnotics in the elderly. Clin Pharmacokinet 1991;21:165.

Hoehns JD, Perry PJ: Zolpidem: a nonbenzodiazepine hypnotic for treatment of insomnia. Clin Pharm 1993;12:814.

Horne AL et al: The influence of the γ2L subunit on the modulation of responses to GABA$_A$ receptor activation. Br J Pharmacol 1993;108:711.

Jonas JM, Cohon MS: A comparison of the safety and efficacy of alprazolam versus other agents in the treatment of anxiety, panic and depression. J Clin Psychiatry 1993;54(Suppl):25.

Kales A et al: Diazepam: Effects on sleep and withdrawal phenomena. J Clin Psychopharmacol 1988;8:340.

Lader M: Rebound insomnia and newer hypnotics. Psychopharmacology 1990;108:248.

Langtry HD, Benfield P: Zolpidem: A review of its pharmacodynamic and pharmacokinetic properties and therapeutic potential. Drugs 1990;40:291.

Lin L-H, Whiting P, Harris RA: Molecular determinants of general anesthetic action: Role of GABA$_A$ receptor structure. J Neurochem 1993;60:1548.

Lucki I: 5HT$_1$ receptors and behaviour. Neurosci Behav Rev 1992;16:83.

Luddens H, Korpi ER: Biological function of GABA$_A$/benzodiazepine receptor heterogeneity. J Psychiatr Res 1995;29:77.

Malizia AL et al: Benzodiazepine receptor function in anxiety disorders. Adv Biochem Psychopharm 1995;48:115.

Melander A et al: Anxiolytic-hypnotic drugs: Relationships between prescribing, abuse and suicide. Eur J Clin Pharmacol 1991;41:525.

Mendelson WB, Jain B: An assessment of short-acting hypnotics. Drug Saf 1995;13:257.

Mihic SJ et al: Pharmacology of recombinant GABA$_A$ receptors. Adv Biochem Psychopharm 1995;48:17.

Napoliello MJ, Domantay AG: Buspirone: A worldwide update. Br J Psychiatry 1991;12:40.

Novas ML et al: Proconvulsant and "anxiogenic" effects of n-butyl-carboline-3-carboxylate, a potent benzodiazepine binding inhibitor. Pharmacol Biochem Behav 1988;30:331.

Patat A et al: Flumazenil antagonizes the central effects of zolpidem, an imidazopyridine hypnotic. Clin Pharmacol Ther 1994;56:430.

Pelissolo A: The benzodiazepine receptor: The enigma of the endogenous ligand. Encéphale 1995;21:133.

Polc P: Involvement of endogenous benzodiazepine ligands in brain disorders; therapeutic potential for benzodiazepine antagonists. Med Hypotheses 1995;44:439.

Prinz PN et al: Geriatrics: Sleep disorders and aging. N Engl J Med 1990;323:520.

Rothschild AJ: Disinhibition, amnestic reactions, and other adverse reactions secondary to triazolam: A review of the literature. J Clin Psychiatry 1992;53:69.

Rothstein JD et al: Purification and characterization of naturally occurring benzodiazepine receptor ligands in rat and human brain. J Neurochem 1992;58:2102.

Salva P, Costa J: Clinical pharmacokinetics and pharmacodynamics of zolpidem: Therapeutic implications. Clin Pharmacokinet 1995;29:142.

Sanger DJ et al: Recent developments in the behavioral pharmacology of benzodiazepine (omega) receptors: Evidence for the functional significance of receptor subtypes. Neurosci Behav Rev 1994;18:355.

Scharf MB, Saschais BA: The pharmacology of disordered sleep. In: Textbook of Clinical Neuropharmacology and Therapeutics. Klawans HL et al (editors). Raven, 1992.

Schoch P et al: Aspects of benzodiazepine receptor structure and function with relevance to drug tolerance and dependence. Biochem Soc Symp 1993;59:121.

Shader RI, Greenblatt DJ: Use of benzodiazepines in anxiety disorders. N Engl J Med 1993;328:1398.

Sheehan DV: Benzodiazepines in panic disorder and agoraphobia. J Affect Disord 1987;13:169.

Sieghart W: GABA$_A$ receptors: Ligand-gated Cl$^-$ ion channels modulated by multiple drug-binding sites. Trends Pharmacol Sci 1992;13:446.

Smith MC, Riskin BJ: The clinical use of barbiturates in neurological disorders. Drugs 1991;42:365.

Sussman N: Treating anxiety while minimizing abuse and dependence. J Clin Psychiatry 1993;54(Suppl):44.

Taylor DP, Moon SL: Buspirone and related compounds as alternative anxiolytics. Neuropeptides 1991;19 (Suppl):15.

Twyman RE et al: Differential regulation of GABA receptor channels by diazepam and phenobarbital. Ann Neurol 1989;25:213.

Unseld E et al: Occurrence of "natural" diazepam in human brain. Biochem Pharmacol 1990;38:2473.

van Laar MW et al: Therapeutic effects and effects on actual driving performance of chronically administered buspirone and diazepam in anxious outpatients. J Clin Psychopharmacol 1992;12:86.

Woods JH et al: Benzodiazepines: Use, abuse, and consequences. Pharmacol Rev 1992;44:151.

Wysowsky DK, Baum C: Outpatient use of prescription sedative-hypnotic drugs in the United States, 1970 through 1989. Arch Intern Med 1991;151:1779.

Zorumsky CF, Isenberg KE: Insights into the structure and function of GABA-benzodiazepine receptors: Ion channels and psychiatry. Am J Psychiatry 1991;148:162.

23

The Alcohols

Susan B. Masters, PhD, & Nancy M. Lee, PhD

Alcohol, primarily in the form of ethyl alcohol (ethanol), has occupied an important place in the history of humankind for at least 8000 years. In Western society, beer and wine were a main staple of daily life until the 19th century. These relatively dilute alcoholic beverages were preferred over water, which was known to be associated with acute and chronic illness. They provided important calories and nutrients in addition to serving as a main source of daily liquid. As systems for improved sanitation and water purification were introduced in the 1800s, beer and wine became less important as components of the human diet, and the consumption of alcoholic beverages, including distilled preparations with higher concentrations of alcohol, shifted toward their present-day role (in many societies) as a socially acceptable form of recreation.

Today, alcohol is widely consumed. Like other sedative-hypnotic drugs, alcohol in low to moderate amounts relieves anxiety and fosters a feeling of well-being or even euphoria. However, alcohol is also the most commonly abused drug in the world, an occasion for vast medical and societal costs. In the United States, approximately 75% of the adult population drinks alcohol regularly. The majority of this drinking population is able to enjoy the pleasurable effects of alcohol without allowing their alcohol consumption to become a health risk. In fact, recent evidence suggests that moderate consumption of ethanol protects some people against cardiovascular disease. However, about 10% of the general population in the United States is unable to limit its ethanol consumption, a condition known as alcohol abuse. People who continue to drink alcohol in spite of adverse medical or social consequences related directly to their alcohol consumption suffer from **alcoholism,** a complex disorder that appears to have genetic as well as environmental determinants. The medical costs of alcohol abuse are staggering; it is estimated that about 30% of all people admitted to hospitals have coexisting alcohol problems. Despite the investment of many resources and much basic research, alcoholism remains a common chronic disease that is difficult to treat.

Ethanol and many other alcohols with potentially toxic effects are used in industry, some in enormous quantities. In addition to ethanol, methanol and ethylene glycol toxicity occur with sufficient frequency to warrant discussion in this chapter.

I. BASIC PHARMACOLOGY OF ETHANOL

Pharmacokinetics

Ethanol is a small water-soluble molecule that is absorbed rapidly from the gastrointestinal tract. After ingestion of alcohol in the fasting state, peak blood alcohol concentrations are reached within 30 minutes. The presence of food in the gut delays absorption by slowing gastric emptying. Distribution is rapid, with tissue levels approximating the concentration in blood. The volume of distribution for ethanol approximates total body water (0.5–0.7 L/kg). For an equivalent oral dose of alcohol, women have a higher peak concentration than men, in part because women have a lower total body water content. In the central nervous system, the concentration of ethanol rises quickly since the brain receives a large proportion of blood flow and ethanol readily crosses biologic membranes.

Over 90% of alcohol consumed is oxidized in the liver; the rest is excreted through the lungs and in the urine. The excretion of a small but consistent proportion of alcohol by the lungs is exploited by breath alcohol tests that serve as a basis for a legal definition of "driving under the influence" in many countries. At levels of ethanol usually achieved in blood, the rate of oxidation follows zero-order kinetics, ie, it is independent of time and concentration of the drug. The amount of alcohol oxidized per unit time is approximately proportionate to body weight or liver weight, and the rate of disappearance of alcohol from the body is markedly reduced by liver damage. The typical adult can metabolize 7–10 g (150–220 mmol) of alcohol per hour, the equivalent of approximately 10 oz of beer, 3.5 oz of wine, or 1 oz of distilled 80 proof spirits.

Two pathways of alcohol metabolism to acetaldehyde have been identified (Figure 23–1). Acetaldehyde is then oxidized by a third metabolic process.

A. Alcohol Dehydrogenase Pathway: The main pathway for alcohol metabolism involves alcohol dehydrogenase (ADH), a cytosolic enzyme that contains zinc and catalyzes the conversion of alcohol to acetaldehyde (Figure 23–1, left). This enzyme is located mainly in the liver, but it can also be found in other organs such as brain and stomach.

A significant amount of ethanol metabolism by gastric ADH occurs in the stomach in men, but a smaller amount occurs in women, who appear to have lower levels of the gastric enzyme (Frezza et al, 1990). This difference in gastric metabolism of alcohol in women probably contributes to the sex-related differences in blood alcohol concentrations noted above. Both male and female alcoholics exhibit lower gastric ADH activity than their nonalcoholic cohorts.

During conversion of ethanol to acetaldehyde, hydrogen ion is transferred from alcohol to the cofactor nicotinamide adenine dinucleotide (NAD⁺) to form NADH. As a net result, alcohol oxidation generates an excess of reducing equivalents in the liver, chiefly as NADH. The excess NADH production appears to underlie a number of metabolic disorders that are described below.

B. Microsomal Ethanol Oxidizing System (MEOS): This enzyme system, also known as the mixed function oxidase system (Chapter 4), uses NADP⁺ instead of NAD⁺ as a cofactor in the metabolism of ethanol (Figure 23–1, right).

At blood concentrations below 100 mg/dL (22 mmol/L), the MEOS system, which has a relatively high K_m for alcohol, contributes little to the metabolism of ethanol. However, when large amounts of ethanol are consumed, the alcohol dehydrogenase system becomes saturated owing to depletion of the required cofactor, NAD⁺. As the concentration of ethanol increases above 100 mg/dL, there is increased contribution from the MEOS system, which does not rely upon NAD⁺ as a cofactor.

During chronic alcohol consumption, MEOS activity increases. As described in Chapter 4, this induction of enzyme activity is associated with an increase in various constituents of the smooth endoplasmic reticulum in the liver. As a result, chronic alcohol consumption can result in significant increases not only in ethanol metabolism but also in the clearance of other drugs that are eliminated by hepatic microsomal enzyme systems. Similarly, other "inducing" drugs such as barbiturates may also enhance the rate of blood alcohol clearance slightly. However, the effect of other drugs on ethanol clearance is less important because the MEOS is not the primary pathway for ethanol metabolism.

C. Acetaldehyde Metabolism: Much of the acetaldehyde formed from alcohol appears to be oxidized in the liver. While several enzyme systems may be responsible for this reaction, observations that acetaldehyde concentrations in the liver after ethanol administration are only 100–350 μmol/L have led to the conclusion that mitochondrial NAD⁺-dependent aldehyde dehydrogenase (the apparent K_m for acetaldehyde is about 10 μmol/L) is the main pathway for acetaldehyde oxidation. The product of this reaction is acetate (Figure 23–1), which can be further metabolized to CO_2 and water. Chronic alcohol consumption results in a decreased rate of acetaldehyde oxidation in intact mitochondria.

Oxidation of acetaldehyde is inhibited by disulfiram, a drug used to deter drinking by alcohol-dependent patients undergoing rehabilitation. When ethanol is consumed in the presence of disulfiram, acetaldehyde accumulates and causes an unpleasant reaction of facial flushing, nausea, dizziness, and headache.

Some people, primarily of Asian descent, have a genetic deficiency in the activity of the mitochondrial form of aldehyde dehydrogenase. When these individuals drink alcohol, they develop high blood acetaldehyde concentrations and experience a flushing reaction similar to that seen with the combination of disulfiram and ethanol.

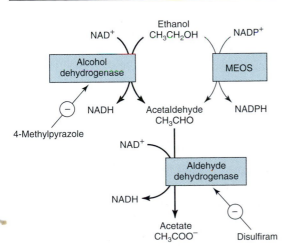

Figure 23–1. Metabolism of ethanol by alcohol dehydrogenase and the microsomal ethanol-oxidizing system (MEOS). Alcohol dehydrogenase and aldehyde dehydrogenase are inhibited by 4-methylpyrazole and disulfiram, respectively.

Pharmacodynamics of Acute Ethanol Consumption

A. Central Nervous System: The central nervous system is markedly affected by acute alcohol consumption. Alcohol causes sedation and relief of anxiety and, at higher concentrations, slurred speech, ataxia, impaired judgment, and disinhibited behavior, a condition usually called **intoxication** or **drunkenness** (Table 23–1). These central nervous system effects are most marked as the blood level is rising, because acute tolerance to the effects of alcohol occurs after a few hours of drinking. For chronic drinkers who are tolerant to the effects of alcohol, much higher concentrations are needed to elicit these central nervous system effects. For example, a chronic alcoholic may appear sober or only slightly intoxicated with a blood alcohol concentration of 300–400 mg/dL, whereas this level is associated with marked intoxication or even coma in a nontolerant individual. The propensity of moderate doses of alcohol to inhibit the attention and information processing skills as well as the motor skills required for operation of motor vehicles has profound effects. Approximately half of all traffic accidents resulting in a fatality in the United States involve at least one person with a blood alcohol near or above the legal level of intoxication, and drunken driving is a leading cause of death in young adults.

Like other sedative-hypnotic drugs, alcohol is a central nervous system depressant. At high blood concentrations, it induces coma, respiratory depression, and death.

No specific receptor for ethanol has been identified. Instead, ethanol has been shown to affect a large number of molecular processes, including neurotransmitter receptors for amines, amino acids, and opioids; enzymes such as Na^+/K^+ ATPase, acetylcholinesterase, adenylyl cyclase, phosphoinositide-specific phospholipase C; the mitochondrial electron transport chain; and ion channels such as those for Ca^{2+} (Lee et al, 1986). Much attention has focused on alcohol's effects upon neurotransmission by GABA and glutamate, the main excitatory and inhibitory neurotransmitters in the central nervous system. Acute ethanol exposure enhances the action of GABA at $GABA_A$ receptors, which is consistent with the ability of GABA-mimetics to intensify many of the acute effects of alcohol and of $GABA_A$ antagonists to attenuate some of the actions of ethanol. Ethanol also inhibits the ability of glutamate to open the cation channel associated with the N-methyl-D-aspartate (NMDA) subtype of glutamate receptors (Tsai et al, 1995). The NMDA receptor is implicated in many aspects of cognitive function, including learning and memory.

For many years it was believed that ethanol's primary effect is disruption of biologic membranes through reduction in lipid viscosity ("fluidization"). This fluidizing effect of ethanol was hypothesized to be responsible for the broad variety of changes observed in membrane function. More recently, it has been suggested that the pharmacologically relevant actions of alcohol result from direct, selective interaction with proteins that mediate transmembrane signaling such as receptor-gated ion channels (Peoples et al, 1995). The main thrust of the argument for moving away from the membrane fluidization theory is that in animals, measures of intoxicating effects of a series of alcohols with an increasing number of carbon atoms exhibit steric limitations whereas membrane fluidization effects do not.

Alcohol has diverse effects at the cellular and tissue levels, particularly in the nervous system. In trigeminal motoneurons, both intracellular and extracellular applications of ethanol depress action potentials and excitatory and inhibitory postsynaptic potentials. In cerebellar Purkinje cells and in the dopamine-containing neurons in the substantia nigra, pars compacta, and striate nucleus, low concentrations of ethanol enhance the firing rate while higher doses inhibit it. In other systems, including the lateral geniculate nucleus, the locus ceruleus, the midbrain raphe nucleus, and hippocampal neurons in culture, only inhibitory effects have been observed. More complex neuronal responses are similarly affected. For example, both the after-discharge following high-frequency stimulation of hippocampal neurons and the frog spinal reflex are enhanced by low doses of ethanol and inhibited by higher doses (Lee et al, 1986).

B. Heart: Significant depression of myocardial contractility has been observed in individuals who acutely consume moderate amounts of alcohol, ie, at a blood concentration above 100 mg/dL. Myocardial biopsies in humans before and after infusion of small amounts of alcohol have shown ultrastructural changes that may be associated with impaired myocardial function. Acetaldehyde is implicated as a cause of heart abnormalities by altering myocardial stores of catecholamines.

C. Smooth Muscle: Ethanol is a vasodilator, probably as a result of both central nervous system effects (depression of the vasomotor center) and direct smooth muscle relaxation caused by its metabolite, acetaldehyde. In cases of severe overdose, hypother-

Table 23–1. Blood alcohol concentration and clinical effects in nontolerant individuals.

Blood Alcohol Concentration (mg/dL)[1]	Clinical Effect
50–100	Sedation, subjective "high," increased reaction times
100–200	Impaired motor function, slurred speech, ataxia
200–300	Emesis, stupor
300–400	Coma
> 500	Respiratory depression, death

[1]In many parts of the USA, a blood level above 80–100 mg/dL for adults or 10 mg/dL for persons under 21 is sufficient for conviction of driving while intoxicated.

mia—caused by vasodilation—may be marked in cold environments. Ethanol also relaxes the uterus and—before the introduction of more effective and safer uterine relaxants (eg, calcium blockers, magnesium ion, NSAIDs, and β_2-adrenoceptor stimulants) —was used intravenously for the suppression of premature labor.

Consequences of Chronic Alcohol Consumption

Chronic alcohol consumption profoundly affects the function of several vital organs, particularly the liver and the nervous, gastrointestinal, and cardiovascular systems. Ethanol has direct toxicity. In addition, since it is a very weak drug that requires concentrations thousands of times higher than other misused drugs (eg, cocaine, opiates, amphetamines) to produce its intoxicating effects, it is often consumed in quantities large enough to qualify it as a food. The disruption in metabolism caused by chronic consumption of such large quantities of this energy-rich drug contributes to the organ toxicity seen during chronic use, as do also the malnutrition and vitamin deficiencies that often accompany alcoholism.

Chronic consumption of large amounts of alcohol is associated with an increased risk of mortality, though light to moderate drinking has a protective effect (see box: The Relationship Between Alcohol Intake & Mortality). Deaths linked to alcohol consumption are caused by liver disease, cancer, accidents, and suicide.

A. Liver and Gastrointestinal Tract: Liver disease is the most common medical complication of alcohol abuse; it is estimated that about 15–30% of chronic heavy drinkers eventually develop severe liver disease. Clinically significant alcoholic liver disease may be insidious in onset and progress without evidence of overt nutritional abnormalities. Alcoholic fatty liver, a reversible condition, may progress to alcoholic hepatitis and finally to cirrhosis and liver failure. In the USA, chronic alcohol abuse is the leading cause of liver cirrhosis and of the need for liver transplantation. The risk of developing liver disease is related both to the average amount of daily consumption and to the duration of alcohol abuse. Women appear to be more susceptible to hepatotoxicity of alcohol than men. Another factor that increases the risk of severe liver disease is concurrent infection with hepatitis B or C virus. Alcoholics with evidence of infection (ie, serum antibody to one of these viruses or measurable viral RNA in their blood) have more severe liver disease than noninfected alcoholics. The contribution of chronic hepatitis B and C viral infection to severe alcoholic liver disease is important because the incidence of these infections is increased in alcoholic populations.

Metabolism of 70 g or more of alcohol (about a six-pack of beer, an amount that alcoholics will often consume daily) places a large load upon the liver and leads to a number of metabolic abnormalities. The increased NADH/NAD$^+$ ratio that results from oxidation of ethanol results in reduced gluconeogenesis, hypoglycemia, and ketoacidosis. It also promotes triglyceride synthesis from free fatty acids, which contributes to accumulation of fat in the liver parenchyma. The excess of acetaldehyde also adversely affects liver function. Since metabolism of acetaldehyde via aldehyde dehydrogenase results in the generation of NADH, some of the acetaldehyde effects may be attributable to NADH excess. Acetaldehyde is itself a very reactive compound that has many toxic effects. Formation of acetaldehyde-protein adducts promotes collagen production and stimulates hepatic inflammation.

In some cases, nutritional factors are critical in alcohol-induced liver disease. It has been suggested that essential factors such as glutathione may be decreased in a malnourished alcoholic, thus removing a valuable scavenger of toxic free radicals that otherwise will injure the liver. Hormonal factors may also contribute to this disease, because female alcoholics are at greater risk for alcohol-induced liver dysfunction than male alcoholics.

Other portions of the gastrointestinal tract may also be injured. Ingestion of alcohol increases gastric and pancreatic secretion and alters mucosal barriers so that the risk of gastritis and pancreatitis is enhanced. The acute effects of alcohol on the stomach are related primarily to the toxic effect of ethanol on the mucosal membranes and have relatively little to do with increased production of gastric acid. Chronic alcoholics are prone to develop gastritis and increased susceptibility to blood and plasma protein loss during drinking, which may contribute to anemia and protein malnutrition. Alcohol also reversibly injures the small intestine, leading to diarrhea, weight loss, and multiple vitamin deficiencies.

The statement sometimes made that malnutrition of alcoholic patients is due simply to dietary deficiency is probably not justified in the vast majority of cases. Malabsorption of vitamins, especially water-soluble ones, contributes to the clinical abnormalities. Although deficiencies in water-soluble vitamins were proposed in the past to account for most of the pathologic effects of alcohol, replacement doses of the vitamins do not completely protect against the injurious effects of alcohol.

B. Nervous System:

1. Tolerance and physical dependence—The consumption of alcohol in high doses over a long period results in tolerance and in physical and psychologic dependence. Tolerance to the intoxicating effects of alcohol is a complex process involving poorly understood changes in the nervous system as well as the metabolic changes described earlier. Although minor degrees of metabolic tolerance after chronic alcohol use have been demonstrated in which the subject's capacity to metabolize the drug increases, the maximal increase in alcohol metabolism is insufficient to account for the magnitude of the observed clinical tolerance. As with other sedative-hypnotic drugs, there is a limit to tolerance, so that only a relatively small increase in the lethal dose occurs with increasing alcohol use.

Chronic alcohol drinkers, when forced to reduce or discontinue alcohol, experience a withdrawal syndrome, which indicates the existence of physical dependence. Alcohol withdrawal symptoms classically consist of hyperexcitability in mild cases and convulsions, toxic psychosis, and **delirium tremens** in severe ones. The dose, rate, and duration of alcohol consumption determine the intensity of the withdrawal syndrome. When consumption has been very high, merely reducing the rate of consumption may lead to signs of withdrawal.

Psychologic dependence upon alcohol is characterized by a compulsive desire to experience the rewarding effects of alcohol and, for current drinkers, a desire to avoid the negative consequences of withdrawal. Detoxified, abstinent alcoholics experience periods of intense craving for alcohol that can be set off by environmental cues associated with drinking in the past, such as familiar places, groups of people, or events.

The molecular basis of alcohol tolerance and dependence is not known. Chronic exposure of animals or cultured cells to alcohol elicits a multitude of adaptive responses involving neurotransmitters and their receptors, ion channels, and enzymes that participate in signal transduction pathways. Up-regulation of the NMDA subtype of glutamate receptors and voltage-sensitive Ca^{+2} channels has been implicated in the seizures than accompany the alcohol withdrawal syndrome (Tsai et al 1995; Hoffman et al, 1994). Based on the ability of sedative-hypnotic drugs that enhance GABAergic neurotransmission to substitute for alcohol during alcohol withdrawal and evidence of down-regulation of $GABA_A$-mediated responses with chronic alcohol exposure, GABA neurotransmission appears to play a central role in the development of tolerance and withdrawal.

Neurotransmission events involved in the sensation of reward are also important. Alcohol causes an acute increase in the local concentrations of serotonin, opioids, and dopamine—neurotransmitters involved in brain reward circuits—whereas chronic use lowers the basal levels of these chemicals. A strong desire for alcohol may represent the brain's effort to bring these neurotransmitters back to normal.

Chronic alcohol use in humans has been reported to alter the activity of two enzymes, monoamine oxidase and adenylyl cyclase, in platelets (Tabakoff et al, 1988). These alterations may be valuable markers of excess alcohol consumption and perhaps of predisposition to alcoholism.

2. Neurotoxicity–Consumption of large amounts of alcohol over extended periods (usually years) can also lead to neurologic deficits. The most frequent neurologic abnormality in chronic alcoholism is a generalized symmetric peripheral nerve injury that begins with distal paresthesias of the hands and feet. Chronic alcoholic patients may also exhibit gait disturbances and ataxia that are due to degenerative changes in the cental nervous system. Other neurologic disturbances associated with alcoholism include dementia and, rarely, demyelinating disease.

Wernicke-Korsakoff syndrome is a relatively uncommon but important entity characterized by paralysis of the external eye muscles, ataxia, and a confused state that can progress to coma and death. It is apparently associated with thiamin deficiency but is rarely seen in the absence of alcoholism. Wernicke's encephalopathy represents the acute phase of this disease; it may be difficult to distinguish from the acute confusional state created by acute alcohol intoxication, which later blends in with the perceptual and behavioral problems associated with alcohol withdrawal. A distinguishing feature of Wernicke's encephalopathy is the longer duration of the confusional state and the relative absence of the agitation that would be expected during withdrawal. Because of the importance of thiamin in this pathologic condition, all patients suspected of having Wernicke-Korsakoff syndrome should receive thiamine therapy (50 mg intravenously once and 50 mg intramuscularly repeated daily until a normal diet is resumed). Often, the ocular signs, ataxia, and confusion improve upon prompt administration of thiamine. However, most patients are left with a chronic disabling memory disorder known as Korsakoff's psychosis.

Alcohol may also impair visual acuity, with painless bilateral blurring that occurs over several weeks of heavy alcohol consumption. Changes are usually bilateral and symmetric and may be followed by optic nerve degeneration. Ingestion of ethanol substitutes such as methanol (see below) causes severe visual disturbances.

C. Cardiovascular System: Alcohol alters the cardiovascular system in many ways. Heavy alcohol consumption of long duration is associated with a dilated cardiomyopathy with ventricular hypertrophy and fibrosis. Direct injury to the myocardium resulting from alcohol abuse was originally thought to be caused by thiamin deficiency or by contaminants in alcoholic beverages. More recent studies indicate that the cardiomyopathy occurs even in the absence of vitamin or other dietary deficiencies. In animals and humans, alcohol induces a number of changes in heart cells that may contribute to cardiomyopathy. They include membrane disruption, depressed function of mitochondria and sarcoplasmic reticulum, intracellular accumulation of phospholipids and fatty acids, and up-regulation of voltage-dependent calcium channels. In many cases of alcohol-induced cardiomyopathy, cessation of drinking is associated with a reduction in cardiac size and improved function.

Heavy drinking—and especially "binge" drinking—are associated with both atrial and ventricular arrhythmias. Patients undergoing alcohol withdrawal syndrome can develop severe arrhythmias that may reflect abnormalities of potassium or magnesium metabolism as well as enhanced release of catecholamines. Seizures, syncope, and sudden death during alcohol withdrawal may be due to these arrhythmias.

A link between heavier alcohol consumption (more than three drinks per day) and hypertension has been firmly established in epidemiologic studies. Alcohol is estimated to be responsible for approximately 5% of cases of hypertension, making it one of the most common causes of reversible hypertension. This association is independent of obesity, salt intake, coffee drinking, or cigarette smoking. The mechanisms responsible for the sustained increase in blood pressure have not been identified. A reduction in alcohol intake appears to be effective in lowering blood pressure in hypertensives who are also heavy drinkers; the hypertension seen in this population is also responsive to standard blood pressure medications.

Curiously, the incidence of coronary heart disease in both men and women has been found to be lower in modest consumers of alcohol (one to three drinks a day) than in those who totally abstain (Suh et al, 1992), an effect that may be responsible for the lower rate of mortality in light to moderate drinkers than in abstainers (see Box: The Relationship Between Alcohol Intake & Mortality). The most plausible mechanism to explain this protective effect is alcohol's ability to raise serum levels of high-density lipoprotein (HDL) cholesterol (Haskell et al, 1984), the form of cholesterol that appears to protect against atherosclerosis by removing free cholesterol from the arterial wall (Chapter 35).

D. Blood: Alcohol indirectly affects hematopoiesis through metabolic and nutritional effects and may also directly inhibit the proliferation of all cellular elements in bone marrow. The most common hematologic disorder seen in chronic drinkers is mild anemia resulting from alcohol-related folic acid deficiency. Iron deficiency anemia may result from gastrointestinal bleeding. Alcohol has also been implicated as a cause of several hemolytic syndromes, some of which are associated with hyperlipidemia and severe liver disease.

THE RELATIONSHIP BETWEEN ALCOHOL INTAKE & MORTALITY

The new "Dietary Guidelines for Americans" announced by the United States government state that part of a healthy lifestyle for women and men is consumption, with a meal, of one alcoholic drink (women) or two (men) alcoholic drinks daily. Why was the reference to alcohol included? While it has long been known that excessive alcohol intake predisposes people to an early death, there is now strong evidence that light to moderate drinkers have a lower mortality rate than abstainers (Poikolainen, 1995). Thus, the relationship between mortality and alcohol intake is J-shaped (or U-shaped in some studies, Figure 23–2). Originally it was proposed that the higher mortality among abstainers might be due to the inclusion in this group of ex-drinkers who had quit because of alcohol-related illness. However, more recent studies have addressed and rejected this simple explanation. The beneficial effect of alcohol has been observed in women as well as men and is thought to be mainly due to protection against coronary heart disease, a major cause of mortality in Western countries. It is not possible to confidently determine the safe limits to drinking because of the difficulty in accurately measuring alcohol intake, but several studies have yielded the same guidelines. Several highly publicized studies suggested that wine, and most notably red wine, is more protective than other forms of ethanol. Further investigation has revealed no major differences between the protective effects of beer, wine, or spirits (Rimm et al, 1996).

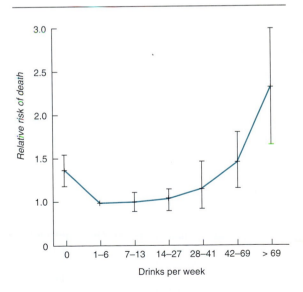

Figure 23–2. Risk of mortality relative to alcohol intake. The graph shows the results of a 10- to 12-year study of 13,000 Danish men and women. The risk of mortality was set at 1.0 for the group with the lowest mortality. (Modified and reproduced, with permission, from Grønbæk et al: Influence of sex, age, body mass index, and smoking on alcohol intake and mortality. Br Med J 1994;308:302.)

Abnormalities in platelets and leukocytes have been described in alcoholics. These effects may account for some of the hemostatic impairment and increased frequency of infection in these individuals.

E. Endocrine System and Electrolyte Balance: Chronic alcohol use has important effects on the endocrine system and on mineral and fluid and electrolyte balance. Clinical reports of gynecomastia and testicular atrophy in alcoholics with cirrhosis suggest a derangement in steroid hormone balance. Gynecomastia and testicular atrophy have also been noted in alcoholics who have little evidence of liver disease.

Alcoholics with chronic liver disease may have disorders of fluid and electrolyte balance, including ascites, edema, and effusions. These factors may be related to decreased protein synthesis and portal hypertension. Alterations of whole body potassium induced by vomiting and diarrhea, as well as severe secondary aldosteronism, may contribute to muscle weakness and can be worsened by diuretic therapy. Some alcoholic patients develop hypoglycemia, probably as a result of impaired hepatic gluconeogenesis. Some alcoholics also develop ketosis, caused by excessive lipolytic factors, especially increased cortisol and growth hormone.

F. Fetal Alcohol Syndrome: Chronic maternal alcohol abuse during pregnancy is associated with important teratogenic effects on the offspring (Abel, 1981; Ernhart et al, 1987), and alcohol appears to be a leading cause of mental retardation and congenital malformation. The abnormalities that have been characterized as fetal alcohol syndrome include (1) retarded body growth, (2) microcephaly, (3) poor coordination, (4) underdevelopment of midfacial region (appearing as a flattened face), and (5) minor joint anomalies. More severe cases may include congenital heart defects and mental retardation. It is likely that heavy drinking in the first trimester of pregnancy has the greatest effect on fetal development; heavy alcohol consumption near term may have a greater effect on fetal nutrition and birth weight. While the level of alcohol intake required for causing serious neurologic deficits appears quite high, the threshold for causing more subtle neurologic deficits is uncertain.

The mechanisms that underlie ethanol's teratogenic effects are unknown. Ethanol rapidly crosses the placenta and reaches concentrations in the fetus that are similar to those in maternal blood. The fetal liver has little or no alcohol dehydrogenase activity, so the fetus must rely upon maternal and placental enzymes for elimination of alcohol. The poorly defined neuroadaptive changes that are responsible for development of tolerance and dependence in adults probably also occur in the fetus and may lead to permanent neurologic changes in the vulnerable developing brain. The neuropathologic abnormalities seen in humans and in animal models of fetal alcohol syndrome indicate that ethanol causes aberrant neuronal and glial migration in the developing nervous system. In tissue culture systems, ethanol causes a striking reduction in neurite outgrowth. Alcohol's toxicity to the developing brain may be due to selective interference with the synthesis or function of molecules that are critical for cell recognition and migration, such as L1, an immunoglobulin cell adhesion molecule (Ramanathan et al, 1996) and gangliosides, major structural components of neuronal plasma membranes (Rosenberg et al, 1994).

G. Immune System: Alcoholics have a higher than normal rate of infection and are especially prone to respiratory infections such as pneumonia and tuberculosis. While secondary effects of alcohol dependence, including nutritional deficiencies and social conditions such as homelessness, contribute to the high rate of infection, a number of studies have indicated that chronic ethanol consumption can directly impair immune function (MacGregor, 1986). This could also be a major factor underlying the increased incidence of certain forms of cancer in alcoholics (see below). The types of immunologic changes reported include alterations in chemotaxis of granulocytes, lymphocyte response to mitogens, T cell numbers, natural killer cell (NK) activity, and levels of tumor necrosis factor (Nelson et al, 1995). Even a single dose of ethanol may alter some of these variables.

H. Increased Risk of Cancer: Chronic alcohol use increases the risk for cancer of the mouth, pharynx, larynx, esophagus, and liver. Some evidence suggests that there is a small increase in the incidence of breast cancer that is alcohol intake-dependent (Schatzkin et al, 1994). Although the methodologic problems of studies relating cancer to alcohol use have been formidable, the consistency of results is impressive. Much more information is required before a threshold level for alcohol consumption as it relates to cancer can be established. In fact, alcohol itself does not appear to be a carcinogen in most test systems. However, alcoholic beverages may carry potential carcinogens produced in fermentation or processing and may alter liver function so that the activity of potential carcinogens is increased.

Alcohol-Drug Interactions

Interactions between ethanol and other drugs can have important clinical effects that result from alterations in the pharmacokinetics or pharmacodynamics of the second drug.

The most frequent pharmacokinetic alcohol-drug interactions occur as a result of alcohol-induced proliferation ("induction") of the smooth endoplasmic reticulum of liver cells as described in Chapter 4. Thus, prolonged intake of alcohol without damage to the liver may enhance the metabolic biotransformation of other drugs. In contrast, *acute* alcohol use may inhibit metabolism of other drugs. This inhibition may be due to decreased metabolism or decreased liver blood flow. This acute alcohol effect may contribute to the commonly recognized danger of mixing alcohol with other drugs when performing activities requiring some skill, especially driving. Phenothiazines, tricyclic antidepressants, and sedative-hypnotic drugs are the most important drugs that may interact with alcohol by this pharmacokinetic mechanism.

Pharmacodynamic alcohol interactions are also of great clinical significance. Additive central nervous system depression with other sedative-hypnotics is most important. Alcohol also potentiates the pharmacologic effects of many nonsedative drugs, including vasodilators and oral hypoglycemic agents. There is some evidence that alcohol also enhances the antiplatelet action of aspirin.

II. CLINICAL PHARMACOLOGY OF ETHANOL

Ethanol is one of the least potent drugs consumed by humans, yet it is the cause of more preventable morbidity and mortality than all other drugs combined with the exception of tobacco. This is true even though moderate consumption of ethanol is associated with sedative-hypnotic effects, reduction of the symptoms and hormonal changes associated with stress, and even with a reduction in mortality.

The search for specific etiologic factors or the identification of significant predisposing variables for alcohol abuse has generally led to disappointing results. Personality type, severe life stresses, psychiatric disorders, and parental role models are not reliable predictors of alcohol abuse. Comparisons of differences in alcohol metabolism are unreliable, and markers of disordered alcohol metabolism are not sufficiently predictive. It is clear that alcohol abuse is not equally distributed in all social groups, and abuse appears to occur at a higher rate among relatives of alcoholics than in the general population (Devor et al, 1989). The rate of alcoholism in persons with an alcoholic biologic parent is almost four times that of a selected control group—a finding that has now been confirmed by several studies. It is difficult to distinguish between contributing factors of familial learning experiences and genetic variables, but current evidence suggests that genetic factors play a role in defining human alcohol use and medical complications. Genetic control of alcohol preference in animals has been clearly established, and, using the abundance of new genetic markers for humans and animals, an intensive search for genes that predispose toward alcohol dependence is under way. One candidate is the A1 allele of the dopamine D_2 receptor gene, which may be associated with a severe form of alcohol dependence (Blum et al, 1990). Since alcohol dependence is a diverse disorder, at least several distinct genes are likely to be able to confer an increased risk of developing alcohol dependence.

MANAGEMENT OF ACUTE ALCOHOL INTOXICATION

Nontolerant individuals who consume alcohol in large quantities develop typical effects of acute sedative-hypnotic drug overdose along with the cardiovascular effects described above (vasodilation, tachycardia) and gastrointestinal irritation. Since tolerance is not absolute, even chronic alcoholics may become severely intoxicated. The degree of intoxication depends upon three factors: the blood ethanol concentration, the rapidity of the rise of the alcohol level, and the time during which the blood level is maintained. The pattern of drinking, the state of the absorptive surface of the gastrointestinal tract, and the presence in the body of other medications also affect the apparent degree of intoxication.

The most important goals in the treatment of acute alcohol intoxication are to prevent severe respiratory depression and aspiration of vomitus. Even with very high blood ethanol levels, survival is probable as long as the respiratory and cardiovascular systems can be supported. The average blood alcohol concentration in fatal cases is above 400 mg/dL; however, the lethal dose of alcohol varies because of varying degrees of tolerance.

Metabolic alterations may require treatment of hypoglycemia and ketosis by administration of glucose. Alcoholic patients who are dehydrated and vomiting should also receive electrolyte solutions. If vomiting is severe, large amounts of potassium may be required as long as renal function is normal. Especially important is recognition of decreased serum concentrations of phosphate, which may be aggravated by glucose administration. Low phosphate stores may contribute to poor wound healing, neurologic deficits, and an increased risk of infection.

MANAGEMENT OF ALCOHOL WITHDRAWAL SYNDROME

Abrupt alcohol withdrawal leads to a characteristic syndrome of motor agitation, anxiety, insomnia, and reduction of seizure threshold. The severity of the syndrome is usually proportionate to the degree and duration of alcohol abuse. However, this can be greatly modified by the use of other sedatives as well as by associated factors (eg, diabetes, injury). In its mildest form, the alcohol withdrawal syndrome of tremor, anxiety, and insomnia occurs 6–8 hours after alcohol is stopped. These effects usually abate in 1–2 days. In some patients, more severe withdrawal reactions occur in which visual hallucinations, total disorientation, and marked abnormalities of vital signs occur. The more severe the withdrawal syndrome, the greater the need for meticulous investigation of possible underlying medical complications. The mortality risks of severe alcohol withdrawal have been overstated in the past. The prognosis is probably related chiefly to the underlying medical complications.

The major objective of drug therapy in the alcohol withdrawal period is prevention of seizures, delirium, and arrhythmias (Romach et al, 1991). Potassium, magnesium, and phosphate balance should be restored as rapidly as is consistent with renal function. Thiamine therapy is initiated in all cases. Persons in mild alcohol withdrawal do not need any other pharmacologic assistance.

Specific drug treatment for detoxification in severe cases involves two basic principles: substituting a long-acting sedative-hypnotic drug for alcohol and then gradually reducing ("tapering") the dose of the long-acting drug. Unfortunately, the most widely used "treatment" for alcohol withdrawal is renewed alcohol intake. Although alcohol can be slowly tapered, it is psychologically undesirable to maintain the patient on alcohol. Barbiturates such as phenobarbital have been used in the past for treatment of the alcohol withdrawal syndrome; however, the benzodiazepines, with their wider margin of safety, are currently preferred for this purpose. Since any benzodiazepine will prevent symptoms of alcohol withdrawal, the choice of a specific agent in this class is generally based upon pharmacokinetic or economic considerations. Long-acting benzodiazepines, including chlordiazepoxide, clorazepate, and diazepam, have the advantage of requiring less frequent dosing. Since their pharmacologically active metabolites are eliminated slowly, the long-acting drugs provide a built-in tapering effect. A disadvantage of the long-acting drugs is that they and their pharmacologically active metabolites may accumulate, especially in patients with compromised liver function. Short-acting drugs such as oxazepam are rapidly converted to inactive water-soluble metabolites that will not accumulate, and for this reason the short-acting drugs are especially useful in alcoholic patients with liver disease. Benzodiazepines can be administered orally in mild or moderate cases, or parenterally for patients with more severe withdrawal reactions.

Phenothiazine medications for alcohol withdrawal have potentially serious adverse effects (eg, increasing seizures) that probably outweigh their benefits. Antihistamine drugs have been used but with little justification.

Phenytoin has been suggested by some to be effective in preventing seizures in alcoholic patients with a history of seizures. Since phenytoin is poorly absorbed from intramuscular sites, the drug should be given intravenously. A loading dose of 12–15 mg/kg is given, and the patient is maintained on 300 mg/d with monitoring of blood levels.

After the alcohol withdrawal syndrome has been treated acutely, sedative-hypnotic medications must be tapered slowly over several weeks. Complete detoxification is not achieved with just a few days of alcohol abstinence. Several months may be required for restoration of normal nervous system function, especially sleep.

PHARMACOTHERAPY OF ALCOHOLISM

Following detoxification, psychosocial therapy either in intensive inpatient or in outpatient rehabilitation programs serves as the primary treatment for alcohol dependence. Since these programs have been only moderately successful, with about 50% of patients relapsing within the first year, there is much interest in finding drugs that can be useful adjuncts to psychosocial counseling. The first approach to pharmacotherapy was to deter drinking with drugs that cause a noxious reaction to alcohol by blocking its metabolism. Disulfiram, an inhibitor of aldehyde dehydrogenase, is the drug most commonly used for this purpose in the USA. More recently, research has focused on identifying drugs that alter brain responses to alcohol, eg, by decreasing the craving of abstinent alcoholics for alcohol or by blunting the pleasurable "high" that comes with renewed drinking. Naltrexone, an inhibitor of opioid receptors, was the first drug of this type to be approved by the FDA for treatment of alcohol dependence.

Other psychiatric problems, most commonly depressive or anxiety disorders, often coexist with alcoholism and, if untreated, can contribute to the tendency of detoxified alcoholics to relapse. Treatment of these associated disorders with counseling and drugs can help decrease the rate of relapse for alcoholic patients.

Disulfiram

Disulfiram (tetraethylthiuram), a widely used antioxidant in the rubber industry, causes extreme discomfort to patients who drink alcoholic beverages. Disulfiram given by itself to nondrinkers has little effect; however, flushing, throbbing headache, nausea, vomiting, sweating, hypotension, and confusion occur within a few minutes after drinking alcohol. The effect may last 30 minutes in mild cases or several hours in severe ones. After the symptoms wear off, the patient is usually exhausted and may sleep for several hours.

Disulfiram acts by inhibiting aldehyde dehydrogenase. Thus, alcohol is metabolized as usual, but acetaldehyde accumulates. The symptoms resulting from disulfiram plus alcohol are typical of acetaldehyde toxicity: the reaction is reproduced by acetaldehyde infusion in humans.

Disulfiram is rapidly and completely absorbed from the gastrointestinal tract; however, a period of 12 hours is required for its full action. Its elimination rate is slow, so that its action may persist for several days after the last dose. The drug inhibits the metabolism of many other therapeutic agents, including phenytoin, oral anticoagulants, and isoniazid.

Disulfiram is used as a pharmacologic adjunct in the treatment of alcoholism and should only be used in concert with behavioral therapies (Chick et al, 1992).

Compliance with disulfiram therapy is often low, and both compliance and clinical outcome can be improved by supervised administration. When the drug is prescribed, the alcohol content of common nonprescription medications should be communicated to the patient; some of these are listed in Table 64–3. Management with disulfiram should be initiated only when the patient has been free of alcohol for at least 24 hours. The drug may cause mild changes in liver function tests. The safety of disulfiram in pregnancy has

not been demonstrated. The duration of disulfiram treatment should be individualized and determined by the patient's responsiveness and clinical improvement. The usual oral dose is 250 mg daily taken at bedtime.

Many other drugs, eg, metronidazole, certain cephalosporins, sulfonylurea hypoglycemic drugs, and chloral hydrate, have disulfiram-like effects on ethanol metabolism (Stockley, 1983). Patients should be warned to avoid drinking ethanol while taking these drugs and for several days after they discontinue them.

MANIPULATING BRAIN NEURO-TRANSMITTER SYSTEMS TO TREAT ALCOHOLISM

Advances in knowledge about the neurochemistry of the brain's reward system have increased the hope that pharmacologic manipulation of brain neurotransmitter systems can help people who become addicted to alcohol and other drugs (Litten et al, 1991). The apparent utility of naltrexone, an opioid antagonist, in preventing craving and relapse in alcoholic patients provides evidence that the opioid system is an important player in the alcohol response system.

Several other neurotransmitter systems are leading targets in studies of drugs to treat alcoholism. Considerable evidence from animal studies indicates that serotonergic and dopaminergic systems participate in the regulation of alcohol consumption. Clinical trials are focusing on selective serotonin reuptake inhibitors (SSRI) such as fluoxetine, as well as selective serotonin receptor antagonists such as buspirone, a 5-HT_{1A} receptor partial agonist; ritanserin, a 5-HT_2 receptor antagonist; and ondansetron, a 5-HT_3 receptor antagonist.

The SSRI drugs have been most thoroughly studied. Results from clinical trials have been mixed, with some studies showing favorable results and others failing to find that SSRIs attenuate alcohol consumption in nondepressed heavy drinkers (Kranzler et al, 1995). A number of dopamine receptor antagonists are also under investigation, including selective antagonists of D_1 and D_2 dopamine receptors. Because of their importance in alcohol-related effects, drugs that modify neurotransmission through GABA and glutamate systems are also under investigation. Alcoholism is a heterogeneous disorder. As efforts to classify alcoholic patients into specific subtypes become more sophisticated, it may be possible to identify the subtypes that respond best to specific pharmacotherapies.

Naltrexone

Naltrexone is an orally available opioid receptor antagonist that blocks the effects of exogenous and, presumably, endogenous opioids. Studies in experimental animals first suggested a link between alcohol consumption and opioids. Injection of small amounts of opioids was followed by an increase in alcohol drinking, whereas administration of opioid antagonists inhibited self-administration of alcohol. Several double-blind, placebo-controlled clinical trials showed that the combination of naltrexone with psychosocial therapy decreased the rate of relapse and reduced alcohol craving (Volpicelli et al, J Clin Psychiatry 1995; O'Malley et al, 1996). The subjects taking naltrexone who "slipped," that is, who sampled alcohol during the trial, were better able to control their drinking and avoid relapsing into heavy drinking. The lower alcohol consumption in naloxone-treated subjects was associated with a diminution of the subjective "high" associated with alcohol (Volpicelli et al, J Clin Psychiatry 1995). The durability of naltrexone's effect in alcoholism is not clear, since the initial clinical trials were only for 12 weeks. In a follow-up study, the decrease in relapse after 12 weeks of treatment continued for only one month after discontinuation of the naltrexone (O'Malley et al, 1996).

Following oral administration, naltrexone undergoes extensive first-pass metabolism to pharmacologically active and inactive metabolites (Chapter 31). Naltrexone is taken once a day in a dose of 50 mg for treatment of alcoholism.

Opioid antagonists have few effects in the absence of exogenous opioids. The most common adverse effects of oral naltrexone are nausea, dizziness, and headache. The incidence of nausea can be reduced by initiating therapy with lower doses. A concern with naltrexone is that high doses, in the range of 300 mg/d, can cause elevations in liver enzymes. Acute hepatitis and liver failure are contraindications to naltrexone's use. The drug should be used with caution in alcoholic patients with evidence of mild abnormalities in serum aminotransferase activity.

The combination of naltrexone plus disulfiram should be avoided since both drugs are potential hepatotoxins. Administration of naltrexone to patients who are physically dependent upon opioids will precipitate an acute withdrawal syndrome so patients must be opioid-free before initiating naltrexone therapy. Naltrexone also blocks the effects of usual doses of opioids.

III. PHARMACOLOGY OF OTHER ALCOHOLS

Other alcohols related to ethanol have wide applications as industrial solvents and occasionally cause severe poisoning (Litovitz, 1986). Of these, **methanol** and **ethylene glycol** are two of the most common causes of intoxication.

Methanol

Methanol (methyl alcohol, wood alcohol) is derived from the destructive distillation of wood. It is used as a gasoline additive, industrial solvent, solvent in xerographic copier solutions, and feedstock for bacterial synthesis of protein. Methanol is most frequently found in the home in the form of "canned heat" or in windshield-washing products. It can be absorbed through the skin or from the respiratory or gastrointestinal tract. It is rapidly absorbed from the gastrointestinal tract and distributed in body water.

The primary mechanism of elimination of methanol in humans is by oxidation to formaldehyde, formic acid, and CO_2:

Animal species show great variability in mean lethal doses of methanol. The special susceptibility of humans to methanol toxicity is probably due to folate-dependent production of formate and not to methanol itself or to formaldehyde, the intermediate metabolite.

Severe methanol poisoning is usually encountered in chronic alcoholics and may not be recognized unless characteristic symptoms are noted in a group of patients. Because methanol and its metabolite formate are much more potent toxins than ethanol, it is essential that patients with methanol poisoning be recognized and treated as soon as possible.

The most characteristic symptom in methanol poisoning is a visual disturbance, frequently described as "like being in a snowstorm." Visual disturbances are a universal complaint in epidemics of methanol poisoning. A complaint of blurred vision with a relatively clear sensorium should strongly suggest the diagnosis of methanol poisoning. Since much of the toxicity is due to metabolites of methanol, there is often a delay of up to 30 hours before development of visual disturbances and other signs of severe intoxication.

Physical findings in methanol poisoning are generally nonspecific. In severe cases, the odor of formaldehyde may be present on the breath or in the urine. Changes in the retina may sometimes be detected on examination, but these are usually late. The development of bradycardia, prolonged coma, seizures, and resistant acidosis all imply a poor prognosis. The cause of death in fatal cases is sudden cessation of respiration.

It is critical that the blood methanol level be determined as soon as possible if the diagnosis is suspected. Methanol concentrations in excess of 50 mg/dL are thought to be an absolute indication for hemodialysis and ethanol treatment, though formate blood levels are a better indication of clinical pathology. Additional laboratory evidence includes metabolic acidosis with an elevated anion gap and osmolar gap (Chapter 59). A decrease in serum bicarbonate is a uniform feature of severe methanol poisoning.

The first treatment for methanol poisoning, as in all critical poisoning situations, is support of respiration, with intubation of the trachea if necessary. Emesis can be induced if the patient is not comatose, is not having seizures, and has not lost the gag reflex. If any of these contraindications exist, gastric lavage should be carried out with a large-bore tube after the airway has been protected by endotracheal intubation. Since methanol is not effectively removed by charcoal, administration of activated charcoal is not useful in methanol poisoning.

There are three "specific" modalities of treatment for severe methanol poisoning: suppression of metabolism by alcohol dehydrogenase to toxic products, dialysis to enhance removal of methanol and its toxic products, and alkalinization to counteract metabolic acidosis.

The enzyme chiefly responsible for methanol oxidation in the liver is alcohol dehydrogenase. Ethanol has a higher affinity than methanol for alcohol dehydrogenase; thus, saturation of the enzyme with ethanol reduces formate production. Ethanol is often used intravenously as a treatment for acute methanol toxicity. The dose-dependent characteristics of ethanol metabolism and the variability of ethanol metabolism induced by chronic ethanol intake require frequent monitoring of blood ethanol levels to ensure appropriate alcohol concentration.

Hemodialysis rapidly eliminates both methanol and formate. However, with initiation of dialysis procedures, ethanol will also be eliminated in the dialysate, requiring alterations in the dose of ethanol. Hemodialysis is discussed in Chapter 59.

Because of profound metabolic acidosis in methanol poisoning, treatment with bicarbonate may be necessary. Quantities of bicarbonate to be administered should be based on estimated sodium intake, potassium balance, cardiovascular status, and changes in blood and urine pH.

Since folate-dependent systems are responsible for the oxidation of formic acid to CO_2 in humans, it is probably useful to administer folic acid to patients poisoned with methanol, though this has never been fully tested in clinical studies.

A special diagnostic problem occurs if a patient has a relatively low methanol level but visual symptoms are present. In this situation, laboratory tests for methanol itself should be repeated and confirmed with osmolality estimates. If visual impairment is present, hemodialysis should be started in spite of low methanol levels.

Ethylene Glycol

Polyhydric alcohols such as ethylene glycol (CH_2OHCH_2OH) are used as heat exchangers, in antifreeze formulations, and as industrial solvents. Owing to the low volatility of the glycols, they produce little vapor hazard at ordinary temperatures. However, since they are used as antifreeze mixtures and as heat exchangers, they may be encountered in vapor or mist form, particularly if the temperature is high. Young children are sometimes attracted by the sweet taste of ethylene glycol and, rarely, it is ingested intentionally as an ethanol substitute. As with other alcohols, ethylene glycol is metabolized by alcohol dehydrogenase to toxic aldehydes and oxalate.

Ethylene glycol appears to be considerably more toxic to humans than to many other animal species. Three stages of ethylene glycol overdose have been recognized. Within the first few hours after exposure or ingestion, there is transient excitation followed by central nervous system depression. After a delay of 4–12 hours, severe metabolic acidosis develops, and finally delayed renal insufficiency occurs due to deposition of oxalate in renal tubules. In severe cases, increased muscle enzyme and decreased calcium have been found in the plasma. The key to the diagnosis of ethylene glycol poisoning is the recognition of anion gap acidosis, osmolar gap, and oxalate crystals in the urine in a patient without visual symptoms. Ethylene glycol-intoxicated patients have no detectable odor of alcohol on their breath, and the ophthalmoscopic examination is usually normal. As with methanol poisoning, early ethanol infusion and dialysis are required. Prompt treatment with 4-methylpyrazole, an inhibitor of alcohol dehydrogenase, may prevent the development of metabolic acidosis (Baud et al, 1986, 1988).

PREPARATIONS AVAILABLE

Drugs for the Treatment of Acute Alcohol Withdrawal Syndrome
Clorazepate (generic, Tranxene)
  Oral: 3.75, 7.5, 15 mg tablets and capsules
Diazepam (generic, Valium, others)
  Oral: 2, 3, 10 mg tablets; 5 mg/5 mL solutions
    (see also Chapter 22)
  Parenteral: 5 mg/mL for injection
Oxazepam (generic, Serax)
  Oral: 10, 15, 30 mg capsules, 15 mg tablets
Thiamine (generic)
  Parenteral: 100 mg/mL for IV injection

Drugs for the Prevention of Alcohol Abuse
Disulfiram (generic, Antabuse)
  Oral: 250, 500 mg tablets
Naltrexone (ReVia)
  Oral: 50 mg tablets

Drugs for the Treatment of Acute Methanol or Ethylene Glycol Poisoning
Ethanol (generic)
  Parenteral: 5% or 10% ethanol and 5% dextrose in water for IV infusion

REFERENCES

Abel EL (editor): *Fetal Alcohol Syndrome.* CRC Press, 1981.

Ballard HS: Hematological complications of alcoholism. Alcohol Clin Exp Res 1989;13:706.

Baud FJ et al: 4-Methylpyrazole may be an alternative to ethanol therapy for ethylene glycol intoxication in man. J Toxicol Clin Toxicol 1986;24:463.

Baud FJ et al: Treatment of ethylene glycol poisoning with intravenous 4-methylpyrazole. N Engl J Med 1988;319:97.

Becker CE: The alcoholic patient is a toxic emergency. Emerg Med Clin North Am 1983;1:51.

Becker CE: Methanol poisoning. J Emerg Med 1983;2:47.

Blum K, Noble EP, Sheridan PJ: Allelic association of human dopamine receptor gene and alcoholism. JAMA 1990;263:2055.

Brien JF, Loomis CW: Pharmacology of acetaldehyde. Can J Physiol Pharmacol 1983;61:1.

Buck KJ, Harris RA: Neuroadaptive responses to chronic ethanol. Alcohol Clin Exp Res 1991;15:460.

Charness ME, Simon RP, Greenberg DA: Ethanol and the nervous system. N Engl J Med 1989;321:442.

Chick J et al: Disulfiram treatment of alcoholism. Br J Psychiatry 1992;161:84.

Devor EJ, Cloninger CR: Genetics of alcoholism. Annu Rev Genet 1989;23:19.

Dietrich RA et al: Mechanism of action of ethanol: Initial central nervous system actions. Pharmacol Rev 1989;41:489.

Ernhart CB et al: Alcohol teratogenicity in the human: A detailed assessment of specificity, critical period, and threshold. Am J Obstet Gynecol 1987;156:33.

Frances RJ, Borg L: The treatment of anxiety in patients with alcoholism. J Clin Psychiatry 1993;54(Suppl):37.

Frezza M et al: High blood alcohol levels in women: The role of decreased gastric alcohol dehydrogenase activity and first-pass metabolism. N Engl J Med 1990; 322:95.

Gandhi CR, Ross DH: Influence of ethanol on calcium, inositol phospholipids, and intracellular signalling mechanisms. Experientia 1989;45:407.

Gaziano JM et al: Moderate alcohol intake, increased levels of high-density lipoprotein and its subfractions, and decreased risk of myocardial infarction. N Engl J Med 1993;329:1829.

Geokas MC (editor): Ethyl alcohol and disease. (Symposium.) Med Clin North Am 1984;68:1.

Grønbæk et al: Influence of sex, age, body mass index, and smoking on alcohol intake and mortality. Br Med J 1994;308:302.

Grogan JR, Kochar MS: Alcohol and hypertension. Arch Fam Med 1994;3:150.

Harris RA, Allan AM: Alcohol intoxication: Ion channels and genetics. FASEB J 1989;3:1689.

Hoffman PL, Tabakoff B: The role of the NMDA receptor in ethanol withdrawal. EXS 1994;71:61.

Holford NH: Clinical pharmacokinetics of ethanol. Clin Pharmacokinet 1987;13:273.

Irwin M et al: Testosterone in chronic alcoholic men. Br J Addict 1988;83:949.

Korpi ER: Role of GABA$_A$ receptors in the actions of alcohol and in alcoholism: recent advances. Alcohol 1994; 29:115.

Kranzler HR et al: Placebo-controlled trial of fluoxetine as an adjunct to relapse prevention in alcoholics. Am J Psychiatry 1995;152:391.

Lee NM, Smith AS: Ethanol. In: *Toxicology of CNS Depressants*. Ho IK (editor). CRC Press, 1986.

Levallois C et al: Effects of ethanol in vitro on some parameters of the immune system. Drug Alcohol Depend 1989;24:239.

Lieber CS: Interaction of ethanol with drugs, hepatotoxic agents, carcinogens, and vitamins. Alcohol 1990;25:157.

Lieber CS: Medical disorders of alcoholism. N Engl J Med 1995;333:1058.

Litovitz T: The alcohols: Ethanol, methanol, isopropanol, ethylene glycol. Pediatr Clin North Am 1986;33:311.

Litten RZ, Allen JP: Pharmacotherapies for alcoholism: Promising agents and clinical issues. Alcoholism: Clin Exp Res 1991;15:620.

MacGregor RR: Alcohol and immune defense. JAMA 1986;256:1474.

Martensson E, Olofsson U, Heath A: Clinical and metabolic features of ethanol-methane poisoning in chronic alcoholics. Lancet 1988;1:327.

Mufti SI, Darban HR, Watson RR: Alcohol, cancer, and immunomodulation. Crit Rev Oncol Hematol 1989;9:243.

Nagy LE et al: Ethanol increases extracellular adenosine by inhibiting adenosine uptake via the nucleoside transporter. J Biol Chem 1990;265:1946.

Naranjo CA et al: Fluoxetine differentially alters alcohol intake and other consummatory behaviors in problem drinkers. Clin Pharmacol Ther 1990;47:490.

Naranjo CA, Ozdemir V, Bremner KE: Diagnosis and pharmacological treatment of alcoholic patients. CNS Drugs 1994;1:330.

Nelson S et al: Alcohol, tumor necrosis factor, and tuberculosis. Alcohol Clin Exp Res 1995;19:17.

O'Malley SS et al: Six-month follow-up of naltrexone and psychotherapy for alcohol dependence. Arch Gen Psychiatry 1996;53:217.

Peoples RW, Weight FF: Cutoff in potency implicates alcohol inhibition of *N*-methyl-D-aspartate receptors in alcohol intoxication. Proc Natl Acad Sci USA 1995; 92: 2825.

Piano MR, Schwertz DW: Alcoholic heart disease: A review. Heart Lung 1994;23:3.

Poikolainen K: Alcohol and mortality: A review. J Clin Epidemiol 1995;48:455. [Erratum appears in J Clin Epidemiol 1995;48(9):i.]

Ramanathan R et al: Alcohol inhibits cell-cell adhesion mediated by human L1. J Cell Biol 1996;133:381.

Rimm EB et al: Review of moderate alcohol consumption and reduced risk of coronary heart disease: Is the effect due to beer, wine, or spirits. Br Med J 1996; 312:731.

Romach MK, Sellers EM: Management of the alcohol withdrawal syndrome. Annu Rev Med 1991;42:323.

Rooney TA et al: Short chain alcohols activate guanine nucleotide-dependent phosphoinositidase C in turkey erythrocyte membranes. J Biol Chem 1989;264:6817.

Rosenberg A, Noble EP: Ethanol attenuation of ganglioside sialylation and neuritogenesis. Alcohol 1994;11:565.

Samson HH, Harris RA: Neurobiology of alcohol abuse [see comments]. Trends Pharmacol Sci 1992;13:206.

Schatzkin A et al: Alcohol consumption and breast cancer in the epidemiologic follow-up study of the First National Health and Nutrition Examination Survey. N Engl J Med 1987;316:1169.

Schatzkin A, Longnecker MP: Alcohol and breast cancer. Where are we now and where do we go from here? Cancer 1994;74(3 Suppl):1101.

Schenker S et al: Fetal alcohol syndrome: Current status of pathogenesis. Alcoholism: Clin Exp Res 1990;14:635.

Sherlock DS: Chronic hepatitis C. Dis Mon 1994;40:117.

Steinberg W, Tenner S: Acute pancreatitis. N Engl J Med 1994;330:1198.

Stockley IH: Drugs, foods, and environmental chemical agents which can initiate Antabuse-like reactions with alcohol. Pharmacy Int 1983;4:12.

Suh I et al: Alcohol use and mortality from coronary heart disease: The role of high-density lipoprotein cholesterol. Ann Intern Med 1992;116:881.

Tabakoff B et al: Differences in platelet enzyme activity between alcoholics and nonalcoholics. N Engl J Med 1988;318:134.

Tsai G, Gastfriend DR, Coyle JT: The glutamatergic basis of human alcoholism. Am J Psychiatry 1995;152:332.

Volpicelli JR et al: Effect of naltrexone on alcohol "high" in alcoholics. Am J Psychiatry 1995;152:613.

Volpicelli JR et al: Naltrexone in the treatment of alcoholism: Predicting response to naltrexone. J Clin Psychiatry 1995;7:39.

Wood WG, Gorka C, Schroeder F: Acute and chronic effects of ethanol on transbilayer membrane domains. J Neurochem 1989;52:1925.

Wright C, Moore RD: Disulfiram treatment of alcoholism. Am J Med 1990;88:647.

24

Antiepileptic Drugs*

Roger J. Porter, MD, & Brian S. Meldrum MB, PhD

Approximately 1% of the world's population has epilepsy, the second most common neurologic disorder after stroke. Although standard therapy permits control of seizures in 80% of these patients, millions (500,000 people in the USA alone) have uncontrolled epilepsy. Epilepsy is a heterogeneous symptom complex—a chronic disorder characterized by recurrent seizures. Seizures are finite episodes of brain dysfunction resulting from abnormal discharge of cerebral neurons. The causes of seizures are many and include the full range of neurologic diseases, from infection to neoplasm and head injury. In a few subgroups, heredity has proved to be a major contributing factor.

The antiepileptic drugs described in this chapter are also used in patients with febrile seizures or with seizures occurring as part of an acute illness such as meningitis, even though the term "epilepsy" is not usually applied to such patients unless they later develop chronic seizures. Seizures are occasionally caused by an acute underlying toxic or metabolic disorder, in which case appropriate therapy should be directed toward the specific abnormality, eg, hypocalcemia. In most cases of epilepsy, however, the choice of medication depends on the empirical seizure classification.

History

Before the antiepileptic drugs were discovered and developed, treatment of epilepsy consisted of trephining, cupping, and the administration of herbal medicines and animal extracts. In 1857, Sir Charles Locock reported the successful use of potassium bromide in the treatment of what is now known as catamenial epilepsy. In 1912, phenobarbital was first used for epilepsy, and in the next 25 years, 35 analogs of phenobarbital were studied as anticonvulsants. In 1938, phenytoin was found to be effective against experimental seizures in cats.

Between 1935 and 1960, tremendous strides were made both in the development of experimental models and in methods for screening and testing new antiepileptic drugs. During that period, 13 new antiepileptic drugs were developed and marketed. Following the enactment of requirements for proof of drug efficacy in 1962, antiepileptic drug development slowed dramatically, and only a few new antiepileptic drugs were marketed in the next 3 decades. However, a series of new compounds have become available in the 1990s.

Present Status of Drug Development for Epilepsy

For a long time it was assumed that a single drug could be developed for treatment of all forms of epilepsy. It now appears unlikely that the wide variety of epileptic seizures can be managed successfully with just one drug. More than one mechanism may be responsible for the various seizures, and drugs useful for one seizure type may occasionally aggravate other types. Drugs used in the treatment of the two major types of seizures (partial and generalized; Table 24–1) are quite distinct in their clinical effects and also fall into two pharmacologic classes, even though seizures may be induced experimentally by a wide variety of methods. The clinical aspects of certain generalized seizures—especially absence seizures—are highly correlated with experimental seizures produced in animals by subcutaneous administration of pentylenetetrazol. Likewise, partial seizures in humans correlate positively with experimental seizures elicited by the maximal electroshock (MES) test. In general, antiepileptic drugs effective against maximal electroshock seizures alter ionic transport across excitable membranes. Phenytoin, for example, is effective against partial seizures and maximal electroshock but with the exception of generalized tonic-clonic seizures is not effective against generalized seizures or those induced

*The authors wish to thank Philip Mayer, PhD, for his assistance in reviewing the pharmacokinetic data in this chapter.

Table 24–1. Classification of seizure types.

Partial seizures
  Simple partial seizures
  Complex partial seizures
  Partial seizures secondarily generalized
Generalized seizures
  Generalized tonic-clonic (grand mal) seizures
  Absence (petit mal) seizures
  Tonic seizures
  Atonic seizures
  Clonic and myoclonic seizures
  Infantile spasms[1]

[1]An epileptic syndrome rather than a specific seizure type; drugs useful in infantile spasms will be reviewed separately.

by subcutaneous pentylenetetrazol. Phenytoin affects cell firing through its action on Na^+ conductance mechanisms. On the other hand, ethosuximide and trimethadione, which are active against pentylenetetrazol and certain generalized seizures, diminish Ca^{2+} entry (through T-type, or low-threshold calcium channels). It is notable that the two distinct classes of antiepileptic drugs have different mechanisms of ac-

tion in spite of marked structural similarities between many of the drugs in the two groups.

New antiepileptic drugs are being sought not only by the screening tests noted above but also by more rational approaches. Compounds are sought that act by one of three mechanisms: (1) enhancement of GABAergic (inhibitory) transmission, (2) diminution of excitatory (usually glutamatergic) transmission, or (3) modification of ionic conductances.

I. BASIC PHARMACOLOGY OF ANTIEPILEPTIC DRUGS

Chemistry

Up to 1990, approximately 16 antiepileptic drugs were available, and 13 of them have been classified into five very similar chemical groups: barbiturates, hydantoins, oxazolidinediones, succinimides, and acetylureas. These groups have in common a similar

MECHANISM OF ACTION OF ANTIEPILEPTIC DRUGS

The ancient Greeks considered epilepsy to be a sign of possession by the gods; other cultures have considered the seizures to be signs of malignant witchcraft. Modern research has done much to dissipate such ideas, but solutions to the questions of the causes and treatment of seizure disorders have been difficult to find.

When the stream of useful drugs discovered through screening methods between 1938 and 1960 came to an end, it became clear that in order to make further progress in the treatment of epilepsy it would be necessary to know more about the cellular pathophysiology of the disease and the mechanisms of action of the successful drugs. In the last 3 decades, considerable progress has been made in the exploration of cerebral synaptic mechanisms in general (Chapter 21) and the actions of currently available antiseizure drugs.

The principal mechanisms of action of antiepileptic drugs have been found to concern voltage-operated ion channels and inhibitory and excitatory synaptic function. Voltage-dependent Na^+ channels enter an inactive state following each action potential (see Chapter 14). Prolongation of this inactive state—with a concomitant prolongation of refractoriness—is thought to be the principal mechanism of action of phenytoin, carbamazepine, and lamotrigine; it may also contribute to the effects of phenobarbital, valproate, and topiramate. This phenomenon is linked to suppression of rapid repetitive firing in isolated

neurons (Figure 24–2) and protection against maximal electroshock in animals and focal seizures in man.

A low-threshold Ca^{2+} current (the T-type Ca^{2+} current) has been found to govern oscillatory responses in thalamic neurons. Reduction of this current by ethosuximide or dimethadione is thought to explain the effect of these compounds in absence seizures.

Effects on synaptic transmission have been sought for many antiepileptic drugs. Enhancement of GABA-mediated inhibition can be produced in many different ways, involving either direct action on the GABA receptor-chloride channel complex (as with benzodiazepines, barbiturates, and possibly topiramate) or actions on the reuptake or metabolism of GABA (as with tiagabine and vigabatrin). This mechanism provides protection against generalized and focal seizures.

Reduction of excitatory glutamatergic neurotransmission is potentially important; AMPA receptor blockade probably contributes to the effect of phenobarbital and topiramate, NMDA receptor blockade to the effect of remacemide, an investigational drug.

These studies of basic mechanisms are beginning to pay dividends. This edition of this book lists 23 antiepileptic drugs compared with the 15 that were listed in the first edition—a 50% increase in little more than a decade.

heterocyclic ring structure with a variety of substituents (Figure 24–1). For drugs with this basic structure, the substituents on the heterocyclic ring determine the pharmacologic class, either anti-MES or antipentylenetetrazol. Very small changes in structure can dramatically alter the mechanism of action and clinical properties of the compound. The remaining drugs—carbamazepine, valproic acid, and the benzodiazepines—are structurally dissimilar, as are the newer compounds of the 1990s, ie, felbamate, gabapentin, lamotrigine, oxcarbazepine, tiagabine, topiramate, and vigabatrin.

Pharmacokinetics

The antiepileptic drugs exhibit many similar pharmacokinetic properties—even those whose structural and chemical properties are quite diverse. Although many of these compounds are only sparingly soluble, absorption is usually good, with 80–100% of the dose reaching the circulation. The oral bioavailability of phenytoin varies from product to product, with both the rate and extent of absorption highly dependent on the formulation.

Except for phenytoin, the benzodiazepines, valproic acid, and tiagabine, antiepileptic drugs are not highly bound to plasma proteins. Phenytoin and valproic acid are able to displace other highly bound drugs, including other anticonvulsants. Benzodiazepine concentrations are too low to affect the binding of other drugs. The relevant data on tiagabine are not yet available.

For disease states with altered serum albumin concentrations (typically hypoalbuminemia), dosing of highly bound drugs may be more appropriately based on free drug concentrations. Whereas free drug concentrations would not generally be altered, total drug concentrations may decrease, leading the clinician to increase the dose; this increase in dose will result in higher free drug levels and possible drug toxicity. Sodium valproate is unique in that the fraction of drug bound is a function of the concentrations of both the drug and the free fatty acids in plasma.

Antiepileptic drugs are cleared chiefly by hepatic mechanisms, though they have low extraction ratios (see Chapter 3). Many, such as primidone and the benzodiazepines, are converted to active metabolites that are also cleared by the liver. The intrinsic ability of the liver to metabolize anticonvulsant drugs is generally low and, with the exception of phenytoin, independent of concentration. These drugs are predominantly distributed into total body water. Plasma clearance is relatively slow; many anticonvulsants are therefore considered to be medium- to long-acting. For most, half-lives are greater than 12 hours. Phenobarbital and carbamazepine are potent inducers of hepatic microsomal enzyme activity.

DRUGS USED IN PARTIAL SEIZURES & GENERALIZED TONIC-CLONIC SEIZURES

The major drugs for partial and generalized tonic-clonic seizures are phenytoin (and congeners), carbamazepine, valproate and the barbiturates. However, the addition of newer drugs—lamotrigine, gabapentin, oxcarbazepine, topiramate, and vigabatrin—is altering clinical practice in countries where these compounds are available.

PHENYTOIN

Phenytoin is the oldest nonsedative antiepileptic drug, introduced in 1938 following a systematic evaluation of compounds such as phenobarbital that altered electrically induced seizures in laboratory animals. It was known for decades as **diphenylhydantoin.**

Chemistry

Phenytoin is a diphenyl-substituted hydantoin with the structure shown below. It has much lower sedative properties than compounds with alkyl substituents at the 5 position. A more soluble prodrug of phenytoin, **fosphenytoin,** has recently been approved for parenteral use. This phosphate ester compound is rapidly converted to phenytoin in the plasma.

Phenytoin

Mechanism of Action

Phenytoin has major effects on several physiologic systems. It alters Na^+, K^+, and Ca^{2+} conductances, membrane potentials, and the concentrations of amino acids and the neurotransmitters norepinephrine,

Figure 24–1. Antiepileptic heterocyclic ring structure. The "X" varies as follows: hydantoin derivatives, –N–; barbiturates, –C–N–; oxazolidinediones, –O–; succinimides, –C–; acetylureas, –NH$_2$ (N connected to C$_2$). R$_1$, R$_2$, and R$_3$ vary within each subgroup.

acetylcholine, and γ-aminobutyric acid (GABA). Phenytoin blocks posttetanic potentiation in spinal cord preparations, but the role of this effect in suppressing seizure spread is not yet defined.

Studies with neurons in cell culture show that phenytoin blocks sustained high-frequency repetitive firing of action potentials (Figure 24–2). This effect is seen at therapeutically relevant concentrations. It is a use-dependent effect (see Chapter 14) on Na^+ conductance, arising from preferential binding to—and prolongation of—the inactivated state of the Na^+ channel (Macdonald et al, 1995). This effect is also seen with therapeutically relevant concentrations of carbamazepine and valproate and probably contributes to their antiepileptic action in the electroshock model and in partial seizures.

At high concentrations, phenytoin also inhibits the release of serotonin and norepinephrine, promotes the uptake of dopamine, and inhibits monoamine oxidase activity. The drug interacts with membrane lipids; this binding might promote the stabilization of the membrane. In addition, phenytoin paradoxically causes excitation in some cerebral neurons. A reduction of calcium permeability, with inhibition of calcium influx across the cell membrane may explain the ability of phenytoin to inhibit a variety of calcium-induced secretory processes, including release of hormones and neurotransmitters. The significance of these biochemical actions and their relationship to phenytoin activity are unclear.

The mechanism of phenytoin's action probably involves a combination of actions at several levels. At therapeutic concentrations, the major action of phenytoin is to block sodium channels and inhibit the generation of repetitive action potentials.

Clinical Use

Phenytoin is one of the most effective drugs against partial seizures and generalized tonic-clonic seizures.

In the latter, it appears to be effective against attacks that are either primary or secondary to another seizure type.

Pharmacokinetics

Absorption of phenytoin is highly dependent on the formulation of the dosage form. Particle size and pharmaceutical additives affect both the rate and extent of absorption. Absorption of phenytoin sodium from the gastrointestinal tract is nearly complete in most patients, though the time to peak may range from 3 hours to 12 hours. Absorption after intramuscular injection is unpredictable, and some drug precipitation in the muscle occurs; this route of administration is not recommended for phenytoin. In contrast, fosphenytoin, a more soluble phosphate prodrug of phenytoin, is well absorbed after intramuscular administration.

Phenytoin is highly bound to plasma proteins. It appears certain that the total plasma level decreases when the percentage that is bound decreases, as in uremia or hypoalbuminemia, but correlation of free levels with clinical states remains uncertain. Drug concentration in cerebrospinal fluid is proportionate to the free plasma level. Phenytoin accumulates in and becomes bound to the endoplasmic reticulum of cells in brain, liver, muscle, and fat.

Phenytoin is metabolized primarily by parahydroxylation to 5-(p-hydroxyphenyl)-5-phenylhydantoin (HPPH), which is subsequently conjugated with glucuronic acid. The metabolites are clinically inactive and are excreted in the urine. Only a very small portion of phenytoin is excreted unchanged. The elimination of phenytoin is dose-dependent. At very low blood levels, phenytoin metabolism is proportionate to the rate at which the drug is presented to the liver, ie, first-order metabolism. However, as blood levels rise within the therapeutic range, the maximum capacity of the liver to metabolize phenytoin is ap-

Figure 24–2. Effects of three antiepileptic drugs on sustained high-frequency firing of action potentials by cultured neurons. Intracellular recordings were made from neurons while depolarizing current pulses, approximately 0.75 s in duration, were applied (on-off step changes indicated by arrows). In the absence of drug, a series of high-frequency repetitive action potentials filled the entire duration of the current pulse. Phenytoin, carbamazepine, and sodium valproate all markedly reduced the number of action potentials elicited by the current pulses. (Modified and reproduced, with permission, from Macdonald RL, Meldrum BS: Principles of antiepileptic drug action. In: *Antiepileptic Drugs*, 4th ed. Levy RH, et al [editors]. Raven Press, 1995.)

proached (Figure 24–3). Further increases in dose, even though relatively small, may produce very large changes in phenytoin concentrations. In such cases, the half-life of the drug increases markedly, steady state is not achieved in routine fashion (since the plasma level continues to rise), and patients quickly develop symptoms of toxicity.

The half-life of phenytoin varies from 12 hours to 36 hours, with an average of 24 hours for most patients in the low- to mid-therapeutic range. Much longer half-lives are observed at higher concentrations. At low blood levels, it takes 5–7 days to reach steady state blood levels after every dosage change; at higher levels it may be 4–6 weeks before blood levels are stable.

Therapeutic Levels & Dosage

The therapeutic plasma level of phenytoin for most patients is between 10 and 20 μg/mL. A loading dose can be given either orally or intravenously; the latter is the method of choice for convulsive status epilepticus (discussed later). When oral therapy is started, it is common to begin adults at a dosage of 300 mg/d regardless of body weight. While this may be acceptable in some patients, it frequently yields steady state blood levels below 10 μg/mL, the minimum therapeutic level for most patients. If seizures continue, higher doses are usually necessary to achieve plasma levels in the upper therapeutic range. Because of its dose-dependent kinetics, some toxicity may occur with

only small increments in dose; the phenytoin dosage should be increased each time by only 25–30 mg in adults, and ample time should be allowed for the new steady state to be achieved before further increasing the dose. A common clinical error is to increase the dosage directly from 300 mg/d to 400 mg/d; toxicity frequently occurs at a variable time thereafter. In children, a dosage of 5 mg/kg/d should be followed by readjustment after steady state plasma levels are obtained.

Two types of oral phenytoin sodium are currently available in the USA, differing in their respective rates of dissolution; one is absorbed rapidly and one more slowly. Only the latter can be given in a single daily dosage, and care must be used when changing brands (see Preparations Available). Although a few patients being given phenytoin on a chronic basis have been proved to have low blood levels either from poor absorption or rapid metabolism, the most common cause of low levels is poor compliance. Fosphenytoin sodium is available only for intravenous or intramuscular use and in the USA will replace intravenous phenytoin sodium, a much less soluble form of the drug.

Drug Interactions & Interference With Laboratory Tests

Drug interactions involving phenytoin are primarily related to protein binding or to metabolism. Since phenytoin is 90% bound to plasma protein, other highly bound drugs, such as phenylbutazone or sulfonamides, can displace phenytoin from its binding site. In theory, such displacement may cause a transient increase in free drug. A decrease in protein binding—eg, in hypoalbuminemia—results in a decrease in the total plasma concentration of drug but not the free concentration; intoxication may occur if efforts are made to maintain total drug levels in the therapeutic range by increasing the dose. The protein binding of phenytoin is decreased in the presence of renal disease. The drug has an affinity for thyroid-binding globulin, which confuses some tests of thyroid function; the most reliable screening test of thyroid function in patients taking phenytoin appears to be measurement of TSH.

Phenytoin has been shown to induce microsomal enzymes responsible for the metabolism of a number of drugs. Autostimulation of its own metabolism, however, appears to be insignificant. Other drugs, notably phenobarbital and carbamazepine, cause decreases in phenytoin steady state concentrations through induction of hepatic microsomal enzymes. On the other hand, isoniazid inhibits the metabolism of phenytoin, resulting in increased steady state concentrations when the two drugs are given together.

Toxicity

Dose-related adverse effects caused by phenytoin are unfortunately similar to other antiepileptic drugs

Figure 24–3. Nonlinear relationship of phenytoin dosage and plasma concentrations. Five different patients (identified by different symbols) received increasing dosages of phenytoin by mouth, and the steady-state serum concentration was measured at each dosage. The curves are not linear, since, as the dosage increases, the metabolism is saturable. Note also the marked variation among patients in the serum levels achieved at any dosage. (Modified, with permission, from Jusko WJ: Bioavailability and disposition kinetics of phenytoin in man. In: *Quantitative Analytic Studies in Epilepsy.* Kellaway P, Peterson I [editors]. Raven Press, 1977.)

in this group, making differentiation difficult in patients receiving multiple drugs. Nystagmus occurs early, as does loss of smooth extraocular pursuit movements, but neither is an indication for decreasing the dose. Diplopia and ataxia are the most common dose-related adverse effects requiring dosage adjustment; sedation usually occurs only at considerably higher levels. Gingival hyperplasia and hirsutism occur to some degree in most patients; the latter can be especially unpleasant in females. Long-term chronic use is associated in some patients with coarsening of facial features and with mild peripheral neuropathy, usually manifested by diminished deep tendon reflexes in the lower extremities. Chronic use may also result in abnormalities of vitamin D metabolism, leading to osteomalacia. Low folate levels and megaloblastic anemia have been reported, but the clinical importance of this observation is unknown.

Idiosyncratic reactions to phenytoin are relatively rare. Most commonly, a typical skin rash heralds the hypersensitivity of the patient to the drug, which is then appropriately discontinued. Fever may also occur, and in rare cases the skin lesions may be severe and exfoliative. Lymphadenopathy may be difficult to distinguish from malignant lymphoma, and although some studies suggest a causal relationship between phenytoin and Hodgkin's disease, the data are far from conclusive. Hematologic complications are exceedingly rare, though agranulocytosis has been reported in combination with fever and rash.

MEPHENYTOIN, ETHOTOIN, & PHENACEMIDE

Many congeners of phenytoin have been synthesized, but only three are marketed in the USA, and these are used to a limited extent. Mephenytoin has a methyl group at the 3 position of the heterocyclic ring, and one of the phenyl groups at the 5 position is replaced by an ethyl group (Figure 24–1). Ethotoin has an ethyl group at the 3 position of the heterocyclic ring and only one phenyl group at the 5 position. The third analog, phenacemide, is similar to phenytoin except that only one phenyl ring is present at carbon 5 and the heterocyclic ring has been opened to form a straight-chain phenylacetylurea compound.

Mephenytoin and ethotoin, like phenytoin, appear to be most effective against generalized tonic-clonic seizures and partial seizures. No well-controlled clinical trials have documented their effectiveness. The incidence of severe reactions such as dermatitis, agranulocytosis, or hepatitis is higher for mephenytoin than for phenytoin.

Ethotoin may be recommended for patients hypersensitive to phenytoin, but larger doses are required. The adverse effects and toxicity are generally less severe than those associated with phenytoin, but the drug appears to be less effective.

Both ethotoin and mephenytoin share with phenytoin the property of saturable metabolism within the therapeutic dosage range. Careful monitoring of the patient during dosage alterations with either drug is essential. Mephenytoin is metabolized to 5,5-ethylphenylhydantoin via demethylation. This metabolite, **nirvanol,** contributes most of the antiepileptic activity of mephenytoin. Both mephenytoin and nirvanol are hydroxylated and undergo subsequent conjugation and excretion. Therapeutic levels for mephenytoin range from 5 to 16 μg/mL, and levels above 20 μg/mL are considered toxic.

Therapeutic blood levels of nirvanol are between 25 and 40 μg/mL. A therapeutic range for ethotoin has not been established.

Phenacemide, the straight-chain analog of phenytoin, is a toxic drug of last resort for refractory partial seizures. It is active against both maximal electroshock and pentylenetetrazol seizures. Its mechanism of action is unknown. It is well absorbed and completely metabolized. The relationship between blood levels and effect has not been established. Serious and sometimes fatal adverse effects have been reported in association with the use of phenacemide. Dose-related effects include behavioral changes, eg, psychosis and depressive reactions. Reactions of an idiosyncratic nature—hepatitis, nephritis, aplastic anemia, and others—appear to be more frequent than with other antiepileptic drugs.

CARBAMAZEPINE

Closely related to imipramine and other antidepressants, carbamazepine is a tricyclic compound effective in treatment of bipolar depression. It was initially marketed for the treatment of trigeminal neuralgia but has proved useful for epilepsy as well.

Chemistry

Although not obvious from a two-dimensional representation of its structure (Figure 24–4), carbamazepine has many similarities to phenytoin. The ureide moiety ($-N-CO-NH_2$) present in the heterocyclic ring of most antiepileptic drugs is also present in carbamazepine. Three-dimensional structural studies indicate that its spatial conformation is similar to that of phenytoin.

Mechanism of Action

The mechanism of action of carbamazepine appears to be similar to that of phenytoin. Like phenytoin, carbamazepine shows activity against maximal electroshock seizures. Studies on membrane permeability indicate that carbamazepine, like phenytoin, blocks sodium channels at therapeutic concentrations and inhibits high-frequency repetitive firing in neurons in culture (Figure 24–2). It also acts presynaptically to decrease synaptic transmission. These effects

Figure 24–4. Carbamazepine and oxcarbazepine and their metabolites. Carbamazepine is oxidized to an epoxy intermediate, which opens to form the dihydroxy derivative. Oxcarbazepine does not have an epoxide metabolite but is rapidly converted to 10-hydroxycarbazepine, which also eventually converts to the same dihydroxy derivative.

probably account for the anticonvulsant action of carbamazepine. Binding studies show that carbamazepine interacts with adenosine receptors, but the functional significance of this observation is not known. Carbamazepine also inhibits uptake and release of norepinephrine from brain synaptosomes but does not influence GABA uptake in brain slices. Recent evidence suggests that the postsynaptic action of GABA can be potentiated by carbamazepine.

Clinical Use

Carbamazepine is considered the drug of choice for partial seizures, and many physicians also use it first for generalized tonic-clonic seizures. It can be used with phenytoin in many patients who are difficult to control. Carbamazepine is not sedative in its usual therapeutic range. The drug is also very effective in some patients with trigeminal neuralgia, though older patients may tolerate higher doses poorly, with ataxia and unsteadiness.

Pharmacokinetics

The rate of absorption of carbamazepine varies widely among different patients, though almost complete absorption apparently occurs in all. Peak levels are usually achieved 6–8 hours after administration. Slowing absorption by giving the drug after meals helps the patient tolerate larger total daily doses. Distribution is slow, and the volume of distribution is roughly 1 L/kg. The drug is only 70% bound to plasma proteins; no displacement of other drugs from protein binding sites has been observed.

Carbamazepine has a very low systemic clearance of approximately 1 L/kg/d at the start of therapy. The drug has a notable ability to induce microsomal enzymes. In several studies of epileptic patients or volunteers on dosage regimens exceeding 1 month, the clearance of carbamazepine increased twofold over initial treatment. Typically, the half-life of 36 hours observed in subjects following an initial single dose decreases to much less than 20 hours in subjects receiving continuous therapy. Considerable dosage adjustments are thus to be expected during the first weeks of therapy. These changes in dose may further alter the microsomal enzyme capacity. Carbamazepine also alters the clearance of other drugs (see below).

Carbamazepine is completely metabolized in humans, in part to the 10,11-dihydro derivative, which is subsequently conjugated. The dihydro derivative is formed by way of a stable epoxide, carbamazepine-10,11-epoxide, which has been shown to have anticonvulsant activity (Figure 24–4). The contribution of this and other metabolites to the clinical activity of carbamazepine is unknown.

Therapeutic Levels & Dosage

Carbamazepine is considered the drug of choice in partial seizures. It is available only in oral form. The drug is effective in children, in whom a dosage of 15–25 mg/kg/d is appropriate. In adults, daily doses of 1 g or even 2 g are tolerated. Higher doses are achieved by giving multiple divided doses daily. In patients receiving three or four daily doses in whom the blood is drawn just before the morning dose (trough level), the therapeutic level is usually 4–8 μg/mL; although many patients complain of diplopia at drug levels above 7 μg/mL, others can tolerate levels above 10 μg/mL, especially with monotherapy. When blood samples are drawn randomly, levels are frequently above 8 μg/mL, but fluctuations related to absorption make long-term comparisons difficult.

Drug Interactions

Drug interactions involving carbamazepine are almost exclusively related to the drug's enzyme-inducing properties. As noted previously, the increased metabolic capacity of the hepatic enzymes may cause a reduction in steady state carbamazepine concentrations and an increased rate of metabolism of primidone, phenytoin, ethosuximide, valproic acid, and clonazepam. Other drugs such as propoxyphene, troleandomycin, and valproic acid may inhibit carbamazepine clearance and increase steady state carbamazepine blood levels. Other anticonvulsants, however, such as phenytoin and phenobarbital, may decrease steady state concentrations of carbamazepine through enzyme induction. No clinically significant protein-binding interactions have been reported.

Toxicity

The most common dose-related adverse effects of carbamazepine are diplopia and ataxia. The diplopia often occurs first and may last less than an hour during a particular time of day. Rearrangement of the divided daily dose can often remedy this complaint. Other dose-related complaints include mild gastrointestinal upsets, unsteadiness, and, at much higher doses, drowsiness. Hyponatremia and water intoxication have occasionally occurred and may be dose-related.

Considerable concern exists regarding the occurrence of idiosyncratic blood dyscrasias with carbamazepine, including fatal cases of aplastic anemia and agranulocytosis. Most of these have been in elderly patients with trigeminal neuralgia, and most have occurred within the first 4 months of treatment. The mild and persistent leukopenia seen in some patients is not necessarily an indication to stop treatment but requires careful monitoring. The most common idiosyncratic reaction is an erythematous skin rash; other responses such as hepatic dysfunction are unusual.

OXCARBAZEPINE

Oxcarbazepine is closely related to carbamazepine and useful in the same seizure types, but it may have an improved toxicity profile. Oxcarbazepine has a half-life of only 1–2 hours. The activity of the drug, therefore, resides almost exclusively in the 10-hydroxy metabolite (Figure 24–4), to which it is rapidly converted and which has a half-life similar to that of carbamazepine, ie, 8–12 hours. The drug is less potent than carbamazepine, both in animal models of epilepsy and in epileptic patients; clinical doses of oxcarbazepine may need to be 50% higher than those of carbamazepine to obtain equivalent seizure control. Some studies report fewer hypersensitivity reactions to oxcarbazepine, and cross-reactivity with carbamazepine does not always occur. Furthermore, the drug appears to induce hepatic enzymes to a lesser extent than carbamazepine, minimizing drug interactions. Those adverse effects—such as hyponatremia—that do occur with oxcarbazepine are similar in character to reactions reported with carbamazepine. The drug is marketed in some countries but not in the USA.

PHENOBARBITAL

Aside from the bromides, phenobarbital is the oldest of the currently available antiepileptic drugs. Although it has long been considered one of the safest of the antiepileptic agents, the use of other medications with lesser sedative effects has been urged. Many consider the barbiturates the drugs of choice for seizures only in infants.

Chemistry

The four derivatives of barbituric acid clinically useful as antiepileptic drugs are phenobarbital, mephobarbital, metharbital, and primidone. The first three are so similar that they will be considered together. Metharbital is methylated barbital, and mephobarbital is methylated phenobarbital; both are demethylated in vivo. The pKa's of these three weak acid compounds range from 7.3 to 7.9. Slight changes in the normal acid-base balance, therefore, can cause significant fluctuation in the ratio of the ionized to the un-ionized species. This is particularly important for phenobarbital, the most commonly used barbiturate, whose pKa is similar to the plasma pH of 7.4.

The three-dimensional conformations of phenobarbital and *N*-methylphenobarbital are similar to that of phenytoin. Both compounds possess a phenyl ring and are active against partial seizures.

Mechanism of Action

The exact mechanism of action of phenobarbital is unknown, but enhancement of inhibitory processes and diminution of excitatory transmission probably contribute importantly. Recent data indicate that phenobarbital may selectively suppress abnormal neurons, inhibiting the spread and suppressing firing from the foci. Like phenytoin, phenobarbital suppresses high-frequency repetitive firing in neurons in culture through an action on Na^+ conductance, but only at high concentrations. Also at high concentrations, barbiturates block some Ca^{2+} currents (L- and N-types). Phenobarbital binds to an allosteric regulatory site on the GABA-benzodiazepine receptor, and it enhances the GABA receptor-mediated current by prolonging the openings of the Cl^- channels. Phenobarbital also blocks excitatory responses induced by glutamate, principally those mediated by activation of the AMPA receptor (see Chapter 21). Both the enhancement of GABA-mediated inhibition and the reduction of glutamate-mediated excitation are seen with therapeutically relevant concentrations of phenobarbital.

Clinical Use

Phenobarbital is useful in the treatment of partial seizures and generalized tonic-clonic seizures, though the drug is often tried for virtually every seizure type, especially when attacks are difficult to control. There is little evidence for its effectiveness in generalized seizures such as absence, atonic attacks, or infantile spasms; it may worsen certain patients with these seizure types.

Some physicians prefer either metharbital or mephobarbital—especially the latter—to phenobarbital because of supposed decreased adverse effects. Only anecdotal data are available to support such comparisons.

Pharmacokinetics

See Chapter 22.

Therapeutic Levels & Dosage

The therapeutic levels of phenobarbital in most patients range from 10 to 40 μg/mL. Documentation of effectiveness is best in febrile seizures, and levels below 15 μg/mL appear ineffective for prevention of febrile seizure recurrence. The upper end of the therapeutic range is more difficult to define, as many patients appear to tolerate chronic levels above 40 μg/mL.

Drug Interactions & Toxicity

See Chapter 22.

PRIMIDONE

Primidone, or 2-desoxyphenobarbital (Figure 24–5), was first marketed in the early 1950s. It was later reported that primidone was metabolized to phenobarbital and phenylethylmalonamide (PEMA). All three compounds are active anticonvulsants.

Mechanism of Action

Although primidone is converted to phenobarbital, the mechanism of action of primidone itself may be more like that of phenytoin.

Clinical Use

Primidone, like its metabolites, is effective against partial seizures and generalized tonic-clonic seizures and may be more effective than phenobarbital. It was previously considered to be the drug of choice for complex partial seizures, but the latest studies of partial seizures in adults strongly suggest that carbamazepine and phenytoin are superior to primidone. Attempts to determine the relative potencies of the parent drug and its two metabolites have been carried out in newborn infants, in whom drug-metabolizing enzyme systems are very immature and in whom primidone is only slowly metabolized. Primidone has been shown to be effective in controlling seizures in this group and in older patients beginning treatment with primidone; the latter show seizure control before phenobarbital

Figure 24–5. Primidone and its active metabolites.

concentrations reach the therapeutic range. Finally, studies of maximal electroshock seizures in animals suggest that primidone has an anticonvulsant action independent of its conversion to phenobarbital and PEMA (the latter is relatively weak).

Pharmacokinetics

Primidone is absorbed completely, usually reaching peak concentrations about 3 hours after oral administration, though considerable variation has been reported. Primidone is generally confined to total body water, with a volume of distribution of 0.6 L/kg. It is not highly bound to plasma proteins; approximately 70% circulates as unbound drug.

Primidone is metabolized by oxidation to phenobarbital, which accumulates very slowly, and by scission of the heterocyclic ring to form PEMA (Figure 24–5). Both primidone and phenobarbital are also hydroxylated at the para position of the phenyl ring and undergo subsequent conjugation and excretion.

Primidone has a larger clearance than most other antiepileptic drugs (2 L/kg/d), corresponding to a half-life of 6–8 hours. PEMA clearance is approximately half that of primidone, but phenobarbital has a very low clearance. The appearance of phenobarbital corresponds to the disappearance of primidone. Phenobarbital therefore accumulates very slowly but eventually reaches therapeutic concentrations in most patients when therapeutic doses of primidone are administered. During chronic therapy, phenobarbital levels derived from primidone are usually two to three times higher than primidone levels. PEMA, which probably makes a minimal contribution to the efficacy of primidone, has a half-life of 8–12 hours and therefore reaches steady state more rapidly than phenobarbital.

Therapeutic Levels & Dosage

Primidone is most efficacious when plasma levels are in the range of 8–12 μg/mL. Concomitant levels of its metabolite, phenobarbital, at steady state will usually vary from 15 to 30 μg/mL. Dosages of 10–20 mg/kg/d are necessary to obtain these levels. It is very important, however, to start primidone at low doses and gradually increase over days to a few weeks to avoid prominent sedation and gastrointestinal complaints. When adjusting doses of the drug, it is important to remember that the parent drug will rapidly reach steady state (30–40 hours), but the active metabolites phenobarbital (20 days) and PEMA (3–4 days) will reach steady state much more slowly.

Toxicity

The dose-related adverse effects of primidone are similar to those of its metabolite, phenobarbital, except that drowsiness occurs early in treatment and may be prominent if the initial dose is too large; gradual increments are indicated when starting the drug in either children or adults.

VIGABATRIN

Current investigations that seek drugs to enhance the effects of GABA include efforts to find GABA agonists and prodrugs, GABA transaminase inhibitors, and GABA uptake inhibitors. Vigabatrin (γ-vinyl-GABA) is among the most promising of these new drugs and has been registered in Europe and South America; its discovery and successful development validates enhancement of the inhibitory effects of GABA as a rational approach to epilepsy treatment. The drug may become available in the USA in 1997.

$$CH_2=CH \diagdown_{CH} \diagup^{CH_2} \diagdown_{CH_2} \diagup^{COOH}$$
$$\underset{NH_2}{|}$$

Vigabatrin

Mechanism of Action

Vigabatrin is an irreversible inhibitor of GABA aminotransferase (GABA-T), the enzyme responsible for the degradation of GABA. It apparently acts by increasing the amount of GABA released at synaptic sites, thereby enhancing inhibitory effects. It is effective in a wide range of seizure models. Vigabatrin is marketed as a racemate; the $S(+)$ enantiomer is active and the $R(-)$ enantiomer appears to be inactive.

Clinical Use

Vigabatrin is indicated particularly for partial seizures and for West's syndrome. In adults, vigabatrin should be started at a dosage of 500 mg twice daily; a total of 1.5 g (or more) daily may be required for full effectiveness. Typical toxicities include drowsiness, dizziness, and weight gain. Less common but more troublesome adverse reactions are agitation, confusion, and psychosis; preexisting mental illness is a relative contraindication. The drug was delayed in its worldwide introduction by the appearance in rats and dogs of a reversible intramyelinic edema. Thousands of patients have now been exposed to vigabatrin; this edema (which may be dose-related) has not been observed in any patient to date.

Pharmacokinetics

Absorption of vigabatrin is rapid, and peak levels are attained in 1–3 hours. Bioavailability appears to be in excess of 60%, and volume of distribution is approximately 0.8 L/kg. The half-life is approximately 6–8 hours, but considerable evidence suggests that the pharmacodynamic activity of the drug is more prolonged and not well correlated with the plasma level. The drug has linear kinetics, no active metabolites, and binds minimally to plasma proteins; elimination is predominantly by the kidneys.

LAMOTRIGINE

Lamotrigine was developed when some investigators thought that the antifolate effects of certain antiepileptic drugs (eg, phenytoin) may contribute to their effectiveness. Several phenyltriazines were developed, and although their antifolate properties were weak, some were active in seizure screening tests, in which this drug resembles phenytoin.

Lamotrigine

Mechanism of Action

Lamotrigine's principal mechanism of action, like that of phenytoin, concerns sodium channels. The drug suppresses sustained rapid firing of neurons and produces a voltage- and use-dependent inactivation of sodium channels (Xie et al, 1995). This action probably explains lamotrigine's efficacy in focal epilepsy. It appears likely that lamotrigine has another as yet unrecognized mechanism of action to account for its efficacy in primary generalized seizures in childhood, including absence attacks.

Clinical Use

Although most controlled studies have evaluated lamotrigine as add-on therapy, a few suggest that the drug is effective as monotherapy for partial seizures. Data in children are sparse and not well controlled, but some authorities feel that the drug is also active against absence and myoclonic seizures in children. Adverse effects include dizziness, headache, diplopia, nausea, somnolence, and rash. The rash is considered a typical hypersensitivity reaction (and can rarely progress to a life-threatening condition), but the risk of rash may be diminished by introducing the drug slowly and at low doses. The drug is now widely marketed.

Pharmacokinetics & Dosage

Lamotrigine is almost completely absorbed and has a volume of distribution in the range of 1–1.4 L/kg. Protein binding is only about 55%. The drug has linear kinetics and is metabolized primarily by glucuronidation to the 2-*N*-glucuronide, which is excreted in the urine. Lamotrigine has a half-life of approximately 24 hours in normal volunteers; this decreases to 13–15 hours in patients taking enzyme-inducing drugs. Lamotrigine is effective against partial seizures in adults, with dosages typically between 100 and 300 mg/d and with a therapeutic blood level near 3 μg/mL. Valproate causes a twofold increase in the drug's half-life; in patients receiving valproate, the initial dosage of lamotrigine must be reduced to 25 mg every other day.

FELBAMATE

Felbamate has been approved and marketed in the USA and in some European countries. Although it is effective in some patients with partial seizures, the drug causes aplastic anemia and severe hepatitis at unexpectedly high rates and has been relegated to a third-line drug for refractory cases. Felbamate has a half-life of 20 hours (somewhat shorter when administered with either phenytoin or carbamazepine) and is metabolized by hydroxylation and conjugation; a significant percentage of the drug is excreted unchanged in the urine. When added to treatment with other antiepileptic drugs, felbamate increases plasma phenytoin and valproic acid levels but decreases levels of carbamazepine.

Felbamate

In spite of the seriousness of the adverse effects, approximately 10,000–15,000 patients in the USA remain on the medication. Usual dosages are 2000–4000 mg/d in adults, and effective plasma levels range from 30 to 100 μg/mL. In addition to its usefulness in partial seizures, felbamate has proved effective against the seizures that occur in Lennox-Gastaut syndrome.

GABAPENTIN

Gabapentin is an amino acid, an analog of GABA, that is effective against partial seizures. Originally planned as a spasmolytic, it was found to be more effective as an antiepileptic.

GABA   **Gabapentin**

Mechanism of Action

In spite of its close structural relationship to GABA, gabapentin appears not to act on GABA receptors. It may, however, alter GABA metabolism or its nonsynaptic release. Gabapentin's anticonvulsant effect in the electroshock model is delayed relative to its peak plasma concentration and appears to depend on its transport into neurons. Its mechanism of action is as yet poorly understood and appears to be different from that of any other antiepileptic drug.

Clinical Use & Dosage

Gabapentin is effective as an adjunct against partial seizures and generalized tonic-clonic seizures at dosages that range up to 2400 mg/d in controlled clinical trials. Open follow-on studies permitted dosages up to 4800 mg/d, but data are lacking on the effectiveness or tolerability of such doses. Monotherapy studies now under way are using dosages in the 1800–3600 mg/d range. Very high dosages have been needed by some clinicians to achieve improvement in seizure control. Effectiveness in other seizure types has not been demonstrated. The most common adverse effects are somnolence, dizziness, ataxia, headache, and tremor.

Pharmacokinetics

The pharmacology of gabapentin is unusual for antiepileptic drugs in that the drug is not metabolized and does not induce hepatic enzymes. Absorption is nonlinear and dose-dependent at very high doses, but otherwise the elimination kinetics are linear. The drug is not bound to plasma proteins. Drug-drug interactions are negligible. Elimination is via renal mechanisms; the drug is excreted unchanged. The half-life is short, ranging from 5 to 8 hours; the drug is typically administered two or three times per day.

TOPIRAMATE

Topiramate is a substituted monosaccharide which is structurally different from all other antiepileptic drugs.

Topiramate

Mechanism of Action

Topiramate blocks repetitive firing of cultured spinal cord neurons as do phenytoin and carbamazepine. Its mechanism of action, therefore, is likely to involve blocking of voltage-dependent sodium channels. Topiramate also appears to potentiate the inhibitory effect of GABA by acting at a site different from the benzodiazepine or barbiturate sites. Topiramate also depresses the excitatory action of kainate on AMPA receptors. It is possible that all three of these actions contribute to topiramate's anticonvulsant effect.

Clinical Use

Clinical trials of topiramate demonstrated a dose-response relationship, and monotherapy trials (using a pseudo placebo) showed the drug to be effective against partial and generalized tonic-clonic seizures. Dosages typically ranged from 200 to 600 mg/d, with a few patients tolerating dosages greater than 1000 mg/d. Most clinicians begin slowly (50 mg/d) and increase slowly to avoid adverse effects. Although no idiosyncratic reactions have been noted, dose-related side effects occur most frequently in the first 4 weeks and include somnolence, fatigue, dizziness, cognitive slowing, paresthesias, nervousness, and confusion. Urolithiasis has also been reported. In spite of this long list, the discontinuation rate is apparently only about 15%. The drug is teratogenic in animal models, but no human fetal deformities have been noted in the very few pregnancies that have occurred concurrent with topiramate administration.

Pharmacokinetics

Topiramate is rapidly absorbed (about 4 hours) and is 80% bioavailable. There is no food effect on absorption, minimal (15%) plasma protein binding, only moderate (20–50%) metabolism, and no active metabolites. The drug is excreted in the urine. The half-life is about 20–30 hours. Although increased levels are seen with renal failure and hepatic impairment, there is no age or gender effect, no autoinduction, no inhibition of metabolism, and kinetics are linear. Drug interactions do occur and can be complex, but the major effect is on topiramate levels rather than on the levels of other antiepileptic drugs. Birth control pills may be less effective in the presence of topiramate, and higher estrogen doses may be required.

TIAGABINE

Tiagabine is a derivative of nipecotic acid and was rationally designed as an inhibitor of GABA uptake. Although other compounds with this mechanism proved too toxic, tiagabine has been successfully developed. The drug increases GABA levels in the brains of animals. It appears to be effective against both partial and generalized tonic-clonic seizures in clinical trials, with an expected adult dosage of approximately 16–48 mg/d. The drug is given three or four times per day. Tiagabine is 100% bioavailable and highly protein-bound. The half-life is 5–8 hours, decreasing to 2–3 hours in the presence of certain other antiepileptic drugs. Food decreases the peak plasma concentration but not the AUC (see Chapter 3). Hepatic impairment causes a slight decrease in clearance, but the drug does not cause inhibition or induction of hepatic enzymes.

Tiagabine

Adverse effects include dizziness, asthenia, nervousness, tremor, depression, and emotional lability. Rash occurs as an idiosyncratic reaction. Psychosis may also occur. Tiagabine does not change the levels of either phenytoin or carbamazepine.

ZONISAMIDE

Zonisamide is a sulfonamide derivative that is marketed in Japan and is under study in other countries worldwide. The drug is effective against partial and generalized tonic-clonic seizures. It has good bioavailability, linear kinetics, low protein binding, renal excretion, and a half-life of 1–3 days. Adverse effects include drowsiness and cognitive impairment. Zonisamide does not interact with other antiepileptic drugs. The major unresolved controversy is the incidence of renal stones; if the incidence proves to be low, the drug will probably be marketed in other countries.

Zonisamide

DRUGS USED IN GENERALIZED SEIZURES

ETHOSUXIMIDE

Ethosuximide was introduced in 1960 as the third of three marketed succinimides in the USA. Ethosuximide has very little activity against maximal electroshock but considerable efficacy against pentylenetetrazol seizures and was introduced as a "pure petit mal" drug. Its popularity continues, based on its safety and efficacy; its role as the "first choice" anti-absence drug remains undiminished, in part because of the idiosyncratic hepatotoxicity of the alternative drug, valproic acid.

Chemistry

Ethosuximide is the last antiepileptic drug to be marketed whose origin is in the cyclic ureide structure. The three antiepileptic succinimides marketed in the USA are ethosuximide, phensuximide, and methsuximide. All three are substituted at the 2 position. (See structure below, and note difference in numbering relative to Figure 24–1.) Methsuximide and phensuximide have phenyl substituents, while ethosuximide is 2-ethyl-2-methylsuccinimide.

Ethosuximide

Mechanism of Action

The mechanism of action of the succinimides probably involves calcium channels. Ethosuximide also inhibits Na^+/K^+ ATPase, depresses the cerebral metabolic rate, and inhibits GABA aminotransferase. However, none of these actions are seen at therapeutic concentrations. Ethosuximide has an important effect on Ca^{2+} currents, reducing the low-threshold (T-type) current. This effect is seen at therapeutically relevant concentrations in thalamic neurons. The T-type calcium currents are thought to provide a pacemaker current in thalamic neurons responsible for generating the rhythmic cortical discharge of an absence attack. Inhibition of this current could therefore account for the specific therapeutic action of ethosuximide.

Clinical Use

Ethosuximide is particularly effective against absence seizures, as predicted from its activity in laboratory models. Documentation of its effectiveness required specific advances in quantitation of absence seizures; this was accomplished in the 1970s, when the characteristic generalized 3/s spike-wave electroencephalographic abnormality was correlated with a decrement in consciousness even when the abnormality occurs for only a few seconds. Long-term electroencephalographic recordings, therefore, provided the necessary quantitative method for determining the frequency of absence attacks and allowed rapid and effective evaluation of the efficacy of anti-absence drugs. Although ethosuximide was marketed in advance of the federal requirements for efficacy, these techniques were applied to later drugs such as clonazepam and valproic acid in documentation of their efficacy. This was accomplished by comparison with ethosuximide.

Pharmacokinetics

Absorption is complete following administration of the oral dosage forms. Peak levels are observed 3–7 hours after oral administration of the capsules. Animal studies indicate that chronic administration of the solution may prove irritating to the gastric mucosa. Ethosuximide is uniformly distributed throughout perfused tissues but does not penetrate fat. The volume of distribution approximates that of total body water, ie, 0.7 L/kg. It is not protein-bound, and spinal fluid concentrations are therefore equal to plasma concentrations.

Ethosuximide is completely metabolized, principally by hydroxylation. Four hydroxylated metabolites have been identified. These metabolites undergo subsequent conjugation and excretion. There is no evidence that they are pharmacologically active. Ethosuximide has a very low total body clearance (0.25 L/kg/d). This corresponds to a half-life of approximately 40 hours, though values from 18 to 72 hours have been reported.

Therapeutic Levels & Dosage

Therapeutic levels of 60–100 μg/mL can be achieved in adults with dosages of 750–1500 mg/d, though lower or higher dosages may be necessary. Some authors report that higher levels (up to 125 μg/mL) are needed in certain patients to achieve efficacy; such patients may tolerate the drug without apparent toxicity at these levels. Ethosuximide has a linear relationship between dose and steady state plasma levels. The drug might be administered as a single daily dose were it not for its adverse gastrointestinal effects; twice-a-day dosage is common. The time of day at which the level is measured is not particularly critical for ethosuximide, as its half-life is relatively long. No parenteral dosage form for ethosuximide is available.

Drug Interactions

Administration of ethosuximide with valproic acid results in a decrease in ethosuximide clearance and higher steady state concentrations due to inhibition of metabolism. No other important drug interactions have been reported for the succinimides.

Toxicity

The most common dose-related adverse effect of ethosuximide is gastric distress, including pain, nausea, and vomiting. This can often be avoided by starting therapy at a low dose, with gradual increases into the therapeutic range. When the adverse effect does occur, temporary dosage reductions may allow adaptation. Ethosuximide is a highly efficacious and safe drug for absence seizures; the appearance of relatively mild, dose-related adverse effects should not immediately call for its abandonment. Other dose-related adverse effects include transient lethargy or fatigue and, much less commonly, headache, dizziness, hiccup, and euphoria. Behavioral changes are usually in the direction of improvement.

Non-dose-related or idiosyncratic adverse effects of ethosuximide are extremely uncommon. Skin rashes have been reported, including at least one case of Stevens-Johnson syndrome. A few patients have had eosinophilia, thrombocytopenia, leukopenia, or pancytopenia; it is not entirely certain that ethosuximide was the causal agent. The development of systemic lupus erythematosus has also been reported, but other drugs may have been involved.

PHENSUXIMIDE & METHSUXIMIDE

Phensuximide and methsuximide are phenylsuccinimides that were developed and marketed before ethosuximide. They are used primarily as anti-absence drugs. Methsuximide is generally considered more toxic—and phensuximide less effective—than ethosuximide. Unlike ethosuximide, these two compounds have some activity against maximal electroshock seizures, and methsuximide has been used for partial seizures by some investigators. The desmethyl metabolite of methsuximide has a half-life of 25 hours or more and exerts the major antiepileptic effect. The toxicity and lack of effectiveness of phensuximide when compared with methsuximide has been investigated, and the failure of the desmethyl metabolite to accumulate in the former probably explains its relatively weak effect.

VALPROIC ACID & SODIUM VALPROATE

Sodium valproate, also used as the free acid, valproic acid, was found to have antiepileptic properties when it was used as a solvent in the search for other drugs effective against seizures. It was marketed in France in 1969 but was not licensed in the USA until 1978. Valproic acid is fully ionized at body pH, thus the active form of the drug may be assumed to be the valproate ion regardless of whether valproic acid or a salt of the acid is administered.

Chemistry

Valproic acid is one of a series of fatty or carboxylic acids that have antiepileptic activity; this activity appears to be greatest for carbon chain lengths of five to eight atoms. Branching and unsaturation do not significantly alter the drug's activity but may increase its lipophilicity, thereby increasing its duration of action. The amides and esters of valproic acid are also active antiepileptic agents.

$$CH_3-CH_2-CH_2 \atop CH_3-CH_2-CH_2 \diagdown CH-COOH$$

Valproic acid

Mechanism of Action

The time course of valproate's anticonvulsant activity appears to be poorly correlated with blood or tissue levels of the parent drug, an observation giving rise to considerable speculation regarding both the active species and the mechanism of action of valproic acid. Valproate is active against both pentylenetetrazol and maximal electroshock seizures. Like phenytoin and carbamazepine, valproate blocks sustained high-frequency repetitive firing of neurons in culture at therapeutically relevant concentrations. Its action against partial seizures is probably a consequence of this effect on Na^+ currents. Much attention, however, has been paid to the effects of valproate on GABA. Several studies have shown increased levels of GABA in the brain after administration of valproate, though the mechanism for this increase remains unclear. Doubt about the relevance of this increase in GABA to the therapeutic effect is raised by the fact that anticonvulsant effects are observed before GABA brain levels are elevated. An effect of valproate to facilitate glutamic acid decarboxylase (GAD, the enzyme responsible for GABA synthesis) has been described. At very high concentrations, valproate inhibits GABA-T in the brain, thus increasing levels of GABA by blocking conversion of GABA to succinic semialdehyde. However, at the relatively low doses of valproate needed to abolish pentylenetetrazol seizures, brain GABA levels may remain unchanged. Valproate produces a reduction in the aspartate content of rodent brain, but the relevance of this effect to its anticonvulsant action is not known.

At high concentrations, valproate has been shown to increase membrane potassium conductance. Furthermore, low concentrations of valproate tend to hyperpolarize membrane potentials. These findings have led to speculation that valproate may exert an action through a direct effect on the potassium channels of the membrane.

Valproate probably owes its broad spectrum of action to more than one molecular mechanism. Its action against absence attacks remains to be explained.

Clinical Use

Valproate is very effective against absence seizures. Although ethosuximide is the drug of choice when absence seizures occur alone, valproate is preferred if the patient has concomitant generalized tonic-clonic attacks. The reason for preferring ethosuximide for uncomplicated absence seizures is valproate's idiosyncratic hepatotoxicity, described below. Valproate is unique in its ability to control certain types of myoclonic seizures; in some cases the effect is very dramatic. The drug is effective in generalized tonic-clonic seizures, especially those which are primarily generalized. A few patients with atonic attacks may also respond, and some evidence suggests that the drug is effective in partial seizures.

Pharmacokinetics

Valproate is well absorbed following an oral dose, with bioavailability greater than 80%. Peak blood levels are observed within 2 hours. Food may delay absorption, and decreased toxicity may result if the drug is given after meals.

Valproic acid has a pKa of 4.7 and is therefore virtually completely ionized at physiologic plasma pH. The drug is also 90% bound to plasma proteins, though the fraction bound is somewhat reduced at blood levels greater than 150 µg/mL. Since it is both highly ionized and highly protein-bound, its distribution is essentially confined to extracellular water, with a volume of distribution of approximately 0.15 L/kg.

Clearance for valproate is very low; its half-life varies from 9 hours to 18 hours. At very high blood levels, the clearance of valproate is dose-dependent. There appear to be offsetting changes in the intrinsic clearance and protein binding at higher doses. Approximately 20% of the drug is excreted as a direct conjugate of valproate. The remainder is metabolized by beta and omega oxidation to a number of compounds; these are also subsequently conjugated and excreted.

The sodium salt of valproate is marketed in Europe as a tablet protected by aluminum foil, as it is quite hygroscopic. In Central and South America, the magnesium salt is available, which is considerably less hygroscopic. The free acid of valproate was first marketed in the USA in a capsule containing corn oil; the sodium salt is also available in syrup, primarily for pediatric use. An enteric-coated tablet of divalproex sodium is also marketed in the USA. This improved product, a 1:1 "coordination compound" of valproic acid and sodium valproate, is as bioavailable as the capsule but is absorbed much more slowly and is preferred by most patients. Peak concentrations following administration of the enteric-coated tablets are seen in 3–4 hours.

Therapeutic Levels & Dosage

Dosages of 25–30 mg/kg/d may be adequate in some patients, but others may require 60 mg/kg or even more. Therapeutic levels of valproate range from 50 to 100 µg/mL. In testing efficacy, this drug should not be abandoned until morning trough levels of at least 80 µg/mL have been attained; some patients may require and tolerate trough levels in excess of 100 µg/mL.

Drug Interactions

As noted above, the clearance of valproate is dose-dependent, caused by changes in both the intrinsic clearance and protein binding. Valproate inhibits its own metabolism at low doses, thus decreasing intrinsic clearance. At higher doses, there is an increased free fraction of valproate, resulting in lower total drug levels than expected. It may be clinically useful, therefore, to measure both total and free drug levels. Valproate also displaces phenytoin from plasma proteins. In addition to binding interactions, valproate inhibits the metabolism of several drugs, including phenobarbital, phenytoin, and carbamazepine, leading to higher steady state concentrations of these agents. The inhibition of phenobarbital metabolism may cause levels of the barbiturate to rise precipitously, causing stupor or coma.

Toxicity

The most common dose-related adverse effects of valproate are nausea, vomiting, and other gastrointestinal complaints such as abdominal pain and heartburn. The drug should be started gradually to avoid these symptoms; a temporary reduction in dose can usually alleviate the problems, and the patient will eventually tolerate higher doses. Sedation is uncommon with valproate alone but may be striking when valproate is added to phenobarbital. A fine tremor is frequently seen at higher levels. Other reversible adverse effects, seen in a small number of patients, include weight gain, increased appetite, and hair loss.

The idiosyncratic toxicity of valproate is largely limited to hepatotoxicity, but this may be severe; there seems little doubt that the hepatotoxicity of valproate has been responsible for more than 50 fatalities in the USA alone. The risk is greatest for patients under the age of 2 years and for those taking multiple medications. Initial AST values may not be elevated in susceptible patients, though these levels do eventually become abnormal. Most fatalities have occurred within 4 months after initiation of therapy. Careful monitoring of liver function is recommended when starting the drug; the hepatotoxicity is reversible in some cases if the drug is withdrawn. The other observed idiosyncratic response with valproate is thrombocytopenia, though documented cases of abnormal bleeding are lacking. It should be noted that valproate is an effective and popular antiepileptic drug and that only a very small number of patients have had severe toxic effects from its use.

Epidemiologic studies of valproate suggest an increased incidence of spina bifida in the offspring of women who took the drug during pregnancy. In addition, an increased incidence of cardiovascular, orofacial, and digital abnormalities has been reported. These observations, although based on a small number of cases, must be strongly considered in the choice of drugs during pregnancy.

OXAZOLIDINEDIONES

Trimethadione, the first oxazolidinedione, was introduced as an antiepileptic drug in 1945 and remained the drug of choice for absence seizures until the introduction of succinimides in the 1950s. The use of the oxazolidinediones (trimethadione, paramethadione, and dimethadione) is now very limited.

Chemistry

The oxazolidinediones contain an oxazolidine heterocyclic ring (Figure 24–1) and are similar in structure to other antiepileptic drugs introduced before 1960. The structure includes only short-chain alkyl substituents on the heterocyclic ring, with no attached phenyl group.

Trimethadione

Mechanism of Action

These compounds are active against pentylenetetrazol-induced seizures. Trimethadione raises the threshold for seizure discharges following repetitive thalamic stimulation. It—or more notably its active metabolite dimethadione—has the same effect on thalamic Ca^{2+} currents as ethosuximide (reducing the T-type calcium current). Thus, suppression of absence seizures is likely to depend on inhibiting the pacemaker action of thalamic neurons.

Pharmacokinetics

Trimethadione is rapidly absorbed, with peak levels reached within an hour after drug administration. It is distributed to all perfused tissues, with a volume of distribution that approximates that of total body water. It is not bound to plasma proteins. Trimethadione is completely metabolized in the liver by demethylation to 5,5-dimethyl-2,4-oxazolidinedione (dimethadione), which may exert the major antiepileptic activity. The drug has a relatively low clearance (1.6 L/kg/d), corresponding to a half-life of approximately 16 hours. The demethylated metabolite, however, is very slowly cleared and accumulates to a much greater extent than the parent drug. The clearance of dimethadione is 0.08 L/kg/d; this metabolite has an extremely long half-life (240 hours).

Therapeutic Levels & Dosage

The therapeutic plasma level range for trimethadione has never been established, though trimethadione blood levels above 20 μg/mL and dimethadione levels above 700 μg/mL have been suggested. A dosage of 30 mg/kg/d of trimethadione is necessary to achieve these levels in adults.

Drug Interactions

Relatively few drug interactions involving the oxazolidinediones have been reported, though trimethadione may competitively inhibit the demethylation of other drugs such as metharbital.

Toxicity

The most common and bothersome dose-related adverse effect of the oxazolidinediones is sedation. An unusual adverse effect is hemeralopia, a glare effect in which visual adaptation is impaired; it is reversible upon withdrawal of the drug. Accumulation of dimethadione has been reported to cause a very mild metabolic acidosis. Trimethadione has been associated with idiosyncratic dermatologic reactions, including rashes and exfoliative dermatitis, as well as toxic reactions involving the blood-forming organs; these have ranged from mild alterations in cell counts to fulminating pancytopenia. Other reactions include reversible nephrotic syndrome, which may involve an immune reaction to the drug, as well as a myasthenic syndrome. These drugs should not be used during pregnancy.

OTHER DRUGS USED IN MANAGEMENT OF EPILEPSY

Some drugs not classifiable by application to seizure type are discussed in this section.

BENZODIAZEPINES
(See also Chapter 22.)

Six benzodiazepines play prominent roles in the therapy of epilepsy. Although many benzodiazepines are quite similar chemically, subtle structural alterations result in differences in activity. They have two different mechanisms of antiepileptic action, which are shown to different degrees by the six compounds. This is evident from the fact that diazepam is relatively more potent against electroshock and clonazepam against pentylenetetrazol (the latter effect correlating with an action at the GABA-benzodiazepine allosteric receptor site). Possible mechanisms of action are discussed in Chapter 22.

Diazepam given intravenously or rectally is highly effective for stopping continuous seizure activity, especially generalized tonic-clonic status epilepticus (see below). The drug is occasionally given orally on a chronic basis, though it is not considered very effective in this application, probably because of the rapid development of tolerance.

Lorazepam is a benzodiazepine that, when given intravenously, appears in some studies to be more effective and longer-acting than diazepam in the treatment of status epilepticus.

Clonazepam is a long-acting drug with documented efficacy against absence seizures; it is one of the most potent antiepileptic agents known. It is also effective in some cases of myoclonic seizures and has been tried in infantile spasms. Sedation is prominent, especially on initiation of therapy; starting doses should be small. Maximal tolerated doses are usually in the range of 0.1–0.2 mg/kg, but many weeks of gradually increasing daily dosage may be needed to achieve these doses in some patients. Therapeutic blood levels are usually less than 0.1 μg/mL and are not routinely measured in most laboratories.

Clorazepate dipotassium is a benzodiazepine approved in the USA as an adjunct to treatment of complex partial seizures in adults. Drowsiness and lethargy are common adverse effects, but as long as the drug is increased gradually, dosages as high as 45 mg/d can be given.

Nitrazepam is not marketed in the USA but is used in many other countries, especially for infantile spasms and myoclonic seizures. It is less potent than clonazepam, and it is not clear that it has any clinical advantages over clonazepam.

Clobazam is not available in the USA but is marketed in most countries and is widely used in a variety of seizure types. It is a 1,5-benzodiazepine (unlike other marketed compounds, all of which are 1,4-benzodiazepines) and reportedly has less sedative potential than marketed benzodiazepines. Whether the drug has significant clinical advantages is not clear. It has a half-life of 18 hours and is effective at dosages of 0.5–1 mg/kg/d. It does interact with some other antiepileptic drugs and causes adverse effects typical of the benzodiazepines; efficacy, in some patients, is limited by the development of tolerance.

Pharmacokinetics

The pharmacokinetic properties of the benzodiazepines in part determine their clinical use. In general, the drugs are well absorbed, widely distributed, and extensively metabolized, with many active metabolites. The rate of distribution of benzodiazepines within the body is different from that of other antiepileptic drugs. Diazepam and lorazepam in particular are rapidly and extensively distributed to the tissues, with volumes of distribution between 1 and 3 L/kg. The onset of action is very rapid. Total body clearances of the parent drug and its metabolites are low, corresponding to half-lives of 20–40 hours.

Limitations

Two prominent aspects of benzodiazepines limit their usefulness. The first is their pronounced sedative effect, which is unfortunate both in the treatment of status epilepticus and in chronic therapy. Children may manifest a paradoxical hyperactivity, as with barbiturates. The second problem is tolerance, in which seizures may respond initially but recur within a few months. The remarkable antiepileptic potency of these compounds often cannot be realized because of these limiting factors.

ACETAZOLAMIDE

Acetazolamide is a diuretic whose main action is the inhibition of carbonic anhydrase (see Chapter 15). The accumulation of carbon dioxide in the brain may be the mechanism by which the drug exerts its antiepileptic activity; alternatively, the depolarizing action of bicarbonate ions moving out of neurons via GABA receptor ion channels will be diminished by carbonic anhydrase inhibition (Staley et al, 1995). Acetazolamide has been used for all types of seizures but is severely limited by the rapid development of tolerance, with return of seizures usually within a few weeks. The drug may have a special role in epileptic women who experience seizure exacerbations at the time of menses; seizure control may be improved and tolerance may not develop because the drug is not administered continuously. The usual dosage is approximately 10 mg/kg/d up to a maximum of 1000 mg/d.

Another carbonic anhydrase inhibitor, **sulthiame,** was not found to be effective in clinical trials in the USA. It is marketed in some other countries.

BROMIDE

Bromide was introduced by Locock in 1857 and was the first antiepileptic drug with any measurable efficacy. Though largely discarded in favor of phenobarbital after the turn of the century, bromide is still occasionally useful, such as in management of epilepsy in patients with porphyria, in whom other drugs may be contraindicated. Its half-life is approximately 12 days, and it is given in dosages of 3–6 g/d in adults to obtain plasma levels of 10–20 meq/L. The mechanism of action of bromide as an antiepileptic agent is unknown. Major toxic problems are unfortunately frequent and include skin rashes, sedation, and behavioral changes. It is not currently available in the USA.

II. CLINICAL PHARMACOLOGY OF ANTIEPILEPTIC DRUGS

SEIZURE CLASSIFICATION

The type of medication utilized for epilepsy is dependent upon the empirical nature of the seizure. For this reason, considerable effort has been made to classify seizures so that clinicians will be able to make a "seizure diagnosis" and thereby prescribe appropriate therapy. Errors in seizure diagnosis cause use of the wrong drugs, and an unpleasant cycle ensues in which poor seizure control is followed by increasing drug doses and medication toxicity. As noted above, seizures are divided into two groups: partial and generalized. Drugs used for partial seizures are more or less the same for the entire group, but drugs used for generalized seizures are determined by the individual seizure type. A shortened version of the international classification of epileptic seizures is presented in Table 24–1.

Partial Seizures

Partial seizures are those in which a localized onset of the attack can be ascertained, either by clinical observation or by electroencephalographic recording; the attack begins in a specific locus in the brain. There are three types of partial seizures, determined to some extent by the degree of brain involvement by the abnormal discharge.

The least complicated partial seizure is the **simple partial** seizure, characterized by minimal spread of the abnormal discharge such that normal consciousness and awareness are preserved. For example, the patient may have a sudden onset of clonic jerking of an extremity lasting 60–90 seconds; residual weakness may last for 15–30 minutes after the attack. The patient is completely aware of the attack and can describe it in detail. The EEG may show an abnormal discharge highly localized to the involved portion of the brain.

The **complex partial** seizure also has a localized onset, but the discharge becomes more widespread (usually bilateral) and almost always involves the limbic system. Most (not all) complex partial seizures arise from one of the temporal lobes, possibly because of the susceptibility of this area of the brain to insults such as hypoxia or infection. Clinically, the patient may have a brief warning followed by an alteration of consciousness during which some patients may stare and others may stagger or even fall. Most, however, demonstrate fragments of integrated motor behavior called automatisms for which the patient has no memory. Typical automatisms are lip smacking, swallowing, fumbling, scratching, or even walking about. After 30–120 seconds, the patient makes a gradual recovery to normal consciousness but may feel tired or ill for several hours after the attack.

The last type of partial seizure is the **secondarily generalized** attack, in which a partial seizure immediately precedes a generalized tonic-clonic (grand mal) seizure. This seizure type is described below.

Generalized Seizures

Generalized seizures are those in which there is no evidence of localized onset. The group is quite heterogeneous. **Generalized tonic-clonic (grand mal)** seizures are the most dramatic of all epileptic seizures and are characterized by tonic rigidity of all extremities, followed in 15–30 seconds by a tremor that is actually an interruption of the tonus by relaxation. As the relaxation phases become longer, the attack enters the clonic phase, with massive jerking of the body. The clonic jerking slows over 60–120 seconds, and the patient is usually left in a stuporous state. The tongue or cheek may be bitten, and urinary incontinence is common. Primary generalized tonic-clonic seizures begin without evidence of localized onset, whereas secondary generalized tonic-clonic seizures are preceded by another seizure type, usually a partial seizure. The medical treatment of both primary and secondary generalized tonic-clonic seizures is the same and utilizes drugs appropriate for *partial* seizures.

The **absence (petit mal)** seizure is characterized by both sudden onset and abrupt cessation. Its duration is usually less than 10 seconds and rarely more than 45 seconds. Consciousness is altered; the attack may also be associated with mild clonic jerking of the eyelids or extremities, with postural tone changes, autonomic phenomena, and automatisms. The occurrence of automatisms can complicate the clinical differentiation from complex partial seizures in some patients. Absence attacks begin in childhood or adolescence and may occur up to hundreds of times a day. The EEG during the seizure shows a highly characteristic 2.5–3.5 Hz spike-and-wave pattern. Atypical absence patients have seizures with postural changes that are more abrupt, and the patients are often mentally retarded; the EEG may show a slower spike-and-wave discharge, and the seizures may be more refractory to therapy.

Myoclonic jerking is seen, to a greater or lesser extent, in a wide variety of seizures, including generalized tonic-clonic seizures, partial seizures, absence seizures, and infantile spasms. Treatment of seizures that include myoclonic jerking should be directed at the primary seizure type rather than at the myoclonus. Some patients, however, have myoclonic jerking as the major seizure type, and some have frequent myoclonic jerking and occasional generalized tonic-clonic seizures without overt signs of neurologic deficit. Many kinds of myoclonus exist, and much effort has gone into attempts to classify this entity.

Atonic seizures are those in which the patient has sudden loss of postural tone. If standing, the patient falls suddenly to the floor and may be injured. If seated, the head and torso may suddenly drop forward. Although most often seen in children, this seizure type is not unusual in adults. Many patients with atonic seizures wear helmets to prevent head injury.

Infantile spasms are an epileptic syndrome and not a seizure type. The attacks, though sometimes fragmentary, are most often bilateral and are included for pragmatic purposes with the generalized seizures. These attacks are most often characterized clinically by brief, recurrent myoclonic jerks of the body with sudden flexion or extension of the body and limbs; the forms of infantile spasms are, however, quite heterogeneous. Ninety percent of affected patients have their first attack before the age of 1 year. Most patients are mentally retarded, presumably from the same cause as the spasms. The cause is unknown in many patients, but such widely disparate disorders as infection, kernicterus, tuberous sclerosis, and hypoglycemia have been implicated. In some cases, the EEG is characteristic. Drugs used to treat infantile spasms are effective only in some patients; there is little evidence that the mental retardation is alleviated by therapy, even when the attacks disappear.

THERAPEUTIC STRATEGY

For most antiepileptic drugs, relationships between blood levels and therapeutic effects have been characterized to a particularly high degree. The same is true for the pharmacokinetics of these drugs. These relationships provide significant advantages in the development of therapeutic strategies for the treatment of epilepsy. The therapeutic index for most antiepileptic drugs is low, and toxicity is not uncommon. Thus, effective treatment of seizures requires an awareness of the therapeutic levels and pharmacokinetic properties as well as the characteristic toxicities of each agent. Measurements of antiepileptic drug plasma levels are extremely useful when combined with clinical observations and pharmacokinetic data (Table 24–2).

MANAGEMENT OF EPILEPSY

PARTIAL SEIZURES & GENERALIZED TONIC-CLONIC SEIZURES

Until recently, the choice of drugs was usually limited to phenytoin, carbamazepine, or barbiturates. There has been a strong tendency in the past few years to limit the use of sedative antiepileptic drugs such as barbiturates and benzodiazepines to patients who cannot tolerate other medications. In the 1980s, the trend was to increase the use of carbamazepine. Although the choice in the 1990s still appears to be divided between carbamazepine and phenytoin, all of the newer drugs have shown effectiveness against these seizures. The exact role of these drugs remains to be determined, making decisions for the individual patient more complex.

GENERALIZED SEIZURES

The drugs used for generalized tonic-clonic seizures are the same as for partial seizures; in addition, valproate is clearly useful.

Three drugs are effective against absence seizures. Two are nonsedating and therefore preferred: etho-

Table 24–2. Effective plasma levels of six antiepileptic drugs.[1]

Drug	Effective Level (μg/mL)	High Effective Level[2] (μg/mL)	Toxic Level (μg/mL)
Carbamazepine	4–12	7	> 8
Primidone	5–15	10	< 12
Phenytoin	10–20	18	> 20
Phenobarbital	10–40	35	> 40
Ethosuximide	50–100	80	> 100
Valproate	50–100	80	> 100

[1]Reprinted, with permission, from Porter RJ: *Epilepsy: 100 Elementary Principles,* 2nd ed. Saunders, 1989.
[2]Level that should be achieved, if possible, in patients with refractory seizures, assuming that the blood samples are drawn before administration of the morning medication. Higher levels are often possible—without toxicity—when the drugs are used alone, ie, as monotherapy.

suximide and valproate. Clonazepam is also highly effective but has disadvantages of dose-related adverse effects and development of tolerance. The drug of choice is ethosuximide, though valproate is effective in some ethosuximide-resistant patients. Lamotrigine may also be useful.

Specific myoclonic syndromes are usually treated with valproate. It is nonsedating and can be dramatically effective. Other patients respond to clonazepam or other benzodiazepines, though high doses may be necessary, with accompanying sedation and drowsiness. A highly specific myoclonic syndrome, "intention myoclonus," which occurs after severe hypoxia, is characterized by myoclonus associated with volitional activity. Improvement in some patients with this unusual disorder has been reported using 5-hydroxytryptophan.

Atonic seizures are often refractory to all available medications, though some reports suggest that valproate may be beneficial, as may lamotrigine. Benzodiazepines have been reported to improve seizure control in some of these patients but may worsen the attacks in others. Felbamate has been demonstrated to be effective in some patients, though the drug's idiosyncratic toxicity limits its use. If the loss of tone appears to be part of another seizure type (such as absence or complex partial seizures), every effort should be made to treat the other seizure type vigorously, hoping for simultaneous alleviation of the atonic component of the seizure.

DRUGS USED IN INFANTILE SPASMS

The treatment of infantile spasms is unfortunately limited to improvement of control of the seizures rather than other features of the disorder, such as re-

tardation. Most patients receive a course of intramuscular corticotropin, though some clinicians note that prednisone may be equally effective and can be given orally. Clinical trials have been unable to settle the matter. In either case, therapy must often be discontinued because of adverse effects. If seizures recur, repeat courses of corticotropin or corticosteroids can be given, or other drugs may be tried. Other drugs widely used are the benzodiazepines such as clonazepam or nitrazepam; their efficacy in this heterogeneous syndrome may be nearly as good as corticosteroids. Vigabatrin may also be effective. The mechanism of action of corticosteroids or corticotropin in the treatment of infantile spasms is unknown.

In spite of more than 30 years experience with corticosteroids and corticotropin for infantile spasms, the optimal dosage and duration of therapy have not been established. Currently, a broad range of dosages are utilized, although most patients are treated with 25–40 units of corticotropin daily. A very few investigators recommend up to 240 units daily. In the 60% of patients who respond, seizure reduction is usually reported within 1–5 weeks. Corticotropin therapy may be continued for 3 months or more unless toxicity requires cessation. For corticosteroids, doses of 2 mg/kg of prednisolone or 0.3 mg/kg of dexamethasone have been utilized. Many clinicians feel that therapy should be initiated early in the course of the illness to enhance the prospect of seizure control.

The toxic effects of corticotropin are characteristic of corticosteroid excess and include hypertension, cushingoid obesity, gastrointestinal disturbances, skin changes, osteoporosis, and electrolyte imbalance.

STATUS EPILEPTICUS

There are many forms of status epilepticus. The most common, generalized tonic-clonic status epilepticus, is a life-threatening emergency, requiring immediate cardiovascular, respiratory, and metabolic management as well as pharmacologic therapy. The latter virtually always requires intravenous administration of antiepileptic medications. Diazepam is the most effective drug in most patients for stopping the attacks and is given directly by intravenous push to a maximum total dose of 20–30 mg in adults. Intravenous diazepam may depress respiration (less frequently cardiovascular function), and facilities for resuscitation must be immediately at hand during its administration. The effect of diazepam is not lasting, but the 30- to 40-minute seizure-free interval allows more definitive therapy to be initiated. For patients who are not actually in the throes of a seizure, diazepam therapy can be omitted and the patient treated at once with a long-acting drug such as phenytoin. Some physicians prefer lorazepam, which is equivalent to diazepam in effect and perhaps somewhat longer-acting.

The mainstay of continuing therapy for status epilepticus has been intravenous phenytoin, which is effective and nonsedating. It should be given as a loading dose of 13–18 mg/kg in adults; the usual error is to give too little. Administration should be at a maximum rate of 50 mg/min. It is safest to give the drug directly by intravenous push, but it can also be diluted in saline; it precipitates rapidly in the presence of glucose. Careful monitoring of cardiac rhythm and blood pressure is necessary, especially in elderly people. At least part of the cardiotoxicity is from the propylene glycol in which the phenytoin is dissolved. With the recent introduction of fosphenytoin, which is freely soluble in intravenous solutions without the need for propylene glycol or other solubilizing agents, these hazards may be lessened. Because of its greater molecular weight, this prodrug is two-thirds to three-quarters as potent as phenytoin on a milligram basis.

In previously treated epileptic patients, the administration of a large loading dose of phenytoin may cause some dose-related toxicity such as ataxia. This is usually a relatively minor problem during the acute status episode and is easily alleviated by later adjustment of plasma levels.

For patients who do not respond to phenytoin, phenobarbital can be given in large doses: 100–200 mg intravenously to a total of 400–800 mg. Respiratory depression is a common complication, especially if benzodiazepines have already been given, and there should be no hesitation in instituting intubation and ventilation.

Although other drugs such as lidocaine have been recommended for the treatment of generalized tonic-clonic status epilepticus, general anesthesia is usually necessary in highly resistant cases.

SPECIAL ASPECTS OF THE TOXICOLOGY OF ANTIEPILEPTIC DRUGS

TERATOGENICITY

The potential teratogenicity of antiepileptic drugs is a controversial and important area. It is important because teratogenicity resulting from chronic drug treatment of millions of people throughout the world may have a profound effect even if the effect occurs in only a small percentage of cases. It is controversial because both epilepsy and antiepileptic drugs are heterogeneous, and few epileptic patients are available for study who are not receiving these drugs. Furthermore, patients with severe epilepsy, in whom genetic factors rather than drug factors may be of greater importance in the occurrence of fetal malformations, are often receiving multiple antiepileptic drugs in high doses.

In spite of these limitations, it appears—from whatever cause—that children born to mothers taking antiepileptic drugs have an increased risk, perhaps twofold, of congenital malformations. One drug, phenytoin, has been implicated in a specific syndrome called **fetal hydantoin syndrome,** though not all investigators are convinced of its existence and a similar syndrome has been attributed both to phenobarbital and to carbamazepine. Valproate, as noted above, has also been implicated in a specific malformation, spina bifida. It is estimated that a pregnant woman taking valproic acid or sodium valproate has a 1–2% risk of having a child with spina bifida (Valproate, 1983). Topiramate, one of the newer antiepileptic drugs, has shown some teratogenicity in animal testing.

In dealing with the clinical problem of a pregnant woman with epilepsy, most epileptologists agree that while it is important to minimize exposure to antiepileptic drugs, both in numbers and dosages, it is also important not to allow maternal seizures to go unchecked.

WITHDRAWAL

Withdrawal of antiepileptic drugs, whether by accident or by design, can cause increased seizure frequency and severity. There are two factors to consider: the effects of the withdrawal itself and the need for continued drug suppression of seizures in the individual patient. In many patients, both factors must be considered. It is important to note, however, that the abrupt discontinuance of antiepileptic drugs ordinarily does not cause seizures in nonepileptic patients provided that the drug levels are not above the usual therapeutic range when the drug is stopped.

Some drugs are more easily withdrawn than others. In general, withdrawal of anti-absence drugs is easier than withdrawal of drugs needed for partial or generalized tonic-clonic seizures. Barbiturates and benzodiazepines are the most difficult to discontinue; weeks or months may be required, with very gradual dosage decrements, to accomplish their complete removal, especially if the patient is not hospitalized.

Because of the heterogeneity of epilepsy, consideration of the complete removal of antiepileptic drugs is an especially difficult problem. If a patient is seizure-free for 3 or 4 years, gradual discontinuance is usually warranted.

OVERDOSE

Antiepileptic drugs are real or potential central nervous system depressants but are rarely lethal. Very high blood levels are usually necessary before overdoses can be considered life-threatening. The most dangerous effect of antiepileptic drugs after large overdoses is respiratory depression, which may be potentiated by other agents, such as alcohol. Treatment of antiepileptic drug overdose is supportive; stimulants should not be used. Efforts to hasten removal of antiepileptic drugs, such as urine alkalinization, are usually ineffective.

PREPARATIONS AVAILABLE

Carbamazepine (generic, Tegretol)
Oral: 200 mg tablets; 100 mg chewable tablets; 100 mg/5 mL suspension
Clonazepam (Klonopin)
Oral: 0.5, 1, 2 mg tablets
Clorazepate dipotassium (generic, Tranxene)
Oral: 3.75, 7.5, 15 mg tablets, capsules
Oral sustained-release (Tranxene-SD): 11.25, 22.5 mg tablets
Diazepam (generic, Valium, others)
Oral: 2, 5, 10 mg tablets; 5 mg/5 mL, 5 mg/mL solutions
Oral sustained-release: 15 mg capsules
Parenteral: 5 mg/mL for injection
Rectal: Diazepam viscous rectal solution
Ethosuximide (Zarontin)
Oral: 250 mg capsules; 250 mg/5 mL syrup
Ethotoin (Peganone)
Oral: 250, 500 mg tablets
Fosphenytoin (Cerebyx)
Parenteral: 150 mg/2 mL, 750 mg/10 mL for injection
Gabapentin (Neurontin)
Oral: 100, 300, 400 mg capsules
Lorazepam (generic, Ativan)
Oral: 0.5, 1, 2 mg tablets
Parenteral: 2, 4 mg/mL for injection
Mephenytoin (Mesantoin)
Oral: 100 mg tablets
Mephobarbital (Mebaral)
Oral: 32, 50, 100 mg tablets
Metharbital (Gemonil)
Oral: 100 mg tablets

Methsuximide (Celontin Kapseals)
Oral: 150, 300 mg capsules
Paramethadione (Paradione)
Oral: 150, 300 mg tablets
Pentobarbital sodium (generic, Nembutal)
Parenteral: 50 mg/mL for injection
Phenacemide (Phenurone)
Oral: 500 mg tablets
Phenobarbital (generic, Luminal Sodium, others)
Oral: 8, 16, 32, 65, 100 mg tablets; 16 mg capsules; 15, 20 mg/5 mL elixirs
Parenteral: 30, 60, 65, 130 mg/mL for injection
Phensuximide (Milontin Kapseals)
Oral: 500 mg capsules
Phenytoin (generic, Dilantin, others)
Oral: 30, 100 mg capsules; 50 mg chewable tablets; 30, 125 mg/5 mL suspension
Oral extended-action: 30, 100 mg capsules
Parenteral: 50 mg/mL for IV injection
Primidone (generic, Mysoline)
Oral: 50, 250 mg tablets; 250 mg/5 mL suspension
Topiramate (Topamax)
Oral: 25, 100, 200 mg tablets
Trimethadione (Tridione)
Oral: 150 mg chewable tablets; 300 mg capsules; 40 mg/mL solution
Valproic acid (generic, Depakene, Myproic Acid)
Oral: 250 mg capsules; 250 mg/5 mL syrup (sodium valproate)
Oral sustained-release (Depakote): 125, 250, 500 mg tablets (as divalproex sodium)

REFERENCES

Ben-Menachem E: Vigabatrin. Epilepsia 1995;36(Suppl 2):S95.

Bialer M: Comparative pharmacokinetics of the newer antiepileptic drugs. Clin Pharmacokinet 1993;24:441.

Brodie MJ: Drug interactions in epilepsy. Epilepsia 1992;33(Suppl):S13.

Brodie MJ, Porter RJ: New and potential anticonvulsants. Lancet 1990;336:425.

Callaghan N, Garrett A, Goggin T: Withdrawal of anticonvulsant drugs in patients free of seizures for two years. N Engl J Med 1988;318:942.

Dalessio DJ: Current concepts: Seizure disorders and pregnancy. N Engl J Med 1985;312:559.

Dreifuss FE, Langer DH: Hepatic considerations in the use of antiepileptic drugs. Epilepsia 1987;28(Suppl 2):S23.

Emerson R, et al: Stopping medication in children with epilepsy: Predictors of outcome. N Engl J Med 1981; 304:1125.

Jones KL, et al: Pattern of malformations in the children of women treated with carbamazepine during pregnancy. N Engl J Med 1989;320:1661.

Loscher W: Effects of the antiepileptic drug valproate on metabolism and function of inhibitory and excitatory amino acids in the brain. Neurochem Res 1993;18:485.

Macdonald RL, Meldrum BS: Principles of antiepileptic drug action. In: *Antiepileptic Drugs,* 4th ed. Levy RH, et al (editors). Raven Press, 1995.

Mattson RH, et al: Comparison of carbamazepine, phenobarbital, phenytoin, and primidone in partial and secondarily generalized tonic-clonic seizures. N Engl J Med 1985;313:145.

Mattson RH et al: A comparison of valproate with carbamazepine for the treatment of complex partial seizures and secondarily generalized tonic-clonic seizures in adults. N Engl J Med 1992;327:765.

McLean MJ: Gabapentin. Epilepsia 1995(Suppl 2);36:S73.

Meldrum BS: Neurotransmission in epilepsy. Epilepsia 1995;36:S30.

Meldrum BS, Porter RJ (editors): *New Anticonvulsant Drugs.* John Libbey, 1986.

Messenheimer JA: Lamotrigine. Epilepsia 1995;36(Suppl 2):S87.

Porter RJ: Recognizing and classifying epileptic seizures and epileptic syndromes. In: *Neurologic Clinics: Epilepsy.* Porter RJ, Theodore WH (editors). Saunders, 1986.

Porter RJ: New antiepileptic agents: Strategies for drug development. Lancet 1990;336:423.

Ramsay RE: Treatment of status epilepticus. Epilepsia 1993;34(Suppl 1):S71.

Rogawski MA: The NMDA receptor, NMDA antagonists and epilepsy therapy: A status report. Drugs 1992; 44:279.

Rogawski MA, Porter RJ: Antiepileptic drugs: Pharmacological mechanisms and clinical efficacy with consideration of promising developmental stage compounds. Pharmacol Rev 1990;42:223.

Shank RP et al: Topiramate: Preclinical evaluation of a structurally novel anticonvulsant. Epilepsia 1994;35:450.

Staley KJ et al: Ionic mechanisms of neuronal excitation by inhibitory GABA-A receptors. Science 1995;269:977.

Suzdak PD, Jansen JA: A review of the preclinical pharmacology of tiagabine: a potent and selective anticonvulsant GABA uptake inhibitor. Epilepsia 1995;35:612.

Theodore WH, Porter RJ: *Epilepsy: 100 Elementary Principles,* 3rd ed. Saunders, 1995.

Theodore WH, Porter RJ, Raubertas RF: Seizures during barbiturate withdrawal: Relation to blood level. Ann Neurol 1987;22:644.

Theodore WH et al: Barbiturates reduce human cerebral glucose metabolism. Neurology 1986;36:60.

Thomson AH, Brodie MJ: Pharmacokinetic optimisation of anticonvulsant therapy. Clin Pharmacokinet 1992; 23:216.

Treiman DM: The role of benzodiazepines in the management of status epilepticus. Neurology 1990;40(Suppl 2):32.

Valproate: A new cause of birth defects: Report from Italy and follow-up from France. MMWR Morb Mortal Wkly Rep 1983;32:438.

Yerby MS: Risks of pregnancy in women with epilepsy. Epilepsia 1992;33(Suppl 1):S23.

Xie X et al: Interaction of the antiepileptic drug lamotrigine with recombinant rat brain IIA Na^+ channels and with native Na^+ channels in rat hippocampal neurones. Pflugers Arch 1995;430:437.

General Anesthetics

25

Anthony J. Trevor, PhD, & Ronald D. Miller, MD

Attempts to suppress the pain of surgical procedures by the use of drugs date from ancient times and have included the oral administration of ethanol and opiates. The first scientific demonstration of drug-induced anesthesia during surgery was in 1846, when William Morton used diethyl ether in Boston. Within a year, chloroform was introduced by James Simpson in Scotland. This was followed 20 years later by the successful demonstration of the anesthetic properties of nitrous oxide, which had been first suggested by Davy in the 1790s. Modern anesthesia dates from the 1930s, when the intravenous barbiturate thiopental was introduced. A decade later, curare was used in anesthesia to achieve skeletal muscle relaxation. The first modern halogenated hydrocarbon, halothane, was introduced as an inhaled anesthetic in 1956 and soon became the standard for comparison for newer inhaled anesthetic drugs.

The state of "general anesthesia" usually includes analgesia, amnesia, loss of consciousness, inhibition of sensory and autonomic reflexes, and, in many cases, skeletal muscle relaxation. The extent to which any individual anesthetic drug can exert these effects varies with the drug, the dosage, and the clinical circumstances.

An ideal anesthetic drug would induce anesthesia smoothly and rapidly and permit rapid recovery as soon as administration ceased. The drug would also possess a wide margin of safety and be devoid of adverse effects. No single anesthetic agent is capable of achieving all of these desirable effects without some disadvantages when used alone. The modern practice of anesthesia most commonly involves the use of combinations of drugs, taking advantage of their individual favorable properties while attempting to minimize their potential for harmful actions.

Anesthesia protocols vary depending on the proposed type of diagnostic, therapeutic, or surgical intervention. For minor procedures, oral sedatives used in conjunction with regional local anesthesia (Chapter 26) may suffice. Conscious sedation protocols involving intravenous benzodiazepines and opioid analgesics can provide profound analgesia, but with retention of the patient's ability to maintain a patent airway and to respond to verbal commands. For major surgical procedures, anesthesia frequently includes the use of preoperative sedatives, the induction of anesthesia with thiopental or other rapidly acting intravenous drug, and the provision of deep anesthesia with inhaled anesthetics alone or in combination with intravenous drugs. In many cases, such protocols include the use of neuromuscular blocking drugs (Chapter 27).

TYPES OF GENERAL ANESTHETICS

General anesthetics are usually given by inhalation or by intravenous injection.

Inhaled anesthetics

The chemical structures of some inhaled anesthetics are shown in Figure 25–1. Nitrous oxide, a gas at ambient temperature and pressure, continues to be an important component of many anesthesia regimens. Halothane, enflurane, isoflurane, desflurane, sevoflurane, and methoxyflurane are volatile liquids. The older inhaled anesthetics such as ether, cyclopropane, and chloroform are no longer used in developed countries for reasons that include potential flammability (ether, cyclopropane) and organ toxicity (chloroform).

Intravenous Anesthetics

Several drugs are used intravenously, alone or with other drugs, to achieve anesthesia, as components of balanced anesthesia, or to sedate patients in intensive care units who must be mechanically ventilated for prolonged periods. They include the following: (1) barbiturates (thiopental, methohexital); (2) benzodiazepines (midazolam, diazepam); (3) opioid analgesics (morphine, fentanyl, sufentanil, alfentanil,

Figure 25–1. Inhaled anesthetics.

remifentanil); (4) propofol; (5) ketamine, an arylcy-clohexylamine that produces a state called dissociative anesthesia; and (6) miscellaneous drugs (droperidol, etomidate, dexmedetomidine). Figure 25–2 shows the structures of commonly used intravenous anesthetics.

SIGNS & STAGES OF ANESTHESIA

Since the introduction of general anesthetics, attempts have been made to correlate their observable effects or signs with the depth of anesthesia. A traditional description of the signs and stages of anesthesia (Guedel's signs) derives mainly from observations of the effects of diethyl ether, which has a slow onset of central action owing to its high solubility in blood. The intermediate stages and signs are rarely observed with the more rapidly acting modern inhaled anesthetics and intravenous agents. Furthermore, most anesthetic protocols for major procedures now consist of a combination of inhaled and intravenous agents. Nevertheless, the signs of diethyl ether anesthesia still provide the basis for assessing anesthetic effect for all general anesthetics. Many of these signs refer to the effects of anesthetics on respiration, reflex activity,

and muscle tone. Traditionally, anesthetic effects are divided into four stages of increasing depth of central nervous system depression.

I. Stage of Analgesia: The patient initially experiences analgesia without amnesia. Later in stage I, both analgesia and amnesia ensue.

II. Stage of Excitement: During this stage, the patient often appears to be delirious and excited but definitely is amnesic. Respiration is irregular both in volume and rate, and retching and vomiting can occur. The patient may struggle and is sometimes incontinent. For these reasons, efforts are made to limit the duration and severity of this stage, which ends with the reestablishment of regular breathing.

III. Stage of Surgical Anesthesia: This stage begins with the recurrence of regular respiration and extends to complete cessation of spontaneous respiration. Four planes of stage III have been described in terms of changes in ocular movements, eye reflexes, and pupil size, which under specified conditions may represent signs of increasing depth of anesthesia.

IV. Stage of Medullary Depression: When spontaneous respiration ceases, stage IV is present. This stage of anesthesia includes severe depression of the vasomotor center in the medulla as well as the res-

Figure 25–2. Intravenous anesthetics.

piratory center. Without full circulatory and respiratory support, death rapidly ensues.

In modern anesthesia practice, the distinctive signs of each of the four stages described above are usually obscured. Reasons for this include the relatively rapid onset of action of many inhaled anesthetics compared to that of diethyl ether and the fact that respiratory activity is often controlled with the aid of a mechanical ventilator. In addition, the presence of other pharmacologic agents given preoperatively or intraoperatively can also influence the signs of anesthesia.

Atropine, used to decrease secretions, also dilates pupils; drugs such as tubocurarine and succinylcholine affect muscle tone; and the opioid analgesics exert depressant effects on respiration. The most reliable indications that stage III (surgical anesthesia) has been achieved are loss of the eyelash reflex and establishment of a respiratory pattern that is regular in rate and depth. The adequacy of ensuing depth of anesthesia for the specific surgical requirements is assessed mainly by changes in respiratory and cardiovascular responses to stimulation.

INHALED ANESTHETICS

PHARMACOKINETICS

Depth of anesthesia is determined by the concentrations of anesthetics in the central nervous system. The rate at which an effective brain concentration is reached (the rate of induction of anesthesia) depends on multiple pharmacokinetic factors that influence the uptake and distribution of the anesthetic. These factors determine the different rates of transfer of the inhaled anesthetic from the lung to the blood and from the blood to the brain and other tissues. These factors also influence the rate of recovery from anesthesia when inhalation of the anesthetic is terminated.

Uptake & Distribution

The concentration of an individual gas in a mixture of gases is proportionate to its **partial pressure** or **tension.** These terms are often used interchangeably in discussing the various transfer processes of anesthetic gases in the body. Achievement of a brain concentration of an anesthetic adequate to cause anesthesia requires transfer of that anesthetic from the alveolar air to blood and then to brain. The rate at which a given concentration of anesthetic in the brain is reached depends on the solubility properties of the anesthetic, its concentration in the inspired air, pulmonary ventilation rate, pulmonary blood flow, and the concentration (partial pressure) gradient of the anesthetic between arterial and mixed venous blood.

A. Solubility: One of the most important factors influencing the transfer of an anesthetic from the lungs to the arterial blood is its solubility. The blood:gas partition coefficient is a useful index of solubility and defines the relative affinity of an anesthetic for the blood compared to air. The partition coefficients for desflurane and nitrous oxide, which are not very soluble in the blood, are low, less than 0.5. At the other extreme, the value may be greater than 10 for agents such as methoxyflurane, an agent that is very soluble in blood (Table 25–1). When an anesthetic with low blood solubility diffuses from the lung into the arterial blood, relatively few molecules are required to raise its partial pressure, and the arterial tension rises quickly (Figure 25–3, top, nitrous oxide). Conversely, for anesthetics with moderate to high solubility, more molecules dissolve before partial pressure changes significantly, and arterial tension of the gas increases less rapidly (Figure 25–3, bottom, halothane). This inverse relationship between the blood solubility of an anesthetic and the rate of rise of its tension in arterial blood is illustrated in Figure 25–4. The blood:gas partition coefficients for nitrous oxide, halothane, and methoxyflurane are 0.47, 2.3, and 12, respectively. Nitrous oxide, with low solubil-

ity in blood, reaches high arterial tensions rapidly, which in turn results in more rapid equilibrium with the brain and faster induction of anesthesia. In contrast, even after 40 minutes, methoxyflurane has reached only 20% of the equilibrium concentration.

B. Anesthetic Concentration in the Inspired Air: The concentration of an inhaled anesthetic in the inspired gas mixture has direct effects on both the maximum tension that can be achieved in the alveoli and the rate of increase in its tension in arterial blood. Increases in the inspired anesthetic concentration will increase the rate of induction of anesthesia by increasing the rate of transfer into the blood according to Fick's law (see Chapter 1). Advantage is taken of this effect in anesthetic practice with inhaled anesthetics of moderate blood solubility such as enflurane, isoflurane, and halothane, which have a relatively slow onset of anesthetic effect. For example, a 3–4% concentration of halothane may be administered initially to increase the rate of induction; this is reduced to 1–2% for maintenance when adequate anesthesia is achieved.

C. Pulmonary Ventilation: The rate of rise of anesthetic gas tension in arterial blood is directly dependent on both the rate and depth of ventilation, ie, minute ventilation. The magnitude of the effect varies according to the blood:gas partition coefficient. An increase in pulmonary ventilation is accompanied by only a slight increase in arterial tension of an anesthetic with low blood solubility or low coefficient but can significantly increase tension of agents with moderate or high blood solubility (Figure 25–5). For example, a fourfold increase in ventilation rate almost doubles the arterial tension of halothane during the first 10 minutes of anesthesia but increases the arterial tension of nitrous oxide by only 15%. Hyperventilation by mechanical control of respiration increases the speed of induction of anesthesia with inhaled anesthetics that would normally have a slow onset. Depression of respiration by other pharmacologic agents, including opioid analgesics, may slow the onset of anesthesia of some inhaled anesthetics if ventilation is not controlled.

D. Pulmonary Blood Flow: Changes in the rates of blood flow to and from the lungs influence transfer processes of the anesthetic gases. An increase in pulmonary blood flow (increased cardiac output) slows the rate of rise in arterial tension, particularly for those anesthetics with moderate to high blood solubility. This is because increased pulmonary blood flow exposes a larger volume of blood to the anesthetic; thus, blood "capacity" increases and tension rises slowly. A decrease in pulmonary blood flow has the opposite effect and increases the rate of rise of arterial tension of inhaled anesthetics. In a patient with circulatory shock, the combined effects of decreased cardiac output (decreased pulmonary flow) and increased ventilation may accelerate the induction of anesthesia with some anesthetics. This is not likely to

Table 25–1. Properties of inhaled anesthetics.

Anesthetic	Blood:Gas Partition Coefficient[1]	Brain:Blood Partition Coefficient[1]	Minimal Alveolar Conc (MAC) (%)[2]	Metabolism	Comments
Nitrous oxide	0.47	1.1	> 100	None	Incomplete anesthetic; rapid onset and recovery
Desflurane	0.42	1.3	6–7	< 0.05%	Low volatility; poor induction agent; rapid recovery
Sevoflurane	0.69	1.7	2.0	2–5% (fluoride)	Rapid onset and recovery; unstable in soda-lime
Isoflurane	1.40	2.6	1.40	< 2%	Medium rate of onset and recovery
Enflurane	1.80	1.4	1.7	8%	Medium rate of onset and recovery
Halothane	2.30	2.9	0.75	> 40%	Medium rate of onset and recovery
Methoxyflurane	12	2.0	0.16	> 70% (fluoride)	Slow onset and recovery

[1]Partition coefficients (at 37 °C) are from multiple literature sources.
[2]MAC is the anesthetic concentration that produces immobility in 50% of patients exposed to a noxious stimulus.

occur with nitrous oxide, desflurane, or sevoflurane because of their low blood solubility.

E. Arteriovenous Concentration Gradient: The anesthetic concentration gradient between arterial and mixed venous blood is dependent mainly on uptake of the anesthetic by the tissues; depending on the rate and extent of tissue uptake, venous blood returning to the lungs may contain significantly less anesthetic than that present in arterial blood. The greater this difference in tensions, the more time it takes to achieve equilibrium. Anesthetic entry into tissues is influenced by factors similar to those that determine transfer from lung to blood, including tissue:blood partition coefficient, rates of blood flow to the tissues, and concentration gradients.

During the induction phase of anesthesia, the tissues that exert greatest influence on the arterial-venous anesthetic concentration gradient are those which are highly perfused. These include the brain, heart, liver, kidneys, and splanchnic bed, which to-

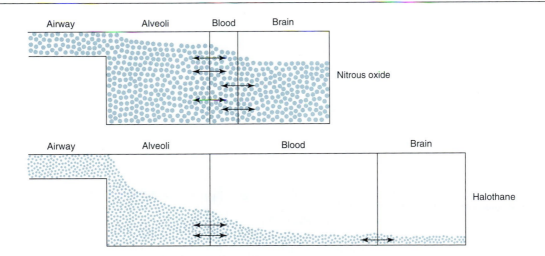

Figure 25–3. Why induction of anesthesia is slower with more soluble anesthetic gases. In this schematic diagram, solubility in blood is represented by the relative size of the blood compartment (the more soluble, the larger the compartment). Relative partial pressures of the agents in the compartments are indicated by the degree of filling of each compartment. For a given concentration or partial pressure of the two anesthetic gases in the inspired air, it will take much longer for the blood partial pressure of the more soluble gas (halothane) to rise to the same partial pressure as in the alveoli. Since the concentration of the anesthetic agent in the brain can rise no faster than the concentration in the blood, the onset of anesthesia will be slower with halothane than with nitrous oxide.

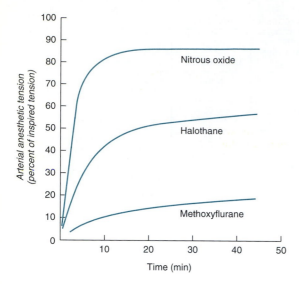

Figure 25–4. Tensions of three anesthetic gases in arterial blood as a function of time after beginning inhalation. Nitrous oxide is relatively insoluble (blood:gas partition coefficient = 0.47); methoxyflurane is much more soluble (coefficient = 12).

gether receive over 75% of the resting cardiac output. In the case of anesthetics with relatively high solubility in these tissues, venous blood concentration will initially be very low, and equilibrium with arterial blood is achieved slowly.

During maintenance of anesthesia with inhaled anesthetics, these drugs may continue to be transferred between various tissues at rates dependent on solubility and blood flow. Muscle and skin, which together constitute 50% of body mass, accumulate anesthetics more slowly than the richly vascularized tissues, since they receive only one-fifth the blood flow of the latter group. Although most anesthetic gases have high solubility in adipose tissues, low blood perfusion rates to these tissues delay accumulation, and equilibrium is unlikely to occur with most anesthetics during the time usually required for surgery.

Elimination

The time to recovery from inhalation anesthesia depends on the rate of elimination of anesthetics from the brain after the inspired concentration of anesthetic has been decreased. Many of the processes of anesthetic transfer during recovery are similar to those that occur during induction of anesthesia. One of the most important factors governing rate of recovery is the blood:gas partition coefficient of the anesthetic agent (see below). Other factors controlling rate of recovery include the pulmonary blood flow, the magnitude of ventilation, and the solubility of the anesthetic in the tissues. Two features of recovery, however, are quite

different from what happens during induction of anesthesia. First, while transfer of an anesthetic from the lungs to blood can be enhanced by increasing its concentration in inspired air, the reverse transfer process cannot be enhanced, since the concentration in the lungs cannot be reduced below zero. Second, at the beginning of recovery, the anesthetic gas tension in different tissues may be quite variable, depending on the specific agent and the duration of anesthesia. With induction of anesthesia, the initial anesthetic tension in all tissues is zero.

Inhaled anesthetics that are relatively insoluble in blood (low blood:gas partition coefficient) and brain are eliminated at faster rates than more soluble anesthetics. The "washout" of nitrous oxide, desflurane, and sevoflurane occurs at a rapid rate, which leads to rapid recovery from their anesthetic effects. Halothane is approximately twice as soluble in brain tissue and five times more soluble in blood than nitrous oxide; its elimination therefore takes place more slowly, and recovery from halothane anesthesia is less rapid. The duration of exposure to the anesthetic can have a marked effect on the time of recovery, especially in the case of more soluble anesthetics such as methoxyflurane. Accumulation of anesthetics in tissues, including muscle, skin, and fat, increases with continuous inhalation, and blood tension may decline slowly during recovery as the anesthetic gradually leaves such tissues. Thus, if exposure to the anesthetic is short, recovery may be rapid. After prolonged anesthesia, recovery may be delayed even with anesthetics of modest solubility such as halothane.

Figure 25–5. Ventilation rate and arterial anesthetic tensions. Increased ventilation (8 versus 2 L/min) has a much greater effect on equilibration of halothane than nitrous oxide.

Clearance of inhaled anesthetics by the lungs into the expired air is the major route of their elimination from the body. However, metabolism by enzymes of the liver and other tissues may also contribute to the elimination of anesthetics. For example, the washout of halothane during recovery is more rapid than that of enflurane, which would not be predicted from their respective solubilities. However, over 40% of inspired halothane is metabolized during an average anesthetic procedure, while less than 10% of enflurane is metabolized over the same period. Oxidative metabolism of halothane results in the formation of trifluoroacetic acid and release of bromide and chloride ions. Under conditions of low oxygen tension, halothane is metabolized to the chlorotrifluoroethyl free radical, which is capable of reacting with hepatic membrane components. Isoflurane and desflurane are the least metabolized of the fluorinated anesthetics, only traces of trifluoroacetic acid appearing in the urine. The metabolism of enflurane and sevoflurane results in the formation of fluoride ion, which does not appear to reach toxic levels under normal circumstances. In addition, sevoflurane is degraded by contact with the carbon dioxide absorbent in anesthesia machines, yielding a vinyl ether called "compound A" that can cause renal damage if high concentrations are absorbed. Over 70% of absorbed methoxyflurane is metabolized by the liver with the release of fluoride ions at concentrations that can be nephrotoxic. Nitrous oxide is probably not metabolized by human tissue. In terms of the extent of metabolism of inhaled anesthetics the rank order is: methoxyflurane > halothane > enflurane > sevoflurane > isoflurane > desflurane > nitrous oxide (Table 25–1).

PHARMACODYNAMICS

Mechanism of Action

An important neurophysiologic action common to most general anesthetics is to increase the cellular threshold for firing (Aloia et al, 1991). With the increase in threshold, there is a decrease in neuronal activity. The inhaled anesthetic agents—as well as the intravenous barbiturates and benzodiazepines—depress spontaneous and evoked activity of neurons in many regions of the brain. Such actions are exerted on both axonal and synaptic transmission, but synaptic processes are more sensitive to the effects. The ionic mechanisms thought to be involved are varied. Inhaled gaseous anesthetics have been reported to cause hyperpolarization of neurons via activation of potassium currents, which leads to decreased ability to initiate action potentials, ie, an increase in threshold. With patch clamp analysis, electrophysiologic studies of cells in culture have shown that isoflurane decreases the duration of opening of nicotinic receptor-activated cation channels—an action that would presumably decrease synaptic transmission at cholinergic synapses. The effects of benzodiazepines and barbiturates on the $GABA_A$ receptor-controlled chloride channel alter channel opening and cause hyperpolarization, again leading to decreased firing (Chapter 21). A similar action to facilitate the inhibitory effects of GABA has also been reported for propofol and certain inhaled anesthetics.

The molecular mechanism by which gaseous anesthetics modify ion currents in neuronal membranes is not clear. Such effects could result from direct interaction between anesthetic molecules and hydrophobic sites on specific membrane protein channels. This type of mechanism has been suggested from studies on gas anesthetic interactions with nicotinic cholinoceptor channels—interactions that appear to stabilize the channel in its closed state. Alternative interpretations, which attempt to take into account the marked structural differences among the anesthetics, invoke less specific interactions of these agents with the lipid matrix of the membrane, with secondary changes in channel function. These interpretations are supported by older observations of the close correlation of anesthetic potency with lipid solubility (Meyer-Overton principle). The concept of indirect interactions mediated via solution in membrane lipid is supported by studies of anesthetics on artificial lipid membranes. These studies show that as an anesthetic gas dissolves in the lipid, there is an increase in membrane fluidity suggestive of a reduction in the "orderliness" of the lipid structure. Such effects on the lipid could be reflected in changes in the function of the channels floating in the lipid membrane.

In experimental animals, general anesthesia can be reversed by placing the animal in a high-pressure chamber. Very high pressures—eg, 50–100 atm—cause reversal of the anesthetic state. High pressure is known to increase the orderliness (decrease the fluidity) of lipid membranes. Such experiments have led to suggestions that solution of anesthetic molecules in the membrane lipid—and the resulting decrease in order—causes a small expansion that distorts ion channels. However, hypotheses based on increased membrane fluidity fail to explain why small elevations of temperature, which increase membrane fluidity to an extent comparable to the effect of clinical concentrations of anesthetics, actually decrease anesthetic potency. In addition, such hypotheses are not congruent with the clinical observation that older patients often have a reduced anesthetic requirement despite the fact that the fluidity of neuronal membranes tends to decrease with age.

The neuropharmacologic basis for the effects that characterize the stages of anesthesia appears to be differential sensitivity to the anesthetic of specific neurons or neuronal pathways. Cells of the substantia gelatinosa in the dorsal horn of the spinal cord are very sensitive to relatively low anesthetic concentration in the central nervous system. A decrease in the activity of neurons in this region interrupts sensory transmission in the spinothalamic tract, including transmission of nociceptive stimuli. These effects contribute to stage I, or analgesia. The disinhibitory effects of general anesthetics (stage II), which occur at higher brain concentrations, result from complex neuronal actions including blockade of many small inhibitory neurons such as Golgi type II cells, together with a paradoxical facilitation of excitatory neurotransmitters. A progressive depression of ascending pathways in the reticular activating system occurs during stage III, or surgical anesthesia, together with suppression of spinal reflex activity, which contributes to muscle relaxation. Neurons in the respiratory and vasomotor centers of the medulla are relatively insensitive to the effects of the general anesthetics, but at high concentrations their activity is depressed, leading to cardiorespiratory collapse (stage IV).

Dose-Response Characteristics: The Minimum Alveolar Anesthetic Concentration (MAC)

Inhaled anesthetics are delivered to the lungs in gas mixtures in which concentrations and flow rates are easy to measure and control. However, dose-response characteristics of gaseous anesthetics are particularly difficult to measure. First, achievement of an anesthetic state depends on the concentration of the anesthetic in the brain, and that concentration is impossible to measure under clinical conditions. Second, neither the lower nor the upper ends of the graded dose-response curve can be ethically determined, since at very low concentrations severe pain might be experienced while at high concentrations there would be a high risk of fatal cardiovascular and respiratory depression. Nevertheless, a useful estimate of anesthetic potency can be obtained using quantal dose-response principles.

During general anesthesia, the partial pressure of an inhaled anesthetic in the brain equals that in the lung when steady state is reached. At a given level of anesthesia, the measurement of the steady state alveolar concentrations of different anesthetics provides a comparison of their relative potencies. The minimum alveolar anesthetic concentration (MAC) of an anesthetic is defined as the concentration (ie, the percentage of the alveolar gas mixture, or partial pressure of the anesthetic as a percentage of 760 mm Hg) that results in immobility in 50% of patients when exposed to a noxious stimulus such as surgical incision. Thus, it represents one point (the ED50) on a conventional quantal dose-response curve (see Figure 2–19). Table 25–1 shows concentrations for the common inhaled anesthetics, permitting comparison of their relative anesthetic potencies. The MAC value greater than 100% for nitrous oxide shows that it is the least potent, since at normal barometric pressure even 760 mm Hg partial pressure of nitrous oxide (100% of the inspired gas) is not equal to 1 MAC.

The dose of anesthetic gas that is administered can be stated in multiples of MAC. While a dose of 1 MAC of any anesthetic prevents movement in response to surgical incision in 50% of patients, individual patients may require 0.5–1.5 MAC. The MAC gives no information about the slope of the dose-response curve. In general, however, the dose-response relationship for inhaled anesthetics is steep; thus, over 95% of patients may fail to respond to a noxious stimulus at 1.1 MAC. The measurement of MAC values under controlled conditions has permitted quantitation of the effects of a number of variables on anesthetic requirements. For example, MAC values decrease in elderly patients but are not affected greatly by sex, height, and weight. Of particular importance is the presence of adjuvant drugs, which can change anesthetic requirements greatly. For example, when drugs such as the opioid analgesics or sedative-hypnotics are present, MAC is decreased, which means that the inspired concentration of anesthetic should be decreased accordingly.

A variety of other techniques, such as measurement of changes in the electroencephalogram, have been tried in an effort to delineate graded dose-response curves for inhaled anesthetics in humans. However, because many other variables unrelated to anesthesia can influence the results, these attempts have not succeeded to date.

Organ System Effects of Inhaled Anesthetics

A. Effects on Cardiovascular System: Halothane, desflurane, enflurane, sevoflurane, and isoflurane all decrease mean arterial pressure in direct proportion to their alveolar concentration. With halothane and enflurane, the reduced arterial pressure appears to be caused by a reduction in cardiac output, because there is little change in systemic vascular resistance despite marked changes in individual vascular beds (eg, increase in cerebral blood flow). In contrast, isoflurane, desflurane, and sevoflurane have a depressant effect on arterial pressure as a result of an endothelium-mediated decrease in systemic vascular resistance; they have little effect on cardiac output.

Inhaled anesthetics change heart rate either by directly altering the rate of sinus node depolarization or by shifting the balance of autonomic nervous system activity. Bradycardia is often seen with halothane and may be a result of direct depression of atrial rate. In contrast, methoxyflurane and enflurane have little effect, and both desflurane and isoflurane increase heart rate. In the case of desflurane, cardiovascular responses include a transient sympathetic activation that can lead to marked increases in heart rate and blood pressure at high inspired gas concentrations.

All inhaled anesthetics tend to increase right atrial pressure in a dose-related fashion, which reflects depression of myocardial function. In general, enflurane and halothane have greater myocardial depressant effects than isoflurane and the newer halogenated anesthetics. Inhaled anesthetics reduce myocardial oxygen consumption, primarily by decreasing those variables that control oxygen demand, such as arterial blood pressure and contractile force. Although certainly less depressant than the other inhaled anesthetics, nitrous oxide has also been found to depress the myocardium in a dose-dependent manner. However, nitrous oxide—alone or in combination with potent inhaled anesthetics—produces sympathetic stimulation that may obscure any cardiac depressant effects of the inhaled anesthetic. The combination of nitrous oxide plus halothane or enflurane, for example, appears to produce less depression at a given level of anesthesia than either of the more potent anesthetics given alone.

Several factors influence the cardiovascular effects of inhaled anesthetics. Surgical stimulation, hypercapnia, and increasing duration of anesthesia will lessen the depressant effects of these drugs. Hypercapnia releases catecholamines, which attenuate the decrease in blood pressure. The blood pressure decrease after 5 hours of anesthesia is less than it is after 1 hour; propranolol blocks this adaptive effect. Halothane sensitizes the myocardium to catecholamines, and ventricular arrhythmias may occur in patients with cardiac disease who are given either direct-acting or indirect-acting sympathomimetic drugs or who have high circulating levels of endogenous catecholamines (eg, patients with pheochromocytoma). Other inhaled anesthetics appear to be less arrhythmogenic than halothane.

B. Effects on Respiratory System: With the exception of nitrous oxide, all inhaled anesthetics in current use cause a decrease in tidal volume and an increase in respiratory rate. However, the increase in rate is insufficient to compensate for the decrease in volume, resulting in a decrease in minute ventilation. All inhaled anesthetics are respiratory depressants, as indicated by the reduced response to various levels of carbon dioxide. The degree of ventilatory depression varies with anesthetic agents, with isoflurane and enflurane being the most depressant. All inhaled anesthetics in current use increase the resting level of $Paco_2$ (the partial pressure of carbon dioxide in arterial blood).

Inhaled anesthetics increase the apneic threshold ($Paco_2$ level below which apnea occurs through lack of CO_2-driven respiratory stimulation) and decrease the ventilatory response to hypoxia. The latter effect is especially important because subanesthetic concentrations (ie, those that exist during recovery) depress the normal compensating increase in ventilation that occurs during hypoxia. All of these respiratory depressant effects of anesthetics are overcome by assisting or controlling ventilation via a mechanical ventilator during surgery. Furthermore, the ventilatory depressant effects of the inhaled anesthetics are lessened by surgical stimulation and increasing duration of anesthesia.

Inhaled anesthetics also depress mucociliary function in the airway. Thus, prolonged anesthesia may lead to pooling of mucus and then result in atelectasis and respiratory infections. However, inhaled anesthetics tend to be bronchodilators. This effect has been used in the treatment of status asthmaticus. Airway irritation, which may provoke coughing or breath holding, is rarely a problem with most inhaled anesthetics. However, it is relatively common with desflurane, and induction is more difficult to accomplish with this anesthetic despite its low blood:gas partition coefficient. Similarly, the pungency of enflurane may elicit breath holding, which can limit speed of induction.

C. Effects on Brain: Inhaled anesthetics decrease the metabolic rate of the brain. Nevertheless, most of them increase cerebral blood flow because they decrease cerebral vascular resistance. The increase in cerebral blood flow is often clinically undesirable. For example, in patients who have an increased intracranial pressure because of brain tumor or head injury, administration of an inhaled anesthetic may increase cerebral blood flow, which in turn will increase cerebral blood volume and further increase intracranial pressure.

Of the inhaled anesthetics, nitrous oxide increases cerebral blood flow the least, although when 60% nitrous oxide is added to halothane anesthesia, cerebral blood flow usually increases more than with halothane alone. At low doses, all of the halogenated agents have similar effects to increase cerebral blood flow. At larger doses, enflurane and isoflurane increase cerebral blood flow less than does halothane. If the patient is hyperventilated before the anesthetic is given (to reduce $Paco_2$), the increase in intracranial pressure from inhaled anesthetics can be minimized.

Halothane, isoflurane, and enflurane have similar effects (eg, burst suppression) on the EEG up to doses of 1–1.5 MAC. At higher doses, the cerebral irritant effects of enflurane may lead to the development of a spike-and-wave pattern during which auditory stimuli can precipitate mild generalized muscle twitching that is augmented by hyperventilation. This seizure activity has never been shown to have any adverse clinical consequences. The effect is not seen clinically with the other inhaled anesthetics. Though nitrous oxide has low anesthetic potency, it does exert marked analgesic and amnesic actions, desirable properties when used in combination with other agents in general anesthesia and dental anesthesia.

D. Effects on the Kidney: To varying degrees, all inhaled anesthetics decrease glomerular filtration rate and effective renal plasma flow and increase filtration fraction. All the anesthetics tend to increase renal vascular resistance. Since renal blood flow decreases during general anesthesia in spite of well-maintained or even increased perfusion pressures, autoregulation of renal flow is probably impaired.

E. Effects on the Liver: All inhaled anesthetics cause a decrease in hepatic blood flow, ranging from 15% to 45% of the preanesthetic flow. Despite transient changes in liver function tests intraoperatively, rarely does permanent change of liver function occur from the use of these agents. The possible hepatotoxicity of halothane is discussed below.

F. Effects on Uterine Smooth Muscle: Nitrous oxide appears to have little effect on uterine musculature. However, the halogenated hydrocarbon anesthetics are potent uterine muscle relaxants. This pharmacologic effect can be used to advantage when profound uterine relaxation is required for intrauterine fetal manipulation during delivery. In contrast, during dilatation and curettage for therapeutic abortion, these anesthetics may cause increased bleeding.

Toxicity

A. Hepatotoxicity (Halothane): Postoperative hepatitis is usually associated with factors such as blood transfusions, hypovolemic shock, and other surgical stresses rather than anesthetic toxicity. However, halocarbon drugs such as halothane can cause liver damage, and chloroform was identified as a hepatotoxin in the first decade of this century. Halothane was introduced into clinical practice in 1956; by 1963, several cases of postoperative jaundice and liver necrosis associated with halothane had been reported. However, several retrospective studies in which halothane was compared with other anesthetics showed no increased incidence in postoperative hepatic damage with halothane. In 1966, the United States National Halothane Study undertook a retrospective review of the incidence of fatal massive hepatic necrosis in a population of about 850,000 surgical patients. Results of the study were inconclusive and did not identify halothane clearly as a hepatotoxin. The incidence of massive necrosis associated with halothane was 7 out of 250,000 halothane administrations, or about 1 in 35,000 (not 1 in 10,000, as sometimes reported). Unlike chloroform and fluroxene, which can produce fatty infiltration, centrilobular necrosis, and elevated aminotransferase concentrations, prolonged exposure of animals to halothane produces little evidence of liver damage. Several animal models have been developed to help define possible halothane-mediated hepatotoxicity. When rats are pretreated with phenobarbital and then exposed to hypoxic conditions with an inspired oxygen concentration of 7–14%, hepatotoxicity from halothane (as well as some other inhaled anesthetics) will occur. The mechanism underlying hepatotoxicity in the animals remains unclear, though these models suggest that it may depend on the production of a reactive metabolite (eg, a free radical) that either causes direct hepatocellular damage or initiates an immune-mediated response. Although this model is reproducible and well defined, its clinical applicability is uncertain because hypoxia is a necessary precondition for production of liver damage.

Recently, it has been found that some individuals have a defect in their hepatic cell membranes that make these cells more susceptible to halothane-induced injury. These individuals are also at a higher risk for halothane-induced hepatic necrosis. A test is being developed that would identify such individuals preoperatively.

B. Nephrotoxicity: In 1966, vasopressin-resistant polyuric renal insufficiency was first reported in 13 of 41 patients receiving methoxyflurane anesthesia for abdominal surgery. Subsequently, the causative agent was shown to be inorganic fluoride, an end product of the extensive biotransformation of methoxyflurane by hepatic and renal enzymes. Metabolism of enflurane and sevoflurane also leads to the formation of fluoride ions, and this has raised questions concerning the potential nephrotoxicity of these anesthetics. Changes in renal concentrating ability have been observed with prolonged exposure to enflurane but not sevoflurane anesthesia. Differences between the two agents may be related to the fact that enflurane (but not sevoflurane) is metabolized in part by renal enzymes, generating fluoride ions intrarenally.

C. Malignant Hyperthermia: Although occurrences are rare, genetically susceptible patients exposed to inhaled anesthetics may develop this potentially lethal syndrome, which includes tachycardia and hypertension progressing to acidosis, hyperkalemia, muscle rigidity, and hyperthermia. The onset is more dramatic if succinylcholine is used for muscle relaxation. Treatment involves intravenous dantrolene with appropriate measures to lower body temperature and to restore electrolyte and acid-base balance.

D. Chronic Toxicity:

1. Mutagenicity–Under normal conditions, most modern and many older inhaled anesthetics are not mutagens and probably not carcinogens. However, older anesthetics that contain the vinyl moiety (fluroxene and divinyl ether) may be mutagens. These agents are rarely or never used.

2. Carcinogenicity–Several epidemiologic studies have suggested an increase in the cancer rate in operating room personnel who may be exposed to trace concentrations of anesthetic agents. However, no study has demonstrated the existence of a cause-and-effect relationship between anesthetics and cancer. Many other factors might account for the questionably positive results seen after a careful review of epidemiologic data. Most operating room theaters remove trace concentrations of anesthetics released from anesthetic machines via vents to the atmosphere.

3. Effects on reproduction–The most consistent finding reported from surveys conducted to determine the reproductive performance of female operating room personnel has been a higher than expected incidence of miscarriages. There are several problems in interpreting these studies, but in general it can be asserted that the evidence is not strong.

However, the association of obstetric problems with surgery and anesthesia in pregnant patients is not open to question. In the USA, at least 50,000 pregnant women each year undergo anesthesia and surgery for indications unrelated to pregnancy. The risk of abortion is clearly higher following this experience. It is not obvious whether the underlying disease, surgery, anesthesia, or a combination of these factors is the cause of the increased risk. Another concern not yet substantiated is that anesthetics during pregnancy may lead to an increased incidence of congenital anomalies. If anesthetics are teratogenic, the risk may be very small.

4. Hematotoxicity—Prolonged exposure to nitrous oxide decreases methionine synthase activity and causes megaloblastic anemia. This is a potential occupational hazard for staff working in poorly ventilated dental operating suites.

Clinical Use of Inhaled Anesthetics

Of the inhaled anesthetics available, nitrous oxide, desflurane, and isoflurane are most commonly used in the USA. Although not often used in adults, halothane is frequently used in pediatric anesthesia. Sevoflurane use is increasing in pediatric and outpatient anesthesia. As indicated previously, nitrous oxide lacks sufficient potency to produce surgical anesthesia by itself and therefore is commonly used with another inhaled or intravenous anesthetic to produce complete anesthesia. Methoxyflurane is occasionally used—especially in obstetric anesthesia—but not for prolonged procedures because of its nephrotoxicity, which is described above. Chloroform is not used because of its hepatotoxicity. Although cyclopropane and diethyl ether were the most commonly used anesthetics before 1960, they are no longer used because of their flammable and explosive characteristics.

Despite the advantages of the inhaled anesthetics now available, there is reason to believe that better ones might be developed (see box: Do We Need Another Inhaled Anesthetic?).

INTRAVENOUS ANESTHETICS

In the last 2 decades there has been increasing use of intravenous drugs in anesthesia, both as adjuncts to gaseous anesthetics and in protocols that do not include inhaled anesthetics. Unlike inhaled anesthetics, intravenous agents do not require specialized equipment for their delivery or expensive facilities for the recovery and disposal of exhaled gases. Intravenous drugs such as thiopental, etomidate, and propofol have an onset of anesthetic action faster than even the newest inhaled gaseous agents such as desflurane and sevoflurane. Such intravenous agents are commonly used for induction of anesthesia. Rates of recovery are fast enough with many intravenous drugs to permit their extensive use in outpatient anesthesia and, in the

DO WE NEED ANOTHER INHALED ANESTHETIC?

For almost 30 years, from its introduction in 1956, halothane was the standard of comparison for inhaled anesthetics. However, the onset of its anesthetic action is slow compared with many intravenous agents, and the rate of recovery from its anesthetic effects is not particularly rapid. In addition, its hepatic metabolism to a reactive compound appears to be a necessary prerequisite in the development of halothane-associated hepatitis.

The newer inhaled anesthetics, desflurane and sevoflurane, have physicochemical characteristics (low blood:gas partition coefficients) favorable to a more rapid onset and a shorter duration of anesthetic actions than older agents such as isoflurane and halothane. However, both of these newer agents also have certain limitations. The low volatility of desflurane necessitates the use of a specialized vaporizer, and the pungency of the drug leads to a high incidence of coughing—and sometimes laryngospasm—such that it cannot be used for induction of anesthesia. In addition, desflurane causes a centrally mediated sympathetic activation leading to elevations of blood pressure and heart rate. Despite its low blood:gas partition coefficient, recovery from desflurane anesthesia, estimated by length of stay in the recovery room, is not consistently more rapid than that with other anesthetics.

In the case of the newest agent, sevoflurane, induction of anesthesia is achieved rapidly and smoothly, and recovery is more rapid than most other inhaled anesthetics including isoflurane. However, sevoflurane is chemically unstable when exposed to carbon dioxide absorbents, degrading to an olefinic compound (fluoromethyl-2,2-difluoro-1-[trifluoromethyl]vinyl ether, compound A) that is potentially nephrotoxic. In addition, sevoflurane is metabolized by the liver to release fluoride ions, raising concerns about possible renal damage similar to that caused by methoxyflurane. Sevoflurane comes close to having the characteristics of an ideal gas anesthetic. A similar compound that has greater chemical stability and resists metabolism could be of value.

case of propofol, are similar to those seen with the shortest-acting inhaled anesthetics. The anesthetic potency of several intravenous anesthetics, including thiopental, ketamine, and propofol, is adequate to permit their use as the sole anesthetic in short surgical procedures. Intravenous opioids (eg, fentanyl) contribute cardiovascular stability, sedation, and marked analgesia to anesthesia protocols, and opioid receptor antagonists can be used to hasten recovery from their actions. Other intravenous agents such as the benzodiazepines (eg, midazolam, diazepam) are too slow in onset to be useful as induction agents but can provide a basal level of sedation for maintenance of anesthesia when used in conjunction with other agents. Benzodiazepines such as lorazepam and midazolam also afford marked anterograde amnesia, a useful action in most patients undergoing anesthesia. Some properties of the intravenous anesthetics are listed in Table 25–2.

ULTRA-SHORT-ACTING BARBITURATES

Although several ultra-short-acting barbiturates are available, thiopental is the one most commonly used for induction of anesthesia, often in combination with inhaled anesthetics. The general pharmacology of the barbiturates is discussed in Chapter 22.

Following intravenous administration, thiopental rapidly crosses the blood-brain barrier and, if given in sufficient dosage, produces hypnosis in one circulation time. Similar effects occur with other ultra-short-acting barbiturates, eg, thiamylal and methohexital. With these barbiturates, plasma:brain equilibrium occurs rapidly (in approximately 1 minute) because of high lipid solubility. Thiopental rapidly diffuses out of the brain and other highly vascular tissues and is redistributed to muscle, fat, and eventually all body tissues (Figure 25–6). It is because of this rapid removal from brain tissue that a single dose of thiopental is so short-acting.

Metabolism of thiopental is much slower than its redistribution and takes place primarily in the liver. Less than 1% of an administered dose of thiopental is excreted unchanged by the kidney. Thiopental is metabolized at the rate of 12–16% per hour in humans following a single dose.

With large doses, thiopental causes dose-dependent decreases in arterial blood pressure, stroke volume, and cardiac output. This is due primarily to its myocardial depressant effect and increased venous capacitance; there is little change in total peripheral resistance. Thiopental, like other barbiturates, is a potent respiratory depressant, lowering the sensitivity of the medullary respiratory center to carbon dioxide.

Cerebral metabolism and oxygen utilization are decreased after thiopental administration in proportion to the degree of cerebral depression. Cerebral blood flow is also decreased, but much less so than oxygen consumption. This makes thiopental a much more desirable drug for use in patients with cerebral swelling than the inhaled anesthetics, since intracranial pressure and blood volume are not increased.

Thiopental may reduce hepatic blood flow and glomerular filtration rate, but it produces no lasting effects on hepatic and renal function. Barbiturates may exacerbate acute intermittent porphyria by inducing the synthesis of hepatic ALA synthase (see Chapter 22). Thiopental has precipitated porphyric crisis when used as an induction agent.

BENZODIAZEPINES

Certain members of this class of sedative-hypnotic drugs, including diazepam, lorazepam, and midazolam, are used in anesthetic procedures. (The basic pharmacology of benzodiazepines is discussed in Chapter 22.) Diazepam and lorazepam are not water-soluble, and their intravenous use necessitates nonaqueous vehicles, which may cause local irritation. Midazolam formulations are water-soluble and thus produce less irritation, but the drug becomes lipid-soluble at physiologic pH and readily crosses the blood-brain barrier.

Compared with intravenous barbiturates, benzodiazepines produce a slower onset of central nervous system effects and induce a plateau of central depression that appears to be below that of a true anesthetic

Table 25–2. Characteristics of intravenous anesthetics.

Drug	Induction and Recovery	Comments
Etomidate	Rapid onset and moderately fast recovery	Cardiovascular stability; decreased steroidogenesis; involuntary muscle movements
Ketamine	Moderately rapid onset and recovery	Cardiovascular stimulation; increased cerebral blood flow; emergence reactions impair recovery
Midazolam	Slow onset and recovery; flumazenil reversal available	Used in balanced anesthesia and conscious sedation; cardiovascular stability; marked amnesia
Propofol	Rapid onset and rapid recovery	Used in induction and for maintenance; hypotension; useful antiemetic action
Thiopental	Rapid onset and rapid recovery (bolus dose)—slow recovery following infusion	Standard induction agent; cardiovascular depression; avoid in porphyrias
Fentanyl	Slow onset and recovery; naloxone reversal available	Used in balanced anesthesia and conscious-sedation; marked analgesia

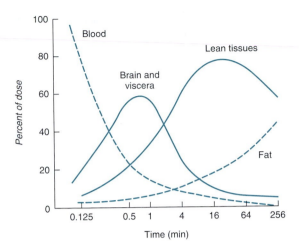

Figure 25–6. Redistribution of thiopental after an intravenous bolus administration. Note that the time axis is not linear.

state. Used intravenously, benzodiazepines prolong the postanesthetic recovery period (an undesirable effect) but also cause a high incidence of anterograde amnesia (amnesia for events occurring after the drug is administered), which is useful. Because it causes a high incidence of amnesia (> 50%), midazolam is frequently given intravenously 15–60 minutes before induction of general anesthesia. Midazolam has a more rapid onset, a shorter elimination half-life (2–4 hours), and a steeper dose-response curve than do the other benzodiazepines used in anesthesia.

The benzodiazepines are useful in anesthesia as premedication; they can also be used for intraoperative sedation and, with other drugs, as part of balanced anesthesia. The benzodiazepine antagonist flumazenil is now used to accelerate recovery from the sedative actions of intravenous benzodiazepines, but its reversal of respiratory depression is less predictable. Its short duration of action may necessitate multiple doses.

OPIOID ANALGESIC ANESTHESIA

Large doses of opioid analgesics have been used to achieve general anesthesia, particularly in patients undergoing cardiac surgery or other major surgery when circulatory reserve is minimal. Intravenous morphine, 1–3 mg/kg, or the high-potency opioid fentanyl, 50–100 µg/kg, have been used in such situations with minimal evidence of circulatory deterioration. More recently, several congeners of fentanyl, including sufentanil, alfentanil, and remifentanil, have also been used. Despite the high doses used (see Table 31–2 for conventional analgesic doses), awareness during anesthesia and unpleasant postoperative recall have occurred.

Intravenous opioids can increase chest wall rigidity, which may impair ventilation, and postoperative respiratory depression may occur, requiring assisted ventilation and the administration of opioid antagonists, eg, naloxone. Postoperative respiratory effects may be reduced by lowering the opioid analgesic dose and simultaneously administering short-acting barbiturates or benzodiazepines, usually with nitrous oxide to achieve balanced anesthesia. Alfentanil and remifentanil, short-acting congeners of fentanyl, are available for use as intravenous agents in shorter surgical procedures. Fentanyl and droperidol (a butyrophenone related to haloperidol) together produce analgesia and amnesia and are sometimes used with nitrous oxide to provide **neuroleptanesthesia.**

Opioid analgesics are also given by the epidural route. While this approach cannot prevent pain caused by surgical incision, it does provide profound postoperative analgesia.

PROPOFOL

2,6-Diisopropylphenol—propofol or disoprofol—is an extremely important intravenous anesthetic. It produces anesthesia at a rate similar to that of the intravenous barbiturates, and recovery is more rapid. In particular, patients are able to ambulate sooner after propofol. Furthermore, patients "feel better" in the immediate postoperative period after propofol as compared with other intravenous anesthetics. Postoperative vomiting is uncommon, and propofol is reported to have antiemetic actions. Propofol is used for both induction and maintenance of anesthesia. The drug does not appear to cause cumulative effects or delayed arousal following prolonged infusion. These favorable properties are responsible for the extensive use of propofol as a component of balanced anesthesia and for its great popularity as an anesthetic for use in "day surgery." The drug is also effective in producing prolonged sedation in patients in critical care settings (see box: Conscious Sedation & Deep Sedation). However, use of propofol for the sedation of children under intensive care has led to severe acidosis in the presence of respiratory infections and possible neurological sequelae on withdrawal.

After intravenous administration, distribution occurs with a half-life ($t_{1/2\,\alpha}$) of 2–8 minutes; the elimination half-life ($t_{1/2\,\beta}$) of propofol is approximately 30–60 minutes. The drug is rapidly metabolized in the liver (ten times faster than thiopental) by conjugation to glucuronide and sulfate and excreted in the urine. Less than 1% of the drug is excreted unchanged. Total body clearance of the anesthetic is greater than hepatic blood flow, suggesting that its elimination includes extrahepatic mechanisms in addition to metabolism by liver enzymes. This property is useful in patients with impaired ability to metabolize other sedative-anesthetic drugs such as midazolam.

CONSCIOUS SEDATION & DEEP SEDATION

Many procedures—diagnostic, therapeutic, and minor surgical—neither require general anesthesia nor the availability of specialized equipment and facilities to effect inhaled anesthesia. Regional anesthesia with local anesthetics, sometimes with orally administered sedatives or opioid analgesics, can often be a more appropriate and safer approach to anesthesia.

A recent approach has been the development of protocols to provide a state of **conscious sedation**—drug-induced alleviation of anxiety and pain, together with an altered level of consciousness, but with retention of the ability of the patient to maintain a patent airway and to respond to verbal commands. Intravenous anesthetic agents have proved to be useful drugs in conscious sedation techniques. For example, intravenous benzodiazepines and opioid analgesics can confer amnestic, sedative, and analgesic effects without complete loss of consciousness. Use of benzodiazepines and opioid analgesics in conscious sedation protocols has the advantage of being reversible by the specific receptor antagonist drugs—flumazenil and naloxone, respectively.

Deep sedation is a controlled state of anesthesia involving decreased consciousness from which the patient is not easily aroused. Since deep sedation is often accompanied by a loss of protective reflexes, an inability to maintain a patent airway, and lack of response to surgical stimuli, the state may be indistinguishable from that of general anesthesia. Intravenous agents used in deep sedation protocols include thiopental, ketamine, propofol, and certain intravenous opioid analgesics.

Effects on respiration are similar to those of thiopental at usual anesthetic doses. However, propofol causes a marked decrease in systemic blood pressure during induction of anesthesia, primarily through decreased peripheral resistance. In addition, propofol has greater negative inotropic effects on the heart than etomidate and thiopental. Apnea and pain at the site of injection also occur. Muscle movements, hypotonus, and (rarely) tremors have also been reported following its use. Hypersensitivity reactions involving hypotension, flushing, and bronchospasm have occurred with preparations of propofol dissolved in the original vehicle (Cremophor), but these do not occur when Intralipid (intravenous fat emulsion) is used as a vehicle. An important disadvantage of prolonged use of propofol is its cost, which greatly exceeds that of the benzodiazepines and barbiturates. Clinical infections due to bacterial contamination of propofol have been reported, possibly associated with reluctance to discard unused quantities of such an expensive drug.

ETOMIDATE

Etomidate is a carboxylated imidazole used for induction of anesthesia and in techniques of balanced anesthesia that do not require its prolonged administration. Its major advantage over other agents is that it causes minimal cardiovascular and respiratory depressant effects. Etomidate produces loss of consciousness within seconds, with slight hypotension, no effect on heart rate, and a low frequency of apnea. The drug has no analgesic effects, and premedication with opioids may be required to decrease cardiac responses during tracheal intubation and to lessen spontaneous muscle movements. Following an induction dose, recovery occurs within 3–5 minutes.

Distribution of etomidate is rapid, with a biphasic plasma concentration curve showing distribution half-lives of 3 and 29 minutes. Redistribution of the drug from brain to highly perfused tissues appears to be responsible for the short duration of its anesthetic effects. Etomidate is hydrolyzed in the liver and plasma to inactive metabolites. Studies in humans indicate that almost 90% of the drug—of which only 2% is unchanged—eventually appears in the urine.

Unfortunately, etomidate causes a high incidence of nausea and vomiting, pain on injection, and myoclonus. The involuntary muscle movements are not associated with epileptiform discharges on the EEG. Etomidate may also cause adrenocortical suppression via inhibitory effects on steroidogenesis, with decreased plasma levels of hydrocortisone after a single dose. Prolonged infusion of etomidate may result in hypotension, electrolyte imbalance, and oliguria.

KETAMINE

Ketamine (Figure 25–2) produces **dissociative anesthesia,** which is characterized by catatonia, amnesia, and analgesia, without actual loss of consciousness. The drug is an arylcyclohexylamine chemically related to phencyclidine (PCP), a drug frequently abused because of its psychoactive properties. The mechanism of action of ketamine may involve blockade of the membrane effects of the excitatory neurotransmitter glutamic acid at the NMDA (N-methyl-D-aspartate) receptor subtype (Chapter 21).

Ketamine, a highly lipophilic drug, is rapidly distributed into highly vascular organs, including the brain, and subsequently redistributed to less perfused tissues with concurrent hepatic metabolism and both urinary and biliary excretion.

Besides being a powerful analgesic, ketamine is the only intravenous anesthetic that routinely produces cardiovascular stimulation. Heart rate, arterial blood pressure, and cardiac output are usually significantly increased. The peak increases in these variables occur 2–4 minutes after intravenous injection and then slowly decline to normal over the next 10–20 minutes. Ketamine produces its cardiovascular stimulation by excitation of the central sympathetic nervous system and possibly by inhibition of the reuptake of norepinephrine at sympathetic nerve terminals. Increases in plasma epinephrine and norepinephrine levels occur as early as 2 minutes after intravenous ketamine and return to control levels 15 minutes later.

Ketamine markedly increases cerebral blood flow, oxygen consumption, and intracranial pressure. In this regard ketamine resembles inhaled anesthetics as a potentially dangerous drug when intracranial pressure is elevated. In most patients, ketamine decreases the respiratory rate slightly for 2–3 minutes. Upper airway muscle tone is well maintained, and upper airway reflexes are usually (not always) active. Ketamine produces little other change in organ systems.

Although it is a desirable anesthetic in many respects, ketamine has been associated with disorientation, sensory and perceptual illusions, and vivid dreams following anesthesia, effects that are termed "emergence phenomena." Diazepam, 0.2–0.3 mg/kg intravenously 5 minutes before administration of ketamine, reduces the incidence of these phenomena. Because of the high incidence of postoperative psychic phenomena associated with its use, ketamine is not commonly used in general surgery in the USA. It is considered useful for poor-risk geriatric patients and patients in shock because of its cardiostimulatory properties. It is also used in outpatient anesthesia and in children undergoing painful procedures such as dressing changes on burns.

PREPARATIONS AVAILABLE

Desflurane (Suprane)
Liquid: 240 mL for inhalation
Diazepam (generic, Valium, others)
Oral: 2, 5, 10 mg tablets; 5 mg/5 mL and 5 mg/mL solution
Oral sustained release: 15 mg capsules
Parenteral: 5 mg/mL for injection
Enflurane (Ethrane)
Liquid: 125, 250 mL for inhalation
Etomidate (Amidate)
Parenteral: 2 mg/mL for injection
Halothane (generic, Fluothane)
Liquid: 125, 250 mL for inhalation
Isoflurane (Forane)
Liquid: 100 mL for inhalation
Ketamine (Ketalar)
Parenteral: 10, 50, 100 mg/mL for injection
Lorazepam (generic, Ativan, Alzapam)
Oral: 0.5, 1, 2 mg tablets
Parenteral: 2, 4 mg/mL for injection
Methohexital (Brevital Sodium)
Parenteral: 0.5, 2.5, 5 g powders to reconstitute for injection

Methoxyflurane (Penthrane)
Liquid: 15, 125 mL for inhalation
Midazolam (Versed)
Parenteral: 1, 5 mg/mL for injection in 1, 2, 5, 10 mL vials
Nitrous oxide (gas, supplied in blue cylinders)
Propofol (Diprivan)
Parenteral: 10 mg/mL in 20 mL vials for injection
Sevoflurane (Ultane)
Liquid: 250 mL for inhalation
Thiamylal (Surital)
Parenteral: solutions for injection in 1, 5, 10 g vials
Thiopental (Pentothal)
Parenteral: 250, 400, 500 mg in preloaded syringes; 500 mg, 1 g solutions with diluent; 1, 2.5, 5 g kits
Rectal: 400 mg solution in preloaded syringes

REFERENCES

Albin MS, Bunegin L, Garcia C: Ketamine and postanesthetic emergence reaction. In: *Status of Ketamine in Anesthesiology.* Domino EF (editor). NPP Books, 1990.

Aloia RC, Curtain CC, Gordon LM (editors): *Drug and Anesthetic Effects on Membrane Structure and Function.* Wiley-Liss, 1991.

Baden JM, Rice, SA: Metabolism and toxicity of inhaled anesthetics. In: *Anesthesia,* 4th ed. Miller RD (editor). Churchill Livingstone, 1994.

Bennett SN et al: Postoperative infections traced to contamination of an intravenous anesthetic, propofol. N Engl J Med 1995;333:147.

Berg-Johnson J, Langmoen IA: Isoflurane hyperpolarizes neurons in rat and human cerebral cortex. Acta Physiol Scand 1987;130:679.

Brett RS, Dilger JP, Yland KF: Isoflurane causes flickering of the acetylcholine receptor channel: Observations using the patch clamp. Anesthesiology 1988;69:161.

Bryson HM et al: Propofol: An update on its use in anaesthesia and conscious sedation. Drugs 1995;50:513.

Caldwell JE: Desflurane clinical pharmacokinetics and pharmacodynamics. Clin Pharmacokinet 1994;27:6.

Clarke JB et al: Halogenated anesthetics form liver adducts and antigens that cross-react with halothane-induced antibodies. Int Arch Allergy & Immunology 1995;108:24.

Dilger JP, Firestone LL: More models described for molecular "target" of anesthetics and alcohols. Trends Pharmacol Sci 1990;11:431.

Ebert TJ et al: Neurocirculatory responses to sevoflurane in humans. A comparison to desflurane. Anesthesiology 1995;83:88.

Eger EI II: New drugs in anesthesia. Int Anesth Clin 1995;33:61.

Eger EI II: Uptake and distribution. In: *Anesthesia,* 4th ed. Miller RD (editor). Churchill Livingstone, 1994.

Eger EI II, Saidman LJ, Brandstater B: Minimum alveolar anesthetic concentration: A standard of anesthetic potency. Anesthesiology 1965;26:756.

Fang ZX et al: Factors affecting production of compound A from the interaction of sevoflurane with baralyme and soda lime. Anesth Analg 1996;82:775.

Franks NP, Lieb WR: Molecular and cellular mechanisms of general anesthesia. Nature 1994;367:607.

Gibbons SJ et al: Inhibition of a fast inwardly rectifying potassium conductance by barbiturates. Anesth Analg 1996;82:1242.

Goldberg ME et al: Sevoflurane versus isoflurane for maintenance of anesthesia: Are serum fluoride ion concentrations of concern? Anesth Analg 1996;82:1268.

Haas DA, Harper DG: Ketamine: A review of its pharmacologic properties and use in ambulatory anesthesia. Anesth Prog 1992;39:61.

Halsey MJ: Molecular interactions of anaesthetics with biological membranes. Gen Pharmacol 1992;23:1013.

Jensen NF et al: Anesthetic considerations in porphyrias. Anesth Analg 1995;90:591.

Kenna JG, Jones RM: The organ toxicity of inhaled anesthetics. Anesth Analg 1995;81(6 Suppl):S51.

Kharasch ED et al: Human kidney methoxyflurane and sevoflurane metabolism: intrarenal fluoride production as a possible mechanism of methoxyflurane nephrotoxicity. Anesthesiology 1995;82:689.

Koblin DD: Mechanisms of action. In: *Anesthesia,* 4th ed. Miller RD (editor). Churchill Livingstone, 1994.

Laster M et al: Comparison of kinetics of sevoflurane and isoflurane in humans. Anesth Analg 1991;72:316.

Nakahiro M et al: General anesthetics modulate GABA receptor channel complex in rat dorsal root ganglions. FASEB J 1989;3:1850.

Nathanson MH et al: Sevoflurane versus desflurane for outpatient anesthesia: A comparison of maintenance and recovery profiles. Anesth Analg 1995;81:1186.

Patel SS, Goa KL: Desflurane: A review of its pharmacodynamic and pharmacokinetic properties and its efficacy in general anesthesia. Drugs 1995;50:742.

Pocock G, Richards CD: Excitatory and inhibitory synaptic mechanisms in anesthesia. Br J Anaesth 1993;71:134.

Smiley RM: An overview of induction and emergence characteristics of desflurane in pediatric, adult, and geriatric patients. Anesth Analg 1992;75(4 Suppl):S38.

Smith I et al: Propofol: An update on its clinical use. Anesthesiology 1994;81:1005.

Sweeney B et al: Toxicity of bone marrow in dentists exposed to nitrous oxide. Br Med J 1985;291:567.

Swerdlow BN, Holley FO: Intravenous anesthetic agents. Pharmacokinetic-pharmacodynamic relationships. Clin Pharmacokinet 1987;12:79.

Uchida H et al: Effect of propofol on spinal dorsal horn neurons. Anesthesiology 1995;83:1312.

Vessey MP: Epidemiological studies of the occupational hazards of anaesthesia. Anaesthesia 1978;33:430.

Weiskopf RB: Implications of chemical and physical properties of desflurane for longer surgery. Anaesthesia 1995;50(Suppl):9.

Young CJ, Apfelbaum JL: Inhalational anesthetics: Desflurane and sevoflurane. J Clin Anesth 1995;7:564.

Zimmerman SA et al: Potentiation of γ-aminobutyric acid$_A$ receptor Cl$^-$ current correlates with in vivo anesthetic potency. J Pharmacol Exp Ther 1994;270:987.

Local Anesthetics

26

Ronald D. Miller, MD

Local anesthetics reversibly block impulse conduction along nerve axons and other excitable membranes that utilize sodium channels as the primary means of action potential generation. This action can be used clinically to block pain sensation from—or sympathetic vasoconstrictor impulses to—specific areas of the body. Cocaine, the first such agent, was isolated by Niemann in 1860. It was introduced into clinical use by Koller in 1884 as an ophthalmic anesthetic. It was soon found to have strongly addicting central nervous system actions but was widely used, nevertheless, for 30 years, since it was the only local anesthetic drug available. In an attempt to improve the properties of cocaine, Einhorn in 1905 synthesized procaine, which became the dominant local anesthetic for the next 50 years. Since 1905, many local anesthetic agents have been synthesized. The goals of these efforts were reduction of local irritation and tissue damage, minimization of systemic toxicity, faster onset of action, and longer duration of action. Lidocaine, still a very popular agent, was synthesized in 1943 by Löfgren and may be considered the prototype local anesthetic agent.

None of the currently available local anesthetics are ideal, and development of newer agents continues. However, while it is relatively easy to synthesize a chemical with local anesthetic effects, it is very difficult to reduce the toxicity significantly below that of the current agents. The major reason for this difficulty is the fact that the most serious toxicity of local anesthetics represents extensions of the therapeutic effect on the brain and the circulatory system. However, new research into the stereoselective aspects of cardiac toxicity, possible alternative mechanisms of local anesthetic action (eg, inhibition of substance P actions), and alternative drug targets for spinal analgesia (eg, α_2 agonists) suggest that it may be possible to find better drugs, at least for spinal anesthesia.

I. BASIC PHARMACOLOGY OF LOCAL ANESTHETICS

Chemistry

Most local anesthetic agents consist of a lipophilic group (frequently an aromatic ring) connected by an intermediate chain (commonly including an ester or amide) to an ionizable group (usually a tertiary amine; Table 26–1). Optimal activity requires a delicate balance between the lipophilic and hydrophilic strengths of these groups. In addition to the general physical properties of the molecules, specific stereochemical configurations can also be important; ie, differences in the potency of stereoisomers have been documented for a few compounds, eg, bupivacaine, ropivacaine (de Jong, 1995; Valenzuela et al, 1995). Since ester links (as in procaine) are more prone to hydrolysis than amide links, esters usually have a shorter duration of action.

Local anesthetics are weak bases. For therapeutic application, they are usually made available as salts for reasons of solubility and stability. In the body, they exist either as the uncharged base or as a cation. The relative proportions of these two forms is governed by their pK_a and the pH of the body fluids according to the Henderson-Hasselbalch equation:

$$\log \frac{\text{Cationic form}}{\text{Unchanged form}} = pK_a - pH$$

Since the pK_a of most local anesthetics is in the range of 8.0–9.0, the larger fraction in the body fluids at physiologic pH will be the charged, cationic form. The cationic form is thought to be the most active form at the receptor site (cationic drug cannot

Table 26–1. Structure and properties of some ester and amide local anesthetics.[1]

	Lipophilic Group	Intermediate Chain	Amine Substituents	Potency (Procaine = 1)	Duration of Action
Esters					
Cocaine				2	Medium
Procaine (Novocain)				1	Short
Tetracaine (Pontocaine)				16	Long
Benzocaine				Surface use only	
Amides					
Lidocaine (Xylocaine, etc)				4	Medium
Mepivacaine (Carbocaine, Isocaine)				2	Medium
Bupivacaine (Marcaine)				16	Long
Etidocaine (Duranest)				16	Long
Prilocaine (Citanest)				3	Medium
Ropivacaine (Naropin)				16	Long

[1]Other chemical types are available including ethers (pramoxine), ketones (dyclonine), and phenetidin derivatives (phenacaine).

readily leave closed channels), but the uncharged form is very important for rapid penetration of biologic membranes: The local anesthetic receptor is not accessible from the external side of the cell membrane (Figure 14–2). This partly explains why dentists and surgeons observe that local anesthetics are much less effective in infected tissues; these tissues have a low extracellular pH, so that a very low fraction of nonionized local anesthetic is available for diffusion into the cell.

Pharmacokinetics

Local anesthetics are usually administered by injection into the area of the nerve fibers to be blocked. Thus, absorption and distribution are not as important in controlling the onset of effect as in determining the rate of offset of anesthesia and the likelihood of central nervous system and cardiac toxicity. Topical application of local anesthetics, however, requires drug diffusion for both onset and offset of anesthetic effect.

A. Absorption: Systemic absorption of injected local anesthetic from the site of administration is modified by several factors, including dosage, site of injection, drug-tissue binding, the presence of vasoconstricting substances, and the physicochemical properties of the drug. Application of a local anesthetic to a highly vascular area such as the tracheal mucosa results in more rapid absorption and thus higher blood levels than if the local anesthetic had been injected into a poorly perfused area, such as tendon. For regional anesthesia involving block of large nerves, maximum blood levels of local anesthetic decrease according to site of administration in the following order: intercostal (highest) > caudal > epidural > brachial plexus > sciatic nerve (lowest).

Vasoconstrictor substances such as epinephrine reduce systemic absorption of local anesthetics from the depot site by decreasing blood flow in these areas. This is especially true for drugs with intermediate and short durations of action such as procaine, lidocaine, and mepivacaine (but not prilocaine). Neuronal uptake of the drug is presumably enhanced by the higher local drug concentration, and the systemic toxic effects of the drug are reduced, since blood levels are lowered by as much as one-third. Furthermore, when used in spinal anesthesia, epinephrine acts directly on the cord to both enhance and prolong local anesthetic-induced spinal anesthesia by acting on α_2 adrenoceptors, which inhibit release of substance P and reduce dorsal horn neuron firing. (Realization of this concept has led to the use of clonidine not only to augment local anesthetic effect spinally but also to produce analgesia in its own right.) The combination of reduced systemic absorption, enhanced local anesthetic uptake by the nerve, and α_2 activation by epinephrine in the CNS is responsible for prolonging the local anesthetic effect by about 50%. Vasoconstrictors are less effective in prolonging anesthetic properties of the more lipid-soluble, long-acting drugs (bupivacaine, etidocaine),

possibly because these molecules are highly tissue-bound. As noted below, cocaine is a special case owing to its sympathomimetic properties (Table 6–5).

B. Distribution: The amide local anesthetics are widely distributed after intravenous bolus administration. There is evidence that sequestration occurs in storage sites, possibly fat tissue. After an initial rapid distribution phase, which probably indicates uptake into highly perfused organs such as the brain, liver, kidney, and heart, a slower distribution phase occurs with uptake into moderately well perfused tissues, such as muscle and gut. Because of the extremely short plasma half-lives of the ester type agents (see below), their tissue distribution has not been studied.

At the nerve fiber level, studies with sciatic nerve block using radioactive lidocaine suggest that only a small fraction of the anesthetic penetrates the fiber. However, the resulting functional block is proportionate to the intraneural concentration.

C. Metabolism and Excretion: The local anesthetics are converted in the liver or in plasma to more water-soluble metabolites and then excreted in the urine. Since local anesthetics in the uncharged form diffuse readily through lipid, little or no urinary excretion of the neutral form occurs. Acidification of urine will promote ionization of the tertiary base to the more water-soluble charged form, which is more readily excreted since it is not so easily reabsorbed by renal tubules.

Ester type local anesthetics are hydrolyzed very rapidly in the blood by butyrylcholinesterase (pseudocholinesterase). Therefore, they typically have very short plasma half-lives, eg, less than 1 minute for procaine and chloroprocaine.

The amide linkage of amide local anesthetics is hydrolyzed by liver microsomal cytochrome P450. There is considerable variation in the rate of liver metabolism of individual amide compounds, the approximate order being prilocaine (fastest) > etidocaine > lidocaine > mepivacaine > bupivacaine (slowest). As a result, toxicity from the amide type of local anesthetic is more likely to occur in patients with liver disease. For example, the average half-life of lidocaine may be increased from 1.8 hours in normal patients to over 6 hours in patients with severe liver disease. Many other drugs used in anesthesia are metabolized by the same P450 isozymes as the local anesthetics. For example, CYP3A4 in human hepatic microsomes metabolizes ropivacaine, a new long-acting agent. The same P450 isozyme metabolizes alfentanil and midazolam, both of which are extensively used in anesthesia. Concomitant use of the two latter agents may slow the metabolism of ropivacaine.

Decreased hepatic removal of local anesthetics should also be anticipated in patients with reduced hepatic blood flow. For example, the hepatic elimination of lidocaine in animals anesthetized with halothane is slower than that measured in animals receiving nitrous oxide and curare. The reduced elimination may be related to decreased hepatic blood flow and to halothane-induced depression of hepatic microsomes.

Pharmacodynamics

A. Mechanism of Action: The primary mechanism of action of local anesthetics—and perhaps the only action in peripheral nerve blockade—is **blockade of voltage-gated sodium channels.** The excitable membrane of nerve axons, like the membrane of cardiac muscle (see Chapter 14) and neuronal cell bodies (see Chapter 21), maintains a transmembrane potential of –90 to –60 mV. During excitation, the sodium channels open, and a fast inward sodium current quickly depolarizes the membrane toward the sodium equilibrium potential (+40 mV). As a result of depolarization, the sodium channels close (inactivate) and potassium channels open. The outward flow of potassium repolarizes the membrane toward the potassium equilibrium potential (about –95 mV); repolarization returns the sodium channels to the rested state. The transmembrane ionic gradients are maintained by the sodium pump. These characteristics are similar to those of heart muscle, and local anesthetics have similar effects in both tissues.

The function of sodium channels can be disrupted in several ways. Biologic toxins such as **batrachotoxin, aconitine, veratridine,** and some **scorpion venoms** bind to receptors within the channel and prevent inactivation. This results in prolonged influx of sodium through the channel rather than block of conduction, with the result that some investigators consider these agents *agonists* at the sodium channel. The marine toxins **tetrodotoxin** and **saxitoxin** block these channels by binding to channel receptors near the extracellular surface. Their clinical effects superficially resemble those of local anesthetics even though their receptor site is quite different. Local anesthetics bind to receptors near the intracellular end of the channel (Figure 14–2) and block the channel in a time- and voltage-dependent fashion (see below). The sodium channel has been cloned and its primary structure identified. However, its three-dimensional structure has not been solved. As a result, the molecular mechanism of local anesthetic binding and blockade has not yet been determined.

When progressively increasing concentrations of a local anesthetic are applied to a nerve fiber, the threshold for excitation increases, impulse conduction slows, the rate of rise of the action potential declines, the action potential amplitude decreases, and, finally, the ability to generate an action potential is abolished. These incremental effects result from binding of the local anesthetic to more and more sodium channels; in each channel, binding results in blockade of the sodium current. If the sodium current is blocked over a critical length of the nerve, propagation across the blocked area is no longer possible. At the minimum dose required to block propagation, the resting potential is not significantly affected.

The blockade of sodium channels by most local anesthetics is *voltage-* and *time-dependent:* Channels in the rested state (which predominate at more negative membrane potentials) have a much lower affinity for local anesthetics than activated (open state) and inactivated channels (which predominate at more positive membrane potentials; Figure 14–8). Thus, the effect of a given drug concentration is more marked in rapidly firing axons than in resting fibers (Figure 26–1).

Between depolarizations of the axon, a portion of the sodium channels recover from local anesthetic block (Figure 14–8). The recovery from drug-induced block is 10–1000 times slower than the recovery of channels from normal inactivation, as shown for the cardiac membrane in Figure 14–4. As a result, the refractory period is lengthened and the nerve can conduct fewer impulses.

Elevated extracellular calcium partially antagonizes the action of local anesthetics. This reversal is caused by the calcium-induced increase of the surface potential on the membrane, which favors the low-affinity rested state. Conversely, increase of extracellular potassium depolarizes the membrane potential and favors the inactivated state (Figure 14–9). This enhances the effect of local anesthetics.

Although local anesthetics can be shown to block a variety of other channels, including chemically gated synaptic channels, there is no convincing evidence that such actions play an important role in the clinical effects of these drugs. However, experimental studies in both nerve fibers and cardiac muscle cells indicate

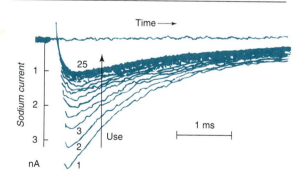

Figure 26–1. Effect of repetitive activity on the block of sodium current produced by a local anesthetic in a myelinated axon. A series of 25 pulses was applied, and the resulting sodium currents are superimposed. Note that the current produced by the pulses rapidly decreased from the first to the 25th pulse. A long rest period following the train resulted in recovery from block, but the block could be reinstated by a subsequent train. (nA, nanoamperes.) (Modified slightly and reproduced, with permission, from Courtney KR: Mechanism of frequency-dependent inhibition of sodium currents in frog myelinated nerve by the lidocaine derivative GEA. J Pharmacol Exp Ther 1975;195:225.)

that drugs which prolong the action potential can significantly increase the sensitivity of sodium channels to local anesthetic blockade (Drachman et al, 1991). This can be explained by the observations described above, ie, that the affinity of activated and inactivated channels for local anesthetics is greater than the affinity of channels in the rested state.

Structure-activity characteristics of local anesthetics. The smaller and more lipophilic the molecule, the faster the rate of interaction with the sodium channel receptor. Potency is also positively correlated with lipid solubility as long as the agent retains sufficient water solubility to diffuse to the site of action. Lidocaine, procaine, and mepivacaine are more water-soluble than tetracaine, etidocaine, and bupivacaine. The latter agents are more potent and have longer durations of action. They also bind more extensively to proteins and will displace or be displaced from these binding sites by other drugs.

Alternative or complementary mechanisms of action may apply to the use of the local anesthetics in spinal anesthesia. The preliminary evidence of inhibition of the postsynaptic actions of substance P has been mentioned (Li et al, 1995) and deserves further investigation.

B. Actions on Nerves: Since local anesthetics are capable of blocking all nerves, their actions are not usually limited to the desired loss of sensation. Although motor paralysis may at times be desirable, it may also limit the ability of the patient to cooperate, eg, during obstetric delivery. During spinal anesthesia, motor paralysis may impair respiratory activity and autonomic nerve blockade may lead to hypotension. However, different types of nerve fibers differ significantly in their susceptibility to local anesthetic blockade on the basis of size and myelination (Table 26–2). Upon application of a local anesthetic to a nerve root, the smaller B and C fibers are blocked first. The small type A delta fibers are blocked next. Thus, pain fibers are blocked first; other sensations disappear next; and motor function is blocked last.

1. Effect of fiber diameter–Local anesthetics preferentially block small fibers because the distance over which such fibers can passively propagate an electrical impulse (related to the space constant) is shorter. During the onset of local anesthesia, when short sections of nerve are blocked, the small-diameter fibers are the first to fail to conduct. For myelinated nerves, three successive nodes must be blocked by the local anesthetic to halt impulse propagation. The thicker the nerve fiber, the farther apart the nodes tend to be—which explains, in part, the greater resistance to block of large fibers. Myelinated nerves tend to become blocked before unmyelinated nerves of the same diameter. For this reason, the preganglionic B fibers may be blocked before the smaller unmyelinated C fibers.

2. Effect of firing frequency–Another important reason for preferential blockade of sensory fibers follows directly from the state-dependent mechanism of action of local anesthetics. Block by these drugs is more marked at higher frequencies of depolarization and with longer depolarizations. Sensory fibers, especially pain fibers, have a high firing rate and a relatively long action potential duration (up to 5 ms). Motor fibers fire at a slower rate and have a shorter action potential duration (< 0.5 ms). A delta and C fibers are small-diameter fibers that participate in high-frequency pain transmission. They therefore are blocked sooner with low concentrations of local anesthetics than are the A alpha fibers.

3. Effect of fiber position in the nerve bundle–An anatomic circumstance that sometimes creates exceptions to the above rules for differential nerve block is the location of the fiber in the peripheral bundle. In large nerve trunks, motor nerves are usually located circumferentially, and for that reason they are exposed first to the drug when it is administered by injection into the tissue surrounding the nerve. Therefore, it is not uncommon that motor nerve block occurs before sensory block in large mixed nerves. In the extremities, proximal sensory fibers are located in the mantle of the nerve trunk, whereas the distal sensory innervation is in the core of the nerve. Thus, during infiltration block of a large nerve, anesthesia first develops proximally and then spreads distally as the drug penetrates the core of the nerve.

Table 26–2. Relative size and susceptibility to block of types of nerve fibers.

Fiber Type	Function	Diameter (μm)	Myelination	Conduction Velocity (m/s)	Sensitivity to Block
Type A					
Alpha	Proprioception, motor	12–20	Heavy	70–120	+
Beta	Touch, pressure	5–12	Heavy	30–70	++
Gamma	Muscle spindles	3–6	Heavy	15–30	++
Delta	Pain, temperature	2–5	Heavy	12–30	+++
Type B	Preganglionic autonomic	< 3	Light	3–15	++++
Type C					
Dorsal root	Pain	0.4–1.2	None	0.5–2.3	++++
Sympathetic	Postganglionic	0.3–1.3	None	0.7–2.3	++++

C. Effects on Other Excitable Membranes:

Local anesthetics have weak neuromuscular blocking effects that are of little clinical importance. However, their effects on cardiac cell membranes are of major clinical significance. Some are useful antiarrhythmic agents (see Chapter 14) at concentrations lower than those required to produce nerve block, and all can *cause* arrhythmias in high enough concentration.

II. CLINICAL PHARMACOLOGY OF LOCAL ANESTHETICS

Local anesthetics can provide temporary but complete analgesia of well-defined parts of the body. The usual routes of administration include topical application, injection in the vicinity of peripheral nerve endings and major nerve trunks, and instillation within the epidural or subarachnoid spaces surrounding the spinal cord (Figure 26–2). In addition, block of autonomic sympathetic fibers can be used to evaluate the role of sympathetic tone in patients with peripheral vasospasm.

The choice of local anesthetic for a specific procedure is usually based on the duration of action required. Procaine and chloroprocaine are short-acting; lidocaine, mepivacaine, and prilocaine have an intermediate duration of action; tetracaine, bupivacaine, etidocaine, and ropivacaine are long-acting drugs (Table 26–1).

As noted above, the anesthetic effect of the agents with short and intermediate durations of action can be prolonged by increasing the dose or by adding a vasoconstrictor agent, such as epinephrine or phenylephrine. The vasoconstrictor retards the removal of drug from the injection site. In addition, it decreases the blood level and hence the chance of toxicity.

The onset of local anesthesia is sometimes accelerated by the use of solutions saturated with carbon dioxide ("carbonated"). The high tissue level of CO_2 results in intracellular acidosis (CO_2 crosses membranes readily), which in turn results in intracellular accumulation of the cationic form of the local anesthetic.

Repeated injection of local anesthetics during epidural anesthesia results in loss of effectiveness (tachyphylaxis). This is probably a consequence of local extracellular acidosis. Local anesthetics are commonly marketed as hydrochloride salts (pH 4.0–6.0). After injection, the salts are buffered in the tissue to physiologic pH, thereby providing sufficient free base for diffusion through axonal membranes. However, repeated injections deplete the local available buffer. The ensuing acidosis increases the extracellular cationic form, which diffuses poorly into axons. The clinical result is apparent tachyphylaxis, especially in areas of limited buffer reserve, such as the cerebrospinal fluid.

Toxicity

Ultimately, local anesthetic agents are absorbed from the site of administration. If blood levels rise too high, effects on several organ systems may be observed.

A. Central Nervous System: Since prehistoric times, the natives of Peru have chewed the leaves of the indigenous plant *Erythroxylon coca,* the source of cocaine, to obtain a feeling of well-being and reduce fatigue. Intense central nervous system effects can be achieved by sniffing cocaine powder and smoking cocaine base. Cocaine has become one of the most widely used drugs of abuse (see Chapter 32).

Other central nervous system effects include sleepiness, light-headedness, visual and auditory disturbances, and restlessness. At higher concentrations, nystagmus and shivering may occur. Finally, overt tonic-clonic convulsions followed by central nervous system depression and death may occur with all local anesthetics, including cocaine. Local anesthetics apparently lead to depression of cortical inhibitory pathways, thereby allowing unopposed activity of excitatory components. This transitional stage of unbalanced excitation may be followed by generalized central nervous system depression if higher blood levels of local anesthetic are reached.

Most serious toxic reactions to local anesthetics are due to convulsions from excessive blood levels. These are best prevented by administering the smallest dose of local anesthetic required for adequate anesthesia. When large doses must be administered, premedication with a benzodiazepine, eg, diazepam, 0.1–0.2 mg/kg parenterally, probably provides significant prophylaxis against seizures. If seizures do occur, it is essential to prevent hypoxemia and acidosis. Although administration of oxygen does not prevent seizure activity, hyperoxemia after onset of seizures appears to be beneficial. Conversely, hypercapnia and acidosis appear to promote the occurrence of seizures. Thus, hyperventilation is recommended during treatment of seizures. Hyperventilation increases blood pH, which in turn lowers extracellular potassium. This hyperpolarizes the transmembrane potential of axons, which favors the rested or low-affinity state of the sodium channels, resulting in decreased local anesthetic toxicity.

Seizures induced by local anesthetics can also be treated with small doses of short-acting barbiturates, eg, thiopental, 1–2 mg/kg intravenously, or diazepam, 0.1 mg/kg intravenously. The muscular manifestations can be suppressed by a short-acting neuromuscular blocking agent, eg, succinylcholine, 0.5–1 mg/kg intravenously. It should be emphasized that succinylcholine does not obliterate cortical manifestations on the EEG. In especially severe cases of convulsions, intubation of the trachea combined with succinylcholine administration and mechanical ventilation can prevent pulmonary aspiration of gastric contents and facilitate hyperventilation therapy.

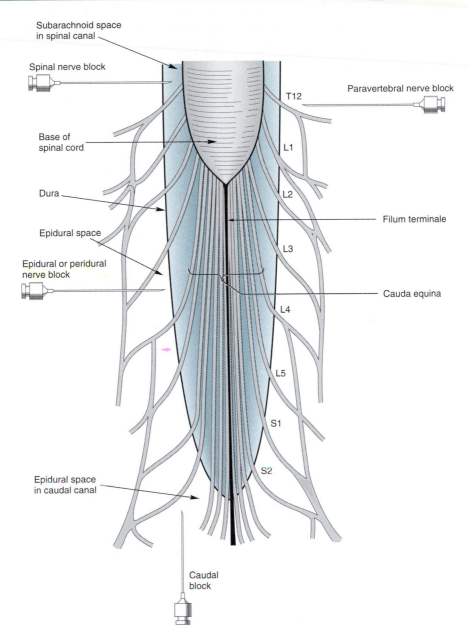

Subarachnoid space
in spinal canal

Spinal nerve block

T12

Paravertebral nerve block

Base of
spinal cord

L1

Dura

L2

Filum terminale

Epidural space

L3

Epidural or peridural
nerve block

Cauda equina

L4

L5

S1

S2

Epidural space
in caudal canal

Caudal
block

Figure 26–2. Schematic diagram of sites of injection of local anesthetics in and near the spinal canal.

B. Peripheral Nervous System (Neurotoxicity): When applied at excessively high concentrations, all local anesthetics can be toxic to nerve tissue. Several case reports document prolonged sensory and motor deficits following accidental spinal anesthesia with large volumes of chloroprocaine. Whether chloroprocaine is more neurotoxic than other local anesthetics has not been determined. More recently, severe neurotoxicity has been reported when lidocaine was used for prolonged spinal anesthesia. It is proposed that this toxicity results from pooling of high concentrations of the local anesthetic in the cauda equina. Although the mechanism of this neurotoxic action is not known, it has been shown that it does not result from excessive sodium channel blockade (Sakura et al, 1995).

C. Cardiovascular System: The cardiovascular effects of local anesthetics result partly from direct effects upon the cardiac and smooth muscle membranes and from indirect effects upon the autonomic nerves. As described in Chapter 14, local anesthetics block cardiac sodium channels and thus depress abnormal cardiac pacemaker activity, excitability, and conduction. With the exception of cocaine, they also depress the strength of cardiac contraction and cause arteriolar dilation, both effects leading to hypotension. Although cardiovascular collapse and death usually occur only after large doses, they may result occasionally from the small amounts used for infiltration anesthesia.

As noted above, cocaine differs from the other local anesthetics in its cardiovascular effects. The blockade of norepinephrine reuptake results in vasoconstriction and hypertension. It may also precipitate cardiac arrhythmias. The vasoconstriction produced by cocaine can lead to ischemia and, in chronic abusers, to ulceration of the mucous membrane and even damage to the nasal septum. This vasoconstrictor property of cocaine can be used clinically to decrease bleeding from mucosal damage in the nasopharynx.

Bupivacaine is more cardiotoxic than other local anesthetics. Several case reports have appeared indicating that accidental intravenous injection of bupivacaine may lead not only to seizures but also to cardiovascular collapse, from which resuscitation may be extremely difficult or unsuccessful. Several experimental animal studies have confirmed the idea that bupivacaine is indeed more toxic when given intravenously than most other local anesthetics. This reflects the fact that bupivacaine block of sodium channels is greatly potentiated by the very long action potential duration of cardiac cells (as compared to nerve fibers) and, unlike lidocaine blockade, cumulates markedly at normal heart rates. Subsequent studies have shown that the most common electrocardiographic finding in patients with bupivacaine intoxication is slow idioventricular rhythm with broad QRS complexes and electromechanical dissociation. Resuscitation has been successful with standard cardiopulmonary support—including the prompt correction of acidosis by hyperventilation and administration of bicarbonate—and aggressive administration of epinephrine, atropine, and bretylium. Local anesthetics, especially bupivacaine, also inhibit basal and epinephrine-stimulated cAMP production. This finding places greater emphasis on aggressive epinephrine therapy during bupivacaine-induced cardiotoxicity. **Ropivacaine** is a new investigational amide local anesthetic with effects similar to those of bupivacaine except for less intense motor block as compared with similar sensory block. It also probably has lower cardiovascular toxicity than bupivacaine, perhaps because ropivacaine is available as the *(S)* stereoisomer (de Jong, 1995), which has inherently less affinity for the cardiac sodium channel.

D. Blood: The administration of large doses (> 10 mg/kg) of prilocaine during regional anesthesia may lead to accumulation of the metabolite *o*-toluidine, an oxidizing agent capable of converting hemoglobin to methemoglobin. When sufficient methemoglobin is present (3–5 mg/dL), the patient may appear cyanotic and the blood chocolate-colored. Such levels of methemoglobinemia are tolerated by healthy individuals but may cause decompensation in patients with cardiac or pulmonary disease and require immediate treatment. Reducing agents such as methylene blue or, less satisfactorily, ascorbic acid may be given intravenously to rapidly convert methemoglobin to hemoglobin.

E. Allergic Reactions: The ester type local anesthetics are metabolized to *p*-aminobenzoic acid derivatives. These metabolites are responsible for allergic reactions in a small percentage of the population. Amides are not metabolized to *p*-aminobenzoic acid, and allergic reactions to agents of the amide group are extremely rare.

PREPARATIONS AVAILABLE

Benzocaine (generic, others)
   Topical: 5, 6% creams; 6, 20% gels; 5% ointments; 0.5% lotion; 20% spray
Bupivacaine (generic, Marcaine, Sensorcaine)
   Parenteral: 0.25, 0.5, 0.75% for injection; 0.25, 0.5, 0.75% with 1:200,000 epinephrine
Butamben picrate (Butesin Picrate)
   Topical: 1% ointment
Chloroprocaine (Nesacaine)
   Parenteral: 1, 2, 3% for injection
Cocaine (generic)
   Topical: 40, 100, mg/mL solutions; 5, 25 g powder; 135 mg soluble tablets
Dibucaine (generic, Nupercainal)
   Topical: 0.5% cream; 1% ointment

Dyclonine (Dyclone)
   Topical: 0.5, 1% solution
Etidocaine (Duranest)
   Parenteral: 1% for injection; 1, 1.5% with 1:200,000 epinephrine for injection
Lidocaine (generic, Xylocaine, others)
   Parenteral: 0.5, 1, 1.5, 2, 4, 10, 20% for injection; 0.5, 1, 1.5, 2% with 1:200,000 epinephrine; 1, 2% with 1:100,000 epinephrine, 2% with 1:50,000 epinephrine
   Topical: 2.5, 5% ointments; 0.5% cream; 2% jelly and solution; 2, 4, 10% solutions
Mepivacaine (generic, Carbocaine, others)
   Parenteral: 1, 1.5, 2, 3% for injection; 2% with 1:20,000 levonordefrin

Pramoxine (Tronothane, Prax)
Topical: 0.5, 1% cream; 1% lotion and gel

Prilocaine (Citanest)
Parenteral: 4% for injection; 4% with 1:200,000 epinephrine

Procaine (generic, Novocain)
Parenteral: 1, 2, 10% for injection

Propoxycaine and procaine (Ravocaine and Novocain)
Parenteral: 7.2 mg propoxycaine with 36 mg procaine and norepinephrine or cobefrin per 1.8 mL dental injection unit

Ropivacaine (Naropin)
Parenteral: 2, 5, 7.5, 10 mg/mL solution for injection

Tetracaine (Pontocaine)
Parenteral: 1% for injection; 0.2, 0.3% with 6% dextrose for spinal anesthesia
Topical: 0.5% ointment; 0.5% solution (ophthalmic); 1% cream; 2% solution for sore throat

REFERENCES

Albright GA: Cardiac arrest following regional anesthesia with etidocaine or bupivacaine. Anesthesiology 1979;51:285.

Arthur GR, Feldman HS, Covino BG: Comparative pharmacokinetics of bupivacaine and proparacaine, a new amide local anesthetic. Anesth Analg 1988;67:1053.

Butterworth JF, Strichartz GR: Molecular mechanisms of local anesthesia: A review. Anesthesiology 1990;72:711.

Catterall WA: Structure and function of voltage-sensitive ion channels. Science 1988;242:50.

Clarkson CW, Hondeghem LM: Evidence for a specific receptor site for lidocaine, quinidine, and bupivacaine associated with cardiac sodium channels in guinea pig ventricular myocardium. Circ Res 1985;56:496.

Concepcion M et al: A new local anesthetic, ropivacaine. Its epidural effects in humans. Anesth Analg 1990;70:80.

Covino BG: Pharmacology of local anaesthetic agents. Br J Anaesth 1986;58:701.

de Jong RH: Ropivacaine. White knight or dark horse? Reg Anesth 1995;20:474.

Drachman D, Strichartz G: Potassium channel blockers potentiate impulse inhibition by local anesthetics. Anesthesiology 1991;75:1051.

Eisenach JC, Lyzak SZ, Viscomi CL: Epidural clonidine analgesia following surgery: Phase I. Anesthesiology 1989;71:640.

Fleming JA, Byck R, Barash PG: Pharmacology and therapeutic applications of cocaine. Anesthesiology 1990;73:518.

Hille B: Local anesthetics: Hydrophilic and hydrophobic pathways for the drug-receptor reactions. J Gen Physiol 1977;69:497.

Kendig JJ, Courtney KR: New modes of nerve block. Anesthesiology 1991;74:207.

Li YM et al: Local anesthetics inhibit substance P binding and evoked increases in intracellular Ca^{2+}. Anesthesiology 1995;82:166.

Oda Y et al: Metabolism of a new local anesthetic, ropivacaine, by human hepatic cytochrome P450. Anesthesiology 1995;82:214.

Popitz-Bergez FA et al: Relation between functional deficit and intraneural local anesthetic during peripheral nerve block: A study in the rat sciatic nerve. Anesthesiology 1995;83:583.

Ragsdale DS et al: Molecular determinants of state-dependent block of Na^+ channels by local anesthetics. Science 1994;265:1724.

Ravindran RS et al: Prolonged neural blockade following regional anesthesia with 2-chloroprocaine. Anesth Analg 1980;59:447.

Reiz S, Nath S: Cardiotoxicity of local anesthetic agents. Br J Anaesth 1986;58:736.

Rigler ML et al: Cauda equina syndrome after continuous spinal anesthesia. Anesth Analg 1991;72:275.

Sakura S et al: Local anesthetic neurotoxicity does not result from blockade of voltage-gated sodium channels. Anesth Analg 1995;81:338.

Scott DB et al: Acute toxicity of ropivacaine compared to that of bupivacaine. Anesth Analg 1989;69:563.

Strichartz GR et al: Fundamental properties of local anesthetics: II. Measured octanol:buffer partition coefficients and pK_a values of clinically used drugs. Anesth Analg 1990;71:158.

Strichartz GR: Pharmacology of local anesthetics. In: *Anesthesia*, 4th ed. Miller RD (editor). Churchill Livingstone, 1994.

Tucker GT: Pharmacokinetics of local anaesthetics. Br J Anaesth 1986;58:717.

Valenzuela C et al: Stereoselective block of cardiac sodium channels by bupivacaine in guinea pig ventricular myocytes. Circulation 1995;92:3014.

27

Skeletal Muscle Relaxants

Ronald D. Miller, MD

Drugs that affect skeletal muscle function fall into two major therapeutic groups: those used during surgical procedures and in intensive care units to cause paralysis, ie, **neuromuscular blockers,** and those used to reduce spasticity in a variety of neurologic conditions, ie, **spasmolytics.** Members of the first group, as their name implies, interfere with transmission at the neuromuscular end plate and are not CNS-active drugs. However, because they are used primarily as adjuncts to general anesthesia, they are often discussed in connection with central nervous system agents. Drugs in the second group have traditionally been called "centrally acting" muscle relaxants. However, at least one of these agents (dantrolene) has no significant central effects, so the traditional name is now inappropriate.

NEUROMUSCULAR BLOCKING DRUGS

History

During the 16th century, European explorers found that natives of the Amazon Basin of South America were using an arrow poison that produced death by skeletal muscle paralysis. This poison later became the subject of intense investigation. **Curare,** the active crude material, formed the basis for some of the earliest scientific studies in pharmacology. The active principle from curare, **tubocurarine** (*d*-tubocurarine), and its synthetic derivatives have had a tremendous influence on the practice of anesthesia and surgery and have been useful also in defining normal neuromuscular physiologic mechanisms.

Normal Neuromuscular Function

Theoretically, muscular relaxation and paralysis can occur from interruption of function at several sites, including the central nervous system, myelinated somatic nerves, unmyelinated motor nerve terminals, nicotinic acetylcholine receptors, the motor end plate, and the muscle membrane or contractile apparatus (Figure 27–1). The mechanism of neuromuscular transmission at the end plate is similar to that described in Chapter 6, with arrival of an impulse at the motor nerve terminal, influx of calcium, and release of acetylcholine. Acetylcholine then diffuses across the synaptic cleft to the nicotinic receptor located on the motor end plate. As noted in Chapter 7, this receptor is composed of five peptides: two alpha peptides, one beta, one gamma, and one delta peptide. Combination of two acetylcholine molecules with receptors on the two alpha subunits causes opening of the channel. The resulting movements of sodium and potassium are associated with depolarization of the end plate membrane. This change in voltage is termed the end plate potential. The magnitude of the end plate potential is directly related to the amount of acetylcholine released. If the potential is small, the permeability and the end plate potential return to normal without an impulse being propagated from the end plate region to the rest of the muscle membrane. However, if the end plate potential is large, the muscle membrane is depolarized to its threshold, and an action potential will be propagated along the entire muscle fiber. Muscle contraction is then initiated by excitation-contraction coupling. The released acetylcholine is removed from the end plate region by diffusion and rapid enzymatic destruction by acetylcholinesterase.

Two additional types of acetylcholine receptors are associated with the neuromuscular apparatus. One is located on the presynaptic motor axon terminal; activation mobilizes additional transmitter for subsequent release, perhaps by mobilizing more acetylcholine vesicles within the ending. The second type of receptor is found on perijunctional cells and not normally involved in transmission. However, under certain conditions, eg, prolonged immobilization, these receptors may proliferate sufficiently to affect neuromuscular transmission.

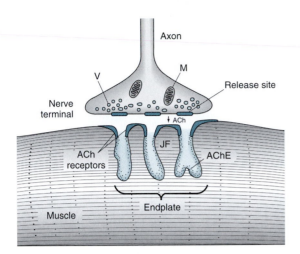

Figure 27–1. Schematic representation of the neuromuscular junction. (V, transmitter vesicle; M, mitochondrion; ACh, acetylcholine; AChE, acetylcholinesterase; JF, junctional folds.) (Reproduced, with permission, from Drachman DB: Myasthenia gravis. N Engl J Med 1978; 298:135.)

Blockade of normal end plate function can occur by two mechanisms. Pharmacologic blockade of the agonist, acetylcholine, is characteristic of *antagonist* drugs. These drugs prevent access of the transmitter to its receptor and prevent depolarization. The prototype of this **nondepolarizing** subgroup is tubocurarine. Block of transmission can also be produced by an excess of depolarizing *agonist*. (This paradoxical effect also occurs at the ganglionic nicotinic acetylcholine receptor.) The prototype **depolarizing** blocking drug is succinylcholine. A similar depolarizing block can be produced by acetylcholine itself if very high local concentrations are reached (eg, in cholinesterase inhibitor intoxication), by nicotine, and by other nicotinic agonists. However, because the block produced by these drugs cannot be controlled adequately, they are of no clinical value in this application.

I. BASIC PHARMACOLOGY OF NEUROMUSCULAR BLOCKING DRUGS

Chemistry

All of the neuromuscular blocking drugs bear a structural resemblance to acetylcholine. In fact, succinylcholine is two acetylcholine molecules linked end-to-end (Figure 27–2). In contrast to the single linear structure of succinylcholine and other depolarizing drugs, the nondepolarizing agents conceal the "double-acetylcholine" structure in one of two types of bulky, relatively rigid ring systems (eg, pancuro-

nium; Figure 27–2). The two major families of nondepolarizing blocking drugs (isoquinoline derivatives and steroids) are shown in Figures 27–3 and 27–4. Another feature common to all useful drugs in this class is the presence of one or two quaternary nitrogens, which makes them poorly soluble in lipid and prevents entry into the central nervous system.

Pharmacokinetics of Neuromuscular Blocking Drugs

All of the neuromuscular blocking drugs are highly polar and inactive when administered by mouth. They are always administered intravenously.

A. Nondepolarizing Drugs: The rate of disappearance of a nondepolarizing neuromuscular block-

Acetylcholine

Succinylcholine

Pancuronium

Figure 27–2. Structural relationship of succinylcholine, a depolarizing agent, and pancuronium, a nondepolarizing agent, to acetylcholine, the neuromuscular transmitter. Succinylcholine, originally called diacetylcholine, is simply two molecules of acetylcholine linked through the acetate methyl groups. Pancuronium may be viewed as two acetylcholine-like fragments *(outlined in blue print)* oriented on a steroid nucleus.

Figure 27–3. Structures of some isoquinoline neuromuscular blocking drugs. These agents are all nondepolarizing in their action.

Figure 27–4. Structures of some steroid neuromuscular blocking drugs. These agents are all nondepolarizing in their action.

ing drug from blood is characterized by a rapid initial distribution phase followed by a slower elimination phase. Because neuromuscular blocking drugs are highly ionized, they do not cross membranes well and have a limited volume of distribution of 80–140 mL/kg—not much larger than blood volume.

The route of elimination is strongly correlated with the duration of action of nondepolarizing relaxants. Drugs that are excreted by the kidney have long half-lives and long durations of action (> 35 minutes). Drugs eliminated by the liver have shorter half-lives and durations of action (Table 27–1). All steroidal muscle relaxants are metabolized to their 3-hydroxy, 17-hydroxy, and 3,17-dihydroxy products, mainly in the liver. The 3-hydroxy metabolites are usually 40–80% as potent as the parent drug. These metabolites are not formed in sufficient quantities to cause significant additional neuromuscular block during surgical anesthesia. However, if the parent compound is being given for several days, as may be done in the intensive care unit, the 3-hydroxy metabolite may accumulate and cause prolonged paralysis (Segredo et al, 1992) because the 3-hydroxy metabolite is more slowly cleared than the parent compound (Caldwell et al, 1994). Although the remaining metabolites also have neuromuscular blocking properties, they are very weak.

The intermediate-duration muscle relaxants (vecuronium and rocuronium) tend to be more dependent on biliary excretion or hepatic metabolism for their elimination. These drugs are more commonly used clinically than the long-acting drugs. Vecuronium has a steroid nucleus like that of pancuronium (Figure 27–4), differing only in that one of the nitrogens is tertiary rather than quaternary. Despite this small structural difference, vecuronium has distinctly different pharmacologic properties. Vecuronium has a shorter duration of action (approximately 20–35 minutes versus 60 minutes) and minimal cardiovascular effects, and is not as dependent upon the kidney for its elimination. Only about 15% of an injected dose of vecuronium is eliminated by the kidney; the remaining 85% is eliminated into the bile as either the unchanged drug or its 3-hydroxy metabolite. Rocuronium is the newest of the steroid derivatives and has a pharmacokinetic profile similar to that of vecuronium. Rocuronium has the most rapid onset time of any nondepolarizing muscle relaxant. It therefore may become the preferred drug for rapid-sequence induction of anesthesia and endotracheal intubation.

Atracurium (Figure 27–3) is an isoquinoline nondepolarizing muscle relaxant with many of the same characteristics as vecuronium. Atracurium is probably inactivated by a form of spontaneous breakdown (Hofmann elimination) rather than being dependent on renal or hepatic mechanisms for the termination of its action. The main breakdown products are laudanosine and a related quaternary acid, neither of which has neuromuscular blocking properties. However, lau-

Table 27–1. Some properties of neuromuscular blocking drugs.

Drug	Elimination via	Clearance (mL/kg/min)	Approximate Duration of Action (minutes)	Approximate Potency Relative to Tubocurarine
Isoquinoline derivatives				
Atracurium	Spontaneous[1]	6.6	20–35	1.5
Cisatracurium	Mostly spontaneous	6	25–44	1.5
Doxacurium	Kidney	2.7	> 35	6
Metocurine	Kidney (40%)	1.2	> 35	4
Mivacurium	Plasma ChE[2]	7.2	10–20	4
Tubocurarine	Kidney (40%)	2.3	> 35	1
Steroid derivatives				
Pancuronium	Kidney (80%)	1.8	> 35	6
Pipecuronium	Kidney (60%) and liver	3.0	> 35	6
Rocuronium	Liver (75–90%) and kidney	2.9	20–35	0.8
Vecuronium	Liver (75–90%) and kidney	5.3	20–35	6
Other agents				
Gallamine	Kidney (100%)	1.3	> 35	0.2
Succinylcholine	Plasma ChE[2] (100%)	Data not found	< 8	Different mechanism[3]

[1]Nonenzymatic and enzymatic hydrolysis of ester bonds.
[2]Butyrylcholinesterase (pseudocholinesterase).
[3]A depolarizing cholinoceptor agonist.

danosine is very slowly metabolized by the liver and has a long elimination half-life (ie, 150 minutes) in comparison with its parent compound, atracurium. It readily crosses the blood-brain barrier and at high blood concentrations may cause seizures. In dogs and rabbits, 17 µg/mL and 3.9 µg/mL blood concentrations of laudanosine, respectively, are required to cause seizures. During surgical procedures in humans, blood levels have ranged from 0.2 to 1 µg/mL. However, with prolonged infusions of atracurium in the intensive care unit, blood levels of laudanosine as high as 5.5 µg/mL have been reported. At much lower blood concentrations (0.2–0.8 µg/mL), laudanosine causes about a 30% increase in anesthetic requirement.

Atracurium has stereoisomers, and some of these have been examined for possible advantages over atracurium itself. One of these, **cisatracurium,** has been approved for use. It has the advantages of atracurium (little dependence on renal or hepatic function and intermediate duration of action) but forms less laudanosine and releases less histamine from tissue stores (Eastwood et al, 1995).

Mivacurium has the shortest duration of action of any nondepolarizing muscle relaxant (Table 27–1). By virtue of its double bond and asymmetric carbons, mivacurium consists of a mixture of isomers (primarily *trans,trans* [52–62%], *cis,trans* [34–40%], and *cis,cis* [4–8%]). Clearance of these forms is rapid (Table 27–1)—by plasma cholinesterase—and is not dependent on the liver or kidney. However, because patients with renal failure have decreased plasma cholinesterase levels, the duration of action of mivacurium may be prolonged in patients with impaired renal function.

B. Depolarizing Drugs: The extremely brief duration of action of succinylcholine (5–10 minutes) is due chiefly to its rapid hydrolysis by plasma cholinesterase (butyrylcholinesterase, pseudocholinesterase), an enzyme of the liver and plasma. Apparently, plasma cholinesterase metabolizes succinylcholine more rapidly than mivacurium, since the duration of action of succinylcholine is shorter than that of mivacurium (Table 27–1). The initial metabolite, succinylmonocholine, is a much weaker neuromuscular blocker. It in turn is metabolized to succinic acid and choline. Plasma cholinesterase has an enormous capacity to hydrolyze succinylcholine at a very rapid rate; as a result, only a small fraction of the original intravenous dose reaches the neuromuscular junction. Since there is little or no plasma cholinesterase at the motor end plate, the neuromuscular blockade of succinylcholine is terminated by its diffusion away from the end plate into extracellular fluid. Plasma cholinesterase, therefore, influences the duration of action of succinylcholine by determining the amount of the drug that reaches the end plate.

Neuromuscular blockade by both succinylcholine and mivacurium may be prolonged in patients with an abnormal variant of plasma cholinesterase of genetic origin. The "dibucaine number"—a test for ability to

metabolize succinylcholine—can be used to identify such patients. Under standardized test conditions, dibucaine inhibits the normal enzyme about 80% and abnormal enzyme only 20%. Many genetic variants of plasma cholinesterase have been identified, although the dibucaine-related variants are the most important.

Mechanism of Action

The interactions of drugs with the acetylcholine receptor and the end plate channel have been described at the molecular level. Several modes of action of drugs on the receptor appear to be possible and are illustrated in Figure 27–5.

A. Nondepolarizing Blocking Drugs: All of the neuromuscular blocking drugs in use in the USA except succinylcholine are classified as nondepolarizing agents. Tubocurarine is the prototype. They produce a surmountable blockade. In small clinical doses and at low frequencies of stimulation, nondepolarizing muscle relaxants act predominantly at the **nicotinic receptor site** to compete with acetylcholine. In larger doses, some of these drugs also enter the pore of the ion channel to cause blockade. This further weakens neuromuscular transmission and diminishes the ability of acetylcholinesterase inhibitors (eg, neostigmine) to antagonize nondepolarizing muscle relaxants. Nondepolarizing relaxants may also block prejunctional sodium—but probably not calcium—channels. As a result, these muscle relaxants also interfere with the mobilization of acetylcholine at the nerve ending.

One consequence of the surmountable nature of the postsynaptic blockade produced by these agents is the fact that tetanic stimulation, by releasing a large quantity of acetylcholine, is followed by a transient post-tetanic breakthrough or relief of the block. An important clinical consequence of the same principle is the ability of cholinesterase inhibitors to reverse the blockade.

The characteristics of a nondepolarizing neuromuscular blockade are summarized in Table 27–2 and Figure 27–6.

B. Depolarizing Drugs:

1. Phase I block (depolarizing)–Succinylcholine is the only depolarizing neuromuscular blocking drug used clinically in the USA. Its neuromuscular effects are like those of acetylcholine, except that succinylcholine produces a longer effect. Succinylcholine reacts with the nicotinic receptor to open the channel and cause depolarization of the end plate, and this in turn spreads to and depolarizes adjacent membranes, causing generalized disorganized contraction of muscle motor units. Results from single-channel recordings indicate that depolarizing blockers can enter the channel to produce a prolonged "flickering" of the ion conductance (Figure 27–7). Because succinylcholine is not metabolized effectively at the synapse, the depolarized membranes remain depolarized and unresponsive to additional impulses. Furthermore, be-

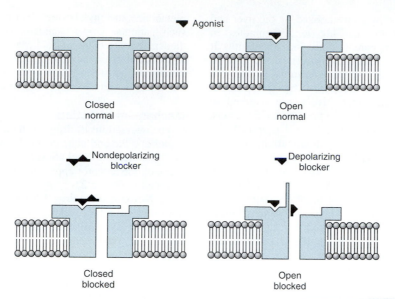

Figure 27–5. Schematic diagram of the interactions of drugs with the acetylcholine receptor on the end plate channel (structures are purely symbolic). *Top:* The action of the normal agonist, acetylcholine, in opening the channel. *Bottom: Left,* A nondepolarizing blocker, eg, tubocurarine, is shown as preventing the opening of the channel when it binds to the receptor. *Right,* a depolarizing blocker, eg, succinylcholine, both occupying the receptor and blocking the channel. Normal closure of the channel gate is prevented. Depolarizing blockers may "desensitize" the end plate by occupying the receptor and causing persistent depolarization. An additional effect of drugs on the end plate channel may occur through changes in the lipid environment surrounding the channel (not shown). General anesthetics and alcohols may impair neuromuscular transmission by this mechanism.

cause excitation-concentration coupling requires end plate repolarization ("repriming") and repetitive firing to maintain muscle tension, a flaccid paralysis results. Phase I block is augmented, not reversed, by cholinesterase inhibitors. The characteristics of a depolarizing neuromuscular blockade are summarized in Table 27–2 and Figure 27–6.

2. Phase II block (desensitizing)—With continued exposure to succinylcholine, the initial end plate depolarization decreases and the membrane becomes repolarized. Despite this repolarization, the membrane cannot be depolarized again by acetylcholine as long as succinylcholine is present. The mechanism for the development of a phase II block is

Table 27–2. Comparison of a typical nondepolarizing muscle relaxant (tubocurarine) and a depolarizing muscle relaxant (succinylcholine).

		Succinylcholine	
	Tubocurarine	**Phase I**	**Phase II**
Administration of tubocurarine	Additive	Antagonistic	Augmented[1]
Administration of succinylcholine	Antagonistic	Additive	Augmented[1]
Effect of neostigmine	Antagonistic	Augmented[1]	Antagonistic
Initial excitatory effect on skeletal muscle	None	Fasciculations	None
Response to a tetanic stimulus	Unsustained	Sustained[2]	Unsustained
Posttetanic facilitation	Yes	No	Yes
Rate of recovery	30–60 min[3]	4–8 min	> 20 min[3]

[1]It is not known whether this interaction is additive or synergistic (superadditive).
[2]The amplitude is decreased, but the response is sustained.
[3]The rate depends on the dose and on the completeness of neuromuscular blockade.

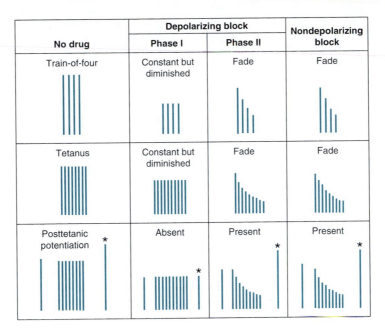

	Depolarizing block		Nondepolarizing block
No drug	**Phase I**	**Phase II**	
Train-of-four	Constant but diminished	Fade	Fade
Tetanus	Constant but diminished	Fade	Fade
Posttetanic potentiation	Absent	Present	Present

Figure 27–6. Muscle responses to different patterns of nerve stimulation used in monitoring skeletal muscle relaxation. The alterations produced by depolarizing and desensitizing blockade by succinylcholine and by a nondepolarizing blocker are shown. (*, posttetanic contraction.) (Modified and reproduced, with permission, from Morgan GE, Mikhail MS: *Clinical Anesthesiology.* Appleton & Lange, 1992.)

4 pA

25 ms

Figure 27–7. Action of succinylcholine on single-channel end plate receptor currents in frog muscle. The upper trace was recorded in the presence of a low concentration of succinylcholine; the downward deflections represent two openings of the channel and passage of inward (depolarizing) current. The lower trace was recorded in the presence of a much higher concentration of succinylcholine and shows prolonged "flickering" of the channel as it repetitively opens and closes or is "plugged" by the drug. (Reproduced, with permission, from Marshall CG, Ogden DC, Colquhoun D: The actions of suxamethonium (succinyldicholine) as an agonist and channel blocker at the nicotinic receptor of frog muscle. J Physiol [Lond] 1990;428:155.)

still unclear, but some evidence (Marshall, 1990) indicates that channel block may become more important than agonist action in this phase of succinylcholine's action. Another hypothesis is that an inexcitable area develops in the muscle membrane immediately surrounding the end plate. This inexcitable area presumably impedes centrifugal spread of impulses initiated by the action of acetylcholine on the receptor. Because the end plate is partially repolarized and still does not respond to acetylcholine, the membrane is said to be desensitized to the effects of acetylcholine. Therefore, this block has also been called a "desensitization block." Whatever the mechanism, the channels behave as if they are in a prolonged closed state (Figure 27–5).

Later in phase II, the characteristics of the blockade become nearly identical to those of a nondepolarizing block, ie, a nonsustained response to a tetanic stimulus (Figure 27–6) and reversal by acetylcholinesterase inhibitors.

II. CLINICAL PHARMACOLOGY OF NEUROMUSCULAR BLOCKING DRUGS

Skeletal Muscle Paralysis

Before the introduction of neuromuscular blocking drugs, adequate skeletal muscle relaxation could only be achieved by deep anesthesia that was often associated with hazardous depressant effects on various organ systems, especially the cardiorespiratory system. The neuromuscular blocking drugs have made it possible to achieve adequate muscle relaxation for all surgical requirements without the depressant effects of deep anesthesia.

Monitoring of the effect of muscle relaxants during surgery may be carried out by means of transdermal stimulation of one of the nerves to the hand and recording of the evoked twitches (Figure 27–6). The "train of four" pattern of stimulation is the one most commonly used.

A. Nondepolarizing Drugs: During anesthesia, the intravenous administration of tubocurarine, 0.12–0.4 mg/kg, will first cause motor weakness; ultimately, skeletal muscles become totally flaccid and inexcitable to stimulation (Figure 27–8). In general, larger muscles (eg, those of the trunk) are more resistant to block and recover more rapidly than smaller ones (eg, muscles of the hand). The diaphragm is the last muscle to be paralyzed. If ventilation is maintained, no adverse effects occur. When the drug is withdrawn, recovery of muscles usually occurs in reverse order, with the diaphragm regaining function first. The effects of the above dose of tubocurarine usually last 30–60 minutes by gross evaluation; more subtle evidence of paralysis may last for another hour. Potency and duration of action of the other nondepolarizing drugs are shown in Table 27–1. Other than the duration of action, the most important property distinguishing the nondepolarizing relaxants is the time to onset of effect, which determines how soon the patient's trachea can be intubated. Of the nondepolarizing drugs currently available or under investigation, rocuronium has the fastest onset (1–2 minutes).

B. Depolarizing Drugs: Following the intravenous administration of succinylcholine, 0.5–1 mg/kg, transient muscle fasciculations occur, especially over the chest and abdomen, though general anesthesia tends to attenuate them. As paralysis de-

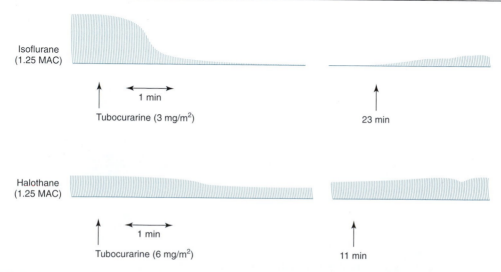

Figure 27–8. Neuromuscular blockade from tubocurarine during isoflurane and halothane anesthesia in patients. Note that at equivalent levels of anesthesia, isoflurane augments the block far more than does halothane.

Figure 27–9. Neuromuscular blockade from succinylcholine during anesthesia in patients. Fasciculations are not seen, because the anesthetic obliterated them.

velops, the arm, neck, and leg muscles are involved at a time when there is only slight weakness of the facial and pharyngeal muscles. Respiratory muscle weakness follows. The onset of neuromuscular blockade from succinylcholine is very rapid, usually within 1 minute (Figure 27–9). Because of its rapid hydrolysis by cholinesterase in the plasma and liver, the duration of neuromuscular block from this dose usually is 5–10 minutes (Table 27–1).

Cardiovascular Effects

Vecuronium, pipecuronium, doxacurium, cisatracurium, and rocuronium have little or no cardiovascular effect. All of the other currently used nondepolarizing muscle relaxants produce some cardiovascular effects. Many of these effects are mediated by autonomic and histamine receptors (Table 27–3). Tubocurarine and, to a much lesser extent, metocurine, mivacurium, and atracurium produce hypotension. This hypotension probably results from the liberation of histamine and, in larger doses, from ganglionic blockade. Premedication with an antihistamine drug will attenuate tubocurarine-induced hy-

potension. Pancuronium causes a moderate increase in heart rate and to a lesser extent cardiac output, with little or no change in systemic vascular resistance. Although the tachycardia is primarily due to a vagolytic action, release of norepinephrine from adrenergic nerve endings and blockade of neuronal uptake of norepinephrine have been suggested as secondary mechanisms. Gallamine increases heart rate by both vagolytic (antimuscarinic) action and sympathetic stimulation. The latter involves the release of norepinephrine from adrenergic nerve endings in the heart by an unknown mechanism.

Succinylcholine causes various cardiac arrhythmias. The drug stimulates all autonomic cholinoceptors: nicotinic receptors in both sympathetic and parasympathetic ganglia and muscarinic receptors in the sinus node of the heart. In low doses, negative inotropic and chronotropic responses occur that can be attenuated by administration of atropine. With large doses, positive inotropic and chronotropic effects may result. Bradycardia has been repeatedly observed when a second dose of the drug is given approximately 5 minutes after the first dose. This bradycardia

Table 27–3. Effects of neuromuscular blocking drugs on other tissues.

Drug	Effect on Autonomic Ganglia	Effect on Cardiac Muscarinic Receptors	Tendency to Cause Histamine Release
Isoquinoline derivatives			
Atracurium	None	None	Slight
Cisatracurium	None	None	None
Doxacurium	None	None	None
Metocurine	Weak block	None	Slight
Mivacurium	None	None	Slight
Tubocurarine	Weak block	None	Moderate
Steroid derivatives			
Pancuronium	None	Moderate block	None
Pipecuronium	None	None	None
Rocuronium	None	Slight	None
Vecuronium	None	None	None
Other agents			
Gallamine	None	Strong block	None
Succinylcholine	Stimulation	Stimulation	Slight

can be prevented by thiopental, atropine, ganglionic blocking drugs, and nondepolarizing muscle relaxants. Direct myocardial effects, increased muscarinic stimulation, and ganglionic stimulation may all be involved in the bradycardia response.

Other Effects

These effects are seen exclusively with depolarizing blockade.

A. Hyperkalemia: Some patients respond to succinylcholine by an exaggerated release of potassium into the blood, occasionally of such magnitude that cardiac arrest occurs. Patients with burns, nerve damage or neuromuscular disease, closed head injury and other trauma, peritoneal infections, and renal failure are especially susceptible. The mechanism of the hyperkalemic response has not been established, but it may be related to the increased number of nicotinic receptors that occur extrajunctionally in a denervated muscle or one that is not used. These extrajunctional receptors tend to be more sensitive to succinylcholine and therefore more prone to release potassium than junctional receptors. Because of cardiac arrests (presumably caused by hyperkalemia), the Food and Drug Administration ruled in 1993 that the use of succinylcholine was contraindicated in children. This contraindication was subsequently modified to a warning.

B. Intraocular Pressure: Administration of succinylcholine is followed by an increase in intraocular pressure that is manifested 1 minute after injection, maximal at 2–4 minutes, and subsides after 5 minutes. The mechanism for this effect has not been clearly defined, but it may involve contraction of tonic myofibrils or transient dilation of choroidal blood vessels. Despite the increase in pressure, the use of succinylcholine for eye operations is not contraindicated unless the anterior chamber is to be opened.

C. Intragastric Pressure: In some patients, especially muscular ones, the fasciculations associated with succinylcholine will cause an increase in intragastric pressure ranging from 5 to 40 cm of water. This may make emesis more likely, with the potential hazard of aspiration of gastric contents.

D. Muscle Pain: This is an important postoperative complaint of patients who have received succinylcholine. Because of subjective factors and differences in study design, the true incidence of this symptom is difficult to establish, but it has been reported in 0.2–20% of patients in different studies. It occurs more frequently in ambulatory than in bedridden patients. The pain is thought to be secondary to damage produced in muscle by the unsynchronized contractions of adjacent muscle fibers just before the onset of paralysis. Muscle damage has been verified by the occurrence of myoglobinuria following the use of succinylcholine.

Interactions With Other Drugs

A. Anesthetics: Inhaled anesthetics augment the neuromuscular blockade from nondepolarizing muscle relaxants in dose-dependent fashion. Of the drugs that have been studied, inhaled anesthetics augment the effects of muscle relaxants in the following order: Isoflurane (Figure 27–8), sevoflurane, desflurane, and enflurane augment more than halothane, which in turn augments more than nitrous oxide-barbiturate-benzodiazepine-opioid anesthesia. The most important factors involved in this interaction are the following: (1) Depression at sites proximal to the neuromuscular junction, ie, the central nervous system. (2) Increased muscle blood flow, which allows a larger fraction of the injected muscle relaxant to reach the neuromuscular junction. This is probably a factor only with isoflurane. (3) Decreased sensitivity of the postjunctional membrane to depolarization.

B. Antibiotics: Over 140 reports of enhancement of neuromuscular blockade by antibiotics, especially aminoglycosides, have appeared in the literature. Many of the antibiotics have been shown to cause a depression of evoked release of acetylcholine similar to that caused by magnesium. The same antibiotics also have postjunctional activity.

C. Local Anesthetics and Antiarrhythmic Drugs: In large doses, most local anesthetics block neuromuscular transmission; in smaller doses, they enhance the neuromuscular block from both nondepolarizing and depolarizing muscle relaxants.

In low doses, local anesthetics depress posttetanic potentiation, and this is thought to be a neural prejunctional effect. With higher doses, local anesthetics block acetylcholine-induced muscle contractions. This stabilizing effect is the result of blockade of the nicotinic receptor ion channels.

Experimentally, similar effects can be demonstrated with antiarrhythmic drugs such as quinidine. However, this interaction is of little or no clinical significance.

D. Other Neuromuscular Blocking Drugs: Depolarizing muscle relaxants are antagonized by nondepolarizing blockers. To prevent the fasciculations associated with succinylcholine administration, a small, nonparalyzing dose of tubocurarine is often given before succinylcholine. While this dose usually reduces fasciculations and postoperative pain, it also increases the amount of succinylcholine required for relaxation by 50–90%.

Effects of Disease & Aging on Drug Response

Several diseases can diminish or augment the neuromuscular blockade produced by nondepolarizing muscle relaxants. Myasthenia gravis markedly augments the neuromuscular blockade from these drugs. Advanced age is often associated with a prolonged duration of action from nondepolarizing relaxants, probably owing to decreased clearance of drugs by the liver and kidneys. As a result, the dose of neuromuscular blocking drugs should probably be reduced in elderly patients.

Conversely, patients with severe burns and those with upper motor neuron disease are resistant to nondepolarizing muscle relaxants. This is probably because of proliferation of extrajunctional receptors, which requires additional nondepolarizing relaxant to block a sufficient number of receptors to produce neuromuscular blockade.

Reversal of Nondepolarizing Neuromuscular Blockade

The cholinesterase inhibitors effectively antagonize the neuromuscular blockade caused by nondepolarizing drugs. Their general pharmacology is discussed in Chapter 7. Neostigmine and pyridostigmine antagonize nondepolarizing neuromuscular blockade by increasing the availability of acetylcholine at the muscle end plate, mainly by inhibition of acetylcholinesterase. To a lesser extent, these agents also increase release of transmitter from the motor nerve terminal. In contrast, edrophonium antagonizes neuromuscular blockade purely by inhibiting acetylcholinesterase.

Neostigmine also decreases the activity of plasma cholinesterase. Because mivacurium is metabolized by plasma cholinesterase, the interaction between these drugs is unpredictable. On one hand, the neuromuscular blockade is antagonized because of increased acetylcholine concentrations in the synapse. On the other hand, mivacurium concentration may be higher because of decreased plasma cholinesterase concentration. The former effect usually dominates clinically.

Other Uses of Neuromuscular Blocking Drugs

A. Control of Ventilation: In patients who have ventilatory failure from various causes, such as obstructive airway disease, it is often desirable to control ventilation to provide adequate volumes and expansion of lungs. Paralysis is sometimes induced by administration of neuromuscular blocking drugs to eliminate chest wall resistance and ineffective spontaneous ventilation.

B. Treatment of Convulsions: Neuromuscular blocking drugs are sometimes used to attenuate or eliminate the peripheral manifestations of convulsions from such causes as epilepsy or local anesthetic toxicity. Although this approach is effective in eliminating the muscular manifestations of the seizures, it has no effect on the central processes involved, since neuromuscular blocking drugs do not cross the blood-brain barrier in significant amounts when used in clinical doses.

SPASMOLYTIC DRUGS

Bertram G. Katzung, MD, PhD

Spasticity is characterized by an increase in tonic stretch reflexes and flexor muscle spasms together with muscle weakness. It is often associated with cerebral palsy, multiple sclerosis, and stroke. These conditions often involve abnormal function of the bowel and bladder as well as of skeletal muscle. In this section, only skeletal muscle spasticity is considered. The mechanisms underlying clinical spasticity appear to involve not the stretch reflex arc itself but higher centers ("upper motor neuron lesion"), with damage to descending pathways that results in hyperexcitability of alpha motoneurons in the cord. Nevertheless, drug therapy may ameliorate some of the symptoms of spasticity by modifying the stretch reflex arc or by interfering directly with skeletal muscle excitation-contraction coupling. The components involved in these processes are shown in Figure 27–10.

Drugs modifying this reflex arc may modulate excitatory or inhibitory synapses (Chapter 21). Thus, to reduce the hyperactive stretch reflex, it is desirable to reduce the activity of the Ia fibers that excite the primary motoneuron or to enhance the activity of the inhibitory internuncial neurons. These structures are shown in greater detail in Figure 27–11.

A variety of compounds used in the past can be loosely described as depressants of spinal "polysynaptic" reflex arcs (barbiturates: phenobarbital; glycerol ethers: mephenesin). A number of similar compounds are still promoted (see Drugs Used For Acute Local Muscle Spasm, below). However, it is clear from Figure 27–11 that nonspecific depression of synapses involved in the stretch reflex could reduce desirable inhibitory activity as well as excitatory transmission. During the past 2–3 decades, more specific therapy has become available. Unfortunately, the lack of a precisely quantifiable measure of clinical response—or, alternatively, an accurate experimental model—has prevented definitive comparison of the agents promoted for use in this heterogeneous group of conditions.

DIAZEPAM

As described in Chapter 22, benzodiazepines facilitate the action of gamma-aminobutyric acid (GABA) in the central nervous system. Diazepam has useful antispastic activity. It apparently acts at all GABA$_A$ synapses, but its site of action in reducing spasticity is at least partly in the spinal cord, because it is effective in patients with cord transection. It can be used in patients with muscle spasm of almost any origin, including local muscle trauma. However, it produces sedation in most patients at the doses required to significantly reduce muscle tone. Dosage is usually begun at 4 mg/d and gradually increased to a maximum of 60 mg/d.

BACLOFEN

Baclofen (*p*-chlorophenyl-GABA) was designed to be an orally active GABA-mimetic agent. The structure is shown below.

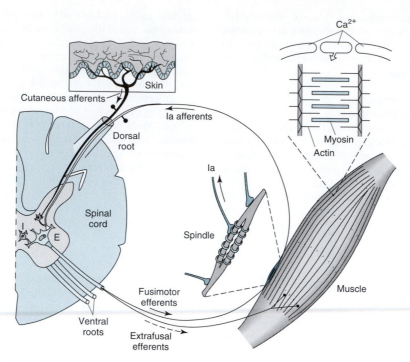

Figure 27–10. Diagram of the structures involved in the stretch reflex arc. *I* is an inhibitory interneuron; *E* indicates an excitatory presynaptic terminal; *Ia* is a primary intrafusal afferent fiber, *Ca²⁺* denotes activator calcium stored in the sarcoplasmic reticulum of skeletal muscle. (Reproduced, with permission, from Young RR, Delwaide PJ: Drug therapy: Spasticity. N Engl J Med 1981;304:28.)

Baclofen is an active spasmolytic and acts as a GABA agonist at $GABA_B$ receptors. Activation of receptors in the brain by baclofen results in hyperpolarization, probably by increased K^+ conductance. It has been suggested that this hyperpolarization (in the cord as well as the brain) serves a presynaptic inhibitory function (Figure 27–11), probably by reducing calcium influx, to reduce the release of excitatory transmitters in both the brain and the spinal cord. Baclofen may also reduce pain in patients with spasticity, perhaps by inhibiting the release of substance P in the spinal cord.

Baclofen

Baclofen is at least as effective as diazepam in reducing spasticity and causes much less sedation. In addition, it does not reduce general muscle strength, as does dantrolene. It is rapidly and completely absorbed after oral administration and has a plasma half-life of 3–4 hours. Dosage is started at 15 mg twice daily, increasing, if tolerated, to as much as 100 mg daily. Toxicity of this drug includes drowsiness, to which the patient may become tolerant. Increased seizure activity has been reported in epileptic patients.

Double-blind studies, using implanted programmable infusion pumps, have shown that in many patients

Figure 27–11. Postulated sites of spasmolytic action of diazepam and baclofen in the spinal cord. (Reproduced, with permission, from Young RR, Delwaide PJ: Drug therapy: Spasticity. N Engl J Med 1981;304:28.)

intrathecal administration of baclofen controls severe spasticity and pain that is not responsive to medication by oral or other parenteral routes. Because of poor egress of baclofen from the spinal cord, peripheral symptoms are few, and higher central concentrations of the drug may be tolerated. Partial tolerance to the effect of the drug may occur after several months of therapy but can be overcome by appropriate dosage adjustment to maintain the beneficial effect (Azouvi et al, 1996). Several cases of somnolence, respiratory depression, and even coma have been recorded, but the major disadvantage of this treatment is the difficulty of maintaining the drug delivery catheter. Careful analyses of long-term intrathecal baclofen therapy suggest that this treatment greatly improves the quality of life of selected patients.

TIZANIDINE

As noted in Chapter 11, clonidine and other imidazoline compounds have a variety of effects in the central nervous system that are not yet been fully understood (see Chapter 11 box: Clonidine: A Pointer to New Receptors & Clinical Applications). Among these effects is the ability to reduce muscle spasm. Tizanidine is the congener of clonidine that has been most thoroughly studied for its spasmolytic actions (Young, 1994). Tizanidine has significant α_2 adrenoceptor agonist effects but reduces spasticity in experimental models at doses that cause less hypotension than clonidine. Neurophysiologic studies in animals and humans suggest that tizanidine reinforces both presynaptic and postsynaptic inhibition in the cord. It also inhibits nociceptive transmission in the spinal dorsal horn.

A number of small and moderate-sized clinical trials, including some double-blind trials, have indicated that tizanidine has significant benefit in patients with several types of spasticity and is probably comparable in efficacy to diazepam, baclofen, and dantrolene, with a different spectrum of adverse effects (Young, 1994). Problems have included drowsiness, hypotension, dry mouth, and asthenia. The dose requirement varies markedly among patients, so that each patient must be titrated to optimal effect. The drug has been in use in Europe for some time, and it was approved by the Food and Drug Administration in 1996.

OTHER DRUGS THAT ACT IN THE SPINAL CORD

Progabide and **glycine** have been found in preliminary studies to reduce spasticity in some patients. Progabide is a $GABA_A$ and $GABA_B$ agonist and has active metabolites, including GABA itself. Glycine is another inhibitory amino acid neurotransmitter (Chapter 21). It appears to be active when given orally and read-

ily passes the blood-brain barrier. These drugs are investigational. **Idrocilamide** is a newer agent also under investigation.

DANTROLENE

Dantrolene is a hydantoin derivative (like phenytoin) but with a unique mechanism of spasmolytic action outside the central nervous system. Its structure is shown below.

Dantrolene

Dantrolene reduces skeletal muscle strength by interfering with excitation-contraction coupling in the muscle fiber. The normal contractile response involves release of activator calcium from its stores in the sarcoplasmic reticulum of the sarcomere. This calcium brings about the tension-generating interaction of actin with myosin. Calcium exits the sarcoplasmic reticulum via a calcium channel, sometimes called the ryanodine receptor channel because the alkaloid **ryanodine** combines with a receptor on the channel protein and, in the case of the skeletal muscle channel, locks it in the open position. Dantrolene interferes with the release of activator calcium via this sarcoplasmic reticulum calcium channel and, in some studies, appears to compete with ryanodine for binding to its site of action.

Thus, the site of action of dantrolene is on the sarcoplasmic reticulum in skeletal muscle. Motor units that contract rapidly are more sensitive to the drug than are slow units. Cardiac muscle and smooth muscle are depressed only slightly, perhaps because the release of calcium from their sarcoplasmic reticulum involves a somewhat different process.

Only about one-third of an oral dose of dantrolene is absorbed; the half-life of the drug is about 8 hours. Treatment is usually begun with 25 mg daily as a single dose, increasing to a maximum of 100 mg four times daily if necessary and tolerated. Major adverse effects are generalized muscle weakness, sedation, and occasionally hepatitis.

A special application of dantrolene is in the treatment of **malignant hyperthermia,** a rare disorder that can be triggered by a variety of stimuli, including general anesthesia and neuromuscular blocking drugs. Patients with this condition have a hereditary impairment of the ability of the sarcoplasmic reticulum to sequester calcium. A trigger event results in sudden and prolonged release of calcium, with massive muscle contraction, lactic acid production, and increased body temperature. Prompt treatment is essential to control acidosis and body temperature and to reduce calcium release. The latter is accomplished with intravenous dantrolene, starting with 1 mg/kg and repeating as necessary to a maximum of 10 mg/kg.

BOTULINUM TOXIN

The therapeutic use of botulinum toxin for ophthalmic purposes and for local muscle spasm was mentioned in Chapter 6. Local injection of botulinum toxin is now finding increased application in the treatment of more generalized spastic disorders due to neurologic injury. Most clinical studies to date have involved administration in one limb, eg, following stroke (Bhakta et al, 1996; Pierson et al, 1996; Simpson et al, 1996). Benefits persist for weeks to months after a single treatment. Although most studies have utilized type A botulinum toxin, types B and F are also available as orphan drugs.

DRUGS USED FOR ACUTE LOCAL MUSCLE SPASM

A large number of drugs (**carisoprodol, chlorphenesin, chlorzoxazone, cyclobenzaprine, metaxalone, methocarbamol,** and **orphenadrine**) are promoted for the relief of acute temporary muscle spasm caused by local trauma or strain. Most act as sedatives or at the level of the spinal cord or brain stem. Cyclobenzaprine may be regarded as the prototype of the group. Cyclobenzaprine is structurally related to the tricyclic antidepressants and has some properties in common with them, eg, antimuscarinic effects. It is believed to act at the level of the brain stem. Cyclobenzaprine is ineffective in muscle spasm due to cerebral palsy or spinal cord injury. The drug has strong antimuscarinic actions and causes significant sedation in most patients and confusion and transient visual hallucinations in some. The dosage of cyclobenzaprine for acute spasm due to injury is 20–40 mg/d in three divided doses.

PREPARATIONS AVAILABLE

Neuromuscular Blocking Drugs

Atracurium (Tracrium)
   Parenteral: 10 mg/mL for injection
Cisatracurium (Nimbex)
   Parenteral: 2, 10 mg/mL for IV injection
Doxacurium (Nuromax)
   Parenteral: 1 mg/mL for IV injection
Gallamine (Flaxedil)
   Parenteral: 20 mg/mL for injection
Metocurine (generic, Metubine Iodide)
   Parenteral: 2 mg/mL for injection
Mivacurium (Mivacron)
   Parenteral: 0.5, 2 mg/mL for injection
Pancuronium (generic, Pavulon)
   Parenteral: 1, 2 mg/mL for injection
Pipecuronium (Arduan)
   Parenteral: 1 mg/mL for IV injection
Rocuronium (Zemuron)
   Parenteral: 10 mg/mL for IV injection
Succinylcholine (Anectine, others)
   Parenteral: 20, 50, 100 mg/mL for injection;
      100, 500 mg per vial powders to reconstitute
      for injection
Tubocurarine (generic)
   Parenteral: 3 mg (20 units)/mL for injection
Vecuronium (Norcuron)
   Parenteral: 10 mg/mL powder to reconstitute for
      injection

Muscle Relaxants (Spasmolytics)

Baclofen (Lioresal, generic)

   Oral: 10, 20 mg tablets
   Intrathecal: 10 mg/20 mL, 10 mg/5 mL ampules
Botulinum toxin type A (Botox)
   Parenteral: Powder for solution, 100 units/vial
Carisoprodol (generic, Soma)
   Oral: 350 mg tablets
Chlorphenesin (Maolate)
   Oral: 400 mg tablets
Chlorzoxazone (generic, Paraflex)
   Oral: 250, 500 mg tablets, caplets
Cyclobenzaprine (Flexeril, generic)
   Oral: 10 mg tablets
Dantrolene (Dantrium)
   Oral: 25, 50, 100 mg capsules
   Parenteral: 20 mg per vial powder to reconstitute for injection
Diazepam (generic, Valium, others)
   Oral: 2, 5, 10 mg tablets; 15 mg sustained-release capsules; 5 mg/5 mL, 5 mg/mL solutions
   Parenteral: 5 mg/mL for injection
Metaxalone (Skelaxin)
   Oral: 400 mg tablets
Methocarbamol (generic, Robaxin)
   Oral: 500, 750 mg tablets
   Parenteral: 100 mg/mL for IM, IV injection
Orphenadrine (generic, Norflex)
   Oral: 100 mg tablets; 100 mg sustained release tablets
   Parenteral: 30 mg/mL for IM, IV injection
Tizanidine (Zanaflex)
   Oral: 4 mg tablets

REFERENCES

Neuromuscular Blockers

Adams PR: Acetylcholine receptor kinetics. J Membr Biol 1981;58:161.

Adt M, Baumert J-H, Reimann H-J: The role of histamine in the cardiovascular effects of atracurium. Br J Anaesth 1992;68:155.

Agoston S et al: Clinical pharmacokinetics of neuromuscular blocking drugs. Clin Pharmacokinet 1992;22:94.

Bartkowski RR et al: Rocuronium onset of action: A comparison with atracurium and vecuronium. Anesth Analg 1993;77:574.

Bevan DR et al: Reversal of neuromuscular blockade. Anesthesiology 1992;77:785.

Caldwell JE et al: The pharmacodynamics and pharmacokinetics of the metabolite desacetylvecuronium (ORG 7268) and its parent compound, vecuronium, in human volunteers. J Pharmacol Exp Ther 1994; 270:1216.

Canfell PC et al: The metabolic disposition of laudanosine in dog, rabbit, and man. Drug Metab Dispos Biol Fate Chem 1986;14:703.

Eastwood NB et al: Pharmacokinetics of 1*R-cis* 1′*R-cis* atracurium besylate (51W89) and plasma laudanosine concentrations in health and chronic renal failure. Br J Anaesth 1995;75:431.

Eldefrawi AT, Miller ER, Eldefrawi ME: Binding of depolarizing drugs to ionic channel sites of the nicotinic acetylcholine receptor. Biochem Pharmacol 1982; 31:1819.

Gibb AJ, Marshall IG: Pre- and postjunctional effects of tubocurarine and other nicotinic antagonists during repetitive stimulation in the rat. J Physiol 1984;351:275.

Hansen-Flaschen JH et al: Use of sedating drugs and neuromuscular blocking agents in patients requiring mechanical ventilation for respiratory failure: A national survey. JAMA 1991;266:2870.

Hunter JM: New neuromuscular blocking drugs. N Engl J Med 1995;332:1691.

Lien CA et al: The pharmacokinetics and pharmacodynamics of the stereoisomers of mivacurium in patients receiving nitrous oxide/opioid/barbiturate anesthesia. Anesthesiology 1994;80:1296.

Marshall CG, Ogden DC, Colquhoun D: The actions of suxamethonium (succinyldicholine) as an agonist and channel blocker at the nicotinic receptor of frog muscle. J Physiol (Lond) 1990;428:155.

Miller RD, Savarese JJ: Pharmacology of muscle relaxants and their antagonists. In: *Anesthesia,* 4th ed. Miller RD (editor). Churchill Livingstone, 1994.

Morita T et al: Inadequate antagonism of vecuronium-induced neuromuscular blockade by neostigmine during sevoflurane or isoflurane anesthesia. Anesth Analg 1995;80:1175.

Nigrovic V, Fox JL: Atracurium decay and the formation of laudanosine in humans. Anesthesiology 1991;74:446.

Owen RT: Resistance to competitive neuromuscular blocking agents in burn patients: A review. Methods Find Exp Clin Pharmacol 1985;7:203.

Phillips BJ, Hunter JM: Use of mivacurium chloride by constant infusion in the anephric patient. Br J Anaesth 1992;68:494.

Scuka M, Mozrzymas JW: Postsynaptic potentiation and desensitization at the vertebrate end-plate receptors. Prog Neurobiol 1992;38:19.

Segredo V et al: Persistent paralysis in critically ill patients after long-term administration of vecuronium. N Engl J Med 1992;327:524.

Stroud RM: Acetylcholine receptor structure. Neurosci Comment 1983;1:124.

Szenshradsky J et al: Pharmacokinetics of rocuronium bromide (ORG 9426) in patients with normal renal function or patients undergoing cadaver renal transplantation. Anesthesiology 1992;77:899.

Spasmolytics

Albright AL, Cervi A, Singletary J: Intrathecal baclofen for spasticity in cerebral palsy. JAMA 1991;265:1418.

Bhakta BB et al: Use of botulinum toxin in stroke patients with severe upper limb spasticity. J Neurol Neurosurg Psychiatry 1996;61:30.

Casale R, Glynn CJ, Buoncore M: Reduction of spastic hypertonia in patients with spinal cord injury: A double-blind comparison of intravenous orphenadrine citrate and placebo. Arch Phys Med Rehabil 1995; 76:660

Davidoff RA: Antispasticity drugs: Mechanisms of action. Ann Neurol 1985;17:107.

Dolphin AC, Scott RH: Activation of calcium channel currents in rat sensory neurons by large depolarizations: Effect of guanine nucleotides and (−)-baclofen. Eur J Neurosci 1990;2:104.

Lazorthes Y et al: Chronic intrathecal baclofen administration for control of severe spasticity. J Neurosurg 1990;72:393.

Lopez JR et al: Effects of dantrolene on myoplasmic free $[Ca^{2+}]$ measured in vivo in patients susceptible to malignant hyperthermia. Anesthesiology 1992;76:711.

Nance P et al: Intrathecal baclofen therapy for adults with spinal spasticity: Therapeutic efficacy and effect on hospital admissions. Can J Neurol Sci 1995;22:22.

Ochs G et al: Intrathecal baclofen for long-term treatment of spasticity: A multi-centre study. J Neurol Neurosurg Psychiat 1989;52:933.

Pierson SH, Katz DI, Tarsy D: Botulinum toxin in the treatment of spasticity: Functional implications and patient selection. Arch Phys Med Rehab 1996;77:717.

Pinder RM et al: Dantrolene sodium: A review of its pharmacological properties and therapeutic efficacy in spasticity. Drugs 1977;3:3.

Simpson DM et al: Botulinum toxin type A in the treatment of upper extremity spasticity: A randomized, double-blind, placebo-controlled trial. Neurology 1996;46:1306.

Steinbok P: Cost analysis of continuous intrathecal baclofen versus selective functional posterior rhizotomy in the treatment of spastic quadriplegia associated with cerebral palsy. Pediatr Neurosurg 1995;22:255.

Young RR (editor): Symposium: Role of tizanidine in the treatment of spasticity. Neurology 1994;44(Suppl 9):1. [Entire issue.]

Young RR, Wiegner AW: Spasticity. Clin Orthop 1987; 219:50.

28

Pharmacologic Management of Parkinsonism & Other Movement Disorders

Michael J. Aminoff, MD, FRCP

Several different types of abnormal movement are recognized. **Tremor** consists of a rhythmic oscillatory movement around a joint and is best characterized by its relation to activity. Tremor present at rest is characteristic of parkinsonism, when it is often associated with rigidity and an impairment of voluntary activity. Tremor may occur during maintenance of sustained posture (postural tremor) or during movement (intention tremor). A conspicuous postural tremor is the cardinal feature of benign essential or familial tremor. Intention tremor occurs in patients with a lesion of the brain stem or cerebellum, especially when the superior cerebellar peduncle is involved, and may also occur as a manifestation of toxicity from alcohol or certain other drugs.

Chorea consists of irregular, unpredictable, involuntary muscle jerks that occur in different parts of the body and impair voluntary activity. In some instances, the proximal muscles of the limbs are most severely affected, and because the abnormal movements are then particularly violent, the term ballismus has been used to describe them. Chorea may be hereditary or may occur as a complication of a number of general medical disorders and of therapy with certain drugs.

Abnormal movements may be slow and writhing in character (**athetosis**) and in some instances are so sustained that they are more properly regarded as abnormal postures (**dystonia**). Athetosis or dystonia may occur with perinatal brain damage, with focal or generalized cerebral lesions, as an acute complication of certain drugs, as an accompaniment of diverse neurologic disorders, or as an isolated phenomenon of uncertain cause known as idiopathic torsion dystonia or dystonia musculorum deformans. Its physiologic basis is uncertain, and treatment is unsatisfactory.

Tics are sudden coordinated abnormal movements that tend to occur repetitively, particularly about the face and head, especially in children, and can be suppressed voluntarily for short periods of time. Common tics include, for example, repetitive sniffing or shoulder shrugging. Tics may be single or multiple

and transient or chronic. Gilles de la Tourette's syndrome is characterized by chronic multiple tics; its pharmacologic management is discussed at the end of this chapter.

Many of the movement disorders have been attributed to disturbances of the basal ganglia, but the precise function of these anatomic structures is not yet fully understood, and it is not possible to relate individual symptoms to involvement at specific sites.

PARKINSONISM (Paralysis Agitans)

Parkinsonism is characterized by a combination of rigidity, bradykinesia, tremor, and postural instability that can occur for a wide variety of reasons but is usually idiopathic. The pathophysiologic basis of the idiopathic disorder may relate to exposure to some unrecognized neurotoxin or to the occurrence of oxidation reactions with the generation of free radicals. Parkinson's disease is generally progressive, leading to increasing disability unless effective treatment is provided. The normally high concentration of dopamine in the basal ganglia of the brain is reduced in parkinsonism, and pharmacologic attempts to restore dopaminergic activity with levodopa and dopamine agonists have been successful in alleviating many of the clinical features of the disorder. An alternative but complementary approach has been to restore the normal balance of cholinergic and dopaminergic influences on the basal ganglia with antimuscarinic drugs. The pathophysiologic basis for these therapies is that in idiopathic parkinsonism, dopaminergic neurons in the substantia nigra that normally inhibit the output of GABAergic cells in the corpus striatum are lost (Figure 28–1). (In contrast, Huntington's chorea involves the loss of some cholinergic neurons and an even greater loss of the GABAergic cells that exit the cor-

450

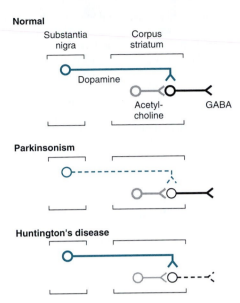

Figure 28–1. Schematic representation of the sequence of neurons involved in parkinsonism and Huntington's chorea. **Top:** Dopaminergic neurons (color) originating in the substantia nigra normally inhibit the GABAergic output from the striatum, whereas cholinergic neurons (gray) exert an excitatory effect. **Middle:** In parkinsonism, there is a selective loss of dopaminergic neurons (dashed, color). **Bottom:** In Huntington's chorea, some cholinergic neurons may be lost (gray), but even more GABAergic neurons (black, dashed) degenerate.

volve the stimulation of adenylyl cyclase or accumulation of cAMP. D_1 receptors stimulate adenylyl cyclase and D_2 receptors inhibit it (Table 6–2).

Dopamine receptors of the D_1 type are located in the zona compacta of the substantia nigra and presynaptically on striatal axons coming from cortical neurons and from dopaminergic cells in the substantia nigra. The D_2 receptors are located postsynaptically on striatal neurons and presynaptically on axons in the substantia nigra belonging to neurons in the basal ganglia. The benefits of dopaminergic antiparkinsonism drugs appear to depend mostly on stimulation of the D_2 receptors, but D_1-receptor stimulation may also be required for maximal benefit. Dopamine agonist or partial agonist ergot derivatives such as lergotrile and bromocriptine that are powerful stimulators of the D_2 receptors have antiparkinsonism properties, whereas certain dopamine blockers that are selective D_2 antagonists can induce parkinsonism.

Chemistry

As discussed in Chapter 6, dopa is the precursor of dopamine and norepinephrine. Its structure is shown in Figure 28–2. Levodopa is the levorotatory stereoisomer of dopa.

Pharmacokinetics

Levodopa is rapidly absorbed from the small intestine, but its absorption depends on the rate of gastric

pus striatum.) Drugs that *induce* parkinsonian syndromes either are dopamine receptor antagonists (eg, antipsychotic agents, Chapter 29) or lead to the destruction of the dopaminergic nigrostriatal neurons (eg, MPTP; see below).

LEVODOPA

Dopamine does not cross the blood-brain barrier and if given into the peripheral circulation has no therapeutic effect in parkinsonism. However, (–)-3-(3,4-dihydroxyphenyl)-L-alanine (levodopa), the immediate metabolic precursor of dopamine, does penetrate the brain, where it is decarboxylated to dopamine (see Figure 6–5). Several dopamine agonists have also been developed and may lead to clinical benefit, as discussed below.

Dopamine receptors can be classified according to various biochemical and pharmacologic features. They have, for example, been subdivided according to whether they are linked to an adenylyl cyclase. Cyclic adenosine monophosphate (cAMP) is formed with activation of this cyclase and is responsible for mediating certain tissue-specific responses to dopamine. Other responses to dopamine apparently do not in-

Dihydroxyphenylalanine (dopa)

Carbidopa

Selegiline

Figure 28–2. Some drugs used in the treatment of parkinsonism.

emptying and the pH of the gastric contents. Food will delay the appearance of levodopa in the plasma. Moreover, certain amino acids from ingested food can compete with the drug for absorption from the gut and for transport from the blood to the brain. Plasma concentrations usually peak between 1 and 2 hours after an oral dose, and the plasma half-life is usually between 1 and 3 hours, though it varies considerably between individuals. About two-thirds of the dose appears in the urine as metabolites within 8 hours of an oral dose, the main metabolic products being 3-methoxy-4-hydroxy-phenylacetic acid (homovanillic acid, HVA) and dihydroxyphenylacetic acid (DOPAC). Unfortunately, only about 1–3% of administered levodopa actually enters the brain unaltered, the remainder being metabolized extracerebrally, predominantly by decarboxylation to dopamine, which does not penetrate the blood-brain

barrier. This means that levodopa must be given in large amounts when it is used alone. However, when it is given in combination with a dopa decarboxylase inhibitor that does not penetrate the blood-brain barrier, the peripheral metabolism of levodopa is reduced, plasma levels of levodopa are higher, plasma half-life is longer, and more dopa is available for entry into the brain (Figure 28–3). Indeed, concomitant administration of a peripheral dopa decarboxylase inhibitor may reduce the daily requirements of levodopa by approximately 75%.

Clinical Use

In considering the use of levodopa in patients with parkinsonism, it is important to appreciate that the best results are obtained in the first few years of treatment. This is sometimes because the daily dose of

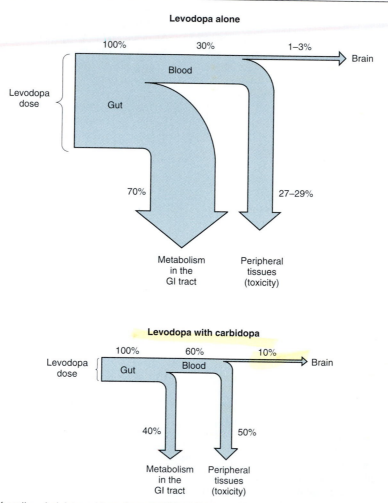

Figure 28–3. Fate of orally administered levodopa and the effect of carbidopa, estimated from animal data. The width of each pathway indicates the absolute amount of the drug present at each site, while the percentages shown denote the relative proportion of the administered dose. The benefits of coadministration of carbidopa include reduction of the amount of levodopa diverted to peripheral tissues and an increase in the fraction of the dose that reaches the brain. (Data from Nutt JG, Fellman JH: Pharmacokinetics of levodopa. Clin Neuropharmacol 1984;7:35.)

levodopa must be reduced with time in order to avoid side effects at doses that were well tolerated at the outset. The reason that adverse effects develop in this way is unclear, but selective denervation or drug-induced supersensitivity may be responsible. Some patients also become less responsive to levodopa, so that previously effective doses eventually fail to produce any therapeutic benefit. It is not clear whether this relates to disease progression or to duration of treatment, although the evidence is increasing that disease progression is primarily responsible for the declining response. Responsiveness to levodopa may ultimately be lost completely, perhaps because of the disappearance of dopaminergic nigrostriatal nerve terminals or some pathologic process directly involving the striatal dopamine receptors. For such reasons, the benefits of levodopa treatment often begin to diminish after about 3 or 4 years of therapy irrespective of the initial therapeutic response. Although levodopa therapy does not stop the progression of parkinsonism, recent evidence suggests that the early initiation of levodopa therapy lowers the mortality rate due to Parkinson's disease. However, long-term therapy may lead to a number of problems in management such as development of the on-off phenomenon discussed below. The most appropriate time to introduce levodopa therapy must therefore be determined individually.

When levodopa is used, it is generally given in combination with carbidopa (Figure 28–2), a peripheral dopa decarboxylase inhibitor, for the reasons set forth above. **Sinemet** is a dopa preparation containing carbidopa and levodopa in fixed proportion (1:10 or 1:4). Treatment is started with a small dose, eg, Sinemet-25/100 (carbidopa 25 mg, levodopa 100 mg) three times daily, and gradually increased depending upon the therapeutic response and development of adverse effects. Most patients ultimately require Sinemet-25/250 (carbidopa 25 mg, levodopa 250 mg) three or four times daily. It may be preferable to keep treatment with this agent at a low level (eg, Sinemet-25/100 three times daily) and to increase dopaminergic therapy by the addition of a dopamine agonist if necessary, in order to reduce the risk of development of response fluctuations, as discussed below. A controlled-release formulation of Sinemet is now available and may be helpful in patients with established response fluctuations or as a means of reducing dosing frequency.

Levodopa can ameliorate all of the clinical features of parkinsonism, but it is particularly effective in relieving bradykinesia and any disabilities resulting from it. When it is first introduced, about one-third of patients respond very well and one-third less well. Most of the remainder either are unable to tolerate the medication or simply fail to respond at all.

Adverse Effects

A. Gastrointestinal Effects: When levodopa is given without a peripheral decarboxylase inhibitor, anorexia and nausea and vomiting occur in about 80% of patients. These adverse effects can be minimized by taking the drug in divided doses, with or immediately after meals, and by increasing the total daily dose very slowly; antacids taken 30–60 minutes before levodopa may also be beneficial. The vomiting has been attributed to stimulation of an emetic center located in the brain stem but outside the blood-brain barrier to dopamine and to peripheral decarboxylase inhibitors. Fortunately, tolerance to this emetic effect develops in many patients after several months. Antiemetics such as phenothiazines are best avoided because they reduce the antiparkinsonism effects of levodopa and may exacerbate the disease.

When levodopa is given in combination with carbidopa to reduce its extracerebral metabolism, adverse gastrointestinal effects are much less frequent and troublesome, occurring in fewer than 20% of cases, so that patients can tolerate proportionately higher doses.

B. Cardiovascular Effects: A variety of cardiac arrhythmias have been described in patients receiving levodopa, including tachycardia, ventricular extrasystoles, and, rarely, atrial fibrillation. This effect has been attributed to increased catecholamine formation peripherally. The incidence of such arrhythmias is low, even in the presence of established cardiac disease, and may be reduced still further if the levodopa is taken in combination with a peripheral decarboxylase inhibitor. In parkinsonism patients who also have heart disease, the anticipated benefits of levodopa, especially when combined with carbidopa, generally outweigh the slight risk of inducing a cardiac arrhythmia.

Postural hypotension is common and often asymptomatic, and tends to diminish with continuing treatment. Hypertension may also occur, especially in the presence of nonselective monoamine oxidase inhibitors or sympathomimetics or when massive doses of levodopa are being taken.

C. Dyskinesias: Dyskinesias occur in up to 80% of patients receiving levodopa therapy for long periods. The form and nature of dopa dyskinesias vary widely in different patients but tend to remain constant in character in individual patients. Chorea, ballismus, athetosis, dystonia, myoclonus, tics, and tremor may occur individually or in any combination in the face, trunk, or limbs. Choreoathetosis of the face and distal extremities is the most common presentation.

The development of dyskinesias is dose-related, but there is considerable individual variation in the dose required to produce them. Dyskinesias seem to occur more commonly in patients receiving levodopa combined with a peripheral decarboxylase inhibitor than in those receiving levodopa alone. Moreover, with continuing treatment, dyskinesias may develop at a dose of levodopa that previously was well tolerated. They can be alleviated or reversed by lowering the daily dose of levodopa, but usually at the expense of reduced antiparkinsonism benefit; many patients are therefore willing to tolerate even a marked dyskinesia, because their mobility is so greatly improved by the medication. In some instances dyskinesias are less marked if levodopa is prescribed alone rather than in combination with carbidopa; in other instances, a drug holiday (see below) may help control the problem. Pharmacologic attempts to counteract the dyskinesia with drugs used to treat chorea have generally not been successful or require the use of drugs that tend to worsen the parkinsonism.

D. Behavioral Effects: A wide variety of adverse mental effects have been reported including depression, anxiety, agitation, insomnia, somnolence, confusion, delusions, hallucinations, nightmares, euphoria, and other changes in mood or personality. Such adverse effects are more common in patients taking levodopa in combination with a decarboxylase inhibitor rather than levodopa alone, presumably because higher levels are reached in the brain. They may be precipitated by intercurrent illness or operation. The only treatment is to reduce or withdraw the medication if necessary. A drug holiday (see below) may also lead to improvement of adverse mental effects.

E. Fluctuations in Response: Certain fluctuations in clinical response to levodopa occur with increasing frequency as treatment continues. In some patients, these fluctuations relate to the timing of levodopa intake, and they are then referred to as wearing-off reactions or end-of-dose akinesia. In other instances, fluctuations in clinical state are unrelated to the timing of doses (on-off phenomenon). In the on-off phenomenon, off-periods of marked akinesia alternate over the course of a few hours with on-periods of improved mobility but often marked dyskinesia. The phenomenon is most likely to occur in patients who responded well to treatment initially. The exact mechanism is unknown, but the off-period can sometimes be shown to relate to falling plasma levels of levodopa. Patients may benefit from taking their medication at more frequent intervals in smaller doses during the day or from the addition of dopamine agonists such as bromocriptine (see below) to the drug regimen. Reduction in dietary intake of protein to the minimum recommended daily allowance and adjustment of the daily routine so that the main protein meal is taken in the evening is also helpful. Controlled-release formulations of Sinemet are sometimes useful. Other strategies include taking Sinemet in liquid form, addition of selegiline (discussed later), and administration of levodopa by intragastric or intraduodenal infusion.

F. Miscellaneous Adverse Effects: Mydriasis may occur and may precipitate an attack of acute glaucoma in some patients. Other reported but rare adverse effects include various blood dyscrasias; a positive Coombs test with evidence of hemolysis; hot flushes; aggravation or precipitation of gout; abnormalities of smell or taste; brownish discoloration of saliva, urine, or vaginal secretions; priapism; and mild—usually transient—elevations of blood urea nitrogen and of serum transaminases, alkaline phosphatase, and bilirubin.

Drug Holidays

A drug holiday may alleviate some of the neurologic and behavioral adverse effects of levodopa but is usually of little help in the management of the on-off phenomenon. Patients must be under close medical supervision. Levodopa medication must be withdrawn gradually, since abrupt cessation of treatment may lead to a severely akinetic state. The optimal duration of a break in treatment with levodopa is unclear but has varied from 3 to 21 days in different studies. Up to two-thirds of patients show temporary improved responsiveness to levodopa when the drug is reinstituted, and—because they can be managed on lower doses than before—adverse mental effects and dyskinesias are less troublesome. The medication can be either restarted at half the previous dose or built up gradually from an even lower level. Fluctuations in response (on-off phenomenon) are reduced in many instances, but any benefit in this regard is usually short-lived. Unfortunately, there is no way of predicting which patients will respond satisfactorily to the holiday. Furthermore, a drug holiday carries the risks of aspiration pneumonia, venous thrombosis, pulmonary embolism, and depression resulting from the immobility accompanying severe parkinsonism. For these reasons and because of the temporary nature of any benefit, drug holidays have generally fallen out of favor.

Drug Interactions

Pharmacologic doses of pyridoxine (vitamin B_6) enhance the extracerebral metabolism of levodopa and may therefore prevent its therapeutic effect unless a peripheral decarboxylase inhibitor is also taken. Levodopa should not be given to patients taking monoamine oxidase A inhibitors or within 2 weeks of their discontinuance, because such a combination can lead to hypertensive crises.

Contraindications

Levodopa should not be given to psychotic patients, as it may exacerbate the mental disturbance. It is also contraindicated in patients with angle-closure glaucoma, but those with chronic open-angle glaucoma may be given levodopa if intraocular pressure is well controlled and can be monitored. It is best given combined with carbidopa to patients with cardiac disease, but even so the risk of cardiac dysrhythmia is slight. Patients with active peptic ulcer must also be managed carefully, since gastrointestinal bleeding has occasionally occurred with levodopa. Because levodopa is a precursor of skin melanin and conceivably may activate malignant melanoma, its use should be avoided in patients with a history of melanoma or with suspicious undiagnosed skin lesions.

DOPAMINE AGONISTS

The enzymes responsible for synthesizing dopamine are depleted in the brains of parkinsonism patients, and drugs acting directly on dopamine receptors may therefore have a beneficial effect additional to that of levodopa. Unlike levodopa, they do not require enzymatic conversion to an active metabolite, have no potentially toxic metabolites, and do not compete with other substances for active transport into the blood and across the blood-brain barrier. Moreover, drugs specifically affecting certain (but not all) dopamine receptors may have more limited adverse effects than levodopa. There are a number of dopamine agonists with antiparkinsonism activity. Some, such as apomorphine, piribedil, and lergotrile, have such serious adverse effects that they cannot be used clinically, but others may have a role in treatment of parkinsonism.

BROMOCRIPTINE

Several ergot derivatives are dopamine agonists (Chapter 16) and have been used in the treatment of parkinsonism; unlike other dopamine-like drugs, these drugs appear to be partial agonists at presynaptic dopamine D_2 receptors. Bromocriptine (structure shown in Table 16–5) is the most widely used in the USA. It has also been used to treat certain endocrinologic disorders, especially hyperprolactinemia (see Chapters 16 and 37), but in lower doses than those required to counteract parkinsonism. The drug is absorbed to a variable extent from the gastrointestinal tract, peak plasma levels being reached within 1–2 hours after an oral dose. It is excreted in the bile and feces.

There is some evidence that bromocriptine has a role as a first-line drug in the treatment of parkinsonism and that its use in this disease is associated with a lower incidence of the response fluctuations and dyskinesias commonly seen with long-term levodopa therapy. In consequence, dopaminergic therapy may best be initiated with a low dose of carbidopa plus levodopa (eg, Sinemet 25/100 three times daily) and then increased by the addition of bromocriptine. Some physicians, however, reserve bromocriptine for parkinsonism patients taking levodopa who have end-of-dose akinesia or on-off phenomena or who are becoming refractory to treatment with levodopa. Partial replacement of levodopa with bromocriptine may then be valuable. Optimal results are obtained by a combination of levodopa and bromocriptine in doses less than the maximum tolerated doses of each. The results of bromocriptine treatment are generally disappointing in patients totally unresponsive to levodopa, and addition of bromocriptine to patients receiving optimal levodopa therapy may cause intolerable adverse effects. Bromocriptine does not complicate treatment with antimuscarinic drugs or amantadine, and these drugs can be continued without change in dosage in patients who are to be given bromocriptine as well.

Clinical Use

The usual daily dose of bromocriptine in parkinsonism is between 7.5 and 30 mg, but in some patients these doses either fail to provide sustained benefit or cannot be tolerated. In order to minimize adverse effects, the dose of bromocriptine should be built up slowly over about 2 or 3 months from a starting level of 1.25 mg twice daily after meals; the daily dose is then increased by 2.5 mg every 2 weeks depending on the response or the development of adverse reactions. The dose of levodopa taken concurrently may have to be gradually lowered to about half of that previously required. However, because occasional patients are very sensitive to the hypotensive effect of bromocriptine and may even collapse within an hour of the first dose, a test dose of 1 mg should be given initially, with food and with the patient in bed. If vascular collapse occurs, recovery is usually rapid and spontaneous, and patients often tolerate subsequent doses well. Treatment with bromocriptine should be stopped if it leads to psychiatric disturbances, cardiac dysrhythmia, erythromelalgia, ergotism, or other intolerable adverse effects.

Adverse Effects

A. Gastrointestinal Effects: Anorexia and nausea and vomiting are especially common when bromocriptine therapy is introduced and can be minimized by taking the medication with meals. Other adverse gastrointestinal effects include constipation, dyspepsia, and symptoms suggestive of reflux esophagitis. Bleeding from peptic ulceration has also been reported.

B. Cardiovascular Effects: Postural hypotension is fairly common, especially at the initiation of therapy. Painless digital vasospasm is a complication of long-term treatment that can be reversed by lowering the dose. Cardiac arrhythmias may also occur with bromocriptine and are an indication for discontinuing treatment.

C. Dyskinesias: Abnormal movements similar to those introduced by levodopa can be produced by bromocriptine. Treatment consists of reducing the total dose of dopaminergic drugs being taken.

D. Mental Disturbances: Confusion, hallucinations, delusions, and other psychiatric reactions are established complications of dopaminergic treatment of parkinsonism. They are more common and severe with bromocriptine than with levodopa itself. Such effects clear on withdrawal of the offending medication.

E. Miscellaneous Adverse Effects: Headache, nasal congestion, increased arousal, pulmonary infiltrates, and erythromelalgia are other reported side effects of bromocriptine. Erythromelalgia consists of red, tender, painful, swollen feet and, occasionally, hands, at times associated with arthralgia; symptoms and signs clear within a few days of withdrawal of bromocriptine.

Contraindications

Bromocriptine treatment is contraindicated in patients with a history of psychotic illness or recent myocardial infarction. It is best avoided in patients with peripheral vascular disease or peptic ulceration.

PERGOLIDE

Pergolide is another dopamine agonist ergot derivative that directly stimulates both D_1 and D_2 receptors. The drug may benefit patients not receiving levodopa, and it also prolongs the response to levodopa in patients with response fluctuations. It is generally well tolerated, but adverse effects are frequent at the initiation of therapy and resemble those of bromocriptine. Pergolide tends to lose its efficacy with time, probably owing to the down-regulation of dopamine receptors. It is not clear whether the use of pergolide at an early stage of Parkinson's disease—either alone or in combination with low-dose levodopa—will delay the onset of dopa-induced adverse effects.

The average therapeutic dose of pergolide is 3 mg daily; patients are generally started on 0.05 mg daily, and the dose is built up by increments until benefit occurs or toxicity limits further increments. The dose of levodopa taken concurrently may have to be reduced.

NEWER DOPAMINE AGONISTS

Several nonergot dopamine agonists have been developed that are more selective than the ergot derivatives and appear quite promising in the treatment of parkinsonism. **Pramipexole** and **ropinirole** are currently in phase III clinical trials.

MONOAMINE OXIDASE INHIBITORS

Two types of monoamine oxidase have been distinguished. Monoamine oxidase A metabolizes norepinephrine and serotonin; monoamine oxidase B metabolizes dopamine. **Selegiline** (deprenyl) (Figure 28–2), a selective inhibitor of monoamine oxidase B, retards the breakdown of dopamine; in consequence, it enhances and prolongs the antiparkinsonism effect of levodopa (thereby allowing the dose of levodopa to be reduced) and may reduce mild on-off or wearing-off phenomena. It is therefore used as adjunctive therapy for patients with a declining or fluctuating response to levodopa. The standard dose is 5 mg with breakfast and 5 mg with lunch. Selegiline may cause insomnia when taken later during the day. It should not be taken by patients receiving meperidine, tricyclic agents, or serotonin reuptake inhibitors because of the risk of acute toxic interactions. The adverse effects of levodopa may be increased by selegiline. Selegiline has only a minor therapeutic effect on parkinsonism when given alone, but studies in animals suggest that it may reduce disease progression. Such an effect of antioxidative therapy on disease progression may be expected if Parkinson's disease is associated with the oxidative generation of free radicals. However, studies to test the effect of selegiline on the progression of parkinsonism in humans have yielded ambiguous results. The findings in a recent large multicenter study have been taken to suggest a beneficial effect in slowing disease progression but may simply have reflected a symptomatic response.

The combined administration of levodopa and an inhibitor of both forms of monoamine oxidase must be avoided, since it may lead to hypertensive crises, probably because of the peripheral accumulation of norepinephrine.

CATECHOL-*O*-METHYLTRANSFERASE INHIBITORS

Inhibition of dopa decarboxylase is associated with compensatory activation of other pathways of levodopa metabolism, especially catechol-*O*-methyltransferase (COMT), and this increases plasma levels of 3-methyldopa (3OMD). Elevated levels of 3OMD have been associated with a poor therapeutic response to levodopa, perhaps in part because 3OMD competes with levodopa for an active carrier mechanism that governs its transport across the intestinal mucosa and the blood-brain barrier. For this reason, selective COMT inhibitors are currently being evaluated as adjunctive therapy for parkinsonian patients receiving levodopa.

AMANTADINE

Amantadine, an antiviral agent, was by chance found to have antiparkinsonism properties. Its mode of action in parkinsonism is unclear, but it may potentiate dopaminergic function by influencing the synthesis, release, or reuptake of dopamine. Release of catecholamines from peripheral stores has been documented.

Pharmacokinetics

Peak plasma concentrations of amantadine are reached 1–4 hours after an oral dose. The plasma half-life is between 2 and 4 hours, most of the drug being excreted unchanged in the urine.

Clinical Use

Amantadine is less potent than levodopa and its benefits may be short-lived, often disappearing after only a few weeks of treatment. Nevertheless, during that time it may favorably influence the bradykinesia, rigidity, and tremor of parkinsonism. The standard dose is 100 mg orally twice daily.

Adverse Effects

Amantadine has a number of undesirable central nervous system effects, all of which can be reversed by stopping the drug. These include restlessness, depression, irritability, insomnia, agitation, excitement, hallucinations, and confusion. Overdosage may produce an acute toxic psychosis. With doses several times higher than recommended, convulsions have occurred.

Livedo reticularis sometimes occurs in patients taking amantadine and usually clears within a month after the drug is withdrawn. Other dermatologic reactions have also been described. Peripheral edema, another well-recognized complication, is not accompanied by signs of cardiac, hepatic, or renal disease and responds to diuretics. Other adverse reactions include headache, congestive heart failure, postural hypotension, urinary retention, and gastrointestinal disturbances (eg, anorexia, nausea, constipation, and dry mouth).

Contraindications

The drug should be used with caution in patients with a history of seizures or congestive heart failure.

ACETYLCHOLINE-BLOCKING DRUGS

A number of centrally acting antimuscarinic preparations are available that differ in their potency and in their efficacy in different patients.

Clinical Use

Treatment is started with a low dose of one of the drugs in this category, the level of medication gradually being increased until benefit occurs or adverse effects limit further increments. Antimuscarinic drugs may improve the tremor and rigidity of parkinsonism but have little effect on bradykinesia. If patients fail to respond to one drug, a trial with another is certainly warranted and may be successful. Some of the more commonly used drugs are listed in Table 28–1.

Adverse Effects

Antimuscarinic drugs have a number of central nervous system effects, including drowsiness, mental slowness, inattention, restlessness, confusion, agitation, delusions, hallucinations, and mood changes.

Table 28–1. Some drugs with antimuscarinic properties used in parkinsonism.

Drug	Usual Daily Dose (mg)
Benztropine mesylate	1–6
Biperiden	2–12
Orphenadrine	150–400
Procyclidine	7.5–30
Trihexyphenidyl	6–20

Such effects are sometimes precipitated by intercurrent infections and usually subside within a few days after withdrawal of the drug. Other common effects include dryness of the mouth, blurring of vision, mydriasis, urinary retention, nausea and vomiting, constipation, tachycardia, tachypnea, increased intraocular pressure, palpitations, and cardiac arrhythmias. Dyskinesias occur in rare cases. Acute suppurative parotitis sometimes occurs as a complication of dryness of the mouth.

If medication is to be withdrawn, this should be accomplished gradually rather than abruptly in order to prevent acute exacerbation of parkinsonism.

Contraindications

Acetylcholine-blocking drugs should be avoided in patients with prostatic hyperplasia, obstructive gastrointestinal disease (eg, pyloric stenosis or paralytic ileus), or angle-closure glaucoma. In parkinsonism patients receiving antimuscarinic medication, concomitant administration of other drugs with antimuscarinic properties (eg, tricyclic antidepressants or antihistamines) may precipitate some of the complications mentioned above.

SURGICAL PROCEDURES

In patients with advanced disease that is poorly responsive to pharmacotherapy, worthwhile benefit may follow thalamotomy (for conspicuous tremor) or posteroventral pallidotomy. Transplantation of dopaminergic tissue (autologous adrenal medullary tissue or fetal substantia nigra tissue) has been reported to confer benefit in some parkinsonism patients, but the results are conflicting and these procedures are best regarded as investigational.

OTHER EXPERIMENTAL APPROACHES TO THE TREATMENT OF PARKINSON'S DISEASE

A therapeutic role has been suggested for vitamin E, a scavenger of free radicals, in slowing disease progression. A recent large multicenter study, however, found no evidence of benefit when tocopherol (2000 IU) was taken daily.

Neurotransmitters other than dopamine and acetylcholine may also be involved in Parkinson's disease. Norepinephrine deficiency has been implicated in the pathogenesis of transient freezing-up, but administration of D, L-*threo*-3, 4-dihydroxyphenylserine (DOPS), a precursor of norepinephrine, has failed to provide consistent benefit. Increased glutamatergic activity from overactivity of the subthalamic nucleus (Figure 28–4) may also occur, and the role of glutamate antagonists in therapy is therefore under investigation.

Several neurotrophic factors, such as muscle-derived differentiation factor and brain-derived neurotrophic factor, are known to influence dopaminergic nigrostriatal cells and may well have a role in therapy once an adequate delivery system has been devised. Similarly, G_{MI} ganglioside has been shown to increase striatal dopamine levels and enhance the dopaminergic innervation of the striatum and may provide a new therapeutic approach.

GENERAL COMMENTS ON DRUG MANAGEMENT OF PATIENTS WITH PARKINSONISM

Parkinson's disease generally follows a progressive course. Moreover, the benefits of levodopa therapy often seem to diminish with time and certain adverse effects may complicate long-term levodopa treatment. Nevertheless, evidence is accumulating that dopaminergic therapy at a relatively early stage may be most effective in alleviating symptoms of parkinsonism and may also favorably affect the mortality rate due to the disease. Symptomatic treatment of mild parkinsonism is probably best avoided until there is some degree of disability or until symptoms begin to have a significant impact on the patient's life-style. When treatment becomes necessary, levodopa is usually prescribed in combination with carbidopa as Sinemet, and amantadine or an antimuscarinic drug (or both) may be necessary as well for optimal benefit. Some of the long-term adverse effects of levodopa (such as response-fluctuations and dyskinesias) can probably be avoided or minimized if the total daily dose of Sinemet is kept low and dopaminergic therapy is increased by adding bromocriptine or pergolide. Physical therapy is helpful in improving mobility. In patients with severe parkinsonism and long-term complications of levodopa therapy, such as the on-off phenomena, a trial of treatment with bromocriptine or pergolide may be worthwhile. Regulation of dietary protein intake may also improve response fluctuations.

Treatment with selegiline of patients who are young or have mild parkinsonism may delay disease progression and merits consideration.

Figure 28–4. Functional circuitry between the cortex, basal ganglia, and thalamus. The involved neurotransmitters are indicated. In Parkinson's disease, there is degeneration of the pars compacta of the substantia nigra, leading to overactivity in the indirect pathway (color) and increased glutamatergic activity by the subthalamic nucleus.

DRUG-INDUCED PARKINSONISM

Reserpine and the related drug tetrabenazine deplete biogenic monoamines from their storage sites, while haloperidol and the phenothiazines block dopamine receptors. These drugs may therefore produce a parkinsonian syndrome, usually within 3 months after introduction, which is related to high dosage and clears over a few weeks or months after withdrawal. If treatment is necessary, antimuscarinic agents are preferred. Levodopa is of no help if neuroleptic drugs are continued and may in fact aggravate the mental disorder for which antipsychotic drugs were prescribed originally.

In 1983, a drug-induced form of parkinsonism was discovered in individuals who attempted to synthesize and use a narcotic drug related to meperidine but actually synthesized and self-administered 1-methyl-4-phenyl-1,2,5,6-tetrahydropyridine, as discussed in the text box: MPTP & Parkinsonism.

MPTP & PARKINSONISM

Reports in the early 1980s of a rapidly progressive form of parkinsonism in young persons opened a new area of research in the etiology and treatment of parkinsonism. The initial report described apparently healthy young people who attempted to support their opioid habit with a meperidine analog synthesized by an amateur chemist. They unwittingly self-administered 1-methyl-4-phenyl-1,2,3,6-tetrahydropyridine (MPTP) and subsequently developed a very severe form of parkinsonism.

MPTP is a protoxin that is converted by monoamine oxidase B to N-methyl-4-phenylpyridinium (MPP$^+$). MPP$^+$ is selectively taken up by cells in the substantia nigra through an active mechanism normally responsible for dopamine reuptake. MPP$^+$ inhibits mitochondrial complex 1, thereby inhibiting oxidative phosphorylation. The interaction of MPP$^+$ with complex I probably leads to cell death and thus to striatal dopamine depletion and parkinsonism.

Recognition of the effects of MPTP suggested that spontaneously occurring Parkinson's disease may result from exposure to an environmental toxin that is similarly selective in its target. However, no such toxin has yet been identified. It also suggested a successful means of producing an experimental model of Parkinson's disease in animals, especially nonhuman primates. This model may assist in the development of new antiparkinsonism drugs. Pretreatment of exposed animals with a monoamine oxidase B inhibitor such as selegiline prevents the conversion of MPTP to MPP$^+$ and thus protects against the occurrence of parkinsonism. This observation has provided one reason to believe that selegiline may retard the progression of Parkinson's disease in humans.

OTHER MOVEMENT DISORDERS

Tremor

Tremor consists of rhythmic oscillatory movements. Physiologic postural tremor, which is a normal phenomenon, is enhanced in amplitude by anxiety, fatigue, thyrotoxicosis, and intravenous epinephrine or isoproterenol. Propranolol reduces its amplitude, and, if administered intra-arterially, prevents the response to isoproterenol in the perfused limb, presumably through some peripheral action. Certain drugs—especially the bronchodilators, tricyclic antidepressants, and lithium—may produce a dose-dependent exaggeration of the normal physiologic tremor that is readily reversed by discontinuing the drug. Although the tremor produced by sympathomimetics such as terbutaline (a bronchodilator) is blocked by propranolol, which antagonizes both β_1 and β_2 receptors, it is not blocked by metoprolol, a β_1-selective antagonist, suggesting that such tremor is mediated mainly by the β_2 receptors.

Essential tremor is a postural tremor, sometimes familial, that is clinically similar to physiologic tremor. Dysfunction of β_1 receptors has been implicated in some instances, since the tremor may respond dramatically to standard doses of metoprolol as well as to propranolol. The most useful approach is with propranolol, but whether the response depends on a central or peripheral action is unclear. The pharmacokinetics, pharmacologic effects, and adverse reactions of propranolol are discussed in Chapter 10. Daily doses of propranolol on the order of 120 mg (range, 60–240 mg) are usually required, and reported adverse effects have been few. Propranolol should be used with caution in patients with congestive cardiac failure, heart block, asthma, and hypoglycemia. Patients can be instructed to take their own pulse and call the physician if significant bradycardia develops. Metoprolol is sometimes useful in treating tremor when patients have concomitant pulmonary disease that contraindicates use of propranolol. Primidone (an antiepileptic drug; see Chapter 24), in gradually increasing doses up to 250 mg three times daily, is also effective in providing symptomatic control in some cases. Patients with tremor are very sensitive to primidone and often cannot tolerate the doses used to treat seizures; they should be started on 50 mg once daily and the daily dose increased by 50 mg every 2 weeks depending on response. Small quantities of alcohol may suppress essential tremor, but only for a short time and by an unknown mechanism. Diazepam, chlordiazepoxide, mephenesin, and antiparkinsonism agents have been advocated in the past but are generally worthless. Alprazolam (in doses up to 3 mg daily) is helpful in occasional patients.

Intention tremor—tremor present during movement but not at rest—sometimes occurs as a toxic manifestation of alcohol or drugs such as phenytoin. Withdrawal or reduction in dosage provides dramatic relief. There is no satisfactory pharmacologic treatment for intention tremor due to other neurologic disorders.

Rest tremor is usually due to parkinsonism.

Huntington's Disease

This dominantly inherited disorder is characterized by progressive chorea and dementia that usually begin in adulthood. The development of chorea seems to be related to an imbalance of dopamine, acetylcholine,

GABA, and perhaps other neurotransmitters in the basal ganglia (Figure 28–1). Pharmacologic studies indicate that chorea results from functional overactivity in dopaminergic nigrostriatal pathways, perhaps because of increased responsiveness of postsynaptic dopamine receptors or deficiency of a neurotransmitter that normally antagonizes dopamine. Drugs that impair dopaminergic neurotransmission, either by depleting central monoamines (eg, reserpine, tetrabenazine) or by blocking dopamine receptors (eg, phenothiazines, butyrophenones), often alleviate chorea, whereas dopamine-like drugs such as levodopa tend to exacerbate it.

Both GABA and the enzyme (glutamic acid decarboxylase) concerned with its synthesis are markedly reduced in the basal ganglia of patients with Huntington's disease, and GABA receptors are usually implicated in inhibitory pathways. There is also a significant decline in concentration of choline acetyltransferase, the enzyme responsible for synthesizing acetylcholine, in the basal ganglia of these patients. These findings may be of pathophysiologic significance and have led to attempts to alleviate chorea by enhancing central GABA or acetylcholine activity. Unfortunately, such pharmacologic manipulations have been disappointing, yielding no consistently beneficial response, and as a consequence the most commonly used drugs for controlling dyskinesia in patients with Huntington's disease are still those that interfere with dopamine activity. With all of the latter drugs, however, reduction of abnormal movements may be associated with iatrogenic parkinsonism.

Reserpine depletes cerebral dopamine by preventing intraneuronal storage; it is introduced in low doses (eg, 0.25 mg daily), and the daily dose is then built up gradually (eg, by 0.25 mg every week) until benefit occurs or adverse effects become troublesome. A daily dose of 2–5 mg is often effective in suppressing abnormal movements, but adverse effects may include hypotension, depression, sedation, diarrhea, and nasal congestion. Tetrabenazine resembles reserpine in depleting cerebral dopamine and has less troublesome adverse effects, but it is not available in the USA. Treatment with postsynaptic dopamine receptor blockers such as phenothiazines and butyrophenones may also be helpful. Haloperidol is started in a small dose, eg, 1 mg twice daily, and increased every 4 days depending upon the response. If haloperidol is not helpful, treatment with increasing doses of perphenazine up to a total of about 20 mg daily sometimes helps. The pharmacokinetics and clinical properties of these drugs are considered in greater detail elsewhere in this book.

Other Forms of Chorea

Treatment is directed at the underlying cause when chorea occurs as a complication of general medical disorders such as thyrotoxicosis, polycythemia vera rubra, systemic lupus erythematosus, hypocalcemia, and hepatic cirrhosis. Drug-induced chorea is managed by withdrawal of the offending substance, which may be levodopa, an antimuscarinic drug, amphetamine, lithium, phenytoin, or an oral contraceptive. Neuroleptic drugs may also produce an acute or tardive dyskinesia (discussed below). Sydenham's chorea is temporary and usually so mild that pharmacologic management of the dyskinesia is unnecessary, but dopamine-blocking drugs are effective in suppressing it.

Ballismus

The biochemical basis of ballismus is unknown, but the pharmacologic approach to management is the same as for chorea. Treatment with haloperidol, perphenazine, or other dopamine-blocking drugs may be helpful.

Athetosis & Dystonia

The pharmacologic basis of these disorders is unknown, and there is no satisfactory medical treatment for them. Occasional patients with dystonia may respond to diazepam, amantadine, antimuscarinic drugs (in high dosage), levodopa, carbamazepine, baclofen, haloperidol, or phenothiazines. A trial of these pharmacologic approaches is worthwhile even though often not successful. Patients with focal dystonias such as blepharospasm or torticollis may benefit from injection of botulinum toxin into the overactive muscles.

Tics

The pathophysiologic basis of tics is unknown. Chronic multiple tics (Gilles de la Tourette's syndrome) may require treatment if the disorder is severe or is having a significant impact on the patient's life. The most effective pharmacologic approach is with haloperidol, and patients are better able to tolerate this drug if treatment is started with a small dosage (eg, 0.25 or 0.5 mg daily) and then increased very gradually over the following weeks. Most patients ultimately require a total daily dose of 3–8 mg. If haloperidol is not helpful, fluphenazine, clonazepam, clonidine, or carbamazepine should be tried. The pharmacologic properties of these drugs are discussed elsewhere in this book. Pimozide, an oral dopamine blocker, may help patients intolerant or unresponsive to haloperidol, but the long-term safety of the drug is unclear.

Drug-Induced Dyskinesias

The pharmacologic basis of the acute dyskinesia or dystonia sometimes precipitated by the first few doses of a phenothiazine is not clear. In most instances, parenteral administration of an antimuscarinic drug such as benztropine (2 mg intravenously), diphenhydramine (50 mg intravenously), or biperiden (2–5 mg intravenously or intramuscularly) is helpful, while in other instances diazepam (10 mg intravenously) alleviates the abnormal movements.

Tardive dyskinesia is a disorder characterized by a variety of abnormal movements that develop after long-term neuroleptic drug treatment. A reduction in dose of the offending medication, a dopamine receptor blocker, commonly worsens the dyskinesia, while an increase in dose may suppress it. These clinical observations, and the exacerbation in the movement disorder that is produced by levodopa, suggest that tardive dyskinesia relates to increased dopaminergic function, but its precise pharmacologic basis is unclear. It would seem, therefore, that phenothiazines cause a short-term reversible blockade of dopamine receptors but that over the long term they increase dopaminergic function. Whether this latter effect depends upon the development of denervation supersensitivity, increased dopamine synthesis, or diminished reuptake of dopamine at central synapses is not known.

There is some evidence that GABA is involved in a striatonigral feedback loop modulating the activity of dopaminergic cells in the substantia nigra, and GABA efferents also pass from the striatum to the globus pallidus and thalamus. GABA-mediated activity may diminish the activity of nigrostriatal dopaminergic cells and thereby decrease involuntary movements. **Muscimol,** a semirigid structural analog of GABA, has been given to a small number of patients with tardive dyskinesia, and at oral doses of 5–9 mg daily consistently attenuated their involuntary movements in one study. However, muscimol has adverse behavioral effects that limit any role for it in the treatment of tardive dyskinesia. Other attempts to increase central GABA activity (eg, with benzodiazepines or sodium valproate) have not yielded consistent benefit. Attempts to restore the balance between dopaminergic and cholinergic activity by increasing the latter with oral choline or lecithin have been helpful in some instances but not in others, and the same was true of treatment with deanol acetamidobenzoate, a drug related to acetylcholine and now discontinued. The drugs most likely to provide immediate symptomatic benefit are those interfering with dopaminergic function, either by depletion (eg, reserpine, tetrabenazine) or receptor blockade (eg, phenothiazines, butyrophenones). Paradoxically, the receptor-blocking drugs are the very ones that also cause the dyskinesia, and they are probably best avoided to prevent the development of a spiral phenomenon in which continuing aggravation of the dyskinesia by the drugs used to control it necessitates increasingly higher doses for its temporary suppression.

Because tardive dyskinesia developing in adults is usually irreversible and has no satisfactory treatment, care must be taken to reduce the likelihood of its occurrence. Antipsychotic medication should be prescribed only when necessary and should be withheld periodically to assess the need for continued treatment and to unmask incipient dyskinesia. Thioridazine, a phenothiazine with a piperidine side chain, is an effective antipsychotic that seems less likely than most to cause extrapyramidal reactions, perhaps because it has little effect on dopamine receptors in the striatal system. Finally, antimuscarinic drugs should not be prescribed routinely in patients receiving neuroleptics, since the combination may increase the likelihood of dyskinesia.

Wilson's Disease

Wilson's disease, a recessively inherited disorder of copper metabolism, is characterized biochemically by reduced serum copper and ceruloplasmin concentrations, pathologically by markedly increased concentration of copper in the brain and viscera, and clinically by signs of hepatic and neurologic dysfunction. Treatment involves the removal of excess copper, followed by maintenance of copper balance. The most satisfactory agent currently available for this purpose is **penicillamine** (dimethylcysteine), a chelating agent that forms a ring complex with copper. It is readily absorbed from the gastrointestinal tract and rapidly excreted in the urine. A common starting dose in adults is 500 mg three or four times daily. After remission occurs, it may be possible to lower the maintenance dose, generally to not less than 1 g daily, which must thereafter be continued indefinitely. Adverse effects include nausea and vomiting, nephrotic syndrome, a lupus-like syndrome, pemphigus, myasthenia, arthropathy, optic neuropathy, and various blood dyscrasias. Treatment should be monitored by frequent urinalysis and complete blood counts. Dietary copper should also be kept below 2 mg daily by the exclusion of chocolate, nuts, shellfish, liver, mushrooms, broccoli, and cereals; and distilled or demineralized water may have to be provided if tap water contains more than 0.1 mg of copper per liter. Potassium disulfide, 20 mg three times daily with meals, reduces the intestinal absorption of copper and should also be prescribed.

For those patients who are unable to tolerate penicillamine, **trientine,** a newer chelating agent, may be used in a daily dose of 1–1.5 g. Trientine appears to have few adverse effects other than mild anemia due to iron deficiency in a few patients.

Zinc acetate administered orally increases the fecal excretion of copper and is sometimes used for maintenance therapy. The dose is 50 mg three times a day. **Zinc sulfate** (200 mg/d orally) has also been used to decrease copper absorption.

PREPARATIONS AVAILABLE

Amantadine (Symmetrel, others)
Oral: 100 mg capsules; 10 mg/mL syrup

Benztropine (Cogentin, others)
Oral: 0.5, 1, 2 mg tablets
Parenteral: 1 mg/mL for injection

Biperiden (Akineton)
Oral: 2 mg tablets
Parenteral: 5 mg/mL for injection

Bromocriptine (Parlodel)
Oral: 2.5 mg tablets; 5 mg capsules

Carbidopa (Lodosyn)
Oral: 25 mg tablets

Carbidopa/levodopa (Sinemet)
Oral: 10 mg carbidopa and 100 mg levodopa, 25 mg carbidopa and 100 mg levodopa, 25 mg carbidopa and 250 mg levodopa tablets
Oral sustained-release (Sinemet CR): 50 mg carbidopa and 200 mg levodopa

Levodopa (Dopar, Larodopa)
Oral: 100, 250, 500 mg tablets, capsules

Orphenadrine (various)
Oral: 100 mg tablets
Oral sustained-release: 100 mg tablets
Parenteral: 30 mg/mL for injection

Penicillamine (Cuprimine, Depen)
Oral: 125, 250 mg capsules; 250 mg tablets

Pergolide (Permax)
Oral: 0.05, 0.25, 1 mg tablets

Procyclidine (Kemadrin)
Oral: 5 mg tablets

Selegiline (deprenyl) (Eldepryl)
Oral: 5 mg tablets

Trientine (Syprine)
Oral: 250 mg capsules

Trihexyphenidyl (Artane, others)
Oral: 2, 5 mg tablets; 2 mg/5 mL elixir
Oral sustained-release (Artane Sequels): 5 mg capsules

REFERENCES

Agid Y: Parkinson's disease: Pathophysiology. Lancet 1991;337:1321.

Aminoff MJ: Treatment of Parkinson's disease. West J Med 1994;161:303.

Brewer JG: Practical recommendations and new therapies for Wilson's disease. Drugs 1995;50:240.

Campanella G et al: Drugs affecting movement disorders. Annu Rev Pharmacol Toxicol 1987;27:113.

Carter JH, et al: Amount and distribution of dietary protein affects clinical response to levodopa in Parkinson's disease. Neurology 1989;39:552.

Cedarbaum JM: Clinical pharmacokinetics of anti-parkinsonian drugs. Clin Pharmacokinet 1987;13:141.

Diamond SG et al: Multi-center study of Parkinson mortality with early versus later dopa treatment. Ann Neurol 1987;22:8.

Edwards RH: Neural degeneration and the transport of neurotransmitters. Ann Neurol 1993;34:638.

Goetz CG et al: Neurosurgical horizons in Parkinson's disease. Neurology 1993;43:1.

Hubble JP et al: Essential tremor. Clin Neuropharmacol 1989;12:453.

Hutton JT et al: Multicenter controlled study of Sinemet CR vs Sinemet (25/100) in advanced Parkinson's disease. Neurology 1989;39(Suppl 2):67.

Hyde TM, Weinberger DR: Tourette's syndrome: A model neuropsychiatric disorder. JAMA 1995;273:498.

Kopin IJ: The pharmacology of Parkinson's disease therapy: An update. Annu Rev Pharmacol Toxicol 1993; 32:467.

Kordower JH et al: Neuropathological evidence of graft survival and striatal reinnervation after the transplantation of fetal mesencephalic tissue in a patient with Parkinson's disease. N Engl J Med 1995;332:1118.

Mouradian MM et al: Modification of central dopaminergic mechanisms by continuous levodopa therapy for advanced Parkinson's disease. Ann Neurol 1990;27:18.

Nakanishi T et al: Second interim report of the nation-wide collaborative study on the long-term effects of bromocriptine in the treatment of parkinsonian patients. Eur Neurol 1989;29(Suppl 1):3.

Nutt JG et al: Effects of peripheral catechol-O-methyltransferase inhibition on the pharmacokinetics and pharmacodynamics of levodopa in parkinsonian patients. Neurology 1994;44:913.

Nutt JG: On-off phenomenon: Relation to levodopa pharmacokinetics and pharmacodynamics. Ann Neurol 1987;22:535.

Nygaard TG et al: Dopa-responsive dystonia: Long-term treatment response and prognosis. Neurology 1991; 41:174.

Obeso JA et al: Overcoming pharmacokinetic problems in the treatment of Parkinson's disease. Mov Disord 1989;4(Suppl 1):70.

Parkinson Study Group: Effects of tocopherol and deprenyl on the progression of disability in early Parkinson's disease. N Engl J Med 1993;328:176.

Quinn N: Drug treatment of Parkinson's disease. Br Med J 1995;310:575.

Riley DE, Lang AK: The spectrum of levodopa-related fluctuations in Parkinson's disease. Neurology 1993;43:1459.

Rinne UK: Long-term combination therapy with bromocriptine and levodopa. In: *Recent Developments in Parkinson's Disease II*. Macmillan, 1987.

Ross RT: Drug-induced parkinsonism and other movement disorders. Can J Neurol Sci 1990;22:155.

Scheinberg IH, Jaffe ME, Sternlieb I: The use of trientine in preventing the effects of interrupting penicillamine therapy in Wilson's disease. N Engl J Med 1987;317:209.

Schneider JS et al: Recovery from experimental parkinsonism in primates with G_{M1} ganglioside treatment. Science 1992;256:843.

Schulzer M et al: The antiparkinson efficacy of deprenyl derives from transient improvement that is likely to be symptomatic. Ann Neurol 1992;32:795.

Shapiro AK et al: Pimozide treatment of tic and Tourette disorders. Pediatrics 1987;79:6.

Stoof JC et al: Regulation of the activity of striatal cholinergic neurons dopamine. Neuroscience 1992;47:755.

29

Antipsychotic Agents & Lithium

William Z. Potter MD, PhD, & Leo E. Hollister, MD

ANTIPSYCHOTIC AGENTS

The terms **antipsychotic** and **neuroleptic** are used interchangeably to denote a group of drugs that have been used mainly for treating schizophrenia but are also effective in some other psychoses and agitated states.

History

Antipsychotic drugs have been used clinically for almost 50 years. Reserpine and chlorpromazine were the first drugs found to be useful in schizophrenia. Although chlorpromazine is still sometimes used for the treatment of psychoses, these forerunner drugs have been superseded by many newer agents. Their impact on psychiatry, however—especially on the treatment of schizophrenia—has been enormous: The number of patients requiring hospitalization in mental institutions has markedly decreased, and psychiatric thinking has shifted to a more biologic basis. Unfortunately, neither of these developments has been as rewarding in human or medical-economic terms as initially hoped.

Nature of Psychosis & Schizophrenia

The term "psychosis" denotes a variety of mental disorders. Schizophrenia is a particular kind of psychosis characterized mainly by a clear sensorium but a marked thinking disturbance.

The pathogenesis of schizophrenia is unknown. Largely as a result of research stimulated by the discovery of antipsychotic drugs, a genetic predisposition has been proposed as a necessary but not always sufficient condition underlying psychotic disorder. To some extent, this assumption has been supported by the familial incidence of schizophrenia. Actual determination of chromosomal linkages using the tech-niques of molecular genetics has been more difficult to establish firmly, mainly because the phenotype is not accurately diagnosable. The molecular basis for schizophrenia still eludes full definition, but a great deal of effort has been expended in attempting to link the disorder with abnormalities of amine neurotransmitter function, especially dopamine function (see accompanying box). The defects of this hypothesis are significant, however, and suggest that the disorder is even more complex than originally supposed.

An additional factor indicating heterogeneity among schizophrenic patients is the presence or absence of anatomic changes. A number of studies using brain imaging techniques (CT or MRI) in living subjects have shown atrophy of various brain structures in some schizophrenics as compared with age-matched normals. Such patients tend to show predominantly "negative" symptoms (emotional blunting, poor socialization, cognitive deficit), which are unresponsive to drugs. Furthermore, positron emission tomography (PET) scanning has shown areas of decreased metabolism in various parts of the brain in some patients.

I. Basic Pharmacology of Antipsychotic Agents

Chemical Types

A number of chemical structures have been associated with antipsychotic properties. The drugs can be classified into several groups as shown in Figures 29–1 and 29–2.

A. Phenothiazine Derivatives: Three subfamilies of phenothiazines, based primarily on the side chain of the molecule, are currently used. Aliphatic derivatives (eg, **chlorpromazine**) and piperidine derivatives (eg, **thioridazine**) are the least potent. Piper-

---

THE DOPAMINE HYPOTHESIS

The dopamine hypothesis for schizophrenia is the most fully developed of several hypotheses and is the basis for much of the rationale for drug therapy. Several lines of circumstantial evidence suggest that excessive dopaminergic activity underlies the disorder: (1) most antipsychotic drugs strongly block postsynaptic D_2 receptors in the central nervous system, especially in the mesolimbic-frontal system; (2) drugs that increase dopaminergic activity, such as levodopa (a precursor), amphetamines (releasers of dopamine), or apomorphine (a direct dopamine receptor agonist), either aggravate schizophrenia or produce it de novo in some patients; (3) dopamine receptor density has been found, postmortem, to be increased in the brains of schizophrenics who have not been treated with antipsychotic drugs; (4) positron emission tomography (PET) has shown increased dopamine receptor density in both treated and untreated schizophrenics when compared with such scans of nonschizophrenic persons; and (5) successful treatment of schizophrenic patients has been reported to change the amount of homovanillic acid (HVA), a metabolite of dopamine, in the cerebrospinal fluid, plasma, and urine.

The dopamine hypothesis is far from complete, however. If an abnormality of dopamine physiology were completely responsible for the pathogenesis of schizophrenia, antipsychotic drugs would do a much better job of treating patients—but they are only partially effective for most and ineffective for some patients. The recent cloning and characterization of multiple dopamine receptor types may permit more widespread acceptance of the dopamine hypothesis if drugs can be developed that act selectively on each receptor type. The traditional antipsychotics bind D_2 50 times more avidly than D_1 or D_3 receptors. Until recently, the main thrust in drug development was to find agents that were more potent and more selective in blocking D_2 receptors. The fact that several of the atypical antipsychotic drugs have much less effect on D_2 receptors and yet are effective in schizophrenia has redirected attention to the role of other dopamine receptors and to nondopamine receptors, especially the $5-HT_2$ receptor. Some studies suggest that even among the traditional phenothiazines, the correlation of clinical efficacy with α-adrenoceptor-blocking potency is better than with dopamine-blocking potency. As a result of these considerations, the direction of research has changed to a greater focus on compounds that may act on several transmitter-receptor systems. The great hope is to produce drugs with greater efficacy and fewer adverse effects, especially extrapyramidal toxicity.

---

azine derivatives are more potent in the sense that they are effective in lower doses. The piperazine derivatives are also more selective in their pharmacologic effects (Table 29–1).

B. Thioxanthene Derivatives: This group of drugs is exemplified primarily by **thiothixene.** In general, these compounds are slightly less potent than their phenothiazine analogs.

C. Butyrophenone Derivatives: This group, of which **haloperidol** is the most widely used, has a very different structure from those of the two preceding groups. Diphenylbutylpiperidines are closely related compounds. These agents tend to be more potent and to have fewer autonomic effects.

D. Miscellaneous Structures: The newer drugs have a variety of structures and include **pimozide, molindone, loxapine, clozapine, olanzapine, quetiapine, risperidone, sertindole,** and **remoxipride** (Figure 29–2).

Pharmacokinetics

A. Absorption and Distribution: Most antipsychotic drugs are readily but incompletely absorbed. Furthermore, many of these drugs undergo significant first-pass metabolism. Thus, oral doses of chlorpromazine and thioridazine have systemic availability from 25% to 35%, while haloperidol, which is less likely to be metabolized, has an average systemic availability of about 65%.

Most antipsychotics are highly lipid-soluble and protein-bound (92–99%). They tend to have large volumes of distribution (usually > 7 L/kg). Probably because these drugs are sequestered in lipid compartments of the body, they generally have a much longer clinical duration of action than would be estimated from their plasma half-lives. Metabolites of chlorpromazine may be excreted in the urine weeks after the last dose of chronically administered drug.

B. Metabolism: Most antipsychotics are almost completely metabolized by a variety of processes. Although some metabolites retain activity, eg, 7-hydroxychlorpromazine and reduced haloperidol, metabolites are not considered to be highly important to the action of these drugs. The sole exception is mesoridazine, the major metabolite of thioridazine, which is more potent than the parent compound and accounts for most of the effect. This compound has been marketed as a separate entity.

C. Excretion: Very little of any of these drugs is excreted unchanged, as they are almost completely

PHENOTHIAZINE DERIVATIVES

THIOXANTHENE DERIVATIVE

Figure 29–1. Structural formulas of some older antipsychotic drugs: phenothiazines, thioxanthenes, and butyrophenones. Only representative members of each type are shown.

metabolized to more polar substances. The elimination half-lives (as determined by metabolic clearance) vary from 10 to 24 hours.

Pharmacologic Effects

The first phenothiazine antipsychotic drugs, with chlorpromazine as the prototype, proved to have a wide variety of central nervous system, autonomic, and endocrine effects. These actions were traced to blocking effects at a remarkable number of receptors. These include dopamine and alpha-adrenoceptor, muscarinic, H_1 histaminic, and serotonin (5-HT$_2$) receptors. Of these, the dopamine receptor effects quickly became the major focus of interest.

A. Dopaminergic Systems: Until 1959, dopamine was not recognized as a neurotransmitter in the central nervous system but was simply regarded as a precursor for norepinephrine. Five important dopaminergic systems or pathways are now recognized in the brain. The first pathway—the one most closely related to behavior—is the **mesolimbic-mesocortical** pathway, which projects from cell bodies near the substantia nigra to the limbic system and neocortex. The second system—the **nigrostriatal** pathway—consists of neurons that project from the substantia nigra to the caudate and putamen; it is involved in the coordination of voluntary movement. The third pathway—the **tuberoinfundibular** system—connects arcuate nuclei and periventricular neurons to the hypothalamus and posterior pituitary. Dopamine released by these neurons physiologically inhibits prolactin secretion. The fourth dopaminergic system—the **medullary-periventricular** pathway—consists of neurons in the motor nucleus of the vagus whose projections are not well defined. This system may be involved in eating behavior. The fifth pathway—the **incertohypothalamic** pathway—forms connections within the hypothalamus and to the lateral septal nuclei. Its functions are not yet defined.

After dopamine was recognized as a neurotransmitter, various experiments showed that its effects on electrical activity in central synapses and on production of cAMP by adenylyl cyclase could be blocked by most antipsychotic drugs. This evidence led to the conclusion in the early 1960s that these drugs should be considered **dopamine antagonists.** The antipsychotic action is now thought to be produced (at least in part) by their ability to block dopamine in the mesolimbic and mesofrontal systems. Furthermore, the antagonism of dopamine in the nigrostriatal system explains the unwanted effect of parkinsonism produced by these drugs. The hyperprolactinemia that follows treatment with antipsychotics is caused by blockade of dopamine's tonic inhibitory effect on prolactin release from the pituitary. Finally, the changes in eating behavior observed in many patients taking antipsychotic drugs may be due to the drugs' effects on the medullary-periventricular pathway. Thus, the

Figure 29–2. Structural formulas of some newer antipsychotic drugs.

same pharmacodynamic action may have distinct psychiatric, neurologic, and endocrinologic consequences.

B. Dopamine Receptors and Their Effects: At present, five different dopamine receptors have been described, consisting of two separate families, the D_1-like and D_2-like receptor groups. The D_1 receptor is coded by a gene on chromosome 5, increases cAMP by activation of adenylyl cyclase, and is located mainly in the putamen, nucleus accumbens, and olfactory tubercle. The second member of this family, D_5, is coded by a gene on chromosome 4, also increases cAMP, and is found in the hippocampus and hypothalamus. The therapeutic potency of antipsy-

chotic drugs does not correlate with their affinity for binding the D_1 receptor (Figure 29–3, top). The D_2 receptor is coded on chromosome 11, decreases cAMP (by inhibition of adenylyl cyclase), and blocks calcium channels but opens potassium channels. It is found both pre- and postsynaptically on neurons in the caudate-putamen, nucleus accumbens, and olfactory tubercle. A second member of this family, the D_3 receptor, is coded by a gene on chromosome 11, is thought to decrease cAMP, and is located in the frontal cortex, medulla, and midbrain. D_4 receptors, the newest members of the D_2-like family, also decrease cAMP. All dopamine receptors have seven-transmembrane domains and are G protein-coupled.

Table 29–1. Antipsychotic drugs: Relation of chemical structure to potency and toxicities.

Chemical Class	Drug	Clinical Potency	Extrapyramidal Toxicity	Sedative Action	Hypotensive Actions
Phenothiazines Aliphatic	Chlorpromazine	Low	Medium	High	High
Piperazine	Fluphenazine	High	High	Low	Very low
Thioxanthene	Thiothixene	High	Medium	Medium	Medium
Butyrophenone	Haloperidol	High	Very high	Low	Very low
Dibenzodiazepine	Clozapine	Medium	Very low	Low	Medium
Benzisoxazole	Risperidone	High	Low[1]	Low	Low
Thienobenzodiazepine	Olanzapine	High	Very low	Medium	Very low
Fluorophenylindole	Sertindole	High	Very low	Very low	Very low

[1]At dosages below 8 mg/d.

The activation of D_2 receptors by a variety of direct or indirect agonists (eg, amphetamines, levodopa, apomorphine) causes increased motor activity and stereotyped behavior in rats, a model that has been extensively used for antipsychotic drug screening. When given to humans, the same drugs aggravate schizophrenia. The antipsychotic agents block D_2 receptors stereoselectively, for the most part, and their binding affinity is very strongly correlated with clinical antipsychotic and extrapyramidal potency (Figure 29–3, bottom), an observation that has led to a profusion of receptor binding studies.

Continuous treatment with antipsychotic drugs has been reported in some studies to produce a transient increase in levels of a dopamine metabolite, homovanillic acid (HVA), in the cerebrospinal fluid, plasma, and urine. After 1–3 weeks, HVA levels decrease to lower than normal levels, and this decrease persists. These changes may be explained as follows: The initial period of receptor blockade causes a compensatory increase in transmitter turnover, resulting in increased levels of HVA. With chronic therapy, feedback inhibition caused by the increased synaptic levels of dopamine results in decreased dopamine release and turnover. Some studies have failed to confirm these findings.

As noted above, these findings have been incorporated into the dopamine hypothesis of schizophrenia. However, many questions have not been satisfactorily answered, and many observations have not been fully confirmed. For example, dopamine receptors exist in both high- and low-affinity forms, and it is not known whether schizophrenia or the antipsychotic drugs alter the proportions of receptors in these two forms. Furthermore, the drug-induced progression of extrapyramidal changes—from diminished function (resembling parkinsonism) to increased activity (manifested by dyskinesias)—often occurs over a period of months to years. This time scale is much longer than that described for other drug-induced changes in receptor function. Most importantly, the most recently introduced drugs, clozapine, olanzapine, and sertin-

dole, are not very potent antagonists at the D_2 receptor, which suggests that additional actions are critical to their antipsychotic effects.

It has not been possible to demonstrate that antagonism of any receptor other than the D_2 receptor plays any role in the action of antipsychotic drugs. Selective D_3 receptor antagonists are not yet available. Specific D_1 receptor antagonists have been developed, and at least one is reputed to have failed in clinical trials. Attempts are under way to assess the effects of D_4 antagonism. Participation of glutamate, GABA, and other receptors in the pathophysiology of schizophrenia or the action of antipsychotic drugs has also been proposed. Definitive answers to these proposals may require a much longer time.

C. Differences Among Antipsychotic Drugs: Although all effective antipsychotic drugs block D_2 receptors, the degree of this blockade in relation to other actions on receptors varies considerably between drugs. Vast numbers of ligand-receptor binding experiments have been performed in an effort to discover a single receptor action that would best predict antipsychotic efficacy. For example, in vitro binding studies indicate that chlorpromazine and thioridazine block α_1 adrenoceptors more potently than D_2 receptors. They also block serotonin 5-HT$_2$ receptors relatively strongly. However, their affinity for D_1 receptors as measured by displacement of a selective D_1 ligand, SCH 23390, is relatively weak (Figure 29–3). Drugs such as perphenazine and haloperidol act mainly on D_2 receptors; they have some effect on 5-HT$_2$ and α_1 receptors but negligible effects on D_1 receptors. Pimozide acts almost exclusively on D_2 receptors. The atypical antipsychotic clozapine, which shows marked clinical differences from the others, binds more to D_4, 5-HT$_2$, α_1, and histamine H_1 receptors than to either D_2 or D_1 receptors. Risperidone is about equally potent in blocking D_2 and 5-HT$_2$ receptors. The recently introduced drug olanzapine is somewhat more potent as an antagonist of 5-HT$_2$ receptors, with lesser and approximately equal potency at D_1, D_2, and α_1 receptors. Sertindole is most potent

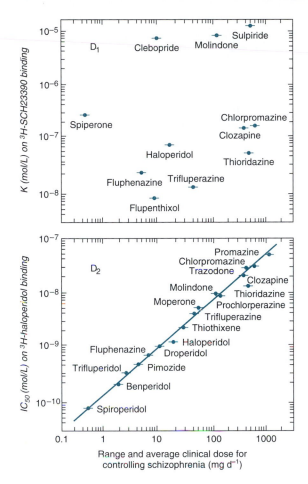

Figure 29–3. Correlations between the therapeutic potency of antipsychotic drugs and their affinity for binding to dopamine D_1 *(top)* or D_2 receptors *(bottom)*. Potency is indicated on the horizontal axes; it decreases to the right. Binding affinity for D_1 receptors was measured by displacing the selective D_1 ligand SCH 23390; affinity for D_2 receptors was similarly measured by displacing the selective D_2 ligand haloperidol. Binding affinity decreases upward. (Modified and reproduced, with permission, from Seeman P: Dopamine receptors and the dopamine hypothesis of schizophrenia. Synapse 1987; 1:133.)

as a 5-HT_2 antagonist and relatively potent as a D_2 and α_1 antagonist. Quetiapine is a lower-potency compound with relatively similar antagonism of 5-HT_2, D_2, α_1, and α_2 receptors. Like clozapine, both olanzapine and quetiapine are also potent inhibitors of H_1 histamine receptors, which is consistent with their sedative properties. A summary of the relative receptor-binding potencies of three key agents in such comparisons illustrates the difficulty in drawing simple conclusions from such experiments:

Chlorpromazine: $\alpha_1 = 5\text{-HT}_2 \geq D_2 > D_1$

Haloperidol: $D_2 > D_1 = D_4 > \alpha_1 > 5\text{-HT}_2$

Clozapine: $D_4 = \alpha_1 > 5\text{-HT}_2 > D_2 = D_1$

It appears that binding to D_1 receptors is the *least* predictive of significant clinical efficacy, but other receptor affinities are more difficult to interpret. Current research is directed toward discovering atypical antipsychotic compounds that are either more selective for the mesolimbic system (to reduce their effects on the extrapyramidal system) or have effects on central neurotransmitter receptors—such as those for acetylcholine and excitatory amino acids—that have not recently been proposed as targets for antipsychotic action.

In contrast to the search for *efficacy,* such differences in the receptor effects of various antipsychotics do explain many of their *toxicities* (Tables 29–1 and 29–2). In particular, extrapyramidal toxicity appears to be associated with high D_2 potency. It is hoped that some combination of various receptor actions may be found to mitigate these unwanted effects as well as increase antipsychotic efficacy.

D. Psychologic Effects: Most antipsychotic drugs cause unpleasant subjective effects in nonpsychotic individuals; the combination of sleepiness, restlessness, and autonomic effects creates experiences unlike those associated with more familiar sedatives or hypnotics. Nonpsychotic persons also experience impaired performance as judged by a number of psychomotor and psychometric tests. Psychotic individuals, however, may actually show improvement in their performance as the psychosis is alleviated.

E. Neurophysiologic Effects: Antipsychotic drugs produce shifts in the pattern of electroencephalographic frequencies, usually slowing them and increasing their synchronization. The slowing (hypersynchrony) is sometimes focal or unilateral, which may lead to erroneous diagnostic interpretations. Both the frequency and the amplitude changes induced by psychotropic drugs are readily apparent and can be quantitated by sophisticated electronic techniques.

Electroencephalographic changes associated with antipsychotic drugs appear first in subcortical electrodes, supporting the view that they exert their main action at subcortical sites. The hypersynchrony produced by these drugs may account for their activating effect on the EEG in epileptic patients as well as their occasional elicitation of seizures in patients with no history of seizures.

F. Endocrine Effects: Antipsychotic drugs produce striking adverse effects on the reproductive system. Amenorrhea-galactorrhea, false-positive pregnancy tests, and increased libido have been reported in women, whereas men have experienced decreased libido and gynecomastia. Some of these effects are secondary to blockade of dopamine's tonic inhibition of prolactin secretion; others may be due to increased peripheral conversion of androgens to estrogens. Absent or minimal increases of prolactin after some of the newer antipsychotics such as olanzapine, quetiapine, and sertindole may be a marker of diminished D_2 antagonism and hence reduced risks of extrapyramidal system dysfunction and tardive dyskinesia as well as endocrine dysfunction.

G. Cardiovascular Effects: Orthostatic hypotension and high resting pulse rates frequently result from use of the "high-dose" (low potency) phenothiazines. Mean arterial pressure, peripheral resistance, and stroke volume are decreased, and pulse rate is increased. These effects are predictable from the autonomic actions of these agents (Table 29–2). Abnormal ECGs have been recorded, especially with thioridazine. Changes include prolongation of QT interval and abnormal configurations of the ST segment and T waves, the latter being rounded, flattened, or notched. These changes are readily reversed by withdrawing the drug.

H. Animal Screening Tests: Inhibition of conditioned (but not unconditioned) avoidance behavior is one of the most predictive tests of antipsychotic action. Another is the inhibition of amphetamine- or apomorphine-induced stereotyped behavior. This inhibition is undoubtedly related to the D_2 receptor-blocking action of the drugs, countering these two dopamine agonists. Other tests that may predict antipsychotic action are reduction of exploratory behavior without undue sedation, induction of a cataleptic state, inhibition of intracranial stimulation of reward areas, and prevention of apomorphine-induced vomiting. Most of these tests are difficult to relate to any model of clinical psychosis.

The psychosis produced by phencyclidine (PCP) is a good model for schizophrenia. As this drug is an antagonist of the NMDA glutamate receptor, attempts have been made to develop antipsychotics that work as NMDA agonists. Sigma opioid and cholecystokinin type b (CCK_b) antagonism have also been suggested as potential targets. Thus far, success has been elusive with these novel models.

Newer models that will provide a means of identifying nondopamine antagonists as potential antipsychotics are the subject of intense investigation.

II. Clinical Pharmacology of Antipsychotic Agents

Indications

A. Psychiatric Indications: Schizophrenia is the primary indication for these drugs, which are presently the mainstay of treatment for this condition. Unfortunately, some patients do not respond at all and virtually none show a complete response. Because some schizophrenics have a favorable course with prolonged remission after an initial episode, most physicians recommend discontinuing drug therapy in this situation after remission has been achieved.

Schizoaffective disorders may be more similar to affective disorders than to schizophrenia. Nonetheless, the psychotic aspects of the illness require treatment with antipsychotic drugs, which may be used with other drugs such as antidepressants, lithium, or valproic acid. The manic episode in bipolar affective disorder often requires treatment with antipsychotic agents, though lithium or valproic acid supplemented with high-potency benzodiazepines (eg, lorazepam or clonopin) may suffice in milder cases. As mania subsides, the antipsychotic drug may be withdrawn. Nonmanic excited states may also be managed by antipsychotics, often in combination with benzodiazepines, but attempts to define the diagnosis should not be abandoned.

Other psychiatric indications for the use of antipsychotics include Tourette's syndrome and the need to control disturbed behavior in patients with senile dementia of the Alzheimer type. The drugs may also be used with antidepressants to control agitation or psychosis in depressed patients. Such patients have been reported to develop tardive dyskinesia more readily, so they must be dosed sparingly. It appears possible that some of the newer drugs such as olanzapine will show "antidepressant" efficacy in schizophrenia, as was reported for thioridazine decades ago. Antipsychotics are not indicated

Table 29–2. Adverse pharmacologic effects of antipsychotic drugs.

Type	Manifestations	Mechanism
Autonomic nervous system	Loss of accommodation, dry mouth, difficulty urinating, constipation	Muscarinic cholinoceptor blockade
	Orthostatic hypotension, failure to ejaculate	Alpha adrenoceptor blockade
Central nervous system	Parkinson's syndrome, akathisia, dystonias	Dopamine receptor blockade
	Tardive dyskinesia	Supersensitivity of dopamine receptors
	Toxic-confusional state	Muscarinic blockade
Endocrine system	Amenorrhea-galactorrhea, infertility, impotence	Dopamine receptor blockade resulting in hyperprolactinemia

for the treatment of various withdrawal syndromes, eg, opioid withdrawal.

Antipsychotics in small doses have been promoted (wrongly) for the relief of anxiety associated with minor emotional disorders. The antianxiety sedatives (see Chapter 21) are far better in every respect, including safety and acceptability to patients.

B. Nonpsychiatric Indications: Most older antipsychotic drugs, with the exception of thioridazine, have a strong antiemetic effect. This action is due to dopamine receptor blockade, both centrally (in the chemoreceptor trigger zone of the medulla) and peripherally (on receptors in the stomach). Some drugs, such as prochlorperazine and benzquinamide, are promoted solely as antiemetics. Phenothiazines with shorter side chains have considerable H_1 receptor-blocking action and have been used for relief of pruritus or, in the case of promethazine, as preoperative sedatives. The butyrophenone droperidol is used in combination with an opioid, fentanyl, in neuroleptanesthesia. The use of these drugs for anesthesia is described in Chapter 25.

Drug Choice

A rational choice of antipsychotic drugs may be based on differences between chemical structures and the attendant pharmacologic differences, since the differences between groups are greater than the differences within groups. Thus, one might choose to be familiar with one member of each of the three subfamilies of phenothiazines, a member of the thioxanthene and butyrophenone group, and perhaps three or four members of the miscellaneous group. A possible selection is shown in Table 29–3.

No basis exists for choosing drugs for use against selected target symptoms, as there is no evidence of specificity in their effects. Although new antipsychotic drugs under development are alleged to be more effective than older ones for treating negative symptoms (emotional blunting, social withdrawal, lack of motivation), such claims have yet to be generally verified. Superiority in terms of general response (positive and negative symptoms) of clozapine and, most recently, olanzapine over haloperidol has been demonstrated, however, in controlled trials. It is not necessary for practitioners to know all of the drugs intimately, but they should be familiar with the effects—including the adverse effects—of one or two drugs in each class. The best guide for selecting a drug for an individual patient is the patient's past responses to drugs. Within the older group, the trend in recent years has been away from "low-potency" agents such as chlorpromazine and thioridazine to the "high-potency" drugs such as thiothixene, haloperi-

Table 29–3. Some representative antipsychotic drugs.

Drug Class	Drug	Advantages	Disadvantages
Phenothiazines Aliphatic	Chlorpromazine[1] (Thorazine)	Generic, inexpensive	Many adverse effects, especially autonomic
Piperidine	Thioridazine[2] (Mellaril)	Slight extrapyramidal syndrome; generic	800 mg/d limit; no parenteral form; cardiotoxicity
Piperazine	Fluphenazine[3] (Permitil, Prolixin)	Depot form also available (enanthate, decanoate)	(?) Increased tardive dyskinesia
Thioxanthene	Thiothixene[4] (Navane)	Parenteral form also available; (?) decreased tardive dyskinesia	Uncertain
Butyrophenone	Haloperidol (Haldol)	Parenteral form also available; generic	Severe extrapyramidal syndrome
Dibenzoxazepine	Loxapine (Loxitane)	(?) No weight gain	Uncertain
Dibenzodiazepine	Clozapine (Clozaril)	May benefit treatment-resistant patients; little extrapyramidal toxicity	May cause agranulocytosis in up to 2% of patients
Benzisoxazole	Risperidone	Broad efficacy; little or no extrapyramidal system dysfunction at low doses	Extrapyramidal system dysfunction, hypotension with higher doses
Thienobenzodiazepine	Olanzapine	Effective against negative as well as positive symptoms; little or no extrapyramidal system dysfunction	Uncertain

[1]Other aliphatic phenothiazines: **promazine, triflupromazine.**
[2]Other piperidine phenothiazines: **piperacetazine, mesoridazine.**
[3]Other piperazine phenothiazines: **acetophenazine, perphenazine, carphenazine, prochlorperazine, trifluoperazine.**
[4]Other thioxanthenes: **chlorprothixene.**

dol, and fluphenazine. At present, use of clozapine is limited to those patients who have failed to respond to substantial doses of conventional antipsychotic drugs or those who have disabling tardive dyskinesia. The agranulocytosis and seizures associated with this drug prevent more widespread use. Risperidone does not appear to substitute for clozapine. Trials are under way to see if olanzapine is comparable to clozapine.

Dosage

The range of effective dosages among various antipsychotics is quite broad. Therapeutic margins are substantial. Assuming that dosages are appropriate, most antipsychotics, with the exception of clozapine and olanzapine, are of equal efficacy in groups of patients. However, some patients who fail to respond to one drug may respond to another, and for this reason several drugs may have to be tried to find the one most effective for an individual patient. Quite possibly, this phenomenon might be due to the differing profiles of receptor actions of the various drugs. Patients who have become refractory to two or three antipsychotics given in substantial doses now become candidates for treatment with clozapine. This drug, in dosages up to 900 mg/d, salvages about 30–50% of patients previously refractory to 60 mg/d of haloperidol. In such cases, the increased risk of clozapine can well be justified. Whether olanzapine, sertindole, or quetiapine will show efficacy similar to that of clozapine remains to be determined. If this is shown to be the case, and if evidence of their safety is sustained, one of these newer agents could emerge as the preferred first-line antipsychotic.

Some dosage relationships between various antipsychotic drugs, as well as possible therapeutic ranges, are shown in Table 29–4.

Plasma Concentrations & Clinical Effects

Attempts to define a therapeutic range of plasma concentrations of antipsychotic agents are beset by many difficulties. Ranges of 2–20 ng/mL have been suggested for haloperidol, though such a wide range is not very helpful clinically. Clinical monitoring of plasma concentrations of these drugs, though technically feasible, is not warranted at this time.

Pharmaceutical Preparations

Well-tolerated parenteral forms of the high-potency older drugs are available for rapid initiation of treatment as well as for maintenance treatment in noncompliant patients. Since the parenterally administered drugs may have much greater bioavailability than the oral forms, doses should be only a fraction of what might be given orally. Fluphenazine decanoate and haloperidol decanoate are suitable for long-term parenteral maintenance therapy in patients who cannot or will not take oral medication.

Dosage Schedules

Antipsychotics may be given in divided daily doses initially while an effective dosage level is being sought. They need not always be equally divided doses, even when given orally. After an effective daily dosage has been defined for an individual patient,

Table 29–4. Dose relationships of antipsychotics.

	Minimum Effective Therapeutic Dose (mg)	Usual Range of Daily Doses (mg)
Chlorpromazine (Thorazine)	100	100–1000
Thioridazine (Mellaril)	100	100–800
Mesoridazine (Lidanar, Serentil)	50	50–400
Piperacetazine (Quide)	10	20–160
Trifluoperazine (Stelazine)	5	5–60
Perphenazine (Trilafon)	10	8–64
Fluphenazine (Permitil, Prolixin)	2	2–60
Thiothixene (Navane)	2	2–120
Haloperidol (Haldol)	2	2–60
Loxapine (Loxitane)	10	20–160
Molindone (Lidone, Moban)	10	20–200
Clozapine (Clozaril)	50	25–600
Olanzapine (Zyprexa)	5	5–20
Sertindole (Serlect)	4	4–24
Quetiapine (Seroquel)	150	150–800
Risperidone (Risperdal)	4	4–16

doses can be given less frequently. Once-daily doses, usually given at night, are feasible for many patients during chronic maintenance treatment. Simplification of dosage schedules leads to better compliance. Maximum dose sizes of many drugs are being increased by manufacturers to meet the needs of once-daily dosing.

Maintenance Treatment

A small minority of schizophrenic patients may remit from an acute episode and require no further drug therapy for prolonged periods. In most cases the choice is between "as needed" treatment for recurrent episodes versus continual maintenance treatment with the smallest possible doses. The choice will depend on social factors such as the availability of family or friends familiar with the symptoms of early relapse and ready access to care.

Drug Combinations

Combining antipsychotic drugs confounds evaluation of the efficacy of the drugs being used. Tricyclic antidepressants may be used with antipsychotics but only for clear symptoms of depression complicating schizophrenia. They are of no proved efficacy for alleviating the social withdrawal and blunted affect of the psychotic patient. Lithium is sometimes added to antipsychotic agents with benefit to patients who fail to respond to the latter drugs alone. It is uncertain whether such instances represent misdiagnosed cases of mania. Sedative drugs may be added for relief of anxiety or insomnia not controlled by antipsychotics.

The drugs most frequently combined with antipsychotics are antiparkinsonism agents (see below).

Adverse Reactions

Most of the unwanted effects of antipsychotics are extensions of their known pharmacologic actions (Tables 29–1 and 29–2), but a few are allergic and some are idiosyncratic.

A. Behavioral Effects: Antipsychotic drugs are unpleasant to take—the more so the less psychotic the patient. Many patients stop taking these drugs because of the adverse effects, which may be mitigated by giving small doses during the day and the major portion at bedtime. A "pseudodepression" that may be due to drug-induced akinesia usually responds to treatment with antiparkinsonism drugs. Other "pseudodepressions" may be due to using higher doses than needed in a partially remitted patient, in which case decreasing the dose may relieve the symptoms. Toxic-confusional states may occur with very high doses of drugs that have prominent antimuscarinic actions.

B. Neurologic Effects: Extrapyramidal reactions occurring early during treatment include typical **Parkinson's syndrome, akathisia** (uncontrollable restlessness), and **acute dystonic reactions** (spastic retrocollis or torticollis). Parkinsonism can be treated,

when necessary, with conventional antiparkinsonism drugs of the antimuscarinic type or, in rare cases, with amantadine. Parkinsonism may be self-limiting, so that an attempt to withdraw antiparkinsonism drugs should be made every 3–4 months. Akathisia and dystonic reactions will also respond to such treatment, but many prefer to use a sedative antihistamine with anticholinergic properties, eg, diphenhydramine, which can be given either parenterally or orally as capsules or elixir.

Tardive dyskinesia, as the name implies, is a late-occurring syndrome of abnormal choreoathetoid movements. It is the most important unwanted effect of antipsychotic drugs. It has been proposed that it is caused by a relative cholinergic deficiency secondary to supersensitivity of dopamine receptors in the caudate-putamen. Older women treated for long periods are most susceptible to the disorder, though it can occur at any age and in either sex. The prevalence varies enormously, but tardive dyskinesia is estimated to occur in 20–40% of chronically treated patients. Early recognition is important, since advanced cases may be difficult to reverse. Many treatments have been proposed, but their evaluation is confounded by the fact that the course of the disorder is variable and sometimes self-limited. Most authorities agree that the first step would be to try to decrease dopamine receptor sensitivity by discontinuing the antipsychotic drug or by reducing the dose. A logical second step would be to eliminate all drugs with central anticholinergic action, particularly antiparkinsonism drugs and tricyclic antidepressants. These two steps are often enough to bring about improvement. If they fail, the addition of diazepam in doses as high as 30–40 mg/d may add to the improvement by enhancing GABAergic activity. The use of reserpine may also be considered, though one runs the risk of increasing receptor sensitivity or precipitating a depressive reaction.

Seizures, while recognized as a complication of chlorpromazine treatment, were so rare with the high-potency older drugs as to merit little consideration. However, de novo seizures may occur in 2–5% of patients treated with clozapine.

C. Autonomic Nervous System Effects: Most patients become tolerant to the antimuscarinic adverse effects of antipsychotic drugs. Those who are made too uncomfortable or who are impaired, as with urinary retention, should be given bethanechol, a peripherally acting cholinomimetic. Orthostatic hypotension or impaired ejaculation—common complications of therapy with chlorpromazine or mesoridazine—should be managed by switching to drugs with less marked adrenoceptor-blocking actions.

D. Metabolic and Endocrine Effects: Weight gain is common and requires monitoring of food intake. Hyperprolactinemia in women results in the amenorrhea-galactorrhea syndrome and infertility; in men, loss of libido, impotence, and infertility may result.

E. Toxic or Allergic Reactions: Agranulocytosis, cholestatic jaundice, and skin eruptions occur rarely with the high-potency antipsychotic drugs currently used.

In contrast to other antipsychotic agents, clozapine causes agranulocytosis in a small but significant number of patients—approximately 1–2% of those treated. This serious, potentially fatal effect can develop rapidly, usually between the sixth and eighteenth weeks of therapy. It is not known whether it represents an immune reaction, but it appears to be reversible upon discontinuance of the drug. *Because of the risk, weekly blood counts are mandatory for patients receiving clozapine.*

F. Ocular Complications: Deposits in the anterior portions of the eye (cornea and lens) are a common complication of chlorpromazine therapy. They may accentuate the normal processes of aging of the lens. Thioridazine is the only antipsychotic drug that causes retinal deposits, which in advanced cases may resemble retinitis pigmentosa. The deposits are usually associated with "browning" of vision. The maximum daily dose of thioridazine has been limited to 800 mg/d to reduce the possibility of this complication.

G. Cardiac Toxicity: Thioridazine in doses exceeding 300 mg daily is almost always associated with minor abnormalities of T waves that are easily reversible. Overdoses of thioridazine are associated with major ventricular arrhythmias, cardiac conduction block, and sudden death; it is not certain whether thioridazine can cause these same disorders when used in therapeutic doses. In view of possible additive antimuscarinic and quinidine-like actions with various tricyclic antidepressants, thioridazine should be combined with the latter drugs only with great care.

H. Use in Pregnancy; Dysmorphogenesis: Although the antipsychotic drugs appear to be relatively safe in pregnancy, a small increase in teratogenic risk could be missed. Questions about whether to use these drugs during pregnancy and whether to abort a pregnancy in which the fetus has already been exposed must be decided individually.

I. Neuroleptic Malignant Syndrome: This life-threatening disorder occurs in patients who are extremely sensitive to the extrapyramidal effects of antipsychotics. The initial symptom is marked muscle rigidity. If sweating is impaired, as it often is during treatment with anticholinergic drugs, fever may ensue, often reaching dangerous levels. The stress leukocytosis and high fever associated with this syndrome may erroneously suggest an infectious process. Autonomic instability, with altered blood pressure and pulse rate, is another midbrain manifestation. Creatine kinase isozymes are usually elevated, reflecting muscle damage. This syndrome is believed to result from an excessively rapid blockade of postsynaptic dopamine receptors. A severe form of extrapyramidal syndrome follows. Early in the course,

vigorous treatment of the extrapyramidal syndrome with antiparkinsonism drugs is worthwhile. Muscle relaxants, particularly diazepam, are often helpful. The use of other muscle relaxants, such as dantrolene, or dopamine agonists, such as bromocriptine, has been reported to be helpful. If fever is present, cooling by physical measures should be tried. Various minor forms of this syndrome are now recognized.

Drug Interactions

Antipsychotics produce more important pharmacodynamic than pharmacokinetic interactions because of their multiple effects. Additive effects may occur when these drugs are combined with others that have sedative effects, α-adrenoceptor-blocking action, anticholinergic effects, and—for thioridazine—quinidine-like action.

A variety of pharmacokinetic interactions have been reported, but none are of major clinical significance.

Overdoses

Poisonings with antipsychotics are rarely fatal, with the exception of those due to mesoridazine and thioridazine. In general, drowsiness proceeds to coma, with an intervening period of agitation. Neuromuscular excitability may be increased and proceed to convulsions. Pupils are miotic, and deep tendon reflexes are decreased. Hypotension and hypothermia are the rule, though fever may be present later in the course. The lethal effects of mesoridazine and thioridazine are related to induction of ventricular tachyarrhythmias. The mild QT_c prolongation observed after therapeutic doses of sertindole suggest that in overdose, this drug may also induce serious arrhythmias.

Patients should be monitored in an intensive care setting for the usual vital signs, venous pressure, arterial blood gases, and electrolytes. Attempts at gastric lavage should be made even if several hours have elapsed since the drug was taken, because gastrointestinal motility is often decreased and tablets may still be present in the stomach. Activated charcoal effectively binds most of these drugs, following which a saline cathartic may be given. Hypotension often responds to fluid replacement. If a pressor agent is to be used, norepinephrine or dopamine is preferred to epinephrine, whose unopposed β-adrenoceptor-stimulant action in the presence of alpha blockade may cause vasodilation. Seizures may be treated with either diazepam or phenytoin, the latter being given with an initial loading dose. Management of overdoses of thioridazine and mesoridazine, which are complicated by cardiac arrhythmias, is similar to that for tricyclic antidepressants (see Chapter 30).

New Approaches

The most recently introduced antipsychotics are at least as potent in inhibiting 5-HT$_2$ receptors as they are in inhibiting D$_2$ receptors. Varying degrees of antagonism of α_1 and α_2 adrenoceptors are also seen with risperidone, clozapine, olanzapine, sertindole, and quetiapine. The clinical relevance of these actions remains to be ascertained.

Unconventional Drugs

The efficacy of propranolol as treatment for schizophrenia remains uncertain after 30 years of study. Patients with marked agitation, hostility, and belligerence may be controlled by the addition of propranolol to a regimen of conventional antipsychotic drugs. High-dose treatment with benzodiazepines may control disturbed behavior, just as barbiturates did 35 years ago. Levodopa, thyrotropin-releasing hormone, endorphins, and apomorphine have been ineffective. Megavitamin therapy has been discredited scientifically, but adherents still persist.

Benefits & Limitations of Drug Treatment

As noted at the beginning of this chapter, these drugs have had a major impact on psychiatric treatment. First, they have shifted the care of patients from mental institutions to the community. For many patients, this shift has provided a better life under more humane circumstances and in some cases has made possible life without constant physical restraints. For others, the tragedy of an aimless existence is now being played out in the streets of our communities rather than in mental institutions.

Second, these drugs have markedly shifted psychiatric thinking to a more biologic orientation. Partly because of research stimulated by the effects of these drugs on schizophrenia, we now know much more about central nervous system physiology and pharmacology than we did before the introduction of these agents. However, despite a great amount of research done by highly competent scientists from many disciplines, schizophrenia remains a scientific mystery and a personal disaster for the patient. While most schizophrenic patients obtain some degree of benefit from these drugs, none are made well by them.

LITHIUM & OTHER MOOD-STABILIZING DRUGS

Lithium carbonate is often referred to as an "antimanic" drug, but in many parts of the world it is considered a "mood-stabilizing" agent because of its primary action of preventing mood swings in patients with bipolar affective (manic-depressive) disorder. Its discovery in 1949 was based on an incorrect hypothesis and extremely good fortune in choosing the correct dosage. Carbamazepine has also been recognized as an effective mood stabilizer in some groups of patients despite not being formally approved for such use. It was introduced during the 1970s, based on the tenuous assumption that since manic attacks, like epilepsy, are episodic, an anticonvulsant might help. Valproate has recently been approved for the treatment of mania and is being evaluated as a mood stabilizer. Clonazepam, a GABAmimetic anticonvulsant, has also been found to be helpful as an adjunct in the treatment of mania.

Nature of Bipolar Affective Disorder

Bipolar affective (manic-depressive) disorder is a frequently diagnosed and very serious psychiatric disorder. Patients with cyclic attacks of mania have many symptoms of paranoid schizophrenia (grandiosity, bellicosity, paranoid thoughts, and overactivity). The gratifying response to lithium therapy of patients with bipolar disorder has made such diagnostic distinctions important.

The episodes of mood swings characteristic of this condition are generally unrelated to life events. The exact biologic disturbance has not been identified, but a preponderance of catecholamine-related activity is thought to be present. Drugs that increase this activity tend to exacerbate mania, whereas those that reduce activity of dopamine or norepinephrine relieve mania. Acetylcholine may also be involved. The nature of the abrupt switch from mania to depression experienced by some patients is uncertain. Bipolar disorder has a strong familial component. Genetic studies have identified at least three possible linkages to different chromosomes.

I. Basic Pharmacology of Lithium

Pharmacokinetics

Lithium is a small monovalent cation. Its pharmacokinetics are summarized in Table 29–5.

Pharmacodynamics

Despite considerable investigation, the mode of action of lithium remains unclear. The major possi-

Table 29–5. Pharmacokinetics of lithium

Absorption	Virtually complete within 6–8 hours; peak plasma levels in 30 minutes to 2 hours.
Distribution	In total body water; slow entry into intracellular compartment. Initial volume of distribution 0.5 L/kg, rising to 0.7–0.9 L/kg; some sequestration in bone. No protein binding.
Metabolism	None.
Excretion	Virtually entirely in urine. Lithium clearance about 20% of creatinine. Plasma half-life about 20 hours.

bilities being investigated include (1) its effects on electrolytes and ion transport; (2) its effects on neurotransmitters and their release; and (3) its effects on second messengers that mediate transmitter action. The last of these three approaches appears to be the most promising.

A. Effects on Electrolytes and Ion Transport: Lithium is closely related to sodium in its properties. It can substitute for sodium in generating action potentials and in Na^+-Na^+ exchange across the membrane. It inhibits the latter process, ie, Li^+-Na^+ exchange is gradually slowed after lithium is introduced into the body. At therapeutic concentrations (around 1 mmol/L), it does not significantly affect the Na^+/Ca^{2+} exchange process or the Na^+/K^+ ATPase sodium pump.

B. Effects on Neurotransmitters: Lithium appears to enhance some of the actions of serotonin, though findings have been contradictory. Its effects on norepinephrine are variable. The drug may decrease norepinephrine and dopamine turnover, and these effects, if confirmed, might be relevant to its antimanic action. Lithium also appears to block the development of dopamine receptor supersensitivity that may accompany chronic therapy with antipsychotic agents. Finally, lithium may augment the synthesis of acetylcholine, perhaps by increasing choline uptake into nerve terminals. Some clinical studies have suggested that increasing cholinergic activity may mitigate mania. However, as noted below, a second-messenger effect of lithium may obviate any effect of increased acetylcholine release.

C. Effects on Second Messengers: Currently, the best-defined effect of lithium is its action on inositol phosphates. Early studies of lithium demonstrated changes in brain inositol phosphate levels, but the significance of these changes was not appreciated until the second-messenger roles of inositol-1,4,5-trisphosphate (IP_3) and diacylglycerol (DAG) were discovered. As described in Chapter 2, IP_3 and DAG are important second messengers for both alpha-adrenergic and muscarinic transmission. Lithium inhibits several important enzymes in the normal recycling of membrane phosphoinositides, including conversion of IP_2 to IP_1 (IP, inositol monophosphate) and the conversion of IP to inositol (Figure 29–4). This block leads to a depletion of phosphatidylinositol-4,5-bisphosphate (PIP_2), the membrane precursor of IP_3 and DAG. Over time, the effects of transmitters on the cell will diminish in proportion to the amount of activity in the PIP_2-dependent pathways. Before therapy, such activity might be greatly increased in mania; thus, lithium could cause a selective depression of the overactive circuits. For example, recent studies suggest that persistent activation of muscarinic receptors can prevent the normal inhibitory action of adenosine on certain hippocampal neurons. This excitatory cholinergic action can be prevented by therapeutic concentrations of lithium, as would be

Figure 29–4. Effect of lithium on the IP_3 and DAG second-messenger system. The schematic diagram shows the synaptic membrane of a neuron. (PIP_2, phosphatidylinositol-4,5-bisphosphate; PLC, phospholipase-C; G, coupling protein; EFFECTS, activation of protein kinase C, mobilization of intracellular Ca^{2+}, etc.) Lithium, by inhibiting the recycling of inositol substrates, may cause depletion of the second-messenger source PIP_2 and therefore reduce the release of IP_3 and DAG. Lithium may also act by other mechanisms.

predicted from the proposed mechanism of selective depression.

Studies of noradrenergic effects in isolated brain tissue indicate that lithium can inhibit norepinephrine-sensitive adenylyl cyclase. Such an effect could relate to both its antidepressant and its antimanic effects. The relationship of these effects to lithium's actions on IP_3 mechanisms is currently unknown.

Since lithium affects second-messenger systems involving both activation of adenylyl cyclase and phosphoinositol turnover, it is not surprising that possible shared components of signal transduction, G proteins, are also found to be affected. Several studies suggest that lithium may uncouple receptors from their G proteins; indeed, two of lithium's most common side effects, polyuria and subclinical hypothyroidism, may be due to uncoupling of the vasopressin and TSH receptors from their G proteins. Recent studies implicate an effect of lithium on specific isozymes of protein kinase C (activated by DAG) as possibly mediating the alteration of G protein function through shifts in phosphorylation.

II. Clinical Pharmacology of Lithium

Bipolar Affective Disorder

Agreement has been universal (until the advent of valproate for this indication) that lithium carbonate is the preferred treatment for bipolar disorder, especially in the manic phase. Because its onset of action is slow, concurrent use of antipsychotic drugs or potent benzodiazepines may be required for severely manic patients. The overall success rate for achieving remission from the manic phase of bipolar disorder has been reported to be 60–80%. However, among patients who require hospitalization, success rates are considerably lower. A similar situation applies to maintenance treatment, which is about 60% effective overall but less in severely ill patients. These considerations have led to increased use of combined treatment in severe cases.

When mania is mild, lithium alone may be effective treatment. In more severe cases, it is almost always necessary to add clonazepam or lorazepam and often to give one of the antipsychotic drugs as well. After mania is controlled, the antipsychotic drug may be stopped, then the benzodiazepine, and lithium continued as maintenance therapy.

The depressive phase of manic-depressive disorder often requires concurrent use of an antidepressant drug (Chapter 30). Tricyclic antidepressant agents have been linked to precipitation of mania, with more rapid cycling of mood swings, although most patients do not show this effect. It is difficult to choose among the newer antidepressants, because most of them may also activate mania. Carbamazepine may be useful in such situations or in patients whose manic episodes are not controlled by lithium alone. For some patients, an MAO inhibitor may be the antidepressant of choice.

Unlike antipsychotic or antidepressant drugs, which exert several actions on the central or autonomic nervous system, lithium ion at therapeutic concentrations is devoid of autonomic blocking effects and of activating or sedating effects, though it can produce nausea and tremor. Since it is a small inorganic ion, lithium is distributed in body water and is not metabolized. It is easily measured in body fluids such as plasma, urine, or saliva. Thus, its kinetics can be studied easily, and plasma or tissue concentrations can be correlated with clinical effects.

Another attribute of considerable interest has been the prophylactic use of lithium in preventing both mania and depression. It is indeed remarkable that a so-called functional psychosis can be controlled so easily by such a simple chemical as lithium carbonate.

Other Applications

Acute endogenous depression is not generally considered to be an indication for treatment with lithium. Alcohol and substance abuse have a high association with bipolar illness. However, recurrent endogenous depressions with a cyclic pattern are controlled by either lithium or imipramine, both of which are superior to a placebo.

Schizoaffective disorders are characterized by a mixture of schizophrenic symptoms and altered affect in the form of depression or excitement. Antipsychotic drugs alone or combined with lithium are used in the excited as well as in the maintenance phases; clozapine may be particularly effective. Various antidepressants are added if depression is present, but none has been adequately studied in this condition.

While lithium alone is rarely successful in treating schizophrenia, adding it to an antipsychotic may salvage an otherwise treatment-resistant patient. Carbamazepine may work equally well when added to an antipsychotic.

An interesting application of lithium that is relatively well supported by controlled studies is as an adjunct to tricyclic antidepressants and selective serotonin reuptake inhibitors in patients with unipolar depression who do not respond fully to monotherapy with the antidepressant. For this application, concentrations of lithium at the lower end of the recommended range for manic depressive illness appear to be adequate.

Dosage Schedules

Before treatment is started, one should obtain laboratory data such as a complete blood count, urinalysis, common biochemical tests, and an ECG in older patients and those with a history of cardiac disorders. These tests serve as baseline measurements in assessing possible complications of treatment.

The patient's age, body weight, and renal function should be considered in determining appropriate initial doses of lithium carbonate. The initial volume of distribution of lithium will be the same as that of body water, or about 0.5–0.6 L/kg body weight for women and 0.55–0.7 L/kg for men. As lithium is excreted solely by the kidneys, the dosage should be reduced if creatinine clearance is impaired, as it will be in most elderly patients.

A daily lithium dose of 0.5 meq/kg will produce the desired serum lithium concentration in the range of 0.6–1.4 meq/L after a week of treatment if renal function is normal. Each 300 mg dose unit of lithium carbonate contains approximately 8 meq of lithium. Daily doses of lithium may range between 600 and 3600 mg among different individuals. The majority require between 1500 and 1800 mg/d.

It is almost always necessary to give lithium in divided doses to avoid gastric distress when initiating treatment. Medication is best taken with or shortly after meals. Slow-release dosage forms may also be tried. Later in treatment, it may be possible to use a single daily dose at bedtime.

Monitoring Treatment

Clinicians have relied heavily on measurements of serum concentrations for assessing both the dosage required for satisfactory treatment of acute mania and the adequacy of maintenance treatment. These measurements are customarily taken 10–12 hours after the last dose, so all data in the literature pertaining to these concentrations reflect this interval.

An initial determination of serum lithium concentration should be obtained about 5 days after the start of treatment, at which time steady state conditions should obtain for the dosage chosen. If the clinical response suggests a change in dosage, simple arithmetic (new dose equals present dose times desired blood level divided by present blood level) should produce the desired level. The serum concentration attained with the adjusted dosage can be checked in another 5 days. Once the desired concentration has been achieved, levels can be measured at increasing intervals unless the schedule is influenced by intercurrent illness or the introduction of a new drug into the treatment program.

Maintenance Treatment

The decision to use lithium as *prophylactic* treatment depends on many factors: the frequency and severity of previous episodes, a crescendo pattern of appearance, and the degree to which the patient is willing to follow a program of indefinite maintenance therapy. If the present attack was the patient's first or if the patient is unreliable, one might prefer to terminate treatment after the attack has subsided. Patients who have one or more episodes of illness per year are candidates for maintenance treatment. While some patients can be maintained with serum levels as low as 0.6 meq/L, the best results in groups of patients have been obtained with higher levels, such as 0.9 meq/L.

Drug Interactions

Renal clearance of lithium is reduced about 25% by diuretics (eg, thiazides), and doses may need to be reduced by a similar amount. A similar reduction in lithium clearance has been noted with several of the newer nonsteroidal anti-inflammatory drugs that block synthesis of prostaglandins. This interaction has not been reported for either aspirin or acetaminophen. All neuroleptics tested to date, with the possible exception of clozapine and the newer antipsychotics, may produce more severe extrapyramidal syndromes when combined with lithium.

Adverse Effects & Complications

Many adverse effects associated with lithium treatment occur at varying times after treatment is started. Some are harmless, but it is important to be alert to adverse effects that may signify impending serious toxic reactions.

A. Neurologic and Psychiatric Adverse Effects: Tremor is one of the most frequent adverse effects of lithium treatment, occurring at therapeutic dosage levels. Propranolol and atenolol, which have been reported to be effective in essential tremor, also alleviate lithium-induced tremor. Other reported neurologic abnormalities include choreoathetosis, motor hyperactivity, ataxia, dysarthria, and aphasia. Psychiatric disturbances at toxic concentrations are generally marked by mental confusion and withdrawal or bizarre motor movements. Appearance of any new neurologic or psychiatric symptoms or signs is a clear indication for temporarily stopping treatment with lithium and close monitoring of serum levels.

B. Effects on Thyroid Function: Lithium probably decreases thyroid function in most patients exposed to the drug, but the effect is reversible or nonprogressive. Few patients develop frank thyroid enlargement, and fewer still show symptoms of hypothyroidism. Although initial thyroid testing with regular monitoring of thyroid function has been proposed, such procedures are not cost-effective. Obtaining a serum TSH concentration every 6–12 months, however, is prudent.

C. Renal Adverse Effects: Polydipsia and polyuria are frequent but reversible concomitants of lithium treatment, occurring at therapeutic serum concentrations. The principal physiologic lesion involved is loss of the ability of the collecting tubule to conserve water under the influence of antidiuretic hormone, resulting in excessive free water clearance (**nephrogenic diabetes insipidus).** Lithium-induced diabetes insipidus is resistant to vasopressin but responds to amiloride.

An extensive literature has accumulated concerning other forms of renal dysfunction during long-term lithium therapy, including **chronic interstitial nephritis** and **minimal change glomerulopathy** with nephrotic syndrome. Some instances of decreased glomerular filtration rate have been encountered but no instances of marked azotemia or renal failure.

Patients receiving lithium should avoid dehydration and the associated increased concentration of lithium in urine. Periodic tests of renal concentrating ability should be performed to detect changes.

D. Edema: Edema is a frequent adverse effect of lithium treatment and may be related to some effect of lithium on sodium retention. Although weight gain may be expected in patients who become edematous, water retention alone probably does not account for all of it.

E. Cardiac Adverse Effects: The bradycardia-tachycardia ("sick sinus") syndrome is a definite contraindication to the use of lithium because the ion further depresses the sinus node. T wave flattening is often observed on the ECG but is of questionable significance.

F. Use During Pregnancy: Renal clearance of lithium increases during pregnancy and reverts to lower levels immediately after delivery. A patient whose serum lithium concentration is in a good therapeutic range during pregnancy may develop toxic levels following delivery. Special care in monitoring lithium levels is needed at these times. Lithium is transferred to nursing infants through breast milk, in which it has a concentration about one-third to one-half that of serum. Lithium toxicity in newborns is manifested by lethargy, cyanosis, poor suck and Moro reflexes, and perhaps hepatomegaly.

The issue of dysmorphogenesis is not settled. An earlier report suggested an increase in the frequency of cardiac anomalies, especially Ebstein's anomaly, in lithium babies, but the most recent data suggest that lithium carries a relatively low risk of teratogenic effects.

G. Miscellaneous Adverse Effects: Transient acneiform eruptions have been noted early in lithium treatment. Some of them subside with temporary discontinuance of treatment and do not recur with its resumption. Folliculitis is less dramatic and probably occurs more frequently. Leukocytosis is always present during lithium treatment, probably reflecting a direct effect on leukopoiesis rather than mobilization from the marginal pool. This "adverse effect" has now become a therapeutic effect in patients with low leukocyte counts.

Overdoses

Therapeutic overdoses are more common than those due to deliberate or accidental ingestion of the drug. Therapeutic overdoses are usually due to accumulation of lithium resulting from some change in the patient's status, such as diminished serum sodium, use of diuretics, fluctuating renal function, or pregnancy. Since the tissues will have already equilibrated with the blood, the plasma concentrations of lithium may not be excessively high in proportion to the degree of toxicity; any value over 2 meq/L must be considered as indicating potential toxicity. As lithium is a small ion, it is dialyzed readily. Both peritoneal dialysis and hemodialysis are effective, though the latter is preferred. Dialysis should be continued until the plasma concentrations fall below the usual therapeutic range.

VALPROIC ACID

Valproic acid (valproate), discussed in detail elsewhere as an antiepileptic (Chapter 24), has recently been demonstrated to have antimanic effects and has been approved for this indication in the USA. Overall, it shows efficacy equivalent to that of lithium during the early weeks of treatment and is currently being evaluated as a maintenance treatment. Importantly, valproic acid has been effective in some patients who have failed to respond to lithium. Moreover, its side effect profile is such that one can rapidly increase the dose over a few days to produce blood levels in the apparent therapeutic range, with nausea being the only limiting factor in some patients.

Combinations of valproic acid with other psychotropic medications likely to be used in the management of either phase of bipolar illness are generally well tolerated. Valproic acid is becoming recognized as an appropriate first-line treatment for mania, though it is not clear that it will be as effective as lithium as a maintenance treatment in all subsets of patients. Many clinicians argue for combining valproic acid and lithium in patients who do not fully respond to either agent alone.

CARBAMAZEPINE

Carbamazepine has been considered to be a reasonable alternative to lithium when the latter is less than optimally efficacious. It may be used to treat acute mania and also for prophylactic therapy. Adverse effects (discussed in Chapter 24) are generally no greater and sometimes are less than those associated with lithium. Carbamazepine may be used alone or, in refractory patients, in combination with lithium or, rarely, valproate. The mode of action of carbamazepine is unclear, but it may reduce the sensitization of the brain to repeated episodes of mood swing. Such a mechanism might be similar to its anticonvulsant effect.

The use of carbamazepine as a mood stabilizer is similar to its use as an anticonvulsant (see Chapter 24). Dosage usually begins with 200 mg twice daily, with increases as needed. Maintenance dosage is similar to that used for treating epilepsy, ie, 800–1200 mg/d. Plasma concentrations between 3 and 14 mg/L are considered desirable, though no therapeutic range has been established. Although blood dyscrasias have figured prominently in the adverse effects of carbamazepine when it is used as an anticonvulsant, they have not been a major problem with its use as a mood stabilizer. Overdoses of the drug are a major emergency and should be managed in general like overdoses of tricyclic antidepressants.

PREPARATIONS AVAILABLE

Antipsychotic Agents

Acetophenazine (Tindal) Oral: 20 mg tablets

Chlorpromazine (generic, Thorazine, others)
Oral: 10, 25, 50, 100, 200 mg tablets; 10 mg/5 mL syrup; 30, 100 mg/mL concentrate
Oral sustained-release: 30, 75, 150, 200, 300 mg capsules
Rectal: 25, 100 mg suppositories
Parenteral: 25 mg/mL for IM injection

Chlorprothixene (Taractan)
Oral: 10, 25, 50, 100 mg tablets; 100 mg/5 mL concentrate
Parenteral: 12.5 mg/mL for IM injection

Clozapine (Clozaril)
Oral: 25, 100 mg tablets

Fluphenazine (generic, Permitil, Prolixin)
Oral: 1, 2.5, 5, 10 mg tablets; 2.5 mg/5 mL elixir; 5 mg/mL concentrate
Parenteral: 2.5 mg/mL for IM injection

Fluphenazine esters (generic [decanoate only], Prolixin Enanthate, Prolixin Decanoate)
Parenteral: 25 mg/mL

Haloperidol (generic, Haldol)
Oral: 0.5, 1, 2, 5, 10, 20 mg tablets; 2 mg/mL concentrate
Parenteral: 5 mg/mL for IM injection

Haloperidol ester (Haldol Decanoate)
Parenteral: 50, 100 mg/mL for IM injection

Loxapine (Loxitane)
Oral: 5, 10, 25, 50 mg capsules; 25 mg/mL concentrate
Parenteral: 50 mg/mL for IM injection

Mesoridazine (Serentil)
Oral: 10, 25, 50, 100 mg tablets; 25 mg/mL concentrate
Parenteral: 25 mg/mL for IM injection

Molindone (Moban)
Oral: 5, 10, 25, 50, 100 mg tablets; 20 mg/mL concentrate

Olanzapine (Zyprexa)
Oral: 5, 7.5, 10 mg tablets

Perphenazine (generic, Trilafon)
Oral: 2, 4, 8, 16 mg tablets; 16 mg/5 mL concentrate
Parenteral: 5 mg/mL for IM or IV injection

Pimozide (Orap)
Oral: 2 mg tablets

Prochlorperazine (generic, Compazine)
Oral: 5, 10, 25 mg tablets; 5 mg/5 mL syrup
Oral sustained-release: 10, 15, 30 mg capsules
Rectal: 2.5, 5, 25 mg suppositories
Parenteral: 5 mg/mL for IM injection

Promazine (generic, Sparine)
Oral: 25, 50, 100 mg tablets
Parenteral: 25, 50 mg/mL for IM injection

Quetiapine (Seroquel)
Oral: Information not yet available

Risperidone (Risperdal)
Oral: 1, 2, 3, 4 mg tablets

Sertindole (Serlect)
Oral: Information not yet available

Thioridazine (generic, Mellaril, others)
Oral: 10, 15, 25, 50, 100, 150, 200 mg tablets; 30, 100 mg/mL concentrate; 25, 100 mg/5 mL suspension

Thiothixene (generic, Navane)
Oral: 1, 2, 5, 10, 20 mg capsules; 5 mg/mL concentrate
Parenteral: 2 mg/mL for IM injection; powder to reconstitute for 5 mg/mL for injection

Trifluoperazine (generic, Stelazine)
Oral: 1, 2, 5, 10 mg tablets; 10 mg/mL concentrate
Parenteral: 2 mg/mL for IM injection

Triflupromazine (Vesprin)
Parenteral: 10, 20 mg/mL for IM injection

Mood Stabilizers

Carbamazepine (generic, Tegretol, others)
Oral: 200 mg tablets, 100 mg chewable tablets; 100 mg/5 mL oral suspension

Divalproex (Depakote)
Oral: 125, 250, 500 mg delayed release tablets

Lithium carbonate (generic, Eskalith) (*Note:* 300 mg lithium carbonate = 8.12 meq Li$^+$.)
Oral: 150, 300, 600 mg capsules; 300 mg tablets; 8 meq/5 mL syrup
Oral sustained-release: 300, 450 mg tablets

Valproic acid (generic, Depakene)
Oral: 250 mg capsules; 250 mg/5 mL syrup

REFERENCES

Antipsychotics

Ad Hoc Committee on Schizophrenia: Friedhoff AJ et al: Report on schizophrenia of the American College of Neuropsychopharmacology. Neuropsychopharmacology 1987;1:89.

Baldessarini RJ, Frankenburg FR: Clozapine: A novel antipsychotic agent. N Engl J Med 1991;324:746.

Beasley CM et al: Olanzapine versus placebo and haloperidol acute phase results of the North American double-blind olanzapine trial. Neuropsychopharmacology 1996;14:111.

Dickey W: The neuroleptic malignant syndrome. Prog Neurobiol 1991;36:423.

Farde L et al: Central D_2-dopamine receptor occupancy in schizophrenic patients treated with antipsychotic drugs. Arch Gen Psychiatry 1987;45:71.

Gerlach J, Peacock L: New antipsychotics: The present status. Int J Psychopharmacol 1995;10:39.

Gingrich JA, Caron MG: Recent advances in the molecular biology of dopamine receptors. Annu Rev Neurosci 1993;16:299.

Grace AA: Phasic versus tonic dopamine release and the modulation of dopamine system responsivity: A hypothesis for the etiology of schizophrenia. Neuroscience 1991;41:1.

Hashimoto F, Sherma CB, Jeffery WH: Neuroleptic malignant syndrome and dopaminergic blockade. Arch Intern Med 1984;144:629.

Healy D: D_1 and D_2 and D_3. Br J Psychiatry 1991;159:319.

Hollister LE, Csernansky JG: Antipsychotic drugs. In: *Clinical Pharmacology of Psychotherapeutic Drugs,* 3rd ed. Churchill Livingstone, 1990.

Jackson DM et al: Preclinical findings with new antipsychotic agents: What makes them atypical? Acta Psychiatr Scand 1994;89(Suppl 380):41.

Jacobsen E: The early history of psychotherapeutic drugs. Psychopharmacology 1986;89:138.

Kane JM et al: Clozapine for the treatment of treatment-resistant schizophrenia: Results of a US multicenter trial. Psychopharmacology 1989;99:560.

Kane JM: Schizophrenia. N Engl J Med 1996;334:445.

Lehmann HE, Wilson WH, Deutsch M: Minimal maintenance medication: Effects of three dose schedules on relapse rates and symptoms in chronic schizophrenic outpatients. Compr Psychiatry 1983;24:293.

Marder SR, Meibach R: Risperidone in the treatment of patients with chronic schizophrenia. Am J Psychiatry 1994;151:825.

McElroy SL et al: Clozapine in the treatment of psychotic mood disorders, schizoaffective disorders, and schizophrenia. J Clin Psychiatry 1991;52:411.

Pickar D et al: Longitudinal measurement of plasma homovanillic acid levels in schizophrenic patients: Correlation with psychosis and response to neuroleptic treatment. Arch Gen Psychiatry 1986;43:669.

Reynolds GP: Beyond the dopamine hypothesis: The neurochemical pathology of schizophrenia. Br J Psychiatry 1989;155:305.

Seeman P: Dopamine receptors and the dopamine hypothesis of schizophrenia. Synapse 1987;1:133.

Seroquel: A putative atypical antipsychotic drug with serotonin- and dopamine-receptor antagonist properties. J Clin Psychiatry 1995;14:438.

Sibley DR, Monsma FJ Jr: Molecular biology of dopamine receptors. Trends Pharmacol Sci 1992; 13:61.

Sokoloff P et al: Molecular cloning and characterization of a novel dopamine receptor (D_3) as a target for neuroleptics. Nature 1990;347:146.

Tarsy D, Baldessarini RJ: The pathophysiologic basis of tardive dyskinesia. Biol Psychiatry 1977;12:431.

Thompson LT, Moran MG, Nies AS: Psychotropic drug use in the elderly. (Two parts.) N Engl J Med 1983; 308:134, 194.

Tricklebank MD, Bristow LJ, Hutson PH: Alternative approaches to the discovery of novel antipsychotic agents. Prog Drug Res 1992;38:299.

Van Kammen DP et al: A randomized, controlled, dose-ranging trial of sertindole in patients with schizophrenia. Psychopharmacology 1996;124:168.

Wong DF et al: Positron emission tomography reveals elevated D_2 dopamine receptors in drug-naive schizophrenics. Science 1986;234:1558.

Mood Stabilizers

Amdisen A: History of lithium. (Letter.) Biol Psychiatry 1987;22:522.

Baraban JM, Worley PF, Snyder SH: Second messenger systems and psychoactive drug action: Focus on the phosphoinositide system and lithium. Am J Psychiatry 1989;146:1251.

Berridge MJ: Inositol trisphosphate, calcium, lithium, and cell signaling. JAMA 1989;262:1834.

Bowden CL et al: Efficacy of divalproex vs lithium, placebo in the treatment of mania. JAMA 1994;271:918.

Bunney WE Jr, Garland-Bunnery BL: Mechanisms of action of lithium in affective illness: Basic and clinical implications. In: *Psychopharmacology: The Third Generation of Progress.* Meltzer HY (editor). Raven Press, 1987.

Consensus Development Conference: *Mood disorder: Pharmacologic Prevention of Recurrences.* Vol 5, No 4. National Institutes of Health, 1984.

Elphick M: The clinical uses and pharmacology of carbamazepine in psychiatry. Int Clin Psychopharmacol 1988;3:185.

Goodwin FK, Jamison KR: *Manic-Depressive Illness.* Oxford Univ Press, 1990.

Hodgkinson S: Molecular genetic evidence for heterogeneity in manic depression. Nature 1987;325:805.

Jefferson JW, Greist JH: *Primer of Lithium Therapy.* Williams & Wilkins, 1977.

Kimmel SE et al: Clozapine in treatment-refractory mood disorders. (Review.) J Clin Psychiatry 1994;55:91.

Kishimoto A et al: Long-term prophylactic effects of carbamazepine in affective disorder. Br J Psychiatry 1983;143:327.

Manji HD: G proteins: Implications for psychiatry. Am J Psychiatry 1992;149:746.

Manji HK, Lenox RH: Long-term action of lithium: A role for transcriptional and posttranscriptional factors regulated by protein kinase C. Synapse 1994;16:11.

McElroy SL et al: Valproate in the treatment of bipolar disorder: Literature review and clinical guidelines. J Clin Psychopharmacol 1992;12(Suppl):42S.

Mitchell PB, Parker GB: Treatment of bipolar disorder. Med J Australia 1991;155:488.

Page C, Benaim S, Lappin F: A long-term retrospective follow-up of patients treated with prophylactic lithium carbonate. Br J Psychiatry 1987;150:175.

Post RM et al: Correlates of antimanic response to carbamazepine. Psychiatry Res 1987;21:71.

Prien RF, Galenberg AJ: Alternatives to lithium for preventive treatment of bipolar disorder. Am J Psychiatry 1989;146:840.

Prien RF, Potter WZ: NIMH workshop report on the treatment of bipolar disorder. Psychopharmacol Bull 1990;26:409.

Sillence DJ, Downes CP: Lithium treatment of affective disorders: Effects of lithium on the inositol phospholipid and cyclic AMP signalling pathways. Biochim Biophys Acta 1992;1138:46.

Suppes T et al: Algorithms for the treatment of bipolar, manic-depressive illness. Psychopharmacol Bull 1995; 31:469.

VanValkenburg C, Kluznik JC, Merrill R: New uses of anticonvulsant drugs in psychosis. Drugs 1992; 44:326.

Vestergaard P, Amdisen A, Schou M: Clinically significant side effects of lithium treatment: A survey of 237 patients in long-term treatment. Acta Psychiatr Scand 1980; 62:193.

Wood A J, Goodwin GM: A review of the biochemical and neuropharmacological actions of lithium. Psychol Med 1987;17:579.

Antidepressant Agents

30

William Z. Potter, MD, PhD, & Leo E. Hollister, MD

Depression is one of the most common psychiatric disorders. At any given moment, about 5–6% of the population is depressed (point prevalence), and an estimated 10% of people may become depressed during their lives (lifetime prevalence). The symptoms of depression are often subtle and unrecognized both by patients and by physicians. Patients with vague complaints that resist explanation as manifestations of somatic disorders and those who might be simplistically called "neurotics" should be suspected of being depressed.

Depression is a heterogeneous disorder that has been characterized and classified in a variety of ways. According to the American Psychiatric Association's fourth edition (1994) of the *Diagnostic and Statistical Manual of Mental Disorders (DSM-IV)*, several diagnoses of affective disorders are possible. Major depression and dysthymia (minor) are pure depressive syndromes, whereas bipolar disorder and cyclothymic disorder signify depression in association with mania. A simplified classification based on presumed origin is as follows: (1) "reactive" or "secondary" depression (most common), occurring in response to real stimuli such as grief, illness, etc; (2) "endogenous" depression, a genetically determined biochemical disorder manifested by inability to cope with ordinary stress; and (3) depression associated with bipolar affective (manic-depressive) disorder. Drugs discussed in this chapter are used chiefly in management of the second type. Table 30–1 indicates how the three types may be differentiated.

An intensive effort to formalize guidelines for the treatment of depression is provided by the cross-disciplinary publication of the Depression Guideline Panel (1993). Pharmacologic treatment with drugs is emphasized, although, their unproved efficacy in milder forms of depression (so-called dysthymia) is noted, as is a remaining role for electroconvulsive therapy for delusional or severe forms of life-threatening depression. Despite intensive research, the mechanisms of action of various pharmacologic treatments are still not understood, though most are believed to involve effects on two monoamine neurotransmitters: serotonin and norepinephrine.

The Pathogenesis of Major Depression: The Amine Hypothesis

Soon after the introduction of reserpine in the early 1950s, it became apparent that the drug could induce depression in patients being treated for hypertension and schizophrenia as well as in normal subjects. Within the next few years, pharmacologic studies revealed that the principal mechanism of action of reserpine was to inhibit the storage of amine neurotransmitters such as serotonin and norepinephrine in the vesicles of presynaptic nerve endings. Reserpine induced depression and depleted stores of amine neurotransmitters; therefore, it was reasoned, depression must be associated with decreased functional amine-dependent synaptic transmission. This simple syllogism provided the basis for what became known as the amine hypothesis of depression. A major puzzle in applying this hypothesis was the fact that although the pharmacologic actions of both tricyclic and MAO inhibitor classes of antidepressants are prompt, the clinical effects require weeks or even months to become manifest. Attempts have been made to explain this observation by invoking slow compensatory responses to the initial blockade of reuptake or MAO inhibition (see below).

While the amine hypothesis is undoubtedly too simplistic, it has provided the major experimental models for the discovery of new antidepressant drugs. As a result, all the currently available antidepressant drugs—except bupropion—are classified as having their primary actions on the metabolism, reuptake, or selective receptor antagonism of serotonin, norepinephrine, or both.

Table 30–1. Differentiation of types of depression.

Type	Diagnostic Features	Comments
Reactive	Loss (adverse life events). Physical illness (myocardial infarct, cancer). Drugs (antihypertensives, alcohol, hormones). Other psychiatric disorders (senility).	More than 60% of all depressions. Core depressive syndrome: depression, anxiety, bodily complaints, tension, guilt. May respond spontaneously or to a variety of ministrations.
Major depressive (endogenous)	Precipitating life event not adequate for degree of depression. Autonomous (unresponsive to changes in life). May occur at any age (childhood to old age). Biologically determined (family history).	About 25% of all depressions. Core depressive syndrome plus "vital" signs: abnormal rhythms of sleep, motor activity, libido, appetite. Usually responds specifically to antidepressants or electroconvulsive therapy. Tends to recur throughout life.
Bipolar affective (manic-depressive)	Characterized by episodes of mania. Cyclic; mania alone, rare; depression alone, occasional; mania-depression, usual.	About 10–15% of all depressions. May be misdiagnosed as endogenous if hypomanic episodes are missed. Lithium carbonate stabilizes mood. Mania may require antipsychotic drugs as well; depression managed with antidepressants.

I. BASIC PHARMACOLOGY OF ANTIDEPRESSANTS

Chemistry

A variety of different chemical structures have been found to have antidepressant activity. The number is constantly growing, but as yet no group has been found to have a clear therapeutic advantage over the others.

A. Tricyclic Antidepressants (TCAs): (Figure 30–1.) Tricyclic antidepressants—so called because of the characteristic three-ring nucleus—have been used clinically for almost four decades. They closely resemble the phenothiazines chemically and, to a lesser extent, pharmacologically. Like the latter drugs, they were first thought to be useful as antihistamines and later as antipsychotics. The discovery of their antidepressant properties was a fortuitous clinical observation. **Imipramine** and **amitriptyline** are the prototypical drugs of the class as mixed norepinephrine and serotonin uptake inhibitors with several other properties.

B. Heterocyclics, Second- and Third-Generation Drugs: Between 1980 and 1996, a number of "second-generation" and "third-generation" or "heterocyclic" antidepressants were introduced. Four of the agents classified as "second-generation" are available for clinical use in the USA and are shown in Figure 30–2. **Amoxapine** and **maprotiline** resemble the structure of the tricyclic agents, while **trazodone** and **bupropion** are distinctive. The heterocyclic agents are not notably different from the older agents in potency. Since 1990, **venlafaxine**, a newer and chemically unique third-generation agent; **mirtazapine**, an analog of a widely used European antidepressant; and **nefazodone**, developed on the basis of trazodone, have been introduced. The structures of these compounds are shown in Figure 30–3.

C. Selective Serotonin Reuptake Inhibitors (SSRIs): One of the major drawbacks of most first-generation antidepressants has been their many "irrelevant" pharmacologic actions, a trait inherited from the phenothiazine antipsychotic agents. As far as has been determined, the antimuscarinic, antihistaminic, and alpha adrenoceptor-blocking actions of tricyclic antidepressants contribute only to the toxicity of these agents. Since the finding that **fluoxetine,** an effective antidepressant with minimal autonomic toxicity, was a highly selective serotonin reuptake inhibitor, a major effort has been under way to find molecules with similar actions. Three selective serotonin reuptake inhibitors are currently available, and more are undergoing clinical trials. All are clearly unlike the tricyclic molecules in regard to their structure, as are the other newer compounds (Figure 30–4).

D. Monoamine Oxidase (MAO) Inhibitors: MAO inhibitors may be classified as hydrazides, exemplified by the C–N–N moiety, as is the case with **phenelzine** and **isocarboxazid;** or nonhydrazides, which lack such a moiety, as with **tranylcypromine** (Figure 30–5). Tranylcypromine closely resembles dextroamphetamine, which is itself a weak inhibitor of MAO. Tranylcypromine retains some of the sympathomimetic characteristics of the amphetamines. The hydrazides appear to combine irreversibly with the enzyme, while tranylcypromine has a prolonged duration of effect even though it is not bound irreversibly. These older MAO inhibitors are nonselective inhibitors of both MAO-A and MAO-B. Moclobemide is an investigational short-acting, selective, reversible inhibitor of MAO-A (RIMA).

Pharmacokinetics

A. Tricyclics: Most tricyclics are incompletely absorbed and undergo significant first-pass metabolism. As a result of high protein binding and relatively high lipid solubility, volumes of distribution tend to be very large. Tricyclics are metabolized by two major routes: transformation of the tricyclic nucleus and

R_1: $-(CH_2)_3N(CH_3)_2$
R_2: H

Imipramine

R_1: = $CH(CH_2)_2N(CH_3)_2$

Amitriptyline

R_1: = $CH(CH_2)_2N(CH_3)_2$

Doxepin

R_1: $-(CH_2)_3NHCH_3$
R_2: H

Desipramine

R_1: = $CH(CH_2)_2NHCH_3$
Nortriptyline

R_1: $-(CH_2)_3N(CH_3)_2$
R_2: $-Cl$

Clomipramine

R_1: $-(CH_2)_3NHCH_3$
Protriptyline

R_1: $-CH_2CH(CH_3)CH_2N(CH_3)_2$
R_2: H

Trimipramine

Figure 30–1. Structural relationships between various tricyclic antidepressants (TCAs).

alteration of the aliphatic side chain. The former route involves ring hydroxylation and conjugation to form glucuronides; the latter, primarily demethylation of the nitrogen. Monodemethylation of tertiary amines leads to active metabolites such as desipramine and nortriptyline (which are themselves available as drugs; Figure 30–1). The proportion of mono-demethylated metabolites that is formed varies from one patient to another. In general, the proportion of amitriptyline to its metabolite nortriptyline favors the

Amoxapine

Maprotiline

Trazodone

Bupropion

Figure 30–2. Some heterocyclic (second-generation) antidepressants.

Figure 30–3. Third-generation heterocyclic antidepressants.

parent drug. The converse is the case with imipramine and its metabolite, desipramine. The pharmacokinetic parameters of various antidepressants are summarized in Table 30–2.

B. Heterocyclics: The pharmacokinetics of these drugs are similar to those of the tricyclics. As can be seen from Table 30–2, data are less complete for these agents. Still, they tend to have variable bioavailability, high protein binding, variable and large volumes of distribution, and, perhaps, active metabolites. Trazodone and venlafaxine have the shortest plasma half-lives, which mandates divided

doses during the day when beginning treatment, though once-a-day dosing may be possible later.

C. Selective Serotonin Reuptake Inhibitors (SSRIs): The pharmacokinetic parameters of these drugs are summarized in Table 30–2. Fluoxetine is well absorbed, and peak plasma concentrations are attained within 4–8 hours. Its demethylated active metabolite, norfluoxetine, has a half-life of 7–9 days at steady state; the parent drug has a slightly shorter half-life. Fluoxetine inhibits various drug-metabolizing enzymes, which has led to a number of significant drug-drug interactions with other antidepressants and

Figure 30–4. Selective serotonin reuptake inhibitors (SSRIs).

Figure 30–5. Some monoamine oxidase inhibitors. Phenelzine is the hydrazide of phenylethylamine (Figure 9–3), while tranylcypromine has a cyclopropyl amine side chain and closely resembles dextroamphetamine (see Figure 9–4). These agents are unselective and produce an extremely long-lasting inhibition of the enzyme. Moclobemide is a new short-acting reversible inhibitor of MAO-A (RIMA) and bears the least structural resemblance to sympathomimetics.

with other drugs as well. Sertraline and paroxetine have pharmacokinetic parameters similar to those of tricyclics.

D. MAO Inhibitors: The MAO inhibitors are readily absorbed from the gastrointestinal tract. The hydrazide inhibitor phenelzine is acetylated in the liver and manifests differences in elimination depending on the acetylation phenotype of the individual (see Chapter 4). However, inhibition of MAO persists even after these drugs are no longer detectable in plasma. Therefore, conventional pharmacokinetic parameters (half-life, etc) are not very helpful in governing dosage. Instead, measuring the inhibition of MAO activity has been used to predict the level of effect, though such measurements are not employed clinically. In practice, it is prudent to assume that the effect will persist for from 7 days (tranylcypromine) to 2 or 3 weeks (phenelzine) after discontinuance of the drug.

Pharmacodynamics

A. Action of Antidepressants on Biogenic Amine Neurotransmitters: The amine hypothesis was buttressed by studies on the mechanism of action of various types of antidepressant drugs (Figure 30–6). Tricyclics block the amine (norepinephrine or serotonin) reuptake pumps, the "off switches" of amine neurotransmission (see Table 30–3 and Chapter

6). Such an action presumably permits a longer sojourn of neurotransmitter at the receptor site. MAO inhibitors block a major degradative pathway for the amine neurotransmitters, which permits more amines to accumulate in presynaptic stores and more to be released. Some of the second-generation antidepressants have similar effects on amine neurotransmitters, while others have mild or minimal effects on reuptake or metabolism. In contrast, trazodone, nefazodone, and mirtazapine stand out as agents in which antagonism of subtypes of serotonin receptors (5-HT$_{2A}$ or 5-HT$_{2C}$) may be important in their action. Mirtazapine is unique in including antagonism of α_2 norepinephrine receptors as presumably contributing to its therapeutic effects. Bupropion has been found to alter the output of norepinephrine in humans following chronic administration through some as yet unidentified primary mechanism. Thus, even the newest antidepressants can still be categorized as working through serotonergic and noradrenergic effects without invoking blockade of neurotransmitter reuptake or metabolism. It is not yet clear whether these biochemical distinctions confer any therapeutic advantage.

B. Receptor and Postreceptor Effects: More attention has been paid recently to the ultimate effects of the increase in neurotransmitter in the synapse acting on postsynaptic receptors. In tests of postsynaptic activity, cAMP concentrations have consistently *decreased* rather than increased, in spite of the presumably longer duration of action of the transmitters. In addition, the number of postsynaptic beta adrenoceptors has shown a measurable decrease that follows the same delayed time course as clinical improvement in patients. Thus, the initial increase in neurotransmitter seen with some antidepressants appears to produce, over time, a compensatory decrease in receptor activity, ie, downregulation of receptors. Decreases in norepinephrine-stimulated cAMP and in beta adrenoceptor binding have been conclusively shown for selective norepinephrine uptake inhibitors, those with mixed action on norepinephrine and serotonin, monoamine oxidase inhibitors, and even electroconvulsive therapy. Such changes do not consistently occur after the selective serotonin uptake inhibitors, α_2 receptor antagonists, and mixed serotonin antagonists. It has been emphasized that enhanced serotonergic transmission, albeit mediated through diverse mechanisms, might be the most common (but not universal) long-term effect of antidepressants. This could occur, for instance, without increasing the concentration of neurotransmitter at the receptor site if there were an increase in serotonin receptor sensitivity. Thus, chronic treatment with tricyclic agents or electroconvulsive shock increases the electrophysiologic response to microiontophoretically applied serotonin in various areas of the rat brain. And selective receptor antagonism of either norepinephrine or serotonin receptors may lead to enhanced extracellular serotonin due to

Table 30–2. Pharmacokinetic parameters of various antidepressants.

Drug	Bioavail-ability (percent)[1]	Protein Binding (percent)[1]	Plasma $t_{1/2}$ (hours)	Active Metabolites	Volume of Distribution (L/kg)[1]	Therapeutic Plasma Concentrations (ng/mL)[1]
Amitriptyline	31–61	82–96	31–46	Nortriptyline	5–10	80–200 total
Amoxapine	nd	nd	8	7-,8-Hydroxy	nd	nd
Bupropion	60–80	85	11–14	nd	20–30	25–100
Clomipramine	nd	nd	22–84	Desmethyl	7–20	240–700
Desipramine	60–70	73–90	14–62	nd	22–59	145[2]
Doxepin	13–45	nd	8–24	Desmethyl	9–33	30–150
Fluoxetine	70	94	24–96	Norfluoxetine	12–97	nd
Fluvoxamine	nd	77	15	None	>5	nd
Imipramine	29–77	76–95	9–24	Desipramine	15–30	>180 total
Maprotiline	66–75	88	21–52	Desmethyl	15–28	200–300
Mirtazapine	nd	nd	20–40	Desmethyl	nd	nd
Nefazodone	15–23	98	2–4	Hydroxy, m-chlorophenyl piperazine	nd	nd
Nortripyline	32–79	93–95	18–93	10-Hydroxy	21–57	50–150
Paroxetine	50	95	24	None	28–31	nd
Protriptyline	77–93	90–95	54–198	nd	19–57	70–170
Sertraline	nd	98	22–35	Desmethyl	20	nd
Trazodone	nd	nd	4–9	m-Chloro-phenyl-piperazine	nd	nd
Venlafaxine	nd	27–30	4–10	O-desmethyl	nd	nd

[1]nd = no data found.
[2]Lower concentrations may be effective.

the complex manner in which these neurotransmitters are interregulated. One current theory holds that enhanced stimulation or responsiveness of postsynaptic 5-HT_{1A} receptors is particularly important in the action of antidepressants.

No clinical studies have directly tested the relevance of these findings from animals for norepinephrine and serotonin function in humans and their relationship to the mode of action of antidepressants. One of the most interesting approaches has been to reduce the amino acid precursor of serotonin, tryptophan, in the diet and, by implication, the amount of available neurotransmitter in the brain, since tryptophan availability can be rate-limiting in the formation of serotonin under certain experimental conditions. Using this approach, it was found that a tryptophan-depleted diet produces low plasma tryptophan and acutely "reverses" antidepressant responses to SSRIs but not to selective or mixed norepinephrine uptake inhibitors. These findings indirectly support the hypothesis that enhanced serotonin throughput is necessary for the antidepressant action of serotonin but not norepinephrine uptake inhibitors. Moreover, tryptophan depletion does not consistently worsen the condition of un-

medicated depressed patients. Thus, there is no clear relationship between serotonin and depression or antidepressant mechanisms in general.

C. Effects of Specific Antidepressants:

1. Tricyclics–The first-generation antidepressants demonstrate varying degrees of selectivity for the reuptake pumps for norepinephrine and serotonin (Table 30–3). They also have numerous autonomic actions, as described below under Adverse Effects.

2. Heterocyclics–Amoxapine is a metabolite of the antipsychotic drug loxapine and retains some of its antipsychotic action and dopamine receptor antagonism. A combination of antidepressant and antipsychotic actions might make it a suitable drug for depression in psychotic patients. However, the dopamine antagonism may cause akathisia, parkinsonism, amenorrhea-galactorrhea syndrome, and perhaps tardive dyskinesia.

Maprotiline (a tetracyclic drug) is most like desipramine in terms of its potent norepinephrine uptake inhibition. Like the latter drug, it has fewer sedative and antimuscarinic actions than the older tricyclics.

Clinical experience with trazodone has indicated unpredictable efficacy for depression though it has

Inhibitory serotonin synapse

Norepinephrine synapse

Figure 30–6. Schematic diagram showing some of the potential sites of action of antidepressant drugs. Chronic therapy with these drugs has been proved to reduce reuptake of norepinephrine or serotonin (or both), reduce the number of postsynaptic beta receptors, and reduce the generation of cAMP. The MAO inhibitors act on MAO in the nerve terminals and cause the same effects on beta receptors and cAMP generation.

proved very useful as a hypnotic, sometimes being combined with MAOIs, which disturb sleep.

3. Selective Serotonin Reuptake Inhibitors—Fluoxetine was the first SSRI to reach general clin-

ical use. Paroxetine and sertraline differ mainly in having shorter half-lives and different potencies as inhibitors of specific P450 isoenzymes. While SSRIs have not been shown to be more effective overall than prior drugs, they lack many of the toxicities of the tricyclic and heterocyclic antidepressants. Thus, patient acceptance has been high despite adverse effects such as nausea, decreased libido, and even decreased sexual function.

A dangerous pharmacodynamic interaction may occur when fluoxetine or one of the newer selective serotonin reuptake inhibitors is used in the presence of a monoamine oxidase inhibitor. The combination of increased stores of the monoamine plus inhibition of reuptake after release are thought to result in marked increases of serotonin in the synapses, leading to a "serotonin syndrome." This syndrome includes hyperthermia, muscle rigidity, myoclonus, and rapid changes in mental status and vital signs.

4. MAO inhibitors—MAO-A is the amine oxidase primarily responsible for norepinephrine, serotonin, and tyramine metabolism. MAO-B is more selective for dopamine. If noradrenergic and serotonergic synapses—but not dopaminergic ones—are involved in depression, selective block of MAO-A might be more selective for this condition. Furthermore, irreversible block of MAO, characteristic of the older MAO inhibitors, allows significant accumulation of tyramine and loss of the first-pass metabolism that protects against tyramine in foods. As a result, the irreversible MAO inhibitors are subject to a very high risk of hypertensive reactions to tyramine ingested in

Table 30–3. Pharmacologic differences among several antidepressants.[1]

Drug	Sedative Action	Antimuscarinic Action	Block of Amine Pump for:		
			Serotonin	Norepinephrine	Dopamine
Amitriptyline	+++	+++	+++	++	0
Amoxapine	++	++	+	++	+
Bupropion	0	0	+,0	+,0	?
Clomipramine	+++	++	+++	+++	0
Desipramine	+	+	0	+++	0
Doxepin	+++	+++	++	+	0
Fluoxetine	0	0	+++	0,+	0,+
Imipramine	++	++	+++	++	0
Maprotiline	++	++	0	+++	0
Mirtazapine[2]	+++	0	0	0	0
Nortriptyline	++	++	++	++	0
Paroxetine	+	0	+++	0	0
Protriptyline	0	++	?	+++	?
Sertraline	+	0	+++	0	0
Trazodone	+++	0	++	0	0
Venlafaxine	0	0	+++	++	0, +

[1] 0 = none; + = slight; ++ = moderate; +++ = high; ? = uncertain.
[2] Significant α_2-adrenoceptor antagonism.

food. From the evidence available to date, the reversible, short-acting MAO inhibitor moclobemide appears to be relatively free of this interaction. (The selective MAO-B inhibitor selegiline loses selectivity at antidepressant dosage. Because its action is on the enzyme that metabolizes dopamine, it is most useful in the treatment of Parkinson's disease [Chapter 28].)

II. CLINICAL PHARMACOLOGY OF ANTIDEPRESSANTS

Clinical Indications

The major indication for these drugs is to treat depression, but a number of other uses have been established by clinical experience and controlled trials.

A. Depression: This indication has been kept broad deliberately, even though evidence from clinical studies strongly suggests that the drugs are specifically useful only in major depressive episodes. Major depressive episodes are diagnosed not so much by their severity as by their quality. Formerly, they were referred to as "endogenous," "vital," or "vegetative"—reflecting the characteristic disturbances of major body rhythms of sleep, hunger and appetite, sexual drive, and motor activity. The diagnosis of major depression may be uncertain in individual patients, so that on balance this condition is underdiagnosed and undertreated.

B. Panic Disorder: Imipramine was first shown in 1962 to have a beneficial effect in the acute episodes of anxiety that have come to be known as panic attacks. Recent studies have shown it to be as effective as MAO inhibitors and benzodiazepines. In general, the latter drugs are preferred, as they are better tolerated and their clinical effects become evident promptly. Recently, it has been demonstrated that SSRIs are also effective in panic disorder.

C. Obsessive-Compulsive Disorders: The serotonin reuptake inhibitors have been shown to be uniquely effective for treating these disorders. Recent studies have focused on fluoxetine and other selective serotonin reuptake-inhibiting drugs, although clomipramine, a mixed serotonin and norepinephrine uptake inhibitor, may be more potent.

D. Enuresis: Enuresis is an established indication for tricyclics. Proof of efficacy for this indication is substantial, but drug therapy is not the preferred approach. The beneficial effect of drug treatment lasts only as long as drug treatment is continued. Institutionalized elderly patients with incontinence are often treated with imipramine. Unfortunately, this age group is also the most sensitive to the anticholinergic hallucinogenic effects of the drug.

E. Chronic Pain: Clinicians in pain clinics have found tricyclics to be especially useful for treating a variety of chronically painful states that often cannot be definitively diagnosed. Whether such painful states represent depressive equivalents or whether such patients become secondarily depressed after some initial pain-producing insult is not clear. It is even possible that the tricyclics work directly on pain pathways. Phenothiazines are also sometimes used in combination. Any role of SSRIs and other newer antidepressants in chronic pain is uncertain.

F. Other Indications: Less well established indications for antidepressants are eating disorders (especially bulimia), cataplexy associated with narcolepsy, school phobia, and attention deficit disorder.

Drug Choice

Controlled comparisons of the available antidepressants have usually led to the conclusion that they are roughly equivalent drugs. Although this may be true for groups of patients, individual patients may for uncertain reasons fare better on one drug than on another. Some European studies show that patients depressed enough to be hospitalized respond better to classic tricyclics than to monotherapy with SSRIs. Thus, finding the right drug for the individual patient must be accomplished empirically. The past history of the patient's drug experience is the most valuable guide. At times such a history may lead to the exclusion of tricyclics, as in the case of patients who have responded well in the past to MAO inhibitors.

Antidepressant drugs are apt to be most successful in patients with clearly "vegetative" characteristics, including psychomotor retardation, sleep disturbance, poor appetite and weight loss, and loss of libido.

Tricyclic and heterocyclic agents differ mainly in the degree of sedation (amitriptyline, doxepin, and trazodone cause the most, protriptyline the least) and the amount of antimuscarinic effects (amitriptyline and doxepin have the greatest, Table 30–3). Although it has been argued that the more sedative drugs are preferable for markedly anxious or agitated depressives while the least sedative drugs are preferable for patients with psychomotor withdrawal, this hypothesis has not been tested.

None of the heterocyclic antidepressants have been shown to be more effective overall than the tricyclics with which they have been compared. The major claims are (1) a faster onset of action, (2) less adverse sedative and autonomic effects, and (3) less toxicity when overdoses are taken. Solid evidence to support a claim of more rapid onset of action has been difficult to obtain. Amoxapine and maprotiline seem to have as many sedative and autonomic actions as most tricyclics; more recently introduced antidepressants such as bupropion and venlafaxine have fewer, although nefazodone and mirtazapine are very sedating. Amoxapine and maprotiline are at least as dangerous as the tricyclics when taken in overdoses; the other newer agents seem to be safer.

No special indications for particular types of depression have been found for the selective serotonin reuptake inhibitors or other newer antidepressants. The popularity of these drugs, despite their higher cost, is due principally to their greater acceptance by patients. A provocative clinical report that fluoxetine use increased suicidal or aggressive ideation was not supported by subsequent analyses of massive data bases. Suicidal thoughts are part of the depressive syndrome.

MAO inhibitors are helpful in patients described as having "atypical" depressions—a nonspecific designation scarcely helpful in their identification. Depressed patients with considerable attendant anxiety, phobic features, and hypochondriasis are the ones who respond best to these drugs.

Few clinicians use lithium, an antimanic agent, as primary treatment for depression. However, some have found that lithium along with one of the other antidepressants may achieve a favorable response not obtained by the antidepressant alone. Another potential use of lithium is to prevent relapses of depression.

Dosages

The usual daily dose ranges of antidepressants are shown in Table 30–4. Doses are almost always determined empirically; the patient's acceptance of adverse effects is the usual limiting factor. Tolerance to some of the objectionable effects may develop, so that the usual pattern of treatment has been to start with small doses, increasing either to a predetermined daily dose, or to one that produces relief of depression, or to the maximum tolerated dose. The effective dose of an antidepressant varies widely depending upon many factors.

Table 30–4. Usual daily doses of antidepressant drugs.

Drug	Dose (mg)
Tricyclics	
Amitriptyline	75–200
Clomipramine	75–300
Desipramine	75–200
Doxepin	75–300
Imipramine	75–200
Nortriptyline	75–150
Protriptyline	20–40
Trimipramine	75–200
Heterocyclics	
Amoxapine	150–300
Bupropion	200–400
Maprotiline	75–300
Mirtazapine	15–60
Nefazodone	200–600
Trazodone	50–600
Venlafaxine	75–225
Monoamine oxidase inhibitors	
Phenelzine	45–75
Tranylcypromine	10–30
Selective serotonin reuptake inhibitors	
Fluoxetine	10–60
Fluvoxamine	100–300
Paroxetine	20–50
Sertraline	50–200

Dosage Schedules for Treating the Acute Episode

When patients are treated as outpatients, as many can be, initial doses of tricyclics may vary from 10 mg to 75 mg on the first day of treatment, depending on the patient's size and tolerance for the acute effects. Such conservative dosing regimens are not required for hospitalized patients, in whom initial doses should be around 100 mg. After 2 or 3 days at these levels, doses may be increased in increments of 25 mg every second or third day until a maximum daily dose of 150 mg is reached. Such a dose will place most patients within the presumed range of therapeutic plasma concentration of the drug. However, for patients who do not respond at this dosage, further increments up to 300 mg/d may be made if tolerated.

A similar pattern may be used with most of the heterocyclic drugs and the selective serotonin reuptake inhibitors. Bupropion, venlafaxine, and nefazodone require divided doses during the day, at least during the first few weeks of treatment. With fluoxetine, it is customary to begin with a dosage of 20 mg/d and maintain this level for several weeks until the patient's response can be estimated. Only infrequently are higher doses needed, and elderly patients may be treated with 20 mg every other day.

Phenelzine has been the most carefully studied of the MAO inhibitors. Approximately 80% inhibition of the enzyme is desirable, a goal usually attained with a dosage of 1 mg/kg/d. Dosages of the other MAO inhibitors should be gradually titrated to levels that produce a mild degree of orthostatic hypotension or sleep disturbance.

MAO inhibitors, bupropion, fluoxetine, sertraline, paroxetine, and venlafaxine are customarily given early in the day when initiating treatment, as they can be somewhat stimulating and may cause insomnia if given late. After a few weeks on drug, however, any such effects should disappear and time of day administered is rarely important. Virtually all the other antidepressants have varying degrees of sedative effects and are best given near bedtime. Autonomic adverse effects also tend to be less troublesome if the dose is given late.

Maintenance Treatment

Whether or not to undertake long-term maintenance treatment of a depressed patient depends entirely on the natural history of the disorder. If the depressive episode was the patient's first and if it responded quickly and satisfactorily to drug therapy, it is rational to gradually withdraw treatment over a period of a few months. If relapse does not occur, drug treatment can be stopped until the next attack occurs, which is unpredictable but nearly certain. However, a patient who has had several previous attacks of depression—especially if each succeeding attack was more severe and more difficult to treat—is a candidate for maintenance therapy. In general, maintenance therapy is more effective if full dosage is used rather than partial dosage. The duration of treatment varies, though many patients require maintenance treatment indefinitely.

Monitoring Plasma Concentrations

Routine monitoring of plasma concentrations of antidepressants, while technically feasible for most drugs, is still of uncertain value. Experience with monitoring of plasma concentrations of tricyclics suggests that about 20% of patients become noncompliant at some time or other. Thus, a "poor response" in a patient for whom an adequate dosage of drug has been prescribed may be shown by measurement of the plasma drug concentration to be due merely to failure to take the drug. Blood for plasma drug level determination should be obtained in the postabsorptive state, about 10–12 hours after the last dose. Even when sampling time is constant, the same patient may show variation in both the total plasma concentration and the proportion of parent drug versus metabolites while on a constant dose at steady state conditions. Under no circumstances should the laboratory test results be permitted to overrule the physician's clinical judgment.

Unresponsive Patients

Almost one-third of patients receiving tricyclic antidepressants fail to respond. In evaluating a patient's resistance to treatment, one should consider the five D's: diagnosis, drug, dose, duration of treatment, and different treatment.

Diagnosis might be reassessed if the patient shows little response over a period of 2–3 weeks of adequate dosage or plasma concentrations. Whether or not the patient is bipolar, lithium might be added (Chapter 29); if psychotic, treatment might be augmented with an antipsychotic. Combination of an SSRI with desipramine or bupropion appears relatively safe and effective for some patients. Use of the newest antidepressants—venlafaxine, nefazodone, and mirtazapine—in various combinations with other drugs has not been reported. Some clinicians believe that several weeks or months of treatment should be tried before giving up on a drug or combination. The morbidity of depression, however, is such that long delays in attaining relief are demoralizing.

A generally accepted strategy is to begin treatment with an SSRI in mild to moderate outpatient depression and then augment by adding a drug of a different class for more impaired patients. Otherwise, switch to a drug of different class. Most clinicians would prefer to move through various antidepressant drug classes in the search for the right drug rather than through various drugs within a class.

Dose and duration of treatment must be considered. Most treatment failures are due to inadequate dosage, which should be pushed to the limits of the patient's tolerance in refractory cases. The duration of treatment before giving up on a drug is a matter of clinical judgment.

Finally, some patients may need a completely different type of treatment, such as electroconvulsive therapy (ECT). ECT is often viewed as a treatment of last resort, but it should not be withheld from patients with this disorder who cannot be helped by drug therapy. For patients with psychotic depression, ECT may be a treatment of first choice.

Noncompliance is an important cause of lack of response. Patients should be warned also that noticeable improvement may be slow, perhaps taking 3 weeks or more. Inability to tolerate adverse effects and discouragement with treatment are two major causes for noncompliance and for failure of antidepressants to show efficacy.

Adverse Effects

Adverse effects of various antidepressants are summarized in Table 30–5. Most common unwanted effects are minor, but they may seriously affect patient compliance; the more seriously depressed the patient is, the more likely it is that unwanted effects will be tolerated. Most normal persons find that even moderate doses of many antidepressants cause disagreeable symptoms, especially the classic tertiary amine tricyclics: amitriptyline, imipramine, and doxepin.

Drug Interactions

A. Pharmacodynamic Interactions: Many of the pharmacodynamic interactions of antidepressants with other drugs have already been discussed. Sedative effects may be additive with other sedatives, especially alcohol. Patients taking tricyclics should be warned that use of alcohol may lead to greater than expected impairment of driving ability. MAO inhibitors, by increasing stores of catecholamines, sensitize the patient to indirectly acting sympathomimetics such as tyramine, which is found in some fermented foods and beverages, and to sympathomimetic drugs that may be administered therapeutically, such as diethylpropion or phenylpropanolamine. Such sensitization can result in dangerous hypertensive emergencies. The serious interaction between MAO inhibitors and selective serotonin reuptake inhibitors has been mentioned; the "serotonin syndrome" is potentially lethal and must be avoided.

B. Pharmacokinetic Interactions: The most likely pharmacokinetic interactions are between the potent inhibitors of P450-2D6, paroxetine and fluoxetine, and those few drugs highly dependent on this pathway for clearance (eg, desipramine, nortriptyline, flecainide). Actual instances of clinically significant interactions are extremely rare, there being only a handful of case reports after cumulative exposure of more than 25 million patients to these SSRI drugs. Inhibition of P450-3A4 could possibly occur at high concentrations of nefazodone and fluvoxamine and block the metabolism of such widely used compounds as terfenadine, astemizole, and cisapride. Because elevations of the concentrations of the parent forms of these drugs can cause fatal arrhythmias, the combina-

Table 30–5. Adverse effects of antidepressants.

Tricyclics	
Sedation	Sleepiness, additive effects with other sedative drugs
Sympathomimetic	Tremor, insomnia
Antimuscarinic	Blurred vision, constipation, urinary hesitancy, confusion
Cardiovascular	Orthostatic hypotension, conduction defects, arrhythmias
Psychiatric	Aggravation of psychosis, withdrawal syndrome
Neurologic	Seizures
Metabolic-endocrine	Weight gain, sexual disturbances
Monoamine oxidase inhibitors	Headache, drowsiness, dry mouth, weight gain, postural hypotension, sexual disturbances
Amoxapine	Similar to the tricyclics with the addition of some effects associated with the antipsychotics (Chapter 29)
Maprotiline	Similar to tricyclics; seizures are dose-related
Trazodone, nefazadone	Drowsiness, dizziness, insomnia, nausea, agitation
Venlafaxine	Nausea, somnolence, sweating, dizziness, anxiety, sexual disturbances, hypertension
Bupropion	Dizziness, dry mouth, sweating, tremor, aggravation of psychosis, potential for seizures at high doses
Fluoxetine and other serotonin reuptake inhibitors	Anxiety, insomnia, tremor, gastrointestinal symptoms, rashes, decreased libido, sexual dysfunction

tion of nefazodone or fluvoxamine with any of these drugs is contraindicated.

Overdoses

A. Tricyclics: Tricyclics are extremely dangerous when taken in overdose quantities, and depressed patients are more likely than others to be suicidal. Prescriptions should therefore be limited to amounts less than 1.25 g, or 50 dose units of 25 mg, on a "no refill" basis. If suicide is a serious possibility, the tablets should be entrusted to a family member. The drugs must be kept away from children. Both accidental and deliberate overdoses are frequent and are a serious medical emergency. Major effects include (1) coma with shock and sometimes metabolic acidosis; (2) respiratory depression with a tendency to sudden apnea; (3) agitation or delirium both before and after consciousness is obtunded; (4) neuromuscular irritability and seizures; (5) hyperpyrexia; (6) bowel and bladder paralysis; and (7) a great variety of cardiac manifestations, including conduction defects and arrhythmias.

Management of cardiac problems is difficult. Antiarrhythmic drugs having the least depressant effect on cardiac conduction should be used. Lidocaine, propranolol, and phenytoin have been used successfully, but quinidine and procainamide are contraindicated. Sodium bicarbonate has been useful in reversing conduction block. Physostigmine given in small (0.5 mg) intravenous boluses to a total dose of 3–4 mg may awaken the patient and reverse a rapid supraventricular arrhythmia. It is unlikely to be effective for ventricular arrhythmias. Poison control centers no longer consider physostigmine to be appropriate treatment for this condition. Continuous cardiac monitoring is essential, and facilities must be at hand for resuscita-

tion if needed. Arterial blood gases and pH should be measured frequently, since both hypoxia and metabolic acidosis predispose to arrhythmias. Sodium bicarbonate and intravenous potassium chloride may be required to restore acid-base balance and to correct hypokalemia. Electrical pacing must be used in refractory cases. Other treatment is entirely supportive. (See Chapter 59.)

B. Heterocyclic Drugs: Overdoses of amoxapine are characterized by severe neurotoxicity, with seizures that are difficult to control. Overdoses of maprotiline also have a tendency to cause seizures as well as cardiotoxicity. Overdoses of the other heterocyclic drugs appear to create only minor problems and can usually be managed with purely supportive measures. For example, in one recorded case even 11 g of nefazodone failed to cause serious injury.

C. MAO Inhibitors: Intoxication with MAO inhibitors is unusual. Agitation, delirium, and neuromuscular excitability are followed by obtunded consciousness, seizures, shock, and hyperthermia. Supportive treatment is usually all that is required, though sedative phenothiazines with alpha adrenoceptor-blocking action, such as chlorpromazine, may be useful.

D. Selective Serotonin Reuptake Inhibitors: A few deaths have occurred during overdosage of SSRIs when other drugs were also being taken. The likelihood of fatalities from SSRI overdoses is extremely low. In case of overdose, only supportive treatment can be offered, since the high volume of distribution, as with other antidepressants, rules out removal of drug by dialysis. As much as 2.6 g of sertraline has been taken with survival. Overdoses of paroxetine are relatively benign: Up to 850 mg has been taken with no evidence of cardiotoxicity.

PREPARATIONS AVAILABLE

Tricyclics

Amitriptyline (generic, Elavil, others)
Oral: 10, 25, 50, 75, 100, 150 mg tablets
Parenteral: 10 mg/mL for IM injection
Clomipramine (Anafranil, labeled only for obsessive-compulsive disorder)
Oral: 25, 50, 75 mg capsules
Desipramine (generic, Norpramin, Pertofrane)
Oral: 10, 25, 50, 75, 100, 150 mg tablets; 25, 50 mg capsules
Doxepin (generic, Sinequan, others)
Oral: 10, 25, 50, 75, 100, 150 mg capsules; 10 mg/mL concentrate
Imipramine (generic, Tofranil, others)
Oral: 10, 25, 50 mg tablets (as hydrochloride); 75, 100, 125, 150 mg capsules (as pamoate)
Parenteral: 25 mg/2 mL for IM injection
Nortriptyline (Aventyl, Pamelor)
Oral: 10, 25, 50, 75 mg capsules; 10 mg/5 mL solution
Protriptyline (Vivactil)
Oral: 5, 10 mg tablets
Trimipramine (Surmontil)
Oral: 25, 50, 100 mg capsules

Heterocyclics

Amoxapine (generic, Asendin)
Oral: 25, 50, 100, 150 mg tablets
Bupropion (Wellbutrin)
Oral: 75, 100 mg tablets

Maprotiline (generic, Ludiomil)
Oral: 25, 50, 75 mg tablets
Mirtazapine (Remeron)
Oral: 15, 30 mg tablets
Nefazodone (Serzone)
Oral: 100, 150, 200, 250 mg tablets
Trazodone (generic, Desyrel)
Oral: 50, 100, 150, 300 mg tablets
Venlafaxine (Effexor)
Oral: 25, 37.5, 50, 75, 100 mg tablets

Selective Serotonin Reuptake Inhibitors

Fluoxetine (Prozac)
Oral: 10, 20 mg pulvules, 20 mg/5 mL liquid
Fluvoxamine (Luvox, labeled only for obsessive-compulsive disorder.)
Oral: 50, 100 mg tablets
Paroxetine (Paxil)
Oral: 20, 30 mg tablets
Sertraline (Zoloft)
Oral: 50, 100 mg tablets

Monoamine Oxidase Inhibitors

Phenelzine (Nardil)
Oral: 15 mg tablets
Tranylcypromine (Parnate)
Oral: 10 mg tablets

REFERENCES

American Psychiatric Association: APA practice guideline for major depressive disorder in adults. Am J Psychiatry 1993;150(Suppl):1.

American Psychiatric Association: *Diagnostic and Statistical Manual of Mental Disorders,* 4th ed. American Psychiatric Association,1994.

APA Task Force on Use of Laboratory Tests in Psychiatry: Tricyclic antidepressants: Blood level measurements and clinical outcome: An APA Task Force Report. Am J Psychiatry 1985;142:155.

Blackwell B: Side effects of antidepressant drugs. In: *American Psychiatric Association Annual Review,* vol 6. Hales RE, Frances AJ (editors). American Psychiatric Association, 1987.

Cesura AM, Pletscher A: The new generation of monoamine oxidase inhibitors. Prog Drug Res 1992;38:171.

Danish University Antidepressant Group: Paroxetine: A selective serotonin reuptake inhibitor showing better tolerance but weaker antidepressant effect than clomipramine in a controlled multicenter study. J Affect Disord 1990;18:289.

Dechant KL, Clissold SP: Paroxetine: A review of its pharmacodynamic and pharmacokinetic properties, and therapeutic potential in depressive illness. Drugs 1991; 41:225.

Depression Guideline Panel: Depression in Primary Care: Volume 2. Treatment of Major Depression. Clinical Practice Guideline, Number 5. Rockville, MD: U.S. Department of Health and Human Services, Public Health Service, Agency for Health Care Policy and Research, AHCPR, Pub. No. 93-0551. April 1993.

Derby LE, Jick H, Dean AD: Antidepressant drugs and suicide. J Clin Psychopharmacol 1992;12:235.

Dzuikas LJ, Vohra J: Tricyclic antidepressant poisoning. Med J Aust 1991;154:344.

Fava M et al: Lithium and tricyclic augmentation of fluoxetine treatment for resistant major depression: A double-blind, controlled study. Am J Psychiatry 1994;151:1372.

Frommer DA et al: Tricyclic antidepressant overdose: A review. JAMA 1987;257:521.

Garver DL, Davis JM: Biogenic amine hypothesis of affective disorders. Life Sci 1979;24:383.

Griest JH et al: Efficacy and tolerability of serotonin transport inhibitors in obsessive-compulsive disorder. Arch Gen Psychiatry 1995;52:53.

Heninger GR, Charney DS: Mechanism of action of antidepressant treatments: Implications for the etiology and treatment of depressive disorders. In: *Psychopharmacology: The Third Generation of Progress.* Meltzer HY (editor). Raven Press, 1987.

Hollister LE, Claghorn JL: New antidepressants. Annu Rev Pharmacol Toxicol 1993;32:165.

Jick SS et al: Antidepressants and convulsions. J Clin Psychopharmacol 1992;12:241.

Liebowitz MR et al: Phenelzine vs. imipramine in atypical depression. Arch Gen Psychiatry 1984;41:669.

McDaniel KD: Clinical pharmacology of monamine oxidase inhibitors. Clin Neuropharmacol 1986;9:207.

McGrath PJ et al: Phenelzine treatment of melancholia. J Clin Psychiatry 1986;47:420.

McGrath PJ et al: A double-blind crossover trial of imipramine and phenelzine for outpatients with treatment-refractory depression. Am J Psychiatry 1993; 150:118.

Murphy DL: Neuropsychiatric disorders and the multiple human brain serotonin receptor subtypes and subsystems. Neuropsychopharmacology 1990;3:457.

Potter WZ: Adrenoceptors and serotonin receptor function: Relevance to antidepressant mechanisms of action. J Clin Psychiatry 1996;57(Suppl 4):4.

Potter WZ: Psychotherapeutic drugs and biogenic amines: Current concepts and therapeutic implications. Drugs 1984;28:127.

Reimherr FW et al: Antidepressant efficacy of sertraline: A double blind placebo and amitriptyline-controlled multicenter comparison study in outpatients with major depression. J Clin Psychiatry 1990;51(Suppl 12B):18.

Rothschild AJ: Biology of depression. Med Clin North Am 1988;72:765.

Rothschild AJ et al: Efficacy of the combination of fluoxetine and perphenazine in the treatment of psychotic depression. J Clin Psychiatry 1993;54:338.

Rudorfer MV, Manji HK, Potter WZ: Comparative tolerability profiles of the newer versus older antidepressants. Drug Saf 1994;10:1846.

Schatzberg AF, Nemeroff CB (editors): *The American Psychiatric Press Textbook of Psychopharmacology.* American Psychiatric Press, 1995.

Schopf J: Treatment of depressions resistant to tricyclic antidepressants, related drugs, or MAO-inhibitors by lithium addition: Review of the literature. Pharmacopsychiatry 1989;22:174.

Shen WW: Cytochrome P450 monooxygenases and interactions of psychotropic drugs: A five-year update. Int J Psychiatry Med 1995;25:277.

Snyder SH: Second messengers and affective illness: Focus on the phosphoinositide cycle. Pharmacopsychiatry 1992;25:25.

Sommi RW, Crismon ML, Bowden CL: Fluoxetine: A serotonin-specific, second-generation antidepressant. Pharmacotherapy 1987;7:1.

Stein DJ, Spadaccini E, Hollander E: Meta-analysis of pharmacotherapy trials for obsessive-compulsive disorder. Int Clin Psychopharmacol 1995;10:11.

Sulser F: Serotonin-norepinephrine receptor interactions in the brain: Implications for the pharmacology and pathophysiology of affective disorders. J Clin Psychiatry 1987;48(Suppl):12.

Thase ME, Rush AJ: Treatment-resistant depression. In: *Psychopharmacology: The Fourth Generation of Progress.* Bloom FE, Kupfer DJ (editors). Raven, 1995.

Weissman MN et al: Cross-national epidemiology of major depression and bipolar disorder. 1996;276:293.

31

Opioid Analgesics & Antagonists

Walter L. Way, MD, Howard L. Fields, MD, PhD, & E. Leong Way, PhD

As recently as 100 years ago, few therapeutically useful drugs existed, but morphine was known to relieve severe pain with remarkable efficacy. In fact, Sir William Osler called morphine "God's own medicine," and to this day it remains the standard of comparison for drugs with strong analgesic action. The term "narcotic," often used in connection with this drug group, is an imprecise one, since "narcosis" connotes a stuporous or somnolent state. The term "opioid analgesic" is more appropriate because it implies the production of analgesia (absence of pain) without causing sleep or loss of consciousness. Opioids are usually understood to include all of the natural and semisynthetic alkaloid derivatives from opium, their pharmacologically similar synthetic surrogates, as well as all other compounds whose opioid-like actions are blocked by the nonselective opioid receptor antagonist naloxone. This definition includes several endogenous peptides that are synthesized by nerve cells and adrenal medullary cells and interact with opioid receptors. Morphine is considered the prototypical opioid agonist.

History

The source of opium, the crude substance, and morphine, one of its active constituents, is the opium poppy, *Papaver somniferum*. The properties of this plant have been known for thousands of years, and accounts of its use may be found in ancient Egyptian, Greek, and Roman documents.

One of the bases of modern pharmacology was established by Sertürner, a German pharmacist, who isolated a pure active alkaline substance from opium in 1803. This was a landmark event in that it made it possible to derive a standardized potency for a natural product. After testing the compound on himself and some friends, Sertürner proposed the name "mor-

phine" for the compound after Morpheus, the Greek god of dreams.

I. BASIC PHARMACOLOGY OF THE OPIOID ANALGESICS

Source

Opium is obtained from the opium poppy by incision of the seed pod after the petals of the flower have dropped. The white latex that oozes out turns brown and hardens on standing. This sticky brown gum is opium. It contains about 20 alkaloids, including morphine, codeine, thebaine, and papaverine. Thebaine and papaverine are not analgesic agents, but thebaine is the precursor of several semisynthetic opiate agonists (eg, etorphine, a veterinary agent 500–1000 times as potent as morphine) and antagonists (naloxone). Papaverine is a vasodilator with no established clinical applications that nevertheless inspired the development of verapamil, an important calcium channel-blocking drug (see Chapter 12).

The principal alkaloid in opium is morphine, present in a concentration of about 10%. Codeine is present in less than 0.5% concentration and is synthesized commercially from morphine. Cultivation of the opium poppy is now restricted by international agreement, but enforcement is difficult and illicit production of opium is widespread.

Classification & Chemistry

Opioid drugs include full agonists, partial agonists, and antagonists (see Chapter 2 for definitions).

Full agonist opioids are also known as high efficacy or strong agonists. As with partial agonists in other drug groups, partial agonist opioids can evoke agonist effects but may also displace full agonists from opioid binding sites and reduce their biologic effect. In this way, partial agonists may act as agonists or antagonists depending on the circumstances in which they are used (see Clinical Pharmacology, below, for some of the therapeutic consequences of these actions).

Because there are different subtypes of opioid receptors, it is possible for a compound to have an agonist effect on one opioid receptor subtype and a partial agonist or antagonist effect at another. Such compounds are known as **agonist-antagonists** or **mixed agonist-antagonists.**

In Table 31–1, some of the opioid compounds used as drugs are listed according to their agonist, mixed agonist-antagonist, or antagonist properties. Minor molecular alterations may drastically change the action of these compounds. For example, partial agonist or antagonist properties are associated with replacement of the methyl substituent on the nitrogen atom with larger groups—allyl in the case of nalorphine and naloxone, methylcyclopropane or methylcyclobutane for several other agents. Recall from Chapter 2 that an antagonist binds to a receptor without producing any of the effects associated with agonist binding. This is typical of naloxone. In contrast, morphine is a full agonist at the mu receptor. A partial (or "weak") agonist such as codeine binds to the receptor but produces less than maximal effect even when it has bound to all of the receptors. A mixed opioid agonist-antagonist, eg, nalbuphine, is capable of producing agonist (or partial agonist) effects at one opioid receptor while acting as an antagonist at another receptor.

Substitutions at the C_3 and C_6 hydroxyl groups of morphine significantly alter pharmacokinetic properties. Methyl substitution at the phenolic hydroxyl at C_3 reduces susceptibility to first-pass hepatic metabolism of the molecule by glucuronide conjugation at this position. Therefore, drugs such as codeine and oxycodone have a higher ratio of oral to parenteral potency. Acetylation of both hydroxyl groups of morphine yields heroin, which penetrates the blood-brain barrier much more rapidly than morphine. Heroin is rapidly hydrolyzed in the brain to monoacetylmorphine and morphine.

Endogenous Opioid Peptides

Opioid alkaloids (eg, morphine) produce analgesia through actions at regions in the brain that contain peptides which have opioid-like pharmacologic properties. The general term currently used for these endogenous substances is *endogenous opioid peptides,* which replaces the previous term *endorphin.* The term "endorphin" is now used to denote β-endorphin and other opioid peptides derived from the same precursor molecule (prepro-opiomelanocortin). Three families of endogenous opioid peptides are shown in Figure 31–1 with their precursor molecules.

The most widely distributed opioid peptides possessing analgesic activity are the pentapeptides methionine-enkephalin (met-enkephalin) and leucine-enkephalin (leu-enkephalin). With the exception of the methionine or leucine terminal group, the amino acid sequences of the enkephalins are identical (Tyr-Gly-Gly-Phe). One or both of these two pentapeptides are contained in each of the three opioid precursor proteins described below.

The three principal precursor proteins are prepro-opiomelanocortin (POMC), preproenkephalin (proenkephalin A), and preprodynorphin (proenkephalin B). POMC contains the met-enkephalin sequence, β-endorphin, and several nonopioid peptides, including ACTH, β-lipotropin, and melanocyte-stimulating hormone. Preproenkephalin contains six copies of met-enkephalin and one copy of leu-enkephalin, the first two opioid peptides to be isolated and purified. Preprodynorphin yields several active opioid peptides that contain the leu-enkephalin sequence. These are dynorphin A, dynorphin B, and alpha and beta neoendorphins.

The endogenous opioid precursor molecules are present at brain sites that have been implicated in pain modulation. Evidence suggests that they can be released during stress such as pain or the anticipation of pain. The precursor peptides are also found in the adrenal medulla and neural plexuses of the gut.

Recent studies indicate that several phenanthrene opioids (morphine, codeine) may also be found as endogenous substances at very low (picomolar) concentrations in mammalian tissue; their role at such sites has not been established.

Pharmacokinetics

Some of the pharmacologic properties of the clinically important opioids are summarized in Table 31–2.

A. Absorption: Most opioid analgesics are well absorbed from subcutaneous and intramuscular sites as well as from the mucosal surfaces of the nose or mouth. Transdermal administration of fentanyl has become an important route for certain indications (see below). Although absorption from the gastrointestinal tract is rapid, some opioids given by this route are subject to first-pass metabolism by glucuronidation in the liver. In such cases, the oral dose required to elicit a therapeutic effect may be much higher than the parenteral dose. Since the enzyme activity responsible for this reaction varies considerably in different individuals, the effective oral dose in a particular patient may be difficult to predict. As noted above, codeine and oxycodone have high oral:parenteral potency ratios because they are partially protected from conjugation by a methyl group on the aromatic hydroxyl group at C_3.

B. Distribution: The uptake of opioids by various organs and tissues is a function of both physiologic and chemical factors. Although all opioids bind to plasma proteins with varying degrees of affinity,

Table 31–1. Chemical structures of opioid analgesics and antagonists.

Basic Structure	Strong Agonists	Mild to Moderate Agonists	Mixed Agonist-Antagonists	Antagonists
Phenanthrenes	Morphine	Codeine	Nalbuphine	Nalorphine[1]
	Hydromorphone	Oxycodone	Buprenorphine	Naloxone
	Oxymorphone	Hydrocodone		Naltrexone
Phenylheptylamines	Methadone	Propoxyphene		

Table 31–1. Chemical structures of opioid analgesics and antagonists (cont'd).

Basic Structure	Strong Agonists	Mild to Moderate Agonists	Mixed Agonist-Antagonists	Antagonists
Phenylpiperidines	Meperidine Fentanyl	Diphenoxylate		
Morphinans	Levorphanol		Butorphanol	Levallorphan[1]
Benzomorphans			Pentazocine	

[1]Not a pure antagonist. See text for explanation.

499

POMC

ACTH

β-lipotropin

γ3-MSH

α-MSH

γ-lipotropin

β-endo (1–31)

Prepro-enk

F

E

B

ME ME

ME

ME-RGL

ME

LE

ME-RF

Prepro-dyn

α-neo-endo

dyno (1–17)

Figure 31–1. Three families of endogenous opioid peptides and their precursors. The endogenous peptide agonists are derived by proteolysis from much larger precursor proteins as shown. Pro-opiomelanocortin is also the precursor of adrenocorticotropin and melanocyte-stimulating hormone. **Key:** Stippled areas, signal peptides; diagonal hatched areas, cleavage products without analgesic actions; colored areas, peptides with analgesic effect. The double vertical lines are common cleavage sites. α-neo-endo, α-neoendorphin; β-endo, β-endorphin; ACTH, adrenocorticotropin; dyno, dynorphin; ME, methionine enkephalin; ME-RGL, ME-RF, B, E, F, extended enkephalins; MSH, melanocyte-stimulating hormone; POMC, pro-opiomelanocortin; Prepro-dyn, Pre-prodynorphin; Prepro-enk, pre-proenkephalin. (Redrawn, with permission, from Fields HL: *Pain.* McGraw-Hill, 1987.)

the drugs rapidly leave the blood and localize in highest concentrations in tissues that are highly perfused such as the lungs, liver, kidneys, and spleen. Although drug concentrations in skeletal muscle may be much lower, this tissue serves as the main reservoir for the drug because of its greater bulk. Accumulation in fatty tissue can also be important, particularly after frequent high-dose administration of highly lipophilic opioids that are slowly metabolized, eg, fentanyl.

Because of the blood-brain barrier, brain concentrations of opioids are usually relatively low in comparison to most other organs. Difficulty in gaining access to the brain appears to be greatest with amphoteric agents (ie, drugs possessing both acidic [a phenolic hydroxyl at C_3] and basic groups [the N_{17} amine) such as morphine. Compounds in which the aromatic hydroxyl at C_3 is substituted, as in heroin and codeine, traverse the blood-brain barrier more readily. In neonates the blood-brain barrier for opioids is effectively lacking. Since the opioid analgesics readily traverse the placenta, their use for obstetric analgesia can result in delivery of an infant with depressed respiration.

C. Metabolism: The opioids are converted in large part to polar metabolites, which are then readily excreted by the kidneys. Compounds with free hydroxyl groups are readily conjugated with glucuronic acid; examples are morphine and levorphanol. Esters (eg, heroin, remifentanil) are rapidly hydrolyzed by common tissue esterases. Heroin (diacetylmorphine) is hydrolyzed to monoacetylmorphine and finally to morphine, which is then conjugated with glucuronic acid. These polar glucuronidated metabolites were originally thought to be inactive, but it is now believed that morphine-6-glucuronide possesses analgesic potency that may be even greater than that of morphine itself. Accumulation of these active metabolites may occur in patients in renal failure and may lead to prolonged and more profound analgesia even though central nervous system entry is limited.

The opioids are also N-demethylated by the liver, but this is a minor pathway. However, accumulation of one such demethylated metabolite of meperidine, normeperidine, may occur in patients with decreased renal function or those receiving multiple high doses of the drug. In sufficiently high concentrations, this metabolite may cause seizures, especially in children. In spite of these exceptions, opioid metabolism usually results in compounds with little or no pharmacologic activity.

Hepatic oxidative metabolism is the primary route of degradation of the phenylpiperidine opioids (fen-

Table 31–2. Common opioid analgesics.

Generic Name	Product Name	Approximate Dose (mg)	Oral:Parenteral Potency Ratio	Duration of Analgesia (hours)	Maximum Efficency	Addiction/Abuse Liability
Morphine		10	Low	4–5	High	High
Hydromorphone	Dilaudid	1.5	Low	4–5	High	High
Oxymorphone	Numorphan	1.5	Low	3–4	High	High
Methadone	Dolophine	10	High	4–6	High	High
Meperidine	Demerol	60–100	Medium	2–4	High	High
Fentanyl	Sublimaze	0.1	Parenteral only	1–1.5	High	High
Sufentanyl	Sufenta	0.02	Parenteral only	1–1.5	High	High
Alfentanil	Alfenta	Titrated	Parenteral only	0.25–0.75	High	High
Levorphanol	Levo-Dromoran	2–3	High	4–5	High	High
Codeine		30–60[2]	High	3–4	Low	Medium
Oxycodone[1]	Percodan	4.5[2]	Medium	3–4	Moderate	Medium
Dihydrocodeine[1]	Drocode	16[2]	Medium	3–4	Moderate	Medium
Propoxyphene	Darvon	60–120[2]	Oral only	4–5	Very low	Low
Pentazocine	Talwin	30–50[2]	Medium	3–4	Moderate	Low
Nalbuphine	Nubain	10	Parenteral only	3–6	High	Low
Buprenorphine	Buprenex	0.3	Parenteral only	4–8	High	Low
Butorphanol	Stadol	2	Parenteral only	3–4	High	Low

[1]Available only in tablets containing aspirin, etc.
[2]Analgesic efficacy at this dose not equivalent to 10 mg of morphine. See text for explanation.

tanyl, alfentanil, sufentanil) and eventually leaves only small quantities of the parent compound unchanged for excretion. A new drug of this group, remifentanil, is a potent opioid that is rapidly metabolized by nonspecific tissue esterases, giving it a very short duration of action.

D. Excretion: The polar metabolites of the opioids are excreted mainly in the urine. Small amounts of unchanged drug may also be found in the urine. Glucuronide conjugates are found in the bile, but enterohepatic circulation represents only a small portion of the excretory process.

Pharmacodynamics

A. Mechanism of Action: Opioid agonists produce analgesia by binding to specific receptors, located primarily in brain and spinal cord regions involved in the transmission and modulation of pain.

1. Receptor types—Three major classes of opioid receptors have been identified in various nervous system sites and in other tissues. The major classes of receptors are μ (mu for morphine), delta (δ), and kappa (κ). The activities of some opioids at these receptors are shown in Table 31–3.

Each of the three major receptors has now been cloned. All are members of the G protein-coupled family of receptors and show significant amino acid sequence homologies. Each receptor type has subtypes:

mu_1, mu_2, $delta_1$, $delta_2$, $kappa_1$, $kappa_2$, and $kappa_3$ are currently the ones best-supported by pharmacologic criteria. Since an opioid drug might function with different potencies as an agonist, partial agonist, or antagonist at more than one receptor class or subtype, it is not surprising that these agents are capable of diverse pharmacologic effects.

2. Relation of physiologic effects to receptor type—Analgesia, as well as the euphoriant, respiratory depressant, and physiologic dependence properties of morphine (typical agonist effects) result principally from actions at mu receptors. Most of the currently available opioid analgesics act primarily at the mu receptor. In fact, the mu receptor was originally defined using the relative potencies for clinical analgesia of a series of opioid alkaloids. Delta and kappa receptors can also contribute to analgesia, particularly at the spinal level. Although morphine does act at kappa and delta sites, it is unclear to what extent this contributes to its analgesic action. The drug pentazocine acts primarily at the kappa receptor but does have some affinity for the mu receptor. The endogenous opioid peptides differ from most of the alkaloids in their affinity for the delta and kappa receptors. For example, leu-enkephalin has a high affinity for the delta receptor and dynorphin for the kappa receptor.

3. Cellular actions—At the molecular level, opioid receptors are linked to G proteins and therefore

Table 31–3. Receptor subtype activity of some representative opioids.[1]

Drug	Receptor Subtype		
	μ (mu)	δ (delta)	κ (kappa)
Opioid peptides			
Enkephalins	Agonist	Agonist	
β-Endorphin	Agonist	Agonist	
Dynorphin	Weak agonist		Agonist
Agonists			
Codeine	Weak agonist	Weak agonist	
Etorphine	Agonist	Agonist	Agonist
Fentanyl	Agonist		
Meperidine	Agonist		
Methadone	Agonist		
Morphine	Agonist	Weak agonist	Weak agonist
Agonist-antagonists			
Buprenorphine	Partial agonist		
Dezocine	Partial agonist	Agonist	
Nalbuphine	Antagonist		Agonist
Pentazocine	Antagonist or partial agonist		Agonist
Antagonists			
Naloxone	Antagonist	Antagonist	Antagonist

[1]Data compiled from various sources. Because of variations in the techniqes used to assign subtype activity, assignments from one source may vary from those of another. See text for additional details.

are able to effect ion gating, intracellular Ca^{2+} disposition, and protein phosphorylation (see Chapter 2). The opioids have two well-established direct actions on neurons: They either close a voltage-gated Ca^{2+} channel on presynaptic nerve terminals and thereby reduce transmitter release, or they hyperpolarize and thus inhibit postsynaptic neurons by opening K^+ channels. Figure 31–2 schematically illustrates the presynaptic action at all three receptor types and the post-synaptic effect at mu receptors on nociceptive afferents in the spinal cord. The presynaptic action—depressed transmitter release—has been demonstrated for release of a large number of neurotransmitters, including acetylcholine, norepinephrine, glutamate, serotonin, and substance P. Figure 31–3 shows electrical recordings of the postsynaptic inhibitory effect—mediated by opening of K^+ channels—of opioids acting at mu receptors in the brain.

4. Receptor distribution and neural mechanisms of analgesia—Opioid receptor binding sites have been localized autoradiographically using high-affinity radioligand binding with antibodies to unique peptide sequences in each receptor subtype. All three major receptors are present in high concentrations in the dorsal horn of the spinal cord (site *B*, Figure 31–4). Receptors are present on both spinal cord pain transmission neurons and on the primary afferents that relay the pain message to them (Figure 31–4, left side). Opioid agonists inhibit the release of excitatory transmitters from these primary afferents, and they directly inhibit the dorsal horn pain transmission neuron. Thus, opioids exert a powerful analgesic effect directly upon the spinal cord. This **spinal action** has been exploited clinically by direct application of opioid agonists to the spinal cord, which provides a regional analgesic effect while minimizing the unwanted respiratory depression, nausea and vomiting, and sedation that may occur from the **supraspinal actions** of systemically administered drugs.

Figure 31–2. Spinal sites of opioid action. Mu, kappa, and delta agonists reduce transmitter release from presynaptic terminals of nociceptive primary afferents. Mu agonists also hyperpolarize second-order pain transmission neurons by increasing K^+ conductance, evoking an inhibitory postsynaptic potential.

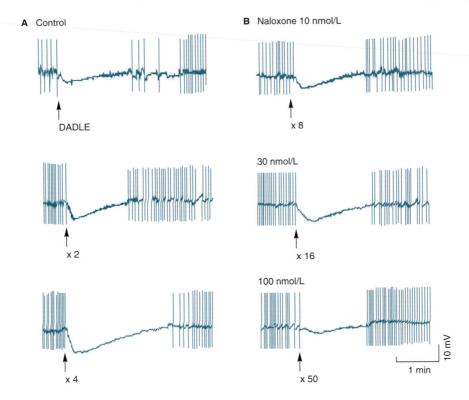

Figure 31–3. Postsynaptic opioid actions in the brain. This drawing shows intracellular recordings from a spontaneously firing locus ceruleus neuron in a tissue slice cut from rat pons and maintained in vitro. Upward deflections are action potentials (truncated); downward deflections are action potential afterhyperpolarizations. [D-Ala^2, D-Leu^5]enkephalin (DADLE) was administered at arrows by applying various numbers of pressure pulses (55 kPa, 24 ms, number indicated) to a micropipette containing the peptide positioned above the slice. **A:** Control responses. **B:** Selected records taken in the presence of different amounts of naloxone (added to the superfusing solution; concentration indicated). (Reproduced, with permission, from Williams JT, Egan TM, North RA: Enkephalin opens potassium channels on mammalian central neurons. Nature [Sept 2] 1982;299:74.)

Under most circumstances, opioids are given systemically and so act concurrently at both spinal and supraspinal sites, and interaction at these two sites tends to increase their overall analgesic efficacy. Different combinations of opioid receptors are found in supraspinal regions implicated in pain transmission and modulation (Figure 31–4). Of particular importance are opioid binding sites in pain-modulating descending pathways (Figure 31–4, right), including the rostral ventral medulla, the locus ceruleus, and the midbrain periaqueductal gray area. At these sites as at others, opioids directly inhibit neurons, yet neurons that send processes to the spinal cord and inhibit pain transmission neurons are activated by the drugs. This activation has been shown to result from the inhibition of inhibitory neurons in several locations (Figure 31–5).

When pain-relieving opioid drugs are given systemically, they act upon brain circuits that contain endogenous opioid peptides.

Part of the pain-relieving action of exogenous opioids involves the release of endogenous opioid peptides. An exogenous opioid agonist (eg, morphine)

may act primarily and directly at the mu receptor, but this action may evoke the release of endogenous opioids that additionally act at delta and kappa receptors. Thus, even a receptor-selective ligand can initiate a complex sequence of events involving multiple synapses and transmitters.

Animal and human clinical studies demonstrate that both endogenous and exogenous opioids can also produce opioid-mediated analgesia at sites *outside* the central nervous system. Pain associated with inflammation seems especially sensitive to these peripheral opioid actions.

5. Tolerance and physiologic dependence—With frequently repeated administration of therapeutic doses of morphine or its surrogates, there is a gradual loss in effectiveness, ie, tolerance. To reproduce the original response, a larger dose must be administered. Along with tolerance, physiologic dependence develops. Physiologic dependence is defined as the occurrence of a characteristic withdrawal or **abstinence syndrome** when the drug is stopped or an antagonist is administered.

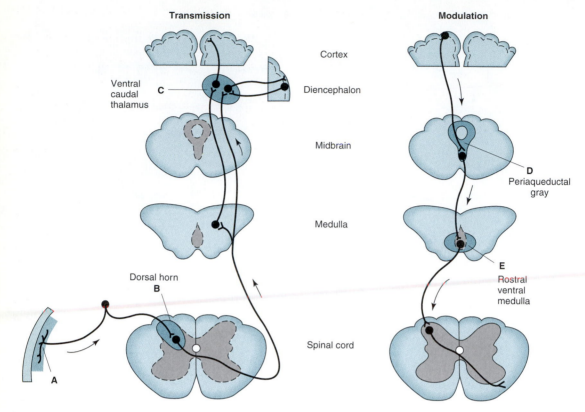

Figure 31–4. Putative sites of action of opioid analgesics (darker color). On the left, sites of action on the pain transmission pathway from the periphery to the higher centers are shown. **A:** Possible direct action of opioids on inflamed peripheral tissues. **B:** Inhibition occurs in the spinal cord. **C:** Possible site of action in the thalamus. On the right, actions on pain-modulating neurons in the midbrain (site **D**) and medulla (site **E**) secondarily affect pain transmission pathways.

The mechanism of development of tolerance and physiologic dependence is not known, but is believed to be a cellular adaptive response that is associated with changes in second messenger systems related to Ca^{2+} flux, adenylyl cyclase inhibition, and protein phosphorylation. Chronic exposure and tolerance to opioids is associated with an elevation of intracellular Ca^{2+} content—unlike acute exposure, which often causes a decrease. The effect appears to be related to a change in the receptor's ability to associate with G coupling proteins, increased amounts of G proteins, and an up-regulated cAMP system. In addition, the number of receptors may be reduced by internalization and by reduced synthesis. The clinical aspects of tolerance and dependence are discussed below.

B. Organ System Effects of Morphine and Its Surrogates: The actions given below for morphine, the prototypic agonist opioid, are also observed with all of the other agonists (Table 31–1). The mixed agonist-antagonist agents, when given to a patient who has not recently received an agonist agent, also produce analgesia but with minor variations in effects as noted below. Characteristics of specific members of these two groups are discussed below. The pure antagonists and the mixed agonist-antagonists, when given to a subject who has received an agonist, will have very different effects, as noted at the end of this chapter.

1. Central nervous system effects–The principal effects of the opioid analgesics with affinity for

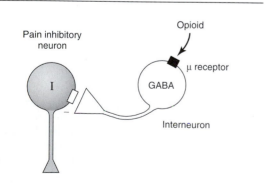

Figure 31–5. Brainstem local circuitry underlying opioid analgesia. The pain inhibitory neuron (I) is indirectly excited by opioids (exogenous or endogenous) that inhibit an inhibitory (GABAergic) interneuron (GABA).

mu receptors are on the central nervous system; the more important ones include analgesia, euphoria, sedation, and respiratory depression. With repeated use, a high degree of tolerance occurs to all of these effects (Table 31–4).

a. Analgesia–Pain consists of both sensory and affective (emotional) components. Opioids can change both aspects of the pain experience. In most cases, these drugs have a relatively greater effect on the affective component.

b. Euphoria–After a dose of morphine, a typical patient in pain or an addict experiences a pleasant floating sensation and freedom from anxiety and distress. However, other patients and some normal subjects (not in pain) experience dysphoric rather than pleasant effects after a dose of opioid analgesic. Dysphoria is a disquieted state characterized by restlessness and a feeling of malaise. In general, if a real indication exists for administration of an opioid analgesic, the most common affective response is euphoria.

c. Sedation–Drowsiness and clouding of mentation are frequent concomitants of opioid action. There is little or no amnesia. Sleep is induced by opiates more frequently in the elderly than in young, healthy individuals. Ordinarily, the patient can be easily aroused from this sleep. However, the combination of morphine with other central depressant drugs such as the sedative-hypnotics may result in very deep sleep. Marked sedation occurs more frequently with compounds closely related to the phenanthrene derivatives and less frequently with the synthetic agents such as meperidine and fentanyl. In standard analgesic doses, morphine (a phenanthrene) disrupts normal REM and NREM sleep patterns. This disrupting effect is probably characteristic of all opioids. In contrast to humans, a number of species (cats, horses, cows, pigs) may manifest excitation rather than sedation when given opioids. These paradoxical effects are at least partially dose-dependent.

d. Respiratory depression–All of the opioid analgesics can produce significant respiratory depression by inhibiting brain stem respiratory mechanisms. Alveolar P_{CO_2} may increase, but the most reliable indicator of this depression is a depressed response to a carbon dioxide challenge. The respiratory depression is dose-related and is influenced significantly by the degree of sensory input occurring at the time. For example, it is possible to partially overcome opioid-induced respiratory depression by stimulation of various sorts. When strongly painful stimuli that have prevented the depressant action of a large dose of an opioid are relieved, respiratory depression may suddenly become marked. A small to moderate decrease in respiratory function, as measured by Pa_{CO_2} elevation, may be well-tolerated in the patient without prior respiratory impairment. However, in individuals with increased intracranial pressure, asthma, chronic obstructive pulmonary dis-

ease, or cor pulmonale, this decrease in respiratory function may not be tolerated.

e. Cough suppression–Suppression of the cough reflex is a well-recognized action of opioids. Codeine in particular has been used to advantage in persons suffering from pathologic cough and in patients in whom it is necessary to maintain ventilation via an endotracheal tube. However, cough suppression by opioids may allow accumulation of secretions and thus lead to airway obstruction and atelectasis. Tolerance develops to the cough suppressant action of opioid analgesics (Table 31–4).

f. Miosis–Constriction of the pupils is seen with virtually all opioid agonists. Miosis is also a pharmacologic action to which little or no tolerance develops; thus, it is valuable in the diagnosis of opioid overdose. Even in highly tolerant addicts, miosis will be seen. This action, which can be blocked by opioid antagonists, is mediated by parasympathetic pathways, which, in turn, can be blocked by atropine.

g. Truncal rigidity–An intensification of tone in the large trunk muscles has been noted with a number of opioids. It was originally believed that truncal rigidity involved a spinal cord action of these drugs, but there is now evidence that it results from an action at supraspinal levels. Truncal rigidity reduces thoracic compliance and thus interferes with ventilation. The effect is most apparent when high doses of the highly lipid-soluble opioids (eg, fentanyl, sufentanil, alfentanil) are rapidly administered intravenously. Truncal rigidity may be overcome by administration of an opioid antagonist, which of course will also antagonize the analgesic action of the opioid. Preventing truncal rigidity while preserving analgesia requires the concomitant use of neuromuscular blocking agents.

h. Nausea and vomiting–The opioid analgesics can activate the brain stem chemoreceptor trigger zone to produce nausea and vomiting. There may also be a vestibular component in this effect because ambulation seems to increase the incidence of nausea and vomiting.

2. Peripheral effects

a. Cardiovascular system–Most opioids have no significant direct effects on the heart and no major effects on cardiac rhythm (except bradycardia) or blood pressure. Exceptions to this generalization will

Table 31–4. Degree of tolerance developed to some of the effects of the opioids.

High	Moderate	Minimal or None
Analgesia Euphoria, dysphoria Mental clouding Sedation Respiratory depression Antidiuresis Nausea and vomiting Cough suppression	Bradycardia	Miosis Constipation Convulsions Antagonist actions

be noted below with the discussion of specific drugs. Blood pressure is usually well maintained in subjects receiving opioids unless the cardiovascular system is stressed, in which case hypotension may occur. This hypotensive effect is probably due to peripheral arterial and venous dilation, which has been attributed to a number of mechanisms including central depression of vasomotor-stabilizing mechanisms and release of histamine. No consistent effect on cardiac output is seen, and the ECG is not significantly affected. However, caution should be exercised in patients with decreased blood volume, since the above mechanisms make these patients quite susceptible to hypotension. Opioid analgesics affect cerebral circulation minimally except when P_{CO_2} rises as a consequence of respiratory depression. Increased P_{CO_2} leads to cerebral vasodilation associated with a decrease in cerebral vascular resistance, an increase in cerebral blood flow, and an increase in intracranial pressure.

b. Gastrointestinal tract—Constipation has long been recognized as an effect of opioids. Opioid receptors exist in high density in the gastrointestinal tract, and the constipating effects of the opioids are mediated through an action on the local enteric nervous system (Chapter 6) as well as the central nervous system. In the stomach, motility (rhythmic contraction and relaxation) may decrease but tone (persistent contraction) may increase—particularly in the central portion; gastric secretion of hydrochloric acid is decreased. Small intestine resting tone is increased, with periodic spasms, but the amplitude of nonpropulsive contractions is markedly decreased. In the large intestine, propulsive peristaltic waves are diminished and tone is increased; this delays passage of the fecal mass and allows increased absorption of water, which leads to constipation. The large bowel actions are the basis for the use of opioids in management of diarrhea. There is a clinical impression that the benzomorphans (eg, pentazocine) cause less constipation than other opioids.

c. Biliary tract—The opioids constrict biliary smooth muscle, which may result in biliary colic. The sphincter of Oddi may constrict, resulting in reflux of biliary and pancreatic secretions and elevated plasma amylase and lipase levels.

d. Genitourinary tract—Renal function is depressed by opioids. It is believed that in humans this is chiefly due to decreased renal plasma flow. This contrasts with animal studies, in which reduced urine output seems to result from increased secretion of antidiuretic hormone as well as reduced renal perfusion. Ureteral and bladder tone are increased by therapeutic doses of the opioid analgesics. Increased sphincter tone may precipitate urinary retention, especially in postoperative patients. Occasionally, ureteral colic caused by a renal calculus is made worse by opioid-induced increase in ureteral tone.

e. Uterus—The opioid analgesics may prolong labor. The mechanism for this action is unclear, but both peripheral and central effects of the opioids can reduce uterine tone.

f. Neuroendocrine—Opioid analgesics stimulate the release of antidiuretic hormone, prolactin, and somatotropin but inhibit the release of luteinizing hormone. These effects suggest that endogenous opioid peptides, through effects in the hypothalamus, play regulatory roles in these systems.

g. Miscellaneous—Therapeutic doses of the opioid analgesics produce flushing and warming of the skin accompanied sometimes by sweating and itching; central effects and histamine release may be responsible for these reactions. The opioids may modulate the actions of the immune system by effects on lymphocyte proliferation, antibody production, and chemotaxis.

C. Effects of Mixed Agonist-Antagonists: Pentazocine and other opioids with agonist actions at some opioid receptors and antagonist actions at others usually produce sedation in addition to analgesia when given in therapeutic doses. At higher doses, sweating, dizziness, and nausea are common, but severe respiratory depression may be less common than with pure agonists. When it does occur, respiratory depression may be reversed by naloxone but not reliably by other agonist-antagonists such as nalorphine. Psychotomimetic effects, with hallucinations, nightmares, and anxiety, have been reported following use of the mixed agonist-antagonist agents.

II. CLINICAL PHARMACOLOGY OF THE OPIOID ANALGESICS

Management of pain is essential to good medical practice and requires careful consideration of proper dose, type of drug, and the disease being treated. There are many situations in which analgesia must be provided before a definitive diagnosis can be reached. Indeed, in some acute situations relief of pain may actually facilitate history taking and physical examination and thus speed the diagnostic process.

Use of opioid drugs in acute situations may be contrasted to their use in chronic pain management, where other factors must be considered–particularly tolerance and physiologic dependence. In all instances, the factors that should enter into the decision about choice of drug include the following: (1) Is analgesia needed? (2) Will the opioid analgesic obscure or alter the signs and symptoms of the underlying disorder? (3) Are the pharmacologic effects of the opioid liable to worsen the condition for which the drug is being used, eg, by increasing cerebrospinal fluid pressure or producing respiratory depression? (4) Do the opioid agent's adverse effects impose a significant hazard? (See Table 31–5.) (5) Is there a possibility of significant drug interaction between the opioid agent and other drugs the patient is receiving? (See Table 31–6.) (6) Are tolerance and drug dependence likely to develop?

Table 31–5. Toxic effects of the opioid analgesics.

Behavioral restlessness, tremulousness, hyperactivity (in dysphoric reactions)
Respiratory depression
Nausea and vomiting
Increased intracranial pressure
Postural hypotension accentuated by hypovolemia
Constipation
Urinary retention
Itching around nose, urticaria (more frequent with parenteral administration)

Table 31–2 shows the range of agonist efficacy of different opioid drugs. It is therefore necessary to select a drug appropriate to the type and severity of pain being treated to make certain that adequate analgesia is provided. The level of pain associated with various disease states also varies; thus, the postoperative pain of a forearm fracture may be adequately treated with codeine; the severe pain of a kidney stone may not. Each drug has a therapeutic ceiling, and to attempt to raise the ceiling with higher doses creates a risk of significant adverse effects and therapeutic failure.

Clinical Use of Opioid Analgesics

A. Analgesia: Severe, *constant* pain is usually relieved with the more efficacious opioids, whereas sharp, intermittent pain does not appear to be as amenable to relief. An attempt should be made to quantify the pain; this information should be used to select the proper agent and to monitor its effects. In this evaluation and selection process, such considerations as route of administration (oral versus parenteral administration), duration of action, ceiling effect (maximal efficacy), duration of therapy, and past experience with opioids are of obvious importance.

The pain associated with cancer and other terminal illnesses must be treated adequately, and concerns about tolerance and dependence should be set aside in favor of making the patient as comfortable as possible. Research by workers in the hospice movement has demonstrated that fixed-interval administration of opioid medication (ie, a regular dose at a regular time)

Table 31–6. Opioid drug interactions.

Drug Group	Interaction With Opioids
Sedative-hypnotics	Increased central nervous system depression, particularly respiratory depression.
Antipsychotic tranquilizers	Increased sedation. Variable effects on respiratory depression. Accentuation of cardiovascular effects (antimuscarinic and alpha-blocking actions).
MAO inhibitors	Relative contraindication to all opioid analgesics because of the high incidence of hyperpyrexic coma; hypertension has also been reported.

is more effective in achieving pain relief than dosing on demand. New dosage forms of morphine that allow slower release of the alkaloid are now available (eg, MS-Contin, Kadian). Their purported advantage is a longer and more stable level of analgesia. In addition, stimulant drugs such as the amphetamines have been shown to enhance the analgesic actions of the opioids and thus may be very useful adjuncts in the patient with chronic pain. Alpha$_2$ adrenoceptor agonists (eg, clonidine) have been shown in both laboratory and clinical studies to produce analgesia when given by a variety of routes of administration, but the place of these drugs in pain management is still unclear.

Opioid analgesics are often employed during obstetric labor. Because opioids cross the placental barrier and reach the fetus, care must be taken to minimize neonatal opioid depression. If this occurs, immediate injection of the antagonist naloxone will reverse the depression. The phenylpiperidine drugs (eg, meperidine) appear to produce less depression, particularly respiratory depression, in newborn infants than does morphine; this may justify their use in obstetric practice.

The acute, severe pain of renal and biliary colic often requires a strong agonist opioid for adequate relief. However, the drug-induced increase in smooth muscle tone may cause a paradoxical *increase* in pain secondary to increased spasm. An increase in the dose of opioid is usually successful in providing adequate analgesia.

B. Acute Pulmonary Edema: The relief produced by intravenous morphine in dyspnea from pulmonary edema associated with left ventricular failure is remarkable. The mechanism is not clear but probably involves reduced *perception* of shortness of breath and reduced patient anxiety as well as reduced cardiac preload (reduced venous tone) and afterload (decreased peripheral resistance).

C. Cough: Suppression of cough can be obtained at doses lower than those needed for analgesia. However, in recent years the use of opioid analgesics to allay cough has diminished largely because a number of effective synthetic compounds have been developed that are neither analgesic nor addictive. These agents are discussed below in the section on antitussives.

D. Diarrhea: Diarrhea from almost any cause can be controlled with the opioid analgesics, but if diarrhea is associated with infection such use must not substitute for appropriate chemotherapy. Crude opium preparations (eg, paregoric) were used in the past to control diarrhea, but now synthetic surrogates with more selective gastrointestinal effects and few or no central nervous system effects are used, eg, diphenoxylate. Phenylpiperidines, cited below, have been prepared specifically for this purpose.

E. Applications in Anesthesia: The opioids are frequently used as premedicant drugs before anesthesia and surgery because of their sedative, anxiolytic, and analgesic properties. The opioids are also used intraoperatively both as adjuncts to other anesthetic agents and, in high doses (eg, 0.02–0.075 mg/kg of fentanyl), as a primary component of the anesthetic regimen (see Chapter 25), most commonly in cardiovascular surgery and other types of high-risk surgery where a primary goal is to minimize cardiovascular depression. In such situations, mechanical respiratory assistance must be provided.

Because of their direct action on the spinal cord, opioids can also be used as regional analgesics by administration into the epidural or subarachnoid spaces of the spinal column. A number of studies have demonstrated that long-lasting analgesia with minimal adverse effects can be achieved by epidural administration of 3–5 mg of morphine, followed by slow infusion through a catheter placed in the epidural space. It was initially assumed that the epidural application of opioids might selectively produce analgesia without impairment of motor, autonomic, or sensory functions other than pain. However, respiratory depression may occur after the drug is injected into the epidural space and may require reversal with naloxone. Other effects such as pruritus and nausea and vomiting are common after epidural and subarachnoid administration of opioids and may also be reversed with naloxone if necessary. Currently, the epidural route is favored because adverse effects are less common. Morphine is the most frequently used agent, but current research is actively aimed at finding compounds that can produce good analgesia with even fewer adverse effects.

F. Alternative Routes of Administration: **Rectal suppositories** of morphine and hydromorphone have long been used when oral and parenteral routes are undesirable. However, rapid progress in newer drug delivery systems has also been adapted to opioid therapy. The epidural route, for action at the spinal level, has been described above. Another example is the **transdermal patch** for systemic effects that provides stable blood levels of drug and better pain control while avoiding the need for repeated parenteral injections. Fentanyl has been the most successful opioid in transdermal application and finds great use in providing pain relief for those with constant pain associated with cancer. The **intranasal** route is another route of administration, utilized on a very limited basis, for patients unable to tolerate oral medications and in whom repeat parenteral drug injections are not practical.

Another type of pain control, called **patient-controlled analgesia (PCA),** is now in widespread use. In this approach, the patient controls a parenteral (usually intravenous) injection device to provide the desired degree of pain control. Claims of better pain control using less opioid are supported by well-designed clinical trials, making this approach very useful in postoperative pain control. A variation of the PCA approach has been used to provide opioid via the subcutaneous route. Some lingering problems with PCA are equipment malfunction and the risk of drug overdosage secondary to improper programming or set-up of the device.

Toxicity & Undesired Effects

Direct toxic effects of the opioid analgesics that are extensions of their acute pharmacologic actions include respiratory depression, nausea, vomiting, and constipation (Table 31–5). In addition, the following must be considered.

A. Tolerance and Dependence: Drug dependence of the opioid type is marked by tolerance, a relatively specific withdrawal or abstinence syndrome reflecting physiologic dependence, and pronounced craving for drug reflecting psychologic dependence. Just as there are pharmacologic differences between the various opioids, there are also differences in abuse potential and the severity of withdrawal effects. For example, withdrawal from dependence upon a strong agonist is associated with more severe withdrawal signs and symptoms than withdrawal from a mild or moderate agonist. Administration of an opioid *antagonist* to an opioid-dependent person is followed by brief but severe withdrawal symptoms (see antagonist-precipitated withdrawal, below). Propoxyphene, a weak opioid agonist, may cause less marked dependence, but the withdrawal syndrome appears to be qualitatively similar to that of other opioids. The addiction liabilities of the mixed agonist-antagonist opioids appear to be less than those of the agonist drugs.

1. Tolerance–Although development of tolerance begins with the first dose of an opioid, tolerance generally does not become clinically manifest until after 2–3 weeks of frequent exposure to ordinary therapeutic doses. Tolerance develops most readily when large doses are given at short intervals and is minimized by giving small amounts of drug with longer intervals between doses.

Depending on the compound and the effect measured, the degree of tolerance may be as great as 35-fold. Marked tolerance usually develops to the analgesic, euphoriant, and respiratory depressant effects. It is possible to produce respiratory arrest in a nontolerant person with a dose of 60 mg of morphine, whereas in addicts maximally tolerant to opioids as much as 2000 mg of morphine taken over a 2- or 3-hour period may not produce significant respiratory depression. Tolerance also develops to the antidiuretic, emetic, and hypotensive effects but not to the miotic, convulsant, and constipating actions (Table 31–4).

Tolerance to the euphoriant and respiratory effects of the opioids dissipates within a few days after the drugs are discontinued. Tolerance to the emetic effects may persist for several months after withdrawal of the drug. The rates at which tolerance appears and disappears, as well as the degree of tolerance, may also differ considerably among the different opioid analgesics. For instance, tolerance to methadone develops more slowly and to a lesser degree than to morphine.

Cross-tolerance is an extremely important characteristic of the opioids, ie, patients tolerant to morphine are also tolerant to other agonist opioids. This is particularly true of those agents with primarily mu activity. Morphine, meperidine, methadone, and their congeners exhibit cross-tolerance not only with respect to their analgesic actions but also to their euphoriant, sedative, and respiratory effects.

Tolerance develops also to the mixed agonist-antagonist analgesics but to a lesser extent than to the agonists. Such effects as hallucinations, sedation, hypothermia, and respiratory depression are reduced after repeated administration of the mixed agonist-antagonist drugs. However, tolerance to agonist-antagonist agents does not generally include cross-tolerance to the agonist opioids. It is also important to note that tolerance does not develop to the antagonist actions of the mixed agonist-antagonists nor to those of the pure antagonists.

2. Physiologic dependence—The development of physiologic dependence is an invariable accompaniment of tolerance to repeated administration of an opioid of the mu type. Failure to continue administering the drug results in a characteristic withdrawal or **abstinence syndrome** that reflects an exaggerated rebound from the acute pharmacologic effects of the opioid. The signs and symptoms of withdrawal include rhinorrhea, lacrimation, yawning, chills, gooseflesh (piloerection), hyperventilation, hyperthermia, mydriasis, muscular aches, vomiting, diarrhea, anxiety, and hostility (see Chapter 32). The number and intensity of the signs and symptoms are largely dependent on the degree of physiologic dependence that has developed. Administration of an opioid at this time suppresses abstinence signs and symptoms almost immediately. The time of onset, the intensity, and the duration of the abstinence effects depend on the drug used and may be related to its biologic half-life. With morphine or heroin, withdrawal signs usually start within 6–10 hours after the last dose. Peak effects are seen at 36–48 hours, after which most of the signs and symptoms gradually subside. By 5 days, most of the effects have disappeared, but some may persist for months. In the case of meperidine, the withdrawal syndrome largely subsides within 24 hours, whereas with methadone several days are required to reach the peak of the abstinence syndrome, and it may last as long as 2 weeks. The slower subsidence of methadone effects is associated with a less intense immediate syndrome, and this is the basis for its use in the detoxification of heroin addicts. After the abstinence syndrome subsides, tolerance also disappears as evidenced by a restoration in sensitivity to the opioid agonist. However, despite the loss of physiologic dependence on the opioid, craving for it may persist for many months.

A transient, explosive abstinence syndrome—**antagonist-precipitated withdrawal**—can be induced in a subject physiologically dependent on opioids by administering naloxone or another antagonist. Within 3 minutes after injection of the antagonist, signs and symptoms similar to those seen after abrupt discontinuance appear, peaking in 10–20 minutes and largely subsiding after 1 hour. Even in the case of methadone, withdrawal of which results in a relatively mild abstinence syndrome, the antagonist-precipitated abstinence syndrome may be very severe.

In the case of the mixed agonist-antagonist agents, withdrawal signs and symptoms can be induced after repeated administration followed by abrupt discontinuance of pentazocine, cyclazocine, or nalorphine, but the syndrome appears to be somewhat different from that produced by morphine and other agonists. Anxiety, loss of appetite and body weight, tachycardia, chills, increase in body temperature, and abdominal cramps have been noted.

3. Psychologic dependence—The euphoria, indifference to stimuli, and sedation usually caused by the opioid analgesics, especially when injected intravenously, tend to promote their compulsive use. In addition, the addict experiences abdominal effects that have been likened to an intense sexual orgasm. These factors constitute the primary reasons for opioid abuse liability and are strongly reinforced by the development of physiologic dependence, since the drug user rationalizes continued use of the drug as the means of preventing abstinence symptoms, ie, to remain "normal."

Obviously, the risk of causing dependence is an important consideration in the therapeutic use of these drugs. *Despite that risk, under no circumstances should adequate pain relief ever be withheld simply because an opioid exhibits potential for abuse or because legislative controls complicate the process of prescribing narcotics.* However, certain principles can be observed by the clinician to minimize problems presented by tolerance and dependence when using opioid analgesics:

a. Establish therapeutic goals before starting opioid therapy. This tends to limit the potential for physiologic dependence. The patient should be included in this process.

b. Once a therapeutic dose is established, attempt to limit dosage to this level.

c. Instead of opioid analgesics—especially in chronic management—consider using other types of analgesics or compounds exhibiting less pronounced withdrawal symptoms on discontinuance.

d. Frequently evaluate continuing analgesic therapy and the patient's need for opioids.

B. Diagnosis and Treatment of Opioid Overdosage: The diagnosis of opioid overdosage may be very simple (known addict, needle marks, miosis, brought to hospital by friends who appear to be using drugs), or it may be very difficult—as in any comatose patient for whom no past history is available. Intravenous injection of naloxone, 0.2–0.4 mg, dramatically reverses coma due to opioid overdose but not that due to other CNS depressants. Treatment is with the same drug, 0.4–0.8 mg given intravenously, and repeated whenever necessary. In using naloxone in the severely depressed newborn, it is important to start with doses of 5–10 µg/kg and to consider a second dose of up to a total of 25 µg/kg if no response is noted. Use of the antagonist should not, of course, delay the institution of other therapeutic measures, especially respiratory support.

C. Contraindications and Cautions in Therapy:

1. Use of pure agonists with mixed agonist-antagonists–When a mixed agonist-antagonist agent such as pentazocine is given to a patient also receiving an agonist (eg, morphine), the possibility of diminishing analgesia or perhaps inducing a state of withdrawal is present; combining agonist with mixed agonist-antagonist opioids should be done cautiously, if at all.

2. Use in patients with head injuries–Carbon dioxide retention caused by respiratory depression results in cerebral vasodilation; in patients with elevated intracranial pressure, this may lead to lethal alterations in brain function.

3. Use during pregnancy–In pregnant women who are chronically using opioids, the fetus may become physiologically dependent in utero and manifest withdrawal symptoms in the early postpartum period. A daily dose as small as 6 mg of heroin (or equivalent) taken by the mother will result in a mild withdrawal syndrome in the infant, and twice that much may result in severe signs and symptoms, including irritability, shrill crying, diarrhea, or even seizures. Recognition of the problem is aided by a careful history and physical examination. When withdrawal symptoms are judged to be relatively mild, treatment is aimed at control of these symptoms with such drugs as diazepam; with more severe withdrawal, camphorated tincture of opium (paregoric; 0.4 mg of morphine/mL) in an oral dose of 0.12–0.24 mL/kg is used. Oral doses of methadone (0.1–0.5 mg/kg) have also been used.

4. Use in patients with impaired pulmonary function–In patients with borderline respiratory reserve, the depressant properties of the opioid analgesics may lead to acute respiratory failure.

5. Use in patients with impaired hepatic or renal function–Because morphine and its congeners are metabolized primarily in the liver, their use in patients in prehepatic coma may be questioned. Half-life is prolonged in patients with impaired renal function, and morphine and its active metabolite, morphine 6-glucuronide, may accumulate; dosage can often be reduced in such patients.

6. Use in patients with endocrine disease–Patients with adrenal insufficiency (Addison's

disease) and those with hypothyroidism (myxedema) may have prolonged and exaggerated responses to opioids.

Drug Interactions

Because seriously ill or hospitalized patients may require a large number of drugs, there is always a possibility of drug interactions when the opioid analgesics are administered. Table 31–6 lists some of these drug interactions and the reasons for not combining the named drugs with opioids.

SPECIFIC AGENTS

The following section describes the most important widely used opioid analgesics, along with features peculiar to specific agents. Data about doses approximately equivalent to 10 mg of intramuscular morphine, oral versus parenteral efficacy, duration of analgesia, maximum efficacy, and addiction and abuse liability are presented in Table 31–2.

STRONG AGONISTS

1. PHENANTHRENES

Morphine, hydromorphone, and **oxymorphone** are strong agonists useful in treating severe pain. These prototypic agents have been described in detail above. **Heroin** is potent and fast-acting, but its use is prohibited in the USA. In recent years there has been considerable agitation to revive its use. However, double-blind studies have not supported the claim that heroin is more effective than morphine in relieving severe chronic pain, at least when given by the intramuscular route.

2. PHENYLHEPTYLAMINES

Methadone has a pharmacodynamic profile very similar to that of morphine but is somewhat longer acting. Acutely, its analgesic potency and efficacy are at least equal to those of morphine. Methadone gives reliable effects when administered orally. Tolerance and physiologic dependence develop more slowly with methadone than with morphine. As noted above, the withdrawal signs and symptoms occurring after abrupt discontinuance of methadone are milder, although more prolonged, than those of morphine. These properties make methadone a useful drug for detoxification and for maintenance of the chronic relapsing heroin addict. For detoxification of a heroin-dependent addict, low doses of methadone (5–10 mg orally) are given two or three times daily for 2 or 3 days. Upon discontinuing methadone, the addict experiences a mild but endurable withdrawal syndrome. For maintenance therapy of the opioid recidivist, tolerance to 50–100 mg/d of oral methadone is deliberately produced; in this state, the addict experiences cross-tolerance to heroin that prevents most of the addiction-reinforcing effects of heroin. A related compound, **levomethadyl acetate** (L-acetylmethadol), which has an even longer half-life than methadone, has been approved by the FDA for use in detoxification clinics. This agent may be given once every two to three days.

The rationale of maintenance programs is that blocking the reinforcement obtained from abuse of illicit opioids removes the drive to obtain them, thereby reducing criminal activity and making the addict more amenable to psychiatric and rehabilitative therapy. The pharmacologic basis for the use of methadone in maintenance programs is sound and the sociologic basis is rational, but some methadone programs fail because nonpharmacologic management is inadequate.

3. PHENYLPIPERIDINES

Meperidine and **fentanyl** are the most widely used agents in this family of synthetic opioids. Meperidine has significant antimuscarinic effects, which may be a contraindication if tachycardia would be a problem. It is also reported to have a negative inotropic action on the heart. The potential for producing seizures secondary to accumulation of normeperidine in patients receiving high doses of meperidine or with renal compromise must be considered. The fentanyl subgroup now includes **sufentanil** and **alfentanil** in addition to the parent compound, fentanyl. These opioids differ mainly in their potency and biodisposition. Sufentanil is five to seven times more potent than fentanyl. Alfentanil is considerably less potent than fentanyl, acts more rapidly, and has a markedly shorter duration of action. The newest addition to this group, **remifentanil,** is metabolized very rapidly by tissue cholinesterases, making its pharmacokinetic and pharmacodynamic half-lives extremely short. It recently received FDA approval for clinical use.

4. MORPHINANS

Levorphanol is a synthetically prepared opioid analgesic closely resembling morphine in its action but offering no advantages.

MILD TO MODERATE AGONISTS

1. PHENANTHRENES

Codeine, oxycodone, dihydrocodeine, and **hydrocodone** are all somewhat less efficacious than mor-

phine or have adverse effects that limit the maximum tolerated dose when one attempts to achieve analgesia comparable to that of morphine. These compounds are rarely used alone but are combined in formulations containing aspirin or acetaminophen and other drugs.

2. PHENYLHEPTYLAMINES

Propoxyphene is chemically related to methadone but has low analgesic activity. Various studies have reported its potency at levels ranging from no better than placebo to half as potent as codeine, ie, 120 mg propoxyphene = 60 mg codeine. Its true potency probably lies somewhere between these extremes, and its analgesic effect is additive to that of an optimal dose of aspirin. However, its low efficacy makes it unsuitable, even in combination with aspirin, for severe pain. Although propoxyphene has a low abuse liability, the increasing incidence of deaths associated with its misuse has caused it to be scheduled as a controlled substance with low potential for abuse.

3. PHENYLPIPERIDINES

Diphenoxylate and its metabolite, **difenoxin,** are not used for analgesia but for the treatment of diarrhea. They are scheduled for minimal control (difenoxin is schedule IV, diphenoxylate schedule V; see inside front cover) because the likelihood of their abuse is remote. The poor solubility of the compounds limits their use for parenteral injection. As antidiarrheal drugs, they are used in combination with atropine. The atropine is added in a concentration too low to have a significant antidiarrheal effect but is presumed to further reduce the likelihood of abuse.

Loperamide is another phenylpiperidine derivative used to control diarrhea. Its potential for abuse is low because of its limited ability to gain access to the brain.

The usual dose with all of these antidiarrheal agents is two tablets to start and then one tablet after each diarrheal stool.

MIXED AGONIST-ANTAGONISTS & PARTIAL AGONISTS

Care should be taken not to administer any agonist-antagonist or partial agonist drug to patients receiving pure agonist drugs because of the unpredictability of both drugs' effects: reduction of analgesia or precipitation of an explosive abstinence syndrome may result.

1. PHENANTHRENES

Nalbuphine acts as a strong kappa receptor *agonist* and is an mu receptor *antagonist;* it is given parenterally. At higher doses there seems to be a definite ceiling—not noted with morphine—to the respiratory depressant effect. Unfortunately, when respiratory depression does occur, it may be relatively resistant to naloxone reversal.

Buprenorphine is a potent and long-acting phenanthrene derivative that is a partial mu receptor agonist. Its long duration of action is due to its slow dissociation from mu receptors. This property renders its effects resistant to naloxone reversal. Its clinical applications are much like those of nalbuphine. In addition, some studies suggest that buprenorphine may be as effective as methadone in the detoxification and maintenance of heroin abusers (eg, Bickel et al, 1988).

2. MORPHINANS

Butorphanol produces analgesia equivalent to nalbuphine and buprenorphine but appears to produce more sedation at equianalgesic doses. Butorphanol is considered to be a kappa agonist.

3. BENZOMORPHANS

Pentazocine is a kappa agonist with weak mu antagonist or partial agonist properties. It is the oldest mixed agonist-antagonist available. It may be used orally or parenterally. However, because of its irritant properties, the injection of pentazocine subcutaneously is not recommended.

Dezocine is a compound structurally related to pentazocine. It has its highest affinity for mu receptors and less interaction with kappa receptors. Although it is said to be equivalent in efficacy to morphine, its use is associated with the same problems observed with all mixed agonist-antagonists.

MISCELLANEOUS

Tramadol is a newer synthetic analgesic drug with weak mu agonist effects and some inhibitory action on norepinephrine and serotonin reuptake in the central nervous system. It is believed to act mainly through an active metabolite that has weak analgesic actions similar to those of propoxyphene. The mechanism of its action may be independent of its opioid receptor effects since it is only partially antagonized by naloxone. The recommended dosage is 50–100 mg orally four times daily. Toxicity includes dependence and withdrawal syndromes, seizures, and, rarely, anaphylactoid reactions. This drug is popular in Europe but has only recently been approved for use in the USA. It is not clear that it offers any advantages over older analgesics.

ANTITUSSIVES

As noted above, the opioid analgesics are among the most effective drugs available for the suppression of cough. This effect is often achieved at doses below those necessary to produce analgesia. The receptors involved in the antitussive effect appear to differ from those associated with the other actions of opioids. For example, the antitussive effect is also produced by stereoisomers of opioid molecules that are devoid of analgesic effects and addiction liability (see below).

The physiologic mechanism of a cough is a complex one, and little is known about the specific mechanism of action of the opioid antitussive drugs. It is likely that both central and peripheral effects play a role.

The opioid derivatives most commonly used as antitussives are dextromethorphan, codeine, levopropoxyphene, and noscapine (levopropoxyphene and noscapine are not available in the USA). While these agents (other than codeine) are largely free of the adverse effects associated with the opioids, they should be used with caution in patients taking MAO inhibitors (see Table 31–6).

Dextromethorphan is the dextrorotatory stereoisomer of a methylated derivative of levorphanol. It is essentially free of analgesic and addictive properties and produces less constipation than codeine. The usual antitussive dose is 15–30 mg three or four times daily. It is available in many over-the-counter products.

Codeine, as noted above, has a useful antitussive action at doses lower than those required for analgesia. Thus, 15 mg is usually sufficient to relieve cough.

Levopropoxyphene is the stereoisomer of the weak opioid agonist dextropropoxyphene. It is devoid of opioid effects, although sedation has been described as a side effect. The usual antitussive dose is 50–100 mg every 4 hours.

Antitussive preparations usually contain expectorants to thin and liquefy respiratory secretions.

THE OPIOID ANTAGONISTS

The pure opioid antagonist drugs **naloxone, naltrexone,** and **nalmefene** are morphine derivatives with bulkier substituents at the N_{17} position. These agents have a relatively high affinity for mu opioid binding sites. They have lower affinity for the other receptors but can also reverse agonists at delta and kappa sites.

Pharmacokinetics

Naloxone has poor efficacy when given by the oral route and a short duration of action (1–2 hours) when given by injection. Metabolic disposition is chiefly by glucuronide conjugation, like that of the agonist opioids with free hydroxyl groups. Naltrexone is well absorbed after oral administration but may undergo rapid first-pass metabolism. It has a half-life of 10 hours, and a single oral dose of 100 mg will block the effects of injected heroin for up to 48 hours. Nalmefene, the newest of these agents, is a derivative of naltrexone but is available only for intravenous administration. Like naloxone, nalmefene is used for opioid overdose but has a longer half-life (8–10 hours).

Pharmacodynamics

When given in the absence of an agonist drug, these antagonists are almost inert at doses that produce marked antagonism of agonist effects.

When given intravenously to a morphine-treated subject, the antagonist will completely and dramatically reverse the opioid effects within 1–3 minutes. In individuals who are acutely depressed by an overdose of an opioid, the antagonist will effectively normalize respiration, level of consciousness, pupil size, bowel activity, etc. In dependent subjects who appear normal while taking opioids, naloxone or naltrexone will almost instantaneously precipitate an abstinence syndrome, as described previously.

There is no tolerance to the antagonistic action of these agents, nor does withdrawal after chronic administration precipitate an abstinence syndrome.

Clinical Use

Naloxone is a pure antagonist and is preferred over older weak agonist-antagonist agents that had been used primarily as antagonists, eg, nalorphine and levallorphan.

The major application of naloxone is in the treatment of acute opioid overdose, as described above (see also Chapter 32). It is very important that the relatively short duration of action of naloxone be borne in mind, because a severely depressed patient may recover after a single dose of naloxone and appear normal, only to relapse into coma after 1–2 hours. The usual dose of naloxone is 0.1–0.4 mg intravenously, repeated as necessary.

Because of its long duration of action, naltrexone has been proposed as a "maintenance" drug for addicts in treatment programs. A single dose given on alternate days blocks virtually all of the effects of a dose of heroin. It might be predicted that this approach to rehabilitation would not be popular with a large percentage of drug users unless they are motivated to become drug-free. More recently, considerable interest has been aroused by reports that naltrexone decreases craving for alcohol in chronic alcoholics, and it was recently approved by the FDA for this purpose (Chapter 23).

PREPARATIONS AVAILABLE
(Antidiarrheal opioid preparations are listed in Chapter 63.)

Analgesic Opioids

Alfentanil (Alfenta)
  Parenteral: 500 μg/mL for injection
Buprenorphine (Buprenex)
  Parenteral: 0.3 mg/mL for injection
Butorphanol (Stadol)
  Parenteral: 1, 2 mg/mL for injection
  Nasal (Stadol NS): 10 mg/mL nasal spray
Codeine (sulfate or phosphate) (generic)
  Oral: 15, 30, 60 mg tablets and soluble tablets
  Parenteral: 30, 60 mg/mL for IM, SC, or IV injection
Dezocine (Dalgan)
  Parenteral: 5, 10, 15 mg/mL for IM or IV injection
Fentanyl (generic, Sublimaze)
  Parenteral: 50 μg/mL for injection
  Fentanyl Transdermal System (Duragesic): 25, 50, 75, 100, μg/h
  Fentanyl Transmucosal System (Fentanyl Oralet): 200, 300, 400 μg oral lozenges
Hydromorphone (generic, Dilaudid)
  Oral: 1, 2, 3, 4 mg tablets
  Parenteral: 1, 2, 3, 4, 10 mg/mL for injection
  Rectal: 3 mg suppositories
Levomethadyl acetate (Orlaam)

  Oral: 10 mg/mL solution. *Note:* Approved only for the treatment of narcotic addiction.
Levorphanol (Levo-Dromoran)
  Oral: 2 mg tablets
  Parenteral: 2 mg/mL for injection
Meperidine (generic, Demerol)
  Oral: 50, 100 mg tablets; 50 mg/5 mL syrup
  Parenteral: 25, 50, 75, 100 mg per dose for SC, IM injection; 10, 50, 100 mg/mL for IV infusion
Methadone (generic, Dolophine)
  Oral: 5, 10 mg tablets; 40 mg dispersible tablets; 1, 2, 10 mg/mL solutions
  Parenteral: 10 mg/mL for injection
Morphine sulfate (generic, others)
  Oral: 10, 15, 30 mg tablets; 10, 20, 100 mg/5 mL solution
  Oral sustained release: 30, 60 mg tablets (MS-Contin); 20, 50, 100 mg capsules (Kadian)
  Parenteral: 0.5, 1, 2, 3, 4, 5, 8, 10, 15 mg/mL for injection
  Rectal: 5, 10, 20, 30 mg suppositories
Nalbuphine (generic, Nubain)
  Parenteral: 10, 20 mg/mL for injection
Oxycodone (generic)
  Oral: 5 mg tablets; 1, 20 mg/mL solutions

Oxymorphone (Numorphan)
Parenteral: 1, 1.5 mg/mL for injection
Rectal: 5 mg suppositories
Pentazocine (Talwin)
Oral: 50 mg tablets
Parenteral: 30 mg/mL for injection
Propoxyphene (generic, Darvon Pulvules, others)
Oral: 32, 65 mg capsules *Note:* This product is not recommended.
Remifentanil (Ultiva)
Parenteral: 1, 2, 5 mL ampules
Sufentanil (Sufenta)
Parenteral: 50 μg/mL for injection
Tramadol (Ultraam)
Oral: 50 mg tablets

Analgesic Combinations*

Codeine/acetaminophen (generic, Tylenol w/Codeine, others)
Oral: 7.5, 15, 30, 60 mg codeine plus 300 mg acetaminophen tablets; 12 mg codeine plus 120 mg acetaminophen tablets
Codeine/aspirin (generic, Empirin Compound, others)
Oral: 30, 60 mg codeine plus 325 mg aspirin tablets
Hydrocodone/acetaminophen (generic, Norcet, Vicodin, Lortab, others)
Oral: 2.5, 5, 7.5, 10 mg hydrocodone plus 500 or 650 mg acetaminophen tablets
Oxycodone/acetaminophen (generic, Percocet, Percodan, Tylox, others)
Oral: 5 mg oxycodone plus 325 or 500 mg

acetaminophen tablets
Note: High-dose acetaminophen has potential for hepatic toxicity with repeated use.
Oxycodone/aspirin (generic, Percodan)
Oral: 4.9 mg oxycodone plus 325 mg aspirin
Propoxyphene/aspirin or acetaminophen (Darvon Compound-65, others)
Oral: 65 mg propoxyphene plus 389 mg aspirin plus 32.4 mg caffeine; 65 mg propoxyphene plus 325 or 650 mg acetaminophen. *Note:* This product is not recommended.

Opioid Antagonists

Nalmefene (Revex)
Parenteral: 0.1, 1 mg/mL ampules for IV administration
Naloxone (Narcan, various)
Parenteral: 0.4, 1 mg/mL; 0.02 mg/mL for neonatal use
Naltrexone (ReVia)
Oral: 50 mg tablets

Antitussives

Codeine (generic, others)
Oral: 15, 30, 60 mg tablets; constituent of many proprietary syrups
Dextromethorphan (generic, Benylin DM, Delsym, others)
Oral: 5 mg lozenges; 5, 7.5, 10, 15 mg/5 mL syrup; 30 mg sustained-action liquid; 15 mg chewy squares; constituent of many proprietary syrups

---

REFERENCES

Barber A, Gottschlich R: Opioid agonists and antagonists: An evaluation of their peripheral actions in inflammation. Med Res Rev 1992;12:525.

Beaver WT (editor): Appropriate management of pain in primary care practice. Symposium. Am J Med 1984;77(Suppl 3A):1.

Beaver WT: Impact of non-narcotic analgesics on pain management. Am J Med 1988;84(Suppl 5A):3.

Benedetti C, Bonica JJ (editors): Recent advances in intraspinal pain therapy. Acta Anaesthesiol Scand 1987;31(Suppl 85):1.

Benedetti C, Premuda L: The history of opium and its derivatives. In: *Advances in Pain Research and Therapy,* vol 14. Benedetti C et al (editors). Raven Press, 1990.

Bickel WK et al: A clinical trial of buprenorphine: Comparison with methadone in the detoxification of heroin addicts. Clin Pharmacol Ther 1988;43:72.

Braga PC: Centrally acting opioid drugs. In: *Cough.* Braga PC, Allegra L (editors). Raven Press, 1989.

Crain SM, Shen K-F: Opioids can evoke direct receptor-mediated excitatory effects on sensory neurons. Trends Pharmacol Sci 1990;11:77.

Evans CJ et al: Cloning of a delta opioid receptor by functional expression. Science 1992;258:1952.

Ferrante FM: Principles of opioid pharmacotherapy: Practical implications of basic mechanisms. J Pain Symptom Manage 1996;11:265.

---

*Dozens of combination products are available; only a few of the most commonly prescribed are listed here. Codeine combination products available in several strengths are usually denoted No. 1 (7.5 mg codeine), No. 2 (15 mg codeine), No. 3 (30 mg codeine), and No. 4 (60 mg codeine). Prescribers should be aware of the possible danger of renal damage with acetaminophen, aspirin, and nonsteroidal anti-inflammatory drugs contained in these analgesic combinations.

Fields HL: Brain stem mechanisms of pain modulation: Anatomy and physiology. In: *Handbook of Experimental Pharmacology. Vol 104: II. Opioids.* Herz A et al (editors). Springer, 1993.

Fields HL, Heinricher MM, Mason P: Neurotransmitters in nociceptive modulatory circuits. Annu Rev Neurosci 1991;14:219.

Foley KM: Misconceptions and controversies regarding the use of opioids in cancer pain. Anticancer Drugs 1995;6(Suppl 3):4.

Frances B et al: Further evidence that morphine-6β-glucuronide is a more potent opioid agonist than morphine. J Pharmacol Exp Ther 1992;262:25.

Galamba JM et al: Continuous subcutaneous infusion of opioids in cancer patients. Ugeskr Laeger 1995; 157:4126.

Goldstein A, Naidu A: Multiple opioid receptors: Ligand selectivity profiles and binding site signatures. Mol Pharmacol 1989;36:265.

Griffin MT, Law PY, Loh HH: Involvement of both inhibitory and stimulatory guanine nucleotide-binding proteins in the expression of chronic opiate regulation of adenylate cyclase activity. J Neurochem 1985;45:1585.

Heijna MH et al: Opioid receptor-mediated inhibition of ^{3}H-dopamine and ^{14}C-acetylcholine release from rat nucleus accumbens slices: A study on the possible involvement of K^+ channels and adenylate cyclase. Naunyn Schmiedebergs Arch Pharmacol 1992;345:627.

Hill CS, Fields WS (editors): *Drug Treatment of Cancer Pain in a Drug Oriented Society. Advances in Pain Research and Therapy,* vol 11. Raven Press, 1989.

Hill HF, Mather LE: Patient-controlled analgesia. Pharmacokinetic and therapeutic considerations. Clin Pharmacokinet 1993;24:124.

Höllt V: Opioid peptide genes: Structure and regulation In: *Neurobiology of Opioids.* Almeida OFX, Shippenberg TS (editors). Springer, 1991.

Irwin RS, Curley FJ, Bennett FM: Appropriate use of antitussives and protussives: A practical review. Drugs 1993;46:80.

Johnson SM, Fleming WW: Mechanisms of cellular adaptive sensitivity changes: Applications to opioid tolerance and dependence. Pharmacol Rev 1989;41:435.

Kaiko, RF et al: Pharmacokinetic-pharmacodynamic relationships of controlled release oxycodone. Clin Pharmacol Ther 1996;59:52.

Kromer W: Endogenous and exogenous opioids in the control of gastrointestinal motility and secretion. Pharmacol Rev 1988;40:121.

Kuhar MJ, Pasternak GW (editors): *Analgesics: Neurochemical, Behavioral, and Clinical Perspectives.* Raven Press, 1984.

Louie AK, Way EL: Overview of opioid tolerance and physical dependence. In: *Neurobiology of Opioids.* Almeida OFX, Shippenberg TS (editors). Springer, 1991.

Millan MJ: κ-Opioid receptors and analgesia. Trends Pharmacol Sci 1990;11:70.

Neil A: Tolerance and dependence. In: *Advances in Pain Research and Therapy.* Benedetti C et al (editors). Raven Press, 1990.

North RA: Opioid receptors and ion channels. In: *Neurobiology of Opioids.* Almeida OFX, Shippenberg TS (editors). Springer, 1991.

Pasternak GW: Pharmacological mechanisms of opioid analgesics. Clin Neuropharmacol 1993;16:1.

Paul D et al: Pharmacological characterization of morphine 6-β glucuronide, a very potent morphine metabolite. J Pharmacol Exp Ther 1989;251:477.

Pechnik RN: Effect of opioids on the hypothalamo-pituitary-adrenal axis. Annu Rev Pharmacol Toxicol 1993;32:353.

Perneger TV et al: Risk of kidney failure associated with use of acetaminophen, aspirin, and nonsteroidal anti-inflammatory drugs. N Engl J Med 1994;331:1675.

Pick CG, Nejat RJ, Pasternak GW: Independent expression of two pharmacologically distinct mu analgesic systems in genetically different mouse strains. J Pharmacol Exp Ther 1993;265:166.

Rasmussen K et al: Opiate withdrawal from the rat locus coeruleus [sic]: Behavioral, electrophysiologic, and biochemical correlates. J Neurosci 1990;10:2308.

Razaka RS, Porreca F: Development of delta opioid peptides as nonaddicting analgesics. Pharm Res 1991;8:1.

Reisine T, Bell GI: Molecular biology of opioid receptors. Trends Neurosci 1993;16:506.

Rouveix B: Opiates and immune function. Therapie 1992;47:503.

Sabinga NES, Goldstein A: Opioid peptides and opioid receptors in cells of the immune system. Annu Rev Immunol 1988;6:29.

Self DW, Nestler E: Molecular mechanisms of drug reinforcement and addiction. Annu Rev Neurosci 1995; 18:463.

Simonds WF: The molecular basis of opioid receptor function. Endocr Rev 1988;9:200.

Smith NT et al: Seizures during opioid anesthetic induction: Are they opioid-induced rigidity? Anesthesiology 1989;71:852.

Stein C: Peripheral mechanisms of opioid analgesia. Anesth Analg 1993;76:182.

Thirlwell MP et al: Pharmacokinetics and clinical efficacy of oral morphine solution and controlled-release morphine tablets in cancer patients. Cancer 1989;63:2275.

Valentino RJ: Neurophysiological and neuropharmacological effects of opiates. Monogr Neural Sci 1987;13:91.

Volpicelli JR et al: Naltrexone in the treatment of alcohol dependence. Arch Gen Psychiatry 1992;49:876.

Way EL, Adler TK: The pharmacologic implications of the fate of morphine and its surrogates. Pharmacol Rev 1968;12:383.

Way EL: Opioid tolerance and physical dependence and their relationship. In: *Handbook of Experimental Pharmacology. Vol 104: II. Opioids.* Herz A et al (editors). Springer, 1993.

Yaksh TL: CNS mechanisms of pain and analgesia. Cancer Surv 1988;7:55.

Yaster M, Deshpande JK: Management of pediatric pain with opioid analgesics. J Pediatr 1988;113:421.

Yeadon M, Kitchen I: Opioids and respiration. Prog Neurobiol 1989;33:1.

32

Drugs of Abuse

Thomas R. Kosten, MD, & Leo E. Hollister, MD

The term "drug abuse" is unfortunate because it connotes social disapproval and may have different meanings to different people. One must also distinguish drug abuse from drug misuse. Abuse of a drug might be construed as any use of a drug for nonmedical purposes, usually for altering consciousness but also for body-building, etc. To misuse a drug might be to take it for the wrong indication, in the wrong dosage, or for too long a period, to mention only a few obvious examples. In the context of drug abuse, the drug itself is of less importance than the pattern of use. For example, taking 50 mg of diazepam to heighten the effect of a daily dose of methadone is an *abuse* of diazepam. On the other hand, taking the same excessive daily dose of the drug but only for its anxiolytic effect is *misusing* diazepam.

Dependence is a biologic phenomenon often associated with "drug abuse." **Psychologic dependence** is manifested by compulsive drug-seeking behavior in which the individual uses the drug repetitively for personal satisfaction, often in the face of known risks to health. Cigarette smoking is an example. **Physiologic dependence** is present when withdrawal of the drug produces symptoms and signs that are frequently the opposite of those sought by the user. It has been suggested that the body adjusts to a new level of homeostasis during the period of drug use and reacts in opposite fashion when the new equilibrium is disturbed. Alcohol withdrawal syndrome is perhaps the best-known example, but milder degrees of withdrawal may be observed in people who drink a lot of coffee every day. Psychologic dependence almost always precedes physiologic dependence but does not inevitably lead to it. **Addiction** is usually taken to mean a state of physiologic and psychologic dependence, but the word is too imprecise to be useful.

Tolerance signifies a decreased response to the effects of the drug, necessitating ever larger doses to achieve the same effect. Tolerance is closely associated with the phenomenon of physiologic dependence. It is largely due to compensatory responses that mitigate the drug's pharmacodynamic action. **Metabolic tolerance** due to increased disposition of the drug after chronic use is occasionally reported. **Behavioral tolerance,** an ability to compensate for the drug's effects, is another possible mechanism of tolerance. **Functional tolerance,** which may be the most common type, is due to compensatory changes in receptors, effector enzymes, or membrane actions of the drug.

A number of experimental techniques have been devised to predict the ability of a drug to produce dependence and to assess its likelihood for abuse. Most of these techniques employ self-administration of the drug by animals. The rates of reinforcement can be altered so as to make the animal work harder for each dose of drug, providing a semiquantitative measure as well. Comparisons are made against a standard drug in the class, eg, morphine among the opioids. Withdrawal of dependent animals from drugs assesses the nature of the withdrawal syndrome and can be used to test drugs that might cross-substitute for the standard drug. Most agents with significant potential for psychologic or physiologic dependence can be readily detected by these techniques. The actual abuse liability, however, is difficult to predict, since many variables enter into the decision to abuse drugs.

Cultural Considerations

Each society accepts certain drugs as licit and condemns others as illicit. In the USA and most of Western Europe, the "national drugs" are caffeine, nicotine, and alcohol. In the Middle East, cannabis may be added to the list of licit drugs, while alcohol is forbidden. Among certain Native American tribes, peyote, a hallucinogen, may be used licitly for religious purposes. In the Andes of South America, cocaine is used to allay hunger and enhance the ability to perform arduous work at high altitudes. Thus, which drugs are licit or illicit or—to use other terminology—"used" or "abused" depends on a social judgment. A major social cost of relegating any substance to the illicit category is the criminal activity that often results, since purveyors of the substance are lured into illegal traffic by the opportunity to make large profits while dependent users may resort to robbery, prostitution, and other types of antisocial behavior to support their habits.

Current USA attitudes to drugs of this type are reflected in the Schedule of Controlled Substances (see Inside Front Cover). This schedule is quite similar to those published by international control bodies. Such schedules affect principally ethical and law-abiding manufacturers of the drugs and have little deterrent effect on illicit manufacturers or suppliers. Such schedules have been circumvented by the synthesis of "designer" drugs that make small modifications of the chemical structures of drugs with little or no change in their pharmacodynamic actions. Thus, schedules must constantly be revised to include these attempts to produce compounds not currently listed.

Because of the high social cost of drug abuse, many countries attempt to interdict their entry across borders. While surveys may indicate that the use of drugs such as cocaine and marijuana is increasing or decreasing, it is difficult to attribute such changes to law enforcement policies. Little progress has been made in decreasing the demand for illicit drugs. Some have argued that the only reasonable solution to the problem is legalization of the drugs. Such proposals are obviously highly controversial.

Any use of mind-altering drugs is based on a complicated interplay between three factors: the user, the setting in which the drug is taken, and the drug. Thus, the personality of the user and the setting may have a strong influence on what the user experiences. Nonetheless, it is usually possible to identify a pharmacologic "core" of drug effects that will be experienced by almost anyone under almost any circumstances if the dosage is adequate.

Neurobiology of Abused Drugs

During the last 20 years, substantial progress has been made elucidating the neurobiology of abused drugs and their effects not only on neurotransmitter receptors and reuptake carriers but also on the cascade of second, third, and fourth intracellular messenger systems (Self et al, 1995). Many abused drugs act through G protein-linked receptors such as the opioid, cannabinoid, and dopamine receptors. These G proteins frequently are coupled to the cAMP second messenger system, and through phosphorylation of various intracellular proteins a cascade of changes occurs in the nucleus and DNA. Immediate early genes such as c-*fos* and c-*jun* are activated followed by regulation of other genes with more sustained effects on protein transcription that may lead to the observed down-regulation of receptor numbers and up-regulation of second messenger systems.

For each of the classes of abused drugs a complex molecular biology has been described, including spe-cific neuroanatomic substrates linked to different neurotransmitters during acute intoxication and during withdrawal after dependence is established. Acute reinforcing effects of abused drugs are clearly a function of specific receptor binding but are also related to the *rate of change* in synaptic levels of dopamine, a key neurotransmitter involved in reinforcement in the nucleus accumbens. The chronic effects of abused drugs include tolerance and sensitization as well as the neurobiologic substrates for withdrawal symptoms. Much has been learned about these neurobiologic substrates for withdrawal in opioid dependence, including the activation of adrenergic brain systems such as the locus ceruleus during withdrawal. The latter findings have important treatment implications, such as the use of clonidine for opioid withdrawal. Other drug classes such as the benzodiazepines have specific receptors on ion-gated chloride channels associated with the neurotransmitter γ-aminobutyric acid (GABA), while other abused drugs such as phencyclidine bind to sites on excitatory amino acid receptors, which are ion-gated channels. The functions of other receptors that bind abused drugs such as opioid and cannabinoid receptors also have been clarified with the identification of endogenous ligands for these receptors, such as β-endorphin for the μ opioid receptor and anandamide for the cannabinoid receptor. These binding sites appear to be critical for the acute effects of these abused drugs, but their relationship to withdrawal after chronic use or even to acute reinforcement is unclear. However, substantial progress has been made in understanding the neurotransmitter basis for reinforcement with stimulants, which directly affect dopamine systems. The dopamine neurons connecting the ventral tegmental area to the nucleus accumbens have been considered the major reinforcement pathway for a wide range of abused drugs, but their role in reinforcement has been most clearly established for cocaine and amphetamine and less clearly for other drugs, particularly hallucinogens.

The neurobiologic findings in animal models have been increasingly confirmed in human studies. These human studies include pharmacologic challenges with neuroendocrine and behavioral outcomes, assessments of endogenous ligands in cerebrospinal fluid from drug-dependent patients, and neuroimaging studies, particularly neuroreceptor imaging. Available radioligands have permitted examination in humans of dopamine receptors and transporters, opioid receptors, and functional brain activity based on blood flow or glucose utilization. These receptor-neuroimaging studies have demonstrated that chronic abuse of drugs which can produce tolerance, dependence, and sensitization may have associated effects on receptor numbers (eg, dopamine D_2 receptors decrease in cocaine abusers) and on transporter numbers (eg, dopamine transporters increase in cocaine abusers). Blood flow and glucose utilization studies have shown that acute drug use is associated with substantial reductions in cerebral metabolic activity and that the rate of change is a correlate of the reinforcing effects of abused drugs.

In the following sections we review current knowledge about the molecular neurobiology of each class of abused drugs and discuss the neuroanatomic substrates that seem most closely linked to the neurotransmitters involved.

OPIOIDS

History

The nepenthe (Gk "free from sorrow") mentioned in the *Odyssey* probably contained opium. Opium smoking was widely practiced in China and the Near East until recently. Isolation of active opium alkaloids as well as the introduction of the hypodermic needle, allowing parenteral use of morphine, increased opioid use in the West. The first of several "epidemics" of opioid use in the USA followed the Civil War. Relief of pain with liberal doses of opiates was one of the few forms of treatment army physicians could offer the gravely wounded, and those lucky enough to survive often found themselves physiologically dependent. About 4% of adults in the USA used opiates regularly during the postbellum period. By the 1900s, the number had dropped to about one in 400 people in the USA, but the problem was still considered serious enough to justify passage of the Harrison Narcotic Act just before World War I. A new epidemic of opioid use started around 1964 and has continued unabated ever since. While fear of AIDS has reduced intravenous use of heroin, recent increases in its purity have led to markedly increased intranasal use. Present estimates are that the number of opioid-dependent people in the USA has recently stabilized at around 750,000.

Chemistry & Pharmacology

The most commonly abused drugs in this group are heroin, morphine, oxycodone, and—among health professionals—meperidine. The chemistry and general pharmacology of these agents are presented in Chapter 31.

Tolerance to the mental effects of opioids develops with chronic use. The need for ever-increasing amounts of drugs to sustain the desired euphoriant effects—as well as to avoid the discomfort of withdrawal—has the expected consequence of strongly reinforcing dependence once it has started. The role of endogenous opioid peptides in opioid dependence is uncertain.

Clinical Aspects

Curiosity and social pressure are the strongest factors in initiating opioid use. Intravenous administration is routine not only because it is the most efficient route but also because it produces a bolus of high concentration of drug that reaches the brain to produce a "rush," followed by euphoria, a feeling of tranquility, and sleepiness ("the nod"). Most doses of heroin available on the street are less than 25 mg and produce effects that last 3–5 hours. Thus, several doses a day are required to forestall manifestations of withdrawal in dependent persons. The trouble and expense of meeting these dose requirements put the dependent person always "on the hustle," either to get money to buy the drug or to find a "connection" with something to sell. Since supplies of heroin are of widely varying potency, the risk of overdosage is always present. And sooner or later in the lives of most heroin abusers, the money runs out or the supplies run out, and the withdrawal syndrome then begins.

Symptoms of opioid withdrawal begin 8–10 hours after the last dose. Many of these symptoms resemble those of increased activity of the autonomic nervous system. Lacrimation, rhinorrhea, yawning, and sweating appear first. Restless sleep followed by weakness, chills, gooseflesh ("cold turkey"), nausea and vomiting, muscle aches, and involuntary movements ("kicking the habit"), hyperpnea, hyperthermia, and hypertension occur in later stages of the withdrawal syndrome. The acute course of withdrawal may last 7–10 days. A secondary phase of protracted abstinence lasts for 26–30 weeks and is characterized by hypotension, bradycardia, hypothermia, mydriasis, and decreased responsiveness of the respiratory center to carbon dioxide.

Heroin users in particular tend to be polydrug users, also using alcohol, sedatives, and stimulants. None of these other drugs serve as substitutes for opioids, but they have desired additive effects. One needs to be sure that the person undergoing a withdrawal reaction is not also withdrawing from alcohol or sedatives, which might be more dangerous and more difficult to manage.

Besides the ever-present risk of fatal overdose, a number of other serious complications are associated with opioid use. Hepatitis B and AIDS are among the many potential complications of sharing contaminated hypodermic syringes. Bacterial infections lead to septic complications such as meningitis, osteomyelitis, and abscesses in various organs. A novel complication of attempts to illicitly manufacture meperidine has been the production of parkinsonism in users of this product. The culprit is a highly specific neurotoxin, MPTP (see Chapter 28). Homicide, suicide, and accidents are more prevalent among heroin abusers than in the general population.

Treatment

Treatment of acute overdoses of opioids may be lifesaving and is described in Chapters 31 and 59. In long-term treatment of opioid-dependent persons, pharmacologic or psychosocial approaches may be used, either separately or together. Widely different opinions have been vigorously expounded about which is the preferred type of treatment. Because each treatment method has a self-selected patient population, it is difficult to compare results. Chronic users tend to prefer pharmacologic approaches; those with shorter histories of drug abuse are more amenable to psychosocial interventions.

Pharmacologic treatment is most often used for detoxification. The principles of detoxification are the same for all drugs: to substitute a longer-acting, orally active, pharmacologically equivalent drug for the abused drug, stabilize the patient on that drug, and then gradually withdraw the substituted drug. Methadone is admirably suited for such use in opioid-dependent persons. More recently, clonidine, a centrally acting sympatholytic agent, has also been used for detoxification. By reducing central sympathetic outflow, clonidine might be expected to mitigate many of the signs of sympathetic overactivity. A presumed advantage of clonidine is that it has no narcotic action and is not addictive.

While it is easy to detoxify patients, the recidivism rate (return to abuse of the agent) is high. Methadone maintenance therapy, which substitutes a long-acting orally active opioid for heroin, has been effective in some settings. A single dose can be given each day, with the possibility of even less frequent than once-a-day dosing for long-term patients. Methadone saturates the opioid receptors and prevents the desired sudden onset of central nervous system effects normally produced by intravenous administration. An even longer-acting methadone analog, L-acetyl-methadol, has been approved and may offer additional technical advantages such as three times a week rather than daily dosing and reduced abuse potential due to slow onset of effects (average of three hours). Another candidate drug for use in this setting is buprenorphine, a partial opioid agonist, that can be given once daily or even less often for maintenance treatment at sublingual doses of 2–20 mg daily depending on the patient. The lower doses are useful for detoxification from heroin, while the higher doses are for longer maintenance treatment.

Use of a narcotic antagonist is rational therapy because blocking the action of self-administered opioids should eventually extinguish the habit. Naltrexone, a long-acting orally active pure opioid antagonist, has been extensively studied. It can be given three times a week once dosage reaches levels of 100–150 mg/d. The greatest drawback is that few addicts will accept naltrexone as permanent treatment. Unlike methadone, on which patients become dependent, naltrexone provides no such "hold" on them. Furthermore, because it is an antagonist, the patient must first be detoxified from opioid dependence before starting naltrexone.

Psychosocial approaches include a variety of techniques. Drug-free communities are based on the assumption that drug use is a symptom of some emotional disturbance or inability to cope with life's stresses. The most common technique employs peer group pressures, emphasizing confrontation. Other techniques include variations on group or individual psychotherapy, didactic approaches, alternative lifestyles through work or communal living, and a variety of types of meditation. Treatment may have to be continued for months or years, with costs depending on the degree to which professional staff is used. Many users eventually tire of their habit or "burn out," even without therapy.

BARBITURATES & OTHER SEDATIVE-HYPNOTICS

History

Ethanol is the sedative-hypnotic with the longest history of both use and abuse; it is discussed in Chapter 23. **Barbiturates** were introduced in 1903; they have been largely replaced in medical practice by newer agents, especially benzodiazepines. Short-acting members of the sedative-hypnotic group have been—and still are—widely abused. Meprobamate was introduced in 1954 as a nonbarbiturate sedative presumably lacking the disadvantages of the older drugs. It turned out to have more similarities to than differences from barbiturates. In fact, some of the nonbarbiturate sedative-hypnotics—examples are glutethimide and methaqualone—were worse than barbiturates in many respects, including abuse potential. The current era of **benzodiazepines** began in 1960. In the opinion of many authorities, these drugs are now the sedative-hypnotics of choice for most medical applications (Chapter 22). Abuse and physiologic dependence definitely occur with benzodiazepines but are probably less frequent than with barbiturates.

Chemistry & Pharmacology

The chemical relationships among this class of drugs are reviewed in Chapter 22. Depending on the dose, these drugs produce sedation, hypnosis, anesthesia, coma, and death. The exact mechanism by which they produce psychologic and physiologic dependence is unclear.

Both barbiturates and benzodiazepines can be classified pharmacokinetically into short- and long-acting compounds. Experience with barbiturates showed that most nonmedical use involved short-acting drugs, eg, secobarbital or pentobarbital sodium, and not long-acting ones, eg, phenobarbital. To some extent, this pattern has been repeated with the benzodiazepines. It is clear that the abruptness of onset of withdrawal syndromes as well as their severity is a function of the half-life of the drug. Drugs with half-lives in the range of 8–24 hours produce a rapidly evolving, severe withdrawal syndrome; those with longer half-lives, eg, 48–96 hours, produce a withdrawal syndrome that is slower in onset and less severe but longer in duration. Drugs with half-lives longer than 96 hours usually have a built-in tapering-off action that reduces the possibility of withdrawal reactions. Drugs with very short half-lives (< 4 hours) generally cannot be taken frequently enough to sustain high concentrations of the drug and are rarely associated with withdrawal reactions.

Clinical Aspects

No one knows how many persons are dependent on sedatives. Much of the presumed dependence is psychologic, perhaps based on the need for these drugs as a form of "replacement therapy." Physiologic dependence of the classic type (see below) has been relatively rare with benzodiazepines considering their extensive use. Such dependence usually occurs following long-term treatment with doses of 40 mg/d or more of diazepam or the equivalent dose of another drug. During the past several years, much interest has developed in the phenomenon of "therapeutic dose dependence." Many patients with this syndrome have never taken more than normal medical doses (15–30 mg/d of diazepam equivalents). Abrupt withdrawal of such doses of benzodiazepines may be followed by some of the same symptoms observed in classic withdrawal but is often characterized by weight loss, changes in perception, paresthesias, and headache. Such a syndrome almost always follows months or years of continual use. This phenomenon may be related to some adaptive change in benzodiazepine receptors following long-term exposure to the drug. All patients who have been taking these drugs for substantial periods of time, regardless of dosage, should have them withdrawn slowly.

Several patterns of sedative abuse have emerged. People with severe emotional disorders may use these drugs to seek escape into oblivion. Most abusers of "medical sedatives" use them to produce an altered mental state with disinhibition in the same way other people—or they themselves—use alcohol. One sometimes sees a pattern of alternating use of sedatives and stimulants, one type of drug being used to counter the effects of the other. A growing trend has been to use sedatives in a pattern of polydrug abuse, which includes most drugs of abuse.

The effects sought by the user are similar to those produced by alcohol—an initial disinhibition followed by drowsiness. Speech may be slurred and incoordination evident. As the goal seems to be to repeat such intoxications frequently, drugs that are eliminated rapidly are preferred.

As these drugs are usually taken orally and the tablets or capsules are consistent in drug content, inadvertent fatal overdoses of single agents are rare. Tolerance may develop to the sedative effect but not to the respiratory depressant effect. Thus, if these drugs are used with large amounts of alcohol, another respiratory depressant, fatalities can occur.

The withdrawal syndrome from medical sedatives is so much like that from alcohol that they are classified together as the alcohol-barbiturate type. Symptoms and signs of chronic intoxication from short-acting drugs may improve during the first 8 hours after withdrawal but are followed by increasing anxiety, tremors, twitches, and nausea and vomiting for the next 16 hours. Propranolol or clonidine may be of value in reducing some of these effects. Convulsions may occur 16–48 hours after withdrawal. Severe cases are associated with delirium, hallucinations, and other psychosis-like manifestations.

In the case of long-acting drugs, the withdrawal syndrome is attenuated. Symptoms may not appear for 2–3 days, and initial symptoms may suggest a recrudescence of those originally treated (nervousness, anxiety). Only by the fourth or fifth day can one be sure that a withdrawal reaction is under way. Convulsions are a late manifestation when they do occur—often not until the eighth or ninth day. Following this, the syndrome subsides. This slow evolution may allow some patients to recognize what is happening and to abort the syndrome by resuming their drug. As withdrawal is generally mild, other patients may go through the syndrome knowing that something is wrong but not being entirely sure what is happening.

Treatment

The time-honored principles of treating abstinence syndromes hold for sedative withdrawal as well. If short-acting drugs have been abused, phenobarbital is substituted as the pharmacologically equivalent agent. If long-acting drugs have been used, the same drug may be continued. The patient is stabilized on whatever dose is required to cause signs and symptoms to abate, and the drug is then gradually withdrawn. The rate of decrement may be 15–25% of the daily dose early in treatment, with later decrements of 5–10%. Complete detoxification can usually be achieved in less than 2 weeks.

No specific treatment programs have been developed for sedative abusers. The problem is so often complicated by abuse of other drugs that it may be more expeditious to enroll the patient in a program designed for alcoholics or opiate-dependent persons. Patients with psychiatric disorders that can be defined, especially those with depression, may be treated with specific drug treatment for the underlying disorder.

Criminal Use

A special form of sedative-hypnotic abuse is the use of such drugs to incapacitate others. Described as a **"Mickey Finn,"** chloral hydrate was the traditional drug slipped into a person's drink without their knowledge to make them incapable of protecting themselves. The Mickey Finn was probably largely restricted to use by criminal elements, and it enjoyed considerable notoriety in crime fiction. More recently, the use of a very rapid onset benzodiazepine has been widely reported as a means of "date rape," a small tasteless dose of the drug making the victim incapable of protecting herself (or himself). The drug most commonly used in this situation has been **flunitrazepam (Rohypnol, "roofies")**. The amnesia-producing effects of the benzodiazepines (Chapter 22) make the victim unable to describe the events after he or she has recovered. This drug is not sold in the USA but is brought in by individuals.

STIMULANTS

History

Caffeine is probably the most widely used social drug worldwide. Most people do not consider it to be a drug, though many, especially as they age, experience disturbing effects on sleep and heart rhythm from too much coffee. A withdrawal syndrome characterized by lethargy, irritability, and headache has been recognized in users of more than 600 mg/d (roughly six cups of coffee).

Nicotine is one of the most widely used licit drugs. It is now considered to be one of the most insidiously addicting substances because most users are not aware of strong feelings of reinforcement when consuming it but have extremely long-lasting cravings for it when trying to quit. Nicotine causes central electroencephalographic activation and euphoriant effects and release of catecholamines from peripheral adrenergic nerves. Tolerance develops rapidly. Despite compelling evidence of serious health hazards involving multiple organ systems, about 28% of adults in the USA still smoke cigarettes because they have become dependent upon nicotine. Deaths directly attributable to smoking account for 20% of all deaths and 30% of cancer deaths in the USA. It is estimated that about 90% of cases of chronic obstructive pulmonary disease in the USA are due to smoking. Various techniques have been used to wean smokers from the drug, including substitution of nicotine in the form of nicotine-containing chewing gum and a slow-release transdermal form of nicotine. These preparations are designed to be used under medical supervision in gradually tapering dosage, so that the patient is gradually withdrawn from the drug. Unfortunately, recruitment of new cigarette smokers seems to equal the number of those who quit. The use of smokeless tobacco products (snuff, chewing tobacco) has increased in recent years, especially in adolescents, apparently in response to new advertising campaigns directed at younger age groups. These products are subject to similar risks of cancer and addiction as smoked tobacco. A brief description of the pharmacology of nicotine is found in Chapter 7.

Cocaine has been used for at least 1200 years in the custom of chewing coca leaves by natives of the South American Andes. Coca was first exported to Europe from the Western Hemisphere in 1580. Cocaine was isolated as the active material in 1860. Its anesthetic properties, especially its topical anesthetic action, were discovered in the 1870s and 1880s. Sigmund Freud was intrigued by the drug and thought it might even be a panacea, but his enthusiasm was dampened by its disastrous effects on a friend who became dependent. A colleague of Freud's, Karl Koller, is credited with first using the drug as a topical anesthetic for eye surgery, a use that continues to this day.

Amphetamine was synthesized in the late 1920s and was introduced into medical practice in 1936. Dextroamphetamine is the major member of the class, though many other amphetamines and amphetamine surrogates, such as methamphetamine (Methedrine, **"speed"**), phenmetrazine (Preludin), and methylphenidate (Ritalin), were subsequently introduced. The number of amphetamine analogs with psychoactive effects continues to multiply. The first of these newer members of the group was 2,5-dimethoxy-4-methylamphetamine (DOM, "STP"), and the list now includes methylenedioxyamphetamine (MDA) and methylenedioxymethamphetamine (MDMA, **"ecstasy"**). The latter drugs have more amphetamine-like than hallucinogenic effects. They have also been shown to be neurotoxic to serotonergic systems in the brains of animals, with uncertain adverse consequences in humans.

A closely related natural alkaloid, **cathinone,** is found in the leaves and stems of *Catha edulis,* or **khat,** a plant found and cultivated in the Middle East and Africa. Chewing of freshly harvested khat results in effects indistinguishable from those of the amphetamines.

Chemistry & Pharmacology

The chemical relationships of the various stimulants are shown in Figure 32–1. Despite their similar actions, caffeine, cocaine, and amphetamine have very different structures.

Caffeine, a methylxanthine compound, appears to exert its central actions (and perhaps some of its peripheral ones as well) by blocking adenosine receptors. Other methylxanthines, eg, theophylline, have the same actions. Adenosine modulates adenylyl cyclase activity, causing contraction of isolated airway smooth muscle as one of its peripheral actions. The same action probably accounts for the central stimulant actions of the methylxanthines. At high concentrations, the methylxanthines inhibit phosphodiesterase, thereby inhibiting the breakdown of cAMP and increasing its concentration inside cells. However, it is doubtful whether this is important at ordinary dosage. Cocaine binds to the dopamine reuptake transporter in the central nervous system, effectively inhibiting dopamine reuptake as well as that of norepinephrine. As noted above (Neurobiology of Abused Drugs), dopamine is very important in the reward system of the brain; its increase probably accounts for the high dependence potential of cocaine.

Figure 32–1. Chemical structures of some popular stimulants.

Amphetamines probably act centrally mainly by increasing release of catecholaminergic neurotransmitters, including dopamine. They are also weak inhibitors of monoamine oxidase and, by virtue of structural similarity, possible direct catecholaminergic agonists in the brain.

Although psychologic dependence is strong for many of these drugs (cocaine is one of the most strongly reinforcing drugs in self-administration paradigms in animals), it was thought for some time that physiologic dependence occurred only rarely. However, recent patterns of abuse of these drugs, especially amphetamine-like agents, have revealed a typical pattern of withdrawal manifested by signs and symptoms opposite to those produced by the drug. Users deprived of the drug become sleepy, have a ravenous appetite, are exhausted, and may suffer mental depression. This syndrome may last for several days after the drug is withdrawn. Tolerance develops quickly, so that abusers may take monumental doses compared with those used medically, eg, as anorexiants.

Clinical Aspects

Amphetamine abuse began in the 1940s. The substance was present in substantial amounts in inhalers promoted as nasal decongestants. During World War II, amphetamines were frequently used by military personnel. A huge supply of amphetamines became available to young people in Japan in the postwar period, resulting in an epidemic of abuse that was ultimately curbed by draconian punishments. Meanwhile, in the USA the drug continued to be used in relatively small oral doses, often alternating with barbiturates. In the 1960s, the pattern changed. Methamphetamine became the preferred drug (largely because it was more easily synthesized illicitly), and the preferred route of administration became intravenous injection.

One pattern of amphetamine abuse is called a "run." Repeated intravenous injections are self-administered to obtain a "rush"—an orgasm-like reaction—followed by a feeling of mental alertness and marked euphoria. Total daily doses as high as 4000 mg have been reported. After several days of such spree use, subjects may enter a paranoid schizophrenia-like state. Typically, they develop delusions that bugs are crawling under their skin, which leads to characteristic discrete excoriations. Finally, the spree is terminated by exhaustion from lack of sleep and lack of food, followed by the withdrawal syndrome mentioned above.

A new pattern of amphetamine abuse has evolved in which methamphetamine base crystals (**"ice"**) are smoked—analogous to the use of **"crack"** cocaine (see below). Smoking delivers a rapid bolus of drug to the brain, somewhat similar to intravenous administration. Since the duration of action of methamphetamine is much longer than that of cocaine, intoxication may last for several hours after a single smoke. It remains to be seen whether "ice" will replace "crack" or merely add another form of abusable drug. It is a curious paradox that efforts to regulate the use of drugs by law often lead to the introduction of more dangerous drugs. With the virtual outlawing of amphetamines from legitimate medical practice (based on adverse effects experienced by using doses two or three orders of magnitude larger than therapeutic doses), cocaine became the substitute. Cocaine may be construed as a highly potent amphetamine ("superspeed") with all of the effects of the latter drug magnified. It is far more likely to lead to dependence than amphetamines, and overdoses leading to death have been widely reported.

Three types of administration of cocaine are current. One may "snuff" or "snort" the drug by sniffing a "line" (a measured amount of drug in a folded piece of paper applied to the nose), or one may smoke "free base." Finally, intravenous use is common, especially among heroin addicts. Cocaine is supplied as a hydrochloride salt, and crack, the free base, is made by alkalinizing the salt and extracting with nonpolar solvents. When free base is smoked, entry through the lungs is almost as fast as by intravenous injection, so that effects are more accentuated than when the drug is snorted (Figure 32–2). The purity and potency of cocaine available to users vary widely.

The plasma half-life of cocaine is short, so that effects following a single dose persist only for an hour or so. Consequently, the euphoric experience may be repeated many times during the course of a day or night.

Cocaine may be used sporadically, as at a party, or regularly by those with a self-imposed high level of activity, such as rock musicians. It may also be part of the repertoire of the polydrug abuser. A **"speedball"** is a combination of cocaine and heroin taken intravenously, presumably doubling the "rush" but extinguishing other effects. Patients in methadone maintenance programs who can no longer get much kick from heroin may turn to cocaine, whose euphoriant effects are not altered by methadone. An epidemic of "cocaine babies" born to mothers who are using cocaine heavily has posed a major new challenge to health care facilities in the inner cities (Volpe, 1992). There are clear-cut deleterious effects on the pregnancy, with increased fetal morbidity and mortality. Whether surviving babies will be impaired in the long term awaits further study.

Besides the paranoid psychosis associated with chronic use of amphetamines, intravenous injection using contaminated syringes leads to the same infectious complications as heroin. A specific lesion associated with chronic amphetamine use is necrotizing arteritis, which may involve many small and medium-sized arteries and lead to fatal brain hemorrhage or renal failure. Overdoses of amphetamines are rarely fatal; they can usually be managed by sedating the patient with haloperidol. The powerful vasoconstrictive action of cocaine has led to a significant number of patients with severe acute hypertensive episodes resulting in myocardial infarcts and strokes. This vasoconstrictive effect may also contribute to the multiple brain perfusion defects that have been described using single photon emission computed tomography (SPECT) blood flow imaging in cocaine abusers. The local anesthetic action of cocaine contributes to the production of seizures. Overdoses of cocaine are usually rapidly fatal, victims dying within minutes from arrhythmias, seizures, or respiratory depression. Those who survive for 3 hours usually recover fully. Intravenous administration of diazepam, propranolol, or calcium channel-blocking drugs may be the best treatment.

Treatment

Subjects with residual emotional disorders, either schizophreniform psychosis or mental depression, may require treatment with antipsychotic or antidepressant drugs before or during weaning from stimu-

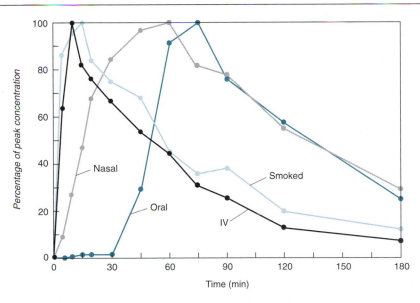

Figure 32–2. Comparison of blood concentrations achieved when cocaine is administered by different routes. Time to peak is nearly as fast by smoking as by intravenous injection. (Modified and reproduced, with permission, from Jones RT: The pharmacology of cocaine smoking in humans. In: *Research Findings on Smoking of Abused Substances. National Institute on Drug Abuse Research Monograph 99.* Chiang CN, Hawks RL [editors]. US Government Printing Office, 1990.)

lants. A number of drugs have been studied to assess their ability to mitigate withdrawal from cocaine, reduce craving during abstinence, and facilitate abstinence. Desipramine, carbamazepine, bromocriptine, amantadine, clonidine, buprenorphine, bupropion, and others are under investigation. No treatment programs have been devised specifically for stimulant users. Those who administer these drugs intravenously have more in common with heroin users than any other group and may be suitable for some of the rehabilitative programs devised for opioid-dependent persons. Nicotine dependence may respond to replacement therapy with either nicotine gum or transdermal patches, and detoxification from nicotine dependence has been described using clonidine.

HALLUCINOGENS

History

Almost every society has found some bark, skin, leaf, vine, berry, fungus, or weed that contains "hallucinogenic" materials. Although the fortuitous discovery of the properties of **lysergic acid diethylamide (LSD)** occurred in a chemical laboratory during the 1940s, this was a case in which scientific art was merely imitating nature. Similar compounds have been found in morning glory seeds, and drugs such as mescaline and psilocybin have long been used by natives of North and Central America in the form of cactus buttons or magical mushrooms. Deliriants, such as the alkaloids in *Atropa belladonna* and *Datura stramonium,* were also known in ancient cultures.

Terminology

Although the term "hallucinogen" will be used here, it is not entirely accurate, since hallucinations may be uncommon effects or only part of the overall effects of these drugs. The term "psychotomimetic" is often used to connote the possible action of these drugs in mimicking naturally occurring psychoses. However, the state induced by these agents does not closely resemble that of schizophrenia. The term "psychedelic" was coined to denote a supposed "mind-revealing" aspect of such drug use, but the insights and revelations achieved are not much different from those that have been claimed with many other disinhibiting drugs, most commonly alcohol.

The drugs we here call hallucinogens are taken for many reasons. The one most widely given by users is that the drugs provide new ways of looking at the world and new insights into personal problems. The former claim implies varying degrees of perceptual distortion, while the latter implies changes in mood and increased introspection. LSD has become the prototypical hallu-

Figure 32–3. Chemical structures of lysergic acid diethylamide (LSD), mescaline, phencyclidine, psilocybin, and the amphetamine analog MDMA.

cinogenic drug because of the extent of its use; because it represents a family of drugs that are similar; and because it has been most extensively studied.

Chemistry & Pharmacology

The LSD-like group of drugs includes **LSD, mescaline, psilocybin,** and their related compounds. Although these substances differ chemically, they share some chemical features and even more pharmacologic ones (Figure 32–3). LSD is a semisynthetic chemical not known to occur in nature. It is related to the ergot alkaloids (Chapter 16). The monoethyl—rather than the diethyl—amide is found in hallucinogenic morning glory seeds. Mescaline, a phenethylamine derivative, and psilocybin, an indolethylamine derivative, are found in nature. These drugs also have chemical resemblances to three major neurotransmitters: norepinephrine, dopamine, and serotonin.

The mode of action of hallucinogens of the LSD type is uncertain despite much experimental study. Measured electroencephalographically, their effects are to produce a state of hyperarousal of the central nervous system. LSD interacts with several serotonin (5-HT) receptor subtypes in the brain. Until recently it was thought to be a potent 5-HT$_2$ receptor antagonist. It appears to alter serotonin turnover, as indicated by increased brain concentrations of its major metabolite, 5-hydroxyindoleacetic acid. In addition, LSD displays agonist activity at 5-HT$_{1A}$ and 5-HT$_{1C}$ receptors. These actions may be more relevant to LSD's hallucinogenic action, because a number of other drugs with good antagonist effects at central 5-HT$_2$ receptors are not hallucinogenic.

The deliriant hallucinogens, exemplified by scopolamine (Chapter 8) and some synthetic centrally acting cholinoceptor-blocking agents, are different chemically as well as pharmacologically from the LSD group. Their effects seem to be entirely explainable by blockade of central muscarinic receptors. Similar mental effects may be seen during therapeutic or deliberate overdoses of commonly used medications with antimuscarinic action, such as anticholinergic antiparkinsonism drugs, tricyclic antidepressants, and antispasmodics. Occasional instances of abuse of these therapeutic agents have occurred.

Phencyclidine (PCP, "angel dust," many other names) is a synthetic phenylcyclohexylamine derivative. There is some question about how it should be classified, since it differs in many ways from other hallucinogens, but its primary use is to obtain hallucinogenic effects. The drug was originally introduced as a "dissociative anesthetic" in 1957. Such anesthetics were presumed to work by making patients insensitive to pain by "separating their bodily functions from their minds" without causing loss of consciousness. Hallucinogenic effects were noted in patients emerging from anesthesia. The drug was withdrawn from use in humans but retained in veterinary practice under the name Sernylan. (The veterinary use has given the drug

one of its street names—"hog.") Ketamine, an analog, replaced phencyclidine as an anesthetic for use in humans (see Chapter 25). It too produces some emergent hallucinogenic effects. The first street use of PCP was in 1967, when it quickly gained a reputation as a bad drug. Over the next several years, it was mislabeled, being sold as LSD, tetrahydrocannabinol (THC), and other hallucinogens. Since the 1970s, PCP has become widely accepted by drug abusers and is now the most commonly used hallucinogenic agent. Phencyclidine may be smoked (by mixing the powder with tobacco), "snorted," taken orally, or injected intravenously. Fortunately, a recent trend toward less frequent use of the drug has been noted.

Some of the early investigators of PCP maintained that it provided a much better model of schizophrenia than LSD, mainly through its action in producing a form of sensory isolation. Receptors for PCP have been identified in the brain that are closely related, if not identical, to the opioid sigma receptor. The drug also acts as an antagonist on the NMDA subtype of glutamate receptors. Earlier work suggested that PCP blocked uptake of dopamine as well. The drug is unique among hallucinogens in that animals will self-administer it.

Clinical Effects

LSD produces a series of somatic, perceptual, and psychologic effects that overlap each other. Dizziness, weakness, tremors, nausea, and paresthesias are prominent somatic symptoms. Blurring of vision, distortions of perspective, organized visual illusions or "hallucinations," less discriminant hearing, and a change in sense of time are common perceptual abnormalities. Impaired memory, difficulty in thinking, poor judgment, and altered mood are prominent psychologic effects. Physiologically, LSD produces signs of overactivity of the sympathetic nervous system and central stimulation, manifested by dilated pupils, increased heart rate, mild elevation of blood pressure, tremor, and alertness. Virtually identical effects are produced by mescaline and psilocybin when they are given in equivalent doses. The onset of effects is fairly rapid, but the duration varies with the dose and is usually measured in hours. Phenomena may vary considerably from one user to another owing to such factors as the personality and expectations of the user and the circumstances under which the drug is taken, but the above effects occur in almost everyone. Waxing and waning of effects is typical.

Usual doses of LSD in humans are approximately 1–2 µg/kg, making it one of the most potent pharmacologic agents known. The drug is equally effective parenterally or orally and consequently is almost always taken by mouth. Psilocybin is usually taken in doses of 250 µg/kg and mescaline in doses of 5–6 mg/kg. Despite these differences in potency, the effects are virtually indistinguishable.

Scopolamine and other antimuscarinic drugs produce delirium with fluctuating levels of awareness, disorientation, marked difficulty in thinking, marked loss of memory, and bizarre delusions. If doses are large, these impairments may last for more than a day, with some subjects claiming that several days may elapse before they once again feel confident about their memory. Most subjects, at least under experimental conditions, find these drugs to be unpleasant and have little desire to repeat the experience. Some become frightened during the period of drug effect. Others deliberately seek out and use such drugs repeatedly.

PCP produces detachment, disorientation, distortions of body image, and loss of proprioception. Somatic symptoms and signs include numbness, nystagmus, sweating, rapid heart rate, and hypertension. Effects are dose-dependent. Overdosage has been fatal, as contrasted with the absence of known fatalities directly caused by drugs of the LSD group.

Use of these hallucinogens has not been associated with dependence or physiologic withdrawal symptoms. This is probably because tolerance develops rapidly, so that closely spaced dosing would be necessary to cause dependence; such frequent dosing is unusual.

Toxicity

Adverse psychologic consequences of hallucinogenic drugs are common. Panic reactions ("bad trips") may be related to excessive doses; they seem to be less common as the doses of street drugs have become more accurate. They are best managed by sedation with a barbiturate or benzodiazepine rather than with a phenothiazine. Simple "talking down" may suffice but is labor-intensive. Acute psychotic or depressive reactions have been precipitated by use of these drugs but usually only in persons with strong predispositions. Acute psychotic reactions are associated with PCP much more commonly than with any of the other hallucinogens. Errors of judgment may lead to reckless acts that threaten life; any person under the influence of one of these drugs should be provided with a nondrugged companion until the effect has dissipated.

Overdoses of the antimuscarinic agents can be treated with infusions of physostigmine, but supportive care is usually preferred.

Overdoses of PCP are dangerous but can be managed if recognized promptly. PCP is secreted into the stomach, so that removal may be hastened by continual nasogastric suction. Excretion of this basic drug may be hastened by acidification of the urine to pH 5.5 (but see Chapter 59). Diazepam can be given to protect against seizures or to curb excitation; antipsychotic drugs aggravate matters at this point. If a prolonged schizophrenia-like illness follows acute intoxication, one may consider antipsychotics on a sustained basis.

Long-Term Treatment

No systematic program of treatment has been devised for abuse of this class of drugs. Users of hallu-cinogens are likely to stick to this class of drugs rather than proceed to a pattern of polydrug abuse. Separation of the user from the drug culture is probably the best treatment, but it must be voluntarily accepted.

Therapeutic Uses

No therapeutic indication has yet been accepted for any hallucinogen. LSD was promoted as a cure for alcoholism, but objective evidence of benefit is totally lacking. Facilitation of psychotherapy was another proposed use, again with no substantiation or comparison with other drugs. Although it has been tried in both schizophrenics and depressed individuals, LSD is more likely to precipitate or aggravate these disorders than to alleviate them. Use of the drug in chronic cancer patients was said to diminish the need for opioids, but this work has not been confirmed.

MARIJUANA

History

Use of **cannabis** has been recorded for thousands of years, especially in Eastern countries such as China and India. It was certainly known to the Greeks at the height of their civilization as well as to Arabic nations somewhat later. It is estimated that about 200–300 million people use cannabis in some form. Thus, it is not only one of the oldest but also one of the most widely used of mind-altering drugs. Since the 1960s, the rise in marijuana use in the USA has been remarkable. Although the drug was known in this country prior to that time, there were only a small number of users. It is estimated now that 30–40 million persons in the USA have used the drug and that a substantial number are regular users. Following a period of steadily increasing use of marijuana by young people, an apparent reversal of this pattern was reported a few years ago. Unfortunately, this favorable development has not lasted; the most recent surveys suggest increasing use of the drug at an earlier age.

Several species of cannabis (hemp) have been named, but botanists do not agree that more than one species of the plant exists; many morphologic variants occur. Some plants are excellent for fiber, being a source of hemp, and rather poor producers of drug; the converse also is true. These properties are due to genetic differences. The flowers and small leaves of *Cannabis sativa* supply most of the drug. Marijuana is a mixture of ground-up plant materials that resembles grass clippings thus the street name "grass." Extraction of the resin from the plant provides a more potent product: hashish.

Chemistry & Pharmacokinetics of Cannabinoids

Three major cannabinoids have been found in cannabis; cannabidiol (CBD), Δ^9-tetrahydrocannabinol (THC), and cannabinol (CBN). The biosynthetic pathway begins with CBD, proceeds to THC, and ends with CBN (Figure 32–4). Thus, one can deduce from the proportions of these cannabinoids in plant material the age of the plant. Many other variants of these structures have been found in cannabis, but with the exception of THC and its analogs no other cannabinoids have definite psychoactivity. The content of THC varies considerably among plants, so that special genetic lines may produce as much as 4–6% THC content in very selected ("manicured") materials. Most plants have a THC content ranging from trace amounts to 1–2%.

The preferred route of administration in Western countries is by smoking. The high lipid solubility of THC causes it to be readily trapped on the surfactant lining of the lungs. Pharmacokinetic studies indicate that smoking is almost equivalent to intravenous administration except that lower peak plasma concentrations of THC are attained. In some Eastern countries, cannabis is taken orally in the form of various confections. The rate of absorption from this route is slow and highly variable, though the duration of action is longer.

THC is extensively metabolized, and new metabolites are still being discovered. One metabolite, 11-hydroxy-THC, is actually more active than the parent compound. However, it is not nearly as abundant, and the major part of the activity of cannabis probably derives from THC itself. The high lipid solubility of the drug leads to extensive sequestration in the lipid compartments of the body, and metabolites may be ex-creted for as long as a week after a single dose. Whether accumulation of unchanged THC can occur is questionable.

Pharmacodynamics of Cannabinoids

The mechanism of action of THC has been the subject of intense investigation (Howlett, 1995). A high degree of enantiomer selectivity—of both the natural and newer cannabinoids—has suggested a highly selective receptor. A putative endogenous ligand, anandamide, has been described (Devane et al, 1992). Synthetic cannabinoid agonists with high potency and stereoselectivity in behavioral assays have been used to characterize the cannabinoid binding site. Their binding affinities correlate closely with their relative potencies in biologic assays, suggesting that the receptor also mediates the pharmacologic effects. Binding sites are most numerous in the outflow nuclei of the basal ganglia, the substantia nigra, pars reticulata, globus pallidus, hippocampus, and brain stem. The receptor has been cloned and is G protein-coupled. Positron emission tomographic (PET) studies have revealed increases in metabolism following THC in the same areas in which receptors are localized, again suggesting that the receptors are closely involved in the clinical actions of the drug. Prostaglandins may play a mediator role in THC activity, but how this might occur is unclear. The high lipophilicity of THC has caused some investigators to propose a nonspecific membrane effect, but that would not explain the stereoselective action.

Figure 32–4. Structures of the three main cannabinoids in marijuana. Only THC has psychoactivity. C_5H_{11} is n-pentyl. Arrows indicate the biosynthetic sequence.

THC has a variety of pharmacologic effects that resemble those of amphetamines, LSD, alcohol, sedatives, atropine, and morphine. Thus, the drug does not fit traditional pharmacologic classifications and must be considered as a separate class.

Clinical Effects

Small doses of THC may be associated with a rather definite placebo effect, but large doses are unequivocal in producing the expected range of effects. The expert smoker of marijuana is usually aware of a drug effect after two or three inhalations. As smoking continues, the effects increase, reaching a maximum about 20 minutes after the smoke has been finished. Most effects of the drug usually have vanished after 3 hours, by which time plasma concentrations are low. Peak effects after oral administration may be delayed until 3–4 hours after drug ingestion but may last for 6–8 hours.

The early stage is one of being "high" and is characterized by euphoria, uncontrollable laughter, alteration of time sense, depersonalization, and sharpened vision. Later, the user becomes relaxed and experiences introspective and dream-like states if not actual sleep. Thinking or concentrating becomes difficult, though by force of will the subject can attend.

Two characteristic physiologic signs of cannabis intoxication are increased pulse rate and reddening of the conjunctiva. The latter correlates well with the presence of detectable plasma concentrations. Pupil size is not changed. The blood pressure may fall, especially in the upright position. An antiemetic effect may be present. Muscle weakness, tremors, unsteadiness, and increased deep tendon reflexes may also be noted. Virtually any psychologic test shows impairment if the doses are large enough and the test difficult enough. No distinctive biochemical changes have been found in humans.

Tolerance has been demonstrated in virtually every animal species that has been tested. It is apparent in humans only among heavy long-term users of the drug. Different degrees of tolerance develop for different effects of the drug, with tolerance for the tachycardiac effect developing fairly rapidly. A mild withdrawal syndrome has been noted following chronic use at very high doses.

Heavy marijuana use, especially by the young, has raised concern about possible adverse effects on the health of users. The hazards of use are still controversial and ambiguous, and there are many problems with the studies themselves. First, it is difficult to prove or disprove an adverse behavioral reaction for humans in an animal model. Second, users thus far have been mostly young people in excellent general health. Third, cannabis is often used in combination with alcohol or tobacco. And fourth, many investigators have biases for or against the drug.

Three epidemiologic studies in developing countries have failed to find definite evidence of impairment among heavy users of cannabis, but field studies may lack sensitivity. Experimental studies in which subjects have smoked heavily for varying periods have shown a lower serum testosterone level in men and airway narrowing. Effects on immune mechanisms, chromosomes, and cell metabolism are often contradictory. Effects on the fetus are still uncertain.

Heavy smokers of marijuana may be subject to some of the same problems of chronic bronchitis, airway obstruction, and squamous cell metaplasia as smokers of tobacco cigarettes. Angina pectoris may be aggravated by the speeding of the heart rate, orthostatic hypotension, and increased carboxyhemoglobin. Driving ability is likely to be impaired but is not easily demonstrated with usual testing. "Amotivational syndrome," in which promising young people with obvious social advantages lose interest in school and career and enter the drug culture, is a real phenomenon, but one cannot be sure whether drug use is the cause of the problem or simply a matter of personal choice. Acute panic reactions, toxic delirium, paranoid states, and frank psychoses are rare. Brain damage has not been confirmed in humans, though some suggestion of ultrastructural damage has been found in animals.

Therapeutic Uses

Cannabis was at one time listed in drug formularies but has not been used medically for some time. Recently, interest in cannabis for therapeutic purposes has revived. A finding of lowered intraocular pressure following oral THC administration has been repeatedly confirmed; it remains to be seen whether preparations of cannabis have any advantages over other forms of treatment for glaucoma. Amelioration of nausea and vomiting associated with cancer chemotherapy has also been studied. THC, now named **dronabinol** (Marinol), has been marketed for this indication. It seems able to reduce nausea and vomiting at doses that are associated with only moderate mental effects. Its major disadvantage is that an oral medication is often useless in a patient who is vomiting. **Levonantradol** is another analog that may have medical use, possibly as an analgesic, as an agent for the relief of muscle spasm, or even as an anticonvulsant. It remains to be proved, however, that any of these analogs have advantages over standard agents.

Treatment

Few users seek treatment, though many who have stopped using the drug have been pleasantly surprised at the increased clarity of their thinking. Although marijuana has been alleged to be a substitute for alcohol, it is more commonly used along with alcohol; alcoholism complicating marijuana use is rare. Marijuana may be used in a pattern of multiple drug use, in which case treatment may be required for the more dangerous drugs being taken.

INHALANTS

History

The modern discovery of the intoxicant effects of inhalants began with Sir Humphry Davy in 1799, who administered nitrous oxide to himself and others. As other anesthetic gases were introduced, such as chloroform and ether, they were also used socially. Such use persists, with occasional instances of halothane inhalation being added to the anesthetic gases previously mentioned. In addition to these agents, three other patterns of inhalant use are now prevalent: (1) industrial solvents, including a variety of hydrocarbons, such as toluene; (2) aerosol propellants, such as various fluorocarbons; and (3) organic nitrites, such as amyl or butyl nitrite.

Chemistry & Pharmacology

The structures of some inhalants are shown in Figure 32–5. The mode of action of the inhalant anesthetics has been discussed in Chapter 25.

Clinical Aspects

Nitrous oxide, formerly not easily available, is now sold openly in so-called "head-shops." When self-administered, it produces difficulty in concentrating, dreaminess, euphoria, numbness and tingling, unsteadiness, and visual and auditory disturbances. It is usually taken as 35% N_2O mixed with oxygen; administration of 100% nitrous oxide may cause asphyxia and death.

Ether and **chloroform** are readily available through chemical supply houses. Cloths soaked with the material are used for inhalation of the fumes. After an initial period of exhilaration, the person often loses consciousness. Ether is highly flammable. Halothane is usually available only to medical or health care personnel.

A variety of **industrial solvents** that can be used as inhalants are on the market and virtually impossible to control. They include gasoline, paint thinner, glue, rubber cement, acrylic paint sprays, shoe polish, and degreasers. The toxic ingredients may be toluene, heptane, hexane, benzene, trichloroethylene, methylethylketone, and others. Because of their ready availability, this group of inhalants is widely used. Aerosol propellants have also been widely available, though manufacturers of products using propellants have recently changed from fluorocarbons to less hazardous materials.

Motives for use of inhalants include peer influence, low cost, ready availability, convenient packaging, quick intoxication of short duration, and mood enhancement. Boys in their early teen years from lower socioeconomic classes are the principal users. They generally also have worse than average problems at

Figure 32–5. Structures of some commonly used inhalants.

school and at home. Psychologic dependence perpetuates the use of inhalants.

The clinical effects of industrial solvent inhalation are short, lasting only 5–15 minutes. Rags or "toques" are soaked in the solvent and the fumes inhaled. Aerosol propellants are usually inhaled from a plastic bag. Euphoria and a relaxed "drunk" feeling are followed by disorientation, slow passage of time, and possibly hallucinations.

Organic nitrites have developed a reputation as a sexual enhancer, a sure avenue to popular acceptance. Amyl nitrite is used medically for angina in the form of fragile glass ampules covered with cloth. When these are broken, they make a popping sound—hence the nickname **"poppers."** Street forms of bottled isobutyl nitrite (Locker Room, Rush) are readily available in some areas. Inhalation causes dizziness, giddiness, rapid heart rate, lowered blood pressure, "speeding," and flushing of the skin. These effects last only a few minutes and can readily be repeated. The main effect of the drug on sexual performance is probably to enhance or prolong erection through the release of nitric oxide in the corpora cavernosa (see Chapter 19). Except for an occasional instance of methemoglobinemia associated with excessive use of nitrites, few significant adverse effects have been reported despite extensive use of this drug.

Toxicity

Chloroform has been implicated in liver and kidney damage. Industrial solvents have produced a variety of adverse effects: liver and kidney damage, peripheral nerve damage and possibly brain damage in animals, bone marrow suppression, and pulmonary disease. In human neuroimaging studies using MRI, demyelination of white matter has been described in chronic abusers. Fluorocarbon inhalation has resulted in sudden deaths, due either to ventricular arrhythmias or to asphyxiation. Nitrites have been rather safe but might pose hazards (especially arrhythmias) for persons with preexisting cardiovascular problems.

REFERENCES

General

Bock GR, Whelan J (editors): *Cocaine: Scientific and Social Dimensions.* (Ciba Foundations Symposium 166.) Wiley, 1992.

Committee on Problems of Drug Dependence: *Testing Drugs for Physical Dependence Potential and Abuse Liability.* Brady JV, Lukas SE (editors). National Institute on Drug Abuse Research Monograph 52, US Government Printing Office, 1984.

Koob GF, Bloom FE: Cellular and molecular mechanisms of drug dependence. Science 1988;242:715.

Kulberg A: Substance abuse: Clinical identification and management. Pediatr Clin North Am 1986;33:325.

Musto DF: Opium, cocaine, and marijuana in American history. Sci Am 1991;265:40.

Nestler EJ: Molecular mechanisms of drug addiction. J Neurosci 1992;12:2439.

Ray OA: *Drugs, Society and Human Behavior,* 6th ed. Mosby, 1993.

Self DW, Nestler EJ: Molecular mechanisms of drug reinforcement and addiction. Annu Rev Neurosci 1995; 18:463.

Opioids

Agren H: Clonidine treatment of the opiate withdrawal syndrome: A review of clinical trials of a theory. Acta Psychiatr Scand 1986(Suppl);327:91.

Collier HOJ: Physiological basis of opiate dependence. Drug Alcohol Depend 1983;11:15.

Dole VP: Implications of methadone maintenance treatment for theories of narcotic addiction. JAMA 1988; 260:3025.

Kleber HD: The use of psychotropic drugs in the treatment of compulsive opiate abusers: The rationale for their use. Adv Alcohol Subst Abuse 1985;51:103.

Sedatives

Allgulander C: History and current status of sedative-hypnotic drug use and abuse. Acta Psychiatr Scand 1986;73:465.

Cowen PJ, Nutt DJ: Abstinence symptoms after withdrawal of tranquilizing drugs: Is there a common neurochemical mechanism? Lancet 1982;2:360.

Stimulants

Bartecchi CE, MacKenzie TD, Schrier RW: The human costs of tobacco use. N Engl J Med 1994;330:907.

Benowitz NL: Clinical pharmacology of caffeine. Annu Rev Med 1990;41:277.

Benowitz NL: Clinical pharmacology and toxicity of cocaine. Pharmacol Toxicol 1993;72:3.

Carroll ME et al: Buprenorphine's effects on self-administration of smoked cocaine base and orally delivered phencyclidine, ethanol, and saccharin in Rhesus monkeys. J Pharmacol Exp Ther 1992;261:26.

Cigarette smoking-attributable mortality and years of potential life lost—United States, 1990. MMWR Morb Mortal Wkly Rep 1993;42:645.

Fiore MC et al: Tobacco dependence and the nicotine patch: Clinical guidelines for effective use. JAMA 1992; 268:2687.

Gourlay SG, Benowitz NL: Is clonidine an effective smoking cessation therapy? Drugs 1995;50:197.

Grabowski J, Dworkin SI: Cocaine: An overview of current issues. Int J Addict 1985;20:1065.

Insel TR et al: 3,4-Methylenedioxymethamphetamine ("ecstasy") selectively destroys brain serotonin terminals in rhesus monkeys. J Pharmacol Exp Ther 1989; 249:713.

Johanson C-E, Fischman MW: The pharmacology of cocaine related to its abuse. Pharmacol Rev 1989;41:3.

Kalix P, Braenden O: Pharmacological aspects of the chewing of khat leaves. Pharmacol Rev 1985;37:149.

Kosten TR, Kleber HD (editors): *Clinician's Guide to Cocaine Addiction: Theory, Research, and Treatment.* Guilford, 1992.

Kuhar MJ, Ritz MC, Boja JW: The dopamine hypothesis of the reinforcing properties of cocaine. Trends Neurosci 1991;14:299.

Mello NK et al: The effects of chronic buprenorphine treatment on cocaine and food self-administration by rhesus monkeys. J Pharmacol Exp Ther 1992;260:1185.

Pomerleau OF: Nicotine and the central nervous system: Biobehavioral effects of cigarette smoking. Am J Med 1992;93(Suppl 1A):1A.

Silverman K et al: Withdrawal syndrome after double-blind cessation of caffeine consumption. N Engl J Med 1992;327:1109.

Smith DE et al (editors): *Amphetamine Use, Misuse and Abuse.* GK Hall, 1979.

Tennant FS, Sagherian AA: Double-blind comparison of amantadine and bromocriptine for ambulatory withdrawal from cocaine dependence. Arch Intern Med 1987;147:109.

Volpe JJ: Effect of cocaine use on the fetus. N Engl J Med 1992;327:399.

Hallucinogens

Dilsaver SC: Antimuscarinic agents as substances of abuse: A review. J Clin Psychopharmacol 1988;8:14.

Hollister LE: *Chemical Psychoses: LSD and Related Drugs.* Thomas, 1968.

Johnson KM, Jones SM: Neuropharmacology of phencyclidine: Basic mechanisms and therapeutic potential. Annu Rev Pharmacol Toxicol 1990;30:707.

Lewin L: *Phantastica, Narcotic and Stimulating Drugs.* Dutton, 1931.

Pierce PA, Peroutka SJ: Antagonist properties of d-LSD at 5-hydroxytryptamine-2 receptors. Neuropsychopharmacology 1990;3:503.

Strassman RJ: Adverse reactions to psychedelic drugs: A review of the literature. J Nerv Ment Dis 1984; 172:577.

Cannabis

Bidaut-Russell M, Devane WA, Howlett AC: Cannabinoid receptors and modulation of cyclic AMP accumulation in the rat brain. J Neurochem 1990;55:21.

Block RI, Ghoneim MM: Effects of chronic marijuana use on human cognition. Psychopharmacology 1993; 110:219.

Devane WA et al: Isolation and structure of a brain constituent that binds to the cannabinoid receptor. Science 1992;258:1946.

Herkenhamer M et al: Cannabinoid receptor localization in brain. Proc Natl Acad Sci USA 1990;87:1932.

Hollister LE: Health aspects of cannabis. Pharmacol Rev 1986;38:1.

Howlett AC: Pharmacology of cannabinoid receptors. Annu Rev Pharmacol Toxicol 1995;35:607.

Thomas H: Psychiatric symptoms in cannabis users. Br J Psychiatry 1993;163:141.

Inhalants

Sharp CW, Carroll LT: *Voluntary Inhalation of Industrial Solvents.* DHEW Publication No. (ADM) 79-779, US Government Printing Office, 1979.

WHO: Report of the advisory group meeting on adverse health consequences of volatile solvents/inhalants. Mexican Institute of Psychiatry, Mexico City, Mexico. 1986;April 21.

Section VI.
Drugs Used to Treat Diseases of the Blood, Inflammation, & Gout

Agents Used in Anemias; Hematopoietic Growth Factors

33

Daniel V. Santi, MD, PhD, & Curt A. Ries, MD

Iron, vitamin B_{12}, and folic acid are chemically unrelated essential nutrients that are required for normal erythropoiesis. Deficiency of any of these substances results in severe anemia. Iron is required for hemoglobin production; in the absence of adequate iron, small red cells with insufficient hemoglobin are formed, giving rise to microcytic hypochromic anemia. Vitamin B_{12} and folic acid are required for normal DNA synthesis, and deficiency of either of these vitamins results in impaired production and abnormal maturation of erythroid precursor cells, giving rise to the characteristic blood and bone marrow picture known as megaloblastic anemia.

Erythropoietin and colony-stimulating factors are hormones that regulate blood cell development and proliferation in the marrow. These substances are found in such minute quantities in human tissues that insufficient amounts were available for study until recently. Recombinant DNA technology has made useful quantities of these substances available and is revolutionizing the treatment of certain disorders.

IRON

Basic Pharmacology

Iron forms the nucleus of the iron-porphyrin ring heme, which when combined with appropriate globin chains forms hemoglobin. Hemoglobin is a protein whose structure allows for reversible binding of oxygen, providing the critical mechanism for oxygen transport from the lungs to other tissues. Although iron is also present in other important proteins (myo-globin, cytochromes, etc), the vast majority is normally present in hemoglobin; therefore, anemia is the most prominent clinical feature of iron deficiency.

Iron distribution in normal adults is shown in Table 33–1. About 70% of the total body iron content is in the form of hemoglobin in red blood cells, and 10–20% is in the form of storage iron as ferritin and hemosiderin. Women in the reproductive age group usually have less storage iron than men because of iron losses from menstruation and pregnancies. About 10% of the iron is in myoglobin, a heme-containing protein in muscle. The remainder (< 1%) is distributed in trace amounts in cytochromes and other iron-containing enzymes and as transport iron or transferrin.

Pharmacokinetics

Iron is normally available in the diet from a wide variety of foods; dietary iron is usually in the form of heme or iron complexed to various organic compounds. Therapeutic iron, on the other hand, is usually given in the form of iron salts or iron complexed to inorganic substances. These different forms of iron differ widely in the amount of iron available for absorption, as discussed below.

A. Absorption: Iron is normally absorbed in the duodenum and proximal jejunum, though more distal small bowel sites can absorb iron if necessary. The average diet in the USA contains 10–15 mg of elemental iron daily. A normal individual without iron deficiency absorbs 5–10% of this iron, or about 0.5–1 mg daily. Iron absorption is increased in response to low iron stores or increased iron requirements. Total iron absorption increases to 1–2 mg/d in normal menstruating women and may be as high as 3–4 mg/d in preg-

Table 33–1. Iron distribution in normal adults.[1,2]

	Iron Content (mg)	
	Men	**Women**
Hemoglobin	3050	1700
Myoglobin	430	30
Enzymes	10	8
Transport (transferrin)	8	6
Storage (ferritin and hemosiderin)	750	300
Total	4248	2314

[1]Adapted, with permission, from Brown EB: Iron deficiency anemia. In: *Cecil Textbook of Medicine,* 16th ed. Wyngaarden JB, Smith LH (editors). Saunders, 1982.
[2]Values are based on data from various sources and assume that "normal" men weigh 80 kg and have a hemoglobin of 16 g/dL and that "normal" women weigh 55 kg and have a hemoglobin of 14 g/dL.

nant women. Infants and adolescents also have increased iron requirements during rapid growth periods. Iron is available in a wide variety of foods but is especially abundant in meat protein. The iron in meat protein is also more available for absorption and can be more efficiently absorbed, since heme iron in meat hemoglobin and myoglobin can be absorbed intact as hemin (the ferric form of heme) without first having to be broken down into elemental iron. Iron in other foods is often tightly bound to phytates or other complexing agents and may be much less available for absorption. Nonheme iron in foods and iron in inorganic iron salts and complexes must be converted to ferrous iron before it can be absorbed by the intestinal mucosal cells. Such absorption is decreased by the presence of chelators or complexing agents in the intestinal lumen and is increased in the presence of hydrochloric acid and vitamin C. Gastric resection decreases iron absorption by decreasing or eliminating hydrochloric acid production—and perhaps, even more importantly, by removing the site where food is digested to make dietary iron more available for absorption by the iron-absorbing areas in the duodenum and proximal jejunum.

Iron is transported across the intestinal mucosal cell by active transport. Absorbed ferrous iron is converted to ferric iron within the mucosal cell. Together with ferric iron split from hemin, the newly absorbed iron can be made available for immediate transport from the mucosal cell to the plasma via transferrin or can be converted to ferritin and stored in the mucosal cell. In general, when total body iron stores are high and iron requirements by the body are low, newly absorbed iron is diverted into ferritin in the intestinal mucosal cells rather than being transported to other sites. When iron stores are low or iron requirements are high, however, newly absorbed iron is immediately transported from the mucosal cells to the bone marrow for the production of hemoglobin.

B. Distribution: Iron is transported in the plasma bound to transferrin, a β-globulin that specifically binds ferric iron. Iron can thus be transported from intestinal mucosal cells or from storage sites in liver or spleen to the developing erythroid cells in bone marrow. The transferrin-ferric iron complex is delivered to maturing erythroid cells by a specific receptor mechanism. Transferrin receptors, which are integral membrane glycoproteins present in large numbers on proliferating erythroid cells, bind the transferrin-iron complex and internalize the iron, releasing it within the cell. The transferrin and transferrin receptor are then recycled, providing an efficient mechanism for incorporating iron into hemoglobin in developing red blood cells.

C. Storage: Iron can be stored in two forms: ferritin and hemosiderin. Ferritin, the most readily available form of storage iron, is a water-soluble complex consisting of a core crystal of ferric hydroxide covered by a protein shell of apoferritin. Hemosiderin is a particulate substance consisting of aggregates of ferric core crystals partially or completely stripped of apoferritin. Both ferritin and hemosiderin are stored in macrophages in the liver, spleen, and bone marrow; ferritin is also present in intestinal mucosal cells and in plasma. Since the ferritin present in plasma is in equilibrium with storage ferritin in reticuloendothelial tissues, the plasma (or serum) ferritin level can be used to estimate total body iron stores.

D. Elimination: There is no mechanism for excretion of iron. Small amounts of iron are lost by exfoliation of intestinal mucosal cells into the stool, and trace amounts are excreted in bile, urine, and sweat. These losses, however, can account for no more than 1 mg of iron per day. Because the body's ability to increase excretion of iron is so limited, regulation of iron balance must be achieved by changing intestinal absorption of iron, depending on the body's needs.

E. Regulation of Iron Pharmacokinetics: Iron absorption is regulated by the amount of storage iron present, especially the amount of ferritin present in the intestinal mucosal cells, and by the rate of erythropoiesis. Increased erythropoiesis is associated with an increase in the number of transferrin receptor sites on developing erythroid cells, and the availability of these receptor sites in some way directly increases the rate of iron absorption. Transferrin and ferritin are both present in intestinal mucosal cells, and both appear to regulate iron absorption. Transferrin is increased and ferritin decreased in iron deficiency, promoting increased iron absorption, while transferrin is decreased and ferritin increased in iron overload states, inhibiting further iron absorption.

Clinical Pharmacology

A. Indications for the Use of Iron: The only clinical indication for the use of iron preparations is the treatment or prevention of iron deficiency anemia. Iron deficiency is commonly seen in infants, especially premature infants; in children during rapid growth periods; and in pregnant and lactating women. These situations are all associated with increased iron requirements, and individuals in these settings are often given dietary supplements of oral iron to meet the increased need. Iron deficiency also occurs frequently after gastrectomy and in patients with severe small bowel disease that results in generalized malabsorption. Iron deficiency in these situations is due to inadequate iron absorption.

The most common cause of iron deficiency in adults, however, is blood loss. Menstruating women lose about 30 mg of iron with each menstrual period; women with heavy menstrual bleeding may lose much more. The most common site of unrecognized or occult blood loss is in the gastrointestinal tract. Patients with unexplained iron deficiency anemia must therefore always be evaluated for occult gastrointestinal bleeding, especially to exclude early gastrointestinal cancer, which may present with occult bleeding and anemia at a time when the cancer is still surgically curable. Simple nutritional iron deficiency due to inadequate diet is rare in adults and should never be accepted as an explanation of iron deficiency in a patient until a careful search has ruled out occult blood loss and other causes of iron deficiency.

Individuals suspected of being iron-deficient should generally have the diagnosis confirmed before being treated with iron preparations. As iron deficiency develops, storage iron decreases and then disappears; next, serum ferritin decreases; and then serum iron decreases and iron-binding capacity increases, resulting in a decrease in iron-binding (transferrin) saturation. Thereafter, anemia begins to develop. Red cell indices (mean corpuscular volume [MCV]: normal = 80–100 fL; mean corpuscular hemoglobin concentration [MCHC]: normal = 32–36 g/dL) are usually low normal when iron deficiency anemia is mild, but cells become progressively more microcytic and hypochromic as anemia becomes more severe. By the time iron deficiency is diagnosed, serum iron is usually less than 40 µg/dL; total iron-binding capacity (TIBC) is greater than 400 µg/dL; iron-binding saturation is less than 10%; and serum ferritin is less than 10 µg/L. One of the most sensitive ways to detect early iron deficiency is to examine bone marrow stained to detect the presence or absence of storage iron.

B. Treatment: The treatment of iron deficiency anemia consists of administration of oral or parenteral iron preparations. Oral iron corrects the deficiency just as rapidly and completely as parenteral iron in most cases if iron absorption from the gastrointestinal tract is normal.

1. Oral iron therapy—A wide variety of oral iron preparations are available. Since ferrous iron is most efficiently absorbed, only ferrous salts should be used. Ferrous sulfate, ferrous gluconate, and ferrous fumarate are all effective and inexpensive and are rec-

ommended for the treatment of most patients. Supplementation with vitamin C and other nutrients is generally not necessary. Sustained-release and enteric-coated iron preparations should not be used, since iron is best absorbed in the duodenum and proximal jejunum.

Different iron salts provide different amounts of elemental iron, as shown in Table 33–2. In an iron-deficient individual, about 50–100 mg of iron can be incorporated into hemoglobin daily, and about 25% of oral iron given as ferrous salt can be absorbed. Therefore, 200–400 mg of elemental iron should be given daily to correct iron deficiency most rapidly. Patients unable to tolerate such large doses of iron can be given lower daily doses of iron, which results in slower but still complete correction of iron deficiency.

Treatment with oral iron should be continued for 3–6 months. This will not only correct the anemia but will replenish iron stores. The first measurable response to successful iron therapy can be seen in less than a week, when brisk reticulocytosis occurs, as newly formed hemoglobin-filled red cells from bone marrow enter the bloodstream. The hemoglobin level should increase significantly in 2–4 weeks and should reach normal levels (men = 14–18 g/dL; women = 12–16 g/dL) in 1–3 months. Failure to respond to oral iron therapy may be due to incorrect diagnosis (anemia due to causes other than iron deficiency), continued iron loss (usually secondary to continued blood loss), concurrent chronic inflammation or other illness that suppresses marrow function, or failure of the patient to take or absorb the oral iron.

Common adverse effects of oral iron therapy include nausea, epigastric discomfort, abdominal cramps, constipation, and diarrhea. These effects are usually dose-related and can often be overcome by lowering the daily dose of iron or by taking the tablets immediately after or with meals. Some patients have less severe gastrointestinal adverse effects with one iron salt than another and benefit from changing preparations. Patients taking oral iron develop black stools; this itself has no clinical significance but may obscure the diagnosis of continued gastrointestinal blood loss.

Table 33–2. Some commonly used oral iron preparations.

Preparation	Tablet Size	Elemental Iron per Tablet	Usual Adult Dosage (Tablets per Day)
Ferrous sulfate, hydrated	325 mg	65 mg	3–4
Ferrous sulfate, desiccated	200 mg	65 mg	3–4
Ferrous gluconate	320 mg	37 mg	3–4
Ferrous fumarate	200 mg	66 mg	3–4
Ferrous fumarate	325 mg	106 mg	2–3

2. Parenteral iron therapy–Parenteral therapy should be reserved for patients with documented iron deficiency unable to tolerate or absorb oral iron and patients with extensive chronic blood loss who cannot be maintained with oral iron alone. This includes patients with various postgastrectomy conditions and previous small bowel resection, inflammatory bowel disease involving the proximal small bowel, malabsorption syndromes, and chronic heavy bleeding from nonresectable lesions, as may occur in hereditary hemorrhagic telangiectasia.

Iron dextran is a stable complex of ferric hydroxide and low-molecular-weight dextran containing 50 mg of elemental iron per milliliter of solution. It can be given either by deep intramuscular injection (using the "Z track" injection technique to avoid local tissue staining) or by intravenous infusion. Adverse effects of parenteral iron therapy include local pain and tissue staining (brown discoloration of the tissues overlying the injection site), headache, light-headedness, fever, arthralgias, nausea and vomiting, back pain, flushing, urticaria, bronchospasm, and, rarely, anaphylaxis and death.

The total amount of parenteral iron required to correct iron deficiency anemia and to replenish iron stores in a 70 kg adult can be calculated as follows: grams of iron required = 0.25 × (normal hemoglobin – patient's hemoglobin). Most adults with iron deficiency anemia thus require 1–2 g of replacement iron, or 20–40 mL of iron dextran. Although this amount of parenteral iron can be given as 10–20 daily intramuscular injections, most physicians now prefer to give the entire calculated dose in a single intravenous infusion in several hundred milliliters of normal saline over 1–2 hours. Intravenous administration eliminates the local pain and tissue staining that often occur with the intramuscular route and allows delivery of the entire dose of iron necessary to correct the iron deficiency at one time. There is no clear evidence that any of the adverse effects, including anaphylaxis, are more likely to occur with intravenous than with intramuscular administration.

A small test dose of iron dextran should always be given before full intramuscular or intravenous doses are given. A dose of 0.25–0.5 mL can be given by deep intramuscular injection or slow intravenous infusion of very dilute solution over 30–60 minutes before proceeding with full therapy. If signs or symptoms of an immediate hypersensitivity reaction occur, additional parenteral iron should not be given, and alternative therapy must be considered. Patients with a strong history of allergy and patients who have previously received parenteral iron are more likely to have hypersensitivity reactions following treatment with parenteral iron dextran than those who have not.

Clinical Toxicity

A. Acute Iron Toxicity: Acute iron toxicity is seen almost exclusively in young children who have ingested a number of iron tablets. Although adults appear to be able to tolerate large doses of oral iron without serious consequences, as few as ten tablets of any of the commonly available oral iron preparations can be lethal in young children. Oral iron preparations should therefore always be stored in "childproof" containers and kept out of the reach of children.

Large amounts of oral iron cause necrotizing gastroenteritis, with vomiting, abdominal pain, and bloody diarrhea followed by shock, lethargy, and dyspnea. Subsequently, improvement is often noted, but this may be followed by severe metabolic acidosis, coma, and death. Urgent treatment of acute iron toxicity is necessary, especially in young children. Gastric aspiration should be performed, followed by lavage with carbonate solutions to form insoluble iron salts. Deferoxamine, a potent iron chelating compound, should be given systemically by intermittent intramuscular injection or by continuous intravenous infusion to bind iron that has already been absorbed and to promote its excretion in urine and feces. Some investigators advise also instilling deferoxamine into the stomach to bind any remaining free iron in the gut, but this is controversial. Appropriate supportive therapy for gastrointestinal bleeding, metabolic acidosis, and shock must also be provided (see Chapter 59).

B. Chronic Iron Toxicity: Chronic iron toxicity (iron overload), also known as hemochromatosis and hemosiderosis, results when excess iron is deposited in the heart, liver, pancreas, and other organs. It can lead to organ failure and death. It most commonly occurs in patients with hemochromatosis, an inherited disorder characterized by excessive iron absorption, and in patients who receive many red cell transfusions (each transfusion containing 250 mg of iron) over a long period of time. It is doubtful that clinically significant iron overload can occur in normal individuals who chronically ingest excess iron, because of the protective mechanisms that normally regulate iron absorption and because of the very large amounts of total body iron needed before clinical iron overload becomes apparent. However, continued ingestion of excess iron probably contributes to the development of iron overload in patients who have a higher than normal baseline iron absorption, whether due to inherited factors (subclinical hemochromatosis, etc) or to the presence of anemias other than those due to iron deficiency (anemia of chronic disease, hemolytic anemias, etc).

Chronic iron overload in the absence of anemia is most efficiently treated by intermittent phlebotomy. One unit of blood (containing 250 mg of iron) can be removed every week or so until all of the excess iron is removed. Iron chelation therapy using parenteral deferoxamine is much less efficient as well as more complicated, expensive, and hazardous, but it can be useful for severe iron overload that cannot be managed by phlebotomy.

VITAMIN B$_{12}$ & FOLIC ACID

Basic Pharmacology

Vitamin B$_{12}$ and folic acid are chemically unrelated vitamins essential for normal DNA synthesis. Deficiencies lead to impaired DNA synthesis, inhibition of normal mitosis, and abnormal maturation and function of the cells produced. These changes are most apparent in tissues where cells undergo rapid cell division, such as the bone marrow and the gastrointestinal epithelium, but all dividing cells are affected to some degree. Severe anemia is the chief finding in patients with vitamin B$_{12}$ or folic acid deficiency, but pancytopenia (diminished production of red blood cells, white blood cells, and platelets) may occur, and gastrointestinal symptoms are common. Neurologic abnormalities may also occur in vitamin B$_{12}$ deficiency but not in folic acid deficiency (see Clinical Pharmacology, below).

Anemias caused by vitamin B$_{12}$ and folic acid deficiency have a characteristic appearance of peripheral blood and bone marrow called megaloblastic anemia. Since the underlying defect in megaloblastic anemias is impaired DNA synthesis, there is diminished cell division in the face of continued RNA and protein synthesis. This leads to production of large (macrocytic) red blood cells that have a high RNA:DNA ratio and are defective in the sense that they are highly susceptible to destruction. Morphologically, the bone marrow is hypercellular, with a marked increase in the number of large abnormal early red cell precursors (megaloblasts) but with very few cells maturing beyond this stage to become circulating red cells. The red cells that do form in the bone marrow characteristically show normal cytoplasmic maturation, including normal hemoglobin formation; it is nuclear maturation and cell division that are impaired in the megaloblastic anemias.

Although megaloblastic anemia can theoretically result from any event that impairs DNA synthesis, in practice almost all cases are due to deficiencies of vitamin B$_{12}$ or folic acid. The biochemical and physiologic bases of these deficiencies are now well understood, and it is possible to describe the mechanisms causing these anemias at the molecular level.

Chemistry

A. Vitamin B$_{12}$: Vitamin B$_{12}$ is made up of a porphyrin-like ring with a central cobalt atom attached to a nucleotide (Figure 33–1). Various ligands may be covalently bound to the cobalt atom, forming different cobalamins. Deoxyadenosylcobalamin and methylcobalamin are the active forms of the vitamin in humans. **Cyanocobalamin** and **hydroxocobalamin** (both available for therapeutic use) and other cobalamins found in food sources must be converted to the above active forms. The ultimate source of vitamin

Figure 33–1. Cobalamin; vitamin B$_{12}$ ($C_{63}H_{88}O_{14}N_{14}PCo$). (Reproduced, with permission, from Murray RK et al: *Harper's Biochemistry*, 24th ed. Appleton & Lange, 1996.)

B_{12} is from microbial synthesis; the vitamin is not synthesized by animals or plants. The chief dietary source of vitamin B_{12} is microbially derived vitamin B_{12} in meat (especially liver), eggs, and dairy products. Vitamin B_{12} is sometimes called **extrinsic factor** to differentiate it from intrinsic factor, a substance normally secreted by the stomach.

B. Folic Acid: Folic acid (pteroylglutamic acid) is a compound composed of a pteridine heterocycle, *p*-aminobenzoic acid, and glutamic acid (Figure 33–2). Various numbers of glutamic acid moieties may be attached to the pteroyl portion of the molecule, resulting in monoglutamates, triglutamates, or polyglutamates. The fully oxidized pteridine ring of folic acid can undergo reduction, catalyzed by the enzyme dihydrofolate reductase, to give 7,8-dihydrofolic acid (H_2folate) and then to the fully reduced 5,6,7,8-tetrahydrofolic acid (H_4folate) (Figure 33–3). H_4folate can subsequently be transformed to folate cofactors possessing one-carbon units attached to the 5-nitrogen (5-CH_3–H_4folate and 5-CHO–H_4folate), the 10-nitrogen (10-CHO–H_4folate), or both positions (5,10-CH_2–H_4folate and 5,10-CH^+–H_4folate) (Figure 33–4). The folate cofactors are interconvertible by various enzymatic reactions and serve the important biochemical function of donating one-carbon units at various levels of oxidation. In most instances, H_4folate is regenerated in these reactions and is available for reutilization. Various forms of folic acid are present in a wide variety of plant and animal tissues; the richest sources are yeast, liver, kidney, and green vegetables.

Pharmacokinetics

A. Vitamin B_{12}: The average diet in the USA contains 5–30 μg of vitamin B_{12} daily, 1–5 μg of which is usually absorbed. The vitamin is avidly stored, primarily in the liver, with an average adult having a total vitamin B_{12} storage pool of 3000–5000 μg. Only

Figure 33–3. The reduction of folic acid to dihydrofolic acid and dihydrofolic acid to tetrahydrofolic acid by the enzyme dihydrofolate reductase. (Modified and reproduced, with permission, from Murray RK et al: *Harper's Biochemistry,* 24th ed. Appleton & Lange, 1996.)

Figure 33–2. The structure and numbering of atoms of folic acid. (Reproduced, with permission, from Murray RK et al: *Harper's Biochemistry,* 24th ed. Appleton & Lange, 1996.)

trace amounts of vitamin B_{12} are normally lost in urine and stool. Since the normal daily requirements of vitamin B_{12} are only about 2 μg, it would take about 5 years for all of the stored vitamin B_{12} to be exhausted and for megaloblastic anemia to develop if B_{12} absorption stopped. Vitamin B_{12} in physiologic amounts is absorbed only after it complexes with intrinsic factor. Intrinsic factor is a glycoprotein with a molecular weight of about 50,000 that is secreted by the parietal cells of the gastric mucosa. Intrinsic factor combines with vitamin B_{12} liberated from dietary sources in the stomach and duodenum, and the intrinsic factor-vitamin B_{12} complex is subsequently absorbed in the distal ileum by a highly specific receptor-mediated transport system. Vitamin B_{12} deficiency in humans most often results from malabsorption of vitamin B_{12}, due either to lack of intrinsic factor or to loss or malfunction of the specific absorptive mechanism in the distal ileum.

Figure 33–4. The interconversions of one-carbon moieties attached to tetrahydrofolate. (Modified and reproduced, with permission, from Murray RK et al: *Harper's Biochemistry*, 24th ed. Lange, 1996.)

Once absorbed, vitamin B_{12} is transported to the various cells of the body bound to a plasma glycoprotein, transcobalamin II. Excess vitamin B_{12} is transported to the liver for storage. Significant amounts of vitamin B_{12} are excreted in the urine only when very large amounts are given parenterally, overcoming the binding capacities of the transcobalamins (50–100 μg).

B. Folic Acid: The average diet in the USA contains 500–700 μg of folates daily, 50–200 μg of which is usually absorbed, depending on metabolic requirements (pregnant women may absorb as much as 300–400 μg of folic acid daily). Normally, 5–20 mg of folates is stored in the liver and other tissues. Folates are excreted in the urine and stool and are also destroyed by catabolism, so serum levels fall within a few days when intake is diminished. Since body stores of folates are relatively low and daily requirements high, folic acid deficiency and megaloblastic anemia can develop within 1–6 months after the intake of folic acid stops, depending on the patient's nutritional status and the rate of folate utilization.

Unaltered folic acid is readily and completely absorbed in the proximal jejunum. Dietary folates, however, consist primarily of polyglutamate forms of 5-CH_3—H_4folate, with very little unmodified folate present. Before absorption, all but one of the glutamyl residues of the polyglutamates must be hydrolyzed by the enzyme α-L-glutamyl transferase ("conjugase") within the brush border of the intestinal mucosa. The monoglutamate 5-CH_3–H_4folate is subsequently transported into the bloodstream, both by active and passive transport, and then widely distributed throughout the body.

Pharmacodynamics

A. Vitamin B_{12}: There are two essential enzymatic reactions in humans that require vitamin B_{12} (Figure 33–5). In one reaction, deoxyadenosylcobalamin is a required cofactor in the conversion of methylmalonyl-CoA to succinyl-CoA by the enzyme methylmalonyl-CoA mutase. In vitamin B_{12} deficiency, this conversion cannot take place, and the substrate, methylmalonyl-CoA, accumulates. As a result, abnormal fatty acids are synthesized and incorporated into cell membranes. It is believed that incorporation of such nonphysiologic fatty acids into cell membranes of the central nervous system is responsible for the neurologic manifestations of vitamin B_{12} deficiency.

The other enzymatic reaction that requires vitamin B_{12} is conversion of 5-CH_3–H_4folate and homocysteine to H_4folate and methionine by the enzyme 5-CH_3–H_4folate-homocysteine methyltransferase (Fig-

A. Methylmalonyl-CoA mutase

B. 5-CH$_3$ — H$_4$folate-homocysteine methyltransferase

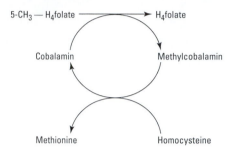

Figure 33–5. Enzymatic reactions that use vitamin B$_{12}$.

ure 33–5B). In this reaction, cobalamin and methyl-cobalamin are interconverted, and the vitamin may be considered a true catalyst. When vitamin B$_{12}$ deficiency occurs, conversion of the major dietary and storage folate, 5-CH$_3$–H$_4$folate, to the precursor of folate cofactors, H$_4$folate, cannot occur. As a result, 5-CH$_3$–H$_4$folate accumulates, and a deficiency of folate cofactors necessary for DNA synthesis develops. This accumulation of the body's folate as 5-CH$_3$–H$_4$folate and the associated inability to form folate cofactors in vitamin B$_{12}$ deficiency have been referred to as the "methylfolate trap." This is the biochemical step whereby vitamin B$_{12}$ and folic acid metabolism are linked and explains why the megaloblastic anemia of vitamin B$_{12}$ deficiency (but not the neurologic abnormalities) can be partially corrected by folic acid.

B. Folic Acid: As noted above, the ultimate role of the folates is the formation of folate cofactors essential for one-carbon transfer reactions necessary for DNA synthesis. The de novo synthesis of the purine heterocycle involves two enzymatic reactions that use folate cofactors. In these, 10-CHO–H$_4$folate and 5,10-CH$^+$–H$_4$folate (Figure 33–4) donate their one-carbon units to ultimately form carbons 2 and 8 of the purine heterocycle. In both of these reactions, H$_4$folate is regenerated and can again accept a one-carbon unit and reenter the H$_4$folate cofactor pool.

Another essential reaction in which a folate cofactor is necessary is the synthesis of thymidylic acid (2′-deoxythymidine monophosphate; dTMP), an essential precursor of DNA. In this reaction, the enzyme thymidylate synthase catalyzes the transfer of the one-carbon unit of 5,10-CH$_2$–H$_4$folate to the 5-position of 2′-deoxyuridine monophosphate (dUMP) to form dTMP (Figure 33–6). Unlike all of the other enzy-

matic reactions that utilize folate cofactors, in this reaction the cofactor is oxidized to H$_2$folate, and for each mole of dTMP produced, a mole of H$_4$folate is consumed. In rapidly proliferating tissues, considerable amounts of H$_4$folate can be consumed in this reaction, and continued DNA synthesis requires continued regeneration of H$_4$folate by reduction of H$_2$folate, catalyzed by the enzyme dihydrofolate reductase. The H$_4$folate thus produced can then re-form the cofactor CH$_2$–H$_4$folate by the action of serine transhydroxymethylase and thus allow for the continued synthesis of dTMP. The combined catalytic activities of dTMP synthetase, dihydrofolate reductase, and serine transhydroxymethylase are often referred to as the **dTMP synthesis cycle** (Figure 33–7).

Clinical Pharmacology

Vitamin B$_{12}$ and folic acid are used mainly to treat or prevent deficiencies of these vitamins. There is no evidence that vitamin B$_{12}$ injections have any benefit in persons who do not have vitamin B$_{12}$ deficiency. Supplemental folic acid, however, may be useful in preventing folic acid deficiency in certain high-risk patients with high folate requirements.

The most characteristic clinical manifestation of vitamin B$_{12}$ and folic acid deficiency is megaloblastic anemia. Any patient with macrocytosis, with or without anemia, should be evaluated for possible vitamin B$_{12}$ or folic acid deficiency. Although most patients with neurologic abnormalities caused by vitamin B$_{12}$ deficiency have full-blown megaloblastic anemia when first seen, occasional patients have few if any hematologic abnormalities, and the diagnosis of vitamin B$_{12}$ deficiency may at first be obscure. It is particularly important to differentiate vitamin B$_{12}$ deficiency from other forms of megaloblastic anemia, since treatment with vitamin B$_{12}$ must be continued for life in most cases and the hematologic abnormalities in vitamin B$_{12}$ deficiency may be partially corrected by treatment with large doses of folic acid while the neurologic damage progresses and may become irreversible.

The typical clinical findings in megaloblastic anemia are macrocytic anemia (MCV usually > 120 fL), often with associated mild or moderate leukopenia or thrombocytopenia (or both), and a characteristic hypercellular bone marrow with megaloblastic maturation of erythroid and other precursor cells. Once a diagnosis of megaloblastic anemia is made, it must be determined whether vitamin B$_{12}$ or folic acid deficiency is the cause. (Other causes of megaloblastic anemia are very rare.) This can usually be accomplished by measuring serum levels of the vitamins, though these measurements occasionally give false-positive or false-negative results. Red blood cell folic acid levels are often of greater diagnostic value than serum levels, since serum folic acid levels tend to be quite labile and do not necessarily reflect tissue levels. The Schilling test, which measures absorption and urinary excretion of radioactively labeled vitamin B$_{12}$,

Figure 33–6. The transfer of a methyl moiety from N^5, N^{10}-methylene-H_4folate to deoxyuridylate to generate deoxythymidylate and dihydrofolate (H_2folate). (Modified and reproduced, with permission, from Murray RK et al: *Harper's Biochemistry*, 24th ed. Lange, 1996.)

can be used to further define the mechanism of vitamin B_{12} malabsorption when this is found to be the cause of the megaloblastic anemia.

A. Vitamin B_{12} Deficiency: Vitamin B_{12} deficiency is almost always caused by malabsorption of vitamin B_{12}, due either to deficiency of intrinsic factor or to defects in the absorption of the vitamin B_{12}-intrinsic factor complex in the distal ileum. The most common causes of vitamin B_{12} deficiency are pernicious anemia, partial or total gastrectomy, and diseases that affect the distal ileum, such as malabsorption syndromes, inflammatory bowel disease, or small bowel resection. Nutritional deficiency of vitamin B_{12} is rare but may be seen in strict vegetarians after many years without meat, eggs, or dairy products.

Pernicious anemia results from defective secretion of **intrinsic factor** by the gastric mucosal cells. It is most common in older individuals of northern European extraction, but it may occur at any age and in all races. Patients with pernicious anemia have gastric atrophy and fail to secrete hydrochloric acid (as well as intrinsic factor). The Schilling test shows diminished absorption of radioactively labeled vitamin B_{12}, which is corrected when hog intrinsic factor is administered with radioactive B_{12}, since the vitamin can then be normally absorbed. Pernicious anemia is a lifelong disease, and treatment with vitamin B_{12} injections must be continued indefinitely.

Total or partial gastrectomy removes the parietal cell-containing portion of the stomach that secretes intrinsic factor, resulting in vitamin B_{12} malabsorption similar to that seen in pernicious anemia. Since vita-

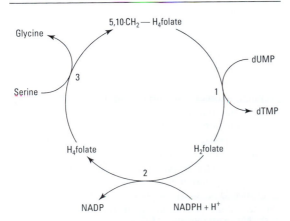

Figure 33–7. dTMP synthesis cycle. (1) dTMP synthetase; (2) H_2folate reductase; (3) serine transhydroxymethylase.

min B_{12} stores may not be exhausted until 5 years after gastrectomy, megaloblastic anemia will not develop until that time; however, many clinicians routinely start patients on vitamin B_{12} injections after gastrectomy to avoid any chance that vitamin B_{12} deficiency will develop later.

Vitamin B_{12} deficiency also occurs when the region of the distal ileum that absorbs the vitamin B_{12}-intrinsic factor complex is damaged, as when the ileum is involved with inflammatory bowel disease or sprue, or when the ileum is surgically resected. In these situations, radioactively labeled vitamin B_{12} is not absorbed in the Schilling test, even when intrinsic factor is added. Other rare causes of vitamin B_{12} deficiency include bacterial overgrowth of the small bowel, blind loop syndrome, fish tapeworm, chronic pancreatitis, and thyroid disease. Rare cases of vitamin B_{12} deficiency in children have been found to be secondary to congenital deficiency of intrinsic factor and congenital selective vitamin B_{12} malabsorption due to defects of the receptor sites in the distal ileum.

Since almost all cases of vitamin B_{12} deficiency are caused by malabsorption of the vitamin, parenteral injections of vitamin B_{12} are required for therapy. For patients with potentially reversible diseases (fish tapeworm, sprue, blind loops), the underlying disease should be treated after initial treatment with parenteral vitamin B_{12}. Most patients, however, do not have curable deficiency syndromes and require lifelong treatment with vitamin B_{12} injections.

Vitamin B_{12} for parenteral injection is available as cyanocobalamin or hydroxocobalamin. Hydroxocobalamin is preferred because it is more highly protein-bound and therefore remains longer in the circulation. Initial therapy should consist of 100–1000 µg of vitamin B_{12} intramuscularly daily or every other day for 1–2 weeks to replenish body stores. Maintenance therapy consists of 100–1000 µg intramuscularly once a month for life. If neurologic abnormalities are present, vitamin B_{12} injections should be given every 1–2 weeks for 6 months before switching to monthly injections. Oral vitamin B_{12}-intrinsic factor mixtures and liver extracts should not be used to treat vitamin B_{12} deficiency; however, oral doses of 1000 µg of vitamin B_{12} daily are usually sufficient to treat patients with pernicious anemia who refuse or cannot tolerate the injections.

The hematologic response to treatment with vitamin B_{12} is rapid. The bone marrow usually returns to normal within 48 hours. Reticulocytosis begins on the second or third day and is usually maximal by the fifth to tenth days. Hemoglobin begins to increase in the first week and returns to normal by 1–2 months. Incomplete correction of the anemia may be due to persistence of other deficiencies (ie, combined vitamin B_{12} and iron deficiency) or the presence of inflammatory disease or other disorders that inhibit erythropoiesis.

B. Folic Acid Deficiency: Folic acid deficiency, unlike vitamin B_{12} deficiency, is often caused by inadequate dietary intake of folates. Elderly patients, poor patients, and food faddists whose diets lack vegetables, eggs, and meat often develop folic acid deficiency. Prolonged cooking of vegetables destroys folates and can lead to folic acid deficiency if this is the only dietary source of this vitamin. Alcoholics and patients with liver disease develop folic acid deficiency because of poor diet and diminished hepatic storage of folates. There is also evidence that alcohol and liver disease interfere with absorption and metabolism of folates. Pregnant women and patients with hemolytic anemia have increased folate requirements and may become folic acid-deficient, especially if their diets are marginal. Recent evidence implicates maternal folic acid deficiency in the occurrence of fetal neural tube defects, eg, spina bifida. Patients with sprue and other malabsorption syndromes also frequently develop folic acid deficiency, perhaps because of a lack of intestinal conjugase. Folic acid deficiency is occasionally associated with cancer, leukemia, myeloproliferative disorders, certain chronic skin disorders, and other chronic debilitating diseases. Patients who require renal dialysis also develop folic acid deficiency, because folates are removed from the plasma each time the patient is dialyzed.

Folic acid deficiency can also be caused by drugs that interfere with folate absorption or metabolism. Phenytoin, some other anticonvulsants, oral contraceptives, and isoniazid can cause folic acid deficiency by interfering with folic acid absorption, possibly by inhibiting intestinal folate conjugases. Other drugs such as methotrexate and, to a lesser extent, trimethoprim and pyrimethamine, inhibit dihydrofolate reductase and may result in a deficiency of folate cofactors and ultimately in megaloblastic anemia (Figure 33–3).

Parenteral administration of folic acid is rarely necessary, since oral folic acid is well absorbed even in patients with malabsorption syndromes. A dose of 1 mg of folic acid orally daily is sufficient to reverse megaloblastic anemia, restore normal serum folate levels, and replenish body stores of folates in almost all patients. Therapy should be continued until the underlying cause of the deficiency is removed or corrected. Therapy may be required indefinitely for patients with malabsorption or dietary inadequacy. Folic acid supplementation to prevent folic acid deficiency should be considered in high-risk patients, including pregnant women, alcoholics, and patients with hemolytic anemia, liver disease, certain skin diseases, and patients on renal dialysis.

The response of patients with folate deficiency to treatment with oral folic acid is rapid and complete and similar to the response of the vitamin B_{12}-deficient patient given parenteral vitamin B_{12}. The hemoglobin level should begin to rise within the first week, and the anemia should be completely corrected in 1–2 months.

C. Miscellaneous Uses:

1. Coronary artery disease—Recent studies have suggested that a high serum concentration of homocysteine (hyperhomocysteinemia) is an independent risk factor for coronary artery disease. Mild elevations of serum homocysteine can easily be reduced by treatment with folic acid and vitamin B_{12}. Clinical studies of this potential risk-reducing therapy are under way.

2. Cyanide poisoning–Hydroxocobalamin is an avid complexing agent for cyanide ion. Several studies show that it is an effective antidote for cyanide poisoning if administered soon enough. The major limitation to this application in the past has been the lack of availability in large-dose formulations. Note that cyanocobalamin is of no value in this application.

3. Prevention of fetal neural tube defects–Several large controlled trials have shown that folic acid supplementation during pregnancy reduces the incidence of neural tube defects, especially spine bifida, in the infant. The United States Public Health Service has therefore recommended that all women capable of becoming pregnant should consume a minimum of 0.4 mg folic acid daily. Unless otherwise indicated, care should be taken to keep daily intake below 1 mg to avoid complicating the diagnosis of pernicious anemia.

Clinical Toxicology

Vitamin B_{12} and folic acid have no known toxic effects even when administered in very large amounts. Large doses of both vitamins are promptly excreted in urine and to a lesser extent in stool, so that prolonged tissue exposure to very high levels does not occur. There is no evidence that cyanocobalamin, even in huge doses, causes cyanide poisoning.

HEMATOPOIETIC GROWTH FACTORS

The hematopoietic growth factors are glycoprotein hormones that regulate the proliferation and differentiation of hematopoietic progenitor cells in the bone marrow. The first growth factors identified were called colony-stimulating factors because they could stimulate the growth of colonies of various bone marrow progenitor cells in vitro. In the past decade, many of these growth factors have been purified and cloned, and their effects on hematopoiesis have been extensively studied (Table 33-3). Quantities of these growth factors sufficient for clinical use have been produced by recombinant DNA technology.

Of the known hematopoietic growth factors, **erythropoietin, granulocyte colony-stimulating factor** (G-CSF), and **granulocyte-macrophage colony-stimulating factor** (GM-CSF) are currently available and in clinical use. Interleukin-3 (IL-3), stem cell factor (SCF), and monocyte-macrophage colony-stimulating factor (M-CSF) are currently undergoing clinical trials and will probably become available in the next year or so. The other potentially useful hematopoietic growth factors listed in Table 33-3 are still in preclinical development.

ERYTHROPOIETIN

Chemistry & Pharmacokinetics

Erythropoietin was the first human hematopoietic growth factor to be isolated. It was first purified from

Table 33–3. Hematopoietic growth factors.

Growth Factor	Progenitor Cell Lines Stimulated				
	Red Cells	Granulocytes	Monocytes-Macrophages	Megakaryocytes-Platelets	Other
Epo	✔				
G-CSF		✔			
M-CSF			✔		
GM-CSF	✔	✔	✔	✔	Eosinophils
IL-3	✔	✔	✔	✔	Eosinophils, basophils
SCF	✔	✔	✔	✔	Eosinophils, basophils, lymphocytes
IL-6		✔	✔	✔	Lymphocytes
IL-9, IL-11				✔	Lymphocytes

Key:
  EPO   = Erythropoietin
  G-CSF   = Granulocyte colony-stimulating factor (filgrastim)
  M-CSF   = Monocyte-macrophage colony-stimulating factor
  GM-CSF = Granulocyte-macrophage colony-stimulating factor (sargramostim)
  IL   = Interleukin
  SCF   = Stem cell factor

the urine of patients with severe anemia. Recombinant human erythropoietin (rHuEpo, epoetin alfa) is produced in a mammalian cell expression system using recombinant DNA technology. It is a heavily glycosylated peptide of 165 amino acids with a molecular weight of 30,400. After intravenous administration, Erythropoietin has a serum half-life of 4–13 hours in patients with chronic renal failure. It is not cleared by dialysis. It is measured in international units (IU).

Pharmacodynamics

Erythropoietin stimulates erythroid proliferation and differentiation by interacting with specific erythropoietin receptors on red cell progenitors in the bone marrow. Endogenous erythropoietin is produced by the kidney in response to tissue hypoxia. When anemia occurs, more erythropoietin is produced by the kidney, signaling the bone marrow to produce more red blood cells. This results in correction of the anemia provided that bone marrow response is not impaired by red cell nutritional deficiency (especially iron deficiency), primary bone marrow disorders (see below), or bone marrow suppression from drugs or chronic diseases.

Normally there is an inverse relationship between the hematocrit or hemoglobin level and the serum erythropoietin level. Nonanemic individuals have serum erythropoietin levels of less than 20 IU/L. As the hematocrit and hemoglobin level fall and anemia becomes more severe, the serum erythropoietin level rises exponentially. Patients with moderately severe anemias usually have erythropoietin levels in the 100–500 IU/L range, and patients with severe anemias may have levels of thousands of IU/L. The most important exception to this inverse relationship is in the anemia of chronic renal failure. In patients with renal disease, erythropoietin levels are usually low because the kidneys cannot produce the growth factor. These patients are the most likely to respond to treatment with exogenous erythropoietin. In most primary bone marrow disorders (aplastic anemia, leukemias, myeloproliferative and myelodysplastic disorders, etc) and most nutritional and secondary anemias, endogenous erythropoietin levels are high, so there is less likelihood of a response to erythropoietin (but see below).

Clinical Pharmacology

Erythropoietin is indicated in the treatment of renal failure patients with significant anemia. Erythropoietin consistently improves the hematocrit and hemoglobin level and usually eliminates the need for transfusions in these patients. An increase in reticulocyte count is usually observed in about 10 days and an increase in hematocrit and hemoglobin levels in 2–6 weeks. Most patients can maintain a hematocrit of about 35% with erythropoietin doses of 50–150 IU/kg intravenously or subcutaneously 3 times a week. Failure to respond to erythropoietin is most commonly due to concurrent iron deficiency, which can be corrected by giving oral iron. Folate supplementation may also be necessary in some patients.

Erythropoietin may also be useful for the treatment of anemia with primary bone marrow disorders and secondary anemias in selected patients. This includes patients with aplastic anemia and other bone marrow failure states, myeloproliferative and myelodysplastic disorders, multiple myeloma and perhaps other chronic bone marrow malignancies, and the anemias associated with chronic inflammation, AIDS, and cancer. Patients with these disorders who have disproportionately low serum erythropoietin levels for their degree of anemia are most likely to respond to treatment with this growth factor. Patients with endogenous erythropoietin levels of less than 100 IU/L have the best chance of response, though patients with erythropoietin levels between 100 and 500 IU/L respond occasionally. These patients generally require higher erythropoietin doses (150–300 IU/kg 3 times a week) to achieve a response, and responses are often incomplete.

Erythropoietin has also been used successfully to offset the anemia produced by zidovudine treatment in patients with HIV infection and in the treatment of the anemia of prematurity. It can also be used to accelerate erythropoiesis after phlebotomies, when blood is being collected for autologous transfusion for elective surgery, or for treatment of iron overload (hemochromatosis).

Toxicity

The most common side effects of erythropoietin are associated with a rapid increase in hematocrit and hemoglobin and include hypertension and thrombotic complications. These difficulties can be minimized by raising the hematocrit and hemoglobin slowly and by adequately monitoring and treating hypertension. Allergic reactions have been infrequent and mild.

MYELOID GROWTH FACTORS

Chemistry & Pharmacokinetics

G-CSF and GM-CSF, the only myeloid growth factors currently available for clinical use, were originally purified from cultured human cell lines. Recombinant human G-CSF (rHuG-CSF; filgrastim) is produced in a bacterial expression system using recombinant DNA technology. It is a nonglycosylated peptide of 175 amino acids, with a molecular weight of 18,800. Recombinant human GM-CSF (rHuGM-CSF; sargramostim) is produced in a yeast expression system using recombinant DNA technology. It is a partially glycosylated peptide of 127 amino acids, with three molecular species with molecular weights of 15,500, 15,800, and 19,500. These preparations have serum half-lives of 2–4 hours after intravenous administration.

Monocyte-macrophage CSF (M-CSF), interleukin-3 (IL-3), stem cell factor (SCF), and the other interleukins with myeloid growth factor activity (Table 33–3) have also been purified, cloned, and produced in various expression systems by recombinant DNA technology. These growth factors are not yet available for clinical use.

Pharmacodynamics

The myeloid growth factors stimulate proliferation and differentiation of their respective cell lines by interacting with specific receptors found on various myeloid progenitor cells. G-CSF and M-CSF are lineage-specific growth factors that support proliferation and differentiation of progenitors already committed to neutrophil and monocyte-macrophage lineages, respectively. GM-CSF and IL-3 are multipotential hematopoietic growth factors that stimulate proliferation and differentiation of early and late granulocytic progenitor cells as well as erythroid and megakaryocyte progenitors. SCF is the earliest hematopoietic growth factor to appear in fetal development, acting on the earliest pluripotent stem cells and early committed granulocytic, erythroid, megakaryocytic, and lymphoid progenitors. The early growth factors potentiate the action of the later growth factors, producing synergy in their proliferative response. Both the early and the late myeloid growth factors (except SCF) also have direct effects on the mature target cells in the blood and tissues, enhancing neutrophil and monocyte-macrophage function.

Clinical Pharmacology

G-CSF and GM-CSF accelerate the rate of granulocyte recovery after dose-intensive myelosuppressive chemotherapy and after bone marrow transplantation. This can result in fewer infections and fewer days of hospitalization for these patients. G-CSF, 5 μg/kg/d, or GM-CSF, 250 μg/m^2/d, is usually started within a few days after completing chemotherapy or the day after bone marrow transplantation and is continued until the absolute neutrophil count is approximately 2000–5000/μL. Although GM-CSF is a multilineage growth factor, it does not significantly accelerate red blood cell or platelet recovery in this setting.

G-CSF and GM-CSF in similar or higher doses may also be effective in treating granulocytopenia associated with myelodysplasia, aplastic anemia, congenital neutropenia, cyclic neutropenia, hairy cell leukemia and other chronic bone marrow malignancies, HIV infection, zidovudine-induced leukopenia, and other neutropenic disorders. Many patients respond with a prompt and sometimes dramatic increase in granulocyte count, and in some cases this results in a decrease in the frequency of infections. Again, few if any patients with anemia or thrombocytopenia have a significant increase in hematocrit and hemoglobin or platelet count.

Combinations of myeloid growth factors, particularly combinations acting on both early and late progenitors, can markedly enhance the proliferative effects on granulocytic as well as on erythroid and megakaryocytic progenitors. IL-3 and SCF will probably be used in this way, and there is hope that this will result in multilineage blood cell recovery. Interleukins-6, 7, and 11 are of particular interest because of their ability to stimulate megakaryocyte proliferation and platelet production. However, the interleukins (except IL-3) also have complex effects on the immune system, which may restrict or preclude their use as megakaryocyte or platelet growth factors in some clinical situations.

Toxicity

The adverse effects of treatment with G-CSF and GM-CSF have generally been infrequent and mild. G-CSF can cause bone pain, which clears when the drug is discontinued. GM-CSF can cause more severe side effects, particularly at higher doses. These include fevers, malaise, arthralgias, myalgias, and a capillary leak syndrome characterized by peripheral edema and pleural or pericardial effusions. Allergic reactions can occur but are infrequent.

PREPARATIONS AVAILABLE

Epoetin alfa (erythropoietin, Epo) (Epogen, Procrit)
Parenteral: 2000, 3000, 4000, and 10,000 IU/mL vials for IV or SC injection

Deferoxamine (Desferal)
Parenteral: 500 mg vials for IM, SC, or IV injection

Filgrastim (G-CSF) (Neupogen)
Parenteral: 300, 480 μg vials for IV or SC injection

Folic acid (folacin, pteroylglutamic acid) (generic)
Oral: 0.1, 0.4, 0.8, 1 mg tablets
Parenteral: 5, 10 mg/mL for injection

Iron (generic)
Oral: See Table 33–2.
Parenteral (Iron Dextran) (InFeD): 50 mg elemental iron/mL

Sargramostim (GM-CSF) (Leukine, Prokine)
Parenteral: 250, 500 μg vials for IV infusion

Vitamin B$_{12}$ (generic cyanocobalamin or hydroxocobalamin)
Oral (cyanocobalamin): 25, 50, 100, 250, 500, 1000 μg tablets
Parenteral (cyanocobalamin): 30, 100, 1000 μg/mL for IM or SC injection
Parenteral (hydroxocobalamin): 1000 μg/mL for IM injection only

REFERENCES

Anthony AC: Megaloblastic anemias. In: *Hematology: Basic Principles and Practice.* Hoffman R et al (editors). Churchill Livingstone, 1991.

Brittenham GM: Disorders of iron metabolism: Iron deficiency and overload. In: *Hematology: Basic Principles and Practice.* Hoffman R et al (editors). Churchill Livingstone, 1991.

Crosier PS, Clark SC: Basic biology of the hematopoietic growth factors. Semin Oncol 1992;19:349.

Dale DC et al: A randomized controlled phase III trial of recombinant human granulocyte colony-stimulating factor (filgrastim) for treatment of severe chronic neutropenia. Blood 1993;81:2496.

Demetri GD, Antman KHS: Granulocyte-macrophage colony stimulating factor (GM-CSF): Preclinical and clinical investigations. Semin Oncol 1992;19:362.

Erslev AJ: Erythropoietin. N Engl J Med 1991;324:1339.

Glaspy JA, Golde DW: Granulocyte colony stimulating factor (G-CSF): Preclinical and clinical studies. Semin Oncol 1992;19:386.

Jandl JH: Iron deficiency anemia. In: *Blood: Textbook of Hematology.* Little, Brown, 1987.

Lieschke GJ, Burgess AW: Granulocyte colony-stimulating factor and granulocyte-macrophage colony-stimulating factor. (Two parts.) N Engl J Med 1992;327:28, 99.

Maier RF et al: The effect of epoetin beta (recombinant human erythropoietin) on the need for transfusion in very low birth weight infants. N Engl J Med 1994;330:1173.

Metcalf D: The Florey lecture, 1991. The colony-stimulating factors: Discovery to clinical use. Philos Trans R Soc Lond B Biol Sci 1991;333:147.

Oski F: Iron deficiency in infancy and childhood. N Engl J Med 1993;329:190.

Singer JW: The role of colony-stimulating factors in bone marrow transplantation. Semin Oncol 1992;19:27.

Drugs Used in Disorders of Coagulation

34

Robert A. O'Reilly, MD

Bleeding and thrombosis are altered states of hemostasis. Impaired hemostasis results in spontaneous bleeding; stimulated hemostasis results in thrombus formation. The drugs used to arrest bleeding and to inhibit thrombosis are the subjects of this chapter.

MECHANISMS OF BLOOD COAGULATION

Thrombogenesis

Hemostasis is the spontaneous arrest of bleeding from a damaged blood vessel. The normal vascular endothelial cell is not thrombogenic, and circulating blood platelets and clotting factors do not adhere to it. The immediate hemostatic response of a damaged vessel is **vasospasm.** Within seconds, platelets stick to the exposed collagen of the damaged endothelium (**platelet adhesion**) and to each other (**platelet aggregation**). Platelets then lose their individual membranes and form a gelatinous mass during **viscous metamorphosis.** This platelet plug quickly arrests bleeding but must be reinforced by fibrin for long-term effectiveness. Fibrin reinforcement results from local stimuli to blood coagulation: the exposed collagen of damaged vessels and the membranes and released contents of platelets (Figure 34–1). The local production of thrombin not only releases platelet ADP, a powerful inducer of platelet aggregation, but also stimulates the synthesis of prostaglandins from the arachidonic acid of platelet membranes. These powerful substances are composed of two groups of eicosanoids (Chapter 18) that have opposite effects on thrombogenesis. **Thromboxane A$_2$** (TXA$_2$) is synthesized within platelets and induces thrombogenesis and vasoconstriction. **Prostacyclin** (PGI$_2$) is synthesized within vessel walls and inhibits thrombogenesis. Serotonin (5-HT) is also released from the platelets, stimulating further aggregation and vasoconstriction.

The **platelet** is central to normal hemostasis and to all thromboembolic disease. A **white thrombus** forms initially in high-pressure arteries by adherence of circulating platelets to areas of abnormal endothelium as described above. The growing thrombus of aggregated platelets reduces arterial flow. This localized stasis triggers fibrin formation, and a red thrombus forms around the nidal white thrombus.

A **red thrombus** can form around a white thrombus as described above or de novo in low-pressure veins, initially by adherence of platelets (as in arteries) but followed promptly by the other processes of hemostasis so that the bulk of the thrombus forms a long tail consisting of a fibrin network in which red cells are enmeshed. These tails become detached easily and travel as emboli to the pulmonary arteries. Although all thrombi are mixed, the platelet nidus dominates the arterial thrombus and the fibrin tail the venous thrombus. Arterial thrombi cause serious disease by producing local occlusive ischemia; venous thrombi, by giving rise to distant embolization.

Blood Coagulation

Blood coagulates by the transformation of soluble fibrinogen into insoluble fibrin. Several circulating proteins interact in a cascading series of limited proteolytic reactions. At each step, a clotting factor zymogen (eg, factor VII) undergoes limited proteolysis and becomes an active protease (eg, factor VIIa). This protease activates the next clotting factor (factor IX), until finally a solid fibrin clot is formed. Fibrinogen (factor I), the soluble precursor of fibrin, is the substrate for the enzyme thrombin (factor IIa). This protease is formed during coagulation by activation of its zymogen, prothrombin (factor II). Prothrombin is bound by calcium to a platelet phospholipid (PL) surface, where activated factor X (Xa), in the presence of factor Va, converts it into circulating thrombin. Several of the blood clotting factors are targets for drug therapy (Table 34–1).

The details of coagulation are still not fully understood. In one theory of blood coagulation, the system is activated by a complex of tissue factor (TF) and factor VII (Figure 34–2). This complex is inhibited and regulated by tissue factor pathway inhibitor (TFPI). Oral anticoagulant drugs inhibit the hepatic

Figure 34–1. Thrombus formation at the site of the damaged vascular wall (EC, endothelial cell) and the role of platelets and clotting factors. Platelet membrane receptors include the glycoprotein (GP) Ia receptor binding to collagen (C), GP Ib receptor binding von Willebrand factor (vWF), and GP IIb/IIIa, which binds fibrinogen and other macromolecules. Antiplatelet prostacyclin (PGI$_2$) is released from the endothelium. Aggregating substances released from the degranulating platelet include ADP, TXA$_2$, and 5-HT. Production of factor Xa is detailed in Figure 34–2. (Redrawn and reproduced, with permission, from Simoons ML, Decker JW: New directions in anticoagulant and antiplatelet treatment. [Editorial.] Br Heart J 1995;74:337.)

synthesis of several clotting factors. Heparin inhibits the activity of several of these *activated* clotting factors. The endogenous anticoagulants protein C and protein S down-regulate the amplification of blood clotting by proteolysis of factors Va, VIIIa, and XIa.

Regulation of Coagulation & Fibrinolysis

Blood coagulation and thrombus formation must be confined to the smallest possible area to achieve local hemostasis in response to bleeding from trauma or surgery without causing disseminated coagulation or impaired blood flow. Two major systems regulate and delimit these processes: **fibrin inhibition** and **fibrinolysis.**

Plasma contains protease inhibitors that rapidly inactivate the coagulation proteins as they escape from the site of vessel injury. The most important proteins of this system are α_1-antiprotease, α_2-macroglobulin, α_2-antiplasmin, and antithrombin III. If this system is overwhelmed, generalized intravascular clotting may occur. This process is called **disseminated intravascular coagulation (DIC)** and may follow massive tissue injury, cell lysis in malignant neoplastic disease, obstetric emergencies such as abruptio placentae, or bacterial sepsis.

The central process of fibrinolysis is conversion of inactive plasminogen to the proteolytic enzyme **plas-**

min. Injured cells release activators of plasminogen. Plasmin remodels the thrombus and limits the extension of thrombosis by proteolytic digestion of fibrin.

Regulation of the fibrinolytic system is useful in therapeutics. Increased fibrinolysis is effective therapy for thrombotic disease. **Tissue plasminogen activator (t-PA), urokinase,** and **streptokinase** all activate the fibrinolytic system (Figure 34–3). Conversely, decreased fibrinolysis protects clots from lysis and reduces the bleeding of hemostatic failure. **Aminocaproic acid** is a clinically useful inhibitor of fibrinolysis. Heparin and the oral anticoagulant drugs do not affect the fibrinolytic mechanism.

I. BASIC PHARMACOLOGY OF THE ANTICOAGULANT DRUGS

HEPARIN

Chemistry & Mechanism of Action

Heparin is a heterogeneous mixture of sulfated mucopolysaccharides. It binds to endothelial cell surfaces. Its biologic activity is dependent upon the plasma protease inhibitor **antithrombin III (ATIII).** Antithrombin inhibits clotting factor proteases by

Table 34–1. Blood clotting factors and drugs that affect them.[1]

Component or Factor	Common Synonym	Target for the Action of:
I	Fibrinogen	
II	Prothrombin	Heparin (IIa); warfarin (synthesis)
III	Tissue thromboplastin	
IV	Calcium	
V	Proaccelerin	
VII	Proconvertin	Heparin (VIIa); warfarin (synthesis)
VIII	Antihemophilic globulin (AHG)	
IX	Christmas factor, plasma thromboplastin component (PTC)	Heparin (IXa); warfarin (synthesis)
X	Stuart-Prower factor	Heparin (IXa); warfarin (synthesis)
XI	Plasma thromboplastin antecedent (PTA)	
XII	Hageman factor	
XIII	Fibrin-stabilizing factor	
Proteins C and S		Warfarin (synthesis)
Plasminogen		Thrombolytic enzymes, aminocaproic acid

[1]See Figure 34–2 and text for additional details.

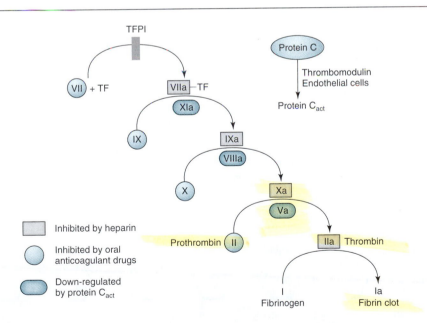

Figure 34–2. A model of blood coagulation. With tissue factor (TF), factor VII forms an activated complex (VIIa-TF) that catalyzes the activation of factor IX to factor IXa. Activated factor XIa also catalyzes this reaction. Tissue factor pathway inhibitor (TFPI) inhibits the catalytic action of the VIIa-TF complex. The cascade proceeds as shown, resulting ultimately in the conversion of fibrinogen to fibrin, an essential component of a functional clot. The two major anticoagulant drugs, heparin and warfarin (an oral anticoagulant), have very different actions. Heparin, acting in the blood, directly activates anticlotting factors—especially antithrombin III, which inactivate the factors enclosed in rectangles. Warfarin, acting in the liver, inhibits the synthesis of the factors enclosed in circles. Proteins C and S exert anticlotting effects by destroying activated factors Va, VIIIa, and XIa.

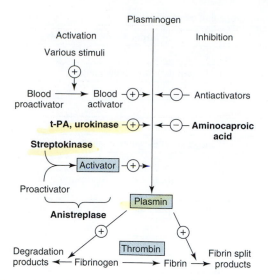

Figure 34–3. Schematic representation of the fibrinolytic system. Plasmin is the active fibrinolytic enzyme. Several clinically useful activators are shown on the left in bold. Anistreplase is a combination of streptokinase and the proactivator plasminogen. Aminocaproic acid (right) inhibits the activation of plasminogen to plasmin and is useful in some bleeding disorders.

complex is formed, heparin is released intact for renewed binding to more antithrombin.

The antithrombin binding region of commercial heparin consists of repeating sulfated disaccharide units composed of D-glucosamine-L-iduronic acid and D-glucosamine-D-glucuronic acid (Figure 34–4). High-molecular-weight (HMW) fractions of heparin with high affinity for antithrombin markedly inhibit blood coagulation. These fractions have an MW range of 5000–30,000. Low-molecular-weight (LMW) fractions of heparin inhibit activated factor X but have less effect on antithrombin and on coagulation in general than the HMW species. **Enoxaparin,** one of many LMW heparin fractions, has been approved by the FDA for the primary prevention of deep venous thrombosis after hip replacement surgery. Enoxaparin has an MW range of 2000–6000. **Dalteparin** and **danaproid,** newer preparations with molecular weights of 2000–9000, have been approved for the same indication. Several LMW heparins, upon comparison with regular heparin, are claimed to have equal efficacy, increased bioavailability from the subcutaneous site of injection, and less frequent dosing requirements (once or twice daily is sufficient). Several of these LMW heparins are undergoing clinical trials for the treatment of thromboembolic disease.

Because commercial heparin consists of a family of molecules of different molecular weights, the correlation between the concentration of a given heparin preparation and its effect on coagulation often is low. Therefore, regular (HMW) heparin is standardized as units of activity by bioassay. Heparin sodium USP must contain at least 120 USP units per milligram. Heparin is generally used as the sodium salt, but calcium heparin is equally effective. Lithium heparin is used in vitro as an anticoagulant for blood samples. Commercial heparin is extracted from porcine intestinal mucosa and bovine lung. Enoxaparin is obtained from the same sources as regular heparin, but doses are specified in milligrams. Dalteparin and danaproid, on the other hand, are specified in anti-factor Xa units.

forming equimolar stable complexes with them. In the absence of heparin, these reactions are slow; in the presence of heparin, they are accelerated 1000-fold. Only about a third of the molecules in commercial heparin preparations have an accelerating effect because the remainder lack the unique polysaccharide needed for high-affinity binding to antithrombin III. The active heparin molecules bind tightly to antithrombin and cause a conformational change in this inhibitor. The conformational change of antithrombin exposes its active site for more rapid interaction with the proteases—the activated clotting factors. Heparin catalyzes the antithrombin-protease reaction without being consumed. Once the antithrombin-protease

Figure 34–4. Structure of heparin. The polymer section illustrates structural features typical of heparin; however, the sequence of variously repeating disaccharide units has been arbitrarily selected. In addition, non-O-sulfated or 3-O-sulfated glucosamines may also occur. Heparin is a strongly acidic molecule because of its high content of anionic sulfate and carboxylic acid. GlcN, glucosamine; IdUA, iduronic acid; GlcUA, glucuronic acid. (Modified, redrawn, and reproduced, with permission, from Lindahl U et al: Structure and biosynthesis of heparinlike polysaccharides. Fed Proc 1977;36:19.)

Toxicity

The major adverse effect of heparin is bleeding. This risk can be decreased by scrupulous patient selection, careful control of dosage, and close monitoring of the partial thromboplastin time (PTT). Elderly women and patients with renal failure are more prone to hemorrhage. Heparin is of animal origin and should be used cautiously in patients with allergy. Increased loss of hair and transient reversible alopecia have been reported. Long-term heparin therapy is associated with osteoporosis and spontaneous fractures. Heparin accelerates the clearing of postprandial lipemia by causing the release of lipoprotein lipase from tissues.

Heparin causes transient thrombocytopenia in 25% of patients and severe thrombocytopenia in 5%. Mild platelet reduction results from heparin-induced aggregation and severe reduction from heparin-induced antiplatelet antibodies. Paradoxical thromboembolism may result from heparin-induced platelet aggregation. The following points should be considered in all patients receiving heparin: Platelet counts should be performed frequently; thrombocytopenia serious enough to cause bleeding should be considered to be heparin-induced; any new thrombus can be the result of heparin; and thromboembolic disease thought to be heparin-induced should be treated by discontinuance of heparin and administration of an oral anticoagulant if clinically warranted.

Contraindications

Heparin is contraindicated in patients who are hypersensitive to the drug, are actively bleeding, or have hemophilia, thrombocytopenia, purpura, severe hypertension, intracranial hemorrhage, infective endocarditis, active tuberculosis, ulcerative lesions of the gastrointestinal tract, threatened abortion, visceral carcinoma, or advanced hepatic or renal disease. Heparin should not be given to patients during or after surgery of the brain, spinal cord, or eye or to patients undergoing lumbar puncture or regional anesthetic blocks. Heparin should be used in pregnant women only when clearly indicated despite the apparent lack of placental transfer.

Administration & Dosage

The indications for the use of heparin are described in the section on clinical pharmacology. A plasma concentration of heparin of 0.2 unit/mL usually prevents pulmonary emboli in patients with established venous thrombosis. This concentration of heparin will prolong the partial thromboplastin time (PTT) to 2–2.5 times that of the control value. This degree of anticoagulant effect should be maintained throughout the course of *continuous* intravenous heparin therapy. When *intermittent* heparin administration is used, the PTT should be measured just before the next heparin dose to adjust this dose so as to maintain prolongation of the PTT to 2–2.5 times that of the control value.

The continuous intravenous administration of heparin is accomplished via an infusion pump. After an initial bolus injection of 5000–10,000 units, a continuous infusion of about 900 units/h or 10–15 units/kg/h is required to maintain the PTT at 2–2.5 times control. Patients with acute pulmonary emboli often require larger doses than these during the first few days because of increased heparin clearance. With intermittent intravenous administration of heparin, 75–100 units/kg is administered every 4 hours. Subcutaneous administration of heparin, as in low-dose prophylaxis, is achieved with 5000 units every 8 or 12 hours. Heparin must never be administered intramuscularly, because of the danger of hematoma formation at the injection site. Enoxaparin is given in a dosage of 30 mg twice daily after hip surgery. The recommended dosage for dalteparin is 2500 units subcutaneously once a day.

Reversal of Heparin Action

Excessive anticoagulant action of heparin is treated by discontinuance of the drug. If bleeding occurs, administration of a specific antagonist such as protamine sulfate is indicated. Protamine is a highly basic peptide that combines with heparin as an ion pair to form a stable complex devoid of anticoagulant activity. For every 100 units of heparin remaining in the patient, administer 1 mg of protamine sulfate intravenously; the rate of infusion should not exceed 50 mg in any 10-minute period. Excess protamine must be avoided; it also has an anticoagulant effect.

HIRUDIN

For a number of years, surgeons have used medicinal leeches (*Hirudo medicinalis*) to prevent thrombosis in the fine vessels of reattached digits. Hirudin is a powerful and specific thrombin inhibitor from the leech which is now being prepared by recombinant DNA technology. Its action is independent of antithrombin III, which means it can reach and inactivate fibrin-bound thrombin in thrombi. Hirudin has little effect on platelets or the bleeding time. Like heparin, it must be administered parenterally and is monitored by the PTT. It has undergone extensive animal testing and is now in clinical trials; it is not yet approved by the FDA.

WARFARIN & THE COUMARIN ANTICOAGULANTS

Chemistry & Pharmacokinetics

The clinical use of the coumarin anticoagulants can be traced to the discovery of an anticoagulant substance formed in spoiled sweet clover silage. It produced a deficiency of plasma prothrombin and a consequent hemorrhagic disease in cattle. The toxic agent was identified as bishydroxycoumarin and synthesized as dicumarol. This drug and its congeners, most notably warfarin (Figure 34–5), are widely used as rodenticides in addition to their application as antithrombotic agents in humans. These drugs are often referred to as **oral anticoagulants** because, unlike heparin, they are administered orally. Warfarin is the most reliable member of this group, and the other coumarin anticoagulants are almost never used in the USA.

Warfarin is generally administered as the sodium salt and has 100% bioavailability. Over 99% of racemic warfarin is bound to plasma albumin, which may contribute to its small volume of distribution (the albumin space), its long half-life in plasma (36 hours), and the lack of urinary excretion of unchanged drug. Warfarin used clinically is a racemic mixture composed of equal amounts of two enantiomorphs. The levorotatory S-warfarin is four times more potent than the dextrorotatory R-warfarin. This observation is useful in understanding the stereoselective nature of several drug interactions involving warfarin.

Mechanism of Action

Coumarin anticoagulants block the γ-carboxylation of several glutamate residues in prothrombin and factors VII, IX, and X as well as the endogenous anticoagulant protein C (Figure 34–2). The blockade results in incomplete molecules that are biologically inactive in coagulation. This protein carboxylation is physiologically coupled with the oxidative deactivation of vitamin K. The anticoagulant prevents the reductive metabolism of the inactive vitamin K epoxide back to its active hydroquinone form (Figure 34–6). Muta-

tional change of the responsible enzyme, vitamin K epoxide reductase, can give rise to genetic resistance to warfarin in humans and especially in rats.

There is an 8- to 12-hour delay in the action of warfarin. Its anticoagulant effect results from a balance between partially inhibited synthesis and unaltered degradation of the four vitamin K-dependent clotting factors. The resulting inhibition of coagulation is dependent on their degradation rate in the circulation (Figure 34–7). These half-lives are 6, 24, 40, and 60 hours for factors VII, IX, X, and II, respectively. Larger initial doses of warfarin—up to about 0.75 mg/kg—hasten the onset of the anticoagulant effect. Beyond this dosage, the speed of onset is independent of the dose size. The only effect of a larger loading dose is to prolong the time that the plasma concentration of drug remains above that required for suppression of clotting factor synthesis. The 1- to 3-day delay between the peak drug concentration in plasma and its maximum hypoprothrombinemic effect can be described by a model based on the relationship of the plasma concentration of drug and the reduced synthesis of clotting factors. The only difference among oral anticoagulants in producing and maintaining hypoprothrombinemia is the half-life of each drug.

Toxicity

Warfarin crosses the placenta readily and can cause a hemorrhagic disorder in the fetus. Furthermore, fetal proteins with γ-carboxyglutamate residues found in bone and blood may be affected by warfarin; the drug can cause a serious birth defect characterized by abnormal bone formation. Thus, warfarin should never be administered during pregnancy. Cutaneous necrosis with reduced activity of protein C sometimes

Dicumarol

Warfarin sodium

Phenindione

Phytonadione (vitamin K₁)

Figure 34–5. Structural formulas of several oral anticoagulant drugs and of vitamin K. The carbon atom of warfarin shown at the asterisk is an asymmetric center.

Figure 34–6. Vitamin K cycle—metabolic interconversions of vitamin K associated with the synthesis of vitamin K-dependent clotting factors. Vitamin K_1 or K_2 is activated by reduction to the hydroquinone form (KH_2). Stepwise oxidation to vitamin K epoxide (KO) is coupled to prothrombin carboxylation by the enzyme carboxylase. The reactivation of vitamin K epoxide is the warfarin-sensitive step (warfarin). The R on the vitamin K molecule represents a 20-carbon phytyl side chain in vitamin K_1 and a 30- to 65-carbon polyprenyl side chain in vitamin K_2.

occurs during the first weeks of therapy. Rarely, the same process causes frank infarction of breast, fatty tissues, intestine, and extremities. The pathologic lesion associated with the hemorrhagic infarction is venous thrombosis, suggesting that it is caused by warfarin-induced depression of protein C synthesis.

Administration & Dosage

Treatment with warfarin should be initiated with small daily doses of 5–10 mg rather than the large loading doses formerly used. The initial adjustment of the prothrombin time takes about 1 week, which usually results in a maintenance dose of 5–7 mg/d. The prothrombin time should be increased to a level representing 25% of normal activity and maintained there for long-term therapy. When the activity is less than 20%, the warfarin dosage should be reduced or omitted until the activity rises above 20%.

The therapeutic range for oral anticoagulant therapy is now defined in terms of an international normalized ratio (INR). The INR is the prothrombin time ratio (test/control) obtained if the more sensitive international reference thromboplastin made from human brain is used rather than the less sensitive rabbit-brain thromboplastin used in North America (Hirsh et al, 1995). Randomized prospective studies with the INR system have resulted in use of lower doses of anticoagulant drug and less bleeding, yet the efficacy is equal to the regimens with higher doses. These less intensive and lower dose regimens are efficacious for many therapeutic indications. Analysis of several clinical trials in patients with artificial heart valves has led

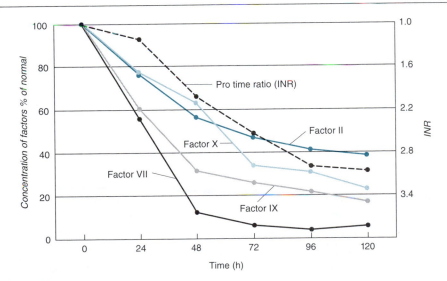

Figure 34–7. The activity of the four vitamin K-dependent clotting factors and the prothrombin time expressed in INR units as a function of time after starting administration of warfarin. True prothrombin, factor II, has a half-life of 60 hours; several days of therapy are required for its activity to reach the therapeutic range. The activity of the natural anticoagulant protein C (which is also vitamin K-dependent and coumarin-sensitive) falls as rapidly as that of factor VII and can contribute to an early *procoagulant* effect of warfarin.

to the recommendation that dosage be adjusted to achieve an INR of 2.5–3.5. (An INR of 3 corresponds to a prothrombin time ratio of 1.6 in the average North American laboratory.)

Drug Interactions

The oral anticoagulants often interact with other drugs and with disease states. These interactions can be broadly divided into **pharmacokinetic** and **pharmacodynamic** effects (Table 34–2). Pharmacokinetic mechanisms for drug interaction with oral anticoagulants are mainly **enzyme induction, enzyme inhibition,** and **reduced plasma protein binding.** Pharmacodynamic mechanisms for interactions with warfarin are **synergism** (impaired hemostasis, reduced clotting factor synthesis, as in hepatic disease), **competitive antagonism** (vitamin K), and an **altered physiologic control loop for vitamin K** (hereditary resistance to oral anticoagulants).

The most serious interactions with warfarin are those that *increase* the anticoagulant effect and the risk of bleeding. The most dangerous of these interactions are the pharmacokinetic interactions with the pyrazolones phenylbutazone and sulfinpyrazone. These drugs not only augment the hypoprothrombinemia but also inhibit platelet function and may induce peptic ulcer disease (Chapter 36). The mechanisms for their hypoprothrombinemic interaction are a stereoselective inhibition of oxidative metabolic transformation of *S*-warfarin and displacement of albumin-bound warfarin, increasing the free fraction. Fortunately, neither phenylbutazone nor sulfinpyrazone is in common use in the USA. Metronidazole, fluconazole, and trimethoprim-sulfamethoxazole also stereoselectively inhibit the metabolic transformation of *S*-warfarin, whereas amiodarone, disulfiram, and cimetidine inhibit metabolism of both enantiomorphs of warfarin. Aspirin, hepatic disease, and hyperthyroidism augment warfarin pharmacodynamically: aspirin by its effect on platelet function and the latter two by increasing the turnover rate of clotting factors. The third-generation cephalosporins eliminate the bacteria in the intestinal tract that produce vitamin K, and, like warfarin, also directly inhibit vitamin K epoxide reductase. Heparin directly prolongs the prothrombin time by inhibiting the activity of several clotting factors.

Barbiturates and rifampin cause a marked *decrease* of the anticoagulant effect by induction of the hepatic enzymes that transform racemic warfarin. Cholestyramine binds warfarin in the intestine and reduces its absorption and bioavailability.

Pharmacodynamic reductions of anticoagulant effect occur with vitamin K (increased synthesis of clotting factors), the diuretics chlorthalidone and spironolactone (clotting factor concentration), hereditary resistance (mutation of vitamin K reactivation cycle molecules), and hypothyroidism (decreased turnover rate of clotting factors).

Drugs with *no* significant effect on anticoagulant therapy include ethanol, phenothiazines, benzodiazepines, acetaminophen, narcotics, indomethacin, and most antibiotics.

Reversal of Action

Excessive anticoagulant effect and bleeding from warfarin can be reversed by stopping the drug and administering large doses of vitamin K_1 (phytonadione) and fresh-frozen plasma or factor IX concentrates such as Konyne 80 and Proplex that also contain large amounts of the prothrombin complex. This disappearance of effect is not correlated with plasma warfarin concentrations but rather with reestablishment of normal activity of the clotting factors. A modest excess of anticoagulant effect without bleeding may require no more than cessation of the drug. Serious bleeding requires large amounts of vitamin K_1 intravenously in 50 mg infusions, factor IX concentrates, and sometimes even transfusion of whole blood.

Analogs & Variants

Vitamin K antagonists other than warfarin are seldom used because they have less favorable pharmacologic properties or greater toxicity. **Dicumarol** is incompletely absorbed and frequently causes gastrointestinal symptoms. **Phenprocoumon** has a long half-life of 6 days. The indanedione group, which includes phenindione and diphenadione, has potentially

Table 34–2. Pharmacokinetic and pharmacodynamic drug and body interactions with oral anticoagulants.

Increased Prothrombin Time		Decreased Prothrombin Time	
Pharmacokinetic	**Pharmacodynamic**	**Pharmacokinetic**	**Pharmacodynamic**
Amiodarone Cimetidine Disulfiram Metronidazole[1] Fluconazole[1] Phenylbutazone[1] Sulfinpyrazone[1] Trimethoprim- sulfamethoxazole	**Drugs** Aspirin (high doses) Cephalosporins, third- generation Heparin **Body factors** Hepatic disease Hyperthyroidism	Barbiturates Cholestyramine Rifampin	**Drugs** Diuretics Vitamin K **Body factors** Hereditary resistance Hypothyroidism

[1]Stereoselectively inhibits the oxidative metabolism of the *(S)*-warfarin enantiomorph of racemic warfarin.

serious adverse effects in the kidney and liver and is of little clinical use.

II. BASIC PHARMACOLOGY OF THE FIBRINOLYTIC DRUGS

Fibrinolytic drugs rapidly lyse thrombi by catalyzing the formation of the serine protease **plasmin** from its precursor zymogen, plasminogen (Figure 34–3). These drugs create a generalized lytic state when administered intravenously. Thus, both protective hemostatic thrombi and target thromboemboli are broken down. The box: Thrombolytic Drugs for Acute Myocardial Infarction describes the use of these drugs in one major application.

STREPTOKINASE, ALTEPLASE, TISSUE PLASMINOGEN ACTIVATOR, RETEPLASE, & UROKINASE

Pharmacology

plasminogen → plasmin

Streptokinase is a protein (but not an enzyme in itself) synthesized by streptococci that combines with the proactivator plasminogen. This enzymatic complex catalyzes the conversion of inactive plasminogen to active plasmin. **Urokinase** is a human enzyme synthesized by the kidney that directly converts plasminogen to active plasmin. While the naturally occurring inhibitors of plasmin in plasma preclude its direct use, the absence of inhibitors for urokinase and the streptokinase-proactivator complex permit their use clinically. Plasmin formed inside a thrombus by these activators is protected from plasma antiplasmins, which allows it to lyse the thrombus from within. **Anistreplase** (anisoylated plasminogen streptokinase activator complex; APSAC) consists of a complex of purified human plasminogen and bacterial streptokinase that has been acylated to protect the enzyme's active site. When administered, the acyl group spontaneously hydrolyzes, freeing the activated streptokinase-proactivator complex. This product allows for rapid intravenous injection, greater clot selectivity (ie, more activity on plasminogen associated with clots than on free plasminogen in the blood), and more thrombolytic activity.

Plasminogen can also be activated endogenously by **tissue plasminogen activators (t-PA).** These activators preferentially activate plasminogen that is bound to fibrin, which (in theory) confines fibrinolysis to the formed thrombus and avoids systemic activation. Human t-PA is manufactured by means of recombinant DNA technology. **Alteplase** is unmodified human t-PA. **Reteplase** is human t-PA from which several amino acid sequences have been deleted.

Indications & Dosage

Use of fibrinolytic drugs by the intravenous route is indicated in cases of **multiple pulmonary emboli** that are not massive enough to require surgical intervention. Intravenous fibrinolytic drugs are also indicated in cases of **central deep venous thrombosis** such as the superior vena caval syndrome and ascending thrombophlebitis of the iliofemoral vein. They have also been used intra-arterially, especially for peripheral vascular disease.

Thrombolytic therapy in the management of **acute myocardial infarction** requires careful patient selection, the use of a specific thrombolytic agent, and the benefit of adjuvant therapy. Considerable controversy surrounds the question of greater safety or efficacy of t-PA compared with the other thrombolytic agents (see the accompanying box).

Streptokinase is administered by intravenous infusion of a loading dose of 250,000 units, followed by 100,000 units/h for 24–72 hours. Patients with antistreptococcal antibodies can develop fever, allergic reactions, and therapeutic resistance. Urokinase requires a loading dose of 300,000 units given over 10 minutes and a maintenance dose of 300,000 units/h for 12 hours. Alteplase (t-PA) is given by intravenous infusion of 60 mg over the first hour and then 40 mg at a rate of 20 mg/h. Reteplase is given as two intravenous bolus injections of 10 units each separated by 30 minutes. Anistreplase is given as a single intravenous injection of 30 units over 3–5 minutes. A course of fibrinolytic drugs is expensive: hundreds of dollars for streptokinase and thousands for urokinase, anistreplase, and t-PA.

III. BASIC PHARMACOLOGY OF ANTITHROMBOTIC DRUGS

Platelet function is regulated by three categories of substances. The first group consists of agents generated outside the platelet that interact with platelet membrane receptors, eg, catecholamines, collagen, thrombin, and prostacyclin. The second category contains agents generated within the platelet that interact with the membrane receptors, eg, ADP, prostaglandin D_2, prostaglandin E_2, and serotonin. The third contains agents generated within the platelet that act within the platelet, eg, prostaglandin endoperoxides and thromboxane A_2, the cyclic nucleotides cAMP and cGMP, and calcium ion. From this list of agents, several targets for platelet inhibitory drugs have been identified (Figure 34–1): inhibition of prostaglandin metabolism (aspirin), inhibition of ADP-induced platelet aggregation (ticlopidine), and blockade of GP IIb/IIIa receptors on platelets (abciximab and integrelin).

tPA → ⊕ plasminogen bound to fibrin

THROMBOLYTIC DRUGS FOR ACUTE MYOCARDIAL INFARCTION

Background: The paradigm shift in 1980 on the causation of acute myocardial infarction to acute coronary occlusion by a thrombus created the rationale for thrombolytic therapy of this common lethal disease. Thrombolytic drugs lyse thrombi by converting inactive plasminogen to active plasmin. At that time—and for the first time—intravenous thrombolytic therapy for acute myocardial infarction in the European Cooperative Study Group trial was found to reduce mortality significantly. But it took later studies, eg, GISSI-2 (see below for acronyms), with thousands of patients in each trial to provide enough statistical power for the 20% reduction in mortality to be considered statistically significant. The additive efficacy of aspirin with the thrombolytic drug streptokinase was shown in ISIS-2.

Patients: The selection of patients for thrombolytic therapy is critical. The diagnosis of acute myocardial infarction is made clinically and is confirmed by electrocardiography. Patients with ST segment elevation and bundle branch block on electrocardiography do best; those with ST segment depression or a normal ECG do less well; and those with non-Q-wave acute myocardial infarction may even be harmed (TIMI-3B). All trials to date show the greatest benefit for thrombolytic therapy when it is given early, within 6 hours after symptomatic onset of acute myocardial infarction.

Clinical trials: ISIS-3 showed that streptokinase plus aspirin performed as well as recombinant tissue-type plasminogen activator (rt-PA) or complex formulations of streptokinase such as anistreplase (APSAC). The GUSTO trial showed a small advantage for the much more expensive t-PA over streptokinase, but with a significantly higher risk of hemorrhagic stroke. The nine clinical trials—each containing over 1000 patients with suspected acute myocardial infarction—reported 11.6% mortality at 35 days in the control group and 9.5% in the treatment group, an 18% reduction in mortality (FTT).

Adjunctive drugs: The best results occur with thrombolytic drugs supplemented by other drugs. Nitroglycerin, given early in acute myocardial infarction for pain relief, had no beneficial effect on mortality in GISSI-3 and ISIS-4. Beta-blocker drugs reduced myocardial ischemia and infarct size, prevented arrhythmias, decreased reinfarction, and improved survival in ISIS-1 and GISSI-1. Aspirin alone and with streptokinase reduced mortality in ISIS-2. Oral anticoagulants are best used in patients with depressed left ventricular function or systemic embolization. Heparin was a necessary adjunct for t-PA in GUSTO but was less useful with streptokinase plus aspirin because of the increased risk of bleeding. ACE inhibitors reduced infarct expansion and arrhythmias and improved survival in GISSI-3. Direct thrombin inhibitors like hirudin are undergoing clinical trial (TIMI-9B and GUSTO-2A).

Summary: Thrombolytic drugs reduce the mortality of acute myocardial infarction. The early and appropriate use of any thrombolytic drug probably transcends individual advantages. Adjunctive drugs like aspirin, beta-blockers, and ACE inhibitors reduce mortality even further. The principles of management are well described in Rawles, 1996.

Glossary of acronyms for the clinical trials: **FTT,** Fibrinolytic Therapy Trialists' Collaborative Group; **GISSI,** Gruppo Italiano per lo Studio della Streptochinasi nell'infarto Miocardico; **GUSTO,** Global Utilization of Streptokinase and Tissue Plasminogen Activator for Occluded Coronary Arteries; **ISIS,** International Study of Infarct Survival; **TIMI,** Thrombolysis and Thrombin Inhibition in Myocardial Infarction. The number after these acronyms indicates multiple trials by that research group.

ASPIRIN

The prostaglandin **thromboxane A$_2$** is an arachidonate product that causes platelets to change shape, to release their granules, and to aggregate (Chapter 18). Drugs that antagonize this pathway interfere with platelet aggregation in vitro and prolong the bleeding time in vivo. **Aspirin** is the prototype of this class of drugs. Drugs that modulate the intraplatelet concentration of cAMP do not prolong the bleeding time. However, dietary therapy can be useful in the prophylaxis of thrombosis. Ingestion of the unsaturated fatty acid **eicosapentaenoic acid,** which is high in cold water fish, generates prostaglandin I$_3$, an effective antiaggregating substance like prostacyclin, and thromboxane A$_3$, which is much less active than TXA$_2$.

Aspirin inhibits the synthesis of thromboxane A$_2$ by irreversible acetylation of the enzyme cyclooxygenase (Chapter 18). Because the anuclear platelet cannot synthesize new proteins, it cannot manufacture new enzyme during its 10-day lifetime. Other salicylates and other nonsteroidal anti-inflammatory drugs also inhibit cyclooxygenase but have a shorter duration of inhibitory action because they cannot acetylate cyclooxygenase, ie, their action is reversible.

Two large prospective, randomized trials in healthy American and British physicians were conducted to evaluate the use of aspirin for 4–5 years in the *primary prophylaxis* of cardiovascular mortality, ie, prevention of first heart attacks. The American study showed a significant reduction in the incidence of nonfatal myocardial infarctions (and was prematurely terminated because of this finding), while the British study showed no significant change. Furthermore, the British study confirmed previous evidence that at a dose of 500 mg/d, aspirin increases the incidence of peptic ulcer disease and gastrointestinal bleeding. Thus, the risk-versus-benefit measure of aspirin as an over-the-counter prophylactic drug is questionable for patients with hypertension or peptic ulcer disease.

The FDA has approved the use of 325 mg/d for *primary* prophylaxis of myocardial infarction but urges caution in this use of aspirin by the general population except when prescribed as an adjunct to risk factor management by smoking cessation and lowering of blood cholesterol and blood pressure. The striking eightfold reduction in expected cardiovascular deaths for both the control and the aspirin groups in the placebo-controlled, double-blinded American study suggested the importance of life-style in highly motivated, health-conscious physicians. Meta-analysis of many published trials of aspirin and other antiplatelet agents confirms the value of this intervention in the *secondary* prevention of vascular events among patients with a history of vascular events.

TICLOPIDINE

Ticlopidine reduces platelet aggregation by inhibiting the ADP pathway of platelets. Unlike aspirin, the drug has no effect on prostaglandin metabolism. Randomized clinical trials with ticlopidine report efficacy in the prevention of vascular events among patients with transient ischemic attacks, completed strokes, and unstable angina pectoris. Adverse effects include nausea, dyspepsia, and diarrhea in up to 20% of patients, hemorrhage in 5%, and, most seriously, leukopenia in 1%. The leukopenia is detected by regular monitoring of the white blood cell count during the first 3 months of treatment. The dosage of ticlopidine is 250 mg twice daily. It is particularly useful in patients who cannot tolerate aspirin. Doses of ticlopidine less than 500 mg/d may be efficacious with fewer adverse effects.

BETA ADRENOCEPTOR-BLOCKING DRUGS

Many clinical trials have been performed with beta-blocking drugs for secondary prophylaxis of myocardial infarction or other cardiac events (eg, arrhythmia) following a first infarction. The Norwegian Multicenter Study of **timolol** was methodologically and statistically sound. It showed that use of timolol resulted in a highly significant reduction of total numbers of deaths (Figure 10–8), and the drug was approved by the FDA for use as a prophylactic agent following myocardial infarction. It is not certain whether these positive results reflect a direct effect on coagulation.

BLOCKADE OF PLATELET GP IIB/IIIA RECEPTORS

A new class of platelet-inhibiting drugs that blocks platelet receptors for integrin and other aggregating substances (Figure 34–1) has been introduced into clinical trials, and the first of these (abciximab) has been approved for use.

Abciximab is a mouse/human chimeric monoclonal antibody that blocks IIb/IIIa receptors. It has been approved by the FDA as adjunctive therapy in patients undergoing high-risk angioplasty and atherectomy. This drug is used along with aspirin and heparin and is given as a 0.25 mg/kg bolus 10 minutes prior to the procedure, followed by infusion of 10 μg/min for 12 hours. The 2100-patient EPIC study demonstrated the efficacy of abciximab as well as its increased bleeding risk versus placebo controls. A pilot study (PROLOG) showed less bleeding when heparin (at adjusted dosage) was combined with abciximab than when heparin was given alone. These results are being tested in a large phase III study (EPILOG).

Integrelin is a synthetic peptide with high affinity for the GP IIb/IIIa integrin receptor protein. Integrelin has undergone successful clinical trial for prevention of thrombosis in percutaneous coronary angioplasty.

IV. CLINICAL PHARMACOLOGY OF DRUGS USED TO TREAT THROMBOSIS

The history of pharmacologic treatment of thromboembolism is one of broken promises resulting from the misuse of antithrombotic drugs. Drugs have been used and discarded before being properly evaluated, eg, oral anticoagulants in management of myocardial infarction and hip surgery. Use of prophylactic low-dose heparin during general surgery was undermined by overuse almost as soon as its efficacy had been rigorously established. The antiplatelet drugs were widely used before any proof of their efficacy was obtained.

VENOUS THROMBOSIS

Risk Factors

A. Resistance to Activated Protein C: The most common genetic risk factor for venous thrombosis is activated protein C resistance. This condition results from mutation of the factor V gene that results in replacement of Arg506 to Gln. This R506Q-factor V mutation is found in 4% of healthy controls and in 20% of patients diagnosed with their first deep venous thrombosis. The relative risk for venous thrombosis is increased eightfold in heterozygotes and 80-fold in homozygotes.

B. Acquired Disease: The increased risk of thromboembolism associated with arrhythmia has long been recognized. Similarly, prolonged bed rest is clearly associated with an increased incidence of deep venous thrombosis and embolism. Many randomized clinical trials in patients with chronic atrial fibrillation have proved the efficacy of long-term prophylaxis with oral anticoagulants in preventing systemic emboli. The evidence is particularly strong in patients over 60.

Antithrombotic Management

A. Prevention: Primary prevention of venous thrombosis reduces the incidence of and mortality rate from pulmonary emboli. Heparin is used to prevent venous thrombosis. Intermittent administration of low-dose heparin subcutaneously provides effective prophylaxis. Oral anticoagulants are also effective, but the risk of bleeding and the necessity for laboratory monitoring of the prothrombin time limit their use for prophylaxis except in patients with chronic atrial fibrillation or prosthetic heart valves.

Early ambulation postoperatively reduces venous stasis. Intermittent external pneumatic compression of the legs also is an effective form of postoperative prophylaxis. At the present time, enoxaparin (LMW heparin) is approved only for prophylaxis in patients undergoing hip replacement. Platelets have a lesser role in venous than in arterial disease; antiplatelet drugs are not consistently effective in prevention of venous disease.

B. Treatment of Established Disease: Established venous thrombosis is treated with maximal dosages of heparin and warfarin. Heparin is used for the first 7–10 days, with a 3- to 5-day overlap with warfarin. Therapy with warfarin is continued after hospital discharge for 6 weeks (first episode) to 6 months (recurrent episodes). Pulmonary embolism is treated the same way. Small thrombi confined to the calf veins are often managed without anticoagulants. The risk, expense, and inconvenience of unnecessary anticoagulant treatment far exceed those of venography, the definitive diagnostic test. Only a third of patients suspected of having deep venous thrombosis actually have the disease.

Deficiencies of proteins C or S are important diagnostic considerations in patients with recurrent thrombi who have a positive family history. Antithrombin III concentrate may be useful in deficient patients. Heparin resistance associated with antithrombin III deficiency can be overcome with this concentrate.

Warfarin readily crosses the placenta. It can cause hemorrhage at any time during pregnancy, as well as developmental defects when administered during the first trimester. Therefore, venous thromboembolic disease in pregnant women should be treated with heparin, best administered by subcutaneous injection. Laboratory monitoring of the anticoagulant effect during pregnancy is mandatory.

Fibrinolytic Therapy

Early treatment with fibrinolytic drugs of a less than massive pulmonary embolus may improve survival and may preserve long-term pulmonary function. The standard course of fibrinolytic therapy should be followed by anticoagulant therapy with heparin and warfarin. Concomitant invasive procedures must be avoided, since bleeding may occur. Therapy is contraindicated after recent surgery or in patients with metastatic cancer, stroke, or underlying hemorrhagic disorders.

ARTERIAL THROMBOSIS

In patients with arterial thrombi, consumption of platelets is excessive. Thus, treatment with platelet-inhibiting drugs such as aspirin and ticlopidine is indicated in patients with transient ischemic attacks and strokes or unstable angina and acute myocardial infarction. In angina and infarction, these drugs are often used in conjunction with beta-blockers or calcium channel blockers and fibrinolytic drugs.

V. DRUGS USED IN BLEEDING DISORDERS

VITAMIN K

Vitamin K confers biologic activity upon prothrombin and factors VII, IX, and X by participating in their postribosomal modification.

Vitamin K is a fat-soluble substance found primarily in leafy green vegetables. The dietary requirement is low, because the vitamin is additionally synthesized by bacteria that colonize the human intestine. Two natural forms exist: vitamins K_1 and K_2. Vitamin K_1 (Figure 34–5) is found in food and is called phytonadione. Vitamin K_2 is found in human tissues, is synthesized by intestinal bacteria, and is called menaquinone (Suttie, 1995).

Vitamins K_1 and K_2 require bile salts for absorption from the intestinal tract. Vitamin K_1 is available clinically in 5 mg tablets and 50 mg ampules. The effect is delayed for 6 hours but is complete by 24 hours when treating depression of prothrombin activity by excess warfarin or vitamin K deficiency. Intravenous administration of vitamin K_1 should be slow, because rapid infusion can produce dyspnea, chest and back pain, and even death. Vitamin K_1 is currently administered to all newborns to prevent the hemorrhagic disease of vitamin K deficiency, which is especially common in premature infants. The water-soluble salt of vitamin K_3 (menadione) should never be used in therapeutics. It is particularly ineffective in the treatment of warfarin overdosage. Vitamin K deficiency frequently occurs in hospitalized patients in intensive care units because of poor diet, parenteral nutrition, recent surgery, multiple antibiotic therapy, and uremia. Severe hepatic failure results in loss of protein synthesis and a hemorrhagic diathesis that is unresponsive to vitamin K.

PLASMA FRACTIONS

Deficiencies in plasma coagulation factors can cause bleeding (Table 34–3). Spontaneous bleeding occurs when factor activity is less than 5% of normal. Factor VIII deficiency (classic hemophilia, or hemophilia A) and factor IX deficiency (Christmas disease, or hemophilia B) account for most of the heritable coagulation defects. Concentrated plasma fractions are available for the treatment of these deficiencies. However, the fear of viral hepatitis and of AIDS is tempering the use of these concentrates in patients with hemophilia. The best use of these therapeutic materials

Table 34–3. Therapeutic products for the treatment of coagulation disorders.[1]

Factor	Deficiency State	Concentration (%) Relative to Normal Plasma Required for Hemostasis[2]	Half-Life (Days) of Infused Factor	Therapeutic Material
I	Afibrinogenemia, defibrination syndrome	40	4	Plasma fibrinogen, cryoprecipitate
II	Prothrombin deficiency	40	3	Concentrate (factor IX-prothrombin complex)
V	Factor V deficiency	20	1	Fresh-frozen plasma
VII	Factor VII deficiency	Unknown	0.25	Concentrate (some preparations of factor IX)
VIII	Hemophilia A (classic)	25–35	0.5	Plasma, cryoprecipitate, and other factor VIII concentrates[3]
	von Willebrand's disease	30	Unknown	
IX	Hemophilia B (Christmas disease)	25	1	Plasma, factor IX-prothrombin complex
X	Stuart-Prower defect	25	1.5	Plasma, concentrate (some preparations of factor IX)
XI	PTA deficiency	Unknown	3	Fresh-frozen plasma
XII	Hageman defect	Not required	Unknown	Treatment not needed
XIII	Fibrin-stabilizing factor deficiency	2	6	Fresh-frozen plasma
AT III	Antithrombin III deficiency	80	3	Concentrate (AT III-specific)

[1]Reproduced, with permission, from Biggs R (editor): *Human Blood Coagulation, Haemostasis, and Thrombosis*, 2nd ed. Blackwell, 1976.
[2]The immediate postinfusion level may need to be much higher and varies according to the degree of trauma.
[3]Highly purified preparations of factor VIII should not be used in the treatment of von Willebrand's disease without specific evidence of their efficacy.

requires diagnostic specificity of the deficient factor and quantitation of its activity in plasma. There are many uncommon inherited and acquired disorders of platelet function. Recombinant factor VIII has been synthesized and has recently been approved for clinical use. Its expense may overbalance the benefit of freedom from risk of transmission of viral disease.

1. FACTOR VIII

Two preparations of concentrated human factor VIII are available. **Cryoprecipitate** is a plasma protein fraction and is obtainable from whole blood. It is used to treat deficiencies of factor VIII in patients with hemophilia and von Willebrand's disease and occasionally to provide fibrinogen. For infusion, the frozen cryoprecipitate unit is thawed and dissolved in a small volume of sterile citrate-saline solution and pooled with other units. Rh-negative women with potential for childbearing should receive only Rh-negative cryoprecipitate because of possible contamination of the product with Rh-positive blood cells. **Lyophilized factor VIII concentrates** are prepared from large pools of plasma. Cryoprecipitate prepared from individual donors is probably safer. Transmission of viral diseases such as hepatitis B and C and AIDS is reduced or eliminated by pasteurization and by extraction of plasma with solvents and detergents. Similarly, treatment of factor VIII concentrates with ultraviolet irradiation may reduce the danger of transmission of AIDS. Ultrapure factor VIII concentrates prepared by monoclonal antibody and recombinant DNA techniques are very expensive. Commercial freeze-dried concentrates may not suffice for treatment of patients with von Willebrand's disease, because the polymeric structure of factor VIII in the von Willebrand protein that supports platelet adhesion may be lost in the manufacturing process.

An uncomplicated hemorrhage into a joint should be treated with sufficient factor VIII replacement to maintain a level of at least 5% of the normal concentration for 24 hours. Soft tissue hematomas require a minimum of 10% activity for 7 days. Hematuria requires at least 10% activity for 3 days. Surgery and major trauma require a minimum of 30% activity for 10 days after an initial loading dose of 50 units/kg of body weight to achieve 100% activity of factor VIII (Table 34–3). Each unit per kilogram of factor VIII raises its activity in plasma 2%. Replacement should be administered every 12 hours.

Desmopressin acetate (arginine vasopressin) increases the factor VIII activity of patients with mild hemophilia A or von Willebrand's disease. It can be used in preparation for minor surgery such as tooth extraction without any requirement for infusion of clotting factor replacement. **Danazol,** an attenuated androgen that also elevates factor VIII activity, has been used experimentally with success in mild hemophiliacs.

Factor VIII concentrates and cryoprecipitate must not be used to treat deficiencies of vitamin K-dependent factors.

2. FACTOR IX

Freeze-dried concentrates of plasma containing prothrombin, factors IX and X, and varied amounts of factor VII (Proplex, etc) are commercially available for treating deficiencies of these factors (Table 34–3). Each unit of factor IX per kilogram of body weight raises its activity in plasma 1.5%. Heparin is often added to inhibit coagulation factors activated by the manufacturing process. However, addition of heparin does not eliminate thromboembolic events. Nevertheless, patients managed with high-purity preparations of factor IX that were virally inactivated by the solvent-detergent method had fewer thrombotic episodes following surgery.

Some preparations of factor IX concentrate contain *activated* clotting factors, which has led to their use in treating patients with inhibitors or antibodies to factor VIII or IX. Two products are available expressly for this purpose: **Autoplex** (with factor VIII correctional activity) and **Feiba** (with factor VIII inhibitor bypassing activity). These products are not uniformly successful in arresting hemorrhage, and the inhibitor titers often rise after treatment with them.

3. FIBRINOGEN

Fibrinogen may be administered to patients as plasma, cryoprecipitate of factor VIII, or lyophilized concentrates of factor VIII. A single unit of cryoprecipitate contains 300 mg of fibrinogen. Lyophilized concentrates of factor VIII are rich in fibrinogen.

FIBRINOLYTIC INHIBITORS: AMINOCAPROIC ACID

Aminocaproic acid (EACA), which is chemically similar to the amino acid lysine, is a synthetic inhibitor of fibrinolysis. It competitively inhibits plasminogen activation (Figure 34–3). It is rapidly absorbed orally and is cleared from the body by the kidney. The usual oral dosage of EACA is 6 g four times a day. When the drug is administered intravenously, a 5 g loading dose should be infused over 30 minutes to avoid hypotension. **Tranexamic acid** is an analog of aminocaproic acid and has the same properties. It is administered orally with a 15 mg/kg loading dose followed by 30 mg/kg every 6 hours.

Clinical uses of aminocaproic acid are as adjunctive therapy in hemophilia, as therapy for bleeding from fibrinolytic therapy, and as prophylaxis for rebleeding from intracranial aneurysms. Treatment success has also been reported in patients with post-surgical gastrointestinal bleeding and postprostatectomy bleeding and bladder hemorrhage secondary to radiation- and drug-induced cystitis. Adverse effects of the drug include intravascular thrombosis from inhibition of plasminogen activator, hypotension, myopathy, abdominal discomfort, diarrhea, and nasal stuffiness.

SERINE PROTEASE INHIBITORS: APROTININ

Aprotinin is a serine protease inhibitor ("serpin") that inhibits fibrinolysis by free plasmin and may have other antihemorrhagic effects as well. It also inhibits the plasmin-streptokinase complex in patients who have received the thrombolytic agent. Aprotinin will reduce bleeding—by as much as 50%—from many types of surgery, especially that involving extracorporeal circulation for open heart procedures (Royston, 1995). It is currently approved for use in patients undergoing coronary artery bypass grafting who are at high risk of excessive blood loss. In placebo-controlled trials, adverse effects of aprotinin were little different from those reported in patients in the placebo group. In larger studies, a possible association with anaphylaxis has been reported in < 0.5% of cases. Therefore, a small test dose is recommended before the full therapeutic dose is given.

PREPARATIONS AVAILABLE

Abciximab (ReoPro)
  Parenteral: 2 mg/mL for IV injection
Alteplase recombinant [t-PA] (Activase)
  Parenteral: 20, 50 mg lyophilized powder to reconstitute for IV injection
Aminocaproic acid (generic, Amicar)
  Oral: 500 mg tablets; 250 mg/mL syrup
  Parenteral: 250 mg/mL for IV injection
Anistreplase (Eminase)
  Parenteral: 30 units lyophilized powder to reconstitute for IV injection
Antihemophilic factor [Factor VIII, AHF] (Hemofil M, Koāte-HP, Kogenate, Monoclate, Recombinate, others)
  Parenteral: in vials
Anti-inhibitor coagulant complex (Autoplex T, Feiba VH Immuno)
  Parenteral: in vials
Antithrombin III (ATnativ)
  500 IU powder to reconstitute for IV injection
Aprotinin (Trasylol)
  Parenteral: 10,000 units/mL in 100 and 200 mL vials
Dalteparin (Fragmin)
  Parenteral: 2500 anti-factor Xa/0.2 mL for SC injection only
Danaproid (Orgaran)
  Parenteral: 750 anti-Xa units/vial
Dipyridamole (Persantine)
  Oral: 25, 50, 75 mg tablets
Enoxaparin (Low-molecular-weight heparin, Lovenox)
  Parenteral: 30 mg/0.3 mL for SC injection only

Factor IX complex, human (Konȳne-80, Profilnine Heat-Treated, Proplex T, Proplex SX-T)
  Parenteral: in vials
Heparin calcium (Calciparine)
  Parenteral: 5000 units/unit dose
Heparin sodium (generic, Liquaemin)
  Parenteral: 1000, 5000, 10,000, 20,000, 40,000 units/mL for injection
Phytonadione [K_1] (Mephyton, AquaMephyton, Konakion)
  Oral: 5 mg tablets
  Parenteral: 2, 10 mg/mL aqueous colloidal solution or suspension for injection
Protamine (generic)
  Parenteral: 10 mg/mL for injection
Reteplase (Retavase)
  Parenteral: 10.8 IU powder for injection
Streptokinase (Kabikinase, Streptase)
  Parenteral: 250,000, 600,000, 750,000, 1,500,000 IU per vial powders to reconstitute for injection
Ticlopidine (Ticlid)
  Oral: 250 mg tablets
Tranexamic acid (Cyklokapron)
  Oral: 500 mg tablets
  Parenteral: 100 mg/mL for injection
Urokinase (Abbokinase)
  Parenteral: 250,000 IU per vial for systemic use; 5000 IU/mL per vial for unblocking central catheters
Warfarin (generic, Coumadin)
  Oral: 1, 2, 2.5, 5, 7.5, 10 mg tablets

REFERENCES

Blood Coagulation

Mann KG, Kalafatis M: Coagulation explosion. Cerebrovasc Dis 1995;5:93.

Rapaport SI, Rao LVM: Tissue factor pathway: How it has become a "prima ballerina." Thromb Haemost 1995;74:7.

Suttie JW: The importance of menaquinones in human nutrition. Annu Rev Nutr 1995;15:399.

Wu KK, Thiagarajan P: Role of endothelium in thrombosis and hemostasis. Annu Rev Med 1996;47:315.

Anticoagulant Drugs

Barrowcliffe TW: Low molecular weight heparin(s). Br J Haematol 1995;90:1.

Blackshear JL et al: Management of atrial fibrillation in adults: Prevention of thromboembolism and symptomatic treatment. Mayo Clin Proc 1996;71:150.

De Valk HW et al: Comparing subcutaneous danaparoid with intravenous unfractionated heparin for the treatment of venous thromboembolism: A randomized controlled trial. Ann Intern Med 1995;123:1.

Fihn SD: Aiming for safe anticoagulation. (Editorial.) N Engl J Med 1995;333:54.

Hirsh J et al: Heparin: Mechanism of action, pharmacokinetics, dosing considerations, monitoring efficacy, and safety. Chest (Suppl) 1995;108:258S.

Hirsh J et al: Oral anticoagulants: Mechanism of action, clinical effectiveness, and optimal therapeutic range. Chest (Suppl) 1995;108:231S.

Mathiesen T et al: Intracranial traumatic and nontraumatic haemorrhagic complications of warfarin treatment. Acta Neurol Scand 1995;91:208.

Fibrinolytic Drugs

Cairns JA et al: Coronary thrombolysis. Chest (Suppl) 1995;108:401S.

European Secondary Prevention Study Group: Translation of clinical trials into practice: A European population-based study of the use of thrombolysis for acute myocardial infarction. Lancet 1996;347:1203.

Heart and Stroke Foundation of Canada et al: Recommendations for ensuring early thrombolytic therapy for acute myocardial infarction. Can Med Assoc J 1996;154:483.

Multicenter Acute Stroke Trial–Europe Study Group: Thrombolytic therapy with streptokinase in acute ischemic stroke. N Engl J Med 1996;335:145.

Rawles J: Magnitude of benefit from earlier thrombolytic treatment in acute myocardial infarction: New evidence from Grampian region early anistreplase trial (GREAT). BMJ 1996;312:212.

Rogers WJ: Contemporary management of acute myocardial infarction. Am J Med 1995;99:195.

Antithrombotic Drugs

Cairns JA et al: Antithrombotic agents in coronary artery disease. Chest (Suppl) 1995;108:380S.

Coller BS: Blockade of platelet GP IIb/IIIa receptors as an antithrombotic strategy. Circulation 1995;92:2373.

Schafer AI: Antiplatelet drugs. Am J Med 1996;101:199.

Simoons ML, Decker JW: New directions in anticoagulant and antiplatelet treatment. (Editorial.) Br Heart J 1995;74:337.

Sweeney JP, Schwartz GG: Applying the results of large clinical trials in the management of acute myocardial infarction. West J Med 1996;164:238.

Tcheng JE et al: Multicenter, randomized, double-blind, placebo-controlled trial of the platelet integrin glycoprotein IIb/IIIa blocker Integrelin in elective coronary intervention. Circulation 1995;91:2151.

Topol EJ: Novel antithrombotic approaches to coronary artery disease. Am J Cardiol 1995;75:27B.

Bleeding Disorders

Brownlee GG: Prospects for gene therapy of haemophilia A and B. Br Med Bull 1995;51:91.

Djulbegovic B et al: Safety and efficacy of purified factor IX concentrate and antifibrinolytic agents for dental extractions in hemophilia B. Am J Hematol 1996;51:168.

Ehmann WC et al: Causes of death in haemophilia. Nature 1995;378:124.

Royston D: Blood-sparing drugs: Aprotinin, tranexamic acid, and epsilon aminocaproic acid. Int Anesthesiol Clin 1995;33:155.

Street AM, Ekert H: Haemophilia—darkest hours before the dawn. (Editorial.) Med J Aust 1996;164:453.

Agents Used in Hyperlipidemia

35

Mary J. Malloy, MD, & John P. Kane, MD, PhD

Virtually all the lipids of human plasma are transported as complexes with proteins. Except for fatty acids, which are bound chiefly to albumin, the lipids are carried in special macromolecular complexes termed **lipoproteins.** A number of metabolic disorders that involve elevations in plasma concentrations of any of the lipoprotein species are thus termed **hyperlipoproteinemias** or **hyperlipidemias.** The term **hyperlipemia** is restricted to conditions that involve increased levels of triglycerides in plasma.

The two major clinical sequelae of the hyperlipoproteinemias are acute pancreatitis and atherosclerosis. Acute pancreatitis occurs in patients with marked hyperlipemia. In such persons, control of triglyceride levels can prevent recurrent attacks of this life-threatening disease.

Atherosclerosis is the leading cause of death for both women and men in the USA and other Western countries. Certain plasma lipoproteins play an essential role in atherogenesis. Those that contain **apolipoprotein (Apo) B-100** have been identified as the vehicles in which cholesterol is transported into the artery wall. These are the **low-density (LDL), intermediate-density (IDL), very low density (VLDL),** and **Lp(a) lipoproteins.**

The characteristic cellular components in atherosclerotic plaques are foam cells, which are transformed macrophages and smooth muscle cells that have become filled with **cholesteryl esters.** This is the result of the endocytosis of chemically modified lipoproteins via as many as four molecular species of scavenger receptors. The massive accumulation of cholesteryl esters is due to the inability of these receptors to be down-regulated by high intracellular levels of cholesterol. The chief chemical modification of lipoproteins that creates ligands for scavenger receptors appears to be free radical-mediated oxidation that occurs in the artery wall. Glycation of lipoproteins in poorly controlled diabetes also contributes to foam cell formation. Arterial hypertension accelerates atherogenesis. It is well established that appropriate treatment of elevated blood pressure helps to prevent coronary disease and stroke. The atheromatous plaque grows over time with the accumulation of increased

numbers of foam cells, and of collagen and fibrin. Cells of neural crest origin can initiate calcification in the lesions. Whereas growing lesions can slowly occlude coronary vessels, clinical symptoms are more frequently precipitated by rupture of the endothelium over active plaques, leading to activation of platelets and formation of occlusive thrombi. These acute events are thought to reflect inflammatory activities of macrophages.

Although treatment of hyperlipidemia causes slow physical regression of plaques, the well-documented reduction in acute coronary events that follows vigorous treatment is attributable chiefly to mitigation of the inflammatory activity of macrophages and is evident within 2–3 months after starting therapy.

High-density lipoproteins (HDL) exert several antiatherogenic effects. They participate in metabolic pathways that retrieve cholesterol from the artery wall, and they inhibit the oxidation of atherogenic lipoproteins. Low levels of HDL (hypoalphalipoproteinemia) are an independent risk factor for coronary disease.

The selection of drugs that increase levels of HDL is indicated in patients with hypoalphalipoproteinemia.

Cigarette smoking is a major risk factor for coronary disease. It is associated with reduced levels of HDL, impairment of cholesterol retrieval, cytotoxic effects on the endothelium, increased oxidation of atherogenic lipoproteins, and stimulation of thrombogenesis. Normally the coronary arteries are able to dilate in response to ischemia and to increased shear stress so as to increase delivery of oxygen to the myocardium. This dilation is mediated by endothelium-derived relaxing factor (EDRF, nitric oxide), which acts upon smooth muscle cells of the arterial media. EDRF function is impaired by high levels of atherogenic lipoproteins in several phenotypes of hyperlipidemias, thus aggravating ischemic manifestations of atherosclerosis. Reductions of the levels of atherogenic lipoproteins in plasma and inhibition of their oxidation—using the natural antioxidants tocopherol and ascorbic acid—helps to restore EDRF function.

Because the process of atherogenesis is multifactorial, therapy should be directed at all the modifiable risk factors, including atherogenic hyperlipidemia. Atherosclerotic disease of both coronary and peripheral arteries is a dynamic process. Trials employing quantitative angiography have conclusively demonstrated that net physical regression of plaques occurs during aggressive lipid-lowering therapy. Large primary and secondary prevention trials have shown significant reduction in mortality from new coronary events. This impact was so large that it also resulted in significant reduction in all-cause mortality. Therefore, the timely diagnosis and treatment of lipoprotein disorders can be expected to decrease morbidity and mortality due to coronary disease.

Many of the hyperlipidemic states are associated with the development of xanthomas. These lesions, which are produced by deposition of lipid in tendons or skin, may be painful or cosmetically unacceptable to the patient. Because xanthomas regress with lipid-lowering therapy, this provides another indication for treatment.

An understanding of the biology of the lipoproteins and the pathophysiology of the various hyperlipidemic states is essential to the rational choice of treatment regimens.

PATHOPHYSIOLOGY OF HYPERLIPOPROTEINEMIA

NORMAL LIPOPROTEIN METABOLISM

Structure

The major lipoproteins of plasma are particles with hydrophobic core regions containing cholesteryl es-

ters and triglycerides. A monolayer of unesterified cholesterol and phospholipids surrounds the core. Specific proteins (apolipoproteins) are located on the surface. Certain lipoproteins contain very high molecular weight apolipoproteins (B proteins) that do not migrate from one particle to another, as do smaller apolipoproteins. There are two primary forms of ApoB: B-48, which is formed in the intestine and found in chylomicrons and their remnants; and B-100, which is synthesized in the liver and found in VLDL, VLDL remnants (intermediate-density lipoproteins, or IDL), LDL (which are formed from VLDL), and the Lp(a) lipoproteins.

Smaller apolipoproteins distribute variably among the lipoproteins. ApoA-I is a cofactor for lecithin: cholesterol acyltransferase (LCAT). ApoC-II is a required cofactor for lipoprotein lipase. Several isoforms of ApoE, based on single amino acid substitutions, are recognized. Isoforms of this protein that are recognized by hepatic receptors are required for uptake of lipoprotein remnants by the liver.

The characteristics of various lipoprotein complexes are shown in Table 35–1.

Synthesis & Catabolism

A. Chylomicrons: Chylomicrons, the largest of the lipoproteins, are formed in the intestine and carry triglycerides of dietary origin. Some cholesteryl esters also appear in the chylomicron core. Phospholipids and free cholesterol—together with newly synthesized ApoB-48, A-I, A-II, and other proteins—form the surface monolayer. The chylomicrons transit the thoracic duct to the bloodstream.

Triglycerides are removed from the chylomicrons in extrahepatic tissues through a pathway shared with VLDL that involves hydrolysis by the lipoprotein lipase (LPL) system. A progressive decrease in particle diameter occurs as triglycerides in the core are depleted. Surface lipids, ApoA-I, ApoA-II, and ApoC are transferred to HDL. The resultant chylomicron "remnants" are taken up by receptor-mediated endocytosis into hepatocytes.

B. Very Low Density Lipoproteins (VLDL): VLDL, secreted by liver, provide a means for export of triglycerides to peripheral tissues (Figure 35–1). VLDL contain ApoB-100 and some ApoC. More ApoC is acquired from HDL in plasma. VLDL triglycerides are hydrolyzed by lipoprotein lipase, yielding free fatty acids for storage in adipose tissue and for oxidation in tissues such as cardiac and skeletal muscle. The resulting depletion of triglycerides produces remnants termed intermediate-density lipoproteins (IDL). Some of the IDL particles are endocytosed directly by the liver. The remainder are converted to LDL by further removal of triglycerides mediated by hepatic lipase. This process explains the clinical phenomenon of the "beta shift," the increase of LDL (beta-lipoprotein) in serum as a hypertriglyceridemic state subsides. Increased levels of LDL in

Table 35–1. Major lipoproteins of human serum.

	Electrophoretic Mobility in Agarose Gel	Density Interval (g/cm³)	Core Lipids	Diameter (nm)	Apolipoproteins in Order of Quantitative Importance
High-density (HDL)	Alpha	1.063–1.21	Cholesteryl esters	7.5–10.5	A-I, A-II, C, E, D
Low-density (LDL)	Beta	1.019–1.063	Cholesteryl esters	21–22	B-100
Intermediate-density (IDL)	Beta	1.006–1.019	Cholesteryl esters, triglycerides	25–30	B-100, E, C
Very low density (VLDL)	Prebeta, some "slow prebeta"	< 1.006	Triglycerides, some cholesteryl esters	39–100	C species, B-100, E
Chylomicrons	Remain at origin	< 1.006	Triglycerides, some cholesteryl esters	80–500	B-48, C, E, A-I, A-II
Lp(a) lipoproteins	Prebeta	1.04–1.08	Cholesteryl esters	21–30	B-100, Lp(a)

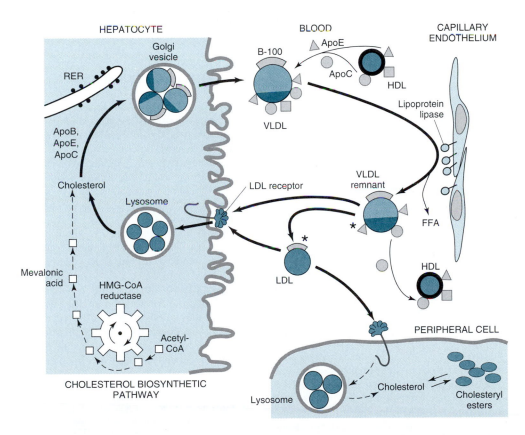

Figure 35–1. Metabolism of lipoproteins of hepatic origin. The heavy arrows show the primary pathways. Nascent VLDL are secreted via the Golgi apparatus. They acquire additional C lipoproteins and ApoE from HDL. VLDL are converted to VLDL remnants (IDL) by lipolysis via lipoprotein lipase in the vessels of peripheral tissues. In the process, C apolipoproteins and a portion of the ApoE are given back to HDL. Some of the VLDL remnants are converted to LDL by further loss of triglycerides and loss of ApoE. A major pathway for LDL degradation involves the endocytosis of LDL by LDL receptors in the liver and the peripheral tissues, for which ApoB-100 is the ligand. (Dark color denotes cholesteryl esters; light color, triglycerides; the asterisk denotes a functional ligand for LDL receptors; triangles indicate apolipoprotein E; circles and squares represent C apolipoproteins; RER denotes rough endoplasmic reticulum.) (Modified and redrawn, with permission, from Kane J, Malloy M: Disorders of lipoproteins. In: *The Molecular and Genetic Basis of Neurological Disease.* Rosenberg RN et al (editors). Butterworth-Heinemann, 1993.)

plasma can result from increased secretion of its precursor VLDL as well as from decreased LDL catabolism.

C. Low-Density Lipoproteins (LDL): A major pathway by which LDL are catabolized in hepatocytes and most other nucleated cells involves high-affinity receptor-mediated endocytosis. Cholesteryl esters from the LDL core are then hydrolyzed, yielding free cholesterol for the synthesis of cell membranes. Cells also obtain cholesterol by de novo synthesis via a pathway involving the formation of mevalonic acid by HMG-CoA reductase. Production of this enzyme and of LDL receptors is regulated at the transcriptional level by the content of cholesterol in the cell. Normally, about half of the removal of LDL from plasma results from endocytosis of LDL into hepatocytes. Even more cholesterol is delivered to liver by endocytosis of the remnants of VLDL and chylomicrons. Thus, the liver plays a major role in the cholesterol economy of the body. Unlike other cells, hepatocytes are capable of eliminating cholesterol from the body by secretion of cholesterol per se in bile and by conversion of cholesterol to bile acids which are also secreted in bile.

D. Lp(a) Lipoprotein: Lp(a) lipoprotein is formed from an LDL-like moiety and the Lp(a) protein linked by a disulfide bridge. Lp(a) protein is highly homologous with plasminogen but lacks the ability to be activated by tissue plasminogen activator. It occurs in a number of isoforms of different molecular weights. The levels of this protein in human serum vary from nil to over 200 mg/dL and appear to be determined in large part by genetic factors. The Lp(a) lipoprotein complex can be found in atherosclerotic plaques and may also contribute to coronary disease by inhibiting thrombolysis.

E. High-Density Lipoproteins (HDL): The apolipoproteins of HDL are secreted by liver and intestine. Much of the lipid in HDL comes from the surface monolayers of chylomicrons and VLDL during lipolysis. HDL also acquire cholesterol from peripheral tissues in a pathway that protects the cholesterol homeostasis of cells. In this process, free cholesterol absorbed from cell membranes is acquired by a small particle termed prebeta-1 HDL. The cholesterol is then esterified by lecithin:cholesterol acyltransferase (LCAT), leading to the formation of larger HDL species. The cholesteryl esters are transferred to VLDL, IDL, LDL, and chylomicron remnants with the aid of cholesteryl ester transfer protein (CETP). Much of the cholesteryl ester thus transferred is ultimately delivered to the liver by endocytosis of the acceptor lipoproteins (Figure 35–1). HDL can also deliver cholesteryl esters directly to liver via a docking receptor (scavenger receptor, SR-BI) that does not endocytose the lipoproteins.

LIPOPROTEIN DISORDERS

Lipoprotein disorders are detected by measuring the content of lipids in serum after a 10-hour fast. The risk of atherosclerotic heart disease increases with concentrations of the atherogenic lipoproteins, is inversely related to levels of HDL, and is modified by other risk factors (Table 35–2). Ideally, triglyceride levels should be below 150 mg/dL. Differentiation requires identification of the species of lipoproteins that account for the observed increases (Table 35–3). Diagnosis of a specific primary lipoprotein disorder usually necessitates gathering further clinical and genetic data as well as ruling out disorders that can cause secondary hyperlipidemia (Table 35–4).

The various patterns of abnormal lipoprotein distribution are described in this section. Drugs mentioned for use in these conditions are described in the following section on basic and clinical pharmacology.

THE PRIMARY HYPERTRIGLYCERIDEMIAS

Hypertriglyceridemia is linked epidemiologically with increased risk of coronary disease and, in some kindreds, may be the only evident risk factor. These patients tend to have cholesterol-rich VLDL of small particle diameter. Hypertriglyceridemic patients with coronary disease or a family history of premature coronary disease should be treated aggressively. In others, treatment decisions should be based on the aggregate of risk factors. Because the clearance of triglycerides by lipoprotein lipase is saturated at about 800 mg/dL of triglycerides, patients with triglycerides above that level should be treated to prevent acute pancreatitis.

Primary Chylomicronemia

Chylomicrons are not normally present in the serum of individuals who have fasted 10 hours. The autosomal recessive traits of lipoprotein lipase deficiency and lipoprotein lipase cofactor deficiency are usually associated with severe lipemia (2000–2500

Table 35–2. National Cholesterol Education Program: Adult Treatment Guidelines (1993).

	Total Cholesterol (mg/dL)	LDL Cholesterol (mg/dL)
Desirable	< 200	< 130
Borderline to high[1]	200–239	130–159
High	≥ 240	≥ 160

[1]Consider as high if coronary heart disease or more than two risk factors are present. A level of HDL cholesterol below 35 mg/dL is considered a major risk factor. The LDL cholesterol goal in patients with coronary artery disease is 100 mg/dL or less.

Table 35–3. The primary hyperlipoproteinemias and their drug treatment.

Disorder	Manifestations	Single Drug[1]	Drug Combination
Primary chylomicronemia (familial lipoprotein lipase or cofactor deficiency)	Chylomicrons, VLDL increased	Dietary management	Niacin, gemfibrozil
Familial hypertriglyceridemia Severe	VLDL, chylomicrons increased	Niacin, gemfibrozil	Niacin plus gemfibrozil
Moderate	VLDL increased; chylomicrons may be increased	Niacin, gemfibrozil	
Familial combined hyperlipoproteinemia	VLDL increased	Niacin, gemfibrozil	
	LDL increased	Niacin, reductase inhibitor, resin	Niacin plus resin or reductase inhibitor
	VLDL, LDL increased	Niacin, reductase inhibitor	Niacin plus resin or reductase inhibitor
Familial dysbetalipoproteinemia	VLDL remnants, chylomicron remnants increased	Gemfibrozil, niacin	Gemfibrozil plus niacin or niacin plus reductase inhibitor
Familial hypercholesterolemia Heterozygous	LDL increased	Resin, reductase inhibitor, niacin	Two or three of the individual drugs
Homozygous	LDL increased	Niacin	Resin plus niacin plus reductase inhibitor
Familial ligand-defective ApoB	LDL increased	Niacin, reductase inhibitor	Niacin plus reductase inhibitor
Lp(a) hyperlipoproteinemia	Lp(a) increased	Niacin	
Unclassified hypercholesterolemia		Resin, niacin, reductase inhibitor, gemfibrozil	

[1]Single-drug therapy should be evaluated before drug combinations are used.

mg/dL triglycerides when the patient is consuming a typical American diet). These disorders may not be diagnosed until an attack of acute pancreatitis occurs. Patients may have eruptive xanthomas, hepatosplenomegaly, hypersplenism, and lipid-laden foam cells in bone marrow, liver, and spleen. The lipemia is aggravated by estrogens, since they stimulate VLDL production in the liver, and pregnancy may cause marked increases in triglyceride levels despite strict dietary control. Although these patients have a predominant chylomicronemia, they may also have moderately elevated VLDL, presenting with a pattern of mixed lipemia (fasting chylomicronemia and elevated VLDL). Lipoprotein lipase deficiency is diagnosed by in vitro assay of lipolytic activity in plasma after intravenous injection of heparin; cofactor deficiency is diagnosed by isoelectric focusing of the VLDL proteins. A presumptive diagnosis of these disorders is made by demonstrating a pronounced decrease in levels of plasma triglycerides a few days after sharp restriction of oral fat intake. Marked restriction of the total fat content in the diet provides effective long-term treatment. No drug treatment is indicated.

Table 35–4. Secondary causes of hyperlipoproteinemia.

Hypertriglyceridemia	Hypercholesterolemia
Diabetes mellitus	Hypothyroidism
Alcohol ingestion	Early nephrosis
Severe nephrosis	Resolving lipemia
Estrogens	Immunoglobulin-lipoprotein
Uremia	complex disorders
Corticosteroid excess	Anorexia nervosa
Hypothyroidism	Cholestasis
Glycogen storage disease	Hypopituitarism
Hypopituitarism	Corticosteroid excess
Acromegaly	
Immunoglobulin-lipoprotein complex disorders	
Lipodystrophy	

Familial Hypertriglyceridemia

A. Severe (Usually Mixed Lipemia): A pattern of mixed lipemia usually results from impaired removal of triglyceride-rich lipoproteins, though factors that increase VLDL production aggravate the lipemia because VLDL and chylomicrons are competing substrates for lipoprotein lipase. The primary mixed lipemias probably represent a variety of modes of inheritance. Most patients have the centripetal pattern of obesity with impaired effectiveness of insulin. In addition to obesity, other factors that lead to increased rate of secretion of VLDL also worsen the lipemia. Eruptive xanthomas, lipemia retinalis, epigastric pain, and overt pancreatitis are variably present, depending on the severity of the lipemia. Treatment is primarily dietary, with restriction of total fat, avoidance of alcohol and exogenous estrogens, and weight reduction to ideal levels. Some patients may require treatment with gemfibrozil or niacin.

B. Moderate (Endogenous Lipemia): Primary increases of VLDL levels probably reflect a number of genetic determinants and are worsened by factors that increase the rate of VLDL secretion from liver, ie, hypertrophic obesity, alcohol ingestion, diabetes, and exogenous estrogens. A major indication for treatment is the presence of atherosclerosis in the patient or the patient's family. Treatment includes weight reduction to ideal levels, restriction of all types of dietary fat, and avoidance of alcohol. Gemfibrozil or niacin usually produces further reduction in triglyceride levels if dietary measures are not sufficient.

Familial Combined Hyperlipoproteinemia

In kindreds with this disorder, individuals may have elevated levels of VLDL, LDL, or both, and the pattern may change with time. The underlying disorder appears to involve an approximately two-fold increase in VLDL secretion. This disorder seems to be transmitted as a semidominant trait. Factors that increase levels of triglycerides in serum in other disorders do so in this one as well. Elevations of serum cholesterol and triglycerides are generally moderate, and xanthomas are usually absent. However, drug treatment is warranted because the risk of coronary atherosclerosis is increased, and diet alone usually does not normalize lipid levels. Patients with elevated VLDL usually respond to niacin. A reductase inhibitor or a resin in combination with niacin may be required to treat elevated levels of LDL.

Familial Dysbetalipoproteinemia

In familial dysbetalipoproteinemia, remnants of chylomicrons and VLDL accumulate. Levels of LDL are usually decreased. Because the remnants are rich in cholesteryl esters, the level of serum cholesterol may be as high as that of triglycerides. Diagnosis is confirmed by the absence of the E3 and E4 isoforms of ApoE. Patients often develop tuberous or tuberoeruptive xanthomas or characteristic planar xanthomas of the palmar creases. They tend to be obese, and some have impaired glucose tolerance. These factors, together with hypothyroidism, can aggravate the lipemia. Coronary and peripheral atherosclerosis occur with increased frequency. A weight reduction diet, together with decreased fat, cholesterol, and alcohol consumption, often is sufficient treatment. Gemfibrozil or niacin is needed in some cases. Frequently, low doses are sufficient. These agents can be given together in more resistant cases.

THE PRIMARY HYPERCHOLESTEROLEMIAS

Familial Hypercholesterolemia

This disorder is transmitted as an autosomal dominant trait. Although levels of LDL tend to increase throughout childhood, the diagnosis can often be made on the basis of elevated umbilical cord blood cholesterol. In most heterozygous adults, serum cholesterol levels commonly range from 260 to 500 mg/dL. Triglyceride levels are usually normal, tendinous xanthomatosis is often present, and arcus corneae and xanthelasma may appear in the third decade. Coronary atherosclerosis tends to occur prematurely. Homozygous familial hypercholesterolemia, which can lead to coronary disease in childhood, is characterized by very high levels of cholesterol in serum (often exceeding 1000 mg/dL) and early tuberous and tendinous xanthomatosis. These patients may also develop elevated plaque-like xanthomas of the aortic valve, digital webs, buttocks, and extremities.

Defects of high-affinity receptors for LDL underlie this disorder. Heterozygotes have about half the usual number, and some individuals have combined heterozygosity for alleles producing nonfunctional and kinetically impaired receptors. Levels of LDL in compliant heterozygous patients can be normalized with combined drug regimens (Figure 35–2).

Individuals whose receptors retain even minimal function may partially respond to resins or reductase inhibitors. Niacin may benefit patients with no receptor function.

Familial Ligand-Defective Apolipoprotein B

Defects in the ligand domain of ApoB-100 (the region that binds to the LDL receptor) impair the endocytosis of LDL, leading to hypercholesterolemia of moderate severity. Tendon xanthomas may occur. It is anticipated that LDL levels will respond to niacin. Response to HMG-CoA reductase inhibitors is variable.

Familial Combined Hyperlipoproteinemia

As described above, some persons in kindreds with this disorder have only an elevation in LDL levels. Levels of serum cholesterol usually are less than 350 mg/dL. Premature onset of coronary disease is common. Dietary and drug treatment, usually with niacin or a reductase inhibitor, is indicated. It is frequently necessary to add niacin to normalize LDL levels or to lower triglycerides if treatment is initiated with a resin.

Lp(a) Hyperlipoproteinemia

This familial disorder, which is associated with increased atherogenesis, appears to be determined in part by genes that dictate increased production of the Lp(a) lipoprotein. Defects that inhibit the removal of LDL seem to augment plasma levels of Lp(a). Preliminary studies indicate that niacin may reduce levels of

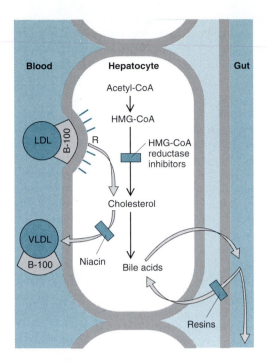

Figure 35–2. Sites of action of HMG-CoA reductase inhibitors, niacin, and resins used in treating hyperlipidemias. LDL receptors (R) are increased by treatment with resins and HMG-CoA reductase inhibitors.

Lp(a) in many patients. Hormone replacement therapy in postmenopausal women mitigates the increase in levels of Lp(a) observed after the menopause.

Unclassified Hypercholesterolemia

Other poorly defined types of hypercholesterolemia occur that are often familial but less severe than the disorders described above. Individuals in some kindreds who have elevated LDL levels have strikingly favorable responses to dietary management.

HDL DEFICIENCY

Certain rare genetic disorders are associated with extremely low levels of HDL in serum. These include Tangier disease and disorders of LCAT. Familial hypoalphalipoproteinemia is a more common disorder of HDL in which levels of HDL cholesterol are usually below 35 mg/dL, with apparent semidominant transmission. These patients tend to have premature atherosclerosis, and the low HDL levels may be the only identified risk factor. Treatment should include special attention to avoidance of other risk factors for coronary disease. Niacin increases HDL cholesterol levels in many of these patients.

In the presence of hypertriglyceridemia, HDL cholesterol levels are low because of exchange of cholesteryl esters from HDL into triglyceride-rich lipopro-

teins. This may contribute to the atherogenic effect of hypertriglyceridemia. In most patients, treatment of the hypertriglyceridemia will result in normalization of HDL cholesterol levels.

SECONDARY HYPERLIPOPROTEINEMIA

Before primary hyperlipoproteinemia can be diagnosed, secondary causes of the specific phenotype must be considered. The more common conditions that may be associated with hyperlipoproteinemia are summarized in Table 35–4. The lipoprotein abnormality usually resolves if the underlying disorder can be treated successfully.

Certain persons, often with a preexisting mild lipemia, develop severe hypertriglyceridemia when given even small doses of estrogens, such as those in oral contraceptives. This effect is smaller when very low doses of estrogen are combined with a progestational agent. If estrogen therapy is clinically necessary, transdermal administration exerts less hypertriglyceridemic effect by avoiding first pass extraction by the liver.

Treatment of the hyperlipidemia associated with chronic nephrotic syndrome is indicated, since coronary vascular disease is prevalent in these patients. Diet has little effect. Gemfibrozil must be used cautiously because it may precipitate myopathy in patients with hypoalbuminemia. Currently, the drugs of choice are bile acid-binding resins combined with niacin. Reductase inhibitors are also useful. Tryptophan supplementation ameliorates hypertriglyceridemia in some nephrotic patients who may be deficient in this amino acid.

The hyperlipidemia associated with cholestasis involves abnormal lipoproteins, including LP-X, vesicular particles rich in unesterified cholesterol and phospholipid. Neuropathy, caused by xanthomatous involvement of nerves, is an indication for treatment of this hyperlipidemia. Although plasmapheresis is most effective, bile acid-binding resins may be of some value. Gemfibrozil is contraindicated, since it can cause an increase in serum cholesterol in these patients.

DIETARY MANAGEMENT OF HYPERLIPOPROTEINEMIA

When the decision is made to treat hyperlipoproteinemia, dietary measures are always initiated first and may obviate the need for drugs. Exceptions are patients with familial hypercholesterolemia or familial combined hyperlipidemia in whom diet and drug therapy should be started simultaneously. Cholesterol and saturated fats are the principal dietary factors that influence LDL levels in plasma whereas total fat restriction is important in management of hypertriglyceridemia. Dietary cholesterol and saturated fats increase the concentration of LDL independently. *Trans* fatty acids formed during hydrogenation of fats and during protracted deep fat frying of food also increase levels of LDL.

Lipoprotein levels are also affected, but to a lesser extent, by other dietary factors. Transient increases in VLDL occur when carbohydrate intake is acutely increased. Sucrose and other simple sugars may raise VLDL levels in an occasional hypertriglyceridemic patient. Some forms of dietary fiber such as oat or rice bran may reduce LDL levels modestly. Alcohol can cause significant hypertriglyceridemia by increasing hepatic secretion of VLDL. Synthesis and secretion of VLDL are increased by excess caloric intake. Caloric restriction, especially in obese subjects, reduces VLDL triglycerides and may also reduce levels of LDL. While the patient is losing weight, LDL and VLDL levels may be much lower than those that can be maintained during neutral caloric balance. Therefore, the conclusion that diet alone suffices for management can only be made after the patient's weight has stabilized for at least 1 month.

Most patients with elevated LDL can be managed appropriately with a diet that is restricted in cholesterol and saturated fat and provides calories to achieve and maintain ideal body weight. Total fat calories should be 20–25%, with saturated fats less than 8% of total calories and cholesterol less than 200 mg/d. Reductions in serum cholesterol range from 10% to 20% on this regimen. Increases in complex carbohydrates and fiber are recommended, and monounsaturated fats should predominate within the fat allowance. Weight reduction and caloric restriction are especially important for patients with elevated VLDL and IDL. Patients with hypertriglyceridemia should avoid alcohol.

The effect of dietary fats in patients with hypertriglyceridemia is highly dependent upon the disposition of double bonds in the fatty acid carbon chain. Omega-3 fatty acids found in fish oils can induce profound lowering of triglycerides in some patients with endogenous or mixed lipemia. In contrast, the omega-6 fatty acids present in vegetable oils may cause levels of triglycerides to rise in these patients.

Patients with primary chylomicronemia and some individuals with mixed lipemia must consume a diet severely restricted in total fat: 10–15 g/d, of which 5 g should be vegetable oils rich in essential fatty acids. Supplementation of fat-soluble vitamins should be given.

BASIC & CLINICAL PHARMACOLOGY OF DRUGS USED IN HYPERLIPIDEMIA

Decisions to use drug therapy for hyperlipidemia must be based on the specific metabolic defect and its potential for causing atherosclerosis or pancreatitis. Suggested drug treatments for the principal lipoprotein disorders are presented in Table 35–3. Diet is a necessary adjunct to drug therapy and should be continued for achievement of the full potential of the drug regimen. Drug treatment of hyperlipidemia should be avoided in women who are likely to become pregnant or who are lactating. Children with heterozygous familial hypercholesterolemia may be treated with a bile acid-binding resin, usually after 7 or 8 years of age, when myelination of the central nervous system is essentially complete. The decision to treat an individual child should be based on the level of plasma LDL, the family history, and the child's age. In general, drug treatment is rarely indicated before age 18.

NIACIN
(Nicotinic Acid)

Niacin (but not niacinamide) decreases VLDL and LDL levels in the plasma of patients with a variety of hyperlipidemias.

Chemistry & Pharmacokinetics

Niacin is a water-soluble vitamin (vitamin B_3). It is converted in the body to the amide, which is incorporated into niacinamide adenine dinucleotide (NAD). It is excreted unmodified in the urine and as niacinamide, *N*-methyl-2-pyridone-3-carboxamide, *N*-methyl-2-pyridone-5-carboxamide, and other less abundant metabolites.

Mechanism of Action

The primary mechanism of action of niacin probably involves inhibition of VLDL secretion, in turn decreasing production of LDL (Figure 35–2). Decreased production of VLDL apolipoproteins has been demonstrated. Increased clearance of VLDL via the lipoprotein lipase pathway contributes to the triglyceride-lowering effect of niacin. The drug has no effect on bile acid production. Excretion of neutral sterols in the stool is increased acutely as cholesterol is mobilized from tissue pools. A new steady state is then reached during chronic administration of the drug. Cholesterogenesis is inhibited, an effect that persists when bile acid-binding resins are given. Decreased synthesis of cholesterol in liver increases hepatic uptake of LDL in support of increased bile acid synthesis induced by the resin. The catabolic rate for HDL is decreased, raising levels of HDL cholesterol and ApoA-I in plasma. The processes of atherogenesis or thrombosis may be influenced by the substantial reduction of circulating fibrinogen levels produced by niacin, and levels of tissue plasminogen activator appear to increase. Niacin is a potent inhibitor of the intracellular lipase system of adipose tissue, possibly reducing VLDL production by decreasing the flux of free fatty acids to liver. Sustained inhibition of lipolysis has not been established, however. Niacin reduces the plasma level of Lp(a) in many subjects by an unknown mechanism.

Therapeutic Uses & Dosage

In combination with a bile acid-binding resin or a reductase inhibitor, niacin has been found to normalize levels of LDL in most patients with heterozygous familial hypercholesterolemia. This drug combination is also indicated in some cases of nephrosis. In severe mixed lipemia that is incompletely responsive to dietary measures, niacin often produces marked reduction of triglyceride levels in plasma. It is also useful in patients with combined hyperlipoproteinemia and in those with familial dysbetalipoproteinemia. It can be used effectively alone or in combination with reductase inhibitors to treat hypercholesterolemia. Niacin is clearly the most effective agent in increasing levels of HDL.

For combined drug treatment of heterozygous familial hypercholesterolemia, most patients require 2–6.5 g of niacin daily; more than this should not be given. For other types of hypercholesterolemia and for hypertriglyceridemia, 1.5–3.5 g daily is often sufficient. The drug should be given in divided doses with meals, starting with 100 mg two or three times daily and increasing gradually.

Toxicity

Most persons experience a harmless cutaneous vasodilation and an uncomfortable sensation of warmth after each dose when the drug is started or the dose is increased. Taking 0.3 g of aspirin about half an hour beforehand blunts this prostaglandin-mediated effect. Ibuprofen, taken once daily, also mitigates the flush. Tachyphylaxis to this adverse effect usually occurs within a few days at any dose level. The physician should warn the patient to expect the flush and should explain that it is a harmless vasodilation of skin capillaries. Pruritus, rashes, dry skin, and acanthosis nigricans have been reported. The appearance of acanthosis contraindicates treatment with niacin because of its association with insulin resistance. Some patients experience nausea and abdominal discomfort. Many can continue the drug at reduced dosage or with the use of antacids not containing aluminum, but niacin should be avoided in patients with severe peptic disease. Moderate elevations in levels of aminotransferases or alkaline phosphatase may occur, usually not associated with serious liver toxicity. However, liver function should be monitored regularly. This effect is reversible and is minimized if the daily dose is increased by no more than 2.5 g in a month. Rarely, severe hepatotoxicity may occur and is an indication for discontinuing the drug. The association of severe hepatic dysfunction—including acute necrosis—with the use of *sustained-release* preparations of niacin contraindicates their use. Carbohydrate tolerance may be moderately impaired, but this is also reversible. In some patients with latent diabetes, however, this effect may be more evident and incompletely reversible. Hyperuricemia occurs in about one-fifth of patients and occasionally precipitates gout. Allopurinol can be given with niacin if needed to treat hyperuricemia. Rarely described conditions associated with the use of niacin include arrhythmias, mostly atrial, and a reversible toxic amblyopia. Patients should be instructed to report blurring of distance vision. Hypotension may occur, especially in patients receiving antihypertensive therapy.

GEMFIBROZIL

Gemfibrozil is a congener of the first-generation fibric acid derivative clofibrate. It resembles the parent drug pharmacologically in reducing VLDL levels and increasing the activity of lipoprotein lipase.

Chemistry & Pharmacokinetics

The gemfibrozil molecule differs from clofibrate in its aliphatic chain and in the presence of two methyl groups rather than a chlorine atom on the phenoxy group. It is supplied as the free carboxylic acid. Gemfibrozil is absorbed quantitatively from the intestine and is tightly bound to plasma proteins. It undergoes enterohepatic circulation and readily passes the placenta. Its plasma half-life is 1.5 hours. Seventy percent is eliminated through the kidneys, mostly unmodified. However, the liver modifies some of the drug at the methyl groups to hydroxymethyl or carboxyl derivatives and some of the compound to a quinol.

Gemfibrozil

Clofibrate

Mechanism of Action

Gemfibrozil appears to increase lipolysis of lipoprotein triglyceride via lipoprotein lipase. Intracellular lipolysis in adipose tissue is decreased. There is a decrease in levels of VLDL in plasma, perhaps in part due to decreased secretion by the liver. Only modest reductions of LDL levels occur in most patients. However, in others—especially those with combined hyperlipidemia—LDL levels often increase as triglycerides are reduced. HDL cholesterol levels increase moderately. Part of the apparent increase of HDL cholesterol levels is a direct consequence of decreasing the content of triglycerides in plasma, with reduction in exchange of triglycerides into HDL in place of cholesteryl esters. Some increase in HDL protein has been reported as well.

Therapeutic Uses & Dosage

This drug is useful in hypertriglyceridemias in which VLDL predominate and in dysbetalipoproteinemia. The usual dose of gemfibrozil is 600 mg orally once or twice daily.

Toxicity

Skin rashes, gastrointestinal symptoms, myopathy, arrhythmias, hypokalemia, and high levels of aminotransferases or alkaline phosphatase in blood have been reported. A few patients show decreases in white blood count or hematocrit. Gemfibrozil potentiates the action of coumarin and indanedione anticoagulants. Doses of these agents should be adjusted during therapy with gemfibrozil. There is an increased risk of myopathy when gemfibrozil is given to patients receiving reductase inhibitors. Rhabdomyolysis has occurred rarely. Gemfibrozil should be avoided in patients with hepatic or renal dysfunction. A modest increase in the incidence of gallstones is associated with this agent. It should be used with caution in patients with biliary tract disease or in those at high risk such as women, obese patients, or Native Americans. Data from the Helsinki Heart Study extension and its ancillary study resulted in the recommendation that gemfibrozil should not be used in patients with combined hyperlipidemia who have symptoms of atherosclerotic heart disease.

OTHER FIBRIC ACID DERIVATIVES

Clofibrate is seldom used because of its association with a small increase in risk of gastrointestinal and hepatobiliary neoplasia.

The following two drugs are not available in the USA. **Fenofibrate** is very similar in action to clofibrate and gemfibrozil, but it may be somewhat more potent in reducing LDL levels. It is hydrolyzed to the anion and is excreted mainly by the kidneys. It is given in doses of 100 mg three times a day. **Bezafibrate** also resembles clofibrate and gemfibrozil in its effect on VLDL, and, like fenofibrate, it may be somewhat more potent in reducing LDL levels. It is given in doses of 200 mg three times daily.

BILE ACID-BINDING RESINS

Colestipol and **cholestyramine** are useful only in hyperlipoproteinemias involving elevated levels of LDL. In patients who have hypertriglyceridemia as well as elevated LDL levels, VLDL levels may be further increased during treatment with the resins.

Chemistry & Pharmacokinetics

Colestipol and cholestyramine are very large polymeric cationic exchange resins that are insoluble in water. They bind bile acids in the intestinal lumen and prevent their reabsorption. Chloride is released from cationic quaternary ammonium binding sites in exchange for bile acids, but the resin itself is not absorbed.

Mechanism of Action

The bile acids, metabolites of cholesterol, are normally reabsorbed in the jejunum and ileum with about 95% efficiency (Figure 35–2). Their excretion is increased up to tenfold when the resins are given. The increased clearance results in enhanced conversion of cholesterol to bile acids in liver via 7α-hydroxylation, normally controlled by negative feedback by bile acids. Increased uptake of LDL from plasma in patients treated with the resins results from up-regulation of high-affinity LDL receptors on cell membranes, particularly in the liver. Hence, the resins are without effect in patients with homozygous familial hypercholesterolemia who have no functioning receptors, but they may be useful in patients with receptor-defective combined heterozygous states.

Therapeutic Uses & Dosage

The resins are used in treatment of patients with heterozygous familial hypercholesterolemia, producing approximately 20% reduction in LDL cholesterol when used in maximal dosage. Larger reductions at lower dosages may be expected in patients with less severe forms of hypercholesterolemia. If the resins are used to treat LDL elevations in persons with combined hyperlipidemia, they may cause an increase in levels of VLDL that would require the addition of a second agent such as niacin. The resins are also used in combination with other drugs to achieve further hypocholesterolemic effect (see below). In addition to their use in hyperlipidemia, they may be helpful in relieving pruritus in patients who have cholestasis and bile salt accumulation. Since they also bind digitalis glycosides, the resins may be used to increase the rate of removal of digitalis from the gastrointestinal tract in severe digitalis toxicity.

Colestipol and cholestyramine are granular preparations available in packets of 5 g and 4 g, respectively, or in bulk. Colestipol is also available in 1 g tablets that must be swallowed whole, precluding their use in children. The maximum daily dose is 16 g. A gradual increase of dosage of granules from 4 or 5 g/d to 20 g/d is recommended. Total dosages of 30–32 g/d may be needed for maximum effect. The usual dosage for a child is 10–20 g/d. Granular resins are mixed with juice or water and allowed to hydrate for 1 minute. Resins should be taken in two or three doses, with meals. Resins taken between meals have no effect.

Toxicity

The most common complaints are constipation and a bloating sensation, usually easily relieved by increasing dietary fiber or mixing psyllium seed with the resin. Heartburn and diarrhea are occasionally reported. In patients who have preexisting bowel disease or cholestasis, steatorrhea may occur. Malabsorption of vitamin K may occur rarely, leading to hypoprothrombinemia. Prothrombin time should be measured frequently in patients who are taking resins and anticoagulants. Malabsorption of folic acid has been reported rarely. Increased formation of gallstones, particularly in obese persons, was an anticipated adverse effect but has rarely occurred in practice. Another occasional problem is dry flaking skin, which is relieved by application of lanolin. Absorption of certain drugs, including those with neutral or cationic charge as well as anions, may be impaired by the resins. These include digitalis glycosides, thiazides, warfarin, tetracycline, vancomycin, thyroxine, iron salts, pravastatin, fluvastatin, folic acid, phenylbutazone, aspirin, and ascorbic acid. Any additional medication (except niacin) should be given 1 hour before or at least 2 hours after the resin to ensure adequate absorption.

COMPETITIVE INHIBITORS OF HMG–COA REDUCTASE (REDUCTASE INHIBITORS)

These compounds are structural analogs of HMG-CoA (3-hydroxy-3-methylglutaryl-coenzyme A). The first drug in this class was compactin. A close congener, **lovastatin,** is widely used (Figure 35–3). **Atorvastatin, fluvastatin, pravastatin,** and **simvastatin** are similar drugs.

Chemistry & Pharmacokinetics

Lovastatin and simvastatin are inactive lactone prodrugs that are hydrolyzed in the gastrointestinal tract to the active beta-hydroxyl derivatives. Atorvastatin, pravastatin, and fluvastatin are active drugs as given. About 30–50% of the ingested dose of lovastatin and pravastatin are absorbed in contrast to fluvastatin, which is almost completely absorbed. All reductase inhibitors have high first pass extraction by the liver. Most of the absorbed dose is excreted in the bile; about 5–20% is excreted in the urine. Itraconazole, a potent inhibitor of hepatic CYP3A4, has been re-

Figure 35–3. Inhibition of HMG-CoA reductase. **Top:** The HMG-CoA intermediate that is the immediate precursor of mevalonate, a critical compound in the synthesis of cholesterol. **Bottom:** The structure of lovastatin and its active form, showing the similarity to the normal HMG-CoA intermediate (shaded areas).

ported to cause a marked elevation in serum levels of lovastatin in some patients.

Mechanism of Action

HMG-CoA reductase mediates the first committed step in sterol biosynthesis. The active forms of lovastatin and its congeners are structural analogs of the HMG-CoA intermediate (Figure 35–3) that is formed by HMG-CoA reductase in the synthesis of mevalonate. These analogs cause partial inhibition of the enzyme and hence theoretically may impair the synthesis of isoprenoids such as ubiquinone and dolichol, and the prenylation of proteins, but it is not known whether this will prove to have biologic significance. However, the reductase inhibitors clearly induce an increase in high-affinity LDL receptors. This effect increases both the fractional catabolic rate of LDL and the liver's extraction of LDL precursors (VLDL remnants), thus reducing the plasma pool of LDL (Figure 35–2). Because of the marked first-pass hepatic extraction of these drugs, the major effect is on the liver. Preferential activity in liver of some congeners appears to be attributable to tissue-specific differences in uptake. Modest decreases in plasma triglycerides and small increases in HDL cholesterol levels also occur during treatment with these agents.

Therapeutic Uses & Dosage

The HMG-CoA inhibitors are useful alone or with bile acid-binding resins or niacin in treating disorders involving elevated plasma levels of LDL. Women who are pregnant, lactating, or likely to become pregnant should not be given these agents. Use in children is restricted to those with heterozygous familial hypercholesterolemia or homozygous familial hypercholesterolemia with some residual receptor activity.

Because of the diurnal pattern of cholesterol biosynthesis, reductase inhibitors should be given in the evening if a single daily dose is used. Absorption is enhanced by taking the dose with food. Daily doses of lovastatin vary from 10 mg to 80 mg. Moderately elevated LDL levels often respond to a single daily dose of 20 mg, preferably in the evening. In patients with heterozygous familial hypercholesterolemia, doses of 20 mg once or twice daily reduce total cholesterol levels by as much as 19% and 34%, respectively. Pravastatin is nearly as potent on a mass basis as lovastatin up to the maximum recommended daily dose, 40 mg. Simvastatin is twice as potent and is given in doses of 5–40 mg daily. Fluvastatin appears to be about half as potent as lovastatin on a mass basis and is given in doses of 10–40 mg daily. Atorvastatin, the most recently released of these agents, is the most potent agent for use in severe hypercholesterolemia. It is given in daily doses of 5–40 mg. Its triglyceride-lowering activity is also greater than that of the other reductase inhibitors, making it useful for treating patients with modestly elevated triglycerides.

The dose-response curves of pravastatin and especially of fluvastatin tend to level off in the upper part of the dosage range in patients with moderate to severe hypercholesterolemia, whereas those of lovastatin, simvastatin, and atorvastatin are more nearly linear.

Toxicity

Mild elevations of serum aminotransferase activity (up to three times the normal level) occur in some patients receiving reductase inhibitors. These increases are often intermittent and are not associated with other evidence of hepatic toxicity. Therapy may be continued in such patients if aminotransferase levels are measured frequently. In about 2% of patients, some of whom have underlying liver disease or a history of alcohol abuse, aminotransferase levels may exceed three times the normal limit. This effect, which may occur at any time after beginning therapy, may portend more severe hepatic toxicity. Medication should be discontinued in patients whose aminotransferase activity is persistently elevated more than three times the normal limit. Dosage of reductase inhibitors should be reduced in patients with hepatic parenchymal disease. In general, aminotransferase activity should be measured at baseline and at 2- to 4-month intervals during therapy.

Minor increases in creatine kinase activity in plasma are observed, usually intermittently, in about 10% of patients receiving reductase inhibitors. Such increases are frequently associated with heavy physical activity. Rarely, patients receiving reductase inhibitors may have marked elevations in kinase activity, often accompanied by generalized pain in skeletal muscles. If the drug is not discontinued, rhabdomyolysis may cause myoglobinuria, which may lead to renal shutdown. Myopathy may occur with monotherapy, but there appears to be an increased incidence in patients receiving a reductase inhibitor concurrently with certain other drugs including cyclosporine, fibric acid derivatives, azole antifungal drugs (especially itraconazole), erythromycin and other macrolides, danazol, and possibly niacin. Most patients receiving cyclosporine may be successfully treated with 5–10 mg of a reductase inhibitor daily. Creatine kinase activity should be measured frequently in such patients. Other drugs used with reductase inhibitors may also precipitate myopathy; general caution is advised until more experience with these combinations is obtained. Creatine kinase levels should be measured before treatment and then about every 4 months during therapy. If significant muscle pain, tenderness, or weakness appears, creatine kinase activity should be measured immediately and the drug should be discontinued if activity exceeds twice normal. The myopathy reverses promptly upon cessation of therapy. If the association is unclear, the patient can be rechallenged under close surveillance. Rarely, hypersensitivity syndromes have been reported that include a lupus-like disorder and peripheral neuropathy. Because of close structural and mechanistic similarities, hypersensitivity syndromes might be expected with all reductase inhibitors.

These drugs should be temporarily discontinued in the event of serious illness, trauma, or major surgery.

TREATMENT WITH DRUG COMBINATIONS

Combined drug therapy is useful when (1) VLDL levels are significantly increased during treatment of hypercholesterolemia with a bile acid-binding resin; (2) LDL and VLDL levels are both elevated initially; (3) LDL or VLDL levels are not normalized with a single agent, or, (4) elevated levels of Lp(a) coexist with other hyperlipidemias.

1. GEMFIBROZIL & BILE ACID-BINDING RESIN

This combination is sometimes useful in treating patients with familial combined hyperlipidemia who are intolerant of niacin. However, it may increase the risk of cholelithiasis.

2. HMG-CoA REDUCTASE INHIBITOR & BILE ACID-BINDING RESIN

HMG-CoA reductase inhibitors work with bile acid-binding resins in a highly synergistic manner. This combination is useful for treatment of familial hypercholesterolemia but may not control levels of VLDL in some patients with familial combined hyperlipidemia. Pravastatin and fluvastatin should be given at least one hour before or four hours after the resin to ensure their absorption.

3. NIACIN & BILE ACID-BINDING RESIN

This combination effectively controls VLDL levels during resin therapy of familial combined hyperlipidemia or other disorders involving both increased VLDL and LDL levels. When VLDL and LDL levels are both initially increased, doses of niacin as low as 1–3 g/d may be sufficient for treatment in combination with a resin.

The niacin-colestipol combination is highly effective for treating heterozygous familial hypercholesterolemia. This probably reflects the combined effects of (1) increased catabolism of LDL due to the resin, (2) decreased synthesis of its precursor VLDL attributable to niacin, and perhaps also (3) the ability of niacin to inhibit cholesterol biosynthesis in the liver. Niacin also significantly elevates levels of HDL cholesterol and frequently decreases levels of Lp(a).

In three major atherosclerosis regression trials, quantitative evidence of reversal of coronary disease was demonstrated with this regimen. Effects on lipoprotein levels are sustained, and no additional adverse effects beyond those encountered when the drugs are used singly have developed. Because the resin has acid-neutralizing properties, the gastric irritation produced by niacin in some patients is relieved when they take the drugs in combination. The drugs may be taken together, because niacin does not bind to the resins. LDL levels in patients with heterozygous familial hypercholesterolemia are usually normalized with daily doses of up to 6.5 g of niacin with 24–30 g of resin.

4. NIACIN & REDUCTASE INHIBITOR

This regimen appears to be more effective than either agent alone in treating familial hypercholesterolemia. Experience indicates that it is the most efficacious and practical combination for treatment of familial combined hyperlipidemia.

5. TERNARY COMBINATION OF RESIN, NIACIN, & REDUCTASE INHIBITOR

These agents act in a complementary fashion to reduce serum cholesterol levels into the low normal range in patients with severe disorders involving elevated LDL levels. The effects are sustained, and little compound toxicity has been observed. Effective doses of the individual drugs may be lower than when each is used alone, eg, as little as 1–2 g of niacin may substantially increase the effects of the other two agents.

PREPARATIONS AVAILABLE

Atorvastatin (Lipitor)
Oral: 10, 20, 40 mg tablets
Cholestyramine (Questran, Questran Light)
Oral: 1, 4 g packets anhydrous granules
cholestyramine resin per packet; 210 g (Questran Light), 378 g (Questran) cans
Colestipol (Colestid)
Oral: 5 g packets granules; 300, 500 g bottles;
1 g tablets
Fluvastatin (Lescol)
Oral: 20, 40 mg capsules

Gemfibrozil (Lopid)
Oral: 600 mg tablets
Lovastatin (Mevacor)
Oral: 10, 20, 40 mg tablets
Niacin, nicotinic acid, vitamin B$_3$ (generic, others)
Oral: 25, 50, 100, 250, 500, 1000 mg tablets
Pravastatin (Pravachol)
Oral: 10, 20, 40 mg tablets
Simvastatin (Zocor)
Oral: 5, 10, 20, 40 mg tablets

REFERENCES

Atherosclerosis: Mechanisms & Epidemiology

Fuster V et al: Mechanisms of disease: The pathogenesis of coronary artery disease and the acute coronary syndrome. (Two parts.) N Engl J Med 1992;326:242, 310.

Kannel WB et al: Overall and coronary heart disease mortality rates in relation to major risk factors in 325,348 men screened for the MRFIT: Multiple Risk Factor Interventional Trial. Am Heart J 1986;112:825.

Kannel WB et al: Serum cholesterol, lipoproteins, and the risk of coronary heart disease: The Framingham Study. Ann Intern Med 1971;74:1.

Ross R, Fuster V: The pathogenesis of atherosclerosis. In: *Atherosclerosis and Coronary Artery Disease.* Fuster V, Ross R, Topol E (editors). Lippincott-Raven, 1996.

Steinberg D et al: Beyond cholesterol: Modifications of low density lipoprotein that increase its atherogenicity. N Engl J Med 1989;320:915.

Atherosclerosis: Regression

Brown BG et al: Impact of management in stabilization in regression of coronary disease. In: *Atherosclerosis and Coronary Artery Disease.* Fuster V, Ross R, Topol E, (editors). Philadelphia, Lippincott-Raven, 1996.

Brown BG et al: Lipid lowering and plaque regression: New insights into prevention of plaque disruption and clinical events in coronary disease. Circulation 1993;87:1781.

Brown G et al: Regression of coronary artery disease as a result of intensive lipid-lowering therapy in men with high levels of apolipoprotein B. N Engl J Med 1990; 323:1289.

Cashin-Hemphill J et al: Beneficial effects of colestipol-niacin on coronary atherosclerosis. A 4-year follow-up. JAMA 1990;264:3013.

Kane JP et al: Regression of coronary atherosclerosis during treatment of familial hypercholesterolemia with combined drug regimens. JAMA 1990;264:3007.

Watts GF et al: Effects on coronary artery disease of lipid-lowering diet, or diet plus cholestyramine in the St. Thomas Atherosclerosis Regression Study. Lancet 1992;339:563.

Outcome Studies

Scandinavian Simvastatin Survival Study: Randomized trial of cholesterol lowering in 4444 patients with coronary heart disease: The Scandinavian Simvastatin Survival Study (4S). Lancet 1994;345:1383.

Shepherd J et al: Prevention of coronary heart disease with pravastatin in men with hypercholesterolemia. N Engl J Med 1995;338:1301.

Sacks FM et al: The effect of pravastatin on coronary events after myocardial infarction in patients with average cholesterol levels. Cholesterol and Recurrent Events Investigators. N Engl J Med 1996;335:1001.

Lipoprotein Metabolism

Havel RJ, Kane JP: Introduction: Structure and metabolism of plasma lipoproteins. In: *The Metabolic and Molecular Bases of Inherited Disease,* 7th ed. Scriver CR et al (editors). McGraw-Hill, 1995.

Kane JP, Havel RJ: Disorders of the biogenesis and secretion of lipoproteins containing the B-apolipoproteins. In: *The Metabolic Basis of Inherited Disease.* 7th ed. Scriver CR et al (editors). McGraw-Hill, 1995.

Hyperlipidemia

Goldstein JL, Hobbs HH, Brown MS: Familial hypercholesterolemia. In: *The Metabolic Bases of Inherited Disease,* 7th ed. Scriver CR et al (editors). McGraw-Hill, 1995.

Kane JP, Havel RJ: Disorders of the biogenesis and secretion of lipoproteins containing the B-apolipoproteins. In: *The Metabolic and Molecular Bases of Inherited Disease,* 7th ed. Scriver CR et al (editors). McGraw-Hill, 1995.

Kane JP, Malloy MJ: Disorders of lipoprotein metabolism. In: *Basic & Clinical Endocrinology,* 5th ed. Greenspan FS, Strewler GJ (editors). Appleton & Lange, 1997.

Mahley RW et al: Type III hyperlipoproteinemia (dysbetalipoproteinemia): The role of apolipoprotein E in normal and abnormal lipoprotein metabolism. In: *The Metabolic and Molecular Bases of Inherited Disease,* 7th ed. Scriver CR et al (editors). McGraw-Hill, 1995.

Dietary Treatment

Grundy SM: Lipids, nutrition, and coronary heart disease, drug treatment. In: *Atherosclerosis and Coronary Artery Disease.* Fuster V, Ross R, Topol E (editors). Lippincott-Raven, 1996.

Drug Treatment

Hunninghake, DG: HMG-CoA reductase inhibitors. Curr Opin Lipidol 1992;3:22.

Malloy MJ et al: Complementarity of colestipol, niacin, and lovastatin in treatment of severe familial hypercholesterolemia. Ann Intern Med 1987;107:616.

Malloy MJ, Kane JP: Aggressive medical therapy and treatment of coronary artery disease. Adv Intern Med 1996;42:1.

National Cholesterol Education Program. Second report of the Expert Panel on Detection, Evaluation, and Treatment of High Blood Cholesterol in Adults (Adult Treatment Panel II). Circulation 1994;89:1329.

36

Nonsteroidal Anti-Inflammatory Drugs; Disease-Modifying Antirheumatic Drugs; Nonopioid Analgesics; Drugs Used in Gout

Bertram G. Katzung, MD, PhD, & Daniel E. Furst, MD

THE INFLAMMATORY RESPONSE

Inflammation is commonly divided into three phases: acute inflammation, the immune response, and chronic inflammation. Acute inflammation is the initial response to tissue injury; it is mediated by the release of autacoids and usually precedes the development of the immune response. Some of the autacoids involved are listed in Table 36–1. The immune response occurs when immunologically competent cells are activated in response to foreign organisms or antigenic substances liberated during the acute or chronic inflammatory response. The outcome of the immune response for the host may be beneficial, as when it causes invading organisms to be phagocytosed or neutralized. On the other hand, the outcome may be deleterious if it leads to chronic inflammation without resolution of the underlying injurious process. Chronic inflammation involves the release of a number of mediators that are not prominent in the acute response. Some of these are listed in Table 36–2. One of the most important conditions involving these mediators is rheumatoid arthritis, in which chronic inflammation results in pain and destruction of bone and cartilage that can lead to severe disability and in which systemic changes occur that can result in shortening of life.

The cell damage associated with inflammation acts on cell membranes to cause leukocytes to release lysosomal enzymes; arachidonic acid is then liberated from precursor compounds, and various eicosanoids are synthesized (see Chapter 18).

Prostaglandins have a variety of effects on blood vessels, on nerve endings, and on cells involved in inflammation. Leukotrienes have a powerful chemotactic effect on eosinophils, neutrophils, and macrophages and promote bronchoconstriction and alter-ations in vascular permeability. Recent evidence suggests that the cyclooxygenase isozyme (COX II) responsible for prostaglandin production by cells involved in inflammation is not identical to the cyclooxygenase present in most other cells in the body (COX I). A selective blocker of COX II might be desirable in the treatment of inflammation since it would leave undisturbed the other functions of the prostaglandins. It has been suggested that the corticosteroids are such selective blockers (see below).

Kinins, neuropeptides, and histamine are also released at the site of tissue injury, as are complement components, cytokines, and other products of leukocytes and platelets. Stimulation of the neutrophil membranes produces oxygen-derived free radicals. Superoxide anion is formed by the reduction of molecular oxygen, which may stimulate the production of other reactive molecules such as hydrogen peroxide and hydroxyl radicals. The interaction of these substances with arachidonic acid results in the generation of chemotactic substances, thus perpetuating the inflammatory process.

THERAPEUTIC STRATEGIES

The treatment of patients with inflammation involves two primary goals: first, the relief of pain, which is often the presenting symptom and the major continuing complaint of the patient; and second, the slowing or—in theory—arrest of the tissue-damaging process. Reduction of inflammation with **nonsteroidal anti-inflammatory** drugs often results in relief of pain for significant periods. Furthermore, most of the nonopioid analgesics (aspirin, etc) also have anti-inflammatory effects, so they are appropriate for the treatment of both acute and chronic inflammatory conditions.

Table 36–1. Some properties of the mediators of acute inflammation.

Mediator	Vasodilation	Vascular Permeability	Chemotaxis	Pain
Histamine	++	↑↑↑	–	–
Serotonin	+/–	↑	–	–
Bradykinin	+++	↑	–	+++
Prostaglandins	+++	↑	+++	+
Leukotrienes	–	↑↑↑	+++	–

The **glucocorticoids** also have powerful anti-inflammatory effects and when first introduced were considered to be the ultimate answer to the treatment of inflammatory arthritis. Unfortunately, the toxicity associated with chronic corticosteroid therapy inhibits their use except in the control of acute flare-ups of joint disease. Therefore, the nonsteroidal anti-inflammatory drugs have assumed a major role in the treatment of arthritis.

Another important group of agents are characterized as **slow-acting antirheumatic drugs (SAARDs)** or **disease-modifying antirheumatic drugs (DMARDs).** Very little is known about their mechanisms of action, but they may slow the bone damage associated with rheumatoid arthritis and are thought to affect more basic inflammatory mechanisms than do the NSAIDs. Unfortunately, they are also more toxic than the nonsteroidal anti-inflammatory agents.

I. NONSTEROIDAL ANTI-INFLAMMATORY DRUGS

Salicylates and other similar agents used to treat rheumatic disease share the capacity to suppress the signs and symptoms of inflammation. These drugs also exert antipyretic and analgesic effects, but it is their anti-inflammatory properties that make them most useful in the management of disorders in which pain is related to the intensity of the inflammatory process. Several of the NSAIDs are used for special indications. These include indomethacin and ketorolac. They are discussed separately.

ASPIRIN & OTHER SALICYLATES

Aspirin and all but one of the other nonsteroidal anti-inflammatory drugs (NSAIDs) (ibuprofen, naproxen, etc) are related chemically in that they are weak organic acids; nabumetone is a ketone prodrug that is metabolized to an acidic active drug. They share the important property of inhibiting prostaglandin biosynthesis. They may also decrease the production of free radicals and of superoxide and may interact with adenylyl cyclase to alter the cellular concentration of cAMP. Although these drugs effectively inhibit inflammation, there is no evidence that—in contrast to drugs such as methotrexate and gold—they alter the course of an arthritic disorder. Aspirin's long history of use and availability without prescription diminishes its glamour compared to that of the newer NSAIDs. However, because of its low cost and long history of safety, aspirin remains the initial drug of choice for treating the majority of articular and musculoskeletal disorders. Aspirin was also the standard against which all anti-inflammatory agents are measured (Table 36–3). Both ibuprofen and naproxen have joined aspirin as over-the-counter NSAIDs in the USA. Both have good to excellent safety records, and ibuprofen especially is now the usual standard against which other NSAIDs are compared.

Table 36–2. Some of the mediators of chronic inflammation, eg, in rheumatoid arthritis.

Mediator	Sources	Primary Effects
Interleukins 1, 2, and 3	Macrophages, T lymphocytes	Lymphocyte activation, prostaglandin production
GM-CSF[1]	T lymphocytes, endothelial cells, fibroblasts	Macrophage and granulocyte activation
TNF-α[2]	Macrophages	Prostaglandin production
Interferons	Macrophages, endothelial cells, T lymphocytes	Many
PDGF[3]	Macrophages, endothelial cells, fibroblasts, platelets	Fibroblast chemotaxis, proliferation

[1]Granulocyte-macrophage colony-stimulating factor.
[2]Tumor necrosis factor alpha.
[3]Platelet-derived growth factor.

History

Quinine from cinchona bark is one of the oldest remedies for relief of mild pain and fever. Willow bark was used in folk medicine for years for similar indications. In 1763, Reverend Edmund Stone, in a letter to the president of the Royal Society, described his success in treating fever with a powdered form of the bark of the willow. He had noted that the bitterness of willow bark was reminiscent of the taste of cinchona bark, the source of quinine. The active ingredient of willow bark, salicin, which on hydrolysis yields salicylic acid, was later found in other natural sources. Acetylsalicylic acid was synthesized in 1853, but the drug was not used until 1899, when it was found to be effective in arthritis and well tolerated. The name aspirin was coined from the German word for the compound, *acetylspir*säure (*Spirea,* the genus of plants from which it was obtained, and *Säure,* the German word for acid). Because of its greater efficacy and lower cost, aspirin rapidly replaced the natural products then in use and has remained one of the most widely employed remedies for over 90 years.

Chemistry & Pharmacokinetics

Salicylic acid is a simple organic acid with a pK_a of 3.0. Aspirin (acetylsalicylic acid; ASA) has a pK_a of 3.5 (see Table 1–1). Sodium salicylate and aspirin are equally effective anti-inflammatory drugs, though aspirin may be more effective as an analgesic.

The salicylates (Figure 36–1) are rapidly absorbed from the stomach and upper small intestine, yielding a peak plasma salicylate level within 1–2 hours. The acid medium in the stomach keeps a large fraction of the salicylate in the nonionized form, promoting absorption. However, when high concentrations of salicylate enter the mucosal cell, the drug may damage the mucosal barrier. If the gastric pH is raised by a suitable buffer to 3.5 or higher, gastric irritation is decreased.

Aspirin is absorbed as such and is rapidly hydrolyzed to acetic acid and salicylate by esterases in tissue and blood. Salicylate is bound to albumin, but, as the serum concentration of salicylate increases, a greater fraction remains unbound and available to tissues. Ingested salicylate and that generated by the hydrolysis of aspirin may be excreted unchanged, but most is converted to water-soluble conjugates that are

Table 36–3. Properties of aspirin and some newer nonsteroidal anti-inflammatory drugs.

Drug	Half-life (hours)	Urinary Excretion of Unchanged Drug	Recommended Anti-inflammatory Dosage
Aspirin	0.25	< 2%	1200–1500 mg tid
Salicylate[1]	2–19	2–30%	See footnote 2
Apazone	15	62%	600 mg bid
Diclofenac	1.1	< 1%	50–75 mg qid
Diflunisal	13	3–9%	500 mg bid
Etodolac	6.5	< 1%	200–300 mg qid
Fenoprofen	2.5	30%	600 mg qid
Flurbiprofen	3.8	< 1%	300 mg tid
Ibuprofen	2	< 1%	600 mg qid
Indomethacin	4–5	16%	50–70 mg tid
Ketoprofen	1.8	< 1%	70 mg tid
Ketorolac	4–10	58%	10 mg qid[3]
Meclofenamate	3	2–4%	100 mg qid
Nabumetone[4]	26	1%	1000–2000 mg qd[5]
Naproxen	14	< 1%	375 mg bid
Oxaprozin	58	1–4%	1200–1800 mg qd[5]
Piroxicam	57	4–10%	20 mg qd[5]
Sulindac	8	7%	200 mg bid
Tolmetin	1	7%	400 mg qid

[1]Major anti-inflammatory metabolite of aspirin.
[2]Salicylate is usually given in the form of aspirin.
[3]Recommended for treatment of acute (eg, surgical) pain only.
[4]Nabumetone is a prodrug; the half-life and urinary excretion are for its active metabolite.
[5]A single daily dose is sufficient because of the long half-life.

Figure 36–1. Structure and metabolism of the salicylates. (Modified and reproduced, with permission, from Meyers FH, Jawetz E, Goldfien A: *Review of Medical Pharmacology,* 7th ed. Lange, 1980.)

rapidly cleared by the kidney (Figure 36–1). When this pathway becomes saturated, a small increase in aspirin dose results in a relatively large increase in plasma levels. Alkalinization of the urine increases the rate of excretion of free salicylate. When aspirin is used in low doses (600 mg), salicylate elimination is in accordance with first-order kinetics and the serum half-life is 3–5 hours. With higher dosage, a mix of capacity-limited and first-order kinetics prevails; at anti-inflammatory dosage (≥ 4 g/d), the half-life increases to 12 hours or more.

Pharmacodynamics

A. Mechanism of Action: The effectiveness of aspirin is due partly to its ability to inhibit cyclooxygenase and partly to the effect of its primary metabolite, salicylate, both to inhibit cyclooxygenase and to act in other ways, eg, as an oxygen radical scavenger (see Chapter 18). Aspirin as such irreversibly blocks the enzyme cyclooxygenase (prostaglandin synthase), which catalyzes the conversion of arachidonic acid to endoperoxide compounds; at appropriate doses, the drug decreases the formation of both the prostaglandins and thromboxane A_2 but not the leukotrienes (Figure 36–2). There is no evidence that aspirin is a selective inhibitor of COX II.

B. Anti-inflammatory Effects: In addition to reducing the synthesis of eicosanoid mediators, aspirin also interferes with the chemical mediators of the kallikrein system (see Chapter 17). As a result, aspirin inhibits granulocyte adherence to damaged vasculature, stabilizes lysosomes, and inhibits the migration of polymorphonuclear leukocytes and macrophages into the site of inflammation.

C. Analgesic Effects: Aspirin is most effective in reducing pain of mild to moderate intensity. It alleviates pain of varying causes, such as that of muscular, vascular, and dental origin, postpartum states, arthritis, and bursitis. Aspirin acts peripherally through its effects on inflammation but probably also inhibits pain stimuli at a subcortical site.

D. Antipyretic Effects: Aspirin reduces elevated temperature, whereas normal body temperature is only slightly affected. The fall in temperature is related to increased dissipation of heat caused by vasodilation of superficial blood vessels. The antipyresis may be accompanied by profuse sweating.

The fever associated with infection is thought to result from two actions. The first is the production of prostaglandins in the central nervous system in response to bacterial pyrogens. The second is the effect of interleukin-1 on the hypothalamus. Interleukin-1 is produced by macrophages and is released during inflammatory responses, when its principal role is to activate lymphocytes (Table 36–2). Aspirin blocks both the pyrogen-induced production of prostaglandins and the central nervous system response to interleukin-1 and so may reset the "temperature control" in the hypothalamus, thereby facilitating heat dissipation by vasodilation.

E. Platelet Effects: Aspirin affects hemostasis. Single low doses of aspirin (about 80 mg) produce a

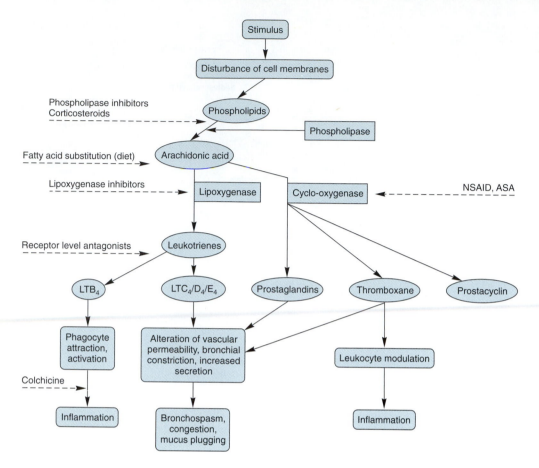

Figure 36–2. Scheme for mediators derived from arachidonic acid and sites of drug action (dashed arrows).

slightly prolonged bleeding time, which doubles if administration is continued for a week. The change is explained by the inhibition of platelet aggregation secondary to inhibition of thromboxane synthesis (see Chapter 34). Because its action is irreversible, aspirin inhibits platelet aggregation for up to 8 days—ie, until new platelets are formed. If potential bleeding complications are a concern in association with surgery, aspirin should be stopped 1 week prior to the operation.

Aspirin has a longer duration of effect than the many other compounds that inhibit platelet aggregation such as ticlopidine and dipyridamole.

Clinical Uses

A. Analgesia and Anti-inflammatory Effects: Aspirin is one of the most frequently employed drugs for relieving mild to moderate pain of varied origin. Aspirin is often combined with other mild analgesics, and over 200 such products may be purchased without prescription. These more costly combinations have never been shown to be more effective or less toxic than aspirin alone, and treating

poisoning due to overdoses of such combinations is more difficult. Furthermore, the phenacetin contained in many such compounds may cause interstitial nephritis with serious renal impairment. Aspirin is not effective in the treatment of severe visceral pain such as that associated with acute abdomen, renal colic, pericarditis, or myocardial infarction. It and other NSAIDs have been combined with opioid analgesics for treatment of cancer pain. In that context, their anti-inflammatory effects act synergistically with the opioids to enhance analgesia.

The anti-inflammatory properties of salicylates in high doses are responsible for their recommendation for treatment of rheumatoid arthritis, rheumatic fever, and other inflammatory joint conditions. In mild arthritis, many patients can be managed using salicylates as their sole medication.

B. Other Indications:

1. Antipyresis—Except for a few diseases (eg, neurosyphilis, chronic brucellosis), there is no evidence that elevation of body temperature is a useful defense mechanism. On the other hand, there is rarely any great need to reduce a mild or moderate fever, especially in adults (Styrt et al, 1990). Aspirin is the best available drug for reducing fever when doing so is desirable and when there are no contraindications to its use (see below).

2. Inhibition of platelet aggregation (see also Chapter 34)—Aspirin has been shown to decrease the incidence of transient ischemic attacks and unstable angina in men and has been used as a prophylactic agent in these conditions. It may also be effective in reducing the incidence of thrombosis in coronary artery bypass grafts. The results of several clinical studies of patients at risk for or recovering from myocardial infarction have provided evidence that aspirin reduces the incidence of coronary artery thrombosis. In one large study, the ingestion of 325 mg of aspirin every other day reduced the incidence of myocardial infarction by over 40% in male physicians.

3. Other uses—Several studies have suggested that aspirin may reduce cataract formation; other studies contradict this finding (Chew et al, 1992). Other epidemiologic studies suggest that long-term use of aspirin at low dosage is associated with a lower incidence of colon cancer (Thun et al, 1991).

Dosage

The optimal analgesic or antipyretic dose of aspirin is less than the 0.6 g oral dose commonly used. Larger doses may prolong the effect. The usual dose may be repeated every 4 hours and smaller doses (0.3 g) every 3 hours. The dose for children is 50–75 mg/kg/d in divided doses.

The average anti-inflammatory dosage of 3.2–4 g daily can be tolerated by most adults. For children, 50–75 mg/kg/d usually produces adequate blood levels. Blood levels of 15–30 mg/dL are associated with anti-inflammatory effects. A simple reliable method for determining salicylate blood levels is available, and the drug can thus be titrated to the proper level. Because of the long half-lives (about 12 hours) of aspirin's active metabolites, frequent dosing is not necessary when daily doses of 4 g or more are required. A convenient method is to give the total amount divided into three doses taken after meals.

The relationship of salicylate blood levels to therapeutic effect and toxicity is illustrated in Figure 36–3.

Drug Selection

Aspirin is available from many different manufacturers, and although it may vary in texture and appearance, the content of aspirin is constant. A disintegration test is part of the official standard, and there is little evidence that differences among tablets have clinical significance. The most popular buffered aspirin does not contain sufficient alkali to modify gastric irritation, and there is no evidence that these more expensive preparations are associated with higher blood levels, greater clinical effectiveness, or a lower incidence of adverse effects. Enteric-coated aspirin may be suitable for pa-

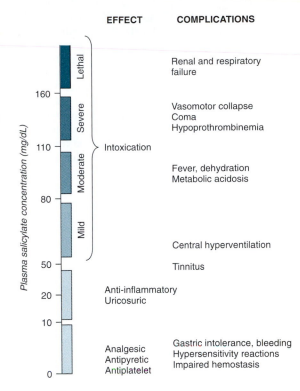

Figure 36–3. Approximate relationships of plasma salicylate levels to pharmacodynamics and complications. (Modified and reproduced, with permission, from Hollander J, McCarty D Jr: *Arthritis and Allied Conditions.* Lea & Febiger, 1972.)

tients in whom buffering fails to control gastritis, since the coating prevents the tablets from dissolving in the stomach and the drug is absorbed adequately in the small intestine. Therapeutic blood levels with this preparation may be similar to those achieved with the same doses of regular aspirin. Enteric coating increases the cost of aspirin, but these products are still less costly than the newer NSAIDs. The concomitant use of H_2 blockers and other drugs (except misoprostol and omeprazol) for the treatment and prevention of acid-peptic disease has not been shown to reduce the incidence of NSAID-induced gastrointestinal damage. Misoprostol, a prostaglandin E_1 derivative, has been shown to reduce NSAID-induced ulceration. Its use is complicated by its cost and some diarrhea, but misoprostol is cost-effective when NSAIDs are necessary in patients at higher risk for gastrointestinal bleeding, eg, elderly women and patients with a history of ulcers.

Adverse Effects

A. Gastrointestinal Effects: At the usual dosage, the main adverse effect is gastric upset (intolerance). This effect can be minimized with suitable buffering (taking aspirin with meals followed by a glass of water or antacids). The gastritis that occurs with aspirin may be due to irritation of the gastric mucosa by the undissolved tablet, to absorption in the stomach of nonionized salicylate, or to inhibition of protective prostaglandins. In animals, ulceration can be produced by the parenteral administration of aspirin, and administration of prostaglandins has prevented aspirin-induced gastric erosions; these observations suggest that the absence of a prostaglandin may make the gastric mucosa more vulnerable. As noted above, misoprostol does reduce the frequency of recurrence of peptic ulceration in patients taking large doses of NSAIDs but causes its own toxicities.

Although aspirin has never been shown to cause peptic ulcers in humans, experimental and epidemiologic studies overwhelmingly document an increased incidence of gastric ulcers and, to a lesser extent, duodenal ulcers with heavy aspirin or newer NSAID use (Ivey, 1986). Upper gastrointestinal bleeding associated with aspirin use is usually related to erosive gastritis. A small increase in fecal blood loss is routinely associated with aspirin administration; about 1 mL of blood normally lost in the stool daily increases to about 4 mL daily in persons using ordinary aspirin doses and more for higher doses. On the other hand, with appropriate therapy, ulcers have been shown to heal while aspirin was taken concomitantly. Nevertheless, aspirin should be avoided or taken with effective buffers or prostaglandins by individuals with peptic ulcer disease.

Vomiting may occur as a result of central nervous system stimulation after absorption of large doses of aspirin.

B. Central Nervous System Effects: With higher doses, patients may experience "salicylism"—tinnitus, decreased hearing, and vertigo—reversible by reducing the dosage. Still larger doses of salicylates cause hyperpnea through a direct effect on the medulla. At low toxic salicylate levels, respiratory alkalosis may occur as a result of the increased ventilation. Later, acidosis supervenes from accumulation of salicylic acid derivatives and depression of the respiratory center.

C. Other Adverse Effects: Aspirin in a daily dose of 2 g or less usually increases serum uric acid levels, whereas doses exceeding 4 g daily decrease urate levels below 2.5 mg/dL. (See Drugs Used in Gout, below.)

Aspirin may cause mild, usually asymptomatic hepatitis, especially in patients with underlying disorders such as systemic lupus erythematosus and juvenile and adult rheumatoid arthritis.

Salicylates may cause reversible decrease of glomerular filtration rate in patients with underlying renal disease, and this may also occur (though rarely) in persons with normal kidneys.

Aspirin in usual doses has a negligible effect on glucose tolerance. Toxic amounts affect the cardiovascular system directly and may depress cardiac function and dilate peripheral blood vessels. Large doses directly affect smooth muscles.

Hypersensitivity reactions may occur after ingestion of aspirin by patients with asthma and nasal polyps and may be associated with bronchoconstriction and shock. These reactions are probably mediated by leukotrienes.

Aspirin is contraindicated in patients with hemophilia. Aspirin is not recommended for pregnant women. However, recent studies have suggested that low-dose aspirin may be valuable in certain pregnant patients with a high risk of hypertension and other complications of pregnancy (Schiff et al, 1989).

Use of aspirin in children during or immediately after a viral infection has been associated with an increase in the incidence of Reye's syndrome (Hurwitz et al, 1987; Hurwitz, 1989), and decreased aspirin use has been associated with a decreased incidence. On the other hand, the incidence of Reye's syndrome decreased in Australia *before* the use of aspirin decreased, so the direct association of Reye's syndrome with aspirin is questioned by some. In any case, acetaminophen should be used in place of aspirin in this situation.

Overdosage Toxicity

Aspirin is such a common household drug that it has been a frequent cause of poisoning in young children. Serious intoxication results when the amount ingested exceeds 150–175 mg/kg of body weight. Since the introduction of child-resistant containers, there has been a significant decrease in fatal aspirin-induced poisonings in children.

Most aspirin is sold and used without prescription. The drug must be kept out of reach of children and in the child-resistant container in which it is dispensed. Colorful, flavored, and liquid preparations should be kept in locked cabinets.

When overdosing occurs, either accidentally or with suicidal intent, gastric lavage is advised (Chapter 59). Hyperthermia may be treated with alcohol sponges or ice packs. It is important to maintain a high urine volume and to treat acid-base abnormalities. In severe toxic reactions, ventilatory assistance may be required. Sodium bicarbonate infusions may be employed to alkalinize the urine, which will increase the amount of salicylate excreted.

Drug Interactions

Drugs that enhance salicylate intoxication include acetazolamide and ammonium chloride. Alcohol increases gastrointestinal bleeding produced by salicylates. Aspirin displaces a number of drugs from protein binding sites in the blood. These include tolbutamide, chlorpropamide, nonsteroidal anti-inflammatory agents, methotrexate, phenytoin, and probenecid. Corticosteroids may decrease salicylate concentration. Aspirin reduces the pharmacologic activity of spironolactone, competes with penicillin G for renal tubular secretion, and inhibits the uricosuric effect of sulfinpyrazone and probenecid.

NONACETYLATED SALICYLATES

These drugs include **magnesium choline salicylate, sodium salicylate,** and **salicylsalicylate.** All nonacetylated salicylates are effective anti-inflammatory drugs, though they may be less effective analgesics than aspirin. Because they are much less effective than aspirin as cyclooxygenase inhibitors, they may be preferable when cyclooxygenase inhibition is undesirable—such as in patients with asthma, those with bleeding tendencies, and even (under close supervision) those with renal dysfunction.

The nonacetylated salicylates are administered in the same dosage as aspirin and can be monitored using serum salicylate measurements.

DIFLUNISAL

Diflunisal is a newer NSAID chemically derived from salicylic acid, although it is not metabolized to salicylate or salicylic acid. The drug has a plasma half-life approaching that of salicylate, and blood levels reach a steady state after several days of dosing. Like aspirin, it has analgesic and anti-inflammatory effects; unlike aspirin, it has little antipyretic activity.

The indications for use of diflunisal include pain, osteoarthritis, and rheumatoid arthritis. Adverse reactions are similar to those of other NSAIDs.

OTHER NONSTEROIDAL ANTI-INFLAMMATORY DRUGS

The adverse effects of aspirin and other salicylates—especially the gastric irritation that occurs when large doses are employed—have led to the search for alternative compounds. Starting with phenylbutazone in 1949, many drugs with aspirin-like properties (designated "newer" nonsteroidal anti-inflammatory drugs) have been approved for use in the USA for the treatment of rheumatoid arthritis or osteoarthritis (Table 36–3). In addition to their use in joint disease, several newer NSAIDs have been approved for other indications as described below.

Chemistry

The NSAIDs are grouped in several chemical classes, some of which are shown in Figure 36–4. This chemical diversity yields such a broad range of pharmacokinetic characteristics that these properties are best discussed in connection with the individual agents.

Pharmacodynamics

The anti-inflammatory activity of the newer NSAIDs is similar in mechanism to that of aspirin and is mediated chiefly through inhibition of biosynthesis of prostaglandins. Various NSAIDs have additional possible mechanisms of action, including inhibition of chemotaxis, down-regulation of interleukin-1 production, and interference with calcium-mediated intracellular events. Unlike aspirin, these drugs are reversible inhibitors of cyclooxygenase. Selectivity for COX I versus COX II is variable and incomplete. For example, in testing against the mouse enzymes, aspirin, indomethacin, piroxicam, and sulindac were considerably more effective in inhibiting COX I; ibuprofen and meclofenamate inhibited the two isozymes about equally; and the active metabolite of nabumetone was somewhat selective for COX II (Meade et al, 1993). Inhibition of lipoxygenase synthesis by the newer NSAIDs, a desirable effect for an anti-inflammatory drug, is limited but may be greater than with aspirin. Benoxaprofen, another newer NSAID, was shown to significantly inhibit leukotriene synthesis but was withdrawn because of toxicity. Of the currently available NSAIDs, indomethacin and diclofenac have been reported to reduce the synthesis of both prostaglandins and leukotrienes. It is likely that development of newer NSAIDs will continue until the clinical significance of inhibition of COX II and of lipoxygenase can be fully evaluated with more selective inhibitors.

During therapy with these drugs, inflammation is reduced by decreasing the release of mediators from granulocytes, basophils, and mast cells. The NSAIDs decrease the sensitivity of vessels to bradykinin and histamine, affect lymphokine production from T lymphocytes, and reverse vasodilation. To varying degrees, all newer NSAIDs are analgesic, anti-inflammatory, and antipyretic, and all inhibit platelet aggregation. They are all gastric irritants as well, though as a group they tend to cause less gastric irritation than aspirin. Nephrotoxicity has been observed for all of the drugs for which extensive experience has been reported, and hepatotoxicity can also occur with any NSAID.

Pharmacokinetics

Although there are many differences in the kinetics of NSAIDs, they have some general properties in common. Most of these drugs are well absorbed, and food does not substantially change their bioavailability. Most of the NSAIDs are highly metabolized, some by phase I and phase II mechanisms and others by direct glucuronidation (phase II) alone. While renal excretion is the most important route, all undergo varying degrees of biliary excretion and reabsorption (enterohepatic circulation). All of the NSAIDs are highly protein-bound ($\geq 98\%$), usually to albumin. Some of the NSAIDs (eg, ibuprofen) are racemic mixtures, while others (eg, naproxen) are provided as a single enantiomer and a few have no chiral center (eg, diclofenac).

All NSAIDs can be found in synovial fluid after repeated dosing. Drugs with short half-lives remain in the joints longer than would be predicted from their

PROPIONIC ACID DERIVATIVE

Ibuprofen

PYRROLEALKANOIC ACID DERIVATIVE

Tolmetin

PHENYLALKANOIC ACID DERIVATIVE

Flurbiprofen

INDOLE DERIVATIVE

Indomethacin

PYRAZOLONE DERIVATIVE

Phenylbutazone

PHENYLACETIC ACID DERIVATIVE

Diclofenac

FENAMATE

Meclofenamic acid

OXICAM

Piroxicam

NAPHTHYLACETIC ACID PRODRUG

Nabumetone

Figure 36–4. Chemical structures of some NSAIDs.

half-lives, while drugs with longer half-lives disappear from the synovial fluid at a rate proportionate to their half-lives.

IBUPROFEN

Ibuprofen is a simple derivative of phenylpropionic acid. In doses of about 2400 mg daily, ibuprofen is equivalent to 4 g of aspirin in anti-inflammatory effect. This drug is rapidly cleared, has a terminal half-life of 1–2 hours, and is more than 99% protein-bound. Ibuprofen is often prescribed in lower doses, at which it is analgesic (but not anti-inflammatory at less than 2400 mg/d). It is available over the counter in lower dosage under several trade names. Ibuprofen is extensively metabolized in the liver, and little is excreted unchanged. Gastrointestinal irritation and bleeding occur, though less frequently than with aspirin. The use of ibuprofen concomitantly with aspirin may decrease the total anti-inflammatory effect. The drug is contraindicated in individuals with nasal polyps, angioedema, and bronchospastic reactivity to aspirin. In addition to the gastrointestinal symptoms (which can be modified by ingestion with meals), rash, pruritus, tinnitus, dizziness, headache, aseptic meningitis particularly in patients with systemic lupus erythematosus), and fluid retention have been reported. Interaction with anticoagulants is uncommon. Rare hematologic effects include agranulocytosis and aplastic anemia. Effects on the kidney (as with all NSAIDs) include acute renal failure, interstitial nephritis, and nephrotic syndrome, again occurring very rarely. Finally, hepatitis has been reported occasionally.

NAPROXEN & FENOPROFEN

Naproxen is a naphthylpropionic acid that binds to plasma protein and has a half-life of 12–15 hours

(Table 36–3). Antacids delay its absorption. Naproxen is excreted in the urine as an inactive glucuronide metabolite. Like ibuprofen, naproxen competes with aspirin for plasma protein binding sites. It also prolongs prothrombin time. It is available over-the-counter, attesting to its relatively good long-term safety profile, though as with other NSAIDs, dyspepsia occurs in 20–40% of patients.

Fenoprofen, another propionic acid derivative, has a half-life of 2–4 hours and is given four times daily. Of all the NSAIDs, this one is most closely associated with the (fortunately very rare) toxicity of interstitial nephritis.

Adverse effects and drug interactions of naproxen and fenoprofen are similar to those of ibuprofen, ie, nephrotoxicity, nausea, dyspepsia, peripheral edema, rash, pruritus, central nervous system and cardiovascular effects, and tinnitus. Also like ibuprofen, these effects are less common than with aspirin.

FLURBIPROFEN

Flurbiprofen is another propionic acid derivative with an intermediate half-life. It is readily absorbed and achieves good synovial concentration like other NSAIDs. Following extensive metabolic degradation, it may undergo some enterohepatic recirculation before it is excreted by the kidneys. The efficacy of flurbiprofen is comparable to that of aspirin and other NSAIDs in clinical trials for patients with rheumatoid arthritis, ankylosing spondylitis, and osteoarthritis. It is also available in a topical ophthalmic formulation for inhibition of intraoperative miosis.

As with other NSAIDs, gastrointestinal symptoms are encountered in 15–20% of patients who take the oral preparation. No significant age-related increase in adverse reactions has been reported.

KETOPROFEN

Ketoprofen is a propionic acid derivative that has some ability to inhibit both cyclooxygenase and lipoxygenase. The drug is rapidly absorbed, and its elimination half-life is 1–3 hours. It is metabolized completely in the liver. Despite being 99% bound to plasma proteins, it does not alter warfarin or digoxin activity. In contrast, concurrent administration of probenecid elevates ketoprofen levels and prolongs its plasma half-life.

The effectiveness of ketoprofen is equivalent to that of other NSAIDs and aspirin in the treatment of rheumatoid arthritis and osteoarthritis. In spite of its dual effect on prostaglandins and leukotrienes, it has not been shown to be superior to other NSAIDs. Its major adverse effects are on the central nervous system and gastrointestinal tract.

OXAPROZIN

Oxaprozin is one of the newest of the propionic acid derivative NSAIDs. As noted in Table 36–3, its major difference from the other members of this subgroup is a very long half-life; it can be given once a day. Because of this long half-life, dosage adjustments should be made at intervals no shorter than 5 days to 2 weeks. The drug appears to have the same benefits and risks associated with other NSAIDs, although it is mildly uricosuric, making it potentially more useful in gout than some other NSAIDs.

DICLOFENAC

Diclofenac is a simple phenylacetic acid derivative that resembles both flurbiprofen and meclofenamate. It is a potent cyclooxygenase inhibitor with anti-inflammatory, analgesic, and antipyretic properties. The drug is rapidly absorbed following oral administration and has a half-life of 1–2 hours. Like flurbiprofen, it accumulates in the synovial fluid. The potency of diclofenac as a cyclooxygenase inhibitor is greater than that of naproxen. The drug is recommended for chronic inflammatory conditions such as rheumatoid arthritis and osteoarthritis and for the treatment of acute musculoskeletal pain. Adverse effects occur in approximately 20% of patients and include gastrointestinal distress, occult gastrointestinal bleeding, and gastric ulceration. Transaminitis (elevation of serum aminotransferase) may occur more commonly with this drug than with other NSAIDs.

An ophthalmic preparation is available that is recommended for prevention of postoperative ophthalmic inflammation. In Europe, diclofenac is available both as a dermatologic preparation and for intramuscular administration.

SULINDAC

Sulindac, a sulfoxide, is a prodrug. Its active metabolite is, like diclofenac, an acetic acid derivative. The drug is effective only after it is converted by liver enzymes to a sulfide, which is excreted in bile and then reabsorbed from the intestine. The enterohepatic cycling prolongs the duration of action to 12–16 hours.

The indications and adverse reactions are similar to those of other NSAIDs. Among the more severe reactions, Stevens-Johnson epidermal necrolysis syndrome, thrombocytopenia, agranulocytosis, and nephrotic syndrome have all been observed. Like diclofenac, sulindac may have some propensity to cause elevation of serum aminotransferase; it is also sometimes associated with cholestatic liver damage.

TOLMETIN

Tolmetin, a pyrroleacetic acid derivative, is similar to aspirin in effectiveness in juvenile and adult rheumatoid arthritis and osteoarthritis. The drug has a short half-life and must be given frequently. Unlike most other NSAIDs, this drug may have minimal or no enterohepatic circulation.

ETODOLAC

Etodolac is newer acetic acid derivative with an intermediate half-life (Table 36–3). Like some other NSAIDs, it is a racemic mixture of R and S forms, the R form being inactive. The drug is well absorbed, with a bioavailability of about 80%, and is strongly bound to plasma proteins (> 90%). There are no data to suggest that etodolac differs significantly from other NSAIDs except in its pharmacokinetic parameters, although it may have slightly less gastric toxicity in terms of ulcer disease than other NSAIDs.

NABUMETONE

Nabumetone is a prodrug. It is given as a ketone (Figure 36–4) and converted to an acetic acid derivative in the body. Its half-life of more than 24 hours (Table 36–3) permits once-daily dosing. Otherwise, its properties are very similar to those of other NSAIDs, though it, like etodolac, may be slightly less gastrotoxic than other NSAIDs when given at a dosage of 1000 mg/d.

MECLOFENAMATE & MEFENAMIC ACID

Meclofenamate, a fenamic acid derivative, reaches a peak plasma level in 30–60 minutes and has a short half-life. It is excreted in the urine, largely as the glucuronide conjugate. Although long-term experience is lacking, meclofenamate appears to have adverse effects similar to those of other newer NSAIDs and to have no advantage over them. This drug enhances the effect of oral anticoagulants. Meclofenamate is contraindicated in pregnancy; its efficacy and safety have not been established for young children.

Mefenamic acid, another fenamate, possesses analgesic properties but is probably less effective than aspirin as an anti-inflammatory agent and is clearly more toxic. It should not be used for longer than 1 week and never in children.

PIROXICAM

Piroxicam, an oxicam, is an NSAID of novel structure (Figure 36–4). It has a half-life of 42–76 hours, permitting once-daily dosing, which should favor compliance. Given its long half-life, it can probably be administered every other day, though no study documenting such a dosing regimen has been published. It is rapidly absorbed in the stomach and upper small intestine and reaches 80% of its peak plasma concentration in 1 hour. It is excreted as the glucuronide conjugate and to a small extent unchanged.

Gastrointestinal symptoms are encountered in 20% of patients. Other adverse reactions include dizziness, tinnitus, headache, and rash. When piroxicam is used in dosages higher than 20 mg/d, an increased incidence of peptic ulcer is encountered. The drug may be used in the treatment of rheumatoid arthritis, ankylosing spondylitis, and osteoarthritis.

AZAPROPAZONE & CARPROFEN

These drugs are available in many other countries but are not sold in the USA. Azapropazone, a pyrazolone derivative, is structurally related to phenylbutazone but appears less likely to cause agranulocytosis. Its half-life is 12–16 hours. In patients with decreased renal function—eg, elderly patients—its half-life may be doubled. Carprofen is a propionic acid derivative with a half-life of 10–16 hours. The indications and adverse effects of azapropazone and carprofen are similar to those of other NSAIDs.

NSAIDS FOR SPECIAL INDICATIONS

INDOMETHACIN

Indomethacin, introduced in 1963, is an indole derivative (Figure 36–4). It is slightly more toxic but in certain circumstances more effective than aspirin. In the laboratory, it is among the most potent of the inhibitors of prostaglandin synthesis. Indomethacin is well absorbed after oral administration and highly bound to plasma proteins. Metabolism occurs in the liver, and unchanged drug and inactive metabolites are excreted in bile and urine.

Clinical Uses

Indomethacin is not suggested for general use as an analgesic. Except for the treatment of patent ductus arteriosus (discussed below), it is not usually used in children. It is useful in special situations, including acute gouty arthritis and ankylosing spondylitis, and has also been effective in extra-articular inflammatory conditions such as pericarditis and pleurisy and in Bartter's syndrome (as one would anticipate other potent cyclooxygenase inhibitors would be). In acute gout, indomethacin often replaces colchicine as the initial medication. (See Drugs Used in Gout, below.)

A special application of indomethacin is in the management of patent ductus arteriosus in premature infants. Because this structure is kept patent in the fetus by the continuous production of prostaglandins, closure can be accelerated in a premature newborn by intravenous infusion of this drug. The production of prostaglandin in this situation is not an inflammatory process and is probably dependent upon COX I rather than COX II. As noted above, indomethacin is relatively selective for COX I. In many cases, surgery can be avoided by the use of indomethacin, though renal toxicity can easily occur.

Indomethacin has been recommended for use as a tocolytic in preterm labor at less than 32 weeks gestation (Morales et al, 1989); inhibition of prostaglandin synthesis reduces the frequency and strength of uterine contractions. However, others dispute this application on the basis of the recognized fetal and maternal toxicity of the drug (Norton et al, 1993). Calcium channel blockers (Chapter 12) are receiving more attention in this application.

Adverse Effects

At higher dosage levels, at least a third of patients have reactions to indomethacin requiring discontinuance of the medication. The gastrointestinal effects may include abdominal pain, diarrhea, gastrointestinal hemorrhage, and pancreatitis. Headache is experienced by 15–25% of patients and may be associated with dizziness, confusion, and depression. Rarely, psychosis with hallucinations has been reported. Hepatic abnormalities are rare. Serious hematologic reactions have been noted, including thrombocytopenia and aplastic anemia. Hyperkalemia has been reported and is related to inhibition of the synthesis of prostaglandins in the kidney. A number of interactions with other drugs have been reported (see Appendix II). Use of indomethacin, like other potent cyclooxygenase inhibitors, should be avoided in patients with nasal polyps or angioedema, in whom asthma may be precipitated. The drug is contraindicated in pregnancy and should be used with caution in persons with psychiatric disorders or peptic ulcer disease.

PHENYLBUTAZONE

Phenylbutazone, a pyrazolone derivative, rapidly gained favor after its introduction in 1949 for the treatment of rheumatoid arthritis, ankylosing spon-

dylitis, acute gouty arthritis, and various musculoskeletal disorders. Its toxicities, particularly the hematologic effects, have resulted in its withdrawal from the North American and most European markets.

Phenylbutazone has a large number of serious adverse effects. The most serious are agranulocytosis and aplastic anemia, which have led to a number of deaths. Phenylbutazone has also caused hemolytic anemia, nephrotic syndrome, optic neuritis, deafness, serious allergic reactions, exfoliative dermatitis, and hepatic and renal tubular necrosis.

KETOROLAC

Ketorolac is an NSAID of intermediate duration of action that is promoted for systemic use mainly as a analgesic, not an anti-inflammatory drug (though it has typical NSAID properties). The drug does appear to have significant analgesic efficacy and has been used successfully to replace morphine in some situations involving mild to moderate postsurgical pain. It is most often given parenterally, but an oral dose-form is available. Longer-term use of ketorolac is associated with a significant incidence of peptic ulceration and renal compromise. This has led to its withdrawal from some European markets, though it is still available in the USA. An ophthalmic preparation is available for anti-inflammatory applications.

CLINICAL PHARMACOLOGY OF THE NSAIDS

Although aspirin is an effective drug, it is less safe than other NSAIDs (at least in the gastrointestinal tract), and it has been largely replaced by ibuprofen since the latter became an over-the-counter medication. As a group, NSAIDs tend to cause less gastric irritation, and the dosing schedule of some is simpler (one tablet once or twice daily). In choosing an agent, it is worth remembering that the cost to the patient is $30–$200 for a 60-day supply of the newer agents compared to about $10–$20 for generic over-the-counter aspirin, ibuprofen, or naproxen. A reliable method for determining salicylate blood levels is available to establish therapeutic range, which is not true for the newer drugs. The cost and follow-up advantages of aspirin must be weighed against easier dosage schedules, better compliance, and lower incidence of gastric irritation with some of the newer agents. Surveys show that most patients with inflammatory arthritis receive NSAIDs without an adequate trial of salicylates, yet none of these newer drugs have proved more effective than aspirin in controlled studies. Moreover, although less gastrointestinal irritation has been shown for most of them, some are proving more toxic in other ways.

Because of the importance of gastric ulceration in patients taking anti-inflammatory doses of the NSAIDs, considerable effort has gone into preventing this complication or reducing its severity. The prostaglandin E_1 analog misoprostol inhibits gastric acid secretion at some doses and probably increases secretion of gastric mucosal protective factors such as bicarbonate at higher doses (see Chapters 18 and 63). Misoprostol is labeled for use with NSAIDs in patients prone to development of peptic ulcers.

The newer NSAIDs have been responsible for instances of acute renal failure and nephrotic syndrome, which develops insidiously and is neither dose-dependent nor related to duration of drug use. Patients rarely have symptoms suggestive of a hypersensitivity reaction, so the condition may go undetected until advanced.

If the decision is made to use a newer NSAID, it is important to consider adverse effects, cost, and dosing schedules. It is not possible to know which patient will respond in a specific way to which NSAID, for some patients derive benefit from one and not from another. How much of this variability of response is related to the agent per se, to individual differences in metabolism of the drug, or to a placebo effect is difficult to evaluate. When compliance is a problem, drugs such as piroxicam, naproxen, sulindac, and oxaprozin are useful because only one or two doses are required daily. If a patient is taking a hypoglycemic agent or warfarin, ibuprofen or tolmetin might be considered, since they do not potentiate the effect of the hypoglycemic drugs or warfarin. Hypersensitivity to one of the phenylpropionic or phenylacetic acids, however, should preclude use of the others in that group. Dosing schedules listed for the drugs are those recommended by the manufacturer, but it is becoming clear that some patients require and may tolerate higher doses. Until blood level assays become available, it is probably safest to use the dosages as listed.

DISEASE-MODIFYING ANTIRHEUMATIC DRUGS (DMARDS)

Careful clinical and epidemiologic studies have shown that rheumatoid arthritis causes significant systemic effects that shorten life in addition to the joint disease that reduces mobility and quality of life. NSAIDs appear to offer mainly symptomatic relief; they reduce inflammation and the pain it causes and often preserve function but have little effect on the progression of bone and cartilage destruction. In recent years, therefore, interest has been renewed in treatments that might arrest—or at least slow—this progression by modifying the disease itself. The ef-fects of disease-modifying drugs may take 6 weeks to 6 months to become evident, ie, they are slow-acting compared with NSAIDs. Members of the group include methotrexate, azathioprine, penicillamine, hydroxychloroquine and chloroquine, organic gold compounds, and sulfasalazine. Considerable controversy surrounds the long-term efficacy of these drugs. The discovery that numerous cytokines are present in joints affected by the disease process (Table 36–2) suggests that one or more of these may be useful targets of disease-modifying drug therapy.

METHOTREXATE & OTHER IMMUNOSUPPRESSIVE DRUGS

The immunosuppressive agents (see Chapter 56) have been employed for many decades in the therapy of rheumatic diseases, but their use has been largely restricted to seriously crippling disease with reversible lesions after conventional therapy has failed. Because of their toxic potential, however, immunosuppressive drugs should be employed only by physicians completely familiar with their actions. Reliable methods of selecting one drug instead of another are not available, and acceptable controlled studies demonstrating efficacy in humans are lacking for most of the drugs. However, several clinical studies suggest that of all the slow-acting antirheumatic drugs, methotrexate has the best benefit-to-risk ratio, ie, fewer patients drop out of therapy with this drug—for reasons of toxicity or lack of benefit—than with any other DMARD (Felson et al, 1990; Wolfe et al, 1990).

Immunosuppressive agents are useful in lupus nephritis, in seropositive progressive rheumatoid arthritis, and occasionally in other rheumatic diseases. They have also been shown to be effective in vasculitis syndromes, such as Wegener's granulomatosis and panarteritis. Because of the severity of toxic effects—especially the oncogenic effects, hepatotoxicity, and bone marrow depression—immunosuppressive drugs should be given only after safer agents have been tried.

Methotrexate at oncologic doses is a potent immunosuppressive drug (Chapter 56). Its principal mechanisms of action at the doses used in the rheumatic diseases probably relate to inhibition of aminoimidazolecarboxamide ribonucleotide (AICAR) transformylase and thymidylate synthase, plus enhanced adenosine release. The drug is approximately 70% absorbed after oral administration, highly polyglutaminated, and excreted in both urine (the major pathway) and bile. It is effective in rheumatoid arthritis at dosages up to 25 mg/wk, though the most common dosage is 15 mg/wk. Nausea and mucosal ulcers were the most common toxicities recorded in a large study comparing DMARDs in rheumatoid arthritis (Singh et al, 1991). Progressive dose-related hepatotoxicity in the form of enzyme changes occur frequently, but cirrhosis is rare (less than 1%), and liver biopsy follow-up is no longer recommended routinely until the patient has taken the drug for 5 years. Some clinicians have expressed concern about a "hypersensitivity" lung reaction and a pseudolymphomatous reaction. Recent evidence suggests that methotrexate toxicity can be reduced without decreasing its efficacy in rheumatoid arthritis by giving leucovorin 24 hours after each weekly dose of methotrexate (Shiroky et al, 1993) or by the use of daily folic acid.

Other immunosuppressive drugs for which there is some experience in the treatment of arthritis include the alkylators **mechlorethamine, cyclophosphamide,** and **chlorambucil** and the purine antagonist **azathioprine,** which is FDA-approved for treatment of rheumatoid arthritis.

Azathioprine is sometimes used for rheumatoid arthritis in dosages up to 2 μg/kg/d. Neither its kinetics nor its mechanism of action in this disease is understood. Its onset of action is slow and its toxicity is considerable, making its use infrequent. Toxicities of particular concern include hematologic and hepatic damage and a slightly increased incidence of non-Hodgkin's lymphoma.

ANTIMALARIAL DRUGS
(Chloroquine, Hydroxychloroquine)

The pharmacology of the 4-aminoquinoline derivatives is more fully discussed in Chapter 53. Chloroquine and hydroxychloroquine have been used in the treatment of rheumatoid arthritis and systemic lupus erythematosus since the 1950s, and their efficacy in inducing remission has been confirmed in carefully controlled studies. Rheumatoid factor, a marker for disease intensity in many patients, declines after prolonged chloroquine use; however, there is no evidence that chloroquine or hydroxychloroquine decreases the progression of erosive bone lesions.

The mechanism of anti-inflammatory action of chloroquine and hydroxychloroquine in rheumatic disorders is unclear. They suppress the responsiveness of T lymphocytes to mitogens, decrease leukocyte chemotaxis, stabilize lysosomal membranes, inhibit DNA and RNA synthesis, and trap free radicals; one or more of these effects might be relevant. The actions of these agents are not apparent until after a latent period of 12–24 weeks. The drugs are often useful as adjuncts to treatment with NSAIDs and have no adverse interactions with other antirheumatic agents.

Indications
Antimalarials are often administered to patients with rheumatoid arthritis who have not responded optimally to salicylates and NSAIDs. In addition to their use in rheumatoid arthritis, antimalarials have been used successfully for their anti-inflammatory effect in juvenile chronic arthritis, Sjögren's syndrome, and systemic lupus erythematosus (in which they have a beneficial effect on both joint and skin findings). The antimalarial drugs should not be used in psoriatic arthritis because of the possible development of exfoliative dermatitis.

Adverse Effects
These are described in detail in Chapter 53.

Dosage
Hydroxychloroquine sulfate is the preferred drug. Initial dosage is up to 6.4 mg/kg/d but not more than 400 mg daily. Once clinical improvement is established, the dose can often be decreased to 200 mg daily.

GOLD

Gold compounds were introduced for treatment of rheumatoid arthritis in the 1920s, but it was not until 1960, in a report of a large double-blind trial, that the gold salts were shown to have a useful effect. Subsequent controlled studies have generally (not universally) supported the view that parenteral gold reduces symptoms and slows progression of the disease. Some studies have demonstrated that these agents retard the progression of bone and articular destruction determined roentgenographically. Further impetus to the popularity of gold salts has been the demonstration that the drug may be continued for years, allaying earlier fears of toxicity from accumulation. A particular disadvantage of gold therapy is the high rate of discontinuance; the probability of remaining on gold therapy is less than 60% after 2 years and less than 10% after 7 years. Most of these dropouts are due to toxicity.

Introduction of an oral gold preparation (auranofin) stimulated a number of large clinical studies during the 1980s. Most of these studies suggest that the oral preparation has modest effects at best and that its benefits may not differ significantly from those of NSAIDs in some types of arthritis, though its toxicity is greater (Carette et al, 1989; Giannini et al, 1990).

Chemistry
The parenterally administered gold preparations available in North America are **aurothiomalate** and **aurothioglucose.** Both are administered intramuscularly as water-soluble gold salts containing 50% elemental gold. **Auranofin** is a substituted gold thioglucose derivative (29% gold) that can be given by mouth.

Pharmacokinetics
Gold salts are approximately 95% bound to plasma protein during transport by the blood. Although they

tend to concentrate in synovial membranes, gold salts are also concentrated in the liver, kidney, spleen, adrenal glands, lymph nodes, and bone marrow. Following intramuscular injection of the parenteral forms, peak serum levels are reached in 2–6 hours; 40% is excreted within a week—about two-thirds in the urine and one-third in the feces. One month after intramuscular injection of 50 mg, 75–80% of the drug has been eliminated from the serum. The total body half-life of intramuscular gold, however, approaches 1 year. After oral administration of auranofin, only about 25% is absorbed. Certain tissue compartments such as the epithelial cells of the renal tubules, which have a particular affinity for gold, show its presence many years after therapy has ceased. Most studies have failed to show a correlation between serum gold concentration and either therapeutic effect or toxicity.

Pharmacodynamics

The precise manner in which gold salts produce their beneficial effects in patients with rheumatoid arthritis and allied disorders is unknown. Gold alters the morphology and functional capabilities of human macrophages; this may be its major mode of action. Other effects ascribed to gold include inhibition of lysosomal enzyme activity, reduction of histamine release from mast cells, inactivation of the first component of complement, suppression of phagocytic activity of the polymorphonuclear leukocytes, inhibition of macrophage function, and inhibition of the Shwartzman phenomenon. In addition, aurothiomalate reduces the number of circulating lymphocytes, and auranofin inhibits the release of prostaglandin E_2 from synovial cells and the release of leukotrienes B_4 and C_4 from polymorphonuclear leukocytes.

Indications & Contraindications

Gold therapy is indicated for active rheumatoid arthritis. Patients who later in the course of their disease show active inflammation and erosive changes are also candidates for gold. Patients with rheumatoid arthritis in the presence of Sjögren's syndrome and those with juvenile rheumatoid arthritis may also be considered, whereas the usefulness of gold in the treatment of psoriatic arthritis is less clear.

The major contraindications to gold are a confirmed history of previous toxicity from the drug, pregnancy, serious impairment of liver or renal function, and blood dyscrasias.

Adverse Effects

Approximately one-third of patients receiving gold salts experience some form of toxicity. Dermatitis, which is usually pruritic, is the most common adverse effect, occurring in 15–20% of patients. Eosinophilia may precede or be associated with cutaneous lesions. Hematologic abnormalities, including thrombocytopenia, leukopenia, and pancytopenia, occur in 1–10% of

patients. Aplastic anemia, although rare, may be fatal. About 8–10% of patients develop proteinuria that may progress to nephrotic syndrome in a few cases. Other adverse effects include stomatitis, a metallic taste in the mouth, skin pigmentation, enterocolitis, cholestatic jaundice, peripheral neuropathy, pulmonary infiltrates, and corneal deposition of gold. Nitritoid reactions (sweating, faintness, flushing, and headaches) may occur, especially with gold thiomalate, and are presumably due to the vehicle rather than the gold salts themselves. Transient aggravation of arthritis symptoms may occur after injections of gold. Gastrointestinal disturbances (especially diarrhea) and dermatitis are the most common adverse effects of oral gold therapy.

Dosage

Parenteral gold is usually given as a 50 mg dose intramuscularly weekly until a total of 1000 mg has been injected (unless there is no response by the time 600–700 mg has been given, in which case the drug can be stopped). If 1 g is given without serious adverse effects and a favorable response is observed, the drug can be continued indefinitely in lengthening intervals of 2, 3, then 4 weeks. Oral gold is given as a 6 mg dose daily, increasing to 9 mg/d if a response is not seen after 3 months. Clinical response usually requires a few months to become evident and may be delayed for as long as 4 months. Careful clinical and laboratory monitoring is mandatory.

PENICILLAMINE

Penicillamine, a metabolite of penicillin, is an analog of the amino acid cysteine. The drug can be resolved into D and L isomers; the D form is used clinically.

$$HS-\underset{\underset{CH_3}{|}}{\overset{\overset{CH_3}{|}}{C}}-\underset{\underset{NH_2}{|}}{\overset{\overset{H}{|}}{C}}-COOH$$

Penicillamine

Pharmacokinetics

About half of an orally administered dose of penicillamine is absorbed. Absorption is enhanced if the drug is administered 1.5 hours after meals. Free penicillamine and its metabolites may be found in urine and feces. About 60% of the drug is excreted in 24 hours. No satisfactory method is available for determining blood levels.

Pharmacodynamics

The mechanism of penicillamine's action in rheumatoid arthritis is unclear. The drug suppresses arthropathy in experimental animal models and has been shown to interact with lymphocyte membrane receptors. It may interfere with the synthesis of DNA, collagen, and mucopolysaccharides. Rheumatoid factor titer falls following administration of drug, probably reflecting disruption of disulfide bonds of macroglobulins but perhaps also reflecting a basic action of the drug on the immune system. Penicillamine is similar to gold in its latency period (3–4 months) and in its anti-inflammatory properties.

Indications

Penicillamine is reserved for patients with active, progressive erosive rheumatoid disease not controlled by conservative therapy. Penicillamine is usually prescribed for patients who have not responded to gold therapy. Penicillamine is not useful in seronegative arthropathies. Caution is required when administering other drugs simultaneously, because penicillamine impedes absorption of many drugs and prevents them from reaching therapeutic levels.

Adverse Effects

The toxic effects of penicillamine limit its usefulness. Animal studies have shown inhibition of wound healing and evidence of muscle and blood vessel damage. In humans, adverse effects are reduced by giving lower doses and by slow progression to maintenance dosages. Proteinuria is encountered in 20% of patients. Immune complex nephritis has been seen in 4% of patients; it is often reversible when the drug is withdrawn. Leukopenia and thrombocytopenia may occur at any time and may herald aplastic anemia. Most deaths related to penicillamine are due to aplastic anemia. Skin and mucous membrane reactions, the most common adverse effects, may occur at any time during therapy and may respond to lowering the dose. Drug fever, which may be seen as an early response to penicillamine, is often associated with cutaneous eruptions.

A variety of autoimmune diseases, including myasthenia gravis, Goodpasture's syndrome, lupus erythematosus, hemolytic anemia, and thyroiditis may be seen. The drug must be discontinued permanently when any of these conditions is encountered.

Loss of taste perception or a metallic taste may develop. The blunting of taste perception relates to zinc chelation. Anorexia, nausea, and vomiting occur. Mammary hyperplasia, alopecia, and psychologic changes have also been observed.

Penicillamine is contraindicated in pregnancy and in the presence of renal insufficiency and should not be given in combination with gold, cytotoxic drugs, or phenylbutazone.

Adverse effects necessitating cessation of the drug occur in about 40% of patients. Blood counts (including platelet count) and urinalysis are performed twice a month for 4–6 months, then monthly. The drug should be stopped if the platelet count falls below 100,000/μL or the white count below 3000/μL. A history of penicillin allergy is not a contraindication to penicillamine. Patients who develop renal involvement, drug fever, autoimmune syndromes, and hematologic problems should not be rechallenged with the drug.

Dosage

Penicillamine is taken orally 1.5 hours after meals. If clinical benefits are to occur, they should be apparent by 6 months. Treatment begins with 125 mg or 250 mg daily for 1–3 months; if no adverse effects are seen and improvement does not occur, the dose is doubled. If therapeutic effects are absent after 3–4 months, the dose is increased at monthly intervals up to 750 mg daily, which it is rarely necessary to exceed. If therapy is discontinued after improvement, most patients relapse within 6 months.

SULFASALAZINE

Sulfasalazine, originally introduced for the treatment of ulcerative colitis, has been shown to be effective in patients with rheumatoid arthritis (Felson et al, 1990). Its pharmacokinetics are somewhat complex, but its primary metabolites are 5-acetylsalicylic acid (5-ASA) and sulfapyridine. While 5-ASA is the active drug in inflammatory bowel disease, it is either the sulfapyridine alone or sulfapyridine and the parent drug that are active in rheumatoid arthritis. The mechanism of action in rheumatoid arthritis is probably *not* that of dihydrofolate inhibitor, though effects on B cell function may be important. Activity in rheumatoid arthritis has been proved, and the drug is approved by the FDA in the USA; it is already a frequently used drug in Europe.

Toxicity, which occurs more frequently in patients with rheumatoid arthritis than in those with ulcerative colitis, includes rashes, gastrointestinal upset, dizziness, and photosensitivity. Rarely, neutropenia may require discontinuation of the drug, and hypersensitivity pneumonitis and sterility have also occurred.

The usual dosage is 2 g/d, given in four divided doses.

GLUCOCORTICOID DRUGS

The pharmacology of corticosteroids and their other applications are discussed in Chapter 39.

The effect of prednisone and other glucocorticoids on rheumatoid arthritis is prompt and dramatic, and recent data suggest that the drug is capable of slowing the appearance of new bone erosions. Glucocorticoids are known to inhibit phospholipase A_2, the enzyme responsible for the liberation of arachidonic acid from membrane lipids (Chapter 18). In addition, glucocorticoids have recently been shown to selectively inhibit the expression of COX II (Kujubu et al, 1992; Winn et al, 1993). However, prolonged use of these drugs leads to serious, disabling toxic effects, including fractures, infections, and cataracts. In predisposed patients, diabetes, hypertension, and accelerated atherosclerotic heart disease may occur. Corticosteroids may be administered for certain serious extra-articular manifestations such as pericarditis or eye involvement or during periods of exacerbation. When prednisone is required for long-term therapy, the dosage should not exceed 10 mg daily, and gradual reduction of the dose should be encouraged. Alternate-day corticosteroid therapy is usually unsuccessful in rheumatoid arthritis, though it can be useful for some vasculitides such as subacute lupus erythematosus. Patients become symptomatic on the day they do not take the drug.

Intra-articular corticosteroids are often helpful to alleviate painful symptoms and, when successful, are preferable to increasing the dosage of systemic medication.

DIETARY MANIPULATION OF INFLAMMATION

Arachidonic acid is an eicosatetraenoic acid metabolized by the cyclooxygenase and lipoxygenase pathways. In this process arachidonic acid is released from membrane phospholipids of stimulated cells, and oxygenated, yielding several mediators. These mediators have potent effects on the development and function of smooth muscles, blood vessels, epithelial surfaces, secretory glands, leukocytes, and elements of the nervous system (Chapter 18).

It may be beneficial to alter or supplement a patient's diet to provide unsaturated fatty acids (such as eicosapentaenoic acid, which is found in marine fish) similar to arachidonic acid. This dietary change causes the alternative fatty acids to be metabolized with arachidonic acid, changing the final products of the process. For example, eicosapentaenoic acid inhibits the uptake and incorporation of arachidonic acid into membrane phospholipids of some cells, and dilutes free arachidonic acid as a substrate for oxygenation. The products of eicosapentaenoic acid oxygenation are less potent than the corresponding mediators derived from arachidonic acid (sometimes by orders of magnitude), and they diminish the activities of these mediators by competing with them for shared target-cell receptors.

Ingestion of unpurified eicosapentaenoic acid by humans causes the attenuation of platelet aggregation and decreased chemotactic activity and adherence of polymorphonuclear leukocytes evoked by leukotriene B_4. The results of clinical studies suggest that therapy with eicosapentaenoic acid decreases both morning stiffness and the number of tender joints in patients with rheumatoid arthritis and erythema associated with psoriasis. The potency of eicosapentaenoic acid approximates that of the NSAIDs. These preliminary results and the near absence of significant adverse effects suggest that dietary alteration or supplementation to provide 1–4 g/d of eicosapentaenoic acid may be a beneficial addition to conventional treatment of these conditions.

II. OTHER ANALGESICS

Acetaminophen is one of the most important drugs used for the treatment of mild to moderate pain when an anti-inflammatory effect is not necessary. Phenacetin, a prodrug that is metabolized to acetaminophen, is more toxic than its active metabolite and has no rational indications.

ACETAMINOPHEN

Acetaminophen is the active metabolite of phenacetin responsible for its analgesic effect. It is a weak prostaglandin inhibitor in peripheral tissues and possesses no significant anti-inflammatory effects.

Pharmacokinetics

Acetaminophen is administered orally. Absorption is related to the rate of gastric emptying, and peak blood concentrations are usually reached in 30–60 minutes. Acetaminophen is slightly bound to plasma proteins and is partially metabolized by hepatic microsomal enzymes and converted to acetaminophen sulfate and glucuronide, which are pharmacologically inactive (Figure 4–4). Less than 5% is excreted unchanged. A minor but highly active metabolite (N-acetyl-p-benzoquinone) is important in large doses because of its toxicity to both liver and kidney. The half-life of acetaminophen is 2–3 hours and is relatively unaffected by renal function. With toxic quantities or liver disease, the half-life may be increased twofold or more.

Indications

Although equivalent to aspirin as an effective analgesic and antipyretic agent (Styrt et al, 1990), acetaminophen differs by its lack of anti-inflammatory properties. It does not affect uric acid levels and lacks platelet-inhibiting properties. The drug is useful in mild to moderate pain such as headache, myalgia, postpartum pain, and other circumstances in which aspirin is an effective analgesic. Acetaminophen alone is inadequate therapy for inflammatory conditions

N-Acetyl-p-aminophenol
(acetaminophen)

Phenacetin
(acetophenetidin)

such as rheumatoid arthritis, though it may be used as an analgesic adjunct to anti-inflammatory therapy. For mild analgesia, acetaminophen is the preferred drug in patients allergic to aspirin or when salicylates are poorly tolerated. It is preferable to aspirin in patients with hemophilia or a history of peptic ulcer and in those in whom bronchospasm is precipitated by aspirin. Unlike aspirin, acetaminophen does not antagonize the effects of uricosuric agents; it may be used concomitantly with probenecid in the treatment of gout. It is preferred to aspirin in children with viral infections.

Adverse Effects

In therapeutic doses, a mild increase in hepatic enzymes may occasionally occur in the absence of jaundice: this is reversible when the drug is withdrawn. With larger doses, dizziness, excitement, and disorientation are seen. Ingestion of 15 g of acetaminophen may be fatal, death being caused by severe hepatotoxicity with central lobular necrosis, sometimes associated with acute renal tubular necrosis (Chapters 4 and 59). Early symptoms of hepatic damage include nausea, vomiting, diarrhea, and abdominal pain. Recent data also implicate acetaminophen in rare cases of renal damage without hepatic damage. This damage has occurred even after usual doses of acetaminophen. Therapy is much less satisfactory than for aspirin overdose. In addition to supportive therapy, measures that have proved extremely useful are the provision of sulfhydryl groups to neutralize the toxic metabolites. Acetylcysteine is used for this purpose (see Chapter 59).

Hemolytic anemia and methemoglobinemia, reported with the use of phenacetin, have rarely been noted with acetaminophen. Interstitial nephritis and papillary necrosis, serious complications of phenacetin, although anticipated with widespread chronic use of acetaminophen, have not occurred despite the fact that about 80% of phenacetin is rapidly metabolized to acetaminophen. Gastrointestinal bleeding does not occur. Caution should be exercised in patients with liver disease.

Dosage

Acute pain and fever may be managed by 325–500 mg four times daily and proportionately less for children. Steady-state conditions are attained within a day.

PHENACETIN

Phenacetin can no longer be prescribed in the USA and has been removed from many over-the-counter analgesic combinations such as Anacin and Empirin Compound. However, it is still present in a number of proprietary analgesics in this country and is in common use in many other parts of the world. The association between the excessive use of analgesic combinations—especially those that contain phenacetin—and the development of renal failure has been recognized for almost 30 years. Estimates of the percentage of patients with end-stage renal disease resulting from this kind of analgesic abuse range from 5% to 15%. After prohibition of the use of phenacetin in proprietary analgesics in Finland, Scotland, and Canada, the number of new cases of analgesic nephropathies in those countries decreased significantly.

III. DRUGS USED IN GOUT

Gout is a familial metabolic disease characterized by recurrent episodes of acute arthritis due to deposits of monosodium urate in joints and cartilage. Formation of uric acid calculi in the kidneys may also occur. Gout is usually associated with high serum levels of uric acid, a poorly soluble substance that is the major end product of purine metabolism. In most mammals, uricase converts uric acid to the more soluble allantoin; this enzyme is absent in humans.

The treatment of gout is aimed at relieving the acute gouty attack and preventing recurrent gouty episodes and urate lithiasis. Therapy for an attack of acute gouty arthritis is based on our current understanding of the pathophysiologic events that occur in this disease (Figure 36–5). Urate crystals are initially phagocytosed by synoviocytes, which then release prostaglandins, lysosomal enzymes, and interleukin-1. Attracted by these chemotactic mediators, polymorphonuclear leukocytes migrate into the joint space and amplify the ongoing inflammatory process. In the later phases of the attack, increased numbers of mononuclear phagocytes (macrophages) appear, ingest the urate crystals, and release more inflammatory mediators. This sequence of events suggests that the most effective agents for the management of acute urate crystal-induced inflammation are those that suppress different phases of leukocyte activation.

Before starting chronic therapy for gout, patients in whom hyperuricemia is associated with gout and

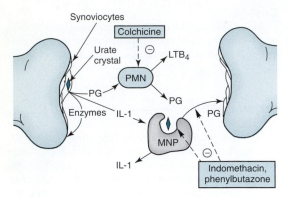

Figure 36–5. Pathophysiologic events in a gouty joint. Synoviocytes phagocytose urate crystals and then secrete inflammatory mediators, which attract and activate polymorphonuclear leukocytes (PMN) and mononuclear phagocytes (MNP) (macrophages). Drugs active in gout inhibit crystal phagocytosis and polymorphonuclear leukocyte and macrophage release of inflammatory mediators. (PG, prostaglandin; IL-1, interleukin-1; LTB$_4$, leukotriene B$_4$.)

Indications

Colchicine has been the traditional drug used for alleviating the inflammation of acute gouty arthritis. Although colchicine is more specific in gout than the NSAIDs, other agents (eg, indomethacin and other NSAIDs [except aspirin]) are often employed because of the troublesome diarrhea associated with colchicine therapy. Colchicine is preferred for the prophylaxis of recurrent episodes of gouty arthritis, is effective in preventing attacks of acute Mediterranean fever, and may have a mild beneficial effect in sarcoid arthritis and in hepatic cirrhosis.

Adverse Effects

Colchicine often causes diarrhea and may occasionally cause nausea, vomiting, and abdominal pain. Colchicine may rarely cause hair loss and bone marrow depression as well as peripheral neuritis and myopathy.

Acute intoxication after ingestion of large (nontherapeutic) doses of the alkaloid is characterized by burning throat pain, bloody diarrhea, shock, hema-

urate lithiasis must be clearly distinguished from those who have only hyperuricemia. In an asymptomatic person with hyperuricemia, the efficacy of long-term drug treatment is unproved. Uric acid levels may be elevated up to 2 standard deviations above the mean for a lifetime without adverse consequences in some individuals.

COLCHICINE

Colchicine is an alkaloid isolated from the autumn crocus, *Colchicum autumnale.* Its structure is shown in Figure 36–6.

Pharmacokinetics

Colchicine is absorbed readily after oral administration and reaches peak plasma levels within 2 hours. Metabolites of the drug are excreted in the intestinal tract and urine.

Pharmacodynamics

Colchicine dramatically relieves the pain and inflammation of gouty arthritis in 12–24 hours without altering the metabolism or excretion of urates and without other analgesic effects. Colchicine produces its anti-inflammatory effects by binding to the intracellular protein tubulin, thereby preventing its polymerization into microtubules and leading to the inhibition of leukocyte migration and phagocytosis. It also inhibits the formation of leukotriene B$_4$. Several of colchicine's adverse effects are produced by its inhibition of tubulin polymerization and cell mitosis.

Colchicine

Probenecid

Sulfinpyrazone

Figure 36–6. Colchicine and uricosuric drugs.

turia, and oliguria. Fatal ascending central nervous system depression has been reported. Treatment is supportive.

Dosage

For terminating an attack of gout, the initial dose of colchicine is usually 0.5 or 1 mg, followed by 0.5 mg every 2 hours until pain is relieved or nausea and diarrhea appear. The total dose can be given intravenously, if necessary, but it should be remembered that as little as 8 mg in 24 hours may be fatal. The prophylactic dose of colchicine is 0.5 mg one to three times daily.

NSAIDS IN GOUT

In addition to inhibiting prostaglandin synthase, indomethacin and other NSAIDs also inhibit urate crystal phagocytosis. Indomethacin may be used as initial treatment of gout or as an alternative drug when colchicine is unsuccessful or causes too much discomfort. Indomethacin is the agent most often used today to treat acute gout. Three to four doses of 50 mg every 6 hours are given; when a response occurs the dosage is reduced to 25 mg three or four times daily for about 5 days.

Other newer NSAIDs are also being used with success in the acute episode. All other NSAIDs except aspirin, salicylates, and tolmetin have been successfully used to treat acute gouty episodes. Oxaprozin, which lowers serum uric acid, is theoretically a good NSAID to use though it should not be given to patients with uric acid stones because it increases uric acid excretion in the urine. These agents appear to be as effective and safe as the older drugs.

URICOSURIC AGENTS

Probenecid and sulfinpyrazone are uricosuric drugs employed to decrease the body pool of urate in patients with tophaceous gout or in those with increasingly frequent gouty attacks. In a patient who excretes large amounts of uric acid, the uricosuric agents should be avoided so as not to precipitate the formation of uric acid calculi.

Chemistry

Uricosuric drugs are organic acids (Figure 36–6) and, as such, act at the anionic transport sites of the renal tubule (Chapter 15). Sulfinpyrazone is a metabolite of an analog of phenylbutazone.

Pharmacokinetics

Probenecid is completely reabsorbed by the renal tubules and is metabolized very slowly. Sulfinpyrazone or its active hydroxylated derivative is rapidly excreted by the kidneys. Even so, the duration of its effect after oral administration is almost as long as that of probenecid.

Pharmacodynamics

Uric acid is freely filtered at the glomerulus. Like many other weak acids, it is also both reabsorbed and secreted in the middle segment of the proximal tubule. Uricosuric drugs—probenecid, sulfinpyrazone, and large doses of aspirin—affect these active transport sites so that net reabsorption of uric acid in the proximal tubule is decreased. Because aspirin in small (analgesic or antipyretic) doses causes net retention of uric acid by inhibiting the secretory transporter, it should not be used for analgesia in patients with gout. The secretion of other weak acids, eg, penicillin, is also reduced by uricosuric agents. Probenecid was originally developed to prolong penicillin blood levels.

As the urinary excretion of uric acid increases, the size of the urate pool decreases, although the plasma concentration may not be greatly reduced. In patients who respond favorably, tophaceous deposits of urate will be reabsorbed, with relief of arthritis and remineralization of bone. With the ensuing increase in uric acid excretion, a predisposition to the formation of renal stones is augmented rather than decreased; therefore, the urine volume should be maintained at a high level and at least early in treatment the urine pH kept above 6.0 by the administration of alkali.

Indications

Uricosuric therapy should be initiated if several acute attacks of gouty arthritis have occurred, when evidence of tophi appears, or when plasma levels of uric acid in patients with gout are so high that tissue damage is almost inevitable. Therapy should not be started until 2–3 weeks after an acute attack.

Adverse Effects

Adverse effects do not provide a basis for preferring one or the other of the uricosuric agents. Both of these organic acids cause gastrointestinal irritation, but sulfinpyrazone is more active in this regard. Probenecid is more likely to cause allergic dermatitis, but a rash may appear after the use of either compound. Nephrotic syndrome has resulted from the use of probenecid. Both sulfinpyrazone and probenecid may (though rarely) cause aplastic anemia.

Contraindications & Cautions

It is essential to maintain a large urine volume to minimize the possibility of stone formation.

Dosage

Probenecid is usually started at a dosage of 0.5 g orally daily in divided doses, progressing to 1 g daily after 1 week. Sulfinpyrazone is started at a dosage of 200 mg orally daily, progressing to 400–800 mg daily. It should be given in divided doses with food to reduce adverse gastrointestinal effects.

ALLOPURINOL

An alternative to increasing uric acid excretion in the treatment of gout is to reduce its synthesis by inhibiting xanthine oxidase with allopurinol.

Chemistry

The structure of allopurinol, an isomer of hypoxanthine, is shown in Figure 36–7.

Pharmacokinetics

Allopurinol is approximately 80% absorbed after oral administration. Like uric acid, allopurinol is itself metabolized by xanthine oxidase. The resulting compound, alloxanthine, retains the capacity to inhibit xanthine oxidase and has a long enough duration of action so that allopurinol need be given only once a day.

Pharmacodynamics

Dietary purines are not an important source of uric acid. The quantitatively important amounts of purine are formed from amino acids, formate, and carbon dioxide in the body. Those purine ribonucleotides not incorporated into nucleic acids and those derived from the degradation of nucleic acids are converted to xanthine or hypoxanthine and oxidized to uric acid (Figure 36–7). When this last step is inhibited by allopurinol, there is a fall in the plasma urate level and a decrease in the size of the urate pool with a concurrent rise in the more soluble xanthine and hypoxanthine.

Indications

Treatment of gout with allopurinol, as with uricosuric agents, is begun with the expectation that it will be continued for years if not for life. Although allopurinol is often the first urate-lowering drug used, its most rational indications are as follows: (1) in chronic tophaceous gout, in which reabsorption of tophi is more rapid than with uricosuric agents; (2) in patients with gout whose 24-hour urinary uric acid on purine-free diet exceeds 600–700 mg; (3) when probenecid or sulfinpyrazone cannot be used because of adverse effects or allergic reactions, or when they are providing less than optimal therapeutic effect; (4) for recurrent renal stones; (5) in patients with renal functional impairment; or (6) when serum urate levels are grossly elevated. One should attempt to lower serum urate levels to less than 6.5 mg/dL. Aside from gout, allopurinol is used as an antiprotozoal (Chapter 53) and is indicated to prevent the massive uricosuria following therapy of blood dyscrasias that could otherwise lead to renal calculi.

Adverse Effects

Acute attacks of gouty arthritis occur early in treatment with allopurinol when urate crystals are being withdrawn from the tissues and plasma levels are below normal. To prevent acute attacks, colchicine should be given during the initial period of therapy with allopurinol unless allopurinol is being used in combination with probenecid or sulfinpyrazone. Gastrointestinal intolerance, including nausea, vomiting, and diarrhea, may occur. Peripheral neuritis and necrotizing vasculitis, depression of bone marrow elements, and, rarely, aplastic anemia may also occur. Hepatic toxicity and interstitial nephritis have been reported. An allergic skin reaction characterized by pruritic maculopapular lesions develops in 3% of patients. Isolated cases of exfoliative dermatitis have been reported. In very rare cases, allopurinol has become bound to the lens, resulting in cataracts.

Figure 36–7. Inhibition of uric acid synthesis by allopurinol. (Modified and reproduced, with permission, from Meyers FH, Jawetz E, Goldfien A: *Review of Medical Pharmacology,* 7th ed. Lange, 1980.)

Interactions & Cautions

When chemotherapeutic mercaptopurines are being given concomitantly, their dose must be reduced to about 25%. Allopurinol may also increase the effect of cyclophosphamide. Allopurinol inhibits the metabolism of probenecid and oral anticoagulants and may increase hepatic iron concentration. Safety in children and during pregnancy has not been established.

Dosage

The initial dosage of allopurinol is 100 mg daily. It may be titrated to 300 mg/d depending on the serum uric acid response.

Colchicine or an NSAID should be given during the first weeks of allopurinol therapy to prevent the gouty arthritis episodes that sometimes occur.

PREPARATIONS AVAILABLE

Salicylates

Aspirin, acetylsalicylic acid (generic, A.S.A. En-
seals, Easprin, others)
Oral (regular or enteric coated): 81, 165, 325,
500, 650, 800, 975 mg tablets; 325, 500 mg
capsules; 650, 800 mg timed-release tablets
Rectal: 200, 300, 600 mg suppositories
Choline salicylate (Arthropan)
Oral: 870 mg/5 mL liquid
Diflunisal (Dolobid)
Oral: 250, 500 mg tablets
Magnesium salicylate (Doan's Pills, Magan, Mo-
bidin)
Oral: 325, 500, 545, 600 mg tablets
Salsalate, salicylsalicylic acid (generic, Disalcid)
Oral: 500, 750 mg tablets; 500 mg capsules
Sodium salicylate (generic, Uracel 5)
Oral: 325, 650 mg enteric-coated tablets
Sodium thiosalicylate (generic, Thiocyl, Tusal)
Parenteral: 50 mg/mL for injection

Other NSAIDs

Diclofenac (Voltaren)
Oral: 25, 50, 75 mg enteric-coated tablets
Ophthalmic: 0.1% solution
Etodolac (Lodine)
Oral: 200, 300 mg capsules
Fenoprofen (generic, Nalfon)
Oral: 200, 300 mg capsules; 600 mg tablets
Flurbiprofen (Ansaid, Ocufen)
Oral: 50, 100 mg tablets
Ophthalmic: 0.03% solution
Ibuprofen (generic, Motrin, Rufen, Advil [OTC],
Nuprin [OTC], others)
Oral: 50, 100, 200, 300, 400, 600, 800 mg
tablets; 100 mg/5 mL suspension; 40 mg/mL
drops
Indomethacin (generic, Indocin, others)
Oral: 25, 50 mg capsules; 75 mg sustained-

release capsules; 25 mg/5 mL suspension
Rectal: 50 mg suppositories
Ketoprofen (Orudis, others)
Oral: 12.5, 25, 50, 75 mg capsules; 100, 150,
200 mg extended-release capsules
Ketorolac (Toradol)
Oral: 10 mg tablets
Parenteral: 15, 30 mg/mL for IM injection
Ophthalmic: 0.5% solution
Meclofenamate sodium (generic, Meclomen)
Oral: 50, 100 mg tablets and capsules
Mefenamic acid (Ponstel)
Oral: 250 mg capsules
Nabumetone (Relafen)
Oral: 500, 750 mg tablets
Naproxen (Naprosyn, Anaprox, Aleve [OTC])
Oral: 200, 250, 375, 500 mg tablets; 375, 550
mg sustained-release tablets; 125 mg/5 mL
suspension
Naproxen sodium (Anaprox)
Oral: 275, 550 mg tablets (250, 500 mg base)
Oxaprozin (Daypro)
Oral: 600 mg tablets
Piroxicam (various, Feldene)
Oral: 10, 20 mg capsules
Sulindac (various, Clinoril)
Oral: 150, 200 mg tablets
Tolmetin (Tolectin)
Oral: 200, 600 mg tablets; 400 mg capsules

Disease-Modifying Antirheumatic Drugs

Auranofin (Ridaura)
Oral: 3 mg capsules
Aurothioglucose (Solganal)
Parenteral: 50 mg/mL suspension for injection
Gold sodium thiomalate (Myochrysine)
Parenteral: 25, 50 mg/mL for injection
Hydroxychloroquine (Plaquenil)
Oral: 200 mg tablets

Methotrexate (generic, Rheumatrex)
Oral: 2.5 mg tablets
Parenteral: 2.5, 25 mg/mL
Penicillamine (Cuprimine, Depen)
Oral: 125, 250 mg capsules; 250 mg tablets
Sulfasalazine (generic, Azulfidine)
Oral: 500 mg tablets, 500 mg enteric coated
tablets, 250 mg/5 mL oral suspension

Drugs Used in Gout
Allopurinol (generic, Zyloprim, others)
Oral: 100, 300 mg tablets
Colchicine (generic)
Oral: 0.5, 0.6 mg tablets
Parenteral: 1 mg/2 mL for injection

Probenecid (generic, Benemid, Probalan)
Oral: 500 mg tablets
Sulfinpyrazone (generic, Anturane)
Oral: 100 mg tablets; 200 mg capsules

Acetaminophen
Acetaminophen (generic, Tylenol, Tempra,
Panadol, Acephen, Acetaminophen, Uniserts,
others)
Oral: 80, 160, 325, 500, 650 mg tablets; 500 mg
capsules; 120, 160, 325 mg/5 mL elixir; 500
mg/15 mL elixir; 100 mg/mL solution; 120
mg/2.5 mL solution
Rectal: 120, 125, 300, 325, 650 mg suppositories

REFERENCES

General

Chandrasoma P, Taylor CR: *Concise Pathology,* 2nd ed. Appleton & Lange, 1994.

Harris ED, Jr: Rheumatoid arthritis. Pathophysiology and implications for therapy. N Engl J Med 1990;322:1277.

Hellman DB: Arthritis and musculoskeletal disorders. In: *Current Medical Diagnosis & Treatment 1994.* Tierney LM, McPhee ST, Papadakis MA (editors). Appleton & Lange, 1994.

Kidd BL et al: Neurogenic influences in arthritis. Ann Rheum Dis 1990;49:649.

Shiroky JB et al: Experimental basis of innovative therapies of rheumatoid arthritis. In: *Therapy of Autoimmune Diseases.* Cruse JM, Lewis RE Jr (editors). Karger, 1989.

Singh G et al: Toxicity profiles of disease modifying antirheumatic drugs in rheumatoid arthritis. J Rheumatol 1991;18:188.

Starkebaum G: Review of rheumatoid arthritis: Recent developments. Immunol Allergy Clin North Am 1993; 13:273.

Symposium: Arachidonic acid metabolism and inflammation. Therapeutic implications. Drugs 1987;33(Suppl):1.

Tsokos GC: Immunomodulatory treatment in patients with rheumatic diseases: Mechanisms of action. Semin Arthritis Rheum 1987;17:24.

Vane J, Botting R: Inflammation and the mechanism of action of anti-inflammatory drugs. FASEB J 1987;1:89.

Walson PD, Mortensen ME: Pharmacokinetics of common analgesics, anti-inflammatories and antipyretics in children. Clin Pharmacokinet 1989;17(Suppl 1):116.

Wilkens RF: New perspectives of secondary and tertiary therapy for rheumatoid arthritis. Drugs 1989;37:739.

Williams KM, Day RO, Briet SN: Biochemical actions and clinical pharmacology of anti-inflammatory drugs. Adv Drug Res 1993;24:121.

Salicylates

Chew EY et al: Aspirin effects on the development of cataracts in patients with diabetes mellitus. Early treatment diabetic retinopathy study report 16. Arch Ophthalmol 1992;110:339.

Gordon IJ et al: Algorithm for modified alkaline diuresis in salicylate poisoning. Br Med J 1984;289:1039.

Henry J, Volans G: ABC of poisoning. Analgesic poisoning: I Salicylates. Br Med J 1984;289:820.

Hurwitz ES et al: Public Health Service Study of Reye's syndrome and medications. Report of the main study. JAMA 1987;257:1905.

Hurwitz ES: Reye's syndrome. Epidemiologic Rev 1989; 11:249.

Ivey KJ: Gastrointestinal intolerance and bleeding with non-narcotic analgesics. Drugs 1986;32(Suppl 4):71.

Miners JO: Drug interactions involving aspirin (acetylsalicylic acid) and salicylic acid. Clin Pharmacokinet 1989;17:327.

Pedersen AK, Fitzgerald GA: Dose-related kinetics of aspirin: Presystemic acetylation of platelet cyclooxygenase. N Engl J Med 1984;311:1206.

Schiff E et al: The use of aspirin to prevent pregnancy-induced hypertension and lower the ratio of thromboxane A_2 to prostacyclin in relatively high risk pregnancies. N Engl J Med 1989;321:351.

Steering Committee of The Physicians' Health Study Research Group: Final report on the aspirin component of the ongoing physicians' health study. N Engl J Med 1989;321:129.

Thun MJ, Namboodiri MM, Heath CW Jr: Aspirin use and reduced risk of fatal colon cancer. N Engl J Med 1991;325:1593.

van Heyningen R, Harding JJ: Do aspirin-like analgesics protect against cataract? Lancet 1986;1:1111.

Other Nonsteroidal Drugs (NSAIDs)

Bonney SL et al: Renal safety of two analgesics used over the counter: ibuprofen and aspirin. Clin Pharmacol Ther 1986;40:373.

Chan WY: Prostaglandins and nonsteroidal anti-inflammatory drugs in dysmenorrhea. Annu Rev Pharmacol Toxicol 1983;23:131.

Douidar SM, Richardson J, Snodgrass WR: Role of indomethacin in ductus closure: An update evaluation. Dev Pharmacol Ther 1988;11:196.

Meade EA, Smith WL, DeWitt DL: Differential inhibition of prostaglandin endoperoxide synthase (cyclooxygenase) isozymes by aspirin and other nonsteroidal anti-inflammatory drugs. J Biol Chem 1993; 268:6610.

Mitchell JA et al: Selectivity of nonsteroidal antiinflammatory drugs as inhibitors of constitutive and inducible cyclooxygenase. Proc Natl Acad Sci USA 1994;90: 11693.

Morales WJ et al: Efficacy and safety of indomethacin versus ritodrine in the management of preterm labor: A randomized study. Obstet Gynecol 1989; 74:567.

Murray MD, Brater DC: Renal toxicity of the nonsteroidal anti-inflammatory drugs. Annu Rev Pharmacol Toxicol 1993;32:435.

Norton ME et al: Neonatal complications after the administration of indomethacin for preterm labor. N Engl J Med 1993;329:1602.

Paulus HE, Furst DE: Aspirin and other non-steroidal anti-inflammatory drugs. In: *Arthritis and Allied Conditions,* 10th ed. McCarty DJ (editor). Lea & Febiger, 1985.

Rainsford KD: Novel non-steroidal anti-inflammatory drugs. Bailliere's Clin Rheumatol 1988;2:485.

Roth SH: Misoprostol in the prevention of NSAID-induced gastric ulcer: A multicenter, double-blind, placebocontrolled trial. J Rheumatol 1990;17(Suppl 20):20.

Verbeeck RK: Pharmacokinetic drug interactions with nonsteroidal anti-inflammatory drugs. Clin Pharmacokinet 1990;19:44.

Eicosapentaenoic Acid

Kremer JM et al: Effects of manipulation of dietary fatty acids on clinical manifestations of rheumatoid arthritis. Lancet 1985;1:184.

Lee TH et al: Effect of dietary enrichment with eicosapentaenoic and docosahexaenoic acids on in vitro neutrophil and monocyte leukotriene generation and neutrophil function. N Engl J Med 1985; 312:1217.

Maurice PDL et al: Effects of dietary supplementation with eicosapentaenoic acid in patients with psoriasis. In: *Advances in Prostaglandin, Thromboxane, and Leukotriene Research.* Samuelsson B, Paoletti R, Ramwell P (editors). Raven Press, 1987.

Disease-Modifying Antirheumatic Drugs & Glucocorticoids

Arend WP, Dayer J-M: Cytokines and cytokine inhibitors or antagonists in rheumatoid arthritis. Arthritis Rheum 1990;33:305.

Arnold M, Schreiber L, Brooks P: Immunosuppressive drugs and corticosteroids in the treatment of rheumatoid arthritis. Drugs 1988;36:340.

Barnes PJ, Adcock I: Anti-inflammatory actions of steroids: Molecular mechanisms. Trends Pharmacol Sci 1993; 14:436.

Carette S et al: A double blind placebo-controlled study of auranofin in patients with psoriatic arthritis. Arthritis Rheum 1989;32:158.

Delamere JP et al: Penicillamine-induced myasthenia in rheumatoid arthritis: Its clinical and genetic features. Ann Rheum Dis 1983;42:500.

Epstein WV et al: Effect of parenterally administered gold therapy on the course of adult rheumatoid arthritis. Ann Intern Med 1991;114:437.

Felson DT, Anderson JJ, Meenan RF: The comparative efficacy and toxicity of second-line drugs in rheumatoid arthritis: Results of two metaanalyses. Arthritis Rheum 1990;33:1449.

Fox DA, McCune WJ: Immunologic and clinical effects of cytotoxic drugs used in the treatment of rheumatoid arthritis and systemic lupus erythematosus. Concepts Immunopathol 1989;7:20.

Fries JF et al: The relative toxicity of disease-modifying antirheumatic drugs. Arthritis Rheum 1993;36:297.

Furst DE: Rational use of disease-modifying antirheumatic drugs. Drugs 1990;39:19.

Giannini EH et al: Auranofin in the treatment of juvenile rheumatoid arthritis. Results of the USA-USSR double blind, placebo-controlled trial. Arthritis Rheum 1990; 33:466.

Hurst NP et al: Chloroquine and hydroxychloroquine inhibit multiple sites in metabolic pathways leading to neutrophil superoxide release. J Rheumatol 1988;15:23.

Iannuzzi L et al: Does drug therapy slow radiographic deterioration in rheumatoid arthritis? N Engl J Med 1983;309:1023.

Kremer JM, Phelps CT: Long-term prospective study of the use of methotrexate in the treatment of rheumatoid arthritis. Update after a mean of 90 months. Arthritis Metab 1992;35:138.

Kujubu DA, Herschman HR: Dexamethasone inhibits the mitogen induction of TIS10 prostaglandin synthase/cyclooxygenase gene. J Biol Chem 1992;267:7991.

Lipsky PE: Remission-inducing therapy in rheumatoid arthritis. Am J Med 1983;75(Suppl 4B):40.

Sharp JT, Lidsky MD, Duffy J: Clinical responses during gold therapy for rheumatoid arthritis: Changes in synovitis, radiologically detectable erosive lesions, serum proteins, and serologic abnormalities. Arthritis Rheum 1982;25:540.

Shiroky JB et al: Low-dose methotrexate with leucovorin (folinic acid) in the management of rheumatoid arthritis. Results of a multicenter randomized, double-blind, placebo-controlled trial. Arthritis Rheum 1993; 36:795.

Tugwell P, Bennett R, Gent M: Methotrexate in rheumatoid arthritis. Ann Int Med 1987;107:358.

Veys EM et al: Levamisole as basic treatment of rheumatoid arthritis: Long-term evaluation. J Rheumatol 1981;8:45.

Weinblatt ME et al: Efficacy of low-dose methotrexate in rheumatoid arthritis. N Engl J Med 1985;312:818.

Winn VD, O'Banion MK, Young DA: Anti-inflammatory action: inhibition of griPGHS, a new cyclooxygenase. J Lipid Mediators 1993;6:101.

Wolfe F, Hawley DJ, Cathey MA: Termination of slow acting antirheumatic therapy in rheumatoid arthritis: A 14-year prospective evaluation of 1017 consecutive starts. J Rheumatol 1990;17:994.

Yocum DE et al: Cyclosporin A in severe, treatment-refractory rheumatoid arthritis. A randomized study. Ann Int Med 1988;109:863.

Other Analgesics

Black M: Acetaminophen hepatotoxicity. Annu Rev Med 1984;35:577.

Linden CH, Rumack BH: Acetaminophen overdose. Emerg Med Clin North Am 1984;2:103.

Styrt B, Sugarman B: Antipyresis and fever. Arch Intern Med 1990;150:1589.

Drugs Used in Gout

Emmerson BT: The management of gout. N Engl J Med 1996;334:445.

Famey JP: Colchicine in therapy: State of the art and new perspectives for an old drug. Clin Exp Rheum 1988; 6:305.

Lerman S, Megaw JM, Gardner K: Allopurinol therapy and cataract progenesis in humans. Am J Ophthalmol 1982;94:141.

Pascual E, Castellano JA: Treatment with colchicine decreases white cell counts in synovial fluid of asymptomatic knees that contain monosodium urate crystals. J Rheumatol 1992;19:600.

Star VL, Hochberg MC: Prevention and management of gout. Drugs 1993;45:212.

Terkeltaub RA: Gout and mechanisms of crystal-induced inflammation. Curr Opinion Rheumatol 1993;5:510.

Section VII.
Endocrine Drugs

Hypothalamic & Pituitary Hormones

37

Paul A. Fitzgerald, MD, & David C. Klonoff, MD

Neuroendocrine control of metabolism, growth, and certain aspects of reproduction is mediated by a combination of neural and endocrine systems located in the hypothalamus and pituitary gland. The pituitary gland weighs an average of about 0.6 g and rests in the bony sella turcica under a layer of dura mater. It is connected to the overlying hypothalamus by a stalk containing neurosecretory fibers surrounded by a complex of blood vessels, including a portal venous system that drains the hypothalamus and perfuses the anterior pituitary.

The pituitary gland consists of an anterior lobe (adenohypophysis) and a posterior lobe (neurohypophysis), which under hypothalamic influence release a number of hormones that either control the secretion of other endocrine glands or affect the metabolic actions of target tissues directly. An intermediate lobe is also present in some species.

The secretion of anterior lobe hormones is regulated by hormones formed in the median eminence of the hypothalamus and carried to the adenohypophysis by the hypothalamic-hypophysial portal venous system (Table 37–1). These hormones are small peptides that function as releasing or inhibiting hormones. The structures of several of these peptides have been determined, thus permitting the synthesis of the natural hormones as well as experimentally modified forms.

The posterior lobe hormones are synthesized in the hypothalamus and transported via the neurosecretory fibers in the stalk of the pituitary to the posterior lobe, from which they are released into the circulation.

The hormones of the intermediate lobe have melanocyte-stimulating properties that are important in animals that utilize skin color changes as adaptive mechanisms. They have not been identified as discrete hormones in humans.

Hypothalamic and pituitary hormones (and their synthetic analogs) have applications in three areas: (1)

ACRONYMS USED IN THIS CHAPTER

ACTH	Adrenocorticotropic hormone
CRH	Corticotropin-releasing hormone
FSH	Follicle-stimulating hormone
GH	Growth hormone
GHBP	Growth hormone-binding protein
GHRH	Growth hormone-releasing hormone
GHRP	Growth hormone-releasing peptide
GnRH	Gonadotropin-releasing hormone
GRH	Growth hormone-releasing hormone
IGF-I	Insulin-like growth factor I
LH	Luteinizing hormone
LHRH	Luteinizing hormone-releasing hormone
β-LPH	β-Lipotropin
PRH	Prolactin-releasing hormone
PRL	Prolactin
SRIH	Somatotropin release-inhibiting hormone (somatostatin)
TRH	Thyrotropin-releasing hormone (protirelin)
TSH	Thyroid-stimulating hormone (thyrotropin)

as replacement therapy for hormone deficiency states; (2) as drug therapy for a variety of disorders using pharmacologic doses to elicit a hormonal effect that is not present at physiologic blood levels; and (3) as diagnostic tools for performing stimulation tests to diagnose hypo- or hyperfunctional endocrine states.

Table 37–1. Links between hypothalamic, pituitary, and target gland hormones.

Hypothalamic Hormone	Pituitary Hormone	Target Organ	Target Organ Hormone
Growth hormone-releasing hormone (GHRH) (+)	Growth hormone (somatotropin, GH)	Liver	Insulin-like growth factors (IGF, somatomedins)
Somatotropin release-inhibiting hormone (SRIH, somatostatin) (–)			
Corticotropin-releasing horrmone (CRH) (+)	Adrenocorticotropin (ACTH)	Adrenal cortex	Glucocorticoids, mineralocorticoids, androgens
Thyrotropin-releasing hormone (TRH) (+)	Thyroid-stimulating hormone (TSH)	Thyroid	Thyroxine, triiodothyronine
Gonadotropin-releasing hormone (GnRH) (+)	Follicle-stimulating hormone (FSH)	Gonads	Estrogen, progesterone, testosterone
	Luteinizing hormone (LH)		
Dopamine (–)	Prolactin (PRL)	Breast	—

(+), stimulant; (–), inhibitor.

HYPOTHALAMIC & ANTERIOR PITUITARY HORMONES

Hypothalamic regulatory hormones that have been identified and (in most cases) synthesized include growth hormone-releasing hormone (GHRH); a growth hormone-inhibiting hormone (somatostatin); thyrotropin-releasing hormone (TRH); corticotropin-releasing hormone (CRH); gonadotropin-releasing hormone (GnRH), also called luteinizing hormone-releasing hormone (LHRH); and prolactin-inhibiting hormone (dopamine).

Six anterior pituitary hormones are recognized: growth hormone (GH), thyrotropin (TSH), follicle-stimulating hormone (FSH), luteinizing hormone (LH), prolactin (PRL), and adrenocorticotropin (ACTH). Another peptide, β-lipotropin (β-LPH), is derived from the same prohormone, pro-opiomelanocortin, as adrenocorticotropin. Beta-lipotropin is secreted from the pituitary along with adrenocorticotropin, but its hormonal function is unknown. It is a precursor of the opioid peptide β-endorphin (see Chapter 30).

MECHANISMS OF HORMONE ACTION

The hypothalamic and pituitary hormones are all peptides that exert their effects by binding to target cell surface membrane receptors with high specificity and affinity.

GHRH, Somatostatin, TRH, TSH, CRH, ACTH, GnRH, FSH, LH, & Dopamine

The receptors for these hormones are typical seven-transmembrane-domain serpentine peptides (Chapter 2). Each hormone acts as a ligand within a receptor pocket, inducing conformational activating changes in the receptor. The conformational changes in the receptor's intracellular third loop and carboxyl terminal tail activate an adjacent intracellular G protein. The G_{14} protein is associated with the receptors for GnRH and TRH, G_i with the dopamine receptor, and G_s protein with the receptors for the other hormones listed above.

A. GHRH, CRH, GnRH, TSH, ACTH, FSH, LH, and Dopamine: The G protein-GTP complexes related to receptors for these hormones activate adenylyl cyclase, which synthesizes the second messenger cAMP. cAMP activates protein kinases, which phosphorylate certain intracellular proteins (eg, enzymes), thus producing the hormonal effect. Conversely, dopamine binding to lactotroph receptors causes conformational changes in its G_i protein that reduce the activity of adenylyl cyclase and inhibit the secretion of prolactin.

B. Growth Hormone: The α-GTP complexes related to somatostatin receptors exert effects on potassium channels, thereby inhibiting GH secretion.

C. Thyrotropin-Releasing Hormone: The G protein complexes related to thyrotrophs' TRH receptors affect phosphoinositide-specific phospholipase C, which increases intracellular cytoplasmic free calcium, thereby stimulating TSH secretion.

Growth Hormone & Prolactin

The receptors for both GH and PRL consist of similar single peptides. The two types of receptors have extracellular amino terminal hormone-binding domains. Both receptors pass through the cell membrane, where an intracellular carboxyl terminal sequence activates a tyrosine kinase, JAK2, causing phosphorylation on tyrosines of intracellular proteins and gene regulation. Fragments of GH receptors circulate in plasma (GH binding protein, GHBP), binding about 50% of the circulating growth hormone.

In the discussion below, the hypothalamic control peptides are paired with their pituitary target hormones in the order in which they are listed in Table 37–1.

GROWTH HORMONE-RELEASING HORMONE (GHRH, Sermorelin) & GROWTH HORMONE-RELEASING PEPTIDES (GHRPs)

Hypothalamic growth hormone-releasing hormone stimulates pituitary secretion of growth hormone (GH). Other hypothalamic growth hormone-releasing peptides also stimulate GH secretion by somatotrophs in pituitaries with intact stalks.

Chemistry, Pharmacokinetics, & Pharmacodynamics

A. Structure: In 1982, separate laboratories isolated a 40-amino-acid peptide and a longer sequence with 44 amino acids, both of which stimulated GH release. The activity of the molecules was found to reside in the first 29 amino acids. $GHRH_{40}$, $GHRH_{44}$, and analogs of $GHRH_{29}$ have all been investigated.

Growth hormone-releasing peptides comprise several groups of small synthetic peptide molecules—currently under clinical investigation—that can stimulate GH secretion in a manner similar to GHRH. GHRP-2 and GHRP-6 have been demonstrated to have clinically significant GH-stimulating properties. Hexarelin, an analog of GHRP-6, also has clinical activity. Several other analogs have been developed that have GH-stimulating properties under laboratory conditions: a pseudotripeptide (G-7502), a tetrapeptide (G-7134), a pentapeptide (G-7039), and a rigid cyclic heptapeptide (G-7203).

B. Absorption, Metabolism, and Excretion: GHRH may be administered intravenously, subcutaneously, or intranasally, and the relative potencies (defined as incremental growth hormone release) by these three routes are 300, 10, and 1, respectively. Intravenous GHRH has a half-life of 7 minutes.

C. Pharmacodynamics: GHRH and GHRPs stimulate anterior pituitary secretion of growth hormone only.

Clinical Pharmacology

A. Diagnostic Uses: GHRH or GHRP (investigational) infusions can be used to evaluate short children with subnormal GH responses to conventional stimuli such as insulin-induced hypoglycemia, oral levodopa, or intravenous arginine. In such children, a normal response suggests GH deficiency due to hypothalamic dysfunction. A subnormal response may occur with dysfunction of either the pituitary or the hypothalamus. A rise in the growth hormone level demonstrates the ability of the somatotroph to produce GH and predicts a favorable response to GHRH therapy.

B. Experimental Therapeutic Uses: A growth hormone-deficient patient whose pituitary somatotrophs are responsive to GHRH could be a candidate for GHRH or GHRP therapy. A potential advantage of GHRH is the probably lower cost of manufacturing GHRH, which is a much smaller molecule than growth hormone. A disadvantage of GHRH therapy is the necessity for at least two injections daily during the course of treatment. In experimental studies with patients with intact pituitary somatotrophs, GHRP stimulated GH release when administered intranasally or orally.

Preparations & Dosage

A single intravenous injection of $GHRH_{1-29}$, 1 μg/kg, with growth hormone measurements at 0, 15, 30, 45, and 60 minutes, will determine the somatotrophs' ability to produce growth hormone. A normal response does not exclude growth hormone deficiency, because such a deficiency is frequently due to hypothalamic dysfunction with intact somatotroph function. GHRH for therapy is investigational. An effective dose is 2–5 μg/kg subcutaneously every 6–12 hours. GHRP-2 administered intranasally in doses of 5–20 μg/kg to patients with responsive pituitary somatotrophs stimulated growth. Hexarelin, a GHRP analog, has clinical activity in doses of 1 μg/kg intravenously or 20 μg/kg intranasally. The bioavailability of hexarelin has been determined to be 77% by the subcutaneous route, 4.8% intranasally, and 0.3% orally.

Toxicity

There may be facial flushing or injection-site pain. Nasal GHRP-2 has been well tolerated.

SOMATOSTATIN (Growth Hormone-Inhibiting Hormone, Somatotropin Release-Inhibiting Hormone)

Somatostatin, a 14-amino-acid peptide, is found in the hypothalamus and other parts of the central nervous system. It has been sequenced (Figure 37–1) and synthesized. It has been shown to inhibit growth hormone release in normal individuals. Somatostatin has also been identified in the pancreas and other sites in the gastrointestinal tract. It has been shown to inhibit the release of glucagon, insulin, and gastrin.

A 28-amino-acid peptide called prosomatostatin isolated from intestine and hypothalamus is believed to be the precursor of somatostatin. It is ten times more potent than somatostatin in inhibiting insulin secretion in rats, but its effect on glucagon secretion is only twice that of somatostatin. Its greater potency and prolonged action make prosomatostatin more useful than somatostatin in testing hormonal control mechanisms.

Exogenously administered somatostatin is rapidly cleared from the circulation, with an initial half-life of 1–3 minutes. The kidney appears to play an important role in its metabolism and excretion.

Peptides have been synthesized that partially separate the various properties of somatostatin. A 7-aminoheptanoic acid derivative containing only four of the 14 amino acids of somatostatin has been found to block the effect of somatostatin.

Clinical Pharmacology of Octreotide (Somatostatin Analog, SMS 201–995)

Somatostatin has limited therapeutic usefulness because of its short duration of action and its multiple effects on many secretory systems. Among several analogs developed, octreotide has been the most effective in management of a variety of clinical disorders (Figure 37–1).

Octreotide is 45 times more potent than somatostatin in inhibiting growth hormone release in intact subjects but only twice as potent in reducing insulin secretion. Because of this relatively reduced effect on pancreatic B cells, octreotide has been particularly useful in treating acromegaly, thyrotropin-secreting pituitary adenomas, and carcinoid tumors without provoking hyperglycemia due to reduced insulin concentrations. Octreotide is also useful for the acute control of bleeding from esophageal varices. The much greater potency of octreotide as compared with somatostatin is not due to differences in affinity for somatostatin receptors. Rather, it appears to be due to octreotide's much lower clearance rate and longer half-life. The plasma elimination half-life of octreotide is about 80 minutes, ie, 30 times longer in humans than the half-life of somatostatin.

Octreotide, in doses of 50–200 µg given subcutaneously every 8 hours, reduces symptoms of a variety of hormone-secreting tumors in patients with acromegaly; the carcinoid syndrome; gastrinoma; glucagonoma; nesidioblastosis; the watery diarrhea, hypokalemia, and achlorhydria (WDHA) syndrome; and of "diabetic diarrhea." Orally administered oc-

treotide has been reported to effectively reduce growth hormone levels in acromegaly, but doses of up to 24 mg/d were required, in contrast to microgram quantities given parenterally.

Adverse effects of therapy include nausea with or without vomiting, abdominal cramps, flatulence, and steatorrhea with bulky bowel movements. Biliary sludge and gallstones may occur after 6 months of use in 20–30% of patients. However, the yearly incidence of symptomatic gallstones is about 1%. Patients may have a transient deterioration in glucose tolerance at the start of therapy, but this subsequently improves.

A prolonged-action form of octreotide has been developed wherein 20–30 mg of the drug is mixed with a polymer matrix; suppression of GH hypersecretion continues for 28–42 days after intramuscular injection.

GROWTH HORMONE (Somatotropin, GH)

Growth hormone is a peptide hormone produced by the anterior pituitary. It produces growth at open epiphyses via stimulation of insulin-like growth factor I (IGF-I, somatomedin C). It also causes lipolysis in adipose tissue and growth of skeletal muscle.

Chemistry & Pharmacokinetics

A. Structure: Growth hormone is a 191-amino-acid peptide with two sulfhydryl bridges. Its structure closely resembles that of prolactin and the placental hormone human chorionic somatomammotropin. Growth hormone for pharmacologic use is produced with recombinant DNA technology and contains either the 191-amino-acid sequence of growth hormone proper (**somatotropin**) or 192 amino acids consisting of the 191 amino acids of growth hormone plus an extra methionine residue at the amino terminal end (**somatrem**).

B. Absorption, Metabolism, and Excretion: Circulating endogenous growth hormone has a half-life of 20–25 minutes and is predominantly cleared by the liver. Human growth hormone can be administered intramuscularly, with peak levels occurring in 2–4 hours and active blood levels persisting for 36 hours.

Pharmacodynamics

Biosynthetic methionyl human growth hormone is equipotent with native and biosynthetic pituitary growth hormone. The metabolic consequence of a pharmacologic dose of growth hormone is an initial insulin-like effect with increased tissue uptake of both glucose and amino acids and decreased lipolysis. Within a few hours, there is a peripheral insulin-antagonistic effect with impaired glucose uptake and increased lipolysis.

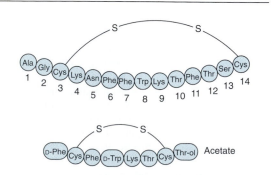

Figure 37–1. Above: Amino acid sequence of somatostatin. **Below:** Sequence of the synthetic analog, octreotide (SMS 201-995).

Pharmacologic doses of growth hormone cause longitudinal growth indirectly via another class of peptide hormones, the somatomedins, or insulin-like growth factors (IGFs). Growth hormone stimulates synthesis of somatomedins IGF-I and IGF-II (predominantly in growth plate cartilage and the liver); somatomedins promote uptake of sulfate into cartilage and are probably the actual mediators of the cellular processes associated with bone growth. This growth can be traced back to the molecular level, where increased incorporation of thymidine into DNA and uridine into RNA occurs (indicating cellular proliferation) along with increased conversion of proline to hydroxyproline (indicating cartilage synthesis).

Growth hormone deficiency leads to inadequate somatomedin production and short stature. Rarely, short stature may be caused by IGF-I deficiency despite high growth hormone levels (Laron dwarfism) or a lack of a pubertal surge of IGF-I (pygmies).

Clinical Pharmacology

A. Growth Hormone Deficiency: Timely growth hormone replacement therapy permits achievement of normal adult height in children with growth hormone deficiency. Criteria for diagnosis of growth hormone deficiency usually include (1) a growth rate below 4 cm per year and (2) the absence of a serum growth hormone response to two growth hormone secretagogues. The prevalence of congenital growth hormone deficiency is approximately 1:4000. Congenital growth hormone deficiency can result from diseases of the hypophysial-pituitary region such as craniopharyngiomas but is most often due to lack of hypothalamic growth hormone-releasing factors, frequently caused by a *pit-I* gene abnormality. In the newborn, hypoglycemia and even seizures can occur if growth hormone is absent.

In addition to isolated growth hormone deficiency, congenital deficiencies of multiple pituitary hormones occur with approximately equal frequency. Such patients—as well as those with acquired growth hormone deficiency, which is often accompanied by multiple hormone deficiencies—may also respond well to growth hormone plus other hormone replacements as needed, provided the underlying disease process can be controlled.

B. Growth Hormone-Responsive States: Some non-growth hormone-deficient short children with a delayed bone age and a slow growth rate achieve increased growth with short-term growth hormone therapy. It is not known whether their adult heights can be increased with prolonged therapy. Selected "normal variant short stature" children can be offered a trial of growth hormone following a baseline period of measurement to confirm a subnormal growth rate. During the first 6 months of treatment, the height velocity must increase by 2 cm per year for treatment to continue. The National Institute for Child Health and Human Development is conducting a 10-year study (to run until 1999) that will evaluate long-term effects and final adult height in growth hormone-treated short children without classic growth hormone deficiency. Girls with Turner's syndrome frequently respond to high-dose growth hormone therapy with increased growth velocity and increased height as adults.

C. Experimental Uses: Growth hormone is currently being tested for production of growth in short children with intrauterine growth retardation and chronic renal failure and for muscle preservation in catabolic states such as corticosteroid therapy, burns, and AIDS.

Short-term treatment of GH-deficient adults has resulted in increased lean body mass, decreased fat mass, increased exercise tolerance, and improved psychologic well-being. Adverse effects often include arthralgias and fluid retention. Doses of GH for adults are considerably lower than in children even when corrected for body weight, and are given three times weekly. The safety of long-term GH treatment of adults is under investigation.

In 1993, the FDA approved the use of recombinant bovine growth hormone (rbGH) in dairy cattle to increase milk production. Although milk and meat from rbGH-treated cows appears to be safe, these cows have a higher frequency of mastitis, which could increase antibiotic use and result in greater antibiotic residues in milk and meat. This potential indirect health effect is being studied.

Dosage

Animal preparations of growth hormone are ineffective in humans. In the past, treatment of children with human growth hormone was limited by the scarcity of the hormone as well as its expense. Until 1985, all commercially available growth hormone (somatropin) was freeze-extracted from human pituitaries. Use of human-derived growth hormone ceased in 1985 because of possible contamination (see below). Biosynthetic growth hormone has replaced these human-derived preparations.

In 1985, somatrem became the second biosynthetic pharmaceutical product (following human insulin) to be approved by the FDA. In 1987, somatropin was also approved by the FDA. The recommended dosage of biosynthetic growth hormone is up to 0.1 mg/kg (0.26 IU/kg) subcutaneously or intramuscularly three times weekly. The two biosynthetic growth hormones have not been studied in comparison to each other, but they appear to have similar potencies. The annual cost of treatment for a GH-deficient child depends upon the child's weight and is typically $10,000–$30,000.

Toxicity & Contraindications

In 1985, the National Hormone and Pituitary Program halted distribution of growth hormone derived from human pituitaries because of a worldwide occurrence of Creutzfeldt-Jakob disease in some patients many years after such treatment. Biosynthetic growth hormone poses no such risk.

Antibody formation may occur in 30% of patients treated with biosynthetic growth hormone; however, these antibodies rarely interfere with the activity of this hormone. Rapid growth induced by successful hormone therapy may rarely result in slipped capital femoral epiphyses, leading to a limp or lower extremity pain. A very slight increase in leukemia incidence has been reported in association with growth hormone therapy; however, it is not clear whether there is a causal relationship.

Patients receiving growth hormone should be screened regularly for hypothyroidism or diabetes. If growth slows in the absence of rising antibody titers, hypopituitarism should be ruled out. Response to growth hormone may be impaired by untreated hypothyroidism, diabetes insipidus, or diabetes mellitus. Excessive glucocorticoid therapy can also impair the response to growth hormone.

THYROTROPIN-RELEASING HORMONE (Protirelin, TRH)

Thyrotropin-releasing hormone, or protirelin, is a tripeptide hormone found in the hypothalamus as well as in other parts of the brain. TRH is secreted into the portal venous system and stimulates the pituitary to produce thyroid stimulating hormone (TSH, thyrotropin), which in turn stimulates the thyroid to produce thyroxine (T_4) and triiodothyronine. TRH stimulation of thyrotropin is blocked by thyroxine and potentiated by lack of thyroxine.

Chemistry & Pharmacokinetics

TRH is (pyro)Glu-His-Pro-NH_2. It is administered intravenously over 1 minute. Rapid plasma inactivation occurs, with a half-life of 4–5 minutes.

Pharmacodynamics

Peak serum thyrotropin levels occur 20–30 minutes after intravenous TRH injection in healthy individuals. In hyperthyroidism, the serum thyrotropin level is suppressed. In primary hypothyroidism, thyrotropin levels are high and the thyrotropin response to TRH may be accentuated. In secondary (pituitary) hypothyroidism, serum thyrotropin levels are "inappropriately" normal or low (using a sensitive TSH assay); TSH often fails to rise after TRH administration. In tertiary (hypothalamic) hypothyroidism, the baseline serum thyrotropin level may be normal or low and the thyrotropin response to TRH may be normal or blunted.

TRH infusion leads to stimulation of prolactin release by the pituitary in healthy individuals but has no effect on cells producing growth hormone or ACTH. In certain types of pituitary tumors, however, the neoplastic cells may respond abnormally to TRH by releasing growth hormone (in acromegaly), by releasing ACTH (in Cushing's disease), or by failing to release prolactin (in prolactinoma). Infusion of TRH or TRH analogs appears to improve the outcome of partial spinal cord injuries (Pitts et al, 1995). This property of TRH is currently being investigated.

Clinical Pharmacology

TRH testing (see above) is now rarely used to diagnose hyperthyroidism or hypothyroidism, having been supplanted by sensitive assays for serum thyrotropin (see below).

A blunted thyrotropin response to TRH may occur in unipolar (contrasted with bipolar) depression and other mental disorders. However, for most psychiatric patients, this test lacks sufficient sensitivity or specificity.

Dosage

The dose of protirelin for diagnostic use is 500 μg for adults and 7 μg/kg for children aged 6 years or older but not to exceed the adult dose. A baseline thyrotropin level should be obtained, followed by three further determinations at 15, 30, and 60 minutes postinfusion.

For experimental treatment of partial spinal cord injuries, TRH has been given as an intravenous bolus of 0.2 mg/kg followed by 0.2 mg/kg/h over 6 hours within 1–7 days after trauma.

Toxicity

Most patients given intravenous TRH note adverse effects lasting for a few minutes: an urge to urinate, a metallic taste, nausea, flushing, or light-headedness. Transient hypertension may occur.

THYROID-STIMULATING HORMONE (Thyrotropin, TSH)

Thyrotropin is an anterior pituitary hormone that regulates thyroid function by stimulating production and secretion of thyroxine and triiodothyronine.

Chemistry & Pharmacokinetics

A. Structure: Thyrotropin consists of two peptides (alpha and beta), both of which contain branched carbohydrate side chains that are important for hormone activity. Therapeutic thyrotropin is prepared from bovine anterior pituitaries. There is 70% homology between human and bovine TSH-α subunits and 90% homology between human and bovine TSH-β subunits. The TSH-α subunit sequence in humans is virtually identical to that of the alpha subunit of FSH, LH, and hCG. The TSH-β subunit confers thyroid specificity.

B. Absorption, Metabolism, and Excretion: Thyrotropin is administered intramuscularly or subcutaneously. Its half-life is approximately 1 hour, with degradation occurring in the kidneys. Little unchanged thyrotropin appears in the urine.

Pharmacodynamics

Thyrotropin stimulates thyroid cell adenylyl cyclase activity. Increased cAMP production causes increased iodine uptake and, ultimately, increased production of thyroid hormones.

Clinical Pharmacology

A. Diagnostic Uses: Synthetic human thyrotropin may prove useful to stimulate radioactive iodine uptake by metastatic thyroid carcinoma, thereby facilitating detection by scanning techniques.

B. Therapeutic Uses: Bovine TSH has proved to be too toxic for therapeutic stimulation of ^{131}I uptake by metastatic differentiated thyroid carcinoma.

Dosage

Thyrotropin derived from beef pituitaries is intended for intramuscular or subcutaneous administration. A dose of 5–10 units/d for 3 days is used for diagnostic purposes; 5–10 units/d for 3–7 days was used in conjunction with ^{131}I for ablation of thyroid carcinoma. Synthetic human thyrotropin requires two or three daily injections to stimulate radioiodine uptake by the thyroid.

Toxicity

Local soreness at the injection site is common. Nausea, vomiting, thyroid tenderness, allergic symptoms, and symptoms of hyperthyroidism may occur. This drug should be used cautiously in the presence of heart disease or adrenocortical insufficiency. Because of these problems, bovine thyrotropin is almost never used clinically.

CORTICOTROPIN-RELEASING HORMONE (CRH)

CRH is a hypothalamic hormone that stimulates release of ACTH and β-endorphin from the pituitary.

Chemistry & Pharmacokinetics

A. Structure: Human CRH is a 41-amino-acid peptide. An analog of human CRH is sheep (ovine) CRH, which also contains 41 amino acids. These molecules differ in seven amino acids.

B. Absorption, Metabolism, and Excretion: CRH is administered intravenously. The first-phase half-lives of human and sheep CRH are 9 minutes and 18 minutes, respectively. The peptide is metabolized in various tissues, and less than 1% is excreted in the urine.

Pharmacodynamics

ACTH released by CRH stimulation of the pituitary subsequently stimulates the adrenal cortex to produce cortisol and androgens.

Clinical Pharmacology

CRH is used only for diagnostic purposes. In Cushing's syndrome, CRH has been used to distinguish Cushing's disease from ectopic ACTH secretion. CRH generally elicits an increase in ACTH and cortisol secretion in Cushing's disease but usually not in the ectopic ACTH syndrome. However, exceptions occur frequently, making this test unreliable. A more reliable test depends on differential concentrations of ACTH. In patients with Cushing's disease, ACTH levels in blood drawn from the inferior petrosal sinuses draining the pituitary are more than 2.5 times higher than levels in simultaneously drawn peripheral venous blood. When tumors are associated with *ectopic* ACTH production, no such difference is observed. Concurrent administration of CRH improves the distinction between blood levels of ACTH further when Cushing's disease is present.

Preparations & Dosage

Synthetic human and sheep CRH are available for investigational use. Sheep CRH is used more frequently because of its longer half-life and slightly greater potency. CRH may be dissolved in water or dilute acid but not in saline. A dose of 1 μg/kg is used for diagnostic testing.

Toxicity

Intravenous bolus doses of 1 μg/kg produce transient facial flushing and, rarely, cause dyspnea.

ADRENOCORTICOTROPIN (Corticotropin, ACTH, ACTH$_{1-24}$)

Adrenocorticotropin is a peptide hormone produced in the anterior pituitary. Its primary endocrine function is to stimulate synthesis and release of cortisol by the adrenal cortex. Corticotropin can be used therapeutically, but a synthetic derivative is more commonly—and almost exclusively—used to assess adrenocortical responsiveness. A substandard adrenocortical response to exogenous corticotropin administration indicates adrenocortical insufficiency.

Chemistry & Pharmacokinetics

A. Structure: Human ACTH is a single peptide chain of 39 amino acids (Figure 37–2). The amino terminal portion containing amino acids 1–24 is necessary for full biologic activity. The remaining amino acids (25–39) confer species specificity. Synthetic human ACTH$_{1-24}$ is known as **cosyntropin.** The amino terminal amino acids 1–13 are identical to

1	2	3	4	5	6	7	8	9	10	11	12	13		25	26	27	28	29	30	31	32	33	34	35	36	37	38	39
Ser	Tyr	Ser	Met	Glu	His	Phe	Arg	Trp	Gly	Lys	Pro	Val	(human)	Asp	Ala	Gly	Glu	Asp	Gln	Ser	Ala	Glu	Ala	Phe	Pro	Leu	Glu	Phe
Ser	Tyr	Ser	Met	Glu	His	Phe	Arg	Trp	Gly	Lys	Pro	Val	(pig)	Asp	Gly	Ala	Glu	Asp	Gln	Leu	Ala	Glu						
Ser	Tyr	Ser	Met	Glu	His	Phe	Arg	Trp	Gly	Lys	Pro	Val	(beef)	Asp	Gly	Glu	Ala	Glu	Asp	Ser	Ala	Gln						
Ser	Tyr	Ser	Met	Glu	His	Phe	Arg	Trp	Gly	Lys	Pro	Val	(sheep)	Ala	Gly	Glu	Asp	Asp	Glu	Ala	Ser	Glu						

Figure 37–2. Amino acid sequences of human, pig, beef, and sheep adrenocorticotropin. Amino acids 1–13 are also present in α-MSH. Amino acids 14–24 (not shown) are identical in all four species.

melanocyte-stimulating hormone (α-MSH), which has been found in animals but not in humans. In states of excessive pituitary ACTH secretion, hyperpigmentation—caused by the α-MSH activity intrinsic to ACTH—may be noted.

ACTH from animal sources is assayed biologically by measuring the depletion of adrenocortical ascorbic acid that follows subcutaneous administration of the ACTH.

B. Absorption, Metabolism, and Excretion: Both porcine and synthetic corticotropin are well absorbed by the intramuscular route. Corticotropin cannot be administered orally because of gastrointestinal proteolysis.

The biologic half-lives of $ACTH_{1-39}$ and $ACTH_{1-24}$ are under 20 minutes. Tissue uptake occurs in the liver and kidneys. $ACTH_{1-39}$ is transformed into a biologically inactive substance, probably by modification of a side chain. ACTH is not excreted in the urine in significant amounts. The effects of long-acting repository forms of porcine corticotropin persist for up to 18 hours with a gelatin complex of the peptide and up to several days with a zinc hydroxide complex.

Pharmacodynamics

ACTH stimulates the adrenal cortex to produce glucocorticoids, mineralocorticoids, and androgens. ACTH increases the activity of cholesterol esterase, the enzyme that catalyzes the rate-limiting step of steroid hormone production: cholesterol → pregnenolone. ACTH also stimulates adrenal hypertrophy and hyperplasia. In pharmacologic doses, corticotropin may cause increased skin pigmentation.

Clinical Pharmacology

A. Diagnostic Uses: ACTH stimulation of the adrenals will fail to elicit an appropriate response in states of adrenal insufficiency. A rapid test for ruling out adrenal insufficiency employs cosyntropin (see below). Plasma cortisol levels are measured before and either 30 or 60 minutes following an intramuscular or intravenous injection of 0.25 mg of cosyntropin. A normal plasma cortisol response is a stimulated peak level exceeding 18 μg/dL. A subnormal response indicates primary or secondary adrenocortical insufficiency that can be differentiated using endogenous plasma ACTH levels (which are increased in primary adrenal insufficiency and decreased in the secondary form). An incremental rise in plasma aldosterone generally occurs in secondary but not primary adrenal insufficiency after cosyntropin stimulation.

ACTH stimulation may distinguish three forms of "late-onset" (nonclassic) congenital adrenal hyperplasia from states of ovarian hyperandrogenism, all of which may be associated with hirsutism. In patients with deficiency of 21-hydroxylase, ACTH stimulation results in an incremental rise in plasma 17-hydroxyprogesterone, the substrate for the deficient enzyme. Patients with 11-hydroxylase deficiency manifest a rise in 11-deoxycortisol, while those with 3β-hydroxy-Δ5 steroid dehydrogenase deficiency show an increase in 17-hydroxypregnenolone in response to ACTH stimulation.

B. Therapeutic Uses: Corticotropin has no therapeutic advantage over direct administration of glucocorticoids. Used in therapeutic doses, cosyntropin causes just as much posttreatment pituitary-adrenal suppression as glucocorticoids.

An $ACTH_{4-9}$ analog (ORG 2766) in doses of 2 mg/d subcutaneously has been reported to reduce neuropathy induced by cisplatin or vincristine used in cancer chemotherapy.

Dosage

Cosyntropin is the preferred preparation for diagnostic use. The standard diagnostic test dose of 0.25 mg is equivalent to 25 units of porcine corticotropin. ACTH is rarely indicated but is available for use in doses of 10–20 units four times daily. Repository ACTH, 40–80 units, may be administered every 24–72 hours.

Toxicity & Contraindications

The toxicity of therapeutic doses of ACTH resembles that of the glucocorticoids (Chapter 39) with the added adverse effect of hyperandrogenism in women. The occasional development of antibodies to animal ACTH or to depot cosyntropin (a preparation not currently available in the USA) has produced anaphylactic reactions or refractoriness to ACTH therapy in a few individuals. Painful swelling occurs at the injection site more often with the zinc hydroxide depot preparation than with the gelatin preparation. Contraindications are similar to those of glucocorticoids. Use of ACTH during pregnancy should be minimized. When immediate effects are desired, glucocorticoids are preferable.

There are virtually no adverse effects from diagnostic doses of cosyntropin.

GONADOTROPIN-RELEASING HORMONE (GNRH; Luteinizing Hormone-Releasing Hormone [LHRH]; Gonadorelin Hydrochloride)

Gonadotropin-releasing hormone is produced in the arcuate nucleus of the hypothalamus and controls release of the gonadotropins FSH and LH. Divergent production of the two gonadotropins is controlled by the frequency of pulsatile GnRH secretion or administration and serum estradiol levels.

Chemistry & Pharmacokinetics

A. Structure: GnRH is a decapeptide found in all mammals. Pharmaceutical GnRH is synthetic. Analogs (eg, leuprolide, nafarelin, buserelin, goserelin, and histrelin) with D-amino acids at position 6 and with ethylamide substituted for glycine at position 10 are more potent and longer-lasting than native GnRH.

5-O-Pro-His-Trp-Ser-Tyr-Gly-Leu-Arg-Pro-Gly-NH$_2$

GnRH (gonadorelin)

5-O-Pro-His-Trp-Ser-Tyr-D-Leu-Leu-Arg-Pro-NHCH$_2$CH$_3$

Leuprolide

5-O-Pro-His-Trp-Ser-Tyr-D-Nal-*Leu-Arg-Pro-Gly-NH$_2$

Nafarelin

5-O-Pro-His-Trp-Ser-Tyr-D-Ser(t-Bu)-Leu-Arg-Pro-NHNHCONH$_2$

Goserelin

5-O-Pro-His-Trp-Ser-Tyr-D-His(N^t-PhCH$_2$)-Leu-Arg-Pro-NHCH$_2$CH$_3$

Histrelin

*D-Nal = D-3-(2-naphthyl)-alanine.

B. Absorption, Metabolism, and Excretion: GnRH may be administered intravenously or subcutaneously. GnRH analogs may be administered subcutaneously, intramuscularly, or via nasal spray. The half-life of intravenous GnRH is 4 minutes, and the half-lives of subcutaneous and intranasal GnRH analogs are 3 hours. Degradation occurs in the hypothalamus and pituitary. GnRH analogs have increased affinity for GnRH receptors and reduced susceptibility to degradation.

Pharmacodynamics

GnRH binds to receptors on pituitary gonadotropes. Pulsatile intravenous administration every 1–4 hours stimulates FSH and LH secretion. In contrast, GnRH administered continuously or GnRH analogs administered in depot formulations *inhibit* gonadotropin release.

Clinical Pharmacology

A. Diagnostic Uses: Delayed puberty in a hypogonadotropic adolescent may be due to a constitutional delay or to hypogonadotropic hypogonadism. The LH response (but not the FSH response) to GnRH can distinguish between these two conditions. Serum LH levels are measured before and then 15, 30, 45, 60, and 120 minutes after a 100 µg intravenous or subcutaneous bolus of GnRH. A peak LH response exceeding 15.6 mIU/mL is normal and suggests impending puberty, whereas an impaired LH response suggests hypogonadotropic hypogonadism due to either pituitary or hypothalamic disease (but may also be seen in constitutional delay of adolescence).

B. Therapeutic Uses:

1. Stimulation–GnRH can stimulate pituitary function and is used to treat infertility caused by hypothalamic hypogonadotropic hypogonadism in both sexes. A portable battery-powered programmable pump and intravenous tubing allows pulsatile GnRH therapy every 90 minutes.

2. Suppression–Leuprolide, nafarelin, goserelin, and histrelin are GnRH analog agonists that induce hypogonadism when given continuously. Such GnRH agonists are used to treat prostate cancer, uterine fibroids, endometriosis, polycystic ovary syndrome, and precocious puberty. Many in vitro fertilization programs sequentially use a GnRH analog to suppress endogenous gonadotropin release, followed by exogenous gonadotropins to achieve synchronous follicular development.

GnRH analog therapy for the purpose of producing pituitary suppression leads to a transient rise in sex hormone concentration during the first 2 weeks of treatment. This can be deleterious in some disorders, such as prostate cancer. Several GnRH analog *antagonists* are under investigation. These agents produce immediate pituitary suppression through complete receptor blockade.

Dosage

A. Prostate Cancer and Endometriosis: The recommended dose of leuprolide is 1 mg/d subcutaneously (Lupron) or 7.5 mg/month intramuscularly (Lupron Depot) for prostate cancer or 3.75 mg/month intramuscularly for endometriosis. Nafarelin is administered as one or two sprays (200 µg/spray) intranasally twice daily. Goserelin is injected from a preloaded syringe subcutaneously as a 3.6 mg implant every 28 days. Histrelin is injected subcutaneously in a dosage of 10 µg/kg daily.

B. Female Infertility: For fertility induction in women, gonadorelin (GnRH) is administered intravenously, 5 µg every 90 minutes from a portable pump. The woman is followed carefully with serum estradiol levels, and an ovarian ultrasound examination is done weekly before refilling the GnRH pump. When an ovarian follicle reaches 14 mm in diameter, ovulation is induced with hCG, 5000 units subcutaneously, and the luteal phase is maintained with hCG, 1500 units every 3 days for 12 days.

C. Male Infertility: For male infertility caused by hypothalamic GnRH deficiency, gonadorelin treatment is begun only after 1 year of preparatory hCG injections in men with prepubertal hypogonadotropic hypogonadism. Gonadorelin is given by intravenous bolus every 90 minutes. Serum testosterone levels and semen analyses must be done regularly. At least 3–6 months of bolus infusions are required before significant numbers of sperm are seen. The alternative to gonadorelin treatment is human menopausal gonadotropins administered subcutaneously.

Toxicity

GnRH used for diagnosis rarely produces headache, abdominal discomfort, or flushing. GnRH analogs can acutely worsen bone pain in prostate cancer patients and causes hot flushes in both sexes. Their use in women should be limited to 6 months because of the risk of osteoporosis. Intravenous GnRH for induction of ovulation is associated with a lower incidence of ovarian hyperstimulation and multiple births than is human menopausal gonadotropins (see below).

FOLLICLE-STIMULATING HORMONE (FSH)

Follicle-stimulating hormone is a glycoprotein hormone produced in the anterior pituitary that, along with LH, regulates gonadal function by increasing cAMP in the target gonadal tissue. It is composed of two linked peptide chains. The principal function of FSH is to stimulate gametogenesis and follicular development in women and spermatogenesis in men. FSH acts on the immature follicular cells of the ovary and induces development of the mature follicle and oocyte. Both LH and FSH are needed for proper ovarian steroidogenesis. LH stimulates androgen production by these cells, and FSH stimulates androgen conversion into estrogens by the granulosa cells. In the testes, FSH acts on the Sertoli cells and stimulates their production of an androgen-binding protein.

A naturally modified form of FSH is available for therapeutic use. The urine of postmenopausal women contains a substance with FSH-like properties (but with 4% of the potency) and an LH-like substance. The FSH-LH combination is known as **menotropins.** Another preparation of human FSH extracted from the urine of postmenopausal women contains virtually no LH and is known as **urofollitropin.** The use of these two gonadotropin preparations is discussed below.

LUTEINIZING HORMONE (LH)

Luteinizing hormone is a glycoprotein hormone consisting of two chains and, like FSH, is produced by the anterior pituitary. LH is primarily responsible for regulation of gonadal steroid hormone production. LH acts on testicular Leydig cells to stimulate testosterone production. In the ovary, LH acts in concert with FSH to stimulate follicular development. LH acts on the mature follicle to induce ovulation, and it stimulates the corpus luteum in the luteal phase of the menstrual cycle to produce progesterone and androgens.

There is no LH preparation presently available for clinical use. **Human chorionic gonadotropin**—with an almost identical structure—is available and can be used as a luteinizing hormone substitute.

GONADOTROPINS (HMG, Menotropins & FSH, Urofollitropin)

Human menopausal gonadotropins (hMG) are a mixture of partially catabolized human FSH and LH extracted from the urine of postmenopausal women. The commercial preparations of hMG, or menotropins, as well as human FSH, or urofollitropin, are biologically standardized for FSH and LH content. They are used in states of infertility to stimulate ovarian follicle development in women and spermatogenesis in men. In both sexes, they must be used in conjunction with a luteinizing hormone, ie, human chorionic gonadotropin (hCG), to permit ovulation and implantation in women and testosterone production and full masculinization in men.

Pharmacokinetics

Over a 7 to 12 day course of daily hMG or urofollitropin administration (intended to mimic the follicular phase of the ovarian cycle in women with hypothalamic amenorrhea), FSH levels gradually rise to twice their baseline level. LH levels increase to 1.5 times their baseline with hMG, but they do not rise with urofollitropin.

Pharmacodynamics

Ovarian follicular growth and maturation will occur during hMG or FSH treatment of gonadotropin-deficient women. Ovulation requires administration of chorionic gonadotropin when adequate follicular maturation has occurred.

In men with gonadotropin deficiencies, pretreatment with chorionic gonadotropin produces external sexual maturation; addition of a subsequent course of hMG will stimulate spermatogenesis and lead to fertility.

Clinical Pharmacology

Human menopausal gonadotropin is indicated for pituitary or hypothalamic hypogonadism with infertility. Anovulatory women with the following conditions may benefit from hMG: primary amenorrhea, secondary amenorrhea, polycystic ovary syndrome, and anovulatory cycles. Both hMG and FSH are used by in vitro fertilization programs for controlled ovarian hyperstimulation.

Over 50% of men with hypogonadotropic hypogonadism become fertile after hMG administration.

Dosage

An ampule of menotropins contains 75 International Units (IU) or 150 IU of FSH and an equal amount of LH. One IU of LH is approximately equivalent to 0.5 IU of hCG. An ampule of urofollitropin contains 75 IU of FSH and less than 1 IU of LH. Human menopausal gonadotropins, FSH, and hCG are administered intramuscularly.

A. Women: In hypothalamic hypogonadism and for in vitro fertilization, 1–2 ampules are administered daily for 5–12 days until evidence of adequate follicular maturation is present. Serum estradiol levels should be measured and a cervical examination performed every 1–2 days. When appropriate follicular maturation has occurred, hMG or FSH is discontinued; the following day, hCG (5000–10,000 IU) is administered intramuscularly to induce ovulation.

B. Men: Following pretreatment with 5000 IU of hCG three times weekly for up to 12 months to achieve masculinization and a normal serum testosterone level, menotropins is administered as 1 ampule (75 units) three times weekly in combination with hCG, 2000 IU twice weekly. At least 4 months of combined treatment are usually necessary before spermatozoa appear in the ejaculate. If there is no response, the menotropins dose may be doubled. When adding menotropins to hCG therapy, the dose of hCG must be reduced to keep serum testosterone in the high normal range and avoid hyperandrogenism.

Toxicity & Contraindications

Overstimulation of the ovary with hMG can lead to uncomplicated ovarian enlargement in approximately 20% of patients. This usually resolves spontaneously. A more serious complication, the "hyperstimulation syndrome," occurs in 0.5–4% of patients. It is characterized by hMG-induced ovarian enlargement, ascites, hydrothorax, and hypovolemia, sometimes to the point of shock. Hemoperitoneum (from a ruptured ovarian cyst), fever, or arterial thromboembolism can occur. The frequency of multiple births is approximately 20%. A reported 25% incidence of spontaneous abortions may be due to earlier diagnosis of pregnancy in treated than in untreated patients, with recognition of very early abortion. There may, however, be abnormal development and premature degeneration of corpus luteum in some treated patients. Gynecomastia occasionally occurs in men. An association between ovarian cancer and fertility drugs has been reported (Spirtas et al, 1993). However, it is not known which, if any, fertility drugs are causally related to cancer.

Human menopausal gonadotropin and urofollitropin should be administered only by a physician experienced in treating infertility. Before treatment of women, a thorough gynecologic evaluation must be performed to rule out uterine, tubal, or ovarian diseases as well as pregnancy. In cases of irregular bleeding, uterine cancer should be ruled out.

HUMAN CHORIONIC GONADOTROPIN (hCG)

Human chorionic gonadotropin is a hormone produced by the human placenta and excreted into the urine, whence it can be extracted and purified. Human chorionic gonadotropin is a glycoprotein consisting of a 92-amino-acid alpha chain virtually identical to that of FSH, LH, and TSH and a beta chain of 145 amino acids that resembles that of LH except for the presence of a carboxyl terminal sequence of 30 amino acids not present in LH.

The function of hCG is to stimulate the ovarian corpus luteum to produce progesterone and maintain the placenta. It is very similar to LH in structure and is used to treat both men and women with LH deficiency.

Pharmacokinetics

Human chorionic gonadotropin is well absorbed after intramuscular administration and has a biologic half-life of 8 hours, compared with 30 minutes for LH. The difference may lie in the high sialic acid content of hCG compared with that of LH. It is apparently modified in the body prior to urinary excretion, because the half-life measured by immunoassay far exceeds that measured by bioassay.

Pharmacodynamics

Human chorionic gonadotropin stimulates production of gonadal steroid hormones. The interstitial and corpus luteal cells of the female produce progesterone, and the Leydig cells of the male produce testosterone. hCG can be used to mimic a midcycle LH surge and trigger ovulation in a hypogonadotropic woman.

Human chorionic gonadotropin has no established effect on appetite or fat mobilization and distribution. It has been advocated without justification as an adjunct to dietary management in obese patients.

Clinical Pharmacology

A. Diagnostic Uses: In prepubertal boys with undescended gonads, hCG can be used to distinguish a truly retained (cryptorchid) testis from a retracted (pseudocryptorchid) one. Testicular descent during a course of hCG administration usually foretells permanent testicular descent at puberty, when circulating

LH levels rise. Lack of descent usually means that orchiopexy will be necessary to preserve spermatogenesis.

Patients with constitutional delay in onset of puberty can be distinguished from those with hypogonadotropic hypogonadism using repeated hCG stimulation. Serum testosterone and estradiol levels rise in the former but not in the latter group.

B. Therapeutic Uses: As described above, hCG can be used in combination with human menotropins to induce ovulation in women with hypogonadotropic hypogonadism or as part of an in vitro fertilization program. hCG stimulates testosterone secretion by the testes of men with hypogonadotropic hypogonadism. In such men, the increased intratesticular testosterone levels promote spermatogenesis, but menotropins are often needed for fertility.

In patients with AIDS-related Kaposi's sarcoma, injection of hCG into the lesions has been reported to cause regression in a dose-related manner. In one study, the Wyeth-Ayerst preparation (A.P.L.) was found to have more activity against the tumor in vitro than other preparations (Gill et al, 1996).

Dosage

The dosages for female and male infertility are described under hMG dosage. For prepubertal cryptorchidism, a dosage of 500–4000 units three times weekly for up to 6 weeks has been advocated.

Toxicity & Contraindications

Reported adverse effects include headache, depression, edema, precocious puberty, gynecomastia, or (rarely) production of antibodies to hCG. Human chorionic gonadotropin should be administered for infertility only by a physician with experience in this field. Androgen-dependent neoplasia and precocious puberty are contraindications to its use.

PROLACTIN

Prolactin is a 198-amino-acid peptide hormone produced in the anterior pituitary. Its structure resembles that of growth hormone. Prolactin is the principal hormone responsible for lactation. Milk production is stimulated by prolactin when appropriate circulating levels of estrogens, progestins, corticosteroids, and insulin are present. A deficiency of prolactin—which can occur in states of pituitary deficiency—is manifested by failure to lactate or by a luteal phase defect. In hypothalamic destruction, prolactin levels may be elevated as a result of impaired transport of prolactin-inhibiting hormone (dopamine) to the pituitary. Hyperprolactinemia can produce galactorrhea and hypogonadism and may be associated with symptoms of a pituitary mass. No preparation is available for use in prolactin-deficient patients. For patients with symptomatic hyperprolactinemia, inhibition of prolactin

secretion can be achieved with bromocriptine and other dopamine agonists.

BROMOCRIPTINE & OTHER DOPAMINE AGONISTS

Although bromocriptine is not a hormone, it has important inhibitory effects on the pituitary that warrant discussion here.

Bromocriptine is an ergot derivative with dopamine agonist properties that lowers circulating prolactin levels and shrinks pituitary prolactin-secreting tumors. Its chemical structure and pharmacokinetic features are presented in Chapter 16.

Bromocriptine decreases pituitary prolactin secretion through a dopamine-mimetic action on the pituitary at two central nervous system loci: (1) It decreases dopamine turnover in the tuberoinfundibular neurons of the arcuate nucleus, generating increased hypothalamic dopamine; and (2) it acts directly on pituitary dopamine receptors to inhibit prolactin release.

Bromocriptine, like L-dopa, stimulates pituitary growth hormone release in normal subjects and—paradoxically—suppresses growth hormone release in acromegalics. Bromocriptine is the drug most widely used and studied for its effectiveness in treating hyperprolactinemia. **Pergolide,** another dopamine agonist for Parkinson's disease, is also used for treatment of hyperprolactinemia and is less costly than bromocriptine.

Clinical Pharmacology

A. Prolactin-Secreting Adenomas: Bromocriptine is the usual initial treatment for prolactinomas. Significant reduction in both tumor size and serum prolactin levels occurs in about 85% of those receiving this drug for 6 months or longer.

B. Amenorrhea-Galactorrhea: Bromocriptine is useful for treating problems caused by hyperprolactinemia: amenorrhea, galactorrhea, infertility, and hypogonadism. Upon cessation of therapy, amenorrhea and galactorrhea generally recur.

C. Physiologic Lactation: Bromocriptine suppresses the prolactin secretion that occurs after parturition or abortion. It has been used to prevent breast engorgement when breast feeding is not desired. Its use for this purpose has been discouraged by several reports of stroke in postpartum women receiving bromocriptine, but a causal relationship has not been established.

D. Acromegaly: Bromocriptine alone or in combination with pituitary surgery, irradiation, or octreotide may be used to treat acromegaly. Acromegalic patients seldom respond adequately to bromocriptine unless the pituitary tumor secretes prolactin as well as growth hormone.

E. Parkinson's Disease: The use of bromocriptine in Parkinson's disease is discussed in Chapter 28.

Preparations & Dosage

Bromocriptine is generally taken after the evening meal at the initial dose of 1.25 mg; the dose is then increased as tolerated. Most patients require 2.5–7.5 mg daily; acromegalics require higher doses, up to 20 mg/d. Bromocriptine tablets may be administered intravaginally to reduce nausea. Long-acting oral bromocriptine formulations (Parlodel SRO) and intramuscular formulations (Parlodel L.A.R.) are available outside the USA.

Cabergoline, another ergot derivative, is administered at a dose of 0.5–1 mg orally or vaginally twice weekly. **Quinagolide** (CV 205502) a nonergot dopamine agonist, is administered orally at a daily dose of 75–600 μg.

Toxicity & Contraindications

Bromocriptine may cause nausea, lightheadedness, orthostatic hypotension, and fatigue. Psychiatric manifestations occasionally occur even at lower doses and may take months to resolve. Erythromelalgia occurs rarely. Dosages above 10 mg/d may cause cold-induced peripheral digital vasospasm. Pulmonary infiltrates may occur with chronic high-dosage therapy.

Bromocriptine therapy during the first 3 weeks of pregnancy has not been associated with an increased risk of spontaneous abortion or congenital malformations. In patients with small pituitary adenomas, bromocriptine is discontinued upon conception since there is usually no growth of the adenoma during pregnancy. Patients with very large adenomas require vigilance for tumor progression and often require bromocriptine throughout pregnancy.

If a woman who is receiving bromocriptine is late in having her menses, a pregnancy test is necessary; if she is amenorrheic, pregnancy tests should be performed regularly because ovulation may occur before menstruation resumes.

POSTERIOR PITUITARY HORMONES

Two posterior pituitary hormones are known: vasopressin and oxytocin. Their structures are very similar. Posterior pituitary hormones are synthesized in the hypothalamus and then transported to the posterior pituitary, where they are stored and then released into the circulation.

OXYTOCIN

Oxytocin is a peptide hormone secreted by the posterior pituitary that elicits milk ejection in lactating women. In pharmacologic doses, oxytocin can be used to induce uterine contractions and maintain labor; however, at physiologic blood levels, the contribution of this hormone to parturition is probably small.

Chemistry & Pharmacokinetics

A. Structure: (Figure 37–3) Oxytocin is a nine amino acid peptide composed of a six amino acid disulfide ring and a three-membered tail. Oxytocin and vasopressin differ from vasotocin—the only posterior pituitary hormone found in nonmammalian vertebrates—by only one amino acid residue each.

B. Absorption, Metabolism, and Excretion: Oxytocin is usually administered intravenously for stimulation of labor. It is also available as a nasal spray to induce lactation postpartum. It is inactive if swallowed, because it is destroyed in the stomach and intestine. Oxytocin is not bound to plasma proteins and is catabolized by the kidneys and liver, with a circulating half-life of 5 minutes.

Pharmacodynamics

Oxytocin alters transmembrane ionic currents in myometrial smooth muscle cells to produce sustained uterine contraction. The sensitivity of the uterus to oxytocin increases during pregnancy. Oxytocin-induced myometrial contractions can be inhibited by β-adrenoceptor agonists, magnesium sulfate, or inhalation anesthetics. Oxytocin also causes contraction of myoepithelial cells surrounding mammary alveoli, which leads to milk ejection. Without oxytocin-induced contraction, normal lactation cannot occur. Oxytocin has weak antidiuretic and pressor activity.

Clinical Pharmacology

A. Diagnostic Uses: Oxytocin infusion near term will produce uterine contractions that decrease the fetal blood supply. The fetal heart rate response to a standardized oxytocin challenge test provides information about placental circulatory reserve. An abnormal response suggests intrauterine growth retardation and may warrant immediate cesarean delivery.

Arginine vasopressin

Oxytocin

Figure 37–3. Posterior pituitary hormones. (Modified and reproduced, with permission, from Ganong WF: *Review of Medical Physiology*, 17th ed. Appleton & Lange, 1995.)

B. Therapeutic Uses: Oxytocin is used to induce labor and augment dysfunctional labor for (1) conditions requiring early vaginal delivery (eg, Rh problems, maternal diabetes, or preeclampsia), (2) uterine inertia, and (3) incomplete abortion. Oxytocin can also be used for control of postpartum uterine hemorrhage. Impaired milk ejection may respond to nasal oxytocin.

Synthetic peptide and nonpeptide oxytocin antagonists that can prevent premature labor are being investigated.

Dosage

For induction of labor, oxytocin should be administered intravenously via an infusion pump with appropriate fetal monitoring. An initial infusion rate of 1 mU/min is gradually increased to 5–20 mU/min until a physiologic contraction pattern is established. For postpartum uterine bleeding, 10–40 units is added to 1 L of 5% dextrose, and the infusion rate is titrated to control uterine atony. Alternatively, 10 units can be given intramuscularly after delivery of the placenta. To induce milk let-down, one puff is sprayed into each nostril in the sitting position 2–3 minutes before nursing.

Toxicity & Contraindications

When oxytocin is used properly, serious toxicity is rare. Among the reported adverse reactions are maternal deaths due to hypertensive episodes, uterine rupture, water intoxication, and fetal deaths. Afibrinogenemia has also been reported.

Contraindications include fetal distress, prematurity, abnormal fetal presentation, cephalopelvic disproportion, and other predispositions for uterine rupture.

VASOPRESSIN (Antidiuretic Hormone, ADH)

Vasopressin is a peptide hormone released by the posterior pituitary in response to rising plasma tonicity or falling blood pressure. Vasopressin possesses antidiuretic and vasopressor properties. A deficiency of this hormone results in diabetes insipidus (see Chapters 15 and 17).

Chemistry & Pharmacokinetics

A. Structure: Vasopressin is a nonapeptide with a six amino acid ring and a three amino acid side chain. The residue at position 8 is arginine in humans and in most other mammals except pigs and related species, whose vasopressin contains lysine at position 8 (Figure 37–3).

B. Absorption, Metabolism, and Excretion: Vasopressin is administered by intravenous, intramuscular, or intranasal routes; oral absorption is slight. The half-life of circulating ADH is approximately 20 minutes, with renal and hepatic catabolism via reduction of the disulfide bond and peptide cleavage. A small amount of vasopressin is excreted as such in the urine.

Pharmacodynamics

Vasopressin interacts with two types of receptors. V_1 receptors are found on vascular smooth muscle cells and mediate vasoconstriction (Chapter 17). V_2 receptors are found on renal tubule cells and mediate antidiuresis through increased water permeability and water resorption in the collecting tubules. Extrarenal V_2-like receptors mediate release of coagulation factor VIII_c and von Willebrand factor.

Desmopressin acetate (DDAVP, 1-desamino-8-D-arginine vasopressin) is a long-acting synthetic analog of vasopressin with minimal V_1 activity and an antidiuretic-to-pressor ratio 4000 times that of vasopressin.

Clinical Pharmacology

Vasopressin and desmopressin are the alternative treatments of choice for pituitary diabetes insipidus. Bedtime desmopressin therapy ameliorates nocturnal enuresis by decreasing nocturnal urine production. Vasopressin infusion is effective in some cases of esophageal variceal bleeding and colonic diverticular bleeding.

Dosage

A. Aqueous Vasopressin: Synthetic aqueous vasopressin is a short-acting preparation for intramuscular, subcutaneous, or intravenous administration. The dose is 5–10 units subcutaneously or intramuscularly every 3–6 hours for transient diabetes insipidus and 0.1–0.5 units/min intravenously for gastrointestinal bleeding.

B. Desmopressin Acetate: This is the preferred treatment for most patients with central diabetes insipidus. Desmopressin may be administered intranasally, intravenously, subcutaneously, or orally. The typical nasal dosage is 10–40 µg (0.1–0.4 mL) daily in one to three divided doses. Nasal desmopressin is available as a unit dose spray that delivers 0.1 mL per spray; it is also available with a calibrated nasal tube that can be made to deliver a more precise dose. Injectable desmopressin is approximately ten times more bioavailable than intranasal desmopressin. The dosage by injection is 1–4 µg (0.25–1 mL) daily every 12–24 hours as needed for polyuria, polydipsia, or hypernatremia.

For nocturnal enuresis, desmopressin, 10–20 µg (0.1–0.2 mL) intranasally at bedtime, is used.

Desmopressin is also available as an oral preparation. The usual dose is 0.1–0.2 mg every 12–24 hours.

Desmopressin is also used for the treatment of coagulopathy in hemophilia A and von Willebrand's disease (see Chapter 34).

Toxicity & Contraindications

Headache, nausea, abdominal cramps, agitation, and allergic reactions occur rarely. Overdosage can result in hyponatremia.

Vasopressin (but not desmopressin) can cause vaso-constriction and should be used cautiously in patients with coronary artery disease. Nasal insufflation of desmopressin may be less effective when nasal congestion is present.

PREPARATIONS AVAILABLE

Bromocriptine (Parlodel)
Oral: 2.5 mg tablets, 5 mg capsules
Chorionic gonadotropin [hCG] (generic, Profasi, A.P.L., Pregnyl, others)
Parenteral: powder to reconstitute for injection: 500, 1000, 2000 units/mL
Corticotropin (generic, ACTH, Acthar, H.P. Acthar Gel, others)
Parenteral: 25, 40 units/vial for SC, IM injection
Repository preparations: 40, 80 units/mL gel for injection; 40 units/mL corticotropin
Cosyntropin (Cortrosyn)
Parenteral: 0.25 mg/vial with diluent for IV or IM injection
Desmopressin (DDAVP, Stimate)
Nasal: 0.1, 1.5 mg/mL solution
Nasal: 100 μg/mL spray pump and rhinal tube delivery system
Parenteral: 4 μg/mL solution for injection
Oral: 0.1, 0.2 mg tablets
Gonadorelin acetate [GnRH] (Lutrepulse)
Parenteral: powder to reconstitute for injection via Lutrepulse pump (0.8, 3.2 mg/vial)
Gonadorelin hydrochloride [GnRH] (Factrel)
Parenteral: powders to reconstitute for injection (100, 500 μg/vial)
Goserelin acetate (Zoladex)
Parenteral: 3.6, 10.8 mg SC implant
Histrelin (Supprelin)
Parenteral: 120, 300, 600 μg in 0.6 mL vials for SC injection
Leuprolide (Lupron)
Parenteral: 5 mg/mL for SC injection
Parenteral depot suspension (Lupron Depot, Depot-Ped, Depot-3): lyophilized micro-spheres to reconstitute for IM injection (3.75, 7.5, 11.25, 15, 22.5 mg/vial)

Menotropins [hMG] (Pergonal, Humegon)
Parenteral: 75 IU FSH and 75 IU LH activity, 150 IU FSH and 150 IU LH activity, each with diluent
Nafarelin (Synarel)
Nasal: 2 mg/mL; 200 μg/spray
Octreotide (Sandostatin)
Parenteral: 0.05, 0.1, 0.2, 0.5, 1.0 mg/mL for SC or IV administration
Oxytocin (generic, Pitocin, Syntocinon)
Parenteral: 10 units/mL for injection
Nasal: 40 units/mL spray
Pergolide (Permax)
Oral: 0.025, 0.25, 1.0 mg tablets
Protirelin (Thypinone, Relefact TRH)
Parenteral: 500 μg/mL for injection
Sermorelin [GHRH] (Geref)
Parenteral: 50 μg powder to reconstitute for injection
Somatrem (Protropin)
Parenteral: 5, 10 mg/vial with diluent for SC or IM injection
Somatropin (Humatrope, Nutropin)
Parenteral: 5, 10 mg/vial with diluent for SC or IM injection
Thyrotropin [TSH] (Thytropar)
Parenteral: 10 IU/vial with diluent for injection
Urofollitropin (Metrodin)
Parenteral: powder to reconstitute for injection (0.83 (75 IU FSH activity), 1.66 mg (150 IU) per ampule
Vasopressin (Pitressin Synthetic)
Parenteral: 20 pressor units/mL for IM or SC administration

REFERENCES

Hypothalamic Releasing & Inhibiting Hormones

Bell GI, Reisine T: Molecular biology of somatostatin receptors. Trends Neurosci 1993;16:34.

Bevan JS et al: Dopamine agonists and pituitary tumor shrinkage. Endocr Rev 1992;13:220.

Catt KJ: Molecular mechanisms of hormone action: Control of target cell function by peptide and catecholamine hormones. In: *Endocrinology and Metabolism,* 3rd ed. Felig P, Baxter JD, Frohman LA (editors). McGraw-Hill, 1995.

Chrousos GP: Regulation and dysregulation of the hypothalamic-pituitary-adrenal axis: The corticotropin-releasing hormone perspective. Endocrinol Metab Clin North Am 1992;21:833.

Duck SC et al: Subcutaneous growth hormone-releasing hormone therapy in growth hormone-deficient children: First year of therapy. J Clin Endocrinol Metab 1992;75:1115.

Elias KA et al: In vitro characterization of four novel classes of growth hormone-releasing peptides. Endocrinology 1995;136:5694.

Ezzat S et al: Octreotide treatment of acromegaly: A randomized, multicenter study. Ann Intern Med 1992; 117:711.

Gill PS et al: The effects of preparations of human chorionic gonadotropin on AIDS-related Kaposi's sarcoma. N Engl J Med 1996;335:1261.

Klingmuller D et al: Hormonal responses to the new potent GnRH antagonist Cetrorelix. Acta Endocrinol 1993; 128:15.

Lamberts SWJ et al: Octreotide. N Engl J Med 1996; 334:246.

Lifshitz F et al: Sustained improvement in growth velocity and recovery from suboptimal growth hormone (GH) secretion after treatment with human pituitary GH-releasing hormone-(1–44)-NH$_2$. J Clin Endocrinol Metab 1992;75:1255.

Marbach P et al: From somatostatin to Sandostatin: Pharmacodynamics and pharmacokinetics. Metabolism 1992;41(Suppl 2):7.

Maton PN, Jensen RT: Use of gut peptide receptor agonists and antagonists in gastrointestinal diseases. Gastroenterol Clin North Am 1992;21:551.

Moghissi KS: Clinical applications of gonadotropin-releasing hormones in reproductive disorders. Endocrinol Metab Clin North Am 1992;21:125.

Molitch ME: Pathologic hyperprolactinemia. Endocrinol Metab Clin North Am 1992;21:877.

Orth DN: Corticotropin-releasing hormone in humans. Endocr Rev 1992;13:164.

Pitts LH et al: Treatment with thyrotropin-releasing hormone (TRH) in patients with traumatic spinal cord injuries. J Neurotrauma 1995;12:235.

Spencer CA et al: Thyrotropin (TSH)-releasing hormone stimulation test responses employing third and fourth generation TSH assays. J Clin Endocrinol Metab 1993; 76:494.

Tjerk WA et al: Clinically monitoring pituitary adenoma and octreotide response to long term high dose treatment and studies in vitro. J Clin Endocrinol Metab 1992;75:1310.

Anterior Pituitary Hormones

Bengtsson B-A et al: Treatment of adults with growth hormone (GH) deficiency with recombinant human GH. J Clin Endocrinol Metab 1993;76:309.

Blacker CM: Ovulation stimulation and induction. Endocrinol Metab Clin North Am 1992;21:57.

Carter-Su C, Schwartz J, Smit LS: Molecular mechanism of growth hormone action. Annu Rev Physiol 1996;58:187.

Chappel SC, Howles C: Reevaluation of the roles of luteinizing hormone and follicle-stimulating hormone in the ovulatory process. Human Reprod 1991;6:1206.

Christiansen P et al: Hormonal treatment of cryptorchidism-hCG or GnRH: A multicentre study. Acta Paediatr 1992;81:605.

Fava M et al: The thyrotropin response to thyrotropin-releasing hormone as a predictor of response to treatment in depressed outpatients. Acta Psychiatr Scand 1992;86:42.

Lavalie C: Prolactin: A hormone with immunoregulatory properties that leads to new therapeutic approaches in rheumatic diseases. J Rheumatol 1992;19:839.

Oelkers W et al: Diagnosis and therapy surveillance in Addison's disease: Rapid adrenocorticotropin (ACTH) test and measurement of plasma ACTH, renin activity, and aldosterone. J Clin Endocrinol Metab 1992;75:259.

Peabody CA et al: Prolactin bioassay and hyperprolactinemia. J Endocrinol Invest 1992;15:497.

Spirtas R et al: Fertility drugs and ovarian cancer: Red alert or red herring? Fertil Steril 1993;59:291.

Tapanainen P, Knip M: Evaluation of growth hormone secretion and treatment. Ann Med 1992;24:237.

Thotakura NR et al: The role of the oligosaccharide chains of thyrotropin α- and β-subunits in hormone action. Endocrinol 1992;131:82.

van Kooten B et al: A pilot study on the influence of a corticotropin (4–9) analog on *Vinca* alkaloid-induced neuropathy. Arch Neurol 1992;49:1027.

Posterior Pituitary Hormones

Blevins LS Jr, Wand GS: Diabetes insipidus. Crit Care Med 1992;20:69.

Chelmow D, Laros RK Jr: Maternal and neonatal outcomes after oxytocin augmentation in patients undergoing a trial of labor after prior cesarean delivery. Obstet Gynecol 1992;80:966.

Evans BE et al: Orally active, nonpeptide oxytocin antagonists. J Med Chem 1992;35:3919.

Key DW et al: Low-dose DDAVP in nocturnal enuresis. Clin Pediatr 1992;31:299.

Thyroid & Antithyroid Drugs

38

Frances S. Greenspan, MD, & Betty J. Dong, PharmD

Because of its anatomic prominence, the thyroid was one of the first of the endocrine glands to be associated with the clinical conditions caused by its malfunction. This gland releases two very different types of hormones. In this chapter we discuss thyroxine and triiodothyronine, which are essential for growth and development and for regulation of energy metabolism. Calcitonin, the second type of thyroid hormone, is important in the regulation of calcium metabolism and is discussed in Chapter 42.

THYROID PHYSIOLOGY

The normal thyroid gland secretes sufficient amounts of the thyroid hormones—triiodothyronine (T_3) and tetraiodothyronine (T_4, thyroxine)—to maintain normal growth and development, normal body temperature, and normal energy levels. These hormones contain 59% and 65% (respectively) of iodine as an essential part of the molecule.

Iodide Metabolism

Nearly all of the iodide (I^-)* intake is via the gastrointestinal tract from food, water, or medication. The recommended daily adult intake is 150 μg. This ingested iodide is rapidly absorbed and enters an extracellular fluid pool. The thyroid gland removes about 75 μg a day from this pool for hormone secretion, and the balance is excreted in the urine. If iodide intake is increased, the fractional iodine uptake by the thyroid is diminished.

Biosynthesis of Thyroid Hormones

Once taken up by the thyroid gland, iodide undergoes a series of enzymatic reactions that convert it into active thyroid hormone (Figure 38–1). The first step is the transport of iodide into the thyroid gland, called **iodide trapping.** This can be inhibited by such anions as SCN^-, TcO_4^-, and ClO_4^-. Iodide is then oxidized by thyroidal peroxidase to iodine, in which form it rapidly iodinates tyrosine residues within the thyroglobulin molecule to form monoiodotyrosine (MIT) and diiodotyrosine (DIT). This process is called **iodide organification.** Thyroidal peroxidase is transiently blocked by high levels of intrathyroidal iodide and blocked by thioamide drugs. Two molecules of DIT combine within the thyroglobulin molecule to form L-thyroxine (T_4). One molecule of MIT and one molecule of DIT combine to form T_3. In addition to thyroglobulin, other proteins within the gland may be iodinated, but these iodoproteins do not have hormonal activity. Thyroid hormones are released from thyroglobulin by **exocytosis** and **proteolysis** of thyroglobulin at the apical colloid border. The colloid droplets of thyroglobulin merge with lysosomes containing proteolytic enzymes, which hydrolyze thyroglobulin and release T_4, T_3, MIT, and DIT. The MIT and DIT are deiodinated within the gland, and the iodine is reutilized. In addition to T_4 and T_3, small amounts of thyroglobulin, tyrosine, and iodide are secreted. This process of proteolysis is also blocked by high levels of intrathyroidal iodide. The ratio of T_4 to T_3 within thyroglobulin is approximately 5:1, so that most of the hormone released is thyroxine. Most of the T_3 circulating in the blood is derived from peripheral metabolism of thyroxine (see below).

Transport of Thyroid Hormones

T_4 and T_3 in plasma are reversibly bound to protein, primarily thyroxine-binding globulin (TBG). About 0.04% of total T_4 and 0.4% of T_3 exist in the free form.

Many physiologic and pathologic states and drugs affect T_4, T_3, and thyroid transport. However, the actual levels of free hormone generally remain normal, reflecting feedback control.

---

*In this chapter, the term "iodine" denotes all forms of the element; the term "iodide" denotes only the ionic form, I^-.

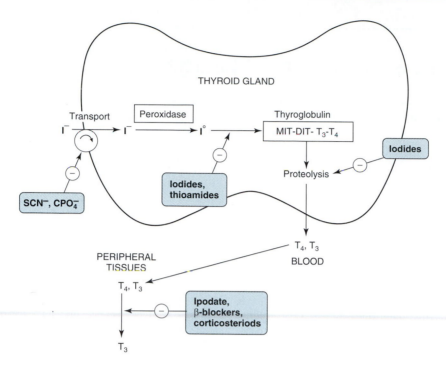

Figure 38–1. Biosynthesis of thyroid hormones. The sites of action of various drugs that interfere with thyroid hormone biosynthesis are shown.

Peripheral Metabolism of Thyroid Hormones

A small amount of thyroxine is biologically inactivated by deamination, decarboxylation, or conjugation and excretion as a glucuronide or sulfate. The primary pathway for the peripheral metabolism of thyroxine, however, is deiodination. Deiodination of T_4 may occur by monodeiodination of the outer ring, producing 3,5,3'-triiodothyronine (T_3), which is three to four times more potent than T_4. Alternatively, deiodination may occur in the inner ring, producing 3,3',5'-triiodothyronine (reverse T_3, or rT_3), which is metabolically inactive (Figure 38–2). Drugs such as ipodate, β-blockers, and corticosteroids and severe illness or starvation inhibit the 5'-deiodinase necessary for the conversion of T_4 to T_3, resulting in low T_3 and high rT_3 levels in the serum (Figure 38–1).

Figure 38–3 shows the amounts of thyroid hormone produced and metabolized per day in normal adults. Normal levels of thyroid hormone in the serum are listed in Table 38–1. The low serum levels of T_3 and rT_3 in normal individuals are due to the high metabolic clearances of these two compounds.

Control of Thyroid Function

The tests used to evaluate thyroid function are listed in Table 38–2.

A. Thyroid-Pituitary Relationships: Control of thyroid function via thyroid-pituitary feedback is also discussed in Chapter 37. Briefly, hypo-

thalamic cells secrete thyrotropin-releasing hormone (TRH) (Figure 38–4). TRH is secreted into capillaries of the pituitary portal venous system, and in the pituitary gland TRH stimulates the synthesis and release of thyroid-stimulating hormone (TSH). TSH in turn stimulates an adenylyl cyclase mechanism in the thyroid cell to increase the synthesis and release of T_4 and T_3. These thyroid hormones, in a negative feedback fashion, act in the pituitary to block the action of TRH and in the hypothalamus to inhibit the synthesis and secretion of TRH. Other hormones or drugs may also affect the release of TRH or TSH.

B. Autoregulation of the Thyroid Gland: The thyroid gland also regulates its uptake of iodide and thyroid hormone synthesis by intrathyroidal mechanisms that are independent of TSH. These mechanisms are primarily related to the level of iodine in the blood. Large doses of iodine inhibit iodide organification (Figure 38–1). In certain disease states (eg, Hashimoto's thyroiditis), this can result in inhibition of thyroid hormone synthesis and hypothyroidism.

C. Abnormal Thyroid Stimulators: In Graves' disease (see below), lymphocytes secrete a TSH receptor-stimulating antibody (TSH-R Ab [stim]), also known as thyroid-stimulating immunoglobulin (TSI). This immunoglobulin binds to the TSH receptor site and turns on the gland in exactly the same fashion as TSH itself. The duration of the effect, however, is much longer than that of TSH.

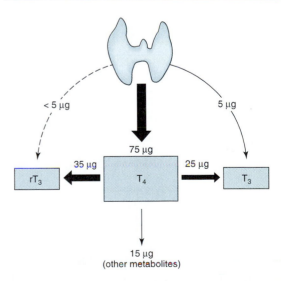

Figure 38–2. Peripheral metabolism of thyroxine. (Modified and reproduced, with permission, from Greenspan FS: Thyroid-gonadal interrelationships. In: *Gynecologic Endocrinology*, 3rd ed. Gold JJ, Josimovich JB [editors]. Harper & Row, 1980.)

I. BASIC PHARMACOLOGY OF THYROID & ANTITHYROID DRUGS

THYROID HORMONES

Chemistry

The structural formulas of thyroxine and triiodothyronine as well as reverse triiodothyronine (rT_3) are shown in Figure 38–2. All of these naturally occurring molecules are levo (L) isomers. The synthetic dextro (D) isomer of thyroxine, dextrothyroxine, has approximately 4% of the biologic activity of the L isomer as evidenced by its ability to suppress TSH secretion and correct hypothyroidism.

Pharmacokinetics

Data on oral absorption of thyroid hormones are derived from administration of exogenous hormones. T_4 is absorbed best in the duodenum and ileum; absorption is modified by intraluminal factors such as food, drugs (eg, aluminum-containing antacids, sucralfate, iron), and intestinal flora. Oral absorption of earlier preparations of L-thyroxine ranged from 35% to 65%; current preparations are better-absorbed, averaging 80% (Table 38–1). In contrast, T_3 is almost completely absorbed (95%) and minimally interfered with by intraluminal binding proteins. T_4 and T_3 absorption appears not to be affected by mild hypothy-

roidism but may be impaired in severe myxedema with ileus. These factors are important in switching from oral to parenteral therapy. For parenteral use, the intravenous route is preferred for both hormones.

In patients with hyperthyroidism, the metabolic clearance rates of T_4 and T_3 are increased and the half-lives decreased; the opposite is true in patients with hypothyroidism. Drugs that induce hepatic microsomal enzymes (eg, rifampin, phenobarbital, carba-

Figure 38–3. Quantitative aspects of thyroid hormone production and metabolism (per day) in normal adults.

Table 38–1. Summary of thyroid hormone kinetics.

Kinetic Variable	T_4	T_3
Volume of distribution	10 L	40 L
Extrathyroidal pool	800 µg	54 µg
Daily production	80 µg	30 µg
Fractional turnover per day	10%	60%
Metabolic clearance per day	1.1 L	24 L
Half-life (biologic)	7 days	1 day
Serum levels Total	5–12 µg/dL (64–154 nmol/L)	88–160 ng/dL (1.4–2.6 nmol/L)
Free	0.7–1.86 ng/dL (9–24 pmol/L)	0.2–0.52 ng/dL (3–8 pmol/L)
Amount bound	99.96%	99.6%
Biologic potency	1	4
Oral absorption	75–90%	95%

mazepine, phenytoin) increase the metabolism of both T_4 and T_3 (see Table 38–3). Despite this change in clearance, the normal hormone concentration is maintained in euthyroid patients as a result of compensatory hyperfunction of the thyroid. However, patients receiving T_4 replacement medication may require in- creased dosages to maintain clinical effectiveness. A similar compensation occurs if binding sites are altered. If TBG sites are increased by pregnancy, estrogens, or oral contraceptives, there is an initial shift of hormone from the free to the bound state and a decrease in its rate of elimination until the normal hor-

Table 38–2. Normal values for thyroid function tests.

Name	Normal Value[1]	Results in Hypothyroidism	Results in Hyperthyroidism
Total thyroxine by RIA (T_4 [RIA])	5–12 µg/dL (64–154 nmol/L)	Low	High
Total triiodothyronine by RIA (T_3 [RIA])	88–160 ng/dL (1.4–2.6 nmol/L)	Normal or low	High
Resin T_3 uptake (RT_3U)	25–35%	Low	High
Free thyroxine index (FT_4I)[1]	1.3–4.2	Low	High
Free T_3 index (FT_3I)	22–56	Normal or low	High
Free T_4 (FT_4)	0.7–1.86 (9–24 pmol/L)	Low	High
Free T_3 (FT_3)	0.2–0.52 ng/dL (3–8 pmol/L)	Low	High
Thyrotropic hormone (TSH)	0.3–5.0 µU/mL (0.3–5.0 mU/L)	High[2]	Low
[123]I uptake at 24 hours	5–35%	Low	High
Thyroglobulin antibodies (Atg-ab)	Titer < 1	Often present	Usually present
Thyroid peroxidase antibodies (TPA)	Titer < 1	Often present	Usually present
Thyrotropin-releasing hormone (TRH)	> 6 µU/mL rise in serum TSH 45 minutes after injection. Blunted TSH response (< 2 µU/mL) in patients over 40 years of age.	Exaggerated rise	No response
Isotope scan with ^{123}I or [99m]TcO_4	Normal pattern	Test not indicated	Diffusely enlarged gland
Thin-needle aspiration biopsy (TNA)	Normal pattern	Test not indicated	Test not indicated
Serum thyroglobulin	< 40 ng/mL	Test not indicated	Test not indicated
Serum calcitonin	Male: < 40 ng/L Female: < 20 ng/L	Test not indicated	Test not indicated

[1]Results may vary with different laboratories.
[2]Exception is central hypothyroidism.

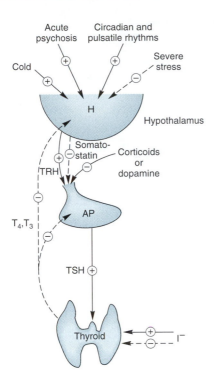

Figure 38–4. The hypothalamic-pituitary-thyroid axis. Acute psychosis or prolonged exposure to cold may activate the axis. Hypothalamic TRH stimulates pituitary TSH release, while somatostatin and dopamine inhibit it. TSH stimulates T4 and T3 synthesis and release from the thyroid, and they in turn inhibit both TRH and TSH synthesis and release. Small amounts of iodide are necessary for hormone production, but large amounts inhibit T3 and T4 production and release. (Solid arrows, stimulatory influence; dashed arrows, inhibitory influence.)

mone concentration is restored. Thus, the concentration of total and bound hormone will increase, but the concentration of free hormone and the steady state elimination will remain normal. The reverse occurs when thyroid binding sites are decreased.

Mechanism of Action

A model of thyroid hormone action is depicted in Figure 38–5, which shows the free forms of thyroid hormones, T_4 and T_3, dissociated from thyroid-binding proteins, entering the cell by diffusion or possibly by active transport. Within the cell, T_4 is converted to T_3 by 5'-deiodinase, and the T_3 enters the nucleus, where T_3 binds to a specific T_3 receptor protein. This protein has been cloned and characterized, and the T_3-binding pocket identified. It is a member of a family of receptors that are homologous with the c-*erb* oncogene. Other members of this family include the steroid hormone receptors and the receptors for vitamins A and D. The T_3 receptor exists in two forms, alpha and beta. Differing concentrations of receptor

forms in different tissues may account for variations in T_3 effect on different tissues.

Most of the effects of thyroid on metabolic processes appear to be mediated by activation of nuclear receptors that lead to increased formation of RNA and subsequent protein synthesis. For example, increased formation of the protein Na^+/K^+ ATPase and the consequent increase in ATP turnover and oxygen consumption are responsible for some of the calorigenic effects of thyroid hormones. This is consistent with the observation that the action of thyroid is manifested in vivo with a time lag of hours or days after its administration.

Large numbers of thyroid hormone receptors are found in the most hormone-responsive tissues (pituitary, liver, kidney, heart, skeletal muscle, lung, and intestine), while few receptor sites occur in hormone-unresponsive tissues (spleen, testes). The brain, which lacks an anabolic response to T_3, contains an intermediate number of receptors. In congruence with their biologic potencies, the affinity of the receptor site for T_4 is about ten times lower than that for T_3. The number of nuclear receptors may be altered to preserve body homeostasis. For example, starvation lowers both circulating T_3 hormone and cellular T_3 receptors.

Effects of Thyroid Hormones

The thyroid hormones are responsible for optimal growth, development, function, and maintenance of all body tissues (Table 38–4). Since T_3 and T_4 are qualitatively similar, they may be considered as one hormone in the discussion that follows.

Thyroid hormone is critical for nervous, skeletal, and reproductive tissues. Its effects depend upon protein synthesis as well as potentiation of the secretion and action of growth hormone. Thyroid deprivation in early life results in irreversible mental retardation and dwarfism—symptoms typical of congenital cretinism.

Effects on growth and calorigenesis are accompanied by a pervasive influence on metabolism of drugs as well as carbohydrates, fats, proteins, and vitamins. Many of these changes are dependent upon or modified by activity of other hormones. Conversely, the secretion and degradation rates of virtually all other hormones, including catecholamines, cortisol, estrogens, testosterone, and insulin, are affected by thyroid status.

Many of the manifestations of thyroid hyperactivity resemble sympathetic nervous system overactivity, though catecholamine levels are not increased. Possible explanations have included an increased number of beta receptor sites or enhanced amplification of the beta receptor signal without an increase in the number of receptor sites. Changes in catecholamine-stimulated adenylyl cyclase activity as measured by cAMP are found with changes in thyroid activity. The most dramatic effects of this catecholamine hyperactivity are seen in the cardiovascular system. Other clinical symptoms reminiscent of excessive epinephrine activ-

Table 38–3. Drug interactions and thyroid function.

Interaction	Drugs
CHANGE IN THYROID HORMONE SYNTHESIS	
Inhibition of TRH or TSH secretion without induction of hypothyroidism	Dopamine, levodopa, corticosteroids, somatostatin
Inhibition of thyroid hormone synthesis or release with the induction of hypothyroidism (or occasionally hyperthyroidism)	Iodides (including amiodarone), lithium, aminoglutethimide
ALTERATION OF THYROID HORMONE TRANSPORT AND SERUM TOTAL T_3 AND T_4 LEVELS, BUT USUALLY NO MODIFICATION OF FT_4 OR TSH	
Increased TBG	Estrogens, tamoxifen, heroin, methadone, mitotane
Decreased TBG	Androgens, glucocorticoids
Displacement of T_3 and T_4 from TBG with transient hyperthyroxinemia	Salicylates, fenclofenac, mefenamic acid, furosemide
ALTERATION OF T_4 AND T_3 METABOLISM WITH MODIFIED SERUM T_3 AND T_4 LEVELS BUT NOT FT_4 OR TSH LEVELS	
Induction of increased hepatic enzyme activity	Phenytoin, carbamazepine, phenobarbital, rifampin, rifabutin
Inhibition of 5′-deiodinase with decreased T_3, increased rT_3	Iopanoic acid, ipodate, amiodarone, β-blockers, corticosteroids, propylthiouracil
OTHER INTERACTIONS	
Interference with T_4 absorption	Cholestyramine, colestipol, aluminum hydroxide, sucralfate, ferrous sulfate
Induction of autoimmune thyroid disease with hypothyroidism or hyperthyroidism	Interferon-α, interleukin-2

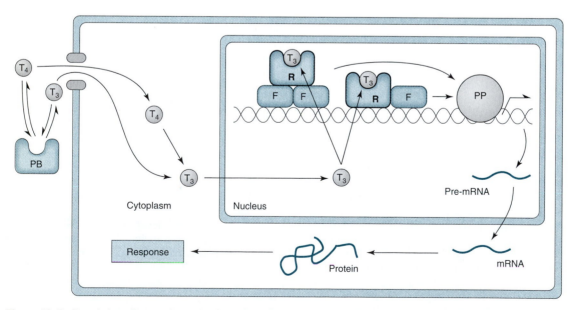

Figure 38–5. Regulation of transcription by thyroid hormones. T_3 and T_4 are triiodothyronine and thyroxine, respectively. PB, plasma binding protein; F, transcription factor; R, receptor; PP, proteins that bind at the proximal promoter. (Reproduced, with permission, from Baxter JD: General concepts of endocrinology. In: *Basic & Clinical Endocrinology,* 4th ed. Greenspan FS, Baxter JD editors. Appleton & Lange, 1994.)

ity (and partially alleviated by adrenoceptor antagonists) include lid lag and retraction, tremor, excessive sweating, anxiety, and nervousness. The opposite constellation of symptoms is seen in hypothyroidism (Table 38–4).

Thyroid Preparations

See the Preparations Available section at the end of this chapter for a list of available preparations. These preparations may be synthetic (levothyroxine, liothyronine, liotrix) or of animal origin (desiccated thyroid).

Synthetic levothyroxine is the preparation of choice for thyroid replacement and suppression therapy because of its stability, content uniformity, low cost, lack of allergenic foreign protein, easy laboratory measurement of serum levels, and long half-life (7 days), which permits once-daily administration. In addition, T_4 is converted to T_3 intracellularly; thus,

administration of T_4 produces both hormones. Generic levothyroxine preparations can be used because they provide comparable efficacy and are more cost-effective than branded preparations.

Although liothyronine is three to four times more active than levothyroxine, it is not recommended for routine replacement therapy because of its shorter half-life (24 hours), which requires multiple daily doses; its higher cost; and the greater difficulty of monitoring its adequacy of replacement by conventional laboratory tests. Furthermore, because of its greater hormone activity and consequent greater risk of cardiotoxicity, T_3 should be avoided in patients with cardiac disease. It is best used for short-term suppression of TSH. Because oral administration of T_3 is unnecessary, use of the more expensive liotrix instead of levothyroxine is never required.

The use of desiccated thyroid rather than synthetic preparations is never justified, since the disadvantages

Table 38–4. Summary of thyroid hormone effects.

System	Thyrotoxicosis	Hypothyroidism
Skin and appendages	Warm, moist skin; sweating; heat intolerance; fine, thin hair; Plummer's nails; pretibial dermopathy (Graves' disease).	Pale, cool, puffy skin; dry and brittle hair; brittle nails.
Eyes, face	Retraction of upper lid with wide stare; periorbital edema; exophthalmos; diplopia (Graves' disease).	Drooping of eyelids; periorbital edema; loss of temporal aspects of eyebrows; puffy, nonpitting facies; large tongue.
Cardiovascular system	Decreased peripheral vascular resistance, increased heart rate, stroke volume, cardiac output, pulse pressure; high-output congestive heart failure; increased inotropic, chronotropic effects; arrhythmias; angina.	Increased peripheral vascular resistance, decreased heart rate, stroke volume, cardiac output, pulse pressure; low-output congestive heart failure; ECG: bradycardia, prolonged PR interval, flat T wave, low voltage; pericardial effusion.
Respiratory system	Dyspnea; decreased vital capacity.	Pleural effusions; hypoventilation and CO_2 retention.
Gastrointestinal system	Increased appetite; increased frequency of bowel movements; hypoproteinemia.	Decreased appetite; decreased frequency of bowel movements; ascites.
Central nervous system	Nervousness; hyperkinesia; emotional lability.	Lethargy; general slowing of mental processes; neuropathies.
Musculoskeletal system	Weakness and muscle fatigue; increased deep tendon reflexes; hypercalcemia; osteoporosis.	Stiffness and muscle fatigue; decreased deep tendon reflexes; increased alkaline phosphatase, LDH, AST.
Renal system	Mild polyuria; increased renal blood flow; increased glomerular filtration rate.	Impaired water excretion; decreased renal blood flow; decreased glomerular filtration rate.
Hematopoietic system	Increased erythropoiesis; anemia.[1]	Decreased erythropoiesis; anemia.[1]
Reproductive system	Menstrual irregularities; decreased fertility; increased gonadal steroid metabolism.	Hypermenorrhea; infertility; decreased libido; impotence; oligospermia; decreased gonadal steroid metabolism.
Metabolic system	Increased basal metabolic rate; negative nitrogen balance; hyperglycemia; increased free fatty acids; decreased cholesterol and triglycerides; increased hormone degradation; increased requirements for fat- and water-soluble vitamins; increased drug detoxification.	Decreased basal metabolic rate; slight positive nitrogen balance; delayed degradation of insulin, with increased sensitivity; increased cholesterol and triglycerides; decreased hormone degradation; decreased requirements for fat- and water-soluble vitamins; decreased drug detoxification.

[1]The anemia of hyperthyroidism is usually normochromic and caused by increased red blood cell turnover. The anemia of hypothyroidism may be normochromic, hyperchromic, or hypochromic and may be due to decreased production rate, decreased iron absorption, decreased folic acid absorption, or to autoimmune pernicious anemia.

of protein antigenicity, product instability, variable hormone concentrations, and difficulty in laboratory monitoring far outweigh the advantage of low cost. Significant amounts of T_3 found in some thyroid extracts and liotrix may produce significant elevations in T_3 levels and toxicity. Equivalent dosages are 100 mg (1.5 gr) of desiccated thyroid, 100 μg of levothyroxine, and 37.5 μg of liothyronine.

The shelf life of synthetic hormone preparations is about 2 years, particularly if they are stored in dark bottles to minimize spontaneous deiodination. The shelf life of desiccated thyroid is not certainly known, but if it is kept dry, its potency is better preserved.

ANTITHYROID AGENTS

Reduction of thyroid activity and hormone effects can be accomplished by agents that interfere with the production of thyroid hormones; by agents that modify the tissue response to thyroid hormones; or by glandular destruction with radiation or surgery. "Goitrogens" are agents that suppress secretion of T_3 and T_4 to subnormal levels and thereby increase TSH, which in turn produces glandular enlargement (goiter). The antithyroid compounds used clinically include the thioamides, iodides, and radioactive iodine, which will be discussed later.

1. THIOAMIDES

The thioamides methimazole and propylthiouracil are major drugs for treatment of thyrotoxicosis. In the United Kingdom, carbimazole, which is converted to methimazole in vivo, is widely used. Methimazole is about ten times more active than propylthiouracil.

The chemical structures of these compounds are shown in Figure 38–6. The thiocarbamide group is essential for antithyroid activity:

Pharmacokinetics

Propylthiouracil is rapidly absorbed, reaching peak serum levels after 1 hour. The bioavailability of 50–80% may be due to incomplete absorption or a large first-pass effect in the liver. The volume of distribution approximates total body water with accumulation in the thyroid gland. Most of an ingested dose of propylthiouracil is excreted by the kidney as the inactive glucuronide within 24 hours.

In contrast, methimazole is completely absorbed but at variable rates. It is readily accumulated by the thyroid gland and has a volume of distribution similar

Figure 38–6. Structure of thioamides.

to that of propylthiouracil. Excretion is slower than with propylthiouracil; 65–70% of a dose is recovered in the urine in 48 hours.

The short plasma half-life of these agents (1.5 hours for propylthiouracil and 6 hours for methimazole) has little influence on the duration of the antithyroid action or the dosing interval because both agents are accumulated by the thyroid gland. For propylthiouracil, giving the drug every 6 hours is reasonable since a single 100 mg dose can inhibit 60% of iodine organification for 7 hours. Since a single 30 mg dose of methimazole exerts an antithyroid effect for longer than 24 hours, a single daily dose is effective in the management of mild to moderate hyperthyroidism.

Both thioamides cross the placental barrier and are concentrated by the fetal thyroid, so that caution must be employed while using these drugs in pregnancy. Of the two, propylthiouracil is preferable in pregnancy because it is more strongly protein-bound and therefore crosses the placenta less readily. In addition, it is not secreted in sufficient quantity in breast milk to preclude breast feeding.

Pharmacodynamics

The thioamides act by multiple mechanisms. The major action is to prevent hormone synthesis by inhibiting the thyroid peroxidase-catalyzed reactions to block iodine organification. In addition, they block coupling of the iodotyrosines. They do not block uptake of iodide by the gland. Propylthiouracil and (to a much lesser extent) methimazole inhibit the peripheral deiodination of T_4 and T_3 (Figure 38–1). Since the synthesis rather than the release of hormones is affected, the onset of these agents is slow, often requiring 3–4 weeks before stores of T_4 are depleted.

Toxicity

Adverse reactions to the thioamides occur in 3–12% of treated patients. Most reactions occur early. The most common adverse effect is a maculopapular pruritic rash, at times accompanied by systemic signs such as fever. Rare adverse effects include an urticarial rash, vasculitis, arthralgia, a lupus-like reaction, cholestatic jaundice, hepatitis, lymphadenopathy, hypoprothrombinemia, and polyserositis. The most dangerous complication is agranulocytosis, an infrequent but potentially fatal adverse reaction. It occurs in 0.3–0.6% of patients taking thioamides, but the risk may be increased in older patients and in those receiving high-dose methimazole therapy (over 40 mg/d). The reaction is usually rapidly reversible when the drug is discontinued, but antibiotic therapy may be necessary for complicating infections. The cross-sensitivity between propylthiouracil and methimazole is about 50%; therefore, switching drugs in patients with severe reactions is not recommended.

2. ANION INHIBITORS

Monovalent anions such as perchlorate (ClO_4^-), pertechnetate (TcO_4^-), and thiocyanate (SCN^-) can block uptake of iodide by the gland through competitive inhibition of the iodide transport mechanism. Since these effects can be overcome by large doses of iodides, their effectiveness is somewhat unpredictable.

The major clinical use for potassium perchlorate is to block thyroidal reuptake of I^- in patients with iodide-induced hyperthyroidism (eg, amiodarone-induced hyperthyroidism). However, potassium perchlorate is rarely used clinically because it has been shown to cause aplastic anemia.

3. IODIDES

Iodides have been known since the 1920s to have multiple effects on the thyroid gland. Prior to the introduction of the thioamides in the 1940s, iodides were the major antithyroid agents; today they are rarely used as sole therapy.

Pharmacodynamics

Iodides have several actions on the thyroid. They inhibit organification and hormone release and decrease the size and vascularity of the hyperplastic gland. In susceptible individuals, iodides can induce hyperthyroidism (jodbasedow) or precipitate hypothyroidism.

In pharmacologic doses (> 6 mg daily), the major action of iodides is to inhibit hormone release, possibly through inhibition of thyroglobulin proteolysis. Rapid improvement in thyrotoxic symptoms occurs within 2–7 days—hence the value of iodide therapy in thyroid storm. In addition, iodides decrease the vascularity, size, and fragility of a hyperplastic gland, making the drugs valuable as preoperative preparation for surgery.

Clinical Use of Iodide

Disadvantages of iodide therapy include an increase in intraglandular stores of iodine, which may delay onset of thioamide therapy or prevent use of radioactive iodine therapy for several weeks. Thus, iodides should be initiated after onset of thioamide therapy and avoided if treatment with radioactive iodine seems likely. Iodide should not be used alone, because the gland will "escape" from the iodide block in 2–8 weeks, and its withdrawal may produce severe exacerbation of thyrotoxicosis in an iodine-enriched gland. Chronic use of iodides in pregnancy should be avoided, since they cross the placenta and can cause fetal goiter.

Toxicity

Adverse reactions to iodine (iodism) are uncommon and in most cases reversible upon discontinuance. They include acneiform rash (similar to that of bromism), swollen salivary glands, mucous membrane ulcerations, conjunctivitis, rhinorrhea, drug fever, metallic taste, bleeding disorders, and, rarely, anaphylactoid reactions.

4. IODINATED CONTRAST MEDIA

The iodinated contrast agents, ipodate and iopanoic acid, are valuable in the treatment of hyperthyroidism, though they are not approved by the FDA for this indication. These drugs rapidly inhibit the conversion of T_4 to T_3 in the liver, kidney, pituitary gland, and brain. This accounts for the dramatic improvement in both subjective and objective parameters. For example, a decrease in heart rate is seen after only 3 days of oral administration of 0.5–1 g/d. T_3 levels often return to normal during this time. The prolonged effect of suppressing T_4 as well as T_3 suggests that inhibition of hormone release due to the iodine released may be an additional mechanism of action. Fortunately, these agents are relatively nontoxic. They provide useful adjunctive therapy in the treatment of thyroid storm and offer valuable alternatives when iodides or thioamides are contraindicated. Surprisingly, these agents may not interfere with ^{131}I retention as much as iodides despite their large iodine content. Their toxicity is similar to that of the iodides, and their safety in pregnancy is undocumented.

5. RADIOACTIVE IODINE

[131]I is the only isotope used for treatment of thyrotoxicosis (others are used in diagnosis). Administered

orally in solution as sodium ^{131}I, it is rapidly absorbed, concentrated by the thyroid, and incorporated into storage follicles. Its therapeutic effect depends on emission of beta rays with an effective half-life of 5 days and a penetration range of 400–2000 μm. Within a few weeks after administration, destruction of the thyroid parenchyma is evidenced by epithelial swelling and necrosis, follicular disruption, edema, and leukocyte infiltration. Advantages of radioiodine include easy administration, effectiveness, low expense, and absence of pain. Fears of radiation-induced genetic damage, leukemia, and neoplasia have caused some clinics to restrict the use of radioiodine in the treatment of hyperthyroidism to adults over some specified age such as 40 years. However, after more than 30 years of clinical experience with radioiodine, these fears have not been realized. Radioactive iodine should not be administered to pregnant women or nursing mothers, since it crosses the placenta and is excreted in breast milk.

6. ADRENOCEPTOR-BLOCKING AGENTS

Many of the symptoms of thyrotoxicosis mimic those associated with sympathetic stimulation, and sympathoplegic agents such as guanethidine or beta-blockers are useful therapeutic adjuncts. Beta-adreno-ceptor-blocking drugs are the agents of choice because they are effective in patients refractory to guanethidine and reserpine. Propranolol has been the drug in this group most widely studied and used in the therapy of thyrotoxicosis.

II. CLINICAL PHARMACOLOGY OF THYROID & ANTITHYROID DRUGS

HYPOTHYROIDISM

Hypothyroidism is a syndrome resulting from deficiency of thyroid hormones and is manifested largely by a reversible slowing down of all body functions (Table 38–4). In infants and children, there is striking retardation of growth and development that results in dwarfism and irreversible mental retardation.

The etiology and pathogenesis of hypothyroidism are outlined in Table 38–5. Hypothyroidism can occur with or without thyroid enlargement (goiter). The laboratory diagnosis of hypothyroidism in the adult is easily made by the combination of a low free thyroxine (or low free thyroxine index) and elevated serum TSH (Table 38–2).

The most common cause of hypothyroidism in the USA at this time is probably Hashimoto's thyroiditis, an immunologic disorder in genetically predisposed individuals. In this condition, there is evidence of humoral immunity in the presence of antithyroid antibodies and lymphocyte sensitization to thyroid antigens.

Management of Hypothyroidism

Except for hypothyroidism caused by drugs (Table 38–5), which can be treated by simply removing the depressant agent, the general strategy of replacement therapy is appropriate. The most satisfactory preparation is levothyroxine. Infants and children require more T_4 per kilogram of body weight than adults. The average dosage for an infant 1–6 months of age is 10–15 μg/kg/d, whereas the average dosage for an adult is about 1.7 μg/kg/d. There is some variability in the absorption of thyroxine, so this dosage may vary from patient to patient. Because of the long half-life of thyroxine, the dose can be given once daily. Children should be monitored for normal growth and development. Serum TSH and the free thyroxine index should be measured at regular intervals and maintained within the normal range. It takes 6–8 weeks after starting a given dose of thyroxine to reach steady state levels in the bloodstream. Thus, dosage changes should be made slowly.

In long-standing hypothyroidism, in older patients, and in patients with underlying cardiac disease, it is imperative to start treatment with reduced dosage. In such adult patients, levothyroxine is given in a dosage of 0.0125–0.025 mg/d for 2 weeks, increasing by 0.025 mg every 2 weeks until euthyroidism or drug toxicity is observed. In older patients, the heart is very sensitive to the level of circulating thyroxine, and if angina pectoris or cardiac arrhythmia develops, it is essential to stop or reduce the dose of thyroxine immediately. In younger patients or those with very mild disease, full replacement therapy may be started immediately.

The toxicity of thyroxine is directly related to the hormone level. In children, restlessness, insomnia, and accelerated bone maturation and growth may be signs of thyroxine toxicity. In adults, increased nervousness, heat intolerance, episodes of palpitation and tachycardia, or unexplained weight loss may be the presenting symptoms of thyroid toxicity. If these symptoms are present, it is important to monitor serum TSH (Table 38–2), which will determine whether the symptoms are due to excess thyroxine blood levels. Chronic overtreatment with T_4, particularly in elderly patients, can increase the risk of atrial fibrillation and accelerated osteoporosis.

Special Problems in Management of Hypothyroidism

A. Myxedema and Coronary Artery Disease: Since myxedema frequently occurs in older persons, it is often associated with underlying coronary artery disease. In this situation, the low levels of circulating thyroid hormone actually protect the heart

Table 38–5. Etiology and pathogenesis of hypothyroidism.

Cause	Pathogenesis	Goiter	Degree of Hypothyroidism
Hashimoto's thyroiditis	Autoimmune destruction of thyroid	Present early, absent later	Mild to severe
Drug-induced[1]	Blocked hormone formation	Present	Mild to moderate
Dyshormonogenesis	Impaired synthesis of T_4 due to enzyme deficiency	Present	Mild to severe
Radiation, ^{131}I, x-ray	Destruction of gland	Absent	Severe
Congenital (cretinism)	Athyreosis or ectopic thyroid, iodine deficiency; TSH receptor blocking antibodies	Absent or present	Severe
Secondary (TSH deficit)	Pituitary or hypothalamic disease	Absent	Mild

[1]Iodides, lithium, fluoride, thioamides, aminosalicylic acid, phenylbutazone, amiodarone, etc.

against increasing demands that could result in angina pectoris or myocardial infarction. Correction of myxedema must be done cautiously to avoid provoking arrhythmia, angina, or acute myocardial infarction. Complete restoration of the euthyroid state may not be possible in patients with severe coronary artery disease unless bypass coronary artery surgery restores a more adequate coronary circulation.

B. Myxedema Coma: Myxedema coma is an end state of untreated hypothyroidism. It is associated with progressive weakness, stupor, hypothermia, hypoventilation, hypoglycemia, hyponatremia, water intoxication, shock, and death. Symptoms usually develop quite slowly, with a gradual onset of lethargy, progressing to stupor or coma.

The pathophysiology of myxedema coma involves three major aspects: (1) CO_2 retention and hypoxia associated with decreased sensitivity of the respiratory center; (2) fluid and electrolyte imbalance with hyponatremia; and (3) marked hypothermia, with body temperatures as low as 24 °C (75 °F). Serum tests are consistent with severe hypothyroidism (see above).

Management of myxedema coma is a medical emergency. The patient should be treated in the intensive care unit, since tracheal intubation and mechanical ventilation may be required. Associated illnesses such as infection or heart failure must be treated by appropriate therapy. It is important to give all preparations intravenously, because patients with myxedema coma absorb drugs poorly from other routes. Intravenous fluids should be administered with caution to avoid excessive water intake. These patients have large pools of empty T_3 and T_4 binding sites in their sera that must be filled before there is adequate free thyroxine to affect tissue metabolism. Accordingly, the treatment of choice in myxedema coma is to give a loading dose of levothyroxine intravenously—usually 300–400 μg initially, followed by 50 μg daily. Intravenous T_3 can also be used but may be more cardiotoxic and more difficult to monitor. Intravenous hydrocortisone is indi-

cated if the patient has associated adrenal or pituitary insufficiency but is probably not necessary in most patients with primary myxedema. Narcotics and sedatives must be used with extreme caution.

Clinically, improvement is evidenced by an increase in body temperature and arousal from the comatose state. Once the patient is able to breathe normally, assisted mechanical ventilation can be removed, and steady improvement will ensue.

C. Hypothyroidism and Pregnancy: Hypothyroid women frequently have anovulatory cycles and are therefore relatively infertile until restoration of the euthyroid state. This has led to the widespread use of thyroid hormone for infertility, though there is no evidence for its usefulness in infertile euthyroid patients. In a pregnant hypothyroid patient receiving thyroxine, it is extremely important that the daily dose of thyroxine be adequate because early development of the fetal brain is dependent on maternal thyroxine. In many hypothyroid patients, a modest increase in the thyroxine dose (about 20–30%) is required to normalize the serum TSH level during pregnancy. Because of the elevated maternal TBG, the free thyroxine index (FT_4I) or free thyroxine (FT_4) and TSH (Table 38–2) must be used to monitor maternal thyroxine dosages.

HYPERTHYROIDISM

Hyperthyroidism (thyrotoxicosis) is the clinical syndrome that results when tissues are exposed to high levels of thyroid hormone.

1. GRAVES' DISEASE

The most common form of hyperthyroidism is Graves' disease, or diffuse toxic goiter. The presenting signs and symptoms of Graves' disease are set forth in Table 38–4.

Pathophysiology

Graves' disease is considered to be an autoimmune disorder in which there is a genetic defect in suppressor T lymphocytes, and helper T lymphocytes stimulate B lymphocytes to synthesize antibodies to thyroidal antigens. One such antibody—TSH receptor-stimulating antibody (TSH-R Ab [stim]), also called thyroid-stimulating immunoglobulin (TSI)—is directed against the TSH receptor site in the thyroid cell membrane and has the capacity to stimulate the thyroid cell.

Laboratory Diagnosis

In most patients with hyperthyroidism, T_3, T_4, RT_3U, FT_4, and FT_4I will all be elevated and TSH is suppressed (Table 38–2). Radioiodine uptake is usually markedly elevated as well. Antithyroglobulin antibodies, thyroid peroxidase antibodies, and TSH-R Ab [stim] are often present.

Management of Graves' Disease

The three primary methods for controlling hyperthyroidism are antithyroid drug therapy, surgical thyroidectomy, and destruction of the gland with radioactive iodine.

A. Antithyroid Drug Therapy: Drug therapy is most useful in young patients with small glands and mild disease. Methimazole or propylthiouracil is administered until the disease undergoes spontaneous remission, which may take from 1 year to 15 years. This is the only therapy that leaves an intact thyroid gland, but it does require a long period of treatment and observation (1–2 years), and there is a 60–70% incidence of relapse. The incidence of relapse is not much lower when antithyroid drugs are used in combination with levothyroxine (see below).

Antithyroid drug therapy is usually begun with large divided doses, shifting to maintenance therapy with single daily doses when the patient becomes clinically euthyroid. However, mild to moderately severe thyrotoxicosis can often be controlled with methimazole given in a single morning dose of 30–40 mg; once-daily dosing may enhance adherence. Maintenance therapy requires 5–15 mg once daily. Alternatively, therapy is started with propylthiouracil, 100–150 mg every 6 hours, followed after 4–8 weeks by gradual reduction of the dose to the maintenance level of 50–150 mg once daily. In addition to inhibiting iodine organification, propylthiouracil also inhibits the conversion of T_4 to T_3, so it brings the level of activated thyroid hormone down more quickly than does methimazole. The best clinical guide to remission is reduction in the size of the goiter. Laboratory tests most useful in monitoring the course of therapy are serum T_3 by RIA, FT_4 or FT_4I, and serum TSH.

Reactivation of the autoimmune process may occur when the dosage of antithyroid drug is lowered during maintenance therapy and TSH begins to drive the gland. TSH release can be prevented by the daily administration of 0.05–0.15 mg of levothyroxine with 5–15 mg of methimazole or 50–150 mg of propylthiouracil for the second year of therapy. When antithyroid drug therapy is discontinued, levothyroxine may be continued for an additional year. The relapse rate with this program is probably comparable to the rate with antithyroid therapy alone but the risk of hypothyroidism and overtreatment is avoided.

Reactions to antithyroid drugs have been described above. A minor rash can often be controlled by antihistamine therapy. Because the more severe reaction of agranulocytosis is often heralded by sore throat or high fever, patients receiving antithyroid drugs must be instructed to discontinue the drug and seek immediate medical attention if these symptoms develop. White cell and differential counts and a throat culture are indicated in such cases, followed by appropriate antibiotic therapy. Rare adverse reactions to antithyroid drugs also requiring cessation of drug therapy include urticaria, cholestatic jaundice, hepatocellular toxicity, exfoliative dermatitis, and acute arthralgia.

B. Thyroidectomy: Subtotal thyroidectomy is the treatment of choice for patients with very large glands or multinodular goiters. Patients are treated with antithyroid drugs until euthyroid (about 6 weeks). In addition, for 2 weeks prior to surgery, they receive saturated solution of potassium iodide, 5 drops twice daily, to diminish vascularity of the gland and simplify surgery. About 50–60% of patients will require thyroid supplementation following subtotal thyroidectomy.

C. Radioactive Iodine: Radioiodine therapy utilizing ^{131}I is the preferred treatment for most patients over 21 years of age. In patients without heart disease, the therapeutic dose may be given immediately in a range of 80–120 μCi/g of estimated thyroid weight corrected for uptake. In patients with underlying heart disease or severe thyrotoxicosis and in elderly patients, it is desirable to treat with antithyroid drugs until the patient is euthyroid. The medication is then stopped for 5–7 days before the appropriate dose of ^{131}I is administered. Iodides should be avoided to ensure maximal ^{131}I uptake. Six to 12 weeks following the administration of radioiodine, the gland will shrink in size and the patient will usually become euthyroid. A second dose may be required in some patients. The major complication of radioiodine therapy is hypothyroidism, which occurs in about 80% of patients. Serum FT_4 and TSH levels should be monitored. When hypothyroidism develops, prompt replacement with levothyroxine, 0.05–0.15 mg orally daily, should be instituted.

D. Adjuncts to Antithyroid Therapy: During the acute phase of thyrotoxicosis, beta-adrenoceptor-blocking agents are extremely helpful. Propranolol, 20–40 mg orally every 6 hours, will control tachycardia, hypertension, and atrial fibrillation. Propranolol is gradually withdrawn as serum thyroxine levels return to normal. Diltiazem, 90–120 mg 3 or 4 times daily, can be used to control tachycardia in patients in whom beta-blockers are contraindicated, eg, those with asthma. Interestingly, other calcium channel blockers may not be effective. Adequate nutrition and vitamin supplements are essential. Barbiturates accelerate T_4 breakdown (by hepatic enzyme induction) and may be helpful both as a sedative and to lower T_4 levels.

2. TOXIC UNINODULAR GOITER & TOXIC MULTINODULAR GOITER

These forms of hyperthyroidism occur often in older women with nodular goiters. FT_4 is moderately elevated or occasionally normal, but T_3 by RIA is strikingly elevated. Single toxic adenomas can be managed with either surgical excision of the adenoma or with radioiodine therapy. Toxic multinodular goiter is usually associated with a large goiter and is best treated by preparation with methimazole or propylthiouracil followed by subtotal thyroidectomy.

3. SUBACUTE THYROIDITIS

During the acute phase of a viral infection of the thyroid gland, there is destruction of thyroid parenchyma with transient release of stored thyroid hormones. A similar state may occur in patients with Hashimoto's thyroiditis. These episodes of transient thyrotoxicosis have been termed "spontaneously resolving hyperthyroidism." Supportive therapy is usually all that is necessary, such as propranolol for tachycardia and aspirin or NSAIDs to control local pain and fever. Corticosteroids may be necessary in severe cases to control the inflammation.

4. THYROTOXICOSIS FACTITIA

This is due to excessive ingestion of thyroid hormones, either accidentally or intentionally. Treatment consists of supportive therapy and discontinuing excessive medication.

5. SPECIAL PROBLEMS

Thyroid Storm

Thyroid storm, or thyrotoxic crisis, is sudden acute exacerbation of all of the symptoms of thyrotoxicosis, presenting as a life-threatening syndrome. The clinical manifestations are variable in intensity but reflect hypermetabolism and excessive adrenergic activity. Fever is present, often associated with flushing and sweating. Tachycardia is common, often with atrial fibrillation, high pulse pressure, and occasionally heart failure. Central nervous system symptoms include marked agitation, restlessness, delirium, and

coma. Gastrointestinal symptoms include nausea, vomiting, diarrhea, and jaundice. Death may occur from heart failure and shock.

Vigorous management is mandatory. Propranolol, 1–2 mg slowly intravenously or 40–80 mg orally every 6 hours, is helpful to control the severe cardiovascular manifestations. If propranolol is contraindicated by the presence of severe heart failure or asthma, hypertension and tachycardia may be controlled with diltiazem, 90–120 mg orally 3 or 4 times daily or 5–10 mg/h by intravenous infusion (asthmatic patients only). Release of thyroid hormones from the gland is retarded by the administration of saturated solution of potassium iodide, 10 drops orally daily, or sodium ipodate, 1 g orally daily. The latter medication will also block peripheral conversion of T_4 to T_3. Hormone synthesis is blocked by the administration of propylthiouracil, 250 mg orally every 6 hours. If the patient is unable to take propylthiouracil by mouth, a rectal formulation can be prepared and administered in a dosage of 400 mg every 6 hours as a retention enema. Methimazole may also be prepared for rectal administration in a dose of 25 mg every 6 hours.* Hydrocortisone, 50 mg intravenously every 6 hours, will protect the patient against shock and will block the conversion of T_4 to T_3, bringing down the level of thyroactive material in the blood quickly.

Supportive therapy is essential to control fever, heart failure, and any underlying disease process that may have precipitated the acute storm. In rare situations, where the above methods are not adequate to control the problem, plasmapheresis or peritoneal dialysis has been used to lower the levels of circulating thyroxine.

Ophthalmopathy

Although severe ophthalmopathy is rare, it is difficult to treat. Management requires effective treatment of the thyroid disease, usually by total surgical excision or ^{131}I ablation of the gland. In addition, local therapy may be necessary, eg, elevation of the head to diminish periorbital edema and artificial tears to relieve corneal drying. Smoking cessation should be advised to prevent progression of the ophthalmopathy. For the severe, acute inflammatory reaction, a short course of prednisone, 60–100 mg orally daily for about a week and then 60–100 mg every other day, tapering the dose over a period of 6–12 weeks, may be effective. If steroid therapy fails or is contraindicated,

---

*Preparation of rectal propylthiouracil: Dissolve 400 mg propylthiouracil in 60 mL of Fleet mineral oil for the first dose and then 400 mg in 60 mL of Fleet Phospho-soda for subsequent enemas. Preparation of rectal methimazole: Dissolve methimazole (1200 mg) in 12 mL water to which has been added a mixture of 2 drops of Span 80 in 52 mL cocoa butter warmed to 37 °C. Stir the mixture to form a water-oil emulsion, pour into 2.6 mL suppository molds, and cool. (Nabil et al, 1982).

irradiation of the posterior orbit, using well-collimated high-energy x-ray therapy, will frequently result in marked improvement of the acute process. Threatened loss of vision is an indication for surgical decompression of the orbit. Eyelid or eye muscle surgery may be necessary to correct residual problems after the acute process has subsided.

Dermopathy

Dermopathy or pretibial myxedema will often respond to topical corticosteroids applied to the involved area and covered with an occlusive dressing.

Thyrotoxicosis During Pregnancy

Ideally, women in the childbearing period with severe disease should have definitive therapy with ^{131}I or subtotal thyroidectomy prior to pregnancy in order to avoid an acute exacerbation of the disease during pregnancy or following delivery. If thyrotoxicosis does develop during pregnancy, radioiodine is contraindicated because it crosses the placenta and may injure the fetal thyroid. In the first trimester, the patient can be prepared with propylthiouracil and a subtotal thyroidectomy performed safely during the mid trimester. It is essential to give the patient a thyroid supplement during the balance of the pregnancy. However, most patients are treated with propylthiouracil during the pregnancy, and the decision regarding long-term management can be made after delivery. The dosage of propylthiouracil must be kept to the minimum necessary for control of the disease (ie, < 300 mg daily), because it may affect the function of the fetal thyroid gland. Methimazole is a potential alternative, though there is concern about a possible risk of fetal scalp defects.

Neonatal Graves' Disease

Graves' disease may occur in the newborn infant, either due to passage of TSH-R Ab [stim] through the placenta, stimulating the thyroid gland of the neonate, or to genetic transmission of the trait to the fetus. Laboratory studies reveal an elevated free thyroxine, a markedly elevated T_3, and a low TSH—in contrast to the normal infant, in whom TSH is elevated at birth. TSH-R Ab [stim] is usually found in the serum of both the child and the mother.

If caused by maternal TSH-R Ab [stim], the disease is usually self-limited and subsides over a period of 4–12 weeks, coinciding with the fall in the infant's TSH-R Ab [stim] level. However, treatment is necessary because of the severe metabolic stress the infant is subjected to. Therapy includes propylthiouracil in a dose of 5–10 mg/kg/d in divided doses at 8-hour intervals; Lugol's solution (8 mg of iodide per drop), 1 drop every 8 hours; and propranolol, 2 mg/kg/d in divided doses. Careful supportive therapy is essential. If the infant is very ill, prednisone, 2 mg/kg/d orally in divided doses, will help block conversion of T_4 to T_3. These medications are gradually reduced as the clinical picture improves and can be discontinued by 6–12 weeks.

NONTOXIC GOITER

Nontoxic goiter is a syndrome of thyroid enlargement without excessive thyroid hormone production. Enlargement of the thyroid gland is usually due to TSH stimulation from inadequate thyroid hormone synthesis. The most common cause of nontoxic goiter worldwide is iodide deficiency, but in the USA it is Hashimoto's thyroiditis. Less common causes include dietary goitrogens, dyshormonogenesis, and neoplasms (see below).

Goiter due to iodide deficiency is best managed by prophylactic administration of iodide. The optimal daily iodide intake is 150–300 μg. Iodized salt and iodate used as preservatives in flour and bread are excellent sources of iodine in the diet. In areas where it is difficult to introduce iodized salt or iodate preservatives, a solution of iodized poppyseed oil has been administered intramuscularly to provide a long-term source of inorganic iodine.

Goiter due to ingestion of goitrogens in the diet is managed by elimination of the goitrogen or by adding sufficient thyroxine to shut off TSH stimulation. Similarly, in Hashimoto's thyroiditis and dyshormonogenesis, adequate thyroxine therapy—0.15–0.2 mg/d orally—will suppress pituitary TSH and result in slow regression of the goiter as well as correction of hypothyroidism.

THYROID NEOPLASMS

Neoplasms of the thyroid gland may be benign (adenomas) or malignant. Thin-needle aspiration biopsy has proved effective for differentiation of benign from malignant disease. Some adenomas will regress following thyroxine therapy; those that do not should be rebiopsied or surgically removed. Management of thyroid carcinoma requires a near-total thyroidectomy, postoperative radioiodine therapy in selected instances, and lifetime replacement with levothyroxine.

PREPARATIONS AVAILABLE

Thyroid Agents

Levothyroxine [T$_4$] (generic, Synthroid, Levothroid, Levoxyl)
Oral: 0.025, 0.05, 0.075, 0.088, 0.1, 0.112, 0.125, 0.137, 0.15, 0.175, 0.2, 0.3 mg tablets
Parenteral: 200, 500 μg per vial (100 μg/mL when reconstituted) for injection

Liothyronine [T$_3$] (generic, Cytomel, Triostat)
Oral: 5, 25, 50 μg tablets
Parenteral: 10 μg/mL

Liotrix [a 4:1 ratio of T$_4$:T$_3$] (Thyrolar)
Oral: tablets containing 12.5, 25, 30, 50, 60, 100, 120, 150, 180 μg T$_4$ and one-fourth as much T$_3$

Thyroid desiccated [USP] (generic, Armour Thyroid, Thyroid Strong, Thyrar, S-P-T)
Oral: tablets containing 15, 30, 60, 90, 120, 180, 240, 300 mg; capsules (S-P-T) containing 120, 180, 300 mg

Antithyroid Agents

Iodide (^{131}I) sodium (Iodotope, Sodium Iodide I 131 Therapeutic)
Oral: available as capsules and solution

Iopanoic acid (Telepaque)
Oral: 500 mg tablets (unlabeled use)

Ipodate sodium (Oragrafin Sodium, Bilivist)
Oral: 500 mg capsules (unlabeled use)

Methimazole (Tapazole)
Oral: 5, 10 mg tablets

Potassium iodide solution
Oral solution (generic, SSKI): 1 g/mL
Oral solution (Lugol's solution): 100 mg/mL potassium iodide plus 50 mg/mL iodine
Oral syrup (Pima): 325 mg/5 mL
Oral controlled action tablets (Iodo-Niacin): 135 mg potassium iodide plus 25 mg niacinamide hydroiodide

Propylthiouracil [PTU] (generic)
Oral: 50 mg tablets

REFERENCES

General

Braverman LE, Utiger RD (editors): *Werner and Ingbar's The Thyroid: A Fundamental and Clinical Text,* 7th ed. Lippincott, 1996.

Greenspan FS: Thyroid gland. In: *Basic & Clinical Endocrinology,* 5th ed. Greenspan FS, Strewler GJ (editors). Appleton & Lange, 1997.

Greenspan FS (editor): Thyroid disease. Med Clin North Am 1991;75:1.

Greer MA (editor): *The Thyroid Gland.* Comprehensive Endocrinology Series. Martini L (editor). Raven Press, 1990.

Larsen PR, Ingbar SH: The thyroid gland. In: *Williams Textbook of Endocrinology,* 8th ed. Wilson JD, Foster DW (editors). Saunders, 1992.

Surks MI et al: American Thyroid Association guidelines for use of laboratory tests in thyroid disorders. JAMA 1990;263:1529.

Utiger RD: The thyroid: physiology, thyrotoxicosis, and the painful thyroid. In: *Endocrinology and Metabolism,* 3rd ed. Felig P, Baxter JD, Frohman LA (editors). McGraw-Hill, 1995.

Wartofsky L et al: The thyroid gland. In: *Principles and Practice of Endocrinology and Metabolism,* 2nd ed. Becker KL (editor). Lippincott, 1995.

Hypothyroidism

Bagchi N, Brown TR, Parish RF: Thyroid dysfunction in adults over age 55 years: A study in an urban US community. Arch Intern Med 1995;150:785.

Fisher DA: Management of congenital hypothyroidism: Clinical review 19. J Clin Endocrinol Metab 1991;72:523.

Jordan RM: Myxedema coma: Pathophysiology, therapy and factors affecting prognosis. Med Clin North Am 1995;79:185.

Lindsay RS, Toft AD. Hypothroidism. Lancet 1997;349:413.

Mandel SJ et al: Increased need for thyroxine during pregnancy in women with primary hypothyroidism. N Engl J Med 1990;323:91.

Mandel SJ, Brent GA, Larsen PR: Levothyroxine therapy in patients with thyroid disease. Ann Intern Med 1993;119:492.

Sawin CT: Subclinical hypothyroidism in older patients. Clin Geriatr Med 1995;11:231.

Singer PA et al: Treatment guidelines for patients with hyperthyroidism and hypothyroidism. JAMA 1995;273:808.

Hyperthyroidism

Aranow WS: The heart and thyroid disease. Clin Geriatr Med 1995;11:219.

Becks GP, Burrow GN: Thyroid disease and pregnancy. Med Clin North Am 1991;75:121.

Farrar JJ, Toft AD: Iodine-131 treatment of hyperthyroidism: Current issues. Clin Endocrinol 1991;35:207.

Feldt-Rassmussen U: Reassessment of antithyroid drug therapy of Graves' disease. Ann Rev Med 1993;44:323.

Franklyn JA: The management of hyperthyroidism. N Engl J Med 1994;330:1731.

Hashizume K et al: Administration of thyroxine in treated Graves' disease: Effects on the level of antibodies to thyroid stimulating hormone receptors and on the risk of recurrence of hyperthyroidism. N Engl J Med 1991;324:947.

Heufelder AE: Pathogenesis of Graves' ophthalmopathy: Recent controversies and progress. Eur J Endocrinol 1995;132:532.

Klein I, Becker DV, Levey GS: Treatment of hyperthyroid disease. Ann Intern Med 1994;121:281.

McDougall IR: Graves' disease: Current concepts. Med Clin North Am 1991;75:79.

Nabil N, Miner DJ, Amatruda JM: Methimazole: An alternative route of administration. J Clin Endocrinol Metab 1982;54:180.

Tietgens ST, Leinuang MC: Thyroid storm. Med Clin North Am 1995;79:169.

Walter RM, Bartle WR: Rectal administration of propylthiouracil in the treatment of Graves' disease. Am J Med 1990;88:69.

Nontoxic Goiter, Nodules, & Cancer

Berghout A et al: Comparison of placebo with L-thyroxine alone or with carbimazole for treatment of sporadic nontoxic goiter. Lancet 1990;336:193.

Burman KD (editor): Thyroid cancer I. Endocrinol Metab Clin North Am 1995;24:663.

Dulgeroff AJ, Hershman JM: Medical therapy for differentiated thyroid carcinoma. Endocr Rev 1994;15:500.

Greenspan FS: The problem of the nodular goiter. Med Clin North Am 1991;75:195.

Lamberg BA: Endemic goiter-iodine deficiency disorders. Ann Med 1991;23:367.

Mazzaferri EL, Jhiang SM: Long term impact of initial surgical and medical therapy on papillary and follicular thyroid cancer. Am J Med 1994;97:418.

The Effects of Drugs on Thyroid Function

Cavalieri RR, Pitt-Rivers R: The effects of drugs on the distribution and metabolism of thyroid hormones. Pharmacol Rev 1981;33:55.

Surks MI, Sievert R: Drugs and thyroid function. N Engl J Med 1995;333:1688.

Adrenocorticosteroids & Adrenocortical Antagonists

39

Alan Goldfien, MD

The natural adrenocortical hormones are steroid molecules produced and released by the adrenal cortex. Both natural and synthetic corticosteroids are used for diagnosis and treatment of disorders of adrenal function. They are also used—more often and in much larger doses—for treatment of a variety of inflammatory and immunologic disorders.

Secretion of adrenocortical steroids is controlled by the pituitary release of corticotropin (ACTH). Secretion of the salt-retaining hormone aldosterone is also under the influence of angiotensin. Corticotropin has some actions that do not depend upon its effect on adrenocortical secretion. However, its pharmacologic value as an anti-inflammatory agent and its use in testing adrenal function depend on its trophic action. Its pharmacology was discussed in Chapter 37 and will be reviewed only briefly here.

Antagonists of the synthesis or action of the adrenocortical steroids are important in the treatment of several tumors. These agents are described at the end of this chapter.

ADRENOCORTICOSTEROIDS

The adrenal cortex releases a large number of steroids into the circulation. Some have minimal biologic activity and function primarily as precursors, and there are some for which no function has been established. The hormonal steroids may be classified as those having important effects on intermediary metabolism (glucocorticoids), those having principally salt-retaining activity (mineralocorticoids), and those having androgenic or estrogenic activity (see Chapter 40). In humans, the major glucocorticoid is cortisol and the most important mineralocorticoid is aldosterone. Quantitatively, dehydroepiandrosterone (DHEA) is the major androgen, since about 20 mg is secreted daily, partly as the sulfate. However, both

DHEA and androstenedione are very weak androgens. A small amount of testosterone is secreted by the adrenal and may be of greater importance as an androgen. Little is known about the estrogens secreted by the adrenal. However, it has been shown that the adrenal androgens such as testosterone and androstenedione can be converted to estrone in small amounts by nonendocrine tissues and that they constitute the major endogenous source of estrogen in women after menopause and in some patients in whom ovarian function is abnormal.

THE NATURALLY OCCURRING GLUCOCORTICOIDS; CORTISOL (Hydrocortisone)

Pharmacokinetics

The major glucocorticoid in humans is cortisol. It is synthesized from cholesterol (as shown in Figure 39–1) by the cells of the zona fasciculata and zona reticularis and released into the circulation under the influence of ACTH. The mechanisms controlling its secretion are discussed in Chapter 37.

In the normal adult in the absence of stress, 10–20 mg of cortisol is secreted daily. The rate of secretion changes in a circadian rhythm governed by irregular pulses of ACTH that peak in the early morning hours and after meals and that are also influenced by light (Figure 39–2). In plasma, cortisol is bound to plasma proteins. Corticosteroid-binding globulin (CBG), an α_2-globulin synthesized by the liver, binds 75% of the circulating hormone under normal circumstances. The remainder is free (about 20%) or loosely bound to albumin (about 5%) and is available to exert its effect on target cells. When plasma cortisol levels exceed 20–30 μg/dL, CBG is saturated, and the concentration of free cortisol rises rapidly. CBG is increased in pregnancy and with estrogen administration, which increases its synthesis by the liver, and in

Figure 39–1. Outline of major pathways in adrenocortical hormone biosynthesis. The major secretory products are underlined. Pregnenolone is the major precursor of corticosterone and aldosterone, and 17-hydroxypregnenolone is the major precursor of cortisol. The enzymes and cofactors for the reactions progressing down each column are shown on the left and from the first to the second column at the top of the figure. When a particular enzyme is deficient, hormone production is blocked at the points indicated by the shaded bars. (Modified after Welikey et al; reproduced, with permission, from Ganong WF: *Review of Medical Physiology,* 17th ed. Appleton & Lange, 1995.)

hyperthyroidism. It is decreased by hypothyroidism, genetic defects in synthesis, and protein deficiency states. Albumin has a large capacity but low affinity for cortisol. Synthetic corticosteroids such as dexamethasone are largely bound to albumin.

The half-life of cortisol in the circulation is normally about 60–90 minutes; half-life may be increased when hydrocortisone (the pharmaceutical preparation of cortisol) is administered in large amounts or when stress, hypothyroidism, or liver disease is present. Only 1% of cortisol is excreted unchanged in the urine; about 20% of cortisol is converted to cortisone by 11-hydroxysteroid dehydrogenase in the kidney and other tissues with mineralocorticoid receptors (see below) before reaching the liver. Most of the cortisone and the remaining cortisol is inactivated in the liver by reduction of the 4,5 dou-

ble bond in the A ring and subsequent conversion to tetrahydrocortisol and tetrahydrocortisone by 3-hydroxysteroid dehydrogenase. (See Figure 39–4 for carbon numbering.) Some is converted to cortol and cortolone by reduction of the C_{20} ketone. There are small amounts of other metabolites. The side chain (C_{20} and C_{21}) is removed from about 5–10% of the cortisol, and the resulting compounds are further metabolized and excreted into the urine as 11-oxy, 17-ketosteroids. These metabolites are then conjugated with glucuronic acid or sulfate at the C_3 and C_{21} hydroxyls, respectively, in the liver; reenter the circulation; and are excreted into the urine.

In some species (eg, the rat), corticosterone is the major glucocorticoid. It is less firmly bound to protein and therefore metabolized more rapidly. The pathways of its degradation are similar to those of cortisol.

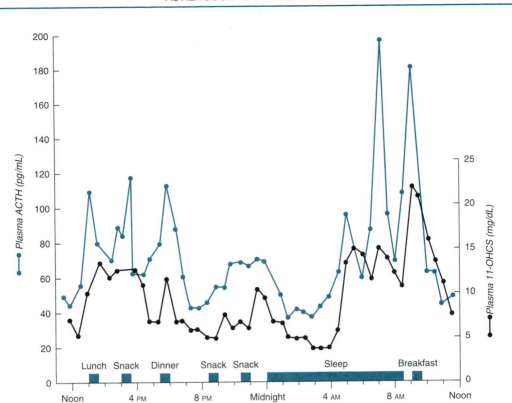

Figure 39–2. Fluctuations in plasma ACTH and glucocorticoids throughout the day in a normal girl (age 16). The ACTH was measured by immunoassay and the glucocorticoids as 11-oxysteroids *(11-OHCS)*. Note the greater ACTH and glucocorticoid rises in the morning, before awakening from sleep. (Reproduced, with permission, from Krieger DT et al: Characterization of the normal temporal pattern of plasma corticosteroid levels. J Clin Endocrinol Metab 1971;32:266.)

Pharmacodynamics

A. Mechanism of Action: Most of the known effects of the glucocorticoids are mediated by widely distributed glucocorticoid receptors. These proteins are members of a superfamily of receptors that includes steroid, thyroid, and many other receptors which regulate the transcription of target genes (Figure 39–3). The function of many of these receptors is unknown, and they are referred to as "orphan receptors."

Two genes for the glucocorticoid receptor have been identified. The receptors are bound to heat shock proteins (Hsp) and other proteins that stabilize them and prevent them from binding to DNA. The most important are the two molecules of Hsp90, though others may be involved. Free hormone in the plasma enters the cell and binds to the receptor, inducing conformational changes that allow dissociation from the heat shock proteins. The hormone-receptor complex forms homodimers and is actively transported to the nucleus, where it binds to glucocorticoid receptor elements (GRE) of the gene.

The GRE is composed of two parts that bind to the hormone receptor dimer, with the alpha helix between the zinc fingers of the receptor fitting into the DNA at the binding site. The receptor complex may also bind to other sites in the promoter region of the gene and form complexes with nuclear proteins (transcription factors), which may also bind to other promoter sites to contribute to the regulation of transcription.

There are estimated to be from 10 to 100 glucocorticoid target genes per cell, but not all of them are expressed in every cell. The number and variety of receptor sites and transcription factors as well as post-transcription events allows specificity of the hormone's actions in various cells. The genomic effects of glucocorticoids are mainly due to proteins synthesized in response to RNA transcribed by the target gene. However, some of the genomic effects may be indirectly mediated by the paracrine effects of hormone-regulated cytokines on neighboring cells.

Rapid effects such as rapid feedback suppression of pituitary ACTH occur in minutes and are too rapid to be explained on the basis of gene transcription and protein synthesis. It is not known how these effects are mediated. Among the mechanisms proposed are direct effects on the cell membrane function and membrane receptors for the hormone or the hormone-receptor complex. These membrane receptors differ from the intracellular receptor, though some may be isoforms that are inserted into the cell membrane.

Figure 39–3. A model of the interaction of a steroid, S (eg, cortisol), and its receptor, R, and the subsequent events in a target cell. The steroid is present in the blood in bound form on the corticosteroid-binding globulin, CBG, but enters the cell as the free molecule. The intracellular receptor is bound to stabilizing proteins, including two molecules of heat shock protein 90 (Hsp90) and several others, denoted as "X" in the figure. This receptor complex is incapable of activating transcription. When the complex binds a molecule of cortisol, an unstable complex is created and the Hsp90 and associated molecules are released. The steroid-receptor complex is able to enter the nucleus, bind to the glucocorticoid response element (GRE) on the gene, and regulate transcription by RNA polymerase II and associated transcription factors. A variety of regulatory factors (not shown) may participate in facilitating (or inhibiting) the steroid response. The resulting mRNA is edited and exported to the cytoplasm for the production of protein that brings about the final hormone response.

B. Physiologic Effects: The glucocorticoids have widespread effects because they influence the function of most cells in the body. The major metabolic consequences of glucocorticoid secretion or administration are due to direct actions of these hormones in the cell. However, some important effects are the result of homeostatic responses by insulin and glucagon. Although many of the effects are dose-related and become magnified when large amounts are administered for therapeutic purposes, there are also "permissive" effects. In other words, many normal reactions that take place at a significant rate only in the presence of corticoids are not further stimulated in the presence of larger amounts of corticoids. For example, the response of vascular and bronchial smooth muscle to catecholamines is diminished in the absence of cortisol and restored by physiologic amounts of this glucocorticoid. The lipolytic responses of fat cells to catecholamines, ACTH, and growth hormone are also attenuated in the absence of glucocorticoid. The mechanisms of these effects have not been determined.

C. Metabolic Effects: The glucocorticoids have important dose-related effects on carbohydrate, protein, and fat metabolism. The same effects are responsible for some of the serious adverse effects associated with their use in therapeutic doses. Glucocorticoids stimulate and are required for gluconeogenesis in the fasted state and in diabetes. Glucocorticoids also increase amino acid uptake by the liver and kidney and increase the activity of enzymes required for gluconeogenesis.

In the liver, glucocorticoids increase glycogen deposition by stimulating glycogen synthase activity and increasing glucose production from protein. The increase in serum glucose levels stimulates insulin release.

Glucocorticoids inhibit the uptake of glucose by fat cells, leading to increased lipolysis. However the increased insulin secretion mentioned above stimulates lipogenesis, leading to a net increase in fat deposition.

The net results of these actions are most apparent in the fasting state, when the supply of glucose from gluconeogenesis, the release of amino acids from muscle catabolism, the inhibition of peripheral glucose uptake, and the stimulation of lipolysis all contribute to the maintenance of an adequate glucose supply to the brain.

D. Catabolic Effects: Although glucocorticoids stimulate protein and RNA synthesis in the liver, they have catabolic effects in lymphoid and connective tissue, muscle, fat, and skin. Supraphysiologic amounts of glucocorticoids lead to decreased muscle mass and weakness. Catabolic effects on bone are the cause of osteoporosis in Cushing's syndrome and constitute a major limitation in the long-term therapeutic use of glucocorticoids. In children, the catabolic effects of excessive amounts of glucocorticoid reduce growth. This effect is not prevented by growth hormone.

E. Anti-inflammatory and Immunosuppressive Effects: Glucocorticoids have the capacity to dramatically reduce the manifestations of inflammation. This is due to their profound effects on the concentration, distribution, and function of peripheral leukocytes. Inflammation, regardless of etiology, is characterized by the extravasation and infiltration of leukocytes into the affected tissue. These events are mediated by a complex series of interactions with cell adhesion molecules, particularly those on endothelial cells, and are inhibited by glucocorticoids. After a single dose of a short-acting glucocorticoid, the concentration of neutrophils increases while the lymphocytes (T and B cells), monocytes, eosinophils, and basophils in the circulation decrease in number. The changes are maximal at 6 hours and are dissipated in 24 hours. The increase in neutrophils is due both to the increased influx into the blood from the bone marrow and decreased migration from the blood vessels, leading to a reduction in the number of cells at the site of inflammation. The reduction in circulating lymphocytes, monocytes, eosinophils, and basophils is the result of their movement from the vascular bed to lymphoid tissue.

Glucocorticoids also inhibit the functions of leukocytes and tissue macrophages. The ability of these cells to respond to antigens and mitogens is reduced. The effect on macrophages is particularly marked and limits their ability to phagocytose and kill microorganisms and to produce interferon-γ, interleukin-1, pyrogen, collagenase, elastase, tumor necrosis factor, and plasminogen activator. Lymphocytes produce less interleukin-2. Although the evidence is conflicting, large doses of glucocorticoids have also been reported to stabilize lysosomal membranes, thereby reducing the concentration of proteolytic enzymes at the site of inflammation.

In addition to their effects on leukocyte function, glucocorticoids influence the inflammatory response by reducing the prostaglandin and leukotriene synthesis that results from activation of phospholipase A_2. Glucocorticoids increase the concentration of certain membrane phospholipids that appear to inhibit prostaglandin and leukotriene synthesis. Cortico-

steroids also increase the concentration of lipocortins, members of the annexin family of proteins that reduce the availability of the phospholipid substrates of phospholipase A_2. Finally, glucocorticoids reduce expression of cyclooxygenase in inflammatory cells, thus reducing the amount of enzyme available to produce prostaglandins. Recent evidence suggests that genes exist for two isoforms of cyclooxygenase: COX I and COX II (Chapter 18). Glucocorticoids inhibit expression of COX II, the enzyme more involved in the inflammatory effects of eicosanoids. They have much less effect on the expression of COX I.

Glucocorticoids cause vasoconstriction when applied directly to vessels. They decrease capillary permeability by inhibiting the activity of kinins and bacterial endotoxins and by reducing the amount of histamine released by basophils.

The anti-immune effect of glucocorticoids is largely due to the effects described above. In humans, complement activation is unaltered, but its effects are inhibited. Antibody production can be reduced by large doses of steroids, though it is unaffected by moderate dosages (eg, 20 mg/d of prednisone). However, inhibition of the production and effects of interleukin-2 and blockade of the effects of migration inhibition factor and macrophage inhibition factor impair delayed hypersensitivity reactions. The efficacy of these steroids in the control of transplant rejection is augmented by their ability to reduce antigen release from the grafted tissue, delay revascularization, and interfere with the sensitization of antibody-forming cells.

The anti-inflammatory and immunosuppressive effects of these agents are widely useful therapeutically but are also responsible for some of their most serious adverse effects (see below).

F. Other Effects: Glucocorticoids have important effects on the nervous system. Adrenal insufficiency causes marked slowing of the alpha rhythm of the EEG. Increased amounts lower the threshold for electrically induced convulsions in rats and often produce behavioral disturbances in humans. Large doses of glucocorticoids may rarely increase intracranial pressure (pseudotumor cerebri).

Glucocorticoids suppress the pituitary release of ACTH and beta-lipotropin but do not decrease circulating levels of beta-endorphin (see Chapter 37). They also reduce secretion of TSH and FSH.

Large doses of glucocorticoids stimulate excessive production of acid and pepsin in the stomach and facilitate the development of peptic ulcer. They promote fat absorption and appear to antagonize the effect of vitamin D on calcium absorption. The glucocorticoids also have important effects on the hematopoietic system. In addition to their effects on leukocytes described above, they increase the number of platelets and red blood cells.

In the absence of physiologic amounts of cortisol, renal function (particularly glomerular filtration) is impaired and there is an inability to excrete a water load normally.

Glucocorticoids also have some effects on the development of the fetus. The structural and functional changes in the lungs near term, including the production of pulmonary surface-active material required for air breathing (surfactant), are stimulated by glucocorticoids.

SYNTHETIC ADRENOCORTICOSTEROIDS

ACTH and steroids having glucocorticoid activity have become important agents for use in the treatment of many inflammatory and allergic disorders. This has stimulated the development of many synthetic steroids with anti-inflammatory activity.

Pharmacokinetics

A. Source: Although the natural corticosteroids can be obtained from animal adrenals, pharmaceutical steroids are usually synthesized from cholic acid (obtained from cattle) or steroid sapogenins, diosgenin in particular, that are found in plants of the Liliaceae and Dioscoreaceae families. Further modifications of these steroids have led to the marketing of a large group of synthetic steroids with special characteristics that are pharmacologically and therapeutically important (Table 39–1; Figure 39–4).

B. Disposition: The metabolism of the naturally occurring adrenal steroids has been discussed above. The synthetic corticosteroids for oral use (Table 39–1) are in most cases rapidly and completely absorbed when given by mouth. Although they are transported and metabolized in a fashion similar to that of the endogenous steroids, important differences exist.

Alterations in the molecule influence its affinity for glucocorticoid and mineralocorticoid receptors as well as its protein-binding avidity, side chain stability, rate of reduction, and metabolic products. Halogenation at the 9 position, unsaturation of the $\Delta1$–2 bond of the A ring, and methylation at the 2 or 16 position will prolong the half-life by more than 50%. The 11-hydroxyl group also appears to inhibit destruction, since the half-life of 11-deoxycortisol is half that of cortisol. The $\Delta1$ compounds are excreted in the free form. In some cases, the agent given is a prodrug—eg, prednisone is rapidly converted to prednisolone in the body.

Pharmacodynamics

The actions of the synthetic steroids are similar to those of cortisol (see above). They bind to the specific intracellular receptor proteins and produce the same

Table 39–1. Some commonly used natural and synthetic corticosteroids for general use.

Agent	Anti-inflam-matory	Activity[1] Topical	Salt-Retaining	Equivalent Oral Dose (mg)	Forms Available
Short- to medium-acting glucocorticoids					
Hydrocortisone (cortisol)	1	1	1	20	Oral, injectable, topical
Cortisone	0.8	0	0.8	25	Oral, injectable, topical
Prednisone	4	0	0.3	5	Oral
Prednisolone	5	4	0.3	5	Oral, injectable, topical
Methylprednisolone	5	5	0	4	Oral, injectable, topical
Meprednisone[2]	5		0	4	Oral, injectable
Intermediate-acting glucocorticoids					
Triamcinolone	5	5[3]	0	4	Oral, injectable, topical
Paramethasone[2]	10		0	2	Oral, injectable
Fluprednisolone	15	7	0	1.5	Oral
Long-acting glucocorticoids					
Betamethasone	25–40	10	0	0.6	Oral, injectable, topical
Dexamethasone	30	10	0	0.75	Oral, injectable, topical
Mineralocorticoids					
Fludrocortisone	10	10	250	2	Oral, injectable, topical
Desoxycorticosterone acetate	0	0	20		Injectable, pellets

[1]Potency relative to hydrocortisone.
[2]Outside USA.
[3]Acetonide: Up to 100.

Figure 39–4. Chemical structures of several glucocorticoids. The acetonide-substituted derivatives (eg, triamcinolone acetonide) have increased surface activity and are useful in dermatology. Dexamethasone is identical to betamethasone except for the configuration of the methyl group at C_{16}: in betamethasone it is beta (projecting *up* from the plane of the rings); in dexamethasone it is alpha.

effects but have different ratios of glucocorticoid to mineralocorticoid potency (Table 39–1).

Clinical Pharmacology

A. Diagnosis and Treatment of Disturbed Adrenal Function:

1. Adrenocortical insufficiency–

a. Chronic (Addison's disease)–Chronic adrenocortical insufficiency is characterized by hyperpigmentation, weakness, fatigue, weight loss, hypotension, and inability to maintain the blood glucose level during fasting. In such individuals, minor noxious, traumatic, or infectious stimuli may produce acute adrenal insufficiency with shock and finally death.

In adrenal insufficiency, whether primary or following adrenalectomy, about 20–30 mg of cortisol must be given daily, with increased amounts during periods of stress. Although cortisol has some mineralocorticoid activity, this must be supplemented by an appropriate amount of salt-retaining hormone such as fludrocortisone. It is for this reason that glucocorticoids devoid of salt-retaining activity are not used in these patients.

b. Acute–When acute adrenocortical insufficiency is suspected, treatment must be instituted immediately. In addition to large amounts of parenteral cortisol, therapy includes correction of fluid and elec-

trolyte abnormalities and treatment of precipitating factors.

Cortisol hemisuccinate or phosphate in doses of 100 mg intravenously is given every 6–8 hours until the patient is stable. The dose is then gradually reduced, achieving maintenance dosage in 5 days. The administration of salt-retaining hormone is resumed when the total cortisol dosage has been reduced to 50 mg/d.

2. Adrenocortical hyperfunction–

a. Congenital adrenal hyperplasia–This group of disorders is characterized by specific defects in the synthesis of cortisol. In pregnancies at high risk for congenital adrenal hyperplasia, fetuses can be protected from genital abnormalities by administration of dexamethasone to the mother. The most common defect is a decrease in or lack of P450c21 (21β-hydroxylase) activity.* As can be seen in Figure 39–1, this would lead to a reduction in cortisol synthesis and produce a compensatory increase in ACTH release. If

---

*Names for the adrenal steroid synthetic enzymes include the following:

P450c11 (11β-hydroxylase)
P450c17 (17α-hydroxylase)
P450c21 (21β-hydroxylase)

sufficient enzyme activity is present, a normal amount of cortisol will be produced in response to the increased level of ACTH, but the gland will become hyperplastic and produce abnormally large amounts of precursors such as 17-hydroxyprogesterone that can be diverted to the androgen pathway, leading to virilization. Metabolism of this compound in the liver leads to pregnanetriol, which is characteristically excreted into the urine in large amounts in this disorder and can be used to make the diagnosis. However, the most reliable method of detecting this disorder is the increased response of plasma 17-hydroxyprogesterone to ACTH stimulation.

If the defect is in 11-hydroxylation, large amounts of desoxycorticosterone are produced and hypertension is prominent. When 17-hydroxylation is defective in the adrenals and gonads, hypogonadism will be present. However, increased amounts of 11-desoxycorticosterone (DOC; see below) are formed, and the signs and symptoms associated with mineralocorticoid excess—such as hypertension and hypokalemia—are also found.

When first seen, the infant with congenital adrenal hyperplasia may be in an acute adrenal crisis and should be treated as described above using an intravenous preparation of cortisol, mineralocorticoid, and appropriate electrolyte solutions as required. Once the patient is stabilized, hydrocortisone, 12–18 mg/m²/d in three divided doses is begun. The dosage is then adjusted to allow normal growth and bone maturation and to prevent androgen excess. Alternate-day therapy with prednisone has also been used to achieve greater ACTH suppression without increasing growth inhibition. Salt-losing patients also require fludrocortisone, 0.05–0.1 mg/d by mouth, and added salt to maintain normal blood pressure, plasma renin activity, and electrolytes.

b. Cushing's syndrome–Cushing's syndrome is usually the result of bilateral adrenal hyperplasia secondary to a pituitary adenoma (Cushing's disease) but occasionally is due to tumors or nodular hyperplasia of the adrenal gland or ectopic production of ACTH by other tumors. The manifestations are those associated with the presence of excessive glucocorticoids. When changes are marked, a rounded, plethoric face and trunk obesity are striking in appearance. The manifestations of protein loss are often found and include muscle wasting, thinning of the skin, striae, easy bruisability, poor wound healing, and osteoporosis. Other serious disturbances include mental disorders, hypertension, and diabetes. This disorder is treated by surgical removal of the tumor producing the hormone, irradiation or removal of a pituitary microadenoma producing ACTH, or resection of hyperplastic adrenals. These patients must receive large doses of cortisol during and following the surgical procedure. Doses of 300 mg of soluble hydrocortisone are given as a continuous intravenous infusion on the day of surgery. The dose must be reduced

slowly to normal replacement levels, since rapid reduction in dose may produce symptoms, including fever and joint pain. If adrenalectomy has been performed, long-term maintenance is similar to that outlined above for adrenal insufficiency.

c. Aldosteronism–Primary aldosteronism usually results from the excessive production of aldosterone by an adrenal adenoma. However, it may also result from abnormal secretion by hyperplastic glands or from a malignant tumor. The clinical findings of hypertension, polyuria, polydipsia, weakness, and tetany are related to the continued renal loss of potassium, which leads to hypokalemia, alkalosis, and hypernatremia. This syndrome can also be produced in disorders of adrenal steroid biosynthesis by excessive secretion of desoxycorticosterone, corticosterone, or 18-hydroxycorticosterone.

In contrast to patients with secondary aldosteronism (see below), these patients have low (suppressed) levels of plasma renin activity and angiotensin II. When treated with desoxycorticosterone acetate (20 mg/d intramuscularly for 3 days) or fludrocortisone (0.2 mg twice daily orally for 3 days), they fail to retain sodium and their secretion of aldosterone is not significantly reduced. When the disorder is mild, it may escape detection when serum potassium levels are used for screening. However, it may be detected by an increased ratio of plasma aldosterone to renin. Patients are generally improved when treated with spironolactone, and the response to this agent is of diagnostic and therapeutic value.

3. Use of glucocorticoids for diagnostic purposes–It is sometimes necessary to suppress the production of ACTH in order to identify the source of a particular hormone or to establish whether its production is influenced by the secretion of ACTH. In these circumstances, it is advantageous to employ a very potent substance such as dexamethasone because the use of small quantities reduces the possibility of confusion in the interpretation of hormone assays in blood or urine. For example, if complete suppression is achieved by the use of 50 mg of cortisol, the urinary 17-hydroxycorticosteroids will be 15–18 mg/24 h, since one-third of the dose given will be recovered in urine as 17-hydroxycorticosteroid. If an equivalent dose of 1.5 mg of dexamethasone is employed, the urinary excretion will be only 0.5 mg/24 h and blood levels will be low.

The **dexamethasone suppression test** is used for the diagnosis of Cushing's syndrome and has also been used in the differential diagnosis of depressive psychiatric states. Dexamethasone, 1 mg, is given orally at 11 PM, and a plasma sample is obtained in the morning. In normal individuals, the morning cortisol concentration is usually less than 5 μg/dL, whereas in Cushing's syndrome the level is usually greater than 10 μg/dL. The results are not reliable in the presence of depression, anxiety, illness, and other stressful conditions. However, in patients in whom the diagnosis of Cushing's syndrome has been established clinically and confirmed by a finding of elevated urine free cortisol, suppression with large doses of dexamethasone will help to distinguish patients with Cushing's disease from those with steroid-producing tumors of the adrenal cortex or with the ectopic ACTH syndrome. Dexamethasone is given in a dosage of 2 mg orally every 6 hours for 2 days and the urine assayed for cortisol or its metabolites—or dexamethasone is given as a single dose of 8 mg at 11 PM and the plasma cortisol is measured at 8 AM the following day. In patients with Cushing's disease, the suppressant effect of dexamethasone will usually produce a 50% reduction in hormone levels. In patients in whom suppression does not occur, the ACTH level will be low in the presence of a cortisol-producing adrenal tumor and elevated in patients with an ectopic ACTH-producing tumor.

Suppression of the adrenal with glucocorticoids and of the ovary with estrogens can be useful in locating the source of androgen production in a hirsute woman if the effect on androgen levels in blood can be measured before and during hormone administration.

B. Adrenocorticosteroids and Stimulation of Lung Maturation in the Fetus:
Lung maturation in the fetus is regulated by the fetal secretion of cortisol. Treatment of the mother with large doses of glucocorticoid reduces the incidence of respiratory distress syndrome in infants delivered prematurely. When delivery is anticipated before 34 weeks of ges-

tation, betamethasone, 12 mg, followed by an additional dose of 12 mg 18–24 hours later, is commonly used. Protein binding of this corticosteroid is less than that of cortisol, allowing increased transfer across the placenta to the fetus. Corticosteroid levels achieved in the fetus are equivalent to those observed when the fetus is stressed.

C. Adrenocorticosteroids and Nonadrenal Disorders:
Cortisol and its synthetic analogs are useful in the treatment of a diverse group of diseases unrelated to any known disturbance of adrenal function (Table 39–2). The usefulness of corticosteroids in these disorders is a function of their ability to suppress inflammatory and immune responses, as described above. In disorders in which host response is the cause of the major manifestations of the disease, these agents are useful. In instances where the inflammatory or immune response is important in controlling the pathologic process, therapy with corticosteroids may be dangerous but justified to prevent irreparable damage from an inflammatory response—if used in conjunction with specific therapy for the disease process.

Since the corticosteroids are not usually curative, the pathologic process may progress while clinical manifestations are suppressed. Therefore, chronic therapy with these drugs should be undertaken with great care and only when the seriousness of the disorder warrants their use and less hazardous measures have been exhausted.

Table 39–2. Some therapeutic indications for the use of glucocorticoids in nonadrenal disorders.

Disorder	Examples
Allergic reactions	Angioneurotic edema, asthma, bee stings, contact dermatitis, drug reactions, allergic rhinitis, serum sickness, urticaria
Collagen-vascular disorders	Giant cell arteritis, lupus erythematosus, mixed connective tissue syndromes, polymyositis, polymyalgia rheumatica, rheumatoid arthritis, temporal arteritis
Eye diseases	Acute uveitis, allergic conjunctivitis, choroiditis, optic neuritis
Gastrointestinal diseases	Inflammatory bowel disease, nontropical sprue, subacute hepatic necrosis
Hematologic disorders	Acquired hemolytic anemia, acute allergic purpura, leukemia, autoimmune hemolytic anemia, idiopathic thrombocytopenic purpura, multiple myeloma
Infections	Gram-negative septicemia; occasionally helpful to suppress excessive inflammation
Inflammatory conditions of bones and joints	Arthritis, bursitis, tenosynovitis
Neurologic disorders	Cerebral edema (large doses of dexamethasone are given to patients following brain surgery to minimize cerebral edema in the postoperative period), multiple sclerosis
Organ transplants	Prevention and treatment of rejection (immunosuppression)
Pulmonary diseases	Aspiration pneumonia, bronchial asthma, prevention of infant respiratory distress syndrome, sarcoidosis
Renal disorders	Nephrotic syndrome
Skin diseases	Atopic dermatitis, dermatoses, lichen simplex chronicus (localized neurodermatitis), mycosis fungoides, pemphigus, seborrheic dermatitis, xerosis
Thyroid diseases	Malignant exophthalmos, subacute thyroiditis
Miscellaneous	Hypercalcemia, mountain sickness

In general, attempts should be made to bring the disease process under control using short-acting glucocorticoids as well as all ancillary measures possible to keep the dose low. Where possible, alternate-day therapy should be utilized (see below). Therapy should not be decreased or stopped abruptly. When prolonged therapy is anticipated, it is helpful to obtain chest x-rays and a tuberculin test. The presence of diabetes, peptic ulcer, osteoporosis, and psychologic disturbances should be excluded, and cardiovascular function should be assessed.

The following supplemental measures should be considered: The diet should be rich in potassium and low in sodium to prevent electrolyte disturbances. Caloric management to prevent obesity should be instituted. High protein intake is required to compensate for the loss due to the increased breakdown of protein from gluconeogenesis. Antacids should be used three or four times daily in patients prone to epigastric distress. Osteoporosis is caused by depressed bone formation in the presence of unaltered ongoing bone resorption, and parathyroid hormone and vitamin D changes are not involved. Physical therapy and androgens have been recommended to limit glucocorticoid-induced osteoporosis but are not of proved value. However, adequate calcium and Vitamin D and treatment with a bisphosphonate such as alendronate may prove useful in the prevention of osteoporosis and should be considered in patients receiving or expected to take high doses of glucocorticoid for more than a few months (see Chapter 42).

Toxicity

The benefits obtained from use of the glucocorticoids vary considerably. They must be carefully weighed in each patient against the widespread effects on every part of the organism. The major undesirable effects of the glucocorticoids are the result of their hormonal actions (see above) and lead to the clinical picture of iatrogenic Cushing's syndrome.

When the glucocorticoids are used for short periods (less than 1 week), it is unusual to see serious adverse effects even with moderately large doses. However, behavioral changes and acute peptic ulcers are occasionally observed even after a few days of treatment.

A. Metabolic Effects: Most patients who are given daily doses of 100 mg of cortisol or more (or the equivalent amount of synthetic steroid) for longer than 2 weeks undergo a series of changes that have been termed iatrogenic Cushing's syndrome. The rate of development is a function of the dose. The appearance of the face is altered by rounding, puffiness, and plethora. Fat tends to be redistributed from the extremities to the trunk and face. There is an increased growth of fine hair over the thighs and trunk and sometimes the face. Acne may increase or appear, and insomnia and increased appetite are noted. In the treatment of dangerous or disabling disorders, these changes may not require cessation of therapy. However, the underlying metabolic changes accompanying them can be very serious by the time they become obvious. The continuing breakdown of protein and diversion of amino acids to glucose production increase the need for insulin and over a period of time result in weight gain; fat deposition; muscle wasting; thinning of the skin, with striae and bruising; hyperglycemia; and eventually the development of osteoporosis, diabetes, and aseptic necrosis of the hip. Wound healing is also impaired under these circumstances. When diabetes occurs, it is treated by diet and insulin. These patients are often resistant to insulin but rarely develop ketoacidosis. In general, patients treated with corticosteroids should be on high-protein diets, and increased potassium and anabolic steroids should be used when required.

B. Other Complications: Other serious complications include the development of peptic ulcers and their complications. The clinical findings associated with other disorders, particularly bacterial and mycotic infections, may be masked by the corticosteroids, and patients must be carefully watched to avoid serious mishap when large doses are used. Some patients develop a myopathy the nature of which is unknown. The frequency of myopathy is greater in patients treated with triamcinolone. The administration of this drug as well as of methylprednisolone has been associated with nausea, dizziness, and weight loss in some patients. It is treated by changing drugs, reducing dosage, and increasing the potassium and protein intake.

Psychosis may occur, particularly in patients receiving large doses of corticosteroids. Long-term therapy is associated with the development of posterior subcapsular cataracts. Periodic slitlamp examination is indicated in such patients. Increased intraocular pressure is common, and glaucoma may be induced. Benign intracranial hypertension also occurs. In dosages of 45 mg/m^2/d or more, growth retardation occurs in children.

When given in greater than physiologic amounts, steroids such as cortisone and hydrocortisone, which have mineralocorticoid effects in addition to glucocorticoid effects, cause some sodium and fluid retention and loss of potassium. In patients with normal cardiovascular and renal function, this leads to a hypokalemic, hypochloremic alkalosis and eventually a rise in blood pressure. In patients with hypoproteinemia, renal disease, or liver disease, edema may also occur. In patients with heart disease, even small degrees of sodium retention may lead to congestive heart failure. These effects can be minimized by sodium restriction and judicious use of potassium supplements.

C. Adrenal Suppression: When corticosteroids are administered for more than a few days, adrenal suppression occurs. If treatment extends over weeks to months, the patient should be given supplementary therapy at times of severe stress such as accidental trauma or surgery. If corticoid dosage is to be reduced, it should be tapered slowly. If therapy is to be stopped, the reduction process should be quite slow when the dose reaches replacement levels. It will take 2–3 months for the pituitary to become responsive, and cortisol levels may not return to normal for another 6–9 months. Treatment with ACTH does not significantly reduce the time required for the return of normal function.

If the dose is reduced too rapidly in such patients, the symptoms of the disorder may reappear or increase in intensity. However, patients without an underlying disorder (eg, with treated Cushing's disease) will also become symptomatic with rapid reductions in corticoid levels. These symptoms include anorexia, nausea or vomiting, weight loss, lethargy, headache, fever, joint or muscle pain, and postural hypotension. Although many of these symptoms suggest adrenal insufficiency, they may occur in the presence of normal or even elevated plasma cortisol levels.

Contraindications & Cautions

A. Special Precautions: Patients receiving these drugs must be observed carefully for the development of hyperglycemia, glycosuria, sodium retention with edema or hypertension, hypokalemia, peptic ulcer, osteoporosis, and hidden infections.

The dosage should be kept as low as possible and intermittent dosage (eg, alternate-day) employed when satisfactory therapeutic results can be obtained on this schedule. Even patients being maintained on relatively low doses of corticosteroids may require supplementary therapy at times of stress such as when surgical procedures are performed or accidents occur.

B. Contraindications: These agents must be used with great caution in patients with peptic ulcer, heart disease or hypertension with congestive heart failure, infections, psychoses, diabetes, osteoporosis, glaucoma, or herpes simplex infection.

Selection of Drug & Dosage Schedule

Since these preparations differ with respect to relative anti-inflammatory and mineralocorticoid effect (Table 39–1), duration of action, cost, and dosage forms available, these factors should be taken into account in selecting the drug to be used.

A. ACTH Versus Adrenocortical Steroids: In patients with normal adrenals, ACTH has been used to induce the endogenous production of cortisol to obtain similar effects. However, except when the increase in androgens is desirable, the use of ACTH as a therapeutic agent is probably unjustified. Instances in which ACTH has been claimed to be more effective than glucocorticoids are probably due to the administration of smaller amounts of corticoids than were produced by the dosage of ACTH.

B. Dosage: In determining the dosage regimen to be used, the physician must consider the seriousness of the disease, the amount of drug likely to be required to obtain the desired effect, and the duration of therapy. In some diseases, the amount required for maintenance of the desired therapeutic effect is less than the dose needed to obtain the initial effect, and the lowest possible dosage for the needed effect should be determined by gradually lowering the dose until an increase in signs or symptoms is noted.

Many types of dosage schedules have been used in administering glucocorticoids. When it is necessary to maintain continuously elevated plasma corticosteroid levels in order to suppress ACTH, a slowly absorbed parenteral preparation or small doses at frequent intervals are required. The opposite situation exists with respect to the use of corticosteroids in the treatment of inflammatory and allergic disorders. The same total quantity given in a few doses may be more effective than when given in many smaller doses or in a slowly absorbed parenteral form.

Severe autoimmune conditions involving vital organs must be treated aggressively, and undertreatment is as dangerous as overtreatment. In order to minimize the deposition of immune complexes and the influx of leukocytes and macrophages, 1 mg/kg/d of prednisone in divided doses is required initially. This dose is maintained until the serious manifestations respond. The dose can then be gradually reduced.

When large doses are required for prolonged periods of time, **alternate-day** administration of the compound may be tried after control is achieved. When used in this manner, very large amounts (eg, 100 mg of prednisone) can sometimes be administered with less marked adverse effects because there is a recovery period between each dose. The transition to an alternate-day schedule can be made after the disease process is under control. It should be done gradually and with additional supportive measures between doses. A typical schedule for a patient maintained on 50 mg of prednisone daily would be as follows:

Day 1: 50 mg	Day 7: 75 mg
2: 40 mg	8: 5 mg
3: 60 mg	9: 70 mg
4: 30 mg	10: 5 mg
5: 70 mg	11: 65 mg
6: 10 mg	12: 5 mg, etc

When selecting a drug for use in large doses, a shorter-acting synthetic steroid with little mineralocorticoid effect is advisable. If possible, it should be given as a single morning dose.

Methylprednisolone in doses of 1 g given intravenously over 30–60 minutes at monthly intervals has been reported to be useful in treatment of rheumatoid arthritis in a few cases. The indications for this mode of therapy are not established.

C. Special Dosage Forms: The use of local therapy such as topical preparations for skin disease, ophthalmic forms for eye disease, intra-articular injections for joint disease, and hydrocortisone enemas for ulcerative colitis provides a means of delivering large amounts of steroid to the diseased tissue with reduced systemic effects.

Similarly, beclomethasone dipropionate and several other glucocorticoids administered as aerosols have been found to be effective in the treatment of asthma (see Chapter 20). The switch from therapy with systemic glucocorticoids to aerosol therapy must be undertaken with caution, since adrenal insufficiency will occur if adrenal function has been suppressed. In such patients, a slow, graded reduction of systemic therapy and monitoring of endogenous adrenal function should accompany the institution of aerosol administration.

Beclomethasone dipropionate, triamcinolone acetonide, and flunisolide are available as nasal sprays for the topical treatment of allergic rhinitis. They are effective at doses (one or two sprays two or three times daily) that in most patients result in plasma levels too low to influence adrenal function.

Corticosteroids incorporated in ointments, creams, lotions, and sprays are used extensively in dermatology. These preparations are discussed in more detail in Chapter 62.

MINERALOCORTICOIDS (Aldosterone, Desoxycorticosterone, Fludrocortisone)

The most important mineralocorticoid in humans is aldosterone. However, small amounts of desoxycorticosterone (DOC) are also formed and released. Although the amounts are normally insignificant, DOC was of some importance therapeutically in the past. Its actions, effects, and metabolism are similar to those described below for aldosterone. Fludrocortisone, a synthetic corticosteroid, is the most commonly prescribed salt-retaining hormone.

1. ALDOSTERONE

Aldosterone is synthesized mainly in the zona glomerulosa of the adrenal cortex. Its structure and synthesis are illustrated in Figure 39–1.

The rate of aldosterone secretion is subject to several influences. ACTH produces a moderate stimulation of its release, but this effect is not sustained for more than a few days in the normal individual. Although aldosterone is no less than one-third as effective as cortisol in suppressing ACTH, the quantities of aldosterone produced by the adrenal cortex are insufficient to participate in any significant feedback control of ACTH secretion.

After hypophysectomy and total elimination of ACTH, aldosterone secretion gradually falls to about half the normal rate, which means that other factors,

eg, angiotensin, are able to maintain and perhaps regulate its secretion (see Chapter 17). Independent variations between cortisol and aldosterone secretion can also be demonstrated by means of lesions in the nervous system such as decerebration, which decreases the secretion of hydrocortisone while increasing the secretion of aldosterone.

Physiologic & Pharmacologic Effects

Aldosterone and other steroids with mineralocorticoid properties promote the reabsorption of sodium from urine by the distal renal tubules, loosely coupled to the secretion of potassium and hydrogen ion. Sodium reabsorption in the sweat and salivary glands, gastrointestinal mucosa, and across cell membranes in general is also increased. Excessive levels of aldosterone produced by tumors or overdosage with other mineralocorticoids lead to hypernatremia, hypokalemia, metabolic alkalosis, increased plasma volume, and hypertension.

Mineralocorticoids act by binding to the mineralocorticoid receptor in the cytoplasm of target cells, especially principal cells of the collecting tubules of the kidney. The drug-receptor complex activates a series of events similar to those described above for the glucocorticoids and illustrated in Figure 39–3. It is of interest that this receptor has the same affinity for cortisol, which is present in higher concentrations in the extracellular fluid. The specificity for mineralocorticoids at this site appears to be conferred, at least in part, by the presence of the enzyme 11β-hydroxysteroid dehydrogenase, which converts cortisol to cortisone, which has low affinity for the receptor.

Metabolism

Aldosterone is secreted at the rate of 100–200 µg/d in normal individuals with a moderate dietary salt intake. The plasma level in males (resting supine) is about 0.007 µg/dL. The half-life of aldosterone injected in tracer quantities is 15–20 minutes, and it does not appear to be firmly bound to serum proteins.

The metabolism of aldosterone is similar to that of cortisol, about 50 µg/24 h appearing in the urine as conjugated tetrahydroaldosterone. Approximately 5–15 µg/24 h is excreted free or as the 3-oxo glucuronide.

2. DESOXYCORTICOSTERONE (DOC)

DOC, which also serves as a precursor of aldosterone (Figure 39–1), is normally secreted in amounts of about 200 µg/d. Its half-life when injected into the human circulation is about 70 minutes. Preliminary estimates of its concentration in plasma are approximately 0.03 µg/dL. The control of its secretion differs from that of aldosterone in that the secretion of DOC is primarily under the control of ACTH. Although the response to ACTH is enhanced by dietary sodium restriction, a low-salt diet does not increase DOC secretion. The secretion of DOC may be markedly increased in abnormal conditions such as adrenal carcinoma and congenital adrenal hyperplasia with reduced P450c11 or P450c17 activity.

3. FLUDROCORTISONE

This compound, a potent steroid with both glucocorticoid and mineralocorticoid activity, is the most widely used mineralocorticoid. Doses of 0.1 mg two to seven times weekly have potent salt-retaining activity and are used in the treatment of adrenocortical insufficiency but are too small to have important anti-inflammatory effects.

ADRENAL ANDROGENS

The adrenal cortex secretes large amounts of dehydroepiandrosterone (DHEA) and smaller amounts of androstenedione and testosterone. Although these androgens are thought to contribute to the normal maturation process, they do not stimulate or support androgen-dependent pubertal changes in humans. Re-

cent studies suggest that DHEA and DHEA sulfate (DHEAS) have other important metabolic effects mediated by liver enzymes. These effects inhibit weight gain and atherosclerosis and prolong life in experimental animals (rabbits). The therapeutic use of DHEA in humans is being explored, but the substance has already been adopted with uncritical enthusiasm by members of the sports drug culture and the vitamin and food supplement culture.

ANTAGONISTS OF ADRENOCORTICAL AGENTS

SYNTHESIS INHIBITORS & GLUCOCORTICOID ANTAGONISTS

1. METYRAPONE

Metyrapone (Figure 39–5) is a relatively selective inhibitor of steroid synthesis. It inhibits 11-hydroxylation, interfering with cortisol and corticosterone

Figure 39–5. Some adrenocortical antagonists. Because of their toxicity, several of these compounds are no longer available in the USA.

synthesis and leading to secretion of 11-deoxycortisol. In the presence of a normal pituitary gland, there is a compensatory increase in 11-deoxycortisol production. This response is a measure of the capacity of the anterior pituitary to produce ACTH and has been adapted for clinical use as a diagnostic test. Although the toxicity of metyrapone is much lower than that of mitotane and amphenone B (see below), the drug does produce transient dizziness and gastrointestinal disturbances. This agent has not been widely used for the treatment of Cushing's syndrome. However, in doses of 0.25 g twice daily to 1 g four times daily, metyrapone can reduce cortisol production to normal levels in some patients with adrenal tumors, ectopic ACTH syndromes, and hyperplasia. It may be useful in the management of severe manifestations of cortisol excess while the cause is being determined or in conjunction with radiation or surgical treatment. The major adverse effects observed are salt and water retention and hirsutism resulting from diversion of precursor to DOC and androgen synthesis.

Metyrapone is most commonly used in tests of adrenal function. The blood levels of 11-deoxycortisol and the urinary excretion of 17-hydroxycorticoids are measured before and after administration of the compound. Normally, there is a twofold or greater increase in the urinary 17-hydroxycorticoid excretion. A dose of 300–500 mg every 4 hours for six doses is commonly used, and urine collections are made on the day before and the day after treatment. In patients with Cushing's syndrome, a normal response to metyrapone indicates that the cortisol excess is not the result of adrenal carcinoma or autonomous adenoma, since secretion by such tumors produces suppression of ACTH and atrophy of normal adrenal cortex.

Adrenal function may also be tested by administering metyrapone, 2–3 g orally at midnight, and measuring the level of ACTH or 11-deoxycortisol in blood drawn at 8 AM, or by comparing the excretion of 17-hydroxycorticosteroids in the urine during the 24-hour periods preceding and following administration of the drug. In patients with suspected or known lesions of the pituitary, this procedure is a means of estimating the ability of the gland to produce ACTH. The response is inhibited by oral contraceptives.

2. AMINOGLUTETHIMIDE

Aminoglutethimide (Figure 39–5) blocks the conversion of cholesterol to pregnenolone and causes a reduction in the synthesis of all hormonally active steroids (Figure 39–1). It has been used in conjunction with dexamethasone or hydrocortisone to reduce or eliminate estrogen and androgen production in patients with carcinoma of the breast. In a dosage of 1 g/d it was well tolerated; however, with higher dosages, lethargy was a common effect. This drug can be used in conjunction with ketoconazole to reduce steroid secretion in patients with Cushing's syndrome due to adrenocortical cancer who do not respond to mitotane.

Aminoglutethimide also apparently increases the clearance of some steroids. It has been shown to enhance the metabolism of dexamethasone, reducing its half-life from 264 minutes to 120 minutes.

3. KETOCONAZOLE

Ketoconazole, an antifungal imidazole derivative, is a potent and rather nonselective inhibitor of adrenal and gonadal steroid synthesis. This compound inhibits the cholesterol side chain cleavage, P450c17, C17,20-lyase, 3β-hydroxysteroid dehydrogenase, and P450c11 enzymes required for glucocorticoid synthesis. The sensitivity of the P450 enzymes to this compound in mammalian tissues is much lower than that of the fungal enzymes, so that the inhibitory effects are seen only at high doses. This inhibition is compensated for by increased ACTH production and leads to increases in 17-deoxy steroids such as progesterone and aldosterone and to suppression of plasma renin activity. Ketoconazole also has other endocrine effects. It displaces estradiol and dihydrotestosterone from sex hormone-binding protein in vitro and increases the estradiol-testosterone ratio in plasma in vivo by a different mechanism. The latter may be responsible for the gynecomastia sometimes seen with ketoconazole therapy.

Ketoconazole has been used for the treatment of patients with Cushing's disease due to several causes. Dosages of 200–1200 mg/d have produced a reduction in hormone levels and impressive clinical improvement in some patients in these preliminary studies.

4. MIFEPRISTONE (RU 486)

Mifepristone is a synthetic partial agonist steroid that binds to glucocorticoid as well as to progesterone receptors and has been used experimentally in the treatment of Cushing's syndrome. Its pharmacology and use in women as a progesterone antagonist are discussed in Chapter 40.

5. MITOTANE

Mitotane (Figure 39–5) produces adrenal atrophy in dogs and interferes with biosynthetic pathways in the human adrenal cortex. This drug was administered orally in divided doses of 6–12 mg daily. About one-third of patients with adrenal carcinoma showed a reduction in tumor mass and steroid production was decreased in two-thirds. In 80% of patients, the toxic effects were sufficiently severe to require dose reduction. These included diarrhea, nausea, vomiting, depression, somnolence, and skin problems. The drug has been withdrawn from the market in the USA.

6. AMPHENONE B

Amphenone B (Figure 39–5) is a more potent inhibitor of synthesis than mitotane, blocking hydroxylation at the 11, 17, and 21 positions. It does not have a destructive effect on the tissue, and the block of steroid synthesis leads to increased production of ACTH and hyperplasia of the gland. Amphenone causes central nervous system depression and gastrointestinal tract and skin disorders and impairs liver and thyroid function. It is considered too toxic for use in humans.

7. TRILOSTANE

Trilostane is also a 3β-17 hydroxysteroid dehydrogenase inhibitor that interferes with the synthesis of adrenal and gonadal hormones and is comparable to aminoglutethimide. Its side effects are predominantly gastrointestinal rather than the rashes and drowsiness seen with aminoglutethimide; side effects occur in about 50% of patients with both agents. There is no cross-resistance or crossover of side effects between these compounds.

MINERALOCORTICOID ANTAGONISTS

In addition to agents that interfere with aldosterone synthesis (see above), there are steroids that compete with aldosterone for binding sites and decrease its effect peripherally. Progesterone is mildly active in this respect.

Spironolactone is a 7α-acetylthiospironolactone. Little is known about its metabolism. The onset of activity is slow, and the effects last for 2–3 days after the drug is discontinued. It is used in the treatment of pri-

mary aldosteronism in dosages of 50–100 mg/d. This agent reverses many of the findings of aldosteronism. It has been useful in establishing the diagnosis in some patients and in ameliorating the signs and symptoms when surgical removal of an adenoma is delayed. When used diagnostically for the detection of aldosteronism in hypokalemic patients with hypertension, dosages of 400–500 mg/d for 4–8 days—with an adequate intake of sodium and potassium—will restore potassium levels to or toward normal. This agent is also useful in preparing these patients for surgery. Dosages of 300–400 mg/d for 2 weeks are used for this purpose and may reduce the incidence of cardiac arrhythmias.

Spironolactone is also used in treatment of hirsutism in women. Dosages of 50–200 mg/d cause a reduction in the density, diameter, and rate of growth of facial hair in patients with idiopathic hirsutism or hirsutism secondary to androgen excess. The effect can usually be seen in 2 months and becomes maximal in about 6 months. It may be due to inhibition of androgen production and an action at the hair follicle.

Spironolactone

The use of spironolactone as a diuretic is discussed in Chapter 15. Adverse effects reported for spironolactone include hyperkalemia, menstrual abnormalities, gynecomastia, sedation, headache, gastrointestinal disturbances, and skin rashes.

Drospirenone, a progestin in a new oral contraceptive, also antagonizes the effects of aldosterone.

PREPARATIONS AVAILABLE

Glucocorticoids for Aerosol Use: See Chapter 20.

Glucocorticoids for Dermatologic Use: See Chapter 62.

Glucocorticoids for Oral & Parenteral Use
  Betamethasone (Celestone)
    Oral: 0.6 mg tablets; 0.6 mg/5 mL syrup
  Betamethasone sodium phosphate (generic, Celestone Phosphate, Cel-U-Jec)
    Parenteral: 4 mg/mL for IV, IM, intralesional, or intra-articular injection
  Cortisone (generic, Cortone Acetate)
    Oral: 5, 10, 25 mg tablets
  Dexamethasone (generic, Decadron, others)
    Oral: 0.25, 0.5, 0.75, 1, 1.5, 2, 4, 6 mg tablets; 0.5 mg/5 mL elixir; 0.5 mg/5 mL, 0.5 mg/0.5 mL solution
  Dexamethasone acetate (generic, Decadron-LA, others)
    Parenteral: 8 mg/mL suspension for IM, intralesional, or intra-articular injection; 16 mg/mL suspension for intra-articular injection only
  Dexamethasone sodium phosphate (generic, Decadron Phosphate, others)
    Parenteral: 4, 10, 20, 24 mg/mL for IV, IM, intralesional, or intra-articular injection
  Hydrocortisone [cortisol] (generic, Cortef)
    Oral: 5, 10, 20 mg tablets
  Hydrocortisone acetate (generic)
    Parenteral: 25, 50 mg/mL suspension for intralesional, soft tissue, or intra-articular injection
  Hydrocortisone cypionate (Cortef)
    Oral suspension: 10 mg/5 mL
  Hydrocortisone sodium phosphate
    Parenteral: 50 mg/mL for IV, IM, or SC injection
  Hydrocortisone sodium succinate (generic, Solu-Cortef, others)
    Parenteral: 100, 250, 500, 1000 mg/vial for IV, IM injection
  Methylprednisolone (generic, Medrol, Meprolone)
    Oral: 2, 4, 8, 16, 24, 32 mg tablets
  Methylprednisolone acetate (generic, Depo-Medrol, others)
    Parenteral: 20, 40, 80 mg/mL for IM, intralesional, or intra-articular injection

  Methylprednisolone sodium succinate (generic, Solu-Medrol, others)
    Parenteral: 40, 125, 500, 1000, 2000 mg/vial for injection
  Prednisolone (generic, Delta-Cortef, Prelone)
    Oral: 5 mg tablets; 15 mg/5 mL syrup
  Prednisolone acetate (generic, others)
    Parenteral: 25, 50 mg/mL for soft tissue or intra-articular injection
  Prednisolone sodium phosphate
    Oral: 5 mg/5 mL solution
    Parenteral: 20 mg/mL for IV, IM, intra-articular, or intralesional injection
  Prednisolone tebutate (generic, Hydeltra-T.B.A., others)
    Parenteral: 20 mg/mL for intra-articular or intralesional injection
  Prednisone (generic, Meticorten, others)
    Oral: 1, 2.5, 5, 10, 20, 50 mg tablets; 1, 5 mg/mL solution and syrup
  Triamcinolone (generic, Aristocort, Kenacort, Atolone)
    Oral: 1, 2, 4, 8 mg tablets; 4 mg/5 mL syrup
  Triamcinolone acetonide (generic, Kenalog, others)
    Parenteral: 3, 10, 40 mg/mL for IM, intra-articular, or intralesional injection
  Triamcinolone diacetate (generic, Aristocort, others)
    Parenteral: 25, 40 mg/mL for IM, intra-articular, or intralesional injection
  Triamcinolone hexacetonide (Aristospan)
    Parenteral: 5, 20 mg/mL for intra-articular, intralesional, or sublesional injection

Mineralocorticoids
  Fludrocortisone acetate (Florinef Acetate)
    Oral: 0.1 mg tablets

Adrenal Steroid Inhibitors
  Aminoglutethimide (Cytadren)
    Oral: 250 mg tablets
  Ketoconazole (Nizoral)
    Oral: 200 mg tablets (unlabeled use)
  Mitotane (Lysodren)
    Oral: 500 mg tablets

REFERENCES

Barnes PJ, Adcock I: Anti-inflammatory actions of steroids: Molecular mechanisms. Trends Pharmacol Sci 1993; 14:436.

Baulieu EE: The steroid hormone antagonist RU486: Mechanism at the cellular level and clinical applications. Endocrinol Metab Clin North Am 1991;20:873.

Baxter JD: Minimizing the effects of glucocorticoid therapy. Adv Intern Med 1990;35:173.

Bentley AM et al: Prednisolone treatment in asthma: Reduction in the numbers of eosinophils, T cells, tryptase-only positive mast cells, and modulation of IL-4, IL-5, and interferon-gamma cytokine gene expression within the bronchial mucosa. Am J Resp Crit Care Med 1996;153:551.

Berdanier CD: Role of the glucocorticoids in the regulation of lipogenesis. FASEB J 1989;3:2179.

Bikle DD et al: Elevated 1,25-dihydroxyvitamin D levels in patients with chronic obstructive pulmonary disease treated with prednisone. J Clin Endocrinol Metab 1993;76:456.

Blalock JE: A molecular basis of bidirectional communication between the immune and neuroendocrine systems. Physiol Rev 1989;69:1.

Bracken MB et al: A randomized, controlled trial of methylprednisolone or naloxone in the treatment of acute spinal-cord injury: Results of the Second National Acute Spinal Cord Injury Study. N Engl J Med 1990;322:1405.

Calandra T et al: MIF as a glucocorticoid-induced modulator of cytokine production. Nature 1995;376:68.

Carella MJ et al: Hypothalamic-pituitary-adrenal function one week after a short burst of steroid therapy. J Clin Endocrinol Metab 1993;76:1188.

Chin R: Adrenal crisis. Crit Care Clin 1991;7:23.

Cleary MP: The antiobesity effect of dehydroepiandrosterone in rats. Proc Soc Exp Biol Med 1991;196:8.

Couch RM et al: Kinetic analysis of inhibition of human adrenal steroidogenesis by ketoconazole. J Clin Endocrinol Metab 1987;65:551.

Cumming DC et al: Treatment of hirsutism with spironolactone. JAMA 1982;247:1295.

Cummings JJ, D'Eugenio DB, Gross SJ: A controlled trial of dexamethasone in preterm infants at high risk for bronchopulmonary dysplasia. N Engl J Med 1989;320:1505.

Davidson FF, Dennis EA: Biological relevance of lipocortins and related proteins as inhibitors of phospholipase A_2. Biochem Pharmacol 1989;38:3645.

Dixon RB, Christy NP: On the various forms of corticosteroid withdrawal syndrome. Am J Med 1980;68:224.

Dorr HG, Sippell WG: Prenatal dexamethasone treatment in pregnancies at risk for congenital adrenal hyperplasia due to 21-hydroxylase deficiency: Effect on midgestational amniotic fluid steroid levels. J Clin Endocrinol Metab 1993;76:117.

Engelhardt D, Weber MM: Therapy of Cushing's syndrome with steroid biosynthesis inhibitors. J Steroid Biochem Mol Biol 1994;49:261.

Farese RV Jr et al: Licorice induced hypermineralocorticoidism. N Engl J Med 1991;325:1223.

Farrell EE et al: Impact of antenatal dexamethasone administration on respiratory distress syndrome in surfactant-treated infants. Am J Obstet Gynecol 1989;161:628.

Feldman D: Ketoconazole and other imidazole derivatives as inhibitors of steroidogenesis. Endocr Rev 1985;7:409.

Findling JW, Aron DC, Tyrell JB: Glucocorticoids and adrenal androgens. In: Basic & Clinical Endocrinology, 5th ed. Greenspan FS, Stewler GS (editors). Appleton & Lange, 1996.

Frey BM, Frey FJ: Clinical pharmacokinetics of prednisone and prednisolone. Clin Pharmacokinet 1990: 19:126.

Funder JW et al: Apparent mineralocorticoid excess, pseudohypoaldosteronism, and urinary electrolyte excretion: Toward a redefinition of mineralocorticoid action. FASEB J 1990;4:3234.

Gardiner P et al: Spironolactone metabolism: Steady-state serum levels of the sulfur-containing metabolites. J Clin Pharmacol 1989;29:324.

Godowski PJ, Picard D, Yamamoto KR: Signal transduction and transcriptional regulation by glucocorticoid receptor-LexA fusion proteins. Science 1988;241:812.

Gordon GB, Bush DE, Weisman HF: Reduction of atherosclerosis by administration of dehydroepiandrosterone: A study in the hypercholesterolemic New Zealand white rabbit with intimal injury. J Clin Invest 1988;82:71.

Graber AL et al: Natural history of pituitary-adrenal recovery following long-term suppression with corticosteroids. J Clin Endocrinol Metab 1965;25:11.

Griffing, GT: Dinosaurs and steroids. (Editorial.) J Clin Endocrinol Metab 1993;77:1450.

Hahn BH, Mazzaferri EL: Glucocorticoid-induced osteoporosis. Hosp Pract (Off Ed) 1995;30(8):45.

Hammond GL: Molecular properties of corticosteroid binding globulin and the sex-steroid binding proteins. Endocr Rev 1990;11:65.

Helfer EL, Rose LI: Corticosteroids and adrenal suppression: Characterising and avoiding the problem. Drugs 1989;38:838.

Henriques HF III, Lebovic D: Defining and focusing perioperative steroid supplementation. Am Surg 1995; 61:809.

Hyams JS, Carey DE: Corticosteroids and growth. J Pediatr 1988;113:249.

James VHT (editor): The Adrenal Gland, 2nd ed. Raven Press, 1992.

Johnson TS et al: Prevention of acute mountain sickness by dexamethasone. N Engl J Med 1984;310:683.

Lamberts SWJ, Koper JW, de Jong FH: The endocrine effects of long-term treatment with mifepristone (RU 486). J Clin Endocrinol Metab 1991;73:187.

LaRocca RV et al: Suramin in adrenal cancer: Modulation of steroid hormone production, cytotoxicity in vitro, and clinical antitumor effect. J Clin Endocrinol Metab 1990; 71:497.

Laue L: Glucocorticoid antagonists: Pharmacological attributes of a prototype antiglucocorticoid (RU 486). In: Anti-inflammatory Steroid Action. Basic and Clinical Aspects. Schleimer RP, Claman HN, Oronsky AL (editors). Academic Press, 1989.

Levine BD et al: Dexamethasone in the treatment of acute mountain sickness. N Engl J Med 1989;321:1707.

Luton J-P et al: Clinical features of adrenocortical carcinoma, prognostic factors, and the effect of mitotane therapy. N Engl J Med 1990;322:1190.

Mao J, Regelson W, Kalimi M: Molecular mechanism of RU486 action: A review. Mol Cellular Biochem 1992;109:1.

Meikle AW, Daynes RA, Araneo BA: Adrenal androgen secretion and biologic effects. Endocrinol Metab Clin North Am 1991;20:381.

Messer J et al: Association of adrenocorticosteroid therapy and peptic-ulcer disease. N Engl J Med 1983;309:21.

Miller WL: Molecular biology of steroid hormone synthesis. Endocr Rev 1988;9:295.

Morales AJ et al: Effects of replacement dose of dehydroepiandrosterone in men and women of advancing age. J Clin Endocrinol Metab 1994;78:1360.

Muller M, Renkawitz R: The glucocorticoid receptor. Biochim Biophys Acta 1991;1088:171.

New ML: Prenatal diagnosis and treatment of congenital adrenal hyperplasia due to 21-hydroxylase deficiency. Development Pharmacol Therap 1990;15:200.

Oelkers W et al: Effects of a new oral contraceptive containing an antimineralocorticoid progestin, drospirenone, on the renin-aldosterone system, body weight, blood pressure, glucose tolerance, and lipid metabolism. J Clin Endocrinol Metab 1995;80:1816.

Ogirala RG et al: High dose intramuscular triamcinolone in severe, chronic, life-threatening asthma. N Engl J Med 1991;324:585.

Prummel MF et al: The course of biochemical parameters of bone turnover during treatment with corticosteroids. J Clin Endocrinol Metab 1991;72:382.

Samaan NA, Hickey RC: Adrenal cortical carcinoma. Semin Oncol 1987;14:262.

Sambrook P et al: Prevention of corticosteroid osteoporosis. N Engl J Med 1993;329:1747.

Sato A et al: Glucocorticoid-induced hypertension in the elderly: Relation to serum calcium and family history of essential hypertension. Am J Hypertens 1995;8:823.

Scheinman RI et al: Role of transcriptional activation of I kappa B alpha in mediation of immunosuppression by glucocorticoids. Science 1995;270:283.

Schobitz B, Reul JM, Holsboer F: The role of the hypothalamic-pituitary-adrenocortical system during inflammatory conditions. Crit Rev Neurobiol 1994;8:263.

Schurmeyer TH et al: Pituitary-adrenal responsiveness to corticotropin-releasing hormone in patients receiving chronic, alternate day glucocorticoid therapy. J Clin Endocrinol Metab 1985;61:22.

Semel JD: Fever on drug-free day of alternate-day steroid therapy. Am J Med 1984;76:315.

Smith DF, Toft DO: Steroid receptors and their associated proteins. Mol Endocrinol 1993;4:7.

Sonino N et al: Ketoconazole treatment in Cushing's syndrome: Experience in 34 patients. Clin Endocrinol 1991;35:347.

Sorenson DK et al: Corticosteroids stimulate an increase in phospholipase A_2 inhibitor in human serum. J Steroid Biochem 1988;2:271.

Tabarin A et al: Use of ketoconazole in the treatment of Cushing's disease and ectopic ACTH syndrome. Clin Endocrinol 1991;34:63.

Tappy L et al: Mechanisms of dexamethasone-induced insulin resistance in healthy humans. J Clin Endocrinol Metab 1994;79:1063.

White PC, New MI, Dupont B: Congenital adrenal hyperplasia. (Two parts.) N Engl J Med 1987;316:1519,1580.

Williams CJ et al: Multicentre cross-over study of aminoglutethimide and trilostane in advanced postmenopausal breast cancer. Clin Oncol 1995;7:87.

The Gonadal Hormones & Inhibitors

40

Alan Goldfien, MD

I. THE OVARY (Estrogens, Progestins, Other Ovarian Hormones, Oral Contraceptives, Inhibitors & Antagonists, & Ovulation-Inducing Agents)

The ovary has important gametogenic functions that are integrated with its hormonal activity. In the human female, the gonad is relatively quiescent during the period of rapid growth and maturation. At puberty, the ovary begins a 30- to 40-year period of cyclic function called the **menstrual cycle** because of the regular episodes of bleeding that are its most obvious manifestation. It then fails to respond to gonadotropins secreted by the anterior pituitary gland, and the cessation of cyclic bleeding that occurs is called the **menopause.**

The mechanism responsible for the onset of ovarian function at the time of puberty is thought to be neural in origin, because the immature gonad can be stimulated by gonadotropins already present in the hypothalamus and because the pituitary is responsive to hypothalamic gonadotropin-releasing hormones. The maturation of centers such as the amygdala in the brain may withdraw an inhibition of the cells in the median eminence of the hypothalamus, allowing them to produce **gonadotropin-releasing hormone (GnRH)** in pulses with the appropriate frequency and amplitude, which stimulates the release of **follicle-stimulating hormone (FSH)** and **luteinizing hormone (LH)** (see Chapter 37). At first, small amounts of these latter two hormones are released, and the limited quantities of estrogen secreted in response cause breast development, alterations in fat distribution, and a growth spurt that culminates in epiphysial closure in the long bones.

After a year or so, sufficient estrogen is produced to induce endometrial changes and periodic bleeding.

After the first few cycles, which may be anovulatory, normal cyclic function is established.

At the beginning of each cycle, a variable number of follicles (vesicular follicles), each containing an ovum, begin to enlarge in response to FSH. After 5 or 6 days, one of the follicles begins to develop more rapidly. The granulosa cells of this follicle multiply and, under the influence of LH, synthesize estrogens and release them at an increasing rate. The estrogens appear to inhibit FSH release and may lead to regression of the smaller, less mature follicles. The ovarian follicle consists of an ovum surrounded by a fluid-filled antrum lined by granulosa and theca cells. The estrogen secretion reaches a peak just before midcycle, and the granulosa cells begin to secrete progesterone. These changes stimulate the brief surge in LH and FSH release that precedes (and causes) ovulation. When the follicle ruptures, the ovum is released into the abdominal cavity near the uterine tube.

Following the above events, the cavity of the ruptured follicle fills with blood (corpus hemorrhagicum), and the luteinized theca and granulosa cells proliferate and replace the blood to form the corpus luteum. The cells of this structure produce estrogens and progesterone for the remainder of the cycle, or longer if pregnancy occurs.

If pregnancy does not occur, the corpus luteum begins to degenerate and ceases hormone production, eventually becoming a corpus albicans. The cause of luteolysis in humans is unknown. Most other hormonal events occurring during the normal ovarian cycle can be explained on the basis of feedback regulation. The endometrium, which proliferated during the follicular phase and developed its glandular structure during the luteal phase, is shed in the process of menstruation. These events are summarized in Figure 40–1.

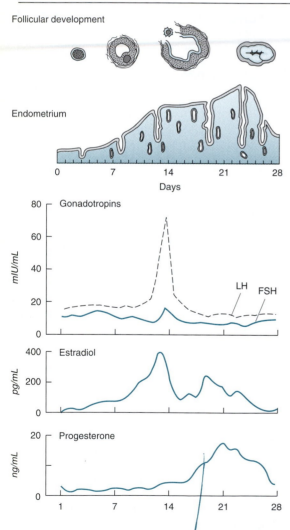

Follicular development

Endometrium

Figure 40–1. The menstrual cycle, showing plasma levels of pituitary and ovarian hormones and histologic changes.

The ovary normally ceases its gametogenic and endocrine function with time. This change is accompanied by a cessation in uterine bleeding (menopause) and occurs at a mean age of 52 years in the USA. Although the ovary ceases to secrete estrogen, significant levels of estrogen persist in many women as a result of conversion of adrenal and ovarian steroids such as androstenedione to estrone and estradiol in adipose and possibly other nonendocrine tissues.

Disturbances in Ovarian Function

Disturbances of cyclic function are common even during the peak years of reproduction. A minority of these result from inflammatory or neoplastic processes that destroy the uterus, ovaries, or pituitary, but the causes of most menstrual problems are poorly understood. Many of the minor disturbances leading to periods of amenorrhea or anovulatory cycles are self-limited. They are often associated with emotional or environmental changes and are thought to represent temporary disorders in the centers in the brain that control the secretion of the hypothalamic releasing factors. Anovulatory disorders are also associated with excessive dieting and with severe exercise such as distance running and swimming. Among the more common organic causes of persistent ovulatory disturbances are pituitary prolactinomas and syndromes and tumors characterized by excessive ovarian or adrenal androgen production. Normal ovarian function can be modified by androgens produced by the adrenal cortex or tumors arising from it. The ovary also gives rise to androgen-producing neoplasms such as arrhenoblastomas and Leydig cell tumors as well as to estrogen-producing granulosa cell tumors.

THE ESTROGENS

Estrogenic activity is shared by a large number of chemical substances. In addition to the variety of steroidal estrogens derived from animal sources, numerous nonsteroidal estrogens have been synthesized. Many phenols are estrogenic, and estrogenic activity has been identified in such diverse forms of life as those found in the sediments of the seas. Estrogens are found in many plants, including soy beans and other foods. However, studies fail to show that eating them produces significant estrogenic effects.

Natural Estrogens

The major estrogens produced by women are estradiol (estradiol-17β, E_2), estrone (E_1), and estriol (E_3) (Figure 40–2). Estradiol appears to be the major secretory product of the ovary. Although some estrone is produced in the ovary, most estrone and estriol are formed in the liver from estradiol or in peripheral tissues from androstenedione and other androgens. As

Figure 40–2. Biosynthesis and metabolism of estrogens.

noted above, during the first part of the menstrual cycle estrogens are produced in the ovarian follicle by the theca cells. After ovulation, the estrogens as well as progesterone are synthesized by the granulosa cells of the corpus luteum, and the pathways of biosynthesis are slightly different.

During pregnancy, a large amount of estrogen is synthesized by the fetoplacental unit. The estriol synthesized by the fetoplacental unit is released into the maternal circulation and excreted into the urine. Repeated assay of maternal urinary estriol excretion has been used in the assessment of fetal well-being.

One of the most prolific natural sources of estrogenic substances is the stallion, which liberates more of this hormone than the pregnant mare or pregnant woman. The equine estrogens—equilenin and equilin—and their congeners are unsaturated in the B as well as the A ring and are excreted in large quantities in urine, from which they can be recovered and used for medicinal purposes.

In normal women, estradiol is produced at a rate that varies during the menstrual cycle, resulting in plasma levels as low as 50 pg/mL in the early follicular phase to as high as 350–850 pg/mL at the time of the preovulatory peak (Figure 40–1).

Synthetic Estrogens

A variety of chemical alterations have been produced in the natural estrogens. The most important effect of these alterations has been to increase the oral effectiveness of the estrogens. Some structures are shown in Figure 40–3. Those with therapeutic use are listed in Table 40–1.

In addition to the steroidal estrogens, a variety of nonsteroidal compounds with estrogenic activity have been synthesized and used clinically. These include

dienestrol, diethylstilbestrol, benzestrol, hexestrol, methestrol, methallenestril, and **chlorotrianisene** (Figure 40–3).

Pharmacokinetics

When released into the circulation, estradiol binds strongly to an α_2-globulin (sex hormone-binding globulin [SHBG]) and to albumin with less affinity. Bound estrogen is relatively unavailable for diffusion into cells, so it is the free fraction that is physiologically active. Estradiol is converted by the liver and other tissues to estrone and estriol (which have low affinity for the estrogen receptor) and their 2-hydroxylated derivatives and conjugated metabolites (which are too insoluble in lipid to cross the cell membrane readily) and excreted in the bile (Figure 40–2). However, the conjugates may be hydrolyzed in the intestine to active, reabsorbable compounds. The catechol estrogens serve as neurotransmitters in the central nervous system. They are converted to the 2- and 4-methoxy compounds by catechol-O methyltransferase

and in high concentrations can inhibit the inactivation of catecholamines by the enzyme. Estrogens are also excreted in small amounts in the breast milk of nursing mothers.

Because significant amounts of estrogens and their active metabolites are excreted in the bile and reabsorbed from the intestine, the resulting enterohepatic circulation ensures that orally administered estrogens will have a high ratio of hepatic to peripheral effects. As noted below, the hepatic effects are thought to be responsible for some undesirable actions such as synthesis of increased clotting factors and plasma renin substrate. When used for their peripheral effects—eg, in postmenopausal women—the hepatic effects can be minimized by routes that avoid first-pass hepatic exposure, ie, vaginal, transdermal, or by injection.

Physiologic Effects

A. Mechanism: Plasma estrogens are bound to sex hormone-binding globulin, from which they dissociate to enter the cell and bind to their receptor. Two

Figure 40–3. Compounds with estrogenic activity.

Table 40–1. Commonly used estrogens.

	Average Replacement Dosage
Ethinyl estradiol	0.005–0.02 mg/d
Micronized estradiol	1–2 mg/d
Estradiol cypionate	2–5 mg every 3–4 weeks
Estradiol valerate	2–20 mg every other week
Estropipate	1.25–2.5 mg/d
Conjugated, esterified, or mixed estrogenic substances:	
Oral	0.3–1.25 mg/d
Injectable	0.2–2 mg/d
Transdermal	Patch
Diethylstilbestrol	0.1–0.5 mg/d
Quinestrol	0.1–0.2 mg/week
Chlorotrianisene	12–25 mg/d
Methallenestril	3–9 mg/d

genes code for estrogen receptors, which are members of the superfamily of steroid and thyroid receptors. The estrogen receptors are found predominantly in the nucleus bound to proteins that stabilize the receptor (Figure 39–3). Binding of the hormone to its receptor alters its conformation and releases the stabilizing proteins (predominantly Hsp90) from the receptor complex. The receptor-hormone complex forms homodimers that bind to a specific sequence of nucleotides called estrogen response elements (EREs) on various genes and regulate their transcription. The ERE is composed of two half-sites arranged as a palindrome separated by a small group of nucleotides called the spacer. The interaction of the receptor dimer with the ERE also involves a number of nuclear proteins (transcription elements). The receptor complex may also bind to other sites in the promoter region of the gene. The number and variety of receptor sites and transcription factors confers the cell specificity of the hormone's actions. The genomic effects of estrogens are mainly due to proteins synthesized in response to RNA transcribed by the gene. Some of the genomic effects are indirect and are mediated by the paracrine effects of cytokines produced by neighboring cells regulated by the target cell proteins that are induced by hormone action. Rapid estrogen-induced effects such as granulosa cell Ca^{2+} uptake and increased uterine blood flow do not require gene activation. These appear to be mediated by membrane receptors that differ from the intracellular receptor.

B. Female Maturation: Estrogens are required for the normal maturation of the female. They stimulate the development of the vagina, uterus, and uterine tubes as well as the secondary sex characteristics. They stimulate stromal development and ductal growth in the breast and are responsible for the accelerated growth phase and the closing of the epiphyses of the long bones that occur at puberty. They contribute to the growth of the axillary and pubic hair and alter the distribution of body fat so as to produce typical female body contours. Larger quantities also

stimulate development of pigmentation in the skin, most prominent in the region of the nipples and areolae and in the genital region.

C. Endometrial Effects: In addition to its growth effects on uterine muscle, estrogen also plays an important role in the development of the endometrial lining. Continuous exposure to estrogens for prolonged periods leads to an abnormal hyperplasia of the endometrium that is usually associated with abnormal bleeding patterns. When estrogen production is properly coordinated with the production of progesterone during the normal human menstrual cycle, regular periodic bleeding and shedding of the endometrial lining occur.

D. Metabolic Effects: Estrogens have a number of important metabolic effects. They seem to be partially responsible for maintenance of the normal structure of the skin and blood vessels in women. Estrogens decrease the rate of resorption of bone by antagonizing the effect of parathyroid hormone on bone but do not stimulate bone formation. Estrogens may have important effects on intestinal absorption because they reduce the motility of the bowel.

In addition to stimulating the synthesis of enzymes and growth factors leading to uterine growth and differentiation, estrogens alter the production and activity of many other proteins in the body. Metabolic alterations in the liver are especially important, so that there is a higher circulating level of proteins such as transcortin (CBG), thyroxine-binding globulin (TBG), sex hormone-binding globulin (SHBG), transferrin, renin substrate, and fibrinogen. This leads to increased circulating levels of thyroxine, estrogen, testosterone, iron, copper, and other substances.

Alterations in the composition of the plasma lipids caused by estrogens are characterized by an increase in the high-density lipoproteins, a slight reduction in the low-density lipoproteins, and a reduction in plasma cholesterol levels. Plasma triglyceride levels are increased. Estrogens decrease oxidation of adipose tissue lipid to ketones and increase synthesis of triglycerides.

E. Effects on Blood Coagulation: Estrogens enhance the coagulability of blood. Many changes in factors influencing coagulation have been reported, including increased circulating levels of factors II, VII, IX, and X and decreased antithrombin III, partially as a result of the hepatic effects mentioned above. Increased plasminogen levels and decreased platelet adhesiveness have also been found (see Hormonal Contraception).

F. Other Effects: Estrogens have many other effects. They induce the synthesis of progesterone receptors. They are responsible for estrous behavior in animals and influence libido in humans. They facilitate the loss of intravascular fluid into the extracellular space, producing edema. The resulting decrease in plasma volume causes a compensatory retention of sodium and water by the kidney. Estrogens also modulate sympathetic nervous system control of smooth muscle function.

Clinical Uses*

A. Primary Hypogonadism: Estrogens have been used extensively for replacement therapy in estrogen-deficient patients. The estrogen deficiency may be due to primary failure of development of the ovaries, castration, or menopause.

Treatment of primary hypogonadism is usually begun at 11–13 years of age in order to stimulate the development of secondary sex characteristics and menses, to stimulate optimal growth, and to avoid the psychologic consequences of delayed puberty. Treatment is initiated with small doses of estrogen (0.3 mg conjugated estrogens or 5–10 μg ethinyl estradiol) on days 1–21 each month. When growth is completed, chronic therapy consists mainly of the administration of estrogens and progestins, as described below.

B. Postmenopausal Hormonal Therapy: In addition to the signs and symptoms that follow closely upon the cessation of normal ovarian function—such as loss of periods, vasomotor symptoms, and genital atrophy—there are longer-lasting changes that influence the health and well-being of postmenopausal women. These include an acceleration of bone loss, which in susceptible women may lead to vertebral, hip, and wrist fractures; and lipid changes, which may contribute to the acceleration of cardiovascular disease noted in postmenopausal women. The effects of estrogens on bone have been extensively studied, and the effects of hormone withdrawal and replacement are well-characterized. However, the role of estrogen and progestins in the cause and prevention of cardiovascular disease, which is responsible for 350,000 deaths per year, and breast cancer, which causes 35,000 deaths per year, is less well understood.

When normal ovulatory function ceases and the estrogen levels fall after the menopause or oophorectomy, there is an accelerated rise in plasma cholesterol and LDL concentrations, and LDL receptors decline. HDL is not much affected, and levels remain higher than in men. VLDL and triglyceride levels are not much different. Since cardiovascular disorders account for most deaths in this age group, the risk for these disorders constitutes a major consideration in deciding whether or not hormonal therapy is indicated and influences the selection of hormones to be administered. The effect of estrogen replacement therapy on circulating lipids and lipoproteins (Figure 40–4) is associated with a reduction in myocardial infarction by about 50% and fatal strokes by as much as 40%. Progestins antagonize estrogen's effects on LDL and HDL to a variable extent. However, a large study has recently shown that the addition of a progestin to estrogen re-

placement therapy does not reduce the cardioprotective effect of the estrogen (Grodstein et al, 1996). Patients at higher risk for cardiovascular disease should be encouraged to quit smoking, exercise, and lose weight if obese. Hypertension and diabetes and lipid disorders should be brought under control if present. Antioxidant vitamins, folic acid (which reduces plasma homocysteine), small amounts of alcohol, and aspirin may also be useful for risk reduction.

Optimal management of the postmenopausal patient requires careful assessment of her symptoms as well as consideration of her age and the risk for cardiovascular disease, osteoporosis, breast cancer, and endometrial cancer. Bearing in mind the effects of the gonadal hormones on each of these disorders, the goals of therapy can then be defined and the risks of therapy assessed and discussed with the patient.

If the main indication for therapy is hot flushes, therapy with the lowest dose of estrogen required for symptomatic relief is recommended. Treatment may be required for only a limited period of time and the possible increased risk for breast cancer avoided. In women who have had a hysterectomy, estrogens alone can be given 5 days per week or continuously, since progestins are not required to reduce the risk for endometrial hyperplasia and cancer. Although hot flushes, sweating, insomnia, and atrophic vaginitis are generally relieved by estrogens and although many patients experience some increased sense of well-being, depression and other psychopathologic states are seldom improved.

The role of estrogens in the prevention and treatment of osteoporosis has been carefully studied (see Chapter 42). The amount of bone present is maximal in the young active adult and begins to decline in middle age in both men and women. The development of osteoporosis also depends on the amount of bone present at the start of this process, on calcium intake, and on the degree of physical activity. The risk of osteoporosis is highest in smokers who are thin, Caucasian, and inactive and have a low calcium intake and a strong family history of osteoporosis.

Estrogens should be used in the smallest dosage consistent with relief of symptoms. In women who have not undergone hysterectomy, it is most convenient to prescribe estrogen on the first 21–25 days of each month. The recommended dosages of estrogen are 0.3–1.25 mg/d of conjugated estrogen or 0.01–0.02 mg/d of ethinyl estradiol. Doses in the middle of this range have been shown to be maximally effective in preventing the decrease in bone density occurring at menopause. From this point of view, it is important to begin therapy as soon as possible after the menopause for maximum effect. In these patients and others not taking estrogen, calcium supplements, bringing the total daily calcium intake up to 1500 mg, are useful.

Patients at low risk of developing osteoporosis who manifest only mild atrophic vaginitis can be treated

---

*The use of estrogens in contraception is discussed below.

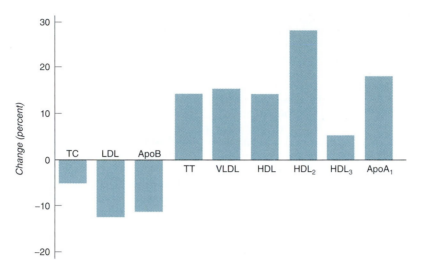

Figure 40–4. Changes in serum lipids and lipoproteins resulting from the use of oral estrogen (equivalent to conjugated estrogens, 0.625 mg/d, for at least 3 months. Redrawn and reproduced, with permission, from Lobo RA: Effects of hormonal replacement on lipids and lipoproteins in postmenopausal women. J Clin Endocrinol Metab 1991;79:925.)

with topical preparations. The vaginal route of application is also useful in the treatment of urinary tract symptoms in these patients. It is important to realize, however, that although locally administered estrogens escape the first-pass effect (so that some undesirable hepatic effects are reduced), they are almost completely absorbed into the circulation, and these preparations should be given cyclically.

As noted below, the administration of estrogen is associated with an increased risk of endometrial carcinoma. The administration of a progestational agent with the estrogen prevents endometrial hyperplasia and markedly reduces the risk of cancer. When estrogen is given for the first 25 days of the month and the progestin medroxyprogesterone (10 mg/d) is added during the last 10–14 days, the risk is only half of that in women not receiving hormone replacement therapy. On this regimen, some women will experience a return of symptoms during the period off estrogen administration. In these patients, the estrogen can be given continuously. If the progestin produces sedation or other undesirable effects, its dose can be reduced to 2.5–5 mg for the last 10 days of the cycle with a slight increase in the risk for endometrial hyperplasia. These regimens are usually accompanied by bleeding at the end of each cycle. Some women experience migraine headaches during the last few days of the cycle. The use of a continuous estrogen regimen will often prevent their occurrence. Women who object to the cyclic bleeding associated with sequential therapy can also consider continuous therapy. Daily therapy with 0.625 mg of conjugated equine estrogens and 2.5–5 mg medroxyprogesterone will eliminate cyclic bleeding, control vasomotor symptoms, prevent genital atrophy, maintain bone density, and show a favorable lipid pro-

file with a small decrease in LDL and an increase in HDL concentrations. These women have endometrial atrophy on biopsy. About half of these patients will experience breakthrough bleeding during the first few months of therapy. Seventy to 80 percent become amenorrheic after the first 4 months, and most remain so. The main disadvantage of continuous therapy is the need for uterine biopsy when bleeding occurs after the first few months.

As noted above, estrogens may also be administered vaginally or transdermally. When estrogens are given by these routes, the liver is bypassed on the first circulation, and the ratio of the liver effects to peripheral effects is reduced.

In patients in whom estrogen replacement therapy is contraindicated, such as those with estrogen-sensitive tumors, relief of vasomotor symptoms may be obtained by the use of progestational agents or clonidine.

C. Other Uses: Estrogens combined with progestins can be used to suppress ovulation in patients with intractable dysmenorrhea or when suppression of ovarian function is used in the treatment of hirsutism and amenorrhea due to excessive secretion of androgens by the ovary. Under these circumstances, greater suppression may be needed, and oral contraceptives containing 50 μg of estrogen or a combination of a low estrogen pill with GnRH suppression may be required.

Estrogens have been used to stop excessive uterine bleeding due to endometrial hyperplasia. Repeated doses of 20 μg of ethinyl estradiol every few hours or the administration of 20 mg of conjugated estrogens intravenously has been useful in arresting blood loss temporarily.

Adverse Effects

Adverse effects of variable severity have been reported with the therapeutic use of estrogens. Many other effects reported in conjunction with hormonal contraceptives may be related to their estrogen content. These are discussed below.

Estrogen therapy is a major cause of **postmenopausal bleeding.** Unfortunately, vaginal bleeding at this time of life may also be due to carcinoma of the endometrium. In order to avoid confusion, patients should be treated with the smallest amount of estrogen possible. It should be given cyclically so that bleeding, if it occurs, will be more likely to occur during the withdrawal period. As noted above, endometrial hyperplasia can be prevented by administration of a progestational agent with estrogen in each cycle.

Nausea and **breast tenderness** are common and can be minimized by using the smallest effective dose of estrogen. **Hyperpigmentation** also occurs. Estrogen therapy is associated with an increase in frequency of **migraine headaches** as well as **cholestasis, hypertension,** and **gallbladder disease.**

The relationship of estrogen therapy to **cancer** continues to be the subject of active investigation. Although no adverse effect of short-term estrogen therapy on the incidence of breast cancer has been demonstrated, a small increase in the incidence of this tumor may occur with prolonged therapy. Although the risk factor is small (1.25), the impact is great since this tumor occurs in 10% of women. The effect of progesterone has not been determined as yet. Studies indicate that following unilateral excision of breast cancer, women receiving tamoxifen show a 35% decrease in contralateral breast cancer compared with controls. These studies also demonstrate that tamoxifen is well tolerated by most patients, produces estrogen-like alterations in plasma lipid levels, and stabilizes bone mineral loss. Studies bearing on the possible efficacy of tamoxifen in postmenopausal women at high risk for breast cancer are under way. Many studies show an increased risk of endometrial carcinoma in patients taking estrogens. The risk seems to vary with the dose and duration of treatment: 15 times as great in patients taking large doses of estrogen for 5 or more years, in contrast with two to four times greater in patients receiving lower doses for short periods. However, as noted above, the concomitant use of a progestin not only prevents this increased risk but actually reduces the incidence of endometrial cancer to less than that in the general population.

There have been a number of reports of adenocarcinoma of the vagina in young women whose mothers were treated with large doses of diethylstilbestrol early in pregnancy. These cancers are most common in young women (ages 14–44). The incidence is less than 1 per 1000 women exposed—too low to establish a cause-and-effect relationship with certainty. However, the risks for infertility, ectopic pregnancy, and premature delivery are also increased. It is now recognized that there is no indication for the use of diethylstilbestrol during pregnancy, and it should be avoided. It is not known whether other estrogens have a similar effect or whether the observed phenomena are peculiar to diethylstilbestrol. This agent should be used only for the treatment of cancer (eg, of the prostate) or as a "morning after" contraceptive (see Table 40–4).

Contraindications

Estrogens should not be used in patients with estrogen-dependent neoplasms such as carcinoma of the endometrium or in those with—or at high risk for—carcinoma of the breast. They should be avoided in patients with undiagnosed genital bleeding, liver disease, or a history of thromboembolic disorder.

Preparations & Dosages

The dosages of commonly used natural and synthetic preparations are listed in Table 40–1. Although the estrogens produce almost the same hormonal effects, their potencies vary both between agents and depending on the route of administration. As noted above, estradiol is the most active endogenous estrogen, and it has the highest affinity for the estrogen receptor. However, its metabolites estrone and estriol have weak uterotropic effects. Another important metabolite of estradiol, 2-hydroxyestrone (a catechol estrogen), has been shown to act as a neurotransmitter in the brain. It also competes with catecholamines for catechol-O-methyltransferase and inhibits tyrosine hydroxylase. Therefore, preparations with estrone and estradiol may produce more central effects than preparations with synthetic estrogens, which are metabolized differently.

For a given level of gonadotropin suppression, oral estrone and estradiol preparations have more effect on the circulating levels of CBG and SHBG than do transdermal preparations. The oral route of administration allows greater concentrations of hormone to reach the liver, thus increasing the synthesis of these binding proteins. Transdermal preparations were developed to avoid this effect. When administered transdermally, 50–100 µg of estradiol has effects similar to those of 0.625–1.25 mg of conjugated oral estrogens on gonadotropin concentrations, endometrium, and vaginal epithelium. Furthermore, the transdermal estrogen preparations do not significantly increase the concentrations of renin substrate, CBG, and TBG and do not produce the characteristic changes in serum lipids. Combined oral preparations containing 0.625 mg of conjugated estrogens and 2.5 mg of medroxyprogesterone acetate are available for menopausal replacement therapy. Tablets containing 0.625 of conjugated estrogens and 5 mg of medroxyprogesterone acetate are available to be used in conjunction with conjugated estrogens in a sequential fashion. Estrogens alone are taken on days 1–14 and the combination on days 15–28.

THE PROGESTINS

Natural Progestins: Progesterone

Progesterone is the most important progestin in humans. In addition to having important hormonal effects, it serves as a precursor to the estrogens, androgens, and adrenocortical steroids. It is synthesized in the ovary, testis, and adrenal from circulating cholesterol. Large amounts are also synthesized and released by the placenta during pregnancy.

In the ovary, progesterone is produced primarily by the corpus luteum. Normal males appear to secrete 1–5 mg of progesterone daily, resulting in plasma levels of about 0.03 μg/dL. The level is only slightly higher in the female during the follicular phase of the cycle, when only a few milligrams per day of progesterone are secreted. During the luteal phase, plasma levels range from 0.5 μg/dL to more than 2 μg/dL (Figure 40–1).

Synthetic Progestins

A variety of progestational compounds have been synthesized. Some are active when given by mouth. They are not a uniform group of compounds, and all of them differ from progesterone in one or more respects. Table 40–2 lists some of these compounds and their effects. In general, the 21-carbon compounds (hydroxyprogesterone, medroxyprogesterone, megestrol, and dimethisterone) are the most closely related, pharmacologically as well as chemically, to progesterone. A new group of "third-generation" synthetic progestins has been introduced, principally as components of oral contraceptives. These "19-nor, 13-ethyl" steroid compounds include gestodene, norgestimate, and desogestrel (Figure 40–5). They are claimed to have lower androgenic activity than older progestins (Bringer, 1992).

Pharmacokinetics

Progesterone is rapidly absorbed following administration by any route. Its half-life in the plasma is approximately 5 minutes, and small amounts are stored temporarily in body fat. It is almost completely metabolized in one passage through the liver, and for that reason it is quite ineffective when administered orally.

In the liver, progesterone is metabolized to pregnanediol and conjugated with glucuronic acid. It is excreted into the urine as pregnanediol glucuronide (Figure 40–6). The amount of pregnanediol in the urine has been used as an index of progesterone secretion. It has been very useful in spite of the fact that the proportion of secreted progesterone converted to this compound varies from day to day and from individual to individ-

Table 40–2. Activities of progestational agents.

	Route	Duration of Action	Activities[1]				
			Estro-genic	Andro-genic	Anties-trogenic	Antian-drogenic	Anabolic
Progesterone and derivatives							
Progesterone	IM	1 day	–	–	+	–	–
Hydroxyprogesterone caproate	IM	8–14 days	sl	sl	–	–	–
Medroxyprogesterone acetate	IM, PO	Tabs: 1–3 days; injection: 4–12 weeks	–	+	+	–	–
Megestrol acetate	PO	1–3 days	–	+	–	+	–
17α-Ethinyl testosterone derivatives							
Testosterone derivatives							
Dimethisterone	PO	1–3 days	–	–	sl	–	–
19-Nortestosterone derivatives							
Desogestrel	PO	1–3 days	–	–	–	–	–
Norethynodrel[2]	PO	1–3 days	+	–	–	–	–
Lynestrenol[3]	PO	1–3 days	+	+	–	–	+
Norethindrone[2]	PO	1–3 days	sl	+	+	–	+
Norethindrone acetate[2]	PO	1–3 days	sl	+	+	–	+
Ethynodiol diacetate[2]	PO	1–3 days	sl	+	+	–	–
L-Norgestrel[2]	PO	1–3 days	–	+	+	–	+

[1]**Interpretation:** + = active; – = inactive; sl = slightly active. Activities have been reported in various species using various end points and may not apply to humans.
[2]See Table 40–3.
[3]Not available in USA.

Figure 40–5. Progesterone and some progestational agents in clinical use. See Table 40–2.

ual. In addition to progesterone, 20α- and 20β-hydroxyprogesterone (20α- and 20β-hydroxy-4-pregnene-3-one) are also found. These compounds have about one-fifth the progestational activity of progesterone in humans and other species. Little is known of their physiologic importance, but 20α-hydroxyprogesterone is produced in large amounts in some species and may be of some importance biologically.

The usual routes of administration and durations of action of the synthetic progestins are listed in Table 40–2. Most of these agents are extensively metabolized to inactive products that are excreted mainly in the urine.

Physiologic Effects

A. Mechanism: The mechanism of action of progesterone is similar to that of other steroid hormones and is described in more detail above (page 612). Progestins enter the cell and bind to progesterone receptors that are distributed between the nucleus and the cytoplasmic domains. The ligand-receptor complex binds to a response element to activate gene transcription. The response element for progesterone appears to be similar to the corticoid response element, and the specificity of the response depends upon which receptor is present in the cell as well as upon other cell-specific transcription factors. The progesterone-receptor complex forms a dimer before binding to DNA. However, in contrast to the estrogen receptor, it can form heterodimers as well as homodimers.

B. Effects of Progesterone: Progesterone has little effect on protein metabolism. It stimulates lipoprotein lipase activity and seems to favor fat deposition. The effects on carbohydrate metabolism are more marked. Progesterone increases basal insulin levels and the insulin response to glucose. There is usually no manifest change in carbohydrate tolerance. In the liver, progesterone promotes glycogen storage, possibly by facilitating the effect of insulin. Progesterone also promotes ketogenesis.

The liganded progesterone receptor can also bind to *glucocorticoid* response elements. Furthermore, progesterone can compete with aldosterone at the renal tubule, causing a decrease in Na^+ reabsorption. This leads to an increased secretion of aldosterone by the adrenal cortex (eg, in pregnancy). Progesterone increases the body temperature in humans. The mechanism of this effect is not known, but an alteration of the temperature-regulating centers in the hypothalamus has been suggested. Progesterone also alters the function of the respiratory centers. The ventilatory response to CO_2 is increased (synthetic progestins with an ethinyl group do not have respiratory effects). This leads to a measurable reduction in arterial and alveolar P_{CO_2} during pregnancy and in the luteal phase of the menstrual cycle. Progesterone and related steroids also have depressant and hypnotic effects on the brain.

Progesterone is responsible for the alveolobular development of the secretory apparatus in the breast. It also causes the maturation and secretory changes in the endometrium that are seen following ovulation (Figure 40–1).

Progesterone decreases the plasma levels of many amino acids and leads to increased urinary nitrogen excretion. It has been found to induce changes in the

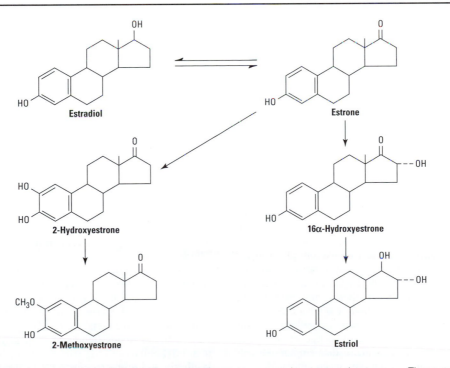

Figure 40–6. Synthetic and degradation pathways for progesterone, androgens, and estrogens. These pathways are similar in the ovary, testis, and adrenal. (Reproduced, with permission, from Greenspan FS [editor]: *Basic & Clinical Endocrinology,* 3rd ed. Appleton & Lange, 1991.)

structure and function of smooth endoplasmic reticulum in experimental animals.

Other effects are noted in the section on Hormonal Contraception.

C. Synthetic Progestins: The 21-carbon progesterone analogs antagonize aldosterone-induced sodium retention (see above) and have slight androgenic or estrogenic effects. The remaining compounds ("19-nortestosterone" third-generation agents) produce a decidual change in the endometrial stroma, do not support pregnancy in test animals, are more effective gonadotropin inhibitors, and may have minimal estrogenic and androgenic or anabolic activity (Table 40–2, Figure 40–5). They are sometimes referred to as "impeded androgens." Progestins without androgenic activity include desogestrel, gestodene, and norgestimate. These compounds are dispensed in combination with ethinyl estradiol for oral contraception (Table 40–3) but are not otherwise available in the USA. Oral contraceptives containing cyproterone (an antiandrogen) or drospirenone (an antimineralocorticoid) in combination with ethinyl estradiol are investigational in the USA.

Clinical Uses of Progestins

A. Therapeutic Applications: The major uses of progestational hormones are for hormone replacement therapy (see above) and hormonal contraception (see below). In addition, they are useful in producing long-term ovarian suppression for other purposes. When used alone in large doses parenterally (eg, medroxyprogesterone acetate, 150 mg intramuscularly every 90 days), prolonged anovulation and amenorrhea result. This therapy has been employed in the treatment of dysmenorrhea, endometriosis, hirsutism, and bleeding disorders when estrogens are contraindicated and for contraception. The major problem with this regimen is the prolonged time required in some patients for ovulatory function to return after cessation of therapy. It should not be used for patients planning a pregnancy in the near future. Similar regimens will relieve hot flushes in some menopausal women and can be used if estrogen therapy is contraindicated.

Medroxyprogesterone acetate, 10–20 mg orally twice weekly–or intramuscularly in doses of 100 mg/m^2 every 1–2 weeks—will arrest accelerated maturation in children with precocious puberty.

Progestins do not appear to have any place in the therapy of threatened or habitual abortion. Early reports of the usefulness of these agents resulted from the unwarranted assumption that after several abortions the likelihood of repeated abortions was over 90%. When progestational agents were administered to patients with previous abortions, a salvage rate of 80% was achieved. It is now recognized that similar patients abort only 20% of the time even when untreated.

Progesterone and medroxyprogesterone have been used in the treatment of women who have difficulty in conceiving and who demonstrate a slow rise in basal body temperature. There is no convincing evidence that this treatment is effective.

Preparations of progesterone and medroxyprogesterone have been used to treat premenstrual syndrome. Controlled studies have not confirmed the effectiveness of such therapy except when doses sufficient to suppress ovulation have been used.

B. Diagnostic Uses: Progesterone can be used as a test of estrogen secretion. The administration of progesterone, 150 mg/d, or medroxyprogesterone, 10 mg/d for 5–7 days, is followed by withdrawal bleeding in amenorrheic patients only when the endometrium has been stimulated by estrogens. A combination of estrogen and progestin can be given to test the responsiveness of the endometrium in patients with amenorrhea.

Contraindications, Cautions, & Adverse Effects

Studies of progestational compounds alone and with combination oral contraceptives indicate that the progestin in these agents may increase blood pressure in some patients. The more androgenic progestins also reduce plasma HDL levels in women. (See Hormonal Contraception, below.)

OTHER OVARIAN HORMONES

The normal ovary produces small amounts of **androgens,** including testosterone, androstenedione, and dehydroepiandrosterone. Of these, only testosterone has a significant amount of biologic activity, though androstenedione can be converted to estrone in peripheral tissues. The normal woman produces less than 200 μg of testosterone in 24 hours, and about one-third of this is probably formed in the ovary directly. The physiologic significance of these small amounts of androgens is not established, but they may be partly responsible for normal hair growth at puberty and may have other important metabolic effects. Androgen production by the ovary may be markedly increased in some abnormal states, usually in association with hirsutism and amenorrhea as noted above.

The ovary also produces **inhibin** and **activin.** These peptides consist of several combinations of α and β subunits. The αβ dimer (inhibin) inhibits FSH secretion while the ββ dimer (activin) increases FSH secretion. Studies in primates indicate that inhibin has no direct effect on ovarian steroidogenesis but that activin modulates the response to LH and FSH. For example, simultaneous treatment with activin and human FSH enhances FSH stimulation of progesterone synthesis and aromatase activity in granulosa cells. When combined with LH, activin suppressed the LH-induced progesterone response by 50% but markedly enhanced basal and LH-stimulated aromatase activity. Activin may also act as a growth factor in other tissues. The physiologic roles of these modulators are not fully understood.

Relaxin is another peptide that can be extracted from the ovary. The three-dimensional structure of relaxin is related to that of the growth-promoting peptides and is similar to that of insulin. Although the amino acid sequence differs from that of insulin, it consists of two chains linked by disulfide bonds, cleaved from a prohormone. It is found in the ovary, placenta, uterus, and blood. Relaxin synthesis has been demonstrated in luteinized granulosa cells of the corpus luteum. It has been shown to increase glycogen synthesis and water uptake by the myometrium and decreases uterine contractility. In some species, it changes the mechanical properties of the cervix and pubic ligaments, facilitating delivery.

In women, relaxin has been measured by immunoassay. Levels were highest immediately after the LH surge and during menstruation. A physiologic role for this hormone has not been established.

Clinical trials with relaxin have been conducted in patients with dysmenorrhea. Relaxin has also been administered to patients in premature labor and during prolonged labor. When applied to the cervix of women at term, it facilitates dilation and shortens labor.

Several other nonsteroidal substances such as follistatin and prostaglandins are produced by the ovary. These probably have paracrine effects within the ovary.

HORMONAL CONTRACEPTION (Oral, Parenteral, & Implanted Contraceptives)

A large number of oral contraceptives containing estrogens or progestins (or both) are now available for clinical use (Table 40–3). These preparations vary chemically and, as might be expected, have many properties in common, but they exhibit definite differences.

Two types of preparations are used for oral contraception: (1) combinations of estrogens and progestins and (2) continuous progestin therapy without concomitant administration of estrogens. The preparations for oral use are all well absorbed, and in combination preparations, the pharmacokinetics of neither drug is significantly altered by the other.

Only one implantable contraceptive preparation is available at present. Norgestrel, also utilized as the progestin component of some oral contraceptive preparations, is an effective suppressant of ovulation when it is released from subcutaneous implants. Intramuscular injection of large doses of medroxypro-gesterone also provides contraceptive action of long duration.

Pharmacologic Effects

A. Mechanism of Action: The combinations of estrogens and progestins exert their contraceptive effect largely through selective inhibition of pituitary function that results in inhibition of ovulation. The combination agents also produce a change in the cervical mucus, in the uterine endometrium, and in motility and secretion in the uterine tubes, all of which decrease the likelihood of conception and implantation. The continuous use of progestins alone does not always inhibit ovulation. The other factors mentioned, therefore, play a major role in the prevention of pregnancy when these agents are used.

B. Effects on the Ovary: Chronic use of combination agents depresses ovarian function. Follicular development is minimal, and corpora lutea, larger follicles, stromal edema, and other morphologic features normally seen in ovulating women are absent. The ovaries usually become smaller even when enlarged before therapy.

The great majority of patients return to normal menstrual patterns when these drugs are discontinued. About 75% will ovulate in the first posttreatment cycle and 97% by the third posttreatment cycle. About 2% of patients remain amenorrheic for periods of up to several years after therapy has been concluded.

The cytologic findings on vaginal smears vary depending on the preparation used. However, with almost all of the combined drugs, a low maturation index is found because of the presence of progestational agents.

C. Effects on the Uterus: After prolonged use, the cervix may show some hypertrophy and polyp formation. There are also important effects on the cervical mucus, making it more like postovulation mucus, ie, thick and less copious.

Agents containing both estrogens and progestins produce a stromal deciduation toward the end of the cycle. The agents containing "19-nor" progestins—particularly those with the smaller amounts of estrogen—tend to produce more glandular atrophy and usually less bleeding.

D. Effects on the Breast: Stimulation of the breasts occurs in most patients receiving estrogen-containing agents. Some enlargement is generally noted. The administration of estrogens and combinations of estrogens and progestins tends to suppress lactation. When the doses are small, the effects on breast feeding are not appreciable. Preliminary studies of the transport of the oral contraceptives into the breast milk suggest that only small amounts of these compounds are found, and they have not been considered to be of importance.

E. Other Effects of Oral Contraceptives:

1. Effects on the central nervous system—The central nervous system effects of the oral

Table 40–3. Some oral and implantable contraceptive agents in use. The estrogen-containing compounds are arranged in order of increasing content of estrogen. (Ethinyl estradiol and mestranol have similar potencies.)

	Estrogen (mg)		Progestin (mg)	
Monophasic combination tablets				
Loestrin 21 1/20	Ethinyl estradiol	0.02	Norethindrone acetate	1.0
Loestrin 21 1.5/30	Ethinyl estradiol	0.03	Norethindrone acetate	1.5
Desogen	Ethinyl estradiol	0.03	Desogestrel	0.15
Lo/Ovral	Ethinyl estradiol	0.03	D,L-Norgestrel	0.3
Nordette	Ethinyl estradiol	0.03	L-Norgestrel	0.15
Brevicon, Modicon	Ethinyl estradiol	0.035	Norethindrone	0.5
Demulen 1/35	Ethinyl estradiol	0.035	Ethynodiol diacetate	1.0
Genora 1/35, Nelova 1/35 E, Norinyl 1/35, Ortho-Novum 1/35	Ethinyl estradiol	0.035	Norethindrone	1.0
Ovcon 35	Ethinyl estradiol	0.035	Norethindrone	0.4
Demulen 1/50	Ethinyl estradiol	0.05	Ethynodiol diacetate	1.0
Ovcon 50	Ethinyl estradiol	0.05	Norethindrone	1.0
Ovral	Ethinyl estradiol	0.05	D,L-Norgestrel	0.5
Genora 1/50, Norinyl 1/50, Ortho-Novum 1/50	Mestranol	0.05	Norethindrone	1.0
Enovid 5 mg	Mestranol	0.075	Norethynodrel	5.0
Enovid 10 mg	Mestranol	0.15	Norethynodrel	9.85
Biphasic combination tablets				
Ortho-Novum 10/11, Nelova 10/11				
Days 1–10	Ethinyl estradiol	0.035	Norethindrone	0.5
Days 11–21	Ethinyl estradiol	0.035	Norethindrone	1.0
Triphasic combination tablets				
Triphasil, Tri-Levlen				
Days 1–6	Ethinyl estradiol	0.03	L-Norgestrel	0.05
Days 7–11	Ethinyl estradiol	0.04	L-Norgestrel	0.075
Days 12–21	Ethinyl estradiol	0.03	L-Norgestrel	0.125
Ortho-Novum 7/7/7				
Days 1–7	Ethinyl estradiol	0.035	Norethindrone	0.5
Days 8–14	Ethinyl estradiol	0.035	Norethindrone	0.75
Days 15–21	Ethinyl estradiol	0.035	Norethindrone	1.0
Tri-Norinyl				
Days 1–7	Ethinyl estradiol	0.035	Norethindrone	0.5
Days 8–16	Ethinyl estradiol	0.035	Norethindrone	1.0
Days 17–21	Ethinyl estradiol	0.035	Norethindrone	0.5
Ortho-Tri-Cyclen				
Days 1–7	Ethinyl estradiol	0.035	Norgestimate	0.18
Days 8–14	Ethinyl estradiol	0.035	Norgestimate	0.215
Days 15–21	Ethinyl estradiol	0.035	Norgestimate	0.25
Daily progestin tablets				
Micronor		. . .	Norethindrone	0.35
Nor-QD		. . .	Norethindrone	0.35
Ovrette		. . .	D,L-Norgestrel	0.075
Implantable progestin preparation				
Norplant System		. . .	L-Norgestrel (6 tubes of 36 mg each)	

contraceptives have not been well studied in humans. A variety of effects of estrogen and progesterone have been noted in animals. Estrogens tend to increase excitability in the brain, whereas progesterone tends to decrease it. The thermogenic action of progesterone and some of the synthetic progestins is also thought to occur in the central nervous system.

It is very difficult to evaluate any behavioral or emotional effects of these compounds in humans. Although the incidence of pronounced changes in mood, affect, and behavior appears to be low, milder changes are commonly reported.

2. Effects on endocrine function–The inhibition of pituitary gonadotropin secretion has been mentioned. Estrogens are known to alter adrenal structure and function. Estrogens increase the plasma concentration of the α_2-globulin that binds hydrocortisone (corticosteroid-binding globulin). This does not appear to lead to any chronic alteration in the rate of secretion of cortisol, but plasma concentrations may be more than double the levels found in untreated individuals. It has also been observed that the ACTH response to the administration of metyrapone is attenuated by estrogens and the oral contraceptives.

These preparations cause alterations in the angiotensin-aldosterone system. Plasma renin activity has been found to increase, and there is an increase in aldosterone secretion.

Thyroxine-binding globulin is increased. As a result, plasma thyroxine (T_4) levels are increased to those commonly seen during pregnancy. Since more of the thyroxine is bound, the free thyroxine level in these patients is normal.

Estrogens also increase the plasma level of SHBG and decrease plasma levels of free androgens by increasing their binding; large amounts of estrogen may decrease androgens by gonadotropin suppression.

3. Effects on blood–Serious thromboembolic phenomena occurring in women taking oral contraceptives have given rise to a great many studies of the effects of these compounds on blood coagulation. A clear picture of such effects has not yet emerged. The oral contraceptives do not consistently alter bleeding or clotting times. The changes that have been observed are similar to those reported in pregnancy. There is an increase in factors VII, VIII, IX, and X and a decrease in antithrombin III. Increased amounts of coumarin derivatives may be required to prolong prothrombin time in patients taking oral contraceptives.

There is an increase in serum iron and total iron-binding capacity similar to that reported in patients with hepatitis.

Significant alterations in the cellular components of blood have not been reported with any consistency. A number of patients have been reported to develop folic acid deficiency anemias.

4. Effects on the liver–These hormones also have profound effects on the function of the liver.

Some of these effects are deleterious and will be considered below in the section on adverse effects.

The effects on serum proteins result from the effects of the estrogens on the synthesis of the various α_2-globulins and fibrinogen. Serum haptoglobins that also arise from the liver are depressed rather than increased by estrogen.

Some of the effects on carbohydrate and lipid metabolism are probably influenced by changes in liver metabolism (see below).

Important alterations in hepatic drug excretion and metabolism also occur. Estrogens in the amounts seen during pregnancy or used in oral contraceptive agents delay the clearance of sulfobromophthalein and reduce the flow of bile. The proportion of cholic acid in bile acids is increased while the proportion of chenodeoxycholic acid is decreased. These changes may cause the observed increase in cholelithiasis associated with the use of these agents.

5. Effects on lipid metabolism–The available studies indicate that estrogens increase serum triglycerides and free and esterified cholesterol. Phospholipids are also increased, as are high-density lipoproteins. Low-density lipoproteins usually decrease. Although the effects are marked with doses of 100 μg of mestranol or ethinyl estradiol, doses of 50 μg or less have minimal effects. The progestins (particularly the 19-nortestosterone derivatives) tend to antagonize these effects of estrogen. Preparations containing small amounts of estrogen and a progestin may slightly decrease triglycerides and high-density lipoproteins.

6. Effects on carbohydrate metabolism–The administration of oral contraceptives produces alterations in carbohydrate metabolism similar to those observed in pregnancy. There is a reduction in the rate of absorption of carbohydrates from the gastrointestinal tract. Progesterone increases the basal insulin level and the rise in insulin induced by carbohydrate ingestion. Preparations with more potent progestins such as norgestrel may cause progressive decreases in carbohydrate tolerance over the years. However, the changes in glucose tolerance are reversible on discontinuing medication.

7. Effects on the cardiovascular system–These agents cause small increases in cardiac output associated with higher systolic and diastolic blood pressure and heart rate. The pressure returns to normal when treatment is terminated. Although the magnitude of the pressure change is small in most patients, it is marked in a few. It is important that blood pressure be followed in each patient. An increase in blood pressure has been reported to occur in few postmenopausal women treated with estrogens alone.

8. Effects on the skin–The oral contraceptives have been noted to increase pigmentation of the skin (chloasma). This effect seems to be enhanced in women who have dark complexions and by exposure to ultraviolet light. Some of the androgen-like progestins may increase the production of sebum, causing acne in some patients. However, since ovarian androgen is suppressed, many patients note decreased sebum production, acne, and terminal hair growth. The sequential oral contraceptive preparations as well as estrogens alone often decrease sebum production.

Clinical Uses

The most important use of combined estrogens and progestins is for oral contraception. A large number of preparations are available for this specific purpose, some of which are listed in Table 40–3. They are specially packaged for ease of administration. In general, they are very effective; when these agents are taken according to directions, the risk of conception is extremely small. The pregnancy rate with combination agents is estimated to be about 0.5–1 per 100 woman years at risk. Contraceptive failure has been observed in some patients taking phenytoin or antibiotics or when one or more doses are missed.

Progestins and estrogens are also useful in the treatment of endometriosis. When severe dysmenorrhea is the major symptom, the suppression of ovulation with estrogen alone may be followed by painless periods. However, in most patients this approach to therapy is inadequate. The long-term administration of large doses of progestins or combinations of progestins and estrogens prevents the periodic breakdown of the endometrial tissue and in some cases will lead to endometrial fibrosis and prevent the reactivation of implants for prolonged periods.

As is true with most hormonal preparations, many of the undesired effects are physiologic or pharmacologic effects that are objectionable only because they are not pertinent to the situation for which they are being used. Therefore, the product containing the smallest effective amounts of hormones should be selected for use.

Adverse Effects

The incidence of serious known toxicities associated with the use of these drugs is low. There are a number of reversible changes in intermediary metabolism. Minor adverse effects are frequent, but most are mild and many are transient. Continuing problems may respond to simple changes in pill formulation. Although it is not often necessary to discontinue medication for these reasons, as many as one-third of all patients started on oral contraception discontinue therapy for reasons other than a desire to become pregnant.

A. Mild Adverse Effects:

1. Nausea, mastalgia, breakthrough bleeding, and edema are related to the amount of estrogen in the preparation. These effects can often be alleviated by a shift to a preparation containing smaller amounts of estrogen or to agents containing progestins with more androgenic effects.

2. Changes in serum proteins and other effects on endocrine function (see above) must be taken into account when thyroid, adrenal, or pituitary function is being evaluated. Increases in sedimentation rate are thought to be due to increased levels of fibrinogen.

3. Headache is mild and often transient. Migraine is often made worse and has been reported to be associated with an increased frequency of cerebrovascular accidents. When this occurs or when migraine has its onset during therapy with these agents, treatment should be discontinued.

4. Withdrawal bleeding sometimes fails to occur— most often with combination preparations—and may cause confusion with regard to pregnancy. If this is disturbing to the patient, a different preparation may be tried or other methods of contraception used.

B. Moderate Adverse Effects: Any of the following may require discontinuance of oral contraceptives:

1. Breakthrough bleeding is the most common problem in using progestational agents alone for contraception. It occurs in as many as 25% of patients. It is more frequently encountered in patients taking low-dose preparations than in those taking combination pills with higher levels of progestin and estrogen. The biphasic and triphasic oral contraceptives (Table 40–3) decrease breakthrough bleeding without increasing the total hormone content.

2. Weight gain is more common with the combination agents containing androgen-like progestins. It can usually be controlled by shifting to preparations with less progestin effect or by dieting.

3. Increased skin pigmentation may occur, especially in dark-skinned women. It tends to increase with time, the incidence being about 5% at the end of the first year and about 40% after 8 years. It is thought to be exacerbated by vitamin B deficiency. It is often reversible upon discontinuance of medication but may disappear very slowly.

4. Acne may be exacerbated by agents containing androgen-like progestins (see Table 40–2), whereas agents containing large amounts of estrogen usually cause marked improvement in acne.

5. Hirsutism may also be aggravated by the "19-nortestosterone" derivatives, and combinations containing nonandrogenic progestins are preferred in these patients.

6. Ureteral dilation similar to that observed in pregnancy has been reported, and bacteriuria is more frequent.

7. Vaginal infections are more common and more difficult to treat in patients who are receiving oral contraceptives.

8. Amenorrhea occurs in some patients. Following cessation of administration of oral contraceptives, 95% of patients with normal menstrual histories resume normal periods and all but a few resume normal cycles during the next few months. However, some patients remain amenorrheic for several years. Many of these patients also have galactorrhea. Patients who have had menstrual irregularities before taking oral contraceptives are particularly susceptible to prolonged amenorrhea when the agents are discontinued. Prolactin levels should be measured in these patients, since many have prolactinomas.

C. Severe Adverse Effects:

1. Vascular disorders–Thromboembolism was one of the earliest of the serious unanticipated effects to be reported and has been the most thoroughly studied.

a. Venous thromboembolic disease–Superficial or deep thromboembolic disease in women not taking oral contraceptives occurs in about one patient per 1000 woman years. The overall incidence of these disorders in patients taking low-dose oral contraceptives is about threefold higher. The risk for this disorder is increased during the first month of contraceptive use and remains constant for several years or more. The risk returns to normal within a month when use is discontinued. The risk of venous thrombosis or pulmonary embolism is increased among women with predisposing conditions such as stasis, altered clotting factors such as antithrombin III, increased levels of homocysteine, or injury. Genetic disorders, including mutations in the genes governing the production of protein C (factor V Leiden), protein S, hepatic cofactor II, and others, markedly increase the risk of venous thromboembolism. The incidence of these disorders is too low for cost-effective screening by current methods, but prior episodes or a family history may be helpful in identifying patients with these conditions.

The incidence of venous thromboembolism is related to the estrogen but not the progestin content of oral contraceptives and is not related to age, parity, mild obesity, or cigarette smoking. Decreased venous blood flow, endothelial proliferation in veins and arteries, and increased coagulability of blood resulting from changes in platelet coagulation and fibrinolytic systems contribute to the increased incidence of thrombosis. The major plasma inhibitor of thrombin, antithrombin III, is substantially decreased during oral contraceptive use. This change occurs in the first month of treatment and lasts as long as treatment persists, reversing within a month thereafter.

b. Myocardial infarction–The use of oral contraceptives is associated with a slightly higher risk of myocardial infarction in women who are obese, have a history of preeclampsia or hypertension, or have hyperlipoproteinemia or diabetes. There is a much higher risk in women who smoke. The risk attributable to oral contraceptives in women 30–40 years of age who do not smoke is about 4 cases per 100,000 users per year, as compared to 185 cases per 100,000 among women 40–44 who smoke heavily. The association with myocardial infarction is thought to involve acceleration of atherogenesis because of decreased glucose tolerance, decreased levels of HDL, increased levels of LDL, and increased platelet aggregation. In addition, facilitation of coronary arterial spasm may also play a role in some of these patients.

The progestational component of oral contraceptives decreases HDL cholesterol levels, in proportion to the androgenic activity of the progestin. The net effect, therefore, will depend on the specific composition of the pill used and the patient's susceptibility to the particular effects. Recent studies suggest that risk of infarction is not increased in past users who have discontinued oral contraceptives.

c. Cerebrovascular disease–The risk of strokes is concentrated in women over age 35. It is increased in current users of oral contraceptives but not in past users. However, subarachnoid hemorrhages have been found to be increased among both current and past users and may increase with time. The risk of thrombotic or hemorrhagic stroke attributable to oral contraceptives (based on older, higher-dose preparations) has been estimated to about 37 cases per 100,000 users per year. Ten percent of these strokes were fatal, and most of the fatal ones were due to subarachnoid hemorrhage. Insufficient data are available on which to base an assessment of the effects of smoking and other risk factors.

Elevations in blood pressure may also increase the risk, since there is a three- to six-fold increase in the incidence of overt hypertension in women taking oral contraceptives.

In summary, available data indicate that oral contraceptives increase the risk of various cardiovascular disorders at all ages and among both smokers and nonsmokers. However, this risk appears to be concentrated in women 35 years of age or older who are heavy smokers. It is clear that these risk factors must be considered in each individual patient for whom oral contraceptives are considered.

2. Gastrointestinal disorders–Many cases of cholestatic jaundice have been reported in patients taking progestin-containing drugs. The differences in incidence of these disorders from one population to another suggest that genetic factors may be involved. The jaundice caused by these agents is similar to that produced by other 17-alkyl-substituted steroids. It is most often observed in the first three cycles and is particularly common in women with a history of cholestatic jaundice during pregnancy. Jaundice and pruritus disappear 1–8 weeks after the drug is discontinued.

These agents have also been found to increase the incidence of symptomatic gallbladder disease, including cholecystitis and cholangitis. This is probably the result of the alterations responsible for jaundice and bile acid changes described above.

It also appears that the incidence of hepatic adenomas is increased in women taking oral contraceptives. Ischemic bowel disease secondary to thrombosis of the celiac and superior and inferior mesenteric arteries and veins has also been reported in women using these drugs.

3. Depression–Depression of sufficient degree to require cessation of therapy occurs in about 6% of patients treated with some preparations.

4. Cancer–The occurrence of malignant tumors in patients taking oral contraceptives has been studied extensively. It is now clear that these compounds *reduce* the risk of endometrial and ovarian cancer. The lifetime risk of breast cancer in the population as a whole does not seem to be affected by oral contraceptive use. Some studies have shown an increased risk in younger women, and it is possible that tumors that develop in younger women become clinically apparent sooner. The relationship of risk of cervical cancer to oral contraceptive use is still controversial.

In addition to the above effects, a number of other adverse reactions have been reported for which a causal relationship has not been established. These include alopecia, erythema multiforme, erythema nodosum, and other skin disorders.

Contraindications & Cautions

These drugs are contraindicated in patients with thrombophlebitis, thromboembolic phenomena, and cerebrovascular disorders or a past history of these conditions. They should not be used to treat vaginal bleeding when the cause is unknown. They should be avoided in patients with known or suspected tumor of the breast or other estrogen-dependent neoplasm. Since these preparations have caused aggravation of preexisting disorders, they should be avoided or used with caution in patients with liver disease, asthma, eczema, migraine, diabetes, hypertension, optic neuritis, retrobulbar neuritis, or convulsive disorders.

The oral contraceptives may produce edema, and for that reason they should be used with great caution in patients in congestive failure or in whom edema is otherwise undesirable or dangerous.

Estrogens may increase the rate of growth of fibroids. Therefore, for women with these tumors, agents with the smallest amounts of estrogen and the most androgenic progestins should be selected. The use of progestational agents alone for contraception might be especially useful in such patients (see below).

These agents are contraindicated in adolescents in whom epiphysial closure has not yet been completed.

Women using oral contraceptives must be made aware of an important interaction that occurs with antimicrobial drugs. Because the normal gastrointestinal flora *increases* the enterohepatic cycling (and bioavailability) of estrogens, antimicrobial drugs that interfere with these organisms may reduce the efficacy of oral contraceptives.

Contraception With Progestins Alone

Small doses of progestins administered orally or by implantation under the skin can be used for contraception. They are particularly suited for use in patients for whom estrogen administration is undesirable. They are about as effective as intrauterine devices or combination pills containing 20–30 μg of ethinyl estradiol. There is a high incidence of abnormal bleeding. Effective contraception can also be achieved by injecting 150 mg of depot medroxyprogesterone acetate (DMPA) every 3 months. After a 150 mg dose, ovulation is inhibited for at least 14 weeks. Almost all users experience episodes of unpredictable spotting and bleeding, particularly during the first year of use. Spotting and bleeding decrease with time, and amenorrhea is common. This preparation is not desirable for women planning a pregnancy soon after cessation of therapy because ovulation suppression can persist for as long as 18 months after the last injection. However, ovulation usually returns in a much shorter time. Long-term DMPA use reduces menstrual blood loss and is associated with a decreased risk of endometrial cancer. Suppression of endogenous estrogen secretion may be associated with a reversible reduction in bone density, and changes in plasma lipids are associated with an increased risk of atherosclerosis.

The use of large doses of oral progestins at the time of intercourse is under study.

Hormonal contraception by progestin implants under the skin is available in the USA. This method utilizes the subcutaneous implantation of capsules containing a progestin (L-norgestrel). These capsules release one-fifth to one-third as much steroid as oral agents, are extremely effective, and last for 5–6 years. The low levels of hormone have little effect on lipoprotein and carbohydrate metabolism or blood pressure. The disadvantages include the need for surgical insertion and removal of capsules and some irregular bleeding rather than predictable menses. An association of intracranial hypertension with implanted norgestrel has been observed in a small number of women. Patients experiencing headache or visual disturbances should be checked for papilledema.

Contraception with progestins is useful in patients with hepatic disease, hypertension, psychosis or mental retardation, or prior thromboembolism. The side effects include headache, dizziness, bloating and weight gain of 1–2 kg, and a reversible reduction of glucose tolerance.

Postcoital Contraceptives

Pregnancy can be prevented following coitus by the administration of estrogens alone or in combination with progestins (**"morning after"** contraception). When treatment is begun within 72 hours, it is effective 99% of the time. Some effective schedules are shown in Table 40–4. The hormones are often administered with antiemetics, since 40% of the patients have nausea or vomiting. Other adverse effects include headache, dizziness, breast tenderness, and abdominal and leg cramps.

Mifepristone (RU 486), an antagonist at progesterone (and glucocorticoid) receptors, has been shown to have a luteolytic effect and is effective as a postcoital contraceptive when combined with a prostaglandin (see below).

Table 40–4. Schedules for use of postcoital contraceptives.

Conjugated estrogens: 10 mg 3 times daily for 5 days

Ethinyl estradiol: 2.5 mg twice daily for 5 days

Diethylstilbestrol: 50 mg daily for 5 days

Norgestrel, 0.5 mg, with ethinyl estradiol, 0.05 mg (eg, Ovral): Two tablets and two in 12 hours

Beneficial Effects of Oral Contraceptives

It has become apparent during the last decade that reduction in the dose of the constituents of oral contraceptives has markedly reduced mild and severe adverse effects, providing a relatively safe and convenient method of contraception for many young women. Treatment with oral contraceptives has now been shown to be associated with many benefits unrelated to contraception. These include a reduced risk of ovarian cysts, ovarian and endometrial cancer, and benign breast disease. There is a lower incidence of pelvic inflammatory disease and ectopic pregnancy. Iron deficiency, duodenal ulcer, and rheumatoid arthritis are less common, and premenstrual symptoms, dysmenorrhea, endometriosis, acne, and hirsutism may be ameliorated with their use.

ESTROGEN & PROGESTERONE INHIBITORS & ANTAGONISTS

TAMOXIFEN

Tamoxifen is a competitive partial agonist inhibitor of estradiol at the estrogen receptor and is extensively used in the palliative treatment of advanced breast cancer in postmenopausal women. It is a nonsteroidal agent (see structure below) that is given orally. Peak plasma levels are reached in a few hours. Tamoxifen has an initial half-life of 7–14 hours in the circulation and is predominantly excreted by the liver. It is used in doses of 10–20 mg twice daily. Hot flushes and nausea and vomiting occur in 25% of patients, and many other minor adverse effects are observed. Studies of patients treated with tamoxifen as adjuvant therapy for early breast cancer have shown a 35% decrease in contralateral breast cancer. However, adjuvant therapy extended beyond 5 years in patients with breast cancer has shown no further improvement in outcome.

Prevention of the expected loss of lumbar spine bone density and plasma lipid changes consistent with a reduction in the risk for atherosclerosis have also been reported in these patients following spontaneous or surgical menopause. However, this agonist activity also affects the uterus and increases the risk of endometrial cancer. Raloxifene, an inhibitor currently undergoing clinical trials, has similar effects on lipids and bone but appears not to stimulate the endometrium.

CLOMIPHENE

Clomiphene citrate is a partial agonist, a weak estrogen that also acts as a competitive inhibitor of endogenous estrogens. It has found use as an ovulation-inducing agent (see below).

MIFEPRISTONE

Mifepristone (RU 486) is a "19-norsteroid" that binds strongly to the progesterone receptor and inhibits the activity of progesterone. The drug has luteolytic properties in 80% of women when given in the midluteal period. The mechanism of this effect is unknown, but it may provide the basis for using mifepristone as a contraceptive (as opposed to an abortifacient). However, the compound has a long half-life; large doses of mifepristone may prolong the follicular phase of the subsequent cycle and so make it difficult to use continuously for this purpose. However, a single dose of 600 mg is an effective emergency postcoital contraceptive, though it may result in a delay in the following cycle. The drug also binds to the glucocorticoid receptor. Limited clinical studies

Tamoxifen

Mifepristone

suggest that mifepristone may be useful in the treatment of endometriosis, Cushing's syndrome, breast cancer, and other neoplasms that contain glucocorticoid or progesterone receptors.

Mifepristone's major use thus far has been to terminate early pregnancies. Doses of 400–600 mg/d for 4 days or 800 mg/d for 2 days successfully terminated pregnancy in 85% of the women studied. The major adverse effect was prolonged bleeding that did not require treatment. The combination of a single oral dose of 600 mg of mifepristone and a vaginal pessary containing 1 mg of prostaglandin E_1 or oral misoprostol has been found to effectively terminate pregnancy in 95% of patients treated during the first 7 weeks after conception. The adverse effects of the medications included vomiting, diarrhea, and pain. As many as 5% of patients have vaginal bleeding requiring intervention.

ZK 98734 is potent experimental progesterone inhibitor and abortifacient in doses of 25 mg twice daily. Like mifepristone, it also appears to have antiglucocorticoid activity.

DANAZOL

Danazol, an isoxazole derivative of ethisterone (17α-ethinyl testosterone) with weak progestational and androgenic activities, is used to suppress ovarian function. Danazol inhibits the midcycle surge of LH and FSH and can prevent the compensatory increase in LH and FSH following castration in animals, but it does not significantly lower or suppress basal LH or FSH levels in normal women. Danazol binds to androgen, progesterone, and glucocorticoid receptors and can translocate the androgen receptor into the nucleus to initiate androgen-specific RNA synthesis. It does not bind to intracellular estrogen receptors, but it does bind to sex hormone-binding globulin and corticosteroid-binding globulins. It inhibits P450scc (the cholesterol side chain-cleaving enzyme), 3α-hydroxysteroid dehydrogenase, 17β-hydroxysteroid dehydrogenase, P450c17 (17α-hydroxylase), P450c11 (11β-hydroxylase), and P450c21 (21-hydroxylase). However, it does not inhibit aromatase, the enzyme required for estrogen synthesis. It increases the mean clearance rate of progesterone, probably by competing with the hormone for binding proteins, and may have similar effects on other active steroid hormones. Ethisterone, a major metabolite of danazol, has both progestational and mild androgenic effects.

Danazol is slowly metabolized in humans, having a half-life of over 15 hours. This results in stable circulating levels when the drug is administered twice daily. It has been found to be highly concentrated in the liver, adrenals, and kidneys and is excreted in both feces and urine.

Danazol has been employed as an inhibitor of gonadal function and has found its major use in the treatment of endometriosis. For this purpose, it can be given in a dosage of 600 mg/d. The dosage is reduced to 400 mg/d after 1 month and to 200 mg/d in 2 months. About 85% of patients show marked improvement in 3–12 months.

Danazol has also been used for the treatment of fibrocystic disease of the breast and hematologic disorders, including hemophilia, Christmas disease, and idiopathic thrombocytopenic purpura.

The major adverse effects are weight gain, edema, decreased breast size, acne and oily skin, increased hair growth, deepening of the voice, headache, hot flushes, changes in libido, and muscle cramps. Although mild adverse effects are very common, it is seldom necessary to discontinue the drug because of them.

Danazol should be used with great caution in patients with hepatic dysfunction, since it has been reported to produce mild to moderate hepatocellular damage in some patients, as evidenced by enzyme changes. It is also contraindicated during pregnancy and breast feeding, as it may produce urogenital abnormalities in the offspring.

OTHER INHIBITORS

Anastrozole, a selective nonsteroidal inhibitor of aromatase (the enzyme required for estrogen synthesis), has been shown to be effective in some women whose breast tumors have become resistant to tamoxifen. It is approved for use in such patients.

Several other aromatase inhibitors are undergoing clinical trials in patients with breast cancer. **Letrozole** and **fadrozole** are newer oral nonsteroidal (triazole) inhibitors of aromatase activity. These compounds appear to be about as effective as tamoxifen. ICI-182780 is a pure antiestrogen that has been somewhat more effective than those with partial agonist effects and is effective in some patients who have become resistant to tamoxifen. ICI-164384 inhibits dimerization of the occupied estrogen receptor and interferes with its binding to DNA. It has also been used experimentally in breast cancer patients who have become resistant to tamoxifen.

GnRH and its analogs (**naferelin, buserelin,** etc) have become important in both stimulating and inhibiting ovarian function. They are discussed in Chapter 37.

OVULATION-INDUCING AGENTS

CLOMIPHENE

Clomiphene citrate, a partial estrogen agonist, is closely related to the estrogen chlorotrianisene (Figure 40–3). This compound is active when taken orally. Very little is known about its metabolism, but about half of the compound is excreted in the feces within 5 days after administration. It has been suggested that clomiphene is slowly excreted from an enterohepatic pool.

Pharmacologic Effects

A. Mechanism of Action: Clomiphene is a partial agonist at estrogen receptors. The estrogenic agonist effects are best demonstrated in animals with marked gonadal deficiency. Clomiphene has also been shown to effectively inhibit the action of stronger estrogens. In humans it leads to an increase in the secretion of gonadotropins and estrogens.

B. Effects: The pharmacologic importance of this compound rests on its ability to stimulate ovulation in women with amenorrhea and other ovulatory disorders. The mechanism by which ovulation is produced is not known. It has been suggested that it blocks an inhibitory influence of estrogens on the hypothalamus and increases the production of gonadotropins.

Clinical Uses

Clomiphene is used for the treatment of disorders of ovulation in patients wishing to become pregnant. In general, a single ovulation is induced by a single course of therapy, and the patient must be treated repeatedly until pregnancy is achieved, since normal ovulatory function does not usually resume. The compound is of no use in patients with ovarian or pituitary failure.

When clomiphene is administered in doses of 100 mg daily for 5 days, a rise in plasma LH and FSH is observed after several days. In patients who ovulate, the initial rise is followed by a second rise of gonadotropin levels just prior to ovulation.

Adverse Effects

The most common adverse effects in patients treated with this drug are hot flushes, which resemble those experienced by menopausal patients. They tend to be mild, and disappear when the drug is discontinued. There have been occasional reports of eye symptoms due to intensification and prolongation of afterimages. These are generally of short duration. Headache, constipation, allergic skin reactions, and reversible hair loss have been reported occasionally.

The effective use of clomiphene is associated with some stimulation of the ovaries and usually with ovarian enlargement. The degree of enlargement tends to be greater and its incidence higher in patients who have enlarged ovaries at the beginning of therapy.

A variety of other symptoms such as nausea and vomiting, increased nervous tension, depression, fatigue, breast soreness, weight gain, urinary frequency, and heavy menses have also been reported. However, these appear to result from the hormonal changes associated with an ovulatory menstrual cycle rather than from the medication. The incidence of multiple pregnancy is approximately 10%. Clomiphene has not been shown to have an adverse effect when inadvertently given to women who are already pregnant.

Contraindications & Cautions

Special precautions should be observed in patients with enlarged ovaries. These women are thought to be more sensitive to this drug and should receive small doses. Any patient who complains of abdominal symptoms should be examined carefully. Maximum ovarian enlargement occurs after the 5-day course has been completed, and many patients can be shown to have a palpable increase in ovarian size by the seventh to tenth days. Treatment with clomiphene for more than a year may be associated with an increased risk for low-grade ovarian cancer; however the evidence for this effect is not conclusive.

Special precautions must also be taken in patients who have visual symptoms associated with clomiphene therapy, since these symptoms may make activities such as driving more hazardous.

Dosages

The recommended dosage of clomiphene citrate at the beginning of therapy is 50 mg/d for 5 days. If ovulation occurs, this same course may be repeated until pregnancy is achieved. If ovulation does not occur, the dosage is doubled to 100 mg/d for 5 days. If ovulation and menses occur, the next course can be started on the fifth day of the cycle. Experience to date suggests that patients who do not ovulate after three courses of 100 mg/d of clomiphene are not likely to respond to continued therapy. However, larger doses are effective in some individuals. Clomiphene is sometimes used in combination with menotropins.

About 80% of patients with anovulatory disorders or amenorrhea can be expected to respond by having ovulatory cycles. Approximately half of these patients will become pregnant.

OTHER DRUGS USED IN OVULATORY DISORDERS

In addition to clomiphene, a variety of other hormonal and nonhormonal agents are used in treating anovulatory disorders. They are discussed in Chapter 37.

II. THE TESTIS (Androgens & Anabolic Steroids, Antiandrogens, & Male Contraception)

The testis, like the ovary, has both gametogenic and endocrine functions. The gametogenic function of the testes is controlled largely by the secretion of FSH by the pituitary. High concentrations of androgens locally are also required for sperm production in the seminiferous tubules. The Sertoli cells in the seminiferous tubules may be the source of the estradiol produced in the testes. With LH stimulation, the androgens are produced in the interstitial or Leydig cells found in the spaces between the seminiferous tubules.

The Sertoli cells in the testis synthesize and secrete a variety of active proteins, including müllerian duct inhibitory factor, inhibin, and activin. As in the ovarian peptides, inhibin and activin appear to be the product of three genes that produce a common alpha subunit and two beta subunits, A and B. Activin is composed of the two beta subunits ($\beta_A\beta_B$). There are two inhibins (A and B), which contain the alpha subunit and one of the beta subunits. Activin stimulates pituitary FSH release and is structurally similar to transforming growth factor-β, which also increases FSH. The inhibins in conjunction with dihydrotestosterone are responsible for the feedback inhibition of pituitary FSH secretion.

ANDROGENS & ANABOLIC STEROIDS

In humans, the most important androgen secreted by the testis is testosterone. The pathways of synthesis of testosterone in the testes are similar to those previously described for the adrenal and ovary (Figures 39–1 and 40–2).

In men, approximately 8 mg of testosterone is produced daily. About 95% is produced by the Leydig cells and only 5% by the adrenal. The testis also secretes small amounts of another potent androgen, dihydrotestosterone, as well as androstenedione and dehydroepiandrosterone, which are weak androgens. Pregnenolone and progesterone and their 17-hydroxylated derivatives are also released in small amounts. Plasma levels of testosterone in males are about 0.6 µg/dL after puberty and appear to decline after age 55. Testosterone is also present in the plasma of women in concentrations of approximately 0.03 µg/dL and is derived in approximately equal parts from the ovaries, the adrenals, and by the peripheral conversion of other hormones.

About 65% of circulating testosterone is bound to sex hormone-binding globulin (SHBG). SHBG is increased in plasma by estrogen, by thyroid hormone, and in patients with cirrhosis of the liver. It is decreased by androgen and growth hormone and is lower in obese individuals. Most of the remaining testosterone is bound to albumin. However, approximately 2% remains free and available to enter cells and bind to intracellular receptors.

Metabolism

In many target tissues, testosterone is converted to dihydrotestosterone by the enzyme 5α-reductase. In these tissues, dihydrotestosterone is the major androgen. The conversion of testosterone to estradiol by P450 aromatase also occurs in some tissues, including adipose tissue, liver, and the hypothalamus, where it may be of importance in regulating gonadal function.

The major pathway for the degradation of testosterone in humans is illustrated in Figure 40–4. In the liver, the reduction of the double bond and ketone in the A ring, as is seen in other steroids with a Δ^4-ketone configuration in the A ring, leads to the production of inactive substances such as androsterone and etiocholanolone that are then conjugated and excreted into the urine.

Androstenedione, dehydroepiandrosterone (DHEA), and dehydroepiandrosterone sulfate (DHEAS) are also produced in significant amounts in humans, though largely in the adrenal rather than in the testes. Although they are thought to contribute to the normal maturation process (adrenarche), they do not stimulate or support other androgen-dependent pubertal changes in the human. Recent studies suggest that DHEA and DHEAS may have other important metabolic effects that inhibit atherosclerosis and prolong life in rabbits and perhaps in men (see Adrenal Androgens, Chapter 39). They are to a large extent metabolized in the same fashion as testosterone. Both steroids—but particularly androstenedione—can be converted by peripheral tissues to estrone in very small amounts (1–5%). The P450 aromatase enzyme responsible for this conversion is also found in the brain and is thought to play an important role in development.

Physiologic Effects

In the normal male, testosterone is responsible for the many changes that occur in puberty. In addition to the general growth-promoting properties of androgens on the body tissues, these hormones are responsible for penile and scrotal growth. Changes in the skin include the appearance of pubic, axillary, and beard hair. The sebaceous glands become more active, and the skin tends to become thicker and oilier. The larynx grows and the vocal cords become thicker, leading to a lower-pitched voice. Skeletal growth is stimulated and epiphysial closure accelerated. Other effects include growth of the prostate and seminal vesicles, darkening of the skin, and increased skin circulation. Androgens play an important role in stimulating and maintaining sexual function in men. Androgens increase lean body mass and stimulate body hair growth and sebum secretion. Metabolic effects include the reduction of hormone binding and other carrier proteins and increased liver synthesis of clotting factors, triglyceride lipase, α_1-antitrypsin, haptoglobin, and sialic acid. They also stimulate renal erythropoietin secretion and decrease high-density lipoprotein levels.

Synthetic Steroids
With Androgenic & Anabolic Action

Testosterone, when administered by mouth, is rapidly absorbed. However, it is largely converted to inactive metabolites, and only about one-sixth of the dose administered is available in active form. Testosterone can be administered parenterally, but it has a more prolonged absorption time and greater activity when esterified to the propionate, enanthate, undecanoate, or cypionate. These derivatives are hydrolyzed to release free testosterone at the site of injection. Testosterone derivatives alkylated at the 17 position, eg, methyltestosterone and fluoxymesterone, are active when given by mouth.

Testosterone and its derivatives have been used for their anabolic effects as well as for the replacement of testosterone deficiency. Although testosterone and other known active steroids can be isolated in pure form and measured by weight, biologic assays are still used in the investigation of new compounds. In some of these studies in animals, the anabolic effects of the compound as measured by trophic effects on muscles or the reduction of nitrogen excretion may be dissociated from the other androgenic effects. This has led to the marketing of compounds claimed to have anabolic activity associated with only weak androgenic effects. Unfortunately, this dissociation is less marked in humans than in the animals used for testing (Table 40–5), and all are potent androgens.

Pharmacologic Effects

A. Mechanism of Action: Like other steroids, testosterone acts intracellularly in target cells. In skin, prostate, seminal vesicles, and epididymis, it is converted to 5α-dihydrotestosterone by the enzyme 5α-reductase. In these tissues, dihydrotestosterone is the dominant androgen. The distribution of this enzyme in the fetus is different and has important developmental implications.

Testosterone and dihydrotestosterone bind to the cytosol androgen receptor, initiating a series of events similar to those described for estradiol and progesterone, leading to growth, differentiation, and synthesis of a variety of enzymes and other functional proteins.

B. Effects: In the male at puberty, androgens cause development of the secondary sex characteristics (see above). In the adult male, large doses of testosterone—when given alone—or its derivatives suppress the secretion of gonadotropins and result in some atrophy of the interstitial tissue and the tubules of the testes. Since fairly large doses of androgens are required to suppress gonadotropic secretion, it has been postulated that inhibin, in combination with androgens, is responsible for the feedback control of secretion. In women, androgens are capable of producing changes similar to those observed in the prepubertal male. These include growth of facial and body hair, deepening of the voice, enlargement of the

Table 40–5. Androgens: Preparations available and relative androgenic:anabolic activity in animals.

	Androgenic: Anabolic Activity
Testosterone	1:1
Testosterone cypionate	1:1
Testosterone enanthate	1:1
Testosterone propionate	1:1
Methyltestosterone	1:1
Fluoxymesterone	1:2
Methandrostenolone (methandienone)	1:3
Oxymetholone	1:3
Ethylestrenol	1:4–1:8
Oxandrolone	1:3–1:13
Nandrolone phenpropionate	1:3–1:6
Nandrolone decanoate	1:2.5–1:4
Stanozolol	1:3–1:6
Dromostanolone propionate	1:3–1:4

clitoris, frontal baldness, and prominent musculature. The natural androgens stimulate erythrocyte production.

The administration of androgens reduces the excretion of nitrogen into the urine, indicating an increase in protein synthesis or a decrease in protein breakdown within the body. This effect is much more pronounced in women and children than in normal men.

Clinical Uses

A. Androgen Replacement Therapy in Men: Androgens are used to replace or augment endogenous androgen secretion in hypogonadal men (Table 40–6). Even in the presence of pituitary deficiency, androgens are used rather than gonadotropin except when normal spermatogenesis is to be achieved. In patients with hypopituitarism, androgens are not added to the treatment regimen until puberty, at which time they are instituted in gradually increasing doses to achieve the growth spurt and the development of secondary sex characteristics. In these patients, therapy should be started with long-acting agents such as testosterone enanthate or cypionate in doses of 200 mg intramuscularly every 1–2 weeks until maturation is complete. The dose can then be reduced to 200 mg at 2- to 3-week intervals. Testosterone propionate, though potent, has a short duration of action and is not practical for long-term use. Testosterone undecanoate can be given orally, administering large amounts of the steroid twice daily (eg, 40 mg/d). Testosterone can also be administered transdermally; skin patches are available for scrotal application and other skin areas. Two patches daily are usually required for replacement therapy. Implanted pellets and other longer-

Table 40–6. Androgen preparations for replacement therapy.

	Route of Administration	Dosage
Methyltestosterone	Oral	25–50 mg/d
	Sublingual (buccal)	5–10 mg/d
Fluoxymesterone	Oral	2–10 mg/d
Testosterone propionate	Sublingual (buccal)	5–20 mg/d
	Intramuscular	10–50 mg 3 times weekly
Testosterone enanthate	Intramuscular	200 mg every 1–2 weeks until matura- tion is complete, then every 2–3 weeks for mainenance
Testosterone cypionate	Intramuscular	

acting preparations are under study. The development of polycythemia or hypertension may require some reduction in dose.

B. Gynecologic Disorders: Androgens are used occasionally in the treatment of certain gynecologic disorders, but the undesirable effects in women are such that they must be used with great caution. Androgens have been used to reduce breast engorgement during the postpartum period, usually in conjunction with estrogens. The weak androgen danazol is used in the treatment of endometriosis (see page 672).

Androgens are sometimes given in combination with estrogens for replacement therapy in the postmenopausal period in an attempt to eliminate the endometrial bleeding that may occur when only estrogens are used. They are also used for chemotherapy of breast tumors in premenopausal women.

C. Use as Protein Anabolic Agents: Androgens and anabolic steroids have been used in conjunction with dietary measures and exercises in an attempt to reverse protein loss after trauma, surgery, or prolonged immobilization and in patients with debilitating diseases.

D. Anemia: In the past, large doses of androgens were employed in the treatment of refractory anemias such as aplastic anemia, Fanconi's anemia, sickle cell anemia, myelofibrosis, and hemolytic anemias. The large doses required prevented this from becoming a useful method of therapy in women. Recombinant erythropoietin has largely replaced androgens for this purpose.

E. Osteoporosis: Androgens and anabolic agents have been used in the treatment of osteoporosis, either alone or in conjunction with estrogens.

F. Use as Growth Stimulators: These agents have been used to stimulate growth in boys with delayed puberty. If the drugs are used carefully, these children will probably achieve their expected adult height (and sooner than normal). If treatment is too vigorous, the patient may grow rapidly at first but will not achieve full stature because of the accelerated epiphysial closure that occurs. It is difficult to control this type of therapy adequately even with frequent

x-ray examination of the epiphyses, since the action of the hormones on epiphysial centers may continue for many months after therapy is discontinued.

G. Anabolic Steroid and Androgen Abuse in Sports: The use of anabolic steroids by athletes has received worldwide attention. Many athletes and their coaches believe that anabolic steroids—in doses 10–200 times larger than normal—increase strength and aggressiveness, thereby improving competitive performance. Although such effects have been demonstrated in women, many studies have failed to unequivocally demonstrate them in men. Placebo effects and the potential impact of minimal changes in championship competitions make evaluation of these studies very difficult. However, the adverse effects of these drugs clearly make their use inadvisable.

H. Aging: Androgen production falls with age in men and may contribute to the decline in muscle mass, strength, and libido. Preliminary studies of androgen replacement in aging males with low androgen levels show an increase in lean body mass and hematocrit and a decrease in bone turnover. Longer studies will be required to assess the usefulness of this therapy.

Adverse Effects

The adverse effects of these compounds are due largely to their masculinizing actions and are most noticeable in women and prepubertal children. In women, the administration of more than 200–300 mg of testosterone per month is usually associated with hirsutism, acne, depression of menses, clitoral enlargement, and deepening of the voice. These effects may occur with even smaller doses in some women. Some of the androgenic steroids exert progestational activity leading to endometrial bleeding. These hormones also alter serum lipids and could conceivably increase susceptibility to atherosclerotic disease in women. Except under the most unusual circumstances, androgen should not be used in infants. Recent studies in animals suggest that administration of androgens in early life may have profound effects on maturation of central nervous system centers governing sexual development, particularly in the female.

Administration of these drugs to pregnant females may lead to masculinization of the external genitalia in the fetus. Although the above-mentioned effects may be less marked with the anabolic agents, they do occur.

Sodium retention and edema are not common but must be carefully watched for in patients with heart and kidney disease.

Most of the synthetic androgens and anabolic agents are 17-alkyl-substituted steroids. Administration of drugs with this structure is often associated with evidence of hepatic dysfunction, eg, increase in sulfobromophthalein retention and aspartate aminotransferase (AST) levels. Alkaline phosphatase values are also elevated. These changes usually occur early in the course of treatment, and the degree is proportionate to the dose. Bilirubin levels occasionally increase until clinical jaundice is apparent. The cholestatic jaundice is reversible upon cessation of therapy, and permanent changes do not occur. In older males, prostatic hyperplasia may develop, causing urinary retention.

Replacement therapy in men may cause acne, sleep apnea, erythrocytosis, gynecomastia, and azoospermia. Supraphysiologic doses of androgens produce azoospermia, acne, and decrease in testicular size— all of which may take months to recover after cessation of therapy. The alkylated androgens in high doses can produce peliosis hepatica, cholestasis, and hepatic failure. They lower plasma HDL_2 and may increase LDL. Hepatic adenomas and carcinomas have also been reported. Behavioral effects include psychologic dependence, increased aggressiveness, and psychotic symptoms.

Contraindications & Cautions

The use of androgenic steroids is contraindicated in pregnant women or women who may become pregnant during the course of therapy.

Androgens should not be administered to male patients with carcinoma of the prostate or breast. Until more is known about the effects of these hormones on the central nervous system in developing children, they should be avoided in infants and young children.

Special caution is required in giving these drugs to children to produce a growth spurt. In most patients, the use of somatotropin is more appropriate (Chapter 37).

Care should be exercised in the administration of these drugs to patients with renal or cardiac disease predisposed to edema. If sodium and water retention occurs, it will respond to diuretic therapy.

Methyltestosterone therapy is associated with creatinuria, but the significance of this finding is not known.

Caution: Several cases of hepatocellular carcinoma have been reported in patients with aplastic anemia treated with androgen anabolic therapy. Colony-stimulating factors (Chapter 33) should be used instead.

ANDROGEN SUPPRESSION & ANTIANDROGENS

ANDROGEN SUPPRESSION

The treatment of advanced prostatic carcinoma often requires orchiectomy or large doses of estrogens to reduce available androgen. The psychologic effects of the former and gynecomastia produced by the latter make these approaches undesirable. As noted in Chapter 37, the gonadotropin-releasing hormone analogs such as goserelin, nafarelin, buserelin, and leuprolide acetate produce gonadal suppression when blood levels are continuous rather than pulsatile (see Chapter 37 and Figure 40–7). **Leuprolide acetate** is injected subcutaneously daily in doses of 1 mg (or depot leuprolide is given once every month or every 3 months) for the treatment of prostatic carcinoma. Goserelin is administered once every 4 weeks as a subcutaneous slow-release injection. Although testosterone levels fall to 10% of their initial values after a month with either of these drugs, they *increase* significantly in the beginning. This increase is usually associated with a flare of tumor activity and an increase in symptoms. The combination of a GnRH agonist and flutamide can prevent the initial stimulation and provide a more effective inhibition of androgenic activity.

GnRH antagonists have also been under study, since they would have the advantage of eliminating the surge of androgen secretion seen at the beginning of GnRH analog therapy. Most of the compounds studied have the capacity to release histamine and are unsuitable for use. However, newer agents with less histamine releasing activity are being studied.

ANTIANDROGENS

The potential usefulness of antiandrogens for the treatment of patients producing excessive amounts of testosterone has led to the search for effective drugs that can be used for this purpose. Several approaches to the problem, especially inhibition of synthesis and receptor antagonism, have met with some success.

Steroid Synthesis

Ketoconazole, used primarily for the treatment of fungal disease, is an inhibitor of adrenal and gonadal steroid synthesis. This compound inhibits P450scc (cholesterol side chain cleavage enzyme), P450c17 (17α-hydroxylase and C17,20-lyase), 3β-hydroxysteroid dehydrogenase, and P450c11 (11β-hydroxylase) enzymes. The sensitivity of the P450 enzymes to this compound in mammalian tissues is much lower than the sensitivity of fungal enzymes, so that the inhibitory effects are seen only at high doses. Keto-conazole also has other endocrine effects. It does not affect ovarian aromatase, but it reduces human placental aromatase activity. It displaces estradiol and dihydrotestosterone from sex hormone-binding protein in vitro and increases the estradiol:testosterone ratio in plasma in vivo by a different mechanism. This compound has been used with some success for the treatment of patients with Cushing's syndrome. However, it does not appear to be clinically useful in women with increased androgens because of the toxicity associated with prolonged use of the 400–800 mg/d required. The drug has also been used experimentally to treat prostatic carcinoma, but the results have not been encouraging. Men treated with keto-conazole often develop reversible gynecomastia during therapy; this may be due to the demonstrated increase in the estradiol:testosterone ratio.

Conversion of Steroid Precursors to Androgens

Several compounds have been developed that inhibit the 17-hydroxylation of progesterone or pregnenolone, thereby preventing the action of the side chain-splitting enzyme and the further transformation of these steroid precursors to active androgens. A few of these compounds have been tested clinically but have been too toxic for prolonged use.

Since dihydrotestosterone—not testosterone—appears to be the essential androgen in the prostate, androgen effects in this and similar dihydrotestosterone-dependent tissues can be reduced by an inhibitor of 5α-reductase (Figure 40–7). **Finasteride,** a steroid-like inhibitor of this enzyme, is orally active and produces a reduction in dihydrotestosterone levels within 8 hours after administration that lasts for about 24 hours. The half-life is about 8 hours (longer in elderly individuals). Forty to 50 percent of the dose is metabolized; more than half is excreted in the feces. It has been reported to be moderately effective in reducing prostate size in men with benign prostatic hyperplasia and is approved for this use in the USA. The dosage is 5 mg/d. Its use in advanced prostatic carcinoma is under study. The drug is not approved for use in women or children, although it has been used successfully in the treatment of hirsutism in women.

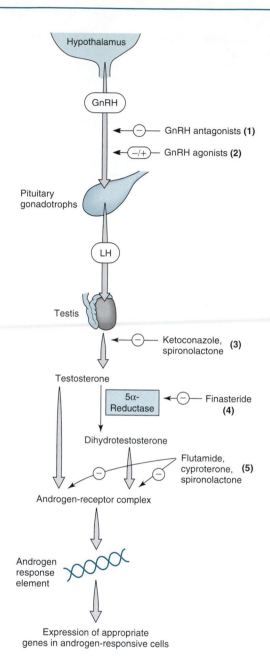

Figure 40–7. Control of androgen secretion and activity and some sites of action of antiandrogens. *(1),* competitive inhibition of GnRH receptors; *(2),* stimulation (+, pulsatile administration) or inhibition via desensitization of GnRH receptors (–, continuous administration); *(3),* decreased synthesis of testosterone in the testis; *(4),* decreased synthesis of dihydrotestosterone by inhibition of 5α-reductase; *(5),* competition for binding to cytosol androgen receptors.

Finasteride

Receptor Inhibitors

Cyproterone and **cyproterone acetate** are effective antiandrogens that inhibit the action of androgens at the target organ. The acetate form has a marked progestational effect that suppresses the feedback enhancement of LH and FSH, leading to a more effective antiandrogen effect. These compounds have been used in women for the treatment of hirsutism and in men to decrease excessive sexual drive and are being studied in other conditions in which the reduction of androgenic effects would be useful. Cyproterone acetate in a dosage of 2 mg/d administered concurrently with an estrogen is used in the treatment of hirsutism in women; it has orphan drug status in the USA.

Flutamide, a substituted anilide, is a potent antiandrogen that has been used in the treatment of prostatic carcinoma. Though not a steroid, it behaves like a competitive antagonist at the androgen receptor. It is rapidly metabolized in humans. It frequently causes mild gynecomastia (probably by increasing testicular estrogen production) and occasionally causes mild reversible hepatic toxicity. Administration of this compound causes some improvement in most patients who have not had prior endocrine therapy. Preliminary studies indicate that flutamide is also useful in the management of excess androgen production in women.

Flutamide

Bicalutamide is a potent orally active antiandrogen that can be administered as a single daily dose. Studies in patients with carcinoma of the prostate indicate that it is well tolerated. It appears to have fewer gastrointestinal side effects than flutamide. A dosage of 150–200 mg/d is required to reduce PSA levels to those achieved by castration.

Spironolactone, a competitive inhibitor of aldosterone (see Chapter 15), also competes with dihydrotestosterone for the androgen receptors in target tissues. It also reduces 17α-hydroxylase activity, lowering plasma levels of testosterone and androstenedione. It is used in dosages of 50–200 mg/d for the treatment of hirsutism in women and appears to be as effective as finasteride, flutamide, or cyproterone.

CHEMICAL CONTRACEPTION IN MEN

Although many studies have been conducted, an effective oral contraceptive for men has not yet been found. For example, various androgens, including testosterone and testosterone enanthate, in a dosage of 400 mg/mo, produced azoospermia in fewer than half the men treated. Minor adverse reactions, including gynecomastia and acne, were encountered. Testosterone in combination with danazol was well tolerated but no more effective than testosterone alone. Androgens in combination with a progestin such as medroxyprogesterone acetate were no more effective. However, preliminary studies indicate that the intramuscular administration of 100 mg of testosterone enanthate weekly together with 500 mg of levonorgestrel daily orally will produce azoospermia in 94% of men.

Cyproterone acetate, a very potent progestin and antiandrogen, will also produce oligospermia but has not produced reliable contraception.

At present, pituitary hormones—and potent antagonist analogs of GnRH—are receiving increased attention. A GnRH antagonist in combination with testosterone has been shown to produce a reversible azoospermia in nonhuman primates.

GOSSYPOL

Extensive trials of this cottonseed derivative have been conducted in China. This compound destroys elements of the seminiferous epithelium but does not alter the endocrine function of the testis.

Gossypol

In Chinese studies, large numbers of men were treated with 20 mg/d of gossypol or gossypol acetic acid for 2 months, followed by a maintenance dosage of 60 mg/wk. On this regimen, 99% of men developed sperm counts below 4 million/mL. Preliminary data indicate that recovery (return of normal sperm count) following discontinuance of gossypol administration is more apt to occur in men whose counts do not fall to extremely low levels and when administration is not continued for more than 2 years. Hypokalemia is the major adverse effect and may lead to transient paralysis. The drug has also been tried as an intravaginal spermicide contraceptive.

PREPARATIONS AVAILABLE
(Oral contraceptives are listed in Table 40–3.)

Estrogens

Chlorotrianisene (TACE)
Oral: 12, 25 mg capsules

Conjugated estrogens (generic, Premarin)
Oral: 0.3, 0.625, 0.9, 1.25, 2.5 mg tablets
Parenteral: 25 mg/5 mL for IM, IV injection
Vaginal: 0.625 mg/g cream base

Dienestrol (Ortho Dienestrol, DV)
Vaginal: 10 mg/g cream

Diethylstilbestrol [DES] (generic)
Oral: 1, 5 mg tablets

Diethylstilbestrol diphosphate (Stilphostrol)
Oral: 50 mg tablets
Parenteral: 50 mg/mL injection

Estradiol cypionate in oil (generic, Depo-Estradiol Cypionate)
Parenteral: 5 mg/mL for IM injection

Estradiol (Estrace)
Oral: 0.5, 1, 2 mg tablets
Vaginal: 0.1 mg/g cream

Estradiol transdermal (Estraderm)
Transdermal: patches with 0.0375, 0.05, 0.075, 0.1 mg/d release rates

Estradiol valerate in oil (generic, others)
Parenteral: 10, 20, 40 mg/mL for IM injection

Estrone aqueous suspension (generic, Theelin Aqueous, others)
Parenteral: 2, 5 mg/mL for injection

Estropipate (Ogen, generic)
Oral: 0.625, 1.25, 2.5 mg tablets
Vaginal: 1.5 mg/g cream base

Ethinyl estradiol (Estinyl)
Oral: 0.02, 0.05, 0.5 mg tablets

Quinestrol (Estrovis)
Oral: 100 μg tablets

Progestins

Hydroxyprogesterone caproate (generic, Dela-lutin, others)
Parenteral: 125, 250 mg/mL for IM injection

Levonorgestrel (Norplant)
Kit for subcutaneous implant: 6 capsules of 36 mg each

Medroxyprogesterone acetate (Provera, others)
Oral: 2.5, 5, 10 mg tablets
Parenteral: 100, 400 mg/mL for IM injection
Parenteral depot: 150 mg/mL for IM injection

Megestrol acetate (generic, Megace)
Oral: 20, 40 mg tablets; 0 mg/mL suspension

Norethindrone (See also Table 40–3)
Oral: 5 mg tablets (Norlutin)
Oral: 0.35 mg tablets (Micronor, Nor-Q.D.)

Norethindrone acetate (Norlutate, Aygestin)
Oral: 5 mg tablets

Norgestrel (Ovrette) (See also Table 40–3)
Oral: 0.075 mg tablets

Progesterone in oil (generic, others)
Parenteral: 50 mg/mL for IM injection

Androgens & Anabolic Steroids

Fluoxymesterone (generic, Halotestin, others)
Oral: 2, 5, 10 mg tablets

Methyltestosterone (generic)
Oral: 10, 25 mg tablets; 10 mg capsules; 10 mg buccal tablets

Nandrolone decanoate (generic, Deca-Durabolin, others)
Parenteral: 50, 100, 200 mg/mL in oil for injection

Nandrolone phenpropionate (generic, Durabolin, others)
Parenteral: 25, 50 mg/mL in oil for IM injection

Oxandrolone (Oxandrin)
Oral: 2.5 mg tablets

Oxymetholone (Androl-50)
Oral: 50 mg tablets

Stanozolol (Winstrol)
Oral: 2 mg tablets

Testolactone (Teslac)
Oral: 50 mg tablets

Testosterone aqueous (generic, others)
Parenteral: 25, 50, 100 mg/mL suspension for IM injection

Testosterone cypionate in oil (generic, others)
Parenteral: 100, 200 mg/mL for IM injection

Testosterone enanthate in oil (generic, others)
Parenteral: 100, 200 mg/mL for IM injection

Testosterone propionate in oil (generic, Testex)
Parenteral: 100 mg/mL for IM injection

Testosterone transdermal system
Patch (Testoderm): 10, 15 mg total content
Patch (Androderm): 12,2 mg total content

Antagonists & Inhibitors (See also Chapter 37)

Anastrozole (Arimidex)
Oral: 1 mg tablets

Bicalutamide (Casodex)
Oral: 50 mg tablets

Clomiphene (Clomid, Serophene, Milophene)
Oral: 50 mg tablets

Danazol (Danocrine)
Oral: 50, 100, 200 mg capsules

Finasteride (Proscar)
Oral: 5 mg tablets

Flutamide (Eulexin)
Oral: 125 mg capsules

Tamoxifen (Nolvadex)
Oral: 10, 20 mg tablets

REFERENCES

Ovarian Hormones

Adashi EY: Intraovarian peptides: Stimulators and inhibitors of follicular growth and differentiation. Endocrinol Metab Clin North Am 1992;21:1.

Belchetz PE: Hormonal treatment of postmenopausal women. N Engl J Med 1994;330:1062.

Bhavnani BR, Cecutti A: Pharmacokinetics of 17β-dihydroequilin sulfate and 17β-dihydroequilin in normal postmenopausal women. J Clin Endocrinol Metab 1994;78:197.

Bikle DD et al: Progestin antagonism of estrogen-stimulated 1,25-dihydroxyvitamin D levels. J Clin Endocrinol Metab 1992;75:519.

Bock GR, Goode JA (editors): *Non-reproductive actions of sex steroids.* Ciba Foundation Symposium 191. Wiley, 1995.

Bringer J: Norgestimate: A clinical overview of a new progestin. Am J Obstet Gynecol 1992;166:1969.

Casper RF, Chapdelaine A: Estrogen and interrupted progestin: A new concept for hormone replacement therapy. Am J Obstet Gynecol 1993;168:1186.

Colditz GA et al: The use of estrogens and progestins and the risk of breast cancer in postmenopausal women. N Engl J Med 1995;332:1589

DiSaia PJ: Estrogen replacement therapy for the breast cancer survivor. J Soc Gynecol Invest 1996;3:57.

Draper MW et al: Antiestrogenic properties of raloxifene. Pharmacology 1995;50:209.

Golditz GA, Egan KM, Stampfer MJ: Hormone replacement therapy and the risk of breast cancer: Results from epidemiologic studies. Am J Obstet Gynecol 1993;168:1473.

Grodstein F et al: Postmenopausal estrogen and progestin use and the risk of cardiovascular disease. N Engl J Med 1996;335:453.

Kaplan SN, Grumbach MM: Pathophysiology and treatment of sexual precocity. J Clin Endocrinol Metab 1990;71:785.

Miller-Bass K, Adashi EY: Current status and future prospects of transdermal estrogen replacement therapy. Fertil Steril 1990;53:961.

Morales AJ et al: Effects of replacement dose of dehydroepiandrosterone in men and women of advancing age. J Clin Endocrinol Metab 1994;78:1360.

Mortola JF, Yen SSC: The effects of oral dehydroepiandrosterone on endocrine-metabolic parameters in postmenopausal women. J Clin Endocrinol Metab 1990;71:696.

Nabulsi AA et al: Association of hormone-replacement therapy with various cardiovascular risk factors in postmenopausal women. N Engl J Med 1993;328:1069.

Rittmaster RS: Medical treatment of androgen-dependent hirsutism. J Clin Endocrinol Metab 1995;80:2559.

Spelsberg TC et al: Nuclear acceptor sites for steroid hormone receptors: Comparisons of steroids and antisteroids. J Steroid Biochem 1988;31:579.

Tesarik J, Mendoza C: Nongenomic effects of 17β-estradiol on maturing oocytes: Relationship to oocyte developmental potential. J Clin Endocrinol Metab 1995; 80:1438.

Venturoli S et al: Ketoconazole therapy for women with acne and/or hirsutism. J Clin Endocrinol Metab 1990; 71:335.

Walsh BW et al: Effects of postmenopausal estrogen replacement on the concentration and metabolism of plasma lipoproteins. N Engl J Med 1991;325:1196.

Weinstein L, Bewtra C, Gallagher JC: Evaluation of a continuous combined low-dose regimen of estrogen-progestin for treatment of the menopausal patient. Am J Obstet Gynecol 1990;162:1534.

Westerveld HT et al: 17β-Estradiol improves postprandial lipid metabolism in postmenopausal women. J Clin Endocrinol Metab 1995;80:249.

Williams SR et al: A study of combined continuous ethinyl estradiol and norethindrone acetate for postmenopausal hormone replacement. Am J Obstet Gynecol 1990; 162:438.

Oral Contraceptives

Azziz R: Leuprolide and estrogen versus oral contraceptive pills for the treatment of hirsutism: A prospective randomized study. J Clin Endocrinol Metab 1995;80:3406.

Baird DT, Glasier AF: Hormonal contraception. N Engl J Med 1993;328:1543.

Brinton LA et al: Oral contraceptive use and the risk of invasive cervical cancer. Int J Epidemiol 1990;19:4.

Burkman RT Jr: The role of oral contraceptives in the treatment of hyperandrogenic disorders. Am J Med 1995; 98:130S.

Darney PD: The androgenicity of progestins. Am J Med 1995;98:104S.

Fotherby K Caldwell AD: New progestogens in oral contraception. Contraception 1994;49:1.

Godsland IF et al: The effects of different formulations of oral contraceptive agents on lipid and carbohydrate metabolism. N Engl J Med 1990;323:1375.

Grimes DA, Mishell DR Jr, Speroff L (editors): Contraceptive choices for women with medical problems. Am J Obstet Gynecol 1993;168(No. 6 Part 2):1979.

Herbst AL, Berek JS: Impact of contraception on gynecologic cancers. Am J Obstet Gynecol 1993;168:1980.

Kaunitz AM: Long-acting injectable contraception with depot medroxyprogesterone acetate. Am J Obstet Gynecol, 1994;170:154.

Kuhl H, Goethe JW (editors): Pharmacokinetics of oral contraceptive steroids and drug interaction. Am J Obstet Gynecol 1990;163:2113.

Leemay A: Attenuation of mild hyperandrogenic activity in postpubertal acne by a triphasic oral contraceptive containing low doses of ethynyl estradiol and DL-norgestrel. J Clin Endocrinol Metab 1990;71:8.

Mishell DR Jr: Noncontraceptive health benefits of oral contraceptives. Am J Obstet Gynecol 1982;142:809.

Oelkers W et al: Effects of a new oral contraceptive containing an antimineralocorticoid progestogen, drospirenone, on the renin-aldosterone system, body weight, blood pressure, glucose tolerance, and lipid metabolism. J Clin Endocrinol Metab 1995;80:1816.

Ortmeier BG et al: A cost-benefit analysis of four hormonal contraceptive methods. Clin Ther 1994;16:707.

Polaneczky M et al: The use of levonorgestrel implants (Norplant) for contraception in adolescent mothers. N Engl J Med 1994;331:1201.

Skouby SO, Jesperson J (editors): Oral contraceptives in the nineties: Metabolic aspects—facts and fiction. Am J Obstet Gynecol 1990;163(Suppl):276.

Wynn V: Effect of duration of low-dose oral contraceptive administration on carbohydrate metabolism. Am J Obstet Gynecol 1982;142(No. 6 Part 2):740.

Androgens

Bagatell CJ, Bremmer WJ: Androgens in men—uses and abuses. N Engl J Med 1996;334:707.

Bagatell CJ et al: Effects of endogenous testosterone and estradiol on sexual behavior in normal young men. J Clin Endocrinol Metab 1993;78:711.

Bardin W, Swerdloff RS, Santen RJ: Androgens: Risks and benefits. J Clin Endocrinol Metab 1991;73:4.

Bebb RA et al: Combined administration of levonorgestrel and testosterone induces more rapid and effective suppression of spermatogenesis than testosterone alone: A promising male contraceptive approach. J Clin Endocrinol Metab 1996;81:757.

Bhasin S: Androgen treatment of hypogonadal men. J Clin Endocrinol Metab 1993;74:1221.

Bremner WJ, Bagatell CJ, Steiner RA: Gonadotropin-releasing hormone antagonist plus testosterone: A potential male contraceptive. J Clin Endocrinol Metab 1991;73:465.

Butler GE et al: Oral testosterone undecanoate in the management of delayed puberty in boys: Pharmacokinetics and effects on sexual maturation and growth. J Clin Endocrinol Metab 1992;75:37.

Cunningham GR, Cordero E, Thornby JI: Testosterone replacement with transdermal therapeutic systems: Physiologic serum testosterone and elevated dihydrotestosterone levels. JAMA 1989;261:2525.

Dallob AL et al: The effect of finasteride, a 5α-reductase inhibition, on scalp skin testosterone and dihydrotestosterone in patients with male pattern baldness. J Clin Endocrinol Metab 1994;79:703.

Kopera H: The history of anabolic steroids and a review of clinical experience with anabolic steroids. Acta Endocrinol 1985;271(Suppl):11.

Malarkey WB et al: Endocrine effects in female weight lifters who self administer testosterone and anabolic steroids. Am J Obstet Gynecol 1991;165:1385.

Marin P, Oden B, Bjorntorp P: Assimilation and mobilization of triglycerides in subcutaneous abdominal and femoral adipose tissue in vivo in men: effects of androgens. J Clin Endocrinol Metab 1995;80:239.

Matsumoto AM: Effects of chronic testosterone administration in normal men: Safety and efficacy of high dosage testosterone and parallel-dose dependent depression of luteinizing hormone, follicle-stimulating hormone, and sperm production. J Clin Endocrinol Metab 1990;70:282.

Meikle W et al: Enhanced transdermal delivery of testosterone across nonscrotal skin produces physiological concentrations of testosterone and its metabolites in hypogonadal men. J Clin Endocrinol Metab 1992;74:623.

Mooradian AD, Morley JD, Korenman SG: Biological action of androgens. Endocr Rev 1987;8:1.

Mortola JF, Yen SSC: The effects of oral dehydroepiandrosterone on endocrine-metabolic parameters in postmenopausal women. J Clin Endocrinol Metab 1990; 71:69.

Tenover JS: Effects of testosterone supplementation in the aging male. J Clin Endocrinol Metab 1992; 75:1092.

Thompson PD et al: Contrasting effects of testosterone and stanozolol on serum lipoprotein levels. JAMA 1989;261:1165.

Wilson JD: Androgen abuse by athletes. Endocr Rev 1988;9:181.

Young NR et al: Body composition and muscle strength in healthy men receiving T enanthate for contraception J Clin Endocrinol Metab 1993;77:1028.

Inhibitors

Bagdade JD et al: Effects of tamoxifen treatment on plasma lipids and lipoprotein lipid concentration. J Clin Endocrinol Metab 1990;70:1132

Baulieu E-E: Contragestion and other clinical applications of RU 486, an antiprogesterone at the receptor. Science 1989;245:1351.

Feldman D: Ketoconazole and other imidazole derivatives as inhibitors of steroidogenesis. Endocr Rev 1985;7:409.

Flack MR et al: Oral gossypol in the treatment of metastatic adrenal cancer. J Clin Endocrinol Metab 1993;76:1019.

Friedman AJ et al: A prospective, randomized trial of gonadotropin-releasing hormone agonist plus estrogen-progestin or progestin "add-back" regimens for women with leiomyomata uteri. J Clin Endocrinol Metab 1993;76:1440.

Fruzzetti F et al: Effects of finasteride, a 5α-reductase inhibitor, on circulating androgen and gonadotropin secretion in hirsute women J Clin Endocrinol Metab 1994;79:811.

Gittes RF: Carcinoma of the prostate. N Engl J Med 1991;324:236.

Glasier A et al: Mifepristone (RU 486) compared with high-dose estrogen and progestogen for emergency postcoital contraception. N Engl J Med 1992; 327:1041.

Gormley GJ et al: Effects of finasteride (MK-906), a 5α-reductase inhibitor, on circulating androgens in male volunteers. J Clin Endocrinol Metab 1990;70:1136.

Grey AB et al: The effect of the anti-estrogen tamoxifen on cardiovascular risk factors in normal postmenopausal women. J Clin Endocrinol Metab 1995;80:8192.

Hill NCW, Ferguson J, MacKenzie IZ: The efficacy of oral mifepristone (RU 38,486) with a prostaglandin E_1 analog vaginal pessary for the termination of early pregnancy: Complications and patient acceptability. Am J Obstet Gynecol 1990:162:414.

Lipton A et al: Letrozole (CGS 20267). A phase I study of a new potent oral aromatase inhibitor of breast cancer. Cancer 1995;75:2132.

Love RR et al: Effects of tamoxifen on bone mineral density in postmenopausal women with breast cancer. N Engl J Med 1992;326:852.

McConnell JD et al: Finasteride, an inhibitor of 5α-reductase, suppresses prostatic dihydrotestosterone in men with benign prostatic hyperplasia. J Clin Endocrinol Metab 1992;74:505.

Miller AA et al: Fadrozole hydrochloride in postmenopausal patients with metastatic breast carcinoma. Cancer 1996;78:789.

Moghetti P et al: Clinical and hormonal effects of the 5α-reductase inhibitor finasteride in idiopathic hirsutism. J Clin Endocrinol Metab 1994;79:1115.

Peyron R et al: Early termination of pregnancy with mifepristone (RU 486) and the orally active prostaglandin misoprostol. N Engl J Med 1993; 328:1509.

Porat O: Effects of gossypol on the motility of mammalian sperm. Mol Reprod Devel 1990;25:400.

Rabinovici J et al: Endocrine effects and pharmacokinetic characteristics of a potent new gonadotropin-releasing hormone antagonist (Ganirelix) with minimal histamine-releasing properties: Studies in postmenopausal women. J Clin Endocrinol Metab 1992;75:1220.

Rittmaster RS: Finasteride. (Drug Therapy.) N Engl J Med 1993;330:120.

Sawaya ME, Hordinsky MK: The antiandrogens: When and how they should be used. Dermatol Ther 1993;11:65.

Silvestre L et al: Voluntary interruption of pregnancy with mifepristone (RU 486) and a prostaglandin analog: A large-scale French experience. N Engl J Med 1990; 322:645.

Spitz IM, Bardin WC: Mifepristone (RU-486)—A modulator of progestin and glucocorticoid action. N Engl J Med 1993;329:404.

Zilembo N et al: Formestane: An effective first-line endocrine treatment for advanced breast cancer. J Cancer Res Clin Oncol 1995;121:378.

41

Pancreatic Hormones & Antidiabetic Drugs

John H. Karam, MD

THE ENDOCRINE PANCREAS

The endocrine pancreas in the adult human consists of approximately 1 million islets of Langerhans interspersed throughout the pancreatic gland. Within the islets, at least four hormone-producing cells have been identified (Table 41–1). Their hormone products include **insulin,** the storage and anabolic hormone of the body; **islet amyloid polypeptide (IAPP, or amylin),** whose metabolic function remains undefined; **glucagon,** the hyperglycemic factor that mobilizes glycogen stores; somatostatin, a universal inhibitor of secretory cells; and **pancreatic peptide,** a small protein that facilitates digestive processes by a mechanism not yet clarified.

Diabetes mellitus is the most important disease involving the endocrine pancreas. Its major manifestations include disordered metabolism and inappropriate hyperglycemia. A therapeutic classification presently recommended by the American Diabetes Association includes two major types: insulin-dependent (IDDM) and non-insulin-dependent (NIDDM) diabetes mellitus. An estimated 12 million people in the USA are known to have diabetes, and at least 1 million have the insulin-dependent type.

Type I diabetes (IDDM) is a severe form associated with ketosis in the untreated state. It occurs most commonly in juveniles but occasionally in adults, especially the nonobese and those who are elderly when hyperglycemia first appears. It is a catabolic disorder in which circulating insulin is virtually absent, plasma glucagon is elevated, and the pancreatic B cells fail to respond to all insulinogenic stimuli. Exogenous insulin is therefore required to reverse the catabolic state, prevent ketosis, and reduce the hyperglucagonemia and the elevated blood glucose level.

Type I diabetes is thought to result from an infectious or toxic environmental insult in people whose immune system is genetically predisposed to develop a vigorous autoimmune response against pancreatic B cell antigens. Extrinsic factors that might affect B cell function include damage caused by viruses such as mumps virus and coxsackievirus B4, by toxic chemical agents, or by destructive cytotoxins and antibodies released from sensitized immunocytes. An underlying genetic defect relating to B cell replication or function may predispose to development of B cell failure after viral infection; in addition, specific HLA genes may increase susceptibility to a diabetogenic virus or may be linked to certain immune response genes that predispose patients to a destructive autoimmune response against their own islet cells (autoaggression). Observations that pancreatic B cell damage appears to be lessened when immunosuppressive drugs such as cyclosporine or azathioprine are given at the initial manifestations of type I diabetes support the importance of autoaggression by the immune system as a major factor in the pathogenesis of this type of diabetes.

Type II diabetes (NIDDM) represents a heterogeneous group comprising milder forms of diabetes that occur predominantly in adults but occasionally in adolescents. Circulating endogenous insulin is sufficient to prevent ketoacidosis but is often either subnormal or relatively inadequate because of tissue insensitivity. Obesity, which generally results in impaired insulin action, is a common risk factor for this type of diabetes, and most patients with NIDDM are obese.

In addition to tissue insensitivity to insulin, which has been noted in most NIDDM patients irrespective of weight, there is an accompanying deficiency of the pancreatic B cell's response to glucose. Both the tissue resistance to insulin and the impaired B cell response to glucose appear to be further aggravated by increased hyperglycemia, and both of these defects are ameliorated by therapeutic maneuvers that reduce the hyperglycemia.

Table 41-1. Pancreatic islet cells and their secretory products.

Cell Types	Approximate Percent of Islet Mass	Secretory Products
A cell (alpha)	20	Glucagon, proglucagon
B cell (beta)	75	Insulin, C-peptide, proinsulin, islet amyloid polypeptide (IAPP)
D cell (delta)	3–5	Somatostatin
F cell (PP cell)[1]	< 2	Pancreatic polypeptide (PP)

[1] Within pancreatic polypeptide-rich lobules of adult islets, located only in the posterior portion of the head of the human pancreas, glucagon cells are scarce (less than 0.5%) and F cells make up as much as 80% of the cells.

When dietary treatment and attempts at weight reduction of obesity fail to correct hyperglycemia, sulfonylurea drugs are usually prescribed. Insulin therapy may be required to achieve satisfactory glycemic control even though it is not needed to prevent ketoacidosis in patients with NIDDM.

INSULIN

Chemistry

Insulin is a small protein with a molecular weight in humans of 5808. It contains 51 amino acids arranged in two chains (A and B) linked by disulfide bridges; there are species differences in the amino acids of both chains. Within the B cell, insulin precursor is produced by DNA- or RNA-directed synthesis. Proinsulin, a long single-chain protein molecule, is processed within the Golgi apparatus and packaged into granules, where it is hydrolyzed into insulin and a residual connecting segment called the C-peptide by removal of four amino acids (shown in dashed circles in Figure 41–1). Insulin and C-peptide are secreted in equimolar amounts in response to all insulin secretagogues; a small quantity of unprocessed or partially hydrolyzed proinsulin is released as well. While proinsulin may have some mild hypoglycemic action, C-peptide has no known physiologic function. Granules within the B cell store the insulin in the form of crystals consisting of two atoms of zinc and six molecules of insulin. The entire human pancreas contains up to 8 mg of insulin, representing approximately 200 biologic "units." Originally, the unit was defined on the basis of the hypoglycemic activity of insulin in rabbits. With improved purification techniques, the unit is presently defined on the basis of weight, and present insulin standards used for assay purposes are 28 units per milligram.

Insulin Secretion

Insulin is released from pancreatic B cells at a low basal rate and at a much higher stimulated rate in response to a variety of stimuli, especially glucose. Other stimulants such as other sugars (eg, mannose), certain amino acids (eg, leucine, arginine), and vagal activity are also recognized. One mechanism of stimulated insulin release is diagrammed in Figure 41–2. As shown in the figure, hyperglycemia results in increased intracellular ATP levels, which close the ATP-dependent potassium channels. Decreased outward potassium current through this channel results in depolarization of the B cell and opening of voltage-gated calcium channels. The resulting increased intracellular calcium triggers secretion of the hormone. The mechanism is undoubtedly more complex than this brief summary suggests, since several intracellular messengers are known to modulate the process (cAMP, inositol trisphosphate, diacylglycerol) and the insulin response to a monophasic rise in glucose is biphasic. As noted below, the sulfonylurea oral hypoglycemic drug group is thought to exploit parts of this mechanism.

Insulin Degradation

The liver and kidney are the two main organs that remove insulin from the circulation, presumably by hydrolysis of the disulfide connections between the A and B chains through the action of glutathione insulin transhydrogenase (insulinase). After this reductive cleavage, further degradation by proteolysis occurs. The liver normally clears the blood of approximately 60% of the insulin released from the pancreas by virtue of its location as the terminal site of portal vein blood flow, with the kidney removing 35–40% of the endogenous hormone. However, in insulin-treated diabetics receiving subcutaneous insulin injections, this ratio is reversed, with as much as 60% of exogenous insulin being cleared by the kidney and the liver removing no more than 30–40%. The half-life of circulating insulin is 3–5 minutes.

Measurement of Circulating Insulin

The radioimmunoassay of insulin permits detection of insulin in picomolar quantities. The assay is based on antibodies developed in guinea pigs against bovine or pork insulin. Because of the similarities between these two insulins and human insulin, the assay successfully measures the human hormone as well.

With this assay, basal insulin values of 5–15 μU/mL (30–90 pmol/L) are found in normal humans, with a peak rise to 60–90 μU/mL (360–540 pmol/L) during meals. Similar assays for measuring all of the known hormones of the endocrine pancreas (including C-peptide and proinsulin) have been developed.

The Insulin Receptor

Once insulin has entered the circulation, it is bound by specialized receptors that are found on the mem-

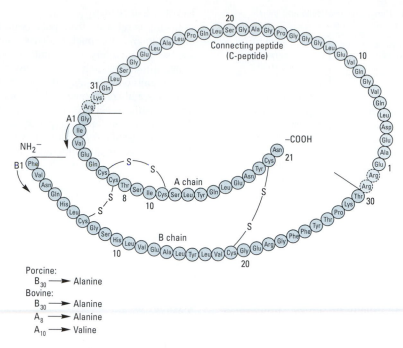

Figure 41–1. Structure of human proinsulin. Insulin is shown as the shaded peptide chains, A and B. Comparisons of human, porcine, and bovine C-peptides show considerable differences between species, with only about 40% homology. Species differences in the A and B chains are noted in the inset.

branes of most tissues. However, the biologic responses promoted by these insulin-receptor complexes have been identified in only a few target tissues, eg, liver, muscle, and adipose tissue. The receptors bind insulin with high specificity and affinity in the picomolar range. The full insulin receptor consists of two heterodimers, each containing an alpha subunit, which is entirely extracellular and constitutes the recognition site, and a beta subunit that spans the membrane (Figure 41–3). The beta subunit contains a tyrosine kinase. When insulin binds to the alpha subunit at the outside surface of the cell, tyrosine kinase activity is stimulated in the beta portion. Although the $\alpha\beta$ dimeric form is capable of binding insulin, it does so with much lower affinity than the tetrameric $\alpha\alpha\beta\beta$ form. Self-phosphorylation of the beta portion of the receptor causes both increased aggregation of $\alpha\beta$ heterodimers and stabilization of the activated state of the receptor tyrosine kinase. The first protein to be phosphorylated by the activated receptor tyrosine kinase has been identified as the docking protein, insulin receptor substrate-1 (IRS-1), which has up to 22 sites for tyrosine phosphorylation. After tyrosine phosphorylation at several sites, IRS-1 binds to and activates other kinases that produce further phosphorylations. This series of phosphorylations within the cell represents insulin's second message and results in translocation of certain proteins such as the glucose transporter from sequestered sites within the cell to exposed locations on the cell surface. Finally, the insulin-receptor complex is internalized. However, it remains controversial whether internalization contributes to further action of insulin or is merely a means of limiting further effects of the hormone by removing insulin and its receptor into scavenger lysosomes.

Various hormonal agents (eg, hydrocortisone) lower the affinity of insulin receptors for insulin; growth hormone in excess increases this affinity slightly. The concentration of these specific receptor molecules as well as their affinity for binding insulin seems to be affected by the concentration of insulin molecules to which they are exposed. Experimentally, desensitization of insulin receptors has been shown to occur with a time course of 4 hours (in vitro) to 24 hours (in vivo). In clinical situations associated with elevated blood levels of circulating insulin, such as obesity or insulinoma, the concentration of insulin receptors is reduced. This down-regulation of insulin receptors seems to provide an intrinsic mechanism whereby target cells limit their response to excessive hormone concentrations.

Effects of Insulin on Its Targets

Insulin promotes the storage of fat as well as glucose (both sources of energy) within specialized target cells (Figure 41–4) and influences cell growth and the metabolic functions of a wide variety of tissues.

A. Action of Insulin on Glucose Transporters: Insulin has an important effect on several

Figure 41–2. One model of control of insulin release from the pancreatic B cell by glucose and by sulfonylurea drugs. In the resting cell with normal (low) ATP levels, potassium diffuses down its concentration gradient through ATP-gated potassium channels (ATP *closes* the channels), maintaining the intracellular potential at a fully polarized, negative level. Insulin release is minimal. If glucose concentration rises, ATP production increases, potassium channels close, and depolarization of the cell results. As in muscle and nerve, voltage-gated calcium channels open in response to depolarization, allowing more calcium to enter the cell. Increased intracellular calcium results in increased insulin secretion. Sulfonylurea hypoglycemic drugs block the ATP-dependent potassium channel, thereby depolarizing the membrane and causing increased insulin release by the same mechanism. (Modified and reproduced, with permission, from *Basic & Clinical Endocrinology,* 4th ed. Greenspan F, Baxter JD [editors]. Appleton & Lange, 1994.)

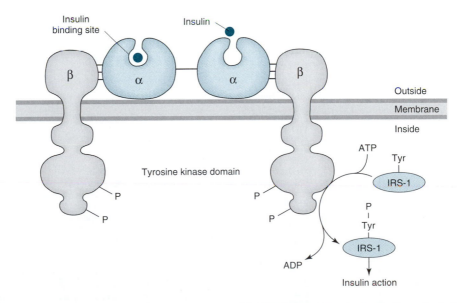

Figure 41–3. Schematic diagram of the probable structure of the insulin receptor tetramer in the activated state. IRS-1, insulin receptor substrate-1; Tyr, tyrosine; P, phosphate.

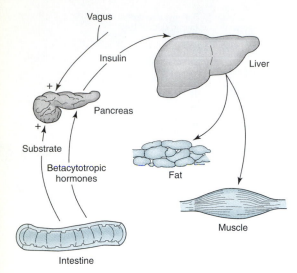

Figure 41–4. Insulin promotes synthesis (from circulating nutrients) and storage of glycogen, triglycerides, and protein in its major target tissues: liver, fat, and muscle. The release of insulin from the pancreas is stimulated by increased blood glucose, vagal nerve stimulation, and other factors (see text).

transport molecules that facilitate glucose movement across cell membranes (Table 41–2). These transporters may play a role in the etiology as well as the manifestations of diabetes. GLUT 4, quantitatively the most important in terms of lowering blood glu-

cose, is inserted into the membranes of muscle and adipose cells from intracellular storage vesicles by insulin. Defects in GLUT 2-mediated transport of glucose into pancreatic B cells may contribute to the reduced insulin secretion that characterizes NIDDM.

B. Action of Insulin on Liver: (Table 41–3.) The first major organ reached by endogenous insulin via the portal circulation is the liver, where it acts to increase storage of glucose as glycogen and to reset the liver to the fed state by reversing a number of catabolic mechanisms associated with the postabsorptive state: glycogenolysis, ketogenesis, and gluconeogenesis. These effects are brought about in part through insulin-induced phosphorylations, which activate pyruvate kinase, phosphofructokinase, and glucokinase, while repressing gluconeogenic enzymes, including pyruvate carboxylase, phosphoenolpyruvate carboxykinase, fructose bisphosphatase, and glucose 6-phosphatase. In addition, insulin decreases urea production, protein catabolism, and cAMP in the liver, promotes triglyceride synthesis, and increases potassium and phosphate uptake by the organ.

C. Effect of Insulin on Muscle: (Table 41–3.) Insulin promotes protein synthesis by increasing amino acid transport and by stimulating ribosomal activity. It also promotes glycogen synthesis to replace glycogen stores expended by muscle activity. This is accomplished by increasing glucose transport into the muscle cell, inducing glycogen synthase, and inhibiting phosphorylase. Approximately 500–600 g of glycogen is stored in muscle tissue of a 70 kg male.

D. Effect of Insulin on Adipose Tissue: (Table 41–3.) The most efficient means of storing en-

Table 41–2. Glucose transporters.

Transporter	Tissues	Glucose K_m (mmol/L)	Function
GLUT 1	All tissues, especially red cells, brain	1–2	Basal uptake of glucose; transport across the blood-brain barrier
GLUT 2	B cells of pancreas, liver, kidney, gut	15–20	Regulation of insulin release, other aspects of glucose homeostasis
GLUT 3	Brain, kidney, placenta, other tissues	< 1	Uptake into neurons, other tissues
GLUT 4	Muscle, adipose	≈ 5	Insulin-mediated uptake of glucose
GLUT 5	Gut, kidney	1–2	Intestinal absorption of fructose

Table 41–3. Endocrine effects of insulin.

Effect on liver:
Reversal of catabolic features of insulin deficiency
  Inhibits glycogenolysis
  Inhibits conversion of fatty acids and amino acids to keto acids
  Inhibits conversion of amino acids to glucose
Anabolic action
  Promotes glucose storage as glycogen (induces glucokinase and glycogen synthase, inhibits phosphorylase)
  Increases triglyceride synthesis and very low density lipoprotein formation
Effect on muscle:
Increased protein synthesis
  Increases amino acid transport
  Increases ribosomal protein synthesis
Increased glycogen synthesis
  Increases glucose transport
  Induces glycogen synthase and inhibits phosphorylase
Effect on adipose tissue:
Increased triglyceride storage
  Lipoprotein lipase is induced and activated by insulin to hydrolyze triglycerides from lipoproteins
  Glucose transport into cell provides glycerol phosphate to permit esterification of fatty acids supplied by lipoprotein transport
  Intracellular lipase is inhibited by insulin

ergy is in the form of triglyceride depots. This provides 9 kcal per gram of stored substrate and, unlike glycogen, does not require water to maintain it within cells. A normal 70 kg man has 12–14 kg of fat in storage, chiefly in adipose tissue.

Insulin acts to reduce circulating free fatty acids and to promote triglyceride storage in adipocytes by three primary mechanisms: (1) induction of lipoprotein lipase, which actively hydrolyzes triglycerides from circulating lipoproteins; (2) glucose transport into cells to generate glycerophosphate as a metabolic product, which permits esterification of fatty acids supplied by lipoprotein hydrolysis; and (3) reduction of intracellular lipolysis of stored triglyceride by a direct inhibition of intracellular lipase. These effects appear to involve suppression of cAMP production and dephosphorylation of the lipases in the fat cell.

Characteristics of Available Insulin Preparations

Commercial insulin preparations differ in a number of ways, including differences in the animal species from which they are obtained; their purity, concentration, and solubility; and the time of onset and duration of their biologic action. In the past 15 years, a number of human insulin preparations have been added to the list of available insulins, and some animal preparations have been removed. As a result, in 1997, approximately 22 different insulin formulations were available for purchase in the USA. If the use of human insulin continues to increase, the number of available insulins from animal sources should decline.

A. Principal Types and Duration of Action of Insulin Preparations: Four principal types of insulins are available: (1) ultra-short-acting, with very rapid onset and short duration; (2) short-acting, with rapid onset of action; (3) intermediate-acting; and (4) long-acting, with slow onset of action (Figure 41–5, Table 41–4). Ultra-short-acting and short-acting insulins are dispensed as clear solutions at neutral pH and contain small amounts of zinc to improve their stability and shelf-life. All other commercial insulins have been modified to provide prolonged action and are dispensed as turbid suspensions at neutral pH with either protamine in phosphate buffer (NPH insulin) or varying concentrations of zinc in acetate buffer (ultralente and lente insulins). Production of protamine zinc insulin and semilente preparations has recently been discontinued, since almost no clinical indications for their use exist. Conventional subcutaneous insulin therapy presently consists of split-dose injections of mixtures of short-acting and intermediate-acting insulins (NPH or lente) or multiple doses of ultra-short-acting or short-acting insulin preprandially in association with any of three insulin suspensions (NPH, lente, or ultralente) whose prolonged duration of action provides overnight basal insulin levels.

1. Ultra-short-acting insulin–Insulin lispro is a new monomeric insulin analog, produced by recom-

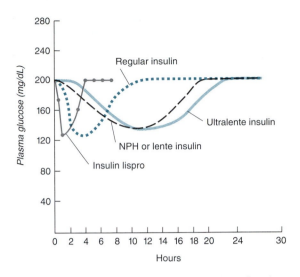

Figure 41–5. Extent and duration of action of various types of insulin (in a fasting diabetic). The durations of action shown are typical of average therapeutic doses; with the exception of insulin lispro, duration increases considerably when dosage is increased. (Reproduced, with permission, from Karam JH: Diabetes mellitus and hypoglycemia. In: *Current Medical Diagnosis & Treatment 1997.* Tierney LM, McPhee SJ, Papadakis MA [editors]. Appleton & Lange, 1997.)

binant technology, wherein two amino acids near the terminal end of the B chain have been reversed in position: proline at position B28 has been moved to B29 and lysine at position B29 has been moved to B28. Reversing these two amino acids does not interfere in any way with insulin lispro's binding to the insulin receptor, its circulating half-life, or its immunogenicity, which are identical with those of human regular insulin. However, the advantage of this analog is its very low propensity—in contrast to human insulin—to form hexamers. When injected subcutaneously, insulin lispro quickly dissociates into monomers and is absorbed very rapidly, reaching peak serum values as early as 1 hour—as compared with human insulin, whose hexameric formulations require considerably more time to dissociate and become absorbed. Clinical trials have demonstrated that optimal time of preprandial subcutaneous injection of comparable doses of insulin lispro and of regular human insulin are 20 minutes and 60 minutes before the meal, respectively, in insulin-dependent diabetics receiving intensive insulin therapy. This ultra-rapid onset of action of insulin lispro has been welcomed as a great convenience by diabetic patients who object to waiting for as long as 60 minutes after injecting regular human insulin before they can begin their meal. Moreover, the duration of insulin lispro, in contrast to regular human insulin, is not prolonged by increasing the dosage of the insulin. Regardless of the dose of insulin lispro injected subcutaneously, its duration is no

Table 41–4. Some insulin preparations available in the USA.[1,2]

Preparation	Species Source	Concentration
Ultra-short-acting insulin		
Insulin lispro, Humalog (Lilly)	Human analog (recombinant)	U100
Short-acting insulins		
Standard[3]		
Regular Iletin (Lilly)	Beef and pork	U100
"Purified"[4]		
Regular (Novo Nordisk)[5]	Pork or human	U100
Regular Humulin (Lilly)	Human	U100, U500
Regular Iletin II (Lilly)	Pork	U100, U500
Velosulin (Novo Nordisk)[6]	Human	U100
Intermediate-acting insulins		
Standard[3]		
Lente Iletin I (Lilly)	Beef and pork	U100
NPH Iletin I (Lilly)	Beef and pork	U100
"Purified"		
Lente Humulin (Lilly)	Human	U100
Lente Iletin II (Lilly)	Pork	U100
Lente (Novo Nordisk)	Pork or human	U100
NPH Humulin (Lilly)	Human	U100
NPH Iletin II (Lilly)	Pork	U100
NPH (Novo Nordisk)	Pork or human	U100
Premixed insulins (% NPH, % regular)		
Novolin 70/30 (Novo Nordisk)	Human	U100
Humulin 70/30 and 50/50 (Lilly)	Human	U100
Long-acting insulins		
"Purified"[4]		
Ultralente Humulin (Lilly)	Human	U100

[1]Modified and reproduced, with permission, from Katzung BG (editor): *Drug Therapy,* 2nd ed. Appleton & Lange, 1991.
[2]All of these agents (except insulin lispro) are available without a prescription. Wholesale prices for all preparations (except insulin lispro) are similar.
[3]Greater than 10 but less than 25 ppm proinsulin.
[4]Less than 10 ppm proinsulin.
[5]Novo Nordisk human insulins are termed Novolin R, L, and N.
[6]Velosulin contains phosphate buffer, which favors its use to prevent insulin aggregation in pump tubing but precludes its being mixed with lente insulin.

more than 3–4 hours, whereas regular human insulin in moderate doses (15–40 units) lasts much longer.

2. Short-acting insulins–Regular insulin is a short-acting soluble crystalline zinc insulin whose effect appears within 30 minutes after subcutaneous injection and generally lasts 5–7 hours. As with all older insulin formulations, the duration of action as well as the intensity of peak action increases with the size of the dose. Short-acting soluble insulin is the only type that should be administered intravenously or by infusion pumps. It is particularly useful for intravenous therapy in the management of diabetic ketoacidosis and when the insulin requirement is changing rapidly, such as after surgery or during acute infections. When used intravenously for hyperglycemic emergencies, insulin lispro has no advantage over regular human insulin, which is 30–40% less costly and is instantly converted to the monomeric form when given by this route.

3. Intermediate-acting and long-acting insulins–Lente insulin is a mixture of 30% semilente (an amorphous precipitate of insulin with zinc ions in acetate buffer that has a relatively rapid onset of action) with 70% ultralente insulin (a poorly soluble crystal of zinc insulin that has a delayed onset and prolonged duration of action). These two components provide a combination of relatively rapid absorption with sustained long action, making lente insulin a useful therapeutic agent. While beef, pork, and human insulins can readily form zinc crystals in acetate buffer under the conditions employed, only beef insulin has the proper hydrophobic alignment within the crystal to provide the delayed, sustained release of insulin characteristic of ultralente. Zinc crystals of pork insulin and human insulin dissolve more rapidly, and while the appearance of the crystals is virtually identical to that of zinc crystals of beef insulin, the onset of action is earlier and the duration shorter.

There has recently been a resurgence of use of ultralente insulin in combination with multiple injections of regular insulin as a means of attempting optimal control in patients with insulin-dependent diabetes. Unfortunately, the Novo Nordisk company has discontinued producing their monospecies beef ultralente, and Eli Lilly has discontinued its beef-pork ultralente insulins; thus, a slightly more soluble ultralente formulation made with human insulin (Humulin U [Lilly]) is the only ultralente insulin available in the USA. Because of its less sustained action compared with beef ultralente (which often achieved satisfactory basal insulin levels with only one injection daily), it is generally recommended that the daily dose of Humulin Ultralente be split into two equal doses given every 12 hours. This is needed in type I patients to achieve basal insulin levels throughout the 24 hours that are comparable to those achieved in normal subjects by basal endogenous secretion or by the overnight infusion rate programmed into insulin pumps. For reasons noted below, ultralente insulin should not be mixed with regular insulin but requires a separate injection.

NPH (neutral protamine Hagedorn, or isophane) insulin is an intermediate-acting insulin wherein the onset of action is delayed by combining appropriate amounts of insulin and protamine so that neither is present in an uncomplexed form ("isophane"). Protamine isolated from the sperm of rainbow trout is a mixture of six major and some minor compounds of similar structure. They appear to be arginine-rich peptides with an average molecular weight of approximately 4400. To form an isophane complex (one in which neither component retains any free binding sites), approximately a 1:10 ratio by weight of protamine to insulin is required, eg, 0.3–0.4 mg of protamine to 4 mg of insulin (100 units). This represents approximately six molecules of insulin per molecule of protamine. After subcutaneous injection, proteolytic enzymes degrade the protamine to permit absorption of insulin.

The onset and duration of action of NPH insulin are comparable to those of lente insulin (Table 41–4); it is usually mixed with regular insulin and given at least twice daily for insulin replacement in patients with insulin-dependent diabetes.

4. Mixtures of insulins–Since intermediate-acting insulins require several hours to reach adequate therapeutic levels, their use in insulin-dependent diabetic patients requires supplements of regular insulin preprandially. For convenience, these are often mixed together in the same syringe and injected subcutaneously in split dosage before breakfast and supper. NPH is preferred to lente insulin as the intermediate-acting component in these mixtures because increased proportions of lente to regular insulin may retard the rapid action of admixed regular insulin, particularly if not injected immediately after mixing. The excess zinc in lente and ultralente insulin can precipitate some of the soluble regular insulin when mixed in vitro (even at equal proportions) and can explain the slight retardation of regular insulin's absorption and biologic effect when mixed with lente or ultralente insulin.

So that NPH insulin does not retard the pharmacokinetic profile of admixed regular insulin, the protamine content of NPH insulin has been reduced by all manufacturers to levels at or below 0.4 mg per 4 mg insulin. NPH insulin is preferable to lente insulin as the intermediate component of a therapeutic mixture containing regular insulin. For this reason, all premixed formulations of insulin contain NPH rather than lente as the intermediate component that is mixed with regular insulin.

With increasing use of ultra-short-acting insulin lispro as a popular and convenient preprandial insulin, it has become evident that combination with a more sustained insulin is essential to maintain postabsorptive control of blood sugar. Insulin lispro can be *acutely* mixed (ie, just before injection) with either NPH or ultralente insulin without affecting its rapid absorption. However, *premixed* preparations have thus far been unstable, since attempts to maintain a 70% NPH and 30% insulin lispro results in a variable loss of soluble insulin lispro as the human insulin in the protamine complex is partially displaced by the insulin lispro. Consequently, over time the soluble component becomes a mixture of regular insulin and insulin lispro at varying ratios. To remedy this, instead of using regular insulin to produce NPH insulin, clinical trials in Europe are going forward with an intermediate insulin composed of isophane complexes of protamine with insulin lispro. This intermediate insulin has been designated as "NPL" (neutral protamine lispro) and it has the same duration of action as NPH insulin. It has the advantage of being able to be dispensed as premixed combinations of NPL and insulin lispro and has been tested in various concentrations of premixed vials, eg, 75% NPL/25% insulin lispro, 50% NPL/50% insulin lispro, and 25% NPL/75% insulin lispro. Preliminary results of clinical trials suggest that the latter given before each meal has served as a valuable premeal insulin to optimize glycemia excursions postprandially while maintaining postabsorptive basal insulin levels. At bedtime, an injection of NPL alone is suggested to maintain overnight basal insulin levels.

Since insulin lispro does not maintain hexamer formation at pharmacologic concentrations, it appears to resist precipitation by high concentrations of zinc and thus cannot be used to make a lente or ultralente formulation. However, this lack of precipitation by zinc allows it to be mixed with any of the lente series—in contrast to regular insulin, which tends to be precipitated by the excess zinc in the lente series when mixed prior to injection.

B. Species of Insulin:

1. Beef and pork insulins–Most commercial insulin in the USA contains beef insulin as its chief component. Beef insulin differs by three amino acids from human insulin, whereas only a single amino acid distinguishes pork and human insulins (Figure 41–1). The beef hormone is slightly more antigenic than pork insulin in humans. The most commonly prescribed preparations in the USA have been standard mixtures containing 70% beef and 30% pork insulin. However, declining production costs for biosynthesis of human insulin have allowed this product to become competitive with animal insulins. It is expected that by 1998, use of human insulin will greatly exceed that of animal insulin throughout most of the world.

Monospecies pork insulin was once advocated as particularly useful in patients with conditions such as allergy or resistance (see below) to the beef insulin found in standard beef-pork insulins. However, human insulin, which is now less expensive than monospecies pork insulin and also less immunogenic, has generally supplanted purified pork insulins, such as Lilly's Iletin II.

2. Human insulins–Mass production of human insulin by recombinant DNA techniques is now carried out by inserting the human proinsulin gene into *E coli* or yeast and treating the extracted proinsulin to form the human insulin molecule.

Human insulin is available for clinical use as Humulin (Lilly) and dispensed as either regular, NPH, lente, or ultralente Humulin. Human insulin prepared biosynthetically in yeast is marketed by Novo Nordisk as human insulin injection in regular, lente, and NPH forms: Novolin R, Monotard Human Insulin (Novolin L), and Novolin N. The same company also produces a human insulin marketed as Velosulin (regular) that contains a phosphate buffer. This reduces aggregation of regular insulin molecules when used in infusion pumps, and it is the only insulin recommended for pump use. However, because of the tendency of phosphate to precipitate zinc ions, Velosulin should not be mixed with any of the lente insulins.

A premixed formulation of 70% NPH and 30% regular human insulin—Novolin 70/30 and Humulin 70/30—is available for use in NIDDM patients and is particularly useful in elderly patients and others who may have difficulties in mixing insulins. Human insulin is also available in a premixed 50/50 formulation of NPH and regular. Human insulins appear to be as effective as conventional animal insulins, and they appear to be considerably less immunogenic in diabetic patients than beef-pork insulins and slightly less immunogenic than pork insulin.

Since threonine contains a hydroxyl group that makes it more polar—and thus more hydrophilic—than alanine, the presence of two threonines in place of two alanines in beef insulin and one such replacement in pork insulin (Figure 41–1) may explain why human insulin tends to be absorbed more rapidly and have a slightly shorter duration of action than animal insulins, regardless of the formulation in which it is administered.

C. Purity of Insulin: Improvements in purification techniques (using gel columns) have greatly reduced contaminating proteins with molecular weights greater than that of insulin. These include proinsulin and partially cleaved proinsulins that are metabolically inactive yet capable of inducing anti-insulin antibodies. Further purification with chromatography can virtually eliminate these larger proteins and markedly lower the concentration of smaller peptide contaminants. Conventional formulations of insulin contain less than 50 ppm of proinsulin. When proinsulin content is less than 10 ppm, manufacturers are entitled by FDA regulations in the USA to label the insulin as "purified."

D. Concentration: Currently, all insulins in the USA and Canada are available in a concentration of 100 units/mL (U100) and are dispensed in 10 mL vials. A limited supply of U500 regular porcine or human insulin is available for use in rare cases of severe insulin resistance in which large quantities of insulin are required.

E. Human Proinsulin: Human proinsulin is now available from recombinant DNA synthesis and shows biologic activity in humans which is 8–12% that of human insulin. Since it has a circulating half-life four to six times longer than that of human insulin, it was proposed for use as an alternative form of longer-acting insulin. It has certain advantages over NPH and lente formulations of human insulin in that it provides prolonged insulin action without need for fish protamine additives or large concentrations of zinc acetate to precipitate the insulin. Moreover, some reports indicate that human proinsulin is less immunogenic than human insulin and has more reproducible absorption characteristics than do precipitated formulations of human insulin (NPH and lente) that have a comparable "intermediate" duration of action. However, clinical trials were suspended because of concern over an increased number of fatal cardiovascular events in a group of diabetic patients receiving human proinsulin. The ultimate role of proinsulin remains to be defined.

F. Insulin Analogs: Among the many variables affecting the absorptive kinetics of insulin, an important one seems to be the tendency of insulin molecules to aggregate in hexameric form when formulated at pharmacologic concentrations. This causes lag periods of up to 30 minutes before insulin absorption is initiated from a subcutaneous depot site and results in a prolonged profile of absorption because the U100 injected regular insulin must be diluted more than 1000-fold by tissue fluids before it becomes monomeric and more readily absorbable into the circulation. Alteration of the insulin peptide provides an opportunity to change the aggregation characteristics and therefore the absorption rate of the molecule. Insulin lispro is the first such analog (of a number under study) to be approved. However, two qualifications were associated with the FDA approval. First, this is the only insulin that must be sold by prescription (all others are over-the-counter) because it was felt that a physician's supervision would be needed until more experience had been obtained with the preparation's novel pharmacokinetics. Second, insulin lispro is not to be used in insulin pumps for subcutaneous infusion until ongoing trials document its safety and efficacy when it is administered by this route.

Insulin Delivery Systems

The standard mode of insulin therapy is subcutaneous injection using conventional disposable needles and syringes. During the last 2 decades, much effort has gone into exploration of other means of administration.

A. Portable Pen Injectors: To facilitate multiple subcutaneous injections of insulin, particularly during intensive insulin therapy, portable pen-sized injectors have been developed (Novo Pen 1.5, B-D Pen). These contain cartridges of U100 human insulin and retractable needles. Human insulin is available for these devices as cartridges of either regular insulin (Novolin R PenFill), NPH insulin (Novolin N PenFill), and premixed 70% NPH and 30% regular (Novolin 70/30 PenFill). These portable injectors have been well accepted by patients because they eliminate the need to carry syringes and bottles of insulin to the workplace and while traveling.

B. Closed-Loop Systems: Automated administration of soluble insulin by "closed-loop" systems (blood glucose-controlled insulin infusion systems) has been successful in acute situations such as management of diabetic ketoacidosis or maintenance of insulin balance in diabetics undergoing surgery. Chronic use of such systems is prevented by the need for uninterrupted aspiration of blood to reach an external glucose sensor and by the size of the computerized insulin pump system used on present models.

C. Open-Loop Systems (Insulin Pumps): Research into smaller "open-loop" methods of insulin delivery (insulin reservoir and pump programmed to deliver regular insulin at a calculated rate without a glucose sensor) has resulted in readily portable pumps for subcutaneous, intravenous, or intraperitoneal infusion. As methods for self-monitoring of blood glucose are increasingly accepted by patients, these pump systems are becoming less "open loop" and therefore potentially more useful for managing insulin-dependent diabetics. However, at present, intensive therapy using conventional daily administration of multiple subcutaneous injections of soluble, rapid-acting insulin and one or two daily injections of long-acting insulin appears to provide blood glucose control as effective as either type of loop system for most patients.

D. Nasal Insulin Delivery: When insulin is combined with a detergent and administered as an aerosol to the nasal mucosa, effective circulating levels of insulin can be achieved almost as rapidly as when an intravenous bolus of insulin is administered. If this route could be shown to produce reliable and reproducible absorption over the long term without toxicity to the nasal mucosa, it might improve insulin delivery to the circulation while reducing the need for injections. However, current formulations have not achieved these goals, particularly because the low efficiency of absorption (less than 8%) makes the method prohibitively expensive.

Treatment With Insulin

The current classification of diabetes mellitus identifies a group of patients who have virtually no insulin secretion and whose survival is dependent on administration of exogenous insulin. This insulin-dependent group (type I) represents about 9% of the diabetic population in the USA. Most type II diabetics do not require exogenous insulin for survival, but many need exogenous supplementation of their endogenous secretion to achieve optimum health. It is estimated that as many as 20% of type II diabetics in the USA (2–2.5 million people) are presently taking insulin.

Benefit of Glycemic Control in Diabetes Mellitus

The consensus of the American Diabetes Association is that intensive insulin therapy associated with comprehensive self-management training should become standard therapy in most IDDM patients after the age of puberty (see box: Benefits of Tight Glycemic Control). Exceptions include patients with advanced renal disease and the elderly, since the detrimental risks of hypoglycemia outweigh the benefit of tight glycemic control in these groups. In children under the age of 7 years, the extreme susceptibility of the developing brain to damage from hypoglycemia contraindicates attempts at tight glycemic control, particularly since diabetic complications do not seem to occur until some years after the onset of puberty.

While patients with NIDDM were not studied in the tight control trial (see box), there is no reason to believe that the effects of better control of blood glucose levels would not also apply to NIDDM. The eye, kidney, and nerve abnormalities are quite similar in both types of diabetes, and it is likely that similar underlying mechanisms apply. However, weight gain may be greater in obese NIDDM patients receiving intensive insulin therapy, and hypoglycemia may be more hazardous in older patients with NIDDM. Data thus far collected are conflicting (see box: Intensive Insulin Therapy in NIDDM: Potential Hazards?). For

BENEFITS OF TIGHT GLYCEMIC CONTROL IN IDDM

A long-term randomized prospective study involving 1441 IDDM patients in 29 medical centers reported in 1993 that "near normalization" of blood glucose resulted in a delay in onset and a major slowing of progression of microvascular and neuropathic complications of diabetes during follow-up periods of up to 10 years (Diabetes Control and Complications Trial [DCCT] Research Group, 1993).

Multiple insulin injections (66%) or insulin pumps (34%) were used in the intensively treated group who were trained to modify their therapy depending on frequent glucose monitoring. The conventionally treated group used no more than two insulin injections, and clinical well-being was the goal with no attempt to modify management based on glycated hemoglobin or their glucose results.

In the intensively treated group a mean glycated hemoglobin of 7.2% (normal, < 6%) and a mean blood glucose of 155 mg/dL were achieved, while in the conventionally treated group, glycated hemoglobin averaged 8.9% with an average blood glucose of 225 mg/dL. Over the study period, which averaged 7 years, there was an approximately 60% reduction in risk in the tight control group compared with the standard control group with regard to diabetic retinopathy, nephropathy, and neuropathy.

As might be predicted, intensively treated patients had a threefold greater risk of serious hypoglycemia; they also showed a greater tendency toward weight gain. However, there were no proven deaths from hypoglycemia in any subjects in the DCCT study, and no evidence of posthypoglycemic neurologic damage was detected.

Because of these dramatic results, tight control of blood glucose is now seen as much more desirable and as more feasible than in the past.

these reasons, common sense and clinical judgment on an individual basis should determine whether intensive insulin therapy is appropriate in NIDDM.

Complications of Insulin Therapy

A. Hypoglycemia:

1. Mechanisms and diagnosis–Hypoglycemic reactions are the most common complication of insulin therapy. They may result from a delay in taking a meal, unusual physical exertion, or a dose of insulin that is too large for immediate needs. With more patients attempting tight control without frequent home monitoring of capillary blood glucose, hypoglycemia is likely to become an even more frequent complication.

It was suggested (Berger et al, 1989) that there is less awareness of hypoglycemia (ie, fewer symptoms are generated) when human insulin rather than pork or beef insulin is used. This would increase the risk of potentially severe hypoglycemic reactions. Considerable controversy was generated by this claim, and some data (Heine et al, 1989; Kern et al, 1990) gave mechanistic support to the clinical impression. However, retrospective data from the extensive DCCT trial—after more than 53,000 patient months of follow-up—showed no substantive differences in the proportion of patients with asymptomatic hypoglycemia who were using human insulin as compared with those receiving nonhuman insulin (Gorden, 1990). The consensus at present is to continue the use of human insulin while awaiting more definitive data from studies specifically directed at the question.

In older diabetics, in those taking longer-acting insulins (regardless of insulin species), and in those exposed to frequent hypoglycemic episodes during tight glycemic control, autonomic warning signals of hypoglycemia are less frequent, and the manifestations of insulin excess are mainly those of impaired function of the central nervous system, eg, mental confusion, bizarre behavior, and ultimately coma. More rapid development of hypoglycemia from the effects of regular insulin causes signs of autonomic hyperactivity, both sympathetic (tachycardia, palpitations, sweating, tremulousness) and parasympathetic (nausea, hunger), that may progress to convulsions and coma if untreated.

An identification bracelet, necklace, or card in the wallet or purse should be carried by every diabetic who is receiving hypoglycemic drug therapy.

2. Treatment of hypoglycemia–All of the manifestations of hypoglycemia are rapidly relieved by glucose administration. In a case of mild hypoglycemia in a patient who is conscious and able to swallow, orange juice, glucose, or any sugar-containing beverage or food may be given. If more severe hypoglycemia has produced unconsciousness or stupor, the treatment of choice is to give 20–50 mL of 50% glucose solution by intravenous infusion over a period of 2–3 minutes. If intravenous therapy is not available, 1 mg of glucagon injected either subcutaneously or intramuscularly will usually restore consciousness within 15 minutes to permit ingestion of sugar. Family members or others in the household should be taught how to give glucagon when the need arises. If the patient is stuporous and glucagon is not available, small amounts of honey or syrup can be inserted into the buccal pouch. In general, however, oral feeding is contraindicated in unconscious patients.

INTENSIVE INSULIN THERAPY IN NIDDM: POTENTIAL HAZARDS?

Recent preliminary data from two clinical trials of tight glycemic control in NIDDM have been conflicting. The differences between the two studies illustrate the difficulty of obtaining a clear answer to a seemingly simple question: Does tight glycemic control benefit patients with NIDDM as much as it does patients with IDDM?

In one pilot study carried out in five hospitals in the USA 153 middle-aged men with NIDDM were randomized into 2 groups: one group received standard insulin therapy to avoid symptoms of hyperglycemia, while the other half of the patients received more intensive insulin therapy to achieve near-normoglycemia (Abraira 1995). The glycemic goals were achieved satisfactorily but significantly more major cardiovascular events occurred during the 30 month study in the intensively treated group. These cardiovascular events could not be accounted for by documented hypoglycemia, increased weight gain, or hypertension and raise questions about other causes for the detrimental effect of insulin during intensive therapy of NIDDM.

Contrasting results have been presented in an interim report from a large ongoing randomized trial in the United Kingdom involving 3942 individuals with NIDDM. Intensive therapy was able to achieve near normoglycemia in these subjects and there have thus far been *no* differences in the rate of cardiovascular complications in the various treatment groups (Turner 1995). Recruitment began in 1977 with the end of the study scheduled for 1998.

The only apparent explanation for differences in the outcomes of the two trials is that the UK study involves a relatively younger population (mean age 52 years) of much milder NIDDM patients, who required less insulin dosage to achieve near-normoglycemia. In fact the control group, which received only diet therapy, also achieved comparable near-normoglycemia despite taking no medications.

B. Immunopathology of Insulin Therapy:

At least five molecular classes of insulin antibodies may be produced during the course of insulin therapy in diabetes: IgA, IgD, IgE, IgG, and IgM. There are two major types of immune disorders in these patients:

1. Insulin allergy–Insulin allergy, an immediate type hypersensitivity, is a rare condition in which local or systemic urticaria results from histamine release from tissue mast cells sensitized by anti-insulin IgE antibodies. In severe cases, anaphylaxis results. A subcutaneous nodule appearing several hours later at the site of insulin injection and lasting for up to 24 hours has been attributed to an IgG-mediated complement-binding Arthus reaction. Because sensitivity is often to noninsulin protein contaminants, the new highly purified insulins have markedly reduced the incidence of insulin allergy, especially local reactions; use of human insulin from the onset of therapy virtually eliminates allergic reactions. When allergy to beef insulin is present, a species change (eg, to pure pork or human insulin) may correct the problem. Antihistamines, corticosteroids, and even desensitization may be required, especially for systemic hypersensitivity. A special kit with serial dilutions of beef or pork insulin for desensitization is available from Eli Lilly.

2. Immune insulin resistance–Most insulin-treated patients develop a low titer of circulating IgG anti-insulin antibodies that neutralize the action of insulin to a small extent. In some diabetic patients, principally those with some degree of tissue insensitivity to insulin (such as occurs in obese diabetics) and a history of interrupted insulin therapy with preparations of less-than-pure beef insulin, a high titer of circulating IgG anti-insulin antibodies develops. This results in extremely high insulin requirements—often more than 200 units daily. With the advent of highly purified insulins, this complication has become exceedingly rare. Switching to a less antigenic (pork or human) purified insulin may make possible a dramatic reduction in insulin dosage or may at least shorten the duration of immune resistance. Other forms of therapy include sulfated beef insulin (a chemically modified form of beef insulin containing an average of six sulfate groups per molecule) and immunosuppression with corticosteroids. In some adults, the foreign insulin can be completely discontinued and the patient maintained on diet alone with oral sulfonylureas. This is possible only when the circulating antibodies do not effectively neutralize the patient's own insulin.

C. Lipodystrophy at Injection Sites:

Atrophy of subcutaneous fatty tissue may occur at the site of injection. This type of immune complication has become rare since the development of highly concentrated, pure pork or human insulin preparations of neutral pH. Injection of these preparations directly into the atrophic area often results in restoration of normal contours. Hypertrophy of subcutaneous fatty tissue remains a problem, even with the purified insulins, if injected repeatedly at the same site. However, this is readily corrected with liposuction.

ORAL HYPOGLYCEMIC AGENTS

A large number of substances are capable of modifying insulin release (Table 41–5), including drugs that are useful in the treatment of diabetes. In the USA, the major oral medications currently available for treating hyperglycemia in non-insulin-dependent diabetics are the class of compounds known as sulfonylureas, which increase the release of endogenous insulin as well as improve its peripheral effectiveness. A wider choice of preparations has been available in other countries, consisting of a second group of compounds, the biguanides. These agents reduce blood glucose even in the absence of pancreatic B cell function. Biguanides were removed from the market in the USA in 1977 because the use of phenformin (the only biguanide available in the USA at the time) was reported to be associated with a relatively high incidence of lactic acidosis. However, clinical trials with metformin, a less toxic biguanide, have been completed in the USA, and the drug became available for clinical use in 1995.

A third class of drugs are competitive inhibitors of intestinal brush-border alpha-glucosidases and decrease absorption of many carbohydrates from the gut. A representative of this class is acarbose, which received FDA approval in December 1995 for use in the USA. It has been used for many years in Europe.

A fourth class of drugs, the thiazolidinediones (eg, troglitazone), act as insulin sensitizers. They are presently in clinical trials and one such drug, troglitazone, has been approved by the FDA.

SULFONYLUREAS

In 1955, sulfonylurea drugs became widely available for treatment of NIDDM. The compounds are arylsulfonylureas with substitutions on the benzene and urea groups. Table 41–6 depicts the chemical structures of the seven sulfonylureas used in the USA, including three "second-generation" preparations.

Mechanism of Action

At least three mechanisms of sulfonylurea action have been proposed: (1) release of insulin from B cells, (2) reduction of serum glucagon levels, and (3) an extrapancreatic effect to potentiate the action of insulin on its target tissues.

A. Insulin Release From Pancreatic B Cells: (Figure 41–2.) Sulfonylureas bind to a specific receptor that is associated with a potassium channel in the B cell membrane. Binding of a sulfonylurea inhibits the efflux of potassium ion through the channel and results in depolarization. Depolarization, in turn, opens a voltage-gated calcium channel and results in calcium influx and the release of pre-

Table 41–5. Regulation of insulin release in humans.[1]

Stimulants of insulin release
Glucose, mannose
Leucine
Vagal stimulation
Sulfonylureas
Amplifiers of glucose-induced insulin release
1. Enteric hormones:
    Glucagon-like peptide 1(7–37)
    Gastrin inhibitory peptide
    Cholecystokinin
    Secretin, gastrin
2. Neural amplifiers:
    β-Adrenoceptor stimulation
3. Amino acids:
    Arginine
Inhibitors of insulin release
Neural: α-Sympathomimetic effect of catecholamines
Humoral: Somatostatin
Drugs: Diazoxide, phenytoin, vinblastine, colchicine

[1]Modified and reproduced, with permission, from Greenspan FS, Baxter JD (editors): *Basic & Clinical Endocrinology,* 4th ed. Lange, 1994.

formed insulin. Calcium channel blockers can prevent the action of sulfonylureas in vitro, but it takes calcium blocker concentrations 100–1000 times the usual therapeutic levels to achieve such blockade, probably because the calcium channels associated with B cells are not identical to the L-type calcium channels of the cardiovascular system (see Chapter 12). Moreover, diazoxide, a thiazide-like potassium channel opener (see Chapter 11), counteracts the insulinotropic effect of sulfonylureas (as well as that of glucose). This observation also provides one explanation for the hyperglycemic effects of thiazide diuretics.

Insulin synthesis is not stimulated and may even be reduced by sulfonylureas. Release of insulin in response to glucose is enhanced. There is some evidence, however, that after prolonged sulfonylurea therapy, serum insulin levels are no longer increased by the drug and may even be decreased. This observation is complicated by the fact that most such data are obtained from oral glucose tolerance testing—an unphysiologic measure of pancreatic response. After mixed meals containing protein as well as carbohydrate, the beneficial effect of chronic sulfonylurea treatment is generally associated with increased levels of serum insulin.

B. Reduction of Serum Glucagon Concentrations: It is now established that chronic administration of sulfonylureas to non-insulin-dependent diabetics reduces serum glucagon levels. This could contribute to the hypoglycemic effect of the drugs. The mechanism for this suppressive effect of sulfonylureas on glucagon levels is unclear but appears to involve indirect inhibition due to enhanced release of both insulin and somatostatin, which inhibit A cell secretion. In the absence of B cells, as in patients with IDDM or in rats with streptozocin-induced diabetes,

Table 41–6. Sulfonylureas.

Sulfonylurea	Chemical Structure	Daily Dose	Duration of Action (hours)
Tolbutamide (Orinase)	H_3C—⬡—SO_2—NH—C(=O)—NH—$(CH_2)_3$—CH_3	0.5–2 g in divided doses	6–12
Tolazamide (Tolinase)	H_3C—⬡—SO_2—NH—C(=O)—NH—N⟨⟩	0.1–1 g as single dose or in divided doses	10–14
Acetohexamide (Dymelor)	H_3C—C(=O)—⬡—SO_2—NH—C(=O)—NH—⬡	0.25–1.5 g as single dose or in divided doses	12–24
Chlorpropamide (Diabinese)	Cl—⬡—SO_2—NH—C(=O)—NH—$(CH_2)_2$—CH_3	0.1–0.5 g as single dose	Up to 60
Glyburide (glibenclamide[1]) (Diaβeta, Micronase)	Cl, ⬡ with OCH$_3$; C(=O)—NH—$(CH_2)_2$—⬡—SO_2—NH—C(=O)—NH—⬡	0.00125–0.02 g	10–24
Glipizide (glydiazinamide[1]) (Glucotrol, Glucotrol XL)	pyrazine (H_3C, N, N)—C(=O)—NH—$(CH_2)_2$—⬡—SO_2—NH—C(=O)—NH—⬡	0.005–0.03 g	10–24[2]
Glimepiride (Amaryl)	H_3C, H_5C_2 ring (N, =O)—CONHCH$_2$CH$_2$—⬡—SO_2NHCONH—⬡—CH_3	0.001–0.008 g	12–24

[1]Outside USA.
[2]Elimination half-life considerably shorter (see text).

sulfonylureas actually produce a slight rise in glucagon secretion. Sulfonylurea receptors have recently been found associated with a potassium ion channel in A cell membranes. Presumably, when sulfonylureas bind to this receptor, the ion channel closes to depolarize the cell, resulting in calcium influx and glucagon release. The presence of adjacent B cells in intact islets prevents this response, since sulfonylureas release considerable insulin that produces a net inhibition of A cells.

C. Potentiation of Insulin Action on Target Tissues: There is evidence that increased binding of insulin to tissue receptors occurs during sulfonylurea administration to patients with type II diabetes. As described in Chapter 2, an increase in receptor number can increase the effect achieved with a given concentration of agonist; such an action by the sulfonylureas would potentiate the effect of the patient's low levels of insulin as well as that of exogenous insulin. However, this in vivo effect has not been found to occur when insulin is added in vitro to insulin target tissues. Moreover, in insulin-dependent diabetics with no endogenous insulin secretion, therapy with sulfonylureas has yet to be shown to improve blood glucose control, enhance sensitivity to administered insulin, or increase receptor binding of insulin.

These observations argue strongly against a direct potentiating effect of sulfonylureas on insulin action. Rather, they suggest a secondary beneficial metabolic effect resulting from reduced glycemia or lower fatty acid levels as sulfonylureas increase insulin release in patients with NIDDM.

Efficacy & Safety of the Sulfonylureas

In 1970, the University Group Diabetes Program (UGDP) reported that the number of deaths due to cardiovascular disease in diabetic patients treated with tolbutamide was excessive compared with either insulin-treated patients or those receiving placebos. Controversy persists about the validity of the conclusions reached by the UGDP, because of the heterogeneity of the population studied and certain features of the experimental design such as the use of a fixed dose of tolbutamide. However, in 1984 a package insert warning of a possible increased risk of death due to cardiovascular disease was placed in all sulfonylureas by order of the FDA. Because of doubts about the study and several qualifying statements in the package insert that considerably weaken the impact of the warning, sulfonylureas continue to be widely prescribed.

1. TOLBUTAMIDE

Tolbutamide is well absorbed but rapidly oxidized in the liver. Its duration of effect is relatively short (6–10 hours), and it is therefore the safest sulfonylurea for use in elderly diabetics. Tolbutamide is best administered in divided doses (eg, 500 mg before each meal and at bedtime); however, some patients require only one or two tablets daily. Acute toxic reactions are rare; skin rash occurs infrequently. Prolonged hypoglycemia has been reported rarely, mostly in patients receiving certain drugs (eg, dicumarol, phenylbutazone, or some of the sulfonamides) that inhibit the metabolism of tolbutamide.

2. CHLORPROPAMIDE

Chlorpropamide has a half-life of 32 hours and is slowly metabolized in the liver to products that retain some biologic activity; approximately 20–30% is excreted unchanged in the urine. Chlorpropamide also interacts with the drugs mentioned above that depend on hepatic oxidative catabolism, and it is contraindicated in patients with hepatic or renal insufficiency. The average maintenance dosage is 250 mg daily, given as a single dose in the morning. Prolonged hypoglycemic reactions are more common than with tolbutamide, particularly in elderly patients, in whom chlorpropamide therapy should be monitored with special care. Dosages in excess of 500 mg daily increase the risk of jaundice, which is uncommon at lower doses. Patients with a genetic predisposition who are taking chlorpropamide may experience a hyperemic flush when alcohol is ingested. Dilutional hyponatremia has been recognized as a complication of chlorpropamide therapy in some patients. This appears to result from both stimulation of vasopressin secretion and potentiation of its action at the renal tubule by chlorpropamide. The antidiuretic effect of chlorpropamide appears to be independent of the sulfonylurea part of its structure, since three other sulfonylureas (acetohexamide, tolazamide, and glyburide) have diuretic effects in humans. Hematologic toxicity (transient leukopenia, thrombocytopenia) occurs in less than 1% of patients.

3. TOLAZAMIDE

Tolazamide is comparable to chlorpropamide in potency but has a shorter duration of action, similar to that of acetohexamide. Tolazamide is more slowly absorbed than the other sulfonylureas, and its effect on blood glucose does not appear for several hours. Its half-life is about 7 hours. Tolazamide is metabolized to several compounds that retain hypoglycemic effects. If more than 500 mg/d is required, the dose should be divided and given twice daily. Dosages larger than 1000 mg daily do not further improve the degree of blood glucose control.

4. ACETOHEXAMIDE

Acetohexamide has a duration of action of 10–16 hours (intermediate between that of tolbutamide and that of chlorpropamide). Therapeutic dosage consists of 0.25–1.5 g daily in one or two doses. The drug is metabolized in the liver to an active metabolite. Adverse effects are similar to those of the other sulfonylurea drugs.

5. SECOND-GENERATION SULFONYLUREAS

Three potent sulfonylurea compounds—glyburide, glipizide, and glimepiride—are considered "second-generation" hypoglycemic agents. Initial use of glyburide in other countries was associated with a high rate of severe hypoglycemic reactions and even some deaths, due probably to lack of familiarity with its potent effects. These drugs should be used with caution in patients with cardiovascular disease or in elderly patients, in whom hypoglycemia would be especially dangerous.

Diabetes patients who have not responded to tolbutamide or tolazamide may respond to the more potent first-generation sulfonylurea chlorpropamide or to one of the second-generation sulfonylureas. It has not been established that the second-generation agents are more efficacious than chlorpropamide, though they have fewer adverse effects (see below). Glyburide and glipizide are also available as less expensive generic formulations in the USA.

Glyburide is metabolized in the liver into products with very low hypoglycemic activity. Although assays specific for the unmetabolized compound suggest a short plasma half-life, the biologic effects of glyburide are clearly persistent 24 hours after a single morning dose in diabetic patients. The usual starting dosage is 2.5 mg/d or less, and the average maintenance dosage is 5–10 mg/d given as a single morning dose; maintenance dosages higher than 20 mg/d are not recommended. A formulation of "micronized" glyburide ("PresTab") is available in a variety of tablet sizes. However, there is some question as to its bioequivalence with nonmicronized formulations, and the FDA recommends careful monitoring to retitrate dosage when switching from standard glyburide doses or from other sulfonylurea drugs.

Glyburide has few adverse effects other than its potential for causing hypoglycemia. Flushing has rarely been reported after ethanol ingestion. Glyburide does not cause water retention—as chlorpropamide does—but it slightly enhances free water clearance. Glyburide is particularly contraindicated in the presence of hepatic impairment and in patients with renal insufficiency.

Glipizide has the shortest half-life (2–4 hours) of the more potent agents. For maximum effect in reducing postprandial hyperglycemia, this agent should be ingested 30 minutes before breakfast, since rapid absorption is delayed when the drug is taken with food. The recommended starting dosage is 5 mg/d, with up to 15 mg/d given as a single dose. When higher daily dosages are required, they should be divided and given before meals. The maximum recommended dosage is 30 mg/d. An extended release preparation (Glucotrol XL) provides 24-hour action after a once-daily morning dose. However, this formulation appears to have sacrificed its lower propensity for severe hypoglycemia compared with longer-acting glyburide without showing any demonstrable therapeutic advantages over the latter (which can be obtained as a generic drug).

Because of its shorter half-life, glipizide is much less likely than glyburide to produce serious hypoglycemia. At least 90% of glipizide is metabolized in the liver to inactive products, and 10% is excreted unchanged in the urine. Glipizide therapy is therefore contraindicated in patients with hepatic or renal impairment, who would therefore be at high risk for hypoglycemia.

Glimepiride has recently been approved by the FDA for "once-daily use as monotherapy or in combination with insulin to lower blood glucose in diabetes patients who cannot control their glucose level through diet and exercise." Glimepiride achieves blood glucose lowering with the lowest dose of any sulfonylurea compound. A single daily dose of 1 mg has been shown to be effective, and the recommended maximal daily dose is 8 mg. It has a long duration of effect with a half-life of 5 hours, allowing once-daily dosing and thereby improving compliance. It is completely metabolized by the liver to inactive products. Further experience is needed to determine whether any safety or efficacy factors favor its use over less expensive generic forms of sulfonylureas.

Secondary Failure & Tachyphylaxis to Sulfonylureas

Secondary failure (ie, failure to maintain a good response to sulfonylurea therapy [tachyphylaxis, tolerance]) remains a disconcerting problem in the management of type II diabetes. While the inability to maintain dietary compliance may be responsible for many of these cases, it is possible that multiple-dose conventional therapy which produces sustained blood levels of long-acting sulfonylureas may induce a refractoriness in responding pancreatic B cells. This phenomenon has been observed during short-term studies of sulfonylurea-induced insulin release and has suggested clinical trials of intermittent or pulse therapy with sulfonylureas in which a single daily dose of a short-acting sulfonylurea is prescribed.

Combined Therapy With Sulfonylureas & Insulin

Since sulfonylurea drugs not only increase the pancreatic B cell secretion of insulin but also might restore peripheral tissue sensitivity to insulin, their use with insulin has been advocated to reduce the total insulin dose required to control hyperglycemia. Moreover, bedtime NPH insulin has been suggested as an adjunct to sulfonylurea therapy in those NIDDM patients who fail to respond adequately to maximal sulfonylurea dosage. Currently, however, data from clinical trials with appropriate controls and crossover studies are too limited to justify the expense of prescribing both insulin and sulfonylureas to treat NIDDM except when severe insulin resistance is present that requires more than 100 units per day.

BIGUANIDES

The structures of some biguanides are shown in Table 41–7. Phenformin was discontinued in the USA because of its association with lactic acidosis and because there was no documentation of any long-term benefit from its use. Metformin, buformin, and phenformin continue to be used elsewhere, though in most areas the indications for therapy with phenformin are being questioned. Clinical trials of metformin in the USA were successfully completed in 1995 and this biguanide is now approved for use in this country.

Mechanism of Action

A full explanation of the biguanides' mechanism of action remains elusive. Their blood glucose-lowering action does not depend on the presence of functioning pancreatic B cells. Glucose is not lowered in normal subjects after an overnight fast, but their postprandial blood glucose levels are lower during biguanide administration. Patients with NIDDM have considerably

Table 41–7. Biguanides.

The general biguanide structure:

$$H_2N-\underset{\underset{NH}{\|}}{C}\quad\overset{\overset{H}{\overset{|}{N}}}{}\quad\underset{\underset{NH}{\|}}{C}-R$$

Biguanide		Daily Dose	Duration of Action (hours)
Phenformin[1]	$-NH-(CH_2)_2-$ (phenyl ring)	0.025–0.15 g as single dose or in divided doses	4–6 8–14[2]
Buformin[1]	$-NH-(CH_2)_3-CH_3$	0.05–0.3 g in divided doses	10–12
Metformin	$-N-(CH_3)_2$	1–2.5 g in divided doses	10–12

[1]In clinical use outside USA.
[2]Timed-disintegration capsules.

less fasting hyperglycemia as well as lower postprandial hyperglycemia after biguanides; however, hypoglycemia during biguanide therapy is essentially unknown. These agents might therefore be more appropriately termed "euglycemic" rather than hypoglycemic agents. Currently proposed mechanisms of action include (1) direct stimulation of glycolysis in tissues, with increased glucose removal from blood; (2) reduced hepatic gluconeogenesis; (3) slowing of glucose absorption from the gastrointestinal tract; and (4) reduction of plasma glucagon levels.

Metabolism & Excretion

Phenformin is about one-third metabolized; the remainder is excreted unchanged in the urine. In patients with renal insufficiency, biguanides accumulate and thereby increase the risk of lactic acidosis, which appears to be a dose-related complication. Metformin has a half-life of 1.5–3 hours, is not bound to plasma proteins, is not metabolized, and is excreted by the kidneys as the active compound.

Clinical Use

Biguanides have been most often prescribed for patients with refractory obesity whose hyperglycemia is due to ineffective insulin action, ie, "insulin resistance syndrome." Because metformin is an insulin-sparing agent and does not increase weight or provoke hypoglycemia, it offers obvious advantages over insulin or sulfonylureas in treating hyperglycemia in such patients. Another indication for their use is in combination with sulfonylureas in non-insulin-dependent diabetics in whom sulfonylurea therapy alone is inadequate.

The dosage of metformin is from 500 mg to a maximum of 2.55 g daily, with the lowest effective dose being recommended. A common schedule would be to begin with a single 500 mg tablet given with breakfast for several days—and, if this is tolerated without gastrointestinal discomfort, to add a second 500 mg tablet with the evening meal if hyperglycemia persists. If further dose increases are required after 1 week, an additional 500 mg tablet can be added to be taken with the midday meal, or the larger (850 mg) tablet can be prescribed twice daily or even three times daily (the maximum recommended dosage) if needed. Dosage should always be divided, since ingestion of more than 850 mg at any one time usually provokes significant gastrointestinal side effects.

The most frequent toxic effects of metformin are gastrointestinal (anorexia, nausea, vomiting, abdominal discomfort, diarrhea) and occur in up to 20% of patients. They are dose related, tend to occur at the onset of therapy, and are often transient. However, use of metformin may have to be discontinued in 3–5% of patients because of persistent diarrhea. Absorption of vitamin B_{12} appears to be reduced during chronic metformin therapy, and annual screening of serum vitamin B_{12} levels and red blood cell parameters has been encouraged by the manufacturer to determine the need for vitamin B_{12} injections. In the absence of hypoxia or renal or hepatic insufficiency, lactic acidosis is less common with metformin therapy than with phenformin therapy.

Biguanides are contraindicated in patients with renal disease, alcoholism, hepatic disease, or conditions predisposing to tissue anoxia (eg, chronic cardiopulmonary dysfunction), because of an increased risk of lactic acidosis induced by biguanide drugs in the presence of these diseases.

ALPHA-GLUCOSIDASE INHIBITORS (Aldose Reductase Inhibitors)

Acarbose has recently been approved by the FDA for use in the USA. It is an oligosaccharide analog that binds 1000 times more avidly than natural carbohydrates to the intestinal disaccharidases such as α-glucosidase. Absorption of most carbohydrates, including starches, dextrins, maltose, and sucrose—but not lactose, which has a beta linkage—is delayed. This competitive inhibition of α-glucosidase limits the postprandial rise of glucose and results in an insulin-sparing action. When acarbose is used to treat hyperglycemic patients, its overall effect is slight, with a reduction of glycated hemoglobin of only 0.5–1% and a reduction of postprandial hyperglycemia by 30–50%. The principal adverse effect, seen in 20–30% of patients, is flatulence. This is caused by undigested carbohydrate reaching the lower bowel, where gases are produced by bacteria. Troublesome diarrhea occurs in 3% of cases. The recommended starting dose of acarbose is 50 mg twice daily, gradually increasing to 100 mg three times a day, which is the maximal recommended dose. For maximum benefit against postprandial hyperglycemia, acarbose should be given with the first mouthful of food ingested. When acarbose is given alone, there is no risk of hypoglycemia. However, if combined with insulin or sulfonylureas, it might increase the risk of hypoglycemia from these agents. Combination therapy with metformin is not recommended because acarbose interferes with absorption of metformin.

THIAZOLIDINEDIONE DERIVATIVES

This new class of oral antidiabetic drugs is presently undergoing clinical trials. The primary mechanism appears to be increased target tissue sensitivity to insulin. Animal studies have documented that these drugs potentiate the action of insulin to increase glucose uptake and glucose oxidation in both muscle and adipose tissue, while reducing hepatic glucose output as well as lipid synthesis in muscle and fat cells. These effects occur in vivo without any increase in insulin release (Hofman et al, 1992; Suter et al, 1992). Included in this class of drugs are **ciglitazone, englitazone, pioglitazone,** and **troglitazone.** One report (Suter et al, 1992) demonstrated the efficacy of troglitazone during a trial of up to 12 weeks in which it lowered insulin resistance, reduced insulinemia, and improved both fasting and postprandial hyperglycemia in NIDDM subjects. Since insulin resistance and hyperinsulinism are considered by some to contribute to the presence of hypertension, hyperlipidemia, and atherosclerosis (Reaven, 1988), this class of agents would seem to offer a welcome therapeutic option for NIDDM therapy. Although most of these agents are in clinical trials, troglitazone (Rezulin) has been approved by the FDA—but only for use in insulin-resistant patients who are receiving insulin.

ALDOSE REDUCTASE INHIBITORS

The aldose reductase inhibitors, eg, tolrestat, are designed to reduce glucose toxicity in tissues such as the eye, the kidney, and nerve trunks. They act by inhibiting the cellular enzyme that converts glucose to fructose and subsequently to sorbitol, both of which may contribute to the toxic effects of hyperglycemia. Several drugs in this class have undergone clinical trials without very impressive results. None of the aldose reductase inhibitors have been documented to prevent progression of nephropathy. Tolrestat has shown some clinical efficacy in improving nerve conduction in a placebo-controlled clinical trial. A long-term retinopathy-prevention trial with tolrestat continues, but as yet there is no evidence that aldose-reductase inhibition can prevent or reduce retinopathy. None of these drugs have been approved for use in the USA.

GLUCAGON

Chemistry & Metabolism

Glucagon is synthesized in the A cells of the pancreatic islets of Langerhans (Table 41–1). Glucagon is a peptide—identical in all mammals—consisting of a single chain of 29 amino acids (Figure 41–6), with a molecular weight of 3485. Selective proteolytic cleavage converts a large precursor molecule of approximately 18,000 MW to glucagon. One of the precursor intermediates consists of a 69-amino-acid peptide called **glicentin,** which contains the glucagon sequence interposed between peptide extensions.

Glucagon is extensively degraded in the liver and kidney as well as in plasma, and at its tissue receptor sites. Because of its rapid inactivation by plasma, chilling of the collecting tubes and addition of inhibitors of proteolytic enzymes are necessary when samples of blood are collected for immunoassay of circulating glucagon. Its half-life in plasma is between 3 and 6 minutes, which is similar to that of insulin.

"Gut Glucagon"

Glicentin immunoreactivity has been found in cells of the small intestine as well as in pancreatic A cells and in effluents of perfused pancreas. The intestinal cells secrete **enteroglucagon,** a family of glucagon-like peptides (Figure 41–6), of which glicentin is a member, along with glucagon-like peptides 1 and 2 (GLP-1 and GLP-2). Unlike the pancreatic A cell, these intestinal cells lack the enzymes to convert glucagon precursors to true glucagon by removing the carboxyl terminal extension from the molecule.

The function of the enteroglucagons has not been clarified, though smaller peptides can bind hepatic glucagon receptors where they exert partial activity. A derivative of the 37-amino-acid form of GLP-1 that lacks the first six amino acids (GLP-1[7–37]) is a potent stimulant of insulin release. It represents the predominant form of GLP in the human intestine and has been termed "insulinotropin." It is being considered

Figure 41–6. The gene for proglucagon (protein shown schematically at top) is found in all tissues. In the pancreatic A cell, the expressed protein is processed as shown, resulting in production of glucagon and other fragments. In the small intestine (bottom), proglucagon is processed in a different way, resulting in the production of glicentin, truncated GLP-1, and GLP-2. Glicentin can be further split as shown. Of the various products, glucagon (from the pancreas) and truncated glucagon-like peptide (GLP-1[7-37]) from the small intestine are therapeutically important.

as a potential therapeutic agent in NIDDM, but only limited data are currently available concerning this application.

Pharmacologic Effects of Glucagon

A. Metabolic Effects: The first six amino acids at the amino terminal of the glucagon molecule bind to specific receptors on liver cells. This leads to a G protein-linked increase in adenylyl cyclase activity and the production of cAMP, which facilitates catabolism of stored glycogen and increases gluconeogenesis and ketogenesis. The immediate pharmacologic result of glucagon infusion is to raise blood glucose at the expense of stored hepatic glycogen. There is no effect on skeletal muscle glycogen, presumably because of the lack of glucagon receptors on skeletal muscle. Pharmacologic amounts of glucagon cause release of insulin from normal pancreatic B cells, catecholamines from pheochromocytoma, and calcitonin from medullary carcinoma cells.

B. Cardiac Effects: Glucagon has a potent inotropic and chronotropic effect on the heart, mediated by the cAMP mechanism described above. Thus, it produces an effect very similar to that of beta-adrenoceptor agonists without requiring functioning beta receptors.

C. Effects on Smooth Muscle: Large doses of glucagon produce profound relaxation of the intestine. In contrast to the above effects of the peptide, this action on the intestine may be due to mechanisms other than adenylyl cyclase activation.

Clinical Uses

A. Severe Hypoglycemia: The major use of glucagon is for emergency treatment of severe hypoglycemic reactions in insulin-dependent patients when unconsciousness precludes oral feedings and use of intravenous glucose is not possible. It is currently available for parenteral use (Glucagon Emergency Kit). Nasal sprays have been developed for this purpose and are presently undergoing clinical trials.

B. Endocrine Diagnosis: Several tests use glucagon to diagnose endocrine disorders. In patients with insulin-dependent diabetes mellitus, a standard test of pancreatic B cell secretory reserve utilizes 1 mg of glucagon administered as an intravenous bolus. Since insulin-treated patients develop circulating anti-insulin antibodies that interfere with radioimmunoassays of insulin, measurements of C-peptide are used to indicate B cell secretion. Normal persons achieve a standard serum concentration of pancreatic C-peptide within 10 minutes after injection, and in insulin-treated diabetics various degrees of B cell insufficiency can be quantitated. Most diabetics with long-standing IDDM show *no* C-peptide response to glucagon.

In patients with suspected endocrine tumors such as insulinoma, pheochromocytoma, or medullary carcinoma of the thyroid, a bolus of 0.5–1 mg of glucagon intravenously is occasionally effective in discharging hormonal products from a tumor, though negative tests may not rule out the diagnosis.

C. Beta-Blocker Poisoning: Glucagon is sometimes useful for reversing the cardiac effects of an overdose of beta-blocking agents because of its ability to increase cAMP production in the heart. However, it is not clinically useful in the treatment of congestive cardiac failure.

D. Radiology of the Bowel: Glucagon has been used extensively in radiology as an aid to x-ray visualization of the bowel because of its ability to relax the intestine.

Adverse Reactions

Transient nausea and occasional vomiting can result from glucagon administration. These are generally mild, and glucagon is relatively free of severe adverse reactions.

ISLET AMYLOID POLYPEPTIDE (IAPP, Amylin)

IAPP is a 37-amino-acid peptide originally derived from islet amyloid deposits in pancreas material from patients with long-standing NIDDM or insulinomas. It is produced by pancreatic B cells, packaged within B cell granules in a concentration 1–2% that of insulin, and secreted in response to B cell secretagogues. A physiologic effect has not been established; however, pharmacologic doses inhibit the action of insulin to promote muscle uptake of glucose. IAPP appears to be a member of the superfamily of neuroregulatory peptides, with 46% homology with the calcitonin gene-related peptide CGRP (see Chapter 17). Whereas CGRP inhibits insulin secretion, this has not been demonstrated at physiologic concentrations of IAPP. Clinical trials have begun to evaluate IAPP and its analogs, eg, pramlintide, as adjuncts to insulin therapy in type I diabetic patients with recurrent episodes of severe insulin-induced hypoglycemia—episodes that are generally refractory to usual preventive measures.

PREPARATIONS AVAILABLE
(See Table 41–4 for insulin preparations.)

Sulfonylureas
Acetohexamide (generic, Dymelor)
Oral: 250, 500 mg tablets
Chlorpropamide (generic, Diabinese)
Oral: 100, 250 mg tablets
Glimepiride (Amaryl)
Oral: 1, 2, 4 mg tablets
Glipizide (generic, Glucotrol, Glucotrol XL)
Oral: 5, 10 mg tablets; 5, 10 mg extended release tablets
Glyburide (generic, Diaβeta, Micronase, Glynase PresTab)
Oral: 1.25, 2.5, 5 mg tablets; 1.5, 3, 6 mg "PresTab, micronized" tablets
Tolazamide (generic, Tolinase)
Oral: 100, 250, 500 mg tablets
Tolbutamide (generic, Orinase)
Oral: 500 mg tablets

Biguanide
Metformin (Glucophage)
Oral: 500, 850 mg tablets

Thiazolidinedione Derivative
Troglitazone (Rezulin)
Oral: 200, 400 mg tablets

Alpha-Glucosidase Inhibitor
Acarbose (Precose)
Oral: 50, 100 mg tablets

Glucagon
Glucagon (generic)
Parenteral: 1, 10 mg lyophilized powders to reconstitute for injection

REFERENCES

Abraira C et al: Veterans Affairs Cooperative Study on glycemic control and complications in type II diabetes, results of the feasibility trial. Diabetes Care 1995;18:1113.

Bailey CJ: Biguanides and NIDDM. Diabetes Care 1992;15:755.

Binder C et al: Insulin pharmacokinetics. Diabetes Care 1984;7:188.

Bloomgarden ZT: NIDDM treatment. Diabetes Care 1995;18:425.

Boyd AE III: Sulfonylurea receptors, ion channels, and fruit flies. Diabetes 1988;37:847.

Brange J et al: Monomeric insulins and their experimental and clinical implications. Diabetes Care 1990;13:923.

Clark CM, Lee DA: Drug therapy: Prevention and treatment of the complications of diabetes mellitus. N Engl J Med 1995;332:1210.

Cohen RD: Lactic acidosis: New perspectives on origins and treatment. Diabetes Rev 1994;2:86.

Coniff RF et al: A double-blind placebo-controlled trial evaluating the safety and efficacy of acarbose for the treatment of patients with insulin-requiring type II diabetes. Diabetes Care 1995;18:928.

Coniff RF et al: Multicenter, placebo-controlled trial comparing acarbose (BAY g 5421) with placebo, tolbutamide, and tolbutamide-plus-Acarbose in NIDDM. Am J Med 1995;98:443.

Cryer PE, Fisher JN, Shamoon H: Hypoglycemia. Diabetes Care 1994;17:734.

DeFronzo RA et al: Efficacy of metformin in patients with non-insulin-dependent diabetes mellitus. N Engl J Med 1995;333:541.

Diabetes Control and Complications Trial Research Group: The effect of intensive treatment of diabetes on the development and progression of long-term complications in insulin-dependent diabetes mellitus. N Engl J Med 1993;329:977.

Diabetes Control and Complications Trial Research Group: Epidemiology of severe hypoglycemia in the diabetes control and complications trial. Am J Med 1991;90:450.

Dunn CJ, Peters DH: Metformin: A review of its pharmacological properties and therapeutic use in non-insulin-dependent diabetes mellitus. Drugs 1995;49:721.

Fehman H-C, Goke R, Goke B: Cell and molecular biology of the incretin hormones glucagon-like peptide I and glucose-dependent insulin-releasing polypeptide. Endocrin Rev 1995;16:390.

Galloway JA et al: Biosynthetic human proinsulin: Review of chemistry, in vitro and in vivo receptor binding, animal and human pharmacology studies, and clinical trial experience. Diabetes Care 1992;15:666.

Genuth S: Management of the adult onset diabetic with sulfonylurea failure. Endocrinol Metab Clin North Am 1992;21:351.

Ghazzi MN et al: Cardiac and glycemic benefits of troglitazone treatment in NIDDM. The Troglitazone Study Group. Diabetes 1997;46:433.

Giugliano D et al: Tolrestat in the primary prevention of diabetic neuropathy. Diabetes Care 1995;18:536.

Gorden P: Human insulin use and hypoglycemia. (Letter.) N Engl J Med 1990;322:1007.

Gray H, O'Rahilly S: Toward improved glycemic control in diabetes; what's on the horizon? Arch Intern Med 1995;155:1137.

Groop L et al: Comparison of pharmacokinetics, metabolic effects and mechanisms of action of glyburide and glipizide during long-term treatment. Diabetes Care 1987;10:671.

Heinemann L et al: Prandial glycemia after a carbohydrate-rich meal in type I diabetic patients. Using the rapid acting insulin analogue [Lys (B28), Pro (B29)] human insulin. Diabetic Med 1996;13:625.

Herman LS et al: Therapeutic comparison of metformin and sulfonylurea, alone and in various combinations: A double blind, controlled study. Diabetes Care 1994;17:1100.

Hofman CA, Colca JR: New oral thiazolidinedione antidiabetic agents act as insulin sensitizers. Diabetes Care 1992;15:1075.

Howey DC et al: [Lys (B28), Pro (B29)]-human insulin: a rapidly absorbed analog of human insulin. Diabetes 1994;43:396.

Kahn BB: Facilitative glucose transporters: Regulatory mechanisms and dysregulation in diabetes. J Clin Invest 1992;89:1367.

Kahn CR: Insulin action, diabetogenes, and the cause of type II diabetes. Diabetes 1994;13:1066.

Kang S et al: Subcutaneous insulin absorption explained by insulin's physicochemical properties. Diabetes Care 1991;14:942.

Karam JH: Type II diabetes and syndrome X: Pathogenesis and glycemic management. Endocrinol Metab Clin North Am 1992;21:329.

Klonoff DC et al: Hypoglycemia following inadvertent and factitious sulfonylurea overdosages. Diabetes Care 1995;18:563.

Kuenhle HF: New therapeutic agents for the treatment of NIDDM. Exp Clin Endocrinol Diabetes 1996;104:93.

Lalau JD et al: Role of metformin accumulation in metformin-associated lactic acidosis. 1995;18:779.

Lebovitz HE, Melander A (editors): Sulfonylurea drugs: Basic and clinical considerations. Diabetes Care 1990;13(Suppl 3):1.

Lefebvre PJ: Glucagon and its family revisited. Diabetes Care 1995;18:715.

Maran A et al: Double blind clinical and laboratory study of hypoglycaemia with human and porcine insulin in diabetic patients reporting hypoglycaemia unawareness after transferring to human insulin. Br Med J 1993;306:167.

Moller DE, Flier JS: Insulin resistance: Mechanism, syndromes, and implications. N Engl J Med 1991;325:938.

Muhlhauser I et al: Hypoglycemic symptoms and frequency of severe hypoglycemia in patients treated with human and animal insulin preparations. Diabetes Care 1991;14:745.

Muhlhauser I, Koch J, Berger M: Pharmacokinetics and bioavailability of injected glucagon: Differences between intramuscular, subcutaneous, and intravenous administration. Diabetes Care 1984;8:39.

Nathan DM et al: Insulinotropic action of glucagon like peptide-1-(7-37) in diabetic and nondiabetic subjects. Diabetes Care 1992;15:270.

Nolan JJ et al: Improvement in glucose tolerance and insulin resistance in obese subjects treated with troglitazone. N Engl J Med 1994;331:1188.

Nolte MS: Insulin therapy in insulin-dependent (type I) diabetes mellitus. Endocrinol Metab Clin North Am 1992;21:281.

Olson PO, Hans A, Henning VS: Miscibility of human semi-synthetic regular and lente insulin and human biosynthetic regular and NPH insulin. Diabetes Care 1987; 10:473.

Pampanelli S et al: Improved postprandial metabolic control after subcutaneous injection of a short-acting insulin analog (lispro) in IDDM of short duration with residual pancreatic beta-cell function. Diabetes Care 1995;18:1452.

Pilch PF, Waugh SM, O'Hare T: The structural basis for insulin receptor function. In: *Advances in Regulation of Cell Growth,* vol 1: *Regulation of Cell Growth and Activation.* Mond JJ, Cambier JC, Weiss A (editors). Raven Press, 1989.

Polonsky KS: The β-cell in diabetes: From molecular genetics to clinical research. Diabetes 1995;44:705.

Rachman J, Turner RC: Drugs on the horizon for treatment of type 2 diabetes. Diabetic Med 1995;12:467.

Rasmussen H et al: Physiology and pathophysiology of insulin secretion. Diabetes Care 1990;13:655.

Reaven GM: Role of insulin resistance in human disease. Diabetes 1988;37:1595.

Resine T, Bell GI: Molecular biology of somatostatin receptors. Endocr Rev 1995;16:427.

Ritzel R et al: Pharmacokinetics, insulinotropic and glucagonostatic properties of GLP-1 (7-36 amide) after subcutaneous injection in healthy volunteers. Diabetologia 1995;38:720.

Rosak C et al: The effect of the timing and the administration of acarbose on postprandial hyperglycemia. Diabetic Med 1995;12:979.

Selam JL, Charles MA: Devices for insulin administration. Diabetes Care 1990;13:955.

Shank ML, DelPrato S, DeFronzo RA: Bedtime insulin/daytime glipizide: effective therapy for sulfonylurea failures in NIDDM. Diabetes 1995;44:165.

Stephens JM, Pilch PF: The metabolic regulation and vesicular transport of GLUT4, the major insulin responsive glucose transporter. Endocr Rev 1995;16:529.

Stumvoll M et al: Metabolic effects of metformin in non-insulin-dependent diabetes mellitus. N Engl J Med 1995;333:550.

Torlone E et al: Pharmacokinetics, pharmacodynamics and glucose counterregulation following subcutaneous injection of the monomeric analogue [Lys (B28), Pro (B29)] in IDDM. Diabetologia 1994;37:713.

Turner RC et al: United Kingdom prospective diabetes study (UKPDS): Relative efficacy of randomly allocated diet, sulphonylurea, insulin or metformin in patients with newly diagnosed non-insulin dependent diabetes followed for 3 years. Br Med J 1995;310:83.

Westermark P et al: Islet amyloid polypeptide: A novel controversy in diabetes research. Diabetologia 1992;35:297.

42

Agents That Affect Bone Mineral Homeostasis

Daniel D. Bikle, MD, PhD

I. BASIC PHARMACOLOGY

Calcium and phosphate, the major mineral constituents of bone, are also two of the most important minerals for general cellular function. Accordingly, the body has evolved a complex set of mechanisms by which calcium and phosphate homeostasis are carefully maintained (Figure 42–1). Approximately 98% of the 1–2 kg of calcium and 85% of the 1 kg of phosphorus in the human adult are found in bone, the principal reservoir for these minerals. These functions are dynamic, with constant remodeling of bone and ready exchange of bone mineral with that in the extracellular fluid. Bone also serves as the principal structural support for the body and provides the space for hematopoiesis. Thus, abnormalities in bone mineral homeostasis can lead not only to a wide variety of cellular dysfunctions (eg, tetany, coma, muscle weakness) but also to disturbances in structural support of the body (eg, osteoporosis with fractures) and loss of hematopoietic capacity (eg, infantile osteopetrosis).

Calcium and phosphate enter the body from the intestine. The average American diet provides 600–1000 mg of calcium per day, of which approximately 100–250 mg is absorbed. This figure represents net absorption, since both absorption (principally in the duodenum and upper jejunum) and secretion (principally in the ileum) occur. The amount of phosphorus in the American diet is about the same as that of calcium. However, the efficiency of absorption (principally in the jejunum) is greater, ranging from 70% to 90% depending on intake. In the steady state, renal excretion of calcium and phosphate balances intestinal absorption. In general, over 98% of filtered calcium and 85% of filtered phosphate is reabsorbed by the kidney. The movement of calcium and phosphate across the intestinal and renal epithelia is closely regulated. Intrinsic disease of the intestine (eg, nontropical sprue) or kidney (eg, chronic renal failure) disrupts bone mineral homeostasis.

Two hormones serve as the principal regulators of calcium and phosphate homeostasis: the peptide parathyroid hormone (PTH) and the steroid vitamin D. Vitamin D is a prohormone rather than a true hormone, since it must be further metabolized to gain biologic activity. Other hormones—calcitonin, prolactin, growth hormone, insulin, thyroid hormone, glucocorticoids, and sex steroids—influence calcium and phosphate homeostasis under certain physiologic circumstances and can be considered secondary regulators. Deficiency or excess of these secondary regulators within a physiologic range does not produce the disturbance of calcium and phosphate homeostasis observed in situations of deficiency or excess of PTH and vitamin D. However, certain of these secondary regulators—especially calcitonin, glucocorticoids, and estrogens—are useful therapeutically and will be discussed in subsequent sections.

In addition to these hormonal regulators, calcium and phosphate themselves, other ions such as sodium and fluoride, and a variety of drugs (bisphosphonates, plicamycin, and diuretics) also alter calcium and phosphate homeostasis.

PRINCIPAL HORMONAL REGULATORS OF BONE MINERAL HOMEOSTASIS

PARATHYROID HORMONE

Parathyroid hormone (PTH) is a single-chain peptide hormone composed of 84 amino acids. It is produced in the parathyroid gland in a precursor form of 115 amino acids, the remaining 31 amino terminal amino acids being cleaved off prior to secretion.

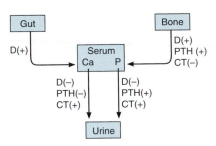

Figure 42–1. Some mechanisms contributing to bone mineral homeostasis. Calcium and phosphorus concentrations in the serum are controlled principally by two hormones, 1,25(OH)2 D₃ *(D)* and parathyroid hormone *(PTH)*, through their action on absorption from the gut and from bone and on excretion in the urine. Both hormones increase input of calcium and phosphorus from bone into the serum; vitamin D also increases absorption from the gut. Vitamin D decreases urinary excretion of both calcium and phosphorus, while PTH reduces calcium but increases phosphorus excretion. Calcitonin *(CT)* is a less critical hormone for calcium homeostasis, but in pharmacologic concentrations CT can reduce serum calcium and phosphorus by inhibiting bone resorption and stimulating their renal excretion. Feedback effects are not shown.

Within the gland is a calcium-sensitive protease capable of cleaving the intact hormone into fragments. Biologic activity resides in the amino terminal region such that synthetic 1–34 PTH is fully active. Loss of the first two amino terminal amino acids eliminates most biologic activity.

The metabolic clearance of intact PTH in dogs has been estimated to be 20 mL/min/kg, with a half-time of disappearance measured in minutes. Most of the clearance occurs in the liver and kidney. The biologically inactive carboxyl terminal fragments produced during metabolism of the intact hormone have a much lower clearance, especially in renal failure. This accounts in part for the very high PTH values often observed in the past in patients with renal failure when measured by radioimmunoassays directed against the carboxyl terminal region of the molecule. However, most PTH assays currently in use measure the intact hormone by a double antibody method, so that this circumstance is less frequently encountered in clinical practice. The appearance of amino terminal fragments of PTH in the blood is difficult to demonstrate—consistent with the observation that only small amounts of such fragments are released into the blood and that their clearance is high.

PTH regulates calcium and phosphate flux across cellular membranes in bone and kidney, resulting in increased serum calcium and decreased serum phosphate. In bone, PTH increases the activity and number of osteoclasts, the cells responsible for bone resorption. However, it appears that this stimulation of osteoclasts is not a direct effect. Rather, PTH acts on the osteoblast (the bone-forming cell), and the osteoblast

somehow regulates the activity of the osteoclast. This action increases bone turnover or bone remodeling, a specific sequence of cellular events initiated by osteoclastic bone resorption and followed by osteoblastic bone formation. In addition, PTH stimulates the differentiation of osteoclast precursors to osteoclasts, thus increasing the number of osteoclasts. Although both bone resorption and bone formation are enhanced by PTH, the net effect of excess PTH is to increase bone resorption. PTH in low doses may actually increase bone formation without first stimulating bone resorption, and analogs of PTH that might exploit this effect are currently under study for the treatment of osteoporosis. Although cAMP is involved in the action of PTH on bone cells, other mediators (including calcium) probably also play a role.

In the kidney, PTH increases the ability of the nephron to reabsorb calcium and magnesium but reduces its ability to reabsorb phosphate, amino acids, bicarbonate, sodium, chloride, and sulfate. Although PTH markedly stimulates the renal production and excretion of cAMP and cAMP reproduces a number of the renal actions of PTH, cAMP may not be the sole mediator of PTH action on the kidney. Another important action of PTH on the kidney is its stimulation of 1,25-dihydroxyvitamin D (1,25[OH]₂D) production.

Recent evidence has called attention to vasoactive and cardiotropic actions of PTH. These observations may explain the ability of PTH to increase the glomerular filtration rate acutely. Whether such actions are involved in the apparent association of hyperparathyroidism and hypertension remains to be determined.

VITAMIN D

Vitamin D is a secosteroid produced in the skin from 7-dehydrocholesterol under the influence of ultraviolet irradiation. Vitamin D is also found in certain foods and is used to supplement dairy products. Both the natural form (vitamin D₃, cholecalciferol) and the plant-derived form (vitamin D₂, ergocalciferol) are present in the diet. These forms differ in that ergocalciferol contains a double bond (C_{22-23}) and an additional methyl group in the side chain (Figure 42–2). In humans this difference apparently is of little physiologic consequence, and the following comments apply equally well to both forms of vitamin D.

Vitamin D is a prohormone that serves as precursor to a number of biologically active metabolites (Figure 42–2). Vitamin D is first hydroxylated in the liver to form 25-hydroxyvitamin D (25[OH]D). This metabolite is further converted in the kidney to a number of other forms, the best-studied of which are 1,25-dihydroxyvitamin D (1,25[OH]₂D) and 24,25-dihydroxyvitamin D (24,25[OH]₂D). Of the natural metabolites, only vitamin D, 25(OH)D (as calcifediol), and 1,25(OH)₂D (as calcitriol), are available for clinical

Figure 42–2. Conversion of 7-dehydrocholesterol to vitamin D_3 and metabolism of D_3 to $1,25(OH)_2D_3$ and $24,25(OH)_2D_3$. Control of the latter step is exerted primarily at the level of the kidney, where low serum phosphorus, low serum calcium, and high parathyroid hormone favor the production of $1,25(OH)_2D_3$. The inset shows the side chain for ergosterol. Ergosterol undergoes similar transformation to vitamin D_2 (ergocalciferol), which, in turn, is metabolized to $25OHD_2$, $1,25(OH)_2D_2$, and $24,25(OH)_2D_2$. In humans, corresponding D_2 and D_3 derivatives have equivalent effects and potency. They are therefore referred to in the text without a subscript.

use (see Table 42–1), though clinical studies with $24,25(OH)_2D$ are under way. Moreover, a number of analogs of $1,25(OH)_2$ are being synthesized in an effort to extend the usefulness of this metabolite to a variety of nonclassic conditions. Calcipotriene (calcipotriol), for example, is currently being used to treat psoriasis, a hyperproliferative skin disorder. Other analogs are being evaluated in the management of hyperparathyroidism and various malignancies. The regulation of vitamin D metabolism is complex, involving calcium, phosphate, and a variety of hormones, the most important of which is PTH.

Vitamin D and its metabolites circulate in plasma tightly bound to a carrier protein, the vitamin D-binding protein. This α-globulin binds $25(OH)D$ and $24,25(OH)_2D$ with comparable high affinity and vitamin D and $1,25(OH)_2D$ with lower affinity. In normal subjects, the terminal half-life of injected calcifediol is 23 days, whereas in anephric subjects it is longer (42 days). The half-life of $24,25(OH)_2D$ is probably similar. Tracer studies with vitamin D have shown a

rapid clearance from the blood. The liver appears to be the principal organ for clearance. Excess vitamin D is stored in adipose tissue. The metabolic clearance of calcitriol in humans indicates a rapid turnover, with a terminal half-life measured in hours. Several of the $1,25(OH)_2$ analogs are bound poorly by the vitamin D-binding protein. As a result, their clearance is very rapid, with a terminal half-life measured in minutes. Such analogs have little of the hypercalcemic, hypercalciuric effects of calcitriol, an important aspect of their use for the management of conditions such as psoriasis.

The mechanism of action of the vitamin D metabolites remains under active investigation. However, calcitriol is well established as the most potent agent with respect to stimulation of intestinal calcium and phosphate transport and bone resorption. Calcitriol appears to act on the intestine both by induction of new proteins (eg, calcium-binding protein) and by modulation of calcium flux across the brush border and mitochondrial membranes by a means that does not require new

Table 42–1. Vitamin D and its clinically available metabolites and analogs.

Chemical Name	Abbreviation	Generic Name
Vitamin D_3	D_3	Cholecalciferol
Vitamin D_2	D_2	Ergocalciferol
25-Hydroxy-vitamin D_3	$25(OH)D_3$	Calciferol
1,25-Dihydroxy-vitamin D_3	$1,25(OH)_2D_3$	Calcitriol
24,25-Dihydroxy-vitamin D_3	$24,25(OH)_2D_3$	Secalcifediol
Dihydrotachysterol	DHT	Dihydrotachysterol

protein synthesis. The molecular action of calcitriol on bone has received less attention. The metabolites $25(OH)D$ and $24,25(OH)_2D$ are far less potent stimulators of intestinal calcium and phosphate transport or bone resorption. However, $25(OH)D$ appears to be more potent than $1,25(OH)_2D$ in stimulating renal reabsorption of calcium and phosphate and may be the major metabolite regulating calcium flux and contractility in muscle. Recent evidence suggests that $24,25(OH)_2D$ stimulates bone formation. Specific receptors for $1,25(OH)_2D$ exist in target tissues. However, the role and even the existence of receptors for $25(OH)D$ and $24,25(OH)_2D$ remain controversial.

The receptor for $1,25(OH)_2D$ exists in a wide variety of tissues—not just bone, gut, and kidney. In these "nonclassic" tissues, $1,25(OH)_2D$ exerts a number of actions including regulation of parathyroid hormone secretion from the parathyroid gland, insulin secretion from the pancreas, cytokine production by macrophages and T cells, and proliferation and differentiation of a large number of cells, including cancer cells. Thus, the clinical utility of $1,25(OH)_2D$ analogs is likely to expand.

INTERACTION OF PTH & VITAMIN D

A summary of the principal actions of PTH and vitamin D on the three main target tissues—intestine, kidney, and bone—is presented in Table 42–2. The net effect of PTH is to raise serum calcium and reduce serum phosphate; the net effect of vitamin D is to raise both. Regulation of calcium and phosphate homeostasis is achieved through a variety of feedback loops. Calcium is the principal regulator of PTH secretion. It binds to a novel ion recognition site that is part of a G_q protein-coupled receptor and links changes in intracellular free calcium concentration to changes in extracellular calcium. As serum calcium levels rise and bind to this receptor, intracellular calcium levels increase and inhibit PTH secretion. Phosphate regulates PTH secretion indirectly by forming complexes with cal-

cium in the serum. Since it is the ionized concentration of calcium that is detected by the parathyroid gland, increases in serum phosphate levels reduce the ionized calcium and lead to enhanced PTH secretion. Such feedback regulation is appropriate to the net effect of PTH to raise serum calcium and reduce serum phosphate levels. Likewise, both calcium and phosphate at high levels reduce the amount of $1,25(OH)_2D$ produced by the kidney and increase the amount of $24,25(OH)_2D$ produced. Since $1,25(OH)_2D$ raises serum calcium and phosphate, whereas $24,25(OH)_2D$ has less effect, such feedback regulation is again appropriate. $1,25(OH)_2D$ itself directly inhibits PTH secretion (independently of its effect on serum calcium) by a direct action on PTH gene transcription. This provides yet another negative feedback loop, because PTH is a major stimulus for $1,25(OH)_2D$ production. This ability of $1,25(OH)_2D$ to inhibit PTH secretion directly is being evaluated using calcitriol analogs that do not raise serum calcium. Such drugs are likely to prove useful in the management of secondary hyperparathyroidism accompanying renal failure or even in selected cases of primary hyperparathyroidism.

SECONDARY HORMONAL REGULATORS OF BONE MINERAL HOMEOSTASIS

A number of hormones modulate the actions of PTH and vitamin D in regulating bone mineral homeo-

Table 42–2. Actions of PTH and vitamin D on gut, bone, and kidney.

	PTH	Vitamin D
Intestine	Increased calcium and phosphate absorption (by increased $1,25[OH]_2D$ production)	Increased calcium and phosphate absorption (by $1,25[OH]_2D$)
Kidney	Decreased calcium excretion, increased phosphate excretion	Calcium and phosphate excretion may be decreased by $25(OH)D$ and $1,25(OH)_2D$
Bone	Calcium and phosphate resorption increased by high doses. Low doses may increase bone formation	Increased calcium and phosphate resorption by $1,25(OH)_2D$; bone formation may be increased by $24,25(OH)_2D$
Net effect on serum levels	Serum calcium increased, serum phosphate decreased	Serum calcium and phosphate both increased

stasis. Compared with that of PTH and vitamin D, the physiologic impact of such secondary regulation on bone mineral homeostasis is minor. However, in pharmacologic amounts, a number of these hormones have actions on the bone mineral homeostatic mechanisms that can be exploited therapeutically.

CALCITONIN

The calcitonin secreted by the parafollicular cells of the mammalian thyroid (and by the ultimobranchial bodies of fish) is a single-chain peptide hormone with 32 amino acids and a molecular weight of 3600. A disulfide bond between positions 1 and 7 is essential for biologic activity. Calcitonin is produced in these glands from a precursor with MW 15,000. The circulating forms of calcitonin are multiple, ranging in size from the monomer (MW 3600) to forms with an apparent molecular weight of 60,000. Whether such heterogeneity includes precursor forms or covalently linked oligomers is not known. Because of its heterogeneity, calcitonin is standardized by bioassay in rats. Activity is compared to a standard maintained by the British Medical Research Council (MRC) and expressed as MRC units.

Human calcitonin monomer has a half-life of about 10 minutes with a metabolic clearance of 8–9 mL/kg/min. Salmon calcitonin has a longer half-life and a reduced metabolic clearance (3 mL/kg/min). Much of the clearance occurs in the kidney, although little intact calcitonin appears in the urine.

The principal effects of calcitonin are to lower serum calcium and phosphate by actions on bone and kidney. Calcitonin inhibits osteoclastic bone resorption. Although bone formation is not impaired at first after calcitonin administration, with time both formation and resorption of bone are reduced. Thus, the early hope that calcitonin would prove useful in restoring bone mass has not been realized. In the kidney, calcitonin reduces both calcium and phosphate reabsorption as well as reabsorption of other ions, including sodium, potassium, and magnesium. Although calcitonin stimulates cAMP formation in both bone and kidney, a requirement for cAMP in mediating its actions is not established. PTH also stimulates cAMP accumulation in these tissues, yet the effects of PTH and calcitonin are generally antagonistic.

Tissues other than bone and kidney are also affected by calcitonin. Calcitonin in pharmacologic amounts decreases gastrin secretion and reduces gastric acid output while increasing secretion of sodium, potassium, chloride, and water in the gut. Pentagastrin is a potent stimulator of calcitonin secretion (as is hypercalcemia), suggesting a possible physiologic relationship between gastrin and calcitonin. In the adult human, no readily demonstrable problem develops in cases of calcitonin deficiency (thyroidectomy) or excess (medullary carcinoma of the thyroid). However,

the ability of calcitonin to block bone resorption and lower serum calcium makes it a useful drug for the treatment of Paget's disease, hypercalcemia, and osteoporosis.

GLUCOCORTICOIDS

Glucocorticoid hormones alter bone mineral homeostasis by antagonizing vitamin D-stimulated intestinal calcium transport, by stimulating renal calcium excretion, by blocking bone collagen synthesis, and by increasing PTH-stimulated bone resorption (although this last action is not universally accepted). Although these observations underscore the negative impact of glucocorticoids on bone mineral homeostasis, these hormones have proved useful in two situations involving bone mineral homeostasis: in the intermediate term treatment of hypercalcemia and as a diagnostic test for determining the cause of hypercalcemia. Prolonged administration of glucocorticoids is a common cause of osteoporosis in adults and stunted skeletal development in children.

ESTROGENS

Estrogens can prevent accelerated bone loss during the immediate postmenopausal period and at least transiently increase bone in the postmenopausal subject. The prevailing hypothesis advanced to explain these observations is that estrogens reduce the bone-resorbing action of PTH. Estrogen administration leads to an increased $1,25(OH)_2D$ level in blood, but estrogens have no direct effect on $1,25(OH)_2D$ production in vitro. The increased $1,25(OH)_2D$ levels in vivo following estrogen treatment may result from decreased serum calcium and phosphate and increased PTH. Estrogen receptors have been found in bone, suggesting that estrogen may have direct effects on bone remodeling. The principal therapeutic application for estrogen administration in disorders of bone mineral homeostasis is the treatment or prevention of postmenopausal osteoporosis.

NONHORMONAL AGENTS AFFECTING BONE MINERAL HOMEOSTASIS

BISPHOSPHONATES

The bisphosphonates are analogs of pyrophosphate in which the P–O–P bond has been replaced with a nonhydrolyzable P–C–P bond (Figure 42–3). Etidro-

Figure 42–3. The structure of pyrophosphate and the three bisphosphonates—etidronate, pamidronate, and alendronate—that are currently approved for use in the USA.

nate, pamidronate, and alendronate are available for clinical use, and newer forms are likely to be available soon. The bisphosphonates owe at least part of their clinical usefulness and toxicity to their ability to retard formation and dissolution of hydroxyapatite crystals within and outside the skeletal system. However, the exact mechanism by which they selectively inhibit bone resorption is not clear.

The results from animal and clinical studies indicate that less than 10% of an oral dose of these drugs is absorbed. Food reduces absorption even further, necessitating their administration on an empty stomach. Because it causes gastric irritation, pamidronate is not available as an oral preparation. Nearly half of the absorbed drug accumulates in bone; the remainder is excreted unchanged in the urine. Decreased renal function is the main contraindication to the use of these drugs. The portion bound to bone is retained for months, depending on the turnover of bone itself.

Etidronate and the other bisphosphonates exert a variety of effects on bone mineral homeostasis. Their physicochemical action of reducing hydroxyapatite formation and dissolution make them clinically useful. In particular, bisphosphonates are being evaluated for the treatment of hypercalcemia associated with malignancy, osteoporosis, and syndromes of ectopic calcification. Their usefulness in the management of Paget's disease is well established, and alendronate has recently been approved for the treatment of osteoporosis

(see box: Bisphosphonates as New Therapy for Osteoporosis). Contrary to expectations, alendronate appears to increase bone mineral density well beyond the 2-year period predicted for a drug whose effects are limited to blocking bone resorption. The bisphosphonates exert a variety of other cellular effects, including inhibition of $1,25(OH)_2D$ production, inhibition of intestinal calcium transport, metabolic changes in bone cells such as inhibition of glycolysis, inhibition of cell growth, and changes in acid and alkaline phosphatase. These effects vary depending on the bisphosphonate being studied and may account for some of the clinical differences observed in the effects of the various bisphosphonates on bone mineral homeostasis. However, with the exception of the induction of a mineralization defect by higher than approved doses of etidronate and gastric irritation by pamidronate and by high doses of alendronate, these drugs have proved to be remarkably free of adverse effects.

PLICAMYCIN (MITHRAMYCIN)

Plicamycin is a cytotoxic antibiotic (see Chapter 55) that has been used clinically for two disorders of bone mineral metabolism: Paget's disease and hypercalcemia. The cytotoxic properties of the drug appear to involve its binding to DNA and interruption of DNA-directed RNA synthesis. The reasons for its usefulness in the treatment of Paget's disease and hypercalcemia are unclear but may relate to the need for protein synthesis to sustain bone resorption. The doses required to treat Paget's disease and hypercalcemia are about one-tenth the amounts required to achieve cytotoxic effects.

THIAZIDES

The chemistry and pharmacology of this family of drugs are covered in Chapter 15. The principal application of thiazides in the treatment of bone mineral disorders is in reducing renal calcium excretion. Thiazides may increase the effectiveness of parathyroid hormone in stimulating reabsorption of calcium by the renal tubules or may act on calcium reabsorption secondarily by increasing sodium reabsorption in the proximal tubule. In the distal tubule, thiazides block sodium reabsorption at the luminal surface, increasing the calcium-sodium exchange at the basolateral membrane and thus enhancing calcium reabsorption into the blood at this site. Thiazides have proved to be quite useful in reducing the hypercalciuria and incidence of stone formation in subjects with idiopathic hypercalciuria. Part of their efficacy in reducing stone formation may lie in their ability to decrease urine oxalate excretion and increase urine magnesium and zinc levels (both of which inhibit calcium oxalate stone formation).

BISPHOSPHONATES AS NEW THERAPY FOR OSTEOPOROSIS

Bone undergoes a continuous remodeling process involving bone resorption and formation. Any process that disrupts this balance by increasing resorption relative to formation results in osteoporosis. Inadequate sex hormone production is the major cause of osteoporosis in men and women. Estrogen replacement therapy at the menopause is a well-established means of preventing osteoporosis in the female, but many women fear its adverse effects, particularly a possible (though not proved) increased risk of breast cancer from continued estrogen use (the well-demonstrated increased risk of endometrial cancer is prevented by cycling with a progestin), or do not like the persistence of menstrual bleeding that often accompanies this form of therapy.

Alternative forms of therapy for osteoporosis with proved efficacy in reducing fracture risk have been limited until recently. Trials with etidronate, the first-generation bisphosphonate, indicated that 5 mg/d for 2 weeks out of every 3 months could increase bone mass and reduce fractures for at least 2 years, though the data beyond the second year were less compelling. More recently, a third-generation bisphosphonate, alendronate, which does not induce the mineralization defect seen with high doses of etidronate, has been conclusively shown to increase bone density and reduce fractures over at least 5 years when used continuously at a dosage of 10 mg/d. Side-by-side trials between alendronate and calcitonin (the other approved nonestrogen drug for osteoporosis) indicated greater efficacy for alendronate.

Alendronate, like other bisphosphonates, is poorly absorbed and must be given on an empty stomach. At the higher doses used in the treatment of Paget's disease, alendronate causes gastric irritation, but this is not a significant problem at the doses recommended for osteoporosis. Ongoing trials suggest that alendronate will be useful in a variety of forms of osteoporosis, including glucocorticoid-induced osteoporosis. Thus, we now have a well-validated, efficacious form of treatment for this common debilitating disease for those who do not need or do not want hormone replacement therapy.

FLUORIDE

Fluoride is well established as effective for the prophylaxis of dental caries and has been under investigation for the treatment of osteoporosis. Both therapeutic applications originated from epidemiologic observations that subjects living in areas with naturally fluoridated water (1–2 ppm) had less dental caries and fewer vertebral compression fractures than subjects living in nonfluoridated water areas. Fluoride is accumulated by bones and teeth, where it may stabilize the hydroxyapatite crystal. Such a mechanism may explain the effectiveness of fluoride in increasing the resistance of teeth to dental caries, but it does not explain new bone growth.

Fluoride in drinking water appears to be most effective in preventing dental caries if consumed prior to the eruption of the permanent teeth. The optimum concentration in drinking water supplies is 0.5–1 ppm. Topical application is most effective if done just as the teeth erupt. There is little further benefit to giving fluoride after the permanent teeth are fully formed. Excess fluoride in drinking water leads to mottling of the enamel proportionate to the concentration above 1 ppm.

Because of the general lack of effectiveness of other agents in stimulating new bone growth in patients with osteoporosis, interest in the use of fluoride for this disorder was renewed (see Osteoporosis, below). Results of earlier studies indicated that fluoride alone without adequate calcium supplementation produced osteomalacia. More recent studies, in which calcium supplementation has been adequate, have demonstrated an improvement in calcium balance, an increase in bone mineral, and an increase in trabecular bone volume. However, two studies of the ability of fluoride to reduce fractures reached opposite conclusions (Pak et al, 1989; Riggs et al, 1990). Adverse effects observed—at the doses used for testing fluoride's effect on bone—include nausea and vomiting, gastrointestinal blood loss, arthralgias, and arthritis in a substantial proportion of patients. Such effects are usually responsive to reduction of the dose or giving fluoride with meals (or both). At present, fluoride is not approved by the Food and Drug Administration for use in osteoporosis, though a slow-release formulation is under consideration.

Acute toxicity, generally due to ingestion of fluoride-containing rat poisons, includes gastrointestinal symptoms and neurologic signs of hypocalcemia presumably related to the calcium-binding properties of fluoride. Fluoride in acutely toxic doses may also cause cardiovascular collapse or respiratory failure. Chronic exposure to very high levels of fluoride dust in the inspired air results in **crippling fluorosis**, characterized by thickening of the cortex of long bones and bony exostoses, especially in the vertebrae.

II. CLINICAL PHARMACOLOGY

Disorders of bone mineral homeostasis generally present with abnormalities in serum or urine calcium levels (or both), often accompanied by abnormal serum phosphate levels. These abnormal mineral concentrations may themselves cause symptoms requiring immediate treatment (eg, coma in malignant hypercalcemia, tetany in hypocalcemia). More commonly, they serve as clues to an underlying disorder in hormonal regulators (eg, primary hyperparathyroidism), target tissue response (eg, chronic renal failure), or drug misuse (eg, vitamin D intoxication). In such cases, treatment of the underlying disorder is of prime importance.

Since bone and kidney play central roles in bone mineral homeostasis, conditions that alter bone mineral homeostasis usually affect either or both of these tissues secondarily. Effects on bone can result in osteoporosis (abnormal loss of bone; remaining bone histologically normal), osteomalacia (abnormal bone formation due to inadequate mineralization), or osteitis fibrosa (excessive bone resorption with fibrotic replacement of resorption cavities). Biochemical markers of skeletal involvement include changes in serum levels of the skeletal isoenzyme of alkaline phosphatase and osteocalcin (reflecting osteoblastic activity) and urine levels of hydroxyproline and pyridinoline cross-links (reflecting osteoclastic activity). The kidney becomes involved when the calcium-times-phosphate product in serum exceeds the point at which ectopic calcification occurs (often in renal parenchyma) or when the calcium-times-oxalate (or phosphate) product in urine exceeds saturation, leading to nephrocalcinosis and nephrolithiasis. Subtle early indicators of such renal involvement include polyuria, nocturia, and hyposthenuria. Radiologic evidence of nephrocalcinosis and stones is not generally observed until later. The degree of the ensuing renal failure is best followed by monitoring the decline in creatinine clearance.

ABNORMAL SERUM CALCIUM & PHOSPHATE LEVELS

HYPERCALCEMIA

Hypercalcemia causes central nervous system depression, including coma, and is potentially lethal. Its major causes (other than thiazide therapy) are hyperparathyroidism and cancer with or without bone metastases. Less common causes are hypervitaminosis D, sarcoidosis, thyrotoxicosis, milk-alkali syndrome, adrenal insufficiency, and immobilization. With the possible exception of hypervitaminosis D, these latter disorders seldom require emergency lowering of serum calcium. A number of approaches are used to manage the hypercalcemic crisis.

Saline Diuresis

In hypercalcemia of sufficient severity to produce symptoms, rapid reduction of serum calcium is required. The first steps include rehydration with saline and diuresis with furosemide. Most patients presenting with severe hypercalcemia have a substantial component of prerenal azotemia owing to dehydration, which prevents the kidney from compensating for the rise in serum calcium by excreting more calcium in the urine. Therefore, the initial infusion of 500–1000 mL/h of saline to reverse the dehydration and restore urine flow can by itself substantially lower serum calcium. The addition of a loop diuretic such as furosemide not only enhances urine flow but also inhibits calcium reabsorption in the ascending limb of the loop of Henle (Chapter 15). Monitoring central venous pressure is important to forestall the development of congestive heart failure and pulmonary edema in predisposed subjects. In many subjects, saline diuresis will suffice to reduce serum calcium levels to a point at which more definitive diagnosis and treatment of the underlying condition can be achieved. If this is not the case or if more prolonged medical treatment of hypercalcemia is required, the following agents are available (discussed in order of preference).

Bisphosphonates

Etidronate, 7.5 mg/kg in 250–500 mL saline, infused over several hours each day for 3 days, has proved quite useful in treating hypercalcemia of malignancy. More recently, pamidronate, 60–90 mg in 500–750 mL saline, infused over 4–24 hours, has been approved for the same indication and appears to be more effective. This form of treatment is remarkably free of toxicity. The effects generally persist for weeks, but treatment can be repeated after a 7-day interval if necessary.

Calcitonin

Calcitonin has proved useful as ancillary treatment in a large number of patients. Calcitonin by itself seldom restores serum calcium to normal, and refractoriness frequently develops. However, its lack of toxicity permits frequent administration at high doses (200 MRC units or more). An effect on serum calcium is observed within 4–6 hours and lasts for 6–10 hours. Calcimar (salmon calcitonin) is available for parenteral and nasal administration.

Gallium Nitrate

Gallium nitrate is approved by the Food and Drug Administration for the management of hypercalcemia of malignancy and is undergoing trials for the treatment of advanced Paget's disease. This drug acts by inhibiting bone resorption. At a dosage of 200 mg/m^2 body surface area per day given as a continuous intravenous infusion in 5% dextrose for 5 days, gallium nitrate proved superior to calcitonin in reducing serum calcium in cancer patients. Because of potential nephrotoxicity, patients should be well-hydrated and have good renal output before starting the infusion.

Plicamycin (Mithramycin)

Because of its toxicity, plicamycin (mithramycin) is not the drug of first choice for the treatment of hypercalcemia. However, when other forms of therapy fail, 25–50 µg/kg given intravenously usually lowers serum calcium substantially within 24–48 hours. This effect can last for several days. This dose can be repeated as necessary. The most dangerous toxic effect is sudden thrombocytopenia followed by hemorrhage. Hepatic and renal toxicity can also occur. Hypocalcemia, nausea, and vomiting may limit therapy. Use of this drug must be accompanied by careful monitoring of platelet counts, liver and kidney function, and serum calcium levels.

Phosphate

Giving intravenous phosphate is probably the fastest and surest way to reduce serum calcium, but it is a hazardous procedure if not done properly. Intravenous phosphate should be used only after other methods of treatment (pamidronate, calcitonin, saline diuresis with furosemide, and plicamycin) have failed to control symptomatic hypercalcemia. Phosphate must be given slowly (50 mmol or 1.5 g elemental phosphorus over 6–8 hours) and the patient switched to oral phosphate (1–2 g/d elemental phosphorus, as one of the salts indicated below) as soon as symptoms of hypercalcemia have cleared. The risks of intravenous phosphate therapy include sudden hypocalcemia, ectopic calcification, acute renal failure, and hypotension. Oral phosphate can also lead to ectopic calcification and renal failure if serum calcium and phosphate levels are not carefully monitored, but the risk is less and the time of onset much longer. Phosphate is available in oral and intravenous forms as the sodium or potassium salt. Amounts required to provide 1 g of elemental phosphorus are as follows:

> **Intravenous:**
> In-Phos: 40 mL
> Hyper-Phos-K: 15 mL
> **Oral:**
> Fleet Phospho-Soda: 6.2 mL
> Neutra-Phos: 300 mL

Glucocorticoids

Glucocorticoids have no clear role in the acute treatment of hypercalcemia. However, the chronic hypercalcemia of sarcoidosis, vitamin D intoxication, and certain cancers may respond within several days to glucocorticoid therapy. Prednisone in oral doses of 30–60 mg daily is generally used, though equivalent doses of other glucocorticoids are effective. The rationale for the use of glucocorticoids in these diseases differs, however. The hypercalcemia of sarcoidosis appears to be secondary to increased production of 1,25(OH)$_2$D, possibly by the sarcoid tissue itself. Glucocorticoid therapy directed at the reduction of sarcoid tissue results in restoration of normal serum calcium and 1,25(OH)$_2$D levels. The treatment of hypervitaminosis D with glucocorticoids probably does not alter vitamin D metabolism significantly but is thought to reduce vitamin D-mediated intestinal calcium transport. An action of glucocorticoids to reduce vitamin D-mediated bone resorption has not been excluded, however. The effect of glucocorticoids on the hypercalcemia of cancer is probably twofold. The malignancies responding best to glucocorticoids (ie, multiple myeloma and related lymphoproliferative diseases) are sensitive to the lytic action of glucocorticoids, so part of the effect may be related to decreased tumor mass and activity. Glucocorticoids have also been shown to inhibit the effectiveness of osteoclast-activating factor, a humoral substance or substances elaborated by multiple myeloma and related cancers that stimulate osteoclastic bone resorption. Other causes of hypercalcemia—particularly primary hyperparathyroidism—do not respond to glucocorticoid therapy.

This difference in response of the various forms of hypercalcemia to glucocorticoids forms the basis for the glucocorticoid suppression test, in which the response of serum calcium to a 10-day course of prednisone, 60 mg orally daily, helps differentiate the hypercalcemia of primary hyperparathyroidism from other causes such as sarcoidosis, vitamin D intoxication, and certain cancers. This test may be misleading and should not be used as a substitute for more specific tests for primary hyperparathyroidism or humoral hypercalcemia of malignancy caused by the secretion of a PTH-like molecule ("PTHrP") by the tumor which can be diagnosed with specific immunoassays for PTH and PTHrP, respectively.

HYPOCALCEMIA

The main features of hypocalcemia are neuromuscular—tetany, paresthesias, laryngospasm, muscle cramps, and convulsions. The major causes of hypocalcemia in the adult are hypoparathyroidism, vitamin D deficiency, renal failure, and malabsorption. Neonatal hypocalcemia is a common disorder that usually resolves without therapy. The roles of PTH, vitamin D, and calcitonin in the neonatal syndrome are under active investigation. Large infusions of citrated blood can produce hypocalcemia by the formation of citrate-calcium complexes. Calcium and vitamin D (or its metabolites) form the mainstay of treatment of hypocalcemia.

Calcium

A number of calcium preparations are available for intravenous, intramuscular, and oral use. Calcium gluceptate (0.9 meq calcium/mL), calcium gluconate (0.45 meq calcium/mL), and calcium chloride (0.68–1.36 meq calcium/mL) are available for intravenous therapy. Calcium gluconate is the preferred form because it is less irritating to veins. Oral preparations include calcium carbonate (40% calcium), calcium lactate (13% calcium), calcium phosphate (25% calcium), and calcium citrate (17% calcium). Calcium carbonate is often the preparation of choice because of its high percentage of calcium, ready availability (eg, Tums), low cost, and antacid properties. In achlorhydric patients, calcium carbonate should be given with meals to increase absorption or the patient switched to calcium citrate, which is somewhat better absorbed. Combinations of vitamin D and calcium are available, but treatment must be tailored to the individual patient and individual disease, a flexibility lost by fixed-dosage combinations. Treatment of severe symptomatic hypocalcemia can be accomplished with slow infusion of 5–20 mL of 10% calcium gluconate. Rapid infusion can lead to cardiac arrhythmias. Less severe hypocalcemia is best treated with oral forms sufficient to provide approximately 400–800 mg of elemental calcium (1–2 g calcium carbonate per day). Dosage must be adjusted to avoid hypercalcemia and hypercalciuria.

Vitamin D

When rapidity of action is required, $1,25(OH)_2D_3$ (calcitriol), 0.25–1 µg daily, is the vitamin D metabolite of choice, since it is capable of raising serum calcium within 24–48 hours. Calcitriol also raises serum phosphate, though this action is usually not observed early in treatment. The combined effects of calcitriol and all other vitamin D metabolites and analogs on both calcium and phosphate make careful monitoring of these mineral levels especially important to avoid ectopic calcification secondary to an abnormally high serum calcium × phosphate product. Since the choice of the appropriate vitamin D metabolite or analog for long-term treatment of hypocalcemia depends on the nature of the underlying disease, further discussion of vitamin D treatment will be found under the headings of the specific diseases.

HYPERPHOSPHATEMIA

Hyperphosphatemia is a frequent complication of renal failure but is also found in all types of hy-poparathyroidism (idiopathic, surgical, and pseudo), vitamin D intoxication, and the rare syndrome of tumoral calcinosis. Emergency treatment of hyperphosphatemia is seldom necessary but can be achieved by dialysis or glucose and insulin infusions. In general, control of hyperphosphatemia involves restriction of dietary phosphate plus the use of phosphate binding gels such as $Al(OH)_3$-containing antacids and of calcium supplements. Because of their potential to induce aluminum-associated bone disease, aluminum-containing antacids should be used sparingly and only when other measures fail to control the hyperphosphatemia.

HYPOPHOSPHATEMIA

A variety of conditions are associated with hypophosphatemia, including primary hyperparathyroidism, vitamin D deficiency, idiopathic hypercalciuria, vitamin D-resistant rickets, various other forms of renal phosphate wasting (eg, Fanconi's syndrome), overzealous use of $Al(OH)_3$-containing antacids, and parenteral nutrition with inadequate phosphate content. Acute hypophosphatemia may lead to a reduction in the intracellular levels of high-energy organic phosphates (eg, ATP), interfere with normal hemoglobin-to-tissue oxygen transfer by decreasing red cell 2,3-diphosphoglycerate levels, and lead to rhabdomyolysis. However, clinically significant acute effects of hypophosphatemia are seldom seen, and emergency treatment is generally not indicated. The long-term effects of hypophosphatemia include proximal muscle weakness and abnormal bone mineralization (osteomalacia). Therefore, hypophosphatemia should be avoided during other forms of therapy and treated in conditions such as vitamin D-resistant rickets of which it is a cardinal feature. Oral forms of phosphate available for use are listed above in the section on hypercalcemia.

SPECIFIC DISORDERS INVOLVING THE BONE MINERAL-REGULATING HORMONES

PRIMARY HYPERPARATHYROIDISM

This rather common disease, if associated with symptoms and significant hypercalcemia, is best treated surgically. Oral phosphate has been tried but cannot be recommended. Asymptomatic patients with mild disease in general do not progress and may be left untreated.

HYPOPARATHYROIDISM

In the absence of PTH (idiopathic or surgical hypoparathyroidism) or a normal target tissue response to PTH (pseudohypoparathyroidism), serum calcium falls and serum phosphate rises. In such patients, $1,25(OH)_2D$ levels are usually low, presumably reflecting the lack of stimulation by PTH of $1,25(OH)_2D$ production. The skeletons of patients with idiopathic or surgical hypoparathyroidism are normal except for a slow turnover rate. A number of patients with pseudohypoparathyroidism appear to have osteitis fibrosa, suggesting that the normal or high PTH levels found in such patients are capable of acting on bone but not on the kidney. The distinction between pseudohypoparathyroidism and idiopathic hypoparathyroidism is made on the basis of normal or high PTH levels but deficient renal response (ie, diminished excretion of cAMP or phosphate) in patients with pseudohypoparathyroidism.

The principal therapeutic concern is to restore normocalcemia and normophosphatemia. Under most circumstances, vitamin D (25,000–100,000 units three times per week) and dietary calcium supplements suffice. More rapid increments in serum calcium can be achieved with calcitriol, though it is not clear that this metabolite offers a substantial advantage over vitamin D itself for long-term therapy. Many patients treated with vitamin D develop episodes of hypercalcemia. This complication is more rapidly reversible with cessation of therapy using calcitriol rather than vitamin D. This would be of importance to the patient in whom such hypercalcemic crises are common. Dihydrotachysterol and 25(OH)D have not received much study as therapy for hypoparathyroidism, though both should be effective. Whether they offer advantages over vitamin D sufficient to justify their added expense remains to be seen.

NUTRITIONAL RICKETS

Vitamin D deficiency, once thought to be rare in this country, is being recognized more often, especially in the pediatric and geriatric populations on vegetarian diets and with reduced sunlight exposure. This problem can be avoided by daily intake of 400 units of vitamin D and treated by somewhat higher dosages (4000 units per day). No other metabolite is indicated. The diet should also contain adequate amounts of calcium and phosphate.

CHRONIC RENAL FAILURE

The major problems of chronic renal failure that impact on bone mineral homeostasis are the loss of $1,25(OH)_2D$ and $24,25(OH)_2D$ production, the retention of phosphate that reduces ionized calcium levels, and the secondary hyperparathyroidism that results. With the loss of $1,25(OH)_2D$ production, less calcium is absorbed from the intestine and less bone is resorbed under the influence of PTH. As a result hypocalcemia usually develops, furthering the development of hyperparathyroidism. The bones show a mixture of osteomalacia and osteitis fibrosa.

In contrast to the hypocalcemia that is more often associated with chronic renal failure, some patients may become hypercalcemic from two causes (in addition to overzealous treatment with calcium). The most common cause of hypercalcemia is the development of severe secondary (sometimes referred to as tertiary) hyperparathyroidism. In such cases, the PTH level in blood is very high. Serum alkaline phosphatase levels also tend to be high. Treatment often requires parathyroidectomy.

A less common circumstance leading to hypercalcemia is development of a form of osteomalacia characterized by a profound decrease in bone cell activity and loss of the calcium buffering action of bone. In the absence of kidney function, any calcium absorbed from the intestine accumulates in the blood. Therefore, such patients are very sensitive to the hypercalcemic action of $1,25(OH)_2D$. These individuals generally have a high serum calcium but nearly normal alkaline phosphatase and PTH levels. The bone in such patients has a high aluminum content, especially in the mineralization front, which may block normal bone mineralization. These patients do not respond favorably to parathyroidectomy. Deferoxamine, an agent used to chelate iron (Chapter 58), also binds aluminum and is being used as therapy for this disorder.

Use of Vitamin D Preparations

The choice of vitamin D preparation to be used in the setting of chronic renal failure in the dialysis patient depends on the type and extent of bone disease and hyperparathyroidism. No consensus has been reached regarding the advisability of using any vitamin D metabolite in the predialysis patient. $1,25(OH)_2D_3$ (calcitriol) will rapidly correct hypocalcemia and at least partially reverse the secondary hyperparathyroidism and osteitis fibrosa. Many patients with muscle weakness and bone pain gain an improved sense of well-being.

Dihydrotachysterol, an analog of $1,25(OH)_2D$, is also available for clinical use. Dihydrotachysterol appears to be as effective as calcitriol, differing principally in its time course of action; calcitriol increases serum calcium in 1–2 days, whereas dihydrotachysterol requires 1–2 weeks. For an equipotent dose (0.2 mg dihydrotachysterol versus 0.5 μg calcitriol), dihydrotachysterol costs about one-fourth as much as calcitriol. A disadvantage of dihydrotachysterol is the inability to measure it in serum. Neither dihydrotachysterol nor calcitriol corrects the osteomalacic component of renal osteodystrophy in the majority of patients, and neither should be used in patients with hypercalcemia, especially if the bone disease is primarily osteomalacic.

Calcifediol (25[OH]D_3) may also be used to advantage. Calcifediol is less effective than calcitriol in stimulating intestinal calcium transport, so that hypercalcemia is less of a problem with calcifediol. Like dihydrotachysterol, calcifediol requires several weeks to restore normocalcemia in hypocalcemic individuals with chronic renal failure. Presumably because of the reduced ability of the diseased kidney to metabolize calcifediol to more active metabolites, high doses (50–100 μg daily) must be given to achieve the supraphysiologic serum levels required for therapeutic effectiveness.

Vitamin D has been used in treating renal osteodystrophy. However, patients with a substantial degree of renal failure who are thus unable to convert vitamin D to its active metabolites usually are refractory to vitamin D. Its use is decreasing as more effective alternatives become available.

Several nonhypercalcemic analogs of calcitriol are being tested for their ability to reduce the secondary hyperparathyroidism of chronic renal failure. Their biggest impact will be in patients in whom the use of calcitriol may lead to unacceptably high serum calcium levels.

Regardless of the drug employed, careful attention to serum calcium and phosphate levels is required. Calcium supplements (dietary and in the dialysate) and phosphate restriction (dietary and with oral ingestion of phosphate binders) should be employed along with the use of vitamin D metabolites. Monitoring serum PTH and alkaline phosphatase levels is useful in determining whether therapy is correcting or preventing secondary hyperparathyroidism. Although not generally available, percutaneous bone biopsies for quantitative histomorphometry may help in choosing appropriate therapy and following the effectiveness of such therapy. Unlike the rapid changes in serum values, changes in bone morphology require months to years. Monitoring serum levels of the vitamin D metabolites is useful to determine compliance, absorption, and metabolism.

INTESTINAL OSTEODYSTROPHY

A number of gastrointestinal and hepatic diseases result in disordered calcium and phosphate homeostasis that ultimately leads to bone disease. The bones in such patients show a combination of osteoporosis and osteomalacia. Osteitis fibrosa does not occur (as it does in renal osteodystrophy). The common features that appear to be important in this group of diseases are malabsorption of calcium and vitamin D. Liver disease may, in addition, reduce the production of 25(OH)D from vitamin D, though the importance of this in all but patients with terminal liver failure remains in dispute. The malabsorption of vitamin D is probably not limited to exogenous vitamin D. The liver secretes into bile a substantial number of vitamin D metabolites and conjugates that are reabsorbed in (presumably) the distal jejunum and ileum. Interference with this process could deplete the body of endogenous vitamin D metabolites as well as limit absorption of dietary vitamin D.

In mild forms of malabsorption, vitamin D (25,000–50,000 units three times per week) should suffice to raise serum levels of 25(OH)D into the normal range. Many patients with severe disease do not respond to vitamin D. Clinical experience with the other metabolites is limited, but both calcitriol and calcifediol have been used successfully in doses similar to those recommended for treatment of renal osteodystrophy. Theoretically, calcifediol should be the drug of choice under these conditions, since no impairment of the renal metabolism of 25(OH)D to 1,25(OH)$_2$D and 24,25(OH)$_2$D exists in these patients. Both calcitriol and 24,25(OH)$_2$D may be of importance in reversing the bone disease. As in the other diseases discussed, treatment of intestinal osteodystrophy with vitamin D and its metabolites should be accompanied by appropriate dietary calcium supplementation and monitoring of serum calcium and phosphate levels.

OSTEOPOROSIS

The estimated cost of fractures in older women and men in the USA was $13.8 billion in 1995 (Incidence and costs, 1996). Osteoporosis is defined as abnormal loss of bone predisposing to fractures. It is most common in postmenopausal women but also occurs in older men. It may occur as a side effect of chronic administration of glucocorticoids or other drugs; as a manifestation of endocrine disease such as thyrotoxicosis or hyperparathyroidism; as a feature of malabsorption syndrome; as a consequence of alcohol abuse; or without obvious cause (idiopathic). The ability of some agents to reverse the bone loss of osteoporosis is shown in Figure 42–4. The postmenopausal form of osteoporosis may be accompanied by lower 1,25(OH)$_2$D levels and reduced intestinal calcium transport. This form of osteoporosis appears to be due to estrogen deficiency and is best treated with cyclic doses of estrogen. It is important to note that the most rapid loss of bone occurs within the first 5 years after menopause and that administration of estrogens after this time may be less effective. Furthermore, if estrogen therapy is discontinued, a period of accelerated bone loss may occur. Thus, treatment with estrogens should be started shortly after the onset of menopause and may need to be continued for life. Since continuous estrogen therapy is associated with increased risk of endometrial carcinoma, among other complications, the recommendation to treat all postmenopausal women with estrogens has not been universally accepted. With the advent of sensitive means of measuring vertebral bone mineral content (CT scan, dual-energy x-ray absorptiometry), estrogen therapy may be reserved for women with reduced bone mineral content at the time of menopause or those who lose bone rapidly in the first year after menopause. Recent evidence, however, indicates that cyclic estrogen therapy in combination with a progestational agent reduces or eliminates this added risk of cancer. Therefore, estrogens should be administered for 21 of 28 days in the lowest effective dosage (eg, 0.625 mg/d of conjugated estrogens or 25–50 µg/d of ethinyl estradiol), with addition of a progestational agent on days 14–21 (eg, 10 mg/d of medroxyprogesterone acetate). This may reinitiate menstrual bleeding, so the patient must be advised of this in advance. Other complications of estrogen therapy such as hypertension and thrombophlebitis must also be kept in mind when such treatment is initiated (Chapter 40). However, the potential complication many women fear most is breast cancer. At present the epidemiologic evidence is mixed, and the small increased risk (if it exists at all) of breast cancer from estrogen therapy is outweighed by the reduced risk of osteoporosis and cardiovascular disease. Nevertheless, many women refuse to consider estrogen replacement therapy or do not tolerate its side effects. Fortunately, several new therapies for osteoporosis are now available.

To counter the reduced intestinal calcium transport associated with osteoporosis, vitamin D therapy is often employed in addition to dietary calcium supplementation. There is no clear evidence that pharmacologic doses of vitamin D are of much additional benefit beyond cyclic estrogens and calcium supplementation. However, calcitriol and its analog 1αOHD$_3$ have been shown to increase bone mass and reduce fractures in several recent studies. Use of these agents for osteoporosis is not FDA-approved, though they are used in other countries.

Despite early promise that fluoride might be useful in the prevention or treatment of postmenopausal osteoporosis, this form of therapy remains controversial. A new formulation of fluoride (slow release, lower dose) appears to avoid much of the toxicity of earlier formulations and may reduce fracture rates. This formulation is under consideration for approval by the FDA. Fluoride is the only known agent that can directly stimulate bone formation and lead to a progressive increase in bone density, at least in the spine (Figure 42–4).

Calcitonin has recently been approved for use in the treatment of postmenopausal osteoporosis. Whether this agent, which reduces bone resorption acutely, will have a long-term effect on bone mass and reduce fracture rates remains uncertain. It has few adverse effects.

Several studies have been published suggesting that intermittent short courses of etidronate (2 weeks per 12-week cycle) improve bone density and reduce spinal fractures (Watts et al, 1990; Storm et al, 1990). Etidronate, however, has not been approved by the FDA for this purpose. Quite recently, a large multicenter study demonstrated that daily administration of alendronate (10 mg/d) could increase bone density and decrease fracture rates over 5 years (Liberman et al, 1995). On the strength of this and other studies, alendronate is now approved by the FDA for the treatment of osteoporosis.

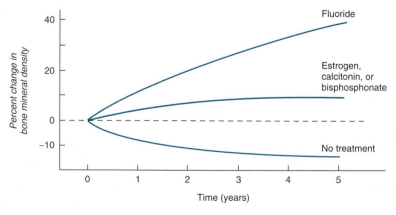

Figure 42–4. Typical changes in bone mineral density with time after the onset of menopause, with and without treatment. In the untreated condition, bone is lost during aging in both men and women. Fluoride promotes new bone formation and can increase bone mineral density in subjects who respond to it throughout the period of treatment. In contrast, estrogen, calcitonin, and bisphosphonates block bone resorption. This leads to a transient increase in bone mineral density because bone formation is not initially decreased. However, with time, both bone formation and bone resorption are decreased and bone mineral density reaches a new plateau.

The cause of idiopathic osteoporosis in men is not known. Treatment usually consists of giving vitamin D and dietary calcium supplements, but little information is available about its efficacy. It is important to exclude more treatable forms of osteoporosis such as that accompanying corticosteroid therapy, alcohol abuse, hyperparathyroidism, thyrotoxicosis, malabsorption, or occult nutritional osteomalacia.

VITAMIN D-RESISTANT RICKETS

This X-linked recessive disorder is manifested by the appearance of rickets and hypophosphatemia in children. The disease can present in adulthood, presumably reflecting either less severe disease or a missed diagnosis in childhood. The main defect appears to be an abnormality in renal phosphate reabsorption. Phosphate is critical to normal bone mineralization; when phosphate stores are deficient, a clinical and pathologic picture resembling vitamin D-deficient rickets develops. However, such children fail to respond to the usual doses of vitamin D employed in the treatment of nutritional rickets. A defect in $1,25(OH)_2D$ production by the kidney has also been suggested by some investigators, because the serum $1,25(OH)_2D$ levels tend to be low relative to the degree of hypophosphatemia observed. This combination of low serum phosphate and low or low-normal serum $1,25(OH)_2D$ provides the rationale for treating such patients with oral phosphate (1–3 g daily) and large doses of vitamin D (25,000–100,000 units daily). Recently, some groups have used calcitriol with good effect (0.25–1 μg daily). Reports of such combination therapy are encouraging in this otherwise debilitating disease.

VITAMIN D-DEPENDENT RICKETS

This entity actually represents two different diseases (types I and II). Both present as childhood rickets that does not respond to conventional doses of vitamin D. Type I vitamin D-dependent rickets is due to an isolated deficiency of $1,25(OH)_2D$ production. This condition can be treated with vitamin D (4000 units daily) or calcitriol (0.25–0.5 μg daily). Type II vitamin D-dependent rickets is caused by a target tissue defect in response to $1,25(OH)_2D$. Studies have shown a number of point mutations in the gene for the $1,25(OH)_2D$ receptor, which disrupt the functions of this receptor and lead to this syndrome (Hughes et al, 1988). The serum levels of $1,25(OH)_2D$ are very high in type II but not in type I. Treatment with large doses of calcitriol has been claimed to be effective in restoring normocalcemia. Such patients are totally refractory to vitamin D. One recent report indicates a reversal of resistance to calcitriol when $24,25(OH)_2D$ was given. These diseases are rare.

NEPHROTIC SYNDROME

Patients with nephrotic syndrome can lose vitamin D metabolites into their urine, presumably by loss of the vitamin D-binding protein. Such patients may have very low 25(OH)D levels. Some of them develop bone disease. It is not yet clear what value vitamin D therapy has in such patients, since this complication of the nephrotic syndrome has only recently been recognized, and therapeutic trials with vitamin D (or any other vitamin D metabolite) have not yet been carried out. Since the problem is not related to vitamin D metabolism, one would not anticipate any advantage in using the more expensive vitamin D metabolites in place of vitamin D itself.

IDIOPATHIC HYPERCALCIURIA

This syndrome, characterized by hypercalciuria and nephrolithiasis with normal serum calcium and PTH levels, has been subdivided into three groups of patients: (1) hyperabsorbers, patients with increased intestinal absorption of calcium, resulting in high-normal serum calcium, low-normal PTH, and a secondary increase in urine calcium; (2) renal calcium leakers, patients with a primary decrease in renal reabsorption of filtered calcium, leading to low-normal serum calcium and high-normal serum PTH; and (3) renal phosphate leakers, patients with a primary decrease in renal reabsorption of phosphate, leading to stimulation of $1,25(OH)_2D$ production, increased intestinal calcium absorption, increased ionized serum calcium, low-normal PTH levels, and a secondary increase in urine calcium. There is some disagreement about this classification, and in many cases patients are not readily categorized. Many such patients present with mild hypophosphatemia, and oral phosphate has been used with some success to reduce stone formation. However, a clear role for phosphate in the treatment of this disorder has not been established. Therapy with hydrochlorothiazide, up to 50 mg twice daily, is recommended, although equivalent doses of other thiazide diuretics work as well. Loop diuretics such as furosemide and ethacrynic acid should not be used, since they increase urinary calcium excretion. The major toxicity of thiazide diuretics, besides hypokalemia, hypomagnesemia, and hyperglycemia, is hypercalcemia. This is seldom more than a biochemical observation unless the patient has a disease such as hyperparathyroidism in which bone turnover is accelerated. Accordingly, one should screen patients for such disorders before starting thiazide therapy and monitor serum and urine calcium when therapy has begun.

An alternative to thiazides is allopurinol. Some studies indicate that hyperuricosuria is associated with idiopathic hypercalcemia and that a small nidus of urate crystals could lead to the calcium oxalate stone formation characteristic of idiopathic hypercalcemia. Allopurinol, 300 mg daily, may reduce stone formation by reducing uric acid excretion.

OTHER DISORDERS OF BONE MINERAL HOMEOSTASIS

PAGET'S DISEASE OF BONE

Paget's disease is a localized bone disease characterized by uncontrolled osteoclastic bone resorption with secondary increases in bone formation. This new bone is poorly organized, however. The cause of Paget's disease is obscure, though recent studies suggest that a slow virus may be involved. The disease is fairly common, though symptomatic bone disease is less common. The biochemical parameters of elevated serum alkaline phosphatase and urinary hydroxyproline are useful for diagnosis. Along with the characteristic radiologic and bone scan findings, these biochemical determinations provide good markers by which to follow therapy. The goal of treatment is to reduce bone pain and stabilize or prevent other problems such as progressive deformity, hearing loss, high-output cardiac failure, and immobilization hypercalcemia. Calcitonin can be used as sole treatment or in combination with bisphosphonates for this disease. Treatment failures may respond to plicamycin. Calcitonin is administered subcutaneously or intramuscularly in doses of 50–100 MRC units every day or every other day. Higher or more frequent doses have been advocated when this initial regimen is ineffective. Improvement in bone pain and reduction in serum alkaline phosphatase and urine hydroxyproline levels require weeks to months. Often a patient who responds well initially will lose the response to calcitonin. This refractoriness is not correlated with the development of antibodies.

Sodium etidronate and alendronate are the bisphosphonates currently approved for clinical use in this condition in the USA. However, other bisphosphonates, including pamidronate, are being used in other countries. The recommended dosage of etidronate is 5 mg/kg/d (typically 400 mg) and of alendronate 40 mg/d by oral administration. Long-term (months to years) remission may be expected in patients who respond to etidronate. Treatment should not exceed 6 months per course but can be repeated after 6 months if necessary. The principal toxicity of etidronate is the development of osteomalacia and an increased incidence of fractures when the dosage is raised substantially above 5 mg/kg/d. Other bisphosphonates such as pamidronate and alendronate do not share this side effect. Some patients treated with etidronate develop bone pain similar in nature to the bone pain of osteomalacia. This subsides after stopping the drug. The principal side effect of alendronate is gastric irritation when used at these high doses. This is reversible on cessation of the drug.

The use of a potentially lethal cytotoxic drug such as plicamycin in a generally benign disorder such as Paget's disease is recommended only when other less toxic agents (calcitonin, alendronate) have failed and the symptoms are debilitating. Insufficient clinical data on long-term use of plicamycin are available to determine its usefulness for extended therapy. However, short courses involving 15–25 µg/kg intravenously for 5–10 days followed by 15 µg/kg intravenously each week have been used to control the disease.

ENTERIC OXALURIA

Patients with short bowel syndromes associated with fat malabsorption can present with renal stones composed of calcium and oxalate. Such patients characteristically have normal or low urine calcium levels but elevated urine oxalate levels. The reasons for the development of oxaluria in such patients are thought to be twofold: first, in the intestinal lumen, calcium (which is now bound to fat) fails to bind oxalate and no longer prevents its absorption; second, enteric flora, acting on the increased supply of nutrients reaching the colon, produce larger amounts of oxalate. Although one would ordinarily avoid treating a patient with calcium oxalate stones with calcium supplementation, this is precisely what is done in patients with enteric oxaluria. The increased intestinal calcium binds the excess oxalate and prevents its absorption. One to 2 g of calcium carbonate can be given daily in divided doses, with careful monitoring of urinary calcium and oxalate to be certain that urinary oxalate falls without a dangerous increase in urinary calcium.

PREPARATIONS AVAILABLE

Vitamin D and Metabolites

Calcifediol (Calderol)
Oral: 20, 50 µg capsules

Calcitriol
Oral (Rocaltrol): 0.25, 0.5 µg capsules
Parenteral (Calcijex): 1, 2 µg/mL for injection

Cholecalciferol [D₃] (vitamin D_3, Delta-D)
Oral: 400, 1000 IU tablets

Dihydrotachysterol [DHT] (DHT, Hytakerol)
Oral: 0.125 mg tablets, capsules; 0.2, 0.4 mg tablets; 0.2 mg/mL intensol solution; 0.25 mg/mL solution in oil

Ergocalciferol [D₂] (vitamin D_2, Calciferol, Drisdol)
Oral: 50,000 IU tablets, capsules; 8000 IU/mL drops
Parenteral: 500,000 IU/mL for injection

Calcium

Calcium acetate [25% calcium] (Phos-Ex, PhosLo)
Oral: 250 mg (62.5 mg calcium, 668 mg (167 mg calcium), 1000 mg (250 mg calcium) tablets; 500 mg (125 mg calcium) capsules

Calcium carbonate [40% calcium] (generic, Tums, Cal-Sup, Os-Cal 500, others)
Oral: Numerous forms available containing 260–600 mg calcium per unit

Calcium chloride [27% calcium] (generic)
Parenteral: 10% solution for IV injection only

Calcium citrate [21% calcium] (generic, Citracal)
Oral: 950 mg (200 mg calcium), 2376 mg (500 mg calcium)

Calcium glubionate [6.5% calcium] (Neo-Calglucon)
Oral: 1.8 g (115 mg calcium)/5 mL syrup

Calcium gluceptate [8% calcium] (Calcium Gluceptate)
Parenteral: 1.1 g/5 mL solution for IM or IV injection

Calcium gluconate [9% calcium] (generic)
Oral: 500 mg (45 mg calcium), 650 mg (58.5 mg calcium), 975 mg (87.75 mg calcium), 1 g (90 mg calcium) tablets
Parenteral: 10% solution for IV or IM injection

Calcium lactate [13% calcium] (generic)
Oral: 325 mg (42.25 mg calcium), 650 mg (84.5 mg calcium) tablets

Dibasic calcium phosphate dihydrate [23% calcium] (generic)
Oral: 486 mg (112 mg calcium) tablets

Tricalcium phosphate [39% calcium] (Posture)
Oral: 1565 mg (600 mg calcium) tablets (as phosphate)

Phosphate

Phosphate (Fleet Phospho-Soda, Neutra-Phos)
Oral: solution containing 645 mg phosphate/5 mL (Fleet Phospho-Soda); capsules containing 250 mg phosphorus, 278 mg potassium, 164 mg sodium (Neutra-Phos); capsules containing 250 mg phosphorus, 556 mg potassium, 0 mg sodium (Neutra-Phos-K)
Parenteral (sodium or potassium phosphate): 3 mM phosphate/mL solution for IV infusion only

Other Drugs

Alendronate (Fosamax)
Oral: 10, 40 mg tablets

Calcitonin-Salmon
Nasal spray (Miacalcin): 200 IU/puff
Parenteral (Calcimar, Miacalcin, Salmonine): 100, 200 IU/mL for injection

Etidronate (Didronel)
Oral: 200, 400 mg tablets
Parenteral: 300 mg/6 mL for IV injection

Gallium nitrate (Ganite)
Parenteral: 500 mg/20 mL vial

Pamidronate (Aredia)
Parenteral: 30, 60, 90 mg/vial

Plicamycin (mithramycin) (Mithracin)
Parenteral: 2.5 mg per vial powder to reconstitute for injection

Sodium fluoride (generic)
Oral: 0.55 mg (0.25 mg F), 1.1 mg (0.5 mg F), 2.2 mg (1.0 mg F) tablets; drops

REFERENCES

Adami S et al: Effects of oral alendronate and intranasal salmon calcitonin on bone mass and biochemical markers of bone turnover in post menopausal women with osteoporosis. Bone 1995;17:383.

Austin LA, Heath HH III: Calcitonin: Physiology and pathophysiology. N Engl J Med 1981;304:269.

Bikle DD: Vitamins D: New actions, new analogs, new therapeutic potential. Endocr Rev 1992;13:765.

Bikle DD et al: Bone disease in alcohol abuse. Ann Intern Med 1985;103:42.

Bilezikian JP: Management of acute hypercalcemia. N Engl J Med 1992;326:1196.

Brown A, Dusso A, Slatopolsky E: Vitamin D. In: *The Kidney: Physiology and Pathophysiology,* 2nd ed. Seldin DW, Giebisch G (editors). Raven, 1992.

Cauley JA et al: Effects of thiazide diuretic therapy on bone mass, fractures, and falls. Ann Intern Med 1993;118:666.

Chapuy MC et al: Vitamin D_3 and calcium to prevent hip fractures in elderly women. N Engl J Med 1992; 327:1637.

Coburn JW, Massry SG (editors): Uses and actions of 1,25-dihydroxyvitamin D_3 in uremia. Contrib Nephrol 1980;18:1.

Dambacher MD, Binswanger U, Fischer JA: Diagnosis and treatment of primary hyperparathyroidism. Urol Res 1979;7:171.

Dawson-Hughes B et al: A controlled trial of the effect of calcium supplementation on bone density in postmenopausal women. N Engl J Med 1990;323:878.

Delmas PD: Biochemical markers of bone turnover: Methodology and clinical use in osteoporosis. Am J Med 1991;91(Suppl 5B):59S.

Ettinger B, Genant HK, Cann CE: Long-term estrogen replacement therapy prevents bone loss and fractures. Ann Intern Med 1985;102:319.

Felson DT et al: The effect of postmenopausal estrogen therapy on bone density in elderly women. N Engl J Med 1993;329:1141.

Fleisch H: Bisphosphonates: Pharmacology and use in the treatment of tumour-induced hypercalcaemic and metastatic bone disease. Drugs 1991;42:919.

Forscher BK, Arnaud CD (editors): The third F. Raymond Keating, Jr., Memorial Symposium: Parathyroid hormone, calcitonin and vitamin D. (Two parts) Am J Med 1974;56:743, 57:1.

Gallagher JC, Goldgar D: Treatment of postmenopausal osteoporosis with high doses of synthetic calcitriol. Ann Intern Med 1990;113:649.

Gucalp R et al: Comparative study of pamidronate disodium and etidronate disodium in the treatment of cancer-related hypercalcemia. J Clin Oncol 1992;10:134.

Hasling C, Charles P, Mosekilde L: Etidronate disodium in the management of malignancy-related hypercalcemia. Am J Med 1987;82(Suppl 2A):51.

Hodsman AB, Drost DJ: The response of vertebral bone mineral density during the treatment of osteoporosis with sodium fluoride. J Clin Endocrinol Metab 1989;69:932.

Hughes MR et al: Point mutations in the human vitamin D receptor gene associated with hypocalcemic rickets. Science 1988;242:1702.

Incidence and costs to Medicare of fractures among Medicare beneficiaries ≥ 65 years—United States, July 1991–June 1992. MMWR Morb Mortal Wkly Rep 1996;45:877.

Kleerkoper M, Balena R: Fluorides and osteoporosis. Annu Rev Nutr 1991;11:309.

Lei DBM, Zawada ET, Kleeman CR: The pathophysiology and clinical aspects of hypercalcemic disorders. West J Med 1978;129:278.

Leyvraz S et al: Pharmacokinetics of pamidronate in patients with bone metastases. J Natl Cancer Inst 1992; 84:788.

Liberman et al: Effect of oral alendronate on bone mineral density and the incidence of fractures in postmenopausal osteoporosis. N Engl J Med 1995;333:1437.

Long RG: Hepatic osteodystrophy: Outlook good but some problems unsolved. Gastroenterology 1980;78:644.

Malluche HH et al: The use of deferoxamine in the management of aluminum accumulation in bone in patients with renal failure. N Engl J Med 1984;311:140.

Okamura WH et al: Vitamin D: Structure-function analyses and the design of analogs. J Cell Biochem 1992;49:10.

Pak CYC (editor): Symposium on urolithiasis. Kidney Int 1978;13:341.

Pak CYC et al: Safe and effective treatment of osteoporosis with intermittent slow release sodium fluoride: Augmentation of vertebral bone mass and inhibition of fracture. J Clin Endocrinol Metab 1989;68:150.

Parfitt AM: Bone and plasma calcium homeostasis. Bone 1987;8(Suppl 1):51.

Popopoulos SE et al: The use of bisphosphonates in the treatment of osteoporosis. Bone 1992;13(Suppl):S41.

Prince RL et al: Prevention of postmenopausal osteoporosis: A comparative study of exercise, calcium supplementation, and hormone-replacement therapy. N Engl J Med 1991;325:1189.

Riggs BL et al: Changes in bone mineral density of the proximal femur and spine with aging: Differences between the postmenopausal and senile osteoporosis syndromes. J Clin Invest 1982;70:716.

Riggs BL et al: Effect of fluoride treatment on the fracture rate in postmenopausal women with osteoporosis. N Engl J Med 1990;322;802.

Riggs BL, Melton LJ III: The prevention and treatment of osteoporosis. N Engl J Med 1992;327:620.

Storm T et al: Effect of intermittent cyclical etidronate treatment on bone mass and fracture rate in women with postmenopausal osteoporosis. N Engl J Med 1990;322:1265.

Suda T, Takahashi N, Abe E: Role of vitamin D in bone resorption. J Cell Biochem 1992;49:53.

Tilyard MW et al: Treatment of postmenopausal osteoporosis with calcitriol or calcium. N Engl J Med 1992; 326:357.

Wallach S: Treatment of Paget's disease. Adv Intern Med 1982;27:1.

Watts NB et al: Intermittent cyclical etidronate treatment of postmenopausal osteoporosis. N Engl J Med 1990; 323:73.

Section VIII.
Chemotherapeutic Drugs

INTRODUCTION TO ANTIMICROBIAL AGENTS

Agents that are active against bacterial, fungal, and viral microorganisms are discussed in the next nine chapters.

The antimicrobial agents developed during the last 60 years are among the most dramatic examples of the advances of modern medicine. Many infectious diseases once considered incurable and lethal are now amenable to treatment with a few pills. The remarkably powerful and specific activity of antimicrobial drugs is due to their selectivity for highly specific targets that are either unique to microorganisms or much more important in them than in humans. Among these targets are specific bacterial and fungal cell wall-synthesizing enzymes (Chapters 43 and 48), the bacterial ribosome (Chapters 44 and 45), the enzymes required for nucleotide synthesis and DNA replication (Chapter 46), and the machinery of viral replication (Chapter 49). The special group of drugs used in mycobacterial infections is discussed in Chapter 47. The much older and less selective cytotoxic antiseptics and disinfectants are discussed in Chapter 50. The clinical uses of all of these agents are presented in Chapter 51.

Microorganisms can adapt to environmental pressures in a variety of effective ways, and their response to antibiotic pressure is no exception. An inevitable consequence of antimicrobial usage is the selection of resistant microorganisms. Thus, an important part of the pharmacology of these drugs is the study of mechanisms of resistance to them. Overuse and inappropriate use of antibiotics has fueled a major increase in prevalence of multidrug-resistant pathogens, leading some to speculate that we are nearing the end of the antibiotic era. Unfortunately, as the need has grown in recent years, development of novel drugs has slowed. The most vulnerable molecular targets of antimicrobial drugs have been identified, and in many cases crystallized and characterized. Pending the identification of new targets and compounds, it seems likely that over the next decade we will have to rely on currently available families of drugs. In the face of continuing development of resistance, considerable effort will be required to maintain the effectiveness of these drug groups.

43

Beta-Lactam Antibiotics & Other Inhibitors of Cell Wall Synthesis

Henry F. Chambers, MD, W. Keith Hadley, MD, PhD,
& Ernest Jawetz, MD, PhD

BETA-LACTAM COMPOUNDS

PENICILLINS

Almost 70 years ago, Alexander Fleming reported his discovery of penicillin (1929). Chain, Florey, and their associates succeeded in producing significant quantities of the first penicillins from cultures of *Penicillium notatum* in 1940. Ten years later, virtually unlimited quantities of penicillin G were available for clinical use. The principal clinical limitations of penicillin G were its instability at acidic pH, susceptibility to destruction by beta-lactamase (penicillinase), and its relative inactivity against gram-negative bacilli. Isolation of the nucleus, 6-aminopenicillanic acid, allowed for the development of numerous semisynthetic penicillins that are stable to acid pH, resistant to beta-lactamase, and active against both gram-positive and gram-negative bacteria.

The penicillins are classified as beta-lactam drugs because of their unique four-membered lactam ring. They share features of chemistry, mechanism of action, pharmacologic and clinical effects, and immunologic characteristics with cephalosporins, monobactams, carbapenems, and beta-lactamase inhibitors, which also are beta-lactam compounds.

Chemistry

All penicillins have the basic structure shown in Figure 43–1. A thiazolidine ring (A) is attached to a beta-lactam ring (B) that carries a secondary amino group (RNH–). Substituents (R; examples shown in Figure 43–2) can be attached to the amino group. Structural integrity of the 6-aminopenicillanic acid nucleus is essential for the biologic activity of these compounds. If the beta-lactam ring is enzymatically cleaved by bacterial beta-lactamases, the resulting product, penicilloic acid, lacks antibacterial activity.

However, it is an antigenic determinant of the penicillins, acting as a sensitizing structure when attached to host proteins. Products of alkaline hydrolysis of the penicillins also contribute to sensitization.

A. Classification: The attachment of different substitutents to 6-aminopenicillanic acid determines the essential pharmacologic and antibacterial properties of the resulting molecules. Penicillins can be assigned to one of three groups:

1. Penicillins (eg, penicillin G)–These have the greatest activity against gram-positive organisms, gram-negative cocci, and non-beta-lactamase-producing anaerobes and little activity against gram-negative rods. They are susceptible to hydrolysis by beta-lactamases.

2. Antistaphylococcal penicillins (eg, nafcillin)–These penicillins are resistant to staphylococcal beta-lactamases. They are active against staphylococci and streptococci but inactive against enterococci, anaerobic bacteria, and gram-negative cocci and rods.

3. Extended-spectrum penicillins (ampicillin and the antipseudomonal penicillins)–These drugs retain the antibacterial spectrum of penicillin and have improved activity against gram-negative organisms, but they are destroyed by beta-lactamases. Within each of these groups are compounds that are relatively stable to gastric acid and suitable for oral administration, eg, penicillin V, dicloxacillin, and amoxicillin. The side chains of some representatives of each group are shown in Figure 43–2, with a few distinguishing characteristics.

B. Penicillin Units and Formulations: The activity of penicillin G was originally defined in units. Crystalline sodium penicillin G contains approximately 1600 units/mg (1 unit = 0.6 μg; 1 million units [1 MU] of penicillin = 0.6 g). Semisynthetic penicillins are prescribed by weight rather than units. Most penicillins are dispensed as the sodium or potassium salt of the free acid. Potassium penicillin G contains about 1.7 meq of K^+ per million units of peni-

Figure 43–1. Core structures of four beta-lactam antibiotic families. The ring marked B in each structure is the beta-lactam ring. The penicillins are susceptible to bacterial metabolism and inactivation by amidases and lactamases at the points shown. Note that the carbapenems have a different stereochemical configuration in the lactam ring that apparently imparts resistance to beta-lactamases. Substituents for the penicillin and cephalosporin families are shown in Figures 43–2 and 43–6, respectively.

cillin (2.8 meq/g). Nafcillin contains Na$^+$, 2.8 meq/g. Procaine salts and benzathine salts of penicillin G provide repository forms for intramuscular injection. In dry crystalline form, penicillin salts are stable for long periods (eg, for years at 4 °C). Solutions lose their activity rapidly (eg, 24 hours at 20 °C) and must be prepared fresh for administration.

Mechanism of Action

Penicillins, like all beta-lactam antibiotics, inhibit bacterial growth by interfering with a specific step in bacterial cell wall synthesis. The cell wall is a rigid outer layer that completely surrounds the cytoplasmic membrane (Figure 43–3). It maintains the shape of the cell and prevents cell lysis that would occur as a result of the high osmotic pressure within the cell compared to its external environment. Cell wall is composed of a complex cross-linked polymer, peptidoglycan (murein, mucopeptide), consisting of polysaccharides and polypeptides. The polysaccharide contains alternating amino sugars, N-acetylglucosamine and N-acetylmuramic acid (Figure 43–4). A five-amino-acid peptide is linked to the N-acetylmuramic acid sugar. This peptide terminates in D-alanyl-D-alanine. Penicillin-binding proteins (PBPs) catalyze the transpeptidase reaction that removes the terminal alanine to form a crosslink with a nearby peptide, which gives cell wall its structural rigidity. Beta-lactam antibiotics are structural analogs of the natural D-Ala-D-Ala substrate and they are covalently bound by PBPs at the active site. After a beta-lactam antibiotic has attached to the PBP, the transpeptidation reaction is inhibited (Figure 43–5), peptidoglycan synthesis is blocked, and the cell dies. The exact mechanism responsible for cell death is not completely understood, but autolysins, bacterial enzymes that remodel and break down cell wall, are involved. Penicillins and cephalosporins are bactericidal only if cells are actively growing and synthesizing cell wall.

Resistance

Resistance to penicillins is due to one of three mechanisms: (1) inactivation of antibiotic by beta-lactamase; (2) alteration in target PBPs; and (3) a permeability barrier preventing penetration of antibiotic to the target. Beta-lactamase production is the most common mechanism of resistance. More than 100 different beta-lactamases have been identified. Some, such as those produced by *Staphylococcus aureus, Haemophilus* species, and *E coli,* are relatively narrow in substrate specificity and will hydrolyze penicillins but not cephalosporins. Other beta-lactamases, such as those produced by *Pseudomonas aeruginosa* and *Enterobacter* species, are much broader in spectrum and will hydrolyze both cephalosporins and penicillins. Carbapenems, which are highly resistant to hydrolysis by penicillinases and cephalosporinases, are hydrolyzed by a metallo-beta-lactamase.

Alteration in target PBPs is responsible for methicillin resistance in staphylococci and penicillin resistance in pneumococci. These resistant organisms produce PBPs that have low affinity for binding beta-lactam antibiotics, and as a result they are not inhibited except at relatively high drug concentrations, which may exceed what is clinically achievable.

Resistance due to inability of drug to penetrate to its cytoplasmic membrane target is due to the outer membrane barrier, which is present in gram-negative

Site of amidase action

6-Aminopenicillanic acid

The following structures can each be substituted at the R to produce a new penicillin.

Penicillin G (benzylpenicillin):
High activity against gram-positive bacteria. Low activity against gram-negative bacteria. Acid-labile. Destroyed by β-lactamase. 60% protein-bound.

Oxacillin (no Cl atoms); cloxacillin (one Cl in structure); dicloxacillin (2 Cls in structure); flucloxacillin (one Cl and one F in structure) (isoxazolyl penicillins):
Similar to methicillin in β-lactamase resistance, but acid-stable. Can be taken orally. Highly protein-bound (95–98%).

Nafcillin (ethoxynaphthamidopenicillin):
Similar to isoxazolyl penicillins. Less strongly protein-bound (90%). Resistant to staphylococcal β-lactamase.

Ampicillin (alpha-aminobenzylpenicillin):
Similar to Penicillin G (destroyed by β-lactamase) but acid-stable and more active against gram-negative bacteria. Carbenicillin has –COONa instead of NH$_2$ group.

Ticarcillin:
Similar to carbenicillin but gives higher blood levels. Piperacillin, azlocillin, and mezlocillin resemble ticarcillin in action against gram-negative aerobes.

Amoxicillin:
Similar to ampicillin but better absorbed, gives higher blood levels.

Figure 43–2. Side chains of some penicillins (R groups of Figure 43–1).

but not gram-positive bacteria. Impaired penetration alone is usually not sufficient to confer resistance, because enough antibiotic eventually enters the cell to inhibit growth. However, this barrier can become important in the presence of a beta-lactamase, which hydrolyzes antibiotic as it slowly enters the cell.

Pharmacokinetics

Absorption of orally administered drug differs greatly for different penicillins, depending in part on their acid stability and protein binding. Methicillin is acid-labile and gastrointestinal absorption of nafcillin is erratic, so neither is suitable for oral administration. Dicloxacillin, ampicillin, and amoxicillin are acid-stable and relatively well absorbed, producing serum concentrations in the range of 4–8 μg/mL following a 500 mg oral dose. Absorption of most oral penicillins (amoxicillin being an exception) is impaired by food, and the drugs should be administered at least 1–2 hours before or after a meal.

After parenteral administration, absorption of most penicillins is complete and rapid. Administration by

Figure 43–3. A highly simplified diagram of the cell envelope of a gram-negative bacterium. The outer membrane, a lipid bilayer, is present in gram-negative but not gram-positive organisms. It is penetrated by porins, proteins that form channels providing hydrophilic access to the cytoplasmic membrane. The peptidoglycan layer is unique to bacteria and is much thicker in gram-positive organisms than in gram-negative ones. Together, the outer membrane and the peptidoglycan layer constitute the cell wall. Penicillin-binding proteins (PBPs) are membrane proteins that cross-link peptidoglycan. Beta-lactamases, if present, reside in the periplasmic space or on the outer surface of the cytoplasmic membrane, where they may destroy beta-lactam antibiotics that penetrate the outer membrane.

the intravenous route is preferred because of irritation and local pain produced by the intramuscular injection of large doses. Serum concentrations 30 minutes after an intravenous injection of 1 g of a penicillin (equivalent to approximately 1.6 million units of penicillin G) are 20–50 μg/mL. Only a fraction of the total drug in serum is present as free drug, the concentration of which is determined by protein binding. Highly protein-bound penicillins (eg, nafcillin) produce lower levels of free drug in serum than less protein-bound penicillins (eg, penicillin G, ampicillin). The relevance of protein binding to clinical efficacy is not fully understood and probably is unimportant unless the protein-bound fraction is 95% or more. Penicillins are widely distributed in body fluids and tissues with the exceptions noted below. They are polar molecules, and the concentration within cells is less than that in extracellular fluids.

Benzathine and procaine penicillins are formulated to delay absorption, resulting in prolonged blood and tissue concentrations. After a single intramuscular injection of 1.2 million units of benzathine penicillin, serum levels in excess of 0.02 μg/mL are maintained for 10 days and levels in excess of 0.003 μg/mL for 3 weeks. The latter is sufficient to protect against beta-hemolytic streptococcal infection and the former to

treat an established infection with these organisms. A 600,000 unit dose of procaine penicillin yields peak concentrations of 1–2 μg/mL and clinically useful concentrations for 12–24 hours after a single intramuscular injection.

Penicillin concentrations in most tissues are equal to those in serum. Penicillin is also excreted into sputum and milk to levels 3–15% of those present in the serum. Penetration into the eye, the prostate, and the central nervous system is poor. However, with active inflammation of the meninges, as in bacterial meningitis, penicillin concentrations of 1–5 μg/mL can be achieved with a daily parenteral dose of 18–24 million units. These concentrations are sufficient to kill susceptible strains of pneumococci and meningococci.

Penicillin is rapidly excreted by the kidneys into the urine; small amounts are excreted by other routes. About 10% of renal excretion is by glomerular filtration and 90% by tubular secretion. The normal half-life of penicillin G is approximately 30 minutes; in renal failure, it may be as long as 10 hours. Ampicillin and the extended-spectrum penicillins are secreted more slowly than penicillin G and have half-lives of 1 hour. For penicillins that are cleared by the kidney, the dose must be adjusted according to renal function, with approximately one-fourth to one-third the normal dose being administered if creatinine clearance is 10 mL/min or less (Table 43–1). Nafcillin is primarily cleared by biliary excretion, and oxacillin, dicloxacillin, and cloxacillin are eliminated by both the kidney and biliary excretion—thus, no dosage adjustment is required for these drugs in renal failure. Because clearance of penicillins is less efficient in the newborn, doses adjusted for weight alone will result in higher systemic concentrations for longer periods than in the adult.

Clinical Uses

Penicillins are by far the most widely effective and the most extensively used antibiotics. Except for amoxicillin, oral penicillins should not be given at mealtimes (instead, give 1–2 hours before or after) to minimize binding to food proteins and acid inactivation. Oxacillin is most strongly bound to food and dicloxacillin somewhat less so. Blood levels of all penicillins can be raised by simultaneous administration of probenecid, 0.5 g (10 mg/kg in children) every 6 hours orally, which impairs tubular secretion of weak acids such as beta-lactam compounds.

A. Penicillin: Penicillin G is the drug of choice for infections caused by streptococci, meningococci, enterococci, penicillin-susceptible pneumococci, non-beta-lactamase-producing staphylococci, *Treponema pallidum* and many other spirochetes, *Bacillus anthracis, Clostridium* species, *Actinomyces,* and other gram-positive rods and non-beta-lactamase-producing gram-negative anaerobic organisms. Depending upon the organism, the site, and the severity of infection, effective doses range between 4 and 24 million units per day administered intravenously in four to six divided doses. Administration of high-dose penicillin G as a continuous intravenous infusion, although infrequently used, is also acceptable. Penicillin G when administered at doses of 18–24 million units is inhibitory for enterococci, but the simultaneous administration of an aminoglycoside is necessary to achieve a bactericidal effect, which is required when treating enterococcal endocarditis.

Penicillin V, the oral form of penicillin, is indicated only in minor infections. Because of its relatively

---

Figure 43–4. The transpeptidation reaction in *Staphylococcus aureus* that is inhibited by beta-lactam antibiotics. The cell wall of gram-positive bacteria is made up of long peptidoglycan polymer chains consisting of the alternating aminohexoses N-acetylglucosamine **(G)** and N-acetylmuramic acid **(M)** with pentapeptide side chains linked (in *S aureus*) by pentaglycine bridges. The exact composition of the side chains varies among species. The diagram illustrates small segments of two such polymer chains and their amino acid side chains. These linear polymers must be cross-linked by transpeptidation of the side chains at the points indicated by the asterisk to achieve the strength necessary for cell viability.

Figure 43–5. The biosynthesis of cell wall peptidoglycan, showing the sites of action of five antibiotics (shaded bars; 1 = fosfomycin, 2 = cycloserine, 3 = bacitracin, 4 = vancomycin, 5 = beta-lactam antibiotics). Bactoprenol (BP) is the lipid membrane carrier that transports building blocks across the cytoplasmic membrane; M = N-acetylmuramic acid; Glc = glucose; NAcGlc or G = N-acetylglucosamine.

poor bioavailability, the need for dosing four times a day, and its narrow antibacterial spectrum, amoxicillin (see below) is often used instead.

Benzathine penicillin and procaine penicillin G for intramuscular injection yield low but prolonged drug levels. A single injection of benzathine penicillin, 1.2 million units intramuscularly, is satisfactory for treatment of beta-hemolytic streptococcal pharyngitis. A similar injection given intramuscularly once every 3–4 weeks provides satisfactory prophylaxis against reinfection with beta-hemolytic streptococci. Penicillin G benzathine, 2.4 million units intramuscularly once a week for 1–3 weeks, is effective in the treatment of syphilis, though its use for treatment of neurosyphilis is controversial. Procaine penicillin G, which in the past was used for treating uncomplicated

pneumococcal pneumonia or gonorrhea, is rarely used nowadays because many strains are penicillin-resistant.

B. Penicillins Resistant to Staphylococcal Beta-Lactamase, Methicillin, Nafcillin, and Isoxazolyl Penicillins: The sole indication for the use of these agents is infection by beta-lactamase-producing staphylococci, though penicillin-susceptible strains of streptococci and pneumococci are also susceptible to these semisynthetic penicillins. Enterococci and methicillin-resistant strains of staphylococci are resistant to antistaphylococcal penicillins.

An isoxazolyl penicillin such as oxacillin, cloxacillin, or dicloxacillin, 0.25–0.5 g orally every 4–6 hours (15–25 mg/kg/d for children), is suitable for treatment of mild localized staphylococcal infec-

Table 43–1. Guidelines for dosing of some commonly used cell wall inhibitor antibiotics.

Antibiotic (Route of Administration)	Adult Dosage	Pediatric Dosage[1]	Neonatal Dosage[2]	Adjusted Dose as a Percentage of Normal Dose for Renal Failure Based on Creatinine Clearance (Cl$_{cr}$)	
				Cl$_{cr}$ Approx 50 mL/min	Cl$_{cr}$ Approx 10 mL/min
PENICILLINS					
Penicillin G (IV)	1–4 mU q4–6h	25,000–400,000 units/kg/d in 4–6 doses	75,000–150,000 units/kg/d in 2–3 doses	50–75%	25%
Penicillin VK (PO)	0.25–0.5 g qid	25–50 mg/kg/d in 4 doses		None	None
ANTISTAPHYLOCOCCAL PENICILLINS					
Cloxacillin, dicloxacillin (PO)	0.25–0.5 g qid	25–50 mg/kg/d in 4 doses		None	None
Nafcillin (IV)	1–2 g q4–6h	50–100 mg/kg/d in 4–6 doses	50–75 mg/kg/d in 2–3 doses	None	None
Oxacillin (IV)	1–2 g q4–6h	50–100 mg/kg/d in 4–6 doses	50–75 mg/kg/d in 2–3 doses	None	None
EXTENDED-SPECTRUM PENICILLINS					
Amoxicillin (PO)	0.25–0.5 g tid	20–40 mg/kg/d in 3 doses		66%	33%
Amoxicillin/potassium clavulanate (PO)	500/125–875/ 125 mg bid–tid	20–40 mg/kg/d in 3 doses		66%	33%
Piperacillin (IV)	3–4 g q4–6h	300 mg/kg/d in 4–6 doses	150 mg/kg/d in 2 doses	50–75%	25–33%
Ticarcillin (IV)	3 g q4–6h	200–300 mg/kg/d in 4–6 doses	150–200 mg/kg/d in 2–3 doses	50–75%	25–33%
FIRST-GENERATION CEPHALOSPORINS					
Cefadroxil (PO)	0.5–1 g qd–bid	30 mg/kg/d in 2 doses		50%	25%
Cephalexin, cephradine (PO)	0.25–0.5 g qid	25–50 mg/kg/d in 4 doses		50%	25%
Cefazolin (IV)	0.5–2 g q8h	25–100 mg/kg/d in 3–4 doses		50%	25%
SECOND-GENERATION CEPHALOSPORINS					
Cefoxitin (IV)	1–2 g q6–8h	75–150 mg/kg/d in 3–4 doses		50–75%	25%
Cefotetan (IV)	1–2 g q12h			50%	25%
Cefuroxime (IV)	0.75–1.5 g q8h	50–100 mg/kg/d in 3–4 doses		66%	25–33%
Cefuroxime axetil (PO)	0.25–0.5 g bid	0.125–0.25 g bid		None	25%
THIRD-GENERATION CEPHALOSPORINS					
Cefotaxime (IV)	1–2 g q6–12h	50–200 mg/kg/d in 4–6 doses	100 mg/kg/d in 2 doses	50%	25%
Ceftazidime (IV)	1–2 g q8–12h	75–150 mg/kg/d in 3 doses	100–150 mg/kg/d in 2–3 doses	50%	25%
Ceftriaxone (IV)	1–4 g q24h	50–100 mg/kg/d in 1–2 doses	50 mg/kg/d once a day	None	None
CARBAPENEMS					
Imipenem (IV)	0.25–0.5 g q6–8h			75%	50%
GLYCOPEPTIDES					
Vancomycin (IV)	30 mg/kg/d in 2–3 doses	40 mg/kg/d in 3–4 doses	15 mg/kg load, then 20 mg/kg/d in 2 doses	40%	10%

[1]The total dose should not exceed the adult dose.
[2]The dose shown is during the first week of life. The daily dose should be increased by approximately 33–50% after the first week of life. The lower dosage range should be used for neonates weighing less than 2 kg. After the first month of life, pediatric doses may be used.

tions. All of these drugs are relatively acid-stable and reasonably well absorbed from the gut. Food interferes with absorption, and the drugs must be administered 1 hour before or after meals.

For serious systemic staphylococcal infections, oxacillin or nafcillin, 8–12 g/d, is given by intermittent intravenous infusion of 1–2 g every 4–6 hours (50–100 mg/kg/d for children). Methicillin is no longer used because of its nephrotoxicity.

C. Extended Spectrum Penicillins, Aminopenicillins, Carboxypenicillins, and Ureidopenicillins:
These drugs, which in general retain the spectrum of activity of penicillin G, differ in having greater activity against gram-negative bacteria due to their enhanced ability to penetrate the gram-negative outer membrane. Like penicillin G, they are inactivated by beta-lactamases.

The aminopenicillins, ampicillin and amoxicillin, have the same spectrum and activity, but amoxicillin is better absorbed from the gut. A dosage of 250–500 mg of amoxicillin three times daily is equivalent to the same amount of ampicillin given four times daily. These drugs are given orally to treat urinary tract infections, sinusitis, otitis, and lower respiratory tract infections. Ampicillin and amoxicillin are the most active of the oral beta-lactam antibiotics against penicillin-resistant pneumococci and are the preferred beta-lactam antibiotics for treating infections suspected to be caused by these resistant strains. Ampicillin (but not amoxicillin) is effective for shigellosis but should not be used to treat uncomplicated *Salmonella* gastroenteritis, as it may prolong the carrier state.

Ampicillin, at dosages of 6–12 g/d intravenously, is useful for treating serious infections caused by penicillin-susceptible organisms, including anaerobes, enterococci, *Listeria monocytogenes,* and susceptible strains of gram-negative cocci and bacilli such as *E coli, H influenzae,* and *Salmonella* species. Unfortunately, many strains of the gram-negative species that formerly were uniformly susceptible now produce beta-lactamases and are therefore resistant to ampicillin, precluding its use for empirical therapy of urinary tract infections, meningitis, and typhoid fever. Ampicillin is not active against *Klebsiella, Enterobacter, Pseudomonas aeruginosa, Citrobacter, Serratia,* indole-positive *Proteus* species, and other gram-negative aerobes that are commonly encountered in hospital-acquired infections.

Carbenicillin, the first antipseudomonal carboxypenicillin, has become obsolete as a parenteral agent with the advent of more active, better tolerated agents. A derivative, carbenicillin indanyl sodium, is acid-stable and can be given orally in urinary tract infections. Ticarcillin, a carboxypenicillin that is similar to carbenicillin in activity but effective in lower doses, extends the ampicillin spectrum of activity (except that it is less active against enterococci) to include *Pseudomonas aeruginosa* and *Enterobacter* species. The ureidopenicillins, piperacillin, mezlocillin, and azlocillin, resemble ticarcillin except that they are also active against selected gram-negative bacilli, such as *Klebsiella pneumoniae.* Because of the propensity of *P aeruginosa* to develop resistance during single drug therapy, an antipseudomonal penicillin generally is used in combination with an aminoglycoside for pseudomonal infections.

Ampicillin, amoxicillin, ticarcillin, and piperacillin are also available in combination with one of several beta-lactamase inhibitors: clavulanic acid, sulbactam, or tazobactam. The addition of a beta-lactamase inhibitor extends the activity of these penicillins to include beta-lactamase-producing strains of *S aureus* as well as some beta-lactamase-producing gram-negative bacteria (see below).

Adverse Reactions

The penicillins are remarkably nontoxic. Most of the serious adverse effects are due to hypersensitivity. All penicillins are cross-sensitizing and cross-reacting. Any preparation containing penicillin, including foods or cosmetics, may induce sensitization. In general, sensitization occurs in direct proportion to the duration and total dose of penicillin received in the past. The responsible antigenic determinants are degradation products of penicillins, particularly penicilloic acid and products of alkaline hydrolysis bound to host protein. A history of a penicillin reaction is not reliable; about 5–8% of people claim such a history, but only 5–10% of these will have an allergic reaction when given penicillin. Fewer than 1% of persons who previously received penicillin without incident will have an allergic reaction when given penicillin. Because of the potential for anaphylaxis, however, penicillin should be administered with caution or a substitute drug given if there is a history of penicillin allergy. The incidence of allergic reactions in small children is negligible.

Allergic reactions include anaphylactic shock (very rare—0.05% of recipients); serum sickness type reactions (now rare—urticaria, fever, joint swelling, angioneurotic edema, intense pruritus, and respiratory embarrassment occurring 7–12 days after exposure); and a variety of skin rashes. Oral lesions, fever, interstitial nephritis (an autoimmune reaction to a penicillin-protein complex), eosinophilia, hemolytic anemia and other hematologic disturbances, and vasculitis may also occur. Most patients allergic to penicillins can be treated with alternative drugs. However, if necessary (eg, treatment of enterococcal endocarditis or neurosyphilis in a highly penicillin-allergic patient), desensitization can be accomplished with gradually increasing doses of penicillin.

In patients with renal failure, penicillin in high doses can cause seizures. Nafcillin is associated with neutropenia; oxacillin can cause hepatitis; and methicillin causes interstitial nephritis. Large doses of penicillins given orally may lead to gastrointestinal upset, particularly nausea, vomiting, and diarrhea. Ampicillin has been associated with pseudomembranous colitis. Secondary infections such as vaginal candidiasis may occur. Ampicillin and amoxicillin can cause skin rashes that are not allergic in nature.

Problems Relating to the Use & Misuse of the Penicillins

The penicillins are by far the most widely used antibiotics. Several thousand tons of these drugs have been administered to humans during the past 40 years. Therefore, penicillins have been responsible for some of the most drastic consequences of antibiotic misuse. The saturation of certain environments (eg, hospitals) with penicillin has produced a selective pressure favoring penicillin-resistant organisms. In the 1950s, use of penicillin in hospitals contributed to selection of beta-lactamase-producing staphylococci. Today, 90% of all staphylococcal strains both in the hospital and in the community are beta-lactamase producers. Beta-lactamase-producing strains of *H influenzae* and *Neisseria gonorrhoeae* are now common, precluding use of penicillins as first-line agents for infections caused by these organisms. The prevalence of penicillin-resistant pneumococci, long considered an example of total and regular susceptibility to penicillins, is 20% or greater in some regions of the United States. Highly resistant strains (eg, those for which the penicillin minimum inhibitory concentration [MIC] exceeds 1 μg/mL) cannot be killed at concentrations of penicillin that are achievable in cerebrospinal fluid, necessitating use of ceftriaxone or vancomycin when treating suspected cases of pneumococcal meningitis. Broad-spectrum penicillins also eradicate normal flora, thereby predisposing the patient to colonization and superinfection with opportunistic, drug-resistant species present within the hospital environment (*Proteus, Pseudomonas, Enterobacter, Serratia*, staphylococci, yeasts, etc).

CEPHALOSPORINS

Cephalosporins are similar to penicillins chemically, in mechanism of action, and toxicity. Cephalosporins are more stable than penicillins to many bacterial beta-lactamases and therefore usually have a broader spectrum of activity. Cephalosporins are not active against enterococci and *Listeria monocytogenes*. Large-scale production of the common nucleus (7-aminocephalosporanic acid) has made possible the synthesis of a vast array of cephalosporins with varying properties. Cephamycins (fermentation products of *Streptomyces*) and some totally synthetic drugs such as moxalactam resemble cephalosporins.

Chemistry

The nucleus of the cephalosporins, 7-aminocephalosporanic acid (Figure 43–6), bears a close resem-

blance to 6-aminopenicillanic acid (Figure 43–1). The intrinsic antimicrobial activity of natural cephalosporins is low, but the attachment of various R_1 and R_2 groups has yielded drugs of good therapeutic activity and low toxicity (Figure 43–6). The cephalosporins have molecular weights of 400–450. They are soluble in water and relatively stable to pH and temperature changes. Cephalosporins can be classified into four major groups or "generations," depending mainly on the spectrum of antimicrobial activity. As a general rule, first-generation compounds have better activity against gram-positive organisms and the later compounds exhibit improved activity against gram-negative aerobic organisms.

FIRST-GENERATION CEPHALOSPORINS

This group includes cefadroxil, cefazolin, cephalexin, cephalothin, cephapirin, and cephradine. These drugs are very active against gram-positive cocci, including pneumococci, streptococci, and staphylococci. Cephalosporins are not active against methicillin-resistant strains of staphylococci. *Escherichia coli, Klebsiella pneumoniae,* and *Proteus mirabilis* are often sensitive, but activity against *Pseudomonas aeruginosa*, indole-positive *Proteus, Enterobacter, Serratia marcescens, Citrobacter,* and *Acinetobacter* is poor. Anaerobic cocci (eg, *Peptococcus, Peptostreptococcus*) are usually sensitive, but *B fragilis* is not.

Pharmacokinetics & Dosage

A. Oral: Cephalexin, cephradine, and cefadroxil are absorbed from the gut to a variable extent. After oral doses of 500 mg, serum levels are 15–20 μg/mL. Urine concentration is usually very high, but in most tissues levels are variable and generally lower than in serum. Cephalexin and cephradine are given orally in dosages of 0.25–0.5 g four times daily (15–30 mg/kg/d) and cefadroxil in dosages of 0.5–1 g twice daily. Excretion is mainly by glomerular filtration and tubular secretion into the urine. Tubular secretory blocking agents, eg, probenecid, may increase serum levels substantially. In patients with impaired renal function, dosage must be reduced (Table 43–1).

B. Parenteral: Cefazolin is almost the only first-generation parenteral cephalosporin now in use. After an intravenous infusion of 1 g, the peak level of cefazolin is 90–120 μg/mL. The usual intravenous dosage of cefazolin for adults is 0.5–2 g intravenously every 8 hours. Cefazolin can also be administered intramuscularly. Excretion is via the kidney, and dose adjustments must be made for impaired renal function.

Clinical Uses

Although the first-generation cephalosporins have a broad spectrum of activity and are relatively non-

7-Aminocephalosporanic acid nucleus. The following structures can each be substituted at R_1 and R_2 to produce the named derivatives.

R_1 **R_2**

"First generation"

Cephalothin

Cephalexin

Cefazolin

Cephradine

Cephapirin

"Second generation"

Cefamandole

Cefoxitin (a cephamycin)

"Third generation"

Cefoperazone

Cefotaxime

Ceftriaxone

Figure 43–6. Structures of some cephalosporins. R_1 and R_2 structures are substituents on the 7-aminocephalosporanic acid nucleus pictured at the top. Other structures (cefoxitin and below) are complete in themselves.

toxic, they are rarely the drug of choice for any infection. Oral drugs may be used for the treatment of urinary tract infections, for minor staphylococcal lesions, or for minor polymicrobial infections such as cellulitis or soft tissue abscess. However, oral cephalosporins should not be relied upon in serious systemic infections.

Cefazolin penetrates well into most tissues. It is the drug of choice for surgical prophylaxis. Second- and third-generation cephalosporins offer no advantage for surgical prophylaxis for most procedures, are far more expensive, and generally should not be used for that purpose. Cefazolin may be a choice in infections for which it is the least toxic drug (eg, *K pneumoniae*) and in persons with staphylococcal or streptococcal infections who have a history of a mild penicillin hypersensitivity reaction but not anaphylaxis. Cefazolin does not penetrate the central nervous system and cannot be used to treat meningitis. Cefazolin is an alternative to an antistaphylococcal penicillin for patients who are allergic to penicillin.

SECOND-GENERATION CEPHALOSPORINS

Members of this group include cefaclor, cefamandole, cefonicid, cefuroxime, cefprozil, loracarbef, and ceforanide and the structurally related cephamycins cefoxitin, cefmetazole, cefotetan, which have activity against anaerobes. This is a heterogeneous group of drugs with marked individual differences in activity, pharmacokinetics, and toxicity. In general, they are active against organisms affected by first-generation drugs, but they have an extended gram-negative coverage. *Klebsiella* (including those resistant to cephalothin) are usually sensitive. Cefamandole, cefuroxime, cefonicid, ceforanide, and cefaclor are active against *H influenzae* but not against *Serratia* or *B fragilis*. In contrast, cefoxitin, cefmetazole, and cefotetan are active against *B fragilis* and some *Serratia* strains but are less active against *H influenzae*. All second-generation cephalosporins are less active against gram-positive bacteria than the first-generation drugs. As with first-generation agents, none are active against enterococci or *P aeruginosa*. Second-generation cephalosporins may exhibit in vitro activity against *Enterobacter* species, but they should not be used to treat infections caused by the organisms because resistant mutants that constitutively express a chromosomal beta-lactamase that hydrolyzes these compounds (as well as third-generation cephalosporins) are readily selected.

Pharmacokinetics & Dosage

A. Oral: Cefaclor, cefuroxime axetil, cefprozil, and loracarbef can be given orally. The usual dosage for adults is 10–15 mg/kg/d in two to four divided dosages; children should be given 20–40 mg/kg/d up to a maximum of 1 g/d. Except for cefuroxime axetil, these drugs are not predictably active against penicillin-resistant pneumococci and should be used cautiously, if at all, to treat suspected or proved pneumococcal infections. Cefaclor is more susceptible to beta-lactamase hydrolysis compared with the other agents, and its utility is correspondingly diminished.

B. Parenteral: After a 1 g intravenous infusion, serum levels are 75–125 μg/mL for most second-generation cephalosporins, but they reach 200–250 μg/mL for cefonicid. There are marked differences among drugs in half-life, protein binding, and interval between doses. Cefonicid is highly protein-bound, a feature that has been implicated as a cause of treatment failures with serious staphylococcal infections. For cefoxitin (50–200 mg/kg/d), the interval is 6–8 hours. Cefotetan is administered every 8–12 hours; cefonicid or ceforanide, every 12–24 hours; and cefprozil, every 24 hours. In general, intramuscular injection is too painful to be used. In renal failure, dosage adjustments are required (Table 43–1).

Clinical Uses

The oral second-generation cephalosporins are active against beta-lactamase-producing *H influenzae* or *Branhamella catarrhalis* and have been primarily used to treat sinusitis, otitis, or lower respiratory tract infections, in which these organisms have an important role. Because of their activity against anaerobes (including *B fragilis*), cefoxitin, cefotetan, or cefmetazole can be useful in such mixed anaerobic infections as peritonitis or diverticulitis. Cefuroxime is used to treat community-acquired pneumonia, particularly in cases where beta-lactamase-producing *H influenzae* or *Klebsiella pneumoniae* is a consideration, but this drug has few other uses. Cefuroxime is the only second-generation drug that crosses the blood-brain barrier, but it is less effective in treatment of meningitis than ceftriaxone or cefotaxime and should not be used.

THIRD-GENERATION CEPHALOSPORINS

Third-generation agents include cefoperazone, cefotaxime, ceftazidime, ceftizoxime, ceftriaxone, cefixime, cefpodoxime proxetil, ceftibuten, and moxalactam.

Antimicrobial Activity

The major features of these drugs (except cefoperazone) are their expanded gram-negative coverage and the ability of some to cross the blood-brain barrier. In addition to the gram-negative bacteria inhibited by other cephalosporins, third-generation drugs are active against *Citrobacter, Serratia marcescens,* and *Providencia* as well as beta-lactamase-producing strains of *Haemophilus* and *Neisseria*. Ceftazidime and cefoperazone are the two third-generation cephalosporins with useful activity against *P aeruginosa*. Like the second-generation drugs, third-generation cephalosporins are hydrolyzable by constitutively produced enterobacter chromosomal beta-lactamase, and they are not reliably active against *Enterobacter* species. Only ceftizoxime and moxalactam have good activity against *B fragilis*. Cefixime, ceftibuten, and cefpodoxime proxetil are oral agents possessing similar activity except that cefixime and ceftibuten are much less active against pneumococci (and completely inactive against penicillin-resistant strains) and have poor activity against *S aureus.*

Pharmacokinetics & Dosage

After intravenous infusion of 1 g of these drugs, serum levels are 60–140 μg/mL. They penetrate body fluids and tissues well and—with the exception of cefoperazone, cefixime, ceftibuten, and cefpodoxime proxetil—achieve levels in the cerebrospinal fluid sufficient to inhibit most pathogens, including gram-negative rods, except perhaps *Pseudomonas.*

The half-lives of these drugs and the necessary dosing intervals vary greatly: Ceftriaxone (half-life 7–8 hours) can be injected once every 24 hours at a dosage of 15–50 mg/kg/d. A single daily 1 g dose is sufficient for most serious infections, with 4 g once daily recommended for treatment of meningitis. Cefoperazone (half-life 2 hours) can be injected every 8–12 hours in a dosage of 25–100 mg/kg/d. The remaining drugs in the group (half-life 1–1.7 hours) can be injected every 6–8 hours in dosages between 2 and 12 g/d, depending on the severity of infection. Cefixime can be given orally (200 mg twice daily or 400 mg once daily) for respiratory or urinary tract infections. Cefpodoxime proxetil and ceftibuten are administered as a 200 mg dose twice daily.

The excretion of cefoperazone and ceftriaxone is mainly through the biliary tract, and no dosage adjustment is required in renal insufficiency. The others are excreted by the kidney and therefore require dosage adjustment in renal insufficiency.

Clinical Uses

Third-generation cephalosporins are used to treat a wide variety of serious infections caused by organisms that are resistant to most other drugs. Ceftriaxone (as a single 125 mg injection) and cefixime (as a single 400 mg oral dose) are first-line drugs for treatment of gonorrhea now that many strains of *N gonorrhoeae* are resistant to penicillin. Unfortunately, these drugs also are widely misused to treat infections that prove to be caused by strains that are susceptible to narrower spectrum agents. They should not be used to treat *Enterobacter* infections even if the clinical isolate appears susceptible in vitro, because of emergence of resistance. Because of their penetration of the central nervous system, third-generation cephalosporins can be used to treat meningitis, including meningitis caused by pneumococci, meningococci, *H influenzae,* and susceptible

enteric gram-negative rods, but not by *Listeria monocytogenes.* They should be used in combination with an aminoglycoside for treatment of meningitis caused by *P aeruginosa.* Ceftriaxone and cefotaxime are the most active cephalosporins against penicillin-resistant strains of pneumococci and are recommended for empirical therapy of serious infections that may be caused by these strains. Meningitis caused by highly penicillin-resistant strains of pneumococci (ie, penicillin MICs > 1 μg/mL) may not respond even to these agents, and addition of rifampin or vancomycin is recommended. Other potential indications include empirical therapy of sepsis of unknown cause in both the immunocompetent and the immunocompromised patient and treatment of infections for which a cephalosporin is the least toxic drug available. In neutropenic, febrile immunocompromised patients, third-generation cephalosporins are often used in combination with an aminoglycoside, but the necessity for including the aminoglycoside in the initial empirical regimen is controversial.

FOURTH-GENERATION CEPHALOSPORINS

Cefepime is an example of a so-called fourth-generation cephalosporin. It is in many ways similar to third-generation agents (and perhaps should be considered as such), but it is more resistant to hydrolysis by chromosomal beta-lactamases (eg, those produced by *Enterobacter*) and some extended-spectrum beta-lactamases that inactivate many of the third-generation cephalosporins. It has good activity against *P aeruginosa,* Enterobacteriaceae, *S aureus,* and *S pneumoniae.* It is highly active against *Haemophilus* and *Neisseria.* In animal models of meningitis, it penetrates well into cerebrospinal fluid. It is cleared by the kidneys and has a half-life of 2 hours, and its pharmacokinetic properties are very similar to those of ceftazidime. The clinical role of cefepime, which remains to be defined, will probably be similar to that of the third-generation cephalosporins except that it may be useful in treatment of infections caused by *Enterobacter.*

Adverse Effects of Cephalosporins

A. Allergy: Cephalosporins are sensitizing and may elicit a variety of hypersensitivity reactions that are identical to those of penicillins, including anaphylaxis, fever, skin rashes, nephritis, granulocytopenia, and hemolytic anemia. However, the chemical nucleus of cephalosporins is sufficiently different from that of penicillins so that some individuals with a history of penicillin allergy may tolerate cephalosporins. The frequency of cross-allergenicity between the two groups of drugs is uncertain but probably is around 5–10%. However, patients with a history of anaphylaxis to penicillins should not receive cephalosporins.

B. Toxicity: Local irritation can produce severe pain after intramuscular injection and thrombophlebitis after intravenous injection. Renal toxicity, including interstitial nephritis and even tubular necrosis, has been demonstrated and has caused the withdrawal of cephaloridine.

Cephalosporins that contain a methylthiotetrazole group (eg, cefamandole, moxalactam, cefmetazole, cefotetan, cefoperazone) frequently cause hypoprothrombinemia and bleeding disorders. Administration of vitamin K, 10 mg twice weekly, can prevent this. Moxalactam can also interfere with platelet function and has induced severe bleeding. It has been largely abandoned. Drugs with the methylthiotetrazole ring can also cause severe disulfiram-like reactions; consequently, alcohol and alcohol-containing medications must be avoided.

C. Superinfection: Many second- and particularly third-generation cephalosporins are ineffective against gram-positive organisms, especially methicillin-resistant staphylococci and enterococci. During treatment with such drugs, these resistant organisms, as well as fungi, often proliferate and may induce superinfection.

OTHER BETA-LACTAM DRUGS

MONOBACTAMS

These are drugs with a monocyclic beta-lactam ring (Figure 43–1). They are relatively resistant to beta-lactamases and active against gram-negative rods (including *Pseudomonas* and *Serratia*). They have no activity against gram-positive bacteria or anaerobes. Aztreonam is the only monobactam available in the USA. It resembles aminoglycosides in its spectrum of activity. Aztreonam is given intravenously every 8 hours in a dose of 1–2 g, providing peak serum levels

of 100 µg/mL. The half-life is 1–2 hours and is greatly prolonged in renal failure.

Penicillin-allergic patients tolerate aztreonam without reaction. Occasional skin rashes and elevations of serum aminotransferases occur during administration of aztreonam, but major toxicity has not yet been reported. The clinical usefulness of aztreonam has not been fully defined.

BETA-LACTAMASE INHIBITORS (Clavulanic Acid, Sulbactam, & Tazobactam)

These substances resemble beta-lactam molecules (Figure 43–7) but themselves have very weak antibacterial action. They are potent inhibitors of many but not all bacterial beta-lactamases and can protect hydrolyzable penicillins from inactivation by these enzymes. Beta-lactamase inhibitors are most active against plasmid-encoded beta-lactamases ("TEM" beta-lactamases in particular), such as those produced by staphylococci, *H influenzae, N gonorrhoeae, Salmonella, Shigella, E coli,* and *K pneumoniae.* They are not good inhibitors of inducible chromosomal beta-lactamases produced by *Enterobacter, Citrobacter, Serratia,* and *Pseudomonas,* but they do inhibit chromosomal beta-lactamases of *Legionella, Bacteroides,* and *Branhamella.*

The three inhibitors differ slightly with respect to pharmacology, stability, potency, and activity, but these differences are of little therapeutic significance. Beta-lactamase inhibitors are available only in fixed combinations with specific penicillins. The antibacterial spectrum of the combination is determined by the companion penicillin, not the beta-lactamase inhibitor. The fixed combinations available in the USA are listed in the Preparations Available section. An inhibitor will extend the spectrum of a penicillin provided that the inactivity of the penicillin is due to destruction by beta-lactamase and that the inhibitor is active against the beta-lactamase that is produced.

Figure 43–7. Structures of beta-lactamase inhibitors.

Thus, ampicillin-sulbactam is active against beta-lactamase-producing *S aureus* and *H influenzae* but not *Serratia,* which produces a beta-lactamase that is not inhibited by sulbactam. Similarly, if a strain of *Pseudomonas aeruginosa* is resistant to piperacillin, it will also be resistant to piperacillin-tazobactam, since tazobactam does not inhibit the chromosomal beta-lactamase.

The indications for penicillin-beta-lactamase inhibitor combinations are empirical therapy for infections caused by a wide range of potential pathogens in both immunocompromised and immunocompetent patients and treatment of mixed aerobic and anaerobic infections, such as intra-abdominal infections. Doses are the same as those used for the single agents except that the recommended dosage of piperacillin in the piperacillin-tazobactam combination is 3 g every 6 hours. This is less than the recommended 3–4 g every 4–6 hours for piperacillin alone, raising concerns about the use of the combination for treatment of suspected pseudomonal infection. Adjustments for renal insufficiency are made based on the penicillin component.

CARBAPENEMS

The carbapenems are structurally related to beta-lactam antibiotics (Figure 43–1). Imipenem and meropenem are the two that are available. Imipenem has a wide spectrum with good activity against many gram-negative rods, gram-positive organisms, and anaerobes. It is resistant to most beta-lactamases but not metallo-beta-lactamases. *Enterococcus faecium,* methicillin-resistant strains of staphylococci, *Clostridium difficile, Burkholderia cepacia,* and *Stenotrophomonas maltophilia* are resistant. Imipenem is inactivated by dehydropeptidases in renal tubules, resulting in low urinary concentrations. Consequently, it is administered together with an inhibitor of renal dehydropeptidase, cilastatin, for clinical use. Meropenem is similar to imipenem but has slightly greater activity against gram-negative aerobes and slightly less activity against gram-positives. It is not significantly degraded by renal dehydropeptidase and does not require an inhibitor.

Imipenem penetrates body tissues and fluids well, including the cerebrospinal fluid. The usual dose is 0.25–0.5 g given intravenously every 6–8 hours (half-life 1 hour). The dose must be reduced in renal insufficiency.

Imipenem is indicated for infections caused by susceptible organisms that are resistant to other available drugs. Imipenem is active against many highly penicillin-resistant strains of pneumococci. Imipenem (or meropenem) is the beta-lactam antibiotic of choice for treatment of *Enterobacter* infections, since it is resistant to destruction by the beta-lactamase produced by these organisms. *Pseudomonas* may rapidly develop resistance to imipenem, so simultaneous use of an aminoglycoside is recommended for infections caused by these organisms. Imipenem with or without an aminoglycoside may be effective treatment for febrile neutropenic patients.

The most common adverse effects of imipenem are nausea, vomiting, diarrhea, skin rashes, and reactions at the infusion sites. Excessive levels in patients with renal failure may lead to seizures. Meropenem is less likely to cause seizures than imipenem. Patients allergic to penicillins may be allergic to carbapenems as well.

OTHER INHIBITORS OF CELL WALL SYNTHESIS

VANCOMYCIN

Vancomycin is an antibiotic produced by *Streptococcus orientalis.* With the single exception of *Flavobacterium,* it is active only against gram-positive bacteria, particularly staphylococci. Vancomycin is a glycopeptide of molecular weight 1500. It is water-soluble and quite stable.

Mechanisms of Action & Basis of Resistance

Vancomycin inhibits cell wall synthesis by binding firmly to the D-Ala-D-Ala terminus of nascent peptidoglycan pentapeptide (Figure 43–5). This inhibits the transglycosylase, preventing further elongation of peptidoglycan and cross-linking. The peptidoglycan is thus weakened and the cell becomes susceptible to lysis. The cell membrane is also damaged, which contributes to the antibacterial effect.

Resistance to vancomycin is due to modification of the D-Ala-D-Ala binding site of the peptidoglycan building block in which the terminal D-Ala is replaced by D-lactate. This results in the loss of a critical hydrogen bond that facilitates high-affinity binding of vancomycin to its target and loss of activity. (For a more complete discussion, see box: Vancomycin Resistance.)

Antibacterial Activity

Vancomycin is bactericidal for gram-positive bacteria in concentrations of 0.5–10 μg/mL. Most pathogenic staphylococci, including those producing beta-lactamase and those resistant to nafcillin and methicillin, are killed by 4 μg/mL or less. Vancomycin kills staphylococci relatively slowly and only if cells are actively dividing; the rate is less than that of the penicillins both in vitro and in vivo. Vancomycin is synergistic with gentamicin and streptomycin against *E faecium* and *E faecalis* strains that do not exhibit high levels of aminoglycoside resistance.

VANCOMYCIN RESISTANCE

Resistance to vancomycin was mainly a laboratory curiosity confined to a few intrinsically resistant, mainly nonpathogenic species (eg, *Lactobacillus, Leuconostoc,* some strains of *Staphylococcus haemolyticus*) and therefore of little clinical consequence. However, *Enterococcus faecium* and *Enterococcus faecalis* strains that are resistant to vancomycin have emerged as a major clinical problem in recent years. Vancomycin-resistant enterococci frequently are resistant to *all* other antibiotics, rendering infections caused by them medically incurable. Acquisition of vancomycin resistance by *S aureus* is a possibility and even more of a concern. Three phenotypes of vancomycin resistance are recognized. The *vanA* phenotype, which confers high-level, inducible resistance to both vancomycin and teicoplanin, is most common and best understood. The resistance determinants are encoded on a transposable element, Tn 1546. Tn 1546 can locate on either chromosomal or plasmid DNA, and it is readily spread by a broad host range conjugative plasmid. Nine genes are encoded on this element. Two genes encode for a transposase and a resolvase, which are responsible for mobilizing and transposing the element. Two other genes, *vanR* and *vanS,* encode regulatory proteins that control expression of the genes directly involved in expression of resistance. In the presence of vancomycin, vanS autophosphorylates and transfers its phosphate to vanR. Phosphorylated vanR is a transcriptional activator that up-regulates expression of five genes: *vanA, vanH,* and *vanX,* which are essential for resistance, and *vanY* and *vanZ,* which are dispensable. VanX is a dipeptidase that hydrolyzes D-Ala-D-Ala, thus eliminating the vancomycin-binding precursor that if incorporated into the cell wall would result in loss of resistance. VanA catalyzes formation of D-Ala-D-lactate, a depsipeptide that is substituted for the D-Ala-D-Ala building block of peptidoglycan precursor. Affinity of vancomycin for binding the D-Ala-D-lactate terminus is 1000-fold less than for D-Ala-D-Ala, which accounts for the observed resistance. However, the terminal D-lactate is even more reactive than D-Ala, and PBP-catalyzed transpeptidation and cross-linking reactions proceed apace. VanH, an alpha-keto acid reductase, is responsible for supplying the D-lactate precursor that is required by vanA for formation of the D-Ala-D-lactate depsipeptide.

The *vanB* phenotype, which is mediated by elements that are genetically similar to those that determine the *vanA* phenotype, confers low-level resistance to vancomycin but not to teicoplanin. Teicoplanin is a poor inducer of resistance, which accounts for susceptibility; however, cells that have been induced with vancomycin or constitutive mutants that have been selected with teicoplanin are also resistant to teicoplanin. The *vanC* phenotype is constitutive and confers resistance to vancomycin only. It is confined to enterococcal species other than *E faecium* and *E faecalis* (eg, *E gallinarum*) and is of little clinical importance.

Pharmacokinetics

Vancomycin is poorly absorbed from the intestinal tract and is administered orally only for the treatment of antibiotic-associated enterocolitis caused by *Clostridium difficile.* Parenteral doses must be administered intravenously. A 1 hour intravenous infusion of 1 g produces blood levels of 15–30 μg/mL for 1–2 hours. The drug is widely distributed in the body. Cerebrospinal fluid levels 7–30% of simultaneous serum concentrations are achieved if there is meningeal inflammation. Ninety percent of the drug is excreted by glomerular filtration. In the presence of renal insufficiency, striking accumulation may occur (Table 43–1). In functionally anephric patients, the half-life of vancomycin is 6–10 days. The drug is not removed by hemodialysis.

Clinical Uses

The main indication for parenteral vancomycin is sepsis or endocarditis caused by methicillin-resistant staphylococci. However, vancomycin is not as effective as an antistaphylococcal penicillin for treatment of serious infections such as endocarditis caused by methicillin-susceptible strains. Vancomycin in combination with gentamicin is an alternative regimen for treatment of enterococcal endocarditis in a patient with serious penicillin allergy. Vancomycin (in combination with cefotaxime, ceftriaxone, or rifampin) is also recommended for treatment of meningitis suspected or known to be caused by a highly penicillin-resistant strain of pneumococcus (ie, MIC > 1 μg/mL). The recommended dosage is 30 mg/kg/d in two or three divided doses. A typical dosing regimen is 1 g every 12 hours for adults with normal renal function. The dosage in children is 40 mg/kg/d in three or four divided doses. Clearance of vancomycin is directly proportionate to creatinine clearance, and the dose is reduced accordingly in patients with renal insufficiency (see Moellering et al, 1981, for guidelines). For functionally anephric adult patients, a 1 g dose administered once a week is usually sufficient. Patients receiving a prolonged course of therapy should have serum concentrations checked. Recommended peak serum concentrations are 20–50 μg/mL, and trough concentrations are 5–15 μg/mL.

Oral vancomycin, 0.125–0.25 g every 6 hours, is used to treat antibiotic-associated enterocolitis caused by *Clostridium difficile*. However, given the emergence of vancomycin-resistant enterococci and the strong selective pressure of oral vancomycin for these resistant organisms, metronidazole is strongly preferred as initial therapy and vancomycin should be reserved for treatment of refractory cases.

Adverse Reactions

Adverse reactions are encountered in about 10% of cases. Most reactions are minor. Vancomycin is irritating to tissue, resulting in phlebitis at the site of injection. Chills and fever may occur. Ototoxicity and nephrotoxicity are uncommon and mild with current preparations. However, administration with another ototoxic or nephrotoxic drug, such as an aminoglycoside, increases the risk of these toxicities. Ototoxicity can be minimized by maintaining peak serum concentrations below 60 μg/mL. Among the more common reactions is the so-called "red man" or "red neck" syndrome. This infusion-related flushing is probably caused by release of histamine. It can be largely prevented by prolonging the infusion period to 1–2 hours or increasing the dosing interval.

TEICOPLANIN

Teicoplanin is a glycopeptide antibiotic that is very similar to vancomycin in mechanism of action and antibacterial spectrum. Unlike vancomycin, it can be given intramuscularly as well as intravenously. Teicoplanin has a long half-life (45–70 hours), permitting once-daily dosing. This drug is available in Europe but has not been approved for use in the United States.

FOSFOMYCIN

Fosfomycin trometamol, a stable salt of fosfomycin **(phosphonomycin)**, inhibits a very early stage of bacterial cell wall synthesis (Figure 43–5). An analog of phosphoenolpyruvate, it is structurally unrelated to any other antimicrobial agent. It inhibits the cytoplasmic enzyme enolpyruvate transferase by covalently binding to the cysteine residue of the active site and blocking the addition of phosphoenolpyruvate to UDP-*N*-acetylglucosamine. This reaction is the first step in the formation of UDP-*N*-acetylmuramic acid, the precursor of *N*-acetylmuramic acid, which is found only in bacterial cell wall. The drug is transported into the bacterial cell by glycerophosphate or glucose 6-phosphate transport systems. Resistance is due to inadequate transport of drug into the cell.

Fosfomycin is active against both gram-positive and gram-negative organisms at concentrations ≥ 125 μg/mL. Susceptibility tests should be performed in growth medium supplemented with glucose 6-phosphate to minimize false-positive indications of resistance. In vitro synergism occurs when fosfomycin is combined with beta-lactam antibiotics, aminoglycosides, or fluoroquinolones.

Fosfomycin trometamol is available in both oral and parenteral formulations, though only the oral preparation is approved for use in the United States. Oral bioavailability is approximately 40%. Peak serum concentrations are 10 μg/mL and 30 μg/mL following a 2 g or 4 g oral dose, respectively. The half-life is approximately 4 hours. The active drug is excreted by the kidney, with urinary concentrations exceeding MICs for most urinary tract pathogens.

Fosfomycin is approved for use as a single 3 g dose for treatment of uncomplicated lower urinary tract infections in women. The drug appears to be safe for use in pregnancy.

BACITRACIN

Bacitracin is a cyclic peptide mixture first obtained from the Tracy strain of *Bacillus subtilis* in 1943. It is active against gram-positive microorganisms. Bacitracin inhibits cell wall formation by interfering with dephosphorylation in cycling of the lipid carrier that transfers peptidoglycan subunits to the growing cell wall (Figure 43–5). There is no cross-resistance between bacitracin and other antimicrobial drugs.

Bacitracin is markedly nephrotoxic if administered systemically, producing proteinuria, hematuria, and nitrogen retention. Hypersensitivity reactions (eg, skin rashes) are rare. Because of its marked toxicity when used systemically, it is limited to topical use. Bacitracin is poorly absorbed. Topical application results in local antibacterial activity without significant systemic toxicity. The small amounts of bacitracin that are absorbed are excreted by glomerular filtration.

Bacitracin, 500 units/g in an ointment base (often combined with polymyxin or neomycin), is useful for the suppression of mixed bacterial flora in surface lesions of the skin, in wounds, or on mucous membranes. Solutions of bacitracin containing 100–200 units/mL in saline can be employed for irrigation of joints, wounds, or the pleural cavity.

CYCLOSERINE

Cycloserine is an antibiotic produced by *Streptomyces orchidaceus*. It is water-soluble and very unstable at acid pH. Cycloserine inhibits many gram-positive and gram-negative organisms, but it is used almost exclusively to treat tuberculosis caused by strains of *M tuberculosis* resistant to first-line agents. Cycloserine is a structural analog of D-alanine and inhibits the incorporation of D-alanine into peptidoglycan pentapeptide by inhibiting alanine racemase, which converts L-alanine to D-alanine, and D-alanyl-D-alanine ligase (Figure 43–5). After ingestion of 0.25 g of cycloserine blood levels reach 20–30 µg/mL—sufficient to inhibit many

strains of mycobacteria and gram-negative bacteria. The drug is widely distributed in tissues. Most of the drug is excreted in active form into the urine. The dosage for treating tuberculosis is 0.5 to 1g/d in two or three divided doses.

Cycloserine causes serious dose-related central nervous system toxicity with headaches, tremors, acute psychosis, and convulsions. If oral dosages are maintained below 0.75 g/d, such effects can usually be avoided.

PREPARATIONS AVAILABLE

PENICILLINS

Amoxicillin (generic, Amoxil, others)
Oral: 125, 250 mg chewable tablets; 250, 500 mg capsules; powder to reconstitute for 25, 50 mg/mL solution

Amoxicillin/potassium clavulanate (Augmentin)
Oral: 250, 500, 875 mg tablets; 125, 250 mg chewable tablets; powder to reconstitute for 125, 250 mg/5 mL suspension

Ampicillin (generic, Omnipen, Polycillin, others)
Oral: 250, 500 mg capsules; powder to reconstitute for 100, 125, 250, 500 mg suspensions
Parenteral: powder to reconstitute for injection (125, 250, 500 mg, 1, 2 g per vial; 1, 2 g per IV piggyback unit; 10 g bulk vials)

Ampicillin/sulbactam sodium (Unasyn)
Parenteral: 1, 2 g powder to reconstitute for IV or IM injection

Bacampicillin (Spectrobid)
Oral: 400 mg tablets (equivalent to 280 mg ampicillin); powder to reconstitute for 125 mg/5 mL suspension

Carbenicillin (Geocillin)
Oral: 382 mg tablets

Cloxacillin (generic, Tegopen)
Oral: 250, 500 mg capsules; powder to reconstitute for 125 mg/5 mL solution

Dicloxacillin (generic, Dynapen, others)
Oral: 125, 250, 500 mg capsules; powder to reconstitute for 62.5 mg/5 mL suspension

Methicillin (Staphcillin)
Parenteral: powder to reconstitute for injection (1, 4, 6 g per vial; 1 g per IV piggyback unit; 10 g bulk package)

Mezlocillin (Mezlin)
Parenteral: powder to reconstitute for injection (in 1, 2, 3, 4 g vials and IV piggyback units, 20 g bulk package)

Nafcillin (generic, Unipen, Nafcil, Nallpen)
Oral: 250 mg capsules; 500 mg tablets
Parenteral: powder to reconstitute for IV, IM injection (0.5, 1, 2 g per vial); 1, 2 g per IV piggyback units; 10 g bulk package

Oxacillin (Bactocill, Prostaphlin)
Oral: 250, 500 mg capsules; powder to reconstitute for 250 mg/5 mL solution
Parenteral: powder to reconstitute for injection (0.25, 0.5, 1, 2, 4 g per vial; 1, 2 g IV piggyback units; 4, 10 g bulk package)

Penicillin G (generic, Pentids, Pfizerpen)
Oral: 0.2, 0.25, 0.4, 0.5, 0.8 million unit tablets; powder to reconstitute 400,000 units/5mL suspension
Parenteral: powder to reconstitute for injection (1, 2, 3, 5, 10, 20 million units)

Penicillin G benzathine (Permapen, Bicillin)
Parenteral: 0.3, 0.6, 1.2, 2.4 million units per dose

Penicillin G procaine (generic)
Parenteral: 0.3, 0.5, 0.6, 1.2, 2.4 million units/mL for IM injection only

Penicillin V (generic, V-Cillin, Pen-Vee K, others)
Oral: 125, 250, 500 mg tablets; powder to reconstitute for 125, 250 mg/5 mL solution

Piperacillin (Pipracil)
Parenteral: powder to reconstitute for injection (2, 3, 4 g per vial or IV piggyback unit; 40 g bulk package)

Piperacillin and tazobactam sodium (Zosyn)
Parenteral: 2,3,4 g powder to reconstitute for IV injection

Ticarcillin (Ticar)
Parenteral: powder to reconstitute for injection (1, 3, 6 g per vial; 3 g per IV piggyback unit; 20, 30 g bulk vials)

Ticarcillin and clavulanate potassium (Timentin)
Parenteral: powder to reconstitute for injection (3 g ticarcillin with 0.1 g clavulanic acid per vial or IV piggyback unit)

CEPHALOSPORINS & OTHER BETA-LACTAM DRUGS

Narrow Spectrum (First-Generation) Cephalosporins

Cefadroxil (generic, Duricef)
Oral: 500 mg capsules; 1 g tablets; 125, 250, 500 mg/5 mL suspension

Cefazolin (Ancef, Kefzol)
Parenteral: powder to reconstitute for injection (0.25, 0.5, 1 g per vial or IV piggyback unit; 5, 10, 20 g per bulk vial)

Cephalexin (generic, Keflex, others)
Oral: 250, 500 mg capsules and tablets; 1 g tablets; 125, 250 mg/5 mL suspension

Cephalothin (generic, Keflin)
Parenteral: powder to reconstitute for injection and solution for injection (1, 2 g per vial or infusion pack; 20 g bulk vials)

Cephapirin (generic, Cefadyl)
Parenteral: powder to reconstitute for injection (0.5, 1, 2, 4 g per vial or IV piggyback unit; 20 g bulk package)

Cephradine (generic, Anspor, Velosef)
Oral: 250, 500 mg capsules; 125, 250 mg/5 mL suspension
Parenteral: powder to reconstitute for injection (0.25, 0.5, 1 g per vial)

Intermediate Spectrum (Second-Generation) Cephalosporins

Cefaclor (Ceclor)
Oral: 250, 500 mg capsules; powder to reconstitute for 125, 187, 250, 375 mg/5 mL suspension

Cefamandole (Mandol)
Parenteral: 0.5, 1, 2, 10 g (in vials) for IM, IV injection

Cefmetazole (Zefazone)
Parenteral: 1, 2 g powder for IV injection

Cefonicid (Monocid)
Parenteral: powder to reconstitute for injection (0.5, 1, 10 g per vial)

Cefoxitin (Mefoxin)
Parenteral: powder to reconstitute for injection (1, 2, 10 g per vial)

Cefpodoxime (Vantin)
Oral: 100, 200 mg tablets; 50, 100 mg granules for suspension in 5 mL

Cefprozil (Cefzil)
Oral: 250, 500 mg tablets; powder to reconstitute 125, 250 mg/5mL suspension

Cefuroxime (Ceftin, Kefurox, Zinacef)
Oral: 125, 250, 500 mg tablets; 125 mg/5 mL suspension
Parenteral: powder to reconstitute for injection (0.75, 1.5, 7.5 g per vial or infusion pack)

Loracarbef (Lorabid)
Oral: 200 mg capsules; powder for 100 mg/5 mL suspension

Broad Spectrum (Third- & Fourth-Generation) Cephalosporins

Cefepime (Maxipime)
Parenteral: powder for injection 0.5, 1, 2 g

Cefixime (Suprax)
Oral: 200, 400 mg tablets; powder for oral suspension, 100 mg/5 mL

Cefoperazone (Cefobid)
Parenteral: powder to reconstitute for injection (1, 2 g per vial)

Cefotaxime (Claforan)
Parenteral: powder to reconstitute for injection (1, 2 g per vial; 10 g bulk package)

Cefotetan (Cefotan)
Parenteral: powder to reconstitute for injection (1, 2, 10 g per vial)

Ceftazidime (Fortaz, Tazidime)
Parenteral: powder to reconstitute for injection (0.5, 1, 2 g per vial; 6, 10 g per bulk package)

Ceftizoxime (Cefizox)
Parenteral: powder to reconstitute for injection and solution for injection (0.5, 1, 2 g per vial; 10 g bulk package)

Ceftriaxone (Rocephin)
Parenteral: powder to reconstitute for injection (0.25, 0.5, 1, 2, 10 g per vial)

Carbapenem & Monobactam

Aztreonam (Azactam)
Parenteral: powder to reconstitute for injection (0.5, 1, 2 g)

Imipenem/cilastatin (Primaxin)
Parenteral: powder to reconstitute for injection (250, 500, 750 mg imipenem per vial)

OTHER DRUGS DISCUSSED IN THIS CHAPTER

Cycloserine (Seromycin Pulvules)
Oral: 250 mg capsules

Fosfomycin (Monurol)
Oral: 3 g packet

Vancomycin (generic, Vancocin, Vancoled)
Oral: 125, 250 mg Pulvules; 1, 10 g powder to reconstitute for solution
Parenteral: 0.5, 1, 5, 10 g powder to reconstitute for IV injection

REFERENCES

Arthur M, Courvalin P: Genetics and mechanisms of gly-copeptide resistance in enterococci. Antimicrob Agents Chemother 1993;37:1563.

Barriere SL, Flaherty JF: Third-generation cephalosporins: A critical evaluation. Clin Pharmacokinet 1984;3:351.

Blanca M et al: Cross-reactivity between penicillins and cephalosporins: Clinical and immunologic studies. J Allergy Clin Immunol 1989;83:381.

Brittain DC, Scully BE, Neu HC: Ticarcillin plus clavulanic acid in the treatment of pneumonia and other infections. Am J Med 1985;79(Suppl 5B):81.

Chow JW et al: *Enterobacter* bacteremia: Clinical features and emergence of antibiotic resistance during therapy. Ann Intern Med 1991;115:585.

Donowitz GR, Mandell GL: Beta lactam antibiotics. (Two parts.) N Engl J Med 1988;318:419, 490.

Eliopoulous GM, Moellering RC Jr: Azlocillin, mezlocillin, and piperacillin: New broad-spectrum penicillins. Ann Intern Med 1982;97:755.

Ellner JJ (editor): Cefixime: A new third generation cephalosporin. Am J Med 1988;85(3A):1.

Erffmeyer JE: Adverse reactions to penicillin. (Two parts.) Ann Allergy 1981;47:288, 294.

Friedland IR, McCracken Jr GH: Management of infections caused by antibiotic-resistant *Streptococcus pneumoniae.* N Engl J Med 1994;331:377.

Ghuysen JM: Serine beta-lactamases and penicillin-binding proteins. Ann Rev Microbiol 1991;45:37.

Handsfiel HH et al: A comparison of single-dose cefixime with ceftriaxone as treatment for uncomplicated gonorrhea. N Engl J Med 1991;325:1337.

Hermans PE, Wilhelm MP: Vancomycin. Mayo Clin Proc 1987;62:901.

Hook EW, Johnson WD: Vancomycin therapy of bacterial endocarditis. Am J Med 1978;65:411.

International Rheumatic Fever Study Group: Allergic reactions to long-term benzathine penicillin prophylaxis for rheumatic fever. Lancet 1991;337:1308.

Johnson AP et al: Resistance to vancomycin and teicoplanin: An emerging clinical problem. Clin Microbiol Rev 1990;3:280.

Kass EH, Lode H (editors): Enzyme-mediated resistance to β-lactam antibiotics: Symposium on sulbactam/ampicillin. Rev Infect Dis 1986;8(Suppl 5):S465.

McHenry MC, Gavan TL: Vancomycin. Pediatr Clin North Am 1983;30:31.

Moellering RC et al: Vancomycin therapy in patients with impaired renal function: A nomogram for dosage. Ann Intern Med 1981;94:343.

Nelson JD: Emerging role of cephalosporins in bacterial meningitis. Am J Med 1985;79(Suppl 2A):47.

Neu HC: Antistaphylococcal penicillins. Med Clin North Am 1982;66:51.

Neu HC: Carbenicillin and ticarcillin. Med Clin North Am 1982;66:61.

Nikaido H: Prevention of drug access to bacterial targets: Role of permeability barriers and active efflux. Science 1994;264:382.

Petz LD: Immunologic cross-reactivity between penicillins and cephalosporins: A review. J Infect Dis 1978; 137(Suppl):S74.

Remington JS (editor): Carbapenems: A new class of antibiotics. (Symposium.) Am J Med 1985;78(Suppl 6A):1.

Rolinson GN: 6-APA and the development of the beta-lactam antibiotics. J Antimicrob Chemother 1979;5:7.

Rolinson GN: Beta-lactam antibiotics. J Antimicrob Chemother 1986;17:5.

Sanders CC: Novel resistance selected by the new expanded-spectrum cephalosporins: A concern. J Infect Dis 1983;147:585.

Schaad UB et al: A comparison of ceftriaxone and cefuroxime for the treatment of bacterial meningitis in children. N Engl J Med 1990;322:141.

Spratt BG: Resistance to antibiotics mediated by target alterations. Science 1994;264:389.

Swan SK, Bennett WM: Drug dosing guidelines in patients with renal failure. West J Med 1992;156:633.

Sykes RB, Bonner DP: Discovery and development of the monobactams. Rev Infect Dis 1985;7(Suppl 4):S579.

Teasley DG et al: Trial of metronidazole vs. vancomycin for *Clostridium difficile:* Associated diarrhea and colitis. Lancet 1983;2:1043.

Walsh CT. Vancomycin resistance: Decoding the molecular logic. Science 1993;261:308.

Wilson WR et al: Antibiotic treatment of adults with infective endocarditis due to streptococci, enterococci, staphylococci, and HACEK microorganisms. JAMA 1995; 274:1706.

Chloramphenicol, Tetracyclines, Macrolides, Clindamycin, & Streptogramins

44

Henry F. Chambers, MD

The drugs described in this chapter all share the property of inhibiting protein synthesis in microorganisms by binding to and interfering with the function of their ribosomes.

CHLORAMPHENICOL

Chloramphenicol was first isolated in 1947 from cultures of *Streptomyces venezuelae*. It was synthesized in 1949, becoming the first completely synthetic antibiotic of importance to be produced commercially.

Crystalline chloramphenicol is a neutral, stable compound with the following structure:

Chloramphenicol

It is soluble in alcohol but poorly soluble in water. Chloramphenicol succinate, which is used for parenteral administration, is highly water-soluble. It is hydrolyzed in vivo with liberation of free chloramphenicol.

Antimicrobial Activity

Chloramphenicol is a potent inhibitor of microbial protein synthesis. It binds reversibly to the 50S subunit of the bacterial ribosome (Figure 44–1). It inhibits the peptidyl transferase step of protein synthesis.

Chloramphenicol is a bacteriostatic broad-spectrum antibiotic that is active against both aerobic and anaerobic gram-positive and gram-negative organisms. It is active also against rickettsiae but not chlamydiae. Most gram-positive bacteria are inhibited at concentrations of 1–10 μg/mL, and many gram-negative bacteria are inhibited by concentrations of 0.2–5 μg/mL. *Haemophilus influenzae, Neisseria meningitidis,* and some strains of *Bacteroides* are highly susceptible, and for them chloramphenicol may be bactericidal.

Low-level resistance may emerge from large populations of chloramphenicol-susceptible cells by selection of mutants that are less permeable to the drug. Clinically significant resistance is due to production of chloramphenicol acetyltransferase, a plasmid-encoded enzyme that inactivates the drug.

Pharmacokinetics

The usual dosage of chloramphenicol is 50–100 mg/kg/d. After oral administration, crystalline chloramphenicol is rapidly and completely absorbed. A 1 g oral dose produces blood levels between 10 and 15 μg/mL. Chloramphenicol palmitate is a prodrug that is hydrolyzed in the intestine to yield free chloramphenicol. The parenteral formulation, chloramphenicol succinate, yields free chloramphenicol by hydrolysis, giving blood levels somewhat lower than those achieved with orally administered drug. After absorption, chloramphenicol is widely distributed to virtually all tissues and body fluids, including the central nervous system and cerebrospinal fluid such that the concentration of chloramphenicol in brain tissue may be equal to that in serum. The drug penetrates cell membranes readily. Most of the drug is inactivated either by conjugation with glucuronic acid (principally in the liver) or by reduction to inactive aryl amines. Excretion of active chloramphenicol (about 10% of the total dose administered) and of inactive degradation products (about 90% of the total) occurs by way of the urine. A small amount of active drug is excreted into bile or feces. The systemic dosage of chloramphenicol need not be altered in renal insufficiency, but it must be reduced markedly in hepatic failure. Newborns less than a week old and premature infants also clear chloramphenicol less well, and the dosage should be reduced to 25 mg/kg/d.

Clinical Uses

Because of potential toxicity, bacterial resistance, and the availability of other effective drugs (eg, cephalosporins), chloramphenicol is all but obsolete as a systemic drug. It may be considered for treatment

743

MECHANISM OF ACTION AND SELECTIVITY OF ANTIBIOTICS THAT INHIBIT PROTEIN SYNTHESIS

Antibiotics discussed in this chapter all act as inhibitors of protein synthesis at the ribosomal level (Figure 44–1). Chloramphenicol, macrolides, clindamycin, and streptogramins bind to nearby sites on the 50S subunit of 70S ribosomal RNA, evidenced by the experimental observation that chloramphenicol competitively inhibits binding of macrolides and clindamycin, and vice versa.

Chloramphenicol blocks binding of the aminoacyl moiety of the charged tRNA molecule to the acceptor site of the ribosomal mRNA complex. The binding of tRNA to its codon is not affected. Failure of the aminoacyl group to associate properly with the acceptor site prevents the transpeptidation reaction catalyzed by peptidyl transferase. The peptide at the donor site on the ribosomal complex is not transferred to its amino acid acceptor, and protein synthesis stops.

Macrolides, clindamycin, and type B streptogramins do not prevent the donor-acceptor transfer reaction but rather prevent translocation of peptidyl tRNA from the acceptor site to the donor site. The incoming tRNA charged with the amino acid that is to be added next cannot access this occupied acceptor site, and protein synthesis stops.

Tetracycline binds to the 30S ribosomal RNA at a site that directly blocks binding of the amino acid-charged tRNA to the acceptor site of the ribosome mRNA complex. Differential susceptibility of bacterial and mammalian cells to chloramphenicol can be explained on the basis of target differences. Mammalian cells contain 80S ribosomal RNA that does not bind chloramphenicol. Mitochondria, which are probably derived from symbiotic bacteria that have taken up residence in mammalian cells, do contain 70S ribosomal RNA. The dose-related bone marrow suppression caused by chloramphenicol may be due its inhibition of mitochondrial ribosome function. Interestingly, tetracycline can inhibit protein synthesis in mammalian cells, but an active efflux mechanism, very similar to that used by tetracycline-resistant bacteria, prevents intracellular accumulation of drug.

of serious rickettsial infections, such as typhus or Rocky Mountain spotted fever, in children for whom tetracyclines are contraindicated, ie, those under 8 years of age. It is an alternative to a beta-lactam antibiotic for treatment of bacterial meningitis caused by a markedly penicillin-resistant strain of pneumococcus or meningococcus occurring in patients who have major hypersensitivity reactions to penicillin. The dosage is 50–100 mg/kg/d in four divided doses.

Chloramphenicol is occasionally used topically in the treatment of eye infections because of its wide antibacterial spectrum and its penetration of ocular tissues and the aqueous humor. It is ineffective for chlamydial infections.

Adverse Reactions

A. Gastrointestinal Disturbances: Adults occasionally develop nausea, vomiting, and diarrhea. This is rare in children. Oral or vaginal candidiasis may occur as a result of alteration of normal microbial flora.

B. Bone Marrow Disturbances: Chloramphenicol commonly causes a dose-related reversible suppression of red cell production at dosages exceeding 50 mg/kg/d after 1–2 weeks. Aplastic anemia is a rare consequence of chloramphenicol administration by any route. It is an idiosyncratic reaction unrelated to dose, though it occurs more frequently with pro-

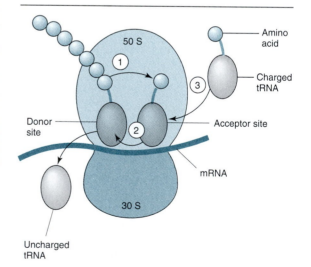

Figure 44–1. Steps in bacterial protein synthesis and sites of action of (1) chloramphenicol; (2) macrolides, clindamycin, and type B streptogramins; and (3) tetracyclines. The 70S ribosomal mRNA complex is shown with its 50S and 30S subunits. The peptidyl tRNA at the donor site donates the growing peptide chain to the aminoacyl tRNA at the acceptor site in a reaction catalyzed by peptidyl transferase. The tRNA, discharged of its peptide, is released from the donor site to make way for translocation of the newly formed peptidyl tRNA. The acceptor site is then free to be occupied by the next "charged" aminoacyl tRNA. (See box opposite for additional details.)

longed use. It tends to be irreversible and can be fatal. Aplastic anemia probably develops in one of every 24,000–40,000 patients who have taken chloramphenicol.

C. Toxicity for Newborn Infants: Newborn infants lack an effective glucuronic acid conjugation mechanism for the degradation and detoxification of chloramphenicol. Consequently, when infants are given dosages above 50 mg/kg/d, the drug may accumulate, resulting in the **gray baby syndrome,** with vomiting, flaccidity, hypothermia, gray color, shock, and collapse. To avoid this toxic effect, chloramphenicol should be used with caution in infants and the dosage limited to 50 mg/kg/d or less (during the first week of life) in full-term infants and 25 mg/kg/d in premature infants.

D. Interaction With Other Drugs: Chloramphenicol inhibits hepatic microsomal enzymes that metabolize several drugs. Half-life is prolonged, and the serum concentrations of phenytoin, tolbutamide, chlorpropamide, and warfarin are increased. Like other bacteriostatic inhibitors of microbial protein synthesis, chloramphenicol can antagonize bactericidal drugs such as penicillins or aminoglycosides.

TETRACYCLINES

The tetracyclines are a large group of drugs with a common basic structure and activity. Chlortetracycline, isolated from *Streptomyces aureofaciens,* was introduced in 1948. Oxytetracycline, derived from *Streptomyces rimosus,* was introduced in 1950. Tetracycline, obtained by catalytic dehalogenation of chlortetracycline, has been available since 1953. Demeclocycline was obtained by demethylation of chlortetracycline.

Chemistry

All of the tetracyclines have the basic structure shown below:

	R_7	R_6	R_5	Renal Clearance (mL/min)
Chlortetracycline	— Cl	— CH$_3$	— H	35
Oxytetracycline	— H	— CH$_3$	— OH	90
Tetracycline	— H	— CH3	— H	65
Demeclocycline	— Cl	— H	— H	35
Methacycline	— H	= CH$_2$*	— OH	31
Doxycycline	— H	— CH$_3$*	— OH	16
Minocycline	— N(CH$_3$)$_2$	— H	— H	10

*There is no — OH at position 6 on methacycline and doxycycline.

Free tetracyclines are crystalline amphoteric substances of low solubility. They are available as hydrochlorides, which are more soluble. Such solutions are acid and, with the exception of chlortetracycline, fairly stable. Tetracyclines chelate divalent metal ions, which can interfere with their absorption and activity.

Antimicrobial Activity

Tetracyclines are broad-spectrum antibiotics that inhibit protein synthesis. They are bacteriostatic for many gram-positive and gram-negative bacteria, including anaerobes, rickettsiae, chlamydiae, mycoplasmas, and L forms, and are active against some protozoa, eg, amebas. The antibacterial activities of most tetracyclines are similar except that tetracycline-resistant strains may remain susceptible to minocycline, which is less rapidly transported by the pump that is responsible for resistance (see below). Differences in clinical efficacy are minor and attributable largely to features of absorption, distribution, and excretion of individual drugs.

Tetracyclines enter microorganisms in part by passive diffusion and in part by an energy-dependent process of active transport. Susceptible cells concentrate the drug intracellularly. Once inside the cell, tetracyclines bind reversibly to the 30S subunit of the bacterial ribosome, blocking the binding of aminoacyl-tRNA to the acceptor site on the mRNA-ribosome complex (Figure 44–1). This prevents addition of amino acids to the growing peptide.

Resistance

Three mechanisms of resistance to tetracycline have been described: (1) decreased intracellular accumulation due to either impaired influx or increased efflux by an active transport protein pump; (2) ribosome protection due to production of proteins that interfere with tetracycline binding to the ribosome; and (3) enzymatic inactivation of tetracyclines. The most important of these is production of an efflux pump. The pump protein is encoded on a plasmid and may be transmitted by transduction or by conjugation. Because these plasmids commonly encode resistance genes for other drugs, eg, aminoglycosides, sulfonamides, and chloramphenicol, tetracycline resistance is a marker for resistance to multiple drugs.

Pharmacokinetics

Tetracyclines mainly differ in their absorption after oral administration and their elimination. Absorption after oral administration is approximately 30% for chlortetracycline; 60–70% for tetracycline, oxytetracycline, demeclocycline, and methacycline; and 95–100% for doxycycline and minocycline. A portion of an orally administered dose of tetracycline remains in the gut lumen, modifies intestinal flora, and is excreted in the feces. Absorption occurs mainly in the upper small intestine and is impaired by food (except doxycycline and minocycline); by divalent cations

(Ca^{2+}, Mg^{2+}, Fe^{2+}) or Al^{3+}; by dairy products and antacids, which contain multivalent cations; and by alkaline pH. Specially buffered tetracycline solutions are formulated for intravenous administration.

Tetracyclines are 40–80% bound by serum proteins. Oral dosages of 500 mg every 6 hours of tetracycline hydrochloride or oxytetracycline produce peak blood levels of 4–6 µg/mL. Peak levels of 2–4 µg/mL are achieved with a 200 mg dose of doxycycline or minocycline. Intravenously injected tetracyclines give somewhat higher levels only temporarily. Tetracyclines are distributed widely to tissues and body fluids except for cerebrospinal fluid, where concentrations are 10–25% of those in serum. Minocycline reaches very high concentrations in tears and saliva, which makes it useful for eradication of the meningococcal carrier state. Tetracyclines cross the placenta to reach the fetus and are also excreted in milk. As a result of chelation with calcium, tetracyclines are bound to—and damage—growing bones and teeth. Carbamazepine, phenytoin, barbiturates, and chronic alcohol ingestion may shorten the half-life of doxycycline 50% by induction of hepatic enzymes that metabolize the drug.

Tetracyclines are excreted mainly in bile and urine. Concentrations in bile exceed those in serum tenfold. Some of the drug excreted in bile is reabsorbed from the intestine (enterohepatic circulation) and contributes to maintenance of serum levels. Ten to 50 percent of various tetracyclines is excreted into the urine, mainly by glomerular filtration. Ten to 40 percent of the drug in the body is excreted in feces. Doxycycline, in contrast to other tetracyclines, is eliminated by nonrenal mechanisms, does not accumulate significantly in renal failure, and requires no dosage adjustment, making it the tetracycline of choice for use in the setting of renal insufficiency.

Tetracyclines are classified as short-acting (chlortetracycline, tetracycline, oxytetracycline), intermediate-acting (demeclocycline and methacycline), or long-acting (doxycycline and minocycline) based on serum half-lives of 6–8 hours, 12 hours, and 16–18 hours, respectively. The almost complete absorption and slow excretion of doxycycline and minocycline allow for once-daily dosing.

Clinical Uses

A tetracycline is the drug of choice in infections with *Mycoplasma pneumoniae*, chlamydiae, rickettsiae, and some spirochetes. They are used in combination regimens to treat gastric and duodenal ulcer disease caused by *Helicobacter pylori*. They may be employed in various gram-positive and gram-negative bacterial infections, including *Vibrio* infections, provided the organism is not resistant. In cholera, tetracyclines rapidly stop the shedding of vibrios, but tetracycline resistance has appeared during epidemics. Tetracyclines remain effective in most chlamydial infections, including sexually transmitted diseases. Tetracyclines are no longer recommended

for treatment of gonococcal disease because of resistance. A tetracycline—usually in combination with an aminoglycoside—is indicated for plague, tularemia, and brucellosis. Tetracyclines are sometimes employed in the treatment of protozoal infections, eg, those due to *Entamoeba histolytica* or *Plasmodium falciparum*. Other uses include treatment of acne, exacerbations of bronchitis, Lyme disease, relapsing fever, leptospirosis, and some nontuberculous mycobacterial infections (eg, *Mycobacterium marinum*). Tetracyclines formerly were used for a variety of common infections, including bacterial gastroenteritis, pneumonia (other than mycoplasmal or chlamydial pneumonia), and urinary tract infections. However, many strains of bacteria causing these infections now are resistant, and other agents have largely supplanted tetracyclines.

Minocycline, 200 mg orally daily for 5 days, can eradicate the meningococcal carrier state, but because of side-effects and resistance of many meningococcal strains, rifampin is preferred. Demeclocycline inhibits the action of ADH in the renal tubule and has been used in the treatment of inappropriate secretion of ADH or similar peptides by certain tumors (see Chapter 15).

A. Oral Dosage: The oral dosage for rapidly excreted tetracyclines, equivalent to tetracycline hydrochloride, is 0.25–0.5 g four times daily for adults and 20–40 mg/kg/d for children (8 years of age and older). For severe systemic infections, the higher dosage is indicated, at least for the first few days. The daily dose is 600 mg for demeclocycline or methacycline, 100 mg once or twice a day for doxycycline, and 100 mg twice a day for minocycline. Doxycycline is the tetracycline of choice because it can be given as a once-daily dose and its absorption is not significantly affected by food. All tetracyclines chelate with metals, and none should be administered with milk, antacids, or ferrous sulfate. To avoid deposition in growing bones or teeth, tetracyclines should be avoided for pregnant women and for children under 8 years of age.

B. Parenteral Dosage: Several tetracyclines are available for intravenous injection in doses of 0.1–0.5 g every 6–12 hours (similar to oral doses), depending on the agent. Intramuscular injection is not recommended because of pain and inflammation at the injection site. Doxycycline is the preferred agent, at a dosage of 100–200 mg every 12–24 hours.

Adverse Reactions

Hypersensitivity reactions (drug fever, skin rashes) to tetracyclines are uncommon. Most adverse effects are due to direct toxicity of the drug or to alteration of microbial flora.

A. Gastrointestinal Adverse Effects: Nausea, vomiting, and diarrhea are the most common reasons for discontinuing tetracycline medication. These effects are attributable to direct local irritation of the intestinal tract. Nausea, anorexia, and diarrhea can usually be controlled by administering the drug with food or carboxymethylcellulose, reducing drug dosage, or discontinuing the drug.

Tetracyclines modify the normal flora, with suppression of susceptible coliform organisms and overgrowth of *Pseudomonas, Proteus,* staphylococci, resistant coliforms, clostridia, and *Candida.* This can result in intestinal functional disturbances, anal pruritus, vaginal or oral candidiasis, or enterocolitis with shock and death. Pseudomembranous enterocolitis associated with *Clostridium difficile* should be treated with metronidazole.

B. Bony Structures and Teeth: Tetracyclines are readily bound to calcium deposited in newly formed bone or teeth in young children. When the drug is given during pregnancy, it can be deposited in the fetal teeth, leading to fluorescence, discoloration, and enamel dysplasia; it can also be deposited in bone, where it may cause deformity or growth inhibition. If the drug is given to children under 8 years of age for long periods, similar changes can result.

C. Liver Toxicity: Tetracyclines can probably impair hepatic function, especially during pregnancy, in patients with preexisting hepatic insufficiency and when high doses are given intravenously. Hepatic necrosis has been reported with daily doses of 4 g or more intravenously.

D. Kidney Toxicity: Renal tubular acidosis and other renal injury resulting in nitrogen retention have been attributed to the administration of outdated tetracycline preparations. Tetracyclines given along with diuretics may produce nitrogen retention. Tetracyclines other than doxycycline may accumulate to toxic levels in patients with impaired kidney function.

E. Local Tissue Toxicity: Intravenous injection can lead to venous thrombosis. Intramuscular injection produces painful local irritation and should be avoided.

F. Photosensitization: Systemic tetracycline administration, especially of demeclocycline, can induce sensitivity to sunlight or ultraviolet light, particularly in fair-skinned persons.

G. Vestibular Reactions: Dizziness, vertigo, nausea, and vomiting have been particularly noted with doxycycline at doses above 100 mg. With dosages of 200–400 mg/d of minocycline, 35–70% of patients will have these reactions.

Medical & Social Implications of Overuse

The widespread use of tetracyclines for minor illnesses has led to the emergence of resistance even among once highly susceptible species, eg, pneumococci, staphylococci, and group A streptococci. Tetracyclines have been extensively used in animal feeds to enhance growth. This practice has contributed to the steadily increasing spread of tetracycline resistance among enteric bacteria and of plasmids that encode tetracycline resistance genes.

MACROLIDES

The macrolides are a group of closely related compounds characterized by a macrocyclic lactone ring (usually containing 14 or 16 atoms) to which deoxy sugars are attached. The prototype drug, erythromycin, which consists of two sugar moieties attached to a 14-atom lactone ring, was obtained in 1952 from *Streptomyces erythreus.* Clarithromycin and azithromycin are semisynthetic derivatives of erythromycin.

Erythromycin (R_1 = CH_3, R_2 = H)
Clarithromycin (R_1, R_2 = CH_3)

ERYTHROMYCIN

Chemistry

The general structure of erythromycin is shown above with the macrolide ring and the sugars desosamine and cladinose. It is poorly soluble in water (0.1%) but dissolves readily in organic solvents. Solutions are fairly stable at 4 °C but lose activity rapidly at 20 °C and at acid pH. Erythromycins are usually dispensed as various esters and salts.

Antimicrobial Activity

Erythromycin is effective against gram-positive organisms, especially pneumococci, streptococci, staphylococci, and corynebacteria, in plasma concentrations of 0.02–2 μg/mL. *Mycoplasma, Legionella, Chlamydia trachomatis, C psittaci, C pneumoniae, Helicobacter, Listeria,* and certain mycobacteria (*Mycobacterium kansasii, Mycobacterium scrofulaceum*) are also susceptible. Gram-negative organisms such as *Neisseria* species, *Bordetella pertussis, Bartonella henselae,* and *B quintana* (etiologic agents of cat-scratch disease and bacillary angiomatosis), some *Rickettsia* species, *Treponema pallidum,* and *Campylobacter* species are susceptible. *Haemophilus influenzae* is somewhat less susceptible.

The antibacterial action of erythromycin may be inhibitory or bactericidal, particularly at higher concentrations, for susceptible organisms. Activity is enhanced at alkaline pH. Inhibition of protein synthesis occurs via binding to the 50S ribosomal RNA. Protein synthesis is inhibited because aminoacyl translocation reactions and the formation of initiation complexes are blocked (Figure 44–1).

Resistance

Resistance to erythromycin is usually plasmid-encoded. Three mechanisms have been identified: (1) reduced permeability of the cell membrane or active efflux; (2) production (by Enterobacteriaceae) of esterases that hydrolyze macrolides; and (3) modification of the ribosomal binding site by chromosomal mutation or by a macrolide-inducible or a constitutive methylase. Methylase production accounts for the vast majority of resistance in gram-positive organisms. Cross-resistance is complete between erythromycin and the other macrolides. Constitutive methylase production also confers resistance to structurally unrelated but mechanistically similar compounds such as clindamycin and streptogramin B (so-called macrolide-lincosamide-streptogramin, or MLS-type B, resistance), which share the same ribosomal binding site. Because nonmacrolides are poor inducers of the methylase, strains expressing an inducible methylase will appear susceptible in vitro. However, constitutive mutants that are resistant can be selected out and emerge during therapy with clindamycin.

Pharmacokinetics

Erythromycin base is destroyed by stomach acid and must be administered with enteric coating. Food interferes with absorption. Stearates and esters are fairly acid-resistant and somewhat better absorbed. The lauryl salt of the propionyl ester of erythromycin (erythromycin estolate) is the best-absorbed oral preparation. Oral dosage of 2 g/d results in serum erythromycin base and ester concentrations of approximately 2 μg/mL. However, only the base is microbiologically active, and its concentration tends to be similar regardless of the formulation. A 500 mg intravenous dose of erythromycin lactobionate produces serum concentrations of 10 μg/mL 1 hour after dosing. The serum half-life is approximately 1.5 h normally and 5 hours in patients with anuria. Adjustment for renal failure is not necessary. Erythromycin is not removed by dialysis. Large amounts of an administered dose are excreted in the bile and lost in feces, and only 5% is excreted in the urine. Absorbed drug is distributed widely except to the brain and cerebrospinal fluid. Erythromycin is taken up by polymorphonuclear leukocytes and macrophages. It traverses the placenta and reaches the fetus.

Clinical Uses

An erythromycin is the drug of choice in corynebacterial infections (diphtheria, corynebacterial sepsis, erythrasma); in respiratory, neonatal, ocular, or genital chlamydial infections; and in treatment of community-acquired pneumonia because its spectrum of activity includes the pneumococcus, *Mycoplasma*, and *Legionella*. Erythromycin is also useful as a penicillin substitute in penicillin-allergic individuals with infections caused by staphylococci (assuming that the isolate is susceptible), streptococci, or pneumococci. Erythromycin has been recommended as prophylaxis against endocarditis during dental procedures in individuals with valvular heart disease, though clindamycin, which is better tolerated, has largely replaced it. Although erythromycin estolate is the best-absorbed salt, it imposes the greatest risk of adverse reactions. Therefore, the stearate or succinate salt may be preferred.

The oral dosage of erythromycin base, stearate, or estolate is 0.25–0.5 g every 6 hours (for children, 40 mg/kg/d). The dosage of erythromycin ethylsuccinate is 0.4–0.6 g every 6 hours. Oral erythromycin base (1 g) is sometimes combined with oral neomycin or kanamycin for preoperative preparation of the colon. The intravenous dosage of erythromycin gluceptate or lactobionate is 0.5–1.0 g every 6 hours for adults and 20–40 mg/kg/d for children. The higher dosage is recommended when treating pneumonia caused by *Legionella* species.

Adverse Reactions

A. Gastrointestinal Effects: Anorexia, nausea, vomiting, and diarrhea occasionally accompany oral administration. Gastrointestinal intolerance, which is due to a direct stimulation of gut motility, is the most frequent reason for discontinuing erythromycin and substituting another antibiotic.

B. Liver Toxicity: Erythromycins, particularly the estolate, can produce acute cholestatic hepatitis (fever, jaundice, impaired liver function), probably as a hypersensitivity reaction. Most patients recover from this, but hepatitis recurs if the drug is readministered. Other allergic reactions include fever, eosinophilia, and rashes.

C. Drug Interactions: Erythromycin metabolites can inhibit cytochrome P450 enzymes and thus increase the serum concentrations of numerous drugs, including theophylline, oral anticoagulants, cyclosporine, methylprednisolone, and antihistamines such as terfenadine and astemizole. The resulting high concentrations of these antihistamines may cause serious cardiac arrhythmias. Erythromycin increases serum concentrations of oral digoxin by increasing its bioavailability.

CLARITHROMYCIN

Clarithromycin is derived from erythromycin by addition of a methyl group to the hydroxyl group at C_6 (see above). This methoxy group improves acid stability and, therefore, oral absorption compared with erythromycin. Its mechanism of action is the same as that of erythromycin. Clarithromycin and erythromycin are virtually identical with respect to antibacterial activity except that clarithromycin is more active against *Mycobacterium avium* complex (see Chapter 47 for its use in treating atypical mycobacterial infections). Clarithromycin also has activity against *M leprae* and *Toxoplasma gondii*. Erythromycin-resistant streptococci and staphylococci are also resistant to clarithromycin.

A 500 mg dose produces serum concentrations of 2–3 µg/mL and an elimination half-life of approximately 6 hours. The longer half-life of clarithromycin compared with erythromycin permits twice-daily dosing. The recommended dosage is 250–500 mg twice daily. Clarithromycin penetrates most tissues well, with concentrations equal to or exceeding serum concentrations. Clarithromycin, like erythromycin, penetrates well into phagocytes.

Clarithromycin is metabolized in the liver. The major metabolite is 14-hydroxyclarithromycin, which also has antibacterial activity. A portion of active drug and this major metabolite is eliminated in the urine, and dosage reduction (eg, a 500 mg loading dose, then 250 mg once or twice daily) is recommended for patients with creatinine clearances less than 30 mL/min. Clarithromycin, having a 14-member lactone ring like that of erythromycin, has drug interactions similar to those described for erythromycin.

The advantages of clarithromycin compared with erythromycin are lower frequency of gastrointestinal intolerance and less frequent dosing. Except for the specific organisms noted above, the two drugs are otherwise therapeutically very similar, and the choice of one over the other usually turns on issues of cost (clarithromycin being much more expensive) and tolerability.

AZITHROMYCIN

Azithromycin, a 15-atom lactone macrolide ring compound, is derived from erythromycin by addition of a methylated nitrogen into the lactone ring of erythromycin. Its spectrum of activity and clinical uses are virtually identical to those of clarithromycin. Azithromycin is active against *M avium* complex and *T gondii*. Azithromycin is slightly less active than erythromycin and clarithromycin against staphylococci and streptococci and slightly more active against *H influenzae*. Azithromycin is highly active against *Chlamydia*.

Azithromycin differs from erythromycin and clarithromycin mainly in pharmacokinetic properties. A 500 mg dose of azithromycin produces relatively low serum concentrations of approximately 0.4 µg/mL. However, azithromycin penetrates into most tissues (except cerebrospinal fluid) and phagocytic cells extremely well, with tissue concentrations exceeding serum concentrations by 10- to 100-fold. Drug is slowly released from tissues (tissue half-life of 2–4 days) to produce an elimination half-life approaching 3 days. These unique properties permit once-daily dosing and shortening of the duration of treatment in many cases. For example, a single 1 g dose of azithromycin is as effective as a 7-day course of doxycycline for chlamydial cervicitis and urethritis. Community-acquired pneumonia can be treated with azithromycin given as a 500 mg loading dose, followed by a 250 mg single daily dose for the next 4 days.

Azithromycin is rapidly absorbed and well tolerated orally. Food decreases bioavailability of azithromycin, which should be administered 1 hour before or 2 hours after meals. Aluminum and magnesium antacids do not alter bioavailability but delay absorption and reduce peak serum concentrations. Because it has a 15-member (not 14-member) lactone ring, azithromycin does not inactivate cytochrome P450 enzymes and therefore is relatively free of the drug interactions that occur with erythromycin and clarithromycin.

CLINDAMYCIN

Clindamycin is a chlorine-substituted derivative of **lincomycin,** an antibiotic that is elaborated by *Streptomyces lincolnensis*. Lincomycin, although structurally distinct, resembles erythromycin in activity, but it is toxic and no longer used.

Clindamycin

Antibacterial Activity

Streptococci, staphylococci, and pneumococci are inhibited by clindamycin, 0.5–5 µg/mL. Enterococci and gram-negative aerobic organisms are resistant (in contrast to their susceptibility to erythromycin). *Bacteroides* species and other anaerobes, both gram-positive and gram-negative, are usually susceptible. *Clostridium difficile,* an important cause of pseudomembranous colitis, is resistant. Clindamycin, like erythromycin, inhibits protein synthesis by interfering with the formation of initiation complexes and with aminoacyl translocation reactions. The binding site for clindamycin on the 50S subunit of the bacterial ribosome is identical with that for erythromycin. Resistance to clindamycin, which generally confers cross-resistance to other macrolides, is due to (1) mutation of the ribosomal receptor site; (2) modification of the receptor by a constitutively expressed methylase (see section on erythromycin resistance, above); and (3) enzymatic inactivation of clindamycin. Gram-negative aerobic species are intrinsically resistant because of poor permeability of the outer membrane.

Pharmacokinetics

Oral dosages of clindamycin, 0.15–0.3 g every 6 hours (10–20 mg/kg/d for children), yield serum levels of 2–3 μg/mL. When administered intravenously, 600 mg of clindamycin every 8 hours gives levels of 5–15 μg/mL. The drug is about 90% protein-bound. Excretion is mainly via the liver, bile, and urine. Clindamycin penetrates well into most tissues, with brain and cerebrospinal fluid being important exceptions. It penetrates well into abscesses and is actively taken up and concentrated by phagocytic cells. Clindamycin is metabolized by the liver, and both active drug and active metabolites are excreted in bile. The half-life is about 2.5 hours in normal individuals, increasing to 6 hours in patients with anuria. No dosage adjustment is required for renal failure.

Clinical Uses

The most important indication for clindamycin is the treatment of severe anaerobic infection caused by *Bacteroides* and other anaerobes that often participate in mixed infections. Clindamycin, sometimes in combination with an aminoglycoside or cephalosporin, is used to treat penetrating wounds of the abdomen and the gut; infections originating in the female genital tract, eg, septic abortion and pelvic abscesses; or aspiration pneumonia. Clindamycin is now recommended instead of erythromycin for prophylaxis of endocarditis in patients with valvular heart disease who are undergoing certain dental procedures. Clindamycin plus primaquine is an effective alternative to trimethoprim-sulfamethoxazole for moderate to moderately severe *Pneumocystis carinii* pneumonia in AIDS patients. It is also used in combination with pyrimethamine for AIDS-related toxoplasmosis of the brain.

Adverse Effects

Common adverse effects are diarrhea, nausea, and skin rashes. Impaired liver function (with or without

jaundice) and neutropenia sometimes occur. Severe diarrhea and enterocolitis have followed clindamycin administration. Antibiotic-associated colitis that has followed administration of clindamycin and other drugs is caused by toxigenic *C difficile.* This organism is infrequently part of the normal fecal flora but is selected out during administration of oral antibiotics. The organism is often acquired nosocomially. It grows to high numbers in the sigmoid colon and secretes a necrotizing toxin that produces a pseudomembranous colitis. This potentially fatal complication must be recognized promptly and treated with metronidazole, 500 mg orally or intravenously three times a day (the preferred therapy), or vancomycin, 125 mg orally four times a day (less desirable given the increasing prevalence of vancomycin-resistant enterococci). Relapse may occur. Variations in the local prevalence of *C difficile* may account for the great differences in incidence of antibiotic-associated colitis. For unknown reasons, neonates given clindamycin may become colonized with toxigenic *C difficile* but do not develop colitis.

STREPTOGRAMINS

No streptogramin antibiotic is currently approved in the United States. RP 59500, an investigational agent, is a combination of two streptogramins—**quinupristin,** a streptogramin B; and **dalfopristin,** a streptogramin A—in a ratio of 3:7. RP 59500 (Synercid) is currently under development for intravenous treatment of streptococcal, staphylococcal, and enterococcal infections, particularly those due to multidrug-resistant strains. RP 59500 inhibits gram-positive cocci at concentrations of 1 μg/mL or less. The mechanism of action of RP 59500 is similar to that of the macrolides except that it is bactericidal for staphylococci. Resistance to quinupristin (but not dalfopristin) results from the same methylase gene that determines resistance to erythromycin and clindamycin. Quinupristin is not an inducer of the methylase, so strains with inducible erythromycin resistance are susceptible. However, if methylase production is constitutive, quinupristin activity and synergism with dalfopristin are lost and treatment failures may occur. Since many multidrug-resistant gram-positive organisms are resistant to erythromycin, this may limit the use of RP 59500. Clinical trials to define the role of RP 59500 in treating infections caused by gram-positive cocci are under way.

PREPARATIONS AVAILABLE

Chloramphenicol
Chloramphenicol (generic, Chloromycetin)
Oral: 250 mg capsules; 150 mg/5 mL suspension
Parenteral: powder to reconstitute 100 mg/mL solution for injection

Tetracyclines
Demeclocycline (Declomycin)
Oral: 150, 300 mg tablets; 150 mg capsules
Doxycycline (generic, Vibramycin, others)
Oral: 50, 100 mg tablets and capsules; powder to reconstitute for 25 mg/5 mL suspension; 50 mg/5 mL syrup
Parenteral: powder to reconstitute for injection (100, 200 mg per vial)
Methacycline (Rondomycin)
Oral: 150, 300 mg capsules
Minocycline (Minocin)
Oral: 50, 100 mg tablets and capsules; 50 mg/5 mL suspension
Parenteral: powder to reconstitute for injection (100 mg per vial)
Oxytetracycline (generic, Terramycin)
Oral: 250 mg capsules
Parenteral: 50, 125 mg/mL for IM injection
Tetracycline (generic, Achromycin V, others)
Oral: 100, 250, 500 mg capsules; 250, 500 mg tablets; 125 mg/5 mL suspension
Parenteral: powder to reconstitute for IM injection, 100, 250 mg/vial; powder to reconstitute for IV injection, 250, 500 mg/vial

Macrolides
Azithromycin (Zithromax)
Oral: 250 mg capsules; powder for 100, 200 mg/5 mL oral suspension
Clarithromycin (Biaxin)
Oral: 250, 500 mg tablets; granules for 125, 250 mg/5 mL oral suspension
Erythromycin (generic, Ilotycin, Ilosone, E-Mycin, Erythrocin, others)
Oral (base): 250, 333, 500 mg enteric-coated tablets
Oral (base) delayed-release: 333 mg tablets, 250 capsules
Oral (estolate): 500 mg tablets; 250 mg capsules; 125, 250 mg/5 mL suspension
Oral (ethylsuccinate): 200, 400 mg film-coated tablets; 200, 400 mg/5 mL suspension
Oral (stearate): 250, 500 mg film-coated tablets
Parenteral: lactobionate, powder to reconstitute for IV injection (0.5, 1 g per vial)

Clindamycin
Clindamycin (generic, Cleocin)
Oral: 75, 150, 300 mg capsules; 75 mg/5 mL granules to reconstitute for solution
Parenteral: 150 mg/mL in 2, 4, 6, 60 mL vials for injection

REFERENCES

Chopra I, Hawkey PM, Hinton M: Tetracyclines, molecular and clinical aspects. J Antimicrob Chemother 1992; 29:245.

Clarithromycin and azithromycin. Med Lett Drugs Ther 1992;34:45.

Derrick CW Jr, Reilly KM: Erythromycin, lincomycin, and clindamycin. Pediatr Clin North Am 1983;30:63.

Falages ME, Gorbach SL: Clindamycin and metronidazole. Med Clin North Am 1995;79:845.

Feder HM Jr, Osier C, Maderazo EG: Chloramphenicol: A review of its use in clinical practice. Rev Infect Dis 1981;3:479.

Jacoby GA: Prevalence and resistance mechanisms of common bacterial respiratory pathogens. Clin Infect Dis 1993;18:951.

Kanatani MS, Guglielmo BJ: The new macrolides azithromycin and clarithromycin. West J Med 1994;160:31.

Klainer AS: Clindamycin. Med Clin North Am 1987; 71:1169.

Martin DH et al: A controlled trial of a single dose of azithromycin for the treatment of chlamydial urethritis and cervicitis. N Engl J Med 1992;327:921.

Periti P et al: Pharmacokinetic drug interactions of macrolides. Clin Pharmacokinet 1992;23:106.

Peters DH, Clissold SP: Clarithromycin: A review of its antimicrobial activity, pharmacokinetic properties and therapeutic potential. Drugs 1992;44:117.

Schlossberg D: Azithromycin and clareithromycin. Med Clin North Am 1995;79:803.

Speer BS, Shoemaker MB, Salyers AA: Bacterial resistance to tetracycline: Mechanism, transfer, and clinical significance. Clin Microbiol Rev 1992;5:387.

Steigbigel NH: Erythromycin, lincomycin, and clindamycin. In: Principles and Practice of Infectious Diseases, 4th ed. Mandell GL, Bennett JE, Dolin R (editors). Churchill Livingstone, 1995.

45

Aminoglycosides & Spectinomycin

Henry F. Chambers, MD, W. Keith Hadley, MD, PhD,
& Ernest Jawetz, MD, PhD

The drugs described in this chapter are, like the drugs described in Chapter 44, protein synthesis inhibitors that interfere with ribosomal function. These agents are useful mainly against aerobic gram-negative microorganisms.

AMINOGLYCOSIDES

Aminoglycosides are a group of bactericidal antibiotics originally obtained from various *Streptomyces* species and sharing chemical, antimicrobial, pharmacologic, and toxic characteristics. The group includes **streptomycin, neomycin, kanamycin, amikacin, gentamicin, tobramycin, sisomicin, netilmicin,** and others.

Aminoglycosides are used most widely against gram-negative enteric bacteria, especially in bacteremia and sepsis, in combination with vancomycin or a penicillin for endocarditis, and for treatment of tuberculosis. Streptomycin is the oldest and best-studied of the aminoglycosides. Gentamicin, tobramycin, and amikacin are the most widely employed aminoglycosides at present. Neomycin and kanamycin are now largely limited to topical or oral use.

General Properties of Aminoglycosides

A. Physical and Chemical Properties: Aminoglycosides have a hexose ring, either streptidine (in streptomycin) or 2-deoxystreptamine (other aminoglycosides), to which various amino sugars are attached by glycosidic linkages (Figures 45–1 and 45–2). They are water-soluble, stable in solution, and more active at alkaline than at acid pH. Aminoglycosides frequently exhibit synergism with beta lactams or vancomycin in vitro. In combination they eradicate organisms more rapidly than would be predicted from the activity of either single agent. However, at high concentrations aminoglycosides may complex with beta-lactam drugs, resulting in loss of activity, and they should not be mixed together for administration.

B. Mechanism of Action: The mode of action of streptomycin has been studied far more than that of other aminoglycosides, but probably all act similarly. Aminoglycosides are irreversible inhibitors of protein synthesis, but the precise mechanism for bactericidal activity is not evident. The initial event is passive diffusion via porin channels across the outer membrane. Drug is then actively transported across the cell membrane into the cytoplasm by an oxygen dependent process. The transmembrane electrochemical gradient supplies the energy for this process and transport is coupled to a proton pump. Low extracellular pH and anaerobic conditions inhibit transport by reducing the gradient. Transport may be enhanced by cell wall-active drugs, such as penicillin or vancomycin; this enhancement may be the basis of the synergism.

Once an aminoglycoside has entered the cell, it binds to specific 30S-subunit ribosomal proteins (S12 in the case of streptomycin). Protein synthesis is inhibited by aminoglycosides in at least three ways (Figure 45–3): (1) They interfere with the "initiation complex" of peptide formation; (2) they induce misreading of mRNA, which causes incorporation of incorrect amino acids into the peptide, resulting in a non-functional or toxic protein; and (3) they cause a breakup of polysomes into nonfunctional monosomes. These activities occur more or less simultaneously, and the overall effect is irreversible and lethal for the cell.

C. Mechanisms of Resistance: Three principal mechanisms have been established: (1) The microorganism produces a transferase enzyme or enzymes that inactivate the aminoglycoside by adenylation, acetylation, or phosphorylation. This is the principal type of resistance encountered clinically. These enzymes are usually plasmid-controlled and their transmission is of great clinical and epidemiologic concern. Specific transferase enzymes are discussed below. (2) Impaired entry of aminoglycoside

Figure 45–1. Structure of streptomycin.

into the cell. This may be genotypic, ie, resulting from mutation or deletion of a porin protein or proteins involved in transport and maintenance of the electrochemical gradient; or phenotypic, eg, resulting from growth conditions under which the oxygen-dependent transport process described above is not functional. (3) The receptor protein on the 30S ribosomal subunit may be deleted or altered as a result of a mutation.

D. Pharmacokinetics: Aminoglycosides are absorbed very poorly from the intact gastrointestinal tract; virtually the entire oral dose is excreted in feces after oral administration. However, the drugs may be absorbed if ulcerations are present. After intramuscular injection, aminoglycosides are well absorbed, giving peak concentrations in blood within 30–90 minutes. Aminoglycosides are usually administered intravenously as a 30–60 minute infusion; after a brief distribution phase this results in serum concentrations that are identical to those following intramuscular injection. Traditionally, aminoglycosides have been administered in two or three equally divided daily doses for patients with normal renal function. However, once-daily aminoglycoside dosing may be preferred in certain clinical situations (see text box: Once-Daily Aminoglycoside Dosing).

Aminoglycosides are highly polar compounds that do not enter cells readily. They are largely excluded from the central nervous system and the eye. In the presence of active inflammation, however, cerebrospinal fluid levels reach 20% of plasma levels, and in neonatal meningitis the levels may be higher. Intrathecal or intraventricular injection is required for high levels in cerebrospinal fluid. Even after parenteral administration, concentrations of aminoglycosides are not high in most tissues except the renal cortex. Concentration in most secretions is also modest; in the bile, it may reach 30% of the blood level. Diffusion into pleural or synovial fluid may result in concentrations 50–90% of that of plasma with prolonged therapy.

Aminoglycosides are cleared by the kidney, and excretion is directly proportionate to creatinine clear-

ance. The normal half-life in serum is 2–3 hours, increasing to 24–48 hours in patients with significant impairment of renal function. Aminoglycosides are only partially and irregularly removed by hemodialysis—eg, 40–60% for gentamicin—and even less effectively by peritoneal dialysis.

Dosage adjustments must be made to avoid accumulation of drug and toxicity in patients with renal insufficiency. Either the dose of drug is kept constant and the interval between doses is increased, or the interval is kept constant and the dose is reduced. Nomograms and formulas have been constructed relating serum creatinine levels to adjustments in treatment regimens. The simplest formula divides the dose (calculated on the basis of normal renal function) by the serum creatinine value (mg/dL). Thus, a 60 kg patient with normal renal function might receive 300 mg/d of gentamicin (maximum daily dose of 5 mg/kg), whereas a 60 kg patient with a serum creatinine of 3 mg/dL would receive 100 mg/d. However, this approach fails to take into account the age and gender of the patient, both of which significantly affect creatinine clearance without necessarily being reflected as a change in serum creatinine. Since aminoglycoside clearance is directly proportionate to the creatinine clearance, a better method for determining the aminoglycoside dose is to estimate creatinine clearance using the Cockcroft-Gault formula described in Chapter 61.

The daily dose of aminoglycoside is calculated by multiplying the maximum daily dose by the ratio of estimated creatinine clearance to normal creatinine clearance, ie, 120 mL/min, which is a typical value for a 70 kg young adult male. For a 60-year-old female weighing 60 kg with a serum creatinine of 3 mg/dL the correct dosage of gentamicin would be approximately 50 mg/d, half the dose calculated by the simplest formula. There is considerable individual variation in aminoglycoside serum levels among patients with similar estimated creatinine clearance values. Therefore, it is mandatory, especially when using higher dosages for more than a few days or when renal function is rapidly changing, to measure serum drug levels in order to avoid severe toxicity. For a traditional twice- or thrice-daily dosing regimen, peak serum concentrations should be determined from a blood sample obtained 30–60 minutes after a dose and trough concentrations from a sample obtained just prior to the next dose.

E. Adverse Effects: All aminoglycosides are ototoxic and nephrotoxic. Ototoxicity and nephrotoxicity are more likely to be encountered when therapy is continued for more than 5 days, at higher doses, in the elderly, and in the setting of renal insufficiency. Concurrent use with loop diuretics (eg, furosemide, ethacrynic acid) or other nephrotoxic antimicrobial agents (eg, vancomycin or amphotericin) can potentiate nephrotoxicity and should be avoided if possible. Ototoxicity can manifest itself either as auditory damage, resulting in tinnitus and high-frequency hearing

Kanamycin R = H

Amikacin R = C—CH—CH_2—CH_2—NH_2 (with O double bond and OH)

Gentamicin, netilmicin

	Ring I			Ring II
	R_1	R_2	C4–C5 bond	R_3
Gentamicin C_1	CH_3	CH_3	Single	H
Gentamicin C_2	CH_3	H	Single	H
Gentamicin C_{1a}	H	H	Single	H
Netilmicin	H	H	Double	C_2H_5

Tobramycin

loss initially; or as vestibular damage, evident by vertigo, ataxia, and loss of balance. Nephrotoxicity results in rising serum creatinine levels or reduced creatinine clearance, though the earliest indication often is an increase in trough serum aminoglycoside concentrations. Neomycin, kanamycin, and amikacin are the most ototoxic agents. Streptomycin and gentamicin are the most vestibulotoxic. Neomycin, tobramycin, and gentamicin are the most nephrotoxic.

In very high doses, aminoglycosides can produce a curare-like effect with neuromuscular blockade that results in respiratory paralysis. This paralysis is usually reversible by calcium gluconate (given promptly) or neostigmine. Hypersensitivity occurs infrequently.

F. Clinical Uses: Aminoglycosides are mostly used against gram-negative enteric bacteria, especially when the isolate may be drug-resistant and when there is suspicion of sepsis. They are almost always used in combination with a beta-lactam antibiotic in order to extend coverage to include potential gram-positive pathogens and to take advantage of the synergism between these two classes of drugs. Penicillin aminoglycoside combinations also are used to achieve bactericidal activity in treatment of enterococcal endocarditis and to shorten duration of therapy for viridans streptococcal and staphylococcal endocarditis. Which aminoglycoside and what dose be used depend upon the infection being treated and susceptibility of the isolate.

STREPTOMYCIN

Streptomycin (Figure 45–1) was isolated from a strain of *Streptomyces griseus* by Waksman and his associates in 1944. The antimicrobial activity of streptomycin is typical of that of other aminoglycosides, as are the mechanisms of resistance. Resistance has emerged in most species, severely limiting the current usefulness of streptomycin, with the exceptions listed below. Ribosomal resistance to streptomycin develops readily, limiting its role as a single agent.

Clinical Uses

A. Mycobacterial Infections: Streptomycin is mainly used as a second-line agent for treatment of tuberculosis. The dosage is 0.5–1 g (7.5–15 mg/kg/d), which is given intramuscularly or intravenously. It

Figure 45–2. Structures of several important aminoglycoside antibiotics. Ring II is 2-deoxystreptamine. The resemblance between kanamycin and amikacin and between gentamicin, netilmicin, and tobramycin can be seen. The circled numerals on the kanamycin molecule indicate points of attack of plasmid-mediated bacterial transferase enzymes that can inactivate this drug. (①, ②, and ③, acetyltransferase; ④, phosphotransferase; ⑤, adenylyltransferase.) Amikacin is resistant to degradation at ②, ③, ④, and ⑤.

Normal bacterial cell

Aminoglycoside-treated bacterial cell

Figure 45–3. Putative mechanisms of action of the aminoglycosides. Normal protein synthesis is shown in the top panel. At least three different aminoglycoside effects have been described, as shown in the bottom panel: block of formation of the initiation complex; miscoding of amino acids in the emerging peptide chain due to misreading of the mRNA; and block of translocation on mRNA. Block of movement of the ribose may occur after the formation of a single initiation complex, resulting in an mRNA chain with only a single ribosome on it, a so-called monosome. (Reproduced, with permission, from Katzung BG, Trevor AT: *Pharmacology: Examination & Board Review,* 4th ed. Appleton & Lange, 1995.)

should be used only in combination with other agents to prevent emergence of resistance. See Chapter 47 for additional information regarding its use in mycobacterial infections.

B. Nontuberculous Infections: In plague, tularemia, and sometimes brucellosis, streptomycin, 1 g/d (15 mg/kg/d for children), is given intramuscularly in combination with an oral tetracycline.

Penicillin plus streptomycin is effective for enterococcal endocarditis and 2-week therapy of viridans streptococcal endocarditis. Gentamicin has largely replaced streptomycin for these indications. Streptomycin remains a useful agent for treating enterococcal infections, however, because approximately 15% of enterococcal isolates that are resistant to gentamicin (and therefore to netilmicin, tobramycin, and amikacin) will be susceptible to streptomycin.

Adverse Reactions

Fever, skin rashes, and other allergic manifestations may result from hypersensitivity to streptomycin. This occurs most frequently upon prolonged contact with the drug, either in patients who receive a prolonged course of treatment (eg, for tuberculosis) or in medical personnel who handle the drug. Desensitization is occasionally successful.

Pain at the injection site is common but usually not severe. The most serious toxic effect is disturbance of vestibular function—vertigo and loss of balance. The frequency and severity of this disturbance are proportionate to the age of the patient, the blood levels of the drug, and the duration of administration. Vestibular dysfunction may follow a few weeks of unusually high blood levels (eg, in individuals with impaired renal function) or months of relatively low blood levels. Vestibular toxicity tends to be irreversible. Streptomycin given during pregnancy can cause deafness in the newborn.

GENTAMICIN

Gentamicin is an aminoglycoside (Figure 45–2) isolated from *Micromonospora purpurea*. It is effective against both gram-positive and gram-negative organisms, and many of its properties resemble those of other aminoglycosides. **Sisomicin** is very similar to the C_{1a} component of gentamicin.

Antimicrobial Activity

Gentamicin sulfate, 2–10 μg/mL, inhibits in vitro many strains of staphylococci and coliforms and other gram-negative bacteria. It is active alone, but also as a synergistic companion with beta-lactam antibiotics, against *Pseudomonas, Proteus, Enterobacter, Klebsiella, Serratia, Stenotrophomonas,* and other gram-negative rods that may be resistant to multiple other antibiotics. Like all aminoglycosides, it has no activity against anaerobes.

Resistance

Streptococci and enterococci are relatively resistant to gentamicin owing to failure of the drug to penetrate into the cell. However, gentamicin in combination with vancomycin or a penicillin produces a potent bactericidal effect, which in part is due to enhanced uptake of drug that occurs with inhibition of cell wall synthesis. Resistance to gentamicin rapidly emerges in staphylococci due to selection of permeability mutants. Ribosomal resistance is rare. Among gram-negative bacteria, resistance is most commonly due to plasmid-encoded aminoglycoside modifying enzymes. Gram-negative bacteria that are gentamicin-resistant usually will be susceptible to amikacin, which is much more resistant to modifying enzyme activity. The enterococcal enzyme that modifies gentamicin is a bifunctional enzyme that also modifies amikacin, netilmicin, and tobramycin, but not streptomycin; the latter is modified by a different enzyme. This is why some gentamicin-resistant enterococci are susceptible to streptomycin.

Clinical Uses

A. Intramuscular or Intravenous Administration: At present, gentamicin is employed mainly in severe infections (eg, sepsis and pneumonia) caused by gram-negative bacteria that are likely to be resistant to other drugs, especially *Pseudomonas, Enterobacter, Serratia, Proteus, Acinetobacter,* and *Klebsiella.* Patients with these infections are often immunocompromised, and the simultaneous action of the aminoglycoside with a cephalosporin or a penicillin may be life-saving. In such situations, 5–6 mg/kg/d of gentamicin is traditionally given intravenously in three equal doses. However, several studies indicate that once-daily administration is just as effective and perhaps less toxic (see box: Once-Daily Aminoglycoside Dosing). Gentamicin is also used concurrently with penicillin G for bactericidal activity in endocarditis due to viridans streptococci or enterococci and in combination with nafcillin in selected cases of staphylococcal endocarditis. Gentamicin should not be used as a single agent to treat staphylococcal infections because resistance develops rapidly. Neither gentamicin nor any other aminoglycoside should be used for single-agent therapy of pneumonia because penetration of infected lung tissue is poor and local conditions of low pH and low oxygen tension contribute to poor activity.

Serum gentamicin concentrations and renal function should be monitored if gentamicin is adminis-

tered for more than a few days or if renal function is changing (eg, in sepsis, which often is complicated by acute renal failure). For patients receiving every-8-hours dosing, target peak concentrations are 5–10 μg/mL and trough concentrations should be less than 1–2 μg/mL. Trough concentrations above 2 μg/mL indicate accumulation of drug and are associated with toxicity; in this case, the dose should be lowered or the interval extended to achieve the target range.

B. Topical Administration: Creams, ointments, or solutions containing 0.1–0.3% gentamicin sulfate have been used for the treatment of infected burns, wounds, or skin lesions and the prevention of intravenous catheter infections. Topical gentamicin is partly inactivated by purulent exudates. Ten milligrams can be injected subconjunctivally for treatment of ocular infections.

C. Intrathecal Administration: Meningitis caused by gram-negative bacteria has been treated by the intrathecal injection of gentamicin sulfate, 1–10 mg/d. However, neither intrathecal nor intraventricular gentamicin was beneficial in neonates with meningitis, and intraventricular gentamicin was toxic, raising questions about the utility of this form of therapy. Moreover, the availability of third-generation cephalosporins for gram-negative meningitis has rendered this therapy obsolete in most cases.

Adverse Reactions

Nephrotoxicity is reversible and usually mild. It occurs in 5–25% of patients receiving the drug for longer than 3–5 days. Nephrotoxicity requires, at the very least, adjustment of the dosing regimen and should prompt reconsideration of the necessity of using the drug, particularly if there is a less toxic alternative agent. Measurement of gentamicin serum levels is essential. Ototoxicity, which tends to be irreversible, manifests itself mainly as vestibular dysfunction, perhaps due to destruction of hair cells by prolonged elevated drug levels. Loss of hearing can also occur. The incidence of ototoxicity is probably 1–5% for patients receiving the drug for more than 5 days. Hypersensitivity reactions to gentamicin are uncommon.

TOBRAMYCIN

This aminoglycoside (Figure 45–2) has an antibacterial spectrum similar to that of gentamicin. While there is some cross-resistance between gentamicin and tobramycin, it is unpredictable in individual strains. Separate laboratory susceptibility tests are therefore necessary.

The pharmacokinetic properties of tobramycin are virtually identical to those of gentamicin. The daily dose of tobramycin is 5–6 mg/kg intramuscularly or intravenously, divided into three equal amounts and given every 8 hours. Monitoring blood levels in renal insufficiency is an essential guide to proper dosing.

ONCE-DAILY AMINOGLYCOSIDE DOSING

Aminoglycosides were originally developed for use in multiple daily dosing regimens. Multiple daily doses are used to maintain serum concentrations above the minimum inhibitory concentration (MIC) for susceptible bacteria for most of the day. While some period of time above MIC clearly is critical for in vivo efficacy of any antibiotic, it is most important for beta-lactams and other antibiotics that cause **time-dependent killing** (see Chapter 51)—ie, antibacterial activity is directly related to time above MIC and becomes independent of concentration once the MIC has been exceeded. Aminoglycosides, on the other hand, have **concentration-dependent killing**—ie, increasing concentrations kill an increasing proportion of bacteria and at a more rapid rate. In addition, aminoglycosides have a significant **postantibiotic effect:** antibacterial activity persists beyond the time that measurable drug is present. The postantibiotic effect of aminoglycosides is significant and can reach several hours (see Chapter 51). Because of these properties, a given total amount of aminoglycoside may have better efficacy when administered as a single large dose than when administered as multiple smaller doses.

Aminoglycoside toxicity is both time- and concentration-dependent. Toxicity is unlikely to occur until a certain threshold concentration is achieved, but once it is achieved the time above this threshold becomes critical. This threshold is imprecisely defined, but a trough concentration above 2 μg/mL is predictive of toxicity. At clinically relevant doses, the time above this threshold will be greater with multiple smaller doses of drug than with a single large dose. Correspondingly, in animal models of aminoglycoside ototoxicity and nephrotoxicity, single-dose regimens are less toxic than multiple-dose regimens for the same total dose.

Numerous clinical studies demonstrate that a single daily dose of aminoglycoside is just as effective and no more (and often less) toxic than multiple smaller doses. Therefore, many authorities now recommend that aminoglycosides be administered as a single daily dose in most clinical situations. The role for once-daily aminoglycoside dosing in combination therapy of enterococcal, streptococcal, and staphylococcal endocarditis remains to be defined, but one study found that a combination of ceftriaxone and netilmicin, each as a single daily dose, was effective for viridans streptococcal endocarditis. Once-daily dosing also has several practical advantages. There is no need to obtain serum concentrations unless the intention is to administer aminoglycoside for more than 4 or 5 days. The most common problem with aminoglycoside usage—ie, subtherapeutic serum concentrations due to underdosing drug because of a legitimate fear of toxicity—is eliminated. Less nursing time is required to give a drug once a day instead of three times a day. Once-a-day dosing lends itself to outpatient therapy.

Use of once-daily dosing does not eliminate responsibility for careful monitoring and dosage adjustment to minimize toxicity. Selection of the appropriate dose is particularly critical if renal insufficiency is present. A single 5 mg/kg dose of gentamicin (or 15 mg/kg of amikacin) given to a patient with a creatinine clearance below 30 mL/min is likely to produce serum concentrations above 5 μg for more than 24 hours, and repeating the error could be disastrous. Rapidly changing renal function, which may occur with acute renal failure in the patient with septic shock, must be anticipated to avoid overdose. Provided these pitfalls are avoided, once-daily aminoglycoside dosing is safe and effective. If the creatinine clearance is 100 mL/min, gentamicin is given as a 5 mg/kg dose (15 mg/kg for amikacin) over 30–60 minutes. If the creatinine clearance is 80 mL/min, the dose is 4 mg/kg (12 mg/kg for amikacin); and if 50 mL/min, the dose is 3 mg/kg (9 mg/kg for amikacin). If the creatinine clearance is less than 50 mL/min, the standard 2 mg/kg gentamicin loading dose is given and subsequent doses are adjusted as would normally be done. Serum concentrations need not be checked until the third to fifth days of therapy depending on the stability of renal function and the anticipated duration of therapy. It is unnecessary to check peak concentrations: they will be high. The goal is to administer drug so that concentrations of less than 1 μg/mL are present between 18 and 24 hours after dosing. This provides a sufficient period of time for washout of drug to occur before the next dose is given. This is most easily determined either by measuring serum concentrations in samples obtained 2 hours and 12 hours after dosing and then adjusting the dose based on the actual clearance of drug, or by measuring the concentration in a sample obtained 8 hours after a dose. If the 8-hour concentration is between 1.5 and 6 μg/mL, the target trough will be achieved at 18 hours.

Tobramycin has almost the same antibacterial spectrum as gentamicin with a few exceptions. Gentamicin is slightly more active against *Serratia,* whereas tobramycin is slightly more active against *Pseudomonas; Enterococcus faecalis* is susceptible to both gentamicin and tobramycin, but *E faecium* is resistant to tobramycin. Gentamicin and tobramycin are otherwise completely interchangeable clinically. Gentamicin is much less expensive, however, and is preferred for this reason.

Like other aminoglycosides, tobramycin is ototoxic and nephrotoxic. Nephrotoxicity of tobramycin may be slightly less than that of gentamicin, but the difference is clinically inconsequential.

AMIKACIN

Amikacin is a semisynthetic derivative of kanamycin; it is less toxic than the parent molecule (Figure 45–2). It is resistant to many enzymes that inactivate gentamicin and tobramycin, and it therefore can be employed against some microorganisms resistant to the latter drugs. Many gram-negative enteric bacteria, including many strains of *Proteus, Pseudomonas, Enterobacter,* and *Serratia,* are inhibited by 1–20 µg/mL amikacin in vitro. After the injection of 500 mg of amikacin every 12 hours (15 mg/kg/d) intramuscularly, peak levels in serum are 10–30 µg/mL.

Strains of multidrug-resistant *Mycobacterium tuberculosis,* including streptomycin-resistant strains, are usually susceptible to amikacin. Kanamycin-resistant strains may be cross-resistant to amikacin. The dosage of amikacin for tuberculosis is 7.5–15 mg/kg/d as a once-daily or two to three times weekly injection, always in combination with other drugs to which the isolate is susceptible.

Like all aminoglycosides, amikacin is nephrotoxic and ototoxic (particularly for the auditory portion of the eighth nerve). Serum concentrations should be monitored. Target peak serum concentrations for an every-12-hours dosing regimen are 20–40 µg/mL, and troughs should be maintained at less than 2 µg/mL.

NETILMICIN

This aminoglycoside became available in the USA in 1983. It shares many characteristics with gentamicin and tobramycin. However, the addition of an ethyl group to the 1-amino position of the 2-deoxystreptamine ring (ring II, Figure 45–2) sterically protects the netilmicin molecule from enzymatic degradation at the 3-amino (ring II) and 2-hydroxyl (ring III) positions. Consequently, netilmicin may not be inactivated by many gentamicin-resistant and tobramycin-resistant bacteria.

The dosage (5–7 mg/kg/d) and the routes of administration are the same as for gentamicin. It is completely therapeutically interchangeable with gentamicin or tobramycin and has similar toxicities.

KANAMYCIN & NEOMYCIN

These drugs are closely related. **Paromomycin** is also a member of this group. All have similar properties.

Antimicrobial Activity & Resistance

Drugs of the neomycin group are active against gram-positive and gram-negative bacteria and some mycobacteria. *Pseudomonas* and streptococci are generally resistant. Mechanisms of antibacterial action and resistance are the same as with other aminoglycosides. The widespread use of these drugs in bowel preparation for elective surgery has resulted in the selection of resistant organisms and some outbreaks of enterocolitis in hospitals. There is complete cross-resistance between kanamycin and neomycin.

Pharmacokinetics

Drugs of the neomycin group are not significantly absorbed from the gastrointestinal tract. After oral administration, the intestinal flora is suppressed or modified and the drug is excreted in the feces. Excretion of any absorbed drug is mainly through glomerular filtration into the urine.

Clinical Uses

Neomycin is too toxic for parenteral use. With the advent of more potent and less toxic aminoglycosides, parenteral administration of kanamycin has also been abandoned. Neomycin and kanamycin are now limited to topical and oral use.

A. Topical Administration: Solutions containing 1–5 mg/mL are used on infected surfaces or injected into joints, the pleural cavity, tissue spaces, or abscess cavities where infection is present. The total amount of drug given in this fashion must be limited to 15 mg/kg/d because at higher doses enough drug may be absorbed to produce systemic toxicity. Whether topical application for active infection adds anything to appropriate systemic therapy is questionable. Ointments, often formulated as a neomycin-polymyxin-bacitracin combination, are applied to infected skin lesions or in the nares for suppression of staphylococci; they are largely ineffective.

B. Oral Administration: In preparation for elective bowel surgery, 1 g of neomycin is given orally every 6–8 hours for 1–2 days, often combined with 1 g of erythromycin base. This reduces the aerobic bowel flora with little effect on anaerobes. In hepatic coma, the coliform flora can be suppressed for prolonged periods by giving 1 g every 6–8 hours together with reduced protein intake, thus reducing ammonia intoxication. Use of neomycin for hepatic coma has been almost entirely supplanted by lactulose, which is much less toxic. Paromomycin, 1 g every 6 hours orally for 2 weeks, has been effective in intestinal amebiasis.

Adverse Reactions

All members of the neomycin group have significant nephrotoxicity and ototoxicity. Auditory function is affected more than vestibular. Deafness has occurred, especially in adults with impaired renal function and prolonged elevation of drug levels.

The sudden absorption of postoperatively instilled kanamycin from the peritoneal cavity (3–5 g) has resulted in curare-like neuromuscular blockade and respiratory arrest. Calcium gluconate and neostigmine can act as antidotes.

While hypersensitivity is not common, prolonged application of neomycin-containing ointments to skin and eyes has resulted in severe allergic reactions.

SPECTINOMYCIN

Spectinomycin is an aminocyclitol antibiotic that is structurally related to aminoglycosides. It lacks amino sugars and glycosidic bonds (Figure 45–4). It is dis-

Spectinomycin

Figure 45–4. Structure of spectinomycin.

pensed as the dihydrochloride pentahydrate for intramuscular injection. While active in vitro against many gram-positive and gram-negative organisms, spectinomycin is used almost solely as an alternative treatment for gonorrhea in patients who are allergic to penicillin or whose gonococci are resistant to other drugs. The vast majority of gonococcal isolates are inhibited by 6 μg/mL of spectinomycin. Strains of gonococci may be resistant to spectinomycin, but there is no cross-resistance with other drugs used in gonorrhea. Spectinomycin is rapidly absorbed after intramuscular injection. A single dose of 2 g (40 mg/kg) is given. There is pain at the injection site and occasionally fever and nausea. Nephrotoxicity and anemia have been observed rarely.

PREPARATIONS AVAILABLE

Amikacin (generic, Amikin)
   Parenteral: 50, 250 mg (in vials) for IM, IV
      injection
Gentamicin (generic, Garamycin, Jenamicin)
   Parenteral: 10, 40 mg/mL vials for IM, IV
      injection; 2 mg/mL vials for intrathecal use
Kanamycin (Kantrex)
   Oral: 500 mg capsules
   Parenteral: 500, 1000 mg for IM, IV injection;
      75 mg for pediatric injection
Neomycin (generic, Mycifradin)
   Oral: 500 mg tablets; 125 mg/5 mL solution
Netilmicin (Netromycin)
   Parenteral: 100 mg/mL for IM, IV injection

Paromomycin (Humatin)
   Oral: 250 mg capsules
Spectinomycin (Trobicin)
   Parenteral: powder to reconstitute for IM
      injection (2, 4 g per vial)
Streptomycin (generic)
   Parenteral: 400 mg/mL for IM injection; also
      available as powder to reconstitute for injection
Tobramycin (generic, Nebcin)
   Parenteral: 10, 30 mg/mL for IM, IV injection;
      powder to reconstitute 30 mg/mL injection

REFERENCES

Appel JB, Neu HC: The nephrotoxicity of antimicrobial agents. (Three parts.) N Engl J Med 1977;296:663, 722, 784.

Blair DC: Inactivation of amikacin and gentamicin by carbenicillin in patients with end-stage renal failure. Antimicrob Agents Chemother 1982;22:376.

Boslego JW et al: Effect of spectinomycin use on the prevalence of spectinomycin-resistant and of penicillinase-producing *Neisseria gonorrhoeae.* N Engl J Med 1987;317:272.

Busse H-J, Wöstmann C, Bakker EP: The bactericidal action of streptomycin: Membrane permeabilization caused by the insertion of mistranslated proteins into the cytoplasmic membrane of *Escherichia coli* and subsequent caging of the antibiotic inside the cells due to degradation of these proteins. J Gen Microbiol 1992; 138:551.

Chan RA et al: Gentamicin therapy in renal failure: A dosage nomogram. Ann Intern Med 1972;76:773.

Edson RS, Terrell CL: The aminoglycosides: Streptomycin, kanamycin, gentamicin, tobramycin, amikacin, netilmicin, and sisomicin. Mayo Clin Proc 1987;62:916.

Gilbert DN: Mini-review: Once-daily aminoglycoside therapy. Antimicrob Agents Chemother 1991;35:399.

Hughes WT et al: Guidelines for the use of antimicrobial agents in neutropenic patients with unexplained fever. J Infect Dis 1990;161:381.

Krogstad DJ et al: Plasmid-mediated resistance to antibiotic synergism in enterococci. J Clin Invest 1978;61:1645.

Love LJ et al: Randomized trial of empiric antibiotic therapy with ticarcillin in combination with gentamicin, amikacin or netilmicin in febrile patients with granulocytopenia and cancer. Am J Med 1979;66:603.

Maigaard S, Frimodt-Moller N, Madsen PO: Comparison of netilmicin and amikacin in treatment of complicated urinary tract infections. Antimicrob Agents Chemother 1978;14:554.

McCormack JP, Jewesson PJ: A critical reevaluation of the "therapeutic range" of aminoglycosides. Clin Infect Dis 1992;14:320.

McCracken GH et al: Intraventricular gentamicin therapy in gram-negative bacillary meningitis of infancy. Lancet 1980;1:787.

Meyer RD: Drugs five years later: Amikacin. Ann Intern Med 1981;95:328.

Moellering RC Jr: Have the new beta-lactams rendered the aminoglycosides obsolete for the treatment of serious nosocomial infections? Am J Med 1986;80(Suppl 6B):44.

Neu HC: New antibiotics: Areas of appropriate use. J Infect Dis 1987;155:403.

Noone M et al: Prospective study of amikacin vs netilmicin in the treatment of severe infections in hospitalized patients. Am J Med 1989;86:809.

Prins JM et al: Once versus thrice daily gentamicin in patients with serious infections. Lancet 1993;341:335.

Rettig PJ et al: Spectinomycin therapy for gonorrhea in prepubertal children. Am J Dis Child 1980;134:359.

Riff LJ, Jackson GG: Conditions for gentamicin inactivation by carbenicillin. Arch Intern Med 1972;130:887.

Sarubbi FA, Hull JH: Amikacin serum concentrations: Prediction of levels and dosage guidelines. Ann Intern Med 1978;89:612.

Smith CR et al: Double blind comparison of the nephrotoxicity and auditory toxicity of gentamicin and tobramycin. N Engl J Med 1980;302:1106.

Snavely SR, Hodges GR: The neurotoxicity of antibacterial agents. Ann Intern Med 1984;101:92.

Spera RV Jr, Farber BF: Multiply-resistant *Enterococcus faecium.* The nosocomial pathogen of the 1990s. JAMA 1992;268:2563.

Swan SK, Bennett WM: Drug dosing guidelines in patients with renal failure. West J Med 1992;156:633.

Swartz MN: Intraventricular use of aminoglycosides in the treatment of gram-negative bacillary meningitis: Conflicting views. J Infect Dis 1981;143:293.

Tablan OC et al: Renal and auditory toxicity of high-dose, prolonged therapy with gentamicin and tobramycin in *Pseudomonas* endocarditis. J Infect Dis 1984;149:257.

Wilson WR et al: Antibiotic treatment of adults with infective endocarditis due to streptococci, enterococci, staphylococci, and HACEK microorganisms. JAMA 1995;274:1706.

Sulfonamides, Trimethoprim, & Quinolones

46

Henry F. Chambers, MD, & Ernest Jawetz, MD, PhD

I. ANTIFOLATE DRUGS

SULFONAMIDES

Chemistry

The basic formula of the sulfonamides and their structural similarity to *p*-aminobenzoic acid (PABA) are shown in Figure 46–1.

Sulfonamides with varying physical, chemical, pharmacologic, and antibacterial properties are produced by attaching substituents to the amido group ($-SO_2-NH-R$) or the amino group ($-NH_2$) of the sulfanilamide nucleus. Sulfonamides tend to be much more soluble at alkaline than at acid pH. Most can be prepared as sodium salts, which are used for intravenous administration.

Antimicrobial Activity

Susceptible microorganisms require extracellular PABA in order to form dihydrofolic acid (Figure 46–2), an essential step in the production of purines and the synthesis of nucleic acids. Sulfonamides are structural analogs of PABA that competitively inhibit dihydropteroate synthase. They inhibit growth by reversibly blocking folic acid synthesis. Accordingly, sulfonamides are bacteriostatic, not bactericidal, drugs.

Sulfonamides inhibit both gram-positive and gram-negative bacteria, *Nocardia*, *Chlamydia trachomatis*, and some protozoa. Some enteric bacteria, such as *E coli*, *Klebsiella*, *Salmonella*, *Shigella*, and *Enterobacter*, are inhibited. Interestingly, rickettsiae are not inhibited by sulfonamides but are actually stimulated in their growth.

Resistance

Mammalian cells (and some bacteria) lack the enzymes required for folate synthesis and depend upon exogenous sources of folate; therefore, they are not susceptible to sulfonamides. Sulfonamide resistance may occur as a result of mutations that cause overproduction of PABA, cause production of a folic acid-synthesizing enzyme that has low affinity for sulfonamides, or cause a loss of permeability to the sulfonamide. Dihydropteroate synthase with low sulfonamide affinity is often encoded on a plasmid that is transmissible and can disseminate rapidly and widely. Sulfonamide-resistant cells may be present in susceptible bacterial populations and can emerge under selective pressure.

Pharmacokinetics

Sulfonamides can be divided into three major groups: (1) oral, absorbable; (2) oral, nonabsorbable; and (3) topical. Sodium salts of sulfonamides in 5% dextrose in water can be given intravenously, but except for sulfamethoxazole-trimethoprim combinations, these are rarely used. The oral, absorbable sulfonamides can be classified as short-, medium-, or long-acting on the basis of their half-lives (Table 46–1). They are absorbed from the stomach and small intestine and distributed widely to tissues and body fluids (including the central nervous system and cerebrospinal fluid), placenta, and fetus. Absorbed sulfonamides become bound to serum proteins to an extent varying from 20% to over 90%. Therapeutic concentrations are in the range of 40–100 μg/mL of blood. Peak blood levels generally occur 2–6 hours after oral administration.

A portion of absorbed drug is acetylated or glucuronidated in the liver. Sulfonamides and inactivated metabolites are then excreted into the urine, mainly by glomerular filtration. In significant renal failure, the dosage of sulfonamide must be reduced.

Sulfanilamide

p-Aminobenzoic acid (PABA)

Sulfadiazine

Sulfisoxazole

Sulfamethoxazole

**Sulfathalidine
(phthalylsulfathiazole)**

Figure 46–1. Structures of some sulfonamides and p-aminobenzoic acid.

Table 46–1. Pharmacokinetic properties of some sulfonamides and trimethoprim.

Drug	Half-Life	Oral Absorption
Sulfonamides		
Sulfacytine	No data	Prompt (peak levels in 1–4 hours)
Sulfisoxazole	Short (6 hours)	Prompt
Sulfamethizole	Short (9 hours)	Prompt
Sulfadiazine	Intermediate (10–17 hours)	Slow (peak levels in 4–8 hours)
Sulfamethox-azole	Intermediate (10–12 hours)	Slow
Sulfapyridine	No data	Slow
Sulfadoxine	Long (7–9 days)	Intermediate
Pyrimidines		
Trimethoprim	Intermediate (11 hours)	Prompt

Clinical Uses

Sulfonamides are infrequently used as single agents. Formerly drugs of choice for infections such as *Pneumocystis carinii* pneumonia, toxoplasmosis, nocardiosis, and occasionally other bacterial infections, they have been largely supplanted by the fixed drug combination of trimethoprim-sulfamethoxazole (see below). Numerous other antimicrobials that are often more effective and less toxic have been introduced into clinical practice during the 60 years since sulfonamides were introduced. Many strains of formerly susceptible species, including meningococci, pneumococci, streptococci, staphylococci, and gonococci, are now resistant. Nevertheless, sulfonamides can be useful for treatment of urinary tract infections due to susceptible organisms and in other special clinical situations discussed below.

A. Oral Absorbable Agents: Sulfisoxazole and sulfamethoxazole are short- to medium-acting agents that are used almost exclusively to treat urinary tract infections. The usual adult dosage is 1 g of sulfisoxazole four times daily or 1 g of sulfamethoxazole two or three times daily. Each is available in combination with phenazopyridine, a urinary tract anesthetic, sold as Azo Gantanol and Azo Gantrisin, respectively. In developing countries, sulfonamides, because they are so inexpensive, continue to be used widely for respiratory tract infections, sinusitis, bronchitis, pneumonia, otitis media, and dysentery.

Sulfadiazine achieves therapeutic concentrations in cerebrospinal fluid and in combination with pyrimethamine is first-line therapy for treatment of acute toxoplasmosis. Pyrimethamine, an antiprotozoal agent, is a potent inhibitor of dihydrofolate reductase. The combination of sulfadiazine and pyrimethamine is synergistic because these drugs block sequential steps in the folate synthetic pathway blockade (Figure 46–2). The dosage of sulfadiazine is 1 g four times daily, with pyrimethamine given as a 75 mg loading dose followed by a 25 mg once-daily dose. Folinic

Figure 46–2. Actions of sulfonamides and trimethoprim.

acid, 10 mg orally each day, should also be administered to minimize bone marrow suppression.

Sulfadoxine, the only long-acting sulfonamide currently available in the United States, is well absorbed after oral intake. Urinary excretion—especially of the free form—is very slow, resulting in prolonged drug levels in serum. The slow renal excretion is due in part to the high protein binding (more than 85%) and in part to the extensive tubular reabsorption of the free drug. Sulfadoxine is available only as Fansidar, a combination formulation with pyrimethamine, which is used as a second-line agent in treatment for malaria.

B. Oral Nonabsorbable Agents: Sulfasalazine (salicylazosulfapyridine) is widely used in ulcerative colitis, enteritis, and other inflammatory bowel disease. This drug is more effective than soluble sulfonamides or other antimicrobials taken orally—all of which may occasionally have a beneficial effect in inflammatory bowel disease. Sulfasalazine is split by intestinal microflora to yield sulfapyridine and 5-aminosalicylate. Salicylate is released in the colon in high concentration and is responsible for an anti-inflammatory effect, the major source of benefit from this drug. Comparably high concentrations of salicylate cannot be achieved in the colon by oral intake of ordinary formulations of salicylates because of severe gastrointestinal toxicity (see Chapter 63). The sulfapyridine is absorbed and may lead to toxic symptoms if more than 4 g of sulfasalazine is taken per day, particularly in persons who are slow acetylators. Olsalazine, a dimer of salicylic acid, is split by bacteria in the colon and is active in ulcerative colitis. It may be better tolerated than sulfasalazine.

C. Topical Agents: Sodium sulfacetamide ophthalmic solution or ointment is effective treatment for bacterial conjunctivitis and as adjunctive therapy for trachoma. Mafenide acetate is used topically to prevent bacterial colonization and infection of burn wounds. Mafenide is absorbed from burn sites, and systemic levels are produced. The drug and its primary metabolite also inhibit carbonic anhydrase and can cause metabolic acidosis, a side effect that limits its usefulness. Silver sulfadiazine is a much less toxic topical sulfonamide and is preferred to mafenide for prevention of infection of burn wounds.

Adverse Reactions

Sulfonamides produce a wide variety of reactions due partly to allergy and partly to toxicity of the active drug and its metabolites. Up to 5% of patients exhibit untoward reactions. All sulfonamides and their derivatives, including carbonic anhydrase inhibitors, thiazides, furosemide, bumetanide, torsemide, diazoxide, and the sulfonylurea hypoglycemic agents, are cross-allergenic.

The most common adverse effects are fever, skin rashes, exfoliative dermatitis, photosensitivity, urticaria, nausea, vomiting, diarrhea, and difficulties referable to the urinary tract (see below). Stevens-Johnson syndrome, although relatively uncommon (ie, fewer than 1% of treatment courses), is a particularly serious and potentially fatal type of skin and mucous membrane eruption associated with sulfonamide use. Other unwanted effects include stomatitis, conjunctivitis, arthritis, hematopoietic disturbances (see below), hepatitis, and, rarely, polyarteritis nodosa and psychosis.

A. Urinary Tract Disturbances: Sulfonamides may precipitate in urine, especially at neutral or acid pH, producing crystalluria, hematuria, or even obstruction. This is rarely a problem with the more soluble sulfonamides (eg, sulfisoxazole). Sulfadiazine when given in large doses, particularly if fluid intake is poor, can cause crystalluria. Crystalluria is treated by administration of sodium bicarbonate to alkalinize the urine and fluids to maintain adequate hydration. Sulfonamides have also been implicated in various types of nephrosis and in allergic nephritis.

B. Hematopoietic Disturbances: Sulfonamides can cause hemolytic or aplastic anemia, granulocytopenia, thrombocytopenia, or leukemoid reactions. Sulfonamides may provoke hemolytic reactions in patients whose red cells are deficient in glucose-6-phosphate dehydrogenase. Sulfonamides taken near the end of pregnancy increase the risk of kernicterus in newborns.

TRIMETHOPRIM & TRIMETHOPRIM-SULFAMETHOXAZOLE MIXTURES

Trimethoprim, a trimethoxybenzylpyrimidine, inhibits bacterial dihydrofolic acid reductase about 50,000 times more efficiently than the same enzyme of mammalian cells. Pyrimethamine, another benzylpyrimidine, inhibits the activity of dihydrofolic acid reductase of protozoa more than that of mammalian cells. Dihydrofolic acid reductases convert dihydrofolic acid to tetrahydrofolic acid, a stage leading to the synthesis of purines and ultimately to DNA. Trimethoprim or pyrimethamine, given together with sulfonamides, produces sequential blocking in this metabolic sequence, resulting in marked enhancement (synergism) of the activity of both drugs (Figure 46–2). The combination often is bactericidal, compared to the bacteriostatic activity of a sulfonamide alone.

Resistance

Resistance to trimethoprim can result from reduced cell permeability, overproduction of dihydrofolate reductase, or production of an altered reductase with reduced drug binding. Resistance can emerge by mutation, though more commonly it is due to plasmid-encoded trimethoprim-resistant dihydrofolate reductases. These resistant enzymes may be located

Trimethoprim

Pyrimethamine

within transposons on conjugative plasmids that exhibit a broad host range, accounting for rapid and widespread dissemination of trimethoprim resistance among numerous bacterial species.

Pharmacokinetics

Trimethoprim is usually given orally, alone or in combination with sulfamethoxazole, the latter chosen because it has a similar half-life. Trimethoprim-sulfamethoxazole can also be given intravenously. Trimethoprim is absorbed well from the gut and distributed widely in body fluids and tissues, including cerebrospinal fluid. Because trimethoprim is more lipid-soluble than sulfamethoxazole, it has a larger volume of distribution than the latter drug. Therefore, when 1 part of trimethoprim is given with 5 parts of sulfamethoxazole (the ratio in the formulation), the peak plasma concentrations are in the ratio of 1:20, which is optimal for the combined effects of these drugs in vitro. About 65–70% of each participant drug is protein-bound, and 30–50% of the sulfonamide and 50–60% of the trimethoprim (or their respective metabolites) are excreted in the urine within 24 hours. The dose should be reduced by half for patients with creatinine clearances of 15 to 30 mL/min.

Trimethoprim (a weak base of pK_a 7.2) concentrates in prostatic fluid and in vaginal fluid, which are more acid than plasma. Therefore, it has more antibacterial activity in prostatic and vaginal fluids than many other antimicrobial drugs.

Clinical Uses

A. Oral Trimethoprim: Trimethoprim can be given alone (100 mg twice daily) in acute urinary tract infections. Most community-acquired organisms tend to be susceptible to the high concentrations that are found in the urine (200–600 µg/mL).

B. Oral Trimethoprim-Sulfamethoxazole: A combination of trimethoprim-sulfamethoxazole is effective treatment for *Pneumocystis carinii* pneumonia, shigellosis, systemic *Salmonella* infections

(caused by ampicillin- or chloramphenicol-resistant organisms), complicated urinary tract infections, prostatitis, some nontuberculous mycobacterial infections, and many others. It is active against many respiratory tract pathogens, including the pneumococcus, *Haemophilus* species, *Moraxella catarrhalis,* and *Klebsiella* (but not *Mycoplasma*) *pneumoniae,* making it a potentially useful alternative to beta-lactam drugs for treatment of upper respiratory tract infections and community-acquired bacterial pneumonia. However. the increasing prevalence of strains of *E coli* (up to 30% or more) and penicillin-resistant pneumococci that are resistant to trimethoprim-sulfamethoxazole must be considered before using this combination for empirical therapy of upper urinary tract infections or pneumonia.

Two double-strength tablets (trimethoprim 160 mg plus sulfamethoxazole 800 mg) given every 12 hours are effective treatment for urinary tract infections and prostatitis. One-half of the regular size (single-strength) tablet given three times weekly for many months may serve as prophylaxis in recurrent urinary tract infections of some women. Two double-strength tablets every 12 hours is effective treatment for infections caused by susceptible strains of *Shigella* and *Salmonella.* The dosage for children treated for shigellosis, urinary tract infection, or otitis media is 8 mg/kg trimethoprim and 40 mg/kg sulfamethoxazole every 12 hours.

Infections with *P carinii* and some other pathogens can be treated orally with high doses of the combination (dosed on the basis of the trimethoprim component at 15–20 mg/kg) or can be prevented in immunosuppressed patients by one double-strength table daily or three times weekly.

C. Intravenous Trimethoprim-Sulfamethoxazole: A solution of the mixture containing 80 mg trimethoprim plus 400 mg sulfamethoxazole per 5 mL diluted in 125 mL of 5% dextrose in water can be administered by intravenous infusion over 60–90 minutes. It is the agent of choice for moderately severe to severe *P carinii* pneumonia, especially in patients with AIDS. It may be used for gram-negative bacterial sepsis, including that caused by some multiple-drug-resistant species such as *Enterobacter* and *Serratia;* shigellosis; typhoid fever; or urinary tract infection caused by a susceptible organism when the patient is unable to take the drug by mouth. The dosage is 10–20 mg/kg/d of the trimethoprim component.

D. Oral Pyrimethamine With Sulfonamide: Pyrimethamine and sulfadiazine have been used for treatment of leishmaniasis and toxoplasmosis. In falciparum malaria, the combination of pyrimethamine with sulfadoxine (Fansidar) has been employed (see Chapter 53).

Adverse Effects

Trimethoprim produces the predictable adverse effects of an antifolate drug, especially megaloblastic anemia, leukopenia, and granulocytopenia. This can be prevented by the simultaneous administration of folinic acid, 6–8 mg/d. In addition, the combination trimethoprim-sulfamethoxazole may cause all of the untoward reactions associated with sulfonamides. Nausea and vomiting, drug fever, vasculitis, renal damage, and central nervous system disturbances occasionally occur also. Patients with AIDS and pneumocystis pneumonia have a particularly high frequency of untoward reactions to trimethoprim-sulfamethoxazole, especially fever, rashes, leukopenia, and diarrhea.

II. DNA GYRASE INHIBITORS

FLUOROQUINOLONES

The important quinolones are synthetic fluorinated analogs of nalidixic acid. They are active against a variety of gram-positive and gram-negative bacteria. Quinolones block bacterial DNA synthesis by inhibiting bacterial topoisomerase II (DNA gyrase) and topoisomerase IV. Inhibition of DNA gyrase prevents the relaxation of positively supercoiled DNA that is required for normal transcription and replication. Inhibition of topoisomerase IV probably interferes with separation of replicated chromosomal DNA into the respective daughter cells during cell division.

Earlier quinolones (nalidixic acid, oxolinic acid, cinoxacin) did not achieve systemic antibacterial levels. These agents were useful only for treatment of lower urinary tract infections (see below); nalidixic acid and cinoxacin are still available. Fluorinated derivatives (ciprofloxacin, ofloxacin, and others; see Figure 46–3 and Table 46–2) have greatly improved

antibacterial activity compared with nalidixic acid and achieve bactericidal levels in blood and tissues.

Antibacterial Activity

Norfloxacin is the least active of the fluoroquinolones. Its MICs are fourfold to eightfold greater than those of ofloxacin or ciprofloxacin for most bacteria. **Sparfloxacin,** a new fluoroquinolone recently approved by the FDA, and **clinafloxacin** and **trovafloxacin,** which are investigational agents, are several times more potent than currently available agents, particularly against gram-positive species. **Ofloxacin** and **ciprofloxacin** inhibit gram-negative cocci and bacilli, including Enterobacteriaceae, *Pseudomonas, Neisseria, Haemophilus,* and *Campylobacter,* at concentrations of 1–2 μg/mL or less. Many staphylococci also are inhibited at concentrations of less than 2 μg/mL. Streptococci, including the pneumococcus, and enterococci tend to be less susceptible than staphylococci, and efficacy of most fluoroquinolones for infections caused by these organisms is limited. Sparfloxacin and **levofloxacin,** the latter being the L-isomer of ofloxacin (an equimolar mixture of D,L-isomers) are more active than ciprofloxacin and ofloxacin against staphylococci and streptococci. Intracellular pathogens such as *Legionella, Chlamydia,* and some mycobacteria, including *M tuberculosis* and *M avium* complex, are inhibited by fluoroquinolones. Anaerobes generally are resistant, though sparfloxacin exhibits some activity in vitro.

Resistance

During fluoroquinolone therapy, resistant organisms emerge with a frequency of about one in 10^7–10^9, especially among staphylococci, *Pseudomonas,* and *Serratia.* Resistance is due to one or more

Figure 46–3. Structures of some fluoroquinolones.

Table 46–2. Pharmacokinetic properties of fluoroquinolones.

Drug	Half-Life (h)	Oral Bioavailability (%)	Peak Serum Concentration (µg/mL)	Oral Dose (mg)
Ciprofloxacin	3–4.5	85	3	500
Enoxacin	3–6	90	4	400
Levofloxacin	5–7	95	8	400
Lomefloxacin	8	95	3	400
Norfloxacin	3.5–5	80	1.5	400
Ofloxacin	5–7	95	8	400
Pefloxacin	10	90	6	400
Sparfloxacin	16–22	—[1]	0.7–1.5	400

[1]Bioavailability is similar to that of other fluoroquinolones.

point mutations in the quinolone binding region of the target enzyme or to a change in the permeability of the organism. DNA gyrase is the primary target in *E coli*, with single-step mutants exhibiting amino acid substitution in the A subunit of gyrase. Topoisomerase IV is a secondary target in *E coli* that is altered in mutants expressing higher levels of resistance. In staphylococci and streptococci, the situation is reversed: topoisomerase IV is the primary target, and gyrase is the secondary target.

Pharmacokinetics (Table 46–2)

After oral administration, the fluoroquinolones are well absorbed (bioavailability of 80–95%) and distributed widely in body fluids and tissues. Serum half-lives range from 3 hours (norfloxacin and ciprofloxacin) up to 10 (pefloxacin and fleroxacin) or even 20 hours (sparfloxacin). The relatively long half-lives of levofloxacin and sparfloxacin permit once-daily dosing. The pharmacokinetics of ofloxacin and levofloxacin are identical. Oral absorption is impaired by divalent cations, including those in antacids. Serum concentrations of intravenously administered drug are similar to those of orally administered drug. Concentrations in prostate, kidney, neutrophils, and macrophages exceed serum concentrations. The fluoroquinolones are excreted mainly by tubular secretion (which can be blocked by probenecid) and by glomerular filtration. Sparfloxacin is metabolized by conjugation to glucuronide, an inactive metabolite that is cleared by the kidney. Up to 20% of the dose is metabolized by the liver. All fluoroquinolones accumulate in renal failure, and dosage adjustment is required at creatinine clearances of 50 mL/min or less.

Clinical Uses

Fluoroquinolones are effective in urinary tract infections even when caused by multidrug-resistant bacteria, eg, *Pseudomonas*. Norfloxacin 400 mg, ciprofloxacin 500 mg, and ofloxacin 400 mg given orally twice daily—all are effective. These agents are also effective for bacterial diarrhea caused by

Shigella, Salmonella, toxigenic *E coli,* or *Campylobacter.* Fluoroquinolones (except norfloxacin, which does not achieve adequate systemic concentrations) have been employed in infections of soft tissues, bones, and joints and in intra-abdominal and respiratory tract infections, including those caused by multidrug-resistant organisms such as *Pseudomonas* and *Enterobacter.* Ciprofloxacin and ofloxacin are effective for gonococcal infection, including disseminated disease, and ofloxacin is effective for chlamydial urethritis or cervicitis. Ciprofloxacin is a second-line agent for legionellosis. Ciprofloxacin or ofloxacin is occasionally used for treatment of tuberculosis and atypical mycobacterial infections. They may be suitable for eradication of meningococci from carriers or for prophylaxis of infection in neutropenic patients.

Owing to their marginal activity against the pneumococcus, fluoroquinolones have not been routinely recommended for empirical treatment of pneumonia and other upper respiratory tract infections. However, levofloxacin, sparfloxacin, and newer investigational fluoroquinolones with enhanced gram-positive activity and activity against atypical pneumonia agents (eg, *Chlamydia, Mycoplasma,* and *Legionella*) are likely to be effective and used increasingly for treatment of upper and lower respiratory tract infections.

Adverse Effects

Fluoroquinolones are extremely well tolerated. The most common effects are nausea, vomiting, and diarrhea. Occasionally, headache, dizziness, insomnia, skin rash, or abnormal liver function tests develop. Photosensitivity has been reported with lomefloxacin and pefloxacin. Concomitant administration of theophylline and quinolones can lead to elevated levels of theophylline with the risk of toxic effects, especially seizures. Fluoroquinolones may damage growing cartilage and cause an arthropathy. Thus, they are not routinely recommended for use in patients under 18 years of age. However, the arthropathy is reversible, and there is a growing consensus that fluoro-

FLUOROQUINOLONES: USE, MISUSE, & RESISTANCE

Fluoroquinolones are extremely useful agents and an important therapeutic advance. They are relatively nontoxic, well tolerated, broad-spectrum agents. Their excellent oral bioavailability permits their use for treatment of a variety of serious bacterial infections such as those caused by *Pseudomonas aeruginosa* or methicillin-resistant *S aureus,* which formerly could be treated only with parenteral agents. As strains of *E coli* and other gram-negative pathogens resistant to trimethoprim-sulfamethoxazole have become more common, fluoroquinolones are increasingly relied on for empirical therapy of urinary tract infections.

Unfortunately, overuse and inappropriate use have already eroded the clinical utility of these agents. The fluoroquinolones currently available should not be used for treatment of routine upper and lower respiratory tract infections or for skin and soft tissue infections. Pneumococci and streptococci, the predominant causes of such infections, are relatively resistant to currently available fluoroquinolones; other agents (eg, beta-lactam or macrolide drugs), should be used. Overuse of the fluoroquinolones, particularly in the hospital setting, has led to selection of resistance, which occurs in a single step. Strains of methicillin-resistant *S aureus,* formerly uniformly susceptible to fluoroquinolones, must now be considered resistant until in vitro susceptibility is demonstrated.

Newer, more potent fluoroquinolones such as clinafloxacin and trovafloxacin are under development. These agents have improved activity against gram-positive organisms and some gram-negatives, including some quinolone-resistant strains. They may have a role in treatment of pneumonia because of their improved activity against the pneumococcus, including penicillin-resistant strains. Emergence of resistance to these newer fluoroquinolones will still be a concern. The challenge is to be better stewards in use of these compounds than has been the case for their predecessors.

quinolones may be used in children in some cases (eg, for treatment of pseudomonal infections in patients with cystic fibrosis). Tendinitis, a rare complication that has been reported in adults, is potentially more serious because of the risk of tendon rupture. Since fluoroquinolones are excreted in breast milk, they are are contraindicated for nursing mothers. They should be avoided during pregnancy in the absence of specific data documenting their safety.

NALIDIXIC ACID & CINOXACIN

Nalidixic acid, the first antibacterial quinolone, was introduced in 1963. It is not fluorinated and is excreted too rapidly to have systemic antibacterial effects. Oxolinic acid and cinoxacin are similar in structure and function to nalidixic acid. Their mechanism of action is the same as for the fluoroquinolones. Because of their relatively weak antibacterial activity, these agents were useful only for the treatment of urinary tract infections. They are rarely used now, having been made obsolete by the more efficacious fluorinated quinolones.

NOVOBIOCIN

Novobiocin is an acidic antibiotic produced by *Streptomyces niveus.* It is an inhibitor of the B subunit of DNA gyrase and is active mainly against gram-positive bacteria. To avoid rapid emergence of resistant variants, novobiocin had to be employed in combination with another drug, and the incidence of adverse effects was high. Although the drug is still available, there appears to be no indication for the use of novobiocin at present.

PREPARATIONS AVAILABLE

General-Purpose Sulfonamides
Multiple sulfonamides, trisulfapyrimidines
(generic)
Oral: 500 mg (total sulfonamide) tablets
Sulfacytine (Renoquid)
Oral: 250 mg tablets
Sulfadiazine (generic)
Oral: 500 mg tablets
Sulfamethizole (Thiosulfil Forte)
Oral: 500 mg tablets
Sulfamethoxazole (generic, Gantanol, others)
Oral: 0.5 g tablets; 500 mg/5 mL suspension
Sulfisoxazole (generic, Gantrisin)
Oral: 500 mg tablets; 500 mg/5 mL syrup
Ophthalmic: 4% solution

Sulfonamides for Special Applications
Mafenide (Sulfamylon)
Topical: 85 mg/g cream
Silver sulfadiazine (generic, Silvadene)
Topical: 10 mg/g cream
Sulfasalazine (generic, Azulfidine)
Oral: 500 mg tablets and enteric-coated tablets;
250 mg/5 mL suspension
Sulfacetamide sodium (generic)
Ophthalmic: 10, 15, 30% solutions; 10% ointment

Trimethoprim
Trimethoprim (generic, Proloprim, Trimpex)
Oral: 100, 200 mg tablets
Trimethoprim-sulfamethoxazole [co-trimoxazole, TMP-SMZ] (generic, Bactrim, Septra, others)
Oral: 80 mg trimethoprim + 400 mg sulfamethoxazole per single-strength tablet; 160 mg trimethoprim + 800 mg sulfamethoxazole per double-strength tablet; 40 mg trimethoprim + 200 mg sulfamethoxazole per 5 mL suspension
Parenteral: 80 mg trimethoprim + 400 mg sulfamethoxazole per 5 mL for infusion (in 5 mL ampules and 5, 10, 20, 30, 50 mL vials)

Quinolones & Fluoroquinolones
Cinoxacin (generic, Cinobac)
Oral: 250, 500 mg capsules
Ciprofloxacin (Cipro, Cipro I.V.)
Oral: 250, 500, 750 mg tablets
Parenteral: 2, 10 mg/mL
Enoxacin (Penetrex)
Oral: 200, 400 mg tablets
Levofloxacin (Levaquin)
Oral: 250, 500 mg tablets
Parenteral: 250, 500 mg for injection
Lomefloxacin (Maxaquin)
Oral: 400 mg tablets
Nalidixic acid (NegGram)
Oral: 250, 500, 1000 mg caplets; 250 mg/5 mL suspension
Norfloxacin (Noroxin)
Oral: 400 mg tablets
Ofloxacin (Floxin)
Oral: 200, 300, 400 mg tablets
Parenteral: 200 mg in 50 mL 5% D/W for IV administration; 20, 40 mg/mL for IV injection
Sparfloxacin (Zagam)
Oral: 200 mg tablets

Miscellaneous
Novobiocin (Albamycin)
Oral: 250 mg capsules

REFERENCES

Ericsson CD et al: Ciprofloxacin or trimethoprim-sulfamethoxazole as initial therapy for travelers' diarrhea: A placebo-controlled, randomized trial. Ann Intern Med 1987;106:216.

Ferrero L, Cameron B, Crouzet J: Analysis of *gyrA* and *grlA* mutations in stepwise-selected ciprofloxacin-resistant mutants of *Staphylococcus aureus.* Antimicrob Agents Chemother 1995;39:1554.

Gordin FM et al: Adverse reactions to trimethoprim-sulfamethoxazole in patients with the acquired immunodeficiency syndrome. Ann Intern Med 1984;100:495.

Heikkila E, Sundstrom L, Huovinen P: Trimethoprim resistance in *Escherichia coli* isolates from a geriatric unit. Antimicrob Agents Chemother 1990;34:2013.

Heikkila E et al: Analysis of localization of the type I trimethoprim resistance gene from *Escherichia coli* isolated in Finland. Antimicrob Agents Chemother 1991;35:1562.

Hooper DC, Wolfson JS: Fluoroquinolone antimicrobial agents. N Engl J Med 1991;324:384.

Lode H: Pharmacokinetics and clinical results of parenterally administered new quinolones in humans. Rev Infect Dis 1989;11(Suppl 5):S996.

Pan XS, Fisher M: Cloning and characteristics of the *parC* and *parE* genes of *Streptococcus pneumoniae* encoding DNA topoisomerase IV: Role in fluoroquinolone resistance. J Bacteriol 1996;178:4060.

Radanst JM et al: Interaction of fluoroquinolones with other drugs: Mechanisms, variability, clinical significance, and management. Clin Infect Dis 1992;14:272.

Rubin RH, Swartz MN: Trimethoprim-sulfamethoxazole. N Engl J Med 1980;303:426.

Smego RA Jr, Moeller MB, Gallis HA: Trimethoprim-sulfamethoxazole therapy for *Nocardia* infections. Arch Intern Med 1983;143:711.

Stamm WE, Hooten TM: Management of urinary tract infections in adults. N Engl J Med 1993;329:1328.

Suh B, Lorber B: Quinolones. Med Clin North Am 1995;79:869.

Then RL, Kohl I, Burdeska A: Frequency and transferability of trimethoprim and sulfonamide resistance in methicillin-resistant *Staphylococcus aureus* and *Staphylococcus epidermidis*. J Chemother 1992;4:67.

47

Antimycobacterial Drugs

Henry F. Chambers, MD, & Ernest Jawetz, MD, PhD

Mycobacterial infections are among the most difficult of all bacterial infections to cure. Mycobacteria are slowly growing organisms, making them relatively resistant to antibiotics, the activity of which tends to depend on how rapidly the cells are dividing. Mycobacterial cells can also be dormant and thus completely resistant to many drugs, or killed only very slowly by the few drugs that are active. The lipid-rich mycobacterial cell wall is impermeable to many agents. A substantial proportion of mycobacterial organisms are intracellular, residing within macrophages, and inaccessible to drugs that penetrate poorly. Finally, mycobacteria are notorious for their ability to develop resistance to any single drug. Combinations of drugs are required to overcome these obstacles and to prevent emergence of resistance during the course of therapy. The response of mycobacterial infections to chemotherapy is slow, and treatment must be administered for months to years depending on which drugs are used. The various drugs used to treat tuberculosis, which is caused by *Mycobacterium tuberculosis* and the closely related *M bovis,* atypical mycobacterial infections, and leprosy, which is caused by *M leprae,* are described in this chapter.

DRUGS USED IN TUBERCULOSIS

Isoniazid (INH), rifampin, pyrazinamide, ethambutol, and **streptomycin** are the five first-line agents for treatment of tuberculosis (Table 47–1). INH and rifampin are the two most active drugs. An INH-rifampin combination administered for 9 months will cure 95–98% of cases of tuberculosis caused by susceptible strains. The addition of pyrazinamide to an INH-rifampin combination for the first 2 months allows the total duration of therapy to be reduced to 6 months without loss of efficacy (Table 47–2). In practice, therapy is initiated with a four-drug regimen of INH, rifampin, pyrazinamide, and either ethambutol or streptomycin until susceptibility of the clinical isolate has been determined. Neither ethambutol nor streptomycin adds substantially to the overall activity of the regimen (ie, the duration of treatment cannot be further reduced if either drug is used), but they do provide additional coverage should the isolate prove to be resistant to INH, rifampin, or both. Unfortunately, such resistance occurs in up to 10% of cases in the United States. The vast majority of patients with tuberculosis can be treated entirely as outpatients, with hospitalization being required only for those who are seriously ill or who require diagnostic evaluation.

ISONIAZID (INH)

INH, introduced in 1952, is the most active drug for the treatment of tuberculosis caused by susceptible strains. INH is the hydrazide of isonicotinic acid. It is a small (MW 137), simple molecule freely soluble in water. The structural similarity to pyridoxine is shown below.

Isoniazid

Pyridoxine

Table 47–1. Antimicrobials used in the treatment of tuberculosis.

Drug	Typical Adult Daily Dosage[1]
First-line agents (in approximate order of preference)	
Isoniazid	300 mg/d
Rifampin	600 mg/d
Pyrazinamide	25 mg/kg/d
Ethambutol	15–25 mg/kg/d
Streptomycin	15 mg/kg/d
Second-line agents	
Amikacin	15 mg/kg/d
Aminosalicylic acid	8–12 g/d
Capreomycin	15 mg/kg/d
Ciprofloxacin	1500 mg/d, divided
Clofazimine	200 mg/d
Cycloserine	500–1000 mg/d, divided
Ethionamide	500–750 mg/d
Ofloxacin	600–800 mg/d
Rifabutin	300 mg/d

[1]Assuming normal renal function.

In vitro, INH inhibits most tubercle bacilli in a concentration of 0.2 µg/mL or less and is bactericidal for actively growing tubercle bacilli. INH is less effective against atypical mycobacterial species. INH is able to penetrate into phagocytic cells and thus is active against both extracellular and intracellular organisms.

Mechanism of Action & Basis of Resistance

INH inhibits synthesis of mycolic acids, which are essential components of mycobacterial cell walls. The precise step at which synthesis is inhibited is not known. Resistance has been associated with overproduction of the product of the *inhA* gene and with mutation or deletion of *katG,* which encodes mycobacterial catalase. The reason why loss of catalase activity leads to resistance to INH is not completely understood, but it may be that catalase is important for an activation step that permits INH to interact with its target protein. *InhA* overproducers express low level resistance and cross-resistance to ethionamide. *KatG* mutants express high-level INH resistance and are not cross-resistant to ethionamide.

Resistant mutants occur in susceptible mycobacterial populations with a frequency of about 1 bacillus in 10^6. Since tuberculous lesions often contain more than 10^8 tubercle bacilli, resistant mutants are readily selected out if INH is given as the sole drug. However, addition of a second independently acting drug, to which resistance also emerges at a frequency of 1 in 10^6 to 10^8, is effective. The odds that a bacillus is resistant to both drugs are approximately 1 in $10^6 \times 10^6$,

or 1 in 10^{12}, which is several orders of magnitude more than the number of infecting organisms. Single drug therapy with INH and failure to use INH plus at least one other drug to which the infecting strain is susceptible (which is tantamount to single drug therapy) has led to the 10–20% prevalence of INH resistance in clinical isolates from the Caribbean and Southeast Asia. Currently, about 8–10% of primary clinical isolates in the United States are INH resistant.

Pharmacokinetics

INH is readily absorbed from the gastrointestinal tract. The administration of a 300 mg oral dose (5 mg/kg in children) results in peak plasma concentrations of 3–5 µg/mL within 1–2 hours. INH diffuses readily into all body fluids and tissues. The concentration in the central nervous system and cerebrospinal fluid ranges between 20% and 100% of simultaneous serum concentrations.

Metabolism of INH, especially acetylation by liver N-acetyltransferase, is genetically determined (see Chapter 4). The average concentration of INH in the plasma of rapid acetylators is about one-third to one-half of that in slow acetylators and average half-lives are less than 1 hour and 3 hours, respectively. Rapid acetylators were once thought to be more prone to hepatotoxicity, but this has not been proved. More rapid clearance of INH by rapid acetylators is of no therapeutic consequence when drug is administered daily, but subtherapeutic concentrations may occur if drug is administered as a once-weekly dose.

INH metabolites and a small amount of unchanged drug are excreted mainly in the urine. The dose need not be adjusted in renal failure, but one third to one half of the normal dose is recommended in severe hepatic insufficiency.

Clinical Uses

The usual dosage of INH is 5–10 mg/kg/d, with a typical adult dose being 300 mg given once daily. Up to 10 mg/kg/d may be used for serious infections, if malabsorption is a problem, or in children. A 15 mg/kg dose, or 900 mg, may be used in a twice-weekly dosing regimen in combination with a second antituberculous agent (eg, rifampin 600 mg). Pyridoxine, 25–50 mg/d is recommended for those with conditions predisposing to neuropathy, an adverse effect of INH. INH is usually given by mouth but can be given parenterally in the same dosage.

INH as a single agent is also indicated for prevention of active tuberculosis in individuals who have been infected with *M tuberculosis,* which is determined by a positive tuberculin skin test. INH is routinely recommended for individuals who are at greatest risk for developing active disease after being infected such as very young children, persons who test positive within 2 years after a documented negative skin test (ie, recent converters), and immunocompromised individuals, especially HIV-infected and AIDS patients. INH is also

COMBINATION CHEMOTHERAPY OF TUBERCULOSIS

The duration of therapy for a patient with tuberculosis depends primarily upon which combination of agents is used (Table 47–2). Provided the isolate is susceptible to both isoniazid (INH) and rifampin, a 9-month course of INH, 300 mg/d (10 mg/kg/d for children up to a maximum of 300 mg), and rifampin, 600 mg/d (10 mg/kg/d to a maximum of 600 mg), is highly effective. Addition of pyrazinamide (PZA), 25 mg/kg/d for the first 2 months, permits shortening the total duration to 6 months. Patients who have a satisfactory response to a daily dosing regimen may be considered for a twice-weekly regimen of INH, 900 mg (20 mg/kg in children to a maximum of 900 mg); rifampin, 600 mg (10 mg/kg in children to a maximum of 600 mg); and PZA, 50 mg/kg to a maximum of 3–4 g. Limited data indicate that AIDS patients can be successfully treated with the 6-month INH-rifampin-pyrazinamide combination regimen.

Extrapulmonary disease is effectively treated with the 6-month regimen. However, some authorities recommend longer courses of therapy (eg, 12 months of INH plus rifampin instead of 9 months) for extrapulmonary disease such as meningitis or bone and joint infections, where drug penetration is an issue, and for disseminated infection. Inability to use an INH-rifampin combination because of intolerance, toxicity, or drug resistance usually requires that therapy be administered for considerably longer periods of time. INH and ethambutol must be administered for 18–24 months and rifampin and ethambutol for 12 months. The rifampin-ethambutol regimen is slightly less efficacious than INH combination regimens, with cure rates of 90–95%. A 6-month regimen of rifampin, pyrazinamide, and ethambutol is effective treatment of tuberculosis caused by an INH-resistant strain. Drug-resistant cases that cannot be treated with these regimens should be treated for 24 months.

Patients being treated for pulmonary tuberculosis who still have positive sputum smears or cultures beyond 3 months are at risk for treatment failure. Directly observed therapy (having the patient take each dose in the presence of a health care worker), if not already in use, should be instituted to exclude noncompliance, and appropriate susceptibility studies should be conducted to determine whether secondary drug resistance has appeared. If a regimen appears to be failing and additional agents are deemed necessary, then not one but at least two new drugs to which the isolate is known or very likely to be susceptible may be added to the regimen pending definitive susceptibility data.

---

indicated for prevention of tuberculosis in close contacts of active cases of pulmonary tuberculosis.

The dosage is 300 mg/d (5–10 mg/kg/d) or 900 mg twice weekly for 6 months in most cases and 12 months for immunocompromised patients or those with an abnormal chest x-ray compatible with prior tuberculosis (once active disease has been ruled out). Some authorities recommend 9 months of INH for children.

Table 47–2. Recommended duration of therapy for tuberculosis.

Regimen (in Approximate Order of Preference)	Duration in Months
Isoniazid, rifampin, pyrazinamide	6
Isoniazid, rifampin	9
Rifampin, ethambutol, pyrazinamide	6
Rifampin, ethambutol	12
Isoniazid, ethambutol	18
All others	≥ 24

Adverse Reactions

The incidence and severity of untoward reactions to INH are related to dosage and duration of administration.

A. Allergic Reactions: Fever and skin rashes are occasionally seen. Drug-induced systemic lupus erythematosus has been reported.

B. Direct Toxicity: INH-induced hepatitis is the most frequent major toxic effect. This is distinct from the minor increases in liver aminotransferases (up to three or four times normal) seen in 10–20% of patients, who usually are asymptomatic. Such increases do not require cessation of the drug. Clinical hepatitis with loss of appetite, nausea, vomiting, jaundice, right upper quadrant pain occurs in 1% of INH recipients and can be fatal, particularly if the drug is not discontinued promptly. There is histologic evidence of hepatocellular damage and necrosis. The risk of hepatitis depends on age. It occurs rarely under age 20, in 0.3% of those from aged 21–35, 1.2% of those aged 36–50, and 2.3% for those aged 50 and above. The risk of hepatitis is greater in alcoholics and possibly during pregnancy and the post-partum period. Development of INH hepatitis contraindicates further use of the drug.

Peripheral neuropathy is observed in 10–20% of patients given dosages greater than 5 mg/kg/d but is infrequently seen with the standard 300 mg adult dose. It is more likely to occur in slow acetylators and patients with predisposing conditions such as malnutrition, alcoholism, diabetes, AIDS, and uremia. Neuropathy is due to a relative pyridoxine deficiency. INH promotes excretion of pyridoxine, and this toxicity is readily reversed by administration of pyridoxine in a dosage as low as 10 mg/d. Central nervous system toxicity, which is less common, includes memory loss, psychosis, and seizures. These may also respond to pyridoxine.

Miscellaneous other reactions include hematologic abnormalities, provocation of pyridoxine deficiency anemia, tinnitus, and gastrointestinal discomfort. INH can reduce the metabolism of phenytoin, increasing its blood level and toxicity.

RIFAMPIN

Rifampin is a large (MW 823), complex semisynthetic derivative of rifamycin, an antibiotic produced by *Streptomyces mediterranei*. It is active in vitro against gram-positive and gram-negative cocci, some enteric bacteria, mycobacteria, and *Chlamydia*. Susceptible organisms are inhibited by less than 1 μg/mL, but resistant mutants are present in all microbial populations at a frequency of approximately $1:10^6$. Administration of rifampin as a single drug selects for these highly resistant organisms. There is no cross-resistance to other classes of antimicrobial drugs, but there is cross-resistance to other rifamycin derivatives, eg, rifabutin.

Antimycobacterial Activity, Resistance, & Pharmacokinetics

Rifampin binds strongly to the β subunit of bacterial DNA-dependent RNA polymerase and thereby inhibits RNA synthesis. Resistance results from one of several possible point mutations that prevent binding of rifampin to RNA polymerase. Human RNA polymerase does not bind rifampin and is not inhibited by it. Rifampin is bactericidal for mycobacteria. It readily penetrates most tissues and into phagocytic cells. It can kill organisms that are poorly accessible to many other drugs, such as intracellular organisms and those sequestered in abscesses and lung cavities.

Rifampin is well absorbed after oral administration and excreted mainly through the liver into bile. It then undergoes enterohepatic recirculation, with the bulk excreted as a deacylated metabolite in feces and a small amount in the urine. Dosage adjustment for renal insufficiency is not necessary. Usual doses result in serum levels of 5–7 μg/mL. Rifampin is distributed widely in body fluids and tissues. Rifampin is relatively highly protein-bound, and consequently adequate cerebrospinal fluid concentrations are achieved only in the presence of meningeal inflammation.

Clinical Uses

A. Mycobacterial Infections: Rifampin, usually 600 mg/d (10 mg/kg/d) orally, is administered together with INH, ethambutol, or another antituberculous drug in order to prevent emergence of drug-resistant mycobacteria. In some short-course therapies, 600 mg of rifampin is given twice weekly. Rifampin also is effective in some atypical mycobacterial infections and in leprosy when used together with a sulfone. Rifampin is an alternative to INH prophylaxis for patients who are unable to take INH or who have had close contact with a case of active tuberculosis caused by an INH-resistant, rifampin-susceptible strain.

B. Other Indications: Rifampin is used in a variety of other clinical situations. An oral dosage of 600 mg twice daily for 2 days can eliminate meningococcal carriage. Rifampin, 20 mg/kg/d for 4 days, is used as prophylaxis in contacts of children with *Haemophilus influenzae* type b disease. Rifampin combined with a second agent is used to eradicate staphylococcal carriage. Rifampin combination therapy is also indicated for treatment of serious staphylococcal infections such as osteomyelitis and prosthetic valve endocarditis. Rifampin has been recommended also for use in combination with ceftriaxone or vancomycin in treatment of meningitis caused by highly penicillin-resistant strains of pneumococci.

Adverse Reactions

Rifampin imparts a harmless orange color to urine, sweat, tears, and contact lenses (soft lenses may be permanently stained). Occasional adverse effects include rashes, thrombocytopenia, and nephritis. It may cause cholestatic jaundice and occasionally hepatitis. Rifampin commonly causes light chain proteinuria. If administered less often than twice weekly, rifampin causes a flu-like syndrome characterized by fever, chills, myalgias, anemia, thrombocytopenia, and sometimes associated with acute tubular necrosis. Rifampin induces microsomal enzymes (eg, cytochrome P450), which increases the elimination of numerous other drugs including methadone, anticoagulants, some anticonvulsants, and contraceptives. Likewise, administration of rifampin with ketoconazole, cyclosporine, or chloramphenicol results in significantly lower serum levels of these drugs. Ketoconazole in turn reduces rifampin serum concentrations.

ETHAMBUTOL

Ethambutol is a synthetic, water-soluble, heat-stable compound, the *dextro* isomer of the structure shown below, dispensed as the dihydrochloride salt.

$$H - \overset{\overset{\displaystyle CH_2OH}{|}}{\underset{\underset{\displaystyle C_2H_5}{|}}{C}} - NH - (CH_2)_2 - NH - \overset{\overset{\displaystyle C_2H_5}{|}}{\underset{\underset{\displaystyle CH_2OH}{|}}{C}} - H$$

Ethambutol

Susceptible strains of *M tuberculosis* and other mycobacteria are inhibited in vitro by ethambutol, 1–5 µg/mL. Ethambutol inhibits synthesis of arabinogalactan, an essential component of mycobacterial cell wall. It enhances the activity of lipophilic drugs such as rifampin and ofloxacin that cross the cell wall primarily in lipid domains of this structure.

Ethambutol is well absorbed from the gut. Following ingestion of 25 mg/kg, a blood level peak of 2–5 µg/mL is reached in 2–4 hours. About 20% of the drug is excreted in feces and 50% in urine in unchanged form. Ethambutol accumulates in renal failure, and the dose should be reduced by half if creatinine clearance is less than 10 mL/min. Ethambutol crosses the blood-brain barrier only if the meninges are inflamed. Concentrations in cerebrospinal fluid are highly variable, ranging from 4% to 64% of serum levels in the setting of meningeal inflammation.

As with all antituberculous drugs, resistance to ethambutol emerges rapidly when the drug is used alone. Therefore, ethambutol is always given in combination with other antituberculous drugs. The mechanism of resistance is unknown.

Clinical Use

Ethambutol hydrochloride, 15–25 mg/kg, is usually given as a single daily dose in combination with INH or rifampin. The higher dose is recommended for treatment of tuberculous meningitis. The dose of ethambutol is 50 mg/kg when a twice-weekly dosing schedule is used.

Adverse Reactions

Hypersensitivity to ethambutol is rare. The most common serious adverse event is retrobulbar neuritis causing loss of visual acuity and red-green color blindness. This dosage-related side effect is more likely to occur at a dosage of 25 mg/kg/d continued for several months. With doses of 15 mg/kg/d or less, visual disturbances are very rare. Periodic visual acuity testing is desirable if the 25 mg/kg/d dosage is used. Ethambutol is relatively contraindicated in children too young to permit assessment of visual acuity and red-green color discrimination.

PYRAZINAMIDE

Pyrazinamide (PZA) is a relative of nicotinamide, stable, slightly soluble in water, and quite inexpensive. At neutral pH, it is inactive in vitro, but at pH 5.5 it kills tubercle bacilli and some other mycobacteria at

concentrations of approximately 20 µg/mL. Drug is taken up by macrophages and kills bacilli residing within this acidic environment.

Pyrazinamide (PZA)

Clinical Use

Serum concentrations of 30–50 µg/mL are achieved with dosages of 25 mg/kg/d. PZA is well absorbed from the gastrointestinal tract and widely distributed in body tissues, including inflamed meninges. The half-life of 12–24 hours permits once-daily dosing. A 50–70 mg/kg dose is used for twice-weekly or thrice-weekly treatment regimens.

Tubercle bacilli develop resistance to pyrazinamide fairly readily, but there is no cross-resistance with isoniazid or other antimycobacterial drugs. For this reason, PZA in combination with either ciprofloxacin or ofloxacin has been recommended for prevention of active disease in close contacts and documented tuberculin skin test converters who have been exposed to a case of multidrug-resistant tuberculosis provided that the isolate of the index case is susceptible to these drugs.

Adverse Reactions

Major adverse effects of pyrazinamide include hepatotoxicity (in 1–5% of patients), nausea, vomiting, drug fever, and hyperuricemia. The latter occurs uniformly and is not a reason to halt therapy. Hyperuricemia may provoke acute gouty arthritis.

STREPTOMYCIN

The mechanism of action and the pharmacologic features of streptomycin have been discussed in Chapter 45. Most tubercle bacilli are inhibited by streptomycin, 1–10 µg/mL, in vitro. Non-tuberculous species of mycobacteria other than *Mycobacterium avium* complex (MAC) and *Mycobacterium kansasii* are resistant. All large populations of tubercle bacilli contain some streptomycin-resistant mutants. On the average, 1 in 10^8 tubercle bacilli can be expected to be resistant to streptomycin at levels of 10–100 µg/mL. Resistance is due to a point mutation that alters the ribosomal binding site.

Streptomycin penetrates into cells poorly, and consequently it is active mainly against extracellular tubercle bacilli. Additional drugs are needed to eliminate intracellular organisms, which constitute a significant proportion of the total mycobacterial burden. Streptomycin crosses the blood-brain barrier and achieves therapeutic concentrations with inflamed meninges.

Clinical Use in Tuberculosis

Streptomycin sulfate remains an important drug in the treatment of tuberculosis. It is employed when an injectable drug is needed or desirable, principally in individuals with severe, possibly life-threatening forms of tuberculosis, eg, meningitis and disseminated disease, and in treatment of infections resistant to other drugs. The usual dosage is 15 mg/kg/d intramuscularly or intravenously daily for adults (20–40 mg/kg/d for children) for several weeks, followed by 1–1.5 g two or three times weekly for several months. Other drugs are always given simultaneously to prevent emergence of resistance.

Adverse Reactions

Streptomycin is ototoxic and nephrotoxic. Vertigo and hearing loss are the most common side effects and may be permanent. Toxicity is dose-related, and the risk is increased in the elderly. As with all aminoglycosides, the dose must be adjusted according to renal function (see Chapter 45). Toxicity can be reduced by limiting therapy to no more than 6 months whenever possible.

ALTERNATIVE SECOND-LINE DRUGS IN TREATMENT OF TUBERCULOSIS

The alternative drugs listed below are usually considered only (1) in the case of resistance to the drugs of first choice (which occurs with increasing frequency); (2) in case of failure of clinical response to conventional therapy; and (3) when expert guidance is available to deal with the toxic effects. For many of the second-line drugs listed below, the dosage, emergence of resistance, and long-term toxicity have not been fully established.

Ethionamide

Ethionamide is chemically related to isoniazid and also blocks the synthesis of mycolic acids. It is poorly water soluble and available only in oral form. It is metabolized by the liver.

Ethionamide

Most tubercle bacilli are inhibited in vitro by ethionamide, 2.5 µg/mL, or less. Some other species of mycobacteria also are inhibited by ethionamide, 10 µg/mL. Serum concentrations in plasma and tissues of approximately 20 µg/mL are achieved by a dosage of 1 g/d. Cerebrospinal fluid concentrations are equal to those in serum. A 1 g/d dosage, although effective in the treatment of tuberculosis, is poorly tolerated because of the intense gastric irritation and neurologic symptoms that commonly occur. Ethionamide is also hepatotoxic. Neurologic symptoms may be alleviated by pyridoxine.

Ethionamide is administered at an initial dosage of 250 mg once daily, which is increased in 250 mg increments to the recommended dosage of 1 g/d (or 15 mg/kg/d) if possible. The 1 g/d dosage, although theoretically desirable, is seldom tolerated, and one often must settle for a total daily dose of 500–750 mg.

Resistance to ethionamide as a single agent develops rapidly in vitro and in vivo. There can be low-level cross-resistance between isoniazid and ethionamide.

Capreomycin

Capreomycin is a peptide antibiotic obtained from *Streptomyces capreolus.* Daily injection of 1 g intramuscularly results in blood levels of 10 µg/mL or more. Such concentrations in vitro are inhibitory for many mycobacteria, including multidrug-resistant strains of *M tuberculosis.*

There is some cross-resistance between capreomycin, kanamycin, and amikacin but not streptomycin. Capreomycin (15 mg/kg/d) is an important injectable agent for treatment of drug-resistant tuberculosis, particularly if the isolate is streptomycin resistant.

Capreomycin is nephrotoxic and ototoxic. Tinnitus, deafness, and vestibular disturbances occur. The injection causes significant local pain, and sterile abscesses may occur.

Dosing of capreomycin is the same as streptomycin. Toxicity is reduced if 1 g is given two or three times weekly after an initial response has been achieved with a daily dosing schedule.

Cycloserine

Cycloserine is an inhibitor of cell wall synthesis and is discussed in Chapter 43. Concentrations of 15–20 µg/mL inhibit many strains of *M tuberculosis.* The dosage of cycloserine in tuberculosis is 0.5–1 g/d in two divided doses. Cycloserine is cleared renally, and the dose should be reduced by half if creatinine clearance is less than 50 mL/min.

The most serious toxic effects are peripheral neuropathy and central nervous system dysfunction, including depression and psychotic reactions. Adverse effects occur in one-fourth or more of patients, particularly at higher doses. These may be minimized by monitoring serum concentrations.

Aminosalicylic Acid (PAS)

PAS is a folate synthesis antagonist that is active almost exclusively against *M tuberculosis.* It is structurally similar to *p*-aminobenzoic aid (PABA) and to the sulfonamides (see Chapter 46).

COOH

OH

NH₂

Aminosalicylic acid (PAS)

Tubercle bacilli are usually inhibited in vitro by PAS, 1–5 µg/mL. PAS is readily absorbed from the gastrointestinal tract. Serum levels are 50 µg/mL or more after a 4 g oral dose. The dosage is 8–12 g/d orally for adults and 300 mg/kg/d for children. The drug is widely distributed in tissues and body fluids except the cerebrospinal fluid. PAS is rapidly excreted in the urine, in part as active PAS and in part as the acetylated compound and other metabolic products. Very high concentrations of PAS are reached in the urine, which can result in crystalluria.

PAS, formerly a first-line agent for treatment of tuberculosis, is used infrequently now because primary resistance is common and other oral drugs are better-tolerated. Gastrointestinal symptoms often accompany full doses of PAS. Anorexia, nausea, diarrhea, and epigastric pain and burning may be diminished by giving PAS with meals and with antacids. Peptic ulceration and hemorrhage may occur. Hypersensitivity reactions manifested by fever, joint pains, skin rashes, hepatosplenomegaly, hepatitis, adenopathy, and granulocytopenia, often occur after 3–8 weeks of PAS therapy, making it necessary to stop PAS administration temporarily or permanently.

Kanamycin & Amikacin

The pharmacology, mode of action, toxicity, and antibacterial properties of kanamycin and amikacin are discussed in Chapter 45. Kanamycin has been used for treatment of tuberculosis caused by streptomycin-resistant strains, but the availability of less toxic alternatives (eg, capreomycin and amikacin) have rendered it obsolete.

The role of amikacin in treatment of tuberculosis has increased with the increasing incidence and prevalence of multidrug-resistant tuberculosis. Prevalence of amikacin-resistant strains is low (less than 5%), and most multidrug-resistant strains remain amikacin-susceptible. *M tuberculosis* is inhibited at concentrations of 1 µg/mL or less. Amikacin is also active against atypical mycobacteria. There is no cross-resistance between streptomycin and amikacin, but kanamycin and capreomycin resistance often indicate resistance to amikacin as well. Serum concentrations of 30–50 µg/mL are achieved 30–60 minutes after a 15 mg/kg intravenous infusion. Amikacin is indicated for treatment of tuberculosis suspected or known to be caused by streptomycin-resistant or multidrug-resistant strains. Amikacin must be used in combination with at least one and preferably two or three other drugs to which the isolate is susceptible for treatment of drug-resistant cases. The recommended dosage is 15 mg/kg/d intramuscularly or intravenously daily for 5 days a week for the first 2 months of therapy and then 1–1.5 g two or three times weekly to complete a 6-month course.

Ciprofloxacin & Ofloxacin

These drugs are discussed in Chapter 46. In addition to their activity against many gram-positive and gram-negative bacteria, ciprofloxacin and ofloxacin inhibit strains of *M tuberculosis* at concentrations less than 2 µg/mL. They are also active against atypical mycobacteria. Ofloxacin tends to be slightly more active in vitro than ciprofloxacin against *M tuberculosis;* ciprofloxacin is slightly more active against atypical mycobacteria. Serum concentrations of 2–4 µg/mL and 4–6 µg/mL are achieved with oral doses of 750 mg of ciprofloxacin and 600 mg of ofloxacin, respectively.

Fluoroquinolones are an important recent addition to the therapeutic armamentarium against tuberculosis, especially strains that are resistant to first-line agents. Resistance, which may result from any one of several single point mutations in the gyrase A subunit, develops rapidly if a fluoroquinolone is used as a single agent; thus, the drug must be used in combination with two or more other active agents. The dosage of ciprofloxacin is 750 mg orally twice a day. That of ofloxacin is 600–800 mg as a single daily dose. A fluoroquinolone plus pyrazinamide may also be used to prevent disease following contact to an active case of multidrug-resistant tuberculosis depending on the susceptibility of the clinical isolate from the index case.

Rifabutin (Ansamycin)

This antibiotic is derived from rifamycin and is related to rifampin. It has significant activity against *M tuberculosis, M avium-intracellulare* and *M fortuitum* (see below). The dosage is 300 mg/d orally. The role of rifabutin in treatment of tuberculosis is not well defined. There is little reason to use rifabutin instead of rifampin for treatment of tuberculosis caused by fully susceptible strains. However, up to 25% of rifampin-resistant strains will be susceptible to rifabutin in vitro, and then rifabutin may be useful. In the remainder of cases, rifabutin is not useful for treatment of drug-resistant tuberculosis because of cross-resistance with rifampin. Rifabutin is effective in prevention and treatment of disseminated atypical mycobacterial infections in patients with advanced AIDS.

Clofazimine

Clofazimine is effective against leprosy and has some activity against *M tuberculosis* in vitro. It is sometimes used as an agent of last resort for treatment of multidrug-resistant tuberculosis, but its efficacy is not well established. The dose is 200 mg orally as a single or divided dose.

DRUGS ACTIVE AGAINST ATYPICAL MYCOBACTERIA

About 10% of mycobacterial infections seen in clinical practice in the USA are caused not by *M tuberculosis* or *M leprae* but by nontuberculous or so-called "atypical" mycobacteria. These organisms have distinctive laboratory characteristics, occur in the environment, and are generally not communicable from person to person. Disease caused by these organisms is often less severe than tuberculosis. As a general rule, these mycobacterial species are less susceptible than *M tuberculosis* to antituberculous drugs. On the other hand, agents such as erythromycin, sulfonamides, or tetracycline, which are not effective against *M tuberculosis*, may be effective against atypical strains. Emergence of resistance during therapy is also a problem with these mycobacterial species, and active infection should be treated with combinations of drugs. *M kansasii* is susceptible to rifampin and ethambutol but relatively resistant to INH and usually completely resistant to pyrazinamide. A three-drug combination of INH, rifampin, and ethambutol is the long-standing conventional treatment for *M kansasii* infection. A few representative pathogens, with the clinical presentation and the drugs to which they are often susceptible, are given in Table 47–3. Satisfactory clinical response correlates directly with susceptibility in vitro, and in vitro resistance often predicts treatment failure.

M avium complex (MAC), which includes both *M avium* and *M intracellulare,* is an important and common cause of disseminated disease in late stages of AIDS (CD4 counts < 50/μL). *Mycobacterium avium* complex is much less susceptible than *M tuberculosis* to most antituberculous drugs; in particular, INH is useless. Combinations of agents are required to suppress the disease. In most cases, disseminated MAC is incurable and therapy is life-long. The need for multidrug therapy frequently leads to side effects that can be difficult to manage. Azithromycin, 500 mg once daily, or clarithromycin, 500 mg twice daily, plus ethambutol, 15 mg/kg/d, is an effective and well-tolerated regimen for treatment of disseminated disease. Some authorities recommend use of a third agent, such as ciprofloxacin 750 mg twice daily or rifabutin, 300 mg once daily. Other agents that may be useful are listed in Table 47–3. Rifabutin in a single daily dose of 300 mg has been shown to reduce the incidence of *M avium* complex bacteremia in AIDS patients with CD4 < 200/μL but may not offer a survival advantage. Clarithromycin also effectively prevents MAC bacteremia in AIDS patients, but if breakthrough bacteremia occurs, the isolate often is resistant to both clarithromycin and azithromycin, precluding the use of the most effective drugs for treatment.

DRUGS USED IN LEPROSY

Mycobacterium leprae has never been grown in vitro but animal models, such as growth in injected mouse footpads, have permitted laboratory evaluation of drugs. Only those drugs that have the widest clini-

Table 47–3. Clinical features and treatment options for mycobacteria other than *M tuberculosis.*

Runyon Group	Species	Clinical Features	Treatment Options
I	M kansasii	Resembles tuberculosis	Ciprofloxacin, clarithromycin, ethambutol, isoniazid, rifampin, trimethoprim-sulfamethoxazole
	M marinum	Granulomatous cutaneous disease	Amikacin, clarithromycin, ethambutol, doxycycline, minocycline, rifampin, trimethoprim-sulfamethoxazole
II	M scrofulaceum	Cervical adenitis in children	Amikacin, erythromycin (or other macrolide), rifampin, streptomycin. (Surgical excision is often curative and the treatment of choice.)
III	M avium complex	Pulmonary disease in patients with chronic lung disease; disseminated infection in AIDS	Amikacin, azithromycin, clarithromycin, ciprofloxacin, ethambutol, ethionamide, rifabutin
IV	M chelonae	Abscess, sinus tract, ulcer; bone, joint, tendon infection	Amikacin, doxycycline, imipenem, macrolides, tobramycin
	M fortuitum	Same as M chelonae	Amikacin, cefoxitin, ciprofloxacin, doxycycline, ofloxacin, trimethoprim-sulfamethoxazole
	M ulcerans	Skin ulcers	Isoniazid, streptomycin, rifampin, minocycline. (Surgical excision may be effective.)

cal use are presented here. Because of increasing reports of dapsone resistance, treatment of leprosy with combinations of the drugs listed below is recommended.

DAPSONE & OTHER SULFONES

Several drugs closely related to the sulfonamides have been used effectively in the long-term treatment of leprosy. The most widely used is dapsone (diaminodiphenylsulfone). Like the sulfonamides, it inhibits folate synthesis. Resistance can emerge in large populations of *M leprae,* eg, in lepromatous leprosy, if very low doses are given. Therefore, the combination of dapsone, rifampin, and clofazimine is recommended for initial therapy. Dapsone may also be used to prevent and treat *Pneumocystis carinii* pneumonia in AIDS.

Dapsone

Sulfones are well absorbed from the gut and widely distributed throughout body fluids and tissues. The serum half-life is 1–2 days, and drug tends to be retained in skin, muscle, liver, and kidney. Skin heavily infected with *M leprae* may contain several times as much of the drug as normal skin. Sulfones are excreted into bile and reabsorbed in the intestine. Excretion into urine is variable, and most excreted drug is acetylated. In renal failure, the dose may have to be adjusted.

The usual adult dosage in leprosy is 100 mg daily. For children, the dose is proportionately less depending on weight.

Dapsone is usually well tolerated. Many patients develop some hemolysis, particularly if they have glucose-6-phosphate dehydrogenase deficiency. Methemoglobinemia is common, but usually is not a problem clinically. Gastrointestinal intolerance, fever, pruritus, and various rashes occur. During dapsone therapy of lepromatous leprosy, erythema nodosum leprosum often develops. It is sometimes difficult to distinguish reactions to dapsone from manifestations of the underlying illness. Erythema nodosum leprosum may be suppressed by corticosteroids or by thalidomide.

RIFAMPIN

This drug (see above) in a dosage of 600 mg daily can be strikingly effective in lepromatous leprosy. Because of the probable risk of emergence of rifampin-resistant *M leprae,* the drug is given in combination with dapsone or another antileprosy drug. A single monthly dose of 600 mg may be beneficial in combination therapy.

CLOFAZIMINE

Clofazimine is a phenazine dye that can be used as an alternative to dapsone. Its mechanism of action is unknown but may involve DNA binding.

Absorption of clofazimine from the gut is variable, and a major portion of the drug is excreted in feces. Clofazimine is stored widely in reticuloendothelial tissues and skin, and its crystals can be seen inside phagocytic reticuloendothelial cells. It is slowly released, so that the serum half-life may be 2 months.

Clofazimine is given for sulfone-resistant leprosy or when patients are intolerant to sulfone. A common dosage is 100 mg/d orally. The most prominent untoward effect is skin discoloration ranging from red-brown to nearly black. Gastrointestinal intolerance occurs occasionally.

PREPARATIONS AVAILABLE

Drugs Used in Tuberculosis

Aminosalicylate sodium (Sodium P.A.S.)
  Oral: 0.5 g tablets
Capreomycin (Capastat Sulfate)
  Parenteral: powder to reconstitute for injection
    (1 g/10 mL vial)
Cycloserine (Seromycin Pulvules)
  Oral: 250 mg capsules
Ethambutol (Myambutol)
  Oral: 100, 400 mg tablets
Ethionamide (Trecator-SC)
  Oral: 250 mg tablets

Isoniazid (generic)
  Oral: 50, 100, 300 mg tablets; syrup,
    50 mg/5 mL
  Parenteral: 100 mg/mL for injection
Pyrazinamide (generic)
  Oral: 500 mg tablets
Rifabutin (Mycobutin)
  Oral: 150 mg capsules
Rifampin (Rifadin, Rimactane)
  Oral: 150, 300 mg capsules
  Parenteral: 600 mg powder for IV injection

Streptomycin (generic)
Parenteral: 400 mg for IM injection; also available as powder to reconstitute for injection

Drugs Used in Leprosy
Dapsone (generic)
Oral: 25, 100 mg tablets
Clofazimine (Lamprene)
Oral: 50, 100 mg capsules

REFERENCES

Bannerjee A et al: *inhA,* a gene encoding a target for isoniazid and ethionamide in *Mycobacterium tuberculosis.* Science 1994;263:227.

Bass JB et al: Treatment of tuberculosis and tuberculosis infection in adults and children. Am J Crit Care Med 1994;149:1359.

Brennan PJ and Nikaido H: The envelope of mycobacteria. Annu Rev Biochem 1995;64:29.

Byrd RB et al: Toxic effects of isoniazid in tuberculosis chemoprophylaxis. JAMA 1979;241:1239.

Carpenter JL et al: Disseminated disease due to *Mycobacterium chelonei* treated with amikacin and cefoxitin. Arch Intern Med 1984;144:2063.

Citron KM: Ocular toxicity from ethambutol. (Editorial.) Thorax 1986;41:737.

Cohn DL et al: A 62 dose, 6 month therapy for pulmonary and extrapulmonary tuberculosis. Ann Intern Med 1990;112:407.

Combs DL et al: USPHS tuberculosis short course chemotherapy trial 21. Ann Intern Med 1990;112:397.

Dutt AK, Moers D, Stead WW: Short-course chemotherapy for extrapulmonary tuberculosis: Nine years' experience. Ann Intern Med 1986;104:7.

Dutt AK, Moers D, Stead WW: Undesirable side effects of isoniazid and rifampin in largely twice-weekly short-course chemotherapy for tuberculosis. Am Rev Respir Dis 1983;128:419.

Ellard GA: Chemotherapy of leprosy. Br Med Bull 1988;44:775.

Farr B, Mandell GL: Rifampin. Med Clin North Am 1982;66:157.

Goble M et al: Treatment of 171 patients with pulmonary tuberculosis resistant to isoniazid and rifampin. N Engl J Med 1993;328:527.

Horsburgh CR: *Mycobacterium avium* complex in AIDS. N Engl J Med 1991;324:1332.

Houston S, Fanning A: Current and potential treatment of tuberculosis. Drugs 1994;48:689.

Iseman MD: Treatment of multidrug-resistant tuberculosis. N Engl J Med 1993;329:784.

Jacobs RF et al: Intensive short course chemotherapy for tuberculous meningitis. Ped Infect Dis J 1992;11:194.

Maddrey WC, Boitnott JK: Isoniazid hepatitis. Ann Intern Med 1973;79:1.

Mitchison DA: The action of antituberculosis drugs in short-course chemotherapy. Tubercle 1985;66:219.

Molavi A, LeFrock JL: Tuberculous meningitis. Med Clin North Am 1985;69:315.

Morris S et al: Molecular mechanisms of multiple drug resistance in clinical isolates of *Mycobacterium tuberculosis.* J Infect Dis 1995;171:954.

Perriens JH et al: Pulmonary tuberculosis in HIV-infected patients in Zaire: A controlled trial of treatment for either 6 months or 12 months. N Engl J Med 1995;332:779.

Quemard A, Lacave C, Laneelle G: Isoniazid inhibition of mycolic acid synthesis by cell extracts of sensitive and resistant strains of *Mycobacterium aurum.* Antimicrob Agents Chemother 1991;35:1035.

Rapp RP et al: New macrolide antibiotics: usefulness in infections caused by mycobacteria other than *Mycobacterium tuberculosis.* Ann Pharmacother 1994;28:1255.

Raviglione MC, Snider DE, Kochi A: Global epidemiology of tuberculosis: Morbidity and mortality of a worldwide epidemic. JAMA 1995;273:220.

Sauret J et al: Treatment of pulmonary disease caused by *Mycobacterium kansasii:* Results of 18 versus 12 months chemotherapy. Tuber Lung Dis 1995;76:104.

Snider DE, Rooper WL: The new tuberculosis. N Engl J Med 1992;326:703.

Snider DE Jr et al: Standard therapy for tuberculosis. Chest 1985;87(Suppl 2):117S.

Waters MF et al: Rifampicin for lepromatous leprosy: Nine years' experience. Br Med J 1978;1:133.

Zhang Y et al: The catalase-peroxidase gene and isoniazid resistance of *Mycobacterium tuberculosis.* Nature 1992;358:591.

48

Antifungal Agents

Don Sheppard, MD, & Harry W. Lampiris, MD

Human fungal infections have increased dramatically in incidence and severity in recent years, due mainly to advances in surgery, cancer treatment, and critical care accompanied by increases in the use of broad-spectrum antimicrobials and the HIV epidemic. These changes have resulted in increased numbers of patients at risk for fungal infections. *Candida albicans* has become the fourth most common organism isolated from blood cultures in the USA. New and unusual organisms are being encountered as we gain experience with this cohort of immunocompromised patients. Furthermore, most fungi are completely resistant to conventional antibacterial drugs.

Pharmacotherapy of fungal disease has been revolutionized by the introduction of the relatively nontoxic oral azole drugs. Combination therapy is being reconsidered, and new formulations of old agents are becoming available.

Unfortunately, the appearance of azole-resistant organisms, as well as the rise in the number of patients at risk for mycotic infections, has created new challenges. Two new classes of antifungals, the echinocandin analogs and the nikkomycins, seem to hold promise. Both classes of agents inhibit enzymes required for fungal cell wall synthesis. They are currently undergoing clinical trials.

The antifungal drugs presently available fall into several categories: systemic drugs (oral or parenteral) for systemic infections, oral drugs for mucocutaneous infections, and topical drugs for mucocutaneous infections.

SYSTEMIC ANTIFUNGAL DRUGS FOR SYSTEMIC INFECTIONS

AMPHOTERICIN B

Amphotericin A and B are antifungal antibiotics produced by *Streptomyces nodosus*. Amphotericin B is the only formulation in clinical use.

Chemistry

Amphotericin B is an amphoteric polyene macrolide (polyene = containing many double bonds; macrolide = containing a large lactone ring of 12 or more atoms). It is nearly insoluble in water, and is there-fore prepared as a colloidal suspension of amphotericin B and sodium desoxycholate for intravenous injection. Several new formulations have been developed in which amphotericin B is packaged in a lipid-associated delivery system (see box: Liposomal Amphotericin B).

Pharmacokinetics

Amphotericin B is poorly absorbed from the gastrointestinal tract. Oral amphotericin B is thus effective only on fungi within the lumen of the tract and cannot be used for treatment of systemic disease. The intravenous injection of 0.6 mg/kg/d of amphotericin B results in average blood levels of 0.3–1 μg/mL and is more than 90% bound by serum proteins. While it is mostly metabolized, some amphotericin B is excreted slowly in the urine over a period of several days. The serum $t_{1/2}$ is approximately 15 days. Hepatic impairment, renal impairment, and dialysis have little impact on drug concentrations and therefore no dose adjustment is required. The drug is widely distributed in tissues, but only 2–3% of the blood level is reached in cerebrospinal fluid, thus occasionally necessitating intrathecal therapy for certain types of fungal meningitis.

Mechanism of Action

Amphotericin B is selective in its fungicidal effect because it exploits the difference in lipid composition of fungal and mammalian cell membranes. **Ergosterol,** a cell membrane sterol, is found in the cell membrane of fungi, whereas the predominant sterol of bacteria and human cells is **cholesterol.** Amphotericin B binds to ergosterol and alters the permeability of the cell by forming amphotericin B-associated pores in the cell membrane. As suggested by its structure, amphotericin B combines avidly with lipids (ergosterol) along the double bond-rich side of its structure and associates with water molecules along the

Amphotericin B

LIPOSOMAL AMPHOTERICIN B

Therapy with amphotericin B is often limited by toxicity, especially drug-induced renal impairment. This has led to the development of lipid drug formulations on the assumption that lipid-packaged drug will bind to the mammalian membrane less readily, permitting the use of effective doses of the drug with lower toxicity. Liposomal amphotericin preparations package the active drug in lipid delivery vehicles, in contrast to the colloidal suspensions currently in use. Amphotericin binds to the lipids in these vehicles with an affinity between that for fungal ergosterol and that for human cholesterol. The lipid vehicle then serves as an amphotericin reservoir, reducing nonspecific binding to human cell membranes. This preferential binding allows for a reduction of toxicity without sacrificing efficacy and permits use of larger doses. Furthermore, some fungi contain lipases that may liberate free amphotericin B directly at the site of infection.

When administered intravenously, these preparations have a short plasma half-life and are rapidly taken up by the reticuloendothelial cells with significant accumulation in liver, spleen, lymph nodes, and lungs. This may offer an additional advantage, since fungal organisms may reside within these cells. Very little drug is detected in the cerebrospinal fluid and the kidney, thus calling into question the efficacy of such treatment for fungal disease at these sites.

Clinical trials have demonstrated a lower incidence of renal and infusion-related toxicities with these preparations compared with standard preparations of amphotericin B, but there are as yet few direct comparative trials in severe fungal infections to demonstrate equivalent efficacy or cost effectiveness. Liposomal amphotericin B is currently approved for treatment of invasive aspergillosis.

hydroxyl-rich side. This amphipathic characteristic facilitates pore formation by multiple amphotericin molecules, with the lipophilic portions around the outside of the pore and the hydrophilic regions lining the inside. The pore allows the leakage of intracellular ions and macromolecules, eventually leading to cell death. Some binding to human membrane sterols does occur, probably accounting for the drug's prominent toxicity.

Resistance to amphotericin B occurs if ergosterol binding is impaired, either by decreasing the membrane concentration of ergosterol or by modifying the sterol target molecule to reduce its affinity for the drug.

Adverse Effects

The toxicity of amphotericin B can be divided into two broad categories: immediate reactions, related to the infusion of the drug, and those occurring more slowly.

A. Infusion-Related Toxicity: These reactions are nearly universal and consist of fever, chills, muscle spasms, vomiting, headache, and hypotension. They can be ameliorated by slowing the infusion rate or decreasing the daily dose. Premedication with antipyretics, antihistamines, meperidine, or corticosteroids can be helpful. When starting therapy, many clinicians administer a test dose of 1 mg intravenously to gauge the severity of the reaction. This can serve as a guide to an initial dosing regimen and premedication strategy.

B. Slower Toxicity: Renal damage is the most significant toxic reaction. Renal impairment occurs in nearly all patients treated with clinically significant doses of amphotericin. The degree of azotemia is variable and often stabilizes during therapy, but can be serious enough to necessitate dialysis. A reversible component is associated with decreased renal perfusion and represents a form of prerenal renal failure. An irreversible component results from renal tubular injury and subsequent dysfunction. Renal toxicity commonly presents with renal tubular acidosis and severe potassium and magnesium wasting. There is some evidence that renal damage can be attenuated with sodium loading, and it is common practice to administer normal saline infusions with the daily doses of amphotericin B.

Abnormalities of liver function tests are occasionally seen, as is a varying degree of anemia due to reduced erythropoietin production by damaged renal tubular cells. After intrathecal therapy with amphotericin, seizures and a chemical arachnoiditis may develop, often with serious neurologic sequelae.

Antifungal Activity

Amphotericin B remains the antifungal agent with the broadest spectrum of action. It has activity against the clinically significant yeasts, including *Candida albicans* and *Cryptococcus neoformans;* the organisms causing endemic mycoses, including *Histoplasma capsulatum, Blastomyces dermatitidis,* and *Coccidioides immitis;* and the pathogenic molds, such as *Aspergillus fumigatus* and *Mucor.* Some fungal organisms such as *Candida lusitaniae* and *Pseudallescheria boydii* display intrinsic amphotericin B resistance.

Clinical Use

Owing to its broad spectrum of activity and fungicidal action, amphotericin B remains the drug of choice for nearly all life-threatening mycotic infections. It is often used as the initial induction regimen for serious fungal infections and is then replaced by one of the newer azole drugs (described below) for chronic therapy or prevention of relapse. Such induction therapy is especially important for immunosuppressed patients and those with severe fungal pneumonia or cryptococcal meningitis with altered mental status. Once a clinical response has been elicited, these patients will then often continue maintenance therapy with an azole; therapy may be lifelong in patients at high risk for disease relapse. Amphotericin has also been used as empiric therapy for selected patients in whom the risks of leaving a systemic fungal infection untreated are high. The most common such patient is the cancer patient with neutropenia who remains febrile on broad-spectrum antibiotics.

For treatment of systemic fungal disease, amphotericin B is given by slow intravenous infusion at a dosage of 0.5–1 mg/kg/d. It is usually continued to a defined total dose (eg, 1–2 g), rather than a defined time span, as used with other antimicrobial drugs.

Intrathecal therapy for fungal meningitis is poorly tolerated and fraught with difficulties related to maintaining cerebrospinal fluid access. Thus, intrathecal therapy with amphotericin B is being increasingly supplanted by other therapies but remains an option in cases of fungal central nervous system infections that have not responded to other agents.

Local administration of amphotericin B has been used with success. Mycotic corneal ulcers and keratitis can be cured with topical drops as well as by direct subconjunctival injection. Fungal arthritis has been treated with adjunctive local injection directly into the joint. Candiduria responds to bladder irrigation with amphotericin B, and this route has been shown to produce no significant systemic toxicity.

FLUCYTOSINE

Flucytosine (5-FC) was discovered in 1957 during a search for novel antineoplastic agents. While devoid of anticancer properties, it became apparent that it was a potent antifungal agent. Flucytosine is a water-soluble pyrimidine analog that is related to the chemotherapeutic agent fluorouracil (5-FU). Its spectrum of action is much narrower than that of amphotericin B.

Flucytosine

Pharmacokinetics

Flucytosine is currently available in North America only in an oral formulation. The dosage is 150 mg/kg/d in patients with normal renal function. It is well (> 90%) absorbed, with serum concentrations peaking 1–2 hours after an oral dose. It is poorly protein-bound and penetrates well into all body fluid compartments, including the cerebrospinal fluid. It is eliminated by glomerular filtration with a half-life of 3–4 hours and is removed by hemodialysis. Levels rise rapidly with renal impairment and can lead to toxicity. Toxicity is more likely to occur in AIDS patients and in the presence of renal insufficiency. Peak serum concentrations should be measured periodically in patients with renal insufficiency and maintained between 50 and 100 µg/mL.

Mechanism of Action

Flucytosine is taken up by fungal cells via the enzyme cytosine permease. It is converted intracellularly first to 5-FU and then to 5-fluorodeoxyuridine monophosphate (F-dUMP) and fluorouridine triphosphate (FUTP), which inhibit DNA and RNA synthesis, respectively. Human cells are unable to convert the parent drug to its active metabolites.

Synergy with amphotericin B has been demonstrated in vitro and in vivo. It may be related to enhanced penetration of the flucytosine through amphotericin-damaged fungal cell membranes. In vitro synergy with azole drugs has also been seen, although the mechanism is unclear.

Resistance is thought to be mediated through altered metabolism of flucytosine, and, while uncommon in primary isolates, it develops rapidly in the course of flucytosine monotherapy.

Adverse Effects

The adverse effects of flucytosine result from metabolism (possibly by intestinal flora) to the toxic antineoplastic compound fluorouracil. Bone marrow toxicity with anemia, leukopenia, and thrombocytopenia are the most common adverse effects, with derangement of liver enzymes occurring less frequently. A form of toxic enterocolitis can occur. There seems to be a narrow therapeutic window, with an increased risk of toxicity at higher drug levels and resistance developing rapidly at subtherapeutic concentrations. The use of drug concentration measurements may be helpful in reducing the incidence of toxic reactions, especially when flucytosine is combined with nephrotoxic agents such as amphotericin B.

Clinical Use

The spectrum of activity of flucytosine is restricted to *Cryptococcus neoformans,* some *Candida* species, and the dematiaceous molds that cause chromoblastomycosis. Flucytosine is not used as a single agent because of its demonstrated synergy with other agents and to avoid the development of secondary resistance. Clinical use at present is confined to combination therapy, either with amphotericin B for cryptococcal meningitis or with itraconazole for chromoblastomycosis. The role of flucytosine with amphotericin B in the treatment of systemic candidal infections remains undefined at present. Despite evidence of in vitro synergy in the treatment of *Aspergillus* infections, it is not usually used for infections with this organism.

AZOLES

The requirement for intravenous administration and the toxicity of the older antifungal agents created a need for antifungal agents with a better therapeutic profile. The relatively nontoxic oral azole medications represent the first major advance in this direction. Since their introduction in the 1980s, these medications have played an increasingly important role in the systemic therapy of fungal disease.

Azoles are synthetic compounds that can be classified as either imidazoles or triazoles according to the number of nitrogen atoms in the five-membered azole ring as indicated below. The imidazoles consist of ketoconazole, miconazole, and clotrimazole (Figure 48–1). The latter two drugs are now used only in topical therapy and will be discussed later. The triazoles include itraconazole and fluconazole, both of which are in common use for systemic treatment of fungal disease.

X = C, imidazole
X = N, triazole

Triazole nucleus

Pharmacology

The pharmacology of each of the azoles is unique and accounts for some of the variations in clinical use. Table 48–1 summarizes the differences between the three commonly prescribed azoles.

Mechanism of Action

The antifungal activity of azole drugs results from the reduction of ergosterol synthesis by inhibition of fungal cytochrome P450 enzymes. The specificity of azole drugs results from their greater affinity for fungal than for human cytochrome P450 enzymes. Imidazoles exhibit a lesser degree of specificity than the triazoles, accounting for their higher incidence of drug interactions and side effects.

Resistance to azoles occurs via multiple mechanisms. Once rare, increasing numbers of resistant strains are being reported, suggesting that increases in the use of these agents for prophylaxis and therapy may be selecting for clinical drug resistance in certain settings.

Clinical Use

The spectrum of action of these medications is quite broad, ranging from many *Candida* species, *Cryptococcus neoformans,* the endemic mycoses (blastomycosis, coccidioidomycosis, histoplasmosis), the dermatophytes, and, in the case of itraconazole, even *Aspergillus* infections. They are also useful in the treatment of intrinsically amphotericin-resistant organisms such as *Pseudallescheria boydii.*

Adverse Effects

As a group, the azoles are relatively nontoxic. The most common adverse reaction is relatively minor gastrointestinal upset. All azoles have been reported to cause abnormalities in liver enzymes and, very rarely, clinical hepatitis. Adverse effects specific to individual agents are discussed below.

Drug Interactions

All azole drugs affect the mammalian cytochrome P450 system of enzymes to some extent, and consequently they are prone to drug interactions. The most significant reactions are indicated below.

1. KETOCONAZOLE

Ketoconazole was the first oral azole introduced into clinical use. It is distinguished from fluconazole and itraconazole by its greater propensity to inhibit mammalian cytochrome P450 enzymes, ie, it is less selective for fungal P450 than are the newer azoles. This phenomenon has two consequences. First, ketoconazole inhibition of human cytochrome P450 enzymes interferes with biosynthesis of adrenal and gonadal steroid hormones, producing significant endocrine effects such as gynecomastia, infertility, and

Figure 48–1. Structural formulas of some antifungal azoles.

menstrual irregularities. Second, the interaction with P450 enzymes can alter the metabolism of other drugs, leading to enhanced toxicity of those agents. The two most significant examples of this are increased cyclosporine levels and enhanced arrhythmogenic effects of the nonsedating antihistamines, astemizole and terfenadine. Furthermore, other drugs can influence the blood levels of ketoconazole. These include H_2 blockers such as cimetidine, which increase gastric pH and thereby interfere with absorption of ketoconazole, and rifamycins (rifampin, rifabutin), which increase hepatic metabolism of the azole.

Clinical use of ketoconazole has been limited not only by the drug interactions and endocrine side ef-

Table 48–1. Pharmacologic properties of the commonly used systemic azole drugs.

	Water Solubility	Absorption	CSF:Serum Concentration Ratio	$t_{1/2}$ (hours)	Elimination	Formulations
Ketoconazole	Low	Variable	< 0.1	7–10	Hepatic	Oral
Itraconazole	Low	Variable	< 0.01	24–42	Hepatic	Oral
Fluconazole	High	High	> 0.7	22–31	Renal	Oral, IV

fects but also because of its narrow therapeutic range. It is available for systemic use in an oral formulation that is best absorbed at a low gastric pH. The drug is used at a dosage of 200–600 mg/d. Adverse effects of ketoconazole are highly dose-dependent and often limit therapy. Ketoconazole remains useful in treatment of mucocutaneous candidiasis and nonmeningeal coccidioidomycosis, since therapy with lower doses is often effective.

2. ITRACONAZOLE

Itraconazole is available in an oral formulation and is used at a dosage of 100–400 mg/d. Like ketoconazole, its absorption is increased by food and by low gastric pH. Like other lipid-soluble azoles, it interacts with hepatic microsomal enzymes, though to a lesser degree than ketoconazole. The principal drug interaction is reduced bioavailability of itraconazole when taken with rifamycins. It does not affect steroid synthesis, and its effects on the metabolism of other hepatically cleared medications are much less than those of ketoconazole. However, the interaction with nonsedating antihistamines remains a concern with itraconazole. Efforts are under way to produce an intravenous formulation of itraconazole and to develop an improved oral formulation with cyclodextran, a molecule that enhances bioavailability by acting as a carrier.

Itraconazole is the most potent of the available azoles, but effectiveness can be limited by reduced bioavailability. Like ketoconazole, it penetrates poorly into the cerebrospinal fluid. Itraconazole is the azole of choice in the treatment of dermatophytoses and onychomycosis and is the only agent with significant activity against *Aspergillus* species. Itraconazole is also the preferred azole for treatment of disease due to the dimorphic fungi *Histoplasma, Blastomyces,* and *Sporothrix.*

3. FLUCONAZOLE

Fluconazole is distinguished from the other azole medications by its water solubility and good cerebrospinal fluid penetration. Not only does its water solubility allow for intravenous administration, but it also results in excellent bioavailability by the oral route. Drug interactions are also less common because of all the azoles, fluconazole has the least effect on hepatic microsomal enzymes. As a result, this drug has a wide therapeutic window, which permits more aggressive dosing than with any other azole.

Fluconazole is the azole of choice in the treatment and secondary prophylaxis of cryptococcal meningitis. The drug is available in oral and intravenous formulations and is used at a dosage of 100–800 mg/d. Intravenous fluconazole has been shown to be equiv-

alent to amphotericin B in treatment of candidemia in ICU patients with normal white blood cell counts. While it is also effective for mucocutaneous candidiasis, ketoconazole is often an acceptable and less expensive alternative. Activity against the dimorphic fungi is limited to coccidioidal disease, and in particular for meningitis, where high doses of fluconazole often obviate the need for intrathecal amphotericin B.

Prophylactic use of fluconazole has been demonstrated to reduce fungal disease in bone marrow transplant recipients and AIDS patients, but the emergence of fluconazole-resistant fungi has raised concerns about this indication.

SYSTEMIC ANTIFUNGAL DRUGS FOR MUCOCUTANEOUS INFECTIONS

GRISEOFULVIN

Griseofulvin is a very insoluble fungistatic drug derived from a species of *Penicillium.* Its only use is in the systemic treatment of dermatophytosis. It is administered in a microcrystalline form at a dosage of 1 g/d. Absorption is improved when it is given with fatty foods. Griseofulvin's mechanism of action at the cellular level is unclear, but it is deposited in newly forming skin where it binds to keratin, protecting the skin from new infection. Since its action is to prevent infection of these new skin structures, it must be administered for 2–6 weeks for skin and hair infections to allow the replacement of infected keratin by the resistant structures. Nail infections may require therapy for months to allow regrowth of the new protected nail and is often followed by relapse. Adverse effects include an allergic syndrome much like serum sickness, hepatitis, and drug interactions with warfarin and phenobarbital. Griseofulvin has been largely replaced by newer antifungal medications such as itraconazole and terbinafine.

TERBINAFINE

Terbinafine is a synthetic allylamine that is available in an oral formulation and is used at a dosage of 250 mg/d. It is used in the treatment of dermatophytoses, especially onychomycosis. Like griseofulvin, it is a keratophilic medication, but unlike griseofulvin, it is fungicidal. Like the azole drugs, it interferes with ergosterol biosynthesis, but rather than interacting with the P450 system, terbinafine inhibits the fungal enzyme squalene epoxidase. This leads to the accumulation of the sterol squalene, which is toxic to the organism. One tablet given daily for 12 weeks achieves an up to 90% cure rate for onychomycosis and is more effective than griseofulvin or itraconazole. Adverse effects are rare, consisting primarily of gastrointestinal upset and headache. Terbinafine does not seem to affect the P450 system and has demonstrated no significant drug interactions to date.

TOPICAL ANTIFUNGAL THERAPY

NYSTATIN

Nystatin is a polyene macrolide much like amphotericin B and has the same pore-forming mechanism of action. It is too toxic for parenteral administration and is only used topically. It is currently available in creams, ointments, suppositories, and other forms for application to skin and mucous membranes. Liposomal formulations for systemic administration are in clinical development. Nystatin is not absorbed to any significant degree from skin, mucous membranes, or the gastrointestinal tract. As a result, it has little significant toxicity, though oral use is often limited by the unpleasant taste.

Nystatin is active against most *Candida* species and is most commonly used for suppression of local candidal infections. Some common indications include oropharyngeal thrush, vaginal candidiasis, and intertriginous candidal infections.

TOPICAL AZOLES

The two azoles most commonly used topically are clotrimazole and miconazole. Both are available over-the-counter and are often used for vulvovaginal candidiasis. Oral clotrimazole troches are available for treatment of oral thrush and are a pleasant-tasting alternative to nystatin. In cream form, both agents are useful for dermatophytic infections, including tinea corporis, tinea pedis, and tinea cruris. Absorption is negligible, and adverse effects are rare.

Topical and shampoo forms of ketoconazole are also available and useful in the treatment of seborrheic dermatitis and pityriasis versicolor. Several other azoles are available for topical use (see Preparations Available).

TOPICAL ALLYLAMINES

Terbinafine and naftifine are allylamines available as topical creams. Both are effective for treatment of tinea cruris and tinea corporis. These are prescription drugs in the USA.

PREPARATIONS AVAILABLE

Amphotericin B (Fungizone Intravenous, Fungizone)
Parenteral: 50 mg per vial solution from lyophilized cake; 5 mg/mL lipid complex suspension for injection
Topical: 3% cream, lotion, ointment
Clotrimazole (Lotrimin, Mycelex)
Topical: 1% cream, solution, lotion
Econazole (Spectazole)
Topical: 1% cream
Fluconazole (Diflucan)
Oral: 50, 100, 150, 200 mg tablets; powder of 10, 40 mg/mL suspension
Parenteral: 2 mg/mL in 200 and 400 mL vials
Flucytosine (Ancobon)
Oral: 250, 500 mg capsules
Griseofulvin (Grifulvin, Grisactin, Fulvin P/G)
Oral microsize: 125, 250 mg capsules; 250, 500 mg tablets, 125 mg/5 mL suspension
Oral ultramicrosize:* 125, 165, 250, 330 mg tablets

Itraconazole (Sporanox)
Oral: 100 mg capsules
Ketoconazole (Nizoral)
Oral: 200 mg tablets
Topical: 2% cream, shampoo
Miconazole (Monistat i.v., Micatin [topical])
Parenteral: 10 mg/mL for injection
Topical: 2% cream, powder, spray
Naftifine (Naftin)
Topical: 1% cream, gel
Nystatin (generic, Mycostatin, others)
Oral: 500,000 unit tablets
Topical: 100,000 units/g cream, ointment, powder
Oxiconazole (Oxistat)
Topical: 1% cream, lotion
Sulconazole (Exelderm)
Topical: 1% cream, lotion
Terbinafine (Lamisil)
Topical: 1% cream

---

*Ultramicrosize formulations of griseofulvin are approximately 1.5 times more potent, mg for mg, than the microsize preparations.

REFERENCES

Aly R, Berger T: Common superficial fungal infections in patients with AIDS. Clin Infect Dis 1996;22(Suppl 2):S128.

Brajtburg J et al: Amphotericin B: Current understanding of mechanisms of action. Antimicrob Agents Chemother 1990;34:183.

Brautigam M, Nolting S, Schopf RE: Randomized, double-blind comparison of terbinafine and itraconazole for treatment of tinea infection. Br Med J 1995;311:919.

Como JA, Dismukes WE: Oral azole drugs as systemic antifungal therapy. N Engl J Med 1994;330:263.

Francis P, Walsh TJ: Evolving role of flucytosine in immunocompromised patients: New insights into safety, pharmacokinetics, and antifungal therapy. Clin Infect Dis 1992;15:1003.

Galgiani J: Coccioidomycosis. West J Med 1996;159:153.

Galgiani JN: Fluconazole, a new antifungal agent. Ann Intern Med 1990;113:177.

Gallis HA, Drew RH, Pickard WW: Amphotericin B: 30 years of clinical experience. Rev Infect Dis 1990;12:308.

Goldman L: Griseofulvin. Med Clin North Am 1970; 54:1339.

Graybill JR: The future of antifungal therapy. Clin Infect Dis 1996;22(Suppl 2):S166.

Hay RJ: Fluconazole. J Infect 1990;21:1.

Hiemenz JW, Walsh TJ: Lipid formulations of amphotericin B: Recent progress and future directions. Clin Infect Dis 1996;22(Suppl 2):S133.

Kauffman CA: Role of azoles in antifungal therapy. Clin Infect Dis 1996;22(Suppl 2):S148.

Petersen D et al: Individualization of 5-fluorocytosine therapy. Chemotherapy 1994;40:149.

Pfaller M: Nosocomial candidiasis: Emerging species, reservoirs and modes of transmission. Clin Infect Dis 1996;22(Suppl 2):S89.

Rezabek GH, Friedman AD: Superficial fungal infections of the skin: Diagnosis and current treatment recommendations. Drugs 1992;43:674.

Saag MS, Dismukes WE: Azole antifungal agents: Emphasis on new triazoles. Antimicrob Agents Chemother 1988;32:1.

Sarosi GA, Davies SF: Therapy for fungal infections. Mayo Clin Proc 1994;69:1111.

Terrell CL, Hermans PE: Antifungal agents used for deep-seated mycotic infections. Mayo Clin Proc 1987; 62:1116.

Uzun O, Anaissie EJ: Problems and controversies in the management of hematogenous candidiasis. Clin Infect Dis 1996;22(Suppl 2):S95.

Viviani MA: Flucytosine–what is its future? J Antimicrob Chemother 1995;35:241.

Zervos M, Silverman J, Meunier F: Fluconazole in fungal infection: a review. Infect Dis Clin Pract 1994;3:94.

49

Antiviral Agents

Sharon Safrin, MD, & Henry F. Chambers, MD

Viruses are obligate intracellular parasites; their replication depends primarily on synthetic processes of the host cell. Consequently, antiviral agents must either block viral entry into the cell or be active inside the host cell to be effective. As a corollary, nonselective inhibitors of virus replication may interfere with host cell function and produce toxicity. The search for chemicals that inhibit virus-specific functions is currently one of the most active areas of pharmacologic investigation.

In many viral infections, replication of the virus peaks at or before the manifestation of clinical symptoms. Optimal clinical efficacy therefore generally depends either on early initiation of therapy (eg, acyclovir for treatment of varicella or zoster infection) or on prevention of infection (eg, chemoprophylaxis against influenza A using amantadine). Viral replication consists of several steps: (1) adsorption to and penetration into susceptible host cells; (2) uncoating of viral nucleic acid; (3) synthesis of early, regulatory proteins, eg, nucleic acid polymerases; (4) synthesis of RNA or DNA; (5) synthesis of late, structural proteins; (6) assembly (maturation) of viral particles; and (7) release from the cell. Antiviral agents can potentially target any of these steps (Figure 49–1).

Research in antiviral chemotherapy began in the early 1950s, when the search for cancer treatments generated several new compounds capable of inhibiting viral DNA synthesis. One such compound was the pyrimidine analog idoxuridine, which subsequently was approved for the topical treatment of herpes keratitis. Since that time, research has focused on both pyrimidine and purine nucleoside analogs, with a goal of identifying agents with greater selectivity, in vivo stability, and lack of toxicity.

With the growth of the AIDS epidemic, research on drugs specifically effective against the human immunodeficiency virus (HIV) became a high priority. Many of the proteins of this retrovirus have been purified and characterized with the goal of designing drugs that would selectively inhibit some critical enzyme in the retrovirus such as reverse transcriptase and the protease that is required for the final packaging of this virus particle. Recent clinical trials suggest that some progress is being made.

ACRONYMS USED IN THIS CHAPTER

ara-A	Vidarabine
AZT	Zidovudine (previously azidothymidine)
CMV	Cytomegalovirus
ddC	Zalcitabine
ddI	Didanosine
d4T	Stavudine
EBV	Epstein-Barr virus
HBV	Hepatitis B virus
HCV	Hepatitis C virus
HHV-6	Human herpes virus, strain 6
HIV	Human immuno-deficiency virus
HSV-1, HSV-2	Herpes simplex virus, strains 1 and 2
IDU, IUDR	Idoxuridine
IFN	Interferon
3TC	Lamivudine
VZV	Varicella-zoster virus

Most of the antiviral agents currently available act on synthesis of purines and pyrimidines (step 4); reverse transcriptase inhibitors block transcription of the HIV RNA genome into DNA, thereby preventing synthesis of viral mRNA and protein. The protease inhibitors act on synthesis of late proteins and packaging (steps 5 and 6).

I. ANTIHERPES AGENTS

ACYCLOVIR

Acyclovir (Figure 49–2) is an acyclic guanosine derivative with clinical activity against herpes simplex

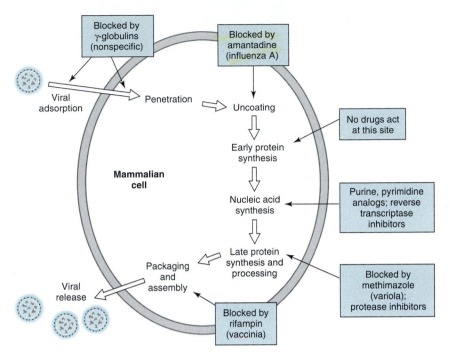

Figure 49–1. The major sites of antiviral drug action. (Modified and reproduced, with permission, from Katzung BG, Trevor AT [editors]: *Pharmacology: Examination & Board Review,* 4th ed. Appleton & Lange, 1995.)

virus-1 and -2 and against varicella-zoster virus. In vitro activity against Epstein-Barr virus, cytomegalovirus, and human herpes virus-6 is present, but comparatively weaker.

Mechanism of Action

Acyclovir requires three phosphorylation steps for activation and is converted first to the monophosphate derivative by the *virus-specified* thymidine kinase and then to the di- and triphosphate compounds by the *host's* cellular enzymes (Figure 49–3). Because it requires the viral kinase for the first phosphorylation, acyclovir is selectively activated and the triphosphate accumulates only in infected cells. Acyclovir triphosphate inhibits viral DNA synthesis by two mechanisms: competitive inhibition of dGTP for the viral DNA polymerase, with binding to the DNA template as an irreversible complex, and chain termination following incorporation into the viral DNA.

Resistance

Resistance to acyclovir can develop in HSV or VZV through alteration in either the viral thymidine kinase or viral DNA polymerase. Most clinical isolates are resistant on the basis of deficient thymidine kinase activity and thus are cross-resistant with valacyclovir, famciclovir, and ganciclovir. Agents such as foscarnet, cidofovir, and trifluridine do not require activation by viral thymidine kinase and thus have preserved activity against acyclovir-resistant strains.

Pharmacokinetics

Acyclovir is available in oral, intravenous, and topical formulations (Table 49–1). The bioavailability of the oral formulation is 15–20%. Serum concentrations peak at approximately 1 µg/mL after a 200 mg oral dose and 1.5–2 µg/mL after an 800 mg dose. Peak serum concentrations are 10 µg/mL and 20 µg/mL after an intravenous infusion of 5 mg/kg and 10 mg/kg over 1 hour, respectively. Topical formulations produce local concentrations that may exceed 10 µg/mL in herpetic lesions, but systemic concentrations are undetectable.

Acyclovir is cleared primarily by glomerular filtration and tubular secretion. The half-life is 3–4 hours in patients with normal renal function and 20 hours in patients with anuria. Dosage adjustment is necessary for patients with creatinine clearances less than 50 mL/min. For intravenous administration, a loading dose of 5–10 mg/kg is given, and the normal total daily maintenance dosage (eg, 15 mg/kg/d) is reduced by one-third for a creatinine clearance of 25–50 mL/min and by two-thirds for clearance of 10–25 mL/min. One-sixth the dosage (eg, 2.5 mg/kg once a day) is recommended for anuric patients. A smaller reduction is recommended for oral acyclovir in the setting of renal insufficiency, with 40% of the usual dosage given when creatinine clearance is less than 10 mL/min. Acyclovir is readily cleared by hemodialysis but not by peritoneal dialysis. The dosage of intravenous acyclovir posthemodialysis is 2.5–5 mg/kg/d.

Figure 49–2. Chemical structures of some representative antiherpes agents.

Acyclovir diffuses into most tissues and body fluids to produce concentrations that are 50–100% of those in serum. Cerebrospinal fluid concentrations are 50% of serum values.

Clinical Uses

Oral acyclovir is effective for treatment of primary infection and recurrences of genital and labial herpes. Acyclovir, 200 mg five times daily, shortens duration of symptoms, time of viral shedding, and time to resolution of lesions by approximately 5 days in primary HSV infections. An alternative dosing option, although less well studied, is 400 mg every 8 hours. Clinical response is less dramatic in treatment of recurrent disease, with shortening of the time course by 1–2 days. Treatment of primary genital herpes does not alter the frequency or severity of recurrent outbreaks. For treatment of HSV proctitis, the recommended oral dosage is 400 mg five times daily. The use of acyclovir in patients with recurrent herpes labialis, 400 mg five times daily, reduces the mean duration of pain but not the time to healing.

Intravenous acyclovir (10 mg/kg every 8 hours) is the treatment of choice for herpes simplex encephalitis and neonatal HSV infection. Intravenous acyclovir (5 mg/kg every 8 hours) also is effective for treatment of primary and recurrent HSV infections but usually is reserved for patients with particularly severe disease and those who cannot ingest oral pills.

Topical acyclovir is much less effective than oral therapy for primary HSV infection. It is of no benefit in treating recurrences.

VZV is less susceptible to acyclovir than HSV (inhibitory concentrations of 1–4 µg/mL). Dosages of 800

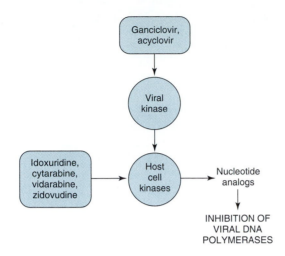

Figure 49–3. Antiviral actions of purine and pyrimidine analogs. Acyclovir and ganciclovir (top) are phosphorylated first by viral kinase to the monophosphate. This intermediate and the drugs shown on the left are then phosphorylated by host cell kinases to the nucleotide analogs that inhibit viral replication. (Modified and reproduced, with permission, from Katzung BG, Trevor AT [editors]: *Pharmacology: Examination & Board Review,* 4th ed. Appleton & Lange, 1995.)

mg five times daily (20 mg/kg every 6 hours in children) shortens the duration of varicella or zoster in immunocompetent patients by 1–2 days. In immunocompromised patients with zoster, intravenous administration of acyclovir (10 mg/kg every 8 hours) reduces the incidence of cutaneous and visceral dissemination. Treatment of zoster with acyclovir does not reduce the frequency of postherpetic neuralgia, though addition of prednisone to the regimen may do so.

Oral acyclovir, 400 mg every 12 hours or 200 mg every 8 hours, is effective for chronic suppression of recurrent genital and labial herpes in patients with frequent outbreaks. Recurrence of outbreaks may resume upon discontinuation of suppressive acyclovir. When given prophylactically to patients undergoing organ transplantation, oral acyclovir (200 mg every 8 hours or 800 mg every 12 hours) or intravenous acyclovir (5 mg/kg every 8 hours) prevents reactivation of HSV infection. The benefit of acyclovir for prevention of CMV infections in transplant patients is controversial.

Adverse Reactions

Acyclovir is generally well-tolerated. Nausea, diarrhea, and headache have occasionally been reported. Intravenous infusion may be associated with renal insufficiency or neurologic toxicity (the latter may include tremors or delirium); however, these are uncommon with adequate hydration and avoidance of rapid infusion rates. Daily use of acyclovir for suppression of genital herpes for more than 10 years has

not been associated with untoward effects. There has been no evidence of teratogenicity to date in the accruing Acyclovir in Pregnancy Registry, and no effect on sperm production was demonstrated in a placebo-controlled trial of patients receiving acyclovir on a daily basis.

VALACYCLOVIR

Valacyclovir is the L-valyl ester of acyclovir. It is rapidly converted to acyclovir when ingested orally, achieving serum levels three to five times greater than those achieved with oral acyclovir and approximating those resulting from administration of acyclovir intravenously. In vitro activity, mechanism of action, emergence of resistance, and pharmacokinetics are identical to those of acyclovir.

Valacyclovir is currently approved in the United States for the treatment of patients with recurrent genital herpes (500 mg every 12 hours) or herpes zoster infections (1 g every 8 hours). Other than less frequent dosing, it appears to offer no advantage over acyclovir except that one controlled study found a reduction in the duration of zoster-associated pain.

Valacyclovir, when used in recommended doses for genital herpes or zoster, is well tolerated; nausea, diarrhea, and headache have occasionally been described. AIDS patients receiving high-dosage valacyclovir (ie, 8 g/d) had an increased incidence of gastrointestinal intolerance as well as thrombotic microangiopathies such as thrombotic thrombocytopenic purpura and hemolytic uremic syndrome.

FAMCICLOVIR

Famciclovir is the diacetyl ester prodrug of 6-deoxy penciclovir, an acyclic guanosine analog (Figure 49–2). Famciclovir is rapidly converted after oral ingestion to penciclovir by first-pass metabolism. Penciclovir, which is the active form of the drug, shares many features with acyclovir. It is active in vitro against HSV-1, HSV-2, VZV, EBV, and hepatitis B virus. Activation by phosphorylation is catalyzed by the virus-specified thymidine kinase in infected cells, followed by competitive inhibition of the viral DNA polymerase to inhibit DNA synthesis. Unlike acyclovir, penciclovir does not cause chain termination. Penciclovir triphosphate has lower affinity for the viral DNA polymerase than acyclovir triphosphate, but it achieves higher intracellular concentrations and has a more prolonged intracellular effect in experimental systems. Typically there is cross-resistance between famciclovir and acyclovir.

Pharmacokinetics

Famciclovir is available as an oral formulation. The bioavailability of penciclovir that is converted

Table 49–1. Recommended uses of currently available antiherpes antiviral agents in adults.

Agent	Route of Administration	Use	Recommended Adult Dosage
Acyclovir	Oral	Genital herpes treatment	200 mg 5 times daily or 400 mg every 8 hours
		Genital herpes suppression	400 mg every 12 hours or 200 mg every 8 hours
		Varicella or zoster; severe genital herpes	800 mg 5 times daily
	Intravenous	Herpes encephalitis	5 mg/kg every 8 hours
		Varicella or zoster in an immunosuppressed host	10 mg/kg every 8 hours
Cidofovir	Intravenous	CMV retinitis	Induction: 5 mg/kg every 7 days Maintenance: 5 mg/kg every 4 days
Famciclovir	Oral	Recurrent genital herpes	125 mg every 12 hours
		Zoster	500 mg every 8 hours
Foscarnet	Intravenous	CMV retinitis	Induction: 60 mg/kg every 8 hours or 90 mg/kg every 12 hours Maintenance: 90–120 mg/kg/d
		Acyclovir-resistant HSV or zoster infection	40 mg/kg every 8 hours
Ganciclovir	Intravenous	CMV retinitis	Induction: 5 mg/kg every 12 hours Maintenance: 5–10 mg/kg/d
	Oral	CMV retinitis treatment, prophylaxis	1 g every 8 hours
Idoxuridine	Ophthalmic solution	Herpes keratitis	1 drop every hour
Sorivudine	Oral	Zoster	40 mg/d
Trifluridine	Ophthalmic solution	Herpes keratitis	1 drop every 2 hours
		Acyclovir-resistant HSV infection	Film covering lesion 5 times daily
Valacyclovir	Oral	Recurrent genital herpes	500 mg every 12 hours
		Zoster	1 g every 8 hours
Vidarabine	Intravenous	HSV encephalitis; VZV infection in immuno-compromised patients	15 mg/kg/d
	Ophthalmic ointment	Herpes keratitis	Apply every 3 hours up to 5 times daily

from orally administered famciclovir is 70%. A peak serum concentration of 2 μg/mL is achieved following a 250 mg oral dose. An intravenous formulation of penciclovir is undergoing clinical evaluation. Clearance of penciclovir and dosage adjustments in renal impairment are similar to those for acyclovir.

Clinical Uses

Famciclovir is approved for the treatment of patients with recurrent genital herpes (125 mg every 12 hours) and for the treatment of patients with herpes zoster infection (500 mg every 8 hours). Comparison with acyclovir in controlled trials in immunocompetent patients with zoster showed no differences in time until healing but more rapid resolution of zoster-associated pain in patients treated with famciclovir.

Adverse Reactions

The drug has been well tolerated in studies to date, though headache, diarrhea, and nausea have been sporadically reported. Testicular toxicity has been demonstrated in animals receiving repeated doses, though men receiving daily famciclovir (250 mg every 12 hours) had no changes in spermatic morphology or motility.

GANCICLOVIR

Ganciclovir (formerly DHPG) is a guanosine analog (Figure 49–2) that requires triphosphorylation for activation prior to inhibiting the viral DNA polymerase. Monophosphorylation is catalyzed by the virus-specified protein kinase phosphotransferase UL97 in CMV-infected cells and by the viral thymidine kinase in HSV-infected cells. The activated compound competitively inhibits viral DNA polymerase, causing an unstable complex, but does not result in chain termination. Ganciclovir has activity against CMV, HSV, VZV, and EBV; its activity against CMV is up to 100 times greater than that of acyclovir. Ganciclovir-resistant isolates of CMV typically have mutations in the *UL97* gene, although DNA polymerase mutations have been described as well. Strains of acyclovir-resistant thymidine kinase-deficient HSV are cross-resistant to ganciclovir.

Pharmacokinetics

Ganciclovir is available in intravenous and oral formulations. The oral bioavailability of ganciclovir is poor (6–9%). A 5 mg/kg dose administered intravenously over 1 hour produces serum concentrations averaging 10 μg/mL. Cerebrospinal fluid concentrations are approximately 50% of those in serum. Intravitreal concentrations average 1 μg/mL. The half-life is 2–4 hours with normal renal function. Clearance of the drug is linearly related to creatinine clearance, and dosage adjustment is recommended for creatinine clearances less than 80 mL/min. The maximum recommended dosage is 1.25 mg/kg/d for patients with creatinine clearance less than 25 mL/min. Ganciclovir is readily cleared by hemodialysis; the daily dose should be given postdialysis.

Clinical Uses

Intravenous ganciclovir (5 mg/kg every 12 hours for induction, then 5 mg/kg/d for maintenance) is indicated for the treatment of CMV retinitis in patients with AIDS. The drug also reduces the incidence of symptomatic CMV disease if administered before organ transplantation. Administration of intravenous ganciclovir to treat CMV pneumonitis in immunocompromised patients is often beneficial, particularly in combination with intravenous cytomegalovirus immunoglobulin. Intravenous ganciclovir has also been used to treat CMV colitis and esophagitis.

Oral ganciclovir (1 g every 8 hours) has recently been approved in the United States for prevention of end-organ CMV disease in AIDS patients and as maintenance therapy of CMV retinitis following induction. Alternative routes of administration of ganciclovir for patients with CMV retinitis (currently under investigation) include intravitreal administration and intraocular implantation.

Adverse Reactions

The most common side effect of treatment with ganciclovir is myelosuppression, particularly neutropenia. Myelosuppression may be additive in patients receiving both ganciclovir and zidovudine. The frequency of myelosuppression is lower with oral than with intravenous ganciclovir. Central nervous system toxicity (headache, changes in mental status, seizures) has been rarely reported. The drug is mitogenic in mammalian cells and carcinogenic and embryotoxic in animals.

CIDOFOVIR

Cidofovir (formerly HPMPC) is a cytosine nucleotide analog with in vitro activity against CMV, HSV-1, HSV-2, VZV, EBV, HHV-6, adenovirus, and human papillomavirus. Phosphorylation of cidofovir to the active diphosphate is independent of virus infection, and the compound has a prolonged intracellular half-life. It has been evaluated in both intravenous and topical gel formulations.

Administration of intravenous cidofovir (5 mg/kg once weekly for 2 weeks, then once every other week) is effective in the treatment of patients with CMV retinitis. Intravitreal administration of cidofovir may be an alternative route for patients with CMV retinitis. Topical 1% cidofovir is under evaluation for the treatment of mucocutaneous herpes simplex infection, including that resistant to acyclovir, and for the treatment of genital warts. Cidofovir is cleared by the kidney, and dosage adjustment is required in renal failure. Nephrotoxicity, the major dose-limiting toxicity associated with use of intravenous cidofovir, is in large part prevented by concomitant administration of oral probenecid (which blocks tubular secretion) and saline hydration. Resistance to cidofovir is due to mutation in the DNA polymerase gene.

FOSCARNET

Foscarnet is an inorganic pyrophosphate compound (Figure 49–2) that inhibits viral DNA polymerase, RNA polymerase, or HIV reverse transcriptase directly, without requirement for activation by phosphorylation. It has in vitro activity against HSV, VZV, CMV, EBV, HHV-6, HBV, and HIV. Resistance to foscarnet in HSV and CMV infection is due to point mutations in the DNA polymerase gene and is typically associated with prolonged or repeated exposure to the drug. Mutations in the HIV-1 reverse transcriptase have also been described.

Pharmacokinetics

The drug is available in an intravenous formulation only. Poor oral bioavailability and gastrointestinal intolerance have so far precluded the production of an oral formulation. Peak serum concentrations averaging 80–100 μg/mL (450–575 μmol/L) are achieved following an infusion of 60 mg/kg. Cerebrospinal fluid concentrations are approximately two-thirds of steady state serum concentrations. Up to 30% of the drug may be deposited in bone, with a half-life of several months; the repercussions of this are unknown.

Clearance of foscarnet is primarily by the kidney and is directly proportionate to creatinine clearance. The initial elimination half-life is 4–8 hours, followed by a prolonged terminal elimination half-life of 3–4 days in patients with normal renal function. Serial adjustment of dose according to calculated creatinine clearance is necessary throughout administration of the drug. Serum drug concentrations are reduced by approximately 50% by a 3-hour hemodialysis.

Clinical Uses

Foscarnet is approved for the treatment of patients with CMV retinitis (60 mg/kg every 8 hours or 90 mg/kg every 12 hours for induction, followed by 90–120 mg/kg/d for maintenance therapy) and acyclovir-resistant HSV infection (40 mg/kg every 8 hours or 40 mg/kg every 12 hours). Controlled comparison with ganciclovir for the treatment of CMV retinitis in AIDS patients demonstrated no significant differences in anti-CMV effect. Controlled comparison with vidarabine for treatment of acyclovir-resistant HSV infection demonstrated superiority of foscarnet. Foscarnet has also been used to treat CMV colitis and esophagitis (90 mg/kg every 12 hours or 60 mg/kg every 8 hours) and acyclovir-resistant VZV infection (40 mg/kg every 8 hours).

Adverse Reactions

Potential adverse effects include renal insufficiency, hypocalcemia or hypercalcemia, and hypo- or hyperphosphatemia. Genital ulcerations associated with foscarnet therapy may be due to high levels of ionized drug in the urine. Central nervous system toxicities include headache, hallucinations, and seizures.

Use of an infusion pump to control the rate of infusion is important to avoid toxicity, and relatively large volumes of fluid are required due to the drug's poor solubility. Saline preloading helps to prevent nephrotoxicity, as does avoidance of concomitant administration of drugs with nephrotoxic potential. Concurrent administration with pentamidine may exacerbate both nephrotoxicity and hypocalcemia.

IDOXURIDINE

Idoxuridine (IDU, IUDR) is a substituted pyrimidine analog that was the first antiviral agent to be approved. It is used topically in the treatment of herpes keratitis (0.1% solution), but because of its lack of selectivity it is too toxic for systemic administration.

SORIVUDINE

Sorivudine (BV-araU) is an investigational pyrimidine nucleoside analog with in vitro activity against VZV, HSV-1, and EBV (Figure 49–2). The concentration of sorivudine that inhibits VZV synthesis is approximately 1000-fold lower than that of acyclovir. It appears to require activation through phosphorylation by the virus-specified thymidine kinase. Sorivudine triphosphate competitively inhibits DNA polymerase but is not incorporated into viral DNA. Although sorivudine-resistant clinical isolates have not yet been evaluated, there is cross-resistance of sorivudine with thymidine kinase-deficient isolates of acyclovir.

An oral formulation is under study but has not yet been approved in the USA. Its long intracellular half-life permits once daily dosing. Sorivudine (40 mg once daily) has efficacy in the treatment of patients with varicella or zoster infection. The principal metabolite, bromovinyl uracil (BVU), inhibits the metabolism of 5-fluorouracil, resulting in severe bone marrow suppression when the two are administered together. Comprehensive evaluations of efficacy and toxicity of this compound are under way.

TRIFLURIDINE

Trifluridine (trifluorothymidine) is a fluorinated pyrimidine nucleoside that inhibits viral DNA synthesis. The compound has in vitro activity against HSV-1, HSV-2, vaccinia, and some adenoviruses. It is phosphorylated intracellularly to its active form by cellular enzymes, then competes with thymidine triphosphate for incorporation by the viral DNA polymerase. Incorporation of trifluridine triphosphate into both viral and cellular DNA prevents its systemic use. Application of a 1% solution is an approved therapy for primary keratoconjunctivitis and recurrent epithelial keratitis due to HSV. Topical application of trifluridine, alone or in combination with interferon-α, has been used successfully in the treatment of acyclovir-resistant HSV infections.

VIDARABINE

Vidarabine (ara-A, adenine arabinoside) is an adenosine analog with in vitro activity against HSV, VZV, and CMV. It is phosphorylated intracellularly by host enzymes to form ara-ATP, then inhibits viral DNA polymerase. Vidarabine triphosphate is incorporated into both viral and cellular DNA; teratogenicity has been demonstrated in animals. In vivo, vidarabine is rapidly metabolized to hypoxanthine arabinoside through removal of the 6-amino group by adenosine deaminase, resulting in markedly reduced antiviral activity. This instability, as well as excessive toxicity, has severely limited its clinical utility.

Vidarabine as a 3% ointment is effective treatment for acute keratoconjunctivitis, superficial keratitis, and recurrent epithelial keratitis due to HSV. Intravenous vidarabine (10–15 mg/kg daily) is effective for treatment of HSV encephalitis, neonatal herpes, and VZV infection in immunocompromised patients. However, acyclovir is generally more effective and less toxic and has become more widely used. Vidarabine has in vitro activity against acyclovir-resistant strains of HSV, but it is less effective and more toxic than foscarnet. The drug is eliminated primarily by renal mechanisms as the hypoxanthine metabolite. A 25% dosage reduction is recommended for patients with significant renal impairment. Owing to its poor solubility in water, it must be administered in large volumes over long periods of time (eg 12 hours). Potential toxicities include gastrointestinal intolerance, neurologic manifestations (confusion, myoclonus, seizures), and myelosuppression.

II. ANTIRETROVIRAL AGENTS (TABLE 49–2)

REVERSE TRANSCRIPTASE INHIBITORS

ZIDOVUDINE

Zidovudine (previously azidothymidine, AZT) is a deoxythymidine analog that requires anabolic phosphorylation for activation to the 5′-triphosphate form (Figure 49–3). After entering the cell by passive diffusion, zidovudine is phosphorylated via three cellular kinases; the triphosphate is a competitive inhibitor of deoxythymidine triphosphate for the reverse transcriptase. Additionally, it acts as a chain terminator in the synthesis of proviral DNA. Zidovudine has in vitro activity against HIV-1, HIV-2, and the human T cell lymphotropic viruses; activity is present but weaker against HBV and EBV.

Resistance

Zidovudine resistance is due to mutations in the reverse transcriptase gene. In vitro resistance typically occurs after prolonged therapy, is more frequent in persons with advanced HIV infection, and is associated with decreased clinical responsiveness. Withdrawal of zidovudine exposure may permit the reversion of HIV-1 isolates to the susceptible (wild-type) phenotype. Mutations at codons 67, 70, 215, and 219 incur a greater than 100-fold reduction in susceptibility when inserted by site-directed mutagenesis. Other sites of mutation have been described as well (eg, codon 41). The effect of such mutations appears to be cumulative, resulting in additive or synergistic reductions in susceptibility.

Pharmacokinetics

Zidovudine is available in intravenous and oral formulations. It is well absorbed from the gut and distributed to most body tissues and fluids, including the cerebrospinal fluid, where drug levels are approximately 60% of those in serum. Substantial first-pass metabolism to an inactive glucuronidated metabolite results in a systemic bioavailability of approximately 65%. The serum half-life is only 1.1 hours, but the intracellular half-life of the active moiety is 3.3 hours. Clearance of zidovudine is reduced by 70% in patients with cirrhosis and by approximately 50% in uremic patients. Therefore, dosage adjustment in the setting of advanced hepatic or renal insufficiency may be warranted.

Table 49–2. Currently available antiretroviral agents.

Agent	Class of Agent	Route of Administration	Recommended Adult Dosage
Didanosine	Nucleoside analog	Oral	200 mg every 12 hours
Indinavir	Protease inhibitor	Oral	800 mg every 8 hours
Lamivudine	Nucleoside analog	Oral	150 mg every 12 hours
Ritonavir	Protease inhibitor	Oral	600 mg every 12 hours
Saquinavir	Protease inhibitor	Oral	600 mg every 8 hours
Stavudine	Nucleoside analog	Oral	40 mg every 12 hours
Zalcitabine	Nucleoside analog	Oral	0.75 mg every 8 hours
Zidovudine	Nucleoside analog	Oral	200 mg every 8 hours, 300 mg every 12 hours, or 100 mg 5 times daily

Clinical Uses

The recommended dosage of zidovudine is 200 mg every 8 hours or 100 mg five times daily; recent data suggest that the dosage of 300 mg every 12 hours is clinically equivalent. Zidovudine inhibits replication of HIV-1 in infected individuals and has been shown to decrease the rate of clinical disease progression and prolong survival. Zidovudine has efficacy in the treatment of HIV-associated encephalopathy and thrombocytopenia, and in the prevention of vertical (mother to newborn) transmission of HIV. Clinical efficacy is limited by the relatively rapid development of resistance, particularly when used as monotherapy. The combination of zidovudine with one or two other agents, such as a second reverse transcriptase inhibitor (eg, lamivudine) or a protease inhibitor, is one strategy to enhance antiviral activity and retard the development of resistance.

Adverse Reactions

The most common adverse effect is myelosuppression, resulting in anemia or neutropenia; this may be additive if zidovudine is coadministered with other drugs that cause bone marrow suppression. Gastrointestinal intolerance, headaches, and insomnia may occur but tend to resolve if ingestion is continued. Less frequent unwanted effects include thrombocytopenia, acute cholestatic hepatitis, and myopathy. Very high doses can cause anxiety, confusion, and tremulousness.

Since zidovudine is eliminated primarily by hepatic glucuronidation, inhibition of this pathway (by drugs such as probenecid, indomethacin, naproxen, beta-lactam antibiotics, phenytoin, phenobarbital, and ethinyl estradiol) may require dosage adjustment. Toxicity may be increased by the concomitant use of drugs that also undergo degradation in the liver, eg, acetaminophen, benzodiazepines, cimetidine, methadone, and sulfonamides. Increased serum levels of zidovudine may occur with concomitant administration of probenecid or fluconazole, and zidovudine levels may decrease when the drug is given with rifampin or clarithromycin. The clinical significance of such interactions has yet to be determined. Zidovudine may decrease phenytoin levels, warranting monitoring of serum levels of the anticonvulsant.

DIDANOSINE

Didanosine (ddI) is a synthetic analog of deoxyadenosine (Figure 49–4). It is metabolized intracellularly by a series of cellular enzymes; its active moiety, 2,3-dideoxyadenosine-5-triphosphate, inhibits viral replication by competitive inhibition of HIV reverse transcriptase and by chain termination. Resis-

Figure 49–4. Chemical structures of some representative antiretroviral agents.

tance to didanosine is typically associated with mutation at codon 74. Appearance of this mutation may partially restore susceptibility to zidovudine but leads to cross-resistance with zalcitabine. High-level resistance (> 100-fold decreased susceptibility) has not been reported to date.

Pharmacokinetics

At acid pH, hydrolysis of the glycosidic bond between the sugar and the base moieties of the nucleoside will inactivate the compound. The original formulation, a buffered powder, has been replaced by chewable/dispersible buffered tablets with greater bioavailability. Absorption is decreased by food. Peak serum concentrations average 1 µg/mL after a 300 mg dose. Cerebrospinal fluid concentrations of the drug are approximately 20% of serum concentrations. The elimination half-life is 0.6–1.5 hours, but the intracellular half-life of the activated compound is approximately 12 hours. The drug is eliminated by glomerular filtration and tubular secretion. Dosage adjustment is required for creatinine clearances less than 60 mL/min.

Clinical Uses

Didanosine in a dosage of 200 mg every 12 hours is effective in slowing clinical progression of disease in HIV-infected individuals when administered as monotherapy or in combination with zidovudine. The dosage should be reduced for low body weight. Didanosine should be taken on an empty stomach and, because of the buffered formulation, should be administered at least 2 hours after drugs requiring acidity for optimal absorption (eg, ketoconazole and dapsone). Fluoroquinolones and tetracyclines should be administered at least 2 hours before or after didanosine in order to avoid decreased antibiotic plasma concentrations due to chelation. Coadministration with ganciclovir results in increased AUC (area under the [plasma concentration] curve) of didanosine and decreased AUC of ganciclovir.

Adverse Reactions

The major clinical toxicity associated with didanosine therapy is dose-dependent pancreatitis. Other risk factors for pancreatitis in a given patient (eg alcoholism, hypertriglyceridemia) are relative contraindications to administration of didanosine, and other drugs with the potential to cause pancreatitis should be avoided. Other reported adverse effects have included peripheral neuropathy, diarrhea, hepatotoxicity, hematocytopenias, and central nervous system toxicity (headache, irritability). A rise in uric acid during therapy with didanosine may precipitate attacks of gout in susceptible individuals.

LAMIVUDINE

Lamivudine (3TC) is a nucleoside analog with in vitro activity against HIV-1, including zidovudine-resistant strains, and HBV. Lamivudine inhibits the reverse transcriptase of HIV-1 and is synergistic with zidovudine against HIV-1. As with zidovudine, lamivudine requires intracellular triphosphorylation for activation. When lamivudine is administered as monotherapy, mutation at codon 184 occurs early and results in high-level resistance. However, this mutation may restore phenotypic sensitivity to zidovudine. Thus, combination therapy with lamivudine and zidovudine may be beneficial. It should be noted, however, that HIV-1 strains resistant to both lamivudine and zidovudine have been isolated.

Lamivudine, administered in combination with zidovudine or another nucleoside analog to retard the emergence of resistance, is indicated for treatment of advanced HIV disease. The recommended dosage of lamivudine is 150 mg every 12 hours orally. Oral bioavailability exceeds 80%. Dosage reduction is recommended in patients with renal insufficiency or low body weight. Potential side effects are headache, insomnia, fatigue, and gastrointestinal discomfort, though these are typically mild. Concomitant administration with trimethoprim-sulfamethoxazole results in an increased AUC of lamivudine, though clinical significance is not yet known.

ZALCITABINE

Zalcitabine (ddC) is a pyrimidine nucleoside that inhibits the replication of HIV-1 (Figure 49–4). Like zidovudine, intracellular activation by triphosphorylation is catalyzed by cellular enzymes; competitive inhibition of the reverse transcriptase and chain termination result. Mutation at codon 65, which emerges after prolonged therapy, is associated with decreased susceptibility to zalcitabine, didanosine, and lamivudine; in contrast, mutation at codon 69 confers resistance to zalcitabine but not to other nucleoside analogs. High-level resistance to zalcitabine has not been reported to date.

The drug is effective as treatment for patients with HIV infection. It is available in oral formulation only and is typically prescribed in combination with zidovudine. The recommended dosage is 0.75 mg every 8 hours. Oral bioavailability is high (> 80%), and cerebrospinal fluid concentrations are approximately 20% of those in the plasma. The intracellular half-life of the active compound is 2.6–10 hours. Dosage adjustment is required for patients with renal insufficiency.

Zalcitabine therapy is associated with a dose-dependent peripheral neuropathy that appears to occur more frequently in patients with low serum cobalamin levels and in those with a history of excessive ethanol consumption. Other reported toxicities include pancreatitis, esophageal ulceration and stomatitis, and arthralgias. Coadministration of drugs that cause either peripheral neuropathy or pancreatitis may increase the frequency of these adverse effects. Headache and nausea may occur but tend to resolve if the drug is continued.

STAVUDINE

Stavudine (d4T) is a thymidine analog (Figure 49–4) that requires intracellular triphosphorylation for activation, acting as a competitive inhibitor of HIV-1 reverse transcriptase and as a chain terminator. When administered orally to patients with HIV-1 infection (dosage, 40 mg every 12 hours), oral bioavailability is high (approximately 80%). The intracellular half-life of stavudine is 3.5 hours, and mean cerebrospinal fluid concentrations are 55% of those of plasma. The major dose-limiting toxicity is peripheral sensory neuropathy. Less common adverse effects include pancreatitis, arthralgias, and elevation in serum transaminases. Daily dosage should be reduced for low body weight or renal insufficiency. Mutation at codon 75 is associated with decreased susceptibility to stavudine, didanosine, and zalcitabine; in contrast, codon 50 mutation is associated with resistance to stavudine alone.

PROTEASE INHIBITORS

INDINAVIR

Indinavir is a specific inhibitor of the HIV-1 protease, an enzyme essential for the production of mature, infectious virions. It is currently approved for the treatment of individuals with HIV-1 infection (dosage, 800 mg every 8 hours) and is recommended for use in combination with a reverse transcriptase inhibitor to delay emergence of resistance. The drug must be consumed on an empty stomach for maximal absorption. Oral bioavailability is excellent.

Resistance

Resistance to indinavir is mediated by the expression of multiple and variable protease amino acid substitutions. At least two-thirds of indinavir-resistant strains are cross-resistant to saquinavir and ritonavir; however, saquinavir-resistant isolates tend to retain susceptibility to indinavir.

Adverse Effects

The most common adverse effects reported thus far are indirect hyperbilirubinemia and nephrolithiasis. Thrombocytopenia, nausea, diarrhea, and irritability have also been reported in some patients. Patients receiving indinavir should take the drug with water and consume at least 48 ounces of water daily to maintain adequate hydration and prevent nephrolithiasis. Indinavir and ritonavir are inhibitors of as well as substrates for cytochrome P450 CPY3A4 (Chapter 4). Thus, numerous complex drug interactions can occur. Serum levels of indinavir will increase in the presence of antifungal azoles (themselves CYP3A4 inhibitors) and decrease in the presence of rifabutin and rifampin (CYP3A4 inducers). Increased levels of rifabutin (also a CYP3A4 substrate) that result from use of indinavir require a reduction in the rifabutin dosage by 50%. Increased levels of antihistamines, cisapride, and benzodiazepines may also occur with potential toxicity from these drugs. More precise delineation of drug interactions is underway.

RITONAVIR

Ritonavir is an inhibitor of HIV-1 protease with a high bioavailability (60–80%). Its recommended dosage is 600 mg every 12 hours taken with meals. The most common adverse effects of ritonavir are gastrointestinal disturbances, circumoral paresthesia, elevated hepatic aminotransferase levels, altered taste, and hypertriglyceridemia. The manufacturer recommends dosage escalation (300 mg every 12 hours for 1 day, then 400 mg every 12 hours for 2 days, then 500 mg every 12 hours for 1 day, then 600 mg every 12 hours) to decrease the frequency of dose-limiting adverse effects. Caution is advised when administering the drug to persons with impaired hepatic function. This drug should be refrigerated for storage. HIV-1 isolates resistant to ritonavir are cross-resistant to indinavir.

A major practical limitation of ritonavir is its numerous drug interactions due to its metabolism by the hepatic P450 cytochrome oxidase system (CYP3A and others). Drugs that increase CYP3A activity (eg, phenobarbital, carbamazepine, dexamethasone, phenytoin, rifampin, rifabutin) will increase the clearance of ritonavir and decrease its plasma concentrations. Tobacco use is associated with an 18% decrease in the area under the curve (AUC) of ritonavir. Ritonavir can also produce large increases in plasma concentrations of certain highly metabolized drugs, including fentanyl, lidocaine, erythromycin, clonazepam, carbamazepine, loratidine, rifampin, nifedipine, verapamil, prednisone, dronabinol, ondansetron, and saquinavir. Dosage adjustments of such agents may be necessary to avoid toxicity. The AUCs of such drugs as oxycodone, amitriptyline, desipramine, fluoxetine, clarithromycin, and methamphetamine are increased also by ritonavir, but to a lesser extent. Ritonavir may cause an increase in AUC of methadone, doxepin, itraconazole, ketoconazole, metronidazole, primaquine, pyrimethamine, cimetidine, and phenobarbital. A decrease in AUC due to increased glucuronidation induced by ritonavir may occur with morphine, ketoprofen, atovaquone, lorazepam, and temazepam, such that dosage alteration may be required to maintain efficacy. The mean AUC of ethinyl estradiol is reduced 40% with ritonavir; thus, dosage increase or alternative contraceptive methods should be considered. Decreases in AUC of zidovudine, didanosine, and sulfamethoxazole have been found but are not felt to be clinically significant.

Because ritonavir contains alcohol, coadministration of disulfiram is contraindicated.

SAQUINAVIR

Saquinavir is a synthetic peptide-like substrate analog that inhibits the activity of HIV-1 protease and prevents the cleavage of viral polyproteins. The in vitro activity of saquinavir against HIV-1 is additive to or synergistic with that of reverse transcriptase inhibitors. As with other agents of this class, it is likely that combination therapy with nucleoside agents will be optimal clinically. To date there is little evidence of cross-resistance between saquinavir and other protease inhibitor compounds or between saquinavir and nucleoside analogs.

Oral saquinavir (600 mg every 8 hours) is poorly bioavailable (approximately 4%) and should be taken within 2 hours of a full meal for enhanced absorption. Reported adverse effects include gastrointestinal discomfort (nausea, diarrhea) and rhinitis. Saquinavir levels increase in the presence of ritonavir or ketoconazole; levels may also increase (due to inhibition of metabolism) when the drug is taken with grapefruit juice. Saquinavir levels decrease when administered with rifampin or rifabutin. Potential increases in plasma concentrations of drugs cleared by the cytochrome P450 system (eg, calcium channel blockers, clindamycin, dapsone, quinidine, triazolam, terfenadine, and astemizole) require further investigation, as does reduced saquinavir levels in the presence of drugs that induce CYP3A4 (eg, phenobarbital, phenytoin, dexamethasone, and carbamazepine).

At the time of writing, many other protease inhibitors are under development. The drug closest to full approval appears to be **nelfinavir.** This drug is currently available to patients unable to take other protease inhibitors through the FDA's "expanded access" program. It has been studied in AIDS patients, and in combination with reverse transcriptase inhibitors it appears able to reduce HIV levels in the blood significantly. The recommended dosage is 750 mg three times daily. The most common toxicity is diarrhea; interactions with other drugs are similar to those of other protease inhibitors.

OTHER ANTIVIRAL AGENTS

AMANTADINE & RIMANTADINE

Amantadine (1-aminoadamantane hydrochloride) and its α-methyl derivative, rimantadine, are cyclic amines that inhibit uncoating of the viral RNA of influenza A within infected host cells, thus preventing

TREATMENT OF HIV-INFECTED INDIVIDUALS: IMPORTANCE OF PHARMACOLOGIC KNOWLEDGE

Initiation of antiretroviral therapy in an HIV-infected individual involves knowledge of clinical efficacy, basic pharmacology, and estimates of the likelihood of emergence of resistance for each drug. A thorough knowledge of potential drug interactions is also important because such individuals are frequently taking multiple medications, including prophylaxis for opportunistic infections, treatment of opportunistic infections, and opioid pain medications or methadone for maintenance therapy.

An example is an HIV-infected patient receiving ganciclovir for treatment of cytomegalovirus retinitis. Such a patient may be unable to tolerate concomitant zidovudine therapy due to additive myelosuppression; addition of colony-stimulating factor therapy for cytopenias or substitution of a different, nonmyelodepressant drug for ganciclovir or zidovudine may ultimately be necessary.

A patient with a history of alcohol abuse is at risk for the development of pancreatitis, a potentially fatal condition, if treated with didanosine. A patient on didanosine who is receiving dapsone for anti-*Pneumocystis* prophylaxis must be cautioned to separate ingestion of the two by at least 2 hours because the buffered formulation of didanosine can interfere with the absorption of dapsone, a drug that requires an acidic environment for maximum bioavailability.

The administration of rifabutin for prophylaxis against *Mycobacterium avium* complex infection could interfere with numerous other therapies because this drug strongly induces hepatic drug-metabolizing P450 enzymes. Indinavir is an inhibitor of this pathway, which also metabolizes rifabutin. Thus, dosage reduction of rifabutin is required when it is coadministered with indinavir. Ritonavir interferes with metabolism of saquinavir, markedly increasing the concentration of the latter. Coadministration of these two protease inhibitors is being investigated as a strategy to improve the activity of saquinavir, which otherwise achieves marginal serum concentrations; the combination might prevent emergence of viral resistance.

its replication (Hay et al, 1985). Both amantadine (200 mg/d) and rimantadine are effective in the prevention of influenza A virus infection in high-risk individuals, reducing the risk of acquisition by 50–90% as well as ameliorating clinical illness in those who acquire the infection. Additionally, both drugs can be used in the treatment of influenza A, effectively reducing the duration of symptoms when administered within 48 hours after their onset. Although de novo resistance is rare, emergence of resistance in clinical isolates of influenza is common in treated individuals (eg, 50% prevalence within 4–6 days) and has been mapped to mutations in the RNA sequence coding for the structural M2 protein. Transmission of resistant virus to household contacts has been documented. The most common side effects are gastrointestinal intolerance and central nervous system effects (eg, nervousness, difficulty in concentrating, lightheadedness); the latter are less frequent with rimantadine than amantadine. The daily dosage of amantadine should be reduced in patients over age 65 and in those with renal insufficiency.

INTERFERONS

Interferons (IFNs) are a group of endogenous proteins that exert virus-nonspecific antiviral activities through cellular metabolic processes involving synthesis of both RNA and protein (Chapter 56). Three major classes of interferons are now recognized, classified on the basis of the cell types from which they were derived: IFN-α (previously type I, leukocyte), IFN-β (previously type I, fibroblast), and IFN-γ (previously type II, immune). Each type is immunologically and physicochemically distinct and each can function as a potent cytokine with complex antiviral, immunomodulatory, and antiproliferative activity. They are not directly antiviral but appear to function by causing elaboration of effector proteins in infected cells, resulting in such effects as inhibition of viral penetration or uncoating, mRNA synthesis and translation, or virion assembly and release. Immunomodulatory effects may be additively antiviral. Three known enzymes are induced by interferons: (1) a protein kinase that ultimately leads to phosphorylation of elongation factor 2, resulting in inhibition of peptide chain initiation; (2) oligoisoadenylate synthase, which ultimately leads to activation of an RNAase and degradation of viral mRNA; and (3) a phosphodiesterase that can degrade the terminal nucleotides of tRNA, inhibiting peptide elongation.

Interferons have been studied for numerous clinical indications. Systemic interferon-α is currently approved in the USA for chronic hepatitis B and C infections, AIDS-associated Kaposi's sarcoma, and laryngeal papillomatosis. IFN-α may be administered by intralesional injection for treatment of external condylomata acuminata and has been studied as an intranasal preparation for prophylaxis against the common cold viruses. Dose-limiting toxicities include neutropenia, anemia, and constitutional symptoms such as fever, malaise, myalgias, and fatigue. A reversible cardiomyopathy associated with interferon-α has also been described.

RIBAVIRIN

Ribavirin is a guanosine analog that is phosphorylated intracellularly by host cell enzymes. Although its mechanism of action has not been fully elucidated, it appears to interfere with synthesis of guanosine triphosphate, to inhibit capping of viral messenger RNA, and to inhibit the viral RNA-dependent RNA polymerase of certain viruses. The triphosphate compound inhibits the replication of a wide range of DNA and RNA viruses, including influenza A and B, parainfluenza, respiratory syncytial virus, paramyxoviruses, HCV, and HIV-1. Ribavirin is administered in aerosolized form (20 mg/mL for 18 hours per day) to children and infants with RSV bronchiolitis or pneumonia, reducing the severity and duration of illness. Aerosolized ribavirin has also been used to treat influenza A and B infection but has not gained widespread use. Intravenous ribavirin decreases mortality in Lassa fever and other viral hemorrhagic fevers if initiated early in the disease. Clinical benefit has been reported in cases of severe measles pneumonitis, and continuous infusion of ribavirin decreased virus shedding in several patients with severe lower respiratory tract influenza or parainfluenza infections. Oral ribavirin (dosage, 1200–1600 mg/d) was not found to be of benefit for the treatment of hepatitis C infection or in patients with HIV infection.

Aerosolized ribavirin is generally well tolerated but may cause conjunctival or bronchial irritation. Health care workers should be protected against extended inhalation exposure. Systemic administration of ribavirin is associated with dose-dependent anemia and bone marrow suppression. The drug is contraindicated in pregnancy due to possible teratogenicity.

PREPARATIONS AVAILABLE

Acyclovir (Zovirax)
Oral: 200 mg capsules, 400, 800 mg tablet; 200 mg/5 mL suspension
Parenteral: powder to reconstitute for injection (500, 1000 mg/vial)

Amantadine (generic, Symmetrel)
Oral: 100 mg capsules; 50 mg/5 mL syrup

Cytomegalovirus immune globulin intravenous (human)
Parenteral: Powder to reconstitute for injection, 2500 mg ± 500 mg.

Didanosine (dideoxyinosine, ddI) (Videx)
Oral: 25, 50, 100, 150 mg tablets; 100, 167, 250, 375 mg powder for oral solution; 2, 4 g powder for pediatric solution.

Famciclovir (Famvir)
Oral: 125, 250, 500 mg tablets

Foscarnet (Foscavir)
Parenteral: 24 mg/mL for IV injection

Ganciclovir (Cytovene)
Oral: 250 mg capsules
Parenteral: 500 mg/vial for IV injection

Hepatitis B immune globulin (HBIG) (H-BIG, others)
Parenteral: 1, 4, 5 mL vials; 0.5 mL prefilled syringe

Idoxuridine (Herplex)
Topical: 0.1% ophthalmic solution

Indinavir (Crixivan)
Oral: 200, 400 mg capsules

Immune globulin intravenous (IGIV) (Gamimune N, others)
Parenteral: 5% in 10, 50, 100 mL vials; 0.5, 1, 2.5, 3, 5, 6 g powder to reconstitute for IV injection

Interferon alfa-2a (Roferon-A)
Parenteral: 3, 6, 36 million IU vials

Interferon alfa-2b (Intron-A)
Parenteral: 3, 5, 10, 18, 25, and 50 million IU vials

Interferon alfa-n3 (Alferon N)
Parenteral: 5 million IU/vial

Lamivudine (Epivir)
Oral: 150 mg tablets, 10 mg/mL oral solution

Nelfinavir (Viracept)
Oral: 250 mg tablets.

Ribavirin (Virazole)
Aerosol: powder to reconstitute for 6 g/dL aerosol

Rimantadine (Flumadine)
Oral: 100 mg tablets; 50 mg/5 mL syrup

Ritonavir (Norvir)
Oral: 100 mg capsules; 80 mg/mL oral solution

Saquinavir (Invirase)
Oral: 200 mg capsules

Stavudine (Zerit)
Oral: 15, 20, 30, 40 mg capsules

Trifluridine (Viroptic)
Topical: 1% ophthalmic solution

Varicella-zoster immune globulin (human)
Parenteral: 125 units globulin in 2.5 mL vial

Valacyclovir (Valtrex)
Oral: 500 mg tablets

Vidarabine (Vira-A)
Topical: 3% ophthalmic ointment

Zalcitabine (dideoxycytidine, ddC) (Hivid)
Oral: 0.375, 0.75 mg tablets

Zidovudine, azidothymidine, AZT (Retrovir)
Oral: 100 mg capsules, 50 mg/5 mL syrup
Parenteral: 10 mg/mL

REFERENCES

Balfour HH et al: Acyclovir halts progression of herpes zoster in immunocompromised patients. N Engl J Med 1983;308:1448.

Beutner KR: Valacyclovir: A review of its antiviral activity, pharmacokinetic properties, and clinical efficacy. Antiviral Res 1995;28:281.

Beutner KR et al: Valaciclovir compared with acyclovir for improved therapy for herpes zoster in immunocompetent adults. Antimicrob Ag Chemother 1995;39:1546.

Browne MJ et al: 2′,3′-didehydro-3′-deoxythymidine (d4T) in patients with AIDS or AIDS-related complex: A phase I trial. J Infect Dis 1993;167:21.

Chrisp P, Clissold SP: Foscarnet: A review of its antiviral activity, pharmacokinetic properties and therapeutic use in immunocompromised patients with cytomegalovirus retinitis. Drugs 1991;41:104.

Cobo M: Reduction of the ocular complications of herpes zoster ophthalmicus by oral acyclovir. Am J Med 1988;85(Suppl 2A):90.

Danner SA et al: A short-term study of the safety, pharmacokinetics, and efficacy of ritonavir, an inhibitor of HIV-1 protease. N Engl J Med 1995;333:1528.

Drew WL et al: Oral ganciclovir as maintenance treatment for cytomegalovirus retinitis in patients with AIDS. N Engl J Med 1995;333:615.

Fichtenbaum CJ et al: Risk factors for dideoxynucleoside-induced toxic neuropathy in patients with the human immunodeficiency virus infection. J Acquir Immune Defic Syndr Hum Retrovirol 1995;10:169.

Fischl MA et al: The efficacy of azidothymidine (AZT) in the treatment of patients with AIDS and AIDS-related complex. N Engl J Med 1987;317:185.

Hall CB et al: Aerosolized ribavirin treatment of infants with respiratory syncytial viral infection: A randomized double-blind study. N Engl J Med 1983;308:1443.

Hayden FG et al: Intravenous ribavirin by constant infusion for serious influenza and parainfluenza infection. Antiviral Ther 1996;1:51.

Huggins JW et al: Prospective, double blind concurrent placebo-controlled trial of intravenous ribavirin therapy of hemorrhagic fever with renal syndrome. J Infect Dis 1991;164:1119.

Kessler HA et al: A pilot study of topical trifluridine for the treatment of acyclovir-resistant mucocutaneous herpes simplex disease in patients with AIDS (ACTG 172). J Acquir Immune Defic Syndr Hum Retrovirol 1996. [In press.]

Lalezari JP et al: (S)-1-[3-Hydroxy-2-(phosphonylmethoxy)propyl]cytosine (cidofovir): Results of a phase I/II study of a novel antiviral nucleotide analogue. J Infect Dis 1995;171:788.

Machida H: Antiviral profile, mode of action, and clinical efficacy of sorivudine. Internat Antiviral News 1993; 1:148.

Matthews T, Boehme R: Antiviral activity and mechanism of action of ganciclovir. Rev Infect Dis 1988;10:S490.

McClung HW et al: Ribavirin aerosol treatment of influenza B virus infection. JAMA 1983;249:2671.

McLeod GX et al: Zidovudine: Five years later. Ann Intern Med 1992;117:487.

Merigan TC: Interferon: The first quarter century. JAMA 1982;248:2513.

Metroka CE et al: Failure of prophylaxis with dapsone in patients taking dideoxyinosine. (Letter.) N Engl J Med 1991;325:737.

New drugs for HIV Infection. Med Lett Drugs Ther 1996;38:35.

Perry CM, Wagstaff AJ: Famciclovir: A review of its pharmacological properties and therapeutic efficacy in herpesvirus infections. Drugs 1995;50:396.

Piscitelli SC et al: Drug interactions in patients infected with human immunodeficiency virus. Clin Infect Dis 1996;23:685.

Prevention and control of influenza. MMWR Morb Mortal Wkly Rep 199 1995;44:1.

Richman DD. Viral resistance to antiretoviral therapy. In: Textbook of AIDS Medicine. Broder S, Merigan TC, Bolognesi D (editors). Williams & Wilkins, 1994.

Rooney JF et al: Oral acyclovir to suppress frequently recurrent herpes labialis: A double-blind, placebo-controlled trial. Ann Intern Med 1993;118:268.

Safrin S et al: A controlled trial comparing foscarnet with vidarabine for acyclovir-resistant mucocutaneous herpes simplex in the acquired immunodeficiency syndrome. N Engl J Med 1991;325:551.

Safrin S et al: Foscarnet therapy in five patients with AIDS and acyclovir-resistant varicella-zoster virus infection. Ann Intern Med 1991;115:19.

Safrin S et al: Foscarnet-resistant herpes simplex virus infection in patients with AIDS. J Infect Dis 1994;169:193.

Snoeck R et al: Successful treatment of progressive mucocutaneous infection due to acyclovir- and foscarnet-resistant herpes simplex virus with (S)-1-(3-hydroxy-2-phosphonylmethoxypropyl)cytosine (HPMPC). Clin Infect Dis 1994;18:570.

Spector SA et al: Pharmacokinetic, safety, and antiviral profiles of oral ganciclovir in persons infected with human immunodeficiency virus: A phase I/II study. J Infect Dis 1995;161:431.

Spruance SL et al: Treatment of recurrent herpes simplex labialis with oral acyclovir. J Infect Dis 1990;161:185.

Studies of Ocular Complications of AIDS Research Group iC: Mortality in patients with the acquired immunodeficiency syndrome treated with either foscarnet or ganciclovir for cytomegalovirus retinitis. N Engl J Med 1992;326:213.

Sullivan V et al: A protein kinase homologue controls phosphorylation of ganciclovir in human cytomegalovirus-infected cells. Nature 1992;358:162.

Tyring S et al: Famciclovir for the treatment of acute herpes zoster: Effects on acute disease and postherpetic neuralgia. A randomized, double-blind, placebo-controlled trial. Ann Intern Med 1995;123:89.

van Leeuwen R et al: Evaluation of safety and efficacy of 3TC (lamivudine) in patients with asymptomatic or mildly symptomatic human immunodeficiency virus infection: A phase I/II study. J Infect Dis 1995;171:1166.

Wallace MR et al: Treatment of adult varicella with oral acyclovir: A randomized, placebo-controlled trial. Ann Intern Med 1992;117:358.

Whitley RJ, Gnann JW Jr: Acyclovir: A decade later. N Engl J Med 1992;327:782.

Miscellaneous Antimicrobial Agents; Disinfectants, Antiseptics, & Sterilants

50

Henry F. Chambers, MD, & W. Keith Hadley, MD, PhD

MISCELLANEOUS ANTIMICROBIAL AGENTS: METRONIDAZOLE, MUPIROCIN, POLYMYXIN, & URINARY ANTISEPTICS

METRONIDAZOLE

Metronidazole is a nitroimidazole antiprotozoal drug (Chapter 53) that also has potent antibacterial activity against anaerobes, including *Bacteroides* and *Clostridium* species. It is well absorbed after oral administration, widely distributed in tissues, and reaches serum levels of 4–6 μg/mL after a 250 mg oral dose. Metronidazole can also be given intravenously or by rectal suppository. The drug penetrates well into the cerebrospinal fluid, reaching levels similar to those in serum. Metronidazole is metabolized in the liver and may accumulate in hepatic insufficiency.

Metronidazole is indicated for treatment of anaerobic or mixed intra-abdominal infections, vaginitis (*Trichomonas,* bacterial vaginosis), antibiotic-associated enterocolitis, and brain abscess. The typical dosage is 500 mg three times daily orally or intravenously (30 mg/kg/d). Vaginitis may respond to a single 2 g dose. A vaginal gel is available for topical use.

Adverse effects include nausea, diarrhea, stomatitis, and peripheral neuropathy with prolonged use. Metronidazole has a disulfiram-like effect, and patients should be instructed to avoid alcohol. Although teratogenic in some animals, metronidazole has not been associated with this effect in humans.

Other properties of metronidazole are discussed in Chapter 53.

MUPIROCIN

Mupirocin (pseudomonic acid) is a natural product produced by *Pseudomonas fluorescens.* It is rapidly inactivated after absorption, and systemic levels are undetectable. It is available as an ointment for topical application.

Mupirocin is active against gram-positive cocci, and its use is directed against *S aureus,* both methicillin-susceptible and methicillin-resistant strains. Mupirocin inhibits and kills staphylococci by inhibiting isoleucyl tRNA synthetase. Low-level resistance, defined as a minimum inhibitory concentration (MIC) of up to 100 μg/mL, is due to point mutation in the gene of the target enzyme. Low-level resistance has been observed after prolonged use, but local concentrations achieved with topical application are well above this MIC, and this level of resistance does not lead to clinical failure. High-level resistance, with MICs exceeding 1000 μg/mL, is due to the presence of a second isoleucyl tRNA synthetase gene, which is plasmid-encoded. High-level resistance results in complete loss of activity. Strains with high-level resistance have caused nosocomial outbreaks of staphylococcal infection and colonization.

Mupirocin is indicated for topical treatment of minor skin infections, such as impetigo. Topical application over large infected areas, such as decubitus ulcers or open surgical wounds, has been identified as an important factor leading to emergence of mupirocin-resistant strains and is not recommended. Mupirocin is also indicated for intranasal application for elimination of methicillin-resistant *S aureus* carriage by patients or health care workers.

POLYMYXINS

The polymyxins are a group of basic peptides active against gram-negative bacteria. Owing to their nephrotoxicity, all but polymyxins B and E have been abandoned. Only polymyxin B is available in the USA.

Polymyxins are cationic, basic peptides with molecular weights of about 1400. All contain the fatty acid D-6-methyloctan-1-oic acid and the amino acids L-threonine and L-diaminobutyric acid. The sulfates are water-soluble and very stable. One microgram of pure polymyxin B sulfate equals 10 units.

Polymyxins are bactericidal for many gram-negative rods, including *Pseudomonas,* in concentrations of 1–5 μg/mL. Polymyxins act like cationic detergents. They attach to and disrupt bacterial cell membranes. They also bind and inactivate endotoxin. Gram-positive organisms, *Proteus,* and *Neisseria* are resistant. In susceptible bacterial populations, resistant mutants are rare.

With availability of numerous alternative antibacterial agents, polymyxins are no longer used for systemic administration because of their poor tissue distribution and their substantial nephrotoxicity and neurotoxicity. Polymyxins are now restricted largely to topical use. Ointments containing polymyxin B, 0.5 mg/g, in mixtures with bacitracin or neomycin (or both) are commonly applied to infected superficial skin lesions. Local reactions and hypersensitivity to topical administration are rare.

URINARY ANTISEPTICS

Urinary antiseptics are agents that exert antibacterial activity in the urine but have little or no systemic antibacterial effect. Their usefulness is limited to lower urinary tract infections. Prolonged suppression of bacteriuria by means of urinary antiseptics may be desirable in chronic urinary tract infections where eradication of infection by short-term systemic therapy has not been possible.

1. NITROFURANTOIN

Nitrofurantoin is bacteriostatic and bactericidal for many gram-positive and gram-negative bacteria. *P aeruginosa* and many strains of *Proteus* are resistant, but in nitrofurantoin-susceptible populations resistant mutants are rare. Clinical drug resistance emerges slowly. There is no cross-resistance between nitrofurantoin and other antimicrobial agents.

The mechanism of action of the nitrofurantoin is not clearly defined. A reduced form of the drug, which is preferentially produced by susceptible bacteria, is probably the active form: it is highly reactive and damages DNA. Activity of nitrofurantoin is greatly enhanced at pH 5.5 or below.

Nitrofurantoin is well absorbed after ingestion. It is metabolized and excreted so rapidly that no systemic antibacterial action is achieved. The drug is excreted into the urine by both glomerular filtration and tubular secretion. With average daily doses, concentrations of 200 μg/mL are reached in urine. In renal failure, urine levels are insufficient for antibacterial action, but high blood levels may cause toxicity.

The average daily dose for urinary tract infection in adults is 100 mg orally taken four times daily with food or milk. Nitrofurantoin is contraindicated in patients with severe renal insufficiency. Oral nitrofurantoin can be given for months for the suppression of chronic urinary tract infection. It is desirable to keep urinary pH below 5.5 (see Acidifying Agents, below). A single daily dose of nitrofurantoin, 100 mg, can prevent recurrent urinary tract infections in some women.

Anorexia, nausea, and vomiting are the principal side effects of nitrofurantoin. Neuropathies and hemolytic anemia occur in glucose-6-phosphate dehydrogenase deficiency. Nitrofurantoin antagonizes the action of nalidixic acid. Rashes, pulmonary infiltration, and other hypersensitivity reactions have been reported.

2. METHENAMINE MANDELATE & METHENAMINE HIPPURATE

Methenamine mandelate is the salt of mandelic acid and methenamine and possesses properties of both of these urinary antiseptics. Methenamine hippurate is the salt of hippuric acid and methenamine. Below pH 5.5, methenamine releases formaldehyde, which is antibacterial. Mandelic acid or hippuric acid taken orally is excreted unchanged in the urine, in which these drugs are bactericidal for some gram-negative bacteria when pH is less than 5.5.

Methenamine mandelate, 1 g four times daily, or methenamine hippurate, 1 g twice daily by mouth (children, 50 mg/kg/d or 30 mg/kg/d, respectively), is used only as a urinary antiseptic. Acidifying agents (eg, ascorbic acid, 4–12 g/d) may be given to lower urinary pH below 5.5. Sulfonamides should not be given at the same time because they may form an insoluble compound with the formaldehyde released by methenamine. Persons taking methenamine mandelate may exhibit falsely elevated tests for catecholamine metabolites.

The action of methenamine mandelate or hippurate is nonspecific against many different microorganisms and consists of the simultaneous effects of formaldehyde and acidity. Microorganisms such as *Proteus* that make a strongly alkaline urine through release of ammonia from urea are usually resistant.

DISINFECTANTS, ANTISEPTICS, & STERILANTS

Disinfectants are chemical agents that inhibit or kill microorganisms (Table 50–1). **Antiseptics** are disinfecting agents with sufficiently low toxicity for host cells that they can be used directly on skin, mucous membranes, or wounds. **Sterilants** kill both vegetative cells and spores when applied to materials

Table 50–1. Activities of disinfectants.

	Bacteria				Viruses		Other		
	Gram-positive	Gram-negative	Acid-fast	Spores	Lipo-philic	Hydro-philic	Fungi	Amebic cysts	Prions
Alcohols (isopropanol, ethanol)	HS	HS	S	R	S	V	—	—	R
Aldehydes (glutaraldehyde, formaldehyde)	HS	HS	MS	S (slow)	S	MS	S	—	R
Chlorhexidine gluconate	HS	MS	R	R	V	R	—	—	R
Sodium hypochlorite, chlorine dioxide	HS	HS	MS	S (pH 7.6)	S	S (at high conc)	MS	S	MS (at high conc)
Hexachlorophene	S (slow)	R	R	R	R	R	R	R	R
Povidone, iodine	HS	HS	S	S (at high conc)	S	R	S	S	R
Phenols, quaternary ammonium compounds	HS	HS	±	R	S	R	—	—	R
Strong oxidizing agents, cresols	HS	MS to R	R	R	S	R	R	R	R

Key: HS, highly susceptible; S, susceptible; MS, moderately susceptible; R, resistant; V, variable; —, no data.

for appropriate times and temperatures. Some of the terms used in this context are defined in Table 50–2.

The process of disinfection prevents infection by reducing the number of potentially infective organisms either by killing, removing, or diluting them. Disinfection can be accomplished by application of chemical agents or use of physical agents such as ionizing irradiation, dry or moist heat, or superheated steam (autoclave, 120 °C) to kill microorganisms. Often a combination of agents is used, eg, water and moderate heat over time (pasteurization); ethylene oxide and moist heat (a sterilant); or addition of disinfectant to a detergent. Prevention of infection also can be achieved by washing, which dilutes the potentially infectious organism, or by establishing a barrier, eg gloves, condom, or respirator, which prevents the pathogen from entry into the host.

Handwashing is the most important means of preventing transmission of infectious agents from person to person or from regions of high microbial load, eg, mouth, nose, or gut, to potential sites of infection. Regular hand washing is best done without disinfectants to minimize drying, irritation, and sensitization of the skin. Soap and warm water efficiently and effectively remove bacteria. Skin disinfectants along with detergent and water are usually used preoperatively as a surgical scrub for surgeons' hands and the patient's surgical incision.

Evaluation of effectiveness of antiseptics, disinfectants, and sterilants, although seemingly simple in principle, is very complex. Factors in any evaluation include the intrinsic resistance of the microorganism, the number of the microorganisms present, mixed populations of organisms, amount of organic material present (eg blood, feces, tissue), concentration and stability of disinfectant or sterilant, time and temperature of exposure, pH, and hydration and binding of the agent to surfaces. Specific, standardized assays of activity are defined for each use. Toxicity for humans also must be evaluated. The Environmental Protection Agency (EPA) regulates disinfectants and sterilants

Table 50–2. Commonly used terms related to chemical and physical killing of microorganisms.

Antisepsis	Application of an agent to living tissue for the purpose of preventing infection
Decontamination	Destruction or marked reduction in number or activity of microorganisms
Disinfection	Chemical or physical treatment that destroys most vegetative microbes or viruses, but not spores, in or on inanimate surfaces
Sanitization	Reduction of microbial load on an inanimate surface to a level considered acceptable for public health purposes
Sterilization	A process intended to kill or remove all types of microorganisms, including spores, and usually including viruses with an acceptable low probability of survival
Pasteurization	A process that kills nonsporulating microorganisms by hot water or steam at 65–100 °C

and the Food and Drug Administration regulates antiseptics.

Users of antiseptics, disinfectants, and sterilants need to consider their short-term and long-term toxicity since they may have general biocidal activity and may accumulate in the environment or in the body of the patient or caregiver using the agent. Disinfectants and antiseptics may also become contaminated by resistant microorganisms—eg spores, *Pseudomonas aeruginosa,* or *Serratia marcescens*—and actually transmit infection. Most topical antiseptics interfere with wound healing to some degree. Simple cleansing with soap and water is less damaging than antiseptics to wounds. Topical antibiotics with a narrow spectrum of action and low toxicity (eg, bacitracin and mupirocin) can be used for temporary control of bacterial growth and are generally preferred to antiseptics. Methenamine mandelate releases formaldehyde in a low antibacterial concentration at acid pH and can be an effective urinary antiseptic for long-term control of urinary tract infections.

Some of the chemical classes of antiseptics, disinfectants, and sterilants are described briefly. The reader is referred to the general references for descriptions of physical disinfection and sterilization methods.

ALCOHOLS

The two alcohols most frequently used for antisepsis and disinfection are ethanol and isopropyl alcohol (isopropanol). They are rapidly active, killing vegetative bacteria, *M tuberculosis,* and many fungi and inactivating lipophilic viruses. The optimum bactericidal concentration is 60–90% by volume in water. They probably act by denaturation of proteins. They are not used as sterilants because they are not sporicidal, do not penetrate protein-containing organic material, may not be active against hydrophilic viruses, and lack residual action because they evaporate completely. The alcohols are useful in situations where sinks with running water are not available for washing with soap and water. Their skin-drying effect can be partially alleviated by addition of emollients to the formulation.

Alcohols are flammable and must be stored in cool, well-ventilated areas. Alcohols must be allowed to evaporate before use of cautery, electrosurgery, or laser surgery. They may be damaging if applied directly to corneal tissue. Therefore, instruments such as tonometers that have been disinfected in alcohol should be rinsed with sterile water or the alcohol allowed to evaporate before they are used.

CHLORHEXIDINE

Chlorhexidine is a cationic biguanide with very low water solubility. Water-soluble chlorhexidine diglu-

conate is used in water-based formulations as an antiseptic. It is active against vegetative bacteria and mycobacteria and has moderate activity against fungi and viruses. It strongly adsorbs to bacterial membranes, causing leakage of small molecules and precipitation of cytoplasmic proteins. It is active at pH 5.5–7.0. Chlorhexidine digluconate is slower in its action than alcohols, but because of its persistence it has residual activity when used repeatedly, producing bactericidal action equivalent to alcohols. It is most effective against gram-positive cocci and less active against gram-positive and gram-negative rods. Spore germination is inhibited by chlorhexidine. Chlorhexidine digluconate is resistant to inhibition by blood and organic materials. Anionic and nonionic agents in moisturizers, neutral soaps, and surfactants may neutralize its action. Chlorhexidine digluconate formulations of 4% concentration have slightly greater antibacterial activity than newer 2% formulations. Chlorhexidine 0.5% in 70% alcohol formulations are available in some countries. Chlorhexidine has a very low skin-sensitizing or irritating capacity. Oral toxicity is low because chlorhexidine is poorly absorbed through the alimentary tract. Chlorhexidine must not be used during surgery on the middle ear because it causes sensorineural deafness. Similar neural toxicity may be encountered during neurosurgery.

HALOGENS

1. Iodine

Iodine in a 1:20,000 solution is bactericidal in 1 minute and kills spores in 15 minutes. Tincture of iodine USP contains 2% iodine and 2.4% sodium iodide in alcohol. It is the most active antiseptic for intact skin. It is not commonly used because of serious hypersensitivity reactions that may occur and because of its staining of clothing and dressings.

2. Iodophors

Iodophors are complexes of iodine with a surface-active agent such as **polyvinyl pyrrolidone (PVP; povidone-iodine).** The amount of free iodine is low, but it is released as the solution is diluted. Iodophors retain the activity of iodine. They kill vegetative bacteria, mycobacteria, fungi, and lipid-containing viruses. They may be sporicidal upon prolonged exposure. Iodophors can be used as antiseptics or disinfectants, the latter containing more free iodine. Dilution may release more free iodine. An iodophor solution must be diluted according to the manufacturer's directions in order to obtain full activity.

Iodophors are less irritating and less likely to produce skin hypersensitivity than tincture of iodine. They act as rapidly as chlorhexidine and have a broader spectrum of action, including sporicidal action, but they lack the persistent action of chlorhexidine.

3. CHLORINE

Chlorine is a strong oxidizing agent and universal disinfectant that is most commonly provided as a 5.25% **sodium hypochlorite** solution, a typical formulation for **household bleach.** As formulations may vary, the exact concentration should be verified on the label. A 1:10 dilution of household bleach provides 5000 ppm of available chlorine. The Centers for Disease Control and Prevention recommends this concentration for disinfection of blood spills. Less than 5 ppm kills vegetative bacteria, whereas up to 5000 ppm is necessary to kill spores. A concentration of 1000–10,000 ppm is tuberculocidal. One hundred ppm kills vegetative fungal cells in 1 hour, but fungal spores require 500 ppm. Viruses are inactivated by 200–500 ppm. Dilutions of 5.25% sodium hypochlorite made up in pH 7.5–8.0 tap water retain their activity for months when kept in tightly closed, opaque containers. Frequent opening and closing of the container reduces the activity markedly.

Because chlorine is inactivated by blood serum, feces, and protein-containing materials, surfaces should be cleaned before chlorine disinfectant is applied. Undissociated hypochlorous acid (HOCl) is the active biocidal agent. When pH is increased, the less active hypochlorite ion, OCl⁻, is formed. When hypochlorite solutions contact formaldehyde, the carcinogen *bis*-chloromethyl is formed. Rapid evolution of irritating chlorine gas occurs when hypochlorite solutions are mixed with acid and urine. Solutions are corrosive to aluminum, silver, and stainless steel.

Alternative chlorine-releasing compounds include **chlorine dioxide** and **chloramine T.** These agents retain chlorine longer and have a prolonged bactericidal action.

PHENOLICS

Phenol itself (perhaps the oldest of the surgical antiseptics) is no longer used even as a disinfectant because of its corrosive effect on tissues, its toxicity upon absorption, and its carcinogenic effect. These adverse actions are diminished by forming derivatives in which a functional group replaces a hydrogen atom in the aromatic ring. The phenolic agents most commonly used are *o*-phenylphenol, *o*-benzyl-*p*-chlorophenol and *p*-tertiary amylphenol. Mixtures of phenolic derivatives are often used. Some of these are derived from coal tar distillates, eg, cresols and xylenols. Skin absorption and skin irritation still occur with these derivatives, and appropriate care is necessary in their use. Detergents are often added to for-

---

HBV & HIV DISINFECTION

Hepatitis B virus (HBV) is highly transmissible upon parenteral or mucous membrane exposure to patients' blood because of the high concentrations of virus in blood. Since HBV cannot be grown in tissue culture, measures of disinfectant activity have been done with the chimpanzee infective dose (CID) test and the morphologic alteration and disintegration (MAD) test, which assumes that physical destruction of virus is correlated with inactivation of infectivity of HBV by the CID test. For disinfection of a direct blood spill on a porous surface which cannot be completely cleaned, a 1:10 dilution of household bleach (0.5% sodium hypochlorite, 500 mg/L available chlorine) for 10 minutes at 24 °C is recommended by CDC. Other standard sterilization systems such as pressurized steam (autoclaving) and room temperature treatment with ethylene oxide, 2% glutaraldehyde (pH 8.6), or high iodine content iodophor (75 mg/L available iodine) in 70% isopropanol for 10 minutes are all effective.

HIV is an enveloped retrovirus. Studies done with 7–10 logs of viral activity from cell cultures (10,000–100,000 times greater than the concentration encountered in the usual clinical situation) have shown persistence of virus for 3 days upon drying and for 15 days at room temperature in an aqueous environment. These studies are significant for a laboratory or manufacturing environment but not for the usual clinical situation. Disinfection procedures used for HBV are also recommended for HIV. HIV is inactivated within 2–10 minutes by many common disinfectants such as phenolics and hydrogen peroxide. Sodium hypochlorite solution (household bleach) in 1:10 dilution and 70% ethanol or isopropanol inactivate HIV within 1 minute of exposure. This is appropriate since many patients with HIV infection may also have HBV, and methods effective against HBV also are effective against HIV, which is present in blood and body fluids in relatively low concentrations.

---

mulations to clean and remove organic material that may decrease the activity of a phenolic compound.

Phenolic compounds disrupt cell wall and membranes, precipitate proteins, and inactivate enzymes. They are bactericidal (including mycobacteria), fungicidal, and capable of inactivating lipophilic viruses. They are not sporicidal. Dilution and time of exposure recommendations of the manufacturer must be followed.

Phenolic disinfectants are used for hard surface decontamination in hospitals and laboratories, eg, floors, beds, and counter or bench tops. They are not recommended for use in nurseries and especially bassinets, where their use has been associated with hyperbilirubinemia. Use of **hexachlorophene** as a skin disinfectant has caused cerebral edema and convulsions in premature infants and occasionally in adults.

QUATERNARY AMMONIUM COMPOUNDS

The quaternary ammonium compounds ("quats") are cationic surface-active detergents. The active cation has at least one long water-repellent hydrocarbon chain, which causes the molecules to concentrate as an oriented layer on the surface of solutions and colloidal or suspended particles. The charged nitrogen portion of the cation has high affinity for water and prevents separation out of solution. The bactericidal action of quaternary compounds has been attributed to inactivation of energy-producing enzymes, denaturation of proteins, and disruption of the cell membrane. These agents are bacteriostatic, fungistatic, sporistatic, and also inhibit algae. They are bactericidal for gram-positive bacteria and moderately active against gram-negative bacteria. Lipophilic viruses are inactivated. They are not tuberculocidal or sporicidal, and they do not inactivate hydrophilic viruses. Quaternary ammonium compounds bind to the surface of colloidal protein in blood, serum, and milk and to fibers present in cotton, mops, cloths, and paper towels used to apply them, which can cause inactivation of the agent by removing it from solution. They are inactivated by anionic detergents (soaps), by many nonionic detergents, and by calcium, magnesium, ferric, and aluminum ions.

Quaternary compounds are used for sanitation of noncritical surfaces (floors, bench tops, etc). Their low toxicity has led to their use as sanitizers in food production facilities. CDC recommends that quaternary ammonium compounds such as **benzalkonium chloride** *not* be used as antiseptics because several outbreaks of infections have occurred that were due to growth of *Pseudomonas* and other gram-negative bacteria in quaternary ammonium antiseptic solutions.

ALDEHYDES

Formaldehyde and **glutaraldehyde** are used for disinfection or sterilization of instruments such as fiberoptic endoscopes, respiratory therapy equipment, hemodialyzers, and dental handpieces that can not withstand exposure to the high temperatures of steam sterilization. They are not corrosive for metal, plastic, or rubber. These agents have a broad spectrum of activity against microorganisms and viruses. They act by alkylation of chemical groups in proteins and nucleic acids. Failures of disinfection or sterilization can occur as a result of dilution below the known effective concentration, the presence of organic material, and the failure of liquid to penetrate into small channels in the instruments. Automatic circulating baths are available that increase penetration of aldehyde solution into the instrument while decreasing exposure of the operator to irritating fumes.

Formaldehyde is available as a 40% w/v solution in water (100% **formalin**). An 8% formaldehyde solution in water has a broad spectrum of activity against bacteria, fungi, and viruses. Sporicidal activity may take as long as 18 hours. Its rapidity of action is increased by solution in 70% isopropanol. Formaldehyde solutions are used for high-level disinfection of hemodialyzers, preparation of vaccines, and preservation and embalming of tissues. The 4% formaldehyde (10% formalin) solutions used for fixation of tissues and embalming may not be mycobactericidal.

Glutaraldehyde is a dialdehyde (1,5-pentanedial). Solutions of 2% w/v glutaraldehyde are most commonly used. The solution must be alkalinized to pH 7.4–8.5 for activation. Activated solutions are bactericidal, sporicidal, fungicidal, and virucidal for both lipophilic and hydrophilic viruses. Glutaraldehyde has greater sporicidal activity than formaldehyde, but its tuberculocidal activity may be less. Lethal action against mycobacteria and spores may require prolonged exposure. Once activated, solutions have a shelf life of 14 days, after which polymerization reduces activity. Other means of activation and stabilization can increase the shelf life. Since glutaraldehyde solutions are frequently reused, the most common reason for loss of activity is dilution and exposure to organic material. Test strips to measure residual activity are recommended.

Formaldehyde has a characteristic pungent odor and is highly irritating to respiratory mucous membranes and eyes at concentrations of 2–5 ppm. OSHA has declared that formaldehyde is a potential carcinogen and has established an employee exposure standard that limits the 8-hour time-weighted average (TWA) exposure to 0.75 ppm. Protection of health care workers from exposure to glutaraldehyde concentrations greater than 0.2 ppm is advisable. Increased air exchange, enclosure in hoods with exhausts, tight-fitting lids on exposure devices, and use of protective personal equipment such as goggles, respirators, and gloves may be necessary to achieve these exposure limits.

PEROXYGEN COMPOUNDS

The peroxygen compounds, **hydrogen peroxide** and **peracetic acid,** have high killing activity and a broad spectrum against bacteria, spores, viruses, and fungi when used in appropriate concentration. They have the advantage that their decomposition products are not toxic and do not injure the environment. They are powerful oxidizers that are used primarily as disinfectants and sterilants.

Hydrogen peroxide is a very effective disinfectant when used for inanimate objects or materials with low organic content such as water. Organisms with the enzymes catalase and peroxidase rapidly degrade hydrogen peroxide. The innocuous degradation products are oxygen and water. Concentrated solutions containing 90% w/v H_2O_2 are prepared electrochemically. When diluted in high-quality deionized water to 6% and 3% and put into clean containers, they remain stable. Hydrogen peroxide has been proposed for disinfection of respirators, acrylic resin implants, plastic eating utensils, soft contact lenses, and cartons intended to contain milk or juice products. Concentrations of 10–25% hydrogen peroxide are sporicidal. Vapor phase hydrogen peroxide (VPHP) is a cold gaseous sterilant that has the potential to replace the toxic or carcinogenic gases ethylene oxide and formaldehyde. VPHP does not require a pressurized chamber and is active at temperatures as low as 4 °C and concentrations as low as 4 mg/L. It is incompatible with liquids and cellulose products. It penetrates the surface of some plastics.

Peracetic acid (CH_3COOOH) is prepared commercially from 90% hydrogen peroxide, acetic acid, and sulfuric acid as a catalyst. It is explosive in the pure form. It is usually used in dilute solution and transported in containers with vented caps to prevent increased pressure as oxygen is released. Peracetic acid is more active than hydrogen peroxide as a bactericidal and sporicidal agent. Concentrations of 250–500 ppm are effective against a broad range of bacteria in 5 minutes at pH 7.0 at 20 °C. Bacterial spores are inactivated by 500–30,000 ppm peracetic acid. Only slightly increased concentrations are necessary in the presence of organic matter. Viruses require variable exposures. Enteroviruses require 2000 ppm for 15–30 minutes for inactivation.

An automated machine has been developed for sterilization of medical, surgical, and dental instruments. It uses buffered peracetic acid liquid of 0.1–0.5% concentration. Peracetic acid sterilization systems have been adopted for hemodialyzers. The food processing and beverage industries use peracetic acid extensively because the breakdown products in high dilution do not produce objectionable odor, taste, or toxicity. Since rinsing is not necessary in this use, time and money are saved.

Peracetic acid is a potent tumor promoter but a weak carcinogen. It is not mutagenic in the Ames test.

HEAVY METALS

Heavy metals, principally mercury and silver, are now rarely used as disinfectants. Mercury is an environmental hazard, and some pathogenic bacteria have developed plasmid-mediated resistance to mercurials. Hypersensitivity to thimerosal is common, possibly in as high as 40% of the population. These compounds are absorbed from solution by rubber and plastic closures. Nevertheless, **thimerosal** 0.001–0.004% is still used as a preservative of vaccines, antitoxins, and immune sera.

Inorganic silver salts are strongly bactericidal. **Silver nitrate**, 1:1000, has been most commonly used, particularly as a preventive for gonococcal ophthalmitis in newborns. Antibiotic ointments have replaced silver nitrate for this indication. **Silver sulfadiazine** slowly releases silver and is used to suppress bacterial growth in burn wounds (see Chapter 46).

STERILANTS

For many years, pressurized steam (**autoclaving**) at 120 °C for 30 minutes has been the basic method for sterilizing instruments and decontaminating materials. If autoclaving was not possible, as is the case with lensed instruments and materials containing plastic and rubber, **ethylene oxide**—diluted with either fluorocarbon or carbon dioxide to diminish explosive hazard—was used at 440–1200 mg/L at 45–60 °C with 30–60% relative humidity. The higher concentrations have been used to increase penetration. Alternatives to ethylene oxide are being sought because it has been classified as a mutagen and carcinogen. The OSHA permissible exposure limit (PEL) for ethylene oxide is 1 ppm calculated as a time-weighted average. Fluorocarbon diluents are under increasing control by the EPA because of their effect on the ozone layer. Medical facilities are under pressure to improve their ventilation systems and modify their sterilizers. Alternative sterilants are being used increasingly.

Alternatives being considered include vapor phase hydrogen peroxide, peracetic acid, ozone, gas plasma, chlorine dioxide, formaldehyde, and propylene oxide. Each of these sterilants has potential advantages and problems. Automated peracetic acid systems are being used increasingly for high-level decontamination and sterilization of endoscopes and hemodialyzers because of their effectiveness, automated features, and the low toxicity of the residual products of sterilization.

PRESERVATIVES

Disinfectants are used as preservatives to prevent the overgrowth of bacteria and fungi in pharmaceutical products, laboratory sera and reagents, cosmetic products, and contact lenses. Multi-use vials of medication that may be reentered through a rubber diaphragm, and eye and nose drops, require preservatives. Preservatives should not be irritant or toxic to tissues to which they will be applied, must be effective in preventing growth of microorganisms likely to contaminate them, and must have sufficient solubility and stability to remain active.

Commonly used preservative agents include organic acids such as **benzoic acid** and salts, the **parabens**, (alkyl esters of *p*-hydroxybenzoic acid), sorbic acid and salts, phenolic compounds, quaternary ammonium compounds, alcohols, and mercurials such as thimerosal in 0.001–0.004% concentration.

PREPARATIONS AVAILABLE

Miscellaneous Antimicrobial Drugs
Methenamine hippurate (Hiprex, Urex)
Oral: 0.5 g tablets
Methenamine mandelate (generic, Mandelamine)
Oral: 0.5, 1 g tablets; 0.25, 0.5, 1 g enteric-coated tablets; 0.25, 0.5 g/5 mL suspension; 0.5, 1 g granules (packets)
Metronidazole (generic, Flagyl, others)
Oral: 250, 500 mg tablets
Parenteral: 500 mg for injection
Nitrofurantoin (generic, Furadantin, others)
Oral: 50, 100 mg capsules and tablets; 25 mg/5 mL suspension; 25, 50, 100 mg macrocrystals (Macrodantin)
Parenteral: 180 mg powder for reconstitution for IV injection
Polymyxin B (Polymyxin B Sulfate, Aerosporin)
Parenteral: 500,000 units per vial for injection
Ophthalmic: 500,000 units per vial

Disinfectants, Antiseptics, & Sterilants
Benzalkonium (generic, Zephiran, others)
Topical: 17% concentrate; 50% solution; 1:750 solution
Chlorhexidine gluconate (Hibiclens, Hibistat, others)
Topical: 2, 4% cleanser, sponge; 0.5% rinse in 70% alcohol (Peridex)
Oral rinse: 0.12%

Hexachlorophene (pHisoHex, Septisol)
Topical: 3% liquid, sponge; 0.25% solution; 0.23% foam
Iodine aqueous (generic, Lugol's Solution)
Topical: 2–5% in water with 2.4% sodium iodide or 10% potassium iodide
Iodine tincture (generic)
Topical: 2% iodine or 2.4% sodium iodide in 47% alcohol, in 15, 30, 120 mL and in larger quantities
Merbromin (Mercurochrome)
Topical: 2% solution
Nitrofurazone (generic, Furacin)
Topical: 0.2% solution, ointment, and cream
Oxychlorosene sodium (Clorpactin)
Topical: 2, 5 g powder for solution for irrigation, instillation, or rinse
Povidone-iodine (generic, Betadine)
Topical: available in many forms, including aerosol, ointment, antiseptic gauze pads, skin cleanser (liquid or foam), solution, and swabsticks
Silver protein (Argyrol S.S. 10%)
Topical: 10% solution
Thimerosal (generic, Merthiolate, Mersol)
Topical: 1:1000 tincture and solution

REFERENCES

Miscellaneous Antimicrobial Agents
Bartlett JG: Anti-anaerobic antibacterial agents. Lancet 1982;2:478.
Cunha BA: Nitrofurantoin—An update. Obstet Gynecol Surv 1989;44:399.
Edwards DI: Nitroimidazole drugs—action and resistance mechanisms. (Two parts.) J Antimicrob Chemother 1993;31:9, 201.
Hamilton-Miller JM, Brumfitt W: Methenamine and its salts as urinary antiseptics. Invest Urol 1977;14:287.
Larson E: Guidelines for use of topical antimicrobial agents. Am J Infect Dis Control 1988;16:233.
Ronald AR, Harding KM: Urinary infection prophylaxis in women. Ann Intern Med 1981;94:268.

Scully BE: Metronidazole. Med Clin North Am 1988; 72:623.
Teasley DG et al: Trial of metronidazole vs vancomycin for *Clostridium difficile:* Associated diarrhea and colitis. Lancet 1983;2:1043.

Antiseptics, Disinfectants, & Sterilants
Alvarado CA et al: Nosocomial infections from contaminated endoscopes: A flawed automated endoscope washer. An investigation using molecular epidemiology. Am J Med 1991;91:272S.
Ascenzi JM (editor): *Handbook of Disinfectants and Antiseptics.* Marcel Dekker, 1996.

Best M et al: Efficacies of selected disinfectants against *Mycobacterium tuberculosis.* J Clin Microbiol 1990;28:2234.

Block SS (editor): *Disinfection, Sterilization and Preservation,* 4th ed. Lea and Febiger, 1991.

Bond WW et al: Inactivation of hepatitis B virus by intermediate to high-level disinfectant chemicals. J Clin Microbiol 1983;18:535.

Craven DE et al: Pseudobacteremia caused by povidone-iodine-solution contaminated with *Pseudomonas cepacia.* N Engl J Med 1981;305:621.

Doebbing BN et al: Comparative efficacy of alternative handwashing agents in reducing infections in intensive care units. N Engl J Med 1992;327:88.

Donowitz LG: Handwashing technique in a pediatric intensive care unit. Am J Dis Child 1987;141:683.

Favero MS, Bond WW: Disinfection and sterilization. In: *Viral Hepatitis, Scientific Basis and Clinical Management.* Zuckerman AJ, Thomas HC (editors) Churchill Livingston, 1993.

Gardner JF, Peel MM: *Introduction to Sterilization, Disinfection and Infection Control,* 2nd ed. Churchill Livingston, 1991.

Guidelines for prevention of transmission of human immunodeficiency virus and hepatitis B virus to health care and public safety workers. MMWR Morb Mortal Wkly Rep 1989;38(S-6):1.

Kaul AF, Jewett JR: Agents and techniques for disinfection of skin. Surg Gynecol Obstet 1981;152:677.

Kaye ET, Kaye KM: Topical antibacterial agents. Infect Dis Clin North Am 1995;9:547.

Kundsin RB, Walter CW: The surgical scrub: Practical considerations. Arch Surg 1973;107:75.

Lewis DL, Arens M: Resistance of microorganisms to dis-infection in dental and medical devices. Nat Med 1995;1:956.

Maki DG et al: Prospective randomized trial of povidone-iodine, alcohol and chlorhexidine for prevention of infection associated with central venous and arterial cath-eters. Lancet 1991;338:339.

Marsik FJ, Denys GA: Sterilization, decontamination and disinfection procedures for the microbiology laboratory. In: *Manual of Clinical Microbiology,* 6th ed. Murray PR (editor). American Society for Microbiology, 1995.

Reams GJ et al: Practical application of infection control in endodontics. J Endodontics 1995;21:281.

Russell AD: Bacterial spores and chemical sporicidal agents. Clin Microbiol Rev 1990;3:99.

Rutala WA et al: Disinfection practices for endoscopes and other semicritical items. Infect Control Hosp Epidemiol 1991;12:282.

Rutula WA: Guidelines for selection and use of disinfectants. Am J Infect Control 1990;18:99.

Satta SA, Springthorpe VS: Survival and disinfectant inactivation of the human immunodeficiency virus: A critical review. Rev Infect Dis 1991;13:430.

United States General Accounting Office: Resources, Community and Economic Development Division. Disinfectants: EPA Lacks Assurance They Work. 1990 GAO/RCE D-90-139 Washington DC 20548.

Viljanto J: Disinfection of surgical wounds without inhibition of normal wound healing. Arch Surg 1980;115:253.

Wood PR: *Cross Infection Control in Dentistry: A Practical Illustrated Guide.* Mosby Year Book, 1992.

51

Clinical Use of Antimicrobial Agents

Harry W. Lampiris, MD, & Daniel S. Maddix, PharmD

The development of antimicrobial drugs represents one of the most important advances in therapeutics, both in the control or cure of serious infections and in the prevention and treatment of infectious complications of other therapeutic modalities such as cancer chemotherapy and surgery. However, there is increasing evidence that antimicrobial agents are vastly overprescribed in many outpatient settings in the United States, and the availability of antimicrobial agents without prescription in many developing countries has—by facilitating the development of resistance—already severely limited therapeutic options in the treatment of life-threatening infections. Therefore, the clinician should first determine whether antimicrobial therapy is warranted for a given patient. The specific questions one should ask include the following:

(1) Is an antimicrobial agent indicated on the basis of clinical findings? Or is it prudent to wait until such clinical findings become apparent?

(2) Have appropriate clinical specimens been obtained to establish a microbiologic diagnosis?

(3) What are the likely etiologic agents for the patient's illness?

(4) What measures should be taken to protect individuals exposed to the index case to prevent secondary cases, and what measures should be implemented to prevent further exposure?

Once a specific cause is identified based upon specific microbiologic tests, the following further questions should be considered:

(1) If a specific microbial pathogen is identified, can a narrower-spectrum agent be substituted for the initial empirical drug?

(2) Is one agent or a combination of agents necessary?

(3) What is the optimal dose, route of administration, and duration of therapy?

(4) What specific tests (eg, susceptibility testing) should be undertaken to identify patients who will not respond to treatment?

(5) What adjunctive measures can be undertaken to eradicate the infection? For example, is surgery feasible for removal of devitalized tissue or foreign bodies—or drainage of an abscess—into which antimicrobial agents may be unable to penetrate? Is it possible to decrease the dosage of immunosuppressive therapy in patients who have undergone organ transplantation or to give immunomodulatory drugs or antitoxins to patients with preexisting immune deficiency?

EMPIRICAL ANTIMICROBIAL THERAPY

Antimicrobial agents are frequently used before the pathogen responsible for a particular illness or the susceptibility to a particular antimicrobial agent is known. This use of antimicrobial agents is called empirical (or presumptive) therapy, and is based upon experience with a particular clinical entity. The usual justification for empirical therapy is the hope that early intervention will improve the outcome, and in the best case this has been established by placebo-controlled, double-blind prospective clinical trials. For example, treatment of febrile episodes in neutropenic cancer patients with empirical antimicrobial therapy has been demonstrated to have impressive morbidity and mortality benefits in placebo-controlled trials even though the specific bacterial agent responsible for fever is determined for only a minority of such episodes. Conversely, there are many clinical situations in which empirical therapy may not be useful or may actually be harmful. For example, neutropenic patients with fever and pulmonary infiltrates may have a wide variety of causes for their clinical illness, including viruses, bacteria, mycobacteria, fungi, protozoa, and noninfectious disorders. In this setting, it may be more prudent to obtain specimens by sputum culture or via bronchoalveolar lavage early in order to offer narrow-spectrum therapy based upon culture results.

Lastly, there are many clinical entities, such as certain episodes of community-acquired pneumonia, in which it is difficult to identify a specific pathogen. In such cases, a clinical response to empirical therapy may be an important clue to the likely pathogen.

Approach to Empirical Therapy

Initiation of empirical therapy should follow a specific and systematic approach.

A. Formulate a Clinical Diagnosis of Microbial Infection: Using all available data, the clinician should conclude that there is anatomic evidence of infection (eg, pneumonia, cellulitis, sinusitis).

B. Obtain Specimens for Laboratory Examination: Examination of stained specimens by microscopy or simple examination of an uncentrifuged sample of urine for white blood cells and bacteria may provide important etiologic clues in a very short time.

C. Formulate a Microbiologic Diagnosis: The history, physical examination, and immediately available laboratory results (eg, Gram's stain of urine or sputum) may provide highly specific information. For example, in a young man with urethritis (usually presenting with urethral discharge and dysuria) and a Gram-stained smear from the urethral meatus demonstrating intracellular gram-negative diplococci in polymorphonuclear leukocytes, the most likely pathogen is *Neisseria gonorrhoeae*. In the latter instance, however, the clinician should be aware that a significant number of patients with gonococcal urethritis have uninformative Gram stains for the organism and that a significant number of patients with gonococcal urethritis, even in the presence of a diagnostic Gram stain, harbor concurrent chlamydial infection that is not demonstrated on the Gram-stained smear.

D. Determine the Necessity for Empirical Therapy: This is an important clinical decision based partly upon experience and partly upon data from clinical trials. Empirical therapy is indicated when there is a significant risk of serious morbidity if therapy is withheld until a specific pathogen is detected by the clinical laboratory.

In other settings, empirical therapy may be indicated for public health reasons rather than for demonstrated superior outcome of therapy in a specific patient. For example, urethritis in a young sexually active male usually requires treatment for *Neisseria gonorrhoeae* and *Chlamydia trachomatis* despite the absence of microbiologic confirmation at the time of diagnosis. Because there is a high risk of noncompliance with follow-up visits in this patient population, empirical therapy is warranted to ensure cure of the infection at the first visit in order to prevent further transmission.

E. Institute Treatment: Selection of empirical therapy may be based upon the microbiologic diagnosis or a clinical diagnosis without available microbiologic clues. If no microbiologic information is available, the antimicrobial spectrum of the agent or agents chosen must necessarily be broader, taking into account the most likely pathogens responsible for the patient's illness.

Choice of Antimicrobial Agent

Selection from among several drugs depends upon host factors. For example, patients with AIDS have a particularly high risk of allergic or toxic reactions to many antimicrobial agents; patients with severe chronic liver disease have an unacceptably high risk of developing nonoliguric renal failure with aminoglycoside therapy. Such host factors may also include prior adverse drug effects and impaired elimination or detoxification of the drug—this may be genetically predetermined but more frequently is associated with impaired renal or hepatic function due to underlying disease. The age of the patient and pregnancy status are other important host factors to be considered. Pharmacologic factors include the kinetics of absorption, distribution, and elimination; the ability of the drug to be delivered to the site of infection; the potential toxicity of an agent; and pharmacokinetic or pharmacodynamic interactions with other drugs. Knowledge of the susceptibility of an organism to a specific agent in a hospital or community setting is important in the selection of empirical therapy. Pharmacokinetic differences among agents with similar antimicrobial spectrums may be exploited to reduce the frequency of dosing (eg, ceftriaxone may be conveniently given every 24 hours). Lastly, increasing consideration is being given to the cost of antimicrobial therapy, especially when multiple agents with comparable efficacy and toxicity are available for a specific infection.

Brief guides to empirical therapy based upon presumptive microbial diagnosis and site of infection are given in Tables 51–1 and 51–2.

ANTIMICROBIAL THERAPY OF INFECTIONS WITH KNOWN ETIOLOGY

INTERPRETATION OF CULTURE RESULTS

Properly obtained and processed specimens for culture frequently yield reliable information about the cause of infection. The lack of a confirmatory microbiologic diagnosis may be due to the following:

(1) Sample error, eg, obtaining cultures after antimicrobial agents have been administered.

(2) Noncultivable or slow-growing organisms, *Histoplasma capsulatum*, *Bartonella* species), where cultures are often discarded before sufficient growth has occurred for detection.

Table 51–1. Empiric antimicrobial therapy based on microbiologic etiology.

Suspected or Proved Disease or Pathogen	Drug(s) of First Choice	Alternative Drug(s)
Gram-negative cocci (aerobic)		
Moraxella (Branhamella) catarrhalis	TMP-SMZ,[1] cephalosporin (second- or third-generation)	Erythromycin, quinolone, clarithromycin, azithromycin
Neisseria gonorrhoeae	Ceftriaxone, cefixime, quinolone	Spectinomycin, cefoxitin
Neisseria meningitidis	Penicillin G	Chloramphenicol, cephalosporin (third-generation)[2]
Gram-negative rods (aerobic)		
E coli, Klebsiella, Proteus	Cephalosporin (first- or second-generation), TMP-SMZ	Quinolone, aminoglycoside
Enterobacter, Citrobacter, Serratia	TMP-SMZ, quinolone, imipenem	Antipseudomonal penicillin[3], aminoglycoside[4]
Shigella	Quinolone	TMP-SMZ, ampicillin, cefixime, ceftriaxone
Salmonella	TMP-SMZ, quinolone, cephalosporin (third-generation)	Chloramphenicol, ampicillin
Campylobacter jejuni	Quinolone, erythromycin	Tetracycline, furazolidone
Brucella species	Doxycycline + rifampin or aminoglycoside[4]	Chloramphenicol + aminoglycoside or TMP-SMZ
Helicobacter pylori	Bismuth + metronidazole + tetracycline or amoxicillin	Omeprazole + amoxicillin or clarithromycin
Vibrio species	Tetracycline, TMP-SMZ	Quinolone
Pseudomonas aeruginosa	Antipseudomonal penicillin + aminoglycoside[4]	Antipseudomonal penicillin + quinolone; ceftazidime, imipenem, or aztreonam ± aminoglycoside
Burkholderia cepacia (formerly Pseudomonas cepacia)	TMP-SMZ	Ceftazidime, chloramphenicol
Stenotrophomonas maltophilia (formerly Xanthomonas maltophilia)	TMP-SMZ	Minocycline, ticarcillin-clavulanate, quinolone
Legionella species	Erythromycin (+ rifampin)	Quinolone (+ rifampin), clarithromycin
Gram-positive cocci (aerobic)		
Streptococcus pneumoniae	Penicillin[5]	Ceftriaxone, cefotaxime, vancomycin, TMP-SMZ, erythromycin, imipenem
Streptococcus pyogenes (group A)	Penicillin, clindamycin	Erythromycin, cephalosporin (first-generation)
Streptococcus agalactiae (group B)	Penicillin (+ aminoglycoside?[4])	Vancomycin
Viridans streptococci	Penicillin	Cephalosporin (first-or third-generation), vancomycin
Staphylococcus aureus Beta-lactamase-negative	Penicillin	Cephalosporin (first-generation), vancomycin
Beta-lactamase-positive	Penicillinase-resistant penicillin[6]	As above
Methicillin-resistant	Vancomycin	TMP-SMZ, minocycline
Enterococcus species[7]	Penicillin + aminoglycoside[4]	Vancomycin + aminoglycoside
Gram-positive rods (aerobic)		
Bacillus species (non-anthracis)	Vancomycin	Imipenem, quinolone, clindamycin
Listeria species	Ampicillin (+ aminoglycoside[4])	TMP-SMZ
Nocardia species	Sulfadiazine, TMP-SMZ	Minocycline, imipenem, amikacin
Anaerobic bacteria		
Gram-positive (clostridia, Peptococcus, Actinomyces, Peptostreptococcus)	Penicillin, clindamycin	Vancomycin, imipenem, chloramphenicol
Clostridium difficile	Metronidazole	Vancomycin, bacitracin

Table 51–1. Empiric antimicrobial therapy based on microbiologic etiology (cont'd).

Suspected or Proved Disease or Pathogen	Drug(s) of First Choice	Alternative Drug(s)
Bacteroides fragilis	Metronidazole, clindamycin	Chloramphenicol, imipenem, beta lactam–beta-lactamase-inhibitor combinations
Fusobacterium, Prevotella, Porphyromonas	Metronidazole, clindamycin	As for *B fragilis*
Mycobacteria *Mycobacterium tuberculosis*	Isoniazid + rifampin + ethambutol + pyrazinamide	Streptomycin, quinolone, amikacin, ethionamide, cycloserine, PAS
Mycobacterium leprae Multibacillary Paucibacillary	Dapsone + rifampin + clofazimine Dapsone + rifampin	
Mycoplasma pneumoniae	Tetracycline, erythromycin	Azithromycin, clarithromycin
Chlamydia *trachomatis*	Tetracycline, erythromycin	Clindamycin, ofloxacin, azithromycin
pneumoniae	Tetracycline, erythromycin	Clarithromycin, azithromycin
psittaci	Tetracycline	Chloramphenicol
Spirochetes *Borrelia recurrentis*	Doxycycline, penicillin	Erythromycin, chloramphenicol
Borrelia burgdorferi Early Late		Azithromycin, clarithromycin Chloramphenicol
Leptospira species	Penicillin	Tetracycline
Treponema species	Penicillin	Tetracycline, erythromycin
Fungi *Aspergillus* species	Amphotericin B	Itraconazole
Blastomyces species	Amphotericin B	Itraconazole, ketoconazole[8]
Candida species, *Torulopsis* species	Amphotericin B	Fluconazole, ketoconazole
Cryptococcus	Amphotericin B ± flucytosine (5-FC)	Fluconazole
Coccidioides immitis	Amphotericin B	Fluconazole, itraconazole, ketoconazole
Histoplasma capsulatum	Amphotericin B	Itraconazole
Mucoraceae *(Rhizopus, Absidia)*	Amphotericin B	
Sporothrix schenkii	Amphotericin B	Itraconazole

[1]Trimethoprim-sulfamethoxazole (TMP-SMZ) is a mixture of one part trimethoprim plus five parts sulfamethoxazole.

[2]**First-generation cephalosporins:** Cephalothin, cephapirin, or cefazolin for parenteral administration; cephalexin or cephradine for oral administration. **Second-generation cephalosporins:** Cefuroxime, cefamandole, cefonicid for parenteral administration; cefaclor, cefuroxime axetil, cefprozil, ceftibuten for oral administration. **Third-generation cephalosporins:** Cefoperazone, cefotaxime, ceftizoxime, ceftriaxone for parenteral administration; cefixime, cefpodoxime for oral administration.

[3]Antipseudomonal penicillin: Carbenicillin, ticarcillin, azlocillin, mezlocillin, piperacillin.

[4]Generally, streptomycin and gentamicin are used to treat infections with gram-positive organisms, whereas gentamicin, tobramycin, and amikacin are used to treat infections with gram-negatives.

[5]See footnote 3 in Table 51–2 for guidelines on the treatment of penicillin-resistant pneumococcal meningitis.

[6]Parenteral nafcillin, oxacillin, or methicillin; oral dicloxacillin, cloxacillin, or oxacillin

[7]There is no regimen that is reliably bactericidal for vancomycin-resistant *Enterococcus*. Regimens that have been reported to be efficacious include single-drug therapy with chloramphenicol, tetracycline, nitrofurantoin (for urinary tract infection); potential regimens for bacteremia include ampicillin + vancomycin and ampicillin + ciprofloxacin + gentamicin.

[8]Ketoconazole does not penetrate the central nervous system and is unsatisfactory for meningitis.

(3) Requesting *bacterial* cultures when infection is due to other organisms.

(4) Not recognizing the need for special media or isolation techniques (eg, charcoal yeast extract agar for isolation of *Legionella* species, shell-vial tissue culture system for rapid isolation of CMV).

Even in the setting of a classic infectious disease for which isolation techniques have been established for decades (eg, pneumococcal pneumonia, pulmonary tuberculosis, streptococcal pharyngitis), the sensitivity of the culture technique may be inadequate to identify all cases of the disease.

Table 51–2. Empiric antimicrobial therapy based on site of infection.

Presumed Site of Infection	Common Pathogens	Drug(s) of First Choice	Alternative Drug(s)
Bacterial endocarditis Acute	Staphylococcus aureus	Penicillinase-resistant peni-cillin[1] + gentamicin	Vancomycin + gentamicin
Subacute	Viridans streptococci, entero-cocci	Penicillin + gentamicin	Vancomycin + gentamicin
Septic arthritis Child	H influenzae, S aureus, β-hemolytic streptococci	Ceftriaxone	Ampicillin-sulbactam
Adult	Gonococcus, S aureus, Enterobacteriaceae	Cefazolin	TMP-SMZ, quinolone
Acute otitis media, sinusitis	H influenzae, S pneumoniae, M catarrhalis	Amoxicillin, TMP-SMZ	Amoxicillin-clavulanate, cefuroxime axetil
Cellulitis	S aureus, group A Strepto-coccus	Penicillinase-resistant penicillin, cephalosporin (first-generation)	Vancomycin
Meningitis Neonate	Group B Streptococcus, E coli, Listeria	Ampicillin + aminoglycoside	Chloramphenicol; ampicillin + cephalosporin (third-genera-tion)
Child	H influenzae, pneumococcus, meningococcus	Ceftriaxone or cefotaxime ± vancomycin[3]	Chloramphenicol
Adult	Pneumococcus, meningo-coccus	Ceftriaxone, cefotaxime	Vancomycin + ceftriaxone or cefotaxime[3]
Peritonitis due to ruptured viscus	Coliforms, B fragilis	Metronidazole + cephalosporin (third-generation), piperacillin-tazobactam	Imipenem
Pneumonia Neonate	As in neonatal meningitis		
Child	Pneumococcus, S aureus, H influenzae	Ceftriaxone, cefuroxime	Ampicillin-sulbactam, TMP-SMZ
Adult (community-acquired)	Pneumococcus, Mycoplasma, Legionella, H influenzae, S aureus, C pneumonia, coliforms	**Outpatient:** Erythromycin, amoxicillin, tetracycline **Inpatient:** Macrolide[4] + cephalosporin (third-generation)	**Outpatient:** Azithromycin, clarithromycin, TMP-SMZ **Inpatient:** Macrolide + piperacillin-tazobactam or ticarcillin-clavulanate
Septicemia	Any	Aminoglycoside + cephalosporin (third-generation) or piperacillin-tazobactam or ticarcillin-clavulanate	
Septicemia with granulocytopenia	Any	Antipseudomonal penicillin + aminoglycoside; ceftazidime + aminoglycoside; imipenem; consider addition of amphotericin B if fever persists beyond 5 days of empiric therapy	

[1]See footnote 6, Table 51–1.
[2]See footnote 2, Table 51–1.
[3]When meningitis with penicillin-resistant pneumococcus is suspected, empiric therapy with this regimen is recommended.
[4]Erythromycin, clarithromycin, or azithromycin (an azalide) may be used.

GUIDING ANTIMICROBIAL THERAPY OF ESTABLISHED INFECTIONS

Susceptibility Testing

Testing bacterial pathogens in vitro for their susceptibility to antimicrobial agents is extremely valuable in confirming susceptibility, ideally to a narrow-spectrum nontoxic antimicrobial drug. Tests measure the concentration of drug required to inhibit growth of the organism (minimal inhibitory concentration [MIC] or to kill the organism (minimum bactericidal concentration [MBC]). The results of these tests can then be correlated with known drug concentrations in various body compartments. Only MICs are routinely measured in most infections, whereas in infections in which bactericidal therapy is required for eradication of infection (eg, meningitis, endocarditis, sepsis in the granulocytopenic host), MBC measurements occasionally may be useful.

Two methods of susceptibility testing in common use are the disk (agar) diffusion (Kirby-Bauer) method and the broth dilution method. In the disk diffusion method, a disk containing a standardized amount of the test antimicrobial agent is placed on an agar plate lightly seeded with a standardized concentration of bacteria. The culture is then placed in an incubator and the bacterial lawn allowed to grow while the antimicrobial agent diffuses out into the agar. The diameter of the visible zone of growth inhibition around the disk correlates with the MIC. In the broth dilution method, the bacteria are inoculated into the liquid medium containing graduated concentrations of the test antimicrobial for direct determination of the MIC. Automated systems that rely on the broth dilution method include VITEK and MICROSCAN, allowing more rapid and automated results, but may be less accurate in determining MICs for certain organisms (eg, methicillin-resistant staphylococci).

Disk diffusion methods are satisfactory for determining susceptibility of many organisms to particular drugs, and they are all that is required when the mechanism of resistance is due to enzymatic degradation of the antimicrobial agent by the organism. However, when there is no sharp dividing line between susceptibility and resistance in the disk test, direct determination of the MIC may be very helpful in guiding therapy. The latter is usually seen in cases where decreased antimicrobial activity is due to alteration in the binding sites of the antimicrobial agent to the organism, as in methicillin-resistant staphylococci.

Specialized Assay Methods

A. Beta-Lactamase Assay: For some bacteria (eg, *Haemophilus* species), the susceptibility patterns of strains are similar except for the production of beta-lactamase. In these cases, extensive susceptibility testing may not be required and a direct test for beta-lactamase utilizing a chromogenic beta-lactam substrate (nitrocephin disk) may be substituted.

B. Synergy Studies: These in vitro tests attempt to measure synergistic, additive, indifferent, or antagonistic drug interactions. In general, these tests have not been standardized and have not correlated well with clinical outcome. (See section on combination chemotherapy for details.)

MONITORING THERAPEUTIC RESPONSE: DURATION OF THERAPY

The therapeutic response may be monitored microbiologically or clinically. Cultures of specimens taken from infected sites should eventually become sterile or demonstrate eradication of the pathogen and are useful for documenting recurrence or relapse. Follow-up cultures may also be useful for detecting superinfections or the development of resistance. Clinically, the patient's systemic manifestations of infection (malaise, fever, leukocytosis) should abate and the clinical findings should improve (eg, as shown by clearing of radiographic infiltrates or lessening hypoxemia in pneumonia). The speed of clinical response is generally directly related to the duration of symptoms prior to the initiation of therapy.

The duration of therapy required for cure depends on the pathogen, the site of infection, and host factors (immunocompromised patients generally require longer courses of treatment). Precise data on duration of therapy exist for specific infections (eg, streptococcal pharyngitis, syphilis, gonorrhea, tuberculosis, cryptococcal meningitis in non-AIDS patients). In many other situations, duration of therapy is determined empirically. For serious infections, continuing therapy for 7–10 days after the patient has become afebrile is a good rule of thumb. For recurrent infections (eg, sinusitis, urinary tract infections), longer courses of antimicrobial therapy are frequently necessary for eradication.

Clinical Failure of Antimicrobial Therapy

When the patient has an inadequate clinical or microbiologic response to antimicrobial therapy selected by in vitro susceptibility testing, systematic investigation should be undertaken to determine the cause of failure. Errors in susceptibility testing are rare, but the original results should be confirmed by repeat testing. Drug dosing and absorption should be scrutinized and tested directly using serum measurements, pill counting, or directly observed therapy.

The clinical data should be reviewed to determine whether the patient's immune function is adequate and, if not, what can be done to maximize it. For example, are adequate numbers of granulocytes present and are HIV infection, malnutrition, or underlying malignancy present? The presence of abscesses or foreign bodies should also be considered. Lastly, culture and susceptibility testing should be repeated to determine if superinfection has occurred with another organism or if the original pathogen has developed drug resistance.

ANTIMICROBIAL PHARMACODYNAMICS

The time course of drug concentration is closely related to the antimicrobial effect at the site of infection and to any toxic effects. Pharmacodynamic factors include pathogen susceptibility testing, drug bactericidal versus bacteriostatic activity, and drug synergism, antagonism, and postantibiotic effects. Together with pharmacokinetics, pharmacodynamic information permits the selection of optimal antimicrobial dosage regimens. Synergism and antagonism will be discussed in the section on antimicrobial combinations.

Bacteriostatic Versus Bactericidal Activity

Antibacterial agents may be classified as bacteriostatic or bactericidal (Table 51–3). For agents that are primarily bacteriostatic, inhibitory drug concentrations are much lower than bactericidal drug concentrations. In contrast, primarily bactericidal agents demonstrate little difference between inhibitory and bactericidal drug concentrations. In general, cell wall-active agents are bactericidal, and drugs that inhibit protein synthesis are bacteriostatic.

The classification of antibacterial agents as bactericidal or bacteriostatic has limitations. Some agents that are considered to be bacteriostatic may be bactericidal against selected organisms. For example, chloramphenicol is often bactericidal against pneumococci, meningococci, and *Haemophilus influenzae.* On the other hand, enterococci are inhibited but not killed by vancomycin, penicillin, or ampicillin used as single agents.

Bacteriostatic and bactericidal agents are equivalent for the treatment of most infectious diseases in immunocompetent hosts. Bactericidal agents should be selected over bacteriostatic ones in circumstances in which local or systemic host defenses are impaired. Bactericidal agents are required for treatment of endocarditis and other endovascular infections, meningitis, and infections in neutropenic cancer patients.

Bactericidal agents can be divided into two groups: agents that exhibit **concentration-dependent killing** (eg, aminoglycosides and quinolones) and agents that exhibit **time-dependent killing** (eg, beta-lactams and vancomycin). For drugs whose killing action is concentration-dependent, the rate and extent of killing increase with increasing drug concentrations. Maximizing peak serum concentrations of such drugs results in increased efficacy and decreased selection of resistant bacteria. Concentration-dependent killing is one of the pharmacodynamic factors responsible for the efficacy of once-daily dosing of aminoglycosides.

Drugs whose killing action is time-dependent do not exhibit increased killing with increasing concentrations above MBC; bactericidal activity continues as long as serum concentrations are greater than the MBC. Drug concentrations of time-dependent killing

agents that lack a postantibiotic effect should be maintained above the MIC for the entire dosage interval.

Postantibiotic Effect

Persistent suppression of bacterial growth after limited exposure to an antimicrobial agent is known as the postantibiotic effect (PAE). The PAE can be expressed mathematically as follows:

$$PAE = T - C$$

where T is the time required for the viable count in the test (in vitro) culture to increase tenfold above the count observed immediately before drug removal and C is the time required for the count in an untreated culture to increase tenfold above the count observed immediately after completion of the same procedure used on the test culture. The PAE reflects the time required for bacteria to return to logarithmic growth.

The exact mechanism of the PAE is unknown. Proposed mechanisms include recovery after reversible nonlethal damage to cell structures, persistence of the drug at a binding site or within the periplasmic space, and the need to synthesize new enzymes before growth. It is believed that the PAE generally represents an extension of the lag phase of bacterial growth.

Most antimicrobials possess significant in vitro PAEs ($\geq$ 1.5 hours) against susceptible gram-positive cocci (Table 51–4). Antimicrobials with significant PAEs against susceptible gram-negative bacilli are limited to carbapenems and agents that inhibit protein or DNA synthesis.

In vivo PAEs are usually much longer than in vitro PAEs. This is thought to be due to **postantibiotic leukocyte enhancement (PALE)** and exposure of bacteria to subinhibitory antibiotic concentrations. PALE reflects the increased susceptibility of bacteria to the phagocytic and bactericidal action of neutrophils. Subinhibitory drug concentrations result in altered bacterial morphology and decreased rate of growth. The lowest drug concentration required to in-

Table 51–3. Bacteriostatic and bactericidal antibacterial agents.

Bactericidal agents	Bacteriostatic agents
Aminoglycosides	Chloramphenicol
Bacitracin	Clindamycin
Beta-lactam antibiotics	Ethambutol
Isoniazid	Macrolides
Metronidazole	Nitrofurantoin
Polymyxins	Novobiocin
Pyrazinamide	Sulfonamides
Quinolones	Tetracyclines
Rifampin	Trimethoprim
Vancomycin	

Table 51–4. Antibacterial agents with in vitro postantibiotic effects $\geq$ 1.5 hours.

Against gram-positive cocci	Against gram-negative bacilli
Aminoglycosides	Aminoglycosides
Carbapenems	Carbapenems
Cephalosporins	Chloramphenicol
Chloramphenicol	Quinolones
Clindamycin	Rifampin
Macrolides	Tetracyclines
Penicillins	
Quinolones	
Rifampin	
Sulfonamides	
Tetracyclines	
Trimethoprim	
Vancomycin	

duce morphologic changes is known as the minimum antibacterial concentration.

The clinical relevance of the PAE is beginning to be appreciated. The efficacy of once-daily dosing regimens is in part due to the PAE. Aminoglycosides and quinolones possess concentration-dependent PAEs; thus, high doses of aminoglycosides given once daily result in enhanced bactericidal activity and extended PAEs. This combination of pharmacodynamic effects allows aminoglycoside serum concentrations that are below the MICs of target organisms to remain effective for extended periods of time. The efficacy of once-daily dosing is also thought to be due to the avoidance of adaptive resistance, a phenomenon in which reduced bactericidal activity occurs following a second antibiotic exposure. Adaptive resistance is probably caused by a reduction in energy-dependent aminoglycoside uptake into bacteria. Once-daily dosing of aminoglycosides is associated with less toxicity and lower monitoring costs than conventional dosing.

PHARMACOKINETIC CONSIDERATIONS

Route of Administration

The absorption of orally or intramuscularly administered antimicrobial agents is unreliable in critically ill patients. The intravenous route is preferred in such patients. Intravenous therapy is also preferred in patients with bacterial meningitis or endocarditis. Parenteral therapy should be selected in patients with nausea, vomiting, gastrectomy, or diseases that may impair oral absorption. The parenteral route is also used for drugs such as vancomycin and antipseudomonal penicillins, which are poorly absorbed from the gastrointestinal tract. On the other hand, many antimicrobial agents have similar pharmacokinetic properties when given orally or parenterally (ie, tetracyclines, trimethoprim-sulfamethoxazole, quinolones, chloramphenicol, metronidazole, clindamycin, rifampin, and fluconazole). In most cases, oral therapy with these drugs is equally effective, less costly, and results in fewer complications than parenteral therapy.

Conditions That Alter Antimicrobial Pharmacokinetics

Various diseases and physiologic states alter the pharmacokinetics of antimicrobial agents. Impairment of renal or hepatic function may result in decreased elimination. Table 51–5 lists drugs that require dosage reduction in patients with renal or hepatic insufficiency. Failure to reduce antimicrobial agent dosage in such patients may cause toxic side effects. Conversely, patients with burns, cystic fibrosis, or trauma may have increased dosage requirements for selected agents. The pharmacokinetics of antimicrobials are also altered in the elderly, in neonates, and in pregnancy.

Drug Concentrations in Body Fluids

Most antimicrobial agents are well distributed to most body tissues and fluids. Penetration into the cerebrospinal fluid is an exception. Most do not penetrate uninflamed meninges to an appreciable extent. In the presence of meningitis, however, the cerebrospinal fluid concentrations of many antimicrobials increase (Table 51–6).

Table 51–5. Antimicrobial agents that require dosage adjustment or are contraindicated in patients with renal or hepatic impairment.

Dosage Adjustment Needed in Renal Impairment	Contraindicated in Renal Impairment	Dosage Adjustment Needed in Hepatic Impairment
Acyclovir	Methenamine	Chloramphenicol
Amantadine	Nalidixic acid	Clindamycin
Aminoglycosides	Nitrofurantoin	Erythromycin
Aztreonam	Sulfonamides (long-acting)	Metronidazole
Cephalosporins[1]	Tetracyclines[2]	Rimantadine
Clarithromycin		
Fluconazole		
Flucytosine		
Foscarnet		
Ganciclovir		
Imipenem		
Penicillins[3]		
Quinolones		
Rimantadine		
Stavudine		
Trimethoprim-sulfamethoxazole		
Vancomycin		
Zalcitabine		
Zidovudine		

[1]Except cefoperazone and ceftriaxone
[2]Except doxycycline and possibly minocycline
[3]Except antistaphylococcal penicillins (eg, nafcillin and dicloxacillin)

Table 51–6. Cerebrospinal fluid (CSF) penetration of selected antimicrobials.

Antimicrobial Agent	CSF Concentration (Uninflamed Meninges) as Percent of Serum Concentration	CSF Concentration (Inflamed Meninges) as Percent of Serum Concentration
Ampicillin	2–3	2–100
Aztreonam	2	5
Cefotaxime	22.5	27–36
Ceftazidime	0.7	20–40
Ceftriaxone	0.8–1.6	16
Cefuroxime	20	17–88
Ciprofloxacin	6–27	26–37
Imipenem	3.1	11–41
Nafcillin	2–15	5–27
Penicillin G	1–2	8–18
Sulfamethoxazole	40	12–47
Trimethoprim	< 41	12–69
Vancomycin	0	1–53

Monitoring Serum Concentration of Antimicrobial Agents

For most antimicrobial agents, the relationship between dose and therapeutic outcome is well established, and serum concentration monitoring is unnecessary for these drugs. To justify routine serum concentration monitoring, it should be established (1) that a direct relationship exists between drug concentrations and efficacy or toxicity; (2) that substantial interpatient variability exists in serum concentrations on standard doses; (3) that a small difference exists between therapeutic and toxic serum concentrations; (4) that the clinical efficacy or toxicity of the drug is delayed or difficult to measure; and (5) that an accurate assay is available.

In clinical practice, serum concentration monitoring is routinely performed on patients receiving aminoglycosides. Despite the lack of supporting evidence for its utility or need, serum vancomycin concentration monitoring is also widespread. Flucytosine serum concentration monitoring has been shown to reduce toxicity when doses are adjusted to maintain peak concentrations below 100 µg/mL.

MANAGEMENT OF ANTIMICROBIAL AGENT TOXICITY

Owing to the large number of antimicrobials available, it is usually possible to select an effective alternative in patients who develop serious drug toxicity (Table 51–1). However, for some infections there are no effective alternatives to the drug of choice. For example, in patients with neurosyphilis who have a history of anaphylaxis to penicillin, it is necessary to perform skin testing and desensitization to penicillin. It is important to obtain a clear history of drug allergy and other adverse drug reactions. A good history may reveal that a patient with a reported allergy to an antimicrobial may have subsequently received the same agent or another agent from the same drug class without a serious reaction. Antimicrobials are often avoided in patients who report a history of antimicrobial allergy but who in fact have had only a mild reaction such as nausea or diarrhea. A patient with a documented antimicrobial allergy should carry a card with the name of the drug and a description of the reaction. Cross-reactivity between penicillins and cephalosporins is less than 10%. Cephalosporins may be administered to patients with penicillin-induced maculopapular rashes but should be avoided in patients with a history of penicillin-induced immediate hypersensitivity reactions. The cross-reactivity between penicillins and imipenem may exceed 50%. On the other hand, aztreonam does not cross-react with penicillins and can be safely administered to patients with a history of penicillin-induced anaphylaxis. Because of the structural similarities between aztreonam and ceftazidime, aztreonam should be avoided in patients with a history of ceftazidime allergy. For mild reactions, it may be possible to continue therapy with use of adjunctive agents or dosage reduction.

Adverse reactions to antimicrobials occur with increased frequency in several groups, including neonates, geriatric patients, renal failure patients, and AIDS patients. Dosage adjustment of the drugs listed in Table 51–5 is essential for the prevention of adverse effects in patients with renal failure. In addition, several agents are contraindicated in patients with renal impairment because of increased rates of serious toxicity (Table 51–5). See the preceding chapters for discussions of specific drugs.

Polypharmacy also predisposes to drug interactions. Although the mechanism is not known, AIDS patients have an unusually high incidence of toxicity to a number of drugs, including clindamycin, aminopenicillins, and sulfonamides. Many of these reactions, including rash and fever, may respond to dosage reduction or treatment with corticosteroids and antihistamines. Other examples are discussed in the preceding chapters and in Appendix II.

ANTIMICROBIAL AGENT COMBINATIONS

RATIONALE FOR COMBINATION ANTIMICROBIAL THERAPY

Most infections should be treated with a single antimicrobial agent. Although indications for combination therapy exist, antimicrobial combinations are often overused in clinical practice. The unnecessary use of antimicrobial combinations increases toxicity and costs and may occasionally result in reduced efficacy due to antagonism of one drug by another. Antimicrobial combinations should be selected for one or more of the following reasons:

(1) To provide broad-spectrum empirical therapy in seriously ill patients. For example, a patient with sepsis of unknown origin may require coverage for gram-positive cocci as well as gram-negative bacilli. In such a patient, it would be reasonable to initiate therapy with an antistaphylococcal agent and an antimicrobial possessing gram-negative activity. Once culture results become available, the unnecessary agents should be discontinued.

(2) To treat polymicrobial infections such as intra-abdominal abscesses. Polymicrobial infections typically involve both aerobic and anaerobic organisms. Following surgical drainage, intra-abdominal abscesses can be treated with a drug with gram-negative activity (eg, an aminoglycoside or third-generation cephalosporin) and a drug with anaerobic activity (eg, metronidazole). The antimicrobial combination chosen should cover the most common known or suspected pathogens but need not cover all possible pathogens. The availability of antimicrobials with excellent polymicrobial coverage (eg, beta-lactamase inhibitor combinations or imipenem) may reduce the need for combination therapy in the setting of polymicrobial infections.

(3) To decrease the emergence of resistant strains. The value of combination therapy in this setting has been clearly demonstrated for tuberculosis. Monotherapy of active tuberculosis predictably results in

emergence of resistance. Resistance develops rapidly in staphylococci when rifampin is used as a single agent but can be prevented by using rifampin in combination with a second antistaphylococcal agent.

(4) To decrease dose-related toxicity by using reduced doses of one or more components of the drug regimen. The use of flucytosine in combination with amphotericin B for the treatment of cryptococcal meningitis in non-HIV-infected patients allows for a reduction in amphotericin B dosage with decreased amphotericin B-induced nephrotoxicity.

(5) To obtain enhanced inhibition or killing. This use of antimicrobial combinations is discussed in the paragraphs that follow.

SYNERGISM & ANTAGONISM

When the inhibitory or killing effects of two or more antimicrobials used together are significantly greater than expected from their effects when used individually, synergism is said to result. Synergism may be marked by a fourfold or greater reduction in the MIC or MBC of each drug when used in combination versus when used alone.

The interaction between two antimicrobial agents can be expressed by the fractional inhibitory concentration (FIC) index:

$$FIC_{index} = FIC_A + FIC_B$$

$$FIC_A = \frac{MIC \text{ of drug A in combination}}{MIC \text{ of drug A alone}}$$

$$FIC_B = \frac{MIC \text{ of drug B in combination}}{MIC \text{ of drug B alone}}$$

The fractional *bactericidal* concentration (FBC) index can be determined by substituting MBCs for MICs in the above equations. Synergism for two drug combinations requires an FIC or FBC index of ≤ 0.5. Antagonism occurs when the combined inhibitory or killing effects of two or more antimicrobials are significantly less than expected when the drugs are used individually. Antibiotic antagonism is marked by an FIC or FBC index of 4 or more.

Mechanisms of Synergistic Action

The need for synergistic combinations of antimicrobials has been clearly established for the treatment of enterococcal endocarditis. Bactericidal activity is essential for the optimal management of bacterial endocarditis. Penicillin or ampicillin in combination with gentamicin or streptomycin is superior to monotherapy with a penicillin or vancomycin. When tested alone, penicillins and vancomycin are only bacteriostatic against susceptible enterococcal isolates. When these agents are combined with an aminoglycoside, however, bactericidal activity results. The addition of gentamicin or streptomycin to penicillin allows for a reduction in the duration of therapy for selected patients with viridans streptococcal endocarditis. Likewise, the addition of gentamicin to nafcillin allows for a reduction in the duration of therapy of right-sided *Staphylococcus aureus* endocarditis in intravenous drug users. There is some evidence that synergistic combinations of antimicrobials (eg, a beta-lactam plus an aminoglycoside) may be of benefit in the treatment of gram-negative bacillary infections in febrile neutropenic cancer patients and in systemic infections caused by *Pseudomonas aeruginosa.*

Other synergistic antimicrobial combinations have been shown to be more effective than monotherapy with individual components. Trimethoprim-sulfamethoxazole has been successfully used for the treatment of bacterial infections and *Pneumocystis carinii* pneumonia. Beta-lactamase inhibitors restore the activity of intrinsically active but hydrolyzable beta-lactams against organisms such as *Staphylococcus aureus* and *Bacteroides fragilis*. Several beta-lactam–beta-lactamase inhibitor combinations (eg, ticarcillin-clavulanic acid; see Chapter 43) have been successful against a variety of bacterial infections, including polymicrobial infections.

Three major mechanisms of antimicrobial synergism have been established:

A. Blockade of Sequential Steps in a Metabolic Sequence: Trimethoprim-sulfamethoxazole is the best-known example of this mechanism of synergy (Chapter 46). Blockade of the two sequential steps in the cyclical folic acid pathway by trimethoprim-sulfamethoxazole results in a much more complete inhibition of growth than achieved by either component alone.

B. Inhibition of Enzymatic Inactivation: Enzymatic inactivation of beta-lactam antibiotics is a major mechanism of antibiotic resistance. Inhibition of beta-lactamase by beta-lactamase inhibitor drugs results in synergism.

C. Enhancement of Antimicrobial Agent Uptake: Penicillins and other cell wall-active agents can increase the uptake of aminoglycosides by a number of bacteria, including staphylococci, enterococci, streptococci, and *Pseudomonas aeruginosa*. It is thought that enterococci are intrinsically resistant to aminoglycosides because of permeability barriers. When an aminoglycoside is combined with a penicillin or glycopeptide against susceptible enterococcal isolates, bactericidal activity results. Similarly, amphotericin B is thought to enhance the uptake of flucytosine by fungi.

Mechanisms of Antagonistic Action

There are few clinically relevant examples of antagonism. The most striking example was reported in a study of patients with pneumococcal meningitis. Patients who were treated with the combination of penicillin and chlortetracycline had a mortality rate of 79% versus a mortality rate of 21% in patients who received penicillin monotherapy (illustrating the first mechanism set forth below).

The use of an antagonistic antimicrobial combination does not preclude other potential beneficial interactions. For example, rifampin may antagonize the action of antistaphylococcal penicillins or vancomycin against staphylococci. However, the aforementioned antimicrobials may prevent the emergence of resistance to rifampin.

Two major mechanisms of antimicrobial antagonism have been established:

A. Inhibition of Cidal Activity by Static Agents: Bacteriostatic agents such as tetracyclines and chloramphenicol can antagonize the action of bactericidal cell wall-active agents (eg, beta-lactam antibiotics). The bactericidal effects of cell wall-active agents require that the bacteria be actively growing and dividing. This antagonistic interaction is thought to be due to inhibition of bacterial growth by the bacteriostatic agent.

Tetracyclines and chloramphenicol have also been shown to antagonize the bactericidal effects of aminoglycosides. The mechanism may involve inhibition of aminoglycoside active transport by susceptible bacteria.

Inhibition of amphotericin B, a fungicidal agent, by the fungistatic azole and triazole antifungal agents has been demonstrated. Azole and triazole antifungal agents act by inhibiting the production of ergosterol in the fungal cell membrane. It is thought that this action prevents the formation of amphotericin B binding sites.

B. Induction of Enzymatic Inactivation: Some gram-negative bacilli, including *Enterobacter* species, *Pseudomonas aeruginosa*, *Serratia marcescens,* and *Citrobacter freundii*, possess inducible beta-lactamases. Beta-lactam antibiotics such as imipenem, cefoxitin, and ampicillin are potent inducers of beta-lactamase production. If an inducing agent is combined with an intrinsically active but hydrolyzable beta-lactam such as piperacillin, antagonism may result.

ANTIMICROBIAL PROPHYLAXIS

Antimicrobial agents are effective in preventing infections in many settings. Antimicrobial prophylaxis should be used in circumstances in which efficacy has been demonstrated and benefits outweigh the risks of prophylaxis. Antimicrobial prophylaxis may be divided into surgical prophylaxis and nonsurgical prophylaxis.

Surgical Prophylaxis

Surgical wound infections are a major category of nosocomial infections. In 1992, surgical wound infections in the USA resulted in an increase in the average length of hospital stay by 7.3 days and added an average of $3152 to each hospital bill. The total annual cost impact of surgical wound infections in the United States is $1.5 billion. In 1992, surgical wound infections directly caused 3251 deaths and contributed to an additional 9726 deaths in the USA (Surveillance, 1992).

The National Research Council (NRC) Wound Classification Criteria have served as the basis for recommending antimicrobial prophylaxis. The NRC criteria consist of four classes, as set forth in the associated box.

The Study of the Efficacy of Nosocomial Infection Control (SENIC) identified four independent risk factors for postoperative wound infections: operations on the abdomen, operations lasting more than 2 hours, contaminated or dirty wound classification, and the presence of at least three medical diagnoses. Patients with at least two SENIC risk factors who undergo clean surgical procedures are at increased risk of developing surgical wound infections and should receive antimicrobial prophylaxis.

Surgical procedures that necessitate the use of antimicrobial prophylaxis include contaminated and clean-contaminated operations, selected operations in which postoperative infection may be catastrophic such as open heart surgery, clean procedures that involve placement of prosthetic materials, and any procedure in an immunocompromised host. The operation should carry a significant risk of postoperative site infection or cause significant bacterial contamination.

General principles of antimicrobial surgical prophylaxis include the following:

(1) The antibiotic should be active against common surgical wound pathogens; unnecessarily broad coverage should be avoided.

(2) The antibiotic should have proved efficacy in clinical trials.

(3) The antibiotic must achieve concentrations greater than the MIC of suspected pathogens, and these concentrations must be present at the time of incision.

(4) The shortest possible course—ideally a single dose—of the most effective and least toxic antibiotic should be used.

(5) The newer broad-spectrum antibiotics should be reserved for therapy of resistant infections.

(6) If all other factors are equal, the least expensive agent should be used.

The proper selection and administration of antimicrobial prophylaxis is of utmost importance. Common indications for surgical prophylaxis are shown in Table 51–7. Cefazolin is the prophylactic agent of choice for head and neck, gastroduodenal, biliary tract, gynecologic, and clean procedures. Local wound infection patterns should be considered when selecting antimicrobial prophylaxis. The selection of vancomycin over cefazolin may be necessary in hospitals with high rates of methicillin-resistant *Staphylococcus aureus* or *S epidermidis* infections. The antibiotic should be present in adequate concentrations at the operative site prior to incision and throughout the procedure; initial dosing is dependent on the volume of distribution, peak levels, clearance, protein binding, and bioavailability. Parenteral agents should be administered during the interval beginning 60 minutes before incision; administration up to the time of incision is preferred. In cesarean section, the antibiotic is administered after umbilical cord clamping. If short-acting agents such as cefoxitin are used, doses should be repeated if the procedure exceeds 3–4 hours in duration. Single-dose prophylaxis is effective for most procedures and results in decreased toxicity and antimicrobial resistance.

Improper administration of antimicrobial prophylaxis leads to excessive surgical wound infection rates. Common errors in antibiotic prophylaxis include selection of the wrong antibiotic, administering the first dose too early or too late, failure to repeat doses during prolonged procedures, excessive duration of prophylaxis, and inappropriate use of broad-spectrum antibiotics.

Nonsurgical Prophylaxis

Nonsurgical prophylaxis includes the administration of antimicrobials to prevent colonization or

---

NATIONAL RESEARCH COUNCIL (NRC) WOUND CLASSIFICATION CRITERIA

Clean: Elective, primarily closed procedure; respiratory, gastrointestinal, biliary, genitourinary, or oropharyngeal tract not entered; no acute inflammation and no break in technique; expected infection rate ≤ 2%.

Clean contaminated: Urgent or emergency case that is otherwise clean; elective, controlled opening of respiratory, gastrointestinal, biliary, or oropharyngeal tract; minimal spillage or minor break in technique; expected infection rate ≤ 10%.

Contaminated: Acute nonpurulent inflammation present; major technique break or major spill from hollow organ; penetrating trauma less than 4 hours old; chronic open wounds to be grafted or covered; expected infection rate about 20%.

Dirty: Purulence or abscess present; preoperative perforation of respiratory, gastrointestinal, biliary, or oropharyngeal tract; penetrating trauma more than 4 hours old; expected infection rate about 40%.

Table 51–7. Recommendations for antimicrobial surgical prophylaxis.

Type of Operation	Common Pathogens	Drug of Choice
Cardiac (with median sternotomy)	Staphylococci, enteric gram-negative rods	Cefazolin
Noncardiac, thoracic	Staphylococci, streptococci, enteric gram-negative rods	Cefazolin
Vascular (abdominal and lower extremity)	Staphylococci, enteric gram-negative rods	Cefazolin
Neurosurgical (craniotomy)	Staphylococci	Cefazolin
Orthopedic (with hardware insertion)	Staphylococci	Cefazolin
Head and neck (with entry into the oropharynx)	S aureus, oral flora	Cefazolin
Gastroduodenal (high-risk patients[1])	S aureus, oral flora, enteric gram-negative rods	Cefazolin
Biliary tract (high-risk patients[2])	S aureus, enterococci, enteric gram-negative rods	Cefazolin
Colorectal (elective surgery)	Enteric gram-negative rods, anaerobes	Oral erythromycin plus neomycin[3]
Colorectal (emergency surgery or obstruction)	Enteric gram-negative rods, anaerobes	Cefoxitin, ceftizoxime, cefotetan, or cefmetazole
Appendectomy	Enteric gram-negative rods, anaerobes	Cefoxitin, ceftizoxime, cefotetan, or cefmetazole
Hysterectomy	Enteric gram-negative rods, anaerobes, enterococci, group B streptococci	Cefazolin
Cesarean section	Enteric gram-negative rods, anaerobes, enterococci, group B streptococci	Cefazolin[4]

[1]Gastric procedures for cancer, ulcer, bleeding, or obstruction; morbid obesity; suppression of gastric acid secretion.
[2]Age > 60, acute cholecystitis, prior biliary tract surgery, common duct stones, jaundice, or diabetes mellitus.
[3]In conjunction with mechanical bowel preparation.
[4]Administer immediately following cord clamping.

asymptomatic infection as well as the administration of drugs following colonization by or inoculation of pathogens but before the development of disease. Nonsurgical prophylaxis is indicated in individuals who are at high risk for temporary exposure to selected virulent pathogens and in patients who are at increased risk for developing infection because of underlying disease (eg, immunocompromised hosts). Prophylaxis is most effective when directed against organisms that are predictably susceptible to antimicrobial agents. Common indications for nonsurgical prophylaxis are listed in Table 51–8.

Table 51–8. Recommendations for nonsurgical antimicrobial prophylaxis.

Infection to Be Prevented	Indication(s)	Drug of Choice	Efficacy
Cholera	Close contacts of a case	Tetracycline	Proposed effective
Diphtheria	Unimmunized contacts	Penicillin or erythromycin	Proposed effective
Endocarditis	Dental, oral, or upper respiratory tract procedures[1] in at-risk patients[2]	Amoxicillin or clindamycin	Proposed effective
	Genitourinary or gastrointestinal procedures[3] in at-risk patients[2]	Ampicillin or vancomycin and gentamicin	Proposed effective
Genital herpes simplex	Recurrent infection (≥ 4 episodes per year)	Acyclovir	Excellent

Table 51–8. Recommendations for nonsurgical antimicrobial prophylaxis (cont'd).

Infection to Be Prevented	Indication(s)	Drug of Choice	Efficacy
Group B streptococcal (GBS) infection	Mothers with cervical or vaginal GBS colonization and their newborns with one or more of the following: (a) onset of labor or membrane rupture before 37 weeks' gestation, (b) prolonged rupture of membranes	Ampicillin or penicillin	Excellent
	(> 12 hours), (c) maternal intrapartum fever, (d) history of GBS bacteriuria during pregnancy. Mothers who have given birth to infants who had early GBS disease		
Haemophilus influenzae type B infection	Close contacts of a case in incompletely immunized children (< 48 months old)	Rifampin	Excellent
HIV infection	Health care workers exposed to blood after needle-stick injury. Pregnant HIV-infected women who are at ≥ 14 weeks of gestation. Newborns of HIV-infected women for the first 6 weeks of life, beginning 8–12 hours after birth	Zidovudine	Good
Influenza A	Unvaccinated geriatric patients, immunocompromised hosts, and health care workers during outbreaks	Amantadine	Good
Malaria	Travelers to areas endemic for chloroquine-susceptible disease	Chloroquine	Excellent
	Travelers to areas endemic for chloroquine-resistant disease	Mefloquine	Excellent
Meningococcal infection	Close contacts of a case	Rifampin	Excellent
Mycobacterium avium complex	HIV-infected patients with CD4 count < 75/μL	Rifabutin	Good
Otitis media	Recurrent infection	Amoxicillin	Good
Pertussis	Close contacts of a case	Erythromycin	Excellent
Plague	Close contacts of a case	Tetracycline	Proposed effective
Pneumococcemia	Children with sickle cell disease or asplenia	Penicillin	Excellent
Pneumocystis carinii pneumonia (PCP)	High-risk patients (eg AIDS, leukemia, transplant)	Trimethoprim-sulfamethoxazole	Excellent
Rheumatic fever	History of rheumatic fever or known rheumatic heart disease	Benzathine penicillin	Excellent
Toxoplasmosis	HIV-infected patients with IgG antibody to *Toxoplasma* and CD4 count < 100/μL	Trimethoprim-sulfamethoxazole	Good
Tuberculosis	Persons with positive tuberculin skin tests and ≥ one of the following: (a) HIV infection, (b) close contacts with newly diagnosed disease, (c) recent skin test conversion, (d) medical conditions that increase the risk of developing tuberculosis, (e) age < 35	Isoniazid	Excellent
Urinary tract infections (UTI)	Recurrent infection	Trimethoprim-sulfamethoxazole	Excellent

[1]Prophylaxis is recommended for the following: dental procedures known to induce gingival or mucosal bleeding, tonsillectomy or adenoidectomy, surgical procedures that involve respiratory mucosa, and rigid bronchoscopy.

[2]Risk factors include the following: prosthetic heart valves, previous bacterial endocarditis, congenital cardiac malformations, rheumatic and other acquired valvular dysfunction, hypertrophic cardiomyopathy, and mitral valve prolapse with valvular regurgitation.

[3]Prophylaxis is recommended for the following: surgical procedures that involve intestinal mucosa, sclerotherapy for esophageal varices, esophageal or urethral dilation, gallbladder surgery, cystoscopy, urethral catheterization or urinary tract surgery in the presence of UTI, prostatic surgery, incision and drainage of infected tissue, vaginal hysterectomy, and vaginal delivery in the presence of infection.

REFERENCES

Allan JD Jr: Antibiotic combinations. Med Clin North Am 1987;71:1079.

American Thoracic Society: Guidelines for the initial management of adults with community-acquired pneumonia: Diagnosis, assessment of severity, and initial antimicrobial therapy. Am Rev Respir Dis 1993;148:1418.

American Thoracic Society: Treatment of tuberculosis and tuberculosis infection in adults and children. Am J Respir Crit Care Med 1994;149:1359.

Antimicrobial prophylaxis in surgery. Med Lett Drugs Ther 1995;37:79.

ASHP therapeutic guidelines on nonsurgical antimicrobial prophylaxis. ASHP Commission on Therapeutics. Clin Pharm 1990;9:423.

Bochner BS et al: Anaphylaxis. N Engl J Med 1991;324:1785.

Classen DC et al: The timing of prophylactic administration of antibiotics and the risk of surgical-wound infection. N Engl J Med 1992;326:281.

Cunha BA: Antimicrobial therapy I. Med Clin North Am 1995;79:463.

Cunha BA: Antimicrobial therapy II. Med Clin North Am 1995;79:679.

Dajani AS et al: Prevention of bacterial endocarditis: Recommendations by the American Heart Association. JAMA 1990;264:2919.

Dellinger EP et al: Quality standard for antimicrobial prophylaxis in surgical procedures. Infect Control Hosp Epidemiol 1994;15:182.

Friedland IR et al: Management of infections caused by antibiotic-resistant *Streptococcus pneumoniae*. N Engl J Med 1994;331:377.

Hyatt JM et al: The importance of pharmacokinetic/pharmacodynamic surrogate markers to outcome: Focus on antibacterial agents. Clin Pharmacokinet 1995;28:143.

Kaye D: Antibacterial agents: Pharmacodynamics, pharmacology, new agents. Infect Dis Clin North Am 1989;3:375.

Kaye D: Antibacterial therapy: In vitro testing, pharmacodynamics, pharmacology, new agents. Infect Dis Clin North Am 1995;9:463.

Lewis DA, Reeves DS: Antibiotics at the extremes of age: Choices and constraints. J Antimicrob Chemother 1994;34(Suppl A):11.

Lorian V: *Antibiotics in Laboratory Medicine,* 3rd ed. Williams & Wilkins, 1991.

MacKenzie FM, Gould IM: The post-antibiotic effect. J Antimicrob Chemother 1993;32:519.

Mandell GL et al: *Principles and Practice of Infectious Diseases,* 4th ed. Churchill Livingstone, 1995.

Manian FA et al: Adverse antibiotic effects associated with renal insufficiency. Rev Infect Dis 1990;12:236.

Neu HC: The crisis in antimicrobial resistance. Science 1992;257:1064.

1993 Sexually Transmitted Diseases Treatment Guidelines. MMWR Morb Mortal Wkly Rep 1993;42:1.

Page CP et al: Antimicrobial prophylaxis for surgical wounds: Guidelines for clinical care. Arch Surg 1993; 128:79.

Recommendations of the U.S. Public Health Service Task Force on the use of zidovudine to reduce perinatal transmission of human immunodeficiency virus: A summary. MMWR Morb Mortal Wkly Rep 1995;43(RR-11):1.

Scheld WM et al: Nosocomial pneumonia: Pathogenesis and recent advances in diagnosis and therapy. Rev Infect Dis 1991;13(Suppl 9):S743.

Stamm WE et al: Management of urinary tract infections in adults. N Engl J Med 1993;329:1328.

Surveillance, prevention, and control of nosocomial infections. MMWR Morb Mortal Wkly Rep 1992;41:783.

USPHS/IDSA guidelines for the prevention of opportunistic infections in persons infected with human immunodeficiency virus: A summary. MMWR Morb Mortal Wkly Rep 1995;44(RR-8):1.

Wenk M et al: Serum level monitoring of antibacterial drugs: A review. Clin Pharmacokinet 1984;9:475.

Wilkowske CJ: General principles of antimicrobial therapy. Mayo Clin Proc 1991;66:931.

Wilson WR et al: Antibiotic treatment of adults with infective endocarditis due to streptococci, enterococci, staphylococci and HACEK microorganisms. JAMA 1995; 274:1706.

Zhanel GG, Craig WA: Pharmacokinetic contributions to postantibiotic effects: Focus on aminoglycosides. Clin Pharmacokinet 1994;27:377.

Zhanel GG et al: The postantibiotic effect: A review of in vitro and in vivo data. DICP, Ann Pharmacother 1991;25:153.

Basic Principles of Antiparasitic Chemotherapy

52

Ching Chung Wang, PhD

In its general scientific sense, the term "parasite" includes all of the known infectious agents such as viruses, bacteria, fungi, protozoa, and helminths. In this and the two following chapters, the term is used in a restricted sense to denote the protozoa and helminths. It has been estimated that 3 billion (3×10^9) humans suffer from parasitic infections, plus a much greater number of domestic and wild animals. Although these diseases constitute the most widespread human health problem in the world today, they have for various reasons also been the most neglected.

In theory, the parasitic infections should be relatively easy to treat because the etiologic agents are known in almost all cases. Furthermore, recent advances in cell culture techniques have made possible in vitro cultivation of many of the important parasites. These advances have not only laid to rest the traditional view that parasites somehow depend on a living host for their existence but have also enabled us to study parasites by methods similar to those employed in investigations of bacteria, including biochemistry, molecular biology, and immunologic pharmacology. However, many problems remain to be solved before effective chemotherapeutic agents will be available for all of the parasitic diseases.

Targets of Chemotherapy

A rational approach to antiparasitic chemotherapy requires comparative biochemical and physiologic investigations of host and parasite to discover differences in essential processes that will permit selective inhibition in the parasite and not in the host. One might expect that the parasite would have many deficiencies in its metabolism associated with its parasitic nature. This is true of many parasites—the oversimplified metabolic pathways are usually indispensable for survival of the parasite and thus represent points of vulnerability. However, oversimplified metabolic pathways are not the only opportunity for attack. Although the parasite lives in a metabolically luxurious environment and may become "lazy," the environment

is not entirely friendly and the parasite must have defense mechanisms in order to survive—ie, to defend itself against immunologic attack, proteolytic digestion, etc, by the host. In some instances, necessary nutrients are not supplied to the parasite from the host, though the latter can obtain the same nutrients from the diet. In this situation, the parasite will have acquired the synthetic activity needed for its survival. Finally, the great evolutionary distance between host and parasite has in some cases resulted in sufficient differences among individual enzymes or functional pathways to allow rather selective inhibition of the parasite. Thus, there can be three major types of potential targets for chemotherapy of parasitic diseases: (1) unique enzymes found only in the parasite; (2) enzymes found in both host and parasite but indispensable only for the parasite; and (3) common biochemical functions found in both parasite and host but with different pharmacologic properties. Examples of specific targets and drugs that act on them are summarized in Table 52–1. This chapter discusses antiparasitic mechanisms based upon these examples and provides background information for the drugs described in Chapters 53 and 54.

ENZYMES FOUND ONLY IN PARASITES

These enzymes would appear to be the cleanest targets for chemotherapy. Like inhibition of the enzymes involved in the synthesis of bacterial cell walls (Chapter 43), inhibition of these enzymes should have no effect on the host. Unfortunately, only a few of these enzymes have been discovered among the parasitic protozoa. Furthermore, their usefulness as chemotherapeutic targets is sometimes limited because of the development of drug resistance. Examples of important target enzymes are discussed in the following pages.

Table 52–1. Identified targets for chemotherapy in parasites.

Targets	Parasites	Inhibitors
Unique enzymes		
Enzymes for dihydropteroate synthesis	Sporozoa	Sulfones and sulfonamides
Glycolipid synthesis	African trypanosomes	None
Pyruvate ferrodoxin oxidoreductase	Anaerobic protozoa	Nitroimidazoles
Pyruvate phosphate dikinase	Anaerobic protozoa	None
Nucleoside phosphotransferase	Flagellated protozoa	Allopurinol riboside and formycin B
Trypanothione reductase	Kinetoplastida	Melarsoprol B and nifurtimox
Sterol synthesis	*Leishmania* and *Trypanosoma cruzi*	Azoles
Indispensable enzymes		
Purine phosphoribosyl transferase	Protozoa	Allopurinol
Ornithine decarboxylase	Protozoa	α-Difluoromethylornithine
Glycolytic enzymes	Kinetoplastida	Glycerol plus salicylhydroxamic acid and suramin
Common biochemical functions with different pharmacologic properties		
Thiamin transporter	Coccidia	Amprolium
Mitochondrial electron transporter	Sporozoa	4-Hydroxyquinolines and 2-hydroxy-naphthoquinones
Microtubules	Helminth	Benzimidazoles
Nervous synaptic transmission	Helminth and ectoparasite	Levamisole, piperazine, the milbe-mycins, and the avermectins

Enzymes for Dihydropteroate Synthesis

The intracellular sporozoan parasites such as *Plasmodium, Toxoplasma,* and *Eimeria* have long been known to respond to sulfonamides and sulfones. This has led to the assumption that sporozoans must synthesize their own folate in order to survive. The reaction of 2-amino-4-hydroxy-6-hydroxymethyl-dihydropteridine diphosphate with *p*-aminobenzoate to form 7,8-dihydropteroate has been demonstrated in cell-free extracts of the rodent malaria parasite *Plasmodium chabaudi.* 2-Amino-4-hydroxy-6-hydroxymethyl-dihydropteridine pyrophosphokinase and 7,8-dihydropteroate synthase have also been identified, isolated, and purified. Sulfathiazole, sulfaguanidine, and sulfanilamide act as competitive inhibitors of *p*-aminobenzoate in this reaction. It has not been possible to demonstrate dihydrofolate synthase activity in the parasites, which raises the possibility that 7,8-dihydropteroate may have substituted for dihydrofolate in malaria parasites. Similar lack of recognition of folate as substrate was also observed in the dihydrofolate reductase of *Eimeria tenella,* a parasite of chickens.

However, lack of utilization of exogenous folate may not fully explain the apparently indispensable nature of the synthesis of 7,8-dihydropteroate in *Plasmodium, Toxoplasma,* and *Eimeria.* It is known that most of the folate molecules in mammalian cells are linked with polyglutamates in the cytoplasm and are transported across cell membranes with difficulty. This additional factor may compound the problem of obtaining 7,8-dihydropteroate or dihydrofolate for the parasite and makes all of the enzymes involved in their synthesis attractive targets for antisporozoan chemotherapy.

The sulfones and sulfonamides synergize with the inhibitors of dihydrofolate reductase, and combina-tions have been effective in controlling malaria, toxoplasmosis, and coccidiosis. Although some incidents of drug resistance, especially among coccidia, have been reported, the combinations remain largely effective against malaria and toxoplasmosis. Fansidar, a combination of sulfadoxine and pyrimethamine, has been successful in controlling some strains of chloroquine-resistant *Plasmodium falciparum* malaria (see Chapter 53).

The pharmacologic properties of parasite 7,8-dihydropteroate synthases may differ from those of the bacterial enzymes. For instance, metachloridine and 2-ethoxy-*p*-aminobenzoate are both ineffective against sulfonamide-sensitive bacteria, but the former has antimalarial activity and the latter is effective against infection by the chicken parasite *Eimeria acervulina;* both activities can be reversed by *p*-aminobenzoate. Recently, the gene encoding this enzyme was cloned from *P falciparum* and found to express a bifunctional enzyme that includes dihydro-6-hydroxymethylpterin pyrophosphokinase at the amino terminal.

Pyruvate: Ferredoxin Oxidoreductase

Certain anaerobic protozoan parasites lack mitochondria and mitochondrial activities for generating ATP. They possess, instead, ferredoxin-like or flavodoxin-like low-redox-potential electron transport proteins to convert pyruvate to acetyl-CoA. In trichomonad flagellates and rumen ciliates, the process takes place in a membrane-limited organelle called the hydrogenosome. By the actions of pyruvate:ferredoxin oxidoreductase and hydrogenase in the hydrogenosome, H_2 is produced by these organisms under anaerobic conditions as the major means of electron disposition. Although *Entamoeba* species and *Giardia lamblia* have no hydrogenosome, a ferredoxin has been isolated from *Entamoeba histolytica,* and the gene encoding pyruvate:ferredoxin oxidoreductase has been isolated from *E histolytica, Trichomonas vaginalis,* and *G lamblia.*

Pyruvate:ferredoxin oxidoreductase has no counterpart in the mammalian system. In contrast to the mammalian pyruvate dehydrogenase complex, pyruvate:ferredoxin oxidoreductase is incapable of reducing pyridine nucleotides because of its low redox potential (approximately –400 mV). However, this low potential can also transfer electrons from pyruvate to the nitro groups of metronidazole and other 5-nitroimidazole derivatives to form cytotoxic reduced products that bind to DNA and proteins. This is apparently why anaerobic protozoal species are highly susceptible to drugs such as metronidazole. Despite the recent development of drug resistance in *Trichomonas vaginalis* and the possibility of carcinogenic properties (see Chapter 53), metronidazole remains the drug of choice for controlling anaerobic protozoal parasite infections.

Pyruvate Phosphate Dikinase

Glycolysis provides the main source of ATP in *E histolytica* and *G lamblia,* but the two organisms do not possess pyruvate kinase. Instead, they rely on the function of a pyruvate phosphate dikinase that is not a homolog of pyruvate kinase but is closely related to phosphoenolpyruvate (PEP) synthase from bacteria. The enzyme catalyzes conversion of PEP to pyruvate accompanied by the synthesis of ATP from AMP and pyrophosphate. Genes encoding the enzyme have been isolated from *E histolytica* and *G lamblia* and have demonstrated considerable structural divergences. No specific inhibitor of this enzyme has yet been identified.

Nucleoside Phosphotransferases

All of the protozoal parasites studied thus far are deficient in de novo synthesis of purine nucleotides. The various purine salvage pathways in these parasites are thus essential for their survival and growth. Among the *Leishmania* species, a unique salvage enzyme has been identified—purine nucleoside phosphotransferase—that can transfer the phosphate group from a variety of monophosphate esters, including *p*-nitrophenylphosphate, to the 5′ position of purine nucleosides. This enzyme also phosphorylates purine nucleoside analogs such as allopurinol riboside, formycin B, 9-deazainosine, and thiopurinol riboside, converting them to the corresponding nucleotides. These nucleotides are either further converted to triphosphates and eventually incorporated into nucleic acid of *Leishmania* or become inhibitors of other essential enzymes in purine metabolism. Consequently, allopurinol riboside, formycin B, 9-deazainosine, and thiopurinol riboside all act as potent antileishmanial agents both in vitro and in vivo. Allopurinol riboside is particularly interesting because it is remarkably nontoxic to the mammalian host.

Trichomonad flagellates appear to be deficient in de novo synthesis of both purines and pyrimidines. Pyrimidine as well as purine salvage thus becomes indispensable for these parasites. Among them, *Trichomonas foetus* (the cow parasite), *T vaginalis,* and *G lamblia* also lack dihydrofolate reductase and thymidylate synthase—a deficiency that enables them to grow normally in the presence of methotrexate, the most potent antifolate, in a concentration of 0.5 mmol/L. This metabolic deficiency leads to apparent isolation of the supply route for thymidine 5′-monophosphate (TMP) from the rest of the pyrimidine ribonucleotides; TMP is provided by a single salvage pathway that converts exogenous thymidine to TMP by the action of a thymidine phosphotransferase (Figure 52–1).

The enzyme activity is not affected by thymidine kinase inhibitors such as acyclovir but is inhibitable by guanosine or 5-fluorodeoxyuridine; both compounds also inhibit the in vitro growth of the parasites. This enzyme is an attractive target for chemotherapeutic treatment of the anaerobic protozoal parasites. One could design either a false substrate or an inhibitor of the thymidine phosphotransferase; DNA synthesis in the parasites may be arrested in either case.

Trypanothione Reductase

Protozoa with kinetoplastids are unusual in that a considerable proportion of their intracellular spermidine and glutathione is found as the unique conjugate N^1-N^8-(glutathionyl)spermidine, which has been assigned the name trypanothione. Kinetoplastids contain neither glutathione reductase nor glutathione peroxidase for maintaining intracellular thiols in the reduced state and removing hydrogen peroxide. Thus, trypanothione plays a central role in Kinetoplastida's defense mechanisms against oxidative damage, and trypanothione reductase is among the essential enzymes for the survival of these parasites. The three-dimensional structure of this enzyme has been solved (Lantwin et al, 1994). Nifurtimox, a nitrofuran derivative effective in treating Chagas' disease (caused by *Trypanosoma cruzi*), has been found to be a potent inhibitor of trypanothione reductase. Other inhibitors are under study (Krauth-Siegel et al, 1995). The antitrypanosomal trivalent arsenicals are taken up by the African trypanosome *Trypanosoma brucei* and complex with trypanothione, forming a product that is also an effective inhibitor of trypanothione reductase.

Sterol Synthesis

Leishmania and *T cruzi* have ergosterol instead of cholesterol in their plasma membrane structures. There is thus a functioning ergosterol biosynthetic pathway in these organisms performing an essential role for their growth and survival. One of the enzymes in this pathway, a cytochrome P450 catalyzing C_{14} demethylation of lanosterol, can be inhibited by a

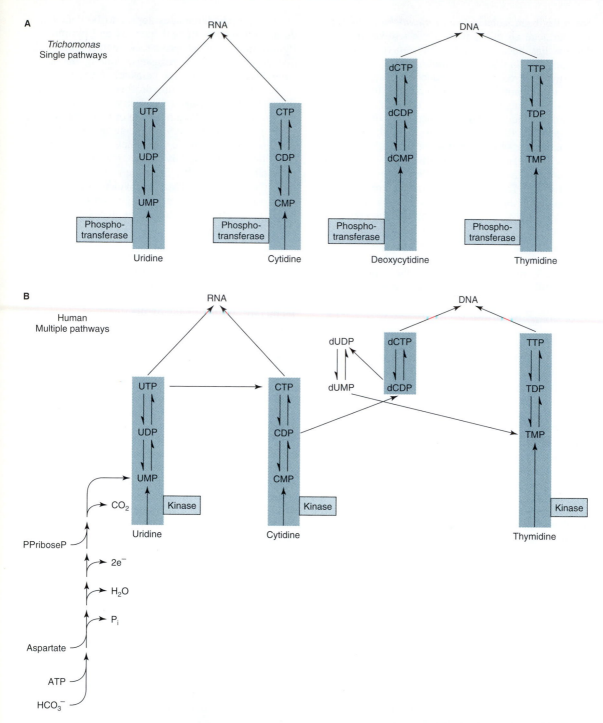

Figure 52–1. Pyrimidine metabolism in *Trichomonas vaginalis* **(A)** and in humans **(B)**. Note that humans have multiple sources for thymidine monophosphate (TMP), an essential precursor for DNA synthesis. The parasite has only one source. (UTP, UDP, UMP, CTP, etc, uridine triphosphate, diphosphate, monophosphate, cytidine triphosphate, etc; PPri-boseP, 1-pyrophosphorylribosyl-5-phosphate; P_i, inorganic phosphate.

number of azole derivatives, including ketoconazole, miconazole, and itraconazole. Some of these drugs have also demonstrated promise against leishmaniasis in recent clinical studies.

Glycolipid Synthesis

The variant surface glycoprotein on the plasma membranes of bloodstream African trypanosomes provides the organisms with the means of evading host immune responses. The glycoprotein is anchored to the cell surface by a glycosyl phosphatidylinositol that contains myristate as its only fatty acid component. Thus, the introduction of a "subversive substrate" to replace myristate from the glycolipid anchor could result in loss of the variant surface glycoprotein, which might suppress development of trypanosomes in mammalian blood. A myristate analog, 10-(propoxy)decanoic acid, was found incorporated into the glycolipid and also active against *T brucei* in in vitro tests. Further validation of this approach to antitrypanosomal chemotherapy must, however, await results of in vivo tests.

ENZYMES INDISPENSABLE ONLY IN THE PARASITES

Because of the many metabolic deficiencies among parasites, there are enzymes whose functions may be essential for the survival of parasites, but the same enzymes are not indispensable to the host—ie, the host may be able to achieve the same result through alternative pathways. This discrepancy opens up opportunities for antiparasitic chemotherapy.

Purine Phosphoribosyl Transferases

The absence of de novo purine nucleotide synthesis in protozoal parasites as well as in the trematode *Schistosoma mansoni* is reflected in the relative importance of hypoxanthine-guanine phosphoribosyl transferase in many species. Hypoxanthine is the obligatory base for purine nucleotide synthesis in *T foetus, S mansoni, G lamblia,* and perhaps other organisms as well. Unusual substrate specificity of the parasite hypoxanthine-guanine phosphoribosyl transferase has been reported. The enzymes in *Leishmania donovani* and *Trypanosoma cruzi* can recognize allopurinol (see Chapter 36) as the substrate and convert it to allopurinol ribotide, which then accumulates in the parasites and becomes aminated, turned into triphosphate, and finally incorporated into the RNA fraction. This abnormal RNA apparently does not support normal growth. Since allopurinol is an extremely poor substrate for the mammalian hypoxanthine-guanine phosphoribosyl transferase, it has selective antileishmanial and antitrypanosomal effects in vivo. Another enzyme in *L donovani,* xanthine phosphoribosyl transferase, has no counterpart in mammalian systems and thus could be another interesting enzyme target for a "subversive substrate" strategy in antileishmanial chemotherapy.

G lamblia has an exceedingly simple scheme of purine salvage. It possesses only two pivotal enzymes: the adenine and guanine phosphoribosyl transferases, which convert exogenous adenine and guanine to the corresponding nucleotides. There is no salvage of hypoxanthine, xanthine, or any purine nucleosides and no interconversion between adenine and guanine nucleotides in the parasite. Functions of the two phosphoribosyl transferases are thus both essential for the survival and development of *G lamblia* (Figure 52–2). The guanine phosphoribosyl transferase is an interesting enzyme because it does not recognize hypoxanthine, xanthine, or adenine as substrate. This substrate specificity distinguishes the *Giardia* enzyme from the mammalian enzyme, which uses hypoxanthine, and the bacterial one, which has xanthine as substrate. Design of a highly specific inhibitor of this enzyme is thus possible. The gene encoding this enzyme has been isolated from *G lamblia* and expressed. It bears little structural resemblance to human hypoxanthine-guanine phosphoribosyltransferase.

T foetus depends primarily on a single enzyme, hypoxanthine-guanine-xanthine phosphoribosyltransferase, for replenishing the needed purine nucleotides. The enzyme-encoding gene has been isolated and expressed, and the detailed structure of the enzyme was recently resolved. It bears significant distinctions in both structure and function when compared with the mammalian enzyme, thus providing an excellent opportunity for specific inhibitor design.

Ornithine Decarboxylase

Polyamines, found in almost all living organisms, are required for cellular proliferation. Ornithine decarboxylase, the enzyme that controls the formation of the polyamine putrescine in numerous eukaryotic cells, is an enzyme characterized by its striking inducibility and very short half-life. In many species of trypanosomatids, putrescine and spermidine form the major pool of polyamines, which are synthesized rapidly from ornithine. Alpha-difluoromethylornithine (DFMO), a suicide inhibitor of ornithine decarboxylase with known antitumor activities, has been found to possess good activity against African trypanosomes in infected animals. The compound is now available for clinical use and has shown good therapeutic activity against *Trypanosoma brucei gambiense* but less activity against *Trypanosoma brucei rhodesiense* infections.

DFMO depletes the intracellular polyamine pool in *T brucei,* and its activity is reversible by putrescine, as predicted by an action on ornithine decarboxylase in the parasite. However, since there is little polyamine in mammalian blood—owing to the high levels of polyamine oxidase, the DMFO effect on blood-resident trypanosomes is not reversed in vivo. Since the African

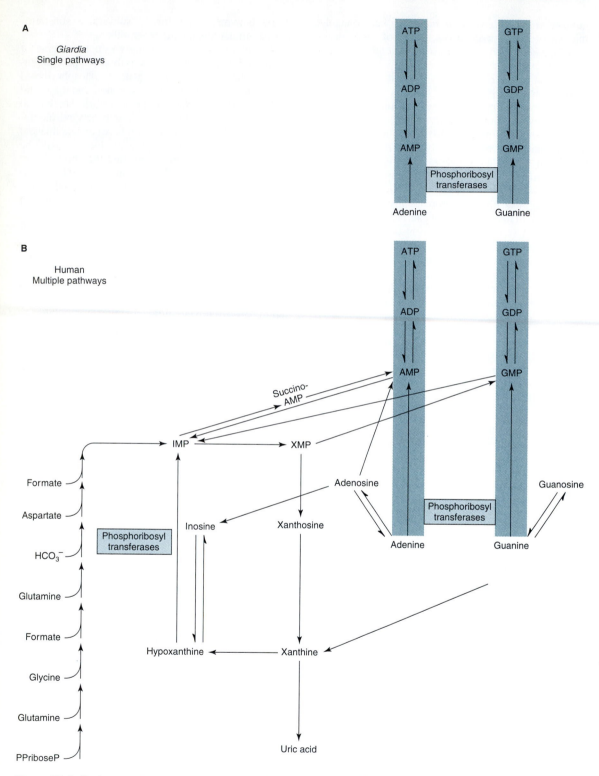

Figure 52–2. Purine metabolism in *Giardia lamblia* **(A)** and in humans **(B)**. *G lamblia* lacks enzymes both for de novo synthesis of essential purine nucleotides and for interconversion of these purine nucleotides. (AMP, GMP, IMP, XMP, etc, adenosine monophosphate, guanosine monophosphate, inosine monophosphate, xanthosine monophosphate, etc.)

trypanosome lives in the blood, DFMO is selectively toxic to it. The physiologic consequence of this action is the transformation of the "long-slender" form of *T brucei* to its nondividing "short-stumpy" form. This nondividing form is apparently incapable of changing its variant surface glycoprotein coat and can eventually be eliminated by the host immune response. In spite of its higher affinity for the mammalian form of ornithine decarboxylase, the drug is less toxic to the host because of more rapid turnover and replacement of the irreversibly inhibited enzyme in the host than in the parasite. Recent studies indicated that *T rhodesiense* ornithine decarboxylase has a much shorter half-life than that of *T gambiense,* which may explain why the former is so much more resistant to DFMO.

Glycolytic Enzymes

In the bloodstream form of African trypanosomes such as *Trypanosoma brucei brucei,* the single mitochondrion has been reduced to a "peripheral canal" lacking both cytochrome and functional Krebs cycle enzymes. The organism is entirely dependent on glycolysis for its production of ATP. Under aerobic conditions, one glucose molecule can generate only two molecules of ATP, with two pyruvate molecules excreted into the host bloodstream as the end product.

This low energy yield makes it necessary to have glycolysis in *T b brucei* proceed at an extremely high rate to enable the trypanosome to divide once every 7 hours. The high glycolytic rate, 50 times that in the mammalian host, is made possible not only by the abundant glucose supply in the host's blood but also by the clustering of most of the glycolytic enzymes of the parasite in membrane-bound microbody organelles, glycosomes (Figure 52–3). Since lactate dehydrogenase is absent from the parasite, the regeneration of NAD from NADH in the glycosome during glycolysis depends on a dihydroxyacetone phosphate:glycerol-3-phosphate shuttle plus a glycerol-3-phosphate oxidase. Thus, under anaerobic conditions, glycerol-3-phosphate cannot be oxidized back to dihydroxyacetone phosphate and accumulates inside the glycosome. This accumulation, together with the accumulation of ADP due to depletion of NAD, eventually drives the reversed glycerol kinase-catalyzed reaction in the glycosome to generate glycerol and ATP. Thus, under anaerobic conditions, *T b brucei* generates only one ATP molecule from each glucose molecule and excretes equimolar pyruvate and glycerol as end products.

This delicate and indispensable glycolytic system appears to be an attractive target for antitrypanosomal

Figure 52–3. Glycolytic pathway in long, slender bloodstream forms of *Trypanosoma brucei brucei.* The principal site of inhibition by trypanocidal drugs in vivo is indicated by the bold arrow. (SHAM, salicylhydroxamic acid; G6P, glucose 6-phosphate; F6P, fructose 6-phosphate; FDP, fructose 1,6-diphosphate; GAP, glyceraldehyde 3-phosphate; DHAP, dihydroxyacetone phosphate; GP, *sn*-glycerol 3-phosphate; DPGA, 1,3-diphosphoglycerate; 3PGA and 2PGA, 3- and 2-phosphoglycerate; PEP, phosphoenolpyruvate.) (Modified and reproduced, with permission, from Fairlamb A: Biochemistry of trypanosomiasis and rational approaches to chemotherapy. Trends Biochem Sci 1982;7:249.)

chemotherapy. It has been shown that glycerol-3-phosphate oxidase can be inhibited in the parasite with salicylhydroxamic acid (SHAM) to bring *T b brucei* into an anaerobic condition. Glycolysis can then be stopped by inhibiting the reversed glycerol kinase-catalyzed reaction with added glycerol. This SHAM plus glycerol combination can lyse the African trypanosome bloodstream forms in vitro within minutes and is very effective in suppressing parasitemia in infected animals.

The systems involved in glycosome biogenesis may also be targets for antitrypanosomal therapy. The drug suramin contains six negatively charged sulfonyl groups and has a molecular weight of 1429. These sulfonyl groups may facilitate binding of the drug to some of the basic amino acids known to be present in several essential glycosomal enzymes. This would result in binding of the enzymes before transport into the glycosome, with a resultant crippling of glycosomal function.

BIOCHEMICAL FUNCTIONS FOUND IN BOTH PARASITE & HOST BUT WITH DIFFERENT PHARMACOLOGIC PROPERTIES

In the parasite, these functions have differentiated sufficiently to become probable targets for antiparasitic chemotherapy, not because of the parasitic nature of the organism but, more likely, because of the long evolutionary distances separating the parasite and the host. It is thus difficult to discover these targets through studying metabolic deficiency or special nutritional requirements of the parasite. They have usually been found by investigating the modes of action of some well-established antiparasitic agents discovered by screening methods in the past. The target of such drugs may not be a single well-defined enzyme but may include transporters, receptors, cellular structural components, or other specific functions essential for the survival of the parasite.

Thiamin Transporter

Carbohydrate metabolism provides the main energy source in coccidia. Diets deficient in thiamin, riboflavin, or nicotinic acid—all cofactors in carbohydrate metabolism—result in suppression of parasitic infestation of chickens by *E tenella* and *E acervulina*. A thiamin analog, amprolium (1-[(4-amino-2-propyl-5-pyrimidinyl)methyl]-2-picolinium chloride), has long been used as an effective anticoccidial agent in chickens and cattle with relatively low host toxicity. The antiparasitic activity of amprolium is reversible by thiamin and is now recognized to involve inhibition of thiamin transport in the parasite. Unfortunately, amprolium has a rather narrow spectrum of antiparasitic activity; it has poor activity against toxoplasmosis, a closely related parasitic infection.

Mitochondrial Electron Transporter

Mitochondria of *E tenella* appear to lack cytochrome c and to contain cytochrome o—a cytochrome oxidase commonly found in the bacterial respiratory chain—as the terminal oxidase. Certain 4-hydroxyquinoline derivatives such as buquinolate, decoquinate, and methyl benzoquate that have long been known to be relatively nontoxic and effective anticoccidial agents have been found to act on the parasites by inhibiting mitochondrial respiration. Direct investigation on isolated intact *E tenella* mitochondria indicated that the 4-hydroxyquinolines have no effect on NADH oxidase or succinoxidase activity but that they are extremely potent inhibitors of NADH- or succinate-induced mitochondrial respiration. On the other hand, the ascorbate-induced *E tenella* mitochondrial respiration was totally insusceptible to these 4-hydroxyquinolines. The block by the anticoccidial agents thus may be located between the oxidases and cytochrome b in the electron transport chain. A certain component at this location must be essential for mediating the electron transport and would appear to be highly sensitive to the 4-hydroxyquinolines. This component must be a very specific chemotherapeutic target in *Eimeria* species, since the 4-hydroxyquinolines have no effect on chicken liver and mammalian mitochondrial respiration and no activity against any parasites other than *Eimeria*.

Many 2-hydroxynaphthoquinones have demonstrated therapeutic activities against sporozoan parasites. Parvaquinone and buparvaquinone have been developed for the treatment of theileriosis in cattle and other domestic animals. Atovaquone is now in clinical trials as an antimalarial drug and is used in the treatment of *Pneumocystis carinii* infections. The 2-hydroxynaphthoquinones are analogs of ubiquinone. The primary site of action of atovaquone in *Plasmodium* is the cytochrome bc_1 complex, where an apparent drug-binding site is present in cytochrome b. In *Plasmodium*, ubiquinone also plays an important role as an electron acceptor for dihydroorotate oxidase. Consequently, pyrimidine biosynthesis in *Plasmodium* is also inhibited by atovaquone.

Microtubules

Microtubules are an important part of the cytoskeleton and the mitotic spindle and consist of α- and β-tubulin subunit proteins. Recent comparisons of α- and β-tubulins from several species of parasitic nematodes indicated the presence of multiple isoforms with varying isoelectric points. This variation is interesting not only in pointing out the evolutionary relations among eukaryotic cells; it is useful also in classifying the tubulins in parasites as potential targets for antiparasitic chemotherapy. A group of benzimidazole derivatives have long been established as highly effective anthelmintics. Mebendazole was among the first such anthelmintics found to act primarily by blocking transport of secretory granules and movement of other subcellular organelles in the parasitic nematode *Ascaris lumbricoides.* This inhibition coincides with the disappearance of cytoplasmic microtubules from the intestinal cells of the worm. The microtubular systems of the host cells are unaffected by the treatment. Mebendazole and fenbendazole, another anthelmintic benzimidazole, have also been shown to compete with colchicine binding to *A lumbricoides* embryonic tubulins with 250–400 times higher potencies than the binding competition to bovine brain tubulins. These differential binding affinities may explain the selective toxicity of the benzimidazoles toward the parasitic nematodes.

Synaptic Transmission

Invertebrate nervous systems in the helminths and the arthropods differ from those of vertebrates in important ways. The motoneurons in invertebrates, for example, are unmyelinated and are thus more susceptible to disturbances of nerve membranes than are the myelinated somatic motor fibers of vertebrates. Muscle fibers in arthropods are innervated by excitatory synapses, in which L-glutamic acid is the neurotransmitter, and by inhibitory nerves, which have γ-aminobutyric acid (GABA) as transmitter. Cholinergic nerves are concentrated in the central nervous system of arthropods. In nematodes, free-living species, eg, *C elegans,* and gastrointestinal parasitic species, eg, *A lumbricoides,* appear to have identical neuronal systems and synaptic transmission. Cholinergic excitatory and GABAergic inhibitory synapses are found at the neuromuscular junctions as well as in the central ventral cords of the worms. The mammalian hosts, on the other hand, have mainly nicotinic receptors at the neuromuscular junctions (see Chapter 6), and the GABA nerves are primarily confined within the central nervous system protected by the blood-brain barrier (Chapter 21).

Neurotoxicant anthelmintics must be administered systemically to mammalian hosts to reach the parasitic nematodes. Therefore, if absorbed, they must be nontoxic to the nervous system of the host. Furthermore, they must penetrate the thick cuticle of the nematodes in order to be effective. It is therefore difficult to find a useful anthelmintic that acts on the nervous system of these parasites. Nevertheless, the majority of presently available anthelmintics do act on the nerves of the nematodes. They can be classified into three groups: (1) those acting as ganglionic nicotinic acetylcholine agonists; (2) those acting directly or indirectly as GABA agonists; and (3) those acting on the chloride ion channel. The first category includes levamisole, pyrantel pamoate, oxantel pamoate, and bephenium. The acetylcholine receptors at the neuromuscular junctions of nematodes are of the ganglionic nicotinic type; these agonists are quite effective in causing muscular contraction of the worms. Experimentally, the ganglionic nicotinic antagonist mecamylamine can reverse the action of these anthelmintics.

The second category consists of only one drug, piperazine, an older agent that apparently acts as a GABA agonist at the neuromuscular junction and causes flaccid paralysis of the nematode.

The third category consists of a family of natural compounds, the milbemycins and avermectins. They act on the ventral cord interneuron and on the motoneuron junction of arthropods to cause paralysis by facilitating the opening of the chloride ion channel (Fritz et al, 1979). Therefore, both the milbemycins and the avermectins are potent anthelmintics, insecticides, and antiectoparasitic agents with no cross-resistance problems with agents acting on the cholinergic systems. Picrotoxin, a specific blocker of the chloride ion channel, can reverse all of the physiologic effects of these drugs (see Chapter 21).

Ivermectin, a simple derivative of the mixture of avermectin B_{1a} and avermectin B_{1b}, is highly effective as an anthelmintic in domestic animals. It is also effective in controlling onchocerciasis by eliminating the microfilariae. It is currently in wide clinical use in West Africa. Avermectins have little effect on the mammalian central nervous system because they do not cross the blood-brain barrier readily. However, when isolated mammalian brain synaptosomes and synaptic membranes are used as models for investigation, specific high-affinity binding sites for the avermectins can be identified in GABAergic nerves. This drug binding stimulates GABA release from the presynaptic end of the GABA nerve and enhances the postsynaptic GABA binding. Avermectins also stimulate benzodiazepine binding to its receptor and enhance diazepam muscle relaxant activity in vivo. There is little doubt that milbemycins and avermectins act on chloride channels associated with GABA receptors and amplify GABA functions in the mammalian central nervous system. In the free-living nematode, *Caenorhabditis elegans,* however, avermectin was found to interact with glutamate-gated chloride ion channels. The complementary DNA encoding an avermectin-sensitive, glutamate-gated chloride channel was recently identified and isolated. This channel may be an attractive target for future studies of antinematode chemotherapy.

Little is known about the nervous systems of cestodes and trematodes except that they probably differ from those of nematodes, since milbemycins and avermectins have no effect on them. However, a highly effective antischistosomal and antitapeworm agent, praziquantel (see Chapter 54), is known to enhance Ca^{2+} influx and induce muscular contraction in those parasites, though it exerts no action on nematodes or insects. Some benzodiazepine derivatives have activities similar to those of praziquantel; these activities are unrelated to the anxiolytic activities in the mammalian central nervous system. The nerves and muscles in schistosomes and tapeworms are thus interesting subjects for future chemotherapeutic studies.

Table 52–2. Some major antiparasitic agents with undefined mechanisms of action.

Antiparasitic Agents	Possibly Relevant Biochemical Activities
Antiamebiasis agents	
Diloxanide furoate	Unknown
Emetine	Inhibitor of eukaryote protein synthesis
Halogenated hydroxyquinolines	Unknown
Paromomycin	Inhibitor of prokaryote protein synthesis
Antifascioliasis agents	
Bithionol	Oxidative phosphorylation uncoupler
Rafoxanide	Oxidative phosphorylation uncoupler
Antifilariasis agent	
Diethylcarbamazine	Inhibitor of lipoxygenase
Antileishmaniasis agents	
Amphotericin B	Voltage-dependent channel maker in cell membrane
Pentavalent antimonials	Unknown
Antimalarials	
Chloroquine	DNA binding, lysosomal neutralization, and hematoporphyrin binding
Primaquine	Its quinoline quinone metabolite is an oxidant
Quinacrine	DNA binding and flavoenzyme inhibition
Quinine	DNA binding and membrane binding
Antischistosomal agents	
Praziquantel	Opening of Ca^{2+} channels
Hycanthone	DNA binding
Metrifonate	Acetylcholinesterase inhibition
Niridazole	Metabolites binding to DNA
Oxamniquine	DNA binding
Trivalent antimonials	Inhibition of phosphofructo-kinase
Antitapeworm agent	
Niclosamide	Oxidative phosphorylation uncoupler
Antitrypanosomiasis agents	
Melarsen oxide	Inhibitor of trypanothione reductase
Aromatic diamidines	Transport can be blocked by polyamines; DNA binding

Drugs for Which the Mechanism Has Not Been Identified

In spite of considerable progress in defining the mechanisms of action of the drugs described above, there are still wide gaps in our understanding of a number of other important antiparasitic agents. These include the compounds presented in Table 52–2. From the biochemical activities that have been identified for them, it appears that many are capable of binding DNA, and some can uncouple oxidative phosphorylation in mammals. These types of activity, which are toxic to the host but could also be involved in the antiparasitic action, may have been preferentially detectable in random screens used for antiparasitic agents in the past.

REFERENCES

Bacchi CJ et al: In vivo effects of α-DL-difluoromethylornithine on the metabolism and morphology of Trypanosoma brucei. Mol Biochem Parasitol 1983;7:209.

Blair KL, Bennett JL, Pax RA: Praziquantel: Physiological evidence for its site(s) of action in magnesium-paralysed Schistosoma mansoni. Parasitology 1992;104(Part 1):59.

Borgers M et al: Influence of the anthelmintic mebendazole on microtubules and intracellular organelle movement in nematode intestinal cells. Am J Vet Res 1975;36:1153.

Bruchhaus I, Tannich E: Primary structure of the pyruvate phosphate dikinase in Entamoeba histolytica. Mol Biochem Parasitol 1993;62:153.

Chin MS, Wang CC: Isolation, sequencing, and expression of the gene encoding hypoxanthine-guanine-xanthine phosphoribosyltransferase of Tritrichomonas foetus. Mol Biochem Parasitol 1994;63:221.

Clarkson AB, Brohn FH: Trypanosomiasis: An approach to chemotherapy by the inhibition of carbohydrate metabolism. Science 1976;194:204.

Del Castillo J, de Mello WC, Morales T: Inhibitory action of γ-aminobutyric acid (GABA) on Ascaris muscle. Experientia 1964;20:141.

Doering TL et al: An analog of myristic acid with selective toxicity for African trypanosomes. Science 1991; 252:1851.

Driscoll M et al: Genetic and molecular analysis of a Caenorhabditis elegans β-tubulin that conveys benzimidazole sensitivity. J Cell Biol 1989;109:2993.

Eads JC et al: The crystal structure of human hypoxanthine-guanine phosphoribosyltransferase with bound GMP. Cell 1994;78:325.

Ellis JE: Coenzyme Q homologs in parasitic protozoa as targets for chemotherapeutic attack. Parasitol Today 1994;10:296.

Fairlamb AH, Henderson GB, Cerami A: Trypanothione is the primary target for arsenical drugs against African trypanosomes. Natl Acad Sci Proc U S A 1989;86:2607.

Ferguson MAJ, Gross GAM: Myristylation of the membrane form of a *Trypanosoma brucei* variant surface glycoprotein. J Biol Chem 1984;259:3011.

Friedman PA, Platzer EG: Interaction of anthelmintic benzimidazoles with *Ascaris suum* embryonic tubulin. Biochim Biophys Acta 1980;630:271.

Fritz LC, Wang CC, Gorio A: Avermectin B_{1a} irreversibly blocks post-synaptic potentials at the lobster neuromuscular junction by reducing muscle membrane resistance. Proc Natl Acad Sci USA 1979;76:2062.

Fry M, Pudney M: Site of action of the antimalarial hydroxynaphthoquinone, 2-[*trans*-4-(chlorophenyl)cyclohexyl]-3-hydroxy-1,4-naphthoquinone (566C80). Biochem Pharmacol 1992;43:1545.

Haughan PA, Goad LJ: Lipid biochemistry of trypanosomatids. In: *Biochemical Protozoology.* Coombs G, North M (editors). Taylor & Francis, 1991.

Hrdý I, Müller M: Primary structure and eubacterial relationships of the pyruvate:ferredoxin oxidoreductase of the amitochondriate eukaryote *Trichomonas vaginalis.* J Mol Evol 1995;41:388.

Hrdý I, Mertens E, Nohynkova E: *Giardia intestinalis:* Detection and characterization of a pyruvate phosphate dikinase. Exp Parasitol 1993;76:438.

Johnson PJ et al: Molecular analysis of the hydrogenosomal ferredoxin of the anaerobic protist *Trichomonas vaginalis.* Natl Acad Sci Proc USA 1990;87:6097.

Kass IS et al: Avermectin B_{1a}, a paralyzing anthelmintic that affects interneurons and inhibitory motor neurons in *Ascaris.* Proc Natl Acad Sci USA 1980;77:6211.

Kohler P, Davies KP, Zahner H: Activity, mechanism of action and pharmacokinetics of 2-*tert*-butylbenzothiazole and CGP 6140 (amocarzine) antifilarial drugs. Acta Trop 1992;51:195.

Krauth-Siegel RL, Schöneck R: Trypanothione reductase and lipoamide dehydrogenase as targets for a structure-based drug design. FASEB J 1995;9:1138.

Lantwin CB et al: The structure of *Trypanosoma cruzei* trypanothione reductase in the oxidized and NADPH reduced state. Proteins 1994;18:161.

Linder E, Thors C: *Schistosoma mansoni:* Praziquantel-induced tegumental lesion exposes actin of surface spines and allows binding of actin depolymerizing factor, gelsolin. Parasitology 1992;105:71.

Marr JJ, Berens RL: Pyrazolopyrimidine metabolism in the pathogenic Trypanosomatidae. Mol Biochem Parasitol 1983;7:339.

Martin RJ, Pennington AJ: A patch-clamp study of effects of dihydroavermectin on *Ascaris* muscle. Br J Pharmacol 1989;98:747.

McCann PP, Pegg AE: Ornithine decarboxylase as an enzyme target for therapy. Pharmacol Ther 1992;54:195.

Müller M: Hydrogenosomes. Symp Soc Gen Microbiol 1980;30:127.

Navin TR et al: Placebo-controlled clinical trial of sodium stibogluconate (Pentostam) versus ketoconazole for treating cutaneous leishmaniasis in Guatemala. J Infect Dis 1992;165:528.

Nevalainen L, Hrdý I, Müller M: Sequence of a *Giardia lamblia* gene coding for the glycolytic enzyme, pyruvate phosphate dikinase. Mol Biochem Parasitol 1996;77:217.

Osinga KA et al: Topogenesis of microbody enzymes: A sequence comparison of the genes for the glycosomal (microbody) and cytosolic phosphoglycerate kinases of *Trypanosoma brucei.* EMBO J 1985;4:3811.

Pax R, Bennett JL, Fetterer R: A benzodiazepine derivative and praziquantel: Effects on musculature of *Schistosoma mansoni* and *Schistosoma japonicum.* Naunyn Schmiedebergs Arch Pharmacol 1978;304:309.

Phillips MA, Coffino P, Wang CC: Cloning and sequencing of the ornithine decarboxylase gene from *Trypanosoma brucei.* Implications for enzyme turnover and selective difluoromethylornithine inhibition. J Biol Chem 1987; 262:8721.

Poulin R et al: Mechanism of the irreversible inactivation of mouse ornithine decarboxylase by α-difluoromethylornithine: Characterization of sequences at the inhibitor and coenzyme binding sites. J Biol Chem 1992;267:150.

Rodigues MA et al: Cloning and characterization of the *Entamoeba histolytica* pyruvate:ferredoxin oxidoreductase gene. Mol Biochem Parasitol 1996;78:273.

Schofield PJ, Edwards MR, Krantz P: Glucose metabolism in *Giardia lamblia.* Mol Biochem Parasitol 1991;45:39.

Sommer JM, Ma H, Wang CC: Cloning, expression, and characterization of an unusual guanine phosphoribosyltransferase from *Giardia lamblia.* Mol Biochem Parasitol 1996;78:185.

Somoza JR et al: The crystal structure of the hypoxanthine-guanine-xanthine phosphoribosyltransferase from the protozoan parasite *Tritrichomonas foetus.* Biochemistry 1996;35:7032.

Tang L, Pritchard RK: Characterization of tubulin from *Brugia malayi* and *Brugia pahangi.* Mol Biochem Parasitol 1989;32:145.

Triglia T, Cowman AF: Primary structure and expression of the dihydropteroate synthetase gene of *Plasmodium falciparum.* Proc Natl Acad Sci U S A 1994;91:7149.

Visser N, Opperdoes FR, Borst P: Subcellular compartmentation of glycolytic intermediates in *Trypanosoma brucei.* Eur J Biochem 1981;118:521.

Wang CC, Aldritt SP: Purine salvage networks in *Giardia lamblia.* J Exp Med 1983;158:1703.

Wang CC, Pong SS: Actions of avermectin B_{1a} on GABA nerves. In: *Membranes and Genetic Disease: Progress in Clinical and Biological Research,* vol 97. Sheppard JR, Anderson VE, Eaton JW (editors). AR Liss, 1982.

Wang CC: A novel suicide inhibitor strategy for antiparasitic drug development. J Cell Biochem 1991;45:49.

Wang CC: Biochemistry and physiology of coccidia. In: *The Biology of the Coccidia.* Long PL (editor). University Park Press, 1982.

Wang CC: Molecular mechanisms and therapeutic approaches to the treatment of African trypanosomiasis. Annu Rev Pharmacol Toxicol 1995;35:93.

53

Antiprotozoal Drugs

Robert S. Goldsmith, MD, DTM&H

TREATMENT OF MALARIA

Four species of *Plasmodium* are responsible for human malaria: *Plasmodium vivax, Plasmodium malariae, Plasmodium ovale,* and *Plasmodium falciparum.* Although all may cause severe illness, *P falciparum* causes most of the serious complications and deaths. The effectiveness of antimalarial agents varies between parasite species and between stages in their life cycles. In addition, parasite resistance to these drugs is an important therapeutic problem.

PARASITE LIFE CYCLE

The mosquito becomes infected by taking human blood that contains parasites in the sexual form. The sporozoites that develop in the mosquito are then inoculated into humans at its next feeding. In the first stage of development in humans, the **exoerythrocytic stage,** the sporozoites multiply in the liver to form tissue schizonts. Later, the parasites escape from the liver into the bloodstream as **merozoites** to initiate the **erythrocytic stage.** In this stage they invade red blood cells, multiply in them to form **blood schizonts,** and finally rupture the cells, releasing a new crop of merozoites. This cycle may be repeated many times. Meanwhile, the **gametocytes** (the sexual stage) form and are released into the circulation, where they may be taken in by another mosquito.

P falciparum and *P malariae* have only one cycle of liver cell invasion and multiplication, and liver infection ceases spontaneously in less than 4 weeks. Thereafter, multiplication is confined to the red blood cells. Thus, treatment that eliminates these species from the red blood cells 4 or more weeks after inoculation of the sporozoites will cure these infections.

In *P vivax* and *P ovale* infections, sporozoites also induce in hepatic cells the dormant stage (the **hypno-** zoite) that causes subsequent recurrences (**relapses**) of the infection. Therefore, treatment that eradicates parasites from both the red cells and the liver is required to cure these infections.

DRUG CLASSIFICATION

Some major antimalarial drugs are shown by chemical group in Figure 53–1. Others include **antibiotics** (tetracycline, doxycycline), halofantrine, and qinghaosu* and its derivatives. Drug combinations used to treat malaria include Fansidar (pyrimethamine plus sulfadoxine) and Maloprim* (pyrimethamine plus dapsone).

The antimalarial drugs can also be classified by their selective actions on different phases of the parasite's life cycle. Drugs that eliminate developing tissue schizonts or latent hypnozoites in the liver (eg, primaquine) are called **tissue schizonticides.** Those that act on blood schizonts are **blood schizonticides** or **suppressive agents** (eg, chloroquine, amodiaquine, proguanil, pyrimethamine, mefloquine, quinine). **Gametocides** are drugs that prevent infection in mosquitoes by destroying gametocytes in the blood (eg, primaquine for *P falciparum* and chloroquine for *P vivax, P malariae,* and *P ovale.*) **Sporonticidal agents** are drugs that render gametocytes noninfective in the mosquito (eg, pyrimethamine, proguanil).

None of these drugs prevent infection (ie, none are true **causal prophylactic drugs**) except for the antifols (pyrimethamine and proguanil), which prevent maturation of the early *P falciparum* hepatic schizonts. However, blood schizonticides do destroy circulating plasmodia, which prevents attacks and, when used for sufficient time (4 weeks), cures *P falciparum*

---

*Not available in the USA.

Figure 53–1. Structural formulas of antimalarial drugs.

and *P malariae* malaria. Primaquine destroys the persisting liver hypnozoites of *P vivax* and *P ovale* and, when given with a blood schizonticide, effects **radical cure** of these infections.

CHEMOPROPHYLAXIS & TREATMENT

Table 53–1 sets forth dosages and regimens for malaria chemoprophylaxis. Table 53–2 outlines treatment, including methods for dealing with infections with *P falciparum* strains resistant to chloroquine. When patients are advised on use of drugs for chemoprophylaxis, they should also be taught methods for preventing mosquito bites.

Individuals who may be exposed to malaria and for whom medical treatment will not be readily available are advised to carry medication for self-treatment if they develop fever or flu-like symptoms. However, *it is imperative that medical follow-up be sought promptly.* Patients should be given written instructions. The choice among available drugs depends on the anticipated exposure to drug-resistant *P falciparum* (see individual drugs regarding geographic distribution of resistance and Table 53–2 for dosages): (1) chloroquine (for 2 days) for persons taking no prophylaxis in chloroquine-sensitive areas, (2) Fansidar (three tablets once only), and (3) quinine plus tetracycline for 7 days (this duration of quinine is toxic for some patients). Mefloquine and halofantrine are not recommended because of their potential for severe toxicity.

Table 53–1. Prevention of malaria in travelers.[1]

TO PREVENT ATTACKS OF ALL FORMS OF MALARIA AND TO ERADICATE *P FALCIPARUM* AND *P MALARIAE* INFECTIONS[2,3,4]

REGIONS WITH CHLOROQUINE-SENSITIVE *P FALCIPARUM* MALARIA: Central America west of the Panama Canal, the Caribbean, North Africa, and parts of the Middle East
Chloroquine[5]
  Dose: Chloroquine phosphate, 500 mg salt (300 mg base). Give a single dose of chloroquine weekly starting 1 week before entering the endemic area, while there, and for 4 weeks after leaving.
REGIONS WITH CHLOROQUINE-RESISTANT *P FALCIPARUM* MALARIA: All other regions of the world; the frequency and intensity of resistance vary by region.
Mefloquine (preferred method)[6]
  Dose: one 250-mg tablet salt (228 mg base). Give a single dose of mefloquine weekly starting 1 week before entering the endemic area, while there, and for 4 weeks after leaving.
Doxycycline (alternative method)[7]
  Dose: 100 mg daily. Give the daily dose for 2 days before entering the endemic area, while there, and for 4 weeks after leaving.
Chloroquine[5] combined with proguanil[5,8] (second alternative method)
  Dose:
    Chloroquine, weekly at the above schedule.
    Proguanil, 200 mg daily while in the endemic area and for 4 weeks after leaving.

TO ERADICATE *P VIVAX* AND *P OVALE* INFECTIONS[2]

Primaquine[9]
  Primaquine is indicated only for persons who have had a high probability of exposure to *P vivax* or *P ovale* (see text). Start primaquine only after returning home, during the last 2 weeks of chemoprophylaxis. Dose: 26.3 mg salt (15 mg base) daily for 14 days.

---

[1]See text for additional information on drug cautions, contraindications, and side effects. For additional information on prophylaxis for specific countries, see the references or call the Centers for Disease Control and Prevention (CDC), Atlanta, GA (404–332–4559; fax 404–332–4565).

[2]The blood schizonticides (chloroquine, mefloquine, and doxycycline), when taken for 4 weeks after leaving the endemic area, are curative for sensitive *P falciparum* and *P malariae* infections; primaquine, however, is needed to eradicate the persistent liver stages of *P vivax* and *P ovale.* Give the drug with meals.

[3]Chloroquine, mefloquine, and doxycycline should be tested about 2 weeks before leaving home. This allows for changing to an alternative drug in the event of significant side effects.

[4]See text for standby drugs for emergency self-treatment of presumptive malaria; such drugs should be used only when a physician is not immediately available. It is imperative, however, that medical follow-up be sought promptly.

[5]Chloroquine and proguanil can be used by pregnant women.

[6]Because of the high frequency of resistance, mefloquine should not be used in Thailand or adjacent countries; it is now the preferred drug for sub-Saharan Africa. Mefloquine is not recommended in the first trimester of pregnancy or under some other conditions (see text).

[7]Doxycycline is used in Thailand and adjacent countries and in other regions by persons who cannot tolerate mefloquine. It is contraindicated in pregnant women. Take with evening meals. See text for side effects.

[8]The combination can be used in countries with a low frequency of chloroquine-resistant falciparum malaria such as southern Asia (not Bangladesh) and parts of the Middle East. Proguanil is not available in the USA but can be purchased in other countries.

[9]Before taking primaquine, patients should be screened to detect glucose-6-phosphate dehydrogenase deficiency. Primaquine is contraindicated in pregnancy. An alternative regimen in regions where chloroquine is effective in prophylaxis is chloroquine phosphate, 500 mg (salt), plus primaquine phosphate, 78.9 mg (salt), weekly for 8 weeks.

Table 53–2. Treatment of malaria in nonimmune adult populations.

Treatment[1] of Infection With All Species (Except Chloroquine-Resistant *P falciparum*)	*Treatment*[1] of Infection With Chloroquine-Resistant *P falciparum* Strains
Oral treatment of *P falciparum*[2] or *P malariae* infection Chloroquine phosphate, 1 g (salt)[3,4] as initial dose, then 0.5 g at 6, 24, and 48 hours. **Oral treatment of *P vivax* or *P ovale* infection** Chloroquine[3,4] as above followed by 0.5 g on days 10 and 17 plus primaquine phosphate, 26.3 mg (salt)[5] daily for 14 days starting about day 4. **Parenteral treatment of severe attacks** Quinine dihydrochloride[6] or quinidine gluconate.[7] Start oral chloroquine therapy as soon as possible; follow with primaquine if the infection is due to *P vivax* or *P ovale.* **or** Chloroquine hydrochloride IM;[13] repeat every 6 hours. Start oral therapy as soon as possible; follow with primaquine if infection is due to *P vivax* or *P ovale.*	**Oral treatment** Quinine sulfate, 10 mg/kg 3 times daily for 3–7 days,[8] plus one of the following: (1) doxycycline,[9] 100 mg twice daily for 7 days, or clindamycin,[9] 900 mg 3 times daily for 3 days; (2) pyrimethamine, 25 mg twice daily for 3 days, and sulfadiazine, 500 mg 4 times daily for 5 days; (3) tetracycline,[9] 250–500 mg 4 times daily for 7 days; (4) once only, pyrimethamine, 75 mg, and sulfadoxine, 1500 mg (= 3 tablets of Fansidar[10]). **or** Mefloquine,[11] 1250 mg (salt) once or 750 mg followed after 6–8 hours by 500 mg. **or** Halofantrine[12] **Parenteral treatment of severe attacks** Quinine dihydrochloride[6] or quinidine gluconate[7] plus intravenous doxycycline or clindamycin. Start oral therapy with quinine sulfate plus the second drug as soon as possible to complete 7 days of treatment.

[1]See text for cautions, contraindications, and side effects of each drug. For advice on management, call the Centers for Disease Control and Prevention (CDC), Atlanta, GA (770-488-7760).

[2]In falciparum malaria, if the patient has not shown a clinical response to chloroquine (48–72 hours for mild infections, 24 hours for severe ones), parasitic resistance to chloroquine should be considered. Chloroquine should be stopped and oral quinine plus doxycycline, or mefloquine, or halofantrine started.

[3]500 mg chloroquine phosphate = 300 mg base.

[4]Chloroquine alone is curative for infection with sensitive strains of *P falciparum* and for *P malariae,* but primaquine is needed to eradicate the persistent liver stages of *P vivax* and *P ovale.* Start primaquine after the patient has recovered from the acute illness; continue chloroquine weekly during primaquine therapy. Patients should be screened for glucose-6-phosphate dehydrogenase deficiency before use of primaquine. An alternative mode for primaquine therapy is combined primaquine, 78.9 mg (salt), and chloroquine, 0.5 g (salt), weekly for 8 weeks.

[5]26.3 mg of primaquine phosphate = 15 mg primaquine base.

[6]Quinine dihydrochloride. Give 10 mg/kg (salt) in 500 mL of 5% glucose solution IV slowly over 4 hours; repeat every 8 hours until oral therapy is possible (maximum, 1800 mg/d). Blood pressure and ECG should be monitored constantly to detect arrhythmias or hypotension. As severe hypoglycemia may occur, blood glucose levels should be monitored. A higher initial loading dose of quinine is given (20 mg/kg) to patients who acquired infections in Southeast Asia if it is known with certainty that they have not already taken the medication. Extreme caution is required in treating patients with quinine who

previously have been taking mefloquine in prophylaxis. In the USA, quinine dihydrochloride is no longer available.

[7]When parenteral quinine is unavailable (as in the USA), quinidine gluconate can be used, administered as a continuous infusion. A loading dose of 10 mg/kg (salt) (maximum, 600 mg) is diluted in 300 mL of normal saline and administered over 1–2 hours, followed by 0.02 mg/kg/min (maximum, 10 mg/kg every 8 hours) by continuous infusion until oral quinine therapy is possible. If more than 48 hours of parenteral treatment is required, some authorities reduce the quinidine dose by one-third to one-half. Fluid status, blood pressure, and ECG should be closely monitored; excessive widening of the QRS interval or lengthening of the QT interval requires discontinuation.

[8]Although quinine sulfate is usually given for 3 days, it should be continued for 7 days in patients who acquired infections in Southeast Asia and South America, where diminished responsiveness to quinine has been noted.

[9]Contraindicated in pregnant women.

[10]Fansidar should not be used for infections acquired in Southeast Asia or the Amazon Basin.

[11]Serious side effects are rare. See text for cautions and contraindications. Mefloquine is hazardous with quinine, quinidine, or halofantrine.

[12]The dosage is 500 mg (salt) every 6 hours for three doses and repeat in 1 week. Possible contraindication is presence of cardiac conduction abnormalities; do not use if mefloquine has been taken in prevous 2–3 weeks. Although halofantrine is approved for use in the USA, it has not been marketed.

[13]To avoid potential severe toxicity, give parenteral chloroquine by low-dose intramuscular injection (maximum, 3.5 mg/kg [salt] every 6 hours).

The rest of this section presents pharmacologic information for selected antimalarial drugs; for further details, see the references. To receive advice in the USA on management of acute attacks of malaria, call the Malarial Branch, CDC, Atlanta (770-488-7760). For recorded information on prophylaxis, call 404-332-4559; fax 404-332-4565. General information for travelers may be downloaded from the CDC World Wide Web page at www.cdc.gov/travel/travel.html.

CHLOROQUINE

Chemistry & Pharmacokinetics

Chloroquine is a synthetic 4-aminoquinoline (Figure 53–1) formulated as the phosphate salt for oral use and as the hydrochloride for parenteral use. It is rapidly and almost completely absorbed from the gastrointestinal tract, reaches maximum plasma concentrations (50–65% protein-bound) in about 3 hours, and is rapidly distributed to the tissues. Because it is concentrated in the tissues, it has a very large apparent volume of distribution of about 13,000 L. From these sites it is slowly released and metabolized. The drug readily crosses the placenta. It is excreted in the urine with a half-life of 3–5 days. Renal excretion is increased by acidification of the urine.

Because of its very large volume of distribution, a loading dose must be given when an effective schizonticidal plasma level of chloroquine is urgently needed in the treatment of acute attacks. To avoid life-threatening toxicity when chloroquine is given parenterally, it should be provided by slow intravenous infusion or by small incremental doses intramuscularly. The therapeutically effective plasma concentration appears to be approximately 30 μg/L against sensitive *P falciparum* and 15 μg/L against *P vivax*.

Antimalarial & Pharmacologic Actions & Resistance

A. Antimalarial Action: Chloroquine is a highly effective blood schizonticide and is the 4-aminoquinoline most widely used in chemoprophylaxis and in treatment of attacks of vivax, ovale, malariae, or sensitive falciparum malaria. It is also moderately effective against gametocytes of *P vivax, P ovale,* and *P malariae* but not against those of *P falciparum.* Chloroquine is not active against the preerythrocytic plasmodium and does not effect radical cures of *P vivax* or *P ovale* infections because it does not eliminate the persisting liver stages of those parasites.

B. Mechanism of Antimalarial Action: The exact mechanism of antimalarial action has not been determined. Chloroquine may act by blocking the enzymatic synthesis of DNA and RNA in both mammalian and protozoal cells and forming a complex with DNA that prevents replication or transcription to RNA. Within the parasite, the drug concentrates in vacuoles and raises the pH of these organelles, interfering with the parasite's ability to metabolize and utilize erythrocyte hemoglobin. Interference with phospholipid metabolism within the parasite has also been proposed. Selective toxicity for malarial parasites depends on a chloroquine-concentrating mechanism in parasitized cells. Chloroquine's concentration in normal erythrocytes is 10–20 times that in plasma; in parasitized erythrocytes, its concentration is about 25 times that in normal erythrocytes.

C. Resistance: Chloroquine-resistant strains of *P falciparum* are now reported from all areas of the world except North America north and west of the Panama Canal, North Africa (including Egypt), and parts of the Middle East. Instances of *P vivax* schizont resistance to chloroquine have been reported from Papua New Guinea and Irian Jaya. Resistance of *P ovale* and *P malariae* to chloroquine has not been observed. Chloroquine-resistant parasites appear to expel chloroquine via a membrane P-glycoprotein pump

similar to that described for multidrug-resistant cancer cells. The pump can be inhibited and resistance reversed (in vitro) by several drugs, including verapamil and desipramine.

D. Pharmacologic Actions: Although chloroquine (and hydroxychloroquine) have anti-inflammatory activity, the mechanism of action in autoimmune disorders is unknown.

Clinical Uses (Tables 53–1, 53–2, 53–3)

A. Acute Malaria Attacks: Chloroquine usually terminates the fever (in 24–48 hours) and clears the parasitemia (in 48–72 hours) of acute attacks of *P vivax, P ovale,* and *P malariae* malaria and of malaria due to nonresistant strains of *P falciparum.* Parenteral treatment should be given if vomiting prevents retention of oral medication, if the peripheral asexual parasitemia is more than 5%, or if there are findings of cerebral malaria. To cure vivax and ovale malaria, primaquine must be given concurrently with chloroquine to eradicate the persistent liver stages. Hydroxychloroquine, a derivative of chloroquine, is almost identical in its properties and can be used if chloroquine is not available.

B. Chemoprophylaxis: Chloroquine is the preferred drug for prophylaxis against all forms of malaria except in regions where *P falciparum* is resistant to 4-aminoquinolines.

C. Amebiasis: Chloroquine is used with emetine as an alternative treatment for amebic liver abscess.

D. Autoimmune Disorders: When used daily at high doses for several months, chloroquine (or hydroxychloroquine) has been useful in the treatment of autoimmune disorders (Chapter 36).

Adverse Effects

Patients usually tolerate chloroquine well when it is used for malaria prophylaxis (including prolonged use) or treatment. Gastrointestinal symptoms, mild headache, pruritus (especially in black persons), anorexia, malaise, blurring of vision, and urticaria are uncommon. Taking the drug after meals may reduce some adverse effects. Rare reactions include hemolysis in G6PD-deficient persons, impaired hearing, confusion, psychosis, convulsions, blood dyscrasias, skin reactions, alopecia, bleaching of hair, and hypotension.

A total cumulative dose of 100 g (base) may, theoretically, contribute to the development of irreversible retinopathy, ototoxicity, and myopathy. Baseline and periodic follow-up ophthalmologic and neuromuscular evaluations are recommended if chloroquine is used more than 5 years. The development of retinal or visual field changes or muscular weakness requires stopping the drug. Chloroquine may cause T wave changes and widening of the QRS complex on the ECG.

Large intramuscular injections (10 mg/kg) or rapid

intravenous infusions can result in severe hypotension and respiratory and cardiac arrest.

Contraindications & Cautions

Chloroquine is contraindicated in patients with psoriasis or porphyria, in whom it may precipitate acute attacks of these diseases. It should not be combined with other drugs known to cause dermatitis. It should not be used in the presence of retinal or visual field abnormalities unless the benefits outweigh the risks.

Chloroquine should be used with caution in patients with a history of liver damage, alcoholism, or neurologic or hematologic disorders. Certain antacids and antidiarrheal agents (kaolin, calcium carbonate, and magnesium trisilicate) interfere with the absorption of chloroquine and should not be taken within about 4 hours before or after chloroquine administration.

Although the safety of chloroquine in pregnancy has not been completely confirmed, extensive experience with the drug during pregnancy with no reports of teratogenic effects has inclined most workers and WHO authorities to the view that the benefits of the drug outweigh its potential fetal risks. Oral chloroquine can be safely taken by young children. A pediatric solution of chloroquine sulfate (Nivaquine) is widely available outside the USA.

MEFLOQUINE

Mefloquine is used in prophylaxis and treatment of chloroquine-resistant and multidrug-resistant falciparum malaria. It is also effective in prophylaxis against *P vivax* and presumably against *P ovale* and *P malariae.*

Pharmacokinetics

Mefloquine hydrochloride is a synthetic 4-quinoline methanol derivative chemically related to quinine. It can only be given orally because intense local irritation occurs with parenteral use. It is well absorbed, and peak plasma concentrations are reached in 7–24 hours. A single oral dose of 250 mg of the salt results in a plasma concentration of 290–340 ng/mL, whereas continuation of this dose daily results in mean steady state plasma concentrations of 560–1250 ng/mL. Plasma levels of 200–300 ng/mL may be necessary to achieve chemosuppression in *P falciparum* infections. The drug is highly bound to plasma proteins, concentrated in red blood cells, and extensively distributed to the tissues, including the central nervous system. Mefloquine is cleared in the liver. Its acid metabolites are slowly excreted, mainly in the feces. Its elimination half-life, which varies from 13 days to 33 days, tends to be shortened in patients with acute malaria. The drug can be detected in the blood for months after dosing ceases.

Antimalarial & Pharmacologic Actions

A. Antimalarial Action: Mefloquine has strong blood schizonticidal activity against *P falciparum* and *P vivax* but is not active against *P falciparum* gametocytes or the hepatic stages of *P vivax.* Insufficient information is available to document effectiveness against *P malariae* or *P ovale,* but theoretically the drug should be effective against circulating schizonts of these species. The mechanism of action of mefloquine is unknown.

B. Resistance: Sporadic and low levels of resistance to mefloquine have been reported from Southeast Asia and Africa. Resistance to the drug can emerge rapidly, and resistant strains have been found in areas where the drug has never been used.

C. Pharmacologic Effects: Mefloquine has quinidine-like effects on the heart.

Clinical Uses

A. Prophylaxis of Chloroquine-Resistant Strains of *P falciparum:* (Table 53–1.) Mefloquine is effective in prophylaxis against most strains of chloroquine-resistant or pyrimethamine-sulfadoxine-resistant *P falciparum* and is curative when taken weekly for 4 weeks after leaving an endemic area. When used for this purpose, the drug also provides prophylaxis against *P vivax* and probably against *P ovale* and *P malariae.* Eradication of *P vivax* and *P ovale,* however, requires a course of primaquine against their hepatic stages (as used with chloroquine in eradicating *P vivax* infections; see above).

Although the drug is effective against chloroquine-sensitive *P falciparum,* it should be reserved for use in malarious areas in which chloroquine is not effective.

B. Treatment of Chloroquine-Resistant *P falciparum* Infection: (Table 53–2.) Mefloquine is indicated in oral treatment of mild to moderate mefloquine-susceptible *P falciparum* infections. Since mefloquine apparently does not act as quickly as quinine or quinidine and cannot be given parenterally, it should not supplant these drugs in management of severely ill patients. (*Caution:* See manufacturer's recommendations before use.)

Adverse Reactions

The frequency and intensity of reactions are dose-related. Most of the symptoms, however, can also occur as a result of malaria itself.

A. Prophylactic Doses: Minor and transient adverse effects include gastrointestinal disturbances (nausea, vomiting, epigastric pain, diarrhea), headache, dizziness, syncope, and extrasystoles, with an incidence not much higher than for placebo or other antimalarials. Transient leukocytosis, thrombocytopenia, and aminotransferase elevations have been reported. Transient neuropsychiatric events (convulsions, depression, psychoses) have been reported rarely.

B. Treatment Doses: Particularly with therapeutic doses over 1000 mg, gastrointestinal symptoms and fatigue are more likely and the incidence of neuropsychiatric symptoms (dizziness, headache, visual disturbances, tinnitus, insomnia, restlessness, anxiety, depression, confusion, acute psychosis, or seizures) may be as high as 1%. Pruritus, skin rash, alopecia, and myalgia are rare. Reactions may occur up to 2–3 weeks after the last dose of mefloquine.

C. Animal Toxicity: Ocular lesions (lens opacity, retinal degeneration) have been reported in animals but not in humans.

D. Mutagenicity, Carcinogenicity, and Teratogenicity: Mutagenicity and carcinogenicity studies have been negative in a variety of assay systems. At high doses, the drug is teratogenic and embryotoxic in experimental animals. Adequate controlled studies in human pregnancy are not available.

Contraindications & Cautions

Mefloquine is contraindicated if there is a history of epilepsy, psychiatric disorders, arrhythmia, cardiac conduction defect, or sensitivity to quinidine or related drugs. The drug should not be used for children under 15 kg or under 2 years of age; in these groups, the drug appears to be poorly tolerated, and efficacy has not been established. Also contraindicated is concurrent administration of mefloquine with quinine, quinidine, or halofantrine. If these agents precede the use of mefloquine, 12 hours should elapse before mefloquine is started. Because of the long half-life of mefloquine, extreme caution is required if quinine or quinidine is used to treat malaria after mefloquine has been taken.

The drug should preferably not be used in the first trimester of pregnancy, and women of childbearing potential who take mefloquine for malarial prophylaxis should use reliable precautions against conception for 3 months after the last dose.

The development of neuropsychiatric symptoms (anxiety, depression, restlessness, confusion) during prophylaxis is an indication to stop mefloquine usage. The drug should not be taken by persons whose work requires fine coordination and spatial discrimination (eg, airline pilots). Patients taking anticonvulsant drugs (particularly valproic acid and divalproex sodium) may have breakthrough seizures; concurrent administration of mefloquine and chloroquine or quinine increases the risk of convulsions.

The safety of mefloquine usage beyond 1 year has not been established. Therefore, if the drug is used for prolonged periods, periodic evaluations, including liver function tests and complete ophthalmologic examinations, are recommended.

PRIMAQUINE

Chemistry & Pharmacokinetics

Primaquine phosphate is a synthetic 8-aminoquinoline derivative (Figure 53–1). After oral administration, the drug is usually well absorbed, reaching peak plasma levels in 1–2 hours, and then is almost completely metabolized and excreted in the urine. Primaquine's plasma half-life is 3–8 hours and its peak serum concentration is 50–66 ng/mL; trace amounts remain at 24 hours. Primaquine is widely distributed to the tissues, but only a small amount is bound there. Its major metabolite is a deaminated derivative, carboxyprimaquine, that reaches plasma concentrations more than ten times greater than those of the parent compound, is eliminated slowly (half-life 22–30 hours), and accumulates with daily dosing; peak serum concentrations after 14 daily doses are 432–1240 ng/mL. Whether primaquine or one of its metabolites is the active compound has not been determined.

Antimalarial & Pharmacologic Actions

A. Antimalarial Action: Primaquine is active against the late hepatic stages (hypnozoites and schizonts) of *P vivax* and *P ovale* and thus effects radical cure of these infections. Primaquine is also highly active against the primary exoerythrocytic stages of *P falciparum*. When used in prophylaxis with chloroquine, it protects against *P vivax* and *P ovale*. Primaquine is highly gametocidal against the four malaria species. When given in nontoxic doses, primaquine's effect on blood schizonts is too slight to be useful in treatment of acute attacks.

B. Mechanism of Action: The mechanism of primaquine's antimalarial action is not well understood. The quinoline-quinone intermediates derived from primaquine are electron-carrying redox compounds that can act as oxidants. These intermediates probably produce most of the hemolysis and methemoglobinemia associated with primaquine's use.

C. Pharmacologic Effects: At high doses, primaquine may suppress myeloid activity. At standard doses, it may affect erythrocytes in genetically susceptible persons (see below).

D. Resistance: Some strains of *P vivax* in New Guinea, Southeast Asia, and perhaps Central and South America are relatively resistant to primaquine and require one or more treatment courses with either 30 mg (base) daily for 14 days or 15 mg (base) daily for 14–21 days.

Clinical Uses (Tables 53–1 and 53–2)

A. Terminal Prophylaxis of Vivax and Ovale Malaria: Because of its effect on the persistent liver stages of *P vivax* and *P ovale,* primaquine and a blood schizonticide, usually chloroquine, are taken together at the end of a period of potential exposure to these parasites to effect radical cure (terminal prophylaxis) (Table 53–1).

B. Radical Cure of Acute Vivax and Ovale Malaria: Primaquine plus chloroquine are used to treat these acute infections (Table 53–2). A 14-day course of primaquine is standard.

C. Gametocidal Action: A single dose of primaquine (45 mg [base]) is occasionally used to render *P falciparum* gametocytes noninfective.

D. *Pneumocystis carinii* Pneumonia: Combined therapy of primaquine with clindamycin is an alternative oral treatment for this infection.

Adverse Effects

Primaquine in recommended doses is generally well tolerated. It infrequently causes nausea, epigastric pain, abdominal cramps, and headache. The more serious adverse effects, leukopenia and agranulocytosis, are rare. Other possible rare reactions are leukocytosis, pruritus, and arrhythmias.

Standard doses of primaquine may cause limited hemolysis, marked hemolysis, or methemoglobinemia (manifested by cyanosis) in persons with some variants of G6PD deficiency or certain other hereditary erythrocytic pentose phosphate pathway defects. Although primaquine can produce methemoglobinemia in normal persons, the effect is more marked in those with congenital deficiency of NADH.

Contraindications & Cautions

Primaquine should not be prescribed concurrently with quinidine or for patients with connective tissue disorders or a history of granulocytopenia or methemoglobinemia. It should not be given during the first trimester of pregnancy and preferably not until after delivery. It is never given parenterally, because it may induce marked hypotension.

When feasible, patients should be tested for G6PD deficiency before primaquine is prescribed.If the test is positive, treatment is based on the risk-versus-benefit relationship. Often, sensitive persons can tolerate and be treated with chloroquine, 0.5 g, plus primaquine, 78.9 mg (45 mg base), once weekly for 8 weeks. The drug should be stopped if there is any evidence of hemolysis (reddening or darkening of the urine) or anemia.

PYRIMETHAMINE & PROGUANIL (Chloroguanide)

Chemistry & Pharmacokinetics

Pyrimethamine and proguanil are dihydrofolate reductase inhibitors (folic acid antagonists, antifols). Pyrimethamine is a 2,4-diaminopyrimidine related to trimethoprim, which is used to treat bacterial infections (Chapter 46). Proguanil is a biguanide derivative. The structures of the two drugs are shown in Figure 53–1.

Both pyrimethamine and proguanil are slowly but adequately absorbed from the gastrointestinal tract. Pyrimethamine reaches peak plasma levels 2–6 hours after an oral dose, is bound to plasma proteins, and has an elimination half-life of about 3.5 days. Proguanil reaches peak plasma levels about 5 hours after an oral dose and has an elimination half-life of about 16 hours. Therefore, in prophylaxis, proguanil must be administered daily, whereas pyrimethamine can be given once a week. Pyrimethamine is extensively metabolized before excretion. Proguanil is a prodrug; only its triazine metabolite, cycloguanil, is active.

Antimalarial & Pharmacologic Actions

A. Antimalarial Action: Pyrimethamine and proguanil are slow-acting blood schizonticides against susceptible strains of all four malarial species. Proguanil (but not pyrimethamine) has a marked effect on the primary tissue stages of susceptible *P falciparum* and therefore may have causal prophylactic action, perhaps effective even when blood schizonts are resistant to the agent. Neither drug is adequately gametocidal nor effective against the persistent liver stages of *P vivax* or *P ovale*.

Pyrimethamine and the triazine metabolite of proguanil have a higher affinity for and more effectively inhibit plasmodial dihydrofolate reductase than the human enzyme; as a result, the reduction of dihydrofolic acid to tetrahydrofolic acid (folinic acid) is selectively inhibited in the parasite.

B. Resistance: Resistance to pyrimethamine and proguanil is found worldwide for *P falciparum* and somewhat less ubiquitously for *P vivax*. Therefore, prophylaxis against falciparum malaria with either drug alone is no longer recommended.

C. Pharmacologic Effects: In dosages used for malaria chemoprophylaxis and treatment, the antifols produce no pharmacologic effects. In the higher doses used for toxoplasmosis, macrocytic anemia and other adverse effects may occur.

Clinical Uses

A. Chemoprophylaxis: In areas of the world where chloroquine resistance is not widespread, and as an alternative to mefloquine, the combination of chloroquine (0.5 g weekly) and proguanil (200 mg daily) is used while in the endemic area and for 4 weeks after leaving. Proguanil is not available in the USA.

B. Treatment of Chloroquine-Resistant Falciparum Malaria: Pyrimethamine in fixed combination with sulfadoxine (Fansidar; see below) is used in single-dose treatment of known or presumptive acute attacks of chloroquine-resistant falciparum malaria (Table 53–2). The combination is no longer used in weekly prophylaxis.

C. Toxoplasmosis Treatment: The treatment of choice is pyrimethamine, 75 mg/d for 3 days, then 25 mg daily, plus either trisulfapyrimidines (2–6 g/d in four divided doses) or sulfadiazine (100 mg/kg/d [maximum 6 g/d] in four divided doses); continue with this treatment for 3–4 weeks. Leucovorin calcium (folinic acid), 10 mg/d in two to four divided doses, is given to avoid the hematologic effects of pyrimethamine-induced folate deficiency. Patients should be screened for a history of sulfonamide sensitivity.

In the treatment of toxoplasmal encephalitis in AIDS, higher doses are used. Primary therapy (for 6 weeks or longer if necessary) is as follows: pyrimethamine, 200 mg as loading dose in two divided doses, then 1–1.5 mg/kg/d; sulfadiazine or trisulfapyrimidines, 4–6 g/d in four divided doses; and leucovorin calcium, 10–50 mg/d in two divided doses. Maintenance therapy is as follows: pyrimethamine, 25–50 mg/d; sulfadiazine or trisulfapyrimidines, 2 g/d in two divided doses; and leucovorin calcium, 5–20 mg/d in two divided doses. In ocular toxoplasmosis, systemic corticosteroids are often added to reduce increased intracranial pressure.

Adverse Effects

In malaria treatment, most patients tolerate pyrimethamine and proguanil well. Gastrointestinal symptoms, skin rashes, and itching are rare. Mouth ulcers and alopecia have been described with proguanil usage.

In the high doses of pyrimethamine used in toxoplasmosis, side effects of folic acid deficiency (megaloblastic anemia, agranulocytosis, thrombocytopenia, atrophic glossitis) are common unless leucovorin calcium is given concurrently. Also with high doses, gastric irritation (reduced if the drug is given with meals) and neurologic symptoms (headache, insomnia, depression, ataxia, tremors, seizures, respiratory depression) may occur.

Cautions & Contraindications

Pyrimethamine should be used cautiously in the presence of renal or hepatic dysfunction. Because pyrimethamine is teratogenic in animals, benefit versus risk must be evaluated and leucovorin supplementation provided if the drug is to be used during pregnancy; generally, pyrimethamine should be avoided during the first trimester. In view of the high dosages used in toxoplasmosis, platelet and white blood cell counts should be performed at least twice weekly. The drug should be discontinued at the first sign of rash, sore throat, purpura, or glossitis.

Proguanil is considered safe in pregnancy, but leucovorin supplementation should be provided.

SULFONAMIDES & SULFONES

Sulfonamides and sulfones have blood schizonticidal action against some strains of *P falciparum* by the same mechanism as in bacteria, namely, inhibition of dihydrofolic acid synthesis (Chapter 46). However, the drugs have only weak effects against the blood schizonts of *P vivax,* and they are not active against the gametocytes or liver stages of *P falciparum* or *P vivax.*

When a sulfonamide or sulfone is combined with an antifol, synergistic blockade of folic acid synthesis occurs in susceptible plasmodia (Figure 46–2). Many combinations have been evaluated for prophylaxis and treatment of chloroquine-resistant *P falciparum*; the most useful are sulfadoxine with pyrimethamine (Fansidar) and dapsone with pyrimethamine (Maloprim). However, in many regions of the world, particularly in Southeast Asia and areas of the Amazon Basin and eastern Africa, *P falciparum* has become resistant to these combinations. In addition to drug resistance, major disadvantages of the sulfonamides and sulfones are the slowness of their blood schizonticidal activity and their numerous and sometimes serious adverse effects.

1. FANSIDAR (Pyrimethamine-Sulfadoxine)

Pharmacokinetics

Fansidar is well absorbed. Its components display peak plasma levels within 2–8 hours and are excreted mainly by the kidneys. Average half-lives are about 170 hours for sulfadoxine and 80–110 hours for pyrimethamine.

Antimalarial Action & Resistance

Fansidar is effective against certain strains of falciparum malaria. However, quinine must be given concurrently in treatment of seriously ill patients, because Fansidar is only slowly active. Fansidar is not effective in vivax malaria, and its usefulness in ovale and malariae malaria has not been adequately studied.

Clinical Uses (Tables 53–1 and 53–2)

A. Treatment of Chloroquine-Resistant Falciparum Malaria: Fansidar (a slow-acting schizonticide) is used in conjunction with quinine (fast-acting) to treat acute attacks of chloroquine-resistant falciparum malaria (Table 53–2).

B. Presumptive Treatment of Chloroquine-Resistant Falciparum Malaria: Fansidar is used in presumptive self-treatment of malaria—ie, when malaria-like symptoms occur that cannot be immediately diagnosed and managed by a local physician, and the patient decides to self-treat with a single dose (three tablets for an adult). *It is imperative, however, that medical follow-up be sought promptly.* This treatment is not effective for vivax, ovale, or malariae malaria but may be effective for susceptible chloroquine-resistant strains of *P falciparum* if the degree of illness does not require a rapidly acting blood schizonticide such as quinine.

Adverse Effects

Rare adverse effects to single-dose Fansidar are those associated with sulfonamide allergy, including the hematologic, gastrointestinal, central nervous system, dermatologic, and renal systems.

Fansidar is no longer used in continuing prophylaxis because of severe reactions, including erythema multiforme, Stevens-Johnson syndrome, and toxic epidermal necrolysis, that occur with a low but significant frequency.

Contraindications & Cautions

Fansidar is contraindicated in patients who have had adverse reactions to sulfonamides. Fansidar should not be used in pregnancy at term, in nursing women, or in children under 2 months of age. Fansidar should be used with caution in the presence of impaired renal or hepatic function, in patients with G6PD deficiency (hemolysis occurs in some), and in those with severe allergic disorders, bronchial asthma, or poor nutritional status.

2. MALOPRIM* (Pyrimethamine-Dapsone)

Because of its potential toxicity (fatal agranulocytosis), this drug is not recommended for prophylaxis.

QUININE & QUINIDINE

1. QUININE

Quinine, the principal alkaloid derived from the bark of the cinchona tree, has been used in malaria suppression and treatment for more than 300 years. Although superseded by other antimalarials, following the development of widespread resistance to chloroquine and other drugs, quinine has again become an important antimalarial.

Pharmacokinetics

Quinine, a bitter-tasting alkaloid, is rapidly absorbed, reaches peak plasma levels in 1–3 hours, and is widely distributed in body tissues. Approximately 80% of plasma quinine is protein-bound; red blood cell levels are about 20% of the plasma level and cerebrospinal fluid concentrations about 7%. The elimination half-life of quinine is 7–12 hours in normal persons but 8–21 hours in malaria-infected persons in proportion to the severity of the disease. Approximately 80% of the drug is metabolized in the liver and excreted for the most part in the urine. Excretion is accelerated in acid urine.

With constant daily doses, plasma concentrations usually reach a plateau on the third day. In normals or in mild infection, standard oral doses result in plasma levels of about 7 μg/mL; in severe malaria, higher plasma levels are reached. A mean plasma concentration of about 5 μg/mL is necessary to eliminate asexual parasites of vivax malaria and a somewhat higher concentration in falciparum malaria. Concentrations lower than 2 μg/mL have little effect, whereas concentrations over 7 μg/mL are generally accompanied by adverse reactions of "cinchonism." Because of this narrow therapeutic range, adverse reactions are common during quinine treatment of falciparum malaria.

Antimalarial & Pharmacologic Actions & Drug Resistance

A. Antimalarial Action: Quinine is a rapidly acting, highly effective blood schizonticide against the four malaria parasites. The drug is gametocidal for *P vivax* and *P ovale* but not very effective against *P falciparum* gametocytes. Quinine has no effect on sporozoites or the liver stages of any of the parasites.

B. Mechanism of Action: The drug's molecular mechanism is unclear. Quinine is known to depress many enzyme systems. It also forms a hydrogen-bonded complex with double-stranded DNA that inhibits strand separation, transcription, and protein synthesis.

C. Pharmacologic Effects: When taken orally, quinine commonly causes gastric irritation. The drug's effect on cardiac muscle is similar to that of its diastereoisomer, quinidine, but less intense. Quinine has a slight oxytocic action on the gravid uterus, especially in the third trimester. In skeletal muscle, quinine has a curare-like effect on the motor endplate; it also appears to lengthen the refractory period of the skeletal muscle membrane. Quinine may diminish tetanic contractions associated with various conditions and has been used to lessen the contractures of myotonia congenita. Use of quinine as an antipyretic or analgesic and as a diagnostic test for myasthenia gravis is now obsolete. Therapeutic doses sometimes cause hypoglycemia through stimulation of pancreatic B cell release of insulin; this is a particular problem in severe infections and in pregnant patients. Severe or even lethal hypotension can follow too-rapid intravenous injections.

D. Resistance: Resistance of quinine when used alone has been increasing in Southeast Asia. However, there is no unequivocal case of a complete failure to respond to quinine when a second drug is also used.

Clinical Uses (Tables 53–1 and 53–2)

A. Parenteral Treatment of Severe Falciparum Malaria: Quinine dihydrochloride, if available, is given *slowly* intravenously when parenteral therapy is required for severe *P falciparum* infections, whether sensitive or resistant to chloroquine. Contrary to earlier views that intramuscular delivery of concentrated quinine was painful and might cause sterile abscess, it is now accepted that a dilute solution (50–100 mg/mL) is well absorbed and can be used without discomfort or tissue necrosis. Dosage regi-

---

*Not available in the USA.

mens are the same as for intravenous use. In the USA, quinine dihydrochloride is not available and quinidine gluconate is used instead.

B. Oral Treatment of Falciparum Malaria Resistant to Chloroquine: Quinine sulfate is used with other drugs for the oral treatment of acute attacks of *P falciparum* malaria resistant to chloroquine. Although quinine effectively reduces parasitemia, combination therapy with another drug is necessary because quinine alone fails to completely eliminate the infection. Quinine, however, is less effective than chloroquine and is therefore not used to treat acute attacks of vivax, ovale, or malariae malaria or chloroquine-sensitive falciparum malaria.

C. Prophylaxis: Because of its potential toxicity, quinine is not generally used in prophylaxis. However, in areas where *P falciparum* is resistant to chloroquine and neither mefloquine nor doxycycline is available, quinine prophylaxis can be considered. The dosage is 325 mg daily while in the endemic area and for 4 weeks after leaving. Eradication of *P vivax* or *P ovale* infection requires a course of primaquine, but quinine and primaquine should not be given concurrently.

D. Other Uses: Quinine sulfate, 200–300 mg, sometimes relieves nighttime leg cramps. Quinine is used concurrently with clindamycin in the treatment of severe babesiosis, caused by *Babesia microti.*

Adverse Effects

A. Gastrointestinal Effects: Quinine is an irritant to the gastric mucosa and often causes nausea, vomiting, or epigastric pain.

B. Cinchonism: A less common effect is cinchonism, a toxic state that usually develops when plasma levels of quinine exceed 7–10 μg/mL; in some patients, however, symptoms may occur at lower plasma levels. Symptoms of mild to moderate cinchonism include headache, nausea, slight visual disturbances, dizziness, and mild tinnitus. They may abate as treatment continues and usually do not require discontinuance of treatment. If the symptoms become severe, the drug should be discontinued temporarily while plasma quinine levels are determined.

C. Hematologic Effects: Hemolysis directly attributable to quinine occurs in 0.05% of people treated for acute malaria; it may also occur in G6PD-deficient persons. Leukopenia, agranulocytosis, thrombocytopenic purpura, Schönlein-Henoch purpura, and hypoprothrombinemia are rare.

D. Hypoglycemia: A decrease in blood sugar may occur at therapeutic doses, as noted above. Administration of glucose may evoke greater insulin release followed by further hypoglycemia.

E. Severe Toxicity: Severe toxicity is rare; findings include fever, skin eruptions, gastrointestinal symptoms, deafness, visual abnormalities, central nervous system effects (syncope, confusion), and quinidine-like effects.

The role of quinine in **blackwater fever** is unclear, but that disorder has been associated with prolonged past use of the drug. In sensitized patients, even a single dose can precipitate the reaction. The syndrome—characterized by massive intravascular hemolysis followed by hemoglobinuria, dark urine, azotemia, intravascular sludging and coagulation, renal failure, and uremia—has a fatality rate of 25–50%.

F. Mutagenicity and Teratogenicity: In humans, large doses of quinine given in failed abortion attempts have resulted in congenital malformations.

G. Other Adverse Effects: Intravenous quinine infrequently causes thrombophlebitis. Excessive rate of infusion may result in moderate to marked hypotension, seizures, ventricular fibrillation, and death.

Contraindications & Cautions

Stop the drug immediately if signs of hemolysis appear. Hypersensitivity reactions (including pruritus, facial edema, asthma) and other severe reactions require permanent discontinuation of the drug. Quinine should not be given subcutaneously and should not be given in pregnancy or to patients with histories of tinnitus, optic neuritis, or myasthenia gravis. Quinine should not be given concurrently with mefloquine (see below) and is contraindicated in patients with G6PD deficiency. In renal insufficiency, determine plasma quinine levels and reduce dosage appropriately. For patients with cardiac arrhythmias, use the same precautions as with quinidine.

Drug Interactions

Aluminum-containing antacids delay the absorption of quinine. Quinine may decrease renal clearance of digoxin and increase serum digoxin concentrations. The action of warfarin and other anticoagulants may be enhanced. Quinine may intensify or reinduce neuromuscular block in patients receiving neuromuscular blockers. Cimetidine slows the elimination of quinine, and acidification of the urine increases quinine clearance.

2. QUINIDINE

Quinidine, the dextrorotatory diastereoisomer of quinine, is formulated as quinidine gluconate for the parenteral treatment of cardiac arrhythmias (see Chapter 14). Quinidine gluconate is also effective in the parenteral treatment of severe malaria and can be used when the parenteral form of quinine, quinine dihydrochloride, is not available, as in the USA.

Intravenous quinidine infrequently causes thrombophlebitis. Quinidine is potentially cardiotoxic (see Chapter 14); the risk-versus-benefit ratio should be considered in the presence of cardiac conduction defects and hepatic or renal dysfunction. Cautions and contraindications for concurrent use of quinidine and other drugs are similar to those for quinine (see above), including concurrent use with mefloquine.

ALTERNATIVE DRUGS

The following alternative drugs are particularly useful in regions where *P falciparum* is resistant to both chloroquine and the antifolate-sulfonamide combinations. Some of these drugs are used in prophylaxis. After the patient has left the endemic area, primaquine can be given (in accordance with the guidelines set forth above) to provide radical cure for *P vivax* and *P ovale* infections.

1. DOXYCYCLINE

Doxycycline, a tetracycline drug (Chapter 44), is generally effective against multidrug-resistant *P falciparum;* for this purpose, it is used prophylactically for up to 3 months in Thailand and adjacent countries (Table 53–1) and in other parts of the world for patients unable to take mefloquine. The drug is also active against the blood stages of the other *Plasmodium* species but not against the liver stages. In the treatment of acute malaria, it is used in conjunction with quinine (Table 53–2). Doxycycline side effects include infrequent gastrointestinal symptoms, candidal vaginitis, and rare photosensitivity. Its safety in long-term prophylaxis has not been evaluated. See Chapter 44 for additional details.

2. HALOFANTRINE*

Halofantrine hydrochloride, a phenanthrene-methanol compound, is an oral schizonticide for all four malarial species. Its use, however, should be restricted to treatment of infection with chloroquine- and multidrug-resistant *P falciparum,* to which halofantrine resistance is also appearing. The drug has no effect on gametocytes or on the intrahepatic stages of the parasites. It should not be used for pre- or post-travel prophylaxis or as a backup drug for presumptive treatment of malaria-like symptoms. Halofantrine's mechanism of action is uncertain.

The dosage is 500 mg given three times at 6-hour intervals and repeated in 1 week. Absorption variability remains a problem. To avoid the increased absorption that occurs with fatty foods (up to sixfold), the drug should not be given from 1 hour before to 3 hours after a meal. Plasma levels of the drug and its main metabolite, *N*-debutyl-halofantrine, peak in 6 and 16 hours, respectively; in malaria-infected patients, half-lives of the compounds are 4–5 days and excretion is mainly in the feces.

In more than three million courses of treatment worldwide, the drug has been well tolerated; rare and mild side effects are abdominal pain, diarrhea, cough, rash, and pruritus. However, the safety of the drug remains a concern as it causes dose-dependent prolongation of QT_c and PR intervals, and rare instances of toxic reactions (syncope, ventricular tachycardia, acute intravascular hemolysis) have occurred. Therefore, treatment should be conducted under electrocardiographic monitoring. The drug is contraindicated in patients with prolongation of the QT interval or in conjunction with another drug that prolongs the interval; it probably should not be used in the presence of other cardiac conduction defects. Halofantrine should not be used in patients who have taken mefloquine within the past 2–3 weeks, as concern remains for potentiation of arrhythmias from their combined use. The drug is embryotoxic in animal studies and is therefore contraindicated in pregnancy unless benefit clearly outweighs risk. The drug is widely available abroad; although approved by FDA, it is not marketed in the USA.

3. QINGHAOSU* (Artemisinin)

Qinghaosu is a sesquiterpene lactone endoperoxide, the active principal of a Chinese herbal medicine *(qing hao)* that has been used as an antipyretic in China for over 2000 years.

Because qinghaosu is only sparingly soluble in water and oils, analogs have been synthesized to increase its solubility: water-soluble artesunate (available as tablets for oral use and as an intravenous formulation) and lipid-soluble artemether (available as tablets and as an intramuscular formulation). Arteether, a lipid-soluble derivative similar to artemether, is also under evaluation. Pharmacologic studies have shown that qinghaosu and its analogs are rapidly absorbed (with peak plasma levels occurring in about 1 hour) and undergo rapid hydrolysis to the biologically active metabolite dihydroqinghaosu, following which the parent compound and metabolite are widely distributed in the tissues and eliminated rapidly (with a half-life of about 4 hours).

Qinghaosu and analogs are effective blood schizonticides against all types of malaria, including chloroquine-resistant falciparum malaria. However, because of their short-half life they are not useful in prophylaxis. They have no effect on the hepatic stages of the parasites and do not cure the relapsing malarias. Their mechanism of action is unknown. The drugs are especially useful in treatment of cerebral falciparum malaria. The recurrence rate is over 40% when therapy is for 1–3 days but considerably less when treatment is extended to 7 days.

The drugs produce few adverse effects (abdominal pain, diarrhea) but are said to be embryotoxic in rats and mice. Therefore, they should not be used in preg-

*Not available in the USA.

nancy. Bone marrow depression has been noted in animals, and depression of reticulocyte counts has been reported in humans. Animal studies suggest a potential for central nervous system toxicity. There are no known qinghaosu-resistant plasmodia.

4. QUINACRINE

Quinacrine, a 9-aminoacridine, is a blood schizonticide that can effectively suppress all four types of human malaria and can effect radical cures of *P malariae* and nonresistant strains of *P falciparum*. Until the introduction of chloroquine in 1945, quinacrine was the principal synthetic drug used for antimalarial prophylaxis, but it is now considered obsolete for this purpose. Its disadvantages include occasional drug deposits that turn the skin yellow and rare psychotic reactions. Quinacrine continues to be used in the treatment of giardiasis.

TREATMENT OF AMEBIASIS

Amebiasis is infection by the protozoan parasite *Entamoeba histolytica*. This pathogen was formerly considered one organism with varying virulence, but the current general view is that there are two distinct though morphologically identical species in the *Entamoeba* complex: (1) *E dispar*, which remains in the colon as a stable commensal that is avirulent and produces an asymptomatic carrier state; and (2) *E histolytica* (about 10% of the complex), which shows varying virulence. *E histolytica* infection may present as a severe intestinal infection (dysentery), a mild to moderate symptomatic intestinal infection, an asymptomatic intestinal infection, or as an ameboma, liver abscess, or other type of extraintestinal infection.

The choice of drug depends on the clinical presentation and on the desired site of drug action, ie, in the intestinal lumen or in the tissues. Table 53–3 outlines a preferred and an alternative method of treatment for each clinical type of amebiasis. Drug dosages are provided in the table footnotes. No drugs are recommended as safe or effective for chemoprophylaxis.

Drugs Used in Treatment

All of the antiamebic drugs act against *Entamoeba histolytica* trophozoites, but most are not effective against the cyst stage.

A. Tissue Amebicides: These drugs eliminate organisms primarily in the bowel wall, liver, and other extraintestinal tissues. They are not effective against organisms in the bowel lumen.

1. Nitroimidazoles–Metronidazole, tinidazole,* and ornidazole* are highly effective against amebas in the bowel wall and other tissues. They are, however,

only partially effective and not adequate as luminal amebicides. For example, metronidazole alone fails to cure up to 50% of intestinal infections.

2. Emetines–Emetine and dehydroemetine† are generally given intramuscularly; in this form, they act on organisms in the bowel wall and other tissues but not on amebas in the bowel lumen.

3. Chloroquine–This drug is active principally against amebas in the liver.

B. Luminal Amebicides: These drugs act primarily in the bowel lumen; they are not effective against organisms in the bowel wall or other tissues.

1. Dichloroacetamides–Diloxanide furoate,† clefamide,* teclozan,* etofamide.*

2. Halogenated hydroxyquinolines–Iodoquinol (diiodohydroxyquin); clioquinol (iodochlorhydroxyquin).*

3. Antibiotics–The oral tetracyclines indirectly affect luminal amebas by inhibiting the bacterial associates of *E histolytica* in the bowel lumen. Paromomycin and erythromycin are directly amebicidal. Except for paromomycin, none of the antibiotics are highly effective against intestinal organisms and therefore should not be used by themselves in treatment. Parenteral antibiotics have little antiamebic activity in any site.

Treatment of Specific Forms of Amebiasis

A. Asymptomatic Intestinal Infection: In endemic areas, asymptomatic carriers generally are not treated because of the frequency of reinfection. In nonendemic areas, the viewpoint of many authorities is—until *E dispar* and *E histolytica* can be conveniently differentiated—to treat asymptomatic carriers with a luminal amebicide. The drugs of choice, diloxanide furoate and iodoquinol, cure about 80–90% of cases in a single course of treatment. Diloxanide causes fewer adverse effects than iodoquinol. In asymptomatic infection, the additional use of a tissue amebicidal drug is not necessary. Other alternatives for treatment or re-treatment are paromomycin or metronidazole plus iodoquinol or diloxanide.

B. Mild to Moderate Intestinal Infection: Metronidazole plus a luminal amebicide is the treatment of choice. Alternative treatments are shown in Table 53–3. The minimum dose of chloroquine needed to destroy trophozoites carried to the liver or to eradicate an undetected early-stage liver abscess is not established.

C. Severe Intestinal Infection (Dysentery): The amebicidal treatment of severe amebic dysentery is the same as in mild to moderate disease. Because of their potential toxicity, the emetines should preferably not be used. Fluid and electrolyte therapy and opioids to control bowel motility are necessary adjuncts.

---

*Not available in the USA.
†In the USA, available only from the Centers for Disease Control and Prevention, Atlanta 30333; telephone 404-639-3356.

Table 53–3. Treatment of amebiasis.

	Drug(s) of Choice	Alternative Drug(s)
Asymptomatic intestinal infection	Diloxanide furoate[1,2]	Iodoquinol (diiodohydroxyquin)[3] or paromomycin[4]
Mild to moderate intestinal infection (nondysenteric colitis)	(1) Metronidazole[5] **plus** (2) Diloxanide furoate,[2] iodoquinol,[3] or paromomycin[4]	(1) Diloxanide furoate[2] or iodoquinol[3] **plus** (2) A tetracycline[6] **followed by** (3) Chloroquine[7] **or** (1) Paromomycin[4] **followed by** (2) Chloroquine[7]
Severe intestinal infection (dysentery)	(1) Metronidazole[8] **plus** (2) Diloxanide furoate[2] or iodoquinol[3] **or, if parenteral therapy is needed initially:** (1) Intravenous metronidazole[9] until oral therapy can be started; (2) Then give oral metronidazole[8] plus diloxanide furoate[2] or iodoquinol[3]	(1) A tetracycline[6] **plus** (2) Diloxanide furoate[2] or iodoquinol[3] **followed by** (3) Chloroquine[10] **or, if parenteral therapy is needed initially:** (1) Dehydroemetine[1,11] or emetine[11] **followed by** (2) A tetracycline[6] plus diloxanide furoate[2] or iodoquinol[3] **followed by** (3) Chloroquine[10]
Hepatic abscess	(1) Metronidazole[8,9] **plus** (2) Diloxanide furoate[2] or iodoquinol[3] **followed by** (3) Chloroquine[10]	(1) Dehydroemetine[1,12] or emetine[12] **followed by** (2) Chloroquine[13] **plus** (3) Diloxanide furoate[2] or iodoquinol[3]
Ameboma or extraintestinal infection	As for hepatic abscess, but not including chloroquine	As for hepatic abscess, but not including chloroquine

[1]Available in the USA only from the Parasitic Disease Drug Service, Centers for Disease Control and Prevention, Atlanta 30333. Telephone requests may be made by calling the central number: 404-639-3670.
[2]Diloxanide furoate, 500 mg three times daily with meals for 10 days.
[3]Iodoquinol (diiodohydroxyquin), 650 mg three times daily for 21 days.
[4]Paromomycin, 25–30 mg/kg (base) (maximum 3 g) in three divided doses after meals daily for 7 days.
[5]Metronidazole, 750 mg three times daily for 10 days. In countries where it is available (not in the USA), tinidazole is preferred over metronidazole as the nitroimidazole component in treatment; although the two drugs are equally effective, tinidazole is given in a shorter course of treatment and is better tolerated. The tinidazole dosage is 800 mg three times daily for 3 days; in severe intestinal disease and hepatic abscess, continue for 5 days.
[6]Tetracycline, 250 mg four times daily for 10 days; in severe dysentery, give 500 mg four times daily for the first 5 days, then 250 mg four times daily for 5 days. Tetracycline should not be used during pregnancy.
[7]Chloroquine, 500 mg (salt) daily for 7 days.
[8]Metronidazole, 750 mg three times daily for 10 days.
[9]An intravenous metronidazole formulation is available; change to oral medication as soon as possible. See manufacturer's recommendation for dosage.
[10]Chloroquine, 500 mg (salt) daily for 14 days.
[11]Dehydroemetine or emetine, 1 mg/kg subcutaneously (preferred) or intramuscularly daily for the least number of days necessary to control severe symptoms (usually 3–5 days) (maximum daily dose for dehydroemetine is 90 mg; for emetine, 65 mg).
[12]Use dosage recommended in footnote 11 for 8–10 days.
[13]Chloroquine, 500 mg (salt) orally twice daily for 2 days and then 500 mg orally daily for 19 days.

D. Hepatic Abscess: Hospitalization and bed rest are usually necessary. The treatment of choice is metronidazole; if given for 10 days, this drug cures over 95% of uncomplicated cases. However, treatment failures occur rarely, either during the course of treatment or after its completion. Some authorities recommend a course of chloroquine to follow. A luminal amebicide such as diloxanide furoate or iodoquinol should also be given to eradicate intestinal infection whether or not organisms are found in the stools. An advantage of metronidazole is its effectiveness against anaerobic bacteria, which are a major cause of bacterial liver abscess. Dehydroemetine and emetine are potentially toxic alternative drugs.

E. Ameboma or Extraintestinal Forms of Amebiasis: Metronidazole is the drug of choice. Dehydroemetine (or emetine) is an alternative drug; chloroquine cannot be used because it does not reach high enough tissue concentrations to be effective (except in the liver). A simultaneous course of a luminal amebicide should also be given.

CHLOROQUINE

Chloroquine reaches high liver concentrations and is highly effective when given with dehydroemetine (or emetine) in the treatment and prevention of amebic liver abscess. Chloroquine is not used, however, in the treatment of intestinal amebiasis, because the drug is not active against luminal organisms. At the dosage levels used in the treatment of amebiasis, the retinopathy sometimes associated with long-term use of chloroquine does not occur.

EMETINE & DEHYDROEMETINE

Chemistry & Pharmacokinetics

Emetine can be derived from ipecac or synthesized. Racemic 2-dehydroemetine dihydrochloride is a synthetic substance.

Emetine and dehydroemetine are administered parenterally, because oral preparations are absorbed erratically, may induce vomiting, and have low effectiveness. When given parenterally, they are stored primarily in the liver, lungs, spleen, and kidneys. The drugs are cumulative; they are eliminated slowly via the kidneys with trace amounts detectable in the urine 1–2 months after the end of therapy.

Pharmacologic Effects

Emetine and dehydroemetine affect almost all tissues. They irreversibly block the synthesis of protein in eukaryotes by inhibiting the movement of the ribosome along messenger RNA; DNA synthesis is blocked secondarily. In experimental animals, emetine given parenterally in toxic doses causes cellular damage in the liver, kidneys, and skeletal and cardiac muscle. Cardiac conduction and contraction are depressed, which may cause a variety of atrial and ventricular arrhythmias, cardiac dilation, and death. Emetine also has adrenoceptor- and cholinoceptor-blocking actions.

Antiamebic Action

These drugs act only against trophozoites, which they directly eliminate.

Clinical Uses

Emetine and dehydroemetine should not be used to treat asymptomatic or mild intestinal infections. When available, dehydroemetine is the preferred drug, since it is equally effective and may be less toxic than emetine. Dosages are listed in Table 53–3.

A. Severe Intestinal Disease (Amebic Dysentery): Parenterally administered emetine and dehydroemetine rapidly alleviate severe intestinal symptoms but are rarely curative even if a full course is given. For this reason and because of their toxicity, they should be given for the minimum period needed to relieve severe symptoms (usually 3–5 days). Marked toxicity is unlikely when the drugs are used for less than 7 days.

B. Other Parasites: Emetine and dehydroemetine have occasionally been useful in the treatment of infections with *Balantidium coli, Fasciola hepatica,* and *Paragonimus westermani,* but safer drugs should be tried first.

Adverse Effects

Few and (usually) mild adverse effects appear if the drugs are given for 3–5 days; additional mild to severe adverse effects appear if they are given for up to 10 days; serious toxicity is common if they are given for more than 10 days. Therefore, use of these drugs for more than 10 days is contraindicated.

Pain, tenderness, and muscle weakness in the area of the injection are frequent. Occasionally, sterile abscesses develop. Nausea and vomiting, which occur infrequently, are thought to be central in origin. However, diarrhea is induced or exacerbated in many patients, generally beginning several days after the onset of therapy. Minor electrocardiographic changes occur frequently, but severe cardiac toxicity with significant conduction defects is rare. The most serious symptoms and findings are tachycardia and other arrhythmias, precordial pain, and congestive heart failure with dyspnea and hypotension. Generalized muscular weakness—sometimes associated with tenderness, stiffness, aching, or tremors—is reported by many patients. Mild paresthesias are often reported.

Contraindications & Cautions

Hospitalization with careful supervision is essential. Considerable effort should be made to avoid dangerous inadvertent intravenous administration.

Emetine and dehydroemetine should not be used in patients with cardiac or renal disease, in those with a recent history of polyneuritis, or in young children unless alternative drugs have not been effective in controlling severe dysentery or liver abscess. They should not be used during pregnancy.

DILOXANIDE FUROATE

Diloxanide furoate is a dichloroacetamide derivative. The drug is directly amebicidal, but its mechanism of action is not known. It has few pharmacologic effects in vertebrates, but at very high doses it has caused abortion in experimental animals. No teratogenic effects have been reported.

Pharmacokinetics

In the gut, diloxanide furoate is split into diloxanide and furoic acid; about 90% of the diloxanide is rapidly absorbed and then conjugated to form the glucuronide, which is rapidly excreted in the urine. The unabsorbed diloxanide is the active antiamebic substance and is not attacked by gut bacteria. The drug's mechanism of action is not understood.

Clinical Uses (Table 53–3)

A. Asymptomatic and Mild Intestinal Amebiasis: Diloxanide furoate used alone is the drug of choice for asymptomatic infections. For the treatment of mild intestinal disease, it is used with another drug.

B. Other Forms of Amebiasis: Diloxanide furoate is not effective as a primary drug in moderate to severe intestinal disease, liver abscess, or extraintestinal disease since it does not affect trophozoites in the bowel wall, liver, or other extraintestinal tissues. Instead, diloxanide is one of several drugs that can be used to eradicate luminal organisms in conjunction with a nitroimidazole that eliminates both tissue and luminal organisms.

Adverse Effects & Contraindications

Diloxanide furoate does not produce serious adverse effects. Flatulence is common, nausea and abdominal cramps are infrequent, and rashes are rare.

The drug should not be used during pregnancy (adequate safety studies have not been done) or administered to children under 2 years of age.

IODOQUINOL

Iodoquinol (diiodohydroxyquin) is a halogenated hydroxyquinoline that is effective against organisms in the bowel lumen but not against trophozoites in the intestinal wall or extraintestinal tissues.

Iodoquinol

Chemistry & Pharmacokinetics

Iodoquinol is the nonproprietary name for 8-hydroxy-5,7-diiodoquinoline. Its pharmacokinetics are poorly understood. Ninety percent of the drug is not absorbed. The remainder enters the circulation, has a half-life of 11–14 hours, and is excreted in the urine as glucuronides.

The drug may interfere with certain thyroid function tests for up to 6 months by increasing protein-bound serum iodine levels, leading to a decrease in ^{131}I uptake.

Antiamebic Action

The mechanism of action of iodoquinol against trophozoites is unknown.

Clinical Uses

A. Intestinal Amebiasis: Iodoquinol is an alternative drug for the treatment of asymptomatic or mild to moderate intestinal amebiasis. The drug is not effective in the initial treatment of severe intestinal disease but is used in the subsequent eradication of the infection. Although it is not effective against amebomas or extraintestinal forms of the disease, including hepatic amebiasis, it is used to eradicate concurrent intestinal infection.

B. Other Intestinal Parasites: Iodoquinol (650 mg three times daily for 10 days) used alone or with a tetracycline (250 mg four times daily for 7 days) provides adequate treatment for *Dientamoeba fragilis* infections. Iodoquinol is used to treat *Balantidium coli* infection (650 mg three times daily for 10 days).

Adverse Effects

The halogenated hydroxyquinolines, including iodoquinol, can produce severe neurotoxicity, particularly if they are given at greater than recommended doses and for long periods of time. The principal findings associated with this level of use are optic atrophy, visual loss, and peripheral neuropathy. Although these reactions usually improve when the drug is discontinued, some patients have experienced irreversible neurologic damage. Use of an analog, clioquinol, is thought to have been responsible for an outbreak of this neurotoxic syndrome, which was given the name **subacute myelo-optic neuropathy (SMON).** Iodoquinol has not been implicated in the production of neurotoxic effects when used at the standard dosage of 650 mg three times daily for 21 days.

Mild and infrequent adverse effects that can occur at the standard dosage include diarrhea, which usually stops after several days, anorexia, nausea and vomiting, gastritis, abdominal discomfort, slight enlargement of the thyroid gland, headache, skin rashes, and perianal itching. Iodoquinol may be more toxic for infants and young children than for adults.

Contraindications & Cautions

Iodoquinol should be taken with meals. It should not be used for the prophylaxis or treatment of travelers' or nonspecific diarrhea. When used to treat amebiasis, it should be taken only for the prescribed period of time at the recommended dosage. The drug should be used with caution in patients with preexisting optic neuropathy, renal or thyroid disease, or hepatic disease other than that due to amebiasis.

The drug should be discontinued if it produces persistent diarrhea or signs of iodine reactions (various skin eruptions, urticaria, pruritus, fever). It is contraindicated in patients with intolerance to iodine or renal and thyroid disease and probably also in those with severe liver disease not caused by amebiasis.

When the drug is used for infants and young children, for whom it may be more toxic, careful ophthalmologic assessment should be made before and during the course of therapy.

METRONIDAZOLE

Metronidazole is extremely useful in the treatment of extraluminal amebiasis. It effectively eradicates amebic tissue infections (liver abscess, intestinal wall and extraintestinal infections), but a luminal amebicide must be used with it to achieve satisfactory cure rates for luminal infections. Metronidazole kills trophozoites but does not kill cysts of *E histolytica*.

The chemistry, pharmacokinetics, adverse effects, contraindications, and cautions of this drug are described below (see Treatment of Trichomoniasis & Giardiasis).

OTHER NITROIMIDAZOLES

Other nitroimidazole derivatives include **tinidazole, nimorazole, secondizole,** and **ornidazole.** They have similar adverse effects and the same mutagenic action in the *Salmonella* test systems as metronidazole. Because of its short half-life, metronidazole must be administered every 8 hours; the other drugs can be administered at longer intervals. However, with the exception of tinidazole, the other nitroimidazoles have produced poorer results than metronidazole in the treatment of amebiasis and are not available in the USA.

PAROMOMYCIN SULFATE

Paromomycin sulfate, a broad-spectrum antibiotic, is an aminoglycoside derived from *Streptomyces rimosus*. It is closely related to neomycin, kanamycin, and streptomycin in properties and structure. Paromomycin by itself is an alternative drug for the treatment of asymptomatic amebiasis. In mild to moderate intestinal disease, it is an alternative luminal drug used concurrently with a drug active against organisms in the tissues, such as metronidazole. Paromomycin is under evaluation in the topical treatment

of cutaneous leishmaniasis and for chronic cryptosporidial diarrhea in AIDS patients. Paromomycin is both directly and indirectly amebicidal; the indirect effect is caused by its inhibition of bowel bacteria.

Because paromomycin is not significantly absorbed from the gastrointestinal tract (nearly 100% is recovered in the stool), it can be used only as a luminal amebicide and has no effect in extraintestinal amebic infections. The small amount absorbed is slowly excreted unchanged, mainly by glomerular filtration; some excretion also occurs in the bile. In the presence of ulcerative lesions of the bowel, however, and perhaps with impaired gastrointestinal motility, increased absorption may occur. In renal insufficiency, the drug may accumulate to a toxic level. Prolonged nontherapeutic use can result in superinfection with strains of bacteria or yeast resistant to the drug.

OTHER ANTIBIOTICS

Although the tetracyclines have very weak direct amebicidal action, their effects on the gut flora make them (especially oxytetracycline) useful with a luminal amebicide in the eradication of mild to severe intestinal disease. However, because of their potential toxicity, the tetracyclines should not be used to treat pregnant women or children under 8 years of age; erythromycin stearate can be used instead, though it is somewhat less effective.

OTHER PROTOZOAL INFECTIONS

For a list of drugs used in the treatment of other protozoal infections, see Table 53–4.

TREATMENT OF LEISHMANIASIS

A variety of diseases (visceral [kala-azar], cutaneous, and mucocutaneous leishmaniasis) are caused by protozoal parasites of the genus *Leishmania*.

Drugs Used

Treatment of leishmaniasis is not satisfactory because of drug toxicity, the long courses required, treatment failures, and the frequent need for hospitalization. The drug of choice is sodium antimony gluconate (sodium stibogluconate). For some forms of infection, alternative drugs, which are generally more toxic, are amphotericin B and pentamidine. Some forms of Old World cutaneous leishmaniasis do not need treatment or can be treated by physical means (cryotherapy, heat therapy, surgery).

A. Sodium Stibogluconate (Sb^5): Treatment is started with a 200 mg test dose, followed by 20 mg

Sb^5/kg/d. Although the drug can be administered intramuscularly, this route may be locally painful; the intravenous route is preferred when the volume to be injected is high. The drug is given on consecutive days: 20 days for the cutaneous form and 28 days for visceral and mucocutaneous leishmaniasis. Although few adverse effects occur initially, they are more likely to occur with cumulative doses. Most common are gastrointestinal symptoms, fever, and rash; hemolytic anemia and liver, renal, and heart damage are rare. Relapses should be treated at the same dosage levels for at least twice the previous duration. In the USA, the drug is available only from the CDC Drug Service, Centers for Disease Control and Prevention, Atlanta 30333 (404-639-3670).

B. Pentamidine Isethionate: See below.

C. Amphotericin B: Amphotericin B is injected slowly intravenously over 6 hours daily or on alternate days. The initial dosage of 0.25 mg/kg/d is increased to 0.5 mg/kg/d and then to 1 mg/kg/d until a total of about 30 mg/kg has been given. Patients must be closely monitored in hospital, because adverse effects may be severe.

For additional information on the pharmacologic effects, pharmacokinetics, and adverse effects of these drugs, see the references.

TREATMENT OF *PNEUMOCYSTIS CARINII* PNEUMONIA & TRYPANOSOMIASIS

PENTAMIDINE

Chemistry & Pharmacokinetics

Pentamidine is an aromatic diamidine, formulated as isethionate and methanesulfonate salts. Only the isethionate is available in the USA.

Pentamidine is administered parenterally because it is not well absorbed from the gastrointestinal tract. The drug leaves the circulation rapidly and is bound avidly by the tissues, especially the liver, spleen, and kidneys. After daily administration of intramuscular 4

Table 53–4. Drugs used in the treatment of other protozoal infections.[1]

Infecting Organism	Drug(s) of Choice	Alternative Drug(s)
Trypanosoma brucei gambiense and *T b rhodesiense* Hemolymphatic stage	Suramin[2] or eflornithine[3]	Pentamidine isethionate[4]
Late disease with CNS involvement	Melarsoprol[2] or eflornithine[3]	Tryparsamide[5] plus suramin[2]
Trypanosoma cruzi	Nifurtimox[2]	Benznidazole[5]
Babesia species	Clindamycin[4,6] plus quinine[4,6]	None
Balantidium coli	Tetracycline[4]	Iodoquinol[4] or metronidazole[4]
Blastocystis hominis	Iodoquinol[4]	Metronidazole[4]
Cryptosporidium species	Paromomycin[4,6]	Azithromycin[4,6]
Dientamoeba fragilis	Iodoquinol[4] or paromomycin	Tetracycline[4]
Giardia lamblia	Metronidazole[4]	Furazolidone or quinacrine
Isosospora belli	Trimethoprim-sulfamethoxazole[4]	None
Leishmania braziliensis	Stibogluconate sodium[2]	Amphotericin B[4]
Leishmania mexicana	Stibogluconate sodium[2]	Amphotericin B[4]
Leishmania donovani	Stibogluconate sodium[2]	Pentamidine isethionate
Leishmania tropica	Stibogluconate sodium[2]	Topical drugs
Pneumocystis carinii	Trimethoprim-sulfamethoxazole	Pentamidine isethionate
Toxoplasma gondii	Pyrimethamine plus trisulfapyrimidines	Spiramycin[7]

[1]Modified and reproduced, with permission, from Katzung B (editor): *Drug Therapy,* 2nd ed. Appleton & Lange, 1991.
[2]Available in the USA only from the Parasitic Disease Drug Service, Centers for Disease Control and Prevention, Atlanta 30333. Telephone 404-639-3356 during the day; 404-639-2888 nights, weekends, and holidays (emergencies only).
[3]Available in the USA only from the manufacturer, Rhône-Poulenc Rorer, Princeton, New Jersey (609-860-4000). Effectiveness in rhodesiense infections is variable.
[4]Available in the USA but not labeled for this indication.
[5]Not available in the USA; available in some other countries.
[6]Effectiveness not established.
[7]Available in the USA only from the manufacturer, Merrell Dow, Cincinnati, Ohio (513-948-9111).

mg/kg doses, plasma concentrations of pentamidine were 0.3–0.5 μg/mL. The drug is excreted slowly and unchanged in the urine; in the first 24 hours after an intramuscular dose, 4–17% is excreted. Daily dosing results in progressive drug accumulation; with discontinuation of treatment, renal excretion continues for about 8 weeks. Pentamidine does not cross the blood-brain barrier but has been shown to cross the placenta in rats. Only trace amounts of pentamidine appear in the central nervous system, so other trypanosomicides must be used to treat the central nervous system involvement in late-stage African trypanosomiasis.

When pentamidine isethionate powder is reconstituted for inhalation, the median diameter of the nebulized particles is reported to be 0.8–1.4 μm by Respirgard II jet ultrasonic nebulizer. Absorption into the systemic circulation after inhalation appears to be 5% or less than levels that follow intravenous administration.

Antiparasitic & Pharmacologic Actions

A. Antiparasitic Action: The mechanisms of pentamidine's antiparasitic action are not well understood. In vitro studies indicate that the drug may interfere with the synthesis of DNA, RNA, phospholipids, and proteins.

B. Pharmacologic Effects: Pentamidine causes mast cells to release histamine, which, with peripheral sympathoplegia, is the probable cause of the marked hypotensive reaction that follows intravenous administration. Pentamidine may cause severe hypotension when given by the intravenous route. In addition, pentamidine appears to be selectively toxic to B cells of the pancreatic islets. This initially produces an inappropriate, nonsuppressible insulin release leading to hypoglycemia; up to several months later, this may be replaced by hyperglycemia and diabetes mellitus.

No studies have evaluated the carcinogenic or mutagenic potential of pentamidine. Limited pregnancy and reproduction studies show embryotoxicity in rabbits.

Clinical Uses

A. Leishmaniasis: Pentamidine provides an alternative to sodium stibogluconate for the treatment of several forms of leishmaniasis. The dosage is 2–4 mg/kg intramuscularly daily or every other day for up to 15 doses. Treatment may be continued or repeated, particularly in some forms of visceral leishmaniasis.

B. Trypanosomiasis: The drug of choice for treatment of American trypanosomiasis (Chagas' disease) is nifurtimox. In African trypanosomiasis (sleeping sickness), pentamidine (4 mg/kg/d for 10 days) is an alternative in the hemolymphatic stage of the disease to (1) suramin in *Trypanosoma brucei gambiense* and *T b rhodesiense* infections or to (2) eflornithine in *T b gambiense* infection.

C. Pneumocystosis: Treatment should always be based on a proved diagnosis. Trimethoprim-sulfamethoxazole and pentamidine isethionate are equally effective, but severe adverse reactions can occur in up to 50% of patients receiving either drug. In non-AIDS patients, the former drug is preferred because of its lower incidence of adverse effects. In AIDS patients, however, adverse effects are equivalent, and the choice of agent therefore depends on other factors (oral drug activity, preexisting renal disease, need for fluid loading, history of sulfonamide sensitivity). Other alternative drugs in treatment are trimethoprim plus dapsone, atovaquone liquid, primaquine plus clindamycin, and trimetrexate plus folinic acid.

For treatment of active pneumocystosis, pentamidine is administered intravenously or intramuscularly as a single daily dose of 4 mg/kg for 14–21 days. (HIV-infected patients are treated for 21 days.) Some workers recommend 3 mg/kg, which may decrease side effects without reducing efficacy.

In primary and secondary prophylaxis, trimethoprim-sulfamethoxazole is the drug of choice. Alternative drugs are dapsone or aerosolized pentamidine (300 mg inhaled monthly via Respirgard II nebulizer, with or without oral pyrimethamine (50 mg twice weekly) and folinic acid (10 mg twice weekly).

D. Blastomycosis: Pentamidine is sometimes used to treat North American blastomycosis.

Adverse Effects

Pain at the injection site is common; infrequently, a sterile abscess develops and ulcerates.

Occasional reactions include rash, metallic taste, gastrointestinal symptoms, neutropenia, abnormal liver function tests, serum folate depression, hyperkalemia, and hypocalcemia. Hypoglycemia (sometimes clinically inapparent) usually appears 5–7 days after onset of treatment; severe hypoglycemia can then persist for days to several weeks. Hyperglycemia, hyponatremia, and delayed nephrotoxicity with azotemia may occur.

Because severe hypotension may develop even after a single dose of pentamidine, the patient should be recumbent when the drug is given. Blood pressure should be followed closely during administration and thereafter until stable. Emergency resuscitation equipment should be immediately available.

Rare adverse reactions include megaloblastic anemia, acute pancreatitis, thrombocytopenia, thrombocytopenic purpura, toxic epidermal necrolysis, hyperkalemia, renal toxicity, and neurotoxicity (mental changes, seizures, neuropathy). Fatalities have occurred from hypotension, hypoglycemia, or arrhythmias.

Adverse effects associated with inhalation therapy include cough, laryngitis, dyspnea, bronchospasm, and rales.

Contraindications & Cautions

Use pentamidine cautiously in the presence of hypotension, hypertension, latent or clinical diabetes, malnutrition, anemia, thrombocytopenia, or renal, cardiac, or hepatic dysfunction. See manufacturer's recommendations for laboratory test monitoring. The risk of marked hypotension is decreased if the drug is given slowly, preferably over 2 hours; throughout administration, the site must be closely observed for venous extravasation.

ATOVAQUONE

Atovaquone, a new quinone derivative, has been approved by the FDA for treatment of mild to moderate *P. carinii* pneumonia. It has not been evaluated, however, in the treatment of severe disease or in prophylaxis. Preliminary studies suggest that atovaquone may also be effective in treatment of babesiosis, cerebral toxoplasmosis in patients with AIDS, and falciparum malaria when combined with proguanil.

The action of atovaquone is not well understood. Its bioavailability is low but is enhanced when the drug is taken with meals; its protein binding is greater than 99%, and its half-life in AIDS patients is 2.2–2.9 days. Most of the drug is eliminated unchanged in the feces. The dosage is 750 mg taken with food three times daily for 21 days. Frequent side effects are fever and rash; less frequent are cough, nausea, vomiting, diarrhea, headache, and insomnia.

TREATMENT OF TRICHOMONIASIS & GIARDIASIS

METRONIDAZOLE

Metronidazole is the drug of choice in treatment of intestinal and extraintestinal amebiasis and urogenital trichomoniasis and an alternative drug in *Giardia lamblia, Balantidium coli, Blastocystis hominis,* and *Dracunculus medinensis* infections. Its uses in the treatment of infection with bacterial anaerobes are described in Chapter 50. The drug is not significantly effective against facultative anaerobes, obligate aerobes, or *Candida albicans.*

Chemistry & Pharmacokinetics

Oral metronidazole is readily absorbed and permeates all tissues by simple diffusion—including cerebrospinal fluid, breast milk, alveolar bone, liver abscesses, vaginal secretions, and seminal fluid. Intracellular concentrations rapidly approach extracellular levels whether administered orally or intravenously. Following 250 mg and 2000 mg oral doses, peak plasma concentrations are reached in 1–3 hours and average 6 and 40 µg/mL, respectively. Protein binding is low (< 20%); the half-life of the unchanged drug is 7.5 hours. The drug and its metabolites are excreted mainly in the urine. Plasma clearance of metronidazole is decreased in patients with impaired liver function.

Metronidazole

Mechanism of Action

Within anaerobic bacteria and sensitive protozoal cells, the nitro group of metronidazole is chemically reduced by ferredoxin (or ferredoxin-linked metabolic processes). The reduction products appear to be responsible for killing the organisms by reacting with various intracellular macromolecules. Thus, reduction is responsible for the drug's bactericidal (not bacteriostatic) action against anaerobic bacteria.

In amebiasis, metronidazole kills *Entamoeba histolytica* trophozoites but not cysts. In dracunculiasis, its action apparently is anti-inflammatory.

Clinical Uses

A. Urogenital Trichomoniasis: The treatment of choice is metronidazole, given in one of several oral dosage regimens: a single dose of 2 g or 250 mg three times daily or 375 mg twice daily for 7 days. The sexual partner should be treated concomitantly whether or not symptomatic or found to be infected. Re-treatment may be necessary. The male partner should use a condom during the course of treatment. In pregnancy, treatment with metronidazole should be delayed until after the first trimester. Metronidazole-resistant strains of *Trichomonas vaginalis* have been described.

B. Giardiasis: The adult dosage of metronidazole is 250 mg orally three times a day for 5 days. Children should receive 5 mg/kg three times a day for 5 days.

C. Amebiasis: See above.

D. Balantidiasis and *Blastocystis hominis* Infection: If tetracycline is ineffective, give metronidazole, 750 mg three times a day for 5 days.

E. Dracunculiasis: 250 three times daily for 10 days.

F. Anaerobic Infections, Phagedenic Leg Ulcers, Acute Ulcerative Gingivitis, Cancrum Oris, Decubitus Ulcers, Bacterial Vaginitis: See Chapter 50.

G. Others: The usefulness of metronidazole in the management of Crohn's disease and *Helicobacter pylori* infection continues under study.

Adverse Effects & Interactions

Nausea, headache, dry mouth, or a metallic taste in the mouth occur commonly. Urine may be dark or reddish-brown. Infrequent adverse effects include vomiting, diarrhea, insomnia, weakness, dizziness, stomatitis, rash, urethral burning, vertigo, and paresthesias. Taking the drug with meals lessens gastrointestinal irritation. Pancreatitis and severe central nervous system toxicity (ataxia, mental changes, seizures, peripheral neuropathy) are rare.

Metronidazole has a disulfiram-like effect, so that nausea and vomiting occur if alcohol is consumed while the drug is still in the body.

Mutagenicity & Carcinogenicity

Metronidazole and its metabolites recovered from the urine of patients taking the drug are mutagenic in certain strains of *Salmonella typhimurium* (Ames test). Chronic oral administration of very large doses to mice has produced a statistically significant increase in the number of lung and liver tumors. This effect has not been found, however, in any nonrodent species. Although the drug has been used in humans for over 20 years, no increase in congenital abnormalities, stillbirths, or low birth weight has been reported.

No increase in frequency of chromosomal aberration has been found in patients receiving large doses.

Contraindications & Cautions

Caution should be used in prescribing the drug in multiple courses or over long periods or for patients with a history of blood dyscrasias, organic brain disease, or severe hepatic dysfunction. Prudence dictates that unless clearly indicated, metronidazole should be avoided in pregnant women (especially in the first trimester), in nursing women, and in young children.

Metronidazole has been reported to potentiate the anticoagulant effect of coumarin-type anticoagulants. Phenytoin and phenobarbital may accelerate elimination of the drug, while cimetidine may decrease plasma clearance. Lithium toxicity may occur when the drug is used with metronidazole. Metronidazole's disulfiram-like effect requires that all patients receiving it be specifically warned not to use alcohol for 24 hours before the first dose and for 48 hours after the last dose.

Parenteral metronidazole should be given by slow intravenous infusion; see manufacturer's recommendation on dosage and the technique of administration.

PREPARATIONS AVAILABLE

Chloroquine hydrochloride [80% chloroquine base] (Aralen HCl)
Parenteral: 50 mg/mL for injection
Chloroquine phosphate [60% chloroquine base] (generic, Aralen; outside the USA: Avloclor, Resochin)
Oral: 250, 500 mg tablets
Note: Chloroquine sulfate is available outside the USA as Nivaquine.
Chloroquine phosphate with primaquine phosphate
Oral: Tablets containing 500 mg chloroquine phosphate (300 mg base) plus primaquine phosphate 79 mg (45 mg base)
Dehydroemetine (Mebadin)
Parenteral: solution for injection in 30, 60 mg ampules
Note: Available in the USA only from the Drug Service, Centers for Disease Control and Prevention, Atlanta, 1-404-639-3670.
Diloxanide furoate (Furamide)
Oral: 500 mg tablets
Note: Available in the USA only from the Drug Service, Centers for Disease Control and Prevention, Atlanta, 1-404-639-3356.

Doxycycline (generic, Vibramycin, others)
Oral: 50, 100 mg tablets and capsules; 100 mg coated pellets; 25, 50 mg/5 mL suspension from powder; 50 mg/5 mL syrup
Parenteral: powder to reconstitute for injection (100, 200 mg per vial)
Emetine (generic)
Parenteral: 65 mg/mL for injection
Iodoquinol [diiodohydroxyquin] (generic, Yodoxin, Moebequin)
Oral: 210, 650 mg tablets; also available as powder
Note: Iodoquinol is available outside the USA as Embequin, Lanodoxin, Savorquin, Sebaquin.
Mefloquine (Lariam)
Oral: 250 mg tablets (228 mg base). In Canada, the tablets contain 274 mg of the salt (250 mg base)
Metronidazole (generic, Flagyl, others)
Oral: 250, 500 mg tablets
Parenteral: powder to reconstitute for injection (500 mg per vial); ready-to-use for injection (in 500 mg/100 mL vials)
Rectal: suppositories *Note:* Not available in the USA.

Paromomycin (Humatin)
Oral: 250 mg capsules
Pentamidine isethionate (Pentam 300)
Parenteral: for injection (300 mg per vial)
Primaquine (generic)
Oral: 26.3 mg tablets (equivalent to 15 mg base)
Proguanil [chloroguanide] (generic, Paludrine)
Oral: 100 mg tablets
Note: Not available in the USA.
Pyrimethamine (Daraprim)
Oral: 25 mg tablets
Pyrimethamine/dapsone (Maloprim)
Oral: tablets containing 100 mg dapsone/12.5
mg pyrimethamine
Note: Not available in the USA.
Quinacrine [mepacrine] (Atabrine HCl)
Oral: 100 mg tablets
Quinidine gluconate (generic)
Parenteral: 80 mg salt (50 mg base) per mL

Quinine dihydrochloride (generic)
Note: Not available in the USA.
Quinine sulfate [83% quinine base] (generic)
Oral: 130, 195, 200, 300, 325 mg capsules; 260,
325 mg tablets
Stibogluconate [sodium antimony gluconate]
(Pentostam)
Note: Available in the USA only from the Drug
Service, Centers for Disease Control and Pre-
vention, Atlanta, 1-404-639-3670.
**Trimethoprim-sulfamethoxazole
[co-trimoxazole, TMP-SMZ]** (generic,
Bactrim, Septra)
Oral: 80 mg TMP/400 mg SMZ single-strength
tablets; 160 mg TMP/800 mg SMZ double-
strength tablets
Parenteral: 80 mg TMP and 400 mg SMZ per 5
mL for infusion

REFERENCES

General

Drugs for parasitic infections. Med Lett Drugs Ther 1995;37:99.

Malaria

Baird JK et al: Primaquine for prophylaxis against malaria among nonimmune transmigrants in Irian Jaya, Indonesia. Am J Trop Med Hyg 1995;52:479.

Bangchang KN et al: Pharmacokinetics of primaquine in G6PD deficient and G6PD normal patients with vivax malaria. Trans R Soc Trop Med Hyg 1994;88:220.

Bartel PR et al: Visual function and long-term chloroquine treatment. S Afr Med J 1994;84:32.

Bhavnani SN, Preston SL: Monitoring of intravenous quinidine infusion in the treatment of *Plasmodium falciparum* malaria. Ann Pharmacother 1995;29:33.

Bouchaud O et al: Clinical efficacy and pharmacokinetics of micronized halofantrine for the treatment of acute uncomplicated falciparum malaria in nonimmune subjects. Am J Trop Med 1994;51:204.

Bradley DJ, Warhurst DC: Malaria prophylaxis: Guidelines for travellers from Britain. Br Med J 1995;310:709.

Centers for Disease Control: Health information for international travel 1992. Atlanta, Georgia: Public Health Service, U.S. Department of Health and Human Services; Publication No. (CDC) 95–8280.

Churchill D et al: Chloroquine and proguanil prophylaxis in travellers to Kenya. Lancet 1992;339:63.

Cook GC: Malarial prophylaxis. Mefloquine toxicity should limit its use to treatment alone. Br Med J 1995;311:190.

Duc DD et al: The pharmacokinetics of a single dose of artemisinin in healthy Vietnamese subjects. Am J Trop Med Hyg 1994;51:785.

Helsby NA et al: The pharmacokinetics and activation of proguanil in man: Consequences of variability in drug metabolism. Br J Clin Pharmacol 1990;30:593.

Hoffman SL: Diagnosis, treatment, and prevention of malaria. Med North Am 1992;76:1327.

Karbwang J et al: A comparative clinical trial of two different regimens of artemether plus mefloquine in multidrug resistant falciparum malaria. Trans R Soc Trop Med Hyg 1995;89:296.

Karbwang J et al: Quinine toxicity when given with doxycycline and mefloquine. Southeast Asian J Trop Med Public Health 1994;25:397.

Karbwang J, Bangchang KN: Clinical application of mefloquine pharmacokinetics in the treatment of *P falciparum* malaria. Clin Pharmacokinet 1994; 8:491.

Karbwang J, Bangchang KN: Clinical pharmacokinetics of halofantrine. Clin Pharmacokinet 1994;27:104.

Krogstad DJ, Schlesinger PH, Gluzman IY: The specificity of chloroquine. Parasitology Today 1992;8:183.

Metzger W et al: High efficiency of short-term quinine-antibiotic combinations for treating adult malaria patients in an area in which malaria is hyperendemic. Antimicrob Agents Chemother 1995;39:245.

Monlum E et al: Cardiac complications of halofantrine: A prospective study of 20 patients. Trans R Soc Trop Med Hyg 1995;89:430.

Na-Bangchang K et al: The pharmacokinetics of chloroquine in healthy Thai subjects and patients with *Plasmodium vivax* malaria. Br J Clin Pharmacol 1994;38:278.

Nosten F et al: Treatment of multidrug-resistant *Plasmodium falciparum* malaria with 3-day artesunate-mefloquine combination. J Infect Dis 1994;170:971.

Price AH, Fletcher KA: The metabolism and toxicity of primaquine. Prog Clin Biol Res 1986;214:261.

Schwartz IK: Prevention of malaria. Infect Dis Clin North Am 1992;6:313.

Slater AFG: Chloroquine: Mechanism of drug action and resistance in *Plasmodium falciparum.* Pharmacol Ther 1993;57:203.

Toma E et al: Clindamycin with primaquine for *Pneumocystis carinii* pneumonia. Lancet 1989;1:1046.

Treatment with quinidine gluconate of persons with severe *Plasmodium falciparum* infection: Discontinuation of parenteral quinine. From CDC Drug Service. MMWR Morb Mortal Wkly Rep 1991;40:21.

van Hensbroek MB et al: A trial of artemether or quinine in children with cerebral malaria. N Engl J Med 1996; 335:69.

White NJ: Antimalarial pharmacokinetics and treatment regimens. Br J Clin Pharmacol 1992;34:1.

WHO: Development of recommendations for the protection of short-stay travellers to malaria endemic areas: Memorandum from two WHO meetings. Bull WHO 1988;66:177.

WHO: Practical chemotherapy of malaria. Tech Report Series 1990b;No. 805.

WHO: Severe and complicated malaria. Trans R Soc Trop Med Hyg 1990a;84(Suppl 2):1.

Amebiasis, Giardiasis, & Trichomoniasis

Burtin P et al: Safety of metronidazole in pregnancy: A meta-analysis. Am J Obstet Gynecol 1995;172:525.

Dooley CP, O'Morain CAO: Recurrence of hepatic amebiasis after successful treatment with metronidazole. J Clin Gastroenterol 1988;10:339.

Hager WD, Rapp RP: Metronidazole. Obstet Gynecol Clin North Am 1992;19:479.

Johnson PJ: Metronidazole and drug resistance. Parasitol Today 1993;9:183.

Kuntzer T et al: Emetine-induced myopathy and carnitine deficiency. J Neurol 1990;237:495.

McAuley JB et al: Diloxanide furoate for treating asymptomatic *Entamoeba histolytica* cyst passers: 14 years' experience in the United States. Clin Infect Dis 1992;15:464.

McAuley JB, Juranek DD: Luminal agents in the treatment of amebiasis. Clin Infect Dis 1992;14:1161.

McAuley JB, Juranek DD: Paromomycin in the treatment of mild-to-moderate intestinal amebiasis. Clin Infect Dis 1992;15:551.

Mengel MB et al: The effectiveness of single-dose metronidazole therapy for patients and their partners with bacterial vaginosis. J Family Pract 1989;28:163.

Plaisance KI, Quintilliani R, Nightingale CM: The pharmacokinetics of metronidazole and its metabolites in critically ill patients. J Antimicrob Chemother 1988;21:195.

Radvin JI: Amebiasis. Clin Infect Dis 1995;20:1453.

Reed S: Amebiasis: An update. Clin Infect Dis 1992;14:385.

Thoren K et al: Treatment of asymptomatic amebiasis in homosexual men: Clinical trials with metronidazole, tinidazole, and diloxanide furoate. Sex Transm Dis 1990; 17:72.

Wright CW et al: Antiamoebic activity of indole analogues of emetine with in-vitro potency greater than that of emetine J Pharm Pharmacol Suppl 1990;42:1.

Leishmaniasis, Pneumocystosis, & Toxoplasmosis

Amantea MA et al: Population pharmacokinetics of pyrimethamine with and without dapsone in patients with HIV. Pharmacotherapy 1994;14:374.

Atovaquone: A review of its pharmacologic properties and therapeutic efficacy in opportunistic infections. Drug Evaluation 1995;50:176.

Black JR et al: Clindamycin and primaquine therapy for mild-to-moderate episodes of *Pneumocystis carinii* pneumonia in patients with AIDS: AIDS clinical trials group 044. Clin Infect Dis 1994;18:905.

Bozzette SA et al: A randomized trial of three antipneumocystis agents in patients with advanced human immunodeficiency virus infection. N Engl J Med 1995;332:693.

Bronner U et al: Pharmacokinetics and adverse reactions after a single dose of pentamidine in patients with *Trypanosoma gambiense* sleeping sickness. Br J Clin Pharmacol 1995;39:289.

Franke ED et al: Efficacy and toxicity of sodium stibogluconate for mucosal leishmaniasis. Ann Intern Med 1990;113:934.

Franke ED et al: Efficacy of 28-day and 40-day regimens of sodium stibogluconate (Pentostam) in the treatment of mucosal leishmaniasis. Am J Trop Med Hyg 1994;51:77.

Giri OP: Treatment of visceral leishmaniasis unresponsive to pentamidine with amphotericin B. J Assoc Physicians India 1994;42:688.

Hepburn NC et al: Hepatotoxicity of sodium stibogluconate therapy for American cutaneous leishmaniasis. Trans R Soc Trop Med Hyg 1994;88:453.

Herwaldt BL, Berman JD: Recommendations for treating leishmaniasis with sodium stibogluconate (Pentostam) and review of pertinent clinical studies. Am J Trop Med Hyg 1992;46:296.

Kovacs JA et al: Efficacy of atovaquone in treatment of toxoplasmosis in patients with AIDS. Lancet 1992;340:637.

Montgomery AB et al: Pentamidine aerosol versus trimethoprim-sulfamethoxazole for *Pneumocystis carinii* in acquired immune deficiency syndrome. Am J Respir Crit Care Med 1995;151:1068.

Murphy K et al: Pyrimethamine alone as long-term suppressive therapy in cerebral toxoplasmosis. Am J Med 1994;96:95.

Neil RA et al: The sensitivity of *Leishmania* species to aminosidine. J Antimicrob Chemother 1995;35:577.

Opravel M et al: Once-weekly administration of dapsone pyrimethamine vs aerosolized pentamidine as combined prophylaxis of *Pneumocystis carinii* pneumonia and toxoplasmic encephalitis in human immunodeficiency virus-infected patients. Clin Infect Dis 1995;20:531.

Opravel M et al: Once-weekly administration of dapsone-pyrimethamine vs. aerosolized pentamidine as combined prophylaxis for *Pneumocystis carinii* pneumonia and toxoplasmotic encephalitis in human immunodeficiency virus-infected patients. Clin Infect Dis 1995;20:531.

Podzamczer D et al: Intermittent trimethoprim-sulfamethoxazole compared with dapsone-pyrimethamine for the simultaneous primary prophylaxis of pneumocystis pneumonia and toxoplasmosis in patients infected with HIV. Ann Intern Med 1995;122:755.

Soto J et al: Successful treatment of New World cutaneous leishmaniasis with a combination of topical paromomycin/methylbenzethonium chloride and injectable meglumine antimonate. Clin Infect Dis 1995;20:47.

Soto J et al: Successful treatment of Colombian cutaneous leishmaniasis with four injections of pentamidine. Am J Trop Med Hyg 1994;50:107.

54

Clinical Pharmacology of the Anthelmintic Drugs

Robert S. Goldsmith, MD, DTM&H

CHEMOTHERAPY OF HELMINTHIC INFECTIONS

Anthelmintic drugs are used to eradicate or reduce the numbers of helminthic parasites in the intestinal tract or tissues of the body. As noted in Chapter 52, these parasites have many biochemical and physiologic processes in common with their human hosts, yet there are subtle differences that are beginning to yield to pharmacologic investigation. Most of the drugs described below were discovered by traditional screening methods; their mechanisms have been clarified only recently. These mechanisms (where known) are described in Chapter 52.

Table 54–1 lists the major helminthic infections and provides a guide to the drug of choice and alternative drugs for each infection. In the text that follows, these drugs are arranged alphabetically.

Most anthelmintics in use today are active against specific parasites, and some are toxic. Therefore, parasites must be identified before treatment is started, usually by finding the parasite, eggs, or larvae in the feces, urine, blood, sputum, or tissues of the host.

Administration of Anthelmintic Drugs

Unless otherwise indicated, oral drugs should be taken with water during or after meals. In posttreatment follow-up for intestinal nematode infections, stools should be reexamined about 2 weeks after the end of treatment.

Dosages for Children

Dosages for infants and children are on a less secure basis than for adults; when not given in milligrams per kilogram of body weight (or otherwise specified), the dosage may be based on surface area or calculated as a fraction of the adult dose based on Clark's rule or Young's rule (see Chapter 60).

Contraindications

Pregnancy and ulcers of the gastrointestinal tract are contraindications for most of the drugs listed. Specific contraindications are given in the discussions that follow.

ALBENDAZOLE

Albendazole, a broad-spectrum oral anthelmintic, is used for pinworm infection, ascariasis, trichuriasis, strongyloidiasis, and infections with both hookworm species. Albendazole is also the drug of choice in hydatid disease and cysticercosis. In the USA, albendazole has been approved for use in hydatid disease and cysticercosis.

Chemistry & Pharmacokinetics

Albendazole is a benzimidazole carbamate.

Albendazole

After oral administration, albendazole is erratically absorbed and then rapidly undergoes first-past metabolism in the liver to albendazole sulfoxide and, to a lesser extent, to other metabolites. About 3 hours after a 400 mg oral dose, the sulfoxide attains a maximum plasma concentration of 250–300 ng/mL; its plasma half-life is 8–9 hours. In large part, the sulfoxide binds to protein and is distributed to the tissues, including bile and cerebrospinal fluid, and en-

Table 54–1. Drugs for the treatment of helminthic infections.

Infecting Organism	Drug of Choice	Alternative Drugs
Roundworms (nematodes)		
Ascaris lumbricoides (roundworm)	Pyrantel pamoate or mebendazole	Albendazole,[2] piperazine, or levamisole[2]
Trichuris trichiura (whipworm)	Mebendazole	Albendazole[2] or oxantel/pyrantel pamoate[1]
Necator americanus (hookworm); *Ancylostoma duodenale* (hookworm)	Pyrantel pamoate[2] or mebendazole	Albendazole[2] or levamisole[2]
Combined infection with *Ascaris, Trichuris,* and hookworm	Mebendazole or albendazole[2]	Oxantel/pyrantel pamoate[1]
Combined infection with *Ascaris* and hookworm	Mebendazole or pyrantel pamoate[2]	Albendazole[2]
Strongyloides stercoralis (threadworm)	Ivermectin[3]	Thiabendazole, albendazole[2,4]
Enterobius vermicularis (pinworm)	Mebendazole or pyrantel pamoate	Albendazole[2]
Trichinella spiralis (trichinosis)	Mebendazole[2,4] or thiabendazole;[4] add corticosteroids for severe infection	Albendazole[4,5]; add corticosteroids for severe infection
Trichostrongylus species	Pyrantel pamoate[2] or mebendazole[2]	Albendazole[2] or levamisole[2]
Cutaneous larva migrans (creeping eruption)	Albendazole[5] or ivermectin[2]	Thiabendazole
Visceral larva migrans	Thiabendazole[8] or albendazole[2]	Mebendazole[2,4] or ivermectin[4]
Angiostrongylus cantonensis	Levamisole[2,4] or thiabendazole[4]	Albendazole[2,4] or mebendazole[2,4]
Wuchereria bancrofti (filariasis); *Brugia malayi* (filariasis); tropical eosinophilia; *Loa loa* (loiasis)	Diethylcarbamazine[6]	Ivermectin[3,7]
Onchocerca volvulus (onchocerciasis)	Ivermectin	Suramin[7]
Dracunculus medinensis (guinea worm)	Metronidazole[2]	Thiabendazole[2] or mebendazole[2]
Capillaria philippinensis (intestinal capillariasis)	Albendazole[1,5]	Mebendazole[2] or thiabendazole[2]
Flukes (trematodes)		
Schistosoma haematobium (bilharziasis)	Praziquantel	Metrifonate[1]
Schistosoma mansoni	Praziquantel	Oxamniquine
Schistosoma japonicum	Praziquantel	
Clonorchis sinensis (liver fluke); *Opisthorchis* species	Praziquantel[2]	Albendazole[2,4] or mebendazole[2,4]
Paragonimus westermani (lung fluke)	Praziquantel[2]	Bithionol[7]
Fasciola hepatica (sheep liver fluke)	Bithionol[7] or triclabendazole[1,4,9]	Praziquantel[2,8] or emetine or dehydroemetine[7]
Fasciolopsis buski (large intestinal fluke)	Praziquantel[2] or niclosamide[2]	Tetrachloroethylene[1]
Heterophyes heterophyes; Metagonimus yokogawai (small intestinal flukes)	Praziquantel[2] or niclosamide[2]	Tetrachloroethylene[1]
Tapeworms (cestodes)		
Taenia saginata (beef tapeworm)	Niclosamide or praziquantel[2]	Mebendazole[2,4]
Diphyllobothrium latum (fish tapeworm)	Niclosamide or praziquantel[2]	
Taenia solium (pork tapeworm)	Niclosamide or praziquantel[2]	
Cysticercosis (pork tapeworm larval stage)	Albendazole	Praziquantel[2]
Hymenolepis nana (dwarf tapeworm)	Praziquantel[2]	Niclosamide

(*continued*)

Table 54–1. Drugs for the treatment of helminthic infections (cont'd).

Infecting Organism	Drug of Choice	Alternative Drugs
Tapeworms (cestodes) *Hymenolepis diminuta* (rat tapeworm); *Dipylidium caninum*	Niclosamide or praziquantel[2]	
Echinococcus granulosus (hydatid disease); *Echinococcus multilocularis*	Albendazole	Mebendazole[2,8]

[1]Not available in the USA but available in some other countries.
[2]Available in the USA but not labeled for this indication (see Unlabeled Use, Chapter 65).
[3]Available in the USA from Merck Sharpe & Dohme. Telephone 610-397-2979.
[4]Effectiveness not established.
[5]Available in the USA.
[6]Available in the USA from Wyeth-Ayerst Laboratories. Telephone 610-971-5772.
[7]Available in the USA only from the Parasitic Disease Drug Service, Parasitic Diseases Branch, Centers for Disease Control and Prevention, Atlanta 30333. Telephone 404-639-3670.
[8]Effectiveness is low.
[9]A veterinary drug, not approved for human use.

ters hydatid cysts. The metabolites are mainly excreted in the urine; only a small amount is excreted in the feces. Absorption of the drug is often about fourfold greater when it is taken with a fatty meal as compared with the fasting state.

Anthelmintic Actions & Pharmacologic Effects

A. Anthelmintic Actions: Albendazole blocks glucose uptake by larval and adult stages of susceptible parasites, depleting their glycogen stores and decreasing formation of ATP. As a result the parasite is immobilized and dies. The drug has larvicidal effects in necatoriasis and ovicidal effects in ascariasis, ancylostomiasis, and trichuriasis. The drug is teratogenic and embryotoxic in some animal species.

B. Pharmacologic Effects: Albendazole does not have pharmacologic effects in humans at therapeutic oral doses (5 mg/kg).

Clinical Uses

Albendazole is probably best administered on an empty stomach when it is used against intraluminal parasites but with a fatty meal when used against tissue parasites.

A. Ascariasis, Trichuriasis, and Hookworm and Pinworm Infections: For pinworm infections, ancylostomiasis, and light ascariasis, necatoriasis, or trichuriasis, the treatment for adults and children over 2 years of age is a single dose of 400 mg orally. In pinworm infection, the dose should be repeated in 2 weeks. This achieves 100% cure rates in pinworm infection and high cure rates for the other infections, or marked reduction in egg counts in those not cured. Although the optimal dosage for achieving high cure rates in heavy ascariasis or satisfactorily reducing worm burden in moderate to heavy necatoriasis and trichuriasis is not established, 400 mg/d for 2–3 days may be tried.

B. Strongyloidiasis: The objective of treatment in strongyloidiasis must be cure. A dosage schedule to

accomplish this is not established; 400 mg twice daily for 7–14 days (with meals) may be tried.

C. Hydatid Disease: A current treatment schedule is 800 mg/kg in divided doses with meals for 3 months. Depending on the clinical results, treatment may need to be extended. Bone cysts may require up to a year of treatment. The duration of treatment for *Echinococcus multilocularis* is not established but is perhaps 5 years to life. Among 253 patients treated in multiple studies, the results among patients with liver cysts were as follows: 33% cured (disappearance or shrinkage), 44% improved, 21% no change, and 2% worse. In patients with lung cysts, 40% were cured, 37% improved, 22% showed no change, and 1% got worse. In follow-ups extending to 7 years, recurrences have been rare. To sterilize cysts at the time of surgery, albendazole should be given at the standard dosage for at least 4 days pre- and 1 month post-surgery. Combined usage of albendazole and praziquantel to enhance effectiveness continues under evaluation since praziquantel is an effective scolicide but has little effect on the germinal membrane.

D. Neurocysticercosis: Medical treatment—usually preferable to surgery—is most effective for parenchymal cysts, less so for intraventricular, subarachnoid, or racemose cysts, and probably has no effect on cysts that show enhancement or calcification. In short-term (3- to 6-month) follow-up of comparative studies with praziquantel, albendazole is more effective and the drug of choice. Other potential advantages of albendazole over praziquantel are that it is less expensive; that it achieves better penetration of cerebrospinal fluid; and that when corticosteroids are given concomitantly, the plasma concentration of albendazole increases but that of praziquantel decreases. A suggested approach is to give a course of albendazole plus steroid; if the response is inadequate, follow with a course of praziquantel. For selected patients, some clinicians wait 3 months to see if cysts will spontaneously disappear. Treatment should be conducted in hospital.

The albendazole dosage schedule of 15 mg/kg/d for 8 days is as effective as a 30-day course. Within a few days after the start of treatment, inflammatory reactions around dying parasites may be manifested by headache (analgesics may be sufficient for mild symptoms), vomiting (try antiemetics), hyperthermia, mental changes, and convulsions; decompensation with death is very rare. It remains controversial whether to give a steroid concomitantly to avoid or diminish this reactive inflammation or to use a steroid only if marked symptoms appear or increase. The inflammatory reaction may occur even when steroids are given in advance. One steroid dosage is prednisone, 30 mg/d in two or three divided doses starting 1–2 days before use of the drug and continuing with diminishing doses for about 14 days afterward. The reaction usually subsides in 48–72 hours, but continuing severity may require steroids in higher dosage and mannitol. Following treatment, 50% cure rates (disappearance of cysts and clearing of symptoms) have been reported. Of the remaining patients, many have amelioration of signs and symptoms, including seizures. Treatment is contraindicated during the acute phase of cysticercotic encephalitis if intracranial hypertension is present.

E. Other Infections: At a dosage of 200–400 mg twice daily, albendazole is the drug of choice in treatment of **cutaneous larval migrans** (give daily for 3–5 days) and in **intestinal capillariasis** (10-day course). With a dosage of 400 mg twice daily for 1 month followed by maintenance therapy, albendazole often results in clinical improvement of chronic diarrhea (it does not eradicate the organism) in *Enterocytozoon bieneusi* and *Septata intestinalis*—AIDS microsporidial infections. At a dosage of 400 mg twice daily, albendazole may be useful in **gnathostomiasis** (21-day course) and **trichinosis** (15-day course); for severe symptoms in the latter infection, prednisolone, 40 mg/d, should be given concurrently for about 3 days and then gradually withdrawn. Cure rates were 90% in **clonorchiasis** and 33% in **opisthorchiasis** at a dosage of 400 mg twice daily for 7 days, with a marked reduction in egg counts in those not cured. There have been isolated reports of some effectiveness in treatment of **toxocariasis** and **loiasis** and conflicting reports of effectiveness in **giardiasis** and **taeniasis.** In experimental animals, the drug showed promise in **fascioliasis** and **angiostrongyliasis.**

Adverse Reactions

When used for 1–3 days, albendazole seems to be nearly free of significant adverse effects. Mild and transient epigastric distress, diarrhea, headache, nausea, dizziness, lassitude, and insomnia have been attributed to the drug in up to 6% of patients, but in two placebo-controlled studies, the incidence of adverse effects was similar in treatment and control groups.

In 3-month treatment courses for hydatid disease, the following toxicities were observed: reversible low-grade aminotransferase elevations in 17% and jaundice in one patient; gastrointestinal symptoms (nausea, vomiting, abdominal pain) in 4%; alopecia in 2%; rash or pruritus in 1%; and leukopenia to under 2900/μL in 2%. In two patients, pronounced eosinophilia appeared, probably related to cyst fluid leakage. Long-term toxicity studies in animals showed diarrhea, anemia, hypotension, marrow depression, and liver function test abnormalities, varying with different species.

Contraindications & Cautions

The safety of albendazole has not been established in children under 2 years of age. Because the drug is teratogenic and embryotoxic in some animal species, it should not be used in pregnancy. It may be contraindicated in the presence of cirrhosis.

ANTIMONY COMPOUNDS

The trivalent antimony compounds were for many years the principal drugs for the treatment of schistosomiasis (bilharziasis), but because of their toxicity and difficulty of administration, they should no longer be used. Pentavalent stibogluconate is still used in the therapy of leishmaniasis (Chapter 53).

BITHIONOL

Bithionol is the drug of choice for the treatment of **fascioliasis (sheep liver fluke),** although relatively little is known about its degree of effectiveness. Of the alternative drugs, emetine and dehydroemetine are toxic and praziquantel is usually not effective.

Bithionol is also an alternative drug in the treatment of pulmonary paragonimiasis. With one course of treatment, cure rates are over 90%. Several courses may be necessary in acute cerebral paragonimiasis, but the drug is not useful in chronic cerebral paragonimiasis. The mode of action of bithionol against *Paragonimus westermani* has not been established.

Pharmacokinetics

After ingestion, bithionol reaches peak blood levels in 4–8 hours. At a daily dosage of 50 mg/kg orally in three divided doses for 5 days, a serum level of 50–200 μg/mL is maintained. Excretion appears to be mainly via the kidney.

Clinical Uses

For treatment of paragonimiasis and fascioliasis, the dosage of bithionol is 30–50 mg/kg in two or three divided doses, given orally after meals on alternate days for 10–15 doses. For pulmonary paragonimiasis, three negative sputum and stool specimens obtained 3 months after completion of treatment indicate eradication of the parasite. Within 4–6 months, chest film abnormalities will disappear in up to 75% of cases.

Adverse Reactions

Adverse effects, which occur in up to 40% of patients, are generally mild and transient, but occasionally their severity requires interruption of therapy. Diarrhea and abdominal cramps are most common; these may diminish or stop after several days of treatment. Anorexia, nausea, vomiting, dizziness, and headache may also occur. Pruritic, urticarial, or papular skin rashes are less frequent and usually begin after a latent period of 1 week or more of therapy; they are probably allergic in nature, resulting from release of antigens from dying worms. Other infrequent reactions are lassitude, pyrexia, tinnitus, insomnia, proteinuria, and leukopenia. Hypersensitivity reactions to the drug itself are rare.

Contraindications & Cautions

Bithionol should be used with caution in children under 8 years of age because of limited experience in that age group. Treatment should be discontinued if serial liver function and hematologic tests suggest development of toxic hepatitis or leukopenia.

Treatment apparently does not worsen the neurologic condition of patients with cerebral paragonimiasis, but this possibility should be kept in mind and steroid therapy initiated if indicated.

DIETHYLCARBAMAZINE CITRATE

Diethycarbamazine is a drug of choice in the treatment of filariasis, loiasis, and tropical eosinophilia. It is an unsatisfactory alternative drug for eradication of microfilariae in onchocerchiasis, and its use should be avoided if ivermectin is available. In bancroftian filariasis, combined therapy with diethylcarbamazine and ivermectin is under evaluation.

Chemistry & Pharmacokinetics

Diethycarbamazine, a synthetic piperazine derivative, is marketed as a citrate salt that contains 51% of the active base. It is rapidly absorbed from the gastrointestinal tract; after a 0.5 mg/kg dose, peak plasma levels of 100–150 ng/mL are reached within 1–2 hours. The plasma half-life is 2–3 hours in the presence of acidic urine but about 10 hours if the urine is alkaline. The drug rapidly equilibrates with all tissues except fat. It is excreted, principally in the urine, as unchanged drug and the N-oxide metabolite. Dosage may have to be reduced in patients with persistent urinary alkalosis or renal impairment.

Anthelmintic Actions & Pharmacologic Effects

Diethycarbamazine immobilizes microfilariae (which results in their displacement in tissues) and alters their surface structure, making them more susceptible to destruction by host defense mechanisms. The mode of action of diethylcarbamazine against adult worms is unknown.

Diethycarbamazine has shown in vivo and in vitro immunosuppressive actions, the mechanism of which is imperfectly understood. The drug has had no teratogenic effects in experimental animals.

Clinical Uses

The drug should be taken after meals.

A. Wuchereria bancrofti, Brugia malayi, Brugia timori, Loa loa: Diethycarbamazine is the drug of choice for treatment of infections with these parasites, given its high order of therapeutic efficacy and lack of serious toxicity. Microfilariae of all species are rapidly killed; adult parasites are killed more slowly, often requiring several courses of treatment. The drug is highly effective against adult *L loa*. The extent to which *W bancrofti* and *B malayi* adults are killed is not known; however, if therapy is adequate, microfilariae do not reappear in the majority of patients, which suggests that adult worms are either killed or permanently sterilized.

These infections are treated with 2 mg/kg three times a day for 3 weeks. For *W bancrofti* infections, to reduce the incidence of allergic reactions to dying microfilariae, a single dose (2 mg/kg) is administered on the first day, two doses on the second day, and three doses on the third day and thereafter. For *L loa* (with its risk of encephalopathy) or *B malayi* infection, the same schedule should be used, but individual doses should start at 1 mg/kg once on the first day and gradually increase over 5–6 days.

Antihistamines may be given for the first 4–5 days of diethylcarbamazine therapy to reduce the incidence of allergic reactions. Corticosteroids should be started and doses of diethylcarbamazine temporarily lowered or interrupted if severe reactions occur.

Blood should be checked for microfilariae several weeks after treatment is completed; a course may be repeated after 3–4 weeks. Cure may require several courses of treatment over 1–2 years.

Spaced treatment doses (weekly to monthly) continue to be evaluated as a macrofilaricide. The drug may also be used in prophylaxis—300 mg weekly or 300 mg on three successive days each month for loiasis and 50 mg monthly for bancroftian and Malayan filariasis.

B. Onchocerca volvulus: Because of its much lower incidence and severity of adverse reactions, ivermectin is the drug of choice and has largely replaced diethylcarbamazine. Both drugs temporarily kill microfilariae but are poorly effective against adult worms. If diethylcarbamazine is used in onchocerciasis treatment, suramin (a toxic drug) must be added to the regimen to kill the adult worms. However, because of the severity of reactions that occur as diethylcarbamazine kills microfilariae, the drug should be administered only by experts and, preferably, treatment should be initiated in hospital. (See references for drug dosages, toxicity, and precautions.)

C. Tropical Eosinophilia: Diethycarbamazine is given orally at a dosage of 2 mg/kg three times daily for 7 days.

D. Other Parasites: Diethylcarbamazine is effective in *Mansonella streptocerca* infections, since it kills both adults and microfilariae. Limited information suggests that the drug is not effective, however, against adult *Mansonella ozzardi* or *M perstans* and that it has only a low order of effectiveness or is inactive against microfilariae of these parasites. Diethylcarbamazine is not active against *Dirofilaria immitis.*

In toxocariasis, diethylcarbamazine may be tried, but its efficacy is not established. The drug has been superseded in treatment of ascariasis and cutaneous larva migrans.

E. Mass Therapy: An important application of diethylcarbamazine therapy has been its use for mass treatment of *W bancrofti* infections to reduce transmission. A common regimen is one dose each week or month for 12 doses. Often, adverse reactions discourage community participation. However, when the drug is administered in low doses in medicated salt, it is stable in cooking, appears to be free of adverse effects, and is active as a microfilaricide and possibly as a macrofilaricide.

Adverse Reactions

A. Drug-Induced Reactions: Reactions to diethylcarbamazine itself are mild and transient and start within 2–4 hours: headache, malaise, anorexia, and weakness are frequent; nausea, vomiting, dizziness, and sleepiness occur less often.

B. Reactions Induced by Dying Parasites: Adverse effects also occur as a result of the release of foreign proteins from dying microfilariae or adult worms in sensitized patients. Eosinophilia and leukocytosis are usually intensified.

1. Reactions in onchocerciasis–Adverse reactions (sometimes after a single dose) affect the skin and eyes in most patients; systemic reactions may also occur (see references for details). The reactions may be severe, especially if infection is heavy, if pruritus is intense, or if microfilariae are near the eyes. Vision can be permanently damaged as a result of dying microfilariae in the optic disks and retina.

2. Reactions in *W bancrofti, B malayi,* and *L loa* infections–Reactions to dying microfilariae are usually mild in *W bancrofti* (in up to 25% of patients), more intense in *B malayi,* and occasionally severe in *L loa* infections. Reactions include fever, malaise, papular rash, headache, gastrointestinal symptoms, cough, chest pains, and muscle or joint pains. Leukocytosis is common; eosinophilia and proteinuria may occur. In *W bancrofti* and *B malayi* infections, symptoms are most likely to occur in patients with heavy loads of microfilariae but may also occur even if the patient is apparently amicrofil-

aremic. In loiasis, severe reactions are more likely to occur if microfilaria counts are greater than 25/µL of blood; in such patients, cytopheresis has been used to reduce parasite loads before starting diethylcarbamazine. Retinal hemorrhages have been described and, rarely, encephalopathy that can be life-threatening.

Between the third and twelfth days of treatment, local reactions may occur in the vicinity of dying adult or immature worms. This includes lymphangitis with localized swellings or nodules or lymph abscesses in *W bancrofti* and *B malayi,* small wheals in the skin in *L loa,* and flat papules in *M streptocerca* infections.

Contraindications & Cautions

There are no absolute contraindications to the use of diethylcarbamazine, but caution is advised in patients with hypertension or renal disease.

Patients suspected of having malaria should be treated before they are given diethylcarbamazine, which may provoke a relapse in asymptomatic malaria infections.

Patients with attacks of lymphangitis due to *W bancrofti* or *B malayi* should be treated during a quiescent period between attacks.

EMETINE HYDROCHLORIDE

Emetine and dehydroemetine (less toxic than emetine) are alternative drugs for the treatment of *Fasciola hepatica* infection. Both drugs are sometimes effective but are more toxic than triclabendazole or bithionol (the drugs of choice). General pharmacologic information, dosage, and precautions in emetine usage are presented in Chapter 53.

IVERMECTIN

Ivermectin is the drug of choice in individual and mass treatment of onchocerciasis and for strongyloidiasis. It is also an alternative drug for scabies. It may also prove useful in the treatment of other forms of filariasis and cutaneous larva migrans.

Chemistry & Pharmacokinetics

Ivermectin, a semisynthetic macrocyclic lactone, is a mixture of avermectin B_{1a} and B_{1b}. It is derived from the soil actinomycete *Streptomyces avermitilis.*

Ivermectin is given only orally in humans. The drug is rapidly absorbed, reaching maximum plasma concentrations (about 50 µg/L) at 4 hours after a 12 mg dose. The drug has a wide tissue distribution and a volume of distribution of about 50 L. It apparently enters the eye slowly and to a limited extent. Its half-life is about 12 hours. Excretion of the drug and its metabolites is almost exclusively in the feces.

Anthelmintic Actions & Pharmacologic Effects

A. Anthelmintic Actions: Ivermectin appears to paralyze nematodes and arthropods (which may lead to their death) by intensifying GABA-mediated transmission of signals in peripheral nerves (see Chapter 52). In onchocerciasis, ivermectin is microfilaricidal and affects embryogenesis. After a single standard dose, microfilariae in the skin diminish rapidly within 2–3 days, remain low for months, and then gradually increase; microfilariae in the anterior chamber of the eye decrease slowly over months, eventually clear, and then gradually return. The single-dose treatment is not effective against adult worms except for its action for some months that blocks release of microfilariae from worm uteri, which is followed by degeneration of microfilariae. With repeated doses of ivermectin at 3-month or yearly intervals, the drug does appear to have a low-level macrofilaricidal action and to permanently reduce microfilarial production. The mode of action of ivermectin on microfilariae is uncertain, ie, whether it paralyzes them, facilitating their removal by the reticuloendothelial system, or kills them directly.

B. Pharmacologic Action: The drug is without known pharmacologic or toxic effects in humans, partly because ivermectin does not readily cross the blood-brain barrier.

In animal studies, ivermectin appears to have a wide margin of safety. However, in mice given high doses, teratogenic effects and occasional unexplained maternal deaths have occurred.

Clinical Uses

A. Onchocerciasis: Treatment is with a single oral dose of 150 μg/kg with water on an empty stomach. The optimum frequency of treatment to control symptoms and prevent disease progression remains to be determined. In one schedule, the dose is repeated at 3-month intervals for 12 months; in another, the dose is repeated monthly three times. Thereafter, treatment is repeated at 12-month intervals until the adult worms die, which may take 10 years or longer. With the first treatment only, patients with microfilariae in the cornea or anterior chamber may benefit from several days of prednisone treatment (1 mg/kg/d) to avoid inflammatory eye reactions.

WHO no longer recommends diethylcarbamazine for treatment of onchocerciasis. In comparison studies, ivermectin is as effective as diethylcarbamazine in reducing the number of microfilariae (which are responsible for the pathologic features of the disease). Moreover, severe systemic and ocular reactions are seen with diethylcarbamazine, and these are much less frequent and severe with ivermectin. In addition, the reduction in microfilariae induced by ivermectin persists longer, and the posttreatment ocular changes seen in diethylcarbamazine-treated patients (including punctate keratitis, chorioretinitis, and optic atrophy) are rare or not seen with ivermectin.

B. Bancroftian Filariasis: In comparisons of ivermectin and diethylcarbamazine, the two drugs appear to be equally efficacious in reducing microfilaria burdens; mild adverse effects (myalgia, headache, fever) are similar in some studies but less for ivermectin in others. However, as ivermectin is not macrofilaricidal, diethylcarbamazine is still needed to kill the adult parasites. Under evaluation and promising in control is combined mass treatment with 400 μg/kg of ivermectin plus 6 mg/kg of diethylcarbamazine; this results in marked reduction in microfilariae (that persists for up to 12 months) with relatively few adverse reactions.

C. Strongyloidiasis: Ivermectin is the drug of choice in treatment of strongyloidiasis; a single dose of 200 μg/kg appears to achieve cure rates of over 80%. Repeat treatments may effect additional cures.

D. Other Parasites: Ivermectin reduces microfilariae in *Brugia malayi* and *Mansonella ozzardi* infections but not in *M perstans*. In **loiasis,** although the drug reduces microfilaria concentrations, it can induce a severe reaction in a small percentage of patients whose microfilaria load is over 3000/mL. Ivermectin is also effective in **scabies** and **cutaneous larva migrans** and in eliminating a large proportion of **ascarid worms.**

Adverse Reactions

The adverse effects of ivermectin are the Mazotti reaction, which starts on the first day after a single oral dose and peaks on the second day. The reaction is due to killing of microfilariae, not to drug toxicity, and its intensity correlates with skin microfilaria loads. In indigenous adults, the reaction occurs in 5–30% of persons, but it is generally mild, well tolerated, of short duration, and controlled by aspirin and antihistamines. The reaction in expatriate adults— perhaps also in indigenous children—may occur more frequently and be more severe.

The Mazotti reaction includes fever (occasionally intermittent for several days), headache, dizziness, somnolence, weakness, rash, increased pruritus, diarrhea, joint and muscle pains, hypotension, tachycardia, lymphadenitis, lymphangitis, and peripheral edema. A more intense Mazotti reaction occurs in 1–3% of persons and a severe reaction in 0.1%, including high fever, hypotension, and bronchospasm. Hypotension can be prevented by advising persons who are weak or dizzy to lie down. The Mazotti reaction diminishes with repeated dosing. Steroids may be necessary for several days. Swellings and abscesses occasionally occur at 1–3 weeks, presumably at sites of adult worms.

Some patients develop punctate corneal opacities several days after treatment. Other uncommon ophthalmologic reactions (all of which can occur with the disease itself) are eyelid edema, anterior uveitis, conjunctivitis, keratitis, optic neuritis, chorioretinitis, and choroiditis. These have rarely been severe or associated with loss of vision and have generally resolved without corticosteroid treatment.

Contraindications & Cautions

Because ivermectin enhances GABA activity, it is best to avoid concomitant use of other drugs with similar effects, eg, barbiturates, benzodiazepines, and valproic acid. Ivermectin should not be used in pregnancy. Safety in children under 5 years has not been established. The proscription against breast feeding by mothers using the drug will probably be reduced to 1 week following the last dose.

The drug should not be administered to patients in whom there may be impairment of the blood-brain barrier, eg, in meningitis and African sleeping sickness. Risks of using the drug during other types of severe illness are being determined. In treatment of expatriates, patients are best observed in hospital for 72 hours after the first ivermectin dose. In AIDS patients, ivermectin treatment of onchocerciasis coinfection did not affect the drug's efficacy or side effects.

LEVAMISOLE

Levamisole hydrochloride is a synthetic imidazothiazole derivative and the L isomer of D,L-tetramisole. It is highly effective in eradicating *Ascaris* and *Trichostrongylus* and moderately effective against both species of hookworm. The drug is marketed in the USA but is approved only for its immunomodulating effect as adjunct therapy with fluorouracil for treatment of colon cancer.

MEBENDAZOLE

Mebendazole is a synthetic benzimidazole that has a wide spectrum of anthelmintic activity and a low incidence of adverse effects.

Mebendazole

Chemistry & Pharmacokinetics

Less than 10% of orally administered mebendazole is absorbed. The absorbed drug is protein-bound (> 90%), rapidly metabolized (primarily in the liver to inactive metabolites), and has a half-life of 2–6 hours. Within 24–48 hours, it is excreted mostly in the urine, either unchanged or as decarboxylated derivatives. In addition, a portion of absorbed drug and its deriva-

tives are excreted in the bile. Absorption is increased if the drug is ingested with a fatty meal.

Anthelmintic Actions & Pharmacologic Effects

Mebendazole inhibits microtubule synthesis in nematodes, thus irreversibly impairing glucose uptake (see Chapter 52). As a result, intestinal parasites are immobilized or die slowly, and their clearance from the gastrointestinal tract may not be complete until several days after treatment. Efficacy of the drug varies with gastrointestinal transit time, with intensity of infection, with whether or not the drug is chewed, and perhaps with the strain of parasite. The drug kills hookworm, *Ascaris,* and *Trichuris* eggs.

In humans, mebendazole is almost inert. No evidence of carcinogenicity or teratogenicity has been found. However, in pregnant rats the drug has embryotoxic and teratogenic activity at single oral doses as low as 10 mg/kg.

Clinical Uses

In the USA, mebendazole has been approved for use in ascariasis, trichuriasis, and hookworm and pinworm infection. It is investigational for other uses.

The drug can be taken before or after meals; the tablets should be chewed before swallowing. No pre- or posttreatment purging is necessary. Cure rates decrease in patients who have gastrointestinal hypermotility. In the treatment of trichinosis, hydatid disease, and dracontiasis, the drug should be taken with food containing fat, which enhances absorption.

A. Pinworm Infection: Give 100 mg once and repeat the dose at 2 and 4 weeks. The same dosage is used for children and adults. Cure rates range between 90% and 100%.

B. *Ascaris lumbricoides,* *Trichuris trichiura,* Hookworm, and *Trichostrongylus:* A dosage of 100 mg twice daily for 3 days is used for adults and for children over 2 years of age. Treatment can be repeated in 2–3 weeks. Cure rates are 90–100% for ascariasis and trichuriasis. Although cure rates are lower for hookworm infections of both species (70–95%), a marked reduction in the worm burden occurs in those not cured. Mebendazole is particularly useful in mixed infections caused by the three parasites.

C. Hydatid Disease: Albendazole is the drug of choice. Mebendazole is the alternative and less satisfactory drug, both with regard to highly variable cure rates and the high daily doses required to overcome poor absorption. Following a course of treatment, subjective improvement is reported for most patients and evidence of regression of cysts in some; in other patients, particularly after long-term follow-up, cysts have continued to grow or have proved viable. Unpredictable plasma levels of the drug (up to 500 ng/L) may contribute to this variability in response. One dosage schedule is 50 mg/kg in three divided doses daily for 3 months. When possible, mebendazole blood levels should be monitored; serum levels in excess of 100 ng/mL 1–3 hours after an oral dose may be necessary for parasite killing.

D. Other Infections: For treatment of **intestinal capillariasis,** mebendazole is an alternative drug at a dosage of 400 mg/d in divided doses for 21 or more days.

In **trichinosis,** limited reports suggest some efficacy against adult worms in the intestinal tract, migrating larvae, and larvae in muscle. The following daily treatment schedule has been recommended for adults: 600 mg initially, increasing stepwise over 3 days to 1200–1500 mg, continuing with the maximum dose for 10 days. Daily doses should be given in three divided portions.

Mebendazole at a dosage of 300 mg twice daily for 3 days has been used in the treatment of **taeniasis** with variable effectiveness; in *Taenia solium* infection, mebendazole has a theoretic advantage over niclosamide in that proglottids are expelled intact.

Cure rates for **strongyloidiasis** using the standard 3-day course of therapy are usually less than 50%; higher doses and longer courses of therapy can be tried.

In **dracontiasis,** the drug's efficacy has been variable. Mebendazole should be further evaluated in **angiostrongyliasis** and **visceral larva migrans** (200–400 mg in divided doses for 5 days) and in **gnathostomiasis** (200 mg every 3 hours for 6 days).

Adverse Reactions

Low-dose mebendazole for 1–3 days for intestinal nematode therapy has been nearly free of adverse effects even in debilitated patients. Mild nausea, vomiting, diarrhea, and abdominal pain have been reported infrequently, more often in children heavily parasitized by *Ascaris.* Slight headache, dizziness, and hypersensitivity reactions (rash, urticaria) are rare. Oral or nasal passage of ascarids in children under 5 years of age has been reported.

Occasional adverse effects associated with high-dose mebendazole treatment of hydatid disease are pruritus, rash, eosinophilia, reversible neutropenia, musculoskeletal pain, fever, and acute pain in the cyst area. Some of these findings may be due to cyst leakage or rupture with release of antigen. Rarely reported are gastric irritation, cough, transient liver function abnormalities, alopecia, glomerulonephritis, and some cases of drug-induced agranulocytosis (with one death).

Contraindications & Cautions

In severe hepatic parenchymal disease, mebendazole is very slowly metabolized and should be used with caution. The drug is contraindicated in the first trimester of pregnancy; alternative drugs are preferred later in pregnancy. Mebendazole should be used with caution in children under 1 year of age because of limited experience and rare reports of convulsions in this age group. Concomitant use of carbamazepine or phenytoin may reduce plasma levels and effectiveness of mebendazole; concomitant use of cimetidine may increase plasma levels. With high-dose hydatid disease therapy, complete blood counts should be done weekly.

METRIFONATE

Metrifonate is a safe, low-cost alternative drug for the treatment of *Schistosoma haematobium* infections. It is not active against *S mansoni* or *S japonicum.* The drug is not available in the USA.

Chemistry & Pharmacokinetics

Metrifonate, an organophosphate compound, is rapidly absorbed after oral administration. Following the standard oral dose, peak blood levels are reached in 1–2 hours; the half-life is about 1.5 hours. Clearance appears to be through nonenzymatic transformation to dichlorvos, its active metabolite. The amount of dichlorvos in the plasma is about 1% of the metrifonate level. Metrifonate and dichlorvos are well distributed to the tissues and are completely eliminated in 24–48 hours.

Anthelmintic Actions & Pharmacologic Effects

The mode of action of dichlorvos against both the mature and immature stages of *S haematobium* is not established but is thought to be related to cholinesterase inhibition. This inhibition temporarily paralyzes the adult worms, resulting in their shift from the bladder venous plexus to small arterioles of the lungs, where they are trapped, encased, and die. The drug is not effective against *S haematobium* eggs; live eggs continue to pass in the urine for several months after all adult worms have been killed.

Therapeutic dosages of metrifonate in humans produce no untoward physiologic or chemical abnormalities except for cholinesterase inhibition. Following oral ingestion of 7.5–12.5 mg/kg of metrifonate by infected persons, there is an almost complete inhibition of plasma butyrylcholinesterase and a marked reduction (about 50%) of erythrocyte acetylcholinesterase. Recovery of plasma cholinesterase is usually 70% (or more) by 2 weeks and is complete by 4 weeks, but erythrocyte enzyme recovery may take up to 15 weeks.

Metrifonate or perhaps impurities associated with its manufacture show weak mutagenicity in the *Salmonella typhimurium* direct test system. It induces mutations in *Escherichia coli* but causes no chromosomal abnormalities in animals or humans. Reproduction toxicity studies showed negative results except for suggestions of impaired spermatogenesis.

Clinical Uses

In the treatment of *S haematobium,* a single dose of 7.5–10 mg/kg is given orally three times at 14-day intervals. Cure rates on this schedule are 44–93%, with marked reductions in egg counts in those not cured.

Metrifonate was also effective as a prophylactic when given monthly to children in a highly endemic area. The drug is used in mass treatment programs. In mixed infections with *S haematobium* and *S mansoni,* metrifonate has been successfully combined with oxamniquine.

Adverse Reactions

Some studies report no adverse effects; others note mild and transient cholinergic symptoms, including nausea and vomiting, diarrhea, abdominal pain, bronchospasm, headache, sweating, fatigue, weakness, dizziness, and vertigo. These symptoms may begin within 30 minutes and persist up to 12 hours. The drug is well tolerated by patients in the advanced hepatosplenic stage of the disease. One case of organophosphate poisoning following a standard dose has been reported; the patient responded well to atropine.

Contraindications & Cautions

Metrifonate should not be used after recent exposure to insecticides or drugs that might potentiate cholinesterase inhibition. The use of muscle relaxants should be avoided for 48 hours after administration of the drug. Metrifonate is contraindicated in pregnancy.

NICLOSAMIDE

Niclosamide is a drug of choice for the treatment of most tapeworm infections.

Chemistry & Pharmacokinetics

Niclosamide is a salicylamide derivative. It appears to be minimally absorbed from the gastrointestinal tract: neither the drug nor its metabolites have been recovered from the blood or urine.

Niclosamide

Anthelmintic Actions & Pharmacologic Effects

Following oral administration in animals and humans, no hematologic, renal, or hepatic abnormalities have been noted.

Scoleces and segments of cestodes—but not ova—are rapidly killed on contact with niclosamide due to the drug's inhibition of oxidative phosphorylation or to its ATPase-stimulating property. With the death of the parasite, digestion of scoleces and segments begins.

The drug has not been fully evaluated for carcinogenic and mutagenic potential. Human peripheral lymphocytes show a dose-related increase in clastogenicity and an increase in chromosome aberrations. Urine from mice fed niclosamide shows mutagenicity in the Ames test.

Clinical Uses

The adult dose is 2 g (four tablets, 500 mg each). Children weighing more than 34 kg are given three tablets; 11–34 kg, two tablets; and under 11 kg, one tablet. Niclosamide should be given in the morning on an empty stomach. The tablets *must be chewed thoroughly* and are then swallowed with water. For small children, pulverize the tablets and then mix with water. The patient may eat 2 hours later. Posttreatment purges to expel the worm are not necessary except for an occasional patient with chronic constipation. In taeniasis, even if a purge and search for the scolex is used to determine cure, the scolex may be partially digested and difficult to find; if the scolex is not found, cure can be presumed only if regenerated segments have not reappeared after 3–5 months. In the absence of a purge, segments may continue to pass with normal peristalsis for several days.

A. *T saginata* (Beef Tapeworm), *T solium* (Pork Tapeworm), and *Diphyllobothrium latum* (Fish Tapeworm): A single 2 g dose of niclosamide results in cure rates of over 85% for *D latum* and about 95% for *T saginata.* It is probably equally effective against *T solium,* but 2 hours after treatment an effective purge (such as 15–30 g of magnesium sulfate) should be given to eliminate all mature segments before ova can be released. The patient should be monitored to ensure that prompt evacuation occurs. Cysticercosis is theoretically possible after treatment of *T solium* infections, since viable ova are released into the gut lumen following digestion of segments. However, after more than 2 decades of use, no cases of cysticercosis have been reported.

B. *Hymenolepis nana* (Dwarf Tapeworm): Praziquantel is the drug of choice. Although niclosamide is effective against the adult parasites in the lumen of the intestine, it is not effective against cysticercoids embedded in the villi. For niclosamide to be successful, it must be given until all of the cysticercoids have emerged (about 4 days). Thus, the minimum course of treatment must be 7 days; some workers repeat the course 5 days later. The overall cure rate is about 75%.

C. Other Tapeworms: Most patients treated for *Hymenolepis diminuta* and *Dipylidium caninum* infections are cured with a 7-day course of treatment; a few require a second course. Niclosamide is not effective against cysticercosis or hydatid disease.

D. Intestinal Fluke Infections: Niclosamide can be used as an alternative drug for the treatment of *Fasciolopsis buski, Heterophyes heterophyes,* and *Metagonimus yokogawai* infections. The standard dose is given every other day for three doses.

Adverse Reactions

Adverse effects are infrequent, mild, and transitory. Nausea, vomiting, diarrhea, and abdominal discomfort occur in less than 4% of patients. Rarely described are headache, skin rash, urticaria, pruritus ani, and vertigo, some of which may be related to release of antigenic material from disintegrating parasites.

Contraindications & Cautions

The consumption of alcohol should be avoided on the day of treatment and for 1 day afterward.

There are no contraindications to the use of niclosamide. In children under 2 years of age, the safety of the drug has not been established. Reproductive studies in animals were negative, but there are no adequate studies in pregnant women.

OXAMNIQUINE

Oxamniquine is a drug of choice for the treatment of *S mansoni* infections. It has also been used extensively for mass treatment. It is not effective against *S haematobium* or *S japonicum.*

Pharmacokinetics

Oxamniquine, a semisynthetic tetrahydroquinoline, is readily absorbed orally. It is not given intramuscularly because this causes intense and prolonged local pain. After therapeutic doses, its plasma half-life is about 2.5 hours. The drug is extensively metabolized to inactive metabolites and excreted in the urine—up to 75% in the first 24 hours. Intersubject variations in serum concentration have been noted, which could explain some treatment failures.

Anthelmintic Actions & Pharmacologic Effects

Oxamniquine is active against both mature and immature stages of *S mansoni* but does not appear to be cercaricidal. Although the exact mechanism is not known, the drug may act by DNA binding. Contraction and paralysis of the worms results in detachment from terminal venules in the mesentery and a shift to the liver, where many die; surviving females return to the mesenteric vessels but cease to lay eggs. The drug has no immunoregulating effect on perioval granuloma formation.

Strains of *S mansoni* in different parts of the world vary in susceptibility. *S mansoni* resistance to oxamniquine can be induced experimentally in mice but has rarely been reported in humans.

Clinical Uses

Oxamniquine is safe and effective in all stages of *S mansoni* disease, including advanced hepatosplenomegaly. In the acute (Katayama) syndrome, treatment results in disappearance of acute symptoms and clearance of the infection.

The drug is generally less effective in children, who require higher doses than adults. It is better tolerated if given with food, although food delays absorption. When divided doses are given in a single day, they should be separated by 6–8 hours.

Optimal dosage schedules vary for different regions of the world. In the Western Hemisphere and western Africa, the adult dosage is 12–15 mg/kg given once (children under 30 kg, 10 mg/kg twice) in 1 day. In northern and southern Africa, give 15 mg/kg twice daily for 2 days (children under 30 kg, twice daily for 2–3 days). In eastern Africa and the Arabian peninsula, give 15–20 mg/kg twice in 1 day (children under 30 kg, twice daily for 1 day). Cure rates are 70–95%, with marked reduction in egg excretion in those not cured.

In mixed infections with *S mansoni* and *S haematobium,* oxamniquine has been successfully used in combination with metrifonate. Oxamniquine's potential for suppressive prophylaxis as shown in animals needs further study in humans.

Adverse Reactions

Experience with the drug in millions of persons has shown it to be nearly free of significant toxicity. However, mild symptoms—starting about 3 hours after a dose, and lasting for several hours—do occur in more than one-third of patients. Central nervous system symptoms (dizziness, headache, drowsiness) are most common; nausea and vomiting, diarrhea, colic, pruritus, and urticaria also occur. Infrequent adverse effects are low-grade fever, an orange to red discoloration of the urine, proteinuria, microscopic hematuria, and a transient decrease in leukocytes and lymphocytes. Seizures are rare and generally occur within hours after ingestion, most often in persons with a history of seizures. Insomnia, amnesia, behavioral changes, and hallucinations are rare.

Liver enzyme elevations, eosinophilia, transient pulmonary infiltrates (sometimes associated with cough and rhonchi), urticaria, and fever (especially in Egypt) that occur from several days to 1 month after treatment have been ascribed to the death of parasites and release of antigens rather than to a direct toxic effect of the drug.

Oxamniquine has shown low mutagenicity in the *S typhimurium* test system and when assayed in mice, but chromosomal abnormalities were not found in other animals or humans. Oxamniquine has also been shown to have an embryocidal effect in rabbits and mice when given in doses ten times the equivalent human dose.

Contraindications & Cautions

It appears prudent to observe patients for about 3 hours after ingestion of the drug for signs of central nervous system disturbances. Patients with a history of epilepsy should be hospitalized for treatment, or an alternative drug used. Since the drug makes many patients dizzy or drowsy, it should be used with caution in patients whose work or activity requires mental alertness (eg, no driving for 24 hours).

Oxamniquine is contraindicated in pregnancy.

OXANTEL PAMOATE & OXANTEL/PYRANTEL PAMOATE

Oxantel pamoate, a tetrahydroxypyrimidine and metaoxyphenol analog of pyrantel pamoate, is effective only in the treatment of trichuriasis infections. Since trichuriasis commonly occurs as a multiple infection with the other soil-transmitted helminths, oxantel is marketed in combination with pyrantel pamoate because the latter is active against *Ascaris* and hookworm infections. Neither oxantel nor oxantel/pyrantel is effective in strongyloidiasis. These drugs are not available in the USA.

PIPERAZINE

The piperazine salts are alternative drugs in the treatment of ascariasis. Cure rates are over 90% when patients are treated for 2 days. Piperazine is not useful for treatment of hookworm infection, trichuriasis, or strongyloidiasis. The drug is no longer recommended in this text in the treatment of pinworm infection, because a 7-day course of treatment is required.

Chemistry & Pharmacokinetics

Piperazine is available as the hexahydrate (which contains about 44% of the base) and as a variety of salts: citrate, phosphate, adipate, tartrate, and others.

Piperazine is readily absorbed from the gastrointestinal tract, and maximum plasma levels are reached in 2–4 hours. Most of the drug is excreted unchanged in the urine in 2–6 hours, and excretion is complete within 24 hours.

Anthelmintic Actions & Pharmacologic Effects

Orally administered piperazine in therapeutic dosage is almost free of pharmacologic action in the host.

The formation of a potentially carcinogenic nitrosamine metabolite, *N*-mononitrosopiperazine, has been reported in gastric contents and urine of volunteers given therapeutic doses of piperazine; the significance of this finding remains to be determined.

Piperazine causes paralysis of *Ascaris* by blocking acetylcholine at the myoneural junction. Piperazine has a similar (but much weaker) myoneural blocking action on mammalian skeletal muscle. When the drug is used in humans, the paralyzed roundworms are unable to maintain their position in the host and are expelled live by normal peristalsis.

Clinical Uses

For ascariasis, the dosage of piperazine (as the hexahydrate) is 75 mg/kg/d orally (maximum dose, 3.5 g) for 2 days in succession, before or after breakfast. For heavy infections, treatment should be continued for 3–4 days or be repeated after 1 week. No pre- or posttreatment cathartics are used. In the nonsurgical management of intestinal obstruction caused by heavy *Ascaris* infection, piperazine syrup is administered via an intestinal drainage tube.

Adverse Reactions

There is a wide range between the therapeutic and toxic doses of piperazine. Mild adverse effects occur occasionally, including nausea, vomiting, diarrhea, abdominal pain, dizziness, and headache. Neurotoxic adverse effects (somnolence, dizziness, ataxia, seizures, chorea, visual disturbances, and others) occur but are rare. Patients with epilepsy may have an exacerbation of seizures. Piperazine is potentially allergenic; serum sickness-like syndromes (urticaria, purpura, fever, eczematous skin reactions, bronchospasm) have rarely been reported 2–4 days after an initial dose.

Contraindications & Cautions

Piperazine compounds should not be given to patients with impaired renal or hepatic function or with a history of epilepsy or chronic neurologic disease. Piperazine and phenothiazines should not be given together. Caution should be exercised in patients with severe malnutrition or anemia. In view of its partial conversion to a nitrosamine (see above), the drug should be given to pregnant women only if clearly indicated and if alternative drugs are not available.

PRAZIQUANTEL

Praziquantel is effective in the treatment of schistosome infections of all species and most other trematode and cestode infections, including cysticercosis. The drug's safety and effectiveness as a single oral dose have also made it useful in mass treatment of several of the infections. Praziquantel is not effective against *Fasciola hepatica* or in hydatid disease. In the USA, although the drug is only labeled for schistosomiasis treatment, it is the drug of choice (as an investigational drug) for many other cestode and trematode infections.

Chemistry & Pharmacokinetics

Praziquantel is a synthetic isoquinoline-pyrazine derivative. It is rapidly absorbed, with a bioavailability of about 80% after oral administration. Peak serum concentrations of 0.2–2 µg/mL of the unchanged drug are reached 1–3 hours after a therapeutic dose. About 80% of the drug is bound to plasma proteins. Cerebrospinal fluid concentrations of praziquantel reach 14–20% of the drug's plasma concentration; estimates for bile, breast milk, and feces are 10–20% of plasma levels. Most of the drug is rapidly metabolized to inactive mono- and polyhydroxylated products after a first pass in the liver; the half-life of the drug is 0.8–1.5 hours, while that of its metabolites is 4–6 hours. Excretion is mainly via the kidneys (60–80%) and bile (15–35%).

Pharmacologic Effects

In humans, no major alterations in biochemical or hematologic tests have been described. Transient elevations in liver function tests and, rarely, minor electrocardiographic changes may occur, but no significant damage to vital organs has been reported. In severe liver dysfunction, plasma levels rise.

In experimental animals, no effects are seen until doses approximately 100 times the therapeutic range are reached; signs of central nervous system toxicity are then noted.

A wide variety of mutagenicity, carcinogenicity, embryotoxicity, and teratogenicity studies have been negative. One laboratory (not confirmed by others) reported that praziquantel and a urinary metabolite acted as a mutagen or comutagen in *S typhimurium* and mammalian cell test systems. On balance, the evidence indicates that praziquantel does not present a genotoxic risk.

Anthelmintic Actions

The threshold serum concentration of praziquantel for therapeutic effect is about 0.3 µg/mL. In spite of its short half-life, praziquantel is the active agent; its metabolites are inactive. However, in vivo evidence suggests that host antibody to the parasite is also essential to eliminate tissue parasites.

Praziquantel's in vitro action on all platyhelminths appears to be the same—the drug increases cell membrane permeability to calcium, resulting in marked contraction, followed by paralysis of worm musculature. Vacuolization and disintegration of the tegmen occur, and parasite death follows. Although *F hepatica* does absorb the drug, no reaction occurs and the infection is not cleared.

In schistosome infections of experimental animals, praziquantel is effective against adult worms and immature stages; adult worms are rapidly immobilized and then passively shift to the liver. In addition, when a single high dose of praziquantel is given concurrently with an infecting dose of cercariae, all immature forms are killed; thus, praziquantel has a prophylactic effect.

Clinical Uses

Praziquantel tablets are taken with liquid after a meal; they should be swallowed immediately without chewing because their bitter taste can induce retching and vomiting. If the drug is taken more than once on the same day, the interval between doses should be no less than 4 hours and no more than 6 hours.

A. Schistosomiasis: Praziquantel is the drug of choice for all forms of schistosomiasis. The dosage is 20 mg/kg at intervals of 4–6 hours for a total of three doses. Other schedules, some with lower total doses, have been effective in some regions: 40 mg/kg once for *S haematobium* and 40 mg/kg in two divided doses for *S mansoni*. High cure rates (75–95%) are achieved when patients are evaluated at 3–6 months; there is marked reduction in egg counts in those not cured. The drug is effective in adults and children and is generally well tolerated by patients in the hepatosplenic stage of advanced disease. It is not clear, however, whether the drug can be safely or effectively used during the acute stage of the disease (Katayama fever) because release of antigens from dying immature worms may exacerbate symptoms. Use of the drug prophylactically has not been established. A recent report indicates reduced susceptibility of *S mansoni* in Senegal.

B. Clonorchiasis and Opisthorchiasis: The dosage of 25 mg/kg three times daily for 1 day for *Opisthorchis* and 2 days for *Clonorchis* infections results in nearly 100% cure rates.

C. Paragonimiasis: When treated with 25 mg/kg three times daily for 2 days, cure rates for pulmonary paragonimiasis are 89–100%.

D. Taeniasis and Diphyllobothriasis: A single dose of praziquantel, 10 mg/kg, results in cure rates of 97–100% for *T saginata* and *T solium*. In cysticercosis-endemic areas, it may be safer but equally effective to use 2.5 mg/kg because at least one instance of an exacerbation of neurocysticercosis symptoms has occurred following low-dose mass treatment for taeniasis. A single dose of 25 mg/kg results in similar cure rates for *D latum* infections. Within 24–48 hours after treatment, a disintegrating worm is usually passed by normal peristalsis. Pre- and posttreatment purges are not necessary. If the scolex is searched for but not found or is not searched for, cure can be presumed only if regenerated segments have not reappeared 3–5 months after treatment. For *T solium,* the recommendation continues that an effective purge (eg, magnesium sulfate, 15–30 g) be given 2 hours after treatment to eliminate all mature segments before eggs can be released from disintegrating segments. Since praziquantel does not kill the eggs, it is theoretically possible that larvae released from eggs in the large bowel could penetrate the intestinal wall and give rise to cysticercosis. However, as with the use of niclosamide, this hazard is probably minimal.

E. Neurocysticercosis: Neurocysticercosis should be treated in hospital by a physician with neurologic expertise. The indications, cautions, use of concomitant corticosteroids, and outcome for praziquantel treatment are similar to those for albendazole use. However, in comparable studies, albendazole (see above) is the preferred drug. The praziquantel dosage is 50 mg/kg/d in three divided doses for 14 days. If appropriate services are available, blood levels should be monitored. Therapy may result in apparent cure, with clearance of symptoms, changes in cysts by cerebral tomograms (disappearance, reduction in size, or calcification), and clearing of abnormal cerebrospinal fluid findings. In other patients, there may be remarkable improvement, including reduction in cerebral hypertension and amelioration of seizures. Still other patients, however, show no change or continued progression of the disease.

F. *H nana:* Praziquantel is the drug of choice for *H nana* infections and the first drug to be highly effective. A single dose of 25 mg/kg is used. Re-treatment may be required.

G. Hydatid Disease: In hydatid disease, praziquantel kills protoscoleces but does not affect the germinal membrane. Praziquantel is being evaluated as an adjunct with albendazole pre- and postsurgery to protect against cyst spillage; in combination, in addition to praziquantel's direct action, the plasma concentration of albendazole sulfoxide (the active metabolite of albendazole) is enhanced.

H. Other Parasites: Limited trials at a dosage of 25 mg/kg three times a day for 1–2 days indicate a high order of effectiveness of praziquantel against **fasciolopsiasis, metagonimiasis,** and other forms of **heterophyiasis.** In **fascioliasis,** however, praziquantel had only a low effectiveness at dosages as high as 25 mg/kg three times daily for 3–7 days.

Adverse Reactions

Mild and transient adverse effects directly attributable to the drug are common. They begin within several hours after ingestion and may persist for hours to 1 day. Most frequent are headache, dizziness, drowsiness, and lassitude; others include nausea, vomiting, abdominal pain, loose stools, pruritus, urticaria, arthralgia, myalgia, and low-grade fever. Minimal to mild transient elevations of liver enzymes have occasionally been reported. Low-grade fever, pruritus, and skin rashes (macular and urticarial), sometimes associated with augmented eosinophilia, may also appear several days after starting the medication and are more likely to be due to the release of foreign proteins from dying worms than to a direct action of the drug.

Praziquantel appears to be better tolerated in children than in adults. Adverse effects may be more frequent in heavily infected patients, especially in *S mansoni* infections. The intensity and frequency of adverse effects also increase with dosage: They are mild and infrequent at dosages of 10 mg/kg given once but occur in up to 50% of patients who receive 25 mg/kg three times in 1 day.

Two types of adverse reactions in treatment of neurocysticercosis are (1) those characteristic of praziquantel usage at high dosage (described above) and (2) new neurologic reactions or exacerbations of existing ones due to inflammatory reactions around dying parasites. Common findings in up to 90% of patients who do not receive corticosteroids are headache, meningismus, nausea, vomiting, mental changes, and seizures (often accompanied by increased cerebrospinal fluid pleocytosis). These occur during or shortly after completion of therapy, last 48–72 hours, and usually are sufficiently mild that they can be ameliorated with analgesics, antiemetics, diuretics, or anticonvulsants. However, arachnoiditis, hyperthermia, and intracranial hypertension may also occur. Many workers give dexamethasone concurrently to decrease the inflammatory reaction; this is controversial, especially with the recent recognition that steroids reduce the plasma level of praziquantel up to 50%. It is not established, however, that the steroidal reduction in plasma levels also reduces the effectiveness of praziquantel.

Drug interactions

As noted above, corticosteroids reduce praziquantel plasma concentration. The bioavailability of praziquantel is reduced by phenytoin and carbamazepine and increased by cimetidine. A digitalis-antagonistic effect has been seen in animal studies.

Contraindications & Cautions

The only specific contraindication is ocular cysticercosis; parasite destruction in the eye may cause irreparable damage. Some workers also caution against use of the drug in spinal neurocysticercosis. In cysticercosis-endemic areas, patients treated with praziquantel for conditions other than cysticercosis should be observed carefully in hospital for about 48 hours after completion of treatment. The drug can be used in the presence of liver impairment, but a reduction in dose may be necessary. Although safety of the drug in children under age 4 years is not established, no pediatric-specific problems have been documented.

Because the drug induces dizziness and drowsiness, patients should not drive and should be warned if their work requires physical coordination or alertness.

The drug should preferably not be taken during pregnancy; an increase in abortion rate was found in rats treated with three times the human dose. In lactating women, although praziquantel appears in milk at about one-fourth of the plasma levels, the drug may be given to the mother provided the infant is not nursed on the day of treatment and for 3 subsequent days.

Patients should be cautioned against chewing the bitter-tasting drug; the retching that results can become a special problem in treatment of *T solium* infection because regurgitation of segments might result, which could be hazardous.

PYRANTEL PAMOATE

Pyrantel pamoate is a broad-spectrum anthelmintic highly effective for the treatment of pinworm, *Ascaris,* and *Trichostrongylus orientalis* infections. It is moderately effective against both species of hookworm but less so against *N americanus.* It is not effective in trichuriasis or strongyloidiasis. Oxantel pamoate, an analog of pyrantel, has been used successfully in the treatment of trichuriasis; the two drugs have been combined for their broad-spectrum anthelmintic activity (see above).

Chemistry & Pharmacokinetics

Pyrantel pamoate is a tetrahydropyrimidine derivative. Because it is poorly absorbed from the gastrointestinal tract, it is active mainly against luminal organisms. Peak plasma levels of 50–130 ng/mL are reached in 1–3 hours. Over half the administered dose is recovered unchanged in the feces; about 7% is excreted in the urine as unchanged drug and metabolites.

Anthelmintic Actions & Pharmacologic Effects

Pyrantel is effective against mature and immature forms of susceptible helminths within the intestinal tract but not against migratory stages in the tissues or against ova. The drug is a depolarizing neuromuscular blocking agent that causes release of acetylcholine and inhibition of cholinesterase; this results in stimulation of ganglionic receptors and worm paralysis, which is followed by expulsion from the host's intestinal tract.

Clinical Uses

The standard dose is 11 mg (base)/kg (maximum, 1 g), given with or without food.

A. Enterobius vermicularis: Pyrantel is given as a single dose and repeated in 2 and 4 weeks. Cure rates are greater than 95%. In the USA, the drug is available for self-medication for this indication.

B. A lumbricoides: Pyrantel is given as a single dose. Cure rates are 85–100%. Treatment should be repeated if eggs are still found 2 weeks later.

C. Hookworm and T orientalis: A single dose produces cures in over 90% of *Ancylostoma duodenale* and *T orientalis* infections and a marked reduction in the worm burden in the remainder. However, for *N americanus* infections, the cure rate depends on the intensity of infection. A single dose may give a satisfactory cure rate in light infections, but for moderate or heavy infections (> 2000 ova per gram of feces), a 3-day course is necessary to reach 90% cure rates. The 3-day course is indicated when the species is unknown. Hookworm burdens should be markedly reduced, but it is not always possible or essential to eradicate the infection. If iron deficiency accompanies the infection, it should be treated with iron medication and a high-protein diet. A course of treatment can be repeated in 2 weeks.

Adverse Reactions; Contraindications & Cautions

Adverse effects, which occur in 4–20% of patients, are infrequent, mild, and transient. They include nausea, vomiting, diarrhea, abdominal cramps, dizziness, drowsiness, headache, insomnia, rash, fever, and weakness. No important effects on hematologic, renal, or hepatic function have been recorded.

There are no contraindications to pyrantel, but it should be used with caution in patients with liver dysfunction, since low, transient transaminase elevations have been noted in a small number of patients. Experience with the drug in children under age 2 years is limited. Although teratogenic studies in animals have been negative, adequate studies in pregnant women have not been done.

QUINACRINE HYDROCHLORIDE

Quinacrine was formerly an alternative drug for the treatment of tapeworm infections. Because of its toxicity, it should no longer be used unless niclosamide or alternative drugs (praziquantel, albendazole, mebendazole, or dichlorophen) are not available.

SURAMIN

Suramin is an alternative drug for the eradication of adult parasites of *Onchocerca volvulus* and a drug of choice in the treatment of the hemolymphatic stage of African trypanosomiasis due to *Trypanosoma brucei gambiense* and *Trypanosoma brucei rhodesiense* The drug is being evaluated as an anticancer agent, including prostate and breast cancer.

Suramin is a nonspecific inhibitor of many enzymes (see Chapter 52). Toxic reactions are frequent and sometimes severe, including nausea, vomiting, urticaria, fever, nephrotoxicity, peripheral neuritis, anemia, jaundice, and exfoliative dermatitis. Some deaths have occurred. The drug should be given only under expert guidance.

TETRACHLOROETHYLENE

Tetrachloroethylene has been used for the treatment of hookworm infections due to *Necator americanus* or *Ancylostoma duodenale.* Other drugs with fewer adverse effects are now preferred, but tetrachloroethylene remains an effective, inexpensive alternative drug, with mild adverse reactions. It is not available in the USA.

THIABENDAZOLE

Thiabendazole is the drug of choice for the treatment of strongyloidiasis and an alternative drug for cutaneous larva migrans. It may also be tried in trichinosis and visceral larva migrans, given the absence of other effective drugs. It is no longer recommended for the treatment of pinworm, ascarid, trichurid, or hookworm infection unless the safer drugs of choice are not available.

Chemistry

Thiabendazole is a benzimidazole compound. It is tasteless and nearly insoluble in water. Although it is a chelating agent that forms stable complexes with a number of metals, including iron, it does not bind calcium.

Pharmacokinetics

Thiabendazole is rapidly absorbed after ingestion. With a standard dose, drug concentrations in plasma peak within 1–2 hours (5 µg/mL) and are barely detectable after 8 hours; the half-life is 1.2 hours. The drug is almost completely metabolized in the liver to the 5-hydroxy form, which appears in the urine largely as the glucuronide or sulfonate conjugate. Ninety percent of the drug is excreted in the urine in 48 hours. Thiabendazole can also be absorbed from the skin. In some clinical situations, it may be useful to monitor serum drug concentrations.

Anthelmintic Actions & Pharmacologic Effects

Thiabendazole has anti-inflammatory properties, which may be an important factor in its ability to relieve symptoms in some parasitic diseases, particularly dracontiasis. It also has immunomodulating effects on T cell function—it appears to be an immunorestorative agent, demonstrating maximum immunopotentiation in the immunosuppressed host. Thiabendazole also has antipyretic and mild antifungal and scabicidal actions. The drug appears to be free of carcinogenic and mutagenic effects. Most studies for teratogenicity were negative, but one study that used high doses in rats and mice was positive.

Thiabendazole's vermicidal action may be a result of interference with microtubule aggregation (see Chapter 52) acting through inhibition of the enzyme fumarate reductase. The drug has ovicidal effects for some parasites.

Clinical Uses

The standard dose is 25 mg/kg (maximum, 1.5 g). The drug should be given after meals. If the tablet formulation is used it should be chewed well. Pre- and posttreatment purges are not necessary.

A. Strongyloides stercoralis: The standard dose is given twice daily for 2 days. Cure rates are 93%. A course can be repeated in 1 week if indicated.

In patients with hyperinfection syndrome, the standard dose is continued twice daily for 5–7 days.

B. Cutaneous Larva Migrans (Creeping Eruption): Thiabendazole is highly effective in the treatment of cutaneous larva migrans. The standard dose is given twice daily for 2 days. If active lesions are still present 2 days after completion of therapy, a second course should be given. Excellent results have also followed daily application, for 5 days, of a cream containing 15% thiabendazole in a hygroscopic base or of a 2% solution in dimethyl sulfoxide.

C. Other Infections: For the treatment of **trichinosis,** the standard dosage is given twice daily for 2–4 days; for **visceral larva migrans,** twice daily for up to 7 days, depending upon the symptomatic response and the drug tolerance by the patient. Information on the effectiveness of the drug for both conditions is limited. During the first 24 hours after ingestion of trichinous pork, the drug may have an effect on adult worms, resulting in a decrease of larvae released. During the invasive stage, thiabendazole provides some symptomatic relief, and biopsy evidence suggests that the drug destroys some (though not all) larvae in muscle. Corticosteroids and ACTH are effective in reducing inflammatory reactions to the larvae and may be lifesaving in severe infections.

Intestinal capillariasis has been successfully treated with thiabendazole at a dose of 12 mg/kg given twice daily for 30 days.

For the treatment of **dracontiasis,** the drug is often effective at a dosage of 50–75 mg/kg/d in two divided doses for 1–3 days. Local inflammation subsides rapidly, and many worms are then spontaneously extruded or can be extracted manually. Re-treatment is occasionally needed.

Several reports have indicated the usefulness of topical thiabendazole for the treatment of **scabies** and **tinea nigra palmaris.**

Adverse Reactions

At the standard dosage of 25 mg/kg twice daily for 2 days, adverse effects occur in 7–50% of patients, generally 3–4 hours after ingestion of the drug, and last 2–8 hours. Higher doses or treatment beyond 2 days increases the frequency and intensity of symptoms. Although toleration may occasionally be improved by reducing the dosage to 25 mg/kg once daily, effectiveness is likely to decrease.

Adverse effects are generally mild and transient but can be severe; the most common are dizziness, anorexia, nausea, and vomiting. Less frequent are epigastric pain, abdominal cramps, diarrhea, pruritus, headache, drowsiness, giddiness, and other neuropsychiatric symptoms. Rarely reported are perianal rashes, tinnitus, paresthesias, bradycardia, hypotension, hyperglycemia, convulsions, transient leukopenia, hematuria, crystalluria, visual disturbances, intrahepatic cholestasis, and parenchymal liver damage; jaundice and liver function abnormalities may result.

In some patients, a medically insignificant asparagine odor is imparted to the urine.

Rare hypersensitivity reactions include fever, chills, skin rashes, pruritus, conjunctival edema, angioedema, lymphadenopathy, toxic epidermal necrolysis, anaphylaxis, and erythema multiforme. Fatal Stevens-Johnson syndrome has occurred in children.

Contraindications & Cautions

Experience with thiabendazole is limited in children weighing less than 15 kg. The drug should not be used in pregnancy, except for life-threatening strongyloidiasis. It may be best to use alternative drugs in pa-tients with hepatic or renal dysfunction. The drug should be used with caution where drug-induced vomiting may be dangerous or in patients with severe malnutrition or anemia. There are a few reports of ascarids becoming hypermotile after treatment and appearing at the nose or mouth.

Since the drug makes some patients dizzy or drowsy, it should not be used during the day for patients whose work or activity requires mental alertness.

Thiabendazole may compete with theophylline for sites of metabolism in the liver. Discontinue the drug immediately if hypersensitivity symptoms appear.

PREPARATIONS AVAILABLE

Albendazole (Albenza Zentel)
Oral: 200 mg tablets
Note: Albendazole is approved in the USA for the treatment of cysticercosis and hydatid disease. See Chapter 65 for its unlabeled use for other indications.

Bithionol (Bitin)
Oral: 200 mg tablets
Note: Bithionol is not marketed in the USA but can be obtained from the Parasitic Disease Drug Service, Centers for Disease Control and Prevention, Atlanta, Georgia; 404-639-3670.

Diethylcarbamazine (Hetrazan)
Oral: 50, 200, 400 mg tablets
Note: Diethylcarbamazine is no longer marketed in the USA but is available upon request from Wyeth-Ayerst Laboratories; 610-971-577.

Ivermectin (Mectizan)
Oral: 6 mg tablets
Note: Ivermectin is approved for use in the USA for the treatment of onchocerciasis. See Chapter 65 for its unlabled use for other indications.

Levamisole (Decaris, Ethnor, Ketrax, Solaskil)
Oral: 50, 150 mg tablets and syrup

Mebendazole (Vermox)
Oral: 100 mg chewable tablets; outside the USA, 100 mg/5 mL suspension

Metrifonate (Bilarcil)
Oral: 100 mg tablets
Note: Metrifonate is not available in the USA.

Niclosamide (Niclocide)
Oral: 500 mg chewable tablets

Oxamniquine (Vansil, Mansil)
Oral: 250 mg capsules; outside the USA, 50 mg/mL syrup

Oxantel pamoate (Quantrel); **oxantel/pyrantel pamoate** (Telopar)
Oral: tablets containing 100 mg (base) of each drug; suspensions containing 20 or 50 mg (base) per mL
Note: Oxantel pamoate and oxantel/pyrantel pamoate are not available in the USA.

Piperazine (generic, Vermizine)
Oral: piperazine citrate tablets equivalent to 250 mg of the hexahydrate; piperazine citrate syrup equivalent to 500 mg of the hexahydrate per 5 mL

Praziquantel (Biltricide; others outside the USA)
Oral: 600 mg tablets (other strengths outside the USA)

Pyrantel pamoate (Antiminth, Combantrin)
Oral: 50 mg (base)/mL suspension; 125 mg tablets are available in Canada and some other countries but not in the USA.

Suramin (Bayer 205, others)
Parenteral: ampules containing 0.5 or 1 g powder to be reconstituted as a 10% solution and used immediately
Note: Suramin is not marketed in the USA but can be obtained from the Parasitic Disease Drug Service, Centers for Disease Control, Atlanta, GA, 404-639-3670.

Thiabendazole (Mintezol)
Oral: 500 mg chewable tablets; suspension, 500 mg/mL

REFERENCES

General

Cook GC (editor): *Manson's Tropical Diseases,* 20th ed. Saunders, 1996.

Drugs for parasitic infections. Med Lett Drugs Ther 1995;37:99.

Edwards G, Winstanley PA, Ward SA: Clinical pharmacokinetics in the treatment of tropical diseases: Some applications and limitations. Clin Pharmacokinet 1994; 27:150.

Rosenblatt JE: Antiparasitic agents. Mayo Clin Proc 1992;67:276.

Tanowitz HB, Weiss LM, Wittner M: Diagnosis and treatment of intestinal helminths. I. Common intestinal cestodes. Gastroenterologist 1993;1:265.

Tanowitz HB, Weiss LM, Wittner M: Diagnosis and treatment of intestinal helminths. II. Common intestinal nematodes. Gastroenterologist 1994;2:39.

Albendazole

Archibald LK et al: Albendazole is effective treatment for chronic strongyloidiasis. Q J Med 1993;86:191.

Bhatia V, Sarin SK: Hepatic visceral larva migrans: Evolution of the lesion, diagnosis, and role of high-dose albendazole therapy. Am J Gastroenterol 1994;89:624.

Cook GC: *Enterobius vermicularis* infection. GUT 1994;35:1159.

Datry A et al: Treatment of *Strongyloides stercoralis* infection with ivermectin compared with albendazole: Results of an open study of 60 cases. Trans R Soc Trop Med Hyg 1994;88:344.

Davies HD, Sakuls P, Keystone JS: Creeping eruption: A review of clinical presentation and management of 60 cases presenting to a tropical disease unit. Arch Dermatol 1993;129:588.

Farbey MD, Reynoldson JA, Thompson RCA: In vitro drug susceptibility of 29 isolates of *Giardia duodenalis* from humans as assessed by an adhesion assay. Int J Parasitol 1995;25:593.

Gunnarsson G et al: Multiorgan microsporidiosis: Report of five case and review. Clin Infect Dis 1995;21:37.

Hall A, Nahar Q: Albendazole and infections with *Ascaris lumbricoides* and *Trichuris trichiura* in children in Bangladesh. Trans R Soc Trop Med Hyg 1994;88:110.

Houston S: Gnathostomiasis: Report of a case and brief review. Can J Infect Dis 1994;5:125.

Jung H et al: Dexamethasone increases plasma levels of albendazole. J Neurol 1990;237:279.

Martinez HR et al: Medical and surgical treatment in neurocysticercosis: A magnetic resonance study of 161 cases. J Neurol Sci 1995;130:25.

Morris DL: Echinococcus of the liver. Gut 1994;35:1517.

Nahmias J et al: Three- to 7-year follow-up after albendazole treatment of 68 patients with cystic echinococcosis (hydatid disease). Ann Trop Med Parasitol 1994;88:295.

Webbe G: Human cysticercosis: Parasitology, pathology, clinical manifestation and available treatment. Pharmacol Ther 1994;64:175.

Bithionol

Bacq Y et al: Successful treatment of acute fascioliasis with bithionol. Hepatology 1991;14:1066.

Bassiouny HK et al: Human fascioliasis in Egypt: Effect of infection and efficacy of bithionol treatment. J Trop Med Hyg 1991;94:333.

Kusner DL, King CH: Cerebral paragonimiasis. Semin Neurol 1993;13:201.

Diethylcarbamazine

Andrade LD et al: Comparative efficacy of three different diethylcarbamazine regimens in lymphatic filariasis. Trans R Soc Trop Med Hyg 1995;89:319.

Awadzi K, Gilles HM: Diethylcarbamazine in the treatment of patients with onchocerciasis. Br J Clin Pharmacol 1992;34:281.

Carme B et al: Five cases of encephalitis during treatment of loiasis with diethylcarbamazine. Am J Trop Med Hyg 1991;44:684.

Klion AD, Ottesen EA, Nutman TBL: Effectiveness of diethylcarbamazine in treating loiasis acquired by expatriate visitors to endemic regions: Long-term follow-up. J Infect Dis 1994;169:604.

Mackenzie CD, Kron MA: Diethylcarbamazine: A review of its action in onchocerciasis, lymphatic filariasis and inflammation. Trop Dis Bull 1985;82:R1.

Magnaval J: Comparative efficacy of diethylcarbamazine and mebendazole for the treatment of toxocariasis. Parasitology 1995;119:529.

Ottesen EA: Efficacy of diethylcarbamazine in eradicating infection with lymphatic-dwelling filariae in humans. Rev Infect Dis 1985;7:341.

Sharma S: Drugs for filariasis. Adv Drug Res 1993; 24:200.

Vijayan VK et al: Tropical eosinophilia: Clinical and physiological response to diethylcarbamazine. Respir Med 1991;85:17.

Ivermectin

Awadzi K et al: The chemotherapy of onchocerciasis XIX: The clinical and laboratory tolerance of high dose ivermectin. Trop Med Parasitol 1995;46:131.

Burnham G: Ivermectin treatment of onchocercal skin lesions: Observations from a placebo-controlled, double-blind trial in Malawi. Am J Trop Med Hyg 1995;52:270.

Churchill DR et al: A trial of three-dose regimen of ivermectin for the treatment of patients with onchocerciasis in the UK. Trans R Soc Trop Med Hyg 1994;88:242.

Datry A et al: Treatment of *Strongyloides stercoralis* infection with ivermectin compared with albendazole: Results of an open study of 60 cases. Trans R Soc Trop Med Hyg 1994;88:344.

Gann PJ, Neva FA, Gam A: A randomized trial of single- and two-dose ivermectin versus thiabendazole for treatment of strongyloidiasis. J Infect Dis 1994;169:1076.

Hovette P et al: Efficacy of ivermectin treatment of *Loa loa* filariasis patients without microfilaraemias. Ann Trop Med Parasitol 1994;88:93.

Meinking TL et al: The treatment of scabies with ivermectin. N Engl J Med 1995;333:26.

Murdoch I et al: Ivermectin and onchocercal optic neuritis: Short-term effects. Eye 1994;8:456.

World Health Organization: WHO Expert Committee on Onchocerciasis Control. Technical Report Series 852. WHO, 1995.

Mebendazole

Ammann RW et al: Effect of chemotherapy on the larval mass and long-term course of alveolar echinococcosis. Hepatology 1994;19:735.

Bartoloni C et al: The efficacy of chemotherapy with mebendazole in human cystic echinococcosis: Long-term follow-up of 52 patients. Ann Trop Med Parasitol 1992;86:249.

Chippaux JP: Mebendazole treatment of dracunculiasis. Trans R Soc Trop Med Hyg 1991;85:280.

Shikiya K et al: Treatment of strongyloidiasis with mebendazole: Long term eradication and new trials. J Japan Assoc Infect Dis 1991;65:433.

Todorov T et al: Chemotherapy of human cystic echinococcosis: Comparative efficacy of mebendazole and albendazole. Ann Trop Med Parasitol 1992;86:59.

Metrifonate

Aden-Abdi Y et al: Metrifonate in healthy volunteers: Interrelationship between pharmacokinetic properties, cho-linesterase inhibition and side effects. Bull World Health Organ 1990;68:731.

Nhachi CFB et al: Effect of single oral dose of metrifonate on human plasma cholinesterase levels. Bull Environ Contam Toxicol 1991;47:641.

Unni LK et al: Pharmacokinetics and pharmacodynamics of metrifonate in humans. Exp Clin Pharmacol 1994; 16:285.

Niclosamide

Botero D et al: Taeniasis and cysticercosis. Infect Dis Clin North Am 1993;7:683.

Jones WE: Niclosamide as a treatment for Hymenolepis diminuta and Dipylidium caninum infection in man. Am J Trop Med Hyg 1979;28:300.

Pearson RD, Hewlett EL: Niclosamide therapy for tapeworm infections. Ann Intern Med 1985;102:550.

Oxamniquine

Foster R: A review of clinical experience with oxamniquine. Trans R Soc Trop Med Hyg 1987;81:55.

Lucey DR, Maguire JH: Schistosomiasis. Infect Dis Clinic North Am 1993;7:635.

Sleigh AC et al: Manson's schistosomiasis in Brazil: 11-year evaluation of successful disease control with oxamniquine. Lancet 1986;1:635.

Piperazine

Ukadgaonkar NG, Bjagwat RB, Kulkarni MU: Transient cerebellar syndrome due to piperazine citrate. Clinician 1982;46:461.

Praziquantel

Botero D: Neurocysticercosis. Curr Opin Infect Dis 1994;7:547.

Fallon PG et al: Short Report: Diminished susceptibility to praziquantel in a Senegal isolate of Schistosoma mansoni. Am J Trop Med Hyg 1995;53:61.

Fernandez J et al: Efficacy and tolerance of praziquantel in patients with dystomatosis due to Fasciola hepatica. Gastroenterology 1993;104:A699.

Flisser A et al: Neurologic symptoms in occult neurocysticercosis after a single taeniacidal dose of praziquantel. Lancet 1993;342:748.

Geerts S: The efficacy of praziquantel for the treatment of cestode and metacestode infections. Int J Antimicrob Agents 1994;4:321.

Herwaldt BL et al: Persistence of Schistosomiasis haematobium infection despite multiple courses of therapy with praziquantel. Clin Infect Dis 1995; 20:309.

Kumar V, Gryseels B: Use of praziquantel against schistosomiasis: A review of current status. Int J Antimicrob Agents 1994;4:313.

Mairiang E, et al: Reversal of biliary-tract abnormalities associated with Opisthorchis viverrini infection following praziquantel treatment. Trans R Soc Trop Med Hyg 1993;87:194.

Pawlowski ZS: Efficacy of low doses of praziquantel in taeniasis. Acta Tropica 1991;48:83.

Rolfs A et al: Clinical and immunologic follow-up of patients with neurocysticercosis after treatment with praziquantel. Neurology 1995;45:532.

Visser LG et al: Outbreak of schistosomiasis among travelers returning from Mali, West Africa. Clin Infect Dis 1995;20:280.

Pyrantel Pamoate

Van Riper G: Pyrantel pamoate for pinworm infestation. Am Pharm 1993;NS33(2):43.

Suramin

Awadzi K et al: The chemotherapy of onchocerciasis XVIII. Aspects of treatment with suramin. Trop Med Parasitol 1995;46:19.

Duke BO: Suramin and the time it takes to kill Onchocerca volvulus. Trop Med Parasitol 1991;42:346.

Stein CA: Suramin: A novel antineoplastic agent with multiple potential mechanisms of action. Cancer Res 1993;53(10 Suppl):2239.

Voogd TE, et al: Recent research on the biologic activity of suramin. Pharmacol Rev 1993;45:177.

Thiabendazole

Boken DJ et al: Treatment of Strongyloidiasis stercoralis hyperinfection with thiabendazole administered per rectum. Clin Infect Dis 1993;16:123.

Gann PH, Neva FA, Gam AA: A randomized trial of single- and two-dose ivermectin versus thiabendazole for treatment of strongyloidiasis. J Infect Dis 1994;169:1076.

Lew G et al: Theophylline-thiabendazole drug interaction. Clin Pharm 1989;8:225.

Liu LX, Weller PF: Strongyloidiasis and other intestinal nematode infections. Infect Dis Clin North Am 1993;7:655.

Cancer Chemotherapy

55

Sydney E. Salmon, MD, & Alan C. Sartorelli, PhD

The incidence, geographic distribution, and behavior of specific types of cancer are related to multiple factors, including sex, age, race, genetic predisposition, and exposure to environmental carcinogens. Of these factors, the last is probably most important. Chemical carcinogens (particularly those in tobacco smoke) as well as agents such as azo dyes, aflatoxins, and benzene have been clearly implicated in cancer induction in humans and animals. Identification of potential carcinogens in the environment has been greatly simplified by the widespread use of the "Ames test" for mutagenic agents. Ninety percent of carcinogens can be shown to be mutagenic on the basis of this assay. Ultimate identification of potential human carcinogens, however, requires testing in at least two animal species.

Certain herpes and papilloma group DNA viruses and type C RNA viruses have also been implicated as causative agents in animal cancers and might be responsible for some human cancers as well. Oncogenic RNA viruses all appear to contain a "reverse transcriptase" enzyme that permits translation of the RNA message of the tumor virus into the DNA code of the infected cell. Thus, the information governing transformation can become a stable part of the genome of the host cell. Expression of virus-induced neoplasia probably also depends on additional host and environmental factors that modulate the transformation process. A specific human T cell leukemia virus (HTLV-I) has been identified as causative of this specific type of leukemia. The virus that causes AIDS (HIV-1) is closely related. Cellular genes are known that are homologous to the transforming genes of the retroviruses, a family of RNA viruses, and induce oncogenic transformation. These mammalian cellular genes, known as **oncogenes,** have been shown to code for specific growth factors and their receptors and may be amplified (increased number of gene copies) or modified by a single nucleotide in malignant cells. The *bcl-2* oncogene may be a generalized "cell death suppressor" gene that directly regulates apoptosis, a pathway of programmed cell death.

Another class of genes, **tumor suppressor genes,** may be deleted or damaged, with resulting neoplastic change. A single gene in this class, the *p53* gene, has been shown to have mutated from a tumor suppressor gene to an oncogene in a high percentage of cases of several human tumors, including liver, breast, colon, lung, cervix, bladder, prostate, and skin. The normal "wild" form of this gene appears to play an important role in suppressing neoplastic transformation; mutation places the cell at high risk of transformation (Harris et al, 1993).

CANCER AS A DISEASE OF CELLS

Whatever the cause, cancer is basically a disease of cells characterized by a shift in the control mechanisms that govern cell proliferation and differentiation. Cells that have undergone neoplastic transformation usually express cell surface antigens that appear to be of normal fetal type, have other signs of apparent "immaturity," and may exhibit qualitative or quantitative chromosomal abnormalities, including various translocations and the appearance of amplified gene sequences. Such cells proliferate excessively and form local tumors that can compress or invade adjacent normal structures. A small subpopulation of cells within the tumor can be described as **tumor stem cells.** They retain the ability to undergo repeated cycles of proliferation as well as to migrate to distant sites in the body to colonize various organs in the process called **metastasis.** Such tumor stem cells thus can express **clonogenic** or colony-forming capability. Tumor stem cells often have chromosome abnormalities reflecting their genetic instability, which leads to progressive selection of subclones that can survive more readily in the multicellular environment of the host. Quantitative abnormalities in various metabolic pathways and cellular components accompany this neoplastic progression. The invasive and metastatic processes as well as a series of metabolic abnormalities resulting from the cancer cause illness and eventual death of the patient unless the neoplasm can be eradicated with treatment.

CANCER THERAPEUTIC MODALITIES

Next to heart disease, cancer is the major cause of death in the USA, causing over 500,000 fatalities annually. With present methods of treatment, one-third of patients are cured with local measures (surgery or radiation therapy), which are quite effective when the tumor has not metastasized by the time of treatment. Earlier diagnosis might lead to increased cure of patients with such local treatment; however, in the remaining cases, early micrometastasis is a characteristic feature of the neoplasm, indicating that a systemic approach such as chemotherapy will be required (often along with surgery or radiation) for effective cancer management. At present, about 50% of patients with cancer can be cured, with chemotherapy contributing to cure in about 17% of patients.

Cancer chemotherapy as currently employed can be curative in certain disseminated neoplasms that have undergone either gross or microscopic spread by the time of diagnosis. These include testicular cancer, diffuse large cell lymphoma, Hodgkin's disease, and choriocarcinoma as well as childhood tumors such as acute lymphoblastic leukemia, Burkitt's lymphoma, Wilms' tumor, and embryonal rhabdomyosarcoma. Of major importance are recent demonstrations that use of chemotherapy along with initial surgery can increase the cure rate in relatively early-stage breast cancer and osteogenic sarcoma. Common carcinomas of the lung and colon are generally refractory to currently available treatment and have usually disseminated by the time of diagnosis.

At present, chemotherapy provides palliative rather than curative therapy for many other forms of disseminated cancer. Effective palliation results in temporary clearing of the symptoms and signs of cancer and prolongation of useful life. In the past decade, advances in cancer chemotherapy have also begun to provide evidence that chemical control of neoplasia may become a reality for many forms of cancer. This will probably be achieved first through combined therapy in which optimal combinations of surgery, radiotherapy, and chemotherapy are used to eradicate both the primary neoplasm and its occult micrometastases before gross spread can be detected on physical or x-ray examination. Use of endocrine agents to modulate tumor growth is playing an increasing role in hormone-responsive tumors thanks to the development of hormone antagonists and partial agonists. Several recombinant biologic agents have recently been identified as being active for cancer therapy. These include interferon and interleukin-2. Gene therapy is the latest investigational approach to cancer treatment and is

now in the earliest stages of clinical investigation. It is too soon to make a judgment about whether it will be useful.

ANTICANCER DRUG DEVELOPMENT

A major effort to develop anticancer drugs through both empirical screening and rational design of new compounds has now been under way for over 3 decades. Recent advances in this field have included the synthesis of peptides and proteins with recombinant DNA techniques and monoclonal antibodies. The drug development program has employed testing in a few well-characterized transplantable animal tumor systems. Simple in vitro assays for measuring drug sensitivity of a battery of human tumor cells augment and shorten the testing program and are used currently as the primary screening tests for new agents by the National Cancer Institute and many pharmaceutical firms. After new drugs with potential anticancer activity are identified, they are subjected to preclinical toxicologic and limited pharmacologic studies in animals as described in Chapter 5. Promising agents that do not have excessive toxicity are then advanced to phase I clinical trials, wherein their pharmacologic and toxic effects are tested in patients with advanced cancer rather than in healthy volunteers. The remainder of clinical testing is similar to that for other drugs but may be accelerated.

Ideal anticancer drugs would eradicate cancer cells without harming normal tissues. Unfortunately, no currently available agents meet this criterion, and clinical use of these drugs involves a weighing of benefits against toxicity in a search for a favorable therapeutic index.

Classes of drugs that have recently entered development include inducers of differentiation, intended to force neoplastic cells past a maturation block to form end-stage cells with little or no proliferative potential; antimetastatic drugs, designed to perturb surface properties of malignant cells and thus alter their invasive and metastatic potential; hypoxic tumor stem cell-specific agents, designed to exploit the greater capacity for reductive reactions in these therapeutically resistant cells created by oxygen deficiency within solid tumors; tumor radiosensitizing and normal tissue radioprotecting drugs, aimed at increased therapeutic effectiveness of radiation therapy; and "biologic response modifiers," which alter tumor-host metabolic and immunologic relationships.

IMPORTANCE OF NEOPLASTIC CELL BURDEN

Patients with widespread cancer (eg, acute leukemia) may have more than 10^{12} tumor cells throughout the

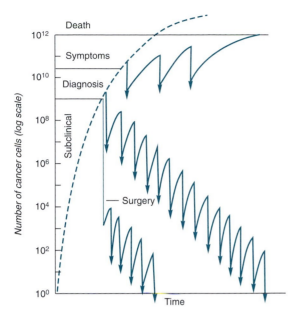

Figure 55–1. The "log-kill hypothesis." Relationship of tumor cell number to time of diagnosis, symptoms, treatment, and survival. Three alternative approaches to drug treatment are shown for comparison with the course of tumor growth when no treatment is given *(dashed line)*. In the protocol diagrammed at top, treatment (indicated by the arrows) is given infrequently and the result is manifested as prolongation of survival but with recurrence of symptoms between courses of treatment and eventual death of the patient. The combination chemotherapy treatment diagrammed in the middle section is begun earlier and is more intensive. Tumor cell kill exceeds regrowth, drug resistance does not develop, and "cure" results. In this example, treatment has been continued long after all clinical evidence of cancer has disappeared (1–3 years). This approach has been established as effective in the treatment of childhood acute leukemia, testicular cancers, and Hodgkin's disease. In the treatment diagrammed near the bottom of the graph, early surgery has been employed to remove the primary tumor and intensive adjuvant chemotherapy has been administered long enough (up to 1 year) to eradicate the remaining tumor cells that comprise the occult micrometastases.

body at the time of diagnosis (Figure 55–1). If tolerable dosing of an effective drug is capable of killing 99.9% of clonogenic tumor cells, this would induce a clinical remission of the neoplasm associated with symptomatic improvement. However, there would still be nine "logs" of tumor cells (10^9) remaining in the body, including some that might be inherently resistant to the drug because of heterogeneity, and others that might reside in pharmacologic sanctuaries (eg, the central nervous system, testes) where effective drug concentrations may be difficult to achieve. When cell cycle-specific drugs are used, the tumor stem cells must also be in the sensitive phase of the cell cycle (not in G_0), so scheduling of these agents is particularly im-

portant. In common bacterial infections, a three-log reduction in microorganisms might be curative because host resistance factors can eliminate residual bacteria through immunologic and microbicidal mechanisms; however, host mechanisms for eliminating moderate numbers of cancer cells appear to be generally ineffective.

Combinations of agents with differing toxicities and mechanisms of action are often employed to overcome the limited "log kill" of individual anticancer drugs. If the drugs do not have too much overlap in toxicity, they can be used at almost full dosage, and at least additive cytotoxic effects can be achieved with combination chemotherapy; furthermore, subclones resistant to only one of the agents can potentially be eradicated. Some combinations of anticancer drugs also appear to exert true synergism, wherein the effect of the two drugs is greater than additive. The efficacy of combination chemotherapy has now been validated in many forms of human cancer, and the scientific rationale appears to be sound. As a result, combination chemotherapy is now the standard approach to curative treatment of testicular cancer and lymphomas and palliative treatment of many other tumor types. This important therapeutic approach was first formulated by Skipper and Schabel and described as the "log-kill hypothesis" (Figure 55–1).

IMPORTANCE OF CELL CYCLE KINETICS

Information on cell and population kinetics of cancer cells in part explains the limited effectiveness of most available anticancer drugs. A schematic summary of cell cycle kinetics is presented in Figure 55–2. This information is relevant to the mode of action, indications, and scheduling of cell cycle-specific (CCS) and cell cycle-nonspecific (CCNS) drugs. Agents falling in these two major classes are summarized in Table 55–1.

In general, CCS drugs have proved most effective in hematologic malignancies and other tumors in which a relatively large proportion of the cells are proliferating or are in the **growth fraction.** CCNS drugs (many of which bind to DNA and damage these macromolecules) are useful in low-growth-fraction "solid tumors" as well as in high-growth-fraction tumors. In all instances, effective agents sterilize or inactivate tumor stem cells, which are often only a small fraction of the cells within a tumor. Non-stem cells (eg, those that have irreversibly differentiated) are considered sterile by definition and are not a significant component of the cancer problem.

Resistance to Cytotoxic Drugs

A major problem in cancer chemotherapy is **drug resistance.** Some tumor types, eg, non-small cell lung cancer and colon cancer, exhibit *primary* resistance,

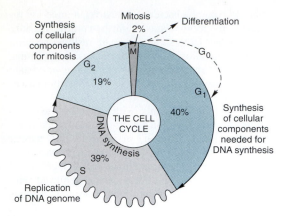

Figure 55–2. The cell cycle and cancer. A conceptual depiction of the cell cycle phases that all cells—normal and neoplastic—must traverse before and during cell division. The percentages given represent the approximate percentage of time spent in each phase by a typical malignant cell; the duration of G_1, however, can vary markedly. Many of the effective anticancer drugs exert their action on cells traversing the cell cycle and are called cell cycle-specific (CCS) drugs (Table 55–1). A second group of agents called cell cycle-nonspecific (CCNS) drugs can sterilize tumor cells whether they are cycling or resting in the G_0 compartment. CCNS drugs can kill both G_0 and cycling cells (although cycling cells are more sensitive).

ie, absence of response on the first exposure, to currently available standard agents. *Acquired* resistance develops in a number of drug-sensitive tumor types. Experimentally, drug resistance can be highly specific to a single drug and usually is based on a change in the tumor cells' genetic apparatus with *amplification* or increased expression of one or more specific genes. In other instances, a multidrug-resistant phenotype occurs—resistance to a variety of natural product anticancer drugs of differing structures developing after exposure to a single agent. This form of multidrug resistance is often associated with increased expression of a normal gene (the *MDR1* gene) for a cell surface glycoprotein (P-glycoprotein) involved in drug efflux.

Table 55–1. Cell cycle relationships of major classes of drugs.

Cell Cycle-Specific (CCS) Agents	Cell Cycle-Nonspecific (CCNS) Agents
Antimetabolites (azacitidine, cytarabine, fluorouracil, mercaptopurine, methotrexate, thioguanine)	Alkylating agents (busulfan, cyclophosphamide, mechlorethamine, melphalan, thiotepa)
Bleomycin peptide antibiotics	Antibiotics (dactinomycin, daunorubicin, doxorubicin, plicamycin, mitomycin)
Podophyllin alkaloids (etoposide, VP-16; teniposide, VM-26)	Cisplatin
Plant alkaloids (vincristine, vinblastine, paclitaxel)	Nitrosoureas (BCNU, CCNU, methyl-CCNU)

This transport molecule (Figure 55–3) uses the energy of ATP to expel a variety of foreign molecules (not limited to antitumor drugs) from the cell. It occurs constitutively in normal tissues such as epithelial cells of the kidney, large intestine, and adrenal gland as well as in a variety of tumors. Multidrug resistance can be reversed experimentally by calcium channel blockers, such as verapamil, and a variety of other drugs, which inhibit the transporter. Preliminary clinical results suggest that reversal of resistance by these drugs may be possible in patients. Other mechanisms of multiple drug resistance involve overexpression of the multidrug resistance-associated protein (MRP), a member of the ATP-binding cassette transmembrane transporter superfamily, that increases resistance to natural product drugs such as anthracyclines, *Vinca* alkaloids, and epipodophyllotoxins; and qualitative or quantitative changes in topoisomerase II, which repairs the lesions created in DNA by antitumor drugs.

I. BASIC PHARMACOLOGY OF CANCER CHEMOTHERAPEUTIC DRUGS

POLYFUNCTIONAL ALKYLATING AGENTS

The major clinically useful alkylating agents (Figure 55–4) have a structure containing a bis(chloroethyl)amine, ethylenimine, or nitrosourea moiety. Among the bis(chloroethyl)amines, cyclophosphamide, mechlorethamine, melphalan, and chlorambucil are the most useful. Ifosfamide is closely related to cyclophosphamide but has a somewhat different spectrum of activity and toxicity. Thiotepa and busulfan are used for specialized purposes for ovarian cancer and chronic myeloid leukemia, respectively. The major nitrosoureas are BCNU (carmustine), CCNU (lomustine), and methyl-CCNU (semustine). A variety of investigational alkylating agents have been synthesized that link various carrier molecules such as amino acids, nucleic acid bases, hormones, or sugar moieties to a group capable of alkylation; however, successful "site-directed" alkylation has not to date been achieved.

As a class, the alkylating agents exert cytotoxic effects via transfer of their alkyl groups to various cellular constituents. Alkylations of DNA within the nucleus probably represent the major interactions that lead to cell death. However, these drugs react chemically with sulfhydryl, amino, hydroxyl, carboxyl, and phosphate groups of other cellular nucleophiles as

Figure 55–3. Schematic concept of the P-glycoprotein drug transport molecule responsible for multidrug resistance in cancer cells. ATP is used to drive the efflux process. The protein consists of 12 transmembrane domains with two ATP binding sites, only one of which must be occupied for drug transport to occur. Verapamil, quinidine, cyclosporine, and certain other drugs are able to inhibit transport at concentrations as low as 3 μmol/L, probably by acting as competitive substrates.

well. The general mechanism of action of these drugs involves intramolecular cyclization to form an **ethyleneimonium ion** that may directly or through formation of a **carbonium ion** transfer an alkyl group to a cellular constituent. In addition to alkylation, a secondary mechanism that occurs with nitrosoureas involves carbamoylation of lysine resi-dues of proteins through formation of isocyanates.

The major site of alkylation within DNA is the N7 position of guanine (Figure 55–5); however, other bases are also alkylated to lesser degrees, including N1 and N3 of adenine, N3 of cytosine, and O6 of guanine, as well as phosphate atoms and proteins associated with DNA. These interactions can occur on a single strand or on both strands of DNA through cross-linking, as most major alkylating agents are bifunctional, with two reactive groups. Alkylation of guanine can result in miscoding through abnormal base pairing with thymine or in depurination by excision of guanine residues. The latter effect leads to DNA strand breakage through scission of the sugar-phosphate backbone of DNA. Cross-linking of DNA appears to be of major importance to the cytotoxic action of alkylating agents, and replicating cells are most susceptible to these drugs. Thus, although alkylating agents are not cell cycle-specific, cells are most susceptible to alkylation in late G_1 and S phases of the cell cycle and express block in G_2.

Drug Resistance

The mechanism of acquired resistance to alkylating agents may involve increased capability to repair DNA lesions, decreased permeability of the cell to the alkylating drug, and increased production of glutathione, which inactivates the alkylating agent through conjugation in a reaction catalyzed by glutathione S-transferase.

Pharmacologic Effects

Active alkylating agents have direct vesicant effects and can damage tissues at the site of injection as well as produce systemic toxicity. Toxicities are generally dose-related and occur particularly in rapidly growing tissues such as bone marrow, gastrointestinal tract, and gonads. After intravenous injection, nausea and vomiting usually occur within 30–60 minutes with mechlorethamine, cyclophosphamide, or BCNU. The emetic effects are of central nervous system origin and can be reduced by pretreatment with phenothiazines or cannabinoids (tetrahydrocannabinol, dronabinol). Subcutaneous injection of mechlorethamine or BCNU leads to tissue necrosis and sloughing. Cyclophosphamide does not have direct vesicant effects and must be activated to cytotoxic forms by microsomal enzymes (Figure 55–6).

The liver microsomal cytochrome P450 mixed-function oxidase system converts cyclophosphamide to 4-hydroxycyclophosphamide, which is in equilibrium with aldophosphamide. These active metabolites are believed to be carried by the bloodstream to tumor and normal tissue, where nonenzymatic cleavage of aldophosphamide to the cytotoxic forms—phosphoramide mustard and acrolein—occurs. The liver appears to be protected through the enzymatic formation of the inactive metabolites 4-ketocyclophosphamide and carboxyphosphamide. The major toxicity of alky-

Figure 55–4. Structures of major classes of alkylating agents.

lating agents is on the bone marrow and results in dose-related suppression of myelopoiesis. The white blood count and absolute granulocyte count reach their low points 10–12 days after injection of mechlorethamine or cyclophosphamide, with subsequent recovery within 21 (cyclophosphamide) to 42 (mechlorethamine) days. The white count nadir with nitrosoureas is delayed to 28 days, with recovery by 42 days. Effects on megakaryocytes and platelets parallel those on granulocytes. Because of the long life span of the erythrocyte, effects on erythropoiesis are minor and the red cell count is usually only mildly reduced. Adverse effects on the bone marrow may be more severe when an alkylating agent is given along with other myelosuppressive drugs or radiation therapy, and dose reductions are often required in such circumstances to avoid excessive toxicity.

Following hematopoietic recovery, these agents may be given again on an intermittent dosage schedule at sufficient intervals to permit blood count recovery. Ovarian or testicular failure is a common late sequel of alkylating agent therapy, while acute

leukemia is a relatively rare complication of use of these mutagenic agents.

Oral dosage forms of alkylating agents have been of great value and have been developed using relatively less reactive alkylating drugs. Oral administration of cyclophosphamide, melphalan, chlorambucil, busulfan, and CCNU represents the most common route of administration of these agents and produces effects similar to those observed with parenteral administration. In general, if a tumor is resistant to one alkylating agent, it will be relatively resistant to other agents of this class (though not necessarily to nitrosoureas); however, there are distinct exceptions to this rule for specific tumor types. Overall, cyclophosphamide is the most useful alkylating agent currently available. The oral drug busulfan has a major degree of specificity for the granulocyte series and therefore is of particular value in therapy of chronic myelogenous leukemia. With all oral alkylating agents, some degree of leukopenia is necessary to provide evidence that the drug has been absorbed adequately. Repeated blood counts are essential during administration of

Figure 55–5. Mechanism of alkylation of DNA guanine. A bis(chloroethyl)amine forms an ethyleneimonium ion and a carbonium ion that react with a base such as N7 of guanine in DNA, producing an alkylated purine. Alkylation of a second guanine residue, through the illustrated mechanism, results in cross-linking of DNA strands.

Figure 55–6. Cyclophosphamide metabolism.

these agents because the development of severe leukopenia or thrombocytopenia necessitates interruption of therapy.

NITROSOUREAS (Carmustine [BCNU], Lomustine [CCNU], & Semustine [Methyl-CCNU])

These drugs appear to be non-cross-reactive (as regards tumor resistance) with other alkylating agents; all appear to require biotransformation, which occurs by nonenzymatic decomposition, to derivatives with both alkylating and carbamoylating activities. The nitrosoureas are highly lipid-soluble and cross the blood-brain barrier, making them useful in the treatment of brain tumors. The nitrosoureas appear to function by cross-linking through alkylation of DNA. The drugs may be more effective against plateau phase cells than exponentially growing cells, though within a cycling cell population the drugs appear to slow cell progression through the DNA synthetic phase. After oral administration of CCNU or methyl-CCNU, peak plasma levels of metabolites appear within 1–4 hours; central nervous system concentrations reach 30–40% of the activity present in the plasma. While the initial plasma half-life is in the range of 6 hours, a second half-life is in the range of 1–2 days. Urinary excretion appears to be the major route of elimination from the body. One naturally occurring sugar-containing nitrosourea, streptozocin, is interesting because it has minimal bone marrow toxicity but is frequently effective in the treatment of insulin-secreting islet cell carcinoma of the pancreas and occasionally in non-Hodgkin's lymphomas.

RELATED DRUGS PROBABLY ACTING AS ALKYLATING AGENTS

A variety of other compounds have mechanisms of action that involve alkylation. These include procarbazine, dacarbazine, altretamine (hexamethylmelamine), and cisplatin.

1. PROCARBAZINE

The oral agent procarbazine is a methylhydrazine derivative with chemotherapeutic activity (particularly in Hodgkin's disease). The drug is also leukemogenic and has teratogenic and mutagenic properties.

The mechanism of action of procarbazine is uncertain; however, the drug inhibits the synthesis of DNA, RNA, and protein; prolongs interphase; and produces chromosome breaks. Oxidative metabolism of this drug by microsomal enzymes generates azoprocarbazine and H_2O_2, which may be responsible for DNA

strand scission. A variety of other metabolites of the drug are formed that may be cytotoxic. One metabolite is a monoamine oxidase (MAO) inhibitor, and adverse side effects can occur when procarbazine is given with other MAO inhibitors. Nausea, vomiting, and myelosuppression are predictable effects; in addition, hemolytic anemia, pulmonary reactions, and adverse responses with alcohol (disulfiram-like) have also been reported, as have skin rashes when procarbazine is given with phenytoin.

Procarbazine is often used in combination chemotherapy of Hodgkin's disease; however, its leukemogenic properties may eventually lead to its replacement with drugs that have lesser carcinogenic potential.

2. DACARBAZINE

Dacarbazine is a synthetic compound that functions as an alkylating agent following metabolic activation by liver microsomal enzymes by oxidative N-demethylation to the monomethyl derivative that spontaneously decomposes to 5-aminoimidazole-4-carboxamide, which is excreted in the urine, and diazomethane. The diazomethane generates a methyl carbonium ion that is believed to be the likely cytotoxic species. Dacarbazine is administered parenterally and is not schedule-dependent. It produces marked nausea, vomiting, and myelosuppression. Its major applications are in melanoma, Hodgkin's disease, and some soft tissue sarcomas. In the latter two tumors, its activity is potentiated by doxorubicin.

3. ALTRETAMINE (Hexamethylmelamine)

Altretamine is structurally similar to triethylenemelamine. It is relatively insoluble and available only in oral form. A related compound, pentamethylmelamine, which is a major metabolite of hexamethylmelamine, is more soluble and is now in clinical trial in an intravenous form. Both agents are rapidly biotransformed by demethylation, presumably to active intermediates. These agents cause nausea, vomiting, and central and peripheral nervous system neuropathies but relatively mild myelosuppression. Altretamine is useful in alkylating agent-resistant ovarian carcinoma.

4. CISPLATIN

Cisplatin (cis-diamminedichloroplatinum [II]) is an inorganic metal complex discovered by Rosenberg and his colleagues, who made the serendipitous observation that neutral platinum complexes inhibit division and induce filamentous growth of Escherichia coli. Many platinum analogs of this very important drug have been synthesized. While the precise mechanism of action of cisplatin is still undefined, it is thought to act analogously to alkylating agents. It kills cells in all stages of the cell cycle, inhibits DNA biosynthesis, and binds DNA through the formation of interstrand cross-links. The primary binding site is the N7 of guanine, but covalent interaction with adenine and cytosine also occurs. The platinum complexes appear to synergize with certain other anticancer drugs. After intravenous administration, the major acute toxicity is nausea and vomiting. Cisplatin has relatively little effect on the bone marrow, but it can induce significant renal dysfunction and occasional acoustic nerve dysfunction. Hydration with saline infusion alone or with mannitol or other diuretics appears to minimize nephrotoxicity.

$$H_3N \diagdown \quad Cl$$
$$Pt$$
$$H_3N \diagup \quad Cl$$

Cisplatin

Cisplatin has major antitumor activity in genitourinary cancers, particularly testicular, ovarian, and bladder cancer. Its use along with vinblastine and bleomycin has been a major advance in the development of curative therapy for nonseminomatous testicular cancers. A platinum analog (carboplatin) with significantly less gastrointestinal and renal toxicity but with myelosuppressive toxicity provides a useful alternative to cisplatin.

Dosage & Toxicity of the Alkylating Agents

The alkylating agents are used in the treatment of a wide variety of hematologic and solid cancers, generally as components of combination chemotherapy. These are discussed along with various specific tumors. Dosages and major toxicities are listed in Table 55–2.

Nausea and vomiting are almost universally reported with intravenously administered mechlorethamine, cyclophosphamide, and carmustine and occur with moderate frequency with oral cyclophosphamide.

The important toxic effect of therapeutic doses of virtually all the alkylating drugs is depression of bone marrow and subsequent leukopenia and thrombocytopenia. Severe infections and septicemia may result, with granulocytopenia below 600 PMNs/μL. Platelet depression below 40,000/μL may be accompanied by induced hemorrhagic phenomena. Cyclophosphamide may produce slight to severe alopecia in up to 30% of patients. It may also cause hemorrhagic cystitis. The cystitis can often be averted with adequate hydration.

The hematopoietic effects of toxic doses of alkylating drugs are treated by discontinuing the agent. Red cell and platelet transfusions and antibiotics to control infections are employed as needed until the marrow has regenerated.

ANTIMETABOLITES (Structural Analogs)

The development of drugs with actions on intermediary metabolism of proliferating cells has been important both clinically and conceptually. While biochemical properties unique to all cancer cells have yet to be discovered, neoplastic cells do have a number of quantitative differences in metabolism from normal cells that render them more susceptible to a number of antimetabolites or structural analogs. Many of these agents have been rationally designed and synthesized, based on knowledge of cellular processes, though a few have been discovered as antibiotics.

Mechanism of Action

The biochemical pathways that have thus far proved to be most exploitable with antimetabolites have been those relating to nucleotide and nucleic acid synthesis. In a number of instances, when an enzyme is known to have a major effect on pathways leading to cell replication, inhibitors of the reaction it catalyzes have proved to be useful anticancer drugs.

These drugs and their doses and toxicities are shown in Table 55–3. The principal drugs are discussed below.

METHOTREXATE

Methotrexate (MTX) is a folic acid antagonist that binds to the active catalytic site of dihydrofolate reductase (DHFR), interfering with the synthesis of the reduced form that accepts one-carbon units. Lack of this cofactor interrupts the synthesis of thymidylate, purine nucleotides, and the amino acids serine and methionine, thereby interfering with the formation of DNA, RNA, and protein. The enzyme binds methotrexate extremely tightly, and at pH 6.0 virtually no dissociation of the enzyme-inhibitor complex occurs (inhibition constant about 1 nmol/L). At physiologic pH, reversible competitive kinetics occur (inhibition constant about 1 μmol/L). Intracellular formation of polyglutamate derivatives appears to be important in the therapeutic action of methotrexate. The polyglutamates of meth-otrexate are retained by cells longer than methotrexate and have increased inhibitory effects on enzymes involved in folate metabolism, making them important determinants of the duration of action of methotrexate.

Table 55–2. Polyfunctional alkylating agents and probable alkylating agents: Dosages and toxicity.

Alkylating Agent	Single-Agent Dosage	Acute Toxicity	Delayed Toxicity
Mechlorethamine (nitrogen mustard; HN2; Mustargen)	0.4 mg/kg IV in single or divided doses	Nausea and vomiting	Moderate depression of peripheral blood count. Excessive doses produce severe bone marrow depression with leukopenia, thrombocytopenia, and bleeding. Alopecia and hemorrhagic cystitis occasionally occur with cyclophosphamide. Cystitis can be prevented with adequate hydration. Busulfan is associated with skin pigmentation, pulmonary fibrosis, and adrenal insufficiency.
Chlorambucil (Leukeran)	0.1–0.2 mg/kg/d orally; 6–12 mg/d	None	
Cyclophosphamide (Cytoxan)	3.5–5 mg/kg/d orally for 10 days; 1 g/m² IV as single dose	Nausea and vomiting	
Melphalan (Alkeran)	0.25 mg/kg/d orally for 4 days every 4–6 weeks		
Thiotepa (triethylenethiophosphoramide)	0.2 mg/kg IV for 5 days	None	
Busulfan (Myleran)	2–8 mg/d orally; 150–250 mg/course	None	
Carmustine (BCNU)	200 mg/m² IV every 6 weeks	Nausea and vomiting	Leukopenia and thrombocytopenia. Rarely hepatitis.
Lomustine (CCNU)	150 mg/m² orally every 6 weeks	Nausea and vomiting	
Semustine (methyl-CCNU)	150 mg/m² orally every 6 weeks	Nausea and vomiting	
Altretamine (hexamethylmelamine)	10 mg/kg/d for 21 days	Nausea and vomiting	Leukopenia, thrombocytopenia, and peripheral neuropathy.
Procarbazine (Matulane)	50–200 mg/d orally	Nausea and vomiting	Bone marrow depression, central nervous system depression.
Dacarbazine	300 mg/m² daily IV for 5 days	Nausea and vomiting	Bone marrow depression.
Cisplatin (Platinol)	20 mg/m²/d IV for 5 days or 50–70 mg/m² as single dose every 3 weeks	Nausea and vomiting	Renal dysfunction. Acoustic nerve dysfunction.
Carboplatin (Paraplatin)	360 mg/m² IV every 4 weeks	Nausea and vomiting	Leukopenia and thrombocytopenia. Rarely neuropathy or hepatic dysfunction.

Drug Resistance

Tumor cell resistance to methotrexate has been attributed to (1) decreased drug transport, (2) altered DHFR with lower affinity for methotrexate, (3) decreased polyglutamate formation, and (4) synthesis of increased levels of DHFR. This occurs through gene amplification and results in a marked increase in DHFR messenger RNA. It remains to be established whether this genetic resistance mechanism is relevant for other drugs or for resistant tumors in patients receiving methotrexate.

Dosage & Toxicity

Methotrexate is administered by the intravenous or oral route (Table 55–3). Up to 90% of an oral dose is excreted in the urine within 12 hours. The drug is not subject to metabolism, and serum levels are therefore proportionate to dose as long as renal function and hydration status are adequate. Toxic effects to proliferating tissues are usually observed in the bone marrow and to a lesser extent in the skin and gastrointestinal mucosa. The effects of methotrexate can be reversed

Folic acid

Methotrexate

Table 55–3. Structural analogs: Dosages and toxicity.

Chemotherapeutic Agent	Single-Agent Dosage	Delayed Toxicity[1]
Azacitidine[2]	200 mg/m^2/d IV for 5 days	Nausea and vomiting, diarrhea, fever, hypotension, prolonged bone marrow hypoplasia.
Cladribine (Leustatin)	0.09 mg/kg/d for 7 days by continuous IV infusion in sterile saline	Severe myelosuppression for about 2 weeks after therapy.
Cytarabine (ara-C, Cytosar-U)	100 mg/m^2/d for 5–10 days, either by continuous IV infusion or SC every 8 hours	Nausea and vomiting, bone marrow depression, megaloblastosis, leukopenia, thrombocytopenia.
Fludarabine (Fludara)	25 mg/m^2/d for 5 days every 28 days (administer IV over 30 minutes)	Myelosuppression. **Note:** High doses can cause serious neurotoxicity.
Fluorouracil (5-FU, Adrucil)	15 mg/kg/d IV for 5 days by 24-hour infusion; 15 mg/kg weekly IV	Nausea, oral and gastrointestinal ulceration, bone marrow depression.
Mercaptopurine (6-MP, Purinethol)	2.5 mg/kg/d orally	Usually well tolerated. Larger dosages may cause bone marrow depression.
Methotrexate (amethopterin, MTX)	2.5–5 mg/d orally (Rheumatrex); 10 mg intrathecally (Folex) once or twice weekly	Oral and gastrointestinal tract ulceration, bone marrow depression, leukopenia, thrombocytopenia.
Thioguanine (6-TG)	2 mg/kg/d orally	Usually well tolerated. Larger dosages may cause bone marrow depression.
Supportive agent with all drugs Allopurinol (Zyloprim)	300–800 mg/d orally for prevention or relief of hyperuricemia	Usually none. Enhances effects and toxicity of mercaptopurine when used in combination.

[1]These drugs do not cause acute toxicity.
[2]For use only in approved treatment protocols.

by administration of leucovorin (citrovorum factor). Leucovorin "rescue" has been used with accidental overdose or experimentally along with high-dose methotrexate therapy in a protocol intended to rescue normal cells while still leaving the tumor cells subject to its cytotoxic action.

Other Applications

Methotrexate also has important applications in the treatment of rheumatoid arthritis (Chapter 36) and psoriasis. It is in clinical trials for the treatment of asthma (Chapter 20). Used with a prostaglandin, methotrexate has proved to be an effective abortifacient.

PURINE ANTAGONISTS

1. 6-THIOPURINES (Mercaptopurine [6-MP] & Thioguanine [6-TG])

Mercaptopurine was the first of the thiopurine series found useful as an anticancer drug. Like other thiopurines, it must be metabolized by hypoxanthine-guanine phosphoribosyl transferase (HGPRT) to the nucleotide form (6-thioinosinic acid), which in turn inhibits a number of the enzymes of purine interconversion. Significant amounts of thioguanylic acid and 6-methylmercaptopurine ribotide (MMPR) also are

formed from 6-MP. These metabolites may also contribute to the action of the mercaptopurine. 6-MP is used primarily in the treatment of childhood acute leukemia, and a closely related analog, azathioprine, is used as an immunosuppressive agent (see Chapter 56).

Thioguanine inhibits several enzymes in the purine nucleotide pathway. A variety of metabolic lesions are associated with the cytotoxic action of the purinethiols. These include inhibition of purine nucleotide interconversion; decrease in intracellular levels of guanine nucleotides, which leads to inhibition of glycoprotein synthesis; interference with the formation of DNA and RNA; and incorporation of purinethiols into both DNA and RNA. 6-TG has a synergistic action when used together with cytarabine in the treatment of adult acute leukemia.

Drug Resistance

Resistance to both 6-MP and 6-TG occurs most commonly by decrease in HGPRT activity; an alternative mechanism in acute leukemia involves elevation of levels of alkaline phosphatase, which results in dephosphorylation of thiopurine nucleotide and cellular loss of the resulting ribonucleoside.

Dosage & Toxicity

Mercaptopurine and thioguanine are both given orally (Table 55–3) and excreted mainly in the urine. However, 6-MP is converted to an inactive metabolite

(6-thiouric acid) by an oxidation catalyzed by xanthine oxidase, whereas 6-TG requires deamination before it is metabolized by this enzyme. This factor is important because the purine analog allopurinol, a potent xanthine oxidase inhibitor, is frequently used with chemotherapy in hematologic cancers to prevent hyperuricemia after tumor cell lysis. It prevents this by blocking purine breakdown, allowing excretion of cellular purines that are relatively more soluble than uric acid. Nephrotoxicity and acute gout produced by excessive uric acid are thereby prevented. Simultaneous therapy with allopurinol and 6-MP results in excessive mercaptopurine toxicity unless the dose of mercaptopurine is reduced to 25–30% of the usual level. This effect does not occur with 6-TG, which can be used in full doses with allopurinol.

Hypoxanthine   **6-Mercaptopurine**   **Allopurinol**

Guanine   **6-Thioguanine**

2. FLUDARABINE PHOSPHATE

Fludarabine phosphate (2-fluoro-arabinofuranosyladenine monophosphate) is rapidly dephosphorylated in vivo to 2-fluoro-arabinofuranosyladenine and then phosphorylated intracellularly by deoxycytidine kinase to the triphosphate. This product interferes with DNA synthesis through inhibition of DNA polymerase and ribonucleotide reductase. Fludarabine phosphate is used chiefly in the treatment of lymphoproliferative diseases. Fludarabine phosphate is given parentally and is excreted primarily in the urine; its dose-limiting toxicity is myelosuppression.

3. CLADRIBINE

Cladribine (2-chlorodeoxyadenosine) achieves high intracellular concentrations because of its resistance to adenosine deaminase; it is phosphorylated by deoxycytidine kinase and is incorporated into DNA. Cladribine causes DNA strand breaks (presumably through interference with DNA repair) and loss of NAD (through activation of poly[ADP-ribose]syn-

thase). Cladribine has been recommended for the treatment of hairy cell leukemia. It is given as a single continuous 7-day infusion; under these conditions its toxicity usually consists of transient severe marrow suppression. Myelosuppression may be associated with infection.

PYRIMIDINE ANTAGONISTS

1. FLUOROURACIL

Fluorouracil (5-FU) undergoes biotransformation to ribosyl and deoxyribosyl nucleotide metabolites. One of these metabolites, 5-fluoro-2'-deoxyuridine 5'-phosphate (FdUMP), forms a covalently bound ternary complex with the enzyme thymidylate synthase and its cofactor $N^{5,10}$-methylenetetrahydrofolate, a reaction critical for the synthesis of thymine nucleotides. This results in inhibition of DNA synthesis through "thymineless death." Fluorouracil is converted to 5-fluorouridine triphosphate and incorporated into RNA, where it interferes with RNA processing and function. Cytotoxicity of fluorouracil is thus due to its effects on both DNA and RNA.

Uracil   **5-FU**

Fluorouracil is normally given intravenously (Table 55–3) and has a short metabolic half-life. Although it is active when given orally, its bioavailability is erratic by that route of administration. Floxuridine (5-fluorodeoxyuridine, FUDR) has an action similar to that of fluorouracil and is used for hepatic artery infusions. A cream incorporating fluorouracil is used topically for treating skin cancers. Fluorouracil is used systemically in the treatment of a variety of adenocarcinomas. Its major toxicities are myelosuppression and mucositis.

2. CYTARABINE

Cytarabine (cytosine arabinoside, ara-C) is an S phase-specific antimetabolite that is converted by deoxycytidine kinase to the 5'-mononucleotide (AraCMP). AraCMP is further metabolized to the triphosphate (AraCTP), which competitively inhibits DNA polymerase. This results in blockade of DNA synthesis while RNA and protein formation continues and leads to unbalanced growth. Cytarabine is also incorporated into RNA and DNA. Incorporation into DNA leads to interference with chain elongation and defective ligation of fragments of newly synthesized DNA. The cellular retention time for AraCTP appears to correlate with its lethality to malignant cells.

Cytosine deoxyriboside

Cytosine arabinoside (cytarabine)

After intravenous administration (Table 55–3), the drug is cleared rapidly, with most of it being deaminated to an inactive form. The ratio of the anabolic enzyme deoxycytidine kinase to the inactivating catalyst cytidine deaminase is important to the cytotoxicity of cytarabine.

In view of cytarabine's S phase specificity, the drug is highly schedule-dependent and must be given either by continuous infusion or every 8–12 hours for 5–7 days. Its activity is limited almost entirely to treatment of acute myelogenous leukemia, for which it is a major drug. Adverse effects include nausea, severe myelosuppression, and varying degrees of stomatitis or alopecia.

3. AZACITIDINE

Azacitidine (5-azacytidine) produces multiple effects associated with its cytotoxicity. It is phosphorylated to the mononucleotide form by uridine-cytidine kinase. Azacytidine 5′-phosphate then inhibits orotidylate decarboxylase, which reduces production of pyrimidine nucleotides. Further metabolism results in incorporation of azacitidine into DNA and RNA and inhibition of DNA, RNA, and protein synthesis.

Azacitidine is administered intravenously (Table 55–3) and must be shielded from light and kept at slightly acid pH, because it is unstable and can undergo ring opening. Nausea and fever are observed during drug administration. The half-life is 3–6 hours, with most of the drug excreted either unchanged or in deaminated form.

Azacitidine is currently an investigational agent in the USA, but it is a recognized second-line agent in the treatment of acute leukemia. Optimal dosage schedules have yet to be developed. The drug can produce profound myelosuppressive toxicity of long duration.

PLANT ALKALOIDS

VINBLASTINE

Vinblastine is an alkaloid derived from *Vinca rosea,* the periwinkle plant. Its mechanism of action involves depolymerization of microtubules, which are an important part of the cytoskeleton and the mitotic spindle. The drug binds specifically to the microtubular protein tubulin in dimeric form; the drug-tubulin complex adds to the forming end of the microtubules to terminate assembly, and depolymerization of the microtubules then occurs. This results in mitotic arrest at metaphase, dissolution of the mitotic spindle, and interference with chromosome segregation. It produces nausea and vomiting and marrow depression as well as alopecia. It has value in the treatment of systemic Hodgkin's disease and other lymphomas. See clinical section below and Table 55–4. Several related agents, including desacetylvinblastine (vindesine) and vinzolidine, are currently in clinical trial as investigational drugs.

Cytidine

5-Azacytidine

Vincristine

R: O $=$ C $-$ H

Vinblastine

R: CH_3

Table 55–4. Natural product cancer chemotherapy drugs: Dosages and toxicity.

Drug	Single-Agent Dosage	Acute Toxicity	Delayed Toxicity
Bleomycin (Blenoxane)	Up to 15 units/m² twice weekly to a total dose of 200 mg/m²	Allergic reactions, fever, hypotension	Edema of hands, pulmonary fibrosis, stomatitis, alopecia
Dactinomycin (actinomycin D, Cosmegen)	0.04 mg/kg IV weekly	Nausea and vomiting	Stomatitis, gastrointestinal tract upset, alopecia, bone marrow depression
Daunorubicin (daunomycin, Cerubidine)	30–60 mg/m² daily IV for 3 days, or 30–60 mg/m² IV weekly	Nausea, fever, red urine (not hematuria)	Cardiotoxicity, bone marrow depression, alopecia
Docetaxel (Taxotere)	100 mg/m² IV over 1 hour every 3 weeks	Hypersensitivity	Neurotoxicity, fluid retention, neutropenia
Doxorubicin (Adriamycin)	60 mg/m² IV every 3 weeks to a maximum total dose of 550 mg/m²	Nausea, red urine (not hematuria)	Cardiotoxicity, alopecia, bone marrow depression, stomatitis
Etoposide (VePesid, VP-16)	50–100 mg/m² daily for 5 days	Nausea, vomiting, hypotension	Alopecia, bone marrow depression
Idarubicin (Idamycin)	12 mg/m² IV daily for 3 days (with cytarabine)	Nausea and vomiting	Bone marrow suppression, mucositis, cardiotoxicity
Irinotecan (Camptosar)	125 mg/m² IV once weekly for 4 weeks; repeat every 6 weeks	Diarrhea, nausea, vomiting	Diarrhea (severe), bone marrow suppression
Mitomycin (Mutamycin)	20 mg/m² every 6 weeks	Nausea	Thrombocytopenia, leukopenia
Paclitaxel (Taxol)	130–170 mg/m² IV over 3 or 24 hours every 3–4 weeks	Nausea, vomiting, hypotension, arrhythmias	Bone marrow suppression
Plicamycin (mithramycin, Mithracin)	25–50 μg/kg IV every other day for up to 8 doses	Nausea and vomiting	Thrombocytopenia, hepatotoxicity
Topotecan (Hycamtin)	1.5 mg/m² IV for 5 days, repeat every 21 days for 4 courses	Nausea and vomiting	Bone marrow suppression
Vinblastine (Velban)	0.1–0.2 mg/kg IV weekly	Nausea and vomiting	Alopecia, loss of reflexes, bone marrow depression
Vincristine (Oncovin)	1.5 mg/m² IV (maximum: 2 mg weekly)	None	Areflexia, muscle weakness, peripheral neuritis, paralytic ileus, mild bone marrow depression, alopecia
Vinorelbine (Navelbine)	30 mg/m² IV weekly	Nausea and vomiting	Fatigue, constipation, hyporeflexia, paresthesias, bone marrow depression

VINCRISTINE

Vincristine, also an alkaloid derivative of *V rosea,* is closely related in structure to vinblastine. Its mechanism of action is considered to be identical to that of vinblastine, and it also appears to be a "spindle poison" and to cause arrest of the mitotic cycle. Despite these similarities to vinblastine, vincristine has a strikingly different spectrum of clinical activity and qualitatively different toxicities.

Vincristine has been used with considerable success in combination with prednisone for remission induction in acute leukemia in children. It is also useful in certain other rapidly proliferating neoplasms. It causes a significant incidence of neurotoxicity (Table 55–4), which limits its use to short courses. It occasionally produces bone marrow depression.

PODOPHYLLOTOXINS (Etoposide & Teniposide)

Two compounds, VP-16 (etoposide) and a related drug, VM-26 (teniposide), are semisynthetic derivatives of podophyllotoxin, which is extracted from the root of the mayapple (*Podophyllum peltatum*). Etoposide is approved for clinical use in the USA; an oral formulation is still investigational.

Etoposide and teniposide are quite similar in chemical structure, both clinically and in their block of cells in the late S-G$_2$ phase of the cell cycle. The mode of action involves inhibition of topoisomerase II, which results in DNA damage through strand breakage induced by the formation of a ternary complex of drug, DNA, and enzyme. The drugs are water-insoluble and require a solubilizing vehicle for clinical formulation. After intravenous administration (Table 55–4), they are protein-bound and distributed throughout the body except for the brain. Excretion is predominantly in the urine, with a lesser amount excreted in bile. In addition to nausea, vomiting, and alopecia, significant toxicity occurs to the hematopoietic and lymphoid systems. Thus far, etoposide has shown activity in monocytic leukemia, testicular cancer, and oat cell carcinoma of the lung; teniposide has activity in various lymphomas.

CAMPTOTHECINS (Topotecan & Irinotecan)

The camptothecins are natural products that interfere with the activity of topoisomerase I, the enzyme responsible for cutting and religating single DNA strands. Inhibition of the enzyme results in DNA damage. Topotecan and irinotecan have been approved recently for clinical use.

Topotecan has been evaluated in several small studies, and preliminary experience indicates that it is valuable in the control of metastatic ovarian cancer, including cisplatin-resistant neoplasms. The drug appears to be as effective as paclitaxel in this disease, though the time to clinical response may be greater. Neutropenia, thrombocytopenia, and anemia are the primary dose-limiting adverse effects. Nausea, vomiting, and alopecia are common.

Irinotecan is a prodrug that is metabolized to an active topoisomerase I inhibitor, SN-38. Irinotecan is indicated in the treatment of patients with colon and rectal cancer, including those whose disease is not responsive to fluorouracil. Diarrhea is the most common adverse effect and can be severe, causing hypovolemia in some cases. The diarrhea that occurs acutely appears to involve a different mechanism from the diarrhea that occurs later. Nausea and vomiting are also common. Myelosuppression is frequently the dose-limiting adverse effect.

TAXANES (Paclitaxel & Docetaxel)

Paclitaxel is an alkaloid ester derived from the Western yew *(Taxus brevifolia)* and the European yew *(Taxus baccata)*. The drug functions as a mitotic spindle poison through the enhancement of tubulin polymerization. This promotion of microtubule assembly by paclitaxel occurs in the absence of microtubule-associated proteins (MAPs) and guanosine triphosphate.

Paclitaxel has significant activity in ovarian and advanced breast cancer. Neutropenia, thrombocytopenia, and peripheral neuropathy are its primary dose-limiting toxicities.

A related drug, docetaxel, has been approved recently. This taxane drug is also approved for use in advanced breast cancer. Its major toxicities are bone marrow suppression, especially in patients with pre-existing hepatic impairment.

ANTIBIOTICS

Screening of microbial products has led to the discovery of a number of growth inhibitors that have proved to be clinically useful in cancer chemotherapy. Many of these antibiotics bind to DNA through intercalation between specific bases and block the synthesis of new RNA or DNA (or both), cause DNA strand scission, and interfere with cell replication. All of the clinically useful anticancer antibiotics now available are products of various strains of the soil fungus *Streptomyces.* These include the anthracyclines, actinomycin, bleomycin, mitomycin, and plicamycin.

ANTHRACYCLINES (Doxorubicin & Daunorubicin)

The anthracycline antibiotics, isolated from *Streptomyces peucetius* var *caesius,* are among the most useful cytotoxic anticancer drugs. Two congeners, doxorubicin and daunorubicin, are FDA-approved and in general use. Their structures are shown below.

R: —C—CH₃ Daunorubicin

R: —C—CH₂OH Doxorubicin

Other anthracyclines are currently being developed, including semisynthetic agents. Daunorubicin (the first agent in this class to be isolated) is used in the treatment of acute leukemia. Doxorubicin has a broad spectrum of potent activity against many different types of cancers.

Mechanism of Action

Three major actions have been documented for the organ and tumor toxicities of the anthracyclines. These include (1) high-affinity binding to DNA through intercalation, with consequent blockade of the synthesis of DNA and RNA, and DNA strand scission through effects on topoisomerase II; (2) binding to membranes to alter fluidity and ion transport; and (3) generation of the semiquinone free radical and oxygen radicals through an enzyme-mediated reductive process. This latter action may be responsible for cardiac toxicity through oxygen radical-mediated damage to membranes.

Pharmacokinetics

In clinical use, anthracyclines are administered by the intravenous route (Table 55–4). Peak blood concentration decreases by 50% within the first 30 minutes after injection, but significant levels persist for up to 20 hours. The anthracyclines are metabolized by the liver, with reduction and hydrolysis of the ring substituents. An alcohol form is an active metabolite, whereas the aglycone is inactive. Most of the drug and its metabolites are excreted in bile, and about one-sixth is excreted in urine. Some metabolites retain antitumor activity. The biliary route of excretion includes enterohepatic recirculation of cytotoxic moieties. In patients with significant elevations of serum bilirubin (> 2.5 mg/dL), the initial dose of anthracyclines must be reduced by 75%.

Clinical Uses

Doxorubicin is one of the most important anticancer drugs, with major clinical application in carcinomas of the breast, endometrium, ovary, testicle, thyroid, and lung and in treatment of many sarcomas, including neuroblastoma, Ewing's sarcoma, osteosarcoma, and rhabdomyosarcoma. It is useful also in hematologic cancers, including acute leukemia, multiple myeloma, Hodgkin's disease, and the diffuse non-Hodgkin's lymphomas. It is used in adjuvant therapy in osteogenic sarcoma and breast cancer. It is generally used in combination with other agents (eg, cyclophosphamide, cisplatin, and nitrosoureas), with which it often synergizes, yielding longer remissions than are observed when it is used as a single agent. This approach can also minimize some of the toxicities that would otherwise be associated with use of higher dosages of doxorubicin.

The major use of daunorubicin is in acute leukemia, and for this purpose the drug may have slightly greater activity than doxorubicin. However, daunorubicin appears to have a far narrower spectrum of utility; its efficacy in solid tumors appears to be limited.

A new anthracycline analog, **idarubicin,** has completed clinical trials and now is approved for use in acute myeloid leukemia. When combined with cytarabine, idarubicin appears to be somewhat more active than daunorubicin in producing complete remissions in patients with acute myelogenous leukemia. There is also some improvement in survival duration with idarubicin plus cytarabine as compared with daunorubicin plus cytarabine.

Adverse Reactions

In common with many other cytotoxic drugs, the anthracyclines cause bone marrow depression, which is of short duration with rapid recovery. Toxicities more pronounced with doxorubicin and daunorubicin than with other agents include a potentially irreversible cumulative, dose-related cardiac toxicity. The mechanism of cardiac toxicity is still under study but appears to involve excessive intracellular production of free radicals within the myocardium by doxorubicin. This is rarely seen at doxorubicin dosages below 500 mg/m^2. Use of lower weekly doses or continuous infusions of doxorubicin that avoid high peak plasma concentrations appear to reduce the frequency of cardiac toxicity as compared with intermittent (every 3–4 weeks) higher dosage schedules.

A second toxicity of doxorubicin and daunorubicin is the almost universal occurrence of severe or total alopecia at standard dosages.

DACTINOMYCIN

Dactinomycin is an antitumor antibiotic isolated from a *Streptomyces* organism.

Mechanism of Action & Pharmacokinetics

Dactinomycin binds tightly to double-stranded DNA through intercalation between adjacent guanine-cytosine base pairs. Dactinomycin inhibits all forms of DNA-dependent RNA synthesis, with ribosomal RNA formation being most sensitive to drug action. DNA replication is much less reduced, but protein synthesis is blocked in affected cells. The degree of responsiveness to dactinomycin appears to be dependent on the cellular capability for accumulation and retention of the antibiotic.

Approximately half of the intravenous dose of dactinomycin (Table 55–4) remains unmetabolized and is excreted in the bile; a small amount is lost by urinary excretion. The plasma half-life is short. Because the drug is irritating to tissues, it is usually administered with caution to avoid extravasation and with flushing with normal saline to wash out the vein.

Clinical Uses

Dactinomycin is used in combination with surgery and vincristine (with or without radiotherapy) in the adjuvant treatment of Wilms' tumor. It is also used along with methotrexate to provide potentially curative treatment for patients with localized or disseminated gestational choriocarcinoma.

Adverse Reactions

Bone marrow depression, the major dose-limiting toxicity of this agent, is usually evident within 7–10 days. All blood elements are affected, but platelets and leukocytes are affected most profoundly, and severe thrombocytopenia sometimes occurs. Nausea and vomiting, diarrhea, oral ulcers, and skin eruptions may also be noted. The agent is also immunosuppressive, and patients receiving this drug should not receive live virus vaccines. Alopecia and various skin abnormalities occur occasionally. As with anthracyclines, dactinomycin can interact with radiation, producing a "radiation recall" skin abnormality associated with inflammation at sites of prior radiation therapy.

PLICAMYCIN

Plicamycin (formerly mithramycin) is one of the chromomycin antibiotics isolated from *Streptomyces plicatus*. Plicamycin's mechanism of action appears to involve its binding to DNA, possibly through an antibiotic-Mg^{2+} complex; this interaction interrupts DNA-directed RNA synthesis. In addition, the drug causes plasma calcium levels to decrease, apparently through an action on osteoclasts that is independent of its action on tumor cells (useful in hypercalcemia; see Chapter 42). The drug has some usefulness in testicular cancers refractory to standard treatment, but it is of more use in reversing severe hypercalcemia associated with malignant disease.

Toxic effects of plicamycin include nausea and vomiting, thrombocytopenia, leukopenia, hypocalcemia, bleeding disorders, and liver toxicity. Aside from its use in management of hypercalcemia, plicamycin currently has few other indications.

MITOMYCIN

Mitomycin (mitomycin C) is an antibiotic isolated from *Streptomyces caespitosus*. It contains quinone, carbamate, and aziridine groups, all of which may contribute to its activity. The drug is a "bioreductive" alkylating agent that undergoes metabolic reductive activation through an enzyme-mediated reduction to generate an alkylating agent that cross-links DNA. Hypoxic tumor stem cells of solid tumors exist in an environment conducive to reductive reactions and are more sensitive to the cytotoxic actions of mitomycin than normal and oxygenated tumor cells. Mitomycin is thought to be a CCNS alkylating agent. While this agent is one of the more toxic drugs available for clinical use, it is the best available drug for use as an adjuvant to x-ray radiation to attack hypoxic tumor cells. It is being used increasingly in combination chemotherapy (with bleomycin and vincristine) for squamous cell carcinoma of the cervix and for adenocarcinomas of the stomach, pancreas, and lung (along with doxorubicin and fluorouracil). The drug also has some usefulness as a second-line agent for metastatic colon cancer. A special application of mitomycin has been in topical intravesical treatment of small bladder papillomas. Instillations of the agent in distilled water are usually held in the bladder for 3 hours, and the procedure is repeated over a course of weeks. Very little of the agent is absorbed systemically, and it can be quite effective at reducing the frequency of such bladder tumors.

Mitomycin

When mitomycin is administered intravenously, it is cleared rapidly from the vascular compartment; it appears to be eliminated primarily by liver metabolism. Mitomycin causes severe myelosuppression with relatively late toxicity against all three formed elements from the bone marrow. Increasingly profound toxicity occurs after repeated doses. This late form of toxicity suggests an action on hematopoietic stem cells as opposed to later progenitors. Nausea, vomiting, and anorexia commonly occur shortly after injection, and occasional instances of renal toxicity and interstitial pneumonitis have been reported.

BLEOMYCIN

The bleomycins are a series of antineoplastic antibiotics produced by *Streptomyces verticillus*. A mixture (Blenoxane) of 11 different glycopeptides is used in therapy, with the major components being bleomycin A_2 and bleomycin B_2. Bleomycin appears to act through binding to DNA, which results in single- and double-strand breaks following free radical formation, and inhibition of DNA biosynthesis. The fragmentation of DNA seems to be due to oxidation of a DNA-bleomycin-Fe(II) complex and leads to chromosomal aberrations. Bleomycin is a CCS drug that causes accumulation of cells in G_2. It appears to be schedule-dependent, and chronic low-dose administration by repeated injection or continuous infusion seems to be the most effective schedule. The drug synergizes with other drugs such as vinblastine and cisplatin in curative treatment for testicular cancers. It is also used in squamous cell carcinomas of the head and neck, cervix, skin, penis, and rectum and in combination chemotherapy for the lymphomas. A special use has been for intracavitary therapy of malignant effusions in ovarian and breast cancer. The drug can be given subcutaneously, intramuscularly, or intravenously as well as by the intracavitary route (Table 55–4). Peak blood levels of bleomycin after intramuscular injection appear within 30–60 minutes. Intravenous injection of similar dosages yields higher peak concentrations and a terminal half-life of about 2.5 hours.

Adverse effects include lethal anaphylactoid reactions and a high incidence of fever, with or without chills, particularly in patients with lymphoma. Fever may result in dehydration and hypotension in susceptible patients, and small test doses of the drug are commonly used to anticipate this potentially serious toxicity. More common toxic effects include anorexia and blistering and hyperkeratosis of the palms. Pulmonary fibrosis is an uncommon but sometimes fatal adverse effect seen particularly in older patients. The drug does not have significant myelosuppressive effects, which means that it may be incorporated into a number of different combination chemotherapy programs with no significant addition to bone marrow toxicity.

HORMONAL AGENTS

STEROID HORMONES & ANTISTEROID DRUGS

The relationship between hormones and hormone-dependent tumors was initially demonstrated in 1896 when Beatson showed that oophorectomy produced improvement in women with advanced breast cancer. Sex hormones and adrenocortical hormones are now employed in the management of several types of neoplastic disease. Since the sex hormones are concerned with the stimulation and control of proliferation and function of certain tissues, including the mammary and prostate glands, cancer arising from these tissues may be inhibited or stimulated by appropriate changes in hormone balance. Cancer of the breast and cancer of the prostate can be palliated with sex hormone therapy or ablation of appropriate endocrine organs.

The adrenal corticosteroids (particularly the glucocorticoid analogs) have been useful in the treatment of acute leukemia, lymphomas, myeloma, and other hematologic cancers as well as in advanced breast cancer and as supportive therapy in the management of hypercalcemia resulting from many types of cancer. These steroids cause dissolution of lymphocytes, regression of lymph nodes, and inhibition of growth of certain mesenchymal tissues.

The steroid hormones and related agents most useful in cancer therapy are listed in Table 55–5.

Pharmacologic Effects

The mechanisms of action of steroid hormones on lymphoid, mammary, or prostatic cancer have been partially clarified. Steroid hormones bind to receptor proteins in cancer cells, and high levels of receptor proteins are predictive for responsiveness of endocrine therapy. Highly specific receptor proteins have been identified for estrogens, progesterone, corticosteroids, and androgens in certain neoplastic cells. As in normal cells, steroid hormones form a mobile steroid-receptor complex that ultimately binds directly to nuclear non-histone protein of DNA to activate transcription of associated clusters of genes (Chapter 39).

Most steroid-sensitive cancers have specific receptors. Prednisone-sensitive lymphomas and estrogen-sensitive breast and prostatic cancers contain, respectively, specific receptors for corticosteroids, estrogens, and androgens. It is now possible to assay biopsy specimens for steroid receptor content and to predict from the results which individual patients are likely to benefit from steroid or antisteroid therapy. Measurement of the estrogen receptor (ER) and progesterone receptor (PR) proteins in breast cancer tissue is now a standard clinical test. ER- or PR-positive results predict responsiveness to endocrine ablation or additive therapy, whereas patients whose tumors are ER-negative generally fail to respond to such treatment.

Clinical Uses

The sex hormones are employed in cancer of the female and male breast, cancer of the prostate, and cancer of the endometrium of the uterus. Extensive studies with the androgenic, estrogenic, and progestational sex hormones have demonstrated their value in these neoplasms (see Clinical Pharmacology, below). In replacement doses, estrogen can stimulate breast and endometrial cancer growth. Surprisingly, high-dose estrogen is useful therapeutically in metastatic breast cancer but has been largely replaced by antiestrogens. In prostate cancer, androgens stimulate growth and estrogen administration results in suppression of androgen production. Drugs that reduce androgen secretion or block androgen receptors are also valuable in prostate cancer.

Adverse Reactions

Androgens, estrogens, and adrenocortical hormones all can produce fluid retention through their sodium-retaining effect. Prolonged use of androgens and estrogens will cause masculinization and feminization, respectively. Extended use of the adrenocortical steroids may result in hypertension, diabetes, increased susceptibility to infection, and cushingoid appearance (Chapter 39 and Table 55–5).

ESTROGEN & ANDROGEN INHIBITORS (Tamoxifen & Flutamide)

The estrogen inhibitor tamoxifen has proved to be extremely useful for the treatment of breast cancer. It also has activity against progesterone-resistant en-

Table 55–5. Hormonally active agents: Dosages and toxicity.

Drug	Usual Adult Dosage	Acute Toxicity	Delayed Toxicity
Androgens Testosterone propionate	100 mg IM 3 times weekly	None	Fluid retention, masculinization. Cholestatic jaundice in some patients receiving fluoxymesterone
Fluoxymesterone (Halotestin)	10–20 mg/d orally	None	
Antiandrogen Flutamide (Eulexin)	500 mg/d orally	None	None
Estrogens Diethylstilbestrol	1–5 mg orally 3 times daily	Occasional nausea and vomiting	Fluid retention, feminization, uterine bleeding
Ethinyl estradiol (Estinyl)	3 mg/d orally		
Antiestrogen Tamoxifen (Nolvadex)	20 mg/d orally	None	None
Progestins Hydroxyprogesterone caproate	1 g IM twice weekly	None	None
Medroxyprogesterone (Provera)	100–200 mg/d orally; 200–600 mg orally twice weekly	None	None
Megestrol acetate (Megace)	40 mg orally 4 times daily	None	Fluid retention
Adrenocorticosteroids Hydrocortisone	40–200 mg/d orally	None	Fluid retention, hypertension, diabetes, increased susceptibility to infection, "moon facies"
Prednisone	20–100 mg/d orally	None	
Gonadotropin-releasing hormone agonists Goserelin acetate (Zoladex)	3.6 mg SC monthly	Transient flare of symptoms	None
Leuprolide (Lupron)	7.5 mg SC monthly	Hot flashes	None
Aromatase inhibitors Aminoglutethimide (Cytadren)	250 mg orally twice daily, with hydrocortisone, 20 mg twice daily	Dizziness, rash	None
Anastrozole (Arimidex)	1 mg orally daily	Diarrhea	Fatigue
Peptide hormone inhibitor Octreotide (Sandostatin)	100–600 μg/d SC in 2–4 divided doses	Nausea and vomiting	None

dometrial cancer. Tamoxifen is also currently undergoing clinical trial as a chemopreventive agent in women at high risk for breast cancer. Tamoxifen functions as a competitive partial agonist-inhibitor of estrogen and binds to the estrogen receptors of estrogen-sensitive tissues and tumors. However, tamoxifen has a tenfold lower affinity constant for ER than does estradiol, indicating the importance of ablation of endogenous estrogen for optimal antiestrogen effect.

High plasma levels of tamoxifen are obtained after oral administration, and the agent has a much longer biologic half-life than estradiol. The usual dosage is 10 mg twice daily (Table 55–5), though doses up to 100 mg/m² have been administered without major toxicity. Because it may take several weeks to achieve a steady state level of the active metabolite (monohydroxytamoxifen) with the dosage of 20 mg/d, it is advisable to give an 80 mg loading dose on the first day to achieve good blood levels rapidly.

Adverse effects in the usual dose range are quite mild. Hot flashes are the most frequent effect. Nausea is observed occasionally, as is fluid retention. Occasional flares of breast cancer are observed that usually subside with continued therapy.

Tamoxifen

In advanced breast cancer, clinical improvement is observed in 40–50% of patients who receive tamoxifen. Patients who show objective benefit with treatment are largely those who (1) lack endogenous estrogens (oophorectomy or postmenopausal state) and (2) have breast cancers in which the cytoplasmic ER or PR protein is demonstrable. Tamoxifen has also been effective at prolonging survival when used as surgical adjuvant therapy for postmenopausal women with ER-positive breast cancer. In addition to its direct antiestrogen effects on tumor cells, tamoxifen also suppresses serum levels of insulin-like growth factor-1 and up-regulates local production of transforming growth factor-beta (TGFβ). These endocrine effects of tamoxifen may account for some of its antitumor actions in other tumor types such as ovarian cancer and melanoma.

An antiandrogen, flutamide, has been approved by the FDA for use in the treatment of prostate cancer. It is used to antagonize residual androgenic effects after orchiectomy or with leuprolide (see below). Finasteride, a nonsteroidal inhibitor of 5α-testosterone reductase (Chapter 40), the enzyme that converts testosterone to dihydrotestosterone, is investigational in the treatment of cancer. It has not proved very valuable in prostate cancer and at present is approved only for the therapy of benign prostatic hyperplasia.

GONADOTROPIN-RELEASING HORMONE AGONISTS (Leuprolide & Goserelin)

Leuprolide acetate and goserelin are synthetic peptide analogs of naturally occurring gonadotropin-releasing hormone (GnRH, LHRH). They are described in Chapters 37 and 40. These analogs are more potent than the natural hormone and function as GnRH agonists, with paradoxic results, when given continuously (or as a depot preparation), on the pituitary—initial stimulation followed by inhibition of the release of follicle-stimulating hormone and luteinizing hormone. This results in reduced testicular androgen synthesis. The latter effect underlies the efficacy of these agents in the treatment of metastatic carcinoma of the prostate.

Leuprolide has been directly compared with standard endocrine therapy of prostatic cancer with diethylstilbestrol (DES). Suppression of androgen synthesis and reductions in serum prostatic acid phosphatase (a marker of metastatic tumor burden) are comparable with both leuprolide and DES. However, painful gynecomastia, nausea, vomiting, edema, and thromboembolism occur significantly less frequently with leuprolide than with DES. Leuprolide and goserelin are more expensive than DES, but that is more than offset by the overall cost of complications of DES or the surgical and hospitalization costs associated with surgical orchiectomy. Long-acting depot formulations of both leuprolide and goserelin are administered once monthly. The endocrine effects of these agents may also prove useful in the management of hormone receptor-positive breast cancer, but this application remains to be established.

AROMATASE INHIBITORS (Aminoglutethimide & Anastrozole)

Aminoglutethimide is an inhibitor of adrenal steroid synthesis at the first step (conversion of cholesterol to pregnenolone; see Chapter 39). Aminoglutethimide also inhibits the extra-adrenal synthesis of estrone and estradiol. Aside from its direct effects on adrenal steroidogenesis, aminoglutethimide is an inhibitor of an aromatase enzyme that converts the adrenal androgen androstenedione to estrone (Figure 40–2). This aromatization of an androgenic precursor into an estrogen can occur in body fat. Since estrogens promote the growth of breast cancer, estrogen synthesis in extragonadal adipose tissue can be important in breast cancer growth in postmenopausal women.

Aminoglutethimide is effective in the treatment of metastatic breast cancer in women whose tumors contain significant levels of estrogen or progesterone receptors. Aminoglutethimide is normally administered with adrenal replacement doses of hydrocortisone to avoid symptoms of adrenal insufficiency. Hydrocortisone is preferable to dexamethasone, because the latter agent accelerates the rate of catabolism of aminoglutethimide. Adverse effects of aminoglutethimide include occasional dizziness, lethargy, visual blurring, and rash.

Aminoglutethimide plus hydrocortisone is normally used as second-line therapy for women who have been treated with tamoxifen, largely because aminoglutethimide causes somewhat more adverse effects than tamoxifen. However, it can be used as primary endocrine therapy also.

Anastrozole is a new selective nonsteroidal inhibitor of aromatase that is claimed to have no detectable effect on glucocorticoid or mineralocorticoid synthesis. It has been approved for the treatment of patients with advanced estrogen- or progesterone-receptor-positive breast cancer that is no longer responsive to tamoxifen. Other purportedly more potent and selective aromatase inhibitors are under investigation (see Chapter 40).

MISCELLANEOUS ANTICANCER DRUGS (See Table 55–6.)

AMSACRINE

Amsacrine is a 9-anilinoacridine derivative that causes chromosome breakage. This drug intercalates between base pairs in DNA, distorts the double helix, and produces single- and double-strand breaks in DNA and DNA-protein cross-links. DNA strand

Table 55–6. Miscellaneous anticancer drugs: Dosages and toxicity.

Drug	Usual Dosage	Acute Toxicity	Delayed Toxicity
Amsacrine	90 mg/m^2 IV for 5 days (leukemia)	Nausea	Bone marrow depression.
Asparaginase (Elspar)	20,000 IU/m^2 daily IV for 5–10 days	Nausea and fever, allergic reactions	Hepatotoxicity, mental depression, pancreatitis.
Hydroxyurea (Hydrea)	300 mg/m^2 orally for 5 days	Nausea and vomiting	Bone marrow depression.
Mitotane (Lysodren)	6–15 g/d orally	Nausea and vomiting	Dermatitis, diarrhea, mental depression.
Mitoxantrone (Novantrone)	10–12 mg/m^2 IV every 3–4 weeks	Nausea	Bone marrow depression, occasional cardiac toxicity, mild alopecia.

breaks appear to be mediated by formation of topo-isomerase II-DNA complexes trapped by amsacrine in the breaking-sealing action of the enzyme.

Amsacrine is predominantly metabolized by the liver with a half-life of 8–9 hours; thus, liver impairment causes considerable prolongation of plasma concentrations. Amsacrine has significant activity against anthracycline- and cytarabine-refractory acute myelogenous leukemia, advanced ovarian carcinomas, and lymphomas. Hematologic toxicity is dose-limiting, and cardiac arrest has been reported during amsacrine infusions.

ASPARAGINASE

Asparaginase (L-asparagine amidohydrolase) is an enzyme that is isolated for clinical use from various bacteria. The drug is used to treat childhood acute leukemia. Asparaginase acts indirectly by catabolic depletion of serum asparagine to aspartic acid and ammonia. Blood glutamine levels are also reduced. This results in inhibition of protein synthesis in neoplastic cells, requiring an external source of asparagine because of low or deficient levels of asparagine synthase, and cell proliferation is blocked. Most normal cells can synthesize asparagine and thus are less susceptible to the action of asparaginase.

HYDROXYUREA

Hydroxyurea (H$_2$NCONHOH) is an analog of urea whose mechanism of action involves the inhibition of DNA synthesis. It exerts its lethal effect on cells in S phase by inhibiting the enzyme ribonucleotide reductase, resulting in the depletion of deoxynucleoside triphosphate pools. The drug is administered orally. Its major uses are in melanoma and chronic myelogenous leukemia; however, it plays a secondary role in both these circumstances. The major adverse effect of this agent is bone marrow depression. At high dosages (> 40 mg/kg/d), megaloblastosis unresponsive to vitamin B$_{12}$ or folic acid may appear. Gastrointestinal

symptoms, including nausea, vomiting, and diarrhea, are common in patients receiving high doses of this drug.

MITOXANTRONE

Mitoxantrone (dihydroxyanthracenedione, DHAD) is an anthracene compound whose structure resembles the anthracycline ring. It binds to DNA to produce strand breakage and inhibits both DNA and RNA synthesis. It was recently approved for treatment of refractory acute leukemia. The plasma half-life of mitoxantrone in patients is approximately 32 hours; it is predominantly excreted in the feces. Mitoxantrone is active in both pediatric and adult acute myelogenous leukemia, non-Hodgkin's lymphomas, and breast cancer. Leukopenia is the dose-limiting toxicity, and mild nausea and vomiting, stomatitis, and alopecia also occur. The drug also produces some cardiac toxicity, usually manifested as arrhythmias.

MITOTANE

This drug (Figure 39–5) is a DDT congener that was first found to be adrenolytic in dogs. Subsequently, it was found to be useful in the treatment of adrenal carcinoma. The drug produces tumor regression and relief of the excessive adrenal steroid secretion that often occurs with this malignancy. Toxicities include skin eruptions, diarrhea, and mental depression. The drug also causes anorexia, nausea, somnolence, and dermatitis.

The utility of mitotane appears to be limited to adrenal carcinoma, and it is labeled for that one indication.

RETINOIC ACID DERIVATIVES

All-*trans*-Retinoic acid (etretinate) produces remissions in patients with acute promyelocytic leukemia (APL) through the induction of terminal differentiation, in which the leukemic promyelocytes lose their ability to proliferate. APL is associated with a t(15;17) chromosomal translocation, which disrupts the gene for the nuclear receptor-α for retinoic acid and fuses it to a gene called *PML*. This chimeric gene, which expresses aberrant forms of the retinoic acid receptor-α, is present in virtually all patients with promyelocytic leukemia and appears to be responsible for sensitivity to all-*trans*-retinoic acid.

13-*cis*-Retinoic acid (isotretinoin) has achieved a significant objective response rate as a chemopreventive adjuvant to prevent second primary tumors in patients with head and neck squamous cell carcinoma.

The most important toxicities of the retinoids include mucocutaneous, skeletal, liver, and teratogenic effects.

BONE MARROW GROWTH FACTORS

Use of bone marrow-stimulating factors with chemotherapy can reduce the frequency and severity of neutropenic sepsis and other complications. Two recombinant bone marrow growth factors that stimulate neutrophil growth are available: granulocyte colony-stimulating factor (G-CSF, filgrastim) and granulocyte-macrophage-stimulating factor (GM-CSF, sargramostim)(Chapter 33). Both sargramostim and filgrastim can shorten hospitalization after bone marrow transplantation. In addition, filgrastim is approved for general use with cancer chemotherapy to shorten the period of neutropenia and prevent infection. Use of filgrastim after induction chemotherapy for acute nonlymphocytic leukemia shortens the period of neutropenia and appears to increase the complete remission rate.

AMIFOSTINE

Amifostine (Ethyol, WH-2721) is an agent designed to produce preferential cytoprotection of normal tissues from cytotoxic therapies. The preferential cytoprotection is due to the metabolism of amifostine to the free thiol, WR-1065, the active form, by membrane-bound alkaline phosphatase at normal tissue sites followed by rapid uptake into the normal tissues by facilitated diffusion. Normal tissues accumulate the free thiol, whereas uptake into neoplastic tissue is relatively slow. The free thiol protects by covalently binding reactive anticancer drugs, such as alkylating

$$NH_2-(CH_2)_3-NH-(CH_2)_2-S-PO_3H_2$$
Amifostine

| Alkaline phosphatase

$$NH_2-(CH_2)_3-NH-(CH_2)_2-SH$$
WR-1065

agents, anthracyclines, and taxanes, to inactivate these agents in normal tissues.

INVESTIGATIONAL AGENTS

Several of the drugs mentioned in the text remain in investigational status in the USA until their efficacy and safety for cancer chemotherapy can be established. In specific instances where treatment with one of these agents seems warranted, it usually can be arranged through a university hospital or cancer center or by contacting the Division of Cancer Treatment of the National Cancer Institute, which can provide further information and identify investigators who are authorized to administer these drugs.

This status applies to gencytabine, amonafide, azacitidine, and amsacrine, agents useful in acute leukemias. Other products still in the investigational phase include suramin, tenizolamide, and many others. All of these drugs have substantial toxicities. Until their pharmacology is more completely understood and their net effects have proved to be beneficial, their use will be restricted to clinical research.

II. CLINICAL PHARMACOLOGY OF CANCER CHEMOTHERAPEUTIC DRUGS (Table 55–7)

Knowledge of the kinetics of tumor cell proliferation as well as information on the pharmacology and mechanism of action of cancer chemotherapeutic agents has become important in designing optimal chemotherapeutic regimens for patients with cancer. The strategy for developing drug regimens requires a knowledge of the particular characteristics of specific tumors—eg, Is there a high growth fraction? Is there a high spontaneous cell death rate? Are most of the cells in G_0? Is a significant fraction of the tumor composed of hypoxic stem cells? Are their normal counterparts under hormonal control? Similarly, knowledge of the pharmacology of specific drugs is equally important—eg, Does the drug have a particular affinity for uptake by the tumor cells (streptozocin)? Are the tumor cells sensitive to the drug? Is the drug cell cycle-specific?

Drugs that affect cycling cells can often be used most effectively after treatment with a cell cycle-non-specific agent (eg, alkylating agents); this principle has been tested in a few human tumors with increasing success. Similarly, recognition of true drug synergism (tumor cell kill by the drug combination greater than the additive effects of the individual drugs) or antagonism is important in the design of combination chemotherapeutic programs. The combination of cy-

Table 55–7. Malignancies responsive to chemotherapy.

Diagnosis	Current Treatment of Choice	Other Valuable Agents
Acute lymphocytic leukemia	Induction: vincristine plus prednisone. Remission maintenance: mercaptopurine, methotrexate, and cyclophosphamide in various combinations	Asparaginase, daunorubicin, carmustine, doxorubicin, cytarabine, allopurinol,[1] craniospinal radiotherapy
Acute myelocytic and myelomonocytic leukemia	Combination chemotherapy: cytarabine and mitoxantrone or daunorubicin or idarubicin	Methotrexate, thioguanine, mercaptopurine, allopurinol,[1] mitoxantrone, asacitidine,[2] amsacrine,[2] etoposide
Chronic lymphocytic leukemia	Chlorambucil and prednisone (if indicated), fludarabine	Chlorambucil and prednisone, allopurinol,[1] doxorubicin, cladribine
Chronic myelogenous leukemia	Busulfan or interferon, allogeneic bone marrow transplantation (selected patients)	Vincristine, mercaptopurine, hydroxyurea, melphalan, interferon, allopurinol[1]
Hodgkin's disease (stages III and IV)	Combination chemotherapy: vinblastine, doxorubicin, dacarbazine, bleomycin	Lomustine, etoposide, ifosfamide, interferon, mechlorethamine, vincristine, procarbazine, prednisone
Non-Hodgkin's lymphomas	Combination chemotherapy: cyclophosphamide, doxorubicin, vincristine, prednisone	Bleomycin, lomustine, carmustine, etoposide, interferon, mitoxantrone, ifosfamide
Multiple myeloma	Melphalan plus prednisone or multiagent combination chemotherapy	Cyclophosphamide, vincristine, carmustine, interferon, doxorubicin, epoetin alfa[1]
Macroglobulinemia	Chlorambucil or fludarabine	Prednisone
Polycythemia vera	Busulfan, chlorambucil, or cyclophosphamide	Radioactive phosphorus 32
Carcinoma of lung	Etoposide plus cisplatin, vinorelbine	Methotrexate, vincristine, vinblastine, doxorubicin, mitomycin C
Carcinomas of head and neck	Fluorouracil plus cisplatin	Methotrexate, bleomycin, hydroxyurea, doxorubicin, vincristine, vinorelbine
Carcinoma of endometrium	Progestins or tamoxifen	Doxorubicin, cisplatin, carboplatin
Carcinoma of ovary	Cisplatin and paclitaxel	Cyclophosphamide, carboplatin, doxorubicin, melphalan, fluorouracil, vincristine, altretamine (hexamethylmelamine), bleomycin
Carcinoma of cervix	Cisplatin, carboplatin	Lomustine, cyclophosphamide, doxorubicin, methotrexate, mitomycin, bleomycin, vincristine, interferon, 13-*cis*-retinoic acid
Breast carcinoma	(1) Adjuvant chemotherapy or tamoxifen after primary breast surgery (2) Combination chemotherapy or hormonal manipulation for late recurrence	Cyclophosphamide, doxorubicin, vincristine, methotrexate, fluorouracil, paclitaxel, mitoxantrone, prednisone,[1] megestrol, androgens,[1] aminoglutethimide
Choriocarcinoma (trophoblastic neoplasms)	Methotrexate alone or etoposide and cisplatin	Vinblastine, mercaptopurine, chlorambucil, doxorubicin
Carcinoma of testis	Combination chemotherapy: cisplatin, bleomycin, and etoposide	Methotrexate, dactinomycin, plicamycin, vinblastine, doxorubicin, cyclophosphamide, etoposide, ifosfamide plus mesna[1]
Carcinoma of prostate	Estrogens or GnRH agonist plus flutamide	Aminoglutethimide, doxorubicin, cisplatin, prednisone,[1] estramustine, fluorouracil, progestins, suramin[2]
Wilms' tumor	Vincristine plus dactinomycin after surgery and radiotherapy	Methotrexate, cyclophosphamide, doxorubicin
Neuroblastoma	Cyclophosphamide plus doxorubicin and vincristine	Dactinomycin, daunorubicin, cisplatin
Carcinoma of thyroid	Radioiodine (^{131}I), doxorubicin, cisplatin	Bleomycin, fluorouracil, melphalan
Carcinoma of adrenal	Mitotane	Suramin[2]
Carcinoma of stomach or pancreas	Fluorouracil plus doxorubicin and mitomycin	Hydroxyurea, lomustine, cisplatin
Carcinoma of colon	Fluorouracil plus leucovorin or interferon (or both)	Cyclophosphamide, mitomycin, nitrosoureas

(continued)

Table 55–7. Malignancies responsive to chemotherapy (cont'd).

Diagnosis	Current Treatment of Choice	Other Valuable Agents
Carcinoid	Doxorubicin plus cyclophosphamide, fluo-rouracil, octreotide	Interferon, dactinomycin, methysergide,[1] streptozocin
Insulinoma	Streptozocin, interferon	Doxorubicin, fluorouracil, mitomycin, strepto-zocin
Osteogenic sarcoma	Doxorubicin, or methotrexate with citrovorum rescue initiated after surgery	Cyclophosphamide, dacarbazine, interferon, ifosfamide plus mesna[1]
Miscellaneous sarcomas	Doxorubicin plus dacarbazine	Methotrexate, dactinomycin, ifosfamide plus mesna,[1] vincristine, vinblastine
Melanoma	Dacarbazine, cisplatin	Lomustine, hydroxyurea, mitomycin, dactino-mycin, interferon, tamoxifen

[1]Supportive agent, not oncolytic.
[2]Investigational agent. Treatment available through qualified investigators and centers authorized by National Cancer Institute and Cooperative Oncology Groups.

tarabine with an anthracycline in acute myelogenous leukemia and the use of vinblastine or etoposide along with cisplatin and bleomycin in testicular tumors are good examples of true drug synergism against cancer cells but not against normal tissues.

In general, it is preferable to use cytotoxic chemotherapeutic agents in intensive "pulse" courses every 3–4 weeks rather than to use continuous daily dosage schedules. This allows for maximum effects against neoplastic cell populations with complete hematologic and immunologic recovery between courses rather than leaving the patient continuously suppressed with cytotoxic therapy. This approach reduces adverse effects but does not reduce therapeutic efficacy.

The application of these principles is well illustrated in the current approach to the treatment of acute leukemia, lymphomas, Wilms' tumor, and testicular neoplasms.

Adjuvant Chemotherapy for Micrometastases: Multimodality Therapy

The most important role for effective cancer chemotherapy is undoubtedly as an adjuvant to initial or "primary field" treatment with other methods such as surgery or radiation therapy. Failures with primary field therapy are due principally to occult micrometastases outside the primary field. With the currently available treatment modalities, this form of multimodality therapy appears to offer the greatest chance of curing patients with solid tumors.

Distant micrometastases are usually present in patients with one or more positive lymph nodes at the time of surgery (eg, in breast cancer) and in patients with tumors having a known propensity for early hematogenous spread (eg, osteogenic sarcoma, Wilms' tumor). The risk of recurrent or metastatic disease in such patients can be extremely high (80%). Only systemic therapy can adequately attack micrometastases. Chemotherapy regimens that are at least moderately effective against advanced cancer

may have curative potential (at the right dosage and schedule) when combined with primary therapy such as surgery. Several studies show that adjuvant chemotherapy prolongs both disease-free and overall survival in patients with osteogenic sarcoma, rhabdomyosarcoma, or breast cancer. Similar comments apply to the use of three cycles of combination chemotherapy (eg, "MOPP") prior to total nodal radiation in stage IIB Hodgkin's disease.

In breast cancer, premenopausal women with positive lymph nodes at the time of mastectomy have benefited from combination chemotherapy. It has been established that several programs of cytotoxic chemotherapy achieve prolonged disease-free and overall survival times; this method of treatment has increased the cure rate in high-risk primary breast cancer. Active regimens have included, in various combinations, the agents cyclophosphamide, methotrexate, fluorouracil, doxorubicin, and vincristine. In general, regimens with at least three active drugs have been useful. The results produced by combination chemotherapy are superior to the results produced by single agents, because combination chemotherapy copes better with tumor cell heterogeneity and produces a greater tumor cell log kill. Full protocol doses of cytotoxic agents are required to maximize the likelihood of efficacy. Clinical trials have proved tamoxifen to be an effective adjuvant in postmenopausal women with positive estrogen receptor tests on the primary tumor. Because it is cytostatic rather than cytocidal, adjuvant therapy with tamoxifen is usually administered for 5 years. A recent trial in women with node-negative disease showed no additional advantage with 10 years of tamoxifen therapy. Tamoxifen adjuvant chemotherapy is now standard in node-positive postmenopausal women with positive ER or PR tests on tumor specimens. Tamoxifen appears to exert an effect on ER-negative tumors as well, perhaps via mechanisms other than the estrogen receptor. For example, tamoxifen administration reduces serum concentrations of insulin-like growth factor-1 and increases concentrations of the growth-suppressing factor TGFβ in stromal cells within a tumor.

Other applications of adjuvant chemotherapy include colorectal (fluorouracil plus levamisole or leucovorin), testicular (vinblastine, bleomycin, and cisplatin), head and neck, and gynecologic neoplasms (various drugs). In a recent large-scale trial in patients with primary melanoma at high risk of metastases of metastase, intensive administration of alpha-interferon improved disease-free survival. Thus, adjuvant chemotherapy (with curative intent) should now be considered for patients who undergo primary surgical staging and therapy and are found to have a stage and histologic type of cancer with a high risk of micrometastasis. This policy is germane to those tumor types for which palliative chemotherapy has already been developed and has been shown to induce complete remissions in advanced stages of the disease. In each instance, the benefit:risk ratio must be closely examined.

Primary chemotherapy (prior to local surgery) is now extensively used in patients with osteogenic sarcoma and has facilitated limb-sparing procedures. Primary chemotherapy is now also being evaluated in breast cancer to "downstage" patients prior to surgery.

THE LEUKEMIAS

1. ACUTE LEUKEMIA

Childhood Leukemia

Acute lymphoblastic leukemia (ALL) is the predominant form of leukemia in childhood and the most common form of cancer in children. Children with this disease now have a relatively good prognosis. A subset of patients with neoplastic lymphocytes expressing surface antigenic features of T lymphocytes have a poor prognosis (see Chapter 56). A cytoplasmic enzyme expressed by normal thymocytes, terminal deoxycytidyl transferase (terminal transferase), is also expressed in many cases of ALL. T cell ALLs also express high levels of the enzyme adenosine deaminase (ADA). This led to interest in the use of ADA inhibitor pentostatin (deoxycoformycin) for treatment of such T cell cases. Until 1948, the median length of survival in ALL was 3 months. With the advent of the folic acid antagonists, the length of survival was greatly increased. Subsequently, corticosteroids, mercaptopurine, cyclophosphamide, vincristine, daunorubicin, and asparaginase were all found to act against this disease. A combination of vincristine and prednisone plus other agents is currently used to initially induce remission. Over 90% of children enter complete remission with this therapy, with only minimal toxicity. However, circulating tumor stem cells often lodge in the brain, and such cells

are not killed by these drugs because they do not cross the blood-brain barrier. The value of "prophylactic" intrathecal methotrexate therapy for prevention of central nervous system leukemia (a major mechanism of relapse) has been clearly demonstrated. Intrathecal therapy with methotrexate should therefore be considered as a standard component of the induction regimen for children with ALL. Alternative approaches for prevention of central nervous system leukemia that also appear to be efficacious are intrathecal cytarabine and craniospinal irradiation. However, radiation therapy to the neuraxis can cause skeletal growth retardation. Once a complete remission has been induced (> three log cell kill), "maintenance" or "consolidation" therapy is always indicated. This usually consists of a combination of oral methotrexate, mercaptopurine, and cyclophosphamide administered either in pulses, simultaneously, or in various sequences. This "total therapy" approach should be considered the standard form of treatment because it has produced a substantial increase in the cure rate of children with acute leukemia. Although many of the clinical trials are still under way, such therapy appears to offer the best hope of cure for an increasing percentage of patients. The median length of survival in childhood acute leukemia is now approaching 4 years. Many centers discontinue intensive chemotherapy in patients who have shown no sign of relapse after 3 years of intensive chemotherapy. Children who survive for 5 years in complete remission have a greater than 60% chance of having a permanent remission or cure (Rivera et al, 1993).

If leukemia does recur in a patient in remission, the same drugs are used again to try to reinduce the remission. If resistance is observed, reinduction is attempted with different agents (daunorubicin, vincristine, asparaginase, methotrexate, etc) in various combinations. The possibility of curing this fatal childhood disease has fueled current investigations into intensive combination chemotherapy with proved agents plus asparaginase, daunorubicin, and other experimental agents and has led to increased interest in combination chemotherapy for other kinds of neoplastic diseases.

Adult Leukemia

Acute leukemia in adults is predominantly myelocytic, though some cases of lymphoblastic leukemia are also seen. Unlike ALL, induction therapy in acute myelogenous leukemia (AML) requires the use of drugs toxic to normal bone marrow cells. The single most active agent for AML is cytarabine; however, it is best used in combination. Recent trials with combinations of anthracyclines with cytarabine have induced complete remissions in about 70% of patients.

The patient often requires intensive supportive care during the toxic period of induction chemotherapy before remission is achieved. Such care includes platelet transfusions to prevent bleeding, filgrastim to shorten periods of neutropenia, and bactericidal antibiotics plus granulocyte transfusions to combat infections. Younger patients (eg, < age 55) who are in complete remission and have an HLA-compatible donor are candidates for allogeneic bone marrow transplantation. The transplant procedure is preceded by high-dose chemotherapy and total body irradiation and followed by immunosuppression. This procedure may cure 40% of eligible acute leukemia patients. Patients over age 60 respond less well to chemotherapy, primarily because their resistance to infection is lower. Remission maintenance is usually with thioguanine and cytarabine courses. Mitoxantrone, azacitidine, and amsacrine are used as secondary agents for patients who develop resistance to standard therapy. The median life expectancy of patients with AML who enter complete remission is now in excess of 1 year, and some patients are in remission for over 3 years. About 20% of adult patients who achieve complete remission with current standard chemotherapy appear to remain free of recurrent leukemia and are probably cured.

2. CHRONIC MYELOGENOUS LEUKEMIA

Chronic myelogenous leukemia (CML) arises from a chromosomally abnormal hematopoietic stem cell. An abnormal chromosome 22 with deletion of a short arm or translocation to the long arm of chromosome 9 is present in 90% of cases. It is called the Philadelphia (Ph[1]) chromosome. The clinical symptoms and course are related to the leukocyte level and its rate of increase. Most patients with leukocyte counts over 50,000/μL should be treated. The goals of treatment are to reduce the granulocytes to normal levels, to raise the hemoglobin concentration to normal, and to relieve metabolic symptoms. The most useful forms of systemic treatment to induce remission are with alpha interferon or busulfan, with other oral alkylating agents, or with hydroxyurea. Local splenic x-ray therapy is occasionally used. In the early stages of the disease, treatment produces a prompt decrease in spleen size, a decrease in the leukocyte count, and an increase in subjective well-being. Recent results obtained with alpha interferon indicate that this agent can reduce or eliminate the expression of the Ph[1] chromosome in bone marrow myeloid progenitors, whereas this rarely occurs with cytotoxic agents. Prolonged chemotherapy relieves symptoms and signs of CML but does not prolong survival. A major advance in the treatment of younger patients with CML has been in the application of allogeneic bone marrow transplantation performed when the patient is in remission and preferably within the first year after the diagnosis has been made. Bone marrow transplantation can be curative in up to 50% of such CML patients.

Patients who are not eligible for bone marrow transplantation (eg, those over age 55 and those who lack an HLA-compatible donor) and those who are not cured by the procedure develop an accelerated or acute leukemic phase 3–5 years after diagnosis. At this point, agents such as hydroxyurea or mercaptopurine may provide temporary improvement. Combination chemotherapy, including cytarabine, asparaginase, and vincristine or hydroxyurea with or without prednisone, may have transient benefit in a subset of patients, but the prognosis for patients with CML in blastic transformation remains grim.

3. CHRONIC LYMPHOCYTIC LEUKEMIA

Treatment of chronic lymphocytic leukemia (CLL) is markedly different from that of CML. Whereas CML is a proliferative neoplasm requiring systemic treatment for symptomatic control, CLL appears to result from a gradual accumulation of monoclonal B lymphocytes rather than from rapid neoplastic cell proliferation. CLL is often detected accidentally long before the development of symptoms. Although the average life expectancy after diagnosis is only 3 years, the disease occurs frequently in elderly patients, which skews the survival data. Many asymptomatic patients may survive for long periods (5–15 years) without any therapy. In patients whose disease is restricted to lymphocytosis in the peripheral blood, it is reasonable to withhold treatment unless the lymphocyte count is well above 150,000/μL. When anemia or thrombocytopenia, immunodeficiency, weight loss, fever, or generalized organ involvement does occur, treatment is indicated.

The therapeutic methods used to treat CLL include corticosteroids, alkylating agent chemotherapy, or use of fludarabine. Prednisone is often quite effective, and after an initial course of 80 mg/d for several weeks the dose can be gradually decreased or switched to an intermittent (every other day) schedule, which virtually eliminates adverse effects. Hemolytic anemia may respond dramatically to prednisone, though thrombocytopenia is often more refractory.

Chlorambucil is probably the most easily administered oral alkylating agent and has the fewest adverse effects. The dosage is usually 0.1 mg/kg/d, with monitoring of blood counts at weekly intervals. Alternatively, cyclophosphamide can be given in pulse courses of 1 g/m² orally over 4 days every 4–6 weeks. Fludarabine is rapidly becoming the treatment of choice in CLL. The goal of therapy is to eliminate the systemic manifestations of the disease; complete normalization of the lymphocyte count is not necessary. Therapy can be discontinued once the patient's condition has stabilized, but maintenance therapy should be considered if symptoms reappear quickly. Local x-ray therapy is useful for shrinking symptomatic enlarged lymph nodes but is only occasionally indicated. It is important not to overtreat these usually elderly patients because of their poor host resistance.

4. HAIRY CELL LEUKEMIA

This rare form of leukemia originates in a specific subset of B cells and has symptoms and signs similar to those of CLL; however, it responds poorly to conventional chemotherapy. Alpha interferon, which is currently the preferred treatment for hairy cell leukemia (HCL), is approved by the FDA for this indication. Approximately 90% of patients with HCL achieve hematologic improvement with alpha interferon. The adenosine deaminase inhibitors cladribine and pentostatin are very active in HCL and can induce complete remissions (indicated by negative biopsies) even in patients who relapse from interferon.

THE LYMPHOMAS

1. HODGKIN'S DISEASE

The treatment of Hodgkin's disease has undergone dramatic improvement over the last 30 years. Hodgkin's disease is a lymphoma with certain unique characteristics in its natural history: (1) its apparent tendency to progress from a single involved node to anatomically adjacent nodes in a somewhat "orderly" fashion, and (2) its tendency to appear confined to the lymphoid system for a long period of time. Extranodal involvement may also occur, and involvement of the liver, bone marrow, lungs, or other sites is taken as evidence of more "malignant" behavior of the tumor. To effectively treat this disorder, the extent of disease must be adequately staged in order to prepare a rational treatment plan. Widespread involvement is manifested by symptoms such as sweats, fever, anorexia, and weight loss and by infiltration of other organs, including the lungs, liver, and bone marrow. Hodgkin's disease is now recognized as being a B cell neoplasm in which the malignant cells (Reed-Sternberg cells) have rearranged *VH* genes and often express components of the Epstein-Barr virus genome.

Intensive x-ray therapy with supervoltage equipment is curative in most cases of early Hodgkin's disease confined to one lymph node area or several adjacent areas above the diaphragm (stages I and II). Radiation therapy is also of some use in asymptomatic patients with stage III Hodgkin's disease, though its use is decreasing. As can be seen in Table 55–7, a variety of chemotherapeutic agents are active in Hodgkin's disease; however, it is now clear that combination chemotherapy produces the best results.

Combination chemotherapy is now indicated in patients presenting with stage III or stage IV Hodgkin's disease. Results in stage IIIA disease with three cycles of chemotherapy (see below) followed by total nodal radiotherapy are clearly superior to those achieved with radiotherapy alone. Standard chemotherapy is with a four-drug combination such as ABVD (Adriamycin [doxorubicin], bleomycin, vinblastine, and dacarbazine) or MOPP (mechlorethamine, Oncovin [vincristine], procarbazine, and prednisone). At present, ABVD is the preferred regimen because it has fewer long-term toxicities. This form of treatment is given repeatedly for at least 6 months and sometimes for as long as 1 year. Over 80% of previously untreated patients with advanced Hodgkin's disease (stages III and IV) go into complete remission, including the disappearance of all symptoms and objective evidence of tumors.

Complex treatment regimens such as these should be under the direction of a medical oncologist who is familiar with the individual and synergistic toxicities of and the contraindications to the drugs involved. After remission induction with at least six courses of ABVD or MOPP, approximately 50% of patients will remain free of all signs of Hodgkin's disease for over 2 years. The ABVD combination has not been associated with the late development of acute leukemia, perhaps because it lacks alkylating agents and procarbazine.

About half of patients who have achieved complete remission with MOPP or ABVD are cured of Hodgkin's disease.

Nitrosoureas such as lomustine are also effective in Hodgkin's disease and have been used with other drugs to reinduce remission in patients who relapse from the standard regimens. New agents observed to be active in Hodgkin's disease include mitoxantrone and isotopically labeled ferritin antibody.

2. NON-HODGKIN'S LYMPHOMAS

The clinical characteristics of non-Hodgkin's lymphomas (NHL) are related to major histopathologic features and the immunologic origin of the neoplastic cells. The simplest useful pathologic classification is one based on cell type plus the presence or absence of nodularity in the lymphomatous tissues. In general, the nodular (or follicular) lymphomas have a far better prognosis (median survival up to 7 years) than do the diffuse ones (median survival about 1–2 years).

Liver and bone marrow, gastrointestinal, and localized extralymphatic involvement are all observed more commonly in NHL than in Hodgkin's disease, and a higher fraction of patients (about one-third) have stage IV disease at presentation—in contrast to 15% of patients with Hodgkin's disease.

Combination chemotherapy is clearly preferred to single-agent therapy for diffuse but not for nodular lymphomas. The nodular lymphomas are "low-grade" indolent tumors and respond much better to palliative treatment with single agents than do the diffuse lymphomas. Some of the diffuse lymphomas are curable with available drugs, whereas nodular lymphomas are not. In fact, there is no evidence that combination chemotherapy is any better than single-agent chlorambucil in the treatment of low-grade nodular lymphomas.

Doxorubicin has been found to be extremely active in the treatment of the diffuse non-Hodgkin's lymphomas. While a number of aggressive drug combinations—including doxorubicin, vincristine, cyclophosphamide, prednisone, cytarabine, bleomycin, methotrexate, and etoposide—have been evaluated, none appear to yield superior results as compared with the four-drug combination of cyclophosphamide, doxorubicin, vincristine, and prednisone ("CHOP"). Current data suggest that one-third to one-half of patients with diffuse large cell lymphomas are cured with intensive combination chemotherapy. For patients with bulky stage I or stage II diffuse NHL, the combination of CHOP plus radiotherapy is preferable to CHOP alone and has a high cure rate. Patients who relapse from unmaintained remission and who are still sensitive to chemotherapy can frequently achieve long-term disease control with high-dose chemotherapy and autologous hematopoietic stem cell rescue with peripheral blood or bone marrow stem cell reinfusion. The new agents mitoxantrone and paclitaxel are also active in non-Hodgkin's lymphomas. Alpha interferon has been observed to cause tumor regression in some nodular lymphomas, and it may have a role for prolonging chemotherapy-induced remissions. Alpha interferon is also useful in peripheral T cell lymphomas. Monoclonal antibodies directed against T or B cell antigens have recently been tested in a few patients with leukemias or lymphomas, and some antitumor effects have been observed.

MULTIPLE MYELOMA

This plasma cell tumor is now one of the "models" of neoplastic disease in humans because the tumor arises from a single tumor stem cell, and the tumor cells produce a marker protein (myeloma immunoglobulin) that allows the total body burden of tumor cells to be quantified. The tumor grows principally in the bone marrow and the surrounding bone, causing bone pain, lytic lesions, bone fractures, and anemia as well as increased susceptibility to infection. Treatment with oral alkylating agents such as melphalan or cyclophosphamide and intermittent high doses of prednisone is effective in most patients with myeloma. Relatively simple combination chemotherapy was therefore developed by combining melphalan and prednisone. Somewhat better results have been obtained in advanced disease with the use of more intensive regimens containing alkylating agents, doxorubicin, a nitrosourea, and a *Vinca* alkaloid. About 75% of myeloma patients improve with this treatment, experiencing significant relief of symptoms and prolonged survival. Resistance to chemotherapy usually develops after 2–3 years of treatment in most responding cases. Allogeneic bone marrow transplants

are a possibility for patients under age 55, and the role of autotransplantation after high-dose chemotherapy as used in the lymphomas is now being explored.

A strategy has been developed that may prolong remission. With this approach, patients who achieve remission with 6–12 months of induction chemotherapy are switched to long-term remission maintenance therapy with alpha interferon. Interferon maintenance has prolonged remission in some studies (but has been ineffective in others) and has not prolonged survival. Given its cost and toxicity, its role in myeloma remains uncertain. For patients who relapse after an initial response to chemotherapy, the combination of vincristine and doxorubicin (VAD) by 4-day infusion with high-dose dexamethasone induces second remissions in about 70% of patients. Patients relapsing again after this program may be "chemosensitized" by the addition of cyclosporine or an investigational chemosensitizer to the regimen. High-dose glucocorticoids alone are also useful in some patients.

CARCINOMA OF THE BREAST

1. STAGE I & STAGE II NEOPLASMS

The management of primary carcinoma of the breast is undergoing remarkable change as a result of major efforts at early diagnosis (through encouragement of self-examination as well as through the use of cancer detection centers) and the implementation of multimodality clinical trials incorporating systemic chemotherapy as an adjuvant to surgery. Women with stage I lateral lesions at the time of breast surgery (small primaries and negative axillary lymph node dissections) are currently treated with surgery and have an 80% chance of cure. The current trend is toward more conservative surgery. While the modified radical mastectomy is still the most common surgical procedure, segmental mastectomy (lumpectomy) plus an axillary lymph node sampling is equally effective in treating primary tumors less than 4 cm in diameter.

Women with one or more positive lymph nodes have a very high risk of systemic recurrence and death from breast cancer. Thus, lymph node status directly indicates the risk of occult distant micrometastasis. In this situation, postoperative use of systemic cytotoxic chemotherapy in six cycles (1 month apart) of cyclophosphamide-methotrexate-fluorouracil (CMF) or of fluorouracil-doxorubicin (Adriamycin)-cyclophosphamide (FAC) reduces the relapse rate and prolongs survival. All these chemotherapy regimens have been of most benefit in women with stage II breast cancer with one to three involved lymph nodes. Women with four or more involved nodes have had limited benefit thus far from adjuvant chemotherapy. High-dose chemotherapy with autologous stem cell rescue and growth factor support is now being evaluated in women with ten or more involved nodes. Long-term analysis has clearly shown improved survival rates in node-positive premenopausal women who have been treated aggressively with multiagent combination chemotherapy. Tamoxifen is useful in postmenopausal women when used alone or with cytotoxic chemotherapy. Tamoxifen is most frequently used for 5 years of continuous therapy after surgery. Longer durations of tamoxifen therapy do not appear to add additional benefit. Results from a number of randomized trials of chemotherapy for breast cancer have established that adjuvant chemotherapy for premenopausal women and adjuvant tamoxifen for postmenopausal women are of benefit to women with stage I (node-negative) breast cancer. While this group of patients has the lowest overall risk of recurrence after surgery alone (about 35–50% over 15 years), this risk can be further reduced with adjuvant therapy. The major benefit of radiotherapy appears to be that it replaces radical surgery, thus allowing the far better cosmetic results obtained with limited breast surgery.

2. STAGE III & STAGE IV NEOPLASMS

Until such multimodality programs as those discussed above are fully effective in the population at risk, the treatment of women with advanced breast cancer remains a major problem. Indeed, some women still present with inoperable "local" lesions with suspected metastases (stage III) or overt distant metastases (stage IV). Currently, most women with local or distant recurrence have had prior breast cancer surgery or surgery plus radiotherapy.

Current treatment of advanced breast cancer is only palliative. Combination chemotherapy or endocrine therapy (or both) modestly prolongs the survival of most patients as well as relieving their symptoms. Biochemically differentiated breast cancers (as determined by the presence of receptors for estrogen or progesterone) retain many of the intrinsic hormonal sensitivities of the normal breast—including the growth stimulatory response to ovarian, adrenal, and pituitary hormones. Oophorectomy or use of tamoxifen is reasonable in premenopausal women with ER- or PR-positive tumors who have skin, lymph node, pleural, or bone metastases. Patients who show improvement with ablative procedures also respond to the addition of tamoxifen. Patients with moderate to severe lung, liver, brain, or visceral involvement rarely benefit from hormonal maneuvers, and initial systemic chemotherapy is indicated in such cases. Irrespective of sites of involvement, if the estrogen receptor is absent, the likelihood of observing a response to hormonal therapy is less than 5%. Males with breast cancer show similar therapeutic responses to castration at almost any age.

Use of Antiestrogens

While both androgens and estrogens are useful in some patients with hormone receptor-positive breast cancer, tamoxifen has proved to be a virtually nontoxic alternative to conventional endocrine therapy of breast cancer and represents the endocrine therapy of first choice for hormone receptor-positive breast cancer in both pre- and postmenopausal patients. Flare of disease is observed occasionally with tamoxifen and can herald the subsequent achievement of an excellent remission, but meticulous supportive care (eg, for bone pain or hypercalcemia) is required. Tamoxifen may slightly increase the risk of developing uterine cancer in a frequency similar to that associated with estrogens.

Use of Aromatase Inhibitors

Aminoglutethimide plus hydrocortisone or anastrozole alone are effective against hormone receptor-positive breast cancers. They are often used in women who have previously responded to tamoxifen or who have ER- or PR-positive breast cancers. Newer aromatase inhibitors with more favorable pharmacologic characteristics are now in clinical trials.

Systemic Chemotherapy

The use of cytotoxic drugs and hormones has become a highly specialized and increasingly effective means of treating breast cancer. Combination chemotherapy has improved considerably for patients with visceral involvement from advanced disease. Doxorubicin and the taxanes (paclitaxel, docetaxel) are the most active cytotoxic drugs. Combination chemotherapy has been found to induce much more durable remissions in 50–80% of patients. Combination regimens based on doxorubicin have generally included cyclophosphamide and fluorouracil (FAC). Combination programs including both doxorubicin and a taxane are now under investigation. With most combination regimens, partial remissions have a median duration of about 10 months and complete remissions a duration of about 15 months. Unfortunately, only 10–20% of patients achieve complete remissions with any of these regimens, and complete remissions are usually not very long-lasting in metastatic breast cancer. The addition of tamoxifen to such programs yields only modest additional improvement. When doxorubicin is used in such combinations, it is generally discontinued before the patient reaches cardiotoxic limits. At that point, other drugs are generally substituted.

CHORIOCARCINOMA OF THE UTERUS

This rare tumor that arises from fetal trophoblastic tissue was the first metastatic cancer cured with chemotherapy. Massive doses of methotrexate—25 mg/d for 4 or 5 days—will produce a high percentage of cures associated with complete regression of metastatic lesions and disappearance of chorionic gonadotropic hormones in the urine. Therapy should be given repeatedly until some months after all evidence of the disease has disappeared. An alternative regimen with a high cure rate (including cures of methotrexate treatment failures) combines etoposide with cisplatin and is now a preferred approach for this rare form of cancer.

CARCINOMA OF THE OVARY

This neoplasm often remains occult until it has metastasized to the peritoneal cavity; it may present with malignant ascites. It is important to stage such neoplasms accurately using laparoscopy, ultrasound, or CT scanning. Patients with stage I tumors appear to benefit from pelvic radiotherapy and might receive additional benefit from combination chemotherapy. Combination chemotherapy is now the standard approach to stage III and stage IV disease. The most useful combination therapy for ovarian cancer is with the use of paclitaxel and cisplatin, which is now preferred over regimens of cisplatin plus cyclophosphamide. Radiotherapy (including whole-abdomen radiotherapy) does not improve the survival rates of patients with higher stages of involvement and is generally not indicated. Multimodality therapy utilizing surgery, radiotherapy, and adjuvant combination chemotherapy in patients with stage I and stage II neoplasms has shown promising signs of efficacy in current clinical trials.

TESTICULAR NEOPLASMS

Single-agent chemotherapy has produced impressive tumor regressions in some advanced nonseminomatous testicular neoplasms, but there have been few complete responses lasting longer than 1 year. The introduction of combination chemotherapy with cisplatin (Platinol), vinblastine, and bleomycin (PVB) has made an impressive change in these statistics. Ninety-five percent of patients respond to chemotherapy, with approximately 90% entering complete remission. It now seems likely that over half of patients achieving complete remission are cured with chemotherapy. Substitution of etoposide for vinblastine yields similar remission and cure rates with significantly less hematologic toxicity and is now the treatment of choice. In advanced disease (patients who have positive lymph nodes), adjuvant use of this treatment is generally not indicated because over half of patients do not relapse after primary surgery that includes retroperitoneal lymphadenectomy and because the salvage rate with chemotherapy in recurrent disease is quite good.

CARCINOMA OF THE PROSTATE

Carcinoma of the prostate was one of the first forms of cancer shown to be responsive to hormonal manipulation. Orchiectomy or low-dose estrogen therapy (or both) has resulted in prolonged improvement in patients with bone lesions. Similar results have also been obtained with the gonadotropin-releasing hormone agonists alone or in combination with an antiandrogen (eg, flutamide). While these agents are less toxic than estrogens, they are much more expensive. There appears to be no survival advantage of "total androgen blockade" (eg, with leuprolide and flutamide) as compared with orchiectomy. Hormonal treatment reduces symptoms in 70–80% of patients and produces a significant degree of regression of established metastases. Subjective relief of bone pain, objective evidence of normalization of involved bones, and reduction of prostate-specific antigen and prostatic alkaline phosphatase are common criteria of response to therapy for this disorder. The antifungal agent ketoconazole inhibits androgenic steroid synthesis and may find increasing application in the treatment of prostate cancer in the future. The growth factor antagonist (and antiparasitic drug) suramin has recently been reported to have anticancer activity in patients with metastatic prostate cancer. It is assumed to act via an endocrine mechanism. Nevertheless, chemotherapy is still of minimal curative value for this disease.

CARCINOMA OF THE THYROID

Until recently, only radioactive iodine (^{131}I) had therapeutic activity in metabolic thyroid cancer, and its effects were limited to well-differentiated tumors that could concentrate iodine. It is now clear that doxorubicin and cisplatin have significant activity against a variety of histologic types of thyroid cancer (particularly anaplastic lesions), induce excellent regressions of tumor, and prolong survival. The use of combination chemotherapy with ^{131}I therapy in thyroid cancer appears promising for high-risk patients who have anaplastic cell characteristics on histologic examination or vascular invasion of the thyroid gland.

GASTROINTESTINAL CARCINOMAS

This group of neoplasms has only limited sensitivity to available chemotherapeutic agents. All these lesions release carcinoembryonic antigen (CEA), and radioimmunoassay can be used to detect recurrence after surgery as well as response to (or relapse from) systemic chemotherapy. Colorectal adenocarcinoma is the most common type, and only 43% of cases are curable with surgery. Patients with micrometastases to regional lymph nodes are candidates for adjuvant chemotherapy with fluorouracil plus levamisole. This combination has been reported to reduce the recurrence rate after surgery by 35% in these patients and clearly improves survival as compared with surgery alone. For patients with rectal carcinoma, surgical adjuvant therapy with protracted intravenous infusion of fluorouracil along with pelvic irradiation have been found to modestly improve both relapse-free and overall survival. Fluorouracil is the most active single agent for patients with metastatic disease, but it induces only a 21% remission rate with virtually no complete remissions. The effects of fluorouracil can be enhanced in patients with metastatic colorectal cancer by coadministration of leucovorin or interferon (or both). Lomustine, mitomycin, and cyclophosphamide all have definite but lesser degrees of activity. Mitomycin or carmustine also acts against these carcinomas when used with fluorouracil. Irinotecan appears to have some benefit in patients who are no longer responding to 5-FU. All of these regimens induce substantial hematologic toxicity. Because these combinations do not induce complete remission, do not prolong survival, and are rather toxic, their use should be limited to patients with symptomatic metastatic disease. Recently, hepatic artery catheterization and repeated arterial infusion of fluorouracil or FUDR have proved useful for treating patients with colorectal cancer that has metastasized only to the liver. Fluorouracil alone has been extensively tried as a surgical adjuvant and has produced a minor reduction in the relapse rate observed with surgery alone.

Gastric carcinoma and pancreatic carcinoma are less common but far more aggressive lesions that usually cannot be completely resected surgically and are generally grossly metastatic at the time of surgery. The combination of fluorouracil, doxorubicin, and mitomycin relieves symptoms in some patients. "Neoadjuvant" chemotherapy with aggressive use of 5-FU prior to surgery appears to have some promise.

Islet cell carcinoma of the pancreas arising from B cells and secreting insulin has been found to be exquisitely sensitive to the antibiotic streptozocin. The results have been good in this rare tumor, and this therapy may be curative in some patients. Streptozocin is often used with several other agents, eg, fluorouracil, doxorubicin, and mitomycin.

BRONCHOGENIC CARCINOMA

The management of epidermoid cancers, large cell cancers, and adenocarcinomas of the lung is very unsatisfactory, and prevention (primarily through avoidance of cigarette smoking) remains the most important means of control. The average life expectancy after diagnosis has been 8 months. The tumor can rarely be cured by surgery, and x-ray therapy is used primarily for palliation of pain, obstruction, or bleeding. However, in most cases of lung cancer, distant metastases have occurred by the time of diagnosis and chemotherapy therefore appears to be the most feasible approach.

Although lung cancer had been notoriously resistant to all conventional forms of cancer chemotherapy, several novel approaches now show promise. Histologic examination of tumor tissue has been found to be important in identifying subgroups of patients who will respond to chemotherapy. Patients with small cell (oat cell) lung cancer (the most rapidly growing type) show the best responses to combination chemotherapy with agents such as cisplatin, etoposide, doxorubicin, cyclophosphamide, vinorelbine, methotrexate, and nitrosoureas. Patients with limited small cell carcinomas respond best to such regimens. They may also require whole brain irradiation to sterilize occult central nervous system metastases, which are often present. However, the role of prophylactic whole brain irradiation remains uncertain because of the significant impairment of brain function that eventually develops in such patients. For non-small cell lung cancer, combinations of etoposide and cisplatin have some limited benefit.

MALIGNANT MELANOMA & MISCELLANEOUS SARCOMAS

Metastatic melanoma is one of the most difficult neoplasms to treat. Most chemotherapeutic agents are reported to induce regression in at least 10% of melanoma patients; however, spontaneous regressions also occur, especially in skin metastases, so regression of cutaneous lesions does not necessarily imply sensitivity to chemotherapy. Immunologic reactivity to the tumor by host lymphocytes may partially explain the evanescent changes in skin lesions, but "spontaneous regression" of visceral disease is rare and metastases occur in virtually every organ in the body. Dacarbazine and cisplatin are the most active cytotoxic agents. Biologic agents, including human leukocyte interferon (natural or recombinant), may have a similar order of activity. Tamoxifen may potentiate the effects of multidrug combinations that include cisplatin.

Osteogenic sarcoma and Ewing's sarcoma respond to doxorubicin, and a combination of doxorubicin and dacarbazine may induce substantial regressions in about 40% of cases of rhabdomyosarcoma, fibrosarcoma, osteogenic sarcoma, and related tumors. The use of adjuvant therapy that includes doxorubicin after primary surgery for osteosarcoma has already lengthened the median survival time. This therapy appears likely to increase the long-term salvage rate for this otherwise almost uniformly fatal neoplasm. Similar results have recently been reported for patients with soft tissue sarcomas of the extremities for whom adjuvant chemotherapy has clearly prolonged disease-free survival. When this approach has been applied together with limb-salvage surgery, it has reduced the need for amputation as part of initial surgery. For grossly metastatic soft tissue sarcomas, first-line therapy uses doxorubicin-based combinations. Patients in relapse from these regimens sometimes benefit from therapy with ifosfamide plus mesna.

BRAIN TUMORS

Stage III and stage IV astrocytomas (predominantly glioblastoma multiforme) are the most common primary brain tumors, and they have been extraordinarily refractory to surgical therapy. Although advances in diagnostic methods such as computerized tomography (CT) scanning have better delineated the site of primary involvement for surgical therapy, the median survival time with surgery alone is still about 20 weeks. The addition of whole brain radiotherapy (approximately 5500 cGy) or carmustine alone (220 mg/m^2 every 6–8 weeks) increases the median survival time to 36 weeks, whereas the use of multimodality therapy (surgery plus radiotherapy plus carmustine) increases it to 50 weeks, with approximately 25% of patients still alive at 18 months. This multimodality approach, although still limited in efficacy, can be recommended as palliation for patients with such tumors until more effective regimens are developed. The experimental agent **tenizolamide** appears to be active in brain tumor therapy and is currently in early clinical trials.

CONTROL OF MALIGNANT EFFUSIONS & ASCITES

The direct injection of mechlorethamine or other anticancer drugs into the involved cavity will eliminate or suppress ascites and effusions caused by carcinoma in about two-thirds of patients. The method is useful irrespective of the type of primary tumor.

The procedure involves withdrawing most of the pleural or ascitic fluid and then injecting the drug into the cavity. The dose of mechlorethamine employed intrapleurally is 0.4 mg/kg, or a total dose of 20–30 mg in the average patient. The solution is prepared immediately before administration so as to avoid loss of potency through hydrolysis. A free flow of fluid from the cavity must be established before the drug is injected to avoid injection into the tissues. Pleural or peritoneal effusions caused by ovarian or breast carcinoma are frequently responsive to an intracavitary dose of 60 units/m^2 of bleomycin. After the drug is injected, the patient is placed in a variety of positions in order to distribute the drug throughout the pleural cavity. On the following day, the remaining fluid is withdrawn.

Pain, nausea, and vomiting sometimes occur following injection of mechlorethamine into the pleural cavity. Nausea and vomiting can often be controlled by giving an intramuscular dose of a phenothiazine immediately before the procedure and at intervals following the injection. Bone marrow depression is mild with this method of administration except in patients who have received extensive radiation therapy. Agents such as bleomycin or thiotepa are preferable to mechlorethamine for intraperitoneal use, since they cause significantly less peritoneal irritation and pain.

Tetracycline was employed intrapleurally with similar therapeutic benefit in the past but is no longer available for this purpose. Local pain and fever were commonly noted, but there was no systemic hematopoietic depression.

EVALUATION OF TUMOR RESPONSE

Since cancer chemotherapy can induce clinical improvement, significant toxicity, or both, it is important to critically assess the effects of treatment to determine that the net effect is beneficial. Preliminary evidence regarding the use of the tumor stem cell assay to determine the appropriate form of chemotherapy is quite encouraging, particularly with respect to rejecting drugs that would probably cause toxicity without compensating clinical benefit. The assay also appears to be relatively accurate (70%) in identifying drugs that will prove useful in the patient.

Shrinkage in tumor size is a useful measure of response and can be demonstrated by physical examination, chest film or other x-ray, or special scanning procedures such as bone scanning (breast, prostate cancer), CT scan, magnetic resonance imaging (MRI), or ultrasonography.

Another sign of therapeutic response is a significant decrease in the quantity of a tumor product or marker substance that reflects the amount of tumor in the body. Examples of such markers include paraproteins in the serum or urine in multiple myeloma and macroglobulinemia, chorionic gonadotropin in choriocarcinoma and testicular tumors, urinary steroids in adrenal carcinoma and paraneoplastic Cushing's syndrome, 5-hydroxyindoleacetic acid in carcinoid syndrome, and prostate-specific antigen in prostatic carcinoma. Secreted tumor antigens such as alpha-fetoprotein can be found in hepatoma, in teratoembryonal carcinoma, and in occasional cases of gastric carcinoma; the carcinoembryonic antigen can be found in carcinomas of the colon, lung, and breast. The tumor antigen CA 125 is very useful in following the response to treatment in women with ovarian cancer.

Normalization of function of organs that were previously impaired by the presence of a tumor is a useful indicator of drug effectiveness. Examples of such improvement include the normalization of liver function (eg, increased serum albumin) in patients known to have liver metastases and improvement in neurologic findings in patients with cerebral metastases. Disappearance of the signs and symptoms of the paraneoplastic syndromes often falls in this general category and can be taken as an indication of tumor response.

A valuable sign of clinical improvement is the general well-being of the patient. Although this finding is a combination of subjective and objective factors and may be subject to placebo effects, it nonetheless serves as an obvious and useful sign of clinical improvement and can be used to reassess some of the objective observations listed above. Factors to be considered in determining general well-being include improved appetite, weight gain, and improved "performance status" (eg, ambulatory versus bedridden). Evaluation of factors such as activity status has the advantage of summarizing beneficial and toxic effects of chemotherapy and enables the physician to judge whether the net effect of chemotherapy is worthwhile palliation. Standardized scales are available (Karnovsky Scale, Eastern Cooperative Oncology Group Scale).

SECOND MALIGNANCIES & CANCER CHEMOTHERAPY

Second malignancy is a late complication of some types of cancer chemotherapy. The most frequent second malignancy is acute myelogenous leukemia (AML). Aside from AML, other second malignancies are sporadic. AML has been observed in up to 15% of patients with Hodgkin's disease who have received radiotherapy plus MOPP and in patients with multiple myeloma, ovarian carcinoma, or breast carcinoma treated with melphalan. Several alkylating agents (as well as ionizing radiation) are considered to be leukemogenic. Additionally, procarbazine (a component of the MOPP combination) is known to be mutagenic to bacteria and carcinogenic in animals. The mechanisms of carcinogenesis with these other agents remain poorly understood. While the risk of AML is relatively small, the benefit of complete remission or cure of Hodgkin's disease or remission of other neoplasms is considerable. As further advances are made in chemical control and cure of cancer, the problem of the second malignant tumor assumes greater importance. There are already hints that certain alkylating agents (eg, cyclophosphamide) may be less carcinogenic than others. Systematic testing of the carcinogenicity of anticancer drugs in several animal species allows less toxic agents to be identified and substituted for other more carcinogenic ones in chemotherapy regimens. In this fashion, the risk of second tumors should be reduced without sacrificing therapeutic benefit.

PREPARATIONS AVAILABLE

The reader is referred to the manufacturers' literature for the most recent information.

REFERENCES

General

Bonadonna G, Zambitti M, Valagussa P: Sequential or alternating doxorubicin and CMF regimens in breast cancer with more than three positive nodes. Ten year results. JAMA 1995;273:542.

Bonadonna GS et al: Adjuvant cyclophosphamide, methotrexate, and fluorouracil in node-positive breast cancer: The results of 20 years of follow-up. N Engl J Med 1995;333:596.

Chabner BA, Collins JM (editors): *Cancer Chemotherapy: Principles and Practice*. Lippincott, 1990.

Cheng KK et al: Pickled vegetables in the aetiology of oesophageal cancer in Hong Kong Chinese. Lancet 1992;339:1314.

DeVita VT Jr, Hellman S, Rosenberg SA (editors): *Cancer: Principles and Practice of Oncology,* 5th ed. Lippincott, 1996.

Dombret H et al: A controlled study of recombinant human granulocyte colony-stimulating factor in elderly patients after treatment for acute myelogenous leukemia. N Engl J Med 1995;332:1678.

Gianni AM et al: High dose chemotherapy and autologous bone marrow transplantation compared with MACOP-B in aggressive B-cell lymphoma. N Engl J Med 1997;336:1290.

Gottesman MM, Pastan I: Biochemistry of multidrug resistance mediated by the multidrug transporter. Ann Rev Biochem 1993;62:385.

Grant CE et al: Overexpression of multidrug resistance-associated protein (MRP) increases resistance to natural product drugs. Cancer Res 1994;54:357.

Harris CC, Hollstein M: Clinical implications of the p53 tumor-suppressor gene. N Engl J Med 1993;329:1318.

Holland JF et al (editors): *Cancer Medicine,* 4th ed. Williams & Wilkins, 1997.

Kaiser HE (editor): *Cancer Growth and Progression.* Kluwer, 1989.

Kontiris TG: Oncogenes. N Engl J Med 1995;333:303.

Koutsky LA et al: A cohort study of the risk of cervical intraepithelial neoplasia grade 2 or 3 in relation to papillomavirus infection. N Engl J Med 1992;27:1272.

Moertel CG: Chemotherapy for colorectal cancer. N Engl J Med 1994;330:1136.

Muindi RF et al: Clinical pharmacology of all-*trans* retinoic acid. Leukemia 1994;8:1807.

O'Connell MJ et al: Improving adjuvant therapy for rectal cancer by combining protracted-infusion fluorouracil with radiation therapy after curative surgery. N Engl J Med 1994;331:502.

Powis G (editor): *Anticancer Drugs: Antimetabolite Metabolism and Natural Anticancer Agents.* Pergamon Press, 1994.

Rinsky RA et al: Benzene and leukemia: An epidemiologic risk assessment. N Engl J Med 1987;316:1044.

Rosenberg SA: The low grade non-Hodgkin's lymphomas: Challenges and opportunities. J Clin Oncol 1985;3:299.

Rozman C, Montserrat E: Chronic lymphocytic leukemia. N Engl J Med 1995;333:1052.

Salmon SE (editor): *Adjuvant Therapy of Cancer VIII.* Lippincott, 1996.

Sartorelli AC: Therapeutic attack on hypoxic cells of solid tumors: Presidential address. Cancer Res 1988;48:775.

Someveld P et al: Modulation of multidrug-resistant multiple myeloma by cyclosporin. Lancet 1992;340:255.

Teicher BF (editor): *Drug Resistance in Oncology.* Marcel Dekker, 1993.

Toguchida J et al: Prevalence and spectrum of germline mutations of the p53 gene among patients with sarcoma. N Engl J Med 1992;326:1301.

Vähäkangas KH et al: Mutations of *p53* and *ras* genes in radon-associated lung cancer from uranium miners. Lancet 1992;339:576.

Vokes EE et al: Head and neck cancer. N Engl J Med 1993;328:184.

Williams SD et al: Immediate adjuvant chemotherapy versus observation with treatment at relapse in pathological stage II testicular cancer. N Engl J Med 1987;317:1433.

Withers HR: Biological basis of radiation therapy for cancer. Lancet 1992;339:156.

Yandell DW et al: Oncogenic point mutations in the human retinoblastoma gene: Their applications to genetic counseling. N Engl J Med 1989;321:1689.

Alkylating Agents

Curtis RE et al: Risk of leukemia after chemotherapy and radiation treatment for breast cancer. N Engl J Med 1992;326:1745.

Antimetabolites

Juliusson G, Elmhorn-Rosenborg A, Liliemark J: Response to 2-chlorodeoxyadenosine in patients with B cell chronic lymphocytic leukemia resistant to fludarabine. N Engl J Med 1992;327:1056.

Koren G et al: Systemic exposure to mercaptopurine as a prognostic factor in acute lymphocytic leukemia in children. N Engl J Med 1990;323:17.

Piro LD et al: Lasting remissions in hairy-cell leukemia induced by a single infusion of 2-chlorodeoxyadenosine. N Engl J Med 1990;322:1117.

Antibiotics & Other Natural Products

Haffty BG et al: Mitomycin C as an adjunct to postoperative radiation therapy in squamous cell carcinoma of the head and neck: Results from two randomized clinical trials. Int J Radiat Oncol Biol Phys 1993; 27:241.

Hudis CA et al: Phase II and pharmacologic study of docetaxel as initial chemotherapy for metastatic breast cancer. J Clin Oncol 1996;14:58.

Ravdin PM, Valero V: Review of docetaxel (Taxotere), a highly active new agent for the treatment of metastatic breast cancer. Semin Oncol 1995;22(Suppl 4):17.

Smith TJ et al: Economic evaluation of a randomized clinical trial comparing vinorelbine, vinorelbine plus cisplatin and vindesine plus cisplatin for non-small-cell lung cancer. J Clin Oncol 1995;13:2166.

Winick NJ et al: Secondary acute myeloid leukemia in children with acute lymphoblastic leukemia treated with etoposide. J Clin Oncol 1993;11:209.

Hormonally Active Agents

Butturini A et al: Use of recombinant granulocyte-macrophage colony-stimulating factor in the Brazil radiation accident. Lancet 1988;2:471.

Fisher B et al: A randomized clinical trial evaluating tamoxifen in the treatment of patients with node-negative breast cancer who have estrogen receptor-positive tumors. N Engl J Med 1989;320:479.

Love RR et al: Effects of tamoxifen on bone mineral density in postmenopausal women with breast cancer. N Engl J Med 1992;326:852.

Prostate Trialists Collaborative Group: Maximum androgen blockade in advanced prostate cancer: An overview of 22 randomized trials with 3283 deaths in 5710 patients. Lancet 1995;346:265.

Biologic Response Modifiers & Immunologic Agents

Gill PS et al: Treatment of adult T-cell leukemia-lymphoma with a combination of interferon alfa and zidovudine. N Engl J Med 1995;332:1744.

Grander D et al: Interferon-induced enhancement of 2',5'-oligoadenylate synthetase in mid-gut carcinoid tumors. Lancet 1990;336:337.

Groopman JE, Molina JM, Scadden DT: Hematopoietic growth factors: Biology and clinical applications. N Engl J Med 1989;321:1449.

Hong WK et al: Prevention of second primary tumors with isotretinoin in squamous cell carcinoma of the head and neck. N Engl J Med 1990;323:795.

Kirkwood JM et al: Interferon alfa-2b adjuvant therapy of high-risk resected melanoma: The Eastern Cooperative Oncology Group Trial EST 1684. J Clin Oncol 1996; 14:7.

Kwak LW et al: Induction of immune responses in patients with B-cell lymphoma against the surface-immunoglobulin idiotype expressed by their tumors. N Engl J Med 1992;327:1209.

Ohno R et al: Effect of granulocyte colony-stimulating factor after intensive induction therapy in relapsed or refractory acute leukemia. N Engl J Med 1990; 323:871.

Salmon SE et al: Combination chemotherapy, glucocorticoids and interferon alpha in the treatment of multiple myeloma. A Southwest Oncology Group Study. J Clin Oncol 1994;12:2405.

Socinski MA et al: Granulocyte-macrophage colony stimulating factor expands the circulating haemopoietic pro-genitor cell compartment in man. Lancet 1988;1:1194.

Vadhan-Raj S et al: Effects of recombinant human granulocyte-macrophage colony-stimulating factor in patients with myelodysplastic syndromes. N Engl J Med 1987; 317:1545.

Combined Modality or Drug Combinations

Al-Sarraf M: Head and neck cancer: Chemotherapy concepts. Semin Oncol 1988;15:70.

Canellos GP et al: Chemotherapy of advanced Hodgkin's disease with MOPP, ABVD, or MOPP alternating with ABVD. N Engl J Med 1992;327:1478.

Champlin R, Gale RP: Acute myelogenous leukemia: Recent advances in therapy. Blood 1987;69:1551.

Coates A et al: Improving the quality of life during chemotherapy for advanced breast cancer: A comparison of intermittent and continuous treatment strategies. N Engl J Med 1987;317:1490.

Early Breast Cancer Trialists' Collaborative Group: Systemic treatment of early breast cancer by hormonal, cytotoxic, or immune therapy. Lancet 1992;339:1.

Fisher B et al: Reanalysis and results after 12 years of followup in a randomized clinical trial comparing total mastectomy with or without irradiation in the treatment of breast cancer. N Engl J Med 1995;333:1456.

Fisher RI et al: Comparison of a standard regimen (CHOP) with three intensive chemotherapy regimens for advanced non-Hodgkin's lymphoma. N Engl J Med 1993;328:1002.

Harris JR et al: Breast cancer. (Three parts.) N Engl J Med 1992;327:319, 390, 473.

Herskovic A et al: Combined chemotherapy and radiotherapy compared with radiotherapy alone in patients with cancer of the esophagus. N Engl J Med 1992;326:1593.

Kaldor JM et al: Leukemia following Hodgkin's disease. N Engl J Med 1990;322:7.

Kaye FJ et al: A randomized trial comparing electron-beam radiation and chemotherapy with topical therapy in the initial treatment of mycosis fungoides. N Engl J Med 1989;321:1784.

Link MP et al: Results of treatment of childhood localized non-Hodgkin's lymphoma with combination chemotherapy with or without radiotherapy. N Engl J Med 1990;322:1169.

McGuire WE, Hoskins WJ, Brady WF: Cyclophosphamide and cisplatin compared with paclitaxel and cisplatin in patients with stage III and stage IV ovarian cancer. N Engl J Med 1996;334:1.

Merlano M et al: Treatment of advanced squamous-cell carcinoma of the head and neck with alternating chemotherapy and radiotherapy. N Engl J Med 1992;327:1115.

Moertel CG et al: Levamisole and fluorouracil for adjuvant therapy of resected colon carcinoma. N Engl J Med 1990;322:352.

Pedersen-Bjergaard J: Carcinoma of the urinary bladder after treatment with cyclophosphamide for non-Hodgkin's lymphoma. N Engl J Med 1988;318:1028.

Rivera GK et al: Treatment of acute lymphoblastic leukemia: 30 years' experience at St. Jude Children's Research Hospital. N Engl J Med 1993;329:1289.

Williams SD et al: Treatment of disseminated germ-cell tumors with cisplatin, bleomycin, and either vinblastine or etoposide. N Engl J Med 1987;316:1435.

Young RC et al: Adjuvant therapy in stage I and stage II epithelial ovarian cancer. N Engl J Med 1990; 322:1021.

Miscellaneous

Byrne TN: Spinal cord compression from epidural metastases. N Engl J Med 1992;327:614.

Chan HSL et al: Immunohistochemical detection of P-glycoprotein: Prognostic correlation in soft tissue sarcoma of childhood. J Clin Oncol 1990;8:689.

Clarkson B: Retinoic acid in acute promyelocytic leukemia: The promise and the paradox. Cancer Cells 1991;3:211.

Cubeddu LX et al: Efficacy of ondansetron (GR 38032F) and the role of serotonin in cisplatin-induced nausea and vomiting. N Engl J Med 1990;322:810.

Gabert J et al: Detection of residual *bcr/abl* translocation by polymerase chain reaction in chronic myeloid leukaemia patients after bone marrow transplantation. Lancet 1989;2:1125.

Hong WK et al: Prevention of second primary tumors with isotretinoin in squamous cell carcinoma of the head and neck. N Engl J Med 1990;323:795.

Luton JP et al: Clinical features of adrenocortical carcinoma, prognostic factors, and the effect of mitotane therapy. N Engl J Med 1990;322:1195.

Ralston SH et al: Comparison of three intravenous bisphosphonates in cancer-associated hypercalcaemia. Lancet 1989;2:1180.

Rifkin MD et al: Comparison of magnetic resonance imaging and ultrasonography in staging early prostate cancer. N Engl J Med 1990;323:621.

Tavorian T et al: Prolonged disease-free survival after autologous bone marrow transplantation in patients with non-Hodgkin's lymphoma with a poor prognosis. N Engl J Med 1987;316:1499.

56

Immunopharmacology

Jose Alexandre M. Barbuto, MD, PhD, Emmanuel T. Akporiaye, PhD,
& Evan M. Hersh, MD

Agents that suppress the immune system play an important role in the retention of organ or tissue grafts and in the treatment of certain diseases that arise from dysregulation of the immune response. While the details of the mechanisms of action of a number of these agents are still obscure, a knowledge of elements of the immune system is useful in understanding their effects. Agents that augment the immune response or selectively alter the balance of various components of the immune system are also becoming important in the management of certain diseases such as cancer and AIDS.

I. ELEMENTS OF THE IMMUNE SYSTEM

NORMAL IMMUNE RESPONSES

The immune system is designed to protect the host from invading pathogens and to eliminate disease. At its functioning best, it is exquisitely responsive to invading pathogens while retaining the capacity to recognize "self" antigens to which it is not responsive. Protection from infection and disease is provided by two major components: the innate and the adaptive (acquired) immune systems.

The Innate Immune System

The innate immune system is the first line of defense against an antigenic insult and includes physical (eg, skin), biochemical (eg, complement, lysozyme), and cellular (macrophages, neutrophils) components. An intact skin or mucosa is the first barrier to infection. When this barrier is breached, bacterial destruction is accomplished by lysozyme, which breaks the peptidoglycan cell wall, and by the split products arising from complement activation. These complement components (Figure 56–1) enhance macrophage and neutrophil

ACRONYMS USED IN THIS CHAPTER	
ADA	Adenosine deaminase
ALG	Antilymphocyte globulin
APC	Antigen presenting cell
ATG	Antithymocyte globulin
CD	Cluster of differentiation
CSF	Colony-stimulating factor
CTL	Cytotoxic T lymphocyte
DTH	Delayed type hypersensitivity
FKBP	FK binding protein
HAMA	Human antimouse antibody
IFN	Interferon
IL	Interleukin
IGIV	Immunoglobulin intravenous
LAK cell	Lymphokine activated killer cell
LFA	Lymphocyte functional antigen
MAb	Monoclonal antibody
MHC	Major histocompatibility complex
NK cell	Natural killer cell
PAF	Platelet activating factor
RA	Rheumatoid arthritis
SCID	Severe combined immunodeficiency disease
SLE	Systemic lupus erythematosus
TCR	T cell receptor
TGFβ	Transforming growth factor-β
T_H1, T_H2	T helper cell types 1 and 2
TNF	Tumor necrosis factor

phagocytosis by acting as opsonins (C3b), attracting immunocytes to inflammatory sites (C3a, C5a) and causing bacterial lysis via the generation of a membrane attack complex. If these mechanisms are successful, the invading pathogen is eliminated and disease is either prevented or is of short duration.

The Adaptive Immune System

When the innate immune response is inadequate to cope with infection, the adaptive immune system is mobilized. The adaptive immune system has a number of distinguishing characteristics that contribute to its success in eliminating pathogens. These include the ability (1) to respond to a variety of antigens, each in a specific manner; (2) to discriminate between foreign ("nonself") antigens and "self" antigens of the host; and (3) to respond to a previously encountered antigen in a learned way by initiating a vigorous memory response. This adaptive response culminates in the production of antibodies, which are the effec-

tors of **humoral immunity;** and the activation of lymphocytes, which are the effectors of **cell-mediated immunity.**

The generation of specific immunity requires the participation of antigen-presenting cells (APCs), which include macrophages, dendritic cells, Langerhans cells, and B lymphocytes. These cells play pivotal roles in the immune response by enzymatically digesting antigens and presenting the derived peptides to the T cell receptor (TCR) in association with class I and class II major histocompatibility complex (MHC) proteins. Activation of these T lymphocytes is dependent on the engagement of both accessory molecules (CD4 on helper T cells, CD8 on cytotoxic T cells, LFA-1 and CD2 on both helper and cytotoxic T cells) and co-stimulatory molecules (B7.1 and B7.2) by cognate receptors on APCs (see inset in Figure 56–4).

The T lymphocytes that respond to foreign antigens are selected in the thymus during fetal development;

Figure 56–1. Role of complement in innate immunity. Complement is made up of nine proteins (C1–C9), which are split into fragments during activation. **A:** Complement components (C3a, C5a) attract phagocytes (1) to inflammatory sites (2), where they ingest and degrade pathogens (3). **B:** Complement components C5b, C6, C7, C8, C9 associate to form a membrane attack complex (MAC) that lyses bacteria, causing their destruction. **C:** Complement component (C3b) is an opsonin that coats bacteria (1) and facilitates their ingestion (2) and digestion (3) by phagocytes.

those that bind with high affinity to "self" antigens present in the thymus undergo apoptosis (negative selection), while those that recognize foreign antigens in the context of self MHC are retained and expanded (positive selection) (Figure 56–2) for export to the periphery (lymph node, spleen, mucosa-associated lymphoid tissue, peripheral blood), where they become activated after encountering MHC-presented peptides (Figure 56–3).

Studies using T cell clones have demonstrated the presence of two subsets of T helper lymphocytes (TH1 and TH2) based on the cytokines they secrete after activation. The TH1 subset characteristically produces interferon-γ (IFNγ), interleukin-2 (IL-2), and tumor necrosis factor-β (TNFβ) and induces cell-mediated immunity by activation of macrophages, cytotoxic T cells (CTL), and natural killer (NK) cells. The TH2 subset produces IL-4, IL-5, and IL-6, which induce B cell proliferation and differentiation into antibody-secreting plasma cells. In addition, these subsets regulate each other, with TH2 cells producing IL-10, which inhibits cytokine production by TH1 via the down-regulation of MHC expression by APCs. Conversely, IFNγ produced by TH1 cells inhibits the proliferation of TH2 cells (Figure 56–4). Although these subsets have been well described in vitro, it is still unclear whether they exist in vivo as distinct populations or as a single T helper population that is capable of exhibit-

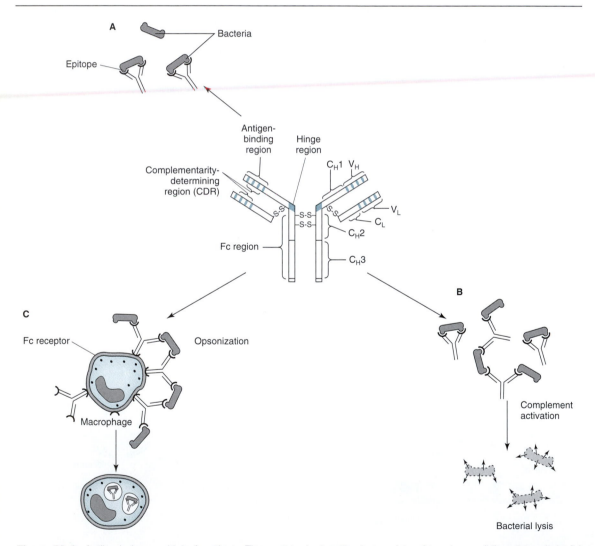

Figure 56–2. Antibody has multiple functions. The prototypical antibody consists of two heavy (H) and two light (L) chains, each subdivided into constant (C_L, C_H) and variable (V_L, V_H) domains. The structure is held together by intra- and interchain disulfide bridges. **A:** The complementarity-determining region (CDR) of the antigen-binding portion of the antibody engages the antigenic determinant (epitope) in a lock and key fashion. **B:** Antigen-antibody complexes activate complement to produce split complement components that cause bacterial lysis. **C:** The Fc portion of antibodies binds to Fc receptors on phagocytes (eg, macrophages, neutrophils) and facilitates uptake of bacteria (opsonization).

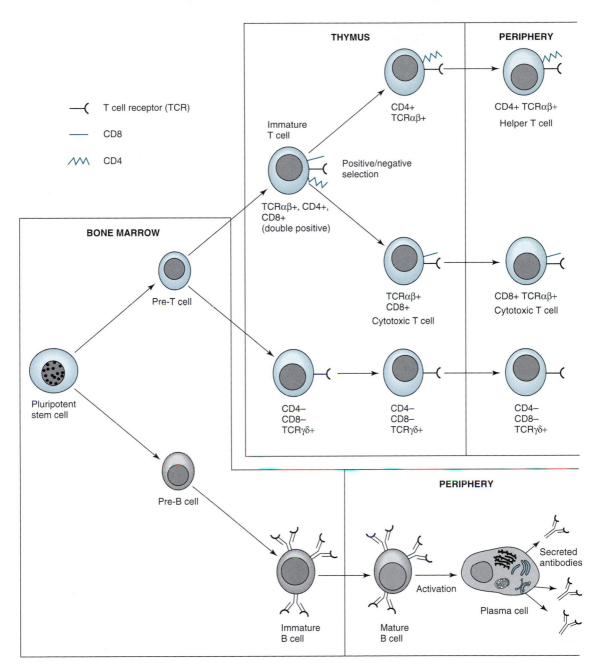

Figure 56–3. Development of cells involved in cell-mediated and humoral immunity. Pluripotent stem cells give rise to pre-T and pre-B lymphocytes in the bone marrow. Under the influence of thymic hormones, pre-T cells migrate to the fetal thymus, where they acquire the T cell receptor and undergo selection to become mature helper CD4+ and cytotoxic CD8+ T cells that are exported to the periphery. B lymphocytes develop in the bone marrow and differentiate into antibody-secreting plasma cells following encounters with specific antigens.

ing either phenotype depending on the nature of the antigenic challenge. Characteristically, extracellular bacteria cause the elaboration of TH2 cytokines, whereas intracellular organisms (eg, *Mycobacterium* species) elicit the production of TH1 cytokines. Another suppressive factor produced by certain tissues is transforming growth factor-β (TGFβ), which downregulates the proliferation of lymphocytes. In addition, the production of prostaglandin E_2 can also downregulate the immune response.

Activated cytotoxic T cells recognize endogenously processed peptides presented by virus-infected cells or tumor cells and induce target cell death via lytic granule enzymes ("granzymes"), perforin, and the Fas-Fas ligand (Fas-Fasl) apoptosis pathways. Nitric oxide may also be released, which inhibits cellular enzyme functions. The presentation of viral antigens by virus-infected cells is as nonapeptide fragments in the groove of the class I MHC molecule (inset in Figure 56–4).

Class I MHC molecules present mainly fragments of cellular antigens (such as virus or tumor antigens) processed through the Golgi apparatus, while MHC II molecules present antigen fragments from internal-

Figure 56–4. Scheme of cellular interactions during the generation of cell-mediated and humoral immune responses (see text). The cell-mediated arm of the immune response involves the ingestion and digestion of antigen by APCs such as macrophages. The resulting processed peptides bound to class II MHC surface proteins are presented to T helper cells. T_H cell activation is optimally achieved when co-stimulatory molecules (B7) and adhesion molecules (ICAM-1, LFA-3) on the APC are bound to their appropriate ligands on the T cell (see inset). Activated T_H cells secrete IL-2, which causes proliferation and activation of CTLs, and T_H1 and T_H2 cell subsets. T_H1 cells also produce IFNγ and TNFβ, which can directly activate macrophages and NK cells. The humoral response is triggered when B lymphocytes bind antigen via their surface immunoglobulin. They are then induced by T_H2-derived IL-4 and IL-5 to proliferate and differentiate into memory cells and antibody-secreting plasma cells. Regulatory cytokines such as IFNγ and IL-10 downregulate T_H2 and T_H1 responses, respectively.

ized and enzymatically digested foreign antigens. In transplant immunity, the major antigen is the MHC molecule itself.

Natural killer (NK) cells (CD16+, 56+, 57+) may play an important role in tumor rejection and viral immunity. NK cells are large granular lymphocytes with azurophilic cytoplasmic granules that are surface immunoglobulin-negative and Fc receptor-positive, with low affinity for sheep red blood cells. Studies with monoclonal antisera originally suggested that NK cells may be of T cell or monocytic origin. More recent studies have shown that they probably belong to an entirely separate lineage of lymphoid cells. NK cells have reactivity against tumor and normal cells without any prior stimulation and may play an important role in host defenses. However, their in vivo relevance remains uncertain. NK cells are also the main precursors of lymphokine-activated killer (LAK) cells. LAK cells are stimulated by high concentrations of IL-2 and are called "promiscuous killers" because they can kill across MHC barriers and can kill target cells that do not express MHC.

B lymphocytes undergo selection in the bone marrow, during which self-reactive B lymphocytes are clonally deleted while B cell clones specific for foreign antigens are retained and expanded. The repertoire of antigen specificities by T cells is genetically determined and arises from T cell receptors; the specificities of B cells arises from immunoglobulin gene rearrangement; for both types of cells, these determinations occur prior to encounters with antigen. Antigen bound to membrane immunoglobulin (IgM or IgD) on B cells is endocytosed, processed, and presented to CD4+ T helper cells, which are stimulated to produce IL-4 and IL-5. These interleukins stimulate B cell proliferation and differentiation into memory B cells and antibody-secreting plasma cells. The primary antibody response consists mostly of IgM-class immunoglobulins. Subsequent antigenic stimulation results in a vigorous "booster" response accompanied by class (isotype) switching to produce IgG, IgA, and IgE antibodies with diverse effector functions. These antibodies also undergo affinity maturation, binding antigen more efficiently. Antibodies mediate their functions by acting as opsonins to enhance phagocytosis and cellular cytotoxicity and by activating complement to elicit an inflammatory response and induce bacterial lysis (Figure 56–2).

ABNORMAL IMMUNE RESPONSES

Whereas the normally functioning immune response can successfully neutralize toxins, inactivate viruses, destroy transformed cells, and eliminate pathogens, clinical instances occur in which an inappropriate response leads to extensive tissue damage (hypersensitivity), reactivity against self antigens (autoimmunity), or impaired reactivity (immunodeficiency).

Hypersensitivity

Hypersensitivity can be classified as immediate or delayed depending on the time required for clinical symptoms to become manifest following exposure of the host to the sensitizing antigen.

A. Immediate Hypersensitivity: Immediate hypersensitivity is usually antibody-mediated, with symptoms occurring within minutes to a few hours following the patient's encounter with antigen. Three categories of immediate hypersensitivity are recognized.

1. Type I–Type I hypersensitivity results from cross-linking of membrane-bound IgE on blood basophils or tissue mast cells by antigen. This interaction causes cells to degranulate, releasing substances (histamine, leukotrienes, etc) that induce asthma, hay fever, or hives in affected individuals (Figure 56–5).

2. Type II–Type II hypersensitivity results from the formation of antigen-antibody complexes between foreign antigen and IgM or IgG immunoglobulins. This type of hypersensitivity occurs during blood transfusion reactions and in hemolytic disease of the newborn. In both cases, antibodies are formed against foreign red blood cell membrane antigens to which they bind. The union activates the complement cascade, generating a membrane attack complex that destroys red blood cells. In hemolytic disease of the newborn, anti-Rh IgG antibodies produced by an Rh-negative mother cross the placenta, bind to red blood cells of an Rh-positive fetus, and damage them. The disease can be prevented by the administration of anti-Rh antibodies to the mother 24–48 hours after delivery of the first Rh+ child (see below). Type II hypersensitivity can also be drug-induced and occurs during the administration of penicillin to allergic patients. In these patients, penicillin binds to red blood cells or other host tissue to form a neoantigen that evokes production of antibodies capable of inducing complement-mediated cell lysis. In these circumstances, subsequent administration of the drug can lead to systemic anaphylaxis.

3. Type III–Type III hypersensitivity is due to the presence of elevated levels of antigen-antibody complexes that cause tissue damage. The formation of these complexes activates complement to produce components with anaphylatoxic and chemotactic activities (C5a, C3a, C4a) that increase vascular permeability and recruit neutrophils to the site of complex deposition. Complex deposition and the action of lytic enzymes released by neutrophils can cause skin rashes, glomerulonephritis, and arthritis in these individuals.

B. Delayed Hypersensitivity: Unlike immediate hypersensitivity, delayed-type hypersensitivity (DTH) is cell-mediated, and responses are manifest 2–3 days after exposure to the sensitizing antigen. Delayed-type hypersensitivity induces a local inflammatory response and causes extensive tissue damage characterized by the influx of antigen-nonspecific

Figure 56–5. Mechanism of type I hypersensitivity. Initial exposure to allergen leads to production of IgE by plasma cells differentiated from allergen-specific B cells (not shown). The secreted IgE binds cognate IgE-specific receptors on blood basophils and tissue mast cells. Re-exposure to allergen leads to cross-linking of membrane-bound IgE. This union causes degranulation of cytoplasmic granules and release of mediators that induce vasodilation, smooth muscle contraction, and increased vascular permeability. These effects lead to the clinical symptoms characteristic of type I hypersensitivity.

Figure 56–6. Mechanism of type IV hypersensitivity (DTH). In the **sensitization phase,** the processed allergen (eg, from poison oak) is presented to CD4+ TH1 cells by antigen-presenting cells (APC) in association with class II MHC. T cells are induced to express IL-2 receptors and are stimulated to proliferate and differentiate into T_DTH cells. Secondary contact with antigen triggers the **effector phase,** in which T_DTH cells release cytokines that attract and activate nonspecific inflammatory macrophages and neutrophils. These cells display increased phagocytic and microbicidal activities and release large quantities of lytic enzymes that cause extensive tissue damage.

inflammatory cells, especially macrophages and neutrophils. These cells are recruited under the influence of TH1-produced cytokines (Figure 56–6), which collectively induce extravasation and chemotaxis of circulating monocytes and neutrophils, induce myelopoiesis, and activate macrophages. The activated macrophages display increased phagocytic, microbicidal, and antigen-presenting functions and release copious amounts of digestive enzymes that contribute to the extensive tissue damage associated with delayed-type hypersensitivity. Although widely considered to be deleterious, delayed-type hypersensitivity responses are very effective in eliminating infections caused by intracellular pathogens such as *M tuberculosis* and *Leishmania* species.

Autoimmunity

Autoimmunity arises when the body mounts an immune response against itself due to failure to distinguish "self" tissues and cells from foreign ("nonself") antigens. This phenomenon derives from the activation of self-reactive T and B lymphocytes that generate cell-mediated or humoral immune responses directed against self antigens. The pathologic consequences of this reactivity constitute autoimmune disease. Examples of autoimmune diseases include rheumatoid arthritis, systemic lupus erythematosus, and insulin-dependent diabetes mellitus. In rheumatoid arthritis, IgM antibodies (rheumatoid factors) are produced that react with the Fc portion of IgG to form immune complexes that activate complement to form split complement components which cause inflammation of the joints and kidneys. In systemic lupus erythematosus, antibodies are made against self DNA, red blood cells, histones, and platelets. In insulin-dependent diabetes, a cell-mediated autoimmune attack destroys insulin-producing B cells of the pancreas. Activated CD4+ T_{DTH} cells that infiltrate the islets of Langerhans and recognize self islet B cell peptides are thought to produce cytokines that stimulate macrophages to produce lytic enzymes which destroy islet B cells. Autoantibodies directed against the islet B cell antigens are also considered to be important in clinical disease.

A number of mechanisms have been proposed to explain autoimmunity: (1) Exposure of self-reactive T lymphocytes to antigens previously sequestered from the immune system (eg, lens protein, myelin basic protein). (2) Molecular mimicry by invading pathogens, in which immune responses are directed at antigenic determinants on pathogens that share identical or similar epitopes with normal host tissue. This phenomenon occurs in rheumatic fever following *Streptococcus pyogenes* infection, in which heart damage is thought to arise from an immune response directed against streptococcal antigenic determinants shared with heart muscle tissue. The suggested viral etiology of autoimmune diseases has been ascribed to immune responses (both cell-mediated and humoral) directed against

virus epitopes that mimic sequestered self antigens. (3) Inappropriate expression of class II MHC molecules on the membranes of cells that normally do not express class II MHC (eg, islet B cells). These cells are now capable of presenting self peptides to T helper cells, which in turn induce CTL, T_{DTH}, and B lymphocyte cells that react against self antigens.

Immunodeficiency Diseases

Immunodeficiency diseases result from abnormalities in the immune system; the consequences of these abnormalities include increased susceptibility to infections and prolonged duration and severity of disease. Immunodeficiency diseases are either congenitally acquired or arise from extrinsic factors such as bacterial or virus infections or drug treatment. The affected individuals frequently succumb to infections caused by opportunistic organisms of low pathogenicity. Examples of congenitally acquired immunodeficiency diseases include X-linked agammaglobulinemia, DiGeorge's syndrome, and severe combined immunodeficiency disease (SCID) due to adenosine deaminase (ADA) deficiency disease. X-linked agammaglobulinemia is a disease affecting males that is characterized by a failure of immature B lymphocytes to mature into antibody-producing plasma cells. These individuals are susceptible to recurrent bacterial infections, though the cell-mediated responses directed against viruses and fungi are preserved. DiGeorge's syndrome is due to a failure of the thymus to develop, resulting in diminished T cell responses (T_{DTH}, CTL), while the humoral response is unaffected. Adenosine deaminase deficiency disease is an inherited disease. The absence of this enzyme, which prevents the accumulation of potentially toxic deoxy-ATP in lymphocytes, leads to death of T and B cells. Infusion of the purified enzyme and transfer of ADA gene-modified lymphocytes have been used successfully to treat this disease.

AIDS represents the classic example of immunodeficiency disease caused by extrinsic factors, in this instance the human immunodeficiency virus (HIV). This virus exhibits a strong tropism for CD4+ helper T cells; these become depleted, giving rise to increased frequency of opportunistic infections and malignancies in infected individuals. This results from the failure of T helper cells to maintain the cytotoxic lymphocyte response. Also in AIDS, the TH1 and TH2 cells become imbalanced, resulting in a loss of cytotoxic lymphocyte activity and delayed hypersensitivity, with concurrent hypergammaglobulinemia.

The clinical conditions that arise when the immune system goes awry demonstrate the importance of immune regulation in ensuring the induction of a successful immune response specific for an invading pathogen without being injurious to the host.

Immunosuppressive agents have proved very useful in minimizing the occurrence or impact of deleterious effects of exaggerated or inappropriate immune responses. Unfortunately, these agents also have the potential to cause disease and to increase the risk of infection and malignancies.

As knowledge of the immune system has grown, we are closer to the development of more immunologically focused approaches to immune suppression and modulation. These approaches would include using transplanted cells or tissues engineered in such as way as not to express MHC or to express self MHC; maneuvers to change the TH1-TH2 balance; administration of molecules specifically targeted to cellular receptors (such as soluble receptors) or to mediator molecules (such as monoclonal antibody [MAb] to IFNγ); or the elimination of specific autoimmune T cell clones (such as the ones responsible for multiple sclerosis).

TESTS OF IMMUNOCOMPETENCE

A wide variety of techniques have been used to test immunologic competence and its drug-induced alteration. The simplest tests that can be used to detect the effects of immunosuppressive or immunostimulating agents include the following. All of them are generally available through the pathology departments of major medical centers.

(1) Delayed hypersensitivity testing with skin test antigens to detect the ability to respond to recall antigens.

(2) Measurement of serum immunoglobulins, serum complement, and specific antibodies to various natural and acquired antigens.

(3) Serial measurements of antibody response after primary immunization or a secondary booster injection.

(4) Total circulating lymphocyte count.

(5) Measurement of the percentages of B cells, T cells, and subsets (eg, with monoclonal antibodies) that comprise the circulating blood lymphocyte count.

(6) In vitro lymphocyte proliferative responses to mitogens such as phytohemagglutinin, concanavalin A, and pokeweed mitogen or to specific antigens of interest. The response may be measured by tritiated thymidine incorporation or by cytokine production.

(7) Mixed lymphocyte reaction, in which the lymphocytes of one individual are mixed with and proliferate in response to allogeneic lymphocytes of another individual.

(8) NK cell cytotoxicity to target tumor cells.

(9) LAK cell generation by in vitro stimulation with IL-2.

RELATIONSHIP BETWEEN IMMUNOSUPPRESSIVE THERAPY & CANCER CHEMOTHERAPY

Although there is definite overlap between the drugs used for immunosuppression (Figure 56–7) and those used in cancer chemotherapy (see Chapter 55), different principles govern their use in these two disease categories. The character and kinetics of cancer cell proliferation are not identical to immune cell proliferation and allow different features to be exploited in immunosuppression. For example, whereas cancer cell proliferation appears to be unstimulated, immune cell proliferation usually occurs in response to the presence of a specific antigen. While division of individual malignant cells within a large cancer cell population appears to occur randomly in an apparently unsynchronized way, immune cell proliferation appears to be partially synchronized in a burst of mitotic division that occurs after introduction of the antigen, with a large fraction of the responding cells going through the generation cycle in order to produce specific immunity. Thus, when cytotoxic drugs are used at the time of initial exposure to foreign antigen (eg, a kidney transplant), a very high percentage of an initially small number of precursor cells can be destroyed, because the antigen stimulates selected relevant clones to proliferate rather than all clones of immune cells. Therefore, some degree of selective toxicity can be initially obtained against the unwanted immune clone, whereas this objective is harder to achieve in cancer chemotherapy. Additionally, when cytotoxic drugs are used for immunosuppression, they are generally administered in a low-dosage daily schedule to block immunoproliferation continuously (because the antigenic stimulus persists). Another reason is the need to kill or inactivate already formed effector cells and to suppress inflammation associated with the tissue immune response. In contrast, when these same drugs (eg, cyclophosphamide) are used for

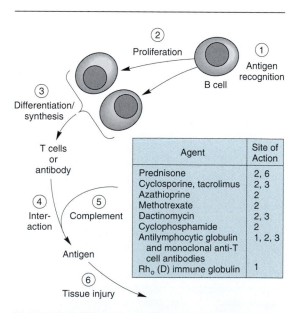

Figure 56–7. The sites of action of immunosuppressive agents on the immune response.

cancer chemotherapy, they are administered intermittently in high-dosage "pulse" courses every 3–6 weeks. Such "pulse" administration permits rapid immune rebound between treatments, which is desirable for augmentation of tumor immunity but undesirable in immunosuppressive therapy.

IMMUNOSUPPRESSIVE AGENTS

CORTICOSTEROIDS

Corticosteroids were the first class of hormonal agents that were recognized to have lympholytic properties. Administration of a glucocorticoid (eg, prednisone, dexamethasone) reduces the size and lymphoid content of the lymph nodes and spleen, though it has essentially no toxic effect on proliferating myeloid or erythroid stem cells in the bone marrow. Glucocorticoids are thought to interfere with the cell cycle of activated lymphoid cells. The mechanism of their action is described in Chapters 39 and 55. Glucocorticoids are quite cytotoxic to certain subsets of T cells, but their immunologic effects are probably due to their ability to modify cellular functions rather than direct cytotoxicity. Glucocorticoids inhibit the production of inflammatory mediators, including PAF, leukotrienes, prostaglandins, histamine, and bradykinin. In monocytes and neutrophils, glucocorticoids cause diminished chemotaxis and impaired bactericidal and fungicidal activities but do not alter their phagocytic ability. Leukocyte distribution is also changed by corticosteroids, which can cause lymphopenia (probably due to lymphoid tissue sequestration) and neutrophilia (due to demargination and impaired extravasation of neutrophils). By inhibiting IL-1 production by monocytes, glucocorticoids also cause a decrease in IL-2 and IFNγ production. Although cellular immunity is more affected than humoral immunity, the primary antibody response can be diminished, and, with continued use, previously established antibody responses are also decreased. Additionally, continuous administration of prednisone increases the fractional catabolic rate of IgG, the major class of antibody immunoglobulins, thus lowering the effective concentration of specific antibodies. Cutaneous delayed hypersensitivity is usually abrogated by corticosteroid therapy.

Glucocorticoids are used in a wide variety of clinical circumstances where it is thought that their immunosuppressive and anti-inflammatory properties account for their beneficial effects. Indications include autoimmune disorders such as autoimmune hemolytic anemia, idiopathic thrombocytopenic purpura, inflammatory bowel disease, lupus erythematosus, and some cases of Hashimoto's thyroiditis. Additionally, corticosteroids also modulate allergic reactions and are useful in bronchial asthma. Corticosteroids are also used liberally in organ transplant recipients and are of particular value during rejection crises because the dosage can be increased without fear of bone marrow toxicity. The usual dosage range for prednisone as an immunosuppressive agent is 10–100 mg orally daily. The potential adverse effects of corticosteroids, including adrenal suppression and serious viral, bacterial, and fungal infections, are also relevant when these agents are used chronically for immunosuppression (Chapter 39).

CYCLOSPORINE

Cyclosporine is an immunosuppressive agent with impressive efficacy in human organ transplantation, in the treatment of **graft-versus-host syndrome** after bone marrow transplantation, and in the treatment of selected autoimmune disorders. Patients in whom it is used as the only immunosuppressant or in combination with prednisone have similar graft survival rates and a lower incidence of rejection and infectious complications than patients treated with combinations of drugs such as azathioprine, prednisone, and antilymphocyte antibodies. Animal studies have also shown excellent results. The drug is a fat-soluble peptide antibiotic that appears to act at an early stage in the antigen receptor-induced differentiation of T cells and blocks their activation. Recent in vitro studies have indicated that cyclosporine inhibits the gene transcription of IL-2, IL-3, IFNγ, and other factors produced by antigen-stimulated T cells, but it does not block the effect of such factors on primed T cells, nor does it block interaction with antigen.

Cyclosporine is given orally at a dosage of 7.5–25 mg/kg/d. Toxicities include nephrotoxicity, hyperglycemia, hyperlipidemia, osteoporosis, some increase in hair growth, and transient liver dysfunction. A significant increase in the incidence of cholelithiasis has been observed in children treated with cyclosporine after heart transplantation. Regular monitoring of blood levels can help in avoiding most of these toxic effects. There is very little bone marrow toxicity. While a slightly increased incidence of lymphoma has been seen in transplant recipients receiving cyclosporine, there is also an increased incidence of lymphoma in other transplant recipients who have received other immunosuppressive agents.

Cyclosporine appears to have sufficient efficacy to obviate the need for simultaneous use of corticosteroids, azathioprine, cyclophosphamide, or other immunosuppressive drugs in some patients, whereas in other patients it must be combined with other immunosuppressive drugs. It has been used with apparent success as the sole immunosuppressant for cadaveric transplants of the kidney, pancreas, and liver, and it has proved extremely useful in cardiac transplants as well. Low-dosage cyclosporine (7.5 mg/kg/d or less) has also proved useful in a variety of autoimmune disorders, including uveitis, rheumatoid arthritis, and the early treatment of type I diabetes. About two-thirds of children with early symptoms of diabetes can discontinue or reduce insulin therapy within 6 weeks after starting cyclosporine therapy. This indicates that nontoxic doses of cyclosporine may be useful in abrogating the anti-islet cell autoimmune process responsible for the genesis of type I diabetes. Cyclosporine may also have potential utility in the clinical management of other conditions, including psoriasis and asthma, where it has been able to significantly improve the pulmonary function of patients suffering from the disease and long-term cortico-steroid toxicity.

Cyclosporine is slowly and incompletely absorbed (20–50%) after oral administration. It has an elimination half-life of 24 hours. The absorbed drug is almost totally metabolized and excreted in the bile.

Cyclosporine appears to be a major step in the direction of a more specific and selective agent that is effective against a subpopulation of lymphocytes. Its adverse effects are still considerable, though perhaps less severe than those of corticosteroids and other cytotoxic agents used for immunosuppression. Its combination with newer agents is showing considerable efficacy in clinical and experimental settings where effective and less toxic immunosuppression is needed.

TACROLIMUS (FK 506)

Tacrolimus is an immunosuppressant macrolide antibiotic produced by *Streptomyces tsukubaensis*. It is not chemically related to cyclosporine, but their mechanisms of action seem to be similar. Both drugs bind to cytoplasmic peptidyl-prolyl isomerases that are abundant in all tissues. Cyclosporine binds to cyclophilin, and tacrolimus binds to FK-binding protein (FKBP). Both complexes inhibit the same cytoplasmic phosphatase, calcineurin, which seems to be necessary for the activation of a T cell-specific transcription factor. This transcription factor, NF-AT, is involved in the synthesis of interleukins by activated T cells.

On a weight basis, tacrolimus is 10–100 times more potent than cyclosporine in inhibiting immune responses. Tacrolimus is currently undergoing clinical trials in heart, kidney, and pancreas transplantation. It is approved for liver transplantion. In kidney transplantation, results obtained with tacrolimus are similar to those obtained with cyclosporine. Although initial studies suggested that tacrolimus might be more effective than cyclosporine for liver transplantation, this was not confirmed in later trials. Multicenter studies in the United States and in Europe indicate that both graft and patient survival are similar for the two drugs. However, episodes of acute, corticosteroid-resistant, or refractory rejection were less frequent in patients treated with tacrolimus. Furthermore, tacrolimus has proved to be

effective as rescue therapy for rejection in patients after failure of standard rejection therapy, including anti-T cell antibodies.

Tacrolimus can be administered orally or intravenously. After oral intake, peak concentrations are reached after 1–4 hours. The half-life of the intravenous form is approximately 9–12 hours, and the drug is metabolized primarily by a P450 enzyme in the liver. Its toxic effects include nephrotoxicity, neurotoxicity, hyperglycemia (requiring insulin therapy), and gastrointestinal dysfunction. The same studies that suggested the higher efficacy of tacrolimus than cyclosporine in the management of liver transplant patients also showed a higher incidence of serious toxicities among patients treated with this drug than among those treated with cyclosporine.

INTERFERONS

The interferons (IFNs) are proteins that can be grouped into three families: **IFNα, IFNβ,** and **IFNγ.** Both IFNα and IFNβ are type I IFNs, ie, acid-stable proteins that act on the same receptor on target cells. IFNγ, a type II IFN, is acid-labile and acts on a separate receptor on target cells. Type I IFNs are usually induced by virus infections, with leukocytes producing IFNα and fibroblasts and epithelial cells producing IFNβ. On the other hand, IFNγ is usually the product of activated T lymphocytes.

As a consequence of IFN interaction with cell receptors—and depending on the cell and IFN types—different effects can be observed. IFNs—mainly IFNγ—display immune-enhancing properties, which include increased antigen presentation and macrophage, natural killer cell, and cytotoxic T lymphocyte activation. IFNs are also able to inhibit cell proliferation. In this respect, IFNα and IFNβ are more potent than IFNγ. Another striking IFN action is the increase in expression of MHC molecules on the cell surface. While all three types of IFN induce MHC class I molecules, only IFNγ induces class II expression. In glial cells, IFNβ antagonizes this effect and may, in fact, decrease antigen presentation within the nervous system.

In clinical practice, IFNs have been used mainly as immunotherapeutic agents in cancer (see below). However, recent clinical trials of IFNβ in patients with multiple sclerosis have shown a very favorable effect of this cytokine in relapsing-remitting multiple sclerosis. Patients treated with this cytokine had a reduced rate of exacerbations and less severe disease; they also showed fewer abnormalities on magnetic resonance imaging. Furthermore, these beneficial effects were accompanied by minimal side effects. The FDA has therefore approved the use of IFNβ in relapsing multiple sclerosis. The mechanism of this cytokine action in multiple sclerosis still needs to be elucidated, and it remains to be determined whether the drug will benefit all patients with progressive disease.

NEW IMMUNOSUPPRESSIVE AGENTS

New immunosuppressive agents are being investigated in an attempt to develop less toxic and more selective drugs.

Mycophenolate Mofetil

Mycophenolate mofetil (RS-61443) is a semisynthetic derivative of mycophenolic acid, isolated from the mold *Penicillium glaucum*. In vitro, it inhibits a series of T and B lymphocyte responses, including mitogen and mixed lymphocyte responses. Its action depends on its ability to inhibit the de novo pathway of purine synthesis. Recently, it has been tested in kidney and liver transplant patients with promising results in rescue therapy for refractory rejections and, in combination with prednisone, as an alternative to cyclosporine or tacrolimus in patients who do not tolerate those drugs. Furthermore, in a recent placebo-controlled multicenter study in Europe, its administration (at 2–3 g/d) to recipients of cadaveric renal allografts, along with cyclosporine and corticosteroids, significantly reduced acute rejection episodes. In the same study, toxic side effects in the group of patients receiving mycophenolate mofetil were mainly gastrointestinal. In heart transplantation, this agent promises to be useful in replacing azathioprine for reducing the incidence of rejection episodes without major side effects. A closely related drug, **mizoribine,** which inhibits the same nucleotide synthesis pathway, is also known to be effective in kidney transplantation. In Japan, it is used as an alternative to the more toxic azathioprine. Another drug in this group, **brequinar sodium,** an inhibitor of the de novo pathway of pyrimidine synthesis, has been used in the treatment of cancer, and clinical trials for its use in transplantation began in 1992. In animal models, it has shown a very potent immunosuppressive effect and synergism with cyclosporine and other agents.

15-Deoxyspergualin

15-Deoxyspergualin, isolated from *Bacillus laterosporus,* has potent antimonocytic effects, including decreased MHC antigen expression, decreased antigen processing and presentation, and inhibition of free radical generation. It also has antilymphocytic effects, inhibiting antibody production after immunization and suppressing cytotoxic cell generation during mixed lymphocyte reactions. Although its mechanism of action is still uncertain, it has been shown to bind to heat shock proteins and could exert its effects through this activity. It appears to act late in the response of T and B cells to activation and to suppress even secondary antibody responses. It has been successful in the treatment of acute rejection in renal transplantation and is showing promising results in pancreas and heart transplantation. In animal models it has demonstrated a greater ability than cyclosporine to reduce atherosclerosis in cardiac allografts. When administered to mice receiving a hamster anti-mouse CD3 monoclonal antibody, it was able to inhibit the mouse anti-hamster antibody response without blocking the immunosuppressive action of the anti-CD3 antibody. This property, which could be of great value in preventing the development of human anti-mouse antibody (HAMA) after mouse monoclonal antibody therapy, is currently being investigated in clinical trials.

Sirolimus

Sirolimus (rapamycin) is a macrolide antibiotic isolated from *Streptomyces hygroscopicus* that shows structural similarity to tacrolimus. Accordingly, it has been shown to bind to FKBP, as does tacrolimus. However, it does not block interleukin production by activated T cells but instead blocks the response of T cells to cytokines. In vitro, it antagonizes tacrolimus for T cell responses but seems to be synergistic with cyclosporine. Furthermore, it is a potent inhibitor of B cell proliferation and immunoglobulin production. Its action seems to depend on blockade of p70 S6 kinase and the cyclin-dependent kinases downstream in cell cycle regulation. Sirolimus also inhibits the mononuclear cell proliferative response to colony-stimulating factors and suppresses hematopoietic recovery after myelotoxic treatment in mice. In contrast, the drug does not inhibit steady state hematopoiesis. In animal studies it has been effective—alone or in combination with other immunosuppressants—in the treatment of kidney and heart allografts. It may also be useful, in combination with cyclosporine, in the management of psoriasis and uveoretinitis.

Thalidomide

Thalidomide is a sedative drug that was withdrawn because of its disastrous teratogenic effects when used during pregnancy. Nevertheless, it has very important immunomodulatory actions and is coming into favor because of its wide spectrum of potential clinical uses. Thalidomide has been used for many years in the treatment of some forms of leprosy reaction; it is very useful in management of the skin manifestations of lupus erythematosus; and in animal models it has been able to replace corticosteroids in producing immunosuppression after lung transplantation. Its mode of action is unknown, but it may be related to a shift in the pattern of T cell responses to antigens and mitogens, favoring a $T_{H}2$ type of response over the $T_{H}1$ response.

CYTOTOXIC AGENTS

Azathioprine

Azathioprine is an imidazolyl derivative of mercaptopurine (6-mercaptopurine; 6-MP) and functions as a structural analog or antimetabolite (Chapter 55). Although its action is presumably mediated by mercaptopurine as the active form, it has been more widely used than mercaptopurine for immunosuppression in humans. These agents represent prototypes of the structural analog group of cytotoxic immunosuppressive drugs, and many other agents that kill proliferative cells appear to work at a similar level in the immune response.

Azathioprine

Azathioprine is well absorbed from the gastrointestinal tract and is metabolized primarily to mercaptopurine (portion below the dashed line in the structure shown). Xanthine oxidase splits much of the active material to 6-thiouric acid prior to excretion in the urine. After administration of azathioprine, small amounts of unchanged drug and mercaptopurine are also excreted by the kidney, and as much as a twofold increase in toxicity may occur in anephric or anuric patients. Since much of the drug's inactivation depends on xanthine oxidase, patients who are also receiving allopurinol (see Chapters 36 and 55) for control of hyperuricemia should have the dose of azathioprine reduced to one-fourth to one-third the usual dose to prevent excessive toxicity.

Immunosuppression with azathioprine or mercaptopurine therapy seems to result from interference with nucleic acid metabolism at steps that are required for the wave of lymphoid cell proliferation which follows antigenic stimulation. The purine analogs are thus cytotoxic agents that destroy stimulated lymphoid cells. Although continued messenger RNA synthesis is necessary for sustained antibody synthesis by plasma cells, these analogs appear to have less effect on this process than on nucleic acid synthesis in proliferating cells. Cellular immunity as well as primary and secondary serum antibody responses can be blocked by these cytotoxic agents.

Azathioprine and mercaptopurine appear to be of definite benefit in maintaining renal allografts and may be of value also in transplantation of other tissues. These analogs have been used with some success in the management of acute glomerulonephritis and in the renal component of systemic lupus erythematosus. They have proved useful as well in some cases of rheumatoid arthritis, Crohn's disease, and multiple sclerosis.

As with mercaptopurine, the chief toxic effect of azathioprine is bone marrow depression, usually manifested as leukopenia, although anemia, thrombocytopenia, and bleeding may occur. Skin rashes, drug fever, nausea and vomiting, and sometimes diarrhea occur, with the gastrointestinal symptoms seen mainly at higher dosages. Hepatic dysfunction, manifested by very high serum alkaline phosphatase levels and mild jaundice, occurs occasionally.

Although these agents are potentially toxic to bone marrow elements, including the megakaryocytes and red cell precursors, the favorable effects often outweigh the toxic effects. The drugs have been of occasional use in prednisone-resistant antibody-mediated idiopathic thrombocytopenic purpura and autoimmune hemolytic anemias.

Cyclophosphamide

The alkylating agent cyclophosphamide has recently been the focus of considerable interest as an immunosuppressive agent in animals and humans. It is perhaps the most potent immunosuppressive drug that has been synthesized. Cyclophosphamide destroys proliferating lymphoid cells but also appears to alkylate some resting cells. It has been observed that very large doses (eg, > 120 mg/kg intravenously over several days) may induce an apparent specific tolerance to a new antigen if the drug is administered simultaneously with, or shortly after, the antigen. In smaller doses, it has been very effective against autoimmune disorders (including systemic lupus erythematosus) and in patients with acquired factor XIII antibodies and bleeding syndromes, autoimmune hemolytic anemia, antibody-induced pure red cell aplasia, and Wegener's granulomatosis.

Although treatment with large doses of cyclophosphamide carries considerable risk of pancytopenia and hemorrhagic cystitis, the drug has aided in "takes" of bone marrow transplants and may have value also in other types of organ transplantation. Although cyclophosphamide appears to induce tolerance for marrow or immune cell grafting, its use does not prevent the subsequent graft-versus-host syndrome, which may be serious or lethal if the donor is a poor histocompatibility match. Specialized medical care and supportive facilities are mandatory for patient survival during the period of intensive therapy.

Other Cytotoxic Agents

Other cytotoxic agents, including vincristine, methotrexate, and cytarabine (Chapter 55), also have immunosuppressive properties. Methotrexate has recently been used extensively in rheumatoid arthritis (Chapter 36). Although the other agents can be used for immunosuppression, they have not received as widespread use as the purine antagonists, and their indications for immunosuppression are less certain. The use of methotrexate (which can be given orally) appears reasonable in patients with idiosyncratic reactions to purine antagonists. The antibiotic dactinomycin has also been used with some success at the time of impending renal transplant rejection. Vincristine appears to be quite useful in idiopathic thrombocytopenic purpura refractory to prednisone. The related *Vinca* alkaloid vinblastine has been shown to prevent mast cell degranulation in vitro by binding to microtubule units within the cell and to prevent release of histamine and other vasoactive compounds.

ANTIBODIES AS IMMUNOSUPPRESSIVE AGENTS

Until recently, development of specific antibodies required immunization and collection of antisera with subsequent purification of the gamma globulin (IgG) fraction. The development of "hybridoma" technology by Milstein and Kohler has revolutionized this field and radically increased the purity and specificity of antibodies used for immunosuppression and other applications. Hybridomas consist of antibody-forming cells fused to immortal plasmacytoma cells. Hybrid cells that are stable and produce the required antibody can be cloned for mass culture for antibody production. Large-scale fermentation facilities are now being used for this purpose in the pharmaceutical industry.

Antilymphocyte & Antithymocyte Antibodies

Antisera directed against lymphocytes have been prepared sporadically since just before the turn of the century. With the advent of human organ transplantation as a therapeutic option, heterologous antilymphocyte globulin (ALG) took on new importance. ALG and antithymocyte globulin (ATG) and monoclonal anti-T cell antibodies are now in clinical use in many medical centers that have organ transplantation programs. The antiserum is usually obtained by immunization of large animals with human lymphoid cells or by the hybridoma technique for monoclonal antibody generation.

Antilymphocyte antibody acts primarily on the small, long-lived peripheral lymphocytes that circulate between the blood and lymph. With continued administration, the "thymus-dependent" lymphocytes from the cuffs of lymphoid follicles are also depleted, as they normally participate in the recirculating pool. Antilymphocyte antibody binds to the surface of these T cells (Figure 56–2) and induces immunosuppression by a variety of mechanisms. Opsonization and phagocytosis of antibody-bound cells takes place in the liver. In the spleen, cytotoxic destruction of the cells—mediated by serum complement—may occur with some polyclonal antibody preparations (but not with murine monoclonal antibodies, since these do not activate human complement); antibody-dependent cell-mediated cytotoxicity is another possible mechanism. Besides cell lysis, an antibody may block immune function by modulating the surface expression of molecules involved in lymphocyte function. This is more readily demonstrated with monoclonal antibodies, especially those directed against the CD3-TCR complex. As a result of destruction or inactivation of the T cells, a rather specific impairment of delayed hypersensitivity and cellular immunity occurs while humoral antibody formation remains relatively intact. Furthermore, antibodies—both polyclonal and monoclonal—are the most selective ways of affecting the immune response and play a definite role in the management of organ transplantation. The use of monoclonal antibodies directed against specific subsets of immune cells further improves the selectivity of the therapy and provides the possibility of use of this approach also for the treatment of autoimmune disorders.

In the management of transplants, ALG and monoclonal antibodies can be used in the induction of immunosuppression, in the treatment of initial rejections, and in the treatment of steroid-resistant rejections. Since such antibodies have not been adequately standardized, only generalizations about dosage and treatment can be given. After transplantation of an organ such as the kidney, ALG is often administered (by intramuscular injection) first on a daily basis and subsequently less often. Because ALG is usually administered along with azathioprine and prednisone, it has not been possible to assess the effect of ALG alone in human kidney transplants. Since cyclosporine has shown an enhanced nephrotoxicity when used shortly after kidney transplantation, ALG and monoclonal antibodies have been used frequently in protocols that avoid the initial use of cyclosporine. Investigators who treat their renal transplant recipients with ALG believe that it reduces the dosage requirements for the other immunosuppressive drugs and improves survival in patients who receive kidneys from unrelated or cadaver donors. There has been some success in the use of ALG for recipient preparation for bone marrow transplantation. In this procedure, the recipient is treated with ALG in large doses for 7–10 days prior to transplantation of bone marrow cells from the donor. Residual ALG appears to destroy the T cells in the donor marrow graft, and the probability of severe graft-versus-host syndrome is reduced.

The adverse effects of ALG are mostly those associated with injection of a foreign protein obtained from heterologous serum. Local pain and erythema often occur at the injection site. Since the humoral antibody mechanism remains active, skin-reactive and precipitating antibodies may be formed against the foreign IgG. Similar reactions occur with monoclonal antibodies of murine origin, and reactions thought to be caused by the release of cytokines by the T cells and monocytes have also been described. With the use of murine monoclonal antibodies, another undesirable effect is the development of human antimouse antibody responses, which cause rapid clearance of the mouse antibodies and preclude their continuous use. For this reason, development of human-to-human hybridomas is a major current research objective. Another recent approach is the "humanization" of murine antibodies using molecular biology techniques, where antigen-binding portions of the murine monoclonal antibody are inserted into a human immunoglobulin framework. These chimeric or hybrid antibodies are less immunogenic than murine monoclonal antibodies. It is now also possible to synthesize entirely human monoclonal antibodies using recombinant techniques and libraries of immunoglobulin variable region genes.

Anaphylactic and serum sickness reactions to ALG and monoclonal antibodies have been observed and usually require cessation of therapy. Complexes of host antibodies with horse ALG may precipitate and localize in the glomerulus of the transplanted kidney. Even more disturbing has been the development of histiocytic lymphoma in the buttock at the site of ALG injection. The incidence of lymphoma as well as other forms of cancer is increased in kidney transplant patients and may be as high as 2% in long-term survivors. It appears likely that part of the increased risk of cancer is related to the suppression of a normally potent defense system against oncogenic viruses or transformed cells. The preponderance of lymphoma in these cancer cases is thought to be related to the concurrence of chronic immune suppression with chronic low-level lymphocyte proliferation.

Standardization of ALG with ATG of monoclonal origin offers considerable promise, because some of these antisera are selective for T cell subsets and are potentially available in unlimited quantities with well-defined specificity. Monoclonal antibodies currently in use or under investigation include mouse and rat antibodies directed against the CD3-TCR complex of T cells, the IL-2 receptor (expressed only on activated T cells), the CD4 molecule, and against lymphokines.

Clinical studies have shown that the murine monoclonal antibody (muromonab-CD3, OKT3) directed against the CD3 molecule on the surface of human thymocytes and mature T cells can also be useful in the treatment of renal transplant rejection. In vitro, OKT3 blocks both killing by cytotoxic human T cells and the generation of other T cell functions. In a prospective randomized multicenter trial with cadaveric renal transplants, use of OKT3 (along with lower doses of steroids or other immunosuppressive drugs) proved more effective at reversing acute rejection than did conventional steroid treatment. This was associated also with a better 1-year graft survival rate (62% with OKT3) as compared with steroid therapy (45%). Accordingly, OKT3 is now marketed for the treatment of renal allograft rejection crises. Another monoclonal antibody preparation, a rat antibody specific to the alpha chain of the IL-2 receptor, has been compared

with ATG in a randomized clinical trial in patients receiving combined pancreas-kidney cadaveric grafts. Though the monoclonal-treated patients experienced a higher frequency of rejection episodes, the long-term survival of patients and grafts was not different between the two treatment groups.

A ricin-conjugated murine monoclonal antibody (xomen H-65) is currently in clinical trials and appears to be quite potent in reversing the graft-versus-host syndrome after allogeneic bone marrow transplantation.

Immune Globulin Intravenous (IGIV)

A quite different approach to immunomodulation is the intravenous use of polyclonal human immunoglobulin. This immunoglobulin preparation is prepared from a pool of thousands of healthy donors, and no specific antigen is the target of the inoculated antibody. Rather, one expects that the pool of different antibodies will have a "normalizing" effect upon the patient's immune network.

IGIV in high doses (2 g/kg) has proved effective in a variety of different conditions ranging from asthma to autoimmune disorders. In patients with Kawasaki syndrome, it has been shown to be safe and effective, reducing systemic inflammation and preventing coronary artery aneurysms. It has also brought about good clinical responses in subacute lupus erythematosus and refractory idiopathic thrombocytopenic purpura. Possible mechanisms of action of intravenous immunoglobulin include diminution of helper T cells, increase in suppressor T cells, and decrease in spontaneous immunoglobulin production and idiotypic-anti-idiotypic interactions with "pathologic antibodies." Though its precise mechanism of action is still controversial, IVIG brings undeniable clinical benefit to many patients and is under active investigation.

$Rh_o(D)$ Immune Globulin Micro-Dose

One of the major advances in immunopharmacology was the development of a technique for preventing Rh hemolytic disease of the newborn. The technique is based on the observation that a primary antibody response to a foreign antigen can be blocked if specific antibody to that antigen is administered passively at the time of exposure to antigen. $Rh_o(D)$ immune globulin is a concentrated (15%) solution of human IgG containing a higher titer of antibodies against the $Rh_o(D)$ antigen of the red cell.

Sensitization of Rh-negative mothers to the D antigen occurs usually at the time of birth of an $Rh_o(D)$-positive or D^u-positive infant, when fetal red cells may leak into the mother's bloodstream. Sensitization might also occur occasionally with miscarriages or ectopic pregnancies. With subsequent pregnancies, maternal antibody against Rh-positive cells is transferred to the fetus during the third trimester, leading to the development of erythroblastosis fetalis, or hemolytic disease of the newborn.

If an injection of $Rh_o(D)$ antibody is administered to the mother within 72 hours after the birth of an Rh-positive baby, the mother's own antibody response to the foreign $Rh_o(D)$-positive cells is suppressed. When the mother has been treated in this fashion, Rh hemolytic disease of the newborn has not been observed in subsequent pregnancies. For this prophylactic treatment to be successful, the mother must be $Rh_o(D)$-negative and D^u-negative and must not already be immunized to the $Rh_o(D)$ factor. Treatment is also often advised for Rh-negative mothers who have had miscarriages, ectopic pregnancies, or abortions, when the blood type of the fetus is unknown. ***Note:*** $Rh_o(D)$ immune globulin is administered to the mother and must not be given to the infant.

The usual dose of $Rh_o(D)$ immune globulin is 2 mL intramuscularly. Adverse reactions are infrequent and consist of local discomfort at the injection site or, rarely, a slight temperature elevation.

The mechanism of suppression of the immune response by administration of specific antibody may consist of prompt elimination of the foreign antigen after combination with the injected antibody or may be a type of feedback immunosuppression in which a change in the antigen results from its combination with antibody, so that it is no longer recognized as foreign. If the antibody produces feedback immunosuppression, it presumably acts on the macrophage, the T lymphocyte, or the B lymphocyte (Figures 56–1 to 56–3).

CLINICAL USES OF IMMUNOSUPPRESSIVE DRUGS

Immunosuppressive agents are currently used in three clinical circumstances: (1) organ transplantation, (2) autoimmune disorders, and (3) isoimmune disorders (hemolytic disease of the newborn, discussed in the previous section). The agents used differ somewhat for the specific disorders treated (see specific agents and Table 56–1), as do administration schedules. Optimal treatment schedules have yet to be established in many clinical situations in which these drugs are used.

Organ Transplantation

In organ transplantation, tissue typing—based on donor and recipient histocompatibility matching with the human leukocyte antigen (HLA) haplotype system

Table 56–1. Clinical uses of immunosuppressive agents.

	Immunosuppressive Agents Used	Response
Autoimmune diseases Idiopathic thrombocytopenic purpura	Prednisone,[1] vincristine, occasionally mercaptopurine or azathioprine, high-dose gamma globulin, plasma immuno-absorption	Usually good
Autoimmune hemolytic anemia	Prednisone,[1] cyclophosphamide, chlorambucil, mercaptopurine, azathioprine, high-dose gamma globulin	Usually good
Acute glomerulonephritis	Prednisone,[1] mercaptopurine, cyclophosphamide	Usually good
Acquired factor XIII antibodies	Cyclophosphamide plus factor XIII	Usually good
Miscellaneous "autoreactive" disorders[2]	Prednisone, cyclophosphamide, azathioprine, cyclosporine	Often good
Isoimmune disease Hemolytic anemia of the newborn	$Rh_o(D)$ immune globulin[1]	Excellent
Organ transplantation Renal	Cyclosporine, azathioprine, prednisone, ALG, OKT3 monoclonal antibody, tacrolimus	Very good
Heart		Good
Liver	Cyclosporine, prednisone, azathioprine, tacrolimus	Fair
Bone marrow (HLA-matched)	Cyclosporine, cyclophosphamide, prednisone, methotrexate, ALG, total body irradiation, donor marrow purging with monoclonal anti-T cell antibodies, immunotoxins	Very good

[1] Drug of choice.
[2] Systemic lupus erythematosus, rheumatoid arthritis, Wegener's granulomatosis, chronic active hepatitis, lipoid nephrosis, inflammatory bowel disease.

and in vitro mixed lymphocyte culture (MLC)—is of definite value. Close histocompatibility matching reduces the likelihood of graft rejection and may also reduce the requirements for intensive immunosuppressive therapy. Response to transplantation and immunosuppressive drugs in renal disease may be dependent on the nature of the primary renal lesions in patients undergoing transplant.

Primary renal disease itself is frequently immunologic in nature. Two major types of glomerular injury, the renal component of systemic lupus erythematosus and acute glomerulonephritis, are mediated by immune mechanisms. Although immunosuppressive therapy may be of benefit in both of these circumstances, the data are incomplete. Since patients with severe glomerulonephritis are often candidates for kidney transplantation, pathologic factors that might persist and also damage the transplanted kidney are of great importance. It has been observed that patients with anti-basement membrane antibody may experience an acute graft rejection when they receive a kidney transplant. Patients with anti-basement membrane antibodies are apt to need immunosuppressive therapy for 6–8 weeks after bilateral nephrectomy, being maintained on a dialysis program, before transplantation of a donor kidney can be considered. Similarly, patients with a disease such as systemic lupus erythematosus are poor candidates for renal transplant until the systemic cause of the renal injury is brought under control.

Even with all these immunologic obstacles, the response to renal transplantation has been increasingly gratifying, including transplants with unmatched kidneys from cadaver donors. Patients who have received prior blood transfusions have a higher success rate with cadaveric renal grafts. The introduction of cyclosporine in the management of transplants has improved graft survival but, more importantly, has decreased the morbidity and increased overall patient survival. At present, over 80% of carefully selected but nonrelated transplanted kidneys survive beyond 2 years after the transplant, and 5-year survival is not an unrealistic hope. As discussed above, use of the monoclonal anti-T cell antibody OKT3 has significantly reduced acute graft rejection.

Recently, increasing success has been achieved with bone marrow transplantation in patients with aplastic anemia, refractory acute leukemia, or severe combined immunodeficiency disease (congenital) who have an HLA- and MLC-matched donor. Patients with aplastic anemia or leukemia require intensive immunosuppression prior to transplantation. Monoclonal antibodies to leukemia-, lymphoma-, and neuroblastoma-associated antigens have been used to "clean up" patients' bone marrow for autologous bone marrow storage and reinfusion after high-dose chemotherapy. Use of monoclonal antibody-immunotoxin conjugates appears most promising in this regard and may broaden the use of autologous bone

marrow transplantation. Patients who do not receive autologous bone marrow or a graft from an identical twin require postengraftment immunosuppression to minimize the graft-versus-host syndrome attributable to donor immunocytes in the marrow graft. Recent investigations indicate that anti-T cell antiserum or cyclosporine can modify or abrogate established graft-versus-host syndrome in a significant proportion of cases.

Cyclosporine has proved to be an effective immunosuppressive drug for use in renal, cardiac, hepatic, and bone marrow transplantation. Together with newer drugs, it is now being evaluated as an alternative to other more complex immunosuppressive regimens.

Autoimmune Disorders

The effectiveness of immunosuppressive drugs in autoimmune disorders varies widely. Nonetheless, with immunosuppressive therapy, remissions can be obtained in many instances of autoimmune hemolytic anemia, idiopathic thrombocytopenic purpura (ITP), type I diabetes mellitus, Hashimoto's thyroiditis, and temporal arteritis. Apparent improvement is also often seen in patients with systemic lupus erythematosus, acute glomerulonephritis, acquired factor VIII inhibitors (antibodies), rheumatoid arthritis, inflammatory myopathy, scleroderma, and certain other autoimmune states.

Some cases of idiopathic aplastic anemia also appear to have an autoimmune basis. In some instances, it appears to be the result of increased activity of CD8+ T suppressor cells. In such instances, IFNγ produced by T suppressor cells may be the humoral mediator of hematopoietic suppression. A recent series of aplastic anemia patients showed significant clinical improvement and prolonged survival when treated with ATG alone. Some prior cases treated with bone marrow transplantation after conditioning with cyclophosphamide, cyclosporine, or ALG have also shown prolonged improvement in blood counts even though there was evidence of graft rejection and recovery of recipient marrow function—again supporting an autoimmune basis for some cases of aplastic anemia. Another new approach to the control of this condition is plasma immunoabsorption using protein A columns. This presumably removes the immunoreactive antibody, particularly in the form of immune complexes.

With our increasing knowledge of mechanisms of action and interactions of the new immunosuppressive agents, it is expected that they will find their way into the management of many autoimmune and even allergic disorders. Immunosuppressive therapy is currently an option in chronic severe asthma, where cyclosporine seems to be an effective drug and rapamycin promises to be another alternative. Tacrolimus is currently under clinical investigation for the management of autoimmune chronic active hepatitis and of multiple sclerosis, where interferon-β has a definitive role.

As discussed above, IGIV has been effective in the treatment of ITP. Another new approach to the control of this condition is plasma immunoabsorption using protein A columns. As in aplastic anemia, this presumably removes the immunoreactive antibody, particularly in the form of immune complexes. This approach is currently FDA-approved for AIDS-related ITP.

In most instances, it is assumed that it is the immunosuppressive properties of drugs such as prednisone, cyclosporine, cyclophosphamide, mercaptopurine, and antilymphocyte globulin that produce these improvements. Anti-inflammatory effects of some of these drugs may also contribute to their efficacy.

IMMUNOMODULATING AGENTS

A new frontier in pharmacology, still in the stage of exploration and debate, is the development of agents that modulate the immune response rather than suppress it. The rationale underlying this research is that such drugs can be used to increase the immune responsiveness of patients who have either selective or generalized immunodeficiency. The major potential uses are in immunodeficiency disorders, chronic infectious diseases, and cancer. At present, all but two of the immunostimulating or immunomodulating agents (BCG and levamisole) are classed as investigational drugs for this purpose. The AIDS epidemic has greatly increased interest in developing more effective immunomodulating drugs.

Thymosin & Other Thymic Peptides

Thymosin consists of a group of protein hormones synthesized by the epithelioid component of the thymus. These proteins have been isolated and purified from bovine and human thymus glands. Thymosin, which has a molecular weight of approximately 10,000, appears to convey T cell specificity to uncommitted lymphoid stem cells. Smaller peptides may have similar activity. Thymosin levels are high through normal childhood and early adulthood, begin to fall in the third to fourth decades, and are low in elderly people. Serum levels are also low in DiGeorge's syndrome of T cell deficiency. In vitro treatment of lymphocytes with thymosin increases the number of cells that manifest T cell surface markers and function.

Mechanistically, thymosin is considered to induce the maturation of pre-T cells. The effects of fetal thymus transplantation in DiGeorge's syndrome are probably attributable to the action of thymosin. The purified hormone therefore has potential therapeutic applications in DiGeorge's syndrome and other T cell deficiency states. A recombinant peptide derived from this hormone, **thymosin α-1,** induces enhanced production of IL-2 and increases the expression of IL-2 receptors on T lymphocytes. This peptide has undergone clinical trials for the treatment of cancer and chronic active hepatitis.

Two other thymus-related peptides, **thymopentin** and **thymic humoral factor,** also have T cell-stimulating properties and have been investigated for the treatment of AIDS as well as cancer and hepatitis. While thymic hormones are licensed in some European countries, their use has not been approved in the USA. Furthermore, most controlled clinical trials of these agents in cancer, AIDS, and hepatitis have been negative.

Cytokines

The cytokines are a large and heterogeneous group of proteins with diverse functions. Some are immunoregulatory proteins synthesized within lymphoreticular cells and play numerous interacting roles in the function of the immune system and in the control of hematopoiesis. The cytokines that have been clearly identified are summarized in Table 56–2. In most instances, cytokines mediate their effects via cell surface receptors on or in relevant target cells and appear to act in a manner similar to the mechanism of action of hormones. In other instances, cytokines may have antiproliferative, antimicrobial, and antitumor effects.

The first group of cytokines discovered, the interferons, were followed by the colony-stimulating factors (CSFs—also discussed in Chapter 33). The latter regulate the proliferation and differentiation of bone marrow progenitor cells. Most of the more recently discovered cytokines have been classified as interleukins and numbered in the order of their discovery. The identification of most interleukins and the production of highly purified cytokines of all types have been greatly facilitated by the development and pharmaceutical application of gene cloning techniques.

Now that they have become available, the cytokines are playing an increasingly important role in immunopharmacology and will probably find a variety of applications in the treatment of infectious, inflammatory, autoimmune, and neoplastic disorders. At present, interferon-α has been approved by the Food and Drug Administration for clinical use in various neoplasms, including hairy cell leukemia, chronic myelogenous leukemia, malignant melanoma, and Kaposi's sarcoma, and for use in hepatitis B and C. It has also shown activity as an anticancer agent in renal cell carcinoma, carcinoid syndrome, and T cell leukemia. Interferon-β has been approved by the FDA for use in relapsing-type multiple sclerosis as discussed above. Interferon-γ has been approved for the treatment of chronic granulomatous disease and IL-2 for metastatic renal cell carcinoma. Numerous clinical investigations of the other cytokines, includ-

Table 56–2. The cytokines.

Cytokine	Properties
Interferon-α (IFNα)	Antiviral, oncostatic, activates NK cells
Interferon-β (IFNβ)	Antiviral, oncostatic, activates NK cells
Interferon-γ (IFNγ)	Antiviral, oncostatic, activates or upregulates TH1 cells, NK cells, CTLs, and macrophages
Interleukin-1 (IL-1)	T cell activation, B cell proliferation and differentiation, HCF[1]
Interleukin-2 (IL-2)	T cell proliferation, TH1, NK and LAK cell activation
Interleukin-3 (IL-3)	Hematopoeitic precursor proliferation and differentiation
Interleukin-4 (IL-4)	TH2 and CTL activation, B cell proliferation
Interleukin-5 (IL-5)	Eosinophil proliferation, B cell proliferation and differentiation
Interleukin-6 (IL-6)	HCF, TH2, CTL and B cell proliferation
Interleukin-7 (IL-7)	CTL, NK, LAK and B cell proliferation, thymic precursor stimulation
Interleukin-8 (IL-8)	Neutrophil chemotaxis, pro-inflammatory
Interleukin-9 (IL-9)	T cell proliferation
Interleukin-10 (IL-10)	TH2 suppression, CTL activation, B cell proliferation
Interleukin-11 (IL-11)	Megakaryocyte proliferation, B cell differentiation
Interleukin-12 (IL-12)	TH1 and CTL proliferation and activation
Interleukin-13 (IL-13)	Macrophage function modulation, B cell proliferation
Interleukin-14 (IL-14)	B cell proliferation and differentiation
Interleukin-15 (IL-15)	TH1, CTL, and NK/LAK activation
Interleukin-16 (IL-16)	T lymphocyte chemotaxis, suppresses HIV replication
Interleukin-17 (IL-17)	Stromal cell cytokine production
Tumor necrosis factor-α (TNFα)	Oncostatic, macrophage activation, proinflammatory
Tumor necrosis factor (TNFβ[LT])	Oncostatic, proinflammatory, chemotactic
Granulocyte colony-stimulating factor (G-CSF)	Granulocyte production
Granulocyte-macrophage colony-stimulating factor (GM-CSF)	Granulocyte, monocyte, eosinophil production
Macrophage colony-stimulating factor (M-CSF)	Monocyte production, macrophage activation
Erythropoietin (epoetin, EPO)	Red cell production
Thymopoietin (TPO)	Platelet production

[1]Hematopoietic cofactor (HCF): Plays some role, but not the central role, in growth and differentiation of bone marrow-derived cells.

ing IL-1, IL-3, IL-4, IL-6, IL-11, and IL-12, are now in progress. Tumor necrosis factor-α (TNFα) has been extensively tested in the therapy of various malignancies, but results have been disappointing. One exception is the use of intra-arterial high-dose TNFα for malignant melanoma and soft tissue sarcoma of the extremities. In these settings, a response rate of over 80% was noted.

Cytokines as adjuvants to vaccines have been under clinical investigation recently. Interferons and IL-2 have shown some positive effects in the response of human subjects to hepatitis B vaccine. However, recombinant cytokines are expensive drugs and may never reach wide use as vaccine adjuvants.

It is important to emphasize that in normal immunophysiology, cytokine interaction with target cells often occurs, with a cascade of different cytokines exerting their effects sequentially or simultaneously. For example, prior IFNγ exposure increases the number of cell surface receptors on target cells for TNFα. Therapy with IL-2 induces the production of TNFα, while therapy with IL-12 induces the production of IFNγ.

Most cytokines (including TNFα, IFNγ, IL-2, G-CSF, and GM-CSF) have very short serum half-lives (measured in minutes). The usual subcutaneous route of administration provides slower release into the circulation. Each cytokine has its own unique toxicity, but some toxicities are shared. Thus, IFNα, IFNβ, IFNγ, IL-2, and TNFα all induce fever, flu-like symptoms, anorexia, fatigue, and malaise.

A more recent approach to immunomodulation involves the use of cytokine inhibitors for the treatment of inflammatory diseases and septic shock, conditions where cytokines such as IL-1 and TNFα are involved in the pathogenesis. Now under investigation are anti-cytokine monoclonal antibodies, soluble cytokine receptors (both soluble IL-1 receptors and soluble TNFα receptors occur naturally in humans), and the IL-1 receptor antagonist IL-1Ra (also a naturally occurring molecule that binds to IL-1 receptors but does not induce biologic responses). These molecules have shown efficacy in animal models of septic shock, experimental arthritis, immune complex-mediated colitis, and diabetes. Phase I clinical studies have demonstrated the safety of monoclonal anti-TNFα and anti-IL-1Ra antibodies in human volunteers. Preliminary data from phase III studies with monoclonal anti-TNFα antibodies suggest that these antibodies may be effective in the treatment of septic shock when bacteremia is present. Furthermore, results from a phase III study of IL-1Ra with 893 patients indicated that among high-risk patients (595 patients with a mortality rate of 24%), treatment with IL-1Ra improved survival significantly. Other clinical trials using IL-1Ra for the treatment of ulcerative colitis, rheumatoid arthritis, and myelogenous leukemia are also being conducted. It is important to point out that none of the anti-cytokines have been approved for the therapy of a human disease.

Levamisole

Levamisole was first synthesized for the treatment of parasitic infections. Later studies suggested that it increases the magnitude of delayed hypersensitivity or T cell-mediated immunity in humans. In immunodeficiency associated with Hodgkin's disease, levamisole has been noted to increase the number of T cells in vitro and to enhance skin test reactivity in vivo. Levamisole has also been widely tested in rheumatoid arthritis and found to have some efficacy. However, it has induced severe agranulocytosis (mainly in HLA-B27-positive patients), which required discontinuation of its use. The drug also potentiates the action of fluorouracil in adjuvant therapy of colorectal cancer, and in this combination it has been approved by the FDA for clinical use in the treatment of Dukes class C colorectal cancer after surgery. Its use in these cases markedly reduces recurrences, and the mechanism probably relates to macrophage activation and the killing of residual tumor cells by activated macrophages.

Roquinimex

Roquinimex is an immunomodulating drug that can augment NK cell numbers and reactivity and can stimulate a variety of T and B cell functions. It was shown to stimulate immune functions when given to post-bone marrow transplant patients. In contrast, in the animal model of chronic relapsing allergic encephalomyelitis, this drug prevented relapses. This led to a clinical trial in patients with multiple sclerosis which showed a marked reduction in relapses, disease activity, and disease progression. If these observations are confirmed in larger studies, this immunomodulator will have an important role in clinical medicine.

BCG (Bacille Calmette-Guérin) & Other Adjuvants

BCG is a viable strain of *Mycobacterium bovis* that has been used for immunization against tuberculosis. It has also been employed as a nonspecific adjuvant or immunostimulant in cancer therapy but has been successful only in intravesical therapy for superficial bladder cancer. BCG appears to act at least in part via activation of macrophages to make them more effective killer cells in concert with lymphoid cells in the efferent limb of the immune response. Lipid extracts of BCG (eg, methanol-extractable residue) as well as nonviable preparations of *Corynebacterium parvum* may have similar nonspecific immunostimulant properties. A chemically defined derivative of the BCG cell wall, [Lys^{18}]-muramyl dipeptide, has been licensed in Japan to induce bone marrow recovery after cancer chemotherapy.

In Japan, a variety of microbial products, including whole organisms and extracts, have been used as immunomodulators as adjuncts to standard cancer treatments. These have included **picibanil** (OK432), **lentinan,** and **pachymaran.** Clinical trials, usually historically controlled, showed a prolongation of remission and survival. In general, these have not been studied or accepted in the West. These agents prepare macrophages for the release of various cytokines, including IL-1, colony-stimulating factors, and TNFα. TNFα is released into the serum of BCG-treated animals after endotoxin challenge. TNFα is also considered an important mediator of the hypotensive reaction observed in patients with endotoxic shock associated with gram-negative bacteremia.

Other Immunomodulators

Inosiplex (isoprinosine) has been found to have immunomodulating activities also, and in various preclinical and clinical settings this agent has increased natural killer cell cytotoxicity as well as T cell and monocyte functional activities. It has been tested in AIDS, with some (slight) benefit observed. Inosiplex is approved in several European countries for the treatment of diverse immunodeficiency diseases but is not approved in the United States.

Other synthetic drugs, including cyanoaziridine compounds (**azimexon, ciamexon,** and **imexon**) and methylinosine monophosphate, have been under investigation for the treatment of AIDS and neoplasia. Several sulfur-containing compounds have also been under investigation as immunomodulators. **Diethyl dithiocarbamate (DTC)** was found to reduce infections and slow progression in patients with advanced but not early asymptomatic HIV infection.

A diverse group of immunomodulators has been targeted toward modulating suppressor cell activity. Low-dose **cyclophosphamide** given prior to immunization with a tumor vaccine can augment the immune response in both animals and humans. **Indomethacin** can nullify the effects of suppressor macrophages, and **cimetidine** or other H$_2$ blockers can reduce the activity of suppressor lymphocytes. At present, none of these have found a definitive niche in any immuno-augmentive therapy.

CANCER IMMUNOTHERAPY

Immunotherapy is an increasingly important component of cancer therapeutics and of immunopharmacology. The approaches to cancer immunotherapy are oriented toward restoring or augmenting antitumor immune responses or to using products of the immune system as anticancer agents. The approaches to cancer immunotherapy include the following:

(1) Active nonspecific immune stimulation, eg, BCG.

(2) Active specific immune stimulation, eg, melacine melanoma vaccine.

(3) Immunomodulators, eg, levamisole.

(4) Cytotoxic cytokines, eg, IFNα.

(5) Immunostimulatory cytokines, eg, IL-2.

(6) Adaptive cellular immunotherapy, eg, LAK cells, TILs.

(7) Monoclonal antibodies, eg, anti-CEA MAb.

Many approaches to cancer immunotherapy are at present experimental. However, more cancer immunotherapeutic options are being developed, and further indications are being identified. Currently, BCG, IFNα, IFNβ, IFNγ, IL-2, and levamisole are approved. Promising immunotherapeutic agents in clinical trials that are likely to be approved for specific indications include TNFα, IL-12, melacine melanoma vaccine, and radiolabeled anti-CD20 monoclonal antibody for the treatment of lymphoma.

GENE THERAPY

Gene therapy will probably play an important role in the treatment of immunologic and other diseases in the future. Human gene transfer can replace a missing gene, replace a gene that has been inactivated through mutation, introduce extra copies of a normally expressed gene, or introduce a gene not normally present. The result is to replace missing functions, amplify existing functions, or confer a new function on a cell or tissue.

For the treatment of immunologic disorders, gene therapy has already been used to treat SCID patients with ADA deficiency by the retroviral transfer of the ADA gene into their lymphocytes. This has normalized their immune response and eliminated their susceptibility to opportunistic infection. It is anticipated that other immunodeficiency diseases will also one day be susceptible to gene transfer therapy.

For cancer therapy, multiple gene therapy approaches are being developed. Those that show promise in immunologic therapy are as follows:

(1) Transfer of cytokine genes for effector molecules such as TNFα into effector lymphocytes such as LAK or tumor-infiltrating lymphocyte (TIL) cells.

(2) DNA vaccines, in which genes encoding tumor rejection antigens are injected and expressed to induce tumor immunity.

(3) Use of gene-modified tumor cells as vaccines, whereby tumors are transduced or transfected in vitro (for subsequent vaccination) or in vivo (to make the tumor more immunogenic). Genes that have been useful for this purpose in animal tumor models include genes encoding IL-1, IL-2, IL-4, IL-6, IL-7, IL-10, and IL-12; TNFα, IFNα, IFNγ, and various cell adhesion molecules such as B7.1 and B7.2. In addition, foreign histocompatibility antigens have been used to "allogenize" the tumor. These maneuvers lead to tumor cells that fail to grow when reintroduced into the mouse model and induce a strong, long-lasting CTL immune response. Immunized animals then reject untransformed tumor.

(4) Use of carrier cells such as fibroblasts transduced with the genes listed above, injected into the tumor or mixed with tumor cells as vaccines. This provides the immunostimulatory gene product adjacent to the immunizing tumor cells.

The principles of these approaches have been established in mouse tumor models, and clinical trials are beginning. Responses have been described in patients with melanoma, breast cancer, renal cancer, and ovarian cancer.

II. IMMUNOLOGIC REACTIONS TO DRUGS & DRUG ALLERGY

The basic immune mechanism and the ways in which it can be suppressed or stimulated by drugs have been discussed in foregoing sections of this chapter. Drugs also activate the immune system in undesirable ways that appear as adverse drug reactions.

These reactions are generally lumped in a broad classification as "drug allergy." Indeed, many drug reactions such as those to penicillin, iodides, phenytoin, and sulfonamides are allergic in nature. These drug reactions are manifested as skin eruptions, edema, anaphylactoid reactions, fever, and eosinophilia. The underlying mechanism of the allergic sensitization to drugs was clarified by the discovery of the IgE class of immunoglobulins and by a better understanding of the process of sensitization and activation of blood basophils and tissue mast cells.

Drug reactions mediated by immune mechanisms may have different mechanisms. Thus, any one of the four major types of hypersensitivity can be associated with an allergic drug reaction:

Type I: IgE-mediated acute allergic reactions to stings, pollens, and drugs, including anaphylaxis, urticaria, and angioedema. IgE is fixed to tissue mast cells and blood basophils.

Type II: Allergic reactions that are complement-dependent and therefore involve IgG or IgM antibodies in which the antibody is fixed to a circulating blood cell subject to complement-dependent lysis.

Type III: Drug reactions that are exemplified by serum sickness, which involves immune complexes containing IgG and is a multisystem complement-dependent vasculitis.

Type IV: Cell-mediated allergy that is the mechanism involved in allergic contact dermatitis from topically applied drugs.

In a number of drug reactions, several of these hypersensitivity reactions may present simultaneously. Some adverse reactions to drugs may be mistakenly classified as allergic or immune when they are in reality genetic deficiency states or are idiosyncratic and not mediated by immune mechanisms (eg, hemolysis due to primaquine in glucose-6-phosphate dehydrogenase deficiency, or aplastic anemia due to chloramphenicol).

MECHANISMS OF IMMEDIATE (TYPE I) DRUG ALLERGY

The mechanisms of immune activation that are operative in drug allergy are similar to the normal humoral antibody responses to foreign macromolecules. These mechanisms can now be placed in a theoretical construct that includes an afferent limb of the immune response (Figure 56–8) as well as an efferent limb that includes the pharmacologic mediators of allergy (Figure 56–9). Landsteiner and his associates first demonstrated that animals could be sensitized to simple chemicals such as picric acid (a hapten) if the chemical was linked to a carrier protein. This linkage can occur in the body, with a normal tissue or serum protein serving as the carrier. The subsequent immune response will be specific for the hapten even though linkage to a carrier is necessary for immune recognition. Surprisingly, carrier recognition is genetically determined even though the host does not produce antibodies against the carrier protein. When drugs serve as haptens, the antibody-forming precursor cells that respond are often the precursors of cells that produce antibodies of the IgE class. IgE class-specific antibody responses are dependent on helper T cells, which secrete IL-4 and promote the differentiation of B cells to IgE-forming cells. This cell population

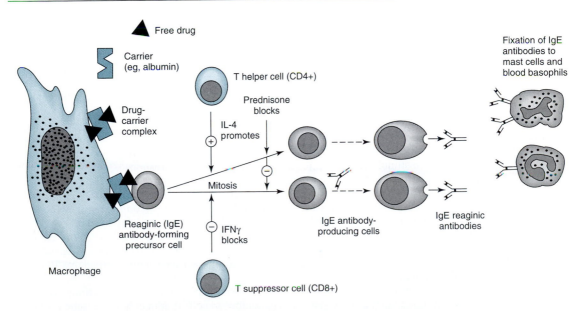

Figure 56–8. Induction of IgE-mediated allergic sensitivity to drugs and other allergens.

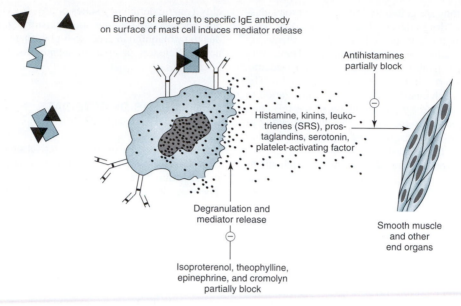

Binding of allergen to specific IgE antibody
on surface of mast cell induces mediator release

Antihistamines
partially block

Histamine, kinins, leuko-
trienes (SRS), pros-
taglandins, serotonin,
platelet-activating factor

Degranulation and
mediator release

Smooth muscle
and other
end organs

Isoproterenol, theophylline,
epinephrine, and cromolyn
partially block

Figure 56–9. Response of IgE-sensitized cells to subsequent exposure to allergens.

could be classified as a TH2 subpopulation. Suppressor T cells secrete IFNγ, which can block B cell differentiation to IgE production and inhibit the IgE response. These cells could actually be classified as TH1 cells, which are suppressor for humoral responses but are the main helpers for cellular responses. In nonallergic individuals, IgE globulin levels are the lowest of any immunoglobulin (<1 μg/mL), whereas in allergy they may be increased tenfold or more. IgE antibodies have the interesting property of fixing to blood basophils and tissue mast cells and are skin-sensitizing or reaginic antibodies.

Fixation of the IgE antibody to high-affinity Fc receptors (Fc_eR) on blood basophils or their tissue equivalent (mast cells) sets the stage for an acute allergic reaction. Among the sites for mast cell distribution and IgE sensitization, the skin, lung, and gastrointestinal tract are most important. When the offending drug is reintroduced into the body, IgE antibody molecules attached to Fc_eR on the surface of sensitized basophilic leukocytes and mast cells bind to the antigenic form of the drug. Sensitized tissue mast cells or blood basophils are stimulated to release mediators (eg, histamine, leukotrienes; Chapters 16 and 18) from granules when IgE molecules on two adjacent Fc_eR are bridged by binding specific antigen. Mediator release is associated with a fall in intracellular cAMP within the mast cell. Many of the drugs that block mediator release appear to act through the cAMP mechanism (eg, catecholamines, corticosteroids, theophylline), with different sites of action in the pathway of cAMP synthesis or degradation. Other vasoactive substances such as kinins may also be generated during histamine release. These mediators initiate immediate skin and smooth muscle responses and thus initiate tissue injury and the inflammatory response. Mediator-induced reactions can be devastating to the patient, especially when they produce laryngospasm, bronchospasm, or hypotension.

Drug Treatment of Immediate Allergy

One can test an individual for possible sensitivity to a drug by a simple scratch test, ie, by applying an extremely dilute solution of the drug to the skin and making a scratch with the tip of a needle. If allergy is present, an immediate wheal and flare will often occur. However, in many instances the skin test may be negative in spite of marked hypersensitivity to a hapten or to a metabolic product of the drug—or, at times, when the antibody may be of a class other than IgE.

Drugs that modify allergic responses act at several links in this chain of events. Prednisone, which is often used in severe allergic reactions, is immunosuppressive and probably blocks proliferation of the IgE-producing clones and inhibits IL-4 production by helper T cells in the IgE response. In the efferent limb of the allergic response, isoproterenol, epinephrine, and theophylline reduce the release of mediators from mast cells and basophils and produce bronchodilation, whereas antihistamines competitively inhibit histamine, which would otherwise produce bronchoconstriction and increased capillary permeability in the end organ. Corticosteroids may also act to reduce tissue injury and edema in the inflamed tissue, as well as "unblocking" beta-blocked cells, thereby facilitating the actions of catecholamines in cells that may have become refractory to epinephrine or isoproterenol. Several agents directed toward the inhibition of leukotriene synthesis are currently in use or in clinical trial, with the view that they may be useful in acute allergic and inflammatory disorders. Cromolyn sodium, a drug that is useful for treatment of allergic asthma, appears to inhibit the liberation of the mediators of anaphylaxis that are released after antibody-antigen interaction (see Chapter 20). However, its complete mechanism of action is still obscure. Ketotifen, an antihistaminic drug that has been used in the prophylaxis of diverse allergic diseases, can prevent allergic reactions by similar mechanisms which are independent from its antihistaminic properties and probably related to its effects on eosinophils.

Desensitization to Drugs

When reasonable alternatives are not available, certain drugs (eg, penicillin, insulin) must be used for life-threatening illnesses even in the presence of known allergic sensitivity. In such cases, desensitization can sometimes be accomplished by starting with very small dosages of the drug and gradually increasing the dose over a period of hours or days to the full therapeutic range. This practice is hazardous, and one must always be ready to manage an episode of acute anaphylactic shock before desensitization has been achieved. This form of desensitization differs from immunosuppression in that the immune mechanism often appears to be stimulated, and reactivity is only predictably diminished while the treatment is continued.

The exact mechanism of desensitization to drugs is complex and incompletely understood. It may be due to controlled anaphylaxis (with gradual depletion of mast cells and basophils), while symptoms are suppressed, or to antigen excess, which can under certain circumstances block mediator release. In some instances, allergic desensitization appears to be accomplished by the stimulation of competing clones of cells that produce "blocking" antibodies, often of the IgG or IgA class. Furthermore, desensitization with antigen could induce the generation of specific suppressor T cells or shift the response to a TH1 pattern of cytokine secretion.

AUTOIMMUNE (TYPE II) REACTIONS TO DRUGS

Certain autoimmune syndromes can be induced by drugs. Examples of this phenomenon include systemic lupus erythematosus following hydralazine or procainamide therapy, "lupoid hepatitis" due to cathartic sensitivity, autoimmune hemolytic anemia resulting from methyldopa administration, thrombocytopenic purpura due to quinidine, and agranulocytosis due to a variety of drugs. In these drug-induced autoimmune states, antibodies to tissue constituents or to the drug can be demonstrated. Immune mecha-

nisms also appear to be involved in many additional cases of so-called idiopathic thrombocytopenic purpura, but it is more difficult to demonstrate the presence of specific antibodies. The blood platelet or granulocyte is sometimes an innocent bystander to an immunologic reaction to a drug but manages to be damaged or activated by antigen-antibody complexes or destroyed by the reticuloendothelial system, leading to the development of "idiopathic" thrombocytopenic purpura or agranulocytosis.

Fortunately, autoimmune reactions to drugs usually subside within several months after the offending drug is withdrawn. Immunosuppressive therapy is warranted only when the autoimmune response is unusually severe.

SERUM SICKNESS & VASCULITIC (TYPE III) REACTIONS

Serum sickness reactions to drugs are more common than immediate anaphylactic responses. The clinical features of serum sickness include urticarial skin eruptions, arthralgia or arthritis, lymphadenopathy, and fever. The reactions generally last 6–12 days and usually subside once the offending drug is eliminated. Although IgE antibodies may play some role, complement-fixing antibodies of the IgM or IgG class are usually involved. Corticosteroids are useful in attenuating severe serum sickness reactions to drugs.

Immune vasculitis can also be induced by drugs. The sulfonamides, penicillin, thiouracil, anticonvulsants, and iodides have all been implicated in the initiation of hypersensitivity angiitis. Erythema multiforme is a relatively mild vasculitic skin disorder that may be secondary to drug hypersensitivity. Stevens-Johnson syndrome is probably a more severe form of this hypersensitivity reaction and consists of erythema multiforme, arthritis, nephritis, central nervous system abnormalities, and myocarditis. It has frequently been associated with sulfonamide therapy.

CLINICAL IDENTIFICATION OF IMMUNOLOGIC REACTIONS TO DRUGS

In view of the multiplicity of drugs taken by outpatients and administered to hospitalized patients, it is not always easy to determine which drug has initiated an allergic or immune syndrome of drug sensitivity. Careful questioning about the history of prior drug sensitivities is an important part of every patient's medical record, and errors of omission can be dangerous. In almost all instances, once an offending drug is identified, its use is discontinued. If an alternative drug is to be used (eg, an antibiotic), it is important to select one from a different class of agents to avoid cross-sensitivity reactions. Since certain commonly used drugs such as the penicillins are among the more common offenders, direct questions about penicillin sensitivity should always be included in the patient's history. Skin testing may be very useful in confirming drug allergy when the history is equivocal and the proper antigens are available. Skin testing is considerably less hazardous than a therapeutic trial and is usually indicated where there is an equivocal allergic history and a strong clinical indication for treatment with the drug. An alternative to skin testing that is increasingly available is the radioallergosorbent test (RAST), a form of radioimmunoassay.

Warnings of known sensitivities should be prominently displayed in the patient's record or hospital chart. When drug intolerance is suspected, an assessment of the patient's anaphylactic potential should be made, since delayed rashes carry a different prognosis from that of urticaria and angioedema. Once a drug allergy is defined, this information should in every case be conveyed to the patient in clear language to prevent repeated challenges with the same agent in the future, when the reaction may be much more severe. In the case of known severe sensitivity to common drugs, the patient should be advised to carry a clearly written notice of the sensitivity to lessen the chance of being given the agent while incapacitated, as after an accident.

PREPARATIONS AVAILABLE*

Azathioprine (Imuran)
  Oral: 50 mg tablets
Bacillus Calmette Guérin, BCG live
  (Thoracys, Tice)
  Parenteral: 27 mg, 3×10^8 organism vial
Cyclophosphamide (Cytoxan, Neosar)
  Oral: 25, 50 mg tablets
  Parenteral: 100 mg/mL for injection (in 20 mL vials); powder to reconstitute or injection (in 100, 200, 500 mg and 1, 2 g vials)
Cyclosporine (Sandimmune)
  Oral: 25, 50 mg capsules; 100 mg/mL solution
  Parenteral: 50 mg/mL for IV administration
Interferon alpha-2a (Roferon), **-2b** (Intron)
  Parenteral: 10–50 million unit powder or solution vials
Interferon beta-1b (Betaseron)
  Parenteral: 0.3 mg vial for SC injection
Interferon gamma-1b (Actimmune)
  Parenteral: 100 μg vials (3 million units)
Interleukin-2, IL-2, Aldesleukin (Proleukin)
  Parenteral: 22 million unit vials

Levamisole (Ergamisol)
  Oral: 50 mg tablets
Lymphocyte immune globulin (Atgam)
  Parenteral: 50 mg/mL for injection (in 5 mL ampules)
Methylprednisolone sodium succinate
  (Solu-Medrol, others)
  Parenteral: 40, 125, 500, 100, 2000 mg
Muromonab-CD3 [OKT3] (Orthoclone OKT3)
  Parenteral: 5 mg/5 mL ampule for injection
Prednisone (generic)
  Oral: 1, 2.5, 10, 20, 50 mg tablets
Rh$_o$(D) immune globulin micro-dose (HypRho-D Mini-Dose, MICRhoGAM, Mini-Gamulin Rh)
  Parenteral: in single-dose and micro-dose vials
Tacrolimus [FK 506] (Prograf)
  Oral: 1, 5 mg capsules
  Parenteral: 5 mg/mL

*Several drugs discussed in this chapter are available as orphan drugs but are not listed here. Other drugs not listed here will be found in other chapters (see Index).

REFERENCES

Current Concepts in Immunology

Abbas AK, Lichtman AH, Pober JS: *Cellular and Molecular Immunology,* 2nd ed. Saunders, 1994.

Adams DH et al: Soluble interleukin-2 receptors in serum and bile of liver transplant recipients. Lancet 1989;1:469.

Ahonen P et al: Clinical variation of autoimmune poly-endocrinopathy-candidiasis-ectodermal dystrophy (APECED) in a series of 68 patients. N Engl J Med 1990;322:1829.

Akira S et al: Biology of multifunctional cytokines: IL 6 and related molecules (IL 1 and TNF). FASEB J 1990; 4:2860.

Banchereau J, Rousset F: Human B lymphocytes: Phenotype, proliferation and differentiation. Adv Immunol 1992;52:125.

Berke G: The binding and lysis of target cells by cytotoxic lymphocytes: Molecular and cellular aspects. Ann Rev Immunol 1994;12:735.

Blaese RM: Development of gene therapy for immunodeficiency: Adenosine deaminase deficiency. Pediatr Res 1993;33(Suppl):S49.

Chatila T et al: An immunodeficiency characterized by defective signal transduction in T lymphocytes. N Engl J Med 1989;320:696.

Ferrara JLM, Deeg HJ: Graft-versus-host disease. N Engl J Med 1991;324:667.

Hall BM et al: Comparison of three immunosuppressive regimens in cadaver renal transplantation: Long-term cyclosporine, short-term cyclosporine followed by azathioprine and prednisolone, and azathioprine and prednisolone without cyclosporine. N Engl J Med 1988;318:1499.

Johnston RB Jr: Current concepts in immunology: Monocytes and macrophages. N Engl J Med 1988; 318:747.

Jones RJ et al: Induction of graft-versus-host disease after autologous bone marrow Transplantation. Lancet 1989;2:754.

Kemp M, Theander TG, Kharazmi A: The contrasting roles of CD4+ cells in intracellular infections in humans: Leishmaniasis as an example. Immunol Today 1996; 17:13.

Kisielow P, von Boehmer H: Development and selection of T cells: Facts and puzzles. Adv Immunol 1995;58:87.

Krensky AM et al: T lymphocyte-antigen interactions in transplant rejection. N Engl J Med 1990;322:510.

Kuby J: *Immunology.* 2nd ed. Freeman, 1994.

Ledbetter J et al: Evolutionary conservation of surface molecules that distinguish T lymphocyte helper/inducer and cytotoxic suppressor subpopulation in mouse and man. J Exp Med 1981;153:310.

Lipsky PE: The control of antibody production by immunomodulatory molecules. Arthritis Rheum 1989;32: 1989.

Liu C-C, Young LHY, Young JD-E: Lymphocyte-mediated cytolysis and disease. N Engl J Med 1996; 335:1651.

Miyajima A et al: Coordinate regulation of immune and inflammatory responses by T cell-derived lymphokines. FASEB J 1988;2:2462.

Nagata S, Golstein P: The Fas death factor. Science 1995; 267:1449.

Nossal GJV: Immunologic tolerance: Collaboration between antigen and lymphokines. Science 1989;245:147.

Ortaldo JR et al: Determination of surface antigens on highly purified human NK cells by flow cytometry with monoclonal antibodies. J Immunol 1981;127: 2401.

Paul W (editor): *Fundamental Immunology,* 3rd ed. Raven Press, 1993.

Rock B et al: The pathogenic effect of IgE4 antibodies in endemic pemphigus foliaceus (fogo selvagem). N Engl J Med 1989;320:1463.

Roitt I, Brostoff J, Male D (editors): *Immunology.* Mosby, 1985.

Schwartz RH: Costimulation of T lymphocytes: The role of CD28 CTLA-4 and B7/BB1 in interleukin-2 production and immunotherapy. Cell 1992;71:1065.

Stites DP, Terr AI (editors): *Basic & Clinical Immunology,* 8th ed. Appleton & Lange, 1994.

Vogelsang G et al: An in vitro predictive test for graft versus host disease in patients with genotypic HLA-identical bone marrow transplants. N Engl J Med 1985; 313:645.

Weinberg K, Parkman R: Severe combined immunodeficiency due to a specific defect in the production of interleukin-2. N Engl J Med 1990;322:1718.

Wilkin TJ: Receptor autoimmunity in endocrine disorders. N Engl J Med 1990;323:1318.

Wirt DP et al: Novel T-lymphocyte population in combined immunodeficiency with features of graft-versus-host disease. N Engl J Med 1989;321:370.

Immunosuppressive Agents

Aagaard Tillery KM, Jelinek DF: Inhibition of human B lymphocyte cell cycle progression and differentiation by rapamycin. Cell Immunol 1994;156:493.

Alegre ML et al: Prevention of the humoral response induced by an anti-CD3 monoclonal antibody by deoxy-spergualin in a murine model. Transplantation 1994; 57:1786.

Armitage JM et al: A clinical trial of FK 506 as primary and rescue immunosuppression in cardiac transplantation. Transplant Proc 1991;23:1149.

Ash RC et al: Successful allogeneic transplantation of T cell-depleted bone marrow from closely HLA-matched unrelated donors. N Engl J Med 1990; 322:485.

Atkinson K et al: Cyclosporin A associated nephrotoxicity in the first 100 days after allogeneic bone marrow transplantation. Br J Haematol 1983;54:59.

Bougneres PF et al: Factors associated with early remission of type I diabetes in children treated with cyclosporine. N Engl J Med 1988;318:663.

Brynskov J et al: A placebo-controlled, double-blind, randomized trial of cyclosporine therapy in active chronic Crohn's disease. N Engl J Med 1989;321:845.

Bumgardner GL, Roberts JP: New immunosuppressive agents. Gastroenterol Clin North Am 1993;22:421.

Cantarovich D et al: Prevention of acute rejection episodes with an anti-interleukin 2 receptor monoclonal antibody. I. Results after combined pancreas and kidney transplantation. Transplantation 1994; 57:198.

Chavin KD et al: Anti-CD2 monoclonal antibodies synergize with FK506 but not with cyclosporine or rapamycin to induce tolerance. Transplantation 1994; 57:736.

Cooper MH et al: Rapamycin but not FK506 inhibits the proliferation of mononuclear phagocytes induced by colony-stimulating factors. Transplantation 1994; 57:433.

Crawford CL: Use of thalidomide in leprosy. Adverse Drug React Toxicol Rev 1994;13:177.

Dhingra K et al: Suppression of human anti-mouse antibody response to murine monoclonal antibody L6 by deoxy-spergualin: A phase I study. Adv Exp Med Biol 1994; 353:193.

Duncan JI: Differential inhibition of cutaneous T cell mediated reactions and epidermal cell proliferation by cyclosporin A, FK506, and rapamycin. J Invest Dermatol 1994;102:84.

Eisen D et al: Effect of topical cyclosporine rinse on oral lichen planus. N Engl J Med 1990;323:290.

Epstein S, Shane E, Bilezikian JP: Organ transplantation and osteoporosis. Curr Opin Rheumatol 1995;7:255.

European FK506 Multicenter Liver Study Group: Randomized trial comparing tacrolimus (FK506) and cyclosporin in prevention of liver allograft rejection. Lancet 1994;344:423.

European Multicentre Trial Group: Cyclosporine in cadaveric renal transplantation. Lancet 1983;2:986.

European Mycophenolate Mofetil Cooperative Study Group: Placebo-controlled study of mycophenolate mofetil combined with cyclosporine and corticosteroids for prevention of acute rejection. Lancet 1995;345:1321.

Fehr J, Hofmann V, Kappeler CM: Transient reversal of thrombocytopenia in idiopathic thrombocytopenia purpura by high-dose intravenous gamma globulin. N Engl J Med 1982;306:1254.

First MR et al: Concomitant administration of cyclosporine and ketoconazole in renal transplant recipients. Lancet 1989;2:1198.

Freda VJ et al: Prevention of Rh hemolytic disease: Ten years' experience with Rh immune globulin. N Engl J Med 1975;292:1014.

Fung J et al: A randomized trial of primary liver transplantation under immunosuppression with FK506 vs cyclosporine. Transplant Proc 1991;23:2977.

Fung J et al: Randomized trial in primary liver trans-plantation under immunosuppression with FK506 or cyclosporine. Transplant Proc 1993;25(1 Part 2):1130.

Gernsheimer T et al: Mechanisms of response to treatment in autoimmune thrombocytopenic purpura. N Engl J Med 1989;320:974.

Group TIMS: Interferon beta-1b is effective in relapsing-remitting multiple sclerosis. I Clinical results of a multicenter randomized double blind placebo-controlled trial. Neurology 1993;43:655.

Hadley S et al: Major infectious complications after orthotopic liver transplantation and comparison of outcomes in patients receiving cyclosporine or FK506 as primary immunosuppression. Transplantation 1995;59:851.

Hayes JM: The immunobiology and clinical use of current immunosuppressive therapy for renal transplantation. J Urol 1993;149:437.

Hoeger PH et al: Immunosuppressant deoxyspergualin inhibits antigen processing in monocytes. J Immunol 1994;153:3908.

Hoffman GS: Immunosuppressive therapy for autoimmune diseases. Ann Allergy 1993;70:263.

Imbach P et al: Intravenous immunoglobulin versus oral corticosteroids in acute immune thrombocytopenic purpura in childhood. Lancet 1985;2:464.

Imamura M et al: In vivo effects of the immunosuppressant 15-deoxyspergualin on hematopoiesis in murine allogeneic bone marrow chimeras: Its thrombopoietic activity and reversal of adverse effects with granulocyte colony-stimulating factor and/or erythropoietin. Transplantation 1994;58:214.

Jacobs I et al: Intrathecally administered natural human fibroblast interferon reduces exacerbations of multiple sclerosis. Arch Neurol 1987;44:589.

Jacobs L et al: Advances in specific therapy for multiple sclerosis. Curr Opin Neurol 1994;7:250.

Jakeman, P Smith WC: Thalidomide in leprosy reaction. Lancet 1994;343:432.

Jenkins MK, Schwartz RH, Pardoll DM: Effects of cyclosporine A on T cell development and clonal deletion. Science 1988;241:1655.

Kahan BD: Cyclosporine. N Engl J Med 1989;321:1725.

Kay AB: Immunosuppressive agents in chronic severe asthma. Allergy Proc 1994;15:147.

Kerr PG et al: Deoxyspergualin suppresses local macrophage proliferation in rat renal allograft rejection. Transplantation 1994;58:596.

Kerstens PJ et al: Purine enzymes in rheumatoid arthritis: A clue to the prediction of the response to azathioprine? Review and hypothesis. Clin Exp Rheumatol 1995;13:107.

Kim HS et al: Effects of cyclosporine and rapamycin on immunoglobulin production by preactivated human B cells. Clin Exp Immunol 1994;94:508.

Kirklin JK et al: Treatment of recurrent heart rejection with mycophenolate mofetil (RS-61443): Initial clinical experience. J Heart Lung Transplant 1994;13:444.

Kornbluth A, George J, Sachar DB: Immunosuppressive drugs in Crohn's disease. Gastroenterologist 1994;2:239.

Larick JW: Potential of monoclonal antibodies as pharmacological agents. Pharmacol Rev 1989;41:539.

Lichtiger S, Present DH: Preliminary report: Cyclosporine in treatment of severe active ulcerative colitis. Lancet 1990;336:16.

Liu J: FK 506 and cyclosporin, molecular probes for studying intracellular signal transduction. Immunol Today 1993;14:290.

Martin DF et al: Synergistic effect of rapamycin and cyclosporin A in the treatment of experimental autoimmune uveoretinitis. J Immunol 1995;154:922.

Matas AJ et al: Pilot evaluation of 15-deoxyspergualin for refractory acute renal transplant rejection. Clin Transplant 1994;8:116.

Mathieson PW et al: Monoclonal antibody therapy in systemic vasculitis. N Engl J Med 1990;323:250.

McCune WJ, Vallance DK, Lynch JP: Immunosuppressive Drug therapy. Curr Opin Rheumatol 1994;6:262.

McDiarmid SV et al: FK506 (tacrolimus) compared with cyclosporine for primary immunosuppression after pediatric liver transplantation: Results from the US Multicenter Trial. Transplantation 1995; 59:530.

McHugh SM et al: The immunosuppressive drug thalidomide induces T helper cell type 2 (TH2) and concomitantly inhibits TH1 cytokine production in mitogen and antigen-stimulated human peripheral blood mononuclear cell cultures. Clin Exp Immunol 1995;99:160.

Monfar M et al: Activation of pp 70/85 S6 kinases in interleukin-2-responsive lymphoid cells is mediated by phosphatidyinositol 3-kinase and inhibited by cyclic AMP. Mol Cell Biol 1995;15:326.

Moran M et al: Prevention of acute graft rejection by the prostaglandin E1 analogue misoprostol in renal-transplant recipients treated with cyclosporine and prednisone. N Engl J Med 1990;322:1183.

Morris RE: Immunopharmacology of new xenobiotic immunosuppressive molecules. Semin Nephrol 1992; 12:304.

Nadeau K et al: Quantitation of the interaction of the immunosuppressant deoxyspergualin and analogs with Hsc70 and Hsp90. Biochemistry 1994;33:2561.

Nair RV, Morris RE: Immunosuppression in cardiac transplantation: A new era in immunopharmacology. Curr Opin Cardiol 1995;10:207.

Nagamine S et al: Effects of cyclosporine and 15-deoxyspergualin on coronary arteriosclerosis after heart transplantation in the rat. J Heart Lung Transplant 1994;13:895.

Ortho Multicenter Transplant Study Group: Randomized trial of OKT3 monoclonal antibody for acute rejection of cadaveric renal transplants. N Engl J Med 1985; 313:337.

Paty DW, Li DK: Interferon beta-1b is effective in relapsing-remitting multiple sclerosis. II. MRI analysis results of a multicenter, randomized, double-blind, placebo-controlled trial. Neurology 1993;43:662.

Prummel MF et al: Prednisone and cyclosporine in the treatment of severe Graves' ophthalmopathy. N Engl J Med 1989;321:1353.

Quesniaux VF et al: The immunosuppressant rapamycin blocks in vitro responses to hematopoietic cytokines and inhibits recovering but not steady-state hematopoiesis in vivo. Blood 1994;84:1543.

Schindler R (editor): *Cyclosporin in Autoimmune Diseases.* Springer, 1985.

Showstack J et al: The effect of cyclosporine on the use of hospital resources for kidney transplantation. N Engl J Med 1989;321:1086.

Schreiber SL, Crabtree GR: The mechanism of action of cyclosporin A and FK506. Immunol Today 1992; 13:136.

Sigal NH, Dumont FJ: Cyclosporin A, FK-506, and rapamycin: Pharmacologic probes of lymphocyte signal transduction. Annu Rev Immunol 1992;10:519.

Snyder HW Jr et al: Experience with protein A-immunoadsorption in treatment-resistant adult immune thrombocytopenic purpura. Blood 1992;79:2237.

Soulillou J-P et al: Randomized controlled trial of monoclonal antibody against the interleukin-2 receptor (33B3.1) as compared with rabbit antithymocyte globulin for prophylaxis against rejection of renal allografts. N Engl J Med 1990;322:1175.

Starzl TE et al: Liver transplantation with the use of cyclosporin A and prednisone. N Engl J Med 1981;305:266.

Taylor DO et al: Mycophenolate mofetil (RS-61443): Preclinical, clinical, and three-year experience in heart transplantation. J Heart Lung Transplant 1994; 13:571.

Tugwell P et al: Low-dose cyclosporine versus placebo in patients with rheumatoid arthritis. Lancet 1990;335: 1051.

The US Multicenter FK506 Liver Study Group: A comparison of tacrolimus (FK 506) and cyclosporine for immunosuppression in liver transplantation. N Engl J Med 1994;331:1110.

Uthoff K et al: Thalidomide as replacement for steroids in immunosuppression after lung transplantation. Ann Thorac Surg 1995;59:277.

Van Oosten BW et al: Multiple sclerosis therapy: A practical guide. Drugs 1995;49:200.

Venkataramanan R et al: Pharmacokinetics of FK506. Transplant Proc 1991;23:2736.

Weinstein S et al: Cholelithiasis in pediatric cardiac transplant patients on cyclosporine. J Pediatr Surg 1995; 30:61.

Yee GC et al: Serum cyclosporine concentration and risk of acute graft-versus-host disease after allogeneic marrow transplantation. N Engl J Med 1988;319:65.

Zachariae H, Steen Olsen T: Efficacy of cyclosporin A (CyA) in psoriasis: An overview of dose/response indications, contraindications, and side-effects. Clin Nephrol 1995;43:154.

Immunomodulating Agents

Atkinson MA et al: 64000 Mr autoantibodies as predictors of insulin-dependent diabetes. Lancet 1990;335:1357.

Audibert FM, Lise LD: Adjuvants: Current status, clinical perspectives and future prospects. Immunol Today 1993;14:281.

Bengtsson M et al: Stimulation of NK cell, T cell, and monocyte functions by the novel immunomodulator linomide after autologous bone marrow transplantation. Transplant 1992;53:882.

Dinarello CA: Modalities for reducing interleukin 1 activity in disease. Immunol Today 1993;14:260.

Dinarello CA, Gelfand JA, Wolff SM: Anticytokine strategies in the treatment of systemic inflammatory response syndrome. JAMA 1993;14:1829.

Ezekowitz AR et al: Partial correction of the phagocyte defect in patients with X-linked chronic granulomatous disease by subcutaneous interferon gamma. N Engl J Med 1988;319:146.

Foon KA: Biological response modifiers: The new immunotherapy. Cancer Res 1989;49:1621.

Gresser I (editor): *Interferon.* Academic Press, 1981.

Hadden JW: Immunostimulants. Immunol Today 1993; 14:275.

Karussis DM et al: Treatment of chronic relapsing experimental autoimmune encephalomyelitis with the synthetic immunomodulator linomide (quinoline-3-carboxamide). Proc Natl Acad Sci U S A 1993;90:6400.

Karussis DM et al: Treatment of secondary progressive multiple sclerosis with the immunomodulator linomide: A double blind, placebo controlled pilot study with monthly MRI evaluation. J Neurol 1995;242(Suppl 7):S24.

Lee B, Ciardelli TL: Clinical applications of cytokines for immunostimulation and immunosuppression. Prog Drug Res 1992;39:167.

Lewis V: Circulating thymic-hormone activity in congenital immunodeficiency. Lancet 1977;2:471.

Norman DJ: Antilymphocyte antibodies in the treatment of allograft rejection: Targets, mechanisms of action, monitoring and efficacy. Semin Nephrol 1992;12:315.

Starzl TE et al: FK 506 for liver, kidney, and pancreas transplantation. Lancet 1989;2:1000.

Starzl TE, Makowka L, Todo S (editors): FK 506: A potential breakthrough in immunosuppression. Transplant Proc 1987;19(Suppl 6):3.

St Georgiev V: New synthetic immunomodulating agents. Trends Pharmacol Sci 1988;9:446.

Vilcek J, Gresser I, Merigan TC (editors): Regulatory functions of interferons. Ann N Y Acad Sci 1980;350:1.

Vitetta ES, Thorpe PE, Uhr JW: Immunotoxins: Magic bullets or misguided missiles? Immunol Today 1993;14:252.

Winter G, Harris WJ: Humanized antibodies. Immunol Today 1993;14:243.

Wybran J: Immunomodulatory properties of isoprinosine in man: In vitro and in vivo data. Int J Immunopharmacol 1980;2:197.

Immunotherapy and Gene Therapy:

Allison AC, Lafferty KJ, Fliri H: Immunosuppressive and anti-inflammatory drugs. Ann N Y Acad Sci 1993; 696.

Aggarwal BB, Puri RK: *Human Cytokines: Their Role in Disease and Therapy.* Cambridge Univ Press, 1995.

Huber BE, Lazo JS (editors): Gene therapy for neoplastic diseases, Ann N Y Acad Sci 1994;716. (Entire issue.)

Uckert W, Walther W: Retrovirus-mediated gene transfer

in cancer therapy. Pharmacol Ther 1994;63:323.

Porgador A, Feldman M, Eisenbach L: Immunotherapy of tumor metastasis via gene therapy. Nat Immunity 1994;13:113.

Miller AR et al: Cytokine mediated gene therapy for cancer. Am Surg Oncol 1994;1:436.

Immunologic Reactions to Drugs and Allergy

Anderson JA, Adkinson NF Jr: Allergic reactions to drugs and biologic agents. JAMA 1987;258:2891.

Askenase PW: Effector and regulatory mechanisms in delayed type hypersensitivity. In: *Allergy Principles and Practice,* 2nd ed. Middleton E Jr, Reed C, Ellis EF (editors). Mosby, 1983.

Goldfine AB, Kathn CR: Insulin allergy and insulin resistance. Curr Ther Endocrinol Metab 1994;5:461.

Morley J: Immunopharmacology of asthma. Immunol Today 1993;14:317.

Nabe M et al: The effect of ketotifen on eosinophils as measured at LTC4 release and by chemotaxis. Allergy Proc 1991;12:267.

Patterson R et al: Drug allergy and protocols for management for drug allergies. Allergy Proc 1994;15:239.

Rieder MJ: Immunopharmacology and adverse drug reactions. J Clin Pharmacol 1993;33:316.

Samuelsson B et al: Leukotrienes and slow reacting substance of anaphylaxis (SRS-A). Allergy 1980;35:375.

Wilson NW. Antibiotic allergy in children. Adv Pediat Infect Dis 1995;10:307.

Introduction to Toxicology: Occupational & Environmental

57

Gabriel L. Plaa, PhD

Humans live in a chemical environment and inhale, ingest, or absorb from the skin many of these chemicals. Estimates indicate that more than 60,000 chemicals are in common use and about 500 new chemicals are said to enter the commercial market annually. Pollution has paralleled technologic advances. Industrialization and the creation of large urban centers have led to the contamination of air, water, and soil. The principal causes of pollution are related to the production and use of energy, the production and use of industrial chemicals, and increased agricultural activity.

TOXICOLOGY & ITS SUBDIVISIONS

Toxicology is concerned with the deleterious effects of chemical and physical agents on all living systems. In the biomedical area, however, the toxicologist is primarily concerned with adverse effects in humans resulting from exposure to drugs and other chemicals as well as the demonstration of safety or hazard associated with their use.

Occupational Toxicology

Occupational toxicology deals with the chemicals found in the workplace. Industrial workers may be exposed to these agents during the synthesis, manufacturing, or packaging of these substances or through their use in an occupational setting. Agricultural workers may be exposed to harmful amounts of pesticides during their application in the field. The major emphasis of occupational toxicology is to identify the agents of concern, define the conditions leading to their safe use, and prevent absorption of harmful amounts. Guidelines have been elaborated to establish safe ambient air concentrations for many chemicals found in the workplace. The American Conference of Governmental Industrial Hygienists periodically prepares lists of recommended **threshold limit values (TLV)** for about 600 such chemicals (Lu, 1991). Three different categories of air concentrations (expressed in parts per million [ppm] or milligrams per cubic meter [mg/m^3]) have been elaborated to cover various exposure conditions: (1) threshold limit value-time-weighted average (TLV-TWA) is the concentration for a normal 8-hour workday or 40-hour workweek to which workers may be repeatedly exposed without adverse effect; (2) threshold limit value-short-term exposure limit (TLV-STEL) is the maximum concentration (a value greater than the TLV-TWA) that should not be exceeded at any time during a 15-minute exposure period; and (3) threshold limit value-ceiling (TLV-C) is the concentration that should not be exceeded even instantaneously. These guidelines are reevaluated as new information becomes available.

Environmental Toxicology

Environmental toxicology deals with the potentially deleterious impact of chemicals, present as pollutants of the environment, to living organisms. The term **environment** includes all the surroundings of an individual organism, but particularly the air, soil, and water. A **pollutant** is a substance that occurs in the environment, at least in part as a result of human activity, and which has a deleterious effect on living organisms. While humans are considered a target species of particular interest, other terrestrial and aquatic species are of considerable importance as potential biologic targets.

Air pollution is a product of industrialization, technologic development, and increased urbanization. Humans may also be exposed to chemicals used in the agricultural environment as pesticides or in food processing that may persist as residues or ingredients in food products. The Food and Agriculture Organization and the World Health Organization (FAO/WHO) Joint Expert Commission on Food Additives adopted the term **acceptable daily intake (ADI)** to denote the daily intake of a chemical which, during an entire lifetime, appears to be without appreciable risk on the basis of all the known facts at the time (Lu, 1991, 1995). After evaluation of the pertinent scientific data, the FAO/WHO periodically lists ADI values (expressed in milligrams per kilogram of body weight per day) for many pesticides and food additives that may enter the human food chain. These guidelines are reevaluated as new information becomes available.

Ecotoxicology

Ecotoxicology has evolved as an extension of environmental toxicology. It is concerned with the toxic effects of chemical and physical agents on living organisms, especially in populations and communities within defined ecosystems; it includes the transfer pathways of those agents and their interactions with the environment. Traditional toxicology is concerned with toxic effects on individual organisms; ecotoxicology is concerned with the impact on populations of living organisms or on ecosystems (Truhaut, 1977). It is possible that an environmental event, exerting severe effects on *individual* organisms, has no important impact on populations or an ecosystem. Thus, the terms "environmental toxicology" and "ecotoxicology" are not interchangeable.

TOXICOLOGIC TERMS & DEFINITIONS

Toxicity, Hazard, & Risk

Toxicity is *the ability of a chemical agent to cause injury.* It is a qualitative term. Whether or not these injuries occur depends on the amount of chemical absorbed (severity of the exposure, dose). Hazard, on the other hand, is *the likelihood that injury will occur in a given situation or setting;* the conditions of use and exposure are primary considerations. To assess hazard, one needs to have knowledge about both the inherent toxicity of the substance (qualitative aspect) and the amounts to which individuals are liable to be exposed (quantitative aspect). Humans can safely use potentially toxic substances when the necessary conditions minimizing absorption are established and respected. The presence of a potentially toxic substance in the workplace or in the environment does not necessarily mean that a hazardous situation exists.

Risk is defined as the *expected frequency of the occurrence of an undesirable effect* arising from exposure to a chemical or physical agent. Estimation of risk makes use of dose-response data and extrapolation from the observed relationships to the expected responses at doses occurring in actual exposure situations. The quality and suitability of the biologic data used in such estimates are major limiting factors. A number of mathematical models have been devised and are often used for calculating risk of carcinogenesis (Ecobichon, 1992); they may also be used to assess the risk involved with other forms of toxicity.

Routes of Exposure

The route of entry for chemicals into the body differs in different exposure situations. In the industrial setting, inhalation is the major route of entry. The transdermal route is also quite important, but oral ingestion is a relatively minor route. Consequently, preventive measures are largely designed to eliminate absorption by inhalation or by topical contact. Atmospheric pollutants gain entry by inhalation, whereas for pollutants of water and soil, oral ingestion is the principal route of exposure for humans.

Duration of Exposure

Toxic reactions may differ qualitatively depending on the duration of the exposure. A single exposure—or multiple exposures occurring over 1 or 2 days—represents **acute exposure.** Multiple exposures continuing over a longer period of time represent a **chronic exposure.** In the occupational setting, both acute (eg, accidental discharge) and chronic (eg, repetitive handling of a chemical) exposures may occur, whereas with chemicals found in the environment (eg, pollutants in ground water), chronic exposure is more likely. Society is also concerned with the possible harmful effects of contact with small concentrations of chemicals over long periods of time; this type of chronic situation is called **low-level, long-term exposure.** The appearance of the toxic effect after acute exposure may appear rapidly or after a variable interval; the latter is called **delayed toxicity.** With chronic exposures, the toxic effect may not be discernible until after several months of repetitive exposure. The harmful effect resulting from either acute or chronic exposure may be reversible or irreversible. The relative reversibility of the toxic effect depends on the recuperative properties of the affected organ.

Presence of Mixtures

Humans normally come in contact with several (or many) different chemicals concurrently or sequentially. This complicates the assessment of potentially hazardous situations encountered in the workplace or in the environment. The resulting biologic effect of combined exposure to several agents can be characterized as **additive, supra-additive (synergistic),** or **infra-additive (antagonistic).** Another type of interaction, **potentiation** (a special form of synergism), may be observed. In cases of potentiation, one of two agents exerts no effect upon exposure; but when exposure to both together occurs, the effect of the active agent is increased. All these types of interactions have been observed in humans. In the absence of contrary evidence, one usually assumes that the toxic effects of mixtures of chemicals are likely to be additive.

ENVIRONMENTAL CONSIDERATIONS

Certain chemical and physical characteristics are known to be important for estimating the potential hazard involved for environmental toxicants. In addition to information regarding effects on different organisms, knowledge about the following properties is essential to predict the environmental impact: The **degradability** of the substance; its **mobility** through air, water, and soil; whether or not **bioaccumulation** occurs; and its transport and **biomagnification** through food chains. Chemicals that are poorly degraded (by abiotic or biotic pathways) exhibit *environmental persistence* and thus can accumulate. Lipophilic substances tend to bioaccumulate in body fat, resulting in tissue residues. When the toxicant is incorporated into the food chain, biomagnification occurs as one species feeds upon others and concentrates the chemical. The pollutants that have the widest environmental impact are poorly degradable; are relatively mobile in air, water, and soil; exhibit bioaccumulation; and also exhibit biomagnification. Attempts have been made to estimate for humans the bioaccumulation potential of organic chemicals found in the environment (Geyer et al, 1986).

In ecotoxicology there are three interacting components; the toxicant, the environment, and the organisms (community, population, or ecosystem). Ecotoxicologic studies are designed to determine emission and entry of the toxicant in the abiotic environment, including distribution and fate; entry and fate of the toxicant in the biosphere; and the qualitative and quantitative toxic consequences to the ecosystem.

SPECIFIC CHEMICALS

AIR POLLUTANTS

Five major substances account for about 98% of air pollution: carbon monoxide (about 52%), sulfur oxides (about 14%), hydrocarbons (about 14%), particulate matter (about 4%), and nitrogen oxides (about 14%) (Costa et al, 1996). The sources of these chemicals include transportation, industry, generation of electric power, space heating, and refuse disposal. Considerable progress has been made in our understanding of the chemistry of urban air pollution (Seinfeld, 1989). The **reducing type** of pollution (sulfur dioxide and smoke resulting from incomplete combustion of coal) has been associated with acute adverse effects, particularly among the elderly and individuals with preexisting cardiac or respiratory disease. The association of acute adverse effects, other than severe irritation of the eyes, is less striking with the **oxidizing or photochemical type** of pollution (hydrocarbons, nitrogen oxides, and photochemical oxidants). Ambient air pollution has been implicated as a contributing factor in bronchitis, obstructive ventilatory disease, pulmonary emphysema, bronchial asthma, and lung cancer (Sarnet et al, 1991).

BIOACCUMULATION & BIOMAGNIFICATION

If the intake of a long-lasting contaminant by an organism exceeds the latter's ability to metabolize or excrete the substance, the chemical accumulates within the tissues of the organism. This is called **bioaccumulation.**

Although the concentration of a contaminant may be virtually undetectable in water, it may be magnified hundreds or thousands of times as the contaminant passes up the food chain. This is called **biomagnification.**

The biomagnification of PCBs in the Great Lakes of North America is illustrated by the following residue values available from *Environment Canada,* a report published by the Canadian government, and other sources.

Source	PCB Concentration (ppm)[1]	Concentration Relative to Phytoplankton
Phytoplankton	0.0025	1
Zooplankton	0.123	49.2
Rainbow smelt	1.04	416
Lake trout	4.83	1,932
Herring gull	124	49,600

[1]Sources: *Environment Canada, The State of Canada's Environment,* 1991. Government of Canada, Ottawa, and other publications.

Thus, the biomagnification for this substance in the food chain, beginning with phytoplankton and ending with the herring gull, is nearly × 50,000. Domesticated animals and humans may eat fish from the Great Lakes, resulting in PCB residues in these species as well.

---

1. CARBON MONOXIDE

Carbon monoxide (CO) is a colorless, tasteless, odorless, and nonirritating gas, a by-product of incomplete combustion. The average concentration of CO in the atmosphere is about 0.1 ppm; in heavy traffic, the concentration may exceed 100 ppm. The recommended 1994–95 threshold limit values (TLV-TWA and TLV-STEL) are shown in Table 57–1.

Mechanism of Action

CO combines reversibly with the oxygen-binding sites of hemoglobin and has an affinity for hemoglobin that is about 220 times that of oxygen. The product formed, carboxyhemoglobin, cannot transport oxygen. Furthermore, the presence of carboxyhemo-globin interferes with the dissociation of oxygen from the remaining oxyhemoglobin, thus reducing the transfer of oxygen to tissues. The brain and the heart are the organs most affected. Normal nonsmoking adults have carboxyhemoglobin levels of less than 1% saturation (1% of total hemoglobin is in the form of carboxyhemoglobin); this level has been attributed to the endogenous formation of CO from heme catabolism. Smokers may exhibit 5–10% saturation, depending on their smoking habits. An individual breathing air containing 0.1% CO (1000 ppm) would have a carboxyhemoglobin level of about 50%.

Clinical Effects

The principal signs of CO intoxication are those of hypoxia and progress in the following sequence: (1) psychomotor impairment; (2) headache and tightness in the temporal area; (3) confusion and loss of visual acuity; (3) tachycardia, tachypnea, syncope, and coma; and (4) deep coma, convulsions, shock, and respiratory failure. Individual variability in response to a given carboxyhemoglobin concentration is quite high. Carboxyhemoglobin levels below 15% rarely produce symptoms; collapse and syncope may appear around 40%; above 60%, death may ensue. Prolonged hypoxia and posthypoxic unconsciousness can result in residual irreversible damage to the brain and the myocardium. The clinical effects may be aggravated by heavy labor, high altitudes, and high ambient temperatures. The presence of cardiovascular disease is considered to increase the risks associated with CO exposure (Folinsbee, 1992).

While CO intoxication is usually thought of as a form of acute toxicity, there is some evidence that chronic exposure to low levels may lead to undesirable effects, including the development of atherosclerotic coronary disease in cigarette smokers. However, convincing experimental evidence is lacking (Penney et al, 1991). The fetus may be quite susceptible to the effects of CO exposure.

Treatment

In cases of acute intoxication, removal of the individual from the exposure source and maintenance of respiration is essential, followed by administration of oxygen—the specific antagonist to CO—within the limits of oxygen toxicity. With room air at 1 atm, the elimination half-time of CO is about 320 minutes; with 100% oxygen, the half-time is about 80 minutes; and with hyperbaric oxygen (2–3 atm), the half-time can be reduced to about 20 minutes. The role of hyperbaric oxygen in the treatment of CO intoxication remains controversial (Ellenhorn et al, 1988).

2. SULFUR DIOXIDE

Sulfur dioxide (SO_2) is a colorless, irritant gas generated primarily by the combustion of sulfur-containing fossil fuels. The 1994–95 threshold limit values are given in Table 57–1.

Mechanism of Action

On contact with moist membranes, SO_2 forms sulfurous acid, which is responsible for its severe irritant effects on the eyes, mucous membranes, and skin. It is estimated that approximately 90% of inhaled SO_2 is absorbed in the upper respiratory tract, the site of its principal effect. The inhalation of SO_2 causes bronchial constriction; altered smooth muscle tone and parasympathetic reflexes appear to be involved in this reaction (Chapter 20). Exposure to 5 ppm for 10 minutes leads to increased resistance to air flow in most humans. Exposures to 5–10 ppm are reported to cause severe bronchospasm; 10–20% of the healthy young adult population is estimated to be reactive to even lower concentrations. The phenomenon of adaptation to irritating concentrations is a recognized occurrence in workers. Asthmatic individuals are especially sensitive to SO_2 (Costa, 1996; Folinsbee, 1992).

Clinical Effects & Treatment

The signs and symptoms of intoxication include irritation of the eyes, nose, and throat and reflex bronchoconstriction. If severe exposure has occurred, delayed onset pulmonary edema may be observed. Cumulative effects from chronic low-level exposure to SO_2 are not striking, particularly in humans. Chronic exposure, however, has been associated with aggravation of chronic cardiopulmonary disease (Ellenhorn et al, 1988). Treatment is not specific for SO_2 but depends on therapeutic maneuvers utilized in the treatment of irritation of the respiratory tract.

Table 57–1. Threshold limit values (TLV) of some common air pollutants and solvents. (NA = none assigned.)

Compound	TLV (ppm)	
	TWA[1]	STEL[2]
Benzene	10	NA
Carbon monoxide	25	NA
Carbon tetrachloride	5	10
Chloroform	10	NA
Nitrogen dioxide	3	5
Ozone	NA	0.1
Sulfur dioxide	2	5
Tetrachloroethylene	25	100
Toluene	50	NA
1,1,1-Trichloroethane	350	450
Trichloroethylene	50	100

[1]TLV-TWA is the concentration for a normal 8-hour workday or 40-hour workweek to which workers may be repeatedly exposed without adverse effects.
[2]TLV-STEL is the maximum concentration that should not be exceeded at any time during a 15-minute exposure period.

3. NITROGEN OXIDES

Nitrogen dioxide (NO_2) is a brownish irritant gas sometimes associated with fires. It is formed also from fresh silage; exposure of farmers to NO_2 in the confines of a silo can lead to **silo-filler's disease.** The 1994–95 threshold limit values are shown in Table 57–1.

Mechanism of Action

NO_2 is a deep lung irritant capable of producing pulmonary edema. The type I cells of the alveoli appear to be the cells chiefly affected on acute exposure. Exposure to 25 ppm is irritating to some individuals; 50 ppm is moderately irritating to the eyes and nose. Exposure for 1 hour to 50 ppm can cause pulmonary edema and perhaps subacute or chronic pulmonary lesions; 100 ppm can cause pulmonary edema and death.

Clinical Effects & Treatment

The signs and symptoms of acute exposure to NO_2 include irritation of the eyes and nose, cough, mucoid or frothy sputum production, dyspnea, and chest pain. Pulmonary edema may appear within 1–2 hours. In some individuals, the clinical signs may subside in about 2 weeks; the patient may then pass into a second stage of abruptly increasing severity, including recurring pulmonary edema and fibrotic destruction of terminal bronchioles (bronchiolitis obliterans). Chronic exposure of laboratory animals to 10–25 ppm NO_2 has resulted in emphysematous changes; thus, chronic effects in humans are of concern. There is no specific treatment for acute intoxication by NO_2; therapeutic measures for the management of deep lung irritation and noncardiogenic pulmonary edema are employed. These measures include maintenance of gas exchange with adequate oxygenation and alveolar ventilation. Drug therapy may include bronchodilators, sedatives, and antibiotics; the use of corticosteroids is controversial (Ellenhorn et al, 1988).

4. OZONE

Ozone (O_3) is a bluish irritant gas that occurs normally in the earth's atmosphere, where it is an important absorbent of ultraviolet light. In the workplace, it can occur around high-voltage electrical equipment and around ozone-producing devices used for air and water purification. It is also an important oxidant found in polluted urban air. The effect of low ambient levels of ozone on admission to Ontario, Canada, hospitals for respiratory problems revealed a near-linear gradient between exposure (1-hour level, 20–100 ppb) and response (Burnett et al, 1994). See Table 57–1 for 1994–95 threshold limit values.

Clinical Effects & Treatment

O_3 is an irritant of mucous membranes. Mild exposure produces upper respiratory tract irritation. Severe exposure can cause deep lung irritation, with pulmonary edema when inhaled at sufficient concentrations. Some of the effects of O_3 resemble those seen with radiation, suggesting that O_3 toxicity may result from the formation of reactive free radicals. The gas causes shallow, rapid breathing and a decrease in pulmonary compliance. Enhanced sensitivity of the lung to bronchoconstrictors is also observed. Exposure around 0.1 ppm for 10–30 minutes causes irritation and dryness of the throat; above 0.1 ppm, one finds changes in visual acuity, substernal pain, and dyspnea. Pulmonary function is impaired at concentrations exceeding 0.8 ppm. Airway hyperresponsiveness and airway inflammation have been observed in humans (Folinsbee, 1992). Animal studies indicate that the response of the lung to O_3 is a dynamic one. The morphologic and biochemical changes are the result of both direct injury and secondary responses to the initial damage (Wright et al, 1990). Long-term exposure in animals results in morphologic and functional pulmonary changes. Chronic bronchitis, bronchiolitis, fibrosis, and emphysematous changes have been reported in a variety of species exposed to concentrations above 1 ppm. There is no specific treatment for acute O_3 intoxication. Management depends on therapeutic measures utilized for deep lung irritation and noncardiogenic pulmonary edema. (See Nitrogen Oxides, above.)

SOLVENTS

1. HALOGENATED ALIPHATIC HYDROCARBONS

These agents find wide use as industrial solvents, degreasing agents, and cleaning agents. The substances include carbon tetrachloride, chloroform, trichloroethylene, tetrachloroethylene (perchloroethylene), and 1,1,1-trichloroethane (methyl chloroform). See Table 57–1 for recommended threshold limit values.

Mechanism of Action & Clinical Effects

In laboratory animals, the halogenated hydrocarbons cause central nervous system depression, liver injury, kidney injury, and some degree of cardiotoxicity. These substances are depressants of the central nervous system in humans, although their relative potencies vary considerably; chloroform is the most potent and was widely used as an anesthetic agent. Chronic exposure to tetrachloroethylene can cause impaired memory and peripheral neuropathy. Recently, evidence has been presented suggesting that 1,1,1-trichloroethane used in some degreasing operations may be associated with peripheral neuropathy (House et al, 1994). This proposed association requires confirmation because of the widespread use of this agent. Hepatotoxicity is also a common toxic effect that can occur in humans after acute or chronic exposures, the severity of the lesion being dependent on the amount absorbed. Carbon tetrachloride is the most potent of the series in this regard. Nephrotoxicity can occur in humans exposed to carbon tetrachloride, chloroform, and trichloroethylene. With chloroform, carbon tetrachloride, trichloroethylene, and tetrachloroethylene, carcinogenicity has been observed in lifetime exposure studies performed in rats or mice. The potential effects of low-level, long-term exposures to humans, however, are yet to be determined.

Treatment

There is no specific treatment for acute intoxication resulting from exposure to halogenated hydrocarbons. Management depends upon the organ system involved (Arena, 1979).

2. AROMATIC HYDROCARBONS

Benzene is widely used for its solvent properties and as an intermediate in the synthesis of other chemicals. The 1994–95 recommended threshold limit values are given in Table 57–1. The acute toxic effect of benzene is depression of the central nervous system. Exposure to 7500 ppm for 30 minutes can be fatal. Exposure to concentrations larger than 3000 ppm may cause euphoria, nausea, locomotor problems, and coma; vertigo, drowsiness, headache, and nausea may occur at concentrations ranging from 250 to 500 ppm. No specific treatment exists for the acute toxic effect of benzene.

Chronic exposure to benzene can result in very serious toxic effects, the most significant being an insidious and unpredictable injury to the bone marrow; aplastic anemia, leukopenia, pancytopenia, or thrombocytopenia may occur. Bone marrow cells in early stages of development appear to be most sensitive to benzene. The early symptoms of chronic benzene intoxication may be rather vague (headache, fatigue, and loss of appetite). Epidemiologic data suggest an association between chronic benzene exposure and an increased incidence of leukemia in workers; such effects have yet to be produced in laboratory animals (Yardley-Jones et al, 1991).

Toluene (methylbenzene) does not possess the myelotoxic properties of benzene, nor has it been associated with leukemia. It is, however, a central nervous system depressant. See Table 57–1 for the threshold limit values. Exposure to 800 ppm can lead to severe fatigue and ataxia; 10,000 ppm can produce rapid loss of consciousness. Chronic effects of long-term toluene exposure are unclear because human studies indicating behavioral effects usually concern exposures to several solvents, not toluene alone (Ellenhorn et al, 1988). In limited occupational studies, however, metabolic interactions and modification of toluene's effects have not been observed in workers also exposed to other solvents (Ukai et al, 1994).

INSECTICIDES

1. CHLORINATED HYDROCARBON INSECTICIDES

These agents are usually classified in four groups: DDT (chlorophenothane) and its analogs, benzene hexachlorides, cyclodienes, and toxaphenes (Table 57–2). They are aryl, carbocyclic, or heterocyclic compounds containing chlorine substituents. The individual compounds differ widely in their biotransformation and capacity for storage in tissues; toxicity and storage are not always correlated. They can be absorbed through the skin as well as by inhalation or oral ingestion. There are, however, important quantitative differences between the various derivatives;

Table 57–2. Chlorinated hydrocarbon insecticides.

Chemical Class	Compounds	Toxicity Rating[1]	ADI[2]
DDT and analogs	Dichlorodiphenyltrichloroethane (DDT)	4	0.005
	Methoxychlor	3	0.1
	Tetrachlorodiphenylethane (TDE)	3	—
Benzene hexachlorides	Benzene hexachloride (BHC; hexachlorocyclohexane)	4	0.008
	Lindane	4	0.008
Cyclodienes	Aldrin	5	0.0001
	Chlordane	4	0.0005
	Dieldrin	5	0.0001
	Heptachlor	5	0.0001
Toxaphenes	Toxaphene (camphechlor)	4	—

[1]Toxicity rating: Probable human oral lethal dosage for class 3 = 500–5000 mg/kg, class 4 = 50–500 mg/kg, and class 5 = 5–50 mg/kg. (See Gosselin et al, 1984 reference.)
[2]ADI = acceptable daily intake (mg/kg/d).

DDT in solution is poorly absorbed through the skin, whereas dieldrin absorption from the skin is very efficient.

Human Toxicology

The acute toxic properties of the chlorinated hydrocarbon insecticides in humans are qualitatively similar. These agents interfere with inactivation of the sodium channel in excitable membranes and cause rapid repetitive firing in most neurons. Calcium ion transport is also inhibited. These events affect repolarization and enhance the excitability of neurons. The major effect is central nervous stimulation. With DDT, tremor may be the first manifestation, possibly continuing on to convulsions, whereas with the other compounds convulsions often appear as the first sign of intoxication. There is no specific treatment for the acute intoxicated state, management being symptomatic. Chronic administration of some of these agents to laboratory animals over long periods has resulted in enhanced tumorigenicity; there is no agreement regarding the potential carcinogenic properties of these substances, and extrapolation of these observations to humans is controversial (Ames et al, 1987; Ames, 1992). Evidence of carcinogenic effects in humans has not been established. In a large epidemiologic study, no relationship was observed between the risk of breast cancer and serum levels of DDE, the major metabolite of DDT (Krieger, 1994; MacMahon, 1994).

Environmental Toxicology

The chlorinated hydrocarbon insecticides are considered persistent chemicals. Degradation is quite slow when compared to other insecticides, and bioaccumulation, particularly in aquatic ecosystems, is well documented. Their mobility in soil depends on the composition of the soil; the presence of organic matter favors the adsorption of these chemicals onto the soil, whereas adsorption is poor in sandy soils. Once adsorbed, they do not readily desorb.

Because of their environmental impact, use of the chlorinated hydrocarbon insecticides has been largely curtailed in North America and Europe. Some of them are still used, however, in tropical countries.

2. ORGANOPHOSPHORUS INSECTICIDES

These agents, some of which are listed in Table 57–3, are utilized to combat a large variety of pests. They are useful pesticides when in direct contact with insects or when used as **plant systemics,** where the agent is translocated within the plant and exerts its effects on insects that feed on the plant. Some of these agents are used in human and veterinary medicine as local or systemic antiparasitics (Chapter 54) or in circumstances in which prolonged inhibition of cholinesterase is indicated (Chapter 7). The com-

Table 57–3. Organophosphorus insecticides.

Compound	Toxicity Rating[1]	ADI[2]
Azinphos-methyl	5	0.005
Chlorfenvinphos	—	0.002
Diazinon	4	0.002
Dichlorvos	—	0.004
Dimethoate	4	0.01
Fenitrothion	—	0.005
Leptophos	—	—
Malathion	4	0.02
Parathion	6	0.005
Parathion-methyl	5	0.02
Trichlorfon	4	0.01

[1]Toxicity rating: Probable human oral lethal dosage for class 4 = 50–500 mg/kg, class 5 = 5–50 mg/kg, and class 6 ≤ 5 mg/kg. (See Gosselin et al, 1984 reference.)
[2]ADI = acceptable daily intake (mg/kg/d).

pounds are absorbed by the skin as well as by the respiratory and gastrointestinal tracts. Biotransformation is rapid, particularly when compared to the rates observed with the chlorinated hydrocarbon insecticides.

Human Toxicology

In mammals as well as insects, the major effect of these agents is inhibition of acetylcholinesterase through phosphorylation of the esteratic site. The signs and symptoms that characterize acute intoxication are due to inhibition of this enzyme and accumulation of acetylcholine; some of the agents also possess direct cholinergic activity. These effects and their treatment are described in Chapters 7 and 8 in this book and in Steenland et al, (1994).

In addition to—and independently of—inhibition of acetylcholinesterase, some of these agents are capable of phosphorylating another enzyme present in neural tissue, the so-called **neuropathy target esterase** (Johnson, 1990; Lotti, 1992). This results in development of a delayed neurotoxicity characterized by polyneuropathy, associated with paralysis and axonal degeneration (organophosphorus ester-induced delayed polyneuropathy; OPIDP); hens are particularly sensitive to these properties and have proved very useful for studying the pathogenesis of the lesion and for identifying potentially neurotoxic organophosphorus derivatives. In humans, neurotoxicity has been observed with **triorthocresyl phosphate (TOCP),** a noninsecticidal organophosphorus compound, and is thought to occur with the insecticides dichlorvos, trichlorfon, leptophos, methamidophos, mipafox, and trichloronat (Lotti, 1992). The polyneuropathy usually begins with burning and tingling sensations, particularly in the feet, with motor weakness following a few days later. Sensory and motor difficulties may extend to the legs and hands.

Gait is affected, and ataxia may be present. There is no specific treatment for this form of delayed neurotoxicity.

Environmental Toxicology

Organophosphorus insecticides are not considered to be persistent pesticides because they are relatively unstable and break down in the environment. As a class they are considered to have a small impact on the environment in spite of their acute effects on organisms.

3. CARBAMATE INSECTICIDES

These compounds (Table 57–4) inhibit acetylcholinesterase by carbamoylation of the esteratic site. Thus, they possess the toxic properties associated with inhibition of this enzyme as described for the organophosphorus insecticides. The effects and treatment are described in Chapters 7 and 8. Generally speaking, the clinical effects due to carbamates are of shorter duration than those observed with organophosphorus compounds. The range between the doses that cause minor intoxication and those which result in lethality is larger with carbamates than that observed with the organophosphorus agents. Spontaneous reactivation of cholinesterase is more rapid after inhibition by the carbamates. While the clinical approach to carbamate poisoning is similar to that for organophosphates, the use of pralidoxime is not recommended (Machemer et al, 1994).

The carbamate insecticides are considered to be nonpersistent pesticides and are thought to exert only a small impact on the environment.

Table 57–4. Carbamate insecticides.

Compound	Toxicity Rating[1]	ADI[2]
Aldicarb	6	0.005
Aminocarb	5	—
Carbaryl	4	0.01
Carbofuran	5	0.01
Dimetan	4	—
Dimetilan	4	—
Isolan	5	—
Methomyl	5	—
Propoxur	4	0.02
Pyramat	4	—
Pyrolan	5	—
Zectran	5	—

[1]Toxicity rating: Probable human oral lethal dosage for class 4 = 50–500 mg/kg, class 5 = 5–50 mg/kg, and class 6 = ≤ 5 mg/kg. (See Gosselin et al, 1984 reference.)
[2]ADI = acceptable daily intake (mg/kg/d).

4. BOTANICAL INSECTICIDES

Insecticides derived from natural sources include **nicotine, rotenone,** and **pyrethrum.** Nicotine is obtained from the dried leaves of *Nicotiana tabacum* and *Nicotiana rustica.* It is rapidly absorbed from mucosal surfaces; the free alkaloid, but not the salt, is readily absorbed from the skin. Nicotine reacts with the acetylcholine receptor of the postsynaptic membrane (sympathetic and parasympathetic ganglia, neuromuscular junction), resulting in depolarization of the membrane. Toxic doses cause stimulation rapidly followed by blockade of transmission. These actions are described in Chapter 7. Treatment is directed toward maintenance of vital signs and suppression of convulsions.

Rotenone (Figure 57–1) is obtained from *Derris elliptica, Derris mallaccensis, Lonchocarpus utilis,* and *Lonchocarpus urucu.* The oral ingestion of rotenone produces gastrointestinal irritation. Conjunctivitis, dermatitis, pharyngitis, and rhinitis can also occur. Treatment is symptomatic.

Pyrethrum consists of six known insecticidal esters: pyrethrin I (Figure 57–1), pyrethrin II, cinerin I, cinerin II, jasmolin I, and jasmolin II. Synthetic pyrethroids account for about 30% of worldwide insecticide usage (Ecobichon, 1996). Pyrethrum may be absorbed after inhalation or ingestion; absorption from the skin is not significant. The esters are extensively biotransformed. Pyrethrum insecticides are not highly toxic to mammals. When absorbed in sufficient quantities, the major site of toxic action is the central nervous system; excitation, convulsions, and tetanic paralysis can occur by a sodium channel mechanism resembling that of DDT. Treatment is with anticonvulsants. The most frequent injury reported in humans results from the allergenic properties of the substance, especially contact dermatitis. Cutaneous paresthesias have been observed in workers spraying synthetic pyrethroids. Severe occupational exposures to synthetic pyrethroids in China resulted in marked effects on the central nervous system, including convulsions (Ecobichon, 1996).

HERBICIDES

1. CHLOROPHENOXY HERBICIDES

2,4-Dichlorophenoxyacetic acid (2,4-D), 2,4,5-trichlorophenoxyacetic acid (2,4,5-T), and their salts and esters are the major compounds of interest as herbicides used for the destruction of weeds (Figure 57–1). They have been assigned toxicity ratings of 4 or 3, respectively, which place the probable human lethal dosages at 50–500 or 500–5000 mg/kg, respectively (Gosselin et al, 1984).

In humans, 2,4-D in large doses can cause coma and generalized muscle hypotonia. Rarely, muscle

Paraquat dichloride

2,3,7,8-Tetrachlorodibenzodioxin (TCDD)

Dichlorodiphenyltrichloroethane (DDT)

2,4-Dichlorophenoxyacetic acid (2,4-D)

Rotenone

2,4,5-Trichlorophenoxyacetic acid (2,4,5-T)

Pyrethrin I

Figure 57–1. Chemical structures of selected herbicides and pesticides.

weakness and marked myotonia may persist for several weeks. With 2,4,5-T, coma may occur, but the muscular dysfunction is less evident. In laboratory animals, signs of liver and kidney dysfunction have also been reported. There is limited evidence that occupational exposure to phenoxy herbicides is associated with an increased risk of non-Hodgkin's lymphoma; the evidence for soft-tissue sarcoma, however, is considered equivocal (Morrison et al, 1992).

The toxicologic profile for these agents, particularly that of 2,4,5-T, has been confusing because of the presence of chemical contaminants (**dioxins**) produced during the manufacturing process (see below). 2,3,7,8-Tetrachlorodibenzo-*p*-dioxin (TCDD) is the most important of these contaminants.

2. BIPYRIDYL HERBICIDES

Paraquat is the most important agent of this class (Figure 57–1). Its mechanism of action is said to be similar in plants and animals and involves single-electron reduction of the herbicide to free radical species. It has been given a toxicity rating of 4, which places the probable human lethal dosage at 50–500 mg/kg. A number of lethal human intoxications (accidental or suicidal) have been reported. Paraquat accumulates slowly in the lung by an active process and causes lung edema, alveolitis, and progressive fibrosis (Sabapathy, 1994).

In humans, the first signs and symptoms after oral exposure are attributable to gastrointestinal irritation (hematemesis and bloody stools). Within a few days, however, respiratory distress may appear (delayed toxicity) with the development of congestive hemorrhagic pulmonary edema accompanied by widespread cellular proliferation. Evidence of hepatic, renal, or myocardial involvement may also be present. The interval between ingestion and death may be several weeks. Because of the delayed pulmonary toxicity, prompt removal of paraquat from the digestive tract is important. Gastric lavage, the use of cathartics, and the use of adsorbents to prevent further absorption have all been advocated; after absorption, treatment is successful in fewer than 50% of cases. Oxygen should be used cautiously to combat dyspnea or cyanosis, as it may aggravate the pulmonary lesions (Arena, 1979). Patients require prolonged observation, because the proliferative phase begins 1–2 weeks after ingestion (Ellenhorn et al, 1988).

ENVIRONMENTAL POLLUTANTS

The **polychlorinated biphenyls (PCBs, coplanar biphenyls)** have been used in a large variety of applications as dielectric and heat transfer fluids, plasticizers, wax extenders, and flame retardants. Their industrial use and manufacture in the USA was terminated by 1977. Unfortunately, they persist in the environment. The products used commercially were actually mixtures of PCB isomers and homologs containing 12–68% chlorine. These chemicals are highly stable and highly lipophilic, poorly metabolized, and very resistant to environmental degradation; they bioaccumulate in food chains. Food is the major source of PCB residues in humans.

A serious exposure to PCBs, lasting several months, occurred in Japan in 1968 as a result of cooking oil contamination with PCB-containing transfer medium (Yusho disease). Possible effects on the fetus and the development of offspring of poisoned women were reported (Yen et al, 1989). It is now known that the contaminated cooking oil contained not only PCBs but also polychlorinated dibenzofurans (PCDFs) and polychlorinated quaterphenyls (PCQs). Consequently, the effects that were initially attributed to the presence of PCBs are now thought to have been largely caused by the other contaminants. Workers occupationally exposed to PCBs have exhibited the following clinical signs: dermatologic problems (chloracne, folliculitis, erythema, dryness, rash, hyperkeratosis, hyperpigmentation), some hepatic involvement, and elevated plasma triglycerides. The effects of PCBs alone on reproduction and development, as well as their carcinogenic effects, have yet to be established in humans, whether workers or the general population, even though some subjects have been exposed to very high levels of PCBs. Some adverse behavioral effects in infants are reported to have been observed in two studies involving subjects from the general population, but the adverse effects observed in the two studies were dissimilar; furthermore, there are a number of uncertainties about the exposure assessments in both studies (Kimbrough, 1995). The bulk of the evidence from human studies indicates that PCBs pose little hazard to human health except in situations where food is contaminated with high concentrations of these congeners.

The **polychlorinated dibenzo-p-dioxins (PCDDs),** or **dioxins,** have been mentioned above as a group of congeners, of which the most important is **2,3,7,8-tetrachlorodibenzo-p-dioxin (TCDD).** In addition, there is a wider group of dioxin-like compounds, including certain **polychlorinated dibenzofurans (PCDFs)** and **coplanar biphenyls.** While PCBs were used commercially, PCDDs and PCDFs are unwanted by-products that appear in the environment as contaminants because of improperly controlled combustion processes. The global PCDD and PCDF contamination of the environment is considered to represent a contemporary problem produced by human activities. These chemicals are very stable and highly lipophilic. They are poorly metabolized and very resistant to environmental degradation.

In laboratory animals, TCDD administered in suitable doses has produced a wide variety of toxic effects, including a wasting syndrome (severe weight loss accompanied by reduction of muscle mass and adipose tissue), thymic atrophy, epidermal changes, hepatotoxicity, immunotoxicity, effects on reproduction and development, teratogenicity, and carcinogenicity. Fortunately, most of these actions have not been observed in humans. The effects observed in workers involved in the manufacture of 2,4,5-T (and therefore presumably exposed to TCDD) consisted primarily of contact dermatitis and chloracne.

The presence of TCDD in 2,4,5-T is believed to be largely responsible also for other human toxicities associated with the herbicide. There is some epidemiologic evidence indicating an association between occupational exposure to the phenoxy herbicides and an excess incidence of non-Hodgkin's lymphoma (Schecter, 1994). The evidence of an association of increased soft tissue sarcomas with herbicides themselves, however, is considered equivocal (Morrison et al, 1992). On the other hand, the TCDD contaminant in these herbicides may play a role in soft tissue sarcomas (Schecter, 1994). A role for TCDD in the etiology of other cancers is suspected but remains to be established (Johnson, 1992, 1993).

REFERENCES

General

Ecobichon DJ: *The Basis of Toxicity Testing.* CRC Press 1992.

Lu FC: *Basic Toxicology: Fundamentals, Target Organs, and Risk Assessment,* 2nd ed. Hemisphere, 1991.

National Research Council: *Complex Mixtures.* National Academy Press, 1988

Air Pollution

Burnett RT et al: Effects of low ambient levels of ozone and sulfates on the frequency of respiratory admissions to Ontario hospitals. Environ Res 1994;65:172.

Costa DL, Amdur MO: Air pollution. In: *Casarett and Doull's Toxicology,* 5th ed. Klaassen CD (editor). Pergamon, 1996.

Folinsbee LJ: Human health effects of air pollution. Environ Health Perspect 1992;100:45.

Penney DG, Howley JW: Is there a connection between carbon monoxide exposure and hypertension? Environ Health Perspect 1991;95:191.

Sarnet JM, Utell MJ: The environment and the lung. JAMA 1991;266:670.

Seinfeld JH: Urban air pollution: State of the science. Science 1989;243:745.

Wright ES, Dziedzic D, Wheeler CS: Cellular, biochemical, and functional effects of ozone: New research and perspectives on ozone health effects. Toxicol Lett 1990; 51:125.

Occupational Toxicology

Cullen MR, Cherniak MG, Rosenstock L: Occupational medicine. (Two parts.) N Engl J Med 1990;322:594,675.

House RA, Liss GM, Wills MC: Peripheral sensory neuropathy associated with 1,1,1-trichlorethane. Arch Environ Health 1994;51:196.

Proctor NH, Hughes JP: *Chemical Hazards of the Workplace,* 3rd ed. Lippincott, 1991.

Ukai H et al: Occupational exposure to solvent mixtures: Effects on health and metabolism. Occup Environ Health 1994;51:523.

Yardley-Jones A, Anderson D, Parke DV: The toxicity of benzene and its metabolism and molecular pathology in human risk assessment. Br J Indust Med 1991;48:437.

Environmental Toxicology & Ecotoxicology

Ames BN: Pollution, pesticides, and cancer. J AOAC Int 1992;75:1.

Ames BN, Magaw R, Gold LS: Ranking possible carcinogenic hazards. Science 1987;236:271.

Geyer H, Scheunert I, Korte F: Bioconcentration potential of organic environmental chemicals in humans. Regul Toxicol Pharmacol 1986;6:313.

Johnson ES: Human exposure to 2,3,7,8-TCDD and risk of cancer. CRC Crit Rev Toxicol 1992;21:451.

Johnson ES: Important aspects of the evidence for TCDD carcinogenicity in man. Environ Health Perspect 1993;99:383.

Kimbrough RD: Polychlorinated biphenyls (PCBs) and human health: An update. CRC Crit Rev Toxicol 1995; 25:133.

Moriarty F: *Ecotoxicology.* Academic Press, 1983.

Reggiani G, Bruppacher R: Symptoms, signs and findings in humans exposed to PCBs and their derivatives. Environ Health Perspect 1985;60:225.

Schecter A: *Dioxins and Health.* Plenum, 1994.

Silberhorn EM, Glauert HP, Robertson LW: Carcinogenicity of polyhalogenated biphenyls: PCBs and PBBs. CRC Crit Rev Toxicol 1990;20:440.

Truhaut R: Ecotoxicology: Objectives, principles and perspectives. Ecotoxicol Environ Saf 1977;1:151.

Yen YY et al: Follow-up study of reproductive hazards of multiparous women consuming PCBs-contaminated rice oil in Taiwan. Bull Environ Contam Toxicol 1989; 43:647.

Pesticides & Herbicides

Ecobichon DJ: Toxic effects of pesticides. In: *Casarett and Doull's Toxicology,* 5th ed. Klaassen CD (editor). Pergamon, 1996.

Johnson MK: Organophosphates and delayed neuropathy: Is NTE alive and well? Toxicol Appl Toxicol 1990;102: 385.

Krieger N et al: Breast cancer and serum organochlorines: A prospective study among white, black anmd Asian women. J Natl Cancer Inst 1994;86:589.

Lotti M: The pathogenesis of organophosphate polyneuropathy. CRC Crit Rev Toxicol 1992;213:465.

Lu FC: A review of the acceptable daily intakes of pesticides assessed by WHO. Regul Toxicol Pharmacol 1995; 21:352.

Machemer LD, Pickel M: Carbamate insecticides. Toxicology 1994;91:29

MacMahon B: Pesticide residues and breast cancer? J Natl Cancer Inst 1994;86:572.

Morrison HI et al: Herbicides and cancer. J Natl Cancer Inst 1992;84:1866

Sabapathy NN: Quaternary ammonium compounds. Toxicology 1994;91:93

Steenland K et al: Chronic neurological sequelae to organophosphate pesticide poisoning. Am J Public Health 1994;84:731.

Clinical Toxicology

Arena JM: *Poisoning,* 4th ed. Thomas, 1979.

Ellenhorn MJ, Barceloux DG: *Medical Toxicology.* Elsevier, 1988.

Gosselin RE, Smith RP, Hodge HC: *Clinical Toxicology of Commercial Products,* 5th ed. Williams & Wilkins, 1984.

58

Chelators & Heavy Metal Intoxication

Michael J. Kosnett, MD, MPH, & Charles E. Becker, MD

Some metals such as iron are essential for life, while others such as lead are present in all organisms but serve no useful biologic purpose. Some of the oldest diseases of humans can be traced to heavy metal poisoning associated with metal mining, refining, and use. Even with the present recognition of the hazards of heavy metals, the incidence of intoxication remains significant and the need for preventive strategies and effective therapy remains high.

PHARMACOLOGY OF CHELATORS

Chelating agents are drugs used to prevent or reverse the toxic effects of a heavy metal on an enzyme or other cellular target or to accelerate the elimination of the metal from the body. Chelating agents are usually flexible molecules with two or more electronegative groups that form stable coordinate-covalent bonds with a cationic metal atom. In some cases, eg, succimer (dimercaptosuccinic acid, DMSA), the parent compound may require in vivo biotransformation to become an active complexing agent. The chelator-metal complexes formed are excreted by the body. The action of these drugs provides an excellent application of the principle of chemical antagonism. Edetate (ethylenediaminetetraacetate; Figure 58–1) is an important example.

The efficiency of the chelator is partly determined by the number of ligands available for metal binding. The greater the number of these ligands, the more stable the metal-chelator complex. Depending on the number of metal-ligand bonds, the complex may be referred to as mono-, bi-, or polydentate. The chelating ligands include functional groups such as –OH, –SH, and –NH, which can donate electrons for coordination with the metal. Such bonding effectively prevents interaction of the metal with similar functional groups of enzymes, coenzymes, cellular nucleophiles, and membranes. Unfortunately, most chelators are nonspecific and may chelate essential metals such as Cu^{2+} and Zn^{2+}, which are vital for body function. Such interactions are determined by the relative affinities for the chelator of the toxic metal and the essential metal. Thus, the toxicity associated with administration of some chelators may be caused by chelation of essential metals. In some cases, this problem may be mitigated by judicious administration of the essential metal during the course of chelation treatment. The relative efficacy of various chelators in facilitating excretion of metals from the body is also determined in part by the pharmacokinetics of the chelator. For any significant metal sequestration to occur, the affinity of the metal for the chelator must be greater than its affinity for endogenous ligands, and the relative rate of exchange of the metal between the endogenous ligands and the chelator must be faster than the rate of elimination of the chelator. If a chelator is eliminated more rapidly than the dissociation of the metal-endogenous ligand complex, it may not be present in sufficient concentrations for effective competition with the endogenous binding sites. This would be particularly critical if sequestration occurred via a ternary complex (endogenous ligand-metal-exogenous chelator). The above considerations also dictate that efficient mobilization can be accomplished only when the physiologic distribution of the chelator includes the body compartment containing the metal. For example, following absorption, lead is initially distributed via the blood stream to heavily vascularized soft tissues such as the liver, kidney, muscle, brain, and gonads and to the subperiosteal surfaces of trabecular and cortical bone. Chelators administered shortly after exposure have access to these sites and may cause significant lead removal (decorporation). However, as lead gradually becomes incorporated into the less vascular bone matrix—which is ultimately the major site of lead accumulation in the body—chelators become less effective.

The most important chelating agents in use today are described below.

DIMERCAPROL
(2,3-Dimercaptopropanol, BAL)

Dimercaprol (Figure 58–2), an oily, colorless liquid with a strong mercaptan-like odor, was developed in Great Britain during World War II as a therapeutic

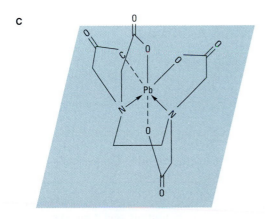

Figure 58–1. Salt and chelate formation with edetate (ethylenediaminetetraacetate, EDTA). **A:** In a solution of the disodium salt of EDTA, the sodium and hydrogen ions are chemically and biologically available. **B:** In solutions of calcium disodium edetate, calcium is bound by coordinate-covalent bonds with nitrogens as well as by the usual ionic bonds. Calcium ions are effectively removed from solution. **C:** In the lead-edetate chelate, lead is incorporated into five heterocyclic rings. (Modified and reproduced, with permission, from Meyers FH, Jawetz E, Goldfien A: *Review of Medical Pharmacology,* 7th ed. Lange, 1980.)

Figure 58–2. Chemical structures of several chelators. Ferroxamine (ferrioxamine) without the chelated iron is deferoxamine. It is represented here to show the functional groups; the iron is actually held in a caged system. The structures of the in vivo metal-chelator complexes for dimercaprol, succimer, and penicillamine are not known and may involve the formation of mixed disulfides with amino acids. (Modified and reproduced, with permission, from Meyers FH, Jawetz E, Goldfien A: *Review of Medical Pharmacology,* 7th ed. Lange, 1980.)

agent for poisoning by the arsenic-containing warfare agent lewisite. It thus became known as British antilewisite, or BAL. Because aqueous solutions of dimercaprol are unstable and oxidize readily, it is dispensed in 10% solution in peanut oil and must be administered by intramuscular injection, which is often painful. In animal models, dimercaprol prevents and reverses arsenic-induced inhibition of sulfhydryl-containing enzymes and, if given soon after exposure, may protect against the lethal effects of inorganic and organic arsenicals. Human data indicate that it can increase the rate of excretion of arsenic and lead and may offer therapeutic benefit in the treatment of acute intoxication by arsenic, lead, and mercury.

Indications & Toxicity

Dimercaprol is FDA-approved as a single-agent treatment of acute poisoning by arsenic and mercury and for the treatment of severe lead poisoning when used in conjunction with edetate calcium disodium (EDTA; see below). Given intramuscularly, it is readily absorbed, metabolized, and excreted by the kidney within 4–8 hours. Animal models indicate that it may also undergo biliary excretion, but the presence of this excretory route in humans—as well as other details of its biotransformation—are uncertain.

When used in therapeutic doses, dimercaprol is associated with a high incidence of adverse side effects, including hypertension, tachycardia, nausea, vomiting, lacrimation, salivation, fever (particularly in children), and pain at the injection site. Its use has also been associated with thrombocytopenia and increased prothrombin time—factors that may limit intramuscular injection because of the risk of hematoma formation at the injection site. Despite its protective effects in acutely intoxicated animals, dimercaprol may redistribute arsenic and mercury to the central nervous system, and it is not advocated for treatment of chronic poisoning. Water-soluble analogs of dimercaprol, succimer (dimercaptosuccinic acid, DMSA) and unithiol (dimercaptopropanesulfonic acid, DMPS), have higher therapeutic indices and have replaced dimercaprol in many settings.

SUCCIMER
(Dimercaptosuccinic Acid, DMSA)

Although originally developed in the late 1950s by Chinese investigators as treatment for poisoning by antimony, arsenic, and lead, succimer was not commercially available in the United States until 1991. Succimer is a water-soluble analog of dimercaprol, and like that agent it has been shown in animal studies to prevent and reverse metal-induced inhibition of sulfhydryl-containing enzymes and to protect against the acute lethal effects of arsenic. In humans, treatment with succimer is associated with an increase in urinary lead excretion and a decrease in blood lead concentration. It may also decrease the mercury content of the kidney, a key target organ of inorganic mercury salts. In the United States, succimer is sold exclusively for oral use, but intravenous formulations have been used successfully in China. It is absorbed rapidly but somewhat variably after oral administration. Peak blood levels occur at approximately 3 hours, with an elimination half-life of 2 hours (Dart et al, 1994). The drug binds in vivo to the amino acid cysteine to form 1:1 and 1:2 mixed disulfides, possibly in the kidney, and it may be these complexes that are the active chelating moieties. The related compound dimercaptopropanesulfonic acid (DMPS; unithiol, Dimaval) is commercially available in some countries (not in the USA) in both oral and parenteral forms. It may be somewhat superior to succimer in the mobilization of mercury.

Indications & Toxicity

Succimer is currently FDA-approved for the treatment of children with blood lead concentrations greater that 45 μg/dL, but it is also commonly used in adults. The usual dosage is 10 mg/kg orally three times a day. Oral administration of succimer is comparable to parenteral EDTA in reducing blood lead concentration and has supplanted EDTA in outpatient treatment of patients capable of absorbing the oral drug. However, despite the demonstrated capacity of both succimer and EDTA to enhance lead elimination, their value in reversing established lead toxicity or in otherwise improving therapeutic outcome has yet to be established by a placebo-controlled clinical trial. Based on its protective effects against arsenic in animals and its ability to mobilize mercury from the kidney, succimer has also been used in the treatment of mercury and arsenic poisoning.

Succimer has been well tolerated in limited clinical trials. It has a negligible impact on body stores of calcium, iron, and magnesium. It induces a mild increase in urinary excretion of zinc and copper that is of minor or no clinical significance. Gastrointestinal disturbances, including anorexia, nausea, vomiting, and diarrhea, are the most common side effects, occurring in less than 10% of patients. Rashes, sometimes requiring discontinuation of the medication, have been reported in less than 5% of patients. Mild, reversible increases in liver aminotransferases have been noted in 6–10% of patients, and mild to moderate neutropenia has occasionally been reported.

PENICILLAMINE
(D-Dimethylcysteine)

Penicillamine (Figure 58–2) is a white crystalline, water-soluble derivative of penicillin. D-Penicillamine is less toxic than the L isomer and consequently is the preferred therapeutic form. Penicillamine is readily absorbed from the gut and is resistant to metabolic degradation.

Indications & Toxicity

Penicillamine is used chiefly for treatment of poisoning with copper or to prevent copper accumulation, as in Wilson's disease. It is also used occasionally in the treatment of severe rheumatoid arthritis (Chapter 36). Its ability to increase urinary excretion of lead and mercury had occasioned its use as outpatient treatment for intoxication with these metals, but succimer, with its stronger metal-mobilizing capacity and lower side effect profile, has generally replaced penicillamine for these purposes.

Adverse effects have been seen in up to a third of patients receiving penicillamine. Hypersensitivity reactions include rash, pruritus, and drug fever, and the drug should be used with extreme caution, if at all, in patients with a history of penicillin allergy. Nephrotoxicity with proteinuria has also been reported, and protracted use of the drug may result in renal insufficiency. Pancytopenia has been associated with prolonged drug intake. Pyridoxine deficiency is a frequent toxic effect of other forms of the drug but is rarely seen with the D form. An acetylated derivative, N-acetylpenicillamine, has been used experimentally in mercury poisoning and may have superior metal-mobilizing capacity, but it is not commercially available.

EDETATE CALCIUM DISODIUM (Ethylenediaminetetraacetate, EDTA)

Ethylenediaminetetraacetic acid (Figure 58–1) is an efficient chelator of many divalent and trivalent metals in vitro. When used in the treatment of lead poisoning, the drug is administered as a calcium disodium salt to prevent potentially life-threatening depletion of calcium.

EDTA penetrates cell membranes relatively poorly and therefore chelates extracellular metal ions much more effectively than intracellular ions.

The highly polar ionic character of EDTA limits its oral absorption. Moreover, oral administration may increase lead absorption from the gut. Consequently, the chelator—as the calcium disodium salt—is administered either by slow intravenous infusion or by the intramuscular route. In patients with normal renal function, EDTA is rapidly excreted by glomerular filtration, with 50% of an injected dose appearing in the urine within 1 hour. Treatment with EDTA induces a marked increase in urinary lead excretion and a corresponding decline in blood lead concentration. In patients with renal insufficiency, excretion of the drug—and its metal-mobilizing effects—may be delayed.

Indications & Toxicity

Edetate calcium disodium is indicated chiefly for the chelation of lead, but it may also have utility in poisoning by zinc, manganese, and certain heavy radionuclides. EDTA has no demonstrated utility in the treatment of atherosclerotic cardiovascular disease.

Because the drug and the mobilized metals are excreted via the urine, the drug is contraindicated in anuric patients. Nephrotoxicity from EDTA has been reported, but in most cases this can be prevented by maintenance of adequate urine flow, avoidance of excessive doses, and limitation of a treatment course to 5 or fewer consecutive days. EDTA may result in temporary zinc depletion that is of uncertain clinical significance. An experimental analog of EDTA, calcium disodium diethylenetriaminepentaacetic acid (DTPA), has been used for decorporation of uranium, plutonium, and other heavy radioisotopes.

TRIENTINE (Triethylenetetramine)

Trientine is a polydentate chelating agent that has affinity for copper and is useful in the treatment of Wilson's disease (hepatolenticular degeneration). It is available for this use in the USA. Early reports suggested that it may be less toxic than penicillamine in

this application. However, it was found to be teratogenic in long-term studies of rats. Another agent, tetrathiomolybdate, an effective and apparently less toxic copper chelator in sheep, is being investigated as a potential replacement for trientine.

DEFEROXAMINE

Deferoxamine is isolated from *Streptomyces pilosus*. It binds iron avidly but essential trace metals poorly. Furthermore, while competing for loosely bound iron in iron-carrying proteins (hemosiderin and ferritin), it fails to compete with biologically chelated iron, as in microsomal and mitochondrial cytochromes and hemoproteins. Consequently, it is the chelator of choice for iron poisoning. It may also be useful in the treatment of aluminum toxicity in renal failure (Jones, 1991).

Deferoxamine is poorly absorbed when administered orally and may increase iron absorption when given by this route. It should therefore be administered intramuscularly or, preferably, intravenously. It is believed to be metabolized, but the pathways are unknown. The iron-chelator complex is excreted in the urine, often turning the urine an orange-red color.

Rapid intravenous administration may result in hypotension. Adverse idiosyncratic responses such as flushing, blotchy erythema, intestinal irritation, and urticaria have also been observed. Pulmonary complications (eg, acute [formerly "adult"] respiratory distress syndrome) have been reported in some patients undergoing deferoxamine infusions lasting longer than 24 hours, and neurotoxicity has been described after long-term therapy of iron overload conditions (eg, hemolytic disease).

Use of deferoxamine in iron poisoning is described in Chapter 33.

TOXICOLOGY OF HEAVY METALS

LEAD

Lead poisoning is one of the oldest occupational diseases in the world. Despite its recognized hazards, lead continues to have widespread commercial application, including the production of storage batteries, pipes, and metal alloys such as brass, bronze, and steel, and the production of ammunition, solder (principally in electronics and automotive radiators), pigments, and industrial paints, glass, and ceramics. Environmental lead exposure, ubiquitous by virtue of the anthropogenic distribution of lead to air, water, and food, has declined considerably in the past 2 decades as a result of diminished use of lead in gasoline, in residential paint, and in the solder used to seal some canned food containers. While these public health measures, together with improved workplace conditions, have decreased the incidence of serious overt lead poisoning, there remains considerable concern over the effects of low-level lead exposure. An extensive body of research indicates that lead may have adverse effects, which are often subclinical, on neurocognitive function—and possibly on cardiovascular function—at blood lead concentrations once considered "normal" or "safe" (Landrigan, 1989). Lead serves no useful purpose in the human body. In key target organs such as the developing central nervous system, no safe threshold of lead exposure has been established.

Pharmacokinetics

Inorganic lead is slowly but consistently absorbed via the respiratory and gastrointestinal tracts. Inorganic lead is poorly absorbed through the skin, but or-

ganic lead compounds are well absorbed by this route. Absorption of lead dust via the respiratory tract is the most common cause of industrial poisoning. The intestinal tract is the primary route of entry in nonindustrial exposure (Table 58–1). Absorption via the gastrointestinal tract varies with the nature of the lead compound, but in general, adults absorb about 10% of the ingested amount while young children absorb closer to 50%. Low dietary calcium, iron deficiency, and ingestion on an empty stomach have all been associated with increased lead absorption.

Once absorbed from the respiratory or gastrointestinal tract, lead is bound to erythrocytes and widely distributed initially to soft tissues such as the bone marrow, brain, kidney, liver, muscle, and gonads; then to the subperiosteal surface of bone; and later to bone matrix. Lead also crosses the placenta and poses a potential hazard to the fetus. The kinetics of lead clearance from the body follows a multi-compartment model, composed predominantly of the blood and soft

Table 58–1. Toxicology of selected arsenic, lead, and mercury compounds.

	Form Entering Body	Major Route of Absorption	Distribution	Major Clinical Effects	Key Aspects of Mechanism	Metabolism and Elimination
Arsenic	Inorganic arsenic salts	Gastrointestinal, skin, respiratory (all mucosal surfaces)	Predominantly soft tissues (highest in liver, kidney). Avidly bound in skin, hair, nails	Multisystemic: Cardiovascular: shock, arrhythmias; CNS: encephalopathy, peripheral neuropathy; gastroenteritis; pancytopenia; cancer (many sites)	Inhibits enzymes via sulfhydryl binding; interferes with oxidative phosphorylation	Methylation. Renal (major); sweat and feces (minor)
Lead	Inorganic lead oxides and salts	Gastrointestinal, respiratory	Soft tissues; redistributed to skeleton (> 90% of adult body burden)	Multisystemic: CNS deficits; peripheral neuropathy; anemia; nephropathy; hypertension (?)	Inhibits enzymes; interferes with essential cations; alters membrane structure	Renal (major); breast milk (minor)
	Organic (tetraethyl lead)	Skin, gastrointestinal, respiratory	Soft tissues, especially liver, CNS	Encephalopathy	Hepatic dealkylation (fast) → trialkymetabolites (slow) → dissociation to lead	Urine and feces (major); sweat (minor)
Mercury	Elemental mercury	Respiratory tract	Soft tissues, especially kidney, CNS	CNS: behavioral (erethism); gingivostomatitis; peripheral neuropathy; acrodynia; pneumonitis (high dose)	Inhibits enzymes; alters membranes	Elemental Hg converted to Hg^{2+}. Urine (major); feces (minor)
	Inorganic: Hg^+ (less toxic); Hg^{2+} (more toxic)	Gastrointestinal, skin (minor)	Soft tissues, especially kidney	Acute tubular necrosis; gastroenteritis; CNS effects (rare)	Inhibits enzymes; alters membranes	Urine
	Organic: alkyl, aryl	Gastrointestinal, skin, respiratory (minor)	Soft tissues	CNS effects, birth defects	Inhibits enzymes; alters neuronal structure	Deacylation. Fecal (alkyl, major); urine (Hg^{2+} after deacylation, minor)

tissues, with a half-life of 1–2 months; and the skeleton, with a half-life of years to decades. Absorbed lead is excreted predominantly in the urine (more than 90%), with lesser amounts excreted through the bile, skin, hair, nails, sweat, and breast milk. The fraction not undergoing prompt excretion, approximately half of the absorbed lead, may be incorporated into the skeleton, the repository of more than 90% of the body lead burden in most adults. In patients with high bone lead burdens, slow release from the skeleton may elevate blood lead concentrations for years after exposure ceases; and pathologic high bone turnover states such as hyperthyroidism or prolonged immobilization may result in frank lead intoxication. The lead burden in bone has been quantitated using noninvasive, in vivo x-ray fluorescence (Kosnett, 1994), a technique that may provide the best measure of long-term, cumulative lead absorption.

Pharmacodynamics

Lead exerts multisystemic toxic effects through at least three mechanisms: by inhibiting enzyme activity, sometimes as a consequence of binding to sulfhydryl groups; by interfering with the action of essential cations, particularly calcium, iron, and zinc; and by altering the structure of cell membranes and receptors. The hematologic, neurologic, renal, reproductive, gastrointestinal, and cardiovascular systems may be adversely affected.

A. Blood: Lead can induce an anemia that may be either normocytic or microcytic and hypochromic. Lead interferes with heme synthesis by blocking the incorporation of iron into protoporphyrin IX and by inhibiting the function of enzymes in the heme synthesis pathway, including aminolevulinic acid dehydratase and ferrochelatase. Within 2–8 weeks after an elevation in blood lead concentration (generally to 30–50 µg/dL or greater), increases in heme precursors, notably free erythrocyte protoporphyrin or its zinc chelate, zinc protoporphyrin, may be detectable in whole blood. Lead also contributes to anemia by increasing erythrocyte membrane fragility and decreasing red cell survival time. Frank hemolysis may occur with high exposure. The presence of basophilic stippling on the peripheral blood smear, thought to be a consequence of lead inhibition of the enzyme 3′,5′-pyrimidine nucleotidase, is sometimes a suggestive—albeit insensitive and nonspecific—diagnostic clue to the presence of lead intoxication.

B. Nervous System: The developing central nervous system of the fetus and young child is the most sensitive target organ for lead's toxic effect. Epidemiologic studies suggest that blood lead concentrations as low as 15 µg/dL may result in subclinical deficits in neurocognitive function in populations of lead-exposed young children, with no demonstrable threshold for a "no effect" level. Hearing acuity may also be diminished. Adults are less sensitive to the CNS effects of lead, but at blood lead concentrations

in excess of 30 µg/dL, subtle behavioral, constitutional, and neurocognitive effects may gradually emerge, producing signs and symptoms such as irritability, fatigue, decreased libido, anorexia, sleep disturbance, impaired visual-motor coordination, and slowed reaction time (Stollery et al, 1989). Headache, arthralgias, and myalgias are also frequent complaints. Tremor occurs but is less common. Lead encephalopathy, usually occurring at blood lead concentrations in excess of 100 µg/dL, is typically accompanied by increased intracranial pressure and may produce ataxia, stupor, coma, convulsions, and death. For reasons that are not well understood, there is wide interindividual variation in the magnitude of lead exposure required to cause overt lead-related signs and symptoms.

Peripheral neuropathy may appear after chronic high-dose lead exposure, usually following months to years of blood lead concentrations in excess of 100 µg/dL. Predominantly motor in character, the neuropathy may present clinically with painless weakness of the extensors, particularly in the upper extremity, resulting in classic wrist-drop. Preclinical signs of lead-induced peripheral nerve dysfunction may be detectable by electrodiagnostic testing.

C. Kidneys: Chronic high-dose lead exposure, usually associated with months to years of blood lead concentrations in excess of 80 µg/dL, may result in renal interstitial fibrosis and nephrosclerosis. Chronic lead nephropathy may have a latency period of years to decades before significant impairment is apparent. Lead may alter uric acid excretion by the kidney, resulting in recurrent bouts of gouty arthritis ("saturnine gout"). Acute high-dose lead exposure sometimes produces reversible acute tubular dysfunction, including a Fanconi-like aminoaciduria in children. Several animal and epidemiologic studies suggest that low-level lead exposure (devoid of any detectable nephrotoxic effect) may be associated with hypertension in susceptible individuals. This may be a consequence of direct effects on vascular smooth muscle (Sharp et al, 1987).

D. Reproductive Organs: Lead is a notorious reproductive toxin. Today, reproductive concerns focus primarily on the effect that relatively low blood lead concentrations in pregnant women (possibly as low as 12–17 µg/dL) may have on in utero neurologic development of the fetus and the subsequent cognitive function of the child. At higher dosage, maternal lead exposure has been associated with an increased rate of miscarriage, decreased gestational age, and low birth weight. In males, blood lead concentrations in excess of 60 µg/dL have been associated with diminished or aberrant sperm production. Paternal-mediated adverse reproductive effects have been less thoroughly studied, however, and the presence of impairment at lower levels of exposure is uncertain.

E. Gastrointestinal Tract: Moderate lead poisoning may cause loss of appetite, constipation, and, less commonly, diarrhea. At high dosage, intermittent bouts of severe colicky abdominal pain ("lead colic") may occur. The mechanism of lead colic is unclear but is believed to involve spasmodic contraction of the smooth muscles of the intestinal wall. In heavily exposed individuals with poor dental hygiene, the reaction of circulating lead with sulfur ions released by microbial action may produce dark deposits of lead sulfide at the gingival margin ("gingival lead lines").

Major Forms of Lead Intoxication

A. Inorganic Lead Poisoning: Lead intoxication exists as a continuum ranging from subtle, subclinical effects at low dosage to life-threatening overt illness at massive exposures.

1. Acute–Acute inorganic lead poisoning is uncommon today. It usually results from industrial inhalation of large quantities of lead oxide fumes or, in small children, from ingestion of a large oral dose of lead in lead-based paints. The abrupt onset of severe symptoms usually requires several days or weeks of recurrent exposure and presents with signs and symptoms of encephalopathy or colic. Evidence of hemolytic anemia (or anemia with basophilic stippling if exposure has been subacute) and elevated hepatic aminotransferases may be present. The diagnosis of acute inorganic lead poisoning may be difficult, and depending on the prominent symptoms, the presentation has sometimes been mistaken for appendicitis, peptic ulcer, pancreatitis, or infectious meningitis. Subacute presentation, featuring headache, fatigue, intermittent abdominal cramps, myalgias, and arthralgias, has often been mistaken for a flu-like viral illness and may not come to medical attention. When there has been recent ingestion of lead-containing paint chips, glazes, or weights, radiopacities may be visible on abdominal radiographs.

2. Chronic–The patient with chronic lead intoxication usually presents with multisystemic findings, including constitutional complaints of anorexia, fatigue, and malaise; neurologic complaints, including headache, difficulty in concentrating, irritability or depressed mood; weakness, arthralgias or myalgias; and gastrointestinal symptoms. Lead poisoning should be strongly suspected in any patient presenting with headache, abdominal pain, and anemia; and less commonly with motor neuropathy, gout, and renal insufficiency. Chronic lead intoxication should be considered in any child with neurocognitive deficits, growth retardation, or developmental delay.

The diagnosis is best confirmed by measuring lead in whole blood. Although this test reflects lead currently circulating in blood and soft tissues and is not a reliable marker of either recent or cumulative lead exposure, most patients with lead-related disease will have blood lead concentrations above the normal range. The geometric mean blood lead concentration in the United States in 1990 was estimated to be 2.8 μg/dL (Pirkle et al, 1994), and levels greater than 10 μg/dL merit investigation for sources other than common background exposure. The concentration of lead in bone assessed by noninvasive in vivo K x-ray fluorescence measurement of lead in bone, an emerging research technique, has been correlated with long-term, cumulative lead exposure, and its relationship to numerous lead-related disorders is a subject of ongoing investigation. Measurement of lead excretion in the urine following a single dose of a chelating agent (sometimes called a "chelation challenge test") is not a totally reliable marker of long-term lead exposure, remote past exposure, or skeletal lead burden.

B. Organolead Poisoning: Organolead poisoning is usually caused by exposure to tetraethyl or tetramethyl lead, used as "antiknock" agents in some gasolines. Although it is no longer sold in the United States, leaded gasoline is still widely available in many countries. Organolead compounds such as lead stearate or lead naphthenate are used in certain commercial chemical processes. Organic lead is highly volatile and lipid-soluble. Thus, it can be readily absorbed through the skin and respiratory tract. Severe poisoning has resulted from deliberate "sniffing" of leaded gasoline. Acute central nervous system disorders result. These can progress rapidly, causing insomnia, hallucinations, delirium, tremors, and convulsions (similar to severe alcohol withdrawal). Fatalities have resulted. Organic lead causes relatively few hematologic abnormalities. Tetraethyl and tetramethyl lead are metabolized by the liver to trialkyl lead and inorganic lead, which are thought to be responsible for the acute poisoning syndrome. Chronic poisoning with organic lead is fortunately uncommon. Most organolead exposures occur in the course of cleaning gasoline storage tanks or from sniffing leaded gasoline. Blood and urine lead levels are relatively unreliable in organolead poisoning but may be elevated.

Treatment

A. Inorganic Lead Poisoning: Treatment of symptomatic inorganic lead poisoning involves immediate termination of exposure, supportive care, and the judicious use of chelation therapy. Encephalopathy is a medical emergency, requiring intensive supportive care and anticonvulsants for seizures. Cerebral edema and elevated intracranial pressure may improve with corticosteroids and mannitol. Adequate urine flow should be maintained, but overhydration should be avoided. Intravenous or intramuscular edetate calcium disodium ($CaNa_2EDTA$) is administered at a dosage of 1500 mg/m^2/d (approximately 30 mg/kg/d) in two or three divided doses for up to 5 days. Some clinicians advocate that chelation treatment for lead encephalopathy be initiated with an intramuscular injection of dimercaprol, followed in 4 hours by concurrent administration of dimercaprol and EDTA. Parenteral chelation is limited to 5 or fewer days, at which time oral treatment with succimer may be instituted. In symptomatic lead intoxication without encephalopathy, treatment may sometimes be initiated with succimer. The end point for chelation is usually resolution of symptoms or return of the blood lead concentration to the premorbid range. In patients with chronic exposure, cessation of chelation may be followed by an upward rebound in blood lead concentration as the lead reequilibrates from elevated bone lead stores.

Because there are no controlled clinical trials in humans or animals demonstrating a beneficial effect of chelation on clinical outcome, the decision to initiate or continue chelation is largely empiric. While most clinicians support chelation for symptomatic patients with elevated blood lead concentrations, the decision to chelate asymptomatic subjects is more controversial. The CDC currently recommends chelation for all children with blood lead concentrations of 45 μg/dL or greater (Preventing, 1991). Prophylactic use of chelating agents in the workplace should never be a substitute for reduction or prevention of excessive exposure.

B. Organic Lead Poisoning: Initial treatment consists of decontaminating the skin and preventing further exposure. Treatment of seizures requires judicious use of anticonvulsants. Empiric chelation may be attempted if high blood lead concentrations are present.

ARSENIC

Arsenic is a naturally occurring element in the earth's crust with a long history of use as a constituent of commercial and industrial products, as a component in pharmaceuticals, and as an agent of deliberate poisoning. Recent commercial applications of arsenic include its use in the manufacture of semiconductors, wood preservatives, herbicides, cotton desiccants, nonferrous alloys, glass, insecticides, and veterinary pharmaceuticals. In some regions of the world, groundwater may contain high levels of arsenic that has leached from natural mineral deposits. Anthropogenic distribution of arsenic may occur via coal fly ash and emissions from nonferrous smelters. Arsine, a hydride gas that is a potent hemolytic agent, is manufactured predominantly for use in the semiconductor industry and may be generated accidentally by the action of acidic agents on some inorganic arsenic compounds.

It is of historical interest that Fowler's solution, which contains 1% potassium arsenite, was widely used as a medicine for many conditions, eg, asthma, from the eighteenth century through the mid-twentieth century. Organic arsenicals were the first pharmaceutical antibiotics* and were widely used for the first

---

* Ehrlich's "magic bullet" for syphilis (arsphenamine; Salvarsan) was an arsenical.

half of the twentieth century until supplanted by penicillin and other more effective and less toxic agents. Other organoarsenicals, most notably lewisite (dichloro[2-chlorovinyl]arsine), were also developed in the twentieth century as chemical warfare agents.

Pharmacokinetics

Soluble arsenic compounds are well absorbed through the respiratory and gastrointestinal tracts. Percutaneous absorption is limited but may be clinically significant after heavy exposure to concentrated arsenic reagents. Most of the absorbed inorganic arsenic undergoes methylation, mainly in the liver, to monomethylarsonic acid and dimethylarsinic acid, which are excreted, along with residual inorganic arsenic, in the urine. When chronic daily absorption is less than 1000 μg of soluble inorganic arsenic, approximately two-thirds of the absorbed dose is excreted in the urine. After massive ingestions, the elimination half-life is prolonged. Inhalation of arsenic compounds of low solubility may result in prolonged retention in the lung and may not be reflected by urinary arsenic excretion. Arsenic binds to sulfhydryl groups present in keratinized tissue, and following cessation of exposure, hair, nails, and skin may contain elevated levels after urine values have returned to normal. However, arsenic present in hair and nails as a result of external deposition may be indistinguishable from that incorporated after internal absorption.

Pharmacodynamics

Arsenic compounds exert multisystemic toxic effects by inhibition of enzymatic reactions. This may involve sulfhydryl group binding (trivalent arsenic) or substitution for phosphate (pentavalent arsenic). Although on a molar basis trivalent arsenic (As^{+3}, or arsenite) is generally two to ten times more toxic than pentavalent arsenic (As^{+5}, or arsenate), in vivo interconversion is known to occur, and the full spectrum of arsenic toxicity has occurred after sufficient exposure to either form. Arsine gas is oxidized in vivo and exerts a potent hemolytic effect associated with depletion of erythrocyte glutathione; however, it also disrupts cellular respiration in other tissues. Arsenic is a recognized human carcinogen and has been associated with cancer of the lung, skin, liver, kidney, and bladder (Bates et al, 1992). Marine organisms may contain large amounts of a well-absorbed trimethylated organoarsenic, arsenobetaine, that exerts no known toxic effects when ingested by mammals and is excreted in the urine unchanged.

Major Forms of Arsenic Intoxication

A. Acute Inorganic Arsenic Poisoning: Within minutes to hours after exposure to high doses (tens to hundreds of milligrams) of soluble inorganic arsenic compounds, many systems are affected. Initial gastrointestinal signs and symptoms include nausea, vomiting, diarrhea, and abdominal pain. Diffuse capillary leak, combined with gastrointestinal fluid loss, may result in hypotension, shock, and death. Cardiopulmonary toxicity, including congestive cardiomyopathy, cardiogenic or noncardiogenic pulmonary edema, and ventricular arrhythmias, may occur promptly or after a delay of several days. Pancytopenia usually develops within a week, and basophilic stippling of erythrocytes may be present soon after. Central nervous system pathology, including delirium, encephalopathy, and coma, may occur within the first few days of intoxication. An ascending sensorimotor peripheral neuropathy that may ultimately include the proximal musculature and result in neuromuscular respiratory failure may begin to develop after a delay of 2–6 weeks. Months after an episode of acute poisoning, transverse white striae (Aldrich-Mees lines) may be visible in the nails.

Acute inorganic arsenic poisoning should be considered in an individual presenting with abrupt onset of gastroenteritis in combination with hypotension and metabolic acidosis. The diagnosis may be confirmed by demonstration of elevated amounts of inorganic arsenic and its metabolites in the urine (typically in the range of several thousand micrograms in the first 2–3 days following acute symptomatic poisoning). Arsenic disappears rapidly from the blood, and except in anuric patients, blood arsenic levels should not be used for diagnostic purposes. Treatment centers on appropriate gut decontamination, intensive supportive care, and prompt chelation with dimercaprol, 3–5 mg/kg intramuscularly every 4–6 hours. In animal studies, the efficacy of dimercaprol has been highest when it is administered within minutes to hours after arsenic exposure; and therefore, if diagnostic suspicion is high, treatment should not be withheld for the several days to weeks often required to obtain laboratory confirmation. Succimer has been effective in animal models and has a higher therapeutic index than dimercaprol. However, because it is available in the United States only for oral administration, its use may not be advisable in the initial treatment of acute arsenic poisoning, when severe gastroenteritis and splanchnic edema may limit absorption by this route.

B. Chronic Inorganic Arsenic Poisoning:
Chronic inorganic arsenic poisoning also results in a constellation of multisystemic signs and symptoms. Overt noncarcinogenic effects may be evident after chronic absorption of more than 500–1000 µg/d. The time to appearance of symptoms will vary with dose and interindividual tolerances. Constitutional symptoms of fatigue, weight loss, and weakness may be present, along with anemia, nonspecific gastrointestinal complaints, and a sensorimotor peripheral neuropathy, particularly featuring a stocking-glove pattern of dysesthesia. Skin changes—among the most characteristic effects—typically develop after years of exposure and include a "raindrop" pattern of hyper-

pigmentation, and hyperkeratoses involving the palms and soles. Peripheral vascular disease and noncirrhotic portal hypertension may also occur. Cancer of the lung, skin, liver, kidney, or bladder may appear years after exposure to doses of arsenic that are not high enough to elicit other acute or chronic effects.

The diagnosis of chronic arsenic poisoning involves integration of the clinical findings with laboratory confirmation of exposure. Urinary levels of total arsenic, usually less than 50 µg/24 h, may return to normal within days to weeks after exposure ceases. Because it may contain large amounts of nontoxic organoarsenic, all seafood should be avoided for 3 days prior to submission of a urine sample for diagnostic purposes. The arsenic content of hair and nails (normally less than 1 ppm) may sometimes reveal past elevated exposure, but results should be interpreted cautiously in view of the potential for external contamination.

C. Arsine Gas Poisoning: Arsine gas poisoning produces a distinctive pattern of intoxication dominated by its profound hemolytic effects. After a latent period that may range from 2 to 24 hours postinhalation (depending on the magnitude of exposure), massive intravascular hemolysis may occur. Initial symptoms may include malaise, headache, dyspnea, weakness, nausea, vomiting, abdominal pain, jaundice, and hemoglobinuria. Oliguric renal failure, a consequence of hemoglobin deposition in the renal tubules, often appears within 1–3 days. In massive exposures, lethal effects on cellular respiration may occur before renal failure develops. Urinary arsenic levels are elevated but will seldom be available to confirm the diagnosis during the critical period of illness. Intensive supportive care—including blood transfusions for hemolytic anemia and forced alkaline diuresis or hemodialysis for renal damage—is the mainstay of therapy. Currently available chelating agents have not been demonstrated to be of value in arsine poisoning.

MERCURY

Metallic mercury as "quicksilver"—the only metal that is liquid under ordinary conditions—has attracted scholarly and scientific interest from antiquity. In early times it was recognized that the mining of mercury was hazardous to health. As industrial use of mercury became common during the past 200 years, new forms of toxicity were recognized that were found to be associated with various transformations of the metal. In the early 1950s, a mysterious epidemic of birth defects and neurologic disease occurred in the Japanese fishing village of Minamata. The causative agent was determined to be methylmercury, formed in ocean water by the metabolic action of aquatic organisms on elemental mercury discharged from a nearby factory. In addition to elemental mercury and alkylmercury (including methylmercury), other key mercurials include inorganic mercury salts and aryl mercury compounds, each of which exerts a relatively unique pattern of clinical toxicity.

Mercury is mined predominantly as HgS in cinnabar ore and is then converted commercially to a variety of chemical forms. Key industrial and commercial applications of mercury are found in the electrolytic production of chlorine and caustic soda; the manufacture of electrical equipment, thermometers, and other instruments; paint and pigment production; dental amalgam; and gold refining. Use in pharmaceuticals and in biocides has declined substantially in recent years, but occasional use in topical antiseptics and folk medicines is still encountered. Environmental exposure to mercury from the burning of fossil fuels—or the bioaccumulation of methylmercury in fish—remains a concern in some regions of the world.

Pharmacokinetics

The absorption of mercury varies considerably depending on the chemical form of the metal. Elemental mercury is quite volatile and can be absorbed from the lungs (Table 58–1). It is poorly absorbed from the intact gastrointestinal tract. Inhaled mercury is the primary source of occupational exposure. Organic short-chain alkylmercury compounds are volatile and potentially harmful by inhalation as well as by ingestion. Percutaneous absorption of all types of mercurials is limited but may be of clinical concern when there is heavy exposure. After absorption, mercury is distributed to the tissues in a few hours, with the highest concentration occurring in the kidney. Inorganic mercury is excreted primarily through the urine. Excretion follows a multicomponent model: Most is excreted within days to weeks, but a fraction may be retained in the kidneys and brain for years. Methylmercury undergoes biliary excretion and enterohepatic circulation, with 90% eventually excreted in the feces. Mercury binds to sulfhydryl groups in keratinized tissue, and, as with lead and arsenic, traces appear in the hair and nails.

Major Forms of Mercury Intoxication

Mercury interacts with sulfhydryl groups in vivo, inhibiting enzymes and altering cell membranes. The pattern of clinical intoxication from mercury depends to a great extent on the chemical form of the metal and the route and severity of exposure.

A. Acute: Acute inhalation of elemental mercury vapors may cause chemical pneumonitis and noncardiogenic pulmonary edema. Acute gingivostomatitis may occur, and neurologic sequelae (see below) may also ensue. Acute ingestion of inorganic mercury salts, such as mercuric chloride, can result in a corrosive, potentially life-threatening hemorrhagic gastroenteritis followed within days by acute tubular necrosis and oliguric renal failure.

B. Chronic: Chronic poisoning from inhalation of mercury vapor results in a classic triad of tremor, neuropsychiatric disturbance, and gingivostomatitis. The tremor usually begins as a fine intention tremor of the hands, but the face may also be involved, and progression to choreiform movements of the limbs may occur. Neuropsychiatric manifestations, including memory loss, fatigue, insomnia, and anorexia, are common. There may be an insidious change in mood to shyness, withdrawal, and depression along with explosive anger or blushing (a behavioral pattern referred to as "erethism"). Recent studies suggest that low-dose exposure may produce subclinical effects (Echeverria et al, 1995). Gingivostomatitis, sometimes accompanied by loosening of the teeth, may be reported. Evidence of peripheral nerve damage may be detected on electrodiagnostic testing, but overt peripheral neuropathy occurs rarely. Acrodynia is an uncommon idiosyncratic reaction to chronic mercury exposure and occurs mainly in children. It is characterized by painful erythema of the extremities and may be associated with hypertension, diaphoresis, anorexia, insomnia, irritability or apathy, and a miliarial rash.

Methylmercury intoxication affects mainly the central nervous system and results in paresthesias, ataxia, hearing impairment, dysarthria, and progressive constriction of the visual fields. Signs and symptoms may first appear several weeks or months after exposure begins. Methylmercury is a reproductive toxin, producing mental retardation and a cerebral palsy-like syndrome in the offspring after prenatal exposure.

As with the other heavy metal intoxications, the diagnosis of mercury intoxication involves careful integration of the history and physical findings with confirmatory laboratory testing. In the absence of occupational exposure, the urine mercury concentration is usually less than 10 μg/L, and whole blood mercury is less than 10 μg/L. In 1990, the Biological Exposure Index (BEI) Committee of the American Conference of Governmental Industrial Hygienists (ACGIH) recommended that workplace exposures should result in urinary mercury concentrations less than 35 μg per gram of creatinine and end-of-work-week whole blood mercury concentrations less than 15 μg/L.

Treatment

A. Acute Exposure: In addition to intensive supportive care, acute chelation with dimercaprol or succimer may be of value in diminishing nephrotoxicity after acute exposure to inorganic mercury salts. While oral succimer is effective, severe gastroenteritis or shock may limit its absorption, and dimercaprol may be preferable as an initial chelating agent. Parenteral dimercaptopropanesulfonic acid appears to be the best agent in this setting, but it is not available in the United States.

B. Chronic Exposure: Succimer, D-penicillamine, and dimercaptopropanesulfonic acid will increase urine mercury excretion following acute or chronic metallic mercury inhalation, but the impact of such treatment on clinical outcome is unknown. Dimercaprol has been shown to redistribute mercury to the central nervous system from other tissue sites, and since the brain is a key target organ, dimercaprol should not be used in treatment of exposure to metallic or organic mercury. Limited data suggest that succimer and dimercaptopropanesulfonic acid may increase body clearance of methylmercury.

PREPARATIONS AVAILABLE

Deferoxamine (Desferal Mesylate)
  Parenteral: Powder to reconstitute 500 mg/vial)
Dimercaprol (BAL, generic)
  Parenteral: 100 mg/mL for injection
Edetate calcium [calcium EDTA] (Calcium Sodium Versenate)
  Parenteral: 200 mg/mL for injection

Penicillamine (Cuprimine, Depen)
  Oral: 125, 250 capsules, tablets
Succimer (Chemet)
  Oral: 100 mg capsules
Trientine (Syprine)
  Oral: 250 mg capsules

REFERENCES

Chelating Agents

Aposhian HV, Aposhian MM: *meso*-2,3-Dimercaptosuccinic acid: Chemical, pharmacological and toxicological properties of an orally effective metal chelating agent. Annu Rev Pharmacol Toxicol 1990;30:279.

Dart RC et al: Pharmacokinetics of *meso*-2,3-dimercaptosuccinic acid in patients with lead poisoning and in healthy adults. J Pediatr 1994;125:309.

Graziano JH: Role of 2,3-dimercaptosuccinic acid in the treatment of heavy metal poisoning. Med Toxicol 1986;1:155.

Graziano JH, Lolacono NJ, Meyer P: Dose-response study of oral 2,3-dimercaptosuccinic acid in children with elevated lead concentrations. J Pediatr 1988;113:751.

Jones MM: New developments in therapeutic chelating agents as antidotes for metal poisoning. Crit Rev Toxicol 1991;21:209.

Kosnett MJ: Unanswered questions in metal chelation. Clin Toxicol 1992;30:529.

Mann KV, Travers JD: Succimer, an oral lead chelator. Clin Pharmacy 1991;10:914.

Netter P et al: Clinical pharmacokinetics of D-penicillamine. Clin Pharmacokinet 1987;13:317.

Walshe JM: Treatment of Wilson's disease with trientine (triethylene tetramine) dihydrochloride. Lancet 1982;1:643.

Heavy Metals, General

Friberg L, Nordberg GF, Vouk V (editors): *Handbook on the Toxicology of Metals,* 2nd ed. Elsevier, 1986.

Greenhouse AH, Glaeske CS: Heavy metal intoxication. In: *Textbook of Clinical Neurotoxicology and Therapeutics,* 2nd ed. Klawans HL et al (editors). Raven Press, 1992.

Landrigan PJ: Occupational and community exposures to toxic metals: Lead, cadmium, mercury and arsenic. West J Med 1982;137:531.

Lead

Baghurst PA et al: Environmental exposure to lead and children's intelligence at the age of seven years. The Port Pirie cohort study. N Engl J Med 1992;327:1279.

Brangstrup-Hanse JP: Chelatable lead burden by calcium disodium EDTA and blood lead concentration in man. J Occup Med 1981;93:39.

Bushnell PJ, Jaeger RJ: Hazards from environmental lead exposure: A review of recent literature. Vet Hum Toxicol 1986;28:255.

Chisolm JJ: The continuing hazard of lead exposure and its effects in children. Neurotoxicology 1985;5:23.

Cory-Slechta DA, Weiss B, Cox C: Mobilization and redistribution of lead over the course of calcium disodium ethylenediamine tetraacetate chelation therapy. J Pharmacol Exp Ther 1987;243:804.

Cory-Slechta DA, Weiss B: Efficacy of the chelating agent CaEDTA in reversing lead-induced changes in behavior. Neurotoxicology 1990;10:685.

Craswell PW et al: Chronic renal failure with gout: A marker of chronic lead poisoning. Kidney Int 1984;26:319.

Ibels LS, Pollock CA: Lead intoxication. Med Toxicol 1986;1:387.

Kosnett MJ et al: Factors influencing bone lead concentration in a suburban community assessed by noninvasive K x-ray fluorescence. JAMA 1994;271:197.

Landrigan PJ: Toxicity of lead at low dose. Br J Ind Med 1989;46:593.

Markowitz ME et al: Effects of calcium disodium versenate (CaNa$_2$EDTA) chelation in moderate childhood lead poisoning. Pediatrics 1993;92:265.

Nadig RJ: Treatment of lead poisoning. JAMA 1990;263:2181.

Needleman HL et al: The long-term effects of exposure to low doses of lead in childhood: An 11-year follow-up report. N Engl J Med 1990;322:83.

Nriagu JO: *Lead and Lead Poisoning in Antiquity.* Wiley, 1983.

O'Connor ME: CaEDTA vs CaEDTA plus BAL to treat children with elevated blood levels. Clin Pediatrics 1992;31:386.

Osterloh JD et al: Body burdens of lead in hypertensive nephropathy. Arch Environ Health 1989;44:304.

Pagliuca A et al: Lead poisoning: clinical, biochemical, and haematological aspects of a recent outbreak. J Clin Pathol 1990;43:277.

Pirkle JL et al: The relationship between blood lead levels and blood pressure and its cardiovascular risk implication. Am J Epidemiol 1985;121:246.

Pirkle JL et al: The decline in blood lead levels in the United States. The National Health and Nutrition Examination Surveys (NHANES). JAMA 1994;272:284.

Preventing lead poisoning in young children. A statement by the Centers For Disease Control, 4th rev. Centers for Disease Control, 1991.

Rempel D: The lead-exposed worker. JAMA 1989;262:532.

Schneitzer L et al: Lead poisoning in adults from renovation of an older home. Ann Emerg Med 1990;19:415.

Schwartz J: Lead, blood pressure, and cardiovascular disease in men and women. Environ Health Perspect 1991;91:71.

Settle DM: Lead in albacore: Guide to lead pollution in America. Science 1980;207:1167.

Sharp DS, Becker CE, Smith AH: Chronic low-level lead exposure: Its role in the pathogenesis of hypertension. Med Toxicol 1987;2:210.

Staessen JA et al: Impairment of renal function with increasing blood lead concentrations in the general population. N Engl J Med 1992;327:151.

Stollery BT et al: Cognitive functioning in lead workers. Br J Ind Med 1989;46:698.

Arsenic

Bates MN, Smith AH, Hopenhayn-Rich C: Arsenic ingestion and internal cancers: A review. Am J Epidemiol 1992;135:462.

Kreppel H et al: Lack of effectiveness of D-penicillamine in experimental arsenic poisoning. Vet Hum Toxicol 1989;31:1.

Martin DW Jr, Woeber KA: Arsenic poisoning. Calif Med (March) 1973;118:13.

Mathieu D et al: Massive arsenic poisoning: Effect of hemodialysis and dimercaprol on arsenic kinetics. Intensive Care Med 1992;18:47.

National Institute of Safety and Health: *Occupational Exposure to Inorganic Arsenic: New Criteria.* US Department of Health, Education, and Welfare Publication No. 75-140, 1975.

Mercury

Agocs MM et al: Mercury exposure from interior latex paint. N Engl J Med 1990;323:1096.

Barregard L: Biological monitoring of exposure to mercury vapor. Scand J Work Environ Health 1993;19(Suppl 1):45.

Done AK: The toxic emergency: The many faces of mercurialism. Emerg Med (Jan) 1980;12:137.

Echeverria D et al: Behavioral effects of low-level exposure to elemental Hg among dentists. Neurotoxical Teratotoxical 1995;17:161.

Jung RC, Aaronson J: Death following inhalation of mercury vapor at home. West J Med 1980;132:539.

Kahn A, Denis R, Blum D: Accidental ingestion of mercuric sulphate in a 4-year-old child. Clin Pediatr 1977;16:956.

Krohn IT et al: Subcutaneous injection of metallic mercury. JAMA 1980;243:548.

Roels H et al: Urinary excretion of mercury after occupational exposure to mercury vapor and influence of the chelating agent *meso*-2,3-dimercaptosuccinic acid (DMSA). Brit J Indust Med 1991;48:247.

Snodgrass W et al: Mercury poisoning from home gold ore processing. JAMA 1981;246:1929.

59

Management of the Poisoned Patient

Kent R. Olson, MD, & Charles E. Becker, MD

Over a million cases of acute poisoning occur each year, though only a small fraction are fatal. Most deaths are due to intentional suicidal overdose by an adolescent or adult. Childhood deaths due to accidental ingestion of a drug or toxic household product have been markedly reduced in the past 20 years as a result of safety packaging and effective poisoning prevention education.

Even with a serious exposure, poisoning is rarely fatal if the victim receives prompt medical attention and good supportive care. Careful management of airway obstruction, respiratory failure, hypotension, seizures, and thermoregulatory disturbances has resulted in improved survival of overdosed patients who reach the hospital alive.

This chapter reviews the basic principles of poisoning, the pathophysiology of lethal poisoning, initial management of the overdose, diagnosis of toxic syndromes, and specialized treatment of poisoning including methods of increasing the elimination of drugs and toxins.

TOXICOKINETICS & TOXICODYNAMICS

Toxicologic problems are best viewed in a classic pharmacologic model. This model is based on the pharmacologic properties of chemical agents and their effects in therapeutic doses. Toxicology extends this information to excessive doses.

The term "toxicokinetics" denotes the absorption, distribution, excretion, and metabolism of toxins, toxic doses of therapeutic agents, and their metabolites. The term "toxicodynamics" is used to denote the injurious effects of these substances on vital function. Although there are many similarities between the pharmacokinetics and toxicokinetics of most substances, there are also important differences. The same caution applies to pharmacodynamics and toxicodynamics.

SPECIAL ASPECTS OF TOXICOKINETICS

Volume of Distribution

The volume of distribution (V_d) is defined as the apparent volume into which a substance is distributed. It is calculated from the dose given and the resulting plasma concentration: V_d = dose/concentration (extrapolated to zero time), as described in Chapter 3. If a chemical is highly tissue-bound or otherwise sequestered outside the plasma, the plasma concentration will be low and the V_d very large. A large V_d implies that the drug is not readily accessible to measures aimed at purifying the blood, such as hemodialysis. Drugs with large volumes of distribution (> 5–10 L/kg) include antidepressants, phenothiazines, propranolol, and verapamil. Drugs with relatively small volumes of distribution (< 1 L/kg) include theophylline, salicylate, phenobarbital, lithium, and phenytoin (Table 3–1).

Clearance

Clearance is a measure of the volume of plasma that is cleared of drug per unit time. For most drugs, the total amount of drug removed per unit time is dependent on the plasma drug concentration as well as the clearance. The body has intrinsic mechanisms for clearing drugs, and the total clearance is the sum of clearances by excretion by the kidneys, metabolism by the liver, and elimination in sweat, feces, and expired air (see Chapter 3). In planning detoxification strategy, it is important to know the contribution of each organ to total clearance. For example, if a drug is 95% cleared by liver metabolism and only 5% cleared by renal excretion, even a dramatic increase in urinary output would have little effect on overall elimination.

Overdosage of a drug can alter the usual pharmacokinetic processes, and this must be considered when applying kinetics to poisoned patients. For example, dissolution of tablets or gastric emptying time may be altered so that absorption and peak toxic effects are delayed. Drugs may injure the gastrointestinal tract and thereby alter absorption. If the capacity of the liver to metabolize a drug is exceeded, more drug will be delivered to the circulation. With a dramatic increase in the concentration of drug in the blood, tissue-binding and protein-binding capacity may be exceeded, resulting in an increased fraction of free drug and greater toxic effect. At normal dosage, most drugs are eliminated at a rate proportionate to the plasma concentration (first-order kinetics). If the plasma concentration is very high and normal metabolism is saturated, the rate of elimination may become fixed (zero-order kinetics). This change in kinetics may markedly prolong the apparent serum half-life and increase toxicity.

SPECIAL ASPECTS OF TOXICODYNAMICS

Knowledge of basic pharmacology may also help the physician anticipate important toxicodynamic problems in the diagnosis and management of the intoxicated patient. The general dose-response principles described in Chapter 2 are of crucial importance in determining the severity of the intoxication. When considering quantal dose-response data, both the therapeutic index and the overlap of therapeutic and toxic response curves must be considered. For instance, as shown in Figure 59–1, drugs A and B have the same therapeutic index. However, drug B is more likely to cause inadvertent intoxication because its toxic response curve overlaps the therapeutic dose range more than is the case with drug A. For some drugs, eg, sedative-hypnotics, the major toxic effect is a direct extension of the therapeutic action, as shown by their graded dose-response curve (Figure 59–2). In the case of a drug with a flat dose-response curve (drug A), lethal effects may require 100 times the normal therapeutic dose. In contrast, a drug with a steeper curve (drug B) may be lethal at ten times the normal dose.

For many drugs, at least part of the toxic effect may be distinct from the therapeutic action. For example, intoxication with drugs that have atropine-like effects (eg, tricyclic antidepressants) will reduce sweating, making it more difficult to dissipate heat. In tricyclic antidepressant intoxication, there may also be increased muscular activity or seizures; the body's production of heat is thus enhanced, and lethal hyperpyrexia may result. Overdoses of drugs that depress the cardiovascular system, eg, β-adrenoceptor-blocking agents or barbiturates, can profoundly alter not only target organ function but all functions that are dependent on blood flow. These include renal and hepatic elimination of the toxin and any other drugs that may be given.

Conversely, lack of tissue perfusion with falling blood pressure may lead to a transient decrease in target organ drug levels. When blood pressure is restored to adequate levels, enhanced delivery of the toxin can lead to an apparent increase in the degree of intoxication. The result may be a confusing waxing and waning of the signs and symptoms.

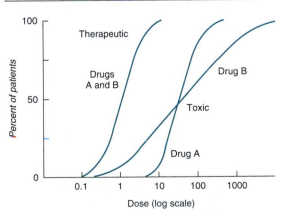

Figure 59–1. Quantal dose-response comparison of two drugs with differing safety margins. Both drugs have the same therapeutic index (TD50/ED50). However, at the dose required for therapeutic effects in 90% of patients, less than 1% of patients receiving drug A have toxicity, but 20% of those taking drug B have toxicity.

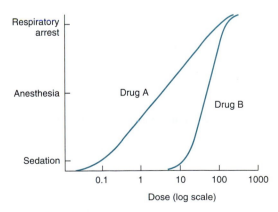

Figure 59–2. Graded dose-response comparison of two sedative-hypnotic drugs. A much larger multiple of the normal prescription dose of drug A is required to cause respiratory arrest, ie, it is safer than drug B.

APPROACH
TO THE POISONED PATIENT

HOW DOES THE POISONED PATIENT DIE?

In the majority of cases of poisoning, supportive measures are the mainstay of treatment. An understanding of common mechanisms of death due to poisoning can help prepare the physician to treat patients effectively.

Many toxins depress the central nervous system, resulting in obtundation or coma. Comatose patients frequently lose their airway protective reflexes and their respiratory drive. Thus, they are likely to die as a result of airway obstruction by the flaccid tongue, aspiration of gastric contents into the tracheobronchial tree, or respiratory arrest. These are the most common causes of death due to overdoses of narcotics, barbiturates, alcohol, and other sedative-hypnotic drugs.

Cardiovascular toxicity is also frequently encountered in poisoning. Hypotension may be due to depression of cardiac contractility; hypovolemia resulting from vomiting, diarrhea, or fluid sequestration; peripheral vascular collapse due to blockade of α-adrenoceptor-mediated vascular tone; or cardiac arrhythmias. Hypotension is common with overdoses of tricyclic antidepressants, phenothiazines, β-adrenoceptor blockers, calcium channel blockers, theophylline, and phenobarbital and other sedative-hypnotic drugs. Hypothermia due to exposure as well as the temperature-dysregulating effects of many drugs can also produce hypotension. Hypothermia may be worsened by rapid infusion of intravenous fluids at room temperature (24 °C). Lethal arrhythmias such as ventricular tachycardia and fibrillation can occur with overdoses of many cardioactive drugs such as amphetamines, cocaine, tricyclic antidepressants, digitalis, and theophylline.

Cellular hypoxia may occur in spite of adequate ventilation and oxygen administration when poisoning is due to cyanide, hydrogen sulfide, carbon monoxide, and other poisons that interfere with transport or utilization of oxygen. In such patients, cellular hypoxia is evident by the development of tachycardia, hypotension, severe lactic acidosis, and signs of ischemia on the ECG.

Seizures, muscular hyperactivity, and rigidity may result in death. Seizures may cause pulmonary aspiration, hypoxia, and brain damage. Hyperthermia may result from sustained muscular hyperactivity and can lead to muscle breakdown and myoglobinuria, renal failure, lactic acidosis, and hyperkalemia. Drugs and poisons that often cause seizures include tricyclic antidepressants, theophylline, isoniazid (INH), diphenhydramine, phenothiazines, cocaine, amphetamines, camphor, and lindane.

Other organ system damage may occur after poisoning, and is sometimes delayed in onset. Paraquat attacks lung tissue, resulting in pulmonary fibrosis several days after ingestion. Massive hepatic necrosis due to poisoning by acetaminophen or certain mushrooms results in hepatic encephalopathy and death 48–72 hours or longer after ingestion.

Finally, some patients may die before hospitalization because the behavioral effects of the ingested drug may result in traumatic injury. Intoxication with alcohol and other sedative-hypnotic drugs is a frequent contributing factor to motor vehicle accidents. Patients under the influence of hallucinogens such as phencyclidine or LSD may die in fights or falls from high places.

INITIAL MANAGEMENT
OF THE POISONED PATIENT

The initial management of a patient with coma, seizures, or otherwise altered mental status should follow the same approach regardless of the poison involved. Attempting to make a specific toxicologic diagnosis only delays the application of supportive measures that form the basis ("ABCDs") of poisoning treatment.

First, the **airway** should be cleared of vomitus or any other obstruction and an oral airway or endotracheal tube inserted if needed. For many patients, simple positioning in the lateral decubitus position is sufficient to move the flaccid tongue out of the airway. **Breathing** should be assessed by observation and by measuring arterial blood gases. Patients with respiratory insufficiency should be intubated and mechanically ventilated. The **circulation** should be assessed by continuous monitoring of pulse rate, blood pressure, urinary output, and evaluation of peripheral perfusion. An intravenous line should be placed and blood drawn for serum glucose and other routine determinations.

At this point, every patient with altered mental status should receive a challenge with concentrated **dextrose,** unless a rapid bedside blood sugar test demonstrates that the patient is not hypoglycemic. Adults are given 25 g (50 mL of 50% dextrose solution) intravenously, children 0.5 g/kg (2 mL/kg of 25% dextrose). This should be routine and immediate, because patients comatose from hypoglycemia are rapidly and irreversibly losing brain cells. Hypoglycemic patients may appear to be intoxicated, and there is no rapid and reliable way to distinguish them from poisoned patients. Alcoholic or malnourished patients should also receive 100 mg of thiamine intramuscularly or in the intravenous infusion solution at this time to prevent Wernicke's syndrome.

The opioid antagonist naloxone (Narcan) may be given in a dose of 0.4–2 mg intravenously. Naloxone will reverse respiratory and central nervous system depression due to all varieties of opioid drugs. It is useful to remember that these drugs cause death primarily by respiratory depression; therefore, if airway and breathing assistance have already been instituted, naloxone may not be necessary. The benzodiazepine antagonist flumazenil (Romazicon; see Chapter 22) may be of value in patients with suspected benzodiazepine overdose, but it should not be used if there is a history of tricyclic antidepressant overdose or a seizure disorder, as it can induce convulsions in such patients.

Management of poisoning requires a thorough knowledge of how to treat hypoventilation, coma, shock, seizures, and psychosis. Sophisticated toxicokinetic considerations are of little value if vital functions are not maintained. Hypoventilation and coma require particular attention to airway management. Arterial blood gases must be checked frequently, and aspiration of gastric contents must be prevented. Fluid and electrolyte management may be complex. With appropriate supportive care, most patients will survive the poisoning.

History & Physical Examination

Once these essential initial interventions have been instituted, one can begin a more detailed evaluation to make a specific diagnosis. This includes gathering any available history and performing a toxicologically oriented physical examination. Other causes of coma or seizures such as head trauma, meningitis, or metabolic abnormalities should be looked for and treated. Table 59–1 lists the characteristics of some important toxic syndromes.

A. History: Oral statements about the amount and even the type of drug ingested in toxic emergencies may be unreliable. Even so, family members, police, and fire department or paramedical personnel should be asked to describe the environment in which the toxic emergency occurred and should bring to the emergency department any syringes, empty bottles, household products, or over-the-counter medications in the immediate vicinity of the possibly poisoned patient.

B. Physical Examination: A brief examination should be performed, emphasizing those areas most likely to give clues to the toxicologic diagnosis. These include vital signs, eyes and mouth, skin, abdomen, and nervous system.

1. Vital signs—Careful evaluation of vital signs (blood pressure, pulse, respirations, and temperature) is essential in all toxicologic emergencies. Hypertension and tachycardia are typical with amphetamines, cocaine, and antimuscarinic (anticholinergic) drugs. Hypotension and bradycardia are characteristic features of overdose with calcium channel blockers, β-adrenoceptor blockers, clonidine, and sedative-hypnotics. Tachycardia and hypotension are common with tricyclic antidepressants, phenothiazines, and theophylline. Rapid respirations are typical of salicylates, carbon monoxide, and other toxins that produce metabolic acidosis or cellular asphyxia. Hyperthermia may be associated with sympathomimetics, anticholinergics, salicylates, and drugs producing seizures or muscular rigidity. Hypothermia can be caused by phenothiazines, and ethanol and other sedative drugs, especially when accompanied by exposure to a cold environment.

2. Eyes—The eyes are a valuable source of toxicologic information. Constriction of the pupils (miosis) is typical of opioids, clonidine, phenothiazines, organophosphate insecticides and other cholinesterase inhibitors, and deep coma due to sedative drugs. Dilation of the pupils (mydriasis) is common with amphetamines, cocaine, LSD, and atropine and other anticholinergic drugs. Horizontal nystagmus is characteristic of intoxication with phenytoin, alcohol, barbiturates, and other sedative drugs. The presence of both vertical and horizontal nystagmus is strongly suggestive of phencyclidine (PCP) poisoning. Ptosis and ophthalmoplegia are characteristic features of botulism.

3. Mouth—The mouth may show signs of burns due to corrosive substances, or soot from smoke inhalation. Typical odors of alcohol, hydrocarbon solvents, or ammonia may be noted. Poisoning due to cyanide can be recognized by some examiners as an odor like bitter almonds. Arsenic and organophosphates have been reported to produce a garlicky odor.

4. Skin—The skin often appears flushed, hot, and dry in poisoning with atropine and other antimuscarinics. Excessive sweating occurs with organophosphates, nicotine, and sympathomimetic drugs. Cyanosis may be caused by hypoxemia or by methemoglobinemia. Icterus may suggest hepatic necrosis due to acetaminophen or *Amanita phalloides* mushroom poisoning.

5. Abdomen—Abdominal examination may reveal ileus, which is typical of poisoning with antimuscarinic, opioid, and sedative drugs. Hyperactive bowel sounds, abdominal cramping, and diarrhea are common in poisoning with organophosphates, iron, arsenic, theophylline, and *A phalloides*.

6. Nervous system—A careful neurologic examination is essential. Focal seizures or motor deficits suggest a structural lesion (such as intracranial hemorrhage due to trauma) rather than toxic or metabolic encephalopathy. Nystagmus, dysarthria, and ataxia are typical of phenytoin, alcohol, barbiturate, and other sedative intoxication. Twitching and muscular hyperactivity are common with atropine and other anticholinergic agents, and cocaine and other sympathomimetic drugs. Muscular rigidity can be caused by haloperidol and other antipsychotic agents and by

Table 59–1. Common toxic syndromes associated with major drug groups.

Drug Group	Clinical Features	Key Interventions
Antidepressants (eg, amitriptyline, doxepin, maprotiline, others)	Anticholinergic features common: dilated pupils, tachycardia, hot, dry skin, decreased bowel sounds. The **three Cs**—coma, convulsions, and cardiac problems—are the most common causes of death. A major diagnostic feature is widening of the QRS complex greater than 0.1 s on ECG (not seen with amoxapine). Hypotension and ventricular arrhythmias are common.	Control seizures, correct acidosis and cardiotoxicity with ventilation and HCO_3^-. Do not use physostigmine or flumazenil. Watch for hyperthermia.
Antimuscarinic drugs (eg, atropine, scopolamine, antihistamines, tricyclic antidepressants, jimsonweed, *Amanita muscaria* mushrooms)	Hallucinations, delirium, coma. Seizures may occur with tricyclic antidepressants, antihistamines. Tachycardia, hypertension. Hyperthermia with hot, dry skin. Mydriasis. Decreased bowel sounds, urinary retention. Delayed gastric emptying is expected.	Control hyperthermia. Physostigmine is of potential value but should not be given for cyclic antidepressants.
Cholinomimetic drugs (eg, organophosphate and carbamate insecticides)	Anxiety, agitation, seizures, coma. May see bradycardia (muscarinic effect) or tachycardia (nicotinic effect). Pinpoint pupils. Excessive salivation, sweating. Bowel sounds hyperactive, with abdominal cramping, diarrhea. Muscle fasciculations and twitching followed by flaccid paralysis. Death due to respiratory muscle paralysis.	Respiratory support, atropine, pralidoxime (2-PAM). Remove clothes, wash skin.
Opioid drugs (eg, morphine, heroin, meperidine, codeine, methadone)	Sleepiness, lethargy, or coma, depending on dose. Blood pressure and heart rate usually decreased. Hypoventilation or apnea. Pinpoint pupils. Skin cool; may show signs of intravenous drug abuse with associated infectious disease complications. Bowel sounds decreased. Muscle tone flaccid; occasionally twitching, rigidity. Clonidine overdose may present with identical syndrome.	Airway support. Frequent supplements of naloxone may be necessary because of its short half-life.
Salicylates	Confusion, lethargy, coma, seizures. Hyperventilation, hyperthermia. Anion gap metabolic acidosis. Dehydration, potassium loss. Acute overdose: 6-hour level over 100 mg/dL (1000 mg/L) very serious. Chronic or accidental overdose: level not reliable; more severe toxicity; often mistakenly diagnosed as upper respiratory infection or gastroenteritis.	Correct acidosis and fluid and electrolyte abnormalities; alkalinize the urine; hemodialysis if pH or CNS symptoms cannot be controlled.
Sedative-hypnotics (eg, benzodiazepines, barbiturates, ethanol)	Highly variable depending on stage of intoxication; initially disinhibition and rowdiness, later lethargy, stupor, coma. With deep coma: hypotension, small pupils. Nystagmus common with moderate intoxication. Bowel sounds decreased in deep coma. Muscle tone usually flaccid. May be associated with hypothermia.	Airway and respiratory support. Avoid fluid overload. Flumazenil may reverse benzodiazepine-induced coma.
Stimulant drugs (eg, amphetamines, cocaine, PCP)	Agitation, psychosis, seizures. Hypertension, tachycardia, arrhythmias. Mydriasis (usually). Vertical and horizontal nystagmus are common with PCP poisoning. Skin warm and sweaty. Muscle tone increased; muscle necrosis is possible. Hyperthermia may be major complication.	Control seizures, blood pressure, and hyperthermia.

strychnine. Seizures are often caused by overdose with tricyclic antidepressants, cocaine, amphetamines, theophylline, isoniazid, and diphenhydramine. Flaccid coma with absent reflexes and even an isoelectric EEG may be seen with deep coma due to opioid or sedative-hypnotic intoxication and may be mistaken for brain death. Table 59–2 lists some common sedative-hypnotic drugs.

Laboratory & X-Ray Procedures

Routine laboratory tests that are valuable in toxicologic diagnosis include the following:

A. Arterial Blood Gases: Hypoventilation will result in an elevated P_{CO_2} (hypercapnia). The P_{O_2} may be low with aspiration pneumonia or drug-induced pulmonary edema. Poor tissue oxygenation due to hypoxia, hypotension, or cyanide poisoning will result in metabolic acidosis. The P_{O_2} measures only oxygen dissolved in the plasma and not total blood oxygen content or oxyhemoglobin saturation, and may appear normal in patients with severe carbon monoxide poisoning. Pulse oximetry may also give falsely normal results in carbon monoxide intoxication.

B. Electrolytes: Sodium, potassium, chloride, and bicarbonate should be measured. The anion gap is then calculated by subtracting the measured anions from cations:

$$\text{Anion gap} = (Na^+ + K^+) - (HCO_3^- + Cl^-)$$

It is normally no greater than 12–16 meq/L. A larger-than-expected anion gap is caused by the presence of unmeasured anions accompanying metabolic acidosis. This may occur with numerous conditions, such as diabetic ketoacidosis, renal failure, or shock-induced lactic acidosis. Drugs that may induce an elevated anion gap metabolic acidosis (Table 59–3) include aspirin, metformin, methanol, ethylene glycol, isoniazid, and iron.

Alterations in the serum potassium level are hazardous because they may result in cardiac arrhythmias. Drugs that may cause hyperkalemia despite normal renal function include potassium itself, β-adrenoceptor blockers, digitalis glycosides, and fluoride. Drugs associated with hypokalemia include barium, β-adrenoceptor agonists, caffeine, theophylline and diuretics.

C. Renal Function Tests: Some toxins have direct nephrotoxic effects; in other cases, renal failure is due to shock or myoglobinuria. Blood urea nitrogen and creatinine levels should be measured and urinalysis performed. Elevated serum creatine kinase (CK) and myoglobin in the urine suggest muscle necrosis due to seizures or muscular rigidity. Oxalate crystals in the urine suggest ethylene glycol poisoning.

D. Serum Osmolality: The calculated serum osmolality is dependent mainly on the serum sodium and glucose and the blood urea nitrogen and can be estimated from the following formula:

$$2 \times Na^+ \text{ (meq/L)} + \frac{\text{Glucose (mg/dL)}}{18} + \frac{\text{BUN (mg/dL)}}{3}$$

This calculated value is normally 280–290 mosm/L. Ethanol and other alcohols may contribute significantly to the measured serum osmolality but, since they are not included in the calculation, cause an "osmolar gap":

Table 59–2. Toxicologic features of some sedative-hypnotic overdoses.

Drug	V_d (L/kg)	Normal Doses $t_{1/2}$ (hours)	Over-doses $t_{1/2}$ (hours)	Maximum Therapeutic Level (mg/L)	Treatment	Comments
Phenobarbital	0.75	60–100	70–120	20	Supportive. Repeat-dose charcoal by gastric tube and urinary alkalinization may enhance elimination.	Avoid fluid overload. Hemoperfusion may be required if serum level > 250 mg/L or if intractable hypotension develops.
Pentobarbital	1–2	20–30	50	50	Supportive	Short-acting
Chloral hydrate	0.6	4–8	19–20	15	Supportive	Gastritis, arrhythmias. Radiopaque pills.
Glutethimide (Doriden)	20–25	8–12	34–40	0.5	Supportive	Cyclic variation in coma; mydriasis
Ethchlorvynol (Placidyl)	3–4	10–20	20–100	100	Supportive	Pink or green aspirate with pungent odor. Prolonged coma with overdose.
Diazepam (Valium)	1–2	30–70	50–140	5	Supportive	Severe overdose uncommon unless combined with other drugs. Flumazenil is a benzodiazepine antagonist.

Osmolar gap =
        Measured osmolality − Calculated osmolality

In the absence of significant levels of an osmotically active intoxicant molecule, the osmolar gap is zero. Table 59–4 lists the concentration and expected contribution to the serum osmolality in ethanol, methanol, ethylene glycol, and isopropanol poisonings.

E. Electrocardiogram: Widening of the QRS complex duration to greater than 0.1 s is typical of tricyclic antidepressant and quinidine overdoses (Figure 59–3). The QT interval may be prolonged in quinidine, phenothiazine, and tricyclic antidepressant poisoning. Variable atrioventricular block and a variety of atrial and ventricular arrhythmias are common with digitalis poisoning. Hypoxemia due to carbon monoxide poisoning may result in ischemic changes on the ECG.

F. X-Ray Findings: A plain film of the abdomen may be useful, since some tablets, particularly iron and potassium, may be radiopaque. Chest x-ray may reveal aspiration pneumonia, hydrocarbon pneumonia, or pulmonary edema. When head trauma is suspected, a CT scan is recommended.

Screening Tests

It is a common misconception that a broad toxicology "screen" is the best way to diagnose and manage an acute poisoning. Unfortunately, toxicology screening is time-consuming, expensive, and often unreliable. Moreover, many highly toxic drugs such as calcium channel blockers, β-blockers, and isoniazid are not even included in the screening process. The clinical examination of the patient and selected routine laboratory tests are usually sufficient to generate a tentative diagnosis and an appropriate treatment plan. While screening tests may be helpful in confirming a suspected intoxication or for ruling out intoxication as a cause of apparent brain death, they should not delay needed treatment.

When a specific antidote or other treatment is under consideration, quantitative laboratory testing may be indicated. For example, determination of the acetaminophen serum level is useful in assessing the need for antidotal therapy with acetylcysteine. Serum lev-

Table 59–3. Drug-induced anion gap acidosis.

Type of Elevation of the Anion Gap	Agents
Organic acid metabolites	Methanol, ethylene glycol, diethylene glycol
Lactic acidosis	Cyanide, carbon monoxide, ibuprofen, isoniazid, metformin, salicylates; any drug-induced seizures, hypoxia, or hypotension

Note: The normal anion gap calculated from $(Na^+ + K^+) - (HCO_3^- + Cl^-)$ is 12–16 meq/L; calculated from $(Na^+) - (HCO_3^- + Cl^-)$, it is 8–12 meq/L.

Table 59–4. Substances that cause osmolar gap.

Substance[1]	Potentially Lethal Level (mg/dL)	Corresponding Osmolar Gap (mosm/kg)
Ethanol	350	75
Methanol	80	25
Ethylene glycol	200	35
Isopropanol	350	60

[1] Other substances than can increase the osmolar gap include acetone, mannitol, and magnesium.
Note: Most laboratories use the freezing point method of determining osmolality. However, if the vaporization point method is used, the alcohols may be driven off and their contribution to osmolality will be lost.

els of theophylline, carbamazepine, lithium, salicylates, phenobarbital, and other drugs may indicate the need for hemodialysis or hemoperfusion (Table 59–5). It is important to consider the time since ingestion when evaluating the plasma level. For example, an aspirin concentration of 60 mg/dL 4–6 hours after ingestion is associated with only mild intoxication; however, the same level obtained 36 hours after ingestion is associated with very severe poisoning. The basis for this relationship lies in the fact that the clinical manifestation of toxic effects in some target organs such as the brain may lag significantly behind the peak levels in the blood.

Decontamination

Decontamination procedures should be undertaken simultaneously with initial stabilization, diagnostic assessment, and laboratory evaluation. Decontamination involves removing toxins from the skin or gastrointestinal tract.

A. Skin: Contaminated clothing should be completely removed and double-bagged to prevent illness in health care providers and for possible laboratory analysis. Percutaneous penetration by toxins has been poorly studied but should be anticipated. Vigorous washing with copious amounts of water and soap should be carried out.

B. Gastrointestinal Tract: There is considerable controversy regarding the efficacy of gut emptying by emesis or gastric lavage, especially when treatment is initiated more than 1 hour after ingestion. Some authorities recommend simple administration of activated charcoal without prior gut emptying in selected patients.

Caution: It is essential to protect the airway. All necessary emergency equipment such as suction must be readily available. Seizures, absence of the gag reflex, and ulcerated oral mucous membranes are contraindications to induced emesis. Gastric lavage is contraindicated if the airway is at risk (eg, unconscious patient with no gag reflex).

1. Emesis–Induce emesis by oral administration of **ipecac syrup,** 30 mL for adults or 10–15 mL for

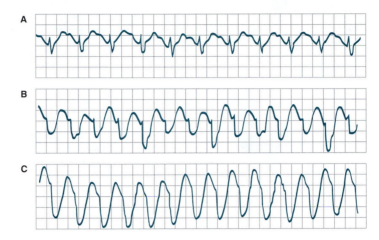

Figure 59–3. Changes in the ECG in tricyclic antidepressant overdosage. ***A:*** Slowed intraventricular conduction results in prolonged QRS interval (0.18 s; normal, 0.08 s). ***B*** and ***C:*** Supraventricular tachycardia with progressive widening of QRS complexes mimics ventricular tachycardia. (Reproduced, with permission, from Benowitz NL, Goldschlager N: Cardiac disturbances in the toxicologic patient. In: *Clinical Management of Poisoning and Drug Overdose.* Haddad LM, Winchester JF [editors]. Saunders, 1983.)

children, repeated once after 15 minutes if necessary. (Ipecac *fluid extract* should be avoided because of its high concentration of emetic and cardiotoxic alkaloids.) Home use of ipecac has been documented to be safe and effective and should be part of the home treatment of children in some ingestions. Ipecac should not be used if the suspected intoxicant is a corrosive agent, a petroleum distillate, or a rapidly-acting convulsant. Previously popular methods of inducing emesis such as fingertip stimulation of the pharynx, salt water, and apomorphine are ineffective or dangerous and should not be used.

2. Gastric lavage–If the patient is awake or if the airway is protected by an endotracheal tube, gastric lavage may be performed using an orogastric or nasogastric tube (Figure 59–4). As large a tube as pos-

sible should be used. Lavage solutions (usually 0.9% saline) should be at body temperature to prevent hypothermia.

3. Activated charcoal–Owing to its large surface area, activated charcoal can adsorb many drugs and poisons. It is most effective if given in a ratio of at least 10:1 of charcoal to estimated dose of toxin by weight. Charcoal does not bind iron, lithium, or potassium, and it binds alcohols and cyanide only poorly. It does not appear to be useful in poisoning due to corrosive mineral acids and alkali, boric acid, ethanol or other alcohols, iron, lithium, methylcarbamate, or tolbutamide. Recent studies suggest that oral activated charcoal given alone may be just as effective as gut emptying followed by charcoal. Also, other studies have shown that repeated doses of oral activated char-

Table 59–5. Indications for hemodialysis (HD) and hemoperfusion (HP).

	Poison	Procedure
Indicated immediately if significant intoxication has occurred	Ethylene glycol	HD
	Methanol	HD
	Salicylate	HD
	Theophylline	HP or HD
	Procainamide	HD or HP
Indicated if supportive measures fail or if prolonged coma is expected	Meprobamate	HP
	Ethchlorvynol	HP
	Phenobarbital	HP
	Lithium	HD
	Carbamazepine	HP
Not indicated	Amphetamines, cocaine	
	Benzodiazepines	
	Chlorpromazine, other antipsychotics	
	Digoxin	
	Opioids	
	Quinidine	
	Tricyclic antidepressants	

Figure 59–4. Positioning of lavage tube and patient for gastric decontamination ("pumping the stomach"). Upper panel shows the relative positions of the endotracheal tube (clear) with cuff in the trachea and the lavage tube (stippled). Lower panel shows the left-lateral position that is optimal for the removal of stomach contents. (Reproduced, with permission, from Olson KR [editor]: *Poisoning & Drug Overdose.* Appleton & Lange, 1990.)

Table 59–6. Usual doses of cathartics in decontamination.[1]

Magnesium citrate (10%) (magnesium = 1.6 meq/mL)	Adult: 100–150 mL Child: 1 mL/kg
Magnesium sulfate (10%) (magnesium = 0.8 meq/mL)	Adult: 150–250 mL Child: 1–2 mL/kg
Sodium sulfate (10%) (sodium = 1.4 meq/mL)	Adult: 150–250 mL Child: 1–2 mL/kg
Sorbitol (70%) (contains no sodium or magnesium)	Adult: 50–100 mL Child: 1 mL/kg

[1]Modified and reproduced, with permission, from Riegel JM, Becker CE: Use of cathartics in toxic ingestions. Ann Emerg Med 1981;10:254.
Note:
1. Avoid magnesium cathartics in renal disease and cases of nephrotoxin ingestion.
2. Avoid sodium cathartics in congestive heart failure and hypertension.
3. Never use oil-based cathartics.

Specific Antidotes

There is a popular misconception that there is an antidote for every poison. Actually, selective antidotes are available for only a few classes of toxins. The major antidotes and their characteristics are listed in Table 59–7.

Methods of Enhancing Elimination of Toxins

After appropriate diagnostic and decontamination procedures and administration of antidotes, it is important to consider measures for enhancing elimination, such as forced diuresis, dialysis, or exchange transfusions. If a patient is able to eliminate a toxin rapidly, the period of coma will be shortened, metabolites removed, and organ damage reduced.

In cases of massive overdose, elimination pathways with limited capacities are often saturated. Drugs that have been demonstrated to exhibit concentration-dependent toxicokinetics in the overdose setting include ethanol, salicylate, phenytoin, chloral hydrate, carbamazepine, theophylline, and acetaminophen. In cases of toxic ingestion of these drugs, methods of enhancing elimination that contribute to total body clearance may significantly improve the clinical outcome.

Drugs or toxins with extremely large volumes of distribution such as tricyclic antidepressants and digoxin are poorly removed by hemodialysis or hemoperfusion. Therefore, critical review of pharmacokinetic parameters is required before undertaking dialysis procedures. Table 59–5 lists intoxications requiring immediate dialysis, those in which it is used only if supportive measures fail, and those for which dialysis is not indicated.

A. Dialysis procedures: (Table 59–5)

1. Peritoneal dialysis–This is a relatively simple and available technique but is inefficient in removing most drugs.

2. Hemodialysis–Hemodialysis is more efficient than peritoneal dialysis and has been well studied. It

coal may enhance systemic elimination of some drugs (including carbamazepine, chlordecone, dapsone, digitoxin, nadolol, phenobarbital, and theophylline) by a mechanism referred to as "gut dialysis."

3. Cathartics–Administration of a cathartic (laxative) agent may hasten removal of toxins from the gastrointestinal tract and reduce absorption, though no controlled studies have been done. Pediatricians have reported finding whole tablets—especially enteric-coated ones—in stools after administration of cathartic agents. Sorbitol (70%) is the preferred cathartic agent. Magnesium sulfate may also be used if renal function is unimpaired. Cathartic agents with an oil base are of no value and are potentially harmful. Table 59–6 lists some common cathartics.

Whole bowel irrigation with a balanced polyethylene glycol-electrolyte solution (GoLYTELY, CoLyte) can enhance gut decontamination after ingestion of iron tablets, enteric-coated medicines, illicit drug-filled packets, and foreign bodies. The solution is administered at 1–2 L/h (500 mL/h in children) for several hours until the rectal effluent is clear.

Table 59–7. Specific antidotes.

Antidote	Poison(s)	Comments
Acetylcysteine (Mucomyst)	Acetaminophen	Best results if given within 8–10 hours of overdose. Follow liver function tests and acetaminophen blood levels. Given orally in the USA. Intravenous acetylcysteine has been used successfully in Europe and is currently under trial in the USA.
Atropine	Anticholinesterases: organophosphates, carbamates	A test dose of 1–2 mg (for children, 0.05 mg/kg) is given IV until symptoms of atropinism appear (tachycardia, dilated pupils, ileus). Dose may be repeated every 10–15 minutes, with decrease of secretions as therapeutic end point.
Bicarbonate, sodium	Membrane-depressant cardiotoxic drugs (tricyclic antidepressants, quinidine, etc)	1–2 meq/kg IV bolus usually reverses cardiotoxic effects (wide QRS, hypotension). Give cautiously in heart failure (avoid sodium overload).
Deferoxamine (Desferal)	Iron salts	If poisoning is severe, give 15 mg/kg/h IV. Urine may become pink. 100 mg of deferoxamine binds 8.5 mg of iron.
Digoxin antibodies (Digibind)	Digoxin and related cardiac glycosides	One vial binds 0.5 mg digoxin; indications include serious arrhythmias, hyperkalemia.
Esmolol	Theophylline, caffeine, metaproterenol	Short-acting beta-blocker reverses β_1-induced tachycardia and β_2-induced vasodilation. Infuse 25–50 μg/kg/min IV.
Ethanol	Methanol, ethylene glycol	Ethanol therapy can be started before laboratory diagnosis is confirmed. A loading dose is calculated so as to give a blood level of at least 100 mg/dL (42 g/70 kg in adults).
Flumazenil (Romazicon)	Benzodiazepines	Adult dose is 0.2 mg IV, repeated as necessary to a maximum of 3 mg. Do not give to patients with seizures, benzodiazepine dependence, or tricyclic overdose.
Glucagon	Beta-adrenoceptor blockers	5–10 mg IV bolus may reverse hypotension and bradycardia that was resistant to beta-agonist drugs. May cause vomiting.
Naloxone (Narcan)	Narcotic drugs, other opioid derivatives	A specific antagonist of opioids; 1–2 mg initially by IV, IM, or subcutaneous injection. Larger doses may be needed to reverse the effects of overdose with propoxyphene, codeine, or fentanyl derivatives. Duration of action (2–3 hours) may be significantly shorter than that of the opioid being antagonized.
Oxygen	Carbon monoxide	Give 100% by high-flow nonrebreathing mask; use of hyperbaric chamber controversial.
Physostigmine salicylate	Suggested for antimuscarinic anticholinergic agents; not for tricyclic antidepressants	Adult dose is 0.5–1 mg IV slowly. The effects are transient (30–60 minutes), and the lowest effective dose may be repeated when symptoms return. May cause bradycardia, increased bronchial secretions, seizures. Have atropine ready to reverse excess effects. *Do not use for tricyclic antidepressant overdose.*
Pralidoxime (2-PAM)	Organophosphate anticholinesterases	Adult dose is 1 g IV, which may be repeated every 3–4 hours as needed or preferably as a constant infusion of 250–400 mg/h. Pediatric dose is approximately 250 mg. No proved benefit in carbamate poisoning.

assists in correction of fluid and electrolyte imbalance and may also enhance removal of toxic metabolites (eg, formate in methanol poisoning, oxalate and glycolate in ethylene glycol poisoning). The efficiency of both peritoneal dialysis and hemodialysis is a function of the molecular weight, water solubility, protein binding, endogenous clearance, and distribution in the body of the specific toxin. Hemodialysis is especially useful in overdose cases in which fluid and electrolyte imbalances are present (eg, salicylate intoxication).

3. Hemoperfusion–Blood is pumped from the patient via a venous catheter through a column of adsorbent material and then recirculated to the patient. Systemic anticoagulation with heparin is required to prevent the blood from clotting in the cartridge. Hemoperfusion does not improve fluid and electrolyte balance. However, it does remove many high-molecular-weight toxins that have poor water solubility because the perfusion cartridge has a large surface area for adsorption that is directly perfused with the blood and is not impeded by a membrane. The rate-limiting factors in removal of toxins by hemoperfusion are the affinity of the adsorbent resin for the drug, the rate of blood flow through the cartridge, and the rate of equilibration of the drug from the peripheral tissues to the blood. Hemoperfusion may enhance whole body clearance of salicylate, phenytoin, ethchlorvynol, phenobarbital, theophylline, and carbamazepine. Complications such as embolization of adsorbed particles, depletion of blood cells, and removal of proteins, solutes, and steroids have been minimized with increasing clinical experience.

B. Forced Diuresis and Urinary pH Manipulation: Previously popular but of unproved value, forced diuresis may cause volume overload and electrolyte abnormalities and is not recommended. Renal elimination of a few toxins can be enhanced by alteration of urinary pH. For example, urinary alkalinization is useful in cases of salicylate or phenobarbital overdose. Acidification may increase the urine concentration of drugs such as phencyclidine and amphetamines but is not advised because it may worsen renal complications from rhabdomyolysis, which often accompanies the intoxication.

RATTLESNAKE ENVENOMATION

In the USA, rattlesnakes are the most common venomous reptiles. Bites are rarely fatal, and 20% do not involve envenomation. However, about 60% of bites cause significant morbidity due to the destructive digestive enzymes found in the venom. Evidence of rattlesnake envenomation includes severe pain, swelling, bruising, hemorrhagic bleb formation, and obvious fang marks. Systemic effects include nausea, vomiting, muscle fasciculations, tingling and metallic taste in the mouth, shock, and systemic coagulopathy with prolonged clotting time and reduced platelet count.

Studies have shown that emergency field remedies such as incision and suction, tourniquets, and ice packs are far more damaging than useful. Avoidance of unnecessary motion, on the other hand, does help to limit the spread of the venom. Definitive therapy relies on intravenous antivenin and should be started as soon as possible.

Before antivenin is administered, blood should be typed and cross-matched. For significant rattlesnake bite, at least five vials of polyvalent crotalid antivenin should be administered; if envenomation is severe, 10–20 vials may be required. After large doses of antivenin, signs of serum sickness often develop 10–12 days after treatment. Skin testing is usually done to determine horse serum sensitivity, but a negative test does not guarantee that anaphylaxis will not occur.

REFERENCES

Ellenhorn MJ, et al (editors): *Ellenhorn's Medical Toxicology. Diagnosis and Treatment of Human Poisoning.* 2nd ed. Williams & Wilkins, 1997.

Goldfrank LR et al (editors): *Goldfrank's Toxicologic Emergencies,* 5th ed. Appleton & Lange, 1994.

Gosselin RE et al: *Clinical Toxicology of Commercial Products,* 6th ed. Williams & Wilkins, 1988.

Haddad LM, Winchester JF (editors): *Clinical Management of Poisoning and Drug Overdose,* 2nd ed. Saunders, 1990.

Hathaway GL et al: *Proctor and Hughes' Chemical Hazards of the Workplace,* 3rd ed. Van Nostrand, Reinhold, 1994.

Klaassen CD, Amdur MO, Doull J (editors): *Casarett and Doull's Toxicology: The Basic Science of Poisons,* 5th ed. Macmillan, 1995.

Olson KR et al (editors): *Poisoning & Drug Overdose,* 2nd ed. Appleton & Lange, 1994.

Rumack BH (editor): *Poisindex.* (Revised Quarterly.) Micromedex, 1997.

Section X.
Special Topics

Special Aspects of Perinatal & Pediatric Pharmacology

60

Gideon Koren, MD

The effects of drugs on the fetus and newborn infant are based on the general principles set forth in Chapters 1–4 of this book. However, the physiologic contexts in which these pharmacologic laws operate are different in pregnant women and in rapidly maturing infants. At present, the special pharmacokinetic factors operative in these patients are beginning to be understood, whereas information regarding pharmacodynamic differences (eg, receptor characteristics and response) is still incomplete. This chapter presents basic principles of pharmacology in the special context of perinatal and pediatric therapeutics.

DRUG THERAPY IN PREGNANCY

Pharmacokinetics

Most drugs taken by pregnant women can cross the placenta and expose the developing embryo and fetus to their pharmacologic and teratogenic effects. Critical factors affecting placental drug transfer and drug effects on the fetus include the following: (1) The physicochemical properties of the drug. (2) The rate at which the drug crosses the placenta and the amount of drug reaching the fetus. (3) The duration of exposure to the drug. (4) Distribution characteristics in different fetal tissues. (5) The stage of placental and fetal development at the time of exposure to the drug. (6) The effects of drugs used in combination.

A. Lipid Solubility: As is true also of other biologic membranes, drug passage across the placenta is dependent on lipid solubility and the degree of drug ionization. Lipophilic drugs tend to diffuse readily across the placenta and enter the fetal circulation. For example, thiopental, a drug commonly used for cesarean sections, crosses the placenta almost immediately and can produce sedation or apnea in the newborn infant. Highly ionized drugs such as succinylcholine and tubocurarine, also used for cesarean sections, cross the placenta slowly and achieve very low concentrations in the fetus. Impermeability of the placenta to polar compounds is relative rather than absolute. If high enough maternal-fetal concentration gradients are achieved, polar compounds cross the placenta in measurable amounts. Salicylate, which is almost completely ionized at physiologic pH, crosses the placenta rapidly. This occurs because the small amount of salicylate that is not ionized is highly lipid-soluble.

B. Molecular Size: The molecular weight of the drug also influences the rate of transfer and the amount of drug transferred across the placenta. Drugs with molecular weights of 250–500 can cross the placenta easily, depending upon their lipid solubility and degree of ionization; those with molecular weights of 500–1000 cross the placenta with more difficulty; and those with molecular weights greater than 1000 cross very poorly. An important clinical application of this property is the choice of heparin as an anticoagulant in pregnant women. Because it is a very large (and polar) molecule, heparin is unable to cross the placenta. Unlike warfarin, which is teratogenic and should be avoided during the first trimester, heparin may be safely given to pregnant women who need anticoagulation. Apparent exceptions to the "size rule" are maternal antibody globulins and certain polypeptides that cross the placenta by some selective mechanism that has not yet been identified.

C. Protein Binding: The degree to which a drug is bound to plasma proteins (particularly albumin) may also affect the rate of transfer and the amount transferred. However, if a compound is very lipid-soluble (eg, some anesthetic gases), it will not be affected greatly by protein binding. Transfer of these more lipid-soluble drugs and their overall rates of equilibration are more dependent on (and proportionate to) placental blood flow. This is because very lipid-soluble drugs diffuse across placental membranes so rapidly that their overall rates of equilibration do not depend on the free drug concentrations becoming equal on both sides. If a drug is poorly lipid-soluble and is ionized, its transfer is slow and will probably be impeded by its binding to maternal plasma proteins. Differential protein binding is also important, since some drugs exhibit greater protein binding in maternal plasma than in fetal plasma because of a lower binding affinity of fetal proteins. This has been shown for sulfonamides, barbiturates, phenytoin, and local anesthetic agents.

D. Placental and Fetal Drug Metabolism: Two mechanisms help to protect the fetus from drugs in the maternal circulation: (1) The placenta itself plays a role both as a semipermeable barrier and as a site of metabolism of some drugs passing through it. Several different types of aromatic oxidation reactions (eg, hydroxylation, *N*-dealkylation, demethylation) have been shown to occur in placental tissue. Pentobarbital is oxidized in this way. Conversely, it is possible that the metabolic capacity of the placenta may lead to creation of toxic metabolites, and the placenta may therefore augment toxicity (eg, ethanol, benzpyrenes). (2) Drugs that have crossed the placenta enter the fetal circulation via the umbilical vein. About 40–60% of umbilical venous blood flow enters the fetal liver; the remainder bypasses the liver and enters the general fetal circulation. A drug that enters the liver may be partially metabolized there before it enters the fetal circulation. In addition, a large proportion of drug present in the umbilical artery (returning to the placenta) may be shunted through the placenta back to the umbilical vein and into the liver again. It should be noted that metabolites of some drugs may be more active than the parent compound and may affect the fetus adversely.

Pharmacodynamics

A. Maternal Drug Actions: The effects of drugs on the reproductive tissues (breast, uterus, etc) of the pregnant woman are sometimes altered by the endocrine environment appropriate for the stage of pregnancy. Drug effects on other maternal tissues (heart, lungs, kidneys, central nervous system, etc) are not changed significantly by pregnancy, though the physiologic context (cardiac output, renal blood flow, etc) may be altered and may require the use of drugs that are not needed in the same woman when she is not pregnant. For example, cardiac glycosides and diuretics may be needed for congestive heart failure precipitated by the increased cardiac workload of pregnancy, or insulin may be required for control of blood glucose in pregnancy-induced diabetes.

B. Therapeutic Drug Actions in the Fetus: Fetal therapeutics is an emerging area in perinatal pharmacology. This involves drug administration to the pregnant woman with the fetus as the target of the drug. At present, corticosteroids are used to stimulate fetal lung maturation when premature birth is expected. Phenobarbital, when given to pregnant women near term, can induce fetal hepatic enzymes responsible for the glucuronidation of bilirubin, and

the incidence of jaundice is lower in newborns when mothers are given phenobarbital than when phenobarbital is not used. Before phototherapy became the preferred mode of therapy for neonatal indirect hyperbilirubinemia, phenobarbital was used for this indication. Recently, administration of phenobarbital to the mother has been shown to decrease the risk of intracranial bleeding in preterm infants. Antiarrhythmic drugs have also been given to mothers for treatment of fetal cardiac arrhythmias, though their efficacy has not yet been established by controlled studies.

C. Predictable Toxic Drug Actions in the Fetus: Chronic use of opioids by the mother may produce dependence in the fetus and newborn. This dependence may be manifested after delivery as a neonatal withdrawal syndrome. A less well understood fetal drug toxicity is caused by the use of angiotensin-converting enzyme inhibitors during pregnancy. These drugs can result in significant and irreversible renal damage in the fetus and are therefore contraindicated in pregnant women. Adverse effects may also be delayed, as in the case of female fetuses exposed to diethylstilbestrol (DES), who may be at increased risk for adenocarcinoma of the vagina after puberty.

D. Teratogenic Drug Actions: A single intrauterine exposure to a drug can affect the fetal structures undergoing rapid development at the time of exposure. Thalidomide is an example of a drug that may profoundly affect the development of the limbs after only brief exposure. This exposure, however, must be at a critical time in the development of the limbs. The thalidomide phocomelia risk occurs during the fourth through the seventh weeks of gestation because it is during this time that the arms and legs develop (Figure 60–1).

1. Teratogenic mechanisms–The mechanisms by which different drugs produce teratogenic effects are poorly understood and are probably multifactorial. For example, drugs may have a direct effect on maternal tissues with secondary or indirect effects on fetal tissues. Drugs may interfere with the passage of oxygen or nutrients through the placenta and therefore have effects on the most rapidly metabolizing tissues of the fetus. Finally, drugs may have important direct actions on the processes of differentiation in developing tissues. For example, vitamin A (retinol) has been shown to have important differentiation-directing actions in normal tissues. Several vitamin A analogs (isotretinoin, etretinate) are powerful teratogens, suggesting that they alter the normal processes of differentiation. Finally, deficiency of a critical substance appears to play a role in some types of abnormalities. For example, folic acid supplementation during pregnancy appears to reduce the incidence of neural tube defects, eg, spina bifida.

Continued exposure to a teratogen may produce cumulative effects or may affect several organs going through varying stages of development. Chronic con-

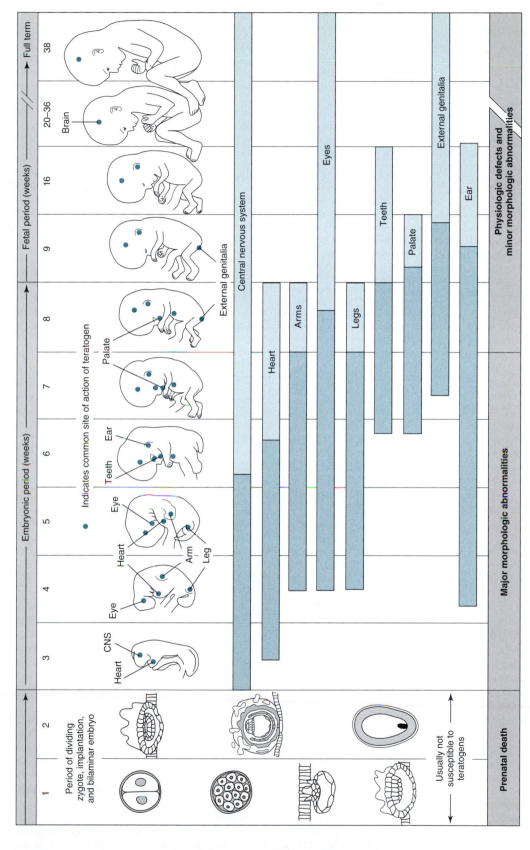

Figure 60–1. Schematic diagram of critical periods of human development. (Reproduced, with permission, from Moore KL: *The Developing Human, Clinically Oriented Embryology*, 4th ed. Saunders, 1988.)

sumption of high doses of ethanol during pregnancy, particularly during the first and second trimesters, may result in the fetal alcohol syndrome (Chapter 23). In this syndrome, the central nervous system, growth, and facial development may be affected.

2. Defining a teratogen–To be considered teratogenic, a candidate substance or process should (1) result in a characteristic set of malformations, indicating a selectivity for certain target organs; (2) exert its effects at a particular stage of fetal development, ie, during the limited time period of organogenesis of the target organs (Figure 60–1); and (3) show a dose-dependent incidence. Some drugs with known teratogenic or other adverse effects in pregnancy are listed in Table 60–1.

3. Counseling women about teratogenic risk–Since the thalidomide disaster, medicine has been practiced as if every drug were a potential human teratogen when, in fact, fewer than 30 such drugs have been identified, with hundreds of agents proved safe for the unborn. Owing to high levels of anxiety among pregnant women—and because half of the pregnancies in North America are unplanned—every year many thousands of women need counseling about fetal exposure to drugs, chemicals, and radiation. In the *Motherrisk* program in Toronto, Canada (Koren et al, 1990), hundreds of women are counseled every month, and the ability of appropriate counseling to prevent unnecessary abortions has been documented. Clinicians who wish to provide such counsel to pregnant women must ensure that their information is up to date and evidence-based and that the woman understands that the baseline teratogenic risk in pregnancy (ie, the risk of a neonatal abnormality in the absence of any known teratogenic exposure) is about 3%.

DRUG THERAPY IN INFANTS & CHILDREN

Physiologic processes that influence pharmacokinetic variables in the infant change significantly in the first year of life, particularly during the first few months. Therefore, special attention must be paid to pharmacokinetics in this age group. Pharmacodynamic differences between pediatric and other patients have not been explored in great detail and are probably small except for those specific target tissues that mature at birth or immediately thereafter, eg, the ductus arteriosus.

Drug Absorption

Drug absorption in infants and children follows the same general principles as in adults. Unique factors that influence drug absorption include blood flow at the site of administration, as determined by the physiologic status of the infant or child; and, for orally administered drugs, gastrointestinal function, which changes rapidly during the first few days after birth.

Age after birth also influences the regulation of drug absorption.

A. Blood Flow at the Site of Administration: Absorption after intramuscular or subcutaneous injection depends mainly, in neonates as in adults, on the rate of blood flow to the muscle or subcutaneous area injected. Physiologic conditions that might reduce blood flow to these areas are cardiovascular shock, vasoconstriction due to sympathomimetic agents, and heart failure. However, sick premature infants requiring intramuscular injections may have very little muscle mass. This is further complicated by diminished peripheral perfusion to these areas. In such cases, absorption becomes irregular and difficult to predict, because the drug may remain in the muscle and be absorbed more slowly than expected. If perfusion suddenly improves, there can be a sudden and unpredictable increase in the amount of drug entering the circulation, resulting in high and potentially toxic concentrations of drug. Examples of drugs especially hazardous in such situations are cardiac glycosides, aminoglycoside antibiotics, and anticonvulsants.

B. Gastrointestinal Function: Significant biochemical and physiologic changes occur in the neonatal gastrointestinal tract shortly after birth. In full-term infants, gastric acid secretion begins soon after birth and increases gradually over several hours. In premature infants, the secretion of gastric acid occurs more slowly, with the highest concentration appearing on the fourth day of life. Therefore, drugs that are partially or totally inactivated by the low pH of gastric contents should not be administered orally.

Gastric emptying time is prolonged (up to 6 or 8 hours) in the first day or so of life. Therefore, drugs that are absorbed primarily in the stomach may be absorbed more completely than anticipated. In the case of drugs absorbed in the small intestine, therapeutic effect may be delayed. Peristalsis in the neonate is irregular and may be slow. The amount of drug absorbed in the small intestine may therefore be unpredictable; more than the usual amount of drug may be absorbed if peristalsis is slowed, and this could result in potential toxicity from an otherwise standard dose. Table 60–2 summarizes data on oral bioavailability of various drugs in neonates as opposed to older children and adults. An increase in peristalsis, as in diarrheal conditions, tends to decrease the extent of absorption, since contact time with the large absorptive surface of the intestine is decreased.

Gastrointestinal enzyme activities tend to be lower in the newborn than in the adult. Activities of α-amylase and other pancreatic enzymes in the duodenum are low in infants up to 4 months of age. Neonates also have low concentrations of bile acids and lipase, which may decrease the absorption of lipid-soluble drugs.

Drug Distribution

As body composition changes with development, the distribution volumes of drugs are also changed.

Table 60–1. Drugs with significant adverse effects on the fetus.

Drug	Trimester	Effect
ACE inhibitors	All, especially second and third	Renal damage.
Aminopterin	First	Multiple gross anomalies.
Amphetamines	All	Abnormal developmental patterns, decreased school performance.
Androgens	Second and third	Masculinization of female fetus.
Antidepressants, tricyclic	Third	Neonatal withdrawal symptoms have been reported with clomipramine, desipramine, and imipramine.
Barbiturates	All	Chronic use can lead to neonatal dependence.
Busulfan	All	Various congenital malformations; low birth weight.
Carbamazepine	First	Neural tube defects
Chlorambucil	All	Genitourinary tract malformations.
Chlorpropamide	All	Prolonged symptomatic neonatal hypoglycemia.
Clomipramine	Third	Neonatal lethargy, hypotonia, cyanosis, hypothermia.
Cocaine	All	Increased risk of spontaneous abortion, abruptio placentae, and premature labor; neonatal cerebral infarction, abnormal development, and decreased school performance.
Cyclophosphamide	First	Various congenital malformations.
Cytarabine	First, second	Various congenital malformations.
Diazepam	All	Chronic use may lead to neonatal dependence.
Diethylstilbestrol	All	Vaginal adenosis, clear cell vaginal adenocarcinoma.
Ethanol	All	Risk of fetal alcohol syndrome in alcoholic mother.
Etretinate	All	High risk of multiple congenital malformations.
Heroin	All	Chronic use leads to neonatal dependence.
Iodide	All	Congenital goiter, hypothyroidism.
Isotretinoin	All	Extremely high risk of congenital anomalies.
Lithium	First	Ebstein's anomaly
Methadone	All	Chronic use leads to neonatal dependence.
Methotrexate	First	Multiple congenital malformations.
Methylthiouracil	All	Hypothyroidism.
Metronidazole	First	May be mutagenic (from animal studies; there is no evidence for mutagenic or teratogenic effects in humans).
Penicillamine	First	Cutis laxa, other congenital malformations.
Phencyclidine	All	Abnormal neurologic examination, poor suck reflex and feeding.
Phenytoin	All	Fetal hydantoin syndrome.
Propylthiouracil	All	Congenital goiter.
Smoking (constituents of tobacco smoke)	All	Intrauterine growth retardation; prematurity; sudden infant death syndrome; perinatal complications.
Streptomycin	All	Eighth nerve toxicity.
Tamoxifen	All	Increased risk of spontaneous abortion or fetal damage.
Tetracycline	All	Discoloration and defects of teeth and altered bone growth.
Thalidomide	First	Phocomelia (shortened or absent long bones of the limbs).
Trimethadione	All	Multiple congenital anomalies.
Valproic acid	All	Neural tube defects.
Warfarin	First	Hypoplastic nasal bridge, chondrodysplasia.
	Second	CNS malformations.
	Third	Risk of bleeding. Discontinue use 1 month before delivery.

Table 60–2. Oral drug absorption (bioavailability) of various drugs in the neonate compared with older children and adults.

Drug	Oral Absorption
Acetaminophen	Decreased
Ampicillin	Increased
Diazepam	Normal
Digoxin	Normal
Penicillin G	Increased
Phenobarbital	Decreased
Phenytoin	Decreased
Sulfonamides	Normal

The neonate has a higher percentage of its body weight in the form of water (70–75%) than does the adult (50–60%). Differences can also be observed between the full-term neonate (70% of body weight as water) and the small premature neonate (85% of body weight as water). Similarly, extracellular water is 40% of body weight in the neonate, compared with 20% in the adult. Most neonates will experience diuresis in the first 24–48 hours of life. Since many drugs are distributed throughout the extracellular water space, the size (volume) of the extracellular water compartment may be important in determining the concentration of drug at receptor sites. This is especially important for water-soluble drugs (such as aminoglycosides) and less crucial for lipid-soluble agents.

Premature infants have much less fat than full-term infants. Total body fat in premature infants is about 1% of total body weight, compared with 15% in full-term neonates. Therefore, organs that generally accumulate high concentrations of lipid-soluble drugs in adults and older children may accumulate smaller amounts of these agents in less mature infants.

Another major factor determining drug distribution is drug binding to plasma proteins. Albumin is the plasma protein with the greatest binding capacity. In general, protein binding of drugs is reduced in the neonate. This has been seen with local anesthetic drugs, diazepam, phenytoin, ampicillin, and phenobarbital. Therefore, the concentration of free (unbound) drug in plasma is increased. Because the free drug exerts the pharmacologic effect, this can result in greater drug effect or toxicity despite a normal or even low plasma concentration of total drug (bound plus unbound). As a practical example, consider a therapeutic dose of a drug, eg, diazepam, given to a patient. The concentration of total drug in the plasma is 300 μg/L. If the drug is 98% protein-bound in an older child or adult, then 6 μg/L is the concentration of free drug. Assume that this concentration of free drug produces the desired effect in the patient without producing toxicity. However, if this drug is given to a premature infant in a dosage adjusted for body weight

and it produces a total drug concentration of 300 μg/L—and protein binding is only 90%—then the free drug concentration will be 30 μg/L, or five times higher! Although the higher free concentration may result in faster elimination (Chapter 3), this concentration may be quite toxic initially.

Some drugs compete with serum bilirubin for binding to albumin. Drugs given to a neonate with jaundice can displace bilirubin from albumin. Because of the greater permeability of the neonatal blood-brain barrier, substantial amounts of bilirubin may enter the brain and cause kernicterus. This was in fact observed when sulfonamide antibiotics were given to premature neonates as prophylaxis against sepsis. Conversely, as the serum bilirubin rises for physiologic reasons or because of a blood group incompatibility, bilirubin can displace a drug from albumin and substantially raise the free drug concentration. This may occur without altering the total drug concentration and would result in greater therapeutic effect or toxicity at normal concentrations. This has been shown to happen with phenytoin.

Drug Metabolism

The metabolism of most drugs occurs in the liver (Chapter 4). The drug-metabolizing activities of the cytochrome P450-dependent mixed-function oxidases and the conjugating enzymes are substantially lower (50–70% of adult values) in early neonatal life than later. The point in development at which enzymatic activity is maximal depends upon the specific enzyme system in question. Glucuronide formation reaches adult values (per kilogram body weight) between the third and fourth years of life. Because of the neonate's decreased ability to metabolize drugs, many drugs have slow clearance rates and prolonged elimination half-lives. If drug doses and dosing schedules are not altered appropriately, this immaturity predisposes the neonate to adverse effects from drugs that are metabolized by the liver. Table 60–3 demonstrates how neonatal and adult drug elimination half-lives can differ and how the half-lives of phenobarbital and phenytoin decrease as the neonate grows older. The process of maturation must be considered when administering drugs to this age group, especially if the drug or drugs are administered over long periods.

Another consideration for the neonate is whether or not the mother was receiving drugs (such as phenobarbital) that can induce early maturation of fetal hepatic enzymes. In this case, the ability of the neonate to metabolize certain drugs will be greater than expected, and one may see less therapeutic effect and lower plasma drug concentrations when the usual neonatal dose is given.

Drug Excretion

The glomerular filtration rate is much lower in newborns than in older infants, children, or adults, and this limitation persists during the first few days of

Table 60–3. Approximate half-lives of various drugs in neonates and adults.

Drug	Neonatal Age	Neonates $t_{1/2}$ (hours)	Adults $t_{1/2}$ (hours)
Acetamino-phen		2.2–5	0.9–2.2
Diazepam		25–100	40–50
Digoxin		60–70	30–60
Phenobar-bital	0–5 days 5–15 days 1–30 months	200 100 50	64–140
Phenytoin	0–2 days 3–14 days 14–50 days	80 18 6	12–18
Salicylate		4.5–11	10–15
Theophylline	Neonate Child	13–26 3–4	5–10

life. Calculated on the basis of surface area, glomerular filtration in the neonate is only 30–40% of the adult value. The glomerular filtration rate is even lower in neonates born before 34 weeks of gestation. Function improves substantially during the first week of life. At the end of the first week, the glomerular filtration rate and renal plasma flow have increased 50% from the first day. By the end of the third week, glomerular filtration is 50–60% of the adult value; by 6–12 months, it reaches adult values (per unit surface area). Therefore, drugs that depend on renal function for elimination are cleared from the body very slowly in the first weeks of life.

Penicillins, for example, are cleared by premature infants at 17% of the adult rate based on comparable surface area and 34% of the adult rate when adjusted for body weight. The dosage of ampicillin for a neonate less than 7 days old is 50–100 mg/kg/d in two doses at 12-hour intervals. The dosage for a neonate over 7 days old is 100–200 mg/kg/d in three doses at 8-hour intervals. A decreased rate of renal elimination in the neonate has also been observed with aminoglycoside antibiotics (kanamycin, gentamicin, neomycin, streptomycin). The dosage of gentamicin for a neonate less than 7 days old is 5 mg/kg/d in two doses at 12-hour intervals. The dosage for a neonate over 7 days old is 7.5 mg/kg/d in three doses at 8-hour intervals. Total body clearance of digoxin is directly dependent upon adequate renal function, and accumulation of digoxin can occur when glomerular filtration is decreased. Since renal function in a sick infant may not improve at the predicted rate during the first weeks and months of life, appropriate adjustments in dosage and dosing schedules may be very difficult. In this situation, adjustments are best made on the basis of plasma drug concentrations determined at intervals throughout the course of therapy.

Special Pharmacodynamic Features in the Neonate

The appropriate use of drugs has made possible the survival of neonates with severe abnormalities who would otherwise die within days or weeks after birth. For example, administration of indomethacin (Chapter 35) causes the rapid closure of a patent ductus arteriosus, which would otherwise require surgical closure in an infant with a normal heart. Infusion of prostaglandin E₁, on the other hand, causes the ductus to remain open, which can be life-saving in an infant with transposition of the great vessels or tetralogy of Fallot (Chapter 18). An unexpected effect of such PGE_1 infusion has recently been described. The drug caused antral hyperplasia with gastric outlet obstruction as a clinical manifestation in 6 of 74 infants who received it (Peled et al, 1992). This phenomenon appears to be dose-dependent.

PEDIATRIC DOSAGE FORMS & COMPLIANCE

The form in which a drug is manufactured and the way in which the parent dispenses the drug to the child determine the actual dose administered. Many drugs prepared for children are in the form of elixirs or suspensions. **Elixirs** are alcoholic solutions in which the drug molecules are dissolved and evenly distributed. No shaking is required, and unless some of the vehicle has evaporated, the first dose from the bottle and the last dose should contain equivalent amounts of drug.

Suspensions contain undissolved particles of drug that must be distributed throughout the vehicle by shaking. If shaking is not thorough each time a dose is given, the first doses from the bottle may contain less drug than the last doses, with the result that less than the expected plasma concentration or effect of the drug may be achieved early in the course of therapy. Conversely, toxicity may occur late in the course of therapy, when it is not expected. This uneven distribution is a potential cause of inefficacy or toxicity in children taking phenytoin suspensions. It is thus essential that the prescriber know the form in which the drug will be dispensed and provide proper instructions to the pharmacist and patient or parent.

Compliance may be more difficult to achieve in pediatric practice than otherwise, since it involves not only the parent's conscientious effort to follow directions but also such practical matters as measuring errors, spilling, and spitting out. For example, the measured volume of "teaspoons" ranges from 2.5 to 7.8 mL. The parents should obtain a calibrated medicine spoon or syringe from the pharmacy. These devices improve the accuracy of dose measurements and simplify administration of drugs to children.

When evaluating compliance, it is often helpful to ask if an attempt has been made to give a further dose after the child has spilled half of what was offered. The parents may not always be able to say with confidence how much of a dose the child actually received. The parents must be told whether or not to wake the baby for its every-6-hour dose day or night. These matters should be discussed and made clear, and no assumptions should be made about what the parents may or may not do. Noncompliance frequently occurs when antibiotics are prescribed to treat otitis media or urinary tract infections and the child feels well after 4 or 5 days of therapy. The parents may not feel there is any reason to continue giving the medicine even though it was prescribed for 10 or 14 days. This common situation should be anticipated so the parents can be told why it is important to continue the medicine for the prescribed period even if the child seems to be "cured."

Practical and convenient dosage forms and dosing schedules should be chosen to the extent possible. The easier it is to administer and take the medicine and the easier the dosing schedule is to follow, the more likely it is that compliance will be achieved.

Consistent with their ability to comprehend and cooperate, children should also be given some responsibility for their own health care and for taking medications. This should be discussed in appropriate terms both with the child and the parents. Possible adverse effects and drug interactions with over-the-counter medicines or foods should also be discussed. Whenever a drug does not achieve its therapeutic effect, the possibility of noncompliance should be considered. There is ample evidence that in such cases parents' or children's reports may be grossly inaccurate. Random measurement of serum concentrations and pill count may help disclose noncompliance. The use of computerized pill containers, which record each lid opening, has been shown to be very effective in measuring compliance.

DRUG USE DURING LACTATION
(Table 60–4)

Drugs should be used conservatively during lactation, and the physician must know which drugs are potentially dangerous to nursing infants (Table 60–4). Most drugs administered to lactating women are detectable in breast milk. Fortunately, the concentration of drugs achieved in breast milk is usually low. Therefore, the total amount the infant would receive in a day is substantially less than what would be considered a "therapeutic dose." If the nursing mother must take medications and the drug is a relatively safe one, she should optimally take it 30–60 minutes after nursing and 3–4 hours before the next feeding. This allows time for many drugs to be cleared from the mother's blood, and the concentrations in breast milk will be relatively low. Drugs for which no data are available on safety during lactation should be avoided or breast feeding discontinued while they are being given.

Most antibiotics taken by nursing mothers can be detected in breast milk. Tetracycline concentrations in breast milk are approximately 70% of maternal serum concentrations and present a risk of permanent tooth staining in the infant. Chloramphenicol concentrations in breast milk are not sufficient to cause the gray baby syndrome, but there is a remote possibility of causing bone marrow suppression, and chloramphenicol should be avoided during lactation. Isoniazid rapidly reaches equilibrium between breast milk and maternal blood. The concentrations achieved in breast milk are high enough so that signs of pyridoxine deficiency may occur in the infant if the mother is not given pyridoxine supplements.

Most sedatives and hypnotics achieve concentrations in breast milk sufficient to produce a pharmacologic effect in some infants. Barbiturates taken in hypnotic doses by the mother can produce lethargy, sedation, and poor suck reflexes in the infant. Chloral hydrate can produce sedation if the infant is fed at peak milk concentrations. Diazepam can have a sedative effect on the nursing infant, but most importantly, its long half-life can result in significant drug accumulation.

Opioids such as heroin, methadone, and morphine enter breast milk in quantities potentially sufficient to prolong the state of neonatal narcotic dependence if the drug was taken chronically by the mother during pregnancy. If conditions are well controlled and there is a good relationship between the mother and the physician, an infant could be breast-fed while the mother is taking methadone. She should not, however, stop taking the drug abruptly; the infant can be tapered off the methadone as the mother's dose is tapered. The infant should be watched for signs of narcotic withdrawal.

Minimal use of alcohol by the mother has not been reported to harm nursing infants. Excessive amounts of alcohol, however, can produce alcohol effects in the infant. Nicotine concentrations in the breast milk of smoking mothers are low and do not produce effects in the infant. Very small amounts of caffeine are excreted in the breast milk of coffee-drinking mothers.

Lithium enters breast milk in concentrations equal to those in maternal serum. Clearance of this drug is almost completely dependent upon renal elimination, and women who are receiving lithium may expose the baby to relatively large amounts of the drug.

Radioactive substances such as iodinated ^{125}I albumin and radioiodine can cause thyroid suppression in infants and may increase the risk of subsequent thyroid cancer as much as tenfold. Breast feeding is contraindicated after large doses and should be withheld for days to weeks after small doses. Similarly, breast feeding should be avoided in mothers receiving cancer chemotherapy or being treated with similar agents for collagen diseases such as lupus erythematosus or post transplant.

Table 60–4. Drugs often used during lactation and possible effects on the nursing infant.

Drug	Effect on Infant	Comments
Ampicillin	Minimal	No significant adverse effects; possible occurrence of diarrhea or allergic sensitization.
Aspirin	Minimal	Occasional doses probably safe; high doses may produce significant concentration in breast milk.
Caffeine	Minimal	Caffeine intake in moderation is safe; concentration in breast milk is about 1% of that in the mother.
Chloral hydrate	Significant	May cause drowsiness if fed at peak concentration in milk.
Chloramphenicol	Significant	Concentrations too low to cause gray baby syndrome; possibility of bone marrow suppression does exist; recommend not taking chloramphenicol while breast feeding.
Chlorothiazide	Minimal	No adverse effects reported.
Chlorpromazine	Minimal	Appears insignificant.
Codeine	Minimal	No adverse effects reported.
Diazepam	Significant	Will cause sedation in breast-fed infants; accumulation can occur in newborns.
Dicumarol	Minimal	No adverse side effects reported; may wish to follow infant's prothrombin time.
Digoxin	Minimal	Insignificant quantities enter breast milk.
Ethanol	Moderate	Moderate ingestion by mother unlikely to produce effects in infant; large amounts consumed by mother can produce alcohol effects in infant.
Heroin	Significant	Enters breast milk and can prolong neonatal narcotic dependence.
Iodine (radioactive)	Significant	Enters milk in quantities sufficient to cause thyroid suppression in infant.
Isoniazid (INH)	Minimal	Milk concentrations equal maternal plasma concentrations. Possibility of pyridoxine deficiency developing in the infant.
Kanamycin	Minimal	No adverse effects reported.
Lithium	Significant	Avoid breast feeding unless levels can be measured.
Methadone	Significant	(See heroin.) Under close physician supervision, breast feeding can be continued. Signs of opiate withdrawal in the infant may occur if mother stops taking methadone or stops breast feeding abruptly.
Oral contraceptives	Minimal	May suppress lactation in high doses.
Penicillin	Minimal	Very low concentrations in breast milk.
Phenobarbital	Moderate	Hypnotic doses can cause sedation in the infant.
Phenytoin	Moderate	Amounts entering breast milk are not sufficient to cause adverse effects in infant.
Prednisone	Moderate	Low maternal doses (5 mg/d) probably safe. Doses 2 or more times physiologic amounts (> 15 mg/d) should probably be avoided.
Propranolol	Minimal	Very small amounts enter breast milk.
Propylthiouracil	Significant	Can suppress thyroid function in infant.
Spironolactone	Minimal	Very small amounts enter breast milk.
Tetracycline	Moderate	Possibility of permanent staining of developing teeth in the infant. Should be avoided during lactation.
Theophylline	Moderate	Can enter breast milk in moderate quantities but not likely to produce significant effects.
Thyroxine	Minimal	No adverse effects in therapeutic doses.
Tolbutamide	Minimal	Low concentrations in breast milk.
Warfarin	Minimal	Very small quantities found in breast milk.

PEDIATRIC DRUG DOSAGE

Because of differences in pharmacokinetics in infants and children, simple proportionate reduction in the adult dose may not be adequate to determine a safe and effective pediatric dose. The most reliable pediatric dose information is usually that provided by the manufacturer in the package insert. However, such information is not available for the majority of products even when studies have been published in the

Table 60–5. Determination of drug dosage from surface area.[1,2]

Weight (kg)	(lb)	Approximate Age	Surface Area (m²)	Percent of Adult Dose
3	6.6	Newborn	0.2	12
6	13.2	3 months	0.3	18
10	22	1 year	0.45	28
20	44	5.5 years	0.8	48
30	66	9 years	1	60
40	88	12 years	1.3	78
50	110	14 years	1.5	90
60	132	Adult	1.7	102
70	154	Adult	1.76	103

[1] Reproduced, with permission, from Silver HK, Kempe CH, Bruyn HB: *Handbook of Pediatrics,* 14th ed. Lange, 1983.
[2] For example, if adult dose is 1 mg/kg, dose for 3-month-old infant would be 2 mg/kg (18% of 70 mg/6 kg).

medical literature—reflecting the reluctance of manufacturers to label their products for children. Recently, the Food & Drug Administration has moved toward more explicit expectations that manufacturers test their new products in infants and children. In the absence of explicit pediatric dose recommendations, an approximation can be made by any of several methods based on age, weight, or surface area. These rules are not precise and should not be used if the manufacturer provides a pediatric dose. Most drugs approved for use in children have recommended pediatric doses, generally stated as milligrams per kilogram or per pound. When pediatric doses are calculated (either from one of the methods set forth below or from a manufacturer's dose), the pediatric dose should never exceed the adult dose.

Surface Area

Calculations of dosage based on age or weight (see below) are conservative and tend to underestimate the required dose. Doses based on surface area (Table 60–5) are more likely to be adequate.

Age (Young's rule):

$$\text{Dose} = \text{Adult dose} \times \frac{\text{Age (years)}}{\text{Age} + 12}$$

Weight (somewhat more precise is Clark's rule):

$$\text{Dose} = \text{Adult dose} \times \frac{\text{Weight (kg)}}{70}$$

or

$$\text{Dose} = \text{Adult dose} \times \frac{\text{Weight (lb)}}{150}$$

REFERENCES

American Academy of Pediatrics, Committee on Drugs: Emergency drug doses for infants and children. Pediatrics 1988;81:462.

Benitz WE, Tatro DS: *The Pediatric Drug Handbook,* 3rd ed. Year Book, 1995.

Besunder JB, Reed MD, Blumer JL: Principles of drug biodisposition in the neonate: A critical evaluation of the pharmacokinetic-pharmacodynamic interface. (Two parts.) Clin Pharmacokinet 1988;14:189, 261.

Briggs GG, Freeman RK, Yaffe SJ: *Drugs in Pregnancy and Lactation. A Reference Guide to Fetal and Neonatal Risk.* 4th ed. Williams & Wilkins, 1994.

Drug toxicity in the newborn. (Symposium.) Fed Proc 1985; 44:2301.

Gilman JT: Therapeutic drug monitoring in the neonate and paediatric age group: Problems and clinical pharmacokinetic implications. Clin Pharmacokinet 1990;19:1.

Hansten PD: *Drug Interactions.* Applied Therapeutics, Lea & Febiger, 1997. [Quarterly.]

Heymann MA: Non-narcotic analgesics: Use in pregnancy and fetal and perinatal effects. Drugs 1986;32(Suppl 4): 164.

Ito S, Koren G: Fetal drug therapy. Perinat Clin North Am 1994;21:1.

Koren G: *Maternal-Fetal Toxicology; A Clinician's Guide,* 2nd ed. Marcel Dekker, 1994.

Koren G, Pastuszak A: Prevention of unnecessary pregnancy terminations by counselling women on drug, chemical, and radiation exposure during the first trimester. Teratology 1990;41:657.

Koren G, Prober C, Gold R: *Antimicrobial Therapy in Infants and Children.* Marcel Dekker, 1987.

Morselli PL: Clinical pharmacology of the perinatal period and early infancy. Clin Pharmacokinet 1989;17(Suppl 1):13.

Nau H: Clinical pharmacokinetics in pregnancy and perinatology: 2. Penicillins. Dev Pharmacol Ther 1987;10:174.

Nottarianni LJ: Plasma protein binding of drugs in pregnancy and in neonates. Clin Pharmacokinet 1990;18:20.

Paap CM, Nahata MC: Clinical pharmacokinetics of antibacterial drugs in neonates. Clin Pharmacokinet 1990;19:280.

Peled N et al: Gastric-outlet obstruction induced by prostaglandin therapy in neonates. N Engl J Med 1992;327:505.

Roberts RJ: *Drug Therapy in Infants: Pharmacologic Principles and Clinical Experience.* Saunders, 1984.

Rousseaux CG, Blakely PM: Fetus. In *Handbook of Toxicologic Pathology.* Haschek WM, Rousseaux CG (editors). Academic Press, 1991.

Safety of antimicrobial drugs in pregnancy. Med Lett Drugs Ther 1987;29:61.

Stewart CF, Hampton EM: Effect of maturation on drug disposition in pediatric patients. Clin Pharm 1987;6:548.

Valdes-Dapena M: Iatrogenic disease in the perinatal period. Pediatr Clin North Am 1989;36:67.

Wilson JT (editor): *Drugs in Breast Milk.* ADIS Press, 1981.

Special Aspects of Geriatric Pharmacology

61

Bertram G. Katzung, MD, PhD

Society often classifies everyone over 65 as "elderly," but most authorities consider the field of geriatrics to apply to persons over 75—even though this too is an arbitrary definition. Furthermore, chronologic age is only one determinant of the changes pertinent to drug therapy that occur in older people. Important changes in responses to some drugs occur with increasing age in many individuals. For other drugs, age-related changes are minimal, especially in the "healthy old." Drug usage patterns also change as a result of the increasing incidence of disease with age and the tendency to prescribe heavily for patients in nursing homes. General changes in the lives of older people have significant effects on the way drugs are used. Among these changes are the increased incidence with advancing age of multiple diseases, nutritional problems, reduced financial resources, and—in some patients—decreased dosing compliance for a variety of reasons.

The health practitioner thus should be aware of the changes in pharmacologic responses that may occur in older people and how to deal with these changes.

PHARMACOLOGIC CHANGES ASSOCIATED WITH AGING

In the general population, measurements of functional capacity of most of the major organ systems show a decline beginning in young adulthood and continuing throughout life. As shown in Figure 61–1, there is no "middle-age plateau" but rather a linear decrease beginning no later than age 45. However, these data reflect the mean and do not apply to every person above a certain age; approximately one-third of healthy subjects have no age-related decrease in, for example, creatinine clearance. Thus, the elderly do not lose specific functions at an accelerated rate compared with young and middle-aged adults but rather accumulate more deficiencies with the passage of time. Some of these changes result in altered pharma-

cokinetics. For the pharmacologist and the clinician, the most important of these is the decrease in renal function. Other changes and concurrent diseases may alter the pharmacodynamic characteristics of the patient.

Pharmacokinetic Changes

A. Absorption: There is little evidence that there is any major alteration in drug absorption with age. However, conditions associated with age may alter the rate at which some drugs are absorbed. Such conditions include altered nutritional habits, greater consumption of nonprescription drugs (eg, antacids, laxatives), and changes in gastric emptying, which is often slower in older persons.

B. Distribution: As noted in Chapters 1 and 3, the distribution of a drug is a function of the chemical characteristics of the drug molecule, blood flow, and the size and composition of the compartments of the body. The elderly have reduced lean body mass, reduced total and percentage body water, and an increase in fat as a percentage of body mass. Some of these changes are shown in Table 61–1. There is usually a decrease in serum albumin, which binds many drugs, especially weak acids. There may be a concurrent increase in serum orosomucoid (α-acid glycoprotein), a protein that binds many basic drugs. Thus, the ratio of bound to free drug may be significantly altered. As explained in Chapter 3, these changes may alter the appropriate loading dose of a drug. However, since both the clearance and the effects of drugs are related to the free concentration, the steady state effects of a maintenance dosage regimen should not be altered by these factors alone. For example, the loading dose of digoxin in an elderly patient with congestive heart failure should be reduced because of the decreased apparent volume of distribution. The maintenance dose may have to be reduced because of reduced clearance of the drug.

C. Metabolism: The capacity of the liver to metabolize drugs does not appear to decline consistently

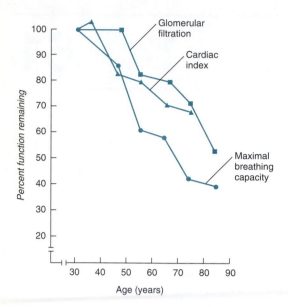

Figure 61–1. Effect of age on some physiologic functions. (Modified and reproduced, with permission, from Kohn RR: *Principles of Mammalian Aging.* Prentice-Hall, 1978.)

Table 61–2. Effects of age on hepatic clearance of some drugs. (1) Phase I metabolism by hepatic mixed function oxidase system; (2) phase II metabolism (conjugation) or phase I metabolism by nonmicrosomal systems.

Age-Related Decrease in Hepatic Clearance Found	No Age Difference Found
Alprazolam (1)	Ethanol (2)
Barbiturates (1)	Isoniazid (2)
Carbenoxolone (1)	Lidocaine (1)
Chlordiazepoxide (1)	Lorazepam (2)
Chlormethiazole (1)	Nitrazepam (2)
Clobazam (1)	Oxazepam (2)
Desmethyldiazepam (1)	Prazosin (1)
Diazepam (1)	Salicylate (2)
Flurazepam (1)	Warfarin (1)
Imipramine (1)	
Meperidine (1)	
Nortriptyline (1)	
Phenylbutazone (1)	
Propranolol (1)	
Quinidine, quinine (1)	
Theophylline (1)	
Tolbutamide (1)	

with age for all drugs. Animal studies and some clinical studies have suggested that certain drugs are metabolized more slowly; some of these drugs are listed in Table 61–2. It would appear that the greatest changes are in phase I reactions, ie, those carried out by the microsomal mixed-function oxidase system; there are much smaller changes in the ability of the liver to carry out conjugation (phase II) reactions (Chapter 4). Some of these changes may be caused by decreased liver blood flow (Table 61–1), an important variable in the clearance of drugs that have a high hepatic extraction ratio. In addition, there is a decline with age of the liver's ability to recover from injury, eg, that caused by alcohol or viral hepatitis. There-

fore, a history of recent liver disease in an older person should lead to caution in dosing with drugs that are cleared primarily by the liver, even after apparently complete recovery from the hepatic insult. Finally, malnutrition and diseases that affect hepatic function—eg, congestive heart failure—are more common in the elderly. Congestive heart failure may dramatically alter the ability of the liver to metabolize drugs and may also reduce hepatic blood flow. Similarly, severe nutritional deficiencies, which occur more often in old age, may impair hepatic function.

D. Elimination: Because the kidney is the major organ for clearance of drugs from the body, the "natural" decline of renal functional capacity referred to above is very important. As shown in Table 61–3, there is an age-related decline in creatinine clearance; this occurs in about two-thirds of the population. It is important to note that this decline is not reflected in

Table 61–1. Some changes related to aging that affect pharmacokinetics of drugs.

Variable	Young Adults (20–30 years)	Geriatric Adults (60–80 years)
Body water (% of body weight)	61	53
Lean body mass (% of body weight)	19	12
Body fat (% of body weight)	26–33 (women) 18–20 (men)	38–45 36–38
Serum albumin (g/dL)	4.7	3.8
Kidney weight (% of young adult)	(100)	80
Hepatic blood flow (% of young adult)	(100)	55–60

Table 61–3. Effects of age on creatinine clearance, serum creatinine concentration, and total body creatinine production.[1]

Age (years)	Creatinine Clearance (mL/min)[2]	Serum Creatinine Concentration (mg/dL)	Creatinine Production (mg/24 h)
17–24	140	0.81	1790
25–34	140	0.81	1862
35–44	133	0.81	1746
45–54	127	0.83	1689
55–64	120	0.84	1580
65–74	110	0.83	1409
75–84	97	0.84	1259

[1] Modified and reproduced, with permission, from Rowe JW et al: The effect of age on creatinine clearance in men: A cross-sectional and longitudinal study. J Gerontol 1976;31:155.
[2] Normalized to 1.73 m² body surface area.

an equivalent rise in serum creatinine because the production of creatinine is also reduced as muscle mass declines with age. The practical result of this change is marked prolongation of the half-life of many drugs (Figure 61–2) and the possibility of accumulation to toxic levels if dosage is not reduced in size or frequency. Dosing recommendations for the elderly often include an allowance for reduced renal clearance. If only the young adult dosage is known for a drug that requires renal clearance, a rough correction can be made by using the Cockcroft-Gault formula (Cockcroft et al, 1976), which is applicable to patients from age 40 through age 80:

Creatine clearence (mL/min) =

$$\frac{(140 - \text{age}) \times (\text{weight in kg})}{72 \times \text{serum creatinine in mg/dL}}$$

For women, the result should be multiplied by 0.85. It must be emphasized that this estimate is, at best, a *population* estimate and may not apply to a particular patient (Goldberg et al, 1987). If the patient has normal renal function (up to one-third of patients), a dose corrected on the basis of this estimate will be too low—but a low dose is initially desirable if one is uncertain of the renal function in any patient. If a precise measure is needed, a standard 12- or 24-hour creatinine clearance determination should be done. As indicated above, nutritional changes alter pharmacokinetic parameters. A patient who is severely dehydrated (not uncommon in patients with stroke or other motor impairment) may have an additional marked reduction in renal drug clearance that is completely reversible by rehydration.

The lungs are important for the excretion of volatile drugs. As a result of reduced respiratory capacity (Figure 61–1) and the increased incidence of active pulmonary disease in the elderly, the use of inhalation anesthesia is less common and parenteral agents more common in this age group. (See Chapter 25.)

Pharmacodynamic Changes

It was long believed that geriatric patients were much more "sensitive" to the action of many drugs, implying a change in the pharmacodynamic interaction of the drugs with their receptors. It is now recognized that many—perhaps most—of these apparent changes result from altered pharmacokinetics or diminished homeostatic responses. Clinical studies have supported the idea that the elderly are more sensitive to *some* sedative-hypnotics and analgesics. In addition, there are some data from animal studies that suggest actual changes with age in the characteristics or numbers of certain receptors. The most extensive studies show a decrease in responsiveness to beta-adrenoceptor stimulants and beta-blockers. Other examples are discussed below.

Certain homeostatic control mechanisms appear to be blunted in the elderly. Since homeostatic responses are often important components of the total response to a drug, these physiologic alterations may change the pattern or intensity of drug response. In the cardiovascular system, the cardiac output increment required by mild or moderate exercise is successfully provided to at least age 75 (in individuals without obvious cardiac disease), but the increase is the result primarily of increased stroke volume in the elderly and not tachycardia, as in young adults. Average blood pressure goes up with age (in most Western countries), but the incidence of symptomatic orthostatic hypotension also increases markedly. Similarly, the average 2-hour postprandial blood sugar increases by about 1 mg/dL for each year of age above 50. Temperature regulation is also impaired, and hypothermia is poorly tolerated in the elderly.

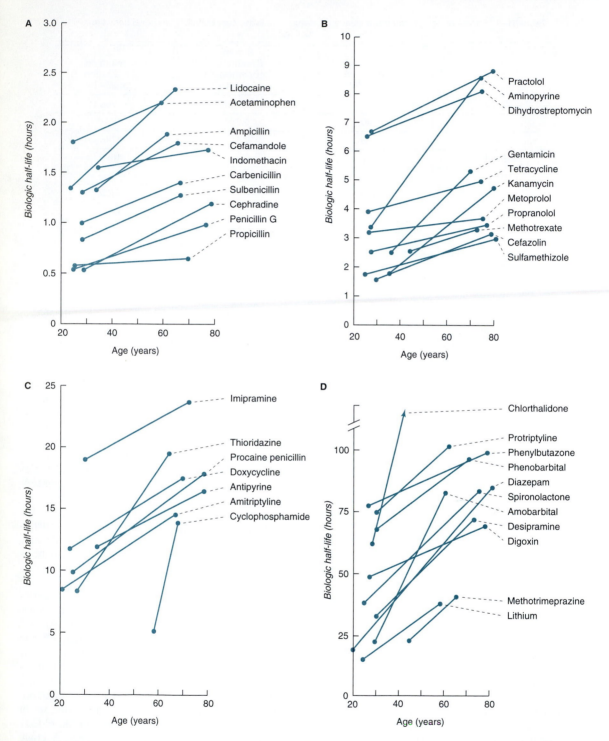

Figure 61–2. Increase in half-life of some drugs with age. The drugs have been grouped on the basis of half-life. **A:** 0.5–3 hours; **B:** 1–10 hours; **C:** 5–25 hours; **D:** 20–370 hours. Note that the lines merely connect the end points of the age range; they do not imply a linear relationship between age and half-life. (Modified and reproduced, with permission, from Ritschel WA: Pharmacokinetics in the aged. In: *Pharmacologic Aspects of Aging.* Pagliaro LA, Pagliaro AM [editors]. Mosby, 1983.)

MAJOR DRUG GROUPS

CENTRAL NERVOUS SYSTEM DRUGS

Sedative-Hypnotics

The half-lives of many benzodiazepines and barbiturates increase 50–150% between age 30 and age 70. Much of this change occurs during the decade from 60 to 70. For many of the benzodiazepines, both the parent molecule and its metabolites (produced in the liver) are pharmacologically active (Chapter 22). The age-related decline in renal function and liver disease, if present, both contribute to the reduction in elimination of these compounds. In addition, an increased volume of distribution has been reported for some of these drugs. Lorazepam and oxazepam may be less affected by these changes than the other benzodiazepines. In addition to these pharmacokinetic factors, it is generally believed that the elderly are more variable in their sensitivity to the sedative-hypnotic drugs on a pharmacodynamic basis as well. Among the toxicities of these drugs, ataxia and other aspects of motor impairment should be particularly watched for in order to avoid accidents (Ray et al, 1987; Ray, 1992).

Analgesics

The opioid analgesics show variable changes in pharmacokinetics with age. However, the elderly are often markedly more sensitive to the respiratory effects of these agents because of age-related changes in respiratory function. Therefore, this group of drugs should be used with caution until the sensitivity of the particular patient has been evaluated, and the patient should then be dosed appropriately for full effect. Studies show that opioids are consistently *underutilized* in patients who require strong analgesics for chronic painful conditions such as cancer (Portenoy et al, 1992). There is no justification for underutilization of these drugs, especially in the care of the elderly, and good pain management plans are readily available (Ashburn et al, 1993; Schug et al, 1992).

Antipsychotic & Antidepressant Drugs

The antipsychotic agents (phenothiazines and haloperidol) have been very heavily used (and probably misused) in the management of a variety of psychiatric diseases in the elderly. There is no doubt that they are useful in the management of schizophrenia in old age, and they are probably useful also in the treatment of some symptoms associated with delirium, dementia, agitation, combativeness, and a paranoid syndrome that appears in some geriatric patients. However, they are not fully satisfactory in these geriatric conditions, and dosage should not be increased on the assumption that full control is possible. There is no evidence that these drugs have any beneficial effects in Alzheimer's dementia, and on theoretical grounds the antimuscarinic effects of the phenothiazines might be expected to worsen memory impairment and intellectual dysfunction (see below). Much of the apparent improvement in agitated and combative patients may simply reflect the sedative effects of the drugs. When a sedative antipsychotic is desired, a phenothiazine such as thioridazine is appropriate. If sedation is to be avoided, haloperidol is more appropriate. The latter drug has increased extrapyramidal toxicity, however, and should be avoided in patients with preexisting extrapyramidal disease. The phenothiazines, especially older drugs such as chlorpromazine, often induce orthostatic hypotension in young adults because of their α-adrenoceptor-blocking effects. They are even more prone to do so in the elderly. (See also Chapter 29.)

Because of increased responsiveness to all these drugs, dosage should usually be started at a fraction of that used in young adults. The half-lives of some phenothiazines are increased in the geriatric population (Figure 61–2). Thioridazine's half-life, for example, is more than doubled. Plasma protein binding of fluphenazine is reduced, which results in an increase of the free drug:total drug ratio.

Lithium is often used in the treatment of mania in the aged. Because it is cleared by the kidneys, dosage must be adjusted appropriately. Concurrent use of thiazide diuretics reduces the clearance of lithium and should be accompanied by further reduction in dosage and more frequent measurement of lithium blood levels.

Psychiatric depression is thought to be underdiagnosed and undertreated in the elderly. The suicide rate in the over-65 age group (twice the national average) supports this view. Unfortunately, the apathy, flat affect, and social withdrawal of major depression may be mistaken for senile dementia. Clinical evidence suggests that the elderly are as responsive to the antidepressants (of all types) as younger patients but are more sensitive to their toxic effects (Preskorn, 1993). This factor along with the reduced clearance of some of these drugs underlines the importance of careful dosing and strict attention to the appearance of toxic effects. If a tricyclic antidepressant is to be used, a drug with reduced antimuscarinic effects should be selected, eg, nortriptyline or desipramine (Table 30–3). To minimize autonomic effects, a selective serotonin reuptake inhibitor may be chosen (Frank et al, 1993).

Drugs Used in Alzheimer's Disease

Alzheimer's disease is characterized by progressive impairment of memory and cognitive functions and may lead to a completely vegetative state. The biochemical defects responsible for these changes have not been identified, but in addition to evidence for abnormalities of neuronal lipoprotein processing (Poirer et al, 1995), there is much evidence for a marked decrease in choline acetyltransferase and other markers of cholinergic neuron activity and for changes in brain glutamate, dopamine, norepinephrine, serotonin, and somatostatin activity. Eventually, cholinergic and perhaps other neurons die or are destroyed. Patients with Alzheimer's disease are often exquisitely sensitive to the central nervous system toxicities of drugs with antimuscarinic effects.

Many methods of treatment of Alzheimer's disease have been explored (Gottlieb et al, 1993). Most attention has been focused on the cholinomimetic drugs because of the evidence for loss of cholinergic neurons noted above. MAO type B inhibition with selegiline (L-deprenyl) has been suggested to have some beneficial effects (Tariot et al, 1987). So-called cerebral vasodilators are ineffective (Thompson et al, 1990). "Ampakines," substances that facilitate synaptic activity at glutamate AMPA* receptors and nerve growth factors, are also under intense study.

Tacrine (tetrahydroaminoacridine, THA), a long-acting cholinesterase inhibitor and muscarinic modulator, has been extensively studied (Schneider, 1993; Knapp et al, 1994; Watkins et al, 1994). Tacrine is an orally active amine that enters the central nervous system readily and has a duration of effect of 6–8 hours. (In contrast, physostigmine has a duration of action of 1–2 hours.) Tacrine blocks both acetylcholinesterase and butyrylcholinesterase and has complex inhibitory effects on M_1 and M_2 cholinoceptors. It is also a weak nicotinic blocker. The drug apparently increases the release of acetylcholine from cholinergic nerve endings as well. Finally, tacrine may inhibit MAO, decrease the release of GABA, and increase the release of norepinephrine, dopamine, and serotonin from nerve endings. Other receptors (NMDA,* adenosine) and potassium channels may also be affected at higher concentrations of tacrine. In spite of its extremely broad range of effects, attention has focused on tacrine's cholinergic actions, and cholinomimetic analogs (eg, **velnacrine**) are currently under investigation. Tacrine causes cholinomimetic adverse effects, including nausea and vomiting, and significant hepatic toxicity. The latter is manifested by a reversible increase in serum AST or ALT levels of sufficient magnitude to require dose reduction or withdrawal in 40–50% of patients. Hepatocellular necrosis with jaundice has been reported (Schneider, 1993).

According to several double-blind trials, tacrine is effective in slowing the progress of Alzheimer's disease in some patients. Less toxic drugs are urgently needed, and the FDA recently approved another

cholinesterase inhibitor, **donepezil,** for use in this disease. Physostigmine is in clinical trials.

CARDIOVASCULAR DRUGS

Antihypertensive Drugs

As noted previously, blood pressure, especially systolic pressure, increases with age in Western countries and in most cultures in which salt intake is high. The increase is especially marked after age 50 in women. The high frequency and sometimes benign course of this form of late-onset systolic hypertension encourage a conservative approach to its treatment. On the other hand, diastolic hypertension and significant elevation of the systolic pressure above the age-corrected norm should be vigorously treated, since they are associated with a marked increase in the incidence of stroke, congestive heart failure, and renal failure (Gifford, 1987) and because effective treatment has been clearly shown to reduce the incidence of these sequelae.

The basic principles of therapy are not different in the geriatric age group from those described in Chapter 11, but the usual cautions regarding altered pharmacokinetics and sensitivity apply. Because of its safety, nondrug therapy (weight reduction in the obese and salt restriction) should be encouraged. Thiazides are a reasonable first step in drug therapy. The hypokalemia, hyperglycemia, and hyperuricemia caused by of these agents are more relevant in the elderly because of the higher incidence in these patients of arrhythmias, non-insulin-dependent diabetes, and gout. Thus, use of low antihypertensive doses—rather than maximum diuretic doses—is important. Calcium channel blockers are effective and safe if titrated to the appropriate response. They are especially useful if the patient also has atherosclerotic angina (Chapter 12). Beta-blockers are potentially hazardous in patients with obstructive airway disease and are considered less useful than calcium channel blockers in the older patient. ACE inhibitors are also considered less useful in the elderly. For more severe hypertension, methyldopa and hydralazine have proved effective and safe. The most powerful drugs, such as guanethidine and minoxidil, are rarely needed.

Positive Inotropic Agents

Congestive heart failure is a common and particularly lethal disease in the elderly. Fear of this condition may be one reason why physicians overuse cardiac glycosides in this age group. In one study, 90% of a group of elderly patients who were withdrawn from digoxin therapy had no recurrence of symptoms or signs of failure, ie, the drug was being used unnecessarily. The toxic effects of this drug group are particularly dangerous in the geriatric population, since the elderly are more susceptible to arrhythmias. The clearance of digoxin appears to be decreased in the older age group, and while the volume of distribution

* See Chapter 21.

is often decreased as well, the half-life of this drug may be increased by 50% or more. Because the drug is cleared by the kidneys, renal function must be considered in designing a dosage regimen. There is no evidence that there is any increase in pharmacodynamic sensitivity to the therapeutic effects of the cardiac glycosides; in fact, animal studies suggest a possible decrease in therapeutic sensitivity. On the other hand, as noted above, there is probably an increase in sensitivity to the toxic arrhythmogenic actions. Hypokalemia, hypomagnesemia, hypoxemia (from pulmonary disease), and coronary atherosclerosis all contribute to the high incidence of digitalis-induced arrhythmias in geriatric patients. The less common toxicities of digitalis such as delirium, visual changes, and endocrine abnormalities (Chapter 13) also occur more often in the elderly than in younger patients.

Antiarrhythmic Agents

The treatment of arrhythmias in the elderly is particularly challenging because of the lack of good hemodynamic reserve, the frequency of electrolyte disturbances, and the high incidence of severe coronary disease. The clearances of quinidine and procainamide decrease and their half-lives increase with age. Disopyramide should probably be avoided in the geriatric population because its major toxicities—antimuscarinic action, leading to voiding problems in men; and negative inotropic cardiac effects, leading to congestive heart failure—are particularly undesirable in these patients. The clearance of lidocaine appears to be little changed, but the half-life is increased in the elderly. Although this observation implies an increase in the volume of distribution, it has been recommended that the loading dose of this drug be reduced in geriatric patients because of their greater sensitivity to its toxic effects.

ANTIMICROBIAL DRUGS

Several age-related changes contribute to the high incidence of infections in geriatric patients. There appears to be a reduction in host defenses in the elderly; this is manifested in the increase in both serious infections and cancer. This may reflect an alteration in T lymphocyte function. In the case of the lungs, a major age- and tobacco-dependent decrease in mucociliary clearance significantly increases susceptibility to infection. In the urinary tract, the incidence of serious infection is greatly increased by urinary retention and catheterization in men.

Since 1940, the antimicrobial drugs have contributed more to the prolongation of life than any other drug group, because they can compensate to some extent for this deterioration in natural defenses. The basic principles of therapy of the elderly with these agents are no different from those applicable in younger patients and have been presented in Chapter 51. The major pharmacokinetic changes relate to decreased renal function; because most of the beta-lactam, aminoglycoside, and fluoroquinolone antibiotics are excreted by this route, important changes in half-life may be expected. This is particularly important in the case of the aminoglycosides, because they cause concentration-dependent toxicity in the kidney and in other organs. For gentamicin, kanamycin, and netilmicin, the half-lives are more than doubled. According to one study, the increase may not be so marked for tobramycin.

ANTI-INFLAMMATORY DRUGS

Osteoarthritis is a very common disease of the elderly. Rheumatoid arthritis is less exclusively a geriatric problem, but the same drug therapy is usually applicable. The basic principles laid down in Chapter 36 and the properties of the anti-inflammatory drugs described there apply fully here.

The nonsteroidal anti-inflammatory agents must be used with special care in the geriatric patient because they cause toxicities to which the elderly are very susceptible. In the case of aspirin, the most important of these is gastrointestinal irritation and bleeding. In the case of the newer NSAIDs, the most important is renal damage, which may be irreversible. Because they are cleared primarily by the kidneys, these drugs will accumulate more rapidly in the geriatric patient and especially in the patient whose renal function is already compromised beyond the average range for his or her age. A vicious cycle is easily set up in which cumulation of the NSAID causes more renal damage, which causes more cumulation, and so on. Benoxaprofen, a very efficacious NSAID, was withdrawn shortly after it was released because several elderly patients died in renal failure as a result of improper dosing. Elderly patients receiving high doses of any NSAID should be carefully monitored for changes in renal function.

Corticosteroids are extremely useful in elderly patients who cannot tolerate full doses of NSAIDs. However, they consistently cause a dose- and duration-related osteoporosis, an especially hazardous toxic effect in the elderly. It is not certain whether this drug-induced effect can be reduced by increased calcium and vitamin D intake, but it would seem prudent to consider these agents and to encourage frequent exercise in any patient taking corticosteroids.

ADVERSE DRUG REACTIONS IN THE ELDERLY

The positive relationship between number of drugs taken and the incidence of adverse reactions to them has been well documented. In long-term care facilities, which have a high population of the elderly, the average number of prescriptions per patient varies between 6.6 and 7.7. Studies have shown that the percentage of patients with adverse reactions increases from about 10% when a single drug is being taken to nearly 100% when ten drugs are taken. Thus, it may be expected that about half of patients in long-term care facilities will have recognized or unrecognized reactions at some time. The overall incidence of drug reactions in geriatric patients is estimated to be at least twice that in the younger population. Reasons for this high incidence undoubtedly include errors in prescribing on the part of the practitioner and errors in drug usage by the patient.

Practitioner errors sometimes occur because the physician does not appreciate the importance of changes in pharmacokinetics with age and age-related diseases. Some errors occur because the practitioner is unaware of incompatible drugs prescribed by other practitioners for the same patient. For example, cimetidine, a drug heavily prescribed to the elderly, has a much higher incidence of untoward effects (eg, confusion, slurred speech) in the geriatric population than in younger patients. It also inhibits the hepatic metabolism of many drugs, including phenytoin, warfarin, beta-blockers, and other agents. A patient who has been taking one of the latter agents without ill effect may develop markedly elevated blood levels and severe toxicity if cimetidine is added to the regimen without adjustment of dosage of the other drugs. Additional examples of drugs that inhibit liver microsomal enzymes and lead to adverse reactions are described in Appendix II.

Patient errors may result from noncompliance for reasons described below. In addition, they often result from use of nonprescription drugs that are taken without the knowledge of the physician. As noted in Chapter 64, many OTC agents contain "hidden ingredients" with potent pharmacologic effects. For example, many antihistamines have significant sedative effects and are inherently more hazardous in patients with impaired cognitive function. Similarly, their antimuscarinic action may precipitate urinary retention in the geriatric male or glaucoma in a patient with a narrow anterior chamber angle. If the patient is also taking a metabolism inhibitor such as cimetidine, the probability of an adverse reaction is greatly increased.

PRACTICAL ASPECTS OF GERIATRIC PHARMACOLOGY

The quality of life in elderly patients can be greatly improved and life can be prolonged by the intelligent use of drugs. However, there are several practical obstacles to compliance that the prescriber must recognize.

The expense of drugs can be a major disincentive in patients receiving marginal retirement incomes who are not covered by health insurance. The prescriber must be aware of the cost of the prescription and of cheaper alternative therapies. For example, the monthly cost of arthritis therapy with newer NSAIDs often exceeds $100, while that for generic aspirin is about $5 and for ibuprofen, an older NSAID, about $20.

Noncompliance may result from forgetfulness or confusion, especially if the patient has several prescriptions and different dosing intervals. A survey carried out in 1986 showed that the population over 65 years of age accounted for 25% of physician visits and 32% of drugs prescribed in the USA though the elderly represented only 11–12% of the population at that time. Since the prescriptions are often written by several different practitioners, there is usually no attempt to design "integrated" regimens that use drugs with similar dosing intervals for the conditions being treated. Patients may forget instructions regarding the need to complete a fixed duration of therapy when a course of anti-infective drug (for example) is being given. The disappearance of symptoms is often regarded as the best reason to halt drug taking, especially if the prescription was expensive.

Noncompliance may also be deliberate. A decision not to take a drug may be based on prior experience with it. There may be excellent reasons for such "intelligent" noncompliance, and the practitioner should try to elicit them. Such efforts may also improve compliance with alternative drugs, because enlisting the patient as a participant in therapeutic decisions tends to increase the motivation to succeed.

Some errors in drug taking are caused by physical disabilities. Arthritis, tremor, and visual problems may all contribute. Liquid medications that are to be measured out "by the spoonful" are especially inappropriate for patients with any type of tremor or motor disability. The use of a pediatric dosing syringe may be helpful in such cases. Because of decreased production of saliva, older patients often have difficulty swallowing large tablets. "Childproof" containers are often "patient-proof" if the patient has arthritis. Cataracts and macular degeneration occur in a large number of patients over 70; therefore, labels on prescription bottles should be large enough for the patient with diminished vision to read, or color-coded if the patient can see but can no longer read.

Drug therapy has considerable potential for both helpful and harmful effects in the geriatric patient. The balance may be tipped in the right direction by adherence to a few principles:

(1) Take a careful drug history. The disease to be treated may be drug-induced, or drugs being taken may lead to interactions with drugs to be prescribed.

(2) Prescribe only for a specific and rational indication. Do not prescribe cimetidine for "dyspepsia."

(3) Define the goal of drug therapy. Then start with

small doses and titrate to the response desired. Wait at least three geriatric half-lives before increasing the dose. If the expected response does not occur at the normal adult dosage, check blood levels. If the expected response does not occur at the appropriate blood level, switch to a different drug.

(4) Maintain a high index of suspicion regarding drug reactions and interactions. Know what other drugs the patient is taking.

(5) Simplify the regimen as much as possible. When multiple drugs are prescribed, try to use drugs that can be taken at the same time of day. Whenever possible, reduce the number of drugs being taken.

REFERENCES

Abrams WB: Cardiovascular drugs in the elderly. Chest 1990;98:980.

Ashburn MA, Lipman AG: Management of pain in the cancer patient. Anesth Analg 1993;76:402.

Avorn J et al: A randomized trial of a program to reduce the use of psychoactive drugs in nursing homes. N Engl J Med 1992;327:168.

Avorn J et al: Use of psychoactive medication and the quality of care in rest homes: Findings and policy implications of a statewide study. N Engl J Med 1989;320:227.

Bambrick LL, Yarowsky PJ, Kreuger BK: Glutamate as a hippocampal neuron survival factor: An inherited defect in the trisomy 16 mouse. Natl Acad Sci Proc 1995; 92:9692.

Bellamy N: Treatment considerations in the elderly rheumatic patient. Gerontology 1988;34(Suppl 1):16.

Birnbaum LS: Pharmacokinetic basis of age-related changes in sensitivity to toxicants. Annu Rev Pharmacol Toxicol 1991;31:101.

Blazer D: Depression in the elderly. N Engl J Med 1989; 320:164.

Chatellier G, Lacomblez L, Groupe Français d' Étude de la Tetrahydroaminoacridine: Tacrine (tetrahydroaminoacridine; THA) and lecithin in senile dementia of the Alzheimer type: A multicentre trial. Br Med J 1990; 300:495.

Cockcroft DW, Gault MH: Prediction of creatinine clearance from serum creatinine. Nephron 1976;16:31.

Cody RJ: Physiologic changes due to age: Implications for drug therapy of congestive heart failure. Drugs Aging 1993;3:320.

Cuello AC, Thoenen H: The pharmacology of neurotrophic factors. In: *Pharmacological Sciences. Perspectives for Research and Therapy in the Late 1990s.* Cuello AC, Collier B (editors). Birkäuser-Verlag, 1995.

Cutler NR, Sramek JJ: Muscarinic M_1-receptor agonists. Potential in the treatment of Alzheimer's disease. CNS Drugs 1995;3:467.

Davis KL et al: A double-blind, placebo-controlled multicenter study of tacrine for Alzheimer's disease. N Engl J Med 1992;327:1253.

Frank E, Karp JF, Rush AJ: Efficacy of treatments for major depression. Psychopharmacol Bull 1993;29:457.

Freeman SE, Dawson RM: Tacrine: A pharmacological review. Prog Neurobiol 1991;36:257.

Gauthier S et al: Tetrahydroaminoacridine-lecithin combination treatment in patients with intermediate-stage Alzheimer's disease. N Engl J Med 1990;322:1272.

Goldberg TH, Finkelstein MS: Difficulties in estimating glomerular filtration rate in the elderly. Arch Intern Med 1987;147:1430.

Gottlieb GL, Kumar A: Conventional pharmacologic treatment for patients with Alzheimer's disease. Neurology 1993;43(Suppl 4):S56.

Greenblatt DJ, Shader RI, Harmatz JS: Implications of altered drug disposition in the elderly: Studies of benzodiazepines. J Clin Pharmacol 1989;29:866.

Greenblatt DJ: Disposition of cardiovascular drugs in the elderly. Med Clin North Am 1989;73:487.

Gurwitz JH, Avorn J: The ambiguous relationship between aging and adverse drug reactions. Ann Intern Med 1991;114:956.

Hayflick L: Theories of biological aging. Exp Gerontol 1985;20:145.

Hospitalizations for the leading causes of death among the elderly: United States, 1987. MMWR Morbid Mortal Wkly Rep 1990;39:777.

Knapp MJ et al: A 30-week randomized controlled trial of high-dose tacrine in patients with Alzheimer's disease. JAMA 1994;271:985.

Kohn RR: *Principles of Mammalian Aging.* Prentice-Hall, 1978.

Lamy PP: The role of cholinesterase inhibitors in Alzheimer's disease. CNS Drugs 1994;1:145.

Lebel M, Bergeron MG: Pharmacokinetics in the elderly. Studies on ciprofloxacin. Am J Med 1987;82(Suppl 4A):108.

Lee CR, Benfield P: Aniracetam: An overview of its pharmacodynamic and pharmacokinetic properties, and a review of its therapeutic potential in senile cognitive disorders. Drugs Aging 1994;4:257.

Lindeman RD, Tobin J, Shock NW: Longitudinal studies on the rate of decline in renal function with age. J Am Geriatr Soc 1985;33:278.

Lipowski ZJ: Delirium in the elderly patient. N Engl J Med 1989;320:578.

Loi CM, Vestal RE: Drug metabolism in the elderly. Pharmacol Ther 1988;36:131.

Massoro EJ: Biology of aging: Facts, thoughts, and experimental approaches. Lab Invest 1991;65:500.

Materson BJ et al: Treatment of hypertension in the elderly: I. Blood pressure and clinical changes. Results of a Department of Veterans Affairs Cooperative Study. Hypertension 1990;15:348.

Meyers BR, Wilkinson P: Clinical pharmacology of antibacterial drugs in the elderly. Implications for selection and dosage. Clin Pharmacokinet 1989;17:385.

Montamat SC, Cusack BJ, Vestal RE: Management of drug therapy in the elderly. N Engl J Med 1989;321:303.

Muller WE, Mutschler E, Riederer P: Noncompetitive NMDA receptor antagonists with fast open-channel blocking kinetics and strong voltage-dependency as potential therapeutic agents for Alzheimer's dementia. Pharmacopsychiatry 1995;28:113.

Ouslander JG, Schnelle JF: Incontinence in the nursing home. Ann Intern Med 1995;122:438.

Pan HY et al: Decline in beta-adrenergic receptor-mediated vascular relaxation with aging in man. J Pharmacol Exp Ther 1986;239:802.

Poirer J, Minnich A, Davignon J: Apolipoprotein E, synaptic plasticity and Alzheimer's disease. Ann Med 1995; 27:663.

Portenoy RK et al: Pain in ambulatory patients with lung or colon cancer: Prevalence, characteristics and impact. Cancer 1992;70:1616.

Preskorn SH: Recent advances in antidepressant therapy for the elderly. Am J Med 1993;95(Suppl 5):2S.

Prinz PN et al: Geriatrics: Sleep disorders and aging. N Engl J Med 1990;323:520.

Ray WA et al: Psychotropic drug use and the risk of hip fracture. N Engl J Med 1987;316:363.

Ray WA: Psychotropic drugs and injuries among the elderly: A review. J Clin Psychopharmacol 1992;12:386.

Roberts J, Tumer N: Age and diet effects on drug action. Pharmacol Ther 1988;37:111.

Schmucker DL: Aging and drug disposition: An update. Pharmacol Rev 1985;37:133.

Schneider EL, Cusack BJ (editors): *Handbook of the Biology of Aging,* 3rd ed. Academic Press, 1990.

Schneider LS, Tariot PN: Emerging drugs for Alzheimer's disease. Mechanisms of action and prospects for cognitive enhancing medications. Med Clin North Am 1994; 78:911.

Schneider LS: Clinical pharmacology of aminoacridines in Alzheimer's disease. Neurology 1993;43(Suppl 4):S64.

Schneider LS: Efficacy of treatment for geropsychiatric patients with severe mental illness. Psychopharmacol Bull 1993;29:501.

Schug SA, Dunlap R, Zech D: Pharmacologic management of cancer pain. Drugs 1992;43:44.

Schwartz JB, Abernethy DR: Cardiac drugs: Adjusting their use in aging patients. Geriatrics 1987;42:31.

Sunderland T et al: Anticholinergic sensitivity in patients with dementia of the Alzheimer type and age-matched controls: A dose-response study. Arch Gen Psychiat 1987;44:418.

Tariot PN et al: L-Deprenyl in Alzheimer's disease. Arch Gen Psychiatry 1987;44:427.

Thompson TL II et al: Lack of efficacy of hydergine in patients with Alzheimer's disease. N Engl J Med 1990; 323:445.

Thompson TL II, Moran MG, Nies AS: Psychotropic drug use in the elderly. (2 parts.) N Engl J Med 1983;308:134, 194.

Tonkin A, Wing L: Aging and susceptibility to drug-induced orthostatic hypotension. Clin Pharmacol Ther 1992; 52:277.

Tsujimoto G, Hashimoto K, Hoffman BB: Pharmacokinetic and pharmacodynamic principles of drug therapy in old age. (Two parts.) Int J Clin Pharmacol Therap Toxicol 1989;27:13, 102.

Tumer N, Scarpace PJ, Lowenthal DT: Geriatric pharmacology: Basic and clinical considerations. Annu Rev Pharmacol Toxicol 1992;32:271.

Watkins PB et al: Hepatotoxic effects of tacrine administration in patients with Alzheimer's disease. JAMA 1994;271:992.

Dermatologic Pharmacology

62

Dirk B. Robertson, MD, & Howard I. Maibach, MD

The skin offers a number of special opportunities to the therapist. For example, the topical route of administration is especially appropriate for diseases of the skin, though some dermatologic diseases respond as well or better to drugs administered systemically.

The general pharmacokinetic principles governing the use of drugs applied to the skin are the same as those involved in other routes of drug administration (Chapters 1 and 3). However, human skin, though often depicted as a simple three-layered structure, is a complex series of diffusion barriers. Quantitation of the flux of drugs and drug vehicles through these barriers is the basis of pharmacokinetic analysis of dermatologic therapy; techniques for making such measurements are rapidly increasing in number and sensitivity.

Major variables that determine pharmacologic response to drugs applied to the skin include the following:

(1) Regional variation in drug penetration: For example, the scrotum, face, axilla, and scalp are far more permeable than the forearm and may require less drug for equivalent effect.

(2) Concentration gradient: Increasing the concentration gradient increases the mass of drug transferred per unit time, just as in the case of diffusion across other barriers (Chapter 1). Thus, resistance to topical corticosteroids can sometimes be overcome by use of higher concentrations of drug.

(3) Dosing schedule: Because of its physical properties, the skin acts as a reservoir for many drugs. As a result, the "local half-life" may be long enough to permit once-daily application of drugs with short systemic half-lives. For example, once-daily application of corticosteroids appears to be just as effective as multiple applications in many conditions.

(4) Vehicles and occlusion: An appropriate vehicle maximizes the ability of the drug to penetrate the outer layers of the skin. In addition, through their physical properties (moistening or drying effects), vehicles may themselves have important therapeutic ef-

fects. Occlusion (application of a plastic wrap to hold the drug and its vehicle in close contact with the skin) is extremely effective in maximizing efficacy.

DERMATOLOGIC VEHICLES

Topical medications usually consist of active ingredients incorporated in a vehicle that facilitates cutaneous application. Important considerations in selection of a vehicle include the solubility of the active agent in the vehicle; the rate of release of the agent from the vehicle; the ability of the vehicle to hydrate the stratum corneum, thus enhancing penetration; the stability of the therapeutic agent in the vehicle; and interactions, chemical and physical, of the vehicle, stratum corneum, and active agent. Vehicles have traditionally been considered pharmacologically inert; however, owing to their unique physical properties, many are therapeutically beneficial themselves.

Depending upon the vehicle, dermatologic formulations may be classified as tinctures, wet dressings, lotions, gels, aerosols, powders, pastes, creams, and ointments. The ability of the vehicle to retard evaporation from the surface of the skin increases in this series, being least in tinctures and wet dressings and greatest in ointments. In general, acute inflammation with oozing, vesiculation, and crusting is best treated with drying preparations such as tinctures, wet dressings, and lotions, while chronic inflammation with xerosis, scaling, and lichenification is best treated with more lubricating preparations such as creams and ointments. Tinctures, lotions, gels, and aerosols are convenient for application to the scalp and hairy areas. Emulsified vanishing type creams may be used in intertriginous areas without causing maceration.

Emulsifying agents are used to provide homogeneous, stable preparations when mixtures of immiscible liquids such as oil-in-water creams are compounded. Some patients develop irritation from these agents. Substituting a preparation that does not contain them or using one containing a lower concentration may resolve the problem.

ANTIBACTERIAL AGENTS

TOPICAL ANTIBACTERIAL PREPARATIONS

Topical antibacterial agents may be useful in preventing infections in clean wounds, in the early treatment of infected dermatoses and wounds, in reducing colonization of the nares by staphylococci, in axillary deodorization, and in the management of acne vulgaris. The efficacy of antibiotics in these topical applications is not uniform. The general pharmacology of the antimicrobial drugs is discussed in Chapters 43–51.

Numerous topical anti-infectives contain corticosteroids in addition to antibiotics. There is no convincing evidence that topical corticosteroids inhibit the antibacterial effect of antibiotics when the two are incorporated in the same preparation. In the treatment of secondarily infected dermatoses, which are usually colonized with streptococci, staphylococci, or both, combination therapy may prove superior to corticosteroid therapy alone. Antibiotic-corticosteroid combinations may be useful in treating diaper dermatitis, otitis externa, and impetiginized eczema.

The selection of a particular antibiotic depends of course upon the diagnosis and, whenever possible, in vitro culture and sensitivity studies of clinical samples. The pathogens isolated from most infected dermatoses are group A beta-hemolytic streptococci, *Staphylococcus aureus,* or both. The pathogens present in surgical wounds will be those resident in the environment. Information about regional epidemiologic data and the prevailing patterns of drug resistance is therefore important in selecting a therapeutic agent. Prepackaged topical antibacterial preparations that contain multiple antibiotics are available in fixed dosages well above the therapeutic threshold. These formulations offer the advantages of efficacy in mixed infections, broader coverage for infections due to undetermined pathogens, and delayed microbial resistance to any single component antibiotic.

1. BACITRACIN & GRAMICIDIN

Bacitracin and gramicidin are peptide antibiotics, active against gram-positive organisms such as streptococci, pneumococci, and staphylococci. In addition, most anaerobic cocci, neisseriae, tetanus bacilli, and diphtheria bacilli are sensitive. Bacitracin is com-

pounded in an ointment base alone or in combination with neomycin, polymyxin B, or both. The use of bacitracin in the anterior nares temporarily decreases colonization by pathogenic staphylococci. Microbial resistance may develop following prolonged use. Bacitracin-induced contact urticaria syndrome, including anaphylaxis, occurs rarely. Allergic contact dermatitis occurs frequently. Bacitracin is poorly absorbed through the skin, so systemic toxicity is rare.

Gramicidin is available only for topical use, in combination with other antibiotics such as neomycin, polymyxin, bacitracin, and nystatin. Systemic toxicity limits this drug to topical use. The incidence of sensitization following topical application is exceedingly low in therapeutic concentrations.

2. MUPIROCIN

Mupirocin (pseudomonic acid A) is structurally unrelated to other currently available topical antibacterial agents. Most gram-positive aerobic bacteria, including methicillin-resistant *S aureus,* are sensitive to mupirocin. It is effective in the treatment of impetigo caused by *S aureus* and group A beta-hemolytic streptococci. Intranasal use for temporarily eliminating nasal carriage of *S aureus* may be associated with irritation of mucous membranes caused by the polyethylene glycol vehicle. Mupirocin is not appreciably absorbed systemically after topical application to intact skin.

3. POLYMYXIN B SULFATE

Polymyxin B is a peptide antibiotic effective against gram-negative organisms, including *Pseudomonas aeruginosa, Escherichia coli, Enterobacter,* and *Klebsiella.* Most strains of *Proteus* and *Serratia* are resistant, as are all gram-positive organisms. Topical preparations may be compounded in either a solution or ointment base. Numerous prepackaged antibiotic combinations containing polymyxin B are available. Detectable serum concentrations are difficult to achieve from topical application, but the total daily dose applied to denuded skin or open wounds should not exceed 200 mg in order to reduce the likelihood of neurotoxicity and nephrotoxicity. Hypersensitivity to topically applied polymyxin B sulfate is uncommon.

4. NEOMYCIN & GENTAMICIN

Neomycin and gentamicin are aminoglycoside antibiotics active against gram-negative organisms, including *E coli, Proteus, Klebsiella,* and *Enterobacter.* Gentamicin generally shows greater activity against *P aeruginosa* than neomycin. Gentamicin is also more active against staphylococci and group A beta-hemolytic streptococci. Widespread topical use of gentamicin, especially in a hospital environment, should be avoided to slow the appearance of gentamicin-resistant organisms.

Neomycin is available in numerous topical formulations, both alone and in combination with polymyxin, bacitracin, and other antibiotics. It is also available as a sterile powder for topical use. Gentamicin is available as an ointment or cream.

Topical application of neomycin rarely results in detectable serum concentrations. However, in the case of gentamicin, serum concentrations of 1–18 $\mu g/mL$ are possible if the drug is applied in a water-miscible preparation to large areas of denuded skin, as in burned patients. Both drugs are water-soluble and are excreted primarily in the urine. Renal failure may permit the accumulation of these antibiotics, with possible nephrotoxicity, neurotoxicity, and ototoxicity.

Neomycin frequently causes sensitization, particularly if applied to eczematous dermatoses or if compounded in an ointment vehicle. When sensitization occurs, cross-sensitivity to streptomycin, kanamycin, paromomycin, and gentamicin is possible.

5. TOPICAL ANTIBIOTICS IN ACNE

Several systemic antibiotics that have traditionally been used in the treatment of acne vulgaris have been shown to be effective when applied topically. Currently, four antibiotics are so utilized: clindamycin phosphate, erythromycin base, metronidazole, and tetracycline hydrochloride. The effectiveness of topical therapy is less than that achieved by systemic administration of the same antibiotic. Therefore, topical therapy is generally suitable in mild to moderate cases of inflammatory acne.

Clindamycin

Clindamycin has in vitro activity against *Propionibacterium (Corynebacterium) acnes;* this has been postulated as the mechanism of its beneficial effect in acne therapy. Approximately 10% of an applied dose is absorbed, and rare cases of bloody diarrhea and pseudomembranous colitis have been reported following topical application. The hydroalcoholic vehicle may cause drying and irritation of the skin, with complaints of burning and stinging. The water-based gel vehicle is well tolerated and less likely to cause dehydration and irritation. Allergic contact dermatitis is uncommon.

Erythromycin

In topical preparations, the base of erythromycin rather than a salt is used to facilitate penetration. Although the mechanism of action of topical erythromycin in inflammatory acne vulgaris is unknown, it is presumed to be due to its inhibitory effects on *P acnes*. One of the possible complications of topical therapy is the development of antibiotic-resistant strains of organisms, including staphylococci. If this occurs in association with a clinical infection, topical erythromycin should be discontinued and appropriate systemic antibiotic therapy started. Adverse local reactions may include a burning sensation at the time of application and drying and irritation of the skin. Allergic hypersensitivity appears to be uncommon. Erythromycin is also available in a fixed combination preparation with benzoyl peroxide (Benzamycin) for topical treatment of acne vulgaris.

Metronidazole

Topical metronidazole is effective in the treatment of acne rosacea. The mechanism of action is unknown, but it may relate to the inhibitory effects of metronidazole on *Demodex brevis*. Oral metronidazole had been shown to be a carcinogen in susceptible rodent species, and topical use during pregnancy and by nursing mothers and children is therefore not recommended.* Adverse local effects include dryness, burning, and stinging. Caution should be exercised when applying metronidazole near the eyes to avoid excessive tearing.

Tetracycline

Two topical tetracycline antibiotics are currently available for treatment of acne vulgaris: (1) tetracycline hydrochloride in a hydroalcoholic base containing *n*-decyl methyl sulfoxide (Topicycline) and (2) meclocycline sulfosalicylate in a cream base (Meclan). Serum levels of tetracycline obtained from continued twice-daily topical use of hydroalcoholic preparations are 0.1 $\mu g/mL$ or less, and no demonstrable absorption has been reported following extensive twice-daily topical application of the meclocycline sulfosalicylate preparation over 4 weeks.

The beneficial effect of these preparations on acne vulgaris has been attributed to their inhibitory action on *P acnes*. Their use is associated with temporary yellow staining of the skin, which is most noticeable in fair-skinned individuals. Although photosensitivity has not been a problem, this hazard should be considered when using these potentially phototoxic antibiotics. As with all tetracycline derivatives, these agents should not be used in patients who are pregnant or have a history of significant renal or hepatic dysfunction.

ANTIFUNGAL AGENTS

The treatment of superficial fungal infections caused by dermatophytic fungi may be accomplished (1) with topical antifungal agents, eg, clotrimazole, miconazole, econazole, ketoconazole, oxiconazole, sulconazole, ciclopirox olamine, naftifine, terbinafine, and tolnaftate;

---

*See Chapter 53 for a more detailed discussion.

or (2) with orally administered agents, ie, griseofulvin, ketoconazole, fluconazole, and itraconazole. Superficial infections caused by *Candida* species may be treated with topical applications of clotrimazole, miconazole, econazole, ketoconazole, oxiconazole, ciclopirox olamine, nystatin, or amphotericin B. Chronic generalized mucocutaneous candidiasis is responsive to long-term therapy with oral ketoconazole.

TOPICAL ANTIFUNGAL PREPARATIONS

1. TOPICAL AZOLE DERIVATIVES

The imidazoles, which currently include clotrimazole, econazole, ketoconazole, miconazole, oxiconazole, and sulconazole, have a wide range of activity against dermatophytes (*Epidermophyton, Microsporum,* and *Trichophyton*) and yeasts, including *Candida albicans* and *Pityrosporum orbiculare,* the cause of tinea versicolor.

Miconazole (Monistat, Micatin) is available for topical application as a cream or lotion and as vaginal cream or suppositories for use in vulvovaginal candidiasis. Clotrimazole (Lotrimin, Mycelex) is available for topical application to the skin as a cream or lotion and as vaginal cream and tablets for use in vulvovaginal candidiasis. Econazole (Spectazole) is available as a cream for topical application. Oxiconazole (Oxistat) is available as a cream and lotion for topical use. Ketoconazole (Nizoral) is available as a cream for topical treatment of dermatophytosis and candidiasis and as a shampoo for the treatment of seborrheic dermatitis. Sulconazole (Exelderm) is available as a solution. Topical antifungal-corticosteroid fixed combinations have recently been introduced on the basis of providing more rapid symptomatic improvement than an antifungal agent alone. Clotrimazole-betamethasone dipropionate cream (Lotrisone) is one such example.

Once- or twice-daily application to the affected area will generally result in clearing of superficial dermatophyte infections in 2–3 weeks, although the medication should be continued until eradication of the organism is confirmed. Paronychial and intertriginous candidiasis can be treated effectively by any of these agents when applied three or four times daily. Seborrheic dermatitis should be treated with twice-daily applications of ketoconazole until clinical clearing is obtained.

Adverse local reactions to the imidazoles may include stinging, pruritus, erythema, and local irritation. Allergic contact dermatitis appears to be uncommon.

2. CICLOPIROX OLAMINE

Ciclopirox olamine is a synthetic broad-spectrum antimycotic agent with inhibitory activity against dermatophytes, *Candida* species, and *P orbiculare.* This agent appears to inhibit the uptake of precursors of macromolecular synthesis; the site of action is probably the cell membrane.

Pharmacokinetic studies indicate that 1–2% of the dose is absorbed when applied as a solution on the back under an occlusive dressing. Ciclopirox olamine is available as a 1% cream and lotion (Loprox) for the topical treatment of dermatomycosis, candidiasis, and tinea versicolor. The incidence of adverse reactions has been low. Pruritus and worsening of clinical disease have been reported. The potential for delayed allergic contact hypersensitivity appears small.

3. NAFTIFINE

Naftifine hydrochloride is an allylamine that is highly active against dermatophytes but less active against yeasts. The antifungal activity derives from selective inhibition of squalene epoxidase, a key enzyme for the synthesis of ergosterol.

Naftifine (Naftin) is available as a 1% cream for the topical treatment of dermatophytosis, to be applied on a twice-daily dosing schedule. Adverse reactions include local irritation, burning sensation, and erythema. Contact with mucous membranes should be avoided.

4. TERBINAFINE

Terbinafine (Lamisil) is an *n*-allylamine with activity similar to that of naftifine hydrochloride. It is available as a 1% cream for the topical treatment of dermatophyte infections. Treatment should be for a minimum of 1 week and should not exceed 4 weeks. Clinical improvement may continue for 2–4 weeks following cessation of therapy. Reported adverse reactions include local irritation with erythema, dryness, and stinging. Contact with eyes and mucous membranes should be avoided.

An oral preparation of terbinafine has been approved for use in the USA. It appears to have efficacy comparable to that of itraconazole (see below) but is less expensive (Terbinafine, 1996).

5. TOLNAFTATE

Tolnaftate is a synthetic antifungal compound that is effective topically against dermatophyte infections caused by *Epidermophyton, Microsporum,* and *Trichophyton.* It is also active against *P orbiculare* but not against *Candida.*

Tolnaftate (Aftate, Tinactin) is available as a cream, solution, powder, or powder aerosol for application twice daily to infected areas. Recurrences following cessation of therapy are common, and infections of the palms, soles, and nails are usually unresponsive to tolnaftate alone. The powder or powder aerosol may be used chronically following initial treatment in patients susceptible to tinea infections. Tolnaftate is generally well tolerated and rarely causes irritation or allergic contact sensitization.

6. NYSTATIN & AMPHOTERICIN B

Nystatin and amphotericin B are useful in the topical therapy of *C albicans* infections but ineffective against dermatophytes. Nystatin is limited to topical treatment of cutaneous and mucosal *Candida* infections because of its narrow spectrum and negligible absorption from the gastrointestinal tract following oral administration. Amphotericin B has a broader antifungal spectrum and is used intravenously in the treatment of many systemic mycoses (Chapter 48) and to a lesser extent in the treatment of cutaneous *Candida* infections.

The recommended dosage for topical preparations of nystatin in treating paronychial and intertriginous candidiasis is application two or three times a day. Oral candidiasis (thrush) is treated by holding 5 mL (infants, 2 mL) of nystatin oral suspension in the mouth for several minutes four times daily before swallowing. An alternative therapy for thrush is to retain a vaginal tablet in the mouth until dissolved four times daily. Recurrent or recalcitrant perianal, vaginal, vulvar, and diaper area candidiasis may respond to oral nystatin, 0.5–1 million units in adults (100,000 units in children) four times daily in addition to local therapy. Vulvovaginal candidiasis may be treated by insertion of 1 vaginal tablet twice daily for 14 days, then nightly for an additional 14–21 days.

Amphotericin B (Fungizone) is available for topical use in cream, ointment, and lotion form. The recommended dosage in the treatment of paronychial and intertriginous candidiasis is application two to four times daily to the affected area.

Adverse effects associated with oral administration of nystatin include mild nausea, diarrhea, and occasional vomiting. Topical application is nonirritating, and allergic contact hypersensitivity is exceedingly uncommon. Topical amphotericin B is well tolerated and only occasionally locally irritating. Hypersensitivity is exceedingly rare. The drug may cause a temporary yellow staining of the skin, especially when the cream vehicle is used.

ORAL ANTIFUNGAL AGENTS

1. GRISEOFULVIN

Griseofulvin is effective orally against dermatophyte infections caused by *Epidermophyton, Mi-crosporum,* and *Trichophyton.* It is ineffective against *Candida* and *P orbiculare.*

Griseofulvin's antifungal activity has been attributed to inhibition of hyphal cell wall synthesis, effects on nucleic acid synthesis, and inhibition of mitosis. Griseofulvin interferes with microtubules of the mitotic spindle and with cytoplasmic microtubules. The destruction of cytoplasmic microtubules may result in impaired processing of newly synthesized cell wall constituents at the growing tips of hyphae. Griseofulvin is active only against growing cells.

Following the oral administration of 1 g of micronized griseofulvin, peak serum levels of 1.5–2 μg/mL are obtained in 4–8 hours. The drug can be detected in the stratum corneum 4–8 hours following oral administration, with the highest concentration in the outermost layers and the lowest in the base. Reducing the particle size of the medication greatly increases absorption of the drug. Formulations that contain the smallest particle size are labeled "ultramicronized." Ultramicronized griseofulvin achieves bioequivalent plasma levels with half the dose of micronized drug. In addition, solubilizing griseofulvin in polyethylene glycol enhances absorption even further. Micronized griseofulvin is available as 250 mg and 500 mg tablets, and ultramicronized drug is available as 125 mg, 165 mg, 250 mg, and 330 mg tablets and as 250 mg capsules.

The usual adult dosage of the micronized ("microsize") form of the drug is 500 mg daily in single or divided doses with meals; occasionally, 1 g/d is indicated in the treatment of recalcitrant infections. The pediatric dosage is 10 mg/kg of body weight daily in single or divided doses with meals. An oral suspension is available for use in children.

Griseofulvin is most effective in treating tinea infections of the scalp and glabrous (nonhairy) skin. In general, infections of the scalp respond to treatment in 4–6 weeks, and infections of glabrous skin will respond in 3–4 weeks. Dermatophyte infections of the nails respond only to prolonged administration of griseofulvin. Fingernails may respond to 6 months of therapy, whereas toenails are quite recalcitrant to treatment and may require 8–18 months of therapy; relapse almost invariably occurs.

Adverse effects seen with griseofulvin therapy include headaches, nausea, vomiting, diarrhea, photosensitivity, peripheral neuritis, and occasionally mental confusion. Griseofulvin is derived from a *Penicillium* mold, and cross-sensitivity with penicillin may occur. It is contraindicated in patients with porphyria or hepatic failure or those who have had hypersensitivity reactions to it in the past. Its safety in pregnant patients has not been established. Leukopenia and proteinuria have occasionally been reported. Therefore, in patients undergoing prolonged therapy, routine evaluation of the hepatic, renal, and hematopoietic systems is advisable. Coumarin anticoagulant activity may be altered by griseofulvin, and anticoagulant dosage may require adjustment.

2. ORAL AZOLE DERIVATIVES

Azole derivatives currently available for oral treatment of systemic mycosis include fluconazole (Diflucan), itraconazole (Sporonax), and ketoconazole (Nizoral). As discussed in Chapter 48, imidazole derivatives act by affecting the permeability of the cell membrane of sensitive cells through alterations of the biosynthesis of lipids, especially sterols, in the fungal cell.

Ketoconazole was the first imidazole derivative used for oral treatment of systemic mycoses. Patients with chronic mucocutaneous candidiasis respond well to a once-daily dose of 200 mg of ketoconazole, with a median clearing time of 16 weeks. Most patients require long-term maintenance therapy. Variable results have been reported in treatment of chromomycosis.

Ketoconazole has been shown to be quite effective in the therapy of cutaneous infections caused by *Epidermophyton, Microsporum,* and *Trichophyton* species. Infections of the glabrous skin often respond within 2–3 weeks to a once-daily oral dose of 200 mg. Palmar-plantar skin is slower to respond, often taking 4–6 weeks at a dosage of 200 mg twice daily. Infections of the hair and nails may take even longer before resolving with low cure rates noted for tinea capitis. Tinea versicolor is very responsive to short courses of a once-daily dose of 200 mg.

Nausea or pruritus has been noted in approximately 3% of patients taking ketoconazole. More significant side effects include gynecomastia, elevations of hepatic enzyme levels, and hepatitis. Caution is advised when using ketoconazole in patients with a history of hepatitis. Routine evaluation of hepatic function is advisable for patients on prolonged therapy.

The newer azole derivatives for oral therapy include fluconazole and itraconazole. Fluconazole is well absorbed following oral administration, with a plasma half-life of 30 hours. In view of this long half-life, daily doses of 100 mg are sufficient to treat mucocutaneous candidiasis; alternate-day doses are sufficient for dermatophyte infections. The plasma half-life of itraconazole is similar to fluconazole, with detectable therapeutic concentrations remaining in the stratum corneum for up to 28 days following termination of therapy. Itraconazole has been demonstrated to be effective for the treatment of onychomycosis in a dosage of 200 mg daily taken with food to ensure maximum absorption for 3 consecutive months.

Coadministration of oral azoles with terfenadine, astemizole, or cisapride may increase the plasma concentration of the latter drugs by inhibiting their metabolism. This may result in severe cardiac dysrhythmias, including ventricular tachycardia and death. Coadministration of oral azoles with midazolam or triazolam has resulted in elevated plasma concentrations and may potentiate and prolong hypnotic and sedative effects of these agents. *Therefore, coadministration of the oral azoles with terfenadine, astemizole,* *cisapride, midazolam, or triazolam is absolutely contraindicated.*

ANTIVIRAL AGENTS

ACYCLOVIR, VALACYCLOVIR, & FAMCICLOVIR

Acyclovir, valacyclovir, and famciclovir are synthetic guanine analogs with inhibitory activity against members of the herpesvirus family, including herpes simplex types 1 and 2. As explained in Chapter 49, these guanine derivatives are phosphorylated preferentially by herpes simplex virus-coded thymidine kinase, and, following further phosphorylation, the resultant triphosphate interferes with herpesvirus DNA polymerase and viral DNA replication. Indications and usage of oral and parenteral acyclovir, valacyclovir, and famciclovir in the treatment of cutaneous infections are discussed in Chapter 49.

Topical acyclovir (Zovirax) is available as a 5% ointment for application to primary cutaneous herpes simplex infections and to limited mucocutaneous herpes simplex virus infections in immunocompromised patients. In primary infections, the use of topical acyclovir shortens the duration of viral shedding and may decrease healing time. In localized, limited mucocutaneous infections in immunocompromised patients, its use may be associated with a decrease in the duration of viral shedding. There is no evidence that the topical use of acyclovir is of any benefit in the treatment of recurrent disease in nonimmunocompromised patients. Indiscriminate use of acyclovir may result in the selection of resistant strains of herpes simplex virus, which are deficient in viral-coded thymidine kinase. This should be considered when contemplating the use of topical acyclovir in other than nonimmunocompromised patients with primary herpes simplex infection. Adverse local reactions to acyclovir may include pruritus and mild pain with transient stinging or burning.

ECTOPARASITICIDES

LINDANE
(Hexachlorocyclohexane)

The gamma isomer of hexachlorocyclohexane was commonly called gamma benzene hexachloride, which was a misnomer, since no benzene ring is present in this compound. Lindane is an effective pediculicide and scabicide.

Percutaneous absorption studies using a solution of

lindane in acetone have shown that almost 10% of a dose applied to the forearm is absorbed, to be subsequently excreted in the urine over a 5-day period. Serum levels following the application of a commercial lindane lotion reach maximum at 6 hours and decline thereafter with a half-life of 24 hours. After absorption, lindane is concentrated in fatty tissues, including the brain.

Lindane (Kwell) is available as a shampoo, lotion, or cream. For pediculosis capitis or pubis, one application of 30 mL of shampoo is worked into a lather and left on the scalp or genital area for 5 minutes and then rinsed off. No additional application is indicated unless living lice are present 1 week after treatment. Then reapplication may be required. Recent concerns about the toxicity of lindane have altered treatment guidelines for its use in scabies; the current recommendation calls for a single application to the entire body from the neck down, left on for 8–12 hours, and then washed off. Patients should be re-treated only if active mites can be demonstrated, and never within 1 week of initial treatment.

Much controversy exists about the possible systemic toxicities of topically applied lindane used for medical purposes. Concerns about neurotoxicity and hematotoxicity have resulted in warnings that lindane should be used with caution in infants, children, and pregnant women. The current USA package insert recommends that it not be used as a scabicide in premature infants and in patients with known seizure disorders. The risk of adverse systemic reactions to lindane appears to be minimal when it is used properly and according to directions in adult patients. However, local irritation may occur, and contact with the eyes and mucous membranes should be avoided.

CROTAMITON

Crotamiton, *N*- ethyl-*o*-crotonotoluidide, is a scabicide with some antipruritic properties. Its mechanism of action is not known, and studies on percutaneous absorption have not been published.

Crotamiton (Eurax) is available as cream or lotion. Suggested guidelines for scabies treatment call for two applications to the entire body from the chin down at 24-hour intervals, with a cleansing bath 48 hours after the last application. Crotamiton is an effective agent that can be used as an alternative to lindane. Allergic contact hypersensitivity and primary irritation may occur, necessitating discontinuance of therapy. Application to acutely inflamed skin or to the eyes or mucous membranes should be avoided.

BENZYL BENZOATE

Benzyl benzoate is effective as a pediculicide and scabicide. It has generally been supplanted by lin-

dane. The mechanism of action of benzyl benzoate is unknown. Although it appears to be relatively nontoxic after topical application, there are no studies of its toxic potential in the treatment of scabies.

SULFUR

Sulfur has a long history of use as a scabicide. Although it is nonirritating, it has an unpleasant odor, is staining, and is thus disagreeable to use. It has been replaced by more esthetic and effective scabicides in recent years, but it remains a possible alternative drug for use in infants and pregnant women. The usual formulation is 5% precipitated sulfur in petrolatum.

PERMETHRIN

Permethrin is neurotoxic to *Pediculus humanus, Pthirus pubis,* and *Sarcoptes scabiei.* Less than 2% of an applied dose is absorbed percutaneously. Residual drug persists up to 10 days following application.

It is recommended that permethrin 1% cream rinse (Nix) be applied undiluted to affected areas of pediculosis for 10 minutes and then rinsed off with warm water. For the treatment of scabies, a single application of 5% cream (Elimite) is applied to the body from the neck down, left on for 8–14 hours, and then washed off. Adverse reactions to permethrin include transient burning, stinging, and pruritus. Cross-sensitization to pyrethrins or chrysanthemums may occur.

AGENTS AFFECTING PIGMENTATION

HYDROQUINONE & MONOBENZONE

Hydroquinone and monobenzone, the monobenzyl ether of hydroquinone, are used to *reduce hyperpigmentation* of the skin. Topical hydroquinone usually results in temporary lightening, whereas monobenzone causes irreversible depigmentation.

The mechanism of action of these compounds appears to involve inhibition of the enzyme tyrosinase, thus interfering with the biosynthesis of melanin. In addition, monobenzone may be toxic to melanocytes, resulting in permanent depigmentation. Some percutaneous absorption of these compounds takes place, because monobenzone may cause hypopigmentation at sites distant from the area of application. Both hydroquinone and monobenzone may cause local irritation. Allergic sensitization to these compounds does occur, and it is advisable to do a patch test on a small area of the body prior to use on the face.

TRIOXSALEN & METHOXSALEN

Trioxsalen and methoxsalen are psoralens used for the *repigmentation* of depigmented macules of vitiligo. With the recent development of high-intensity long-wave ultraviolet fluorescent lamps, photochemotherapy with oral methoxsalen for psoriasis and with oral trioxsalen for vitiligo has been under intensive investigation.

Psoralens must be photoactivated by long-wavelength ultraviolet light in the range of 320–400 nm (UVA) to produce a beneficial effect. Psoralens intercalate with DNA and, with subsequent UVA irradiation, cyclobutane adducts are formed with pyrimidine bases. Both monofunctional and bifunctional adducts may be formed, the latter causing interstrand cross-links. These DNA photoproducts may inhibit DNA synthesis. The major long-term risks of psoralen photochemotherapy are cataracts and skin cancer.

SUNSCREENS

Topical medications useful in protecting against sunlight contain either chemical compounds that absorb ultraviolet light, called **sunscreens;** or opaque materials such as titanium dioxide that reflect light, called **sunshades.** The three classes of chemical compounds most commonly used in sunscreens are *p*-aminobenzoic acid (PABA) and its esters, the benzophenones, and the dibenzoylmethanes.

Most sunscreen preparations are designed to absorb ultraviolet light in B ultraviolet wavelength range from 280 to 320 nm, which is the range responsible for most of the erythema and tanning associated with sun exposure. Chronic exposure to light in this range induces aging of the skin and photocarcinogenesis. Para-aminobenzoic acid and its esters are the most effective available absorbers in the B region.

The benzophenones include oxybenzone, dioxybenzone, and sulisobenzone. These compounds provide a broader spectrum of absorption from 250 to 360 nm, but their effectiveness in the UVB erythema range is less than that of *p*-aminobenzoic acid. The dibenzoylmethanes include Parasol and Eusolex. These compounds absorb wavelengths throughout the longer ultraviolet A range, 320 nm to 400 nm, with maximum absorption at 360 nm. Patients particularly sensitive to ultraviolet A wavelengths include individuals with polymorphous light eruption, cutaneous lupus erythematosus, and drug-induced photosensitivity. In these patients, butyl-methoxydibenzoylmethane-containing sunscreen (UVA Guard) may provide superior photoprotection.

The protection factor (PF) of a given sunscreen is a measure of its effectiveness in absorbing erythrogenic ultraviolet light. It is determined by measuring the minimal erythema dose (MED) with and without the sunscreen in a group of normal people. The ratio of the minimal erythema dose with sunscreen to the minimal erythema dose without sunscreen is the protection factor. Fair-skinned individuals who sunburn easily are advised to use a product with a high protection factor of 15 or greater; those with darker skins may use a sunscreen with a lower protection factor of 10–15.

ACNE PREPARATIONS

RETINOIC ACID & ADAPALENE

Retinoic acid, also known as tretinoin or all-*trans*-retinoic acid, is the acid form of vitamin A. It is an effective topical treatment for acne vulgaris. Several analogs of vitamin A, eg, 13-*cis*-retinoic acid (isotretinoin), have been shown to be effective in various dermatologic diseases when given *orally*. Vitamin A alcohol is the physiologic form of vitamin A. The topical therapeutic agent, retinoic acid, is formed by the oxidation of the alcohol group, with all four double bonds in the side chain in the *trans* configuration as shown.

Retinoic acid

Retinoic acid is insoluble in water but soluble in many organic solvents. It is susceptible to oxidation and ester formation, particularly when exposed to light. Topically applied retinoic acid remains chiefly in the epidermis, with less than 10% absorption into the circulation. The small quantities of retinoic acid absorbed following topical application are metabolized by the liver and excreted in bile and urine.

Retinoic acid has several effects on epithelial tissues. It stabilizes lysosomes, increases ribonucleic acid polymerase activity, increases prostaglandin E_2, cAMP, and cGMP levels, and increases the incorporation of thymidine into DNA. Its action in acne has been attributed to decreased cohesion between epidermal cells and increased epidermal cell turnover. This is thought to result in the expulsion of open comedones and the transformation of closed comedones into open ones.

Topical retinoic acid (Retin-A) is applied initially in a concentration sufficient to induce slight erythema with mild peeling. The concentration or frequency of application may be decreased if too much irritation is produced. Topical retinoic acid should be applied to dry skin only, and care should be taken to avoid contact with the corners of the nose, eyes, mouth, and mucous membranes. During the first 4–6 weeks of therapy, comedones not previously evident may appear and give the impression that the acne has been aggravated by the retinoic acid. However, with continued therapy, the lesions will clear, and in 8–12 weeks optimal clinical improvement should occur.

The most common adverse effects of topical retinoic acid are the erythema and dryness that occur in the first few weeks of use, but these can be expected to resolve with continued therapy. Animal studies suggest that this drug may increase the tumorigenic potential of ultraviolet radiation. In light of this, patients using retinoic acid should be advised to avoid or minimize sun exposure and use a protective sunscreen. Allergic contact dermatitis to topical retinoic acid is rare.

Adapalene (Differin) resembles retinoic acid in structure and effects. It is applied as a 0.1% lotion or gel once daily. Hypopigmentation is claimed to be less likely than with retinoic acid.

ISOTRETINOIN

Isotretinoin (Accutane) is a synthetic retinoid currently restricted to the treatment of severe cystic acne that is recalcitrant to standard therapies. The precise mechanism of action of isotretinoin in cystic acne is not known, although it appears to act by inhibiting sebaceous gland size and function. The drug is well absorbed, extensively bound to plasma albumin, and has an elimination half-life of 10–20 hours.

Most cystic acne patients respond to 1–2 mg/kg, given in two divided doses daily for 4–5 months. If severe cystic acne persists following this initial treatment, after a period of 2 months, a second course of therapy may be initiated. Common adverse effects resemble hypervitaminosis A and include dryness and itching of the skin and mucous membranes. Less common side effects are headache, corneal opacities, pseudotumor cerebri, inflammatory bowel disease, anorexia, alopecia, and muscle and joint pains. These effects are all reversible on discontinuance of therapy. Skeletal hyperostosis has been observed in patients receiving isotretinoin with premature closure of epiphyses noted in children treated with this medication. Lipid abnormalities (triglycerides, HDL) are frequent; their clinical relevance is unknown at present.

Teratogenicity is a significant risk in patients taking isotretinoin; therefore, women of childbearing potential *must* use an effective form of contraception for at least 1 month before, throughout isotretinoin therapy, and for one or more menstrual cycles following discontinuance of treatment. A serum pregnancy test *must* be obtained within 2 weeks before starting therapy in these patients, and therapy should be initiated only on the second or third day of the next normal menstrual period.

BENZOYL PEROXIDE

Benzoyl peroxide is an effective topical agent in the treatment of acne vulgaris. It penetrates the stratum corneum or follicular openings unchanged and is converted metabolically to benzoic acid within the epidermis and dermis. Less than 5% of an applied dose is absorbed from the skin in an 8-hour period.

It has been postulated that the mechanism of action of benzoyl peroxide in acne is related to its antimicrobial activity against P acnes and to its peeling and comedolytic effects.

To decrease the likelihood of irritation, application should be limited to a low concentration (2.5%) once daily for the first week of therapy and increased in frequency and strength if the preparation is well tolerated. A fixed combination formulation of 5% benzoyl peroxide with 3% erythromycin base (Benzamycin) appears more effective than either agent alone.

Benzoyl peroxide is a potent contact sensitizer in experimental studies, and this adverse effect may occur in up to 1% of acne patients. Care should be taken to avoid contact with the eyes and mucous membranes. Benzoyl peroxide is an oxidant and may rarely cause bleaching of the hair or colored fabrics.

AZELAIC ACID

Azelaic acid (Azelex) is a straight-chain saturated dicarboxylic acid that has been demonstrated to be effective in the treatment of acne vulgaris. Its mechanism of action has not been fully determined, but preliminary studies demonstrate antimicrobial activity against *P acnes* as well as an in vitro inhibitory effect on the conversion of testosterone to dihydrotestosterone. Initial therapy is begun with once-daily applications of the 20% cream to the affected areas for 1 week and twice daily thereafter. Most patients will experience mild irritation with redness and dryness of the skin during the first week of treatment. Clinical improvement is noted in 6–8 weeks of continuous therapy.

DRUGS FOR PSORIASIS

ETRETINATE

Etretinate (Tegison) is an aromatic retinoid that is quite effective in the treatment of psoriasis, especially pustular forms. It is given orally at a dosage of 1–5 mg/kg/d, starting with 0.5 mg/kg/d in patients with erythrodermic psoriasis. Chronic dosing studies reveal a slow terminal elimination phase of several months' duration. Adverse effects attributable to etretinate therapy are similar to those seen with isotretinoin and resemble hypervitaminosis A. Lipid abnormalities are not frequently seen with etretinate; however, transient liver enzyme elevations have been reported. Etretinate is more teratogenic than isotretinoin in the animal species studied to date, which is of special concern in view of the drug's prolonged elimination time after chronic administration. Etretinate should not be taken by women with childbearing potential.

It is anticipated that, in the near future, etretinate will most likely be replaced by its active metabolite etretin because of latter's shorter elimination half-life.

CALCIPOTRIENE

Calcipotriene is a synthetic vitamin D_3 derivative that has been shown to be effective in the treatment of plaque type psoriasis vulgaris of moderate severity. Approximately 6% of the 0.005% topically applied ointment is absorbed through psoriatic plaques, resulting in a transient elevation of serum calcium in less than 1% of subjects treated in clinical trials. Improvement of psoriasis was generally noted following 2 weeks of therapy, with continued improvement for up to 8 weeks of treatment. Less than 10% of patients demonstrate total clearing while on calcipotriene as single-agent therapy. Adverse effects include burning, itching, and mild irritation, with dryness and erythema of the treatment area. Care should be taken to avoid facial contact, which may cause ocular irritation.

ANTI-INFLAMMATORY AGENTS

TOPICAL CORTICOSTEROIDS

The remarkable efficacy of topical corticosteroids in the treatment of inflammatory dermatoses was noted soon after the introduction of hydrocortisone in 1952. Subsequently, numerous analogs have been developed that offer extensive choices of potencies, concentrations, and vehicles. The therapeutic effectiveness of topical corticosteroids is based primarily on their anti-inflammatory activity. Definitive explanations of the effects of corticosteroids on endogenous mediators of inflammation such as histamine, kinins, lysosomal enzymes, prostaglandins, and leukotrienes await further experimental clarification. The antimitotic effects of corticosteroids on human epidermis may account for an additional mechanism of action in psoriasis and other dermatologic diseases associated with increased cell turnover. The general pharmacology of these endocrine agents is discussed in Chapter 39.

Chemistry & Pharmacokinetics

The original topical glucocorticosteroid was hydrocortisone, the natural glucocorticosteroid of the adrenal cortex. Prednisolone and methylprednisolone are as active topically as hydrocortisone. The 9α-fluoro derivatives of hydrocortisone were active topically, but their salt-retaining properties made them undesirable even for topical use. The 9α-fluorinated steroids dexamethasone and betamethasone subsequently developed did not have any advantage over hydrocortisone. However, triamcinolone and fluocinolone, the acetonide derivatives of the fluorinated steroids, have a distinct advantage in topical therapy. Similarly, betamethasone is not very active topically, but attaching a 5-carbon valerate chain to the 17-hydroxyl position results in a compound over 300 times as active as hydrocortisone for topical use. Fluocinonide is the 21-acetate derivative of fluocinolone acetonide; the addition of the 21-acetate enhances the topical activity about fivefold. Fluorination of the steroid is not required for high potency; hydrocortisone valerate and butyrate have activity similar to that of triamcinolone acetonide.

Corticosteroids are only minimally absorbed following application to normal skin; for example, approximately 1% of a dose of hydrocortisone solution applied to the ventral forearm is absorbed. Long-term occlusion with an impermeable film such as plastic wrap is an effective method of enhancing penetration, yielding a tenfold increase in absorption. There is a marked regional anatomic variation in corticosteroid penetration. Compared with the absorption from the forearm, hydrocortisone is absorbed 0.14 times as well through the plantar foot arch, 0.83 times as well through the palm, 3.5 times as well through the scalp, 6 times as well through the forehead, 9 times as well through vulvar skin, and 42 times as well through scrotal skin. Penetration is increased severalfold in the inflamed skin of atopic dermatitis; and in severe exfoliative diseases, such as erythrodermic psoriasis, there appears to be little barrier to penetration.

Experimental studies on the percutaneous absorption of hydrocortisone fail to reveal a significant increase in absorption when applied on a repetitive basis compared to a single dose, and a single daily application may be effective in most conditions. Ointment bases tend to give better activity to the corticosteroid than do cream or lotion vehicles. Increasing the concentration of a corticosteroid increases the penetration but not to the same degree. For example, approximately 1% of a 0.25% hydrocortisone solution is absorbed from the forearm. A tenfold increase in concentration causes only a fourfold increase in absorption. Solubility of the corticosteroid in the vehicle is a significant determinant of the percutaneous absorption of a topical steroid. Marked increases in efficacy are noted when optimized vehicles are used, as demonstrated by newer formulations of betamethasone dipropionate and diflorasone diacetate.

Table 62–1 groups topical corticosteroid formulation according to approximate relative efficacy. Table 62–2 lists major dermatologic diseases in order of their responsiveness to these drugs. In the first group of diseases, low- to medium-efficacy corticosteroid preparations often produce clinical remission. In the second group, it is often necessary to use high-efficacy preparations, occlusion therapy, or both. Once a remission has been achieved, every effort should be made to maintain the patient with a low-efficacy corticosteroid.

The limited penetration of topical corticosteroids can be overcome in certain clinical circumstances by the intralesional injection of relatively insoluble corticosteroids, eg, triamcinolone acetonide, triamcinolone diacetate, triamcinolone hexacetonide, and betamethasone acetate-phosphate. When these agents are injected into the lesion, measurable amounts remain in place and are gradually released for 3–4 weeks. This form of therapy is often effective for the lesions listed in Table 62–2 that are generally unresponsive to topical corticosteroids. The dosage of the triamcinolone salts should be limited to 1 mg per treatment site, ie, 0.1 mL of 10 mg/mL suspension, to decrease the incidence of local atrophy (see below).

Adverse Effects

All absorbable topical corticosteroids possess the potential to suppress the pituitary-adrenal axis (Chapter 39). Although most patients with pituitary-adrenal axis suppression demonstrate only a laboratory test abnormality, cases of severely impaired stress response can occur. Iatrogenic Cushing's syndrome may occur as a result of protracted use of topical corticosteroids in large quantities. Applying potent corticosteroids to extensive areas of the body for prolonged periods, with or without occlusion, increases the likelihood of systemic side effects. Fewer of these factors are required to produce adverse systemic effects in children, and growth retardation is of particular concern in the pediatric age group.

Adverse local effects of topical corticosteroids include the following: atrophy, which may present as depressed, shiny, often wrinkled "cigarette paper"-appearing skin with prominent telangiectases and a tendency to develop purpura and ecchymosis; steroid rosacea, with persistent erythema, telangiectatic vessels, pustules, and papules in central facial distribu-

tion; perioral dermatitis, steroid acne, alterations of cutaneous infections, hypopigmentation, hypertrichosis, and increased intraocular pressure; and allergic contact dermatitis, which may be confirmed by patch testing with high concentrations of corticosteroids, ie, 1% in petrolatum, because topical corticosteroids are not irritating. Screening for allergic contact dermatitis potential is performed with tixicortol pivalate, budesonide, and hydrocortisone valerate or butyrate. Topical corticosteroids are contraindicated in individuals who demonstrate hypersensitivity to them. Some sensitized subjects develop a generalized flare when dosed with ACTH or oral prednisone.

TAR COMPOUNDS

Coal tar, the principal by-product of the destructive distillation of bituminous coal, is an exceedingly complex mixture, containing about 10,000 compounds. These include naphthalene, phenanthrene, fluoranthrene, benzene, xylene, toluene, phenol, cresols, other aromatic compounds, pyridine bases, ammonia, and peroxides. Coal tar is available in many over-the-counter preparations in the form of bath additives, shampoos, and hydroalcoholic base gels. Coal tar may also be compounded in accordance with *United States Pharmacopeia, National Formulary,* or other formulations in concentrations ranging from 2% to 10%.

Liquor carbonis detergens (LCD) is a coal tar solution prepared by extracting coal tar with alcohol and an emulsifying agent, such as polysorbate 80. This solution contains 20 g of coal tar per 100 mL and may be compounded in concentrations of 2–10% in creams, ointments, or shampoos.

Tar preparations are used mainly in the treatment of psoriasis, dermatitis, and lichen simplex chronicus. The phenolic constituents endow these compounds with antipruritic properties, making them particularly valuable in the treatment of chronic lichenified dermatitis. Acute dermatitis with vesiculation and oozing may be irritated by even weak tar preparations, which should be avoided. However, in the subacute and chronic stages of dermatitis and psoriasis, these preparations are quite useful and offer an alternative to the use of topical corticosteroids.

The most common adverse reaction to coal tar compounds is an irritant folliculitis, necessitating discontinuance of therapy to the affected areas for a period of 3–5 days. Phototoxicity and allergic contact dermatitis may also occur. Tar preparations should be avoided in patients who have previously exhibited sensitivity to them. Care should be exercised when using tar compounds in patients with erythrodermal or generalized pustular psoriasis, because of the risk of total body exfoliation.

Table 62–1. Relative efficacy of some topical corticosteroids in various formulations.

Lowest efficacy 0.25–2.5%	Hydrocortisone
0.25%	Methylprednisolone acetate (Medrol)
0.04%	Dexamethasone[1] (Hexadrol)
0.1%	Dexamethasone[1] (Decaderm)
1.0%	Methylprednisolone acetate (Medrol)
0.5%	Prednisolone (Meti-Derm)
0.2%	Betamethasone[1] (Celestone)
Low efficacy 0.01%	Fluocinolone acetonide[1] (Fluonid, Synalar)
0.01%	Betamethasone valerate[1] (Valisone)
0.025%	Fluorometholone[1] (Oxylone)
0.05%	Aclometasone dipropionate (Aclovate)
0.025%	Triamcinolone acetonide[1] (Aristocort, Kenalog, Triacet)
0.1%	Clocortolone pivalate[1] (Cloderm)
0.03%	Flumethasone pivalate[1] (Locorten)
Intermediate efficacy 0.2%	Hydrocortisone valerate (Westcort)
0.1%	Mometasone furoate (Elocon)
0.1%	Hydrocortisone butyrate (Locoid)
0.025%	Betamethasone benzoate[1] (Uticort)
0.025%	Flurandrenolide[1] (Cordran)
0.1%	Betamethasone valerate[1] (Valisone)
0.1%	Prednicarbate (Dermatop)
0.05%	Fluticasone propionate (Cutivate)
0.05%	Desonide (Desowen)
0.025%	Halcinonide[1] (Halog)
0.05%	Desoximetasone[1] (Topicort L.P.)
0.05%	Flurandrenolide[1] (Cordran)
0.1%	Triamcinolone acetonide[1]
0.025%	Fluocinolone acetonide[1]
High efficacy 0.05%	Fluocinolide[1] (Lidex)
0.05%	Betamethasone dipropionate[1] (Diprosone, Maxivate)
0.1%	Amcinonide[1] (Cyclocort)
0.25%	Desoximetasone[1] (Topicort)
0.5%	Triamcinolone acetonide[1]
0.2%	Fluocinolone acetonide[1] (Synalar-HP)
0.05%	Diflorasone diacetate[1] (Florone, Maxiflor)
0.1%	Halcinonide[1] (Halog)
Highest efficacy 0.05%	Betamethasone dipropionate in optimized vehicle (Diprolene)[1]
0.05%	Diflorasone diacetate[1] in optimized vehicle (Psorcon)
0.05%	Halobetasol propionate[1] (Ultravate)
0.05%	Clobetasol propionate[1] (Temovate)

[1]Fluorinated steroids.

Table 62–2. Dermatologic disorders responsive to topical corticosteroids ranked in order of sensitivity.

Very responsive
Atopic dermatitis
Seborrheic dermatitis
Lichen simplex chronicus
Pruritus ani
Later phase of allergic contact dermatitis
Later phase of irritant dermatitis
Nummular eczematous dermatitis
Stasis dermatitis
Psoriasis, especially of genitalia and face

Less responsive
Discoid lupus erythematosus
Psoriasis of palms and soles
Necrobiosis lipoidica diabeticorum
Sarcoidosis
Lichen striatus
Pemphigus
Familial benign pemphigus
Vitiligo
Granuloma annulare

Least responsive: intralesional injection required
Keloids
Hypertrophic scars
Hypertrophic lichen planus
Alopecia areata
Acne cysts
Prurigo nodularis
Chondrodermatitis nodularis chronica helicis

KERATOLYTIC & DESTRUCTIVE AGENTS

SALICYLIC ACID

Salicylic acid was chemically synthesized in 1860 and has been extensively used in dermatologic therapy as a keratolytic agent. It is a white powder quite soluble in alcohol but only slightly soluble in water.

Salicylic acid

Salicylic acid is absorbed percutaneously and distributed in the extracellular space, with maximum plasma levels occurring 6–12 hours after application. Since 50–80% of salicylate is bound to albumin, transiently increased serum levels of free salicylates are found in patients with hypoalbuminemia. The urinary metabolites of topically applied salicylic acid include salicyluric acid and acyl and phenolic glucuronides of salicylic acid; only 6% of the total recovered is unchanged salicylic acid. About 95% of a single dose of salicylate is excreted in the urine within 24 hours after its absorption.

The mechanism by which salicylic acid produces its keratolytic and other therapeutic effects is poorly understood. The drug may solubilize cell surface proteins that keep the stratum corneum intact, thereby resulting in desquamation of keratotic debris. Salicylic acid is keratolytic in concentrations of 3–6%. In concentrations greater than 6%, it can be destructive to tissues.

Salicylism and death have occurred following topical application. In an adult, 1 g of a topically applied 6% salicylic acid preparation will raise the serum salicylate level not more than 0.5 mg/dL of plasma; the threshold for toxicity is 30–50 mg/dL. Higher serum levels are possible in children, who are therefore at a greater risk to develop salicylism. In cases of severe intoxication, hemodialysis is the treatment of choice (see Chapter 59). It is advisable to limit both the total amount of salicylic acid applied and the frequency of application. Urticarial, anaphylactic, and erythema multiforme reactions may occur in patients allergic to salicylates. Topical use may be associated with local irritation, acute inflammation, and even ulceration with the use of high concentrations of salicylic acid. Particular care must be exercised when using the drug on the extremities of diabetics or patients with peripheral vascular disease.

PROPYLENE GLYCOL

Propylene glycol is extensively used in topical preparations because it is an excellent vehicle for organic compounds. Propylene glycol has recently been used alone as a keratolytic agent in 40–70% concentrations, with plastic occlusion, or in gel with 6% salicylic acid.

Only minimal amounts of a topically applied dose are absorbed through normal stratum corneum. Percutaneously absorbed propylene glycol is oxidized by the liver to lactic acid and pyruvic acid, with subsequent utilization in general body metabolism. Approximately 12–45% of the absorbed agent is excreted unchanged in the urine.

Propylene glycol is an effective keratolytic agent for the removal of hyperkeratotic debris. Propylene glycol is also an effective humectant and increases the water content of the stratum corneum. The hygroscopic characteristics of the agent may help it to develop an osmotic gradient through the stratum corneum, thereby increasing hydration of the outermost layers by drawing water out from the inner layers of the skin.

Propylene glycol is used under polyethylene occlusion or with 6% salicylic acid for the treatment of ichthyosis, palmar and plantar keratodermas, psoriasis, pityriasis rubra pilaris, keratosis pilaris, and hypertrophic lichen planus.

In concentrations greater than 10%, propylene glycol may act as an irritant in some patients; those with eczematous dermatitis may be more sensitive. Allergic contact dermatitis occurs with propylene glycol, and a 4% aqueous propylene glycol solution is recommended for the purpose of patch testing.

UREA

Urea in a compatible cream vehicle or ointment base has a softening and moisturizing effect on the stratum corneum. It has the ability to make creams and lotions feel less greasy, and this has been utilized in dermatologic preparations to decrease the oily feel of a preparation that otherwise might feel unpleasant. It is a white crystalline powder with a slight ammonia odor when moist.

Urea is absorbed percutaneously, although the precise amount absorbed is not well documented. It is distributed predominantly in the extracellular space and excreted in urine. Urea is a natural product of metabolism, and systemic toxicities with topical application do not occur.

Urea allegedly increases the water content of the stratum corneum, presumably as a result of the hygroscopic characteristics of this naturally occurring molecule. Urea is also keratolytic. The mechanism of action appears to involve alterations in prekeratin and keratin, leading to increased solubilization. In addition, urea may break hydrogen bonds that keep the stratum corneum intact.

As a humectant, urea is used in concentrations of 2–20% in creams and lotions. As a keratolytic agent, it is used in 20% concentration in diseases such as ichthyosis vulgaris, hyperkeratosis of palms and soles, xerosis, and keratosis pilaris. Concentrations of 30–50% in ointment base applied to the nail plate under occlusion have been useful in softening the nail prior to avulsion. Concentrations of 10–20% applied to the diaper area, groin, or areas of eczematous dermatitis may be associated with an unpleasant stinging sensation that may necessitate discontinuance.

PODOPHYLLUM RESIN & PODOFILOX

Podophyllum resin, an alcoholic extract of *Podophyllum peltatum,* commonly known as mandrake root or May apple, is used in the treatment of condyloma acuminatum and other verrucae. It is a mixture of podophyllotoxin, alpha and beta peltatin, desoxypodophyllotoxin, dehydropodophyllotoxin, and other compounds. It is soluble in alcohol, ether, chloroform, and compound tincture of benzoin.

Percutaneous absorption of podophyllum resin occurs, particularly in intertriginous areas and from applications to large moist condylomas. It is soluble in lipids and therefore is distributed widely throughout the body, including the central nervous system.

The major use of podophyllum resin is in the treatment of condyloma acuminatum. Podophyllotoxin and its derivatives are active cytotoxic agents with specific affinity for the microtubule protein of the mitotic spindle. Normal assembly of the spindle is prevented, and epidermal mitoses are arrested in metaphase. A 25% concentration of podophyllum resin in compound tincture of benzoin is recommended for the treatment of condyloma acuminatum. Application should be restricted to wart tissue only, to limit the total amount of medication used and to prevent severe erosive changes in adjacent tissue. In treating cases of large condylomas, it is advisable to limit application to sections of the affected area to minimize systemic absorption. The patient is instructed to wash off the preparation 2–3 hours after the initial application, since the irritant reaction is variable. Depending on the individual patient's reaction, this period can be extended to 6–8 hours on subsequent applications. If three to five applications have not resulted in significant resolution, other methods of treatment should be considered.

Toxic symptoms associated with excessively large applications include nausea, vomiting, alterations in sensorium, muscle weakness, neuropathy with diminished tendon reflexes, coma, and even death. Local irritation is common, and inadvertent contact with the eye may cause severe conjunctivitis. Use during pregnancy is contraindicated in view of possible cytotoxic effects on the fetus.

Pure podophyllotoxin (podofilox) is approved for use as a 0.5% podophyllotoxin preparation (Condylox) for application by the patient in the treatment of genital condylomas. The low concentration of podofilox significantly reduces the potential for systemic toxicity. Most men with penile warts may be treated with less than 70 μL per application. At this dose, podofilox is not routinely detected in the serum. Treatment is self administered in treatment cycles of twice-daily application for 3 consecutive days followed by a 4-day drug-free period. Local adverse effects include inflammation, erosions, burning pain, and itching.

CANTHARIDIN

Cantharidin is the active irritant isolated from cantharides, or dried blister beetles (*Lytta [Cantharis] vesicatoria,* also known as Russian fly or Spanish fly). The ability of insects of the *Cantharis* type to produce vesicles and bullae on human skin led to the investigation of possible therapeutic uses of the vesicant cantharidin in dermatology. The major clinical use is in the treatment of molluscum contagiosum and verruca vulgaris, particularly periungual warts.

The amount of cantharidin absorbed following cutaneous application is unknown. It is excreted by the kidney, and in cases of oral ingestion of significant amounts, marked irritation of the entire urinary tract has resulted, with pain, urinary urgency, and priapism.

Cantharidin acts on mitochondrial oxidative enzymes, resulting in decreased ATP levels. This leads to changes in the epidermal cell membranes, acantholysis, and blister formation. This effect is entirely intraepidermal, and no scarring ensues.

The main use of cantharidin is in the treatment of verruca vulgaris. Periungual warts are treated by applying cantharidin to the wart surface, allowing it to dry, and occluding it with a nonporous plastic tape. A blister will form that will resolve in 7–14 days, at which time the area is debrided and any remaining wart is re-treated. Several applications may be required to effect a cure. Plantar warts are treated by paring and then applying several layers of cantharidin. An occlusive plastic tape is then applied. The resulting blister is removed in 10–14 days, and any residual wart is re-treated. Molluscum contagiosum will often respond to a single application without occlusion. Painless application and lack of residual scarring make cantharidin ideally suited for treatment of children.

A ring of warts may develop at the periphery of a cantharidin-treated wart as a result of intraepidermal inoculation. These may be re-treated with cantharidin or by an alternative method. Systemic toxic effects have not been observed with topical therapy, although ingestion of as little as 10 mg has resulted in abdominal pain, nausea, vomiting, and shock.

FLUOROURACIL

Fluorouracil is a fluorinated pyrimidine antimetabolite that resembles uracil, with a fluorine atom substituted for the 5-methyl group. Its systemic pharmacology is described in Chapter 55. Fluorouracil is used topically for the treatment of multiple actinic keratoses and intralesionally for keratoacanthomas.

The pharmacokinetics of intralesional therapy have not been determined. Approximately 6% of a topically applied dose is absorbed—an amount insufficient to produce adverse systemic effects. Most of the absorbed drug is metabolized and excreted as carbon dioxide, urea, and α-fluoro-β-alanine. A small percentage is eliminated unchanged in the urine. Fluorouracil inhibits thymidylate synthetase activity, interfering with the synthesis of deoxyribonucleic acid and to a lesser extent ribonucleic acid. These effects are most marked in atypical, rapidly proliferating cells.

The response to treatment begins with erythema and progresses through vesiculation, erosion, superficial ulceration, necrosis, and finally reepithelialization. Fluorouracil should be continued until the inflammatory reaction reaches the ulceration and necrosis stage, usually in 3–4 weeks, at which time treatment should be terminated. The healing process may continue for 1–2 months after therapy is discontinued. Local adverse reactions may include pain, pruritus, a burning sensation, tenderness, and residual postinflammatory hyperpigmentation. Excessive exposure to sunlight during treatment may increase the intensity of the reaction and should be avoided. Allergic contact dermatitis to fluorouracil has been reported, and its use is contraindicated in patients with known hypersensitivity. Intralesional injections of keratoacanthomas with a 5% aqueous solution of fluorouracil have recently been advocated. Weekly injections of 25–50 mg are given until 70–80% involution of the lesion is noted. If the lesion does not involute after five injections, excisional surgery is performed. Local reactions include erythema, inflammation, and subsequent necrosis of the tumor. Systemic adverse effects have not been observed and are not anticipated in view of the comparatively small amounts of fluorouracil administered on a weekly basis. Trials demonstrated similar effectiveness of 10% masoprocol cream (Actinex), but usage has been limited because of frequency of allergic contact dermatitis.

ANTIPRURITIC AGENTS

DOXEPIN

Topical doxepin hydrochloride 5% cream (Zonalon) may provide significant antipruritic activity when utilized in the treatment of pruritus associated with atopic dermatitis or lichen simplex chronicus. The precise mechanism of action is unknown but may relate to the potent H_1 and H_2 receptor antagonist properties of dibenzoxepin tricyclic compounds. Percutaneous absorption is variable and may result in significant drowsiness in some patients. In view of the anticholinergic effect of doxepin, topical use is contraindicated in patients with untreated narrow-angle glaucoma or a tendency to urinary retention.

Plasma levels of doxepin similar to those achieved during oral therapy may be obtained with topical application; the usual drug interactions associated with tricyclic antidepressants may occur. Therefore, MAO inhibitors must be discontinued at least 2 weeks prior to the initiation of doxepin cream. Topical application of the cream should be performed four times daily for up to 8 days of therapy. The safety and efficacy of chronic dosing has not been established. Adverse local effects include marked burning and stinging of the treatment site which may necessitate discontinuation of the cream in some patients. Allergic contact dermatitis appears to be frequent, and patients should be monitored for symptoms of hypersensitivity.

PRAMOXINE

Pramoxine hydrochloride is a topical anesthetic that can provide temporary relief from pruritus associated with mild eczematous dermatoses. Pramoxine is available as a 1% cream, lotion, or gel and in combination with hydrocortisone acetate. Application to the affected area two to four times daily may provide short-term relief of pruritus. Local adverse effects include transient burning and stinging. Care should be exercised to avoid contact with the eyes.

TRICHOGENIC AGENTS

MINOXIDIL

Topical minoxidil (Rogaine) is effective in reversing the progressive miniaturization of terminal scalp hairs associated with androgenic alopecia. Vertex balding is more responsive to therapy than frontal balding. The mechanism of action of minoxidil on hair follicles is unknown. Chronic dosing studies have demonstrated that the effect of minoxidil is not permanent, and cessation of treatment will lead to hair loss in 4–6 months. Percutaneous absorption of minoxidil in normal scalp is minimal, but possible systemic effects on blood pressure (Chapter 11) should be monitored in patients with cardiac disease.

ANTISEBORRHEA AGENTS

Table 62–3 lists topical formulations for the treatment of seborrheic dermatitis. These are of variable efficacy and may necessitate concomitant treatment with topical corticosteroids for severe cases.

Table 62–3. Antiseborrhea agents.

Chloroxine shampoo (Capitrol)
Coal tar shampoo (Ionil-T, Pentrax, Theraplex-T, T-Gel)
Fluocinolone acetonide shampoo (FS Shampoo)
Ketoconazole shampoo (Nizoral)
Selenium sulfide shampoo (Selsun, Exsel)
Zinc pyrithione shampoo (DHS-Zinc, Theraplex-Z)

MISCELLANEOUS MEDICATIONS

A number of drugs used primarily for other conditions also find use as oral therapeutic agents for dermatologic conditions. A few such preparations are listed in Table 62–4.

Interferon has been evaluated in controlled studies in melanoma (Chapter 55).

Table 62–4. Miscellaneous oral medications and the dermatologic conditions in which they are used.

Drug or Group	Conditions	
Antihistamines	Pruritus (any cause)	See also Chapter 16.
Antimalarials	Lupus erythematosus, photosensitization	See also Chapter 36.
Antimetabolites	Psoriasis, pemphigus, pemphigoid	See also Chapter 55.
Dapsone	Dermatitis herpetiformis, erythema elevatum diutinum, pemphigus, pemphigoid, bullous lupus erythematosus	See also Chapter 47.
Corticosteroids	Pemphigus, pemphigoid, lupus erythematosus, allergic contact dermatoses, and certain other dermatoses	See also Chapter 39.

REFERENCES

General

Baran R, Maibach HI: *Cosmetic Dermatology.* Martin Dunitz, 1994.

Braun-Falco O, Korting H, Maibach HI: *Liposome Dermatics.* Springer, 1992.

Bronaugh R, Maibach HI: *Percutaneous Penetration: Principles and Practices,* 2nd ed. Marcel Dekker, 1991.

Lorette G, Vaillant L: Pruritus: Current concepts in pathogenesis and treatment. Drugs 1990;39:218.

Orkin M, Maibach HI, Dahl MV (editors): *Dermatology.* Appleton & Lange, 1991.

Phillips TJ, Dover JS: Recent advances in dermatology. N Engl J Med 1992;326:167.

Reeves J, Maibach HI: *Clinical Dermatology, Illustrated.* Williams & Wilkins, 1994.

Steigleder G, Maibach HI: *Pocket Atlas of Dermatology.* Thieme, 1994.

Antibacterial Drugs

Aly R, Beutner K, Maibach HI: *Cutaneous Microbiology.* Marcel Dekker, 1996.

Eady EA, Holland KT, Cunliffe WJ: Topical antibiotics in acne therapy. J Am Acad Dermatol 1981;5:455.

Hirschmann JV: Topical antibiotics in dermatology. Arch Dermatol 1988;124:1691.

Leyden JJ et al: Topical antibiotics and topical antimicrobial agents in acne therapy. Acta Derm Venereol (Stockh) 1980;89(Suppl):75.

Milstone EM, McDonald AJ, Scholhamer CF: Pseudomembranous colitis after topical application of clindamycin. Arch Dermatol 1981;117:154.

Wachs GN, Maibach HI: Cooperative double blind trial of an antibiotic corticoid combination in impetiginized atopic dermatitis. Br J Dermatol 1976;95:323.

Antifungal Drugs

Borgers M: Mechanism of action of antifungal drugs with special reference to the imidazole derivatives. Rev Infect Dis 1980;2:250.

Graybill JR et al: Ketoconazole treatment of chronic mucocutaneous candidiasis. Arch Dermatol 1980;116:1137.

Heel RC et al: Econazole: A review of its antifungal activity and therapeutic efficacy. Drugs 1978;16:177.

Jones HE: Ketoconazole. Arch Dermatol 1982;118:217.

Jones HE, Simpson JG, Artis WW: Oral ketoconazole: An effective and safe treatment for dermatophytosis. Arch Dermatol 1981;117:129.

Knight AG: The activity of various griseofulvin preparations and the appearance of oral griseofulvin in the stratum corneum. Br J Dermatol 1974;91:49.

Sakurai K et al: Mode of action of 6-cyclohexyl-1-hydroxy-4-methyl-2(1H)-pyridone ethanolamine salt (ciclopirox olamine). Chemotherapy 1978;25:68.

Terbinafine for onychomycosis. Med Lett Drugs Ther 1996;38:72.

Urcuyo FG, Zaias N: The successful treatment of pityriasis versicolor by systemic ketoconazole. J Am Acad Dermatol 1982;6:24.

Weber K, Wehland J, Herzog W: Griseofulvin interacts with microtubules both in vivo and in vitro. J Mol Biol 1976;102:817.

Antiviral Agents

Corey L et al: A trial of topical acyclovir in genital herpes simplex virus infection. N Engl J Med 1982;306:1313.

Douglas JM et al: A double-blind study of oral acyclovir for suppression of recurrences of genital herpes simplex virus infection. N Engl J Med 1984;310:1551.

Mertz GJ et al: Double-blind placebo-controlled trial of oral acyclovir in first episode genital herpes simplex virus infection. JAMA 1984;252:1147.

Pagano JS: Acyclovir comes of age. J Am Acad Dermatol 1982;6:396.

Ectoparasiticides

Cubela V, Yawalkar SJ: Clinical experience with crotamiton cream and lotion in the treatment of infants with scabies. Br J Clin Pract 1978;32:229.

Konstantinou D, Stanoeva L, Yawalkar SJ: Crotamiton cream and lotion in the treatment of infants and young children with scabies. J Int Med Res 1979;7:443.

Orkin M et al (editors): *Scabies and Pediculosis.* CRC Press, 1990.

Rasmussen JE: The problem of lindane. J Am Acad Dermatol 1981;5:507.

Schacter B: Treatment of scabies and pediculosis with lindane preparation: An evaluation. J Am Acad Dermatol 1981;5:517.

Agents Affecting Pigmentation

Engasser PG, Maibach HI: Cosmetics and dermatology: Bleaching creams. J Am Acad Dermatol 1981;5:143.

Epstein JH et al: Current status of oral PUVA therapy for psoriasis. J Am Acad Dermatol 1979;1:106.

Kaidbey KH, Kligman AM: An appraisal of the efficacy and substantivity of the new high-potency sunscreens. J Am Acad Dermatol 1981;4:566.

Mosher DB, Parrish JA, Fitzpatrick TB: Monobenzylether of hydroquinone: A retrospective study of treatment of 18 vitiligo patients and a review of the literature. Br J Dermatol 1977;97:669.

Pathak MA, Kramer DM, Fitzpatrick TB: Photobiology and photochemistry of furocoumarins (psoralens). In: *Sunlight and Man: Normal and Abnormal Photobiologic Responses.* Tokyo Univ Press, 1974.

Stolk LML, Siddiqui AH: Biopharmaceutics, pharmacokinetics, and pharmacology of psoralens. Gen Pharmacol 1988;19:649.

Thompson SC et al: Reduction of solar keratoses by regular sunscreen use. N Engl J Med 1993;329:1147.

Retinoids & Other Acne Preparations

Allen JG, Bloxham DP: The pharmacology and pharmacokinetics of the retinoids. Pharmacol Ther 1989;40:1.

Bigby M, Stern RS: Adverse reactions to isotretinoin. J Am Acad Dermatol 1988;18:543.

Ehmann CW, Voorhees JJ: International studies of the efficacy of etretinate in the treatment of psoriasis. J Am Acad Dermatol 1982;6:692.

Ellis CN et al: Etretinate therapy reduces inpatient treatment of psoriasis. J Am Acad Dermatol 1987;17:787.

Lammer EJ et al: Retinoic acid embryopathy. N Engl J Med 1985;313:837.

Larsen FG et al: Pharmacokinetics and therapeutic efficacy of retinoids in skin diseases. Clin Pharmacokinetic 1992;23:42.

Lever L, Marks R: Current views on the aetiology, pathogenesis, and treatment of acne vulgaris. Drugs 1990;39: 681.

Lippman SM, Meyskens FL Jr: Results of the use of vitamin A and retinoids in cutaneous malignancies. Pharmacol Ther 1989;40:107.

Nacht S et al: Benzoyl peroxide: Percutaneous penetration and metabolic disposition. J Am Acad Dermatol 1981;4:31.

Nazzaro-Porro M et al: Beneficial effect of 15% azelaic acid cream on acne vulgaris. Br J Dermatol 1983; 109:45.

Orfanos CE, Ehlert R, Gollnick H: The retinoids: A review of their clinical pharmacology and therapeutic use. Drugs 1987;34:459.

Weinstein GD et al: Topical tretinoin for treatment of photodamaged skin. Arch Dermatol 1991;127:659.

Weiss JS et al: Topical tretinoin improves photoaged skin: A double-blind vehicle-controlled study. JAMA 1988; 259:527.

Anti-inflammatory Agents

Grupper C: The chemistry, pharmacology and use of tar in the treatment of psoriasis. In: *Psoriasis: Proceedings of the International Symposium,* Stanford University. Farber E, Cos AJ (editors). Stanford Univ Press, 1971.

Jackson DB et al: Bioequivalence (bioavailability) of generic topical corticosteroids. J Am Acad Dermatol 1989;20:791.

Korting HC, Maibach HI: *Topical Corticosteroids.* Karger, 1994.

Maibach HI, Stoughton RB: Topical corticosteroids. In: *Steroid Therapy.* Arzanoff DL (editor). Saunders, 1975.

Miller JA, Munro DD: Topical corticosteroids: Clinical pharmacology and therapeutic use. Drugs 1980; 19:119.

Robertson DB, Maibach HI: Topical corticosteroids: A review. Int J Dermatol 1982;21:59.

Surber C, Maibach HI: *Topical Corticosteroids.* Karger, 1994.

Keratolytic & Destructive Agents

Ashton H, Frenk E, Stevenson CJ: Urea as a topical agent. Br J Dermatol 1971;84:194.

Chamberlain MJ, Reynolds AL, Yeoman WB: Toxic effects of podophyllum applications in pregnancy. Br Med J 1972;3:391.

Epstein WL, Kligman AM: Treatment of warts with cantharidin. Arch Dermatol 1958;77:508.

Fine JD, Arndt KA: *Propylene Glycol: A Review.* Excerpta Medica, 1980.

Geotte DK: Topical chemotherapy with 5-fluorouracil. J Am Acad Dermatol 1981;4:633.

Geotte DK, Odom RB: Successful treatment of keratoacanthoma with intralesional fluorouracil. J Am Acad Dermatol 1980;2:212.

Roenigk H, Maibach HI (editors) : *Psoriasis.* Marcel Dekker, 1985.

Taylor JR, Halprin KM: Percutaneous absorption of salicylic acid. Arch Dermatol 1975;111:740.

Antipruritic Agents

Drake LA, Millikan LE:The antipruritic effect of 5% doxepin cream in patients with eczematous dermatitis. Arch Dermatol 195;131:1403.

Dermatotoxicology

Elsner P, Besedesco E, Maibach HI: *Bioengineering of Skin: Water and Stratum Corneum.* CRC Press, 1995.

Elsner P, Maibach HI: *Irritant Dermatitis.* Karger, 1995.

Marzolli F, Maibach H (editors): *Dermatotoxicology,* 5th ed. Hemisphere Press, 1996.

Menne T, Maibach HI: *Exogenous Dermatoses: Environmental Dermatitis.* CRC Press, 1991.

Rougier A, Goldberg A, Maibach H: *In Vitro Skin Toxicology.* M Liebert, 1994.

Van der Valk P, Maibach HI: *Irritant Dermatitis Syndrome.* CRC Press, 1995.

Wang R, Knaak J, Maibach HI: *Dermal Inhalation, Exposure, and Absorption of Toxicants.* CRC Press, 1993.

Drugs Used in Gastrointestinal Diseases

63

David F. Altman, MD

Many drugs discussed elsewhere in this book have applications in the treatment of gastrointestinal diseases. Antimuscarinic drugs inhibit the food-stimulated secretion of gastric acid and also affect intestinal smooth muscle; these drugs are useful in some forms of functional bowel disease. Muscarinic agonists stimulate smooth muscle and are used to promote gastrointestinal motility. Nicotine from tobacco smoke is one of the strongest risk factors for ulcer recurrence; conversely, nicotine (from nicotine chewing gum or a transdermal patch) may have beneficial effects in ulcerative colitis. Some phenothiazines have excellent antiemetic properties, and narcotic analgesics and some of their derivatives are useful antidiarrheal medications by virtue of their ability to inhibit intestinal motility. Several other groups of medications are used almost exclusively in gastrointestinal disease; these are grouped and discussed below according to their therapeutic uses.

DRUGS USED IN ACID-PEPTIC DISEASE

Acid-peptic disease includes peptic ulcer (gastric and duodenal), gastroesophageal reflux, and pathologic hypersecretory states such as Zollinger-Ellison syndrome. The pathogenesis of peptic ulcer is not completely understood. It is clear that gastric acid and pepsin secretion are necessary for the development of a peptic ulcer. However, factors relating to mucosal resistance to acid, particularly the production of gastroduodenal mucus and secretion of bicarbonate by epithelial cells, may be equally important. A principal role for the bacterium *Helicobacter pylori* in ulcer pathogenesis is now widely accepted. Salicylates and other nonsteroidal anti-inflammatory drugs may not only cause dyspepsia but may also cause or exacerbate peptic ulcers and their complications. Currently, drugs are available that may neutralize gastric acid, reduce gastric acid secretion, or enhance mucosal defenses through "cytoprotective" or possibly antimicrobial activities. Most clinicians treat all patients with recurrent ulcers, as well as those in whom *H pylori* infection has been established, with antimicrobial drugs to eradicate *H pylori* colonization.

ANTACIDS

Gastric antacids are weak bases that react with gastric hydrochloric acid to form a salt and water. Their usefulness in peptic ulcer disease appears to lie in their ability to reduce gastric acidity and, since pepsin is inactive in solutions above pH 4.0, to reduce peptic activity. However, trials demonstrating ulcer healing with the administration of relatively low daily doses of antacid suggest that this may not be the only reason for their effectiveness. Animal studies have demonstrated mucosal protection by antacids, either through the stimulation of prostaglandin production or the binding of an unidentified injurious substance. The roles played by these various mechanisms remain to be determined.

Most antacids in current use have as their principal constituent magnesium or aluminum hydroxide, alone or in combination, and occasionally in combination with sodium bicarbonate or a calcium salt. The chemical activities, neutralizing capacity, solubility, and side effects of some of these ingredients are summarized in Table 63–1. The net buffering capacity of any compound is determined by its ability to neutralize gastric acid and the duration of the medication's residence in the stomach. Thus, the combinations available for administration (Table 63–2) have been developed in an effort to maximize effectiveness and minimize inconvenience. Antacids also vary significantly in palatability and price.

Clinical Use of Antacids

After a meal, gastric acid is produced at a rate of about 45 meq/h. A single dose of 156 meq of antacid

Table 63–1. Major constituents of antacids.

Constituent	Neutralizing Capacity	Salt Formed in Stomach	Solubility of Salt	Adverse Effects
$NaHCO_3$	High	NaCl	High	Systemic alkalosis, fluid retention
$CaCO_3$	Moderate	$CaCl_2$	Moderate	Hypercalcemia, nephrolithiasis, milk-alkali syndrome
$Al(OH)_3$	High	$AlCl_3$	Low	Constipation, hypophosphatemia; drug adsorption reduces bioavailability
$Mg(OH)_2$	High	$MgCl_2$	Low	Diarrhea, hypermagnesemia (in patients with renal insufficiency)

given 1 hour after a meal effectively neutralizes gastric acid for 2 hours. A second dose given 3 hours after eating maintains the effect for over 4 hours after the meal. The dose-response relationship of antacids is variable, depending on the gastric secretory capacity (some individuals are "hypersecretors," some "hyposecretors") and the rate at which the antacid is emptied from the stomach. In addition, as implied by the discussion of the individual antacid compounds, antacids vary widely in their potency. The relative amounts of the various compounds and their reactivity will not be clear on the product label. However, commercially available antacids vary as much as sevenfold in in vitro acid-neutralizing capacity. Antacids can be effective in promoting healing of duodenal ulcers; their benefit in gastric ulcers is less clear. In the best-controlled trial of antacid therapy for duodenal ulcer, 140 meq of antacid given 1 and 3 hours after each meal and at bedtime accelerated the healing of duodenal ulcers, though pain relief was not much better than that seen with placebo. Different doses of antacid are required to achieve this degree of neutralizing capability, depending on the commercial product used (Table 63–2). Tablet antacids are generally weak in their neutralizing capability, and a large number of tablets would be required for this high-dose regimen. They are not recommended for the treatment of active peptic ulcer.

Table 63–2. Representative liquid antacids.

Proprietary Preparation	Ingredients	Acid-Neutralizing Capability (meq/mL)	Volume Required to Neutralize 140 meq (mL)	Sodium Content (mg/dose)	Cost of High-Dose Regimen[1]
Alternagel	Aluminum hydroxide	3.2	44	17	$146
Amphojel	Aluminum hydroxide	2.0	70	98	$232
Gelusil	Aluminum hydroxide, magnesium hydroxide, simethicone	4.8	29	7.5	$99
Maalox	Aluminum hydroxide, magnesium hydroxide	2.7	52	14	$127
Maalox HRF	Aluminum hydroxide, magnesium hydroxide	5.7	25	4.0	$195
Mylanta-DS	Aluminum hydroxide, magnesium hydroxide, simethicone	5.1	27	6.2	$95

[1]Cost to the pharmacist of 1 month's treatment with high-dose regimen (see text) based on manufacturers' listings in *Drug Topics Red Book 1996.*

As noted earlier, some studies suggest that accelerated healing may also occur with tablet or liquid antacids at doses far lower than those necessary to neutralize gastric acid. It is possible that the beneficial effects of antacids reflect something other than simple neutralization of gastric acid. Aluminum compounds may act via a direct cytoprotective action or by binding injurious substances.

Adverse reactions to antacids often include a change in bowel habits. As indicated in Table 63–1, magnesium salts often have a cathartic effect, and aluminum hydroxide may be constipating. These problems can be managed by either combining or alternating compounds with these effects. Other potential problems with antacids relate to cation absorption (sodium, magnesium, aluminum, calcium) and systemic alkalosis. Fortunately, these become clinical problems only in patients with renal impairment. In large doses, the sodium content of some antacids may become an important factor in patients with congestive heart failure. Antacids have long been a mainstay of therapy for gastroesophageal reflux. However, they appear to have little impact on the natural history of the disease. Antacid in combination with alginic acid (Gaviscon) does lead to reduced acid reflux and symptomatic improvement. Antacids have been used for pain relief from esophagitis, gastric ulcer, and duodenal ulcer. However, placebo-controlled trials have shown no effect of a single "effective" antacid dose for pain relief in any of these conditions.

GASTRIC ANTISECRETORY DRUGS

Gastric acid secretion is under the control of three principal agonists: histamine, acetylcholine, and gastrin (Figure 63–1). The final common pathway is through the proton pump, H^+/K^+ ATPase. Inhibitors of the activities of the first two secretagogues and of the proton pump have been developed.

H₂-Receptor Antagonists

Since their introduction in the mid 1970s, these compounds have gained wide acceptance. The four drugs in use in the USA are **cimetidine, ranitidine, famotidine,** and **nizatidine** (see Chapter 16). These agents are capable of over 90% reduction in basal, food-stimulated, and nocturnal secretion of gastric acid after a single dose. Many trials have demonstrated their effectiveness in promoting the healing of duodenal and gastric ulcers and preventing their recurrence. It is also apparent that these medications are essentially equally effective in treating these conditions. In addition, they are important in the medical management of Zollinger-Ellison syndrome and gastric hypersecretory states seen in systemic mastocytosis.

Figure 63–1. Schematic diagram of one model of the physiologic control of hydrogen ion secretion by the gastric parietal cell. ECL cell, enterochromaffin-like cell; G(CCK-B), gastrin-cholecystokinin-B receptor; H, histamine; H_2, histamine H_2 receptor; M_1, M_3, muscarinic receptors; ST_2, somatostatin₂ receptor; ATPase, K^+/H^+ ATPase proton pump. Some investigators place histamine receptors—and possibly cholinoceptors—on nearby tissue cells rather than on the parietal cell itself. (Modified and redrawn from Sachs et al, 1996, and other sources.)

A. Dosage: Suppression of nocturnal acid secretion appears to be the most important determinant of the rate of healing of duodenal ulcers. Whereas previous recommendations were to administer these agents at least twice a day, a single bedtime dose may be just as effective and may elicit better compliance. For active ulcer, cimetidine can be given twice daily in doses of 400–600 mg or 800 mg at bedtime; ranitidine and nizatidine can be given in a dosage of 150 mg twice daily or 300 mg at bedtime; and famotidine can be given in a dosage of 20 mg twice daily or 40 mg at bedtime. To prevent recurrence, half of the above bedtime doses can be given daily at bedtime.

B. Toxicity: All of the H_2-receptor antagonists have been generally well tolerated, with few side effects reported. The longest clinical experience has been with cimetidine; there have been reports relating this drug to confusional states, particularly in elderly patients. Cimetidine therapy, particularly when prolonged and at high doses, may cause reversible gynecomastia. This has been reported only rarely with ranitidine and famotidine. Cimetidine is known to cause a dose-dependent elevation in serum prolactin and may alter estrogen metabolism in men. Headache occurs in 34% of people taking famotidine or ranitidine. Reversible hematologic abnormalities have been a rare occurrence with all members of this class of drugs. Cimetidine also slows hepatic microsomal metabolism of some drugs, such as warfarin, theophylline, diazepam, and phenytoin. Ranitidine appears to have less effect and famotidine and nizatidine no effect on hepatic drug metabolism.

C. Combination Therapy: Although combinations of H_2-receptor antagonists and antacids are widely prescribed, there is little rationale for this potentially expensive practice. Although higher 24-hour intragastric pH has been reported in patients receiving this combination, no benefit with respect to either accelerated healing or the promotion of pain relief has been demonstrated. Combining H_2-receptor antagonists with a proton pump inhibitor such as omeprazole appears to inhibit the efficacy of the latter drug.

D. Refractory Disease: Intractability (lack of response to H_2 blockers or antacids) of peptic ulcers remains a problem, especially among older people and cigarette smokers, and as many as 20% of ulcers will fail to heal with 4 weeks of conventional therapy. Alternative pharmacologic approaches to failure of a course of an H_2-blocker include using a higher dose or prolonged course of the initial agent, switching to another H_2-receptor antagonist, or switching to a proton pump inhibitor. All have been shown to be effective in small trials. In patients who are demonstrated to have *H pylori* infection, intractability warrants a trial of the combination of antibiotics and bismuth (see below). Patients with Zollinger-Ellison syndrome often require higher dosages of an H_2-blocker, eg, up to 2400 mg/d of cimetidine.

E. Over-the-Counter H_2-Blockers: OTC versions of all four H_2-blockers are now available in the USA. They are labeled for short-term use in heartburn and dyspepsia.

Antimuscarinic Agents

Cholinoceptor antagonists (discussed in greater detail in Chapter 8) are now rarely used and only as adjuncts to H_2-receptor antagonists, especially in patients refractory to treatment with the latter or those with nocturnal pain. **Pirenzepine,** an antimuscarinic agent with activity relatively selective for gastric M_1 muscarinic receptors, is under investigation and may prove more useful in ulcer therapy.

Proton Pump Inhibitors

Omeprazole is a substituted benzimidazole that irreversibly inhibits the gastric parietal cell proton pump, (H^+/K^+ ATPase; Figure 63–1). The drug requires activation in the acid environment of the secretory canaliculus of the parietal cell, ie, it is a prodrug and probably acts from the external side of the membrane. A single daily dose can inhibit essentially 100% of gastric acid secretion. Omeprazole is approved for the short-term treatment (4–8 weeks) of gastric and duodenal ulcers and for severe gastroesophageal disease. It is also used for pathologic hypersecretory syndromes such as Zollinger-Ellison syndrome, multiple endocrine neoplasias, and systemic mastocytosis. The initial dose is 20 mg once daily. Omeprazole given 3 days per week has been shown to prevent recurrence of duodenal ulcers. Duodenal ulcer prevention and prophylaxis for reflux disease are not yet approved indications for this drug, however. Safety concerns with omeprazole relate to the effects of prolonged complete suppression of acid secretion on bacterial colonization of the stomach and on hypergastrinemia. In rats, chronic administration of large doses of omeprazole causes development of gastric carcinoid tumors. This has not been reported in humans, and omeprazole appears to be safe in trials to date. A second drug of this class, **lansoprazole,** has also been approved for these indications. A daily dose of 30 mg has been shown to be effective in inducing ulcer healing.

Octreotide

Octreotide is a long-acting synthetic somatostatin analog. It has been found to significantly inhibit the secretion of several circulating peptide hormones and to inhibit gastric and pancreatic secretion. Although no controlled prospective trials have been reported, several patients with Zollinger-Ellison syndrome have been treated with octreotide, with some reporting symptomatic improvement and others reporting decreased size of metastases or slowed tumor growth. There is also evidence that in patients with portal hypertension due to chronic liver disease, octreotide can lower portal pressures and reduce the risk of variceal hemorrhage—though renal function may be impaired in some individuals. Because the drug requires parenteral administration, its use for these indications will be limited. However, its apparent effectiveness will further stimulate the search for orally active somatostatin analogs.

MUCOSAL PROTECTIVE AGENTS

Sucralfate

Sucralfate, or aluminum sucrose sulfate, is a sulfated disaccharide developed for use in peptic ulcer disease. Its mechanism of action is thought to involve polymerization and selective binding to necrotic ulcer tissue, where it may act as a barrier to acid, pepsin, and bile. In addition, sucralfate may directly adsorb bile salts. Finally, the drug may stimulate endogenous prostaglandin synthesis. Whatever the mechanism, sucralfate has been shown to be effective in the healing of duodenal ulcers. It is poorly absorbed systemically (though rising blood levels have been documented in patients with renal failure), and few adverse effects have been reported. The dosage is 1 g four times daily on an empty stomach (at least 1 hour before meals). Sucralfate also requires an acid pH to be activated and so should not be administered simultaneously with antacids, H_2-receptor antagonists, or proton pump inhibitors.

Colloidal Bismuth Compounds

Like sucralfate, bismuth compounds also appear to work by selective binding to an ulcer, coating it and protecting it from acid and pepsin. Other postulated mechanisms of action include inhibition of pepsin activity, stimulation of mucous production, and increased prostaglandin synthesis. They may also have some antimicrobial activity against *H pylori,* though this has been disputed. When combined with antibiotics such as metronidazole and tetracycline, ulcer healing rates of up to 98% have been seen. **Bismuth subsalicylate** (Pepto-Bismol) has been used in these trials in the USA. **Tripotassium dicitrato bismuthate** has been extensively tested in Europe and shown to be superior to placebo in the healing of both duodenal and gastric ulcers. Adverse effects have been minimal, and the encephalopathy reported with long-term use of other bismuth compounds has not been noted.

Carbenoxolone

Carbenoxolone is a synthetic derivative of glycyrrhizic acid (an agent extracted from licorice) and has been shown to be effective in healing both gastric and duodenal ulcers. The mechanism of action of carbenoxolone is not clear but is thought to involve an increase in the production, secretion, and viscosity of intestinal mucus. Although its ulcer-healing properties are evident, the drug has a major aldosterone-like side effect, so that hypertension, fluid retention, and hypokalemia have limited its clinical usefulness. The concurrent administration of spironolactone controls the fluid retention but also abolishes the ulcer-healing effect; thiazides prevent sodium retention without abolishing the beneficial effect in peptic disease. Although it has been widely used in Europe, carbenoxolone is still investigational in the USA.

Prostaglandins

These derivatives of arachidonic acid are discussed in detail in Chapter 18. **Misoprostol,** a methyl analog of prostaglandin E_1, is now approved for the prevention of ulcers induced by the administration of nonsteroidal anti-inflammatory drugs (NSAIDs). Although prostaglandins are produced by the gastric mucosa and are thought to have a cytoprotective effect, at the doses needed in experimental animals to prevent or heal ulcers, the principal mechanism of action of prostaglandins appears to be inhibition of gastric secretion. This effect may be mediated through inhibition of histamine-stimulated cAMP production. cAMP is thought to be the major second messenger for histamine-induced acid secretion. Misoprostol causes a dose-dependent diarrhea, and its stimulant effect on the uterus makes it contraindicated in women with childbearing potential. The optimal role of misoprostol in ulcer treatment is difficult to define. Routine clinical prophylaxis of NSAID-induced ulcers may not be justified. However, in patients with rheumatoid arthritis requiring NSAID therapy, prophylaxis with misoprostol may be cost-effective. A fixed-ratio combination of misoprostol with an NSAID is currently under investigation for use in patients thought to be at high risk for development of NSAID gastropathy.

DRUGS PROMOTING GASTROINTESTINAL MOTILITY

Cholinergic mechanisms are responsible for modulating motor phenomena in the gut; thus it is not surprising that cholinomimetic agents such as **bethanechol** are effective in promoting gastrointestinal motility.

Metoclopramide and **cisapride** are promoted as more selective motility stimulants (prokinetic agents). In addition to its cholinomimetic properties, metoclopramide is a potent dopamine antagonist. Both drugs apparently release acetylcholine from cholinergic neurons in the enteric nervous system's myenteric plexus. They may also sensitize intestinal smooth muscle cells to the action of acetylcholine. They do not increase gastric or pancreatic secretion. These drugs hasten esophageal clearance, raise lower esophageal sphincter pressure, accelerate gastric emptying, and shorten small bowel transit time. Metoclopramide's central dopamine antagonist effect is thought to be responsible for its significant antiemetic properties, an action that cisapride appears to lack. Cisapride increases the motility of the colon in some patients.

Clinical applications follow these effects. Metoclopramide is useful for facilitating small bowel intubation. In addition, in patients with gastric motor failure—particularly diabetic gastroparesis but possibly also after vagotomy and in other disorders of gastric emptying—metoclopramide and cisapride can produce significant symptomatic relief (Drenth et al, 1992). In patients with chronic gastroesophageal reflux disease, both agents are effective in decreasing the incidence of heartburn, though long-term effects are uncertain. Finally, metoclopramide is an effective antiemetic, particularly useful in association with cancer chemotherapy and in emergency surgery or labor and delivery to prevent aspiration of gastric contents. Both drugs are rapidly absorbed, with peak concentrations after a single oral dose seen in 40–120 minutes. Their plasma half-lives are 2–4 hours.

The usual dose of metoclopramide is 10 mg four times daily with meals and at bedtime. Larger doses (up to 1–2 mg/kg) have been used in conjunction with cancer chemotherapy. A dose of 20 mg given by slow intravenous infusion is used for small bowel intubation. The most common side effects of metoclopramide are somnolence, nervousness, and dystonic reactions. Parkinsonism and tardive dyskinesia have also been reported. The frequency of the adverse extrapyramidal effects has been underreported, especially in the elderly. The drug also causes increased pituitary prolactin release, and galactorrhea and menstrual disorders have been reported. Cisapride is currently labeled only for use in gastroesophageal reflux, and the recommended dosage is 10 mg four times a day. In clinical trials in patients with diabetic gastroparesis, 5–10 mg of cisapride appeared to improve gastric emptying significantly.

Erythromycin, a macrolide antibiotic described elsewhere, has prokinetic activity in the stomach as a motilin agonist. It appears to be clinically effective in conditions such as diabetic gastroparesis and intestinal pseudo-obstruction.

ANTIEMETIC DRUGS

Nausea and vomiting may be manifestations of a wide variety of conditions, including pregnancy, motion sickness, gastrointestinal obstruction, peptic ulcer, drug toxicity, myocardial infarction, renal failure, and hepatitis. In cancer chemotherapy, drug-induced nausea and vomiting may occur so regularly that anticipatory vomiting occurs when patients return for treatment—before the chemotherapeutic agent is given. If not controlled, the discomfort associated with drug-induced emesis may cause a patient to refuse further chemotherapy.

The physiologic mechanisms responsible for nausea and vomiting are not fully understood. Coordination of the complex motor activity of the stomach and abdominal musculature takes place in the "vomiting center," which is located in the reticular formation in the medulla. The vomiting center receives input from the chemoreceptor trigger zone located on the floor of the fourth ventricle, the vestibular apparatus, and other areas. The trigger zone responds to chemical stimuli such as cancer chemotherapeutic agents, apparently through activation of dopamine or serotonin receptors.

The major categories of antiemetic agents include H_1 antihistamines, phenothiazines, metoclopramide, ondansetron, marijuana, and corticosteroids.

The antihistamines with good antiemetic activity (eg, **diphenhydramine, hydroxyzine**) possess significant antimuscarinic and sedative effects (see Chapter 16). It appears probable that both of these actions and the H_1-blocking effect contribute to the antiemetic efficacy. They are particularly effective for the nausea and vomiting associated with motion sickness, perhaps because of specific depression of conduction in the vestibulocerebellar pathway. Anticholinergic agents, especially scopolamine, are also used to prevent motion sickness (Chapter 8).

The phenothiazines block dopamine receptors in the chemoreceptor trigger zone as well as other areas of the brain (see Chapter 29). **Prochlorperazine** and **promethazine** are often used as antiemetics. Although nearly all phenothiazines possess some antiemetic activity, their use is limited by the degree of sedation associated with the antiemetic action. Extrapyramidal symptoms, especially dystonias, can be severe when large doses are used to combat the nausea and vomiting associated with chemotherapy. The dystonias can usually be reversed by intravenous administration of 50 mg of diphenhydramine.

Metoclopramide also acts as a dopamine antagonist (see above) and has been used in the prevention and treatment of nausea and vomiting. **Ondansetron,** a 5-HT$_3$ inhibitor, is also approved for use in the prevention of chemotherapy-induced and postoperative nausea and vomiting (see Chapter 16). **Marijuana** derivatives, including **tetrahydrocannabinol (THC, dronabinol)** itself, are effective antiemetics in some patients, including some in whom other antiemetics are ineffective. Dronabinol is approved for this indication. The mechanism of action of this drug is not known but appears to involve receptors in the chemoreceptor trigger zone. Corticosteroids, eg, **dexamethasone,** are antiemetics, but their mechanism is unknown. Finally, sedative-hypnotics such as the **benzodiazepines** are often used to control anticipatory nausea and vomiting.

PANCREATIC ENZYME REPLACEMENT PRODUCTS

Steatorrhea occurs in pancreatic insufficiency when lipase output is reduced below 10% of normal. It is estimated that in the postprandial period, approximately 100,000 units of lipase are delivered to the intestinal lumen per hour. Thus, the goal of pancreatic enzyme replacement should be to deliver at least 10,000 units per hour. However, because of inactivation of the enzyme below pH 4.0, only about 8% of the ingested lipase activity reaches the distal duodenum. Different pancreatic enzyme preparations vary markedly in enzyme activity. Manufacturers' listings of enzyme content may not always match a well-standardized in vitro laboratory assay. Two major types of preparation in use are **pancreatin,** an alcoholic extract of hog pancreas, and **pancrelipase,** a lipase-enriched hog pancreas preparation. The enzyme content of several pancreatic enzyme preparations as measured by in vitro assay is given in Table 63–3. As indicated in the table, variation in enzyme content can be partly compensated for by increases in dosage; the in vivo response—measured as reduction in stool fat and nitrogen—can be appreciable. Various dosage schedules have been recommended for pancreatic enzyme replacement, but there appears to be little difference between giving the medication with meals and giving it every 2 hours through the day. Because individual dosage requirements vary, it is essential that the result of therapy—the daily stool fat excretion—be monitored and the number of capsules or tablets increased until a therapeutic effect is seen. Supplementing the regimen with cimetidine enhances the effectiveness of the enzymes, presumably by decreasing the destruction of enzyme activity by gastric acid. Because the enzyme preparations have a high purine content, uric acid renal stones may be seen as a side effect. Also, the lactose in the pills may be sufficient to cause symptoms in lactose-intolerant patients. Finally, pancreatic enzyme replacement is expensive, costing up to $1500 per year for adequate therapy. Ineffectiveness of generic brands of enzyme preparations has been reported; bioequivalence studies have not been required of these products (Hendeles et al, 1990).

LAXATIVES

Laxatives of various types are widely prescribed and more widely purchased without prescription, indicating a cultural preoccupation with "regularity." These drugs are generally classified by simplified mechanism of action as irritants or stimulants, bulking agents, and stool softeners. However, laxatives work through more complex actions such as the interaction of osmotic effects with epithelial transport, changes in the enteric nervous system, and the release of extracellular regulators such as prostaglandins.

IRRITANT OR STIMULANT LAXATIVES

Castor oil is hydrolyzed in the upper small intestine to ricinoleic acid, a local irritant that increases intestinal motility. The onset of action is prompt and continues until the compound is excreted via the colon. **Cascara, senna,** and **aloes** contain emodin alkaloids that are liberated after absorption from the intestine and are excreted into the colon, where peristalsis is stimulated. Thus, their onset of activity is delayed for 6–8 hours. Chronic stimulation of the colon is thought to lead to chronic colonic distention and perpetuation of the perceived need for laxatives. **Phenolphthalein** and **bisacodyl,** which are chemically similar, are also potent colonic stimulants. Their action may be prolonged by an enterohepatic circulation.

BULKING LAXATIVES

Hydrophilic colloids, prepared from the indigestible parts of fruits, vegetables, and seeds, form gels within the large intestine, distending the intestine and thereby stimulating its peristaltic activity. **Agar, psyllium seed,** and **methylcellulose** all act in this manner as well. **Bran** and other forms of vegetable fiber have the same effect. **Saline cathartics** such as magnesium citrate and magnesium hydroxide also

Table 63–3. Enzyme activities in some pancreatic enzyme replacement products.

Proprietary Preparation	Amount (Units per Tablet or Capsule)			Number of Tablets or Capsules per Meal	Percentage Reduction in Feces	
	Lipase	Trypsin	Amylase		Fat	Nitrogen
Ilozyme	3600	3444	329,600	3	48	nd
Cotazyme	2014	1797	499,200	5	nd	35
Pancrease	2005	nd	nd	3	73	40
Viokase	1636	1828	277,333	6	49	40

nd = data not available

distend the bowel and stimulate its contractions. These nonabsorbable salts hold water in the intestine by osmotic force and cause distention. Isosmotic electrolyte solutions containing polyethylene glycol serve as colonic lavage solutions, chiefly in preparation for radiologic or endoscopic procedures and for removal of ingested toxins. **Lactulose** is a synthetic disaccharide (galactose-fructose) that is not absorbed, thus acting as an osmotic laxative when given in doses of 10–20 g up to four times daily. **Sorbitol** is also nonabsorbable and when given as a solution, 15–30 mL once or twice a day, can be effective when used three times a week.

STOOL SOFTENERS

Agents that become emulsified with stool serve to soften it and make passage easier. Examples are **mineral oil, glycerin suppositories,** and detergents such as **dioctyl sodium sulfosuccinate (docusate).**

ANTIDIARRHEAL DRUGS

The two most widely used prescription drugs for diarrhea are **diphenoxylate** (with atropine), a weak analog of meperidine, and **loperamide,** which is chemically related to haloperidol. Loperamide is also available without prescription. **Difenoxin** is the active metabolite of diphenoxylate and is available as a prescription medication. Their mechanism of action on the gut is similar to that of the opioids (see Chapter 31) and involves inhibition of acetylcholine release through presynaptic opioid receptors in the enteric nervous system. Loperamide may not cross the blood-brain barrier and thus may cause less sedation and be less addicting than diphenoxylate (although few central effects are noted with either drug). None of these drugs should be used in patients with severe ulcerative colitis, since toxic megacolon may be precipitated. It has been suggested that these drugs may prolong the duration of diarrhea in patients with *Shigella* or *Salmonella* infection. On the other hand, in patients with irritable bowel syndrome with predominant diarrhea, loperamide in doses of 2–4 mg four times a day may lead to substantial clinical improvement, especially when combined with increased dietary fiber, use of anticholinergic agents as antispasmodics, and supportive counseling. Adsorbents such as **kaolin** and **pectin** are also widely used. Their action is through their ability to adsorb compounds from solution, presumably binding potential intestinal toxins. Overall, however, they are much less effective than the drugs mentioned above, and they may also interfere with the absorption of other medications. Experimental and clinical observations indicate that α_2-adrenoceptor agonists such as clonidine can reduce electrolyte secretion by the bowel in conditions such as diabetic diarrhea (Fedorak et al, 1985). Similar α_2-selective drugs with reduced transport into the central nervous system are being investigated for this purpose.

DRUGS USED FOR THE DISSOLUTION OF GALLSTONES

Cholesterol is solubilized in aqueous bile by the combined effect of bile acids and lecithin, which, together with cholesterol, form the mixed micelle. When cholesterol is secreted in bile in relative excess to lecithin and bile acids, cholesterol crystals precipitate and may coalesce into cholesterol gallstones. Patients with these stones may have impaired bile salt secretion, excess cholesterol secretion, or some combination of both.

Oral Therapy

Chenodiol, a primary bile acid in man, and **ursodiol,** the 7β epimer of chenodiol, are both effective in dissolving cholesterol stones in some patients. Both compounds expand the total bile salt pool, but their principal effect appears to be more complicated. Chenodiol inhibits the rate-limiting enzyme of the conversion of bile salts to cholesterol, HMG-CoA reductase, thus causing an increase in bile salt excretion and a decrease in cholesterol secretion. Ursodiol causes the transport of cholesterol in a liquid crystal form, and it appears also to stabilize the canalicular membrane of hepatocytes. In addition, as 7β epimers do not appear to suppress 7α-hydroxylase, the rate-limiting enzyme for bile acid synthesis, the addition of ursodiol to the bile acid pool does not cause hepatic bile acid synthesis to be down-regulated. These physicochemical differences between the two compounds probably account for some of the differences in their toxicities.

The use of chenodiol is limited by adverse effects. A dose-related diarrhea is seen in up to 30% of patients, and a similar percentage will have increased serum aminotransferase or cholesterol levels. Ursodiol appears to have substantially fewer adverse effects, but it is more expensive. Studies are now in progress to determine whether a combination of ursodiol with chenodiol can be effective at reduced cost and toxicity.

These agents are most effective in dissolving small (< 5 mm) floating stones in a functioning gallbladder. They cannot dissolve stones that are more than 4% calcium by weight; unfortunately, stones with lower calcium concentrations are not often radiopaque and will not be discovered. Thus, many patients will be poor candidates or will not respond with complete dissolution of their stones even with 2 years of therapy. In addition, the recurrence rate after therapy is stopped is sufficiently high that lifelong therapy may be considered for patients who respond well to an initial course of treatment. However, given that recurrent stones may only infrequently cause symptoms, it might be best to reserve additional courses of dissolution therapy only for symptomatic recurrences. An alternative to pharmacologic treatment—shock wave lithotripsy—may have its benefits enhanced by the concurrent administration of chenodiol or ursodiol. This combination is under investigation.

Other conditions in which these agents have been tried include cholestatic disorders of the liver and biliary tree. Some studies have indicated that ursodiol is effective in primary biliary cirrhosis and sclerosing cholangitis. The exact mechanism is unknown, but it is postulated that by modifying the endogenous bile acid pool, ursodiol reverses the intracellular accumulation of toxic bile acids. Therapeutic trials show an improvement in both hepatic enzyme levels and histopathology.

Other Drugs

Methyl *tert*-**butyl ether** can dissolve cholesterol stones in the gallbladder and bile ducts when it is infused via a catheter directly into the gallbladder or bile duct lumen. The ether has a boiling point of 52.2 °C and thus remains liquid at body temperature. Ethers are excellent solvents for lipids, and dissolution of stones can usually be accomplished within hours. The exact therapeutic role of methyl *tert*-butyl ether remains to be defined, and it is likely that for now it will be reserved for selected patients who are not surgical candidates. **Monoctanoin** (glyceryl-1-monooctanoate) is another agent that is infused into the common bile duct through a catheter or T tube to dissolve retained bile duct stones. Stones may be completely dissolved or sufficiently reduced in size to facilitate their subsequent removal.

DRUGS USED IN THE TREATMENT OF CHRONIC INFLAMMATORY BOWEL DISEASE

The principal drugs used in the treatment of chronic inflammatory bowel disease (ulcerative colitis, Crohn's disease) are corticosteroids and other immunosuppressive agents and salicylate derivatives.

Salicylates

Most evidence suggests that nonabsorbed **5-aminosalicylic acid (5-ASA, mesalamine)** is an active anti-inflammatory agent in inflammatory bowel disease. 5-Aminosalicylic acid can affect multiple sites in the arachidonic acid pathway critical in the pathogenesis of inflammation. Although its interrup-

tion of the cyclooxygenase pathway would inhibit prostaglandin production, some studies suggest that leukotriene formation is also inhibited and may be more important. The drug may also act as a free radical scavenger. Further studies are needed to answer these questions.

Unfortunately, 5-aminosalicylic acid itself cannot be taken orally in sufficient dosage to produce a useful effect in the colon without excessive upper gastrointestinal tract irritation and systemic toxicity. **Sulfasalazine** combines sulfapyridine with 5-aminosalicylic acid linked by an azo bond. The drug is poorly absorbed from the intestine, and the azo linkage is broken down by the bacterial flora in the distal ileum and colon to release 5-aminosalicylic acid. Sulfasalazine was first introduced in the 1940s for the treatment of rheumatoid arthritis. It was subsequently shown to be effective in mildly to moderately active ulcerative colitis and Crohn's colitis but less so in Crohn's disease of the small intestine. In ulcerative colitis, it is more effective in maintaining than in achieving clinical remission.

The usual therapeutic dosage of sulfasalazine is 3–4 g/d in divided doses. Smaller dosages, usually 2 g/d, are needed to maintain remission in ulcerative colitis. Dose-related adverse effects such as malaise, nausea, abdominal discomfort, or headache occur in up to 20% of patients given 4 g/d. Some of these effects may be avoided by beginning at a lower dosage and slowly increasing to the desired dosage level or by using enteric-coated or liquid suspension preparations. The inhibition of folic acid absorption by sulfasalazine has been reported, so supplemental folate should be administered. Finally, as with other sulfonamides, serum sickness-like reactions and severe bone marrow suppression have occasionally been seen.

Three other oral forms of 5-aminosalicylate have been developed that can deliver the active moiety to the distal bowel while avoiding the toxicity of sulfapyridine as well as excessive systemic absorption of 5-aminosalicylic acid. **Olsalazine** links two 5-aminosalicylic acid molecules via a diazo bond that is broken down by bacterial action in the colon, releasing the active agent. **Balsalazide** (investigational) links 5-aminosalicylic acid to an inert carrier via a diazo bond, which can be similarly broken down in the colon. 5-Aminosalicylic acid itself is available in two forms: as an enema (see below) and in slow-release microspheres for oral administration. Controlled trials have shown encouraging results in mild to moderate ulcerative colitis and Crohn's disease. Currently, mesalamine is approved only for treatment of active colitis, and olsalazine is approved only for maintenance of remission. These drugs all appear to be well tolerated. The most frequent adverse effect is watery diarrhea, which occurs in 15–35% of patients receiving olsalazine and is thought to be caused by the drug's secretagogue properties. In addition, 5-aminosalicylic acid appears to be responsible for the rarely observed exacerbation of ulcerative colitis associated with sulfasalazine. All of these newer preparations are more expensive than sulfasalazine, and their clinical advantages in patients who tolerate this drug remain to be demonstrated. Topical 5-aminosalicylic acid, delivered in a retention enema or as a suppository, has proved effective in the treatment of active distal colitis and is approved for that use. A full response may require months, however, and enemas will reach, at best, only to the splenic flexure. Oral and rectal forms of 5-aminosalicylic acid may be used in combination to good effect. Fortunately, topical therapy has also proved effective as prophylaxis against recurrence in patients who have achieved remission.

Immunosuppressive Agents

Immunosuppressive agents applied in inflammatory bowel disease include the corticosteroids, which have been used for many years to control acute episodes, and cytotoxic drugs. Both ACTH and standard corticosteroids such as hydrocortisone and prednisone have been used with comparable clinical efficacy. Topical corticosteroids given in enema form are effective for patients with distal colitis, but over the long term their use may be associated with the same side effects as are seen with systemic corticosteroids. Studies of newer topical preparations with the same anti-inflammatory effects but no systemic effects, such as tixocortol pivalate, have been promising. However, none of these compounds are yet available in the USA. Cytotoxic agents, particularly azathioprine and mercaptopurine, are being used more often in the treatment of inflammatory bowel disease. Their steroid-sparing properties can be beneficial to patients with Crohn's disease and ulcerative colitis, and they seem to be particularly helpful in the treatment of fistulas complicating Crohn's disease. Both drugs appear to be more effective than corticosteroids as prophylaxis in patients with Crohn's disease. The dosages are relatively low, beginning at 50 mg/d and usually not exceeding 1.5 mg/kg daily. At these dose levels, hematologic complications are minimized, though careful monitoring is still essential. In addition, the long-term risk of drug-induced malignancy would seem to be minimal at these doses. Drug-induced pancreatitis occurs in 3–15% of patients but typically resolves spontaneously with drug withdrawal. Cyclosporine may also be of value in these conditions, but its toxicity may limit its application in chronic therapy. It is probably best used in patients with severe refractory disease when surgery cannot be tolerated.

DRUGS USED IN THERAPY OF PORTAL-SYSTEMIC ENCEPHALOPATHY

The broad-spectrum, nonabsorbable antibiotic neomycin (see Chapter 45) has been combined with dietary restriction of protein for the treatment of portal-systemic encephalopathy. **Lactulose** is also effective in this condition. The mechanism of action of lactulose is unclear. It is apparently degraded by intestinal bacteria to lactic acid, acetic acid, and other organic acids. It is thought that this may facilitate the "trapping" of ammonium ion or other putative central nervous system toxins in the intestinal tract. Modification of the normal intestinal flora by lactulose has been suggested as another mechanism of action, but this has not been demonstrated with certainty. Lactulose is available as a syrup and is given in doses of 15–30 mL four times daily or until the patient has four or five soft bowel movements daily. The drug is well tolerated and may be given in combination with neomycin, though this combination has no clear advantage over lactulose alone. Lactulose may also be administered as an enema.

PREPARATIONS AVAILABLE
(See Table 63–2 for antacid preparations.)

H₂ Histamine Receptor Blockers
  Cimetidine (generic, Tagamet)
    Oral: 75,* 100, 200, 300, 400, 800 mg tablets; 300 mg/5 mL liquid
    Parenteral: 300 mg/2 mL, 300 mg/50 mL for injection
  Famotidine (Pepcid)
    Oral: 10,* 20, 40 mg tablets; powder to reconstitute for 40 mg/5 mL suspension
    Parenteral: 10 mg/mL for injection
  Nizatidine (Axid)
    Oral: 75,* 150, 300 mg tablets
  Ranitidine (Zantac)
    Oral: 75,* 150, 300 mg tablets; 150 mg

effervescent tablets; 150, 300 mg capsules; 15 mg/mL syrup
    Parenteral: 0.5, 25 mg/mL for injection

Anticholinergic Drugs
  Anisotropine (generic, Valpin)
    Oral: 50 mg tablets
  Atropine (generic)
    Oral: 0.4, 0.6 mg tablets
    Parenteral: 0.05, 0.1, 0.3, 0.4, 0.5, 0.8, 1, mg/mL for injection

*Over-the-counter formulation.

Belladonna alkaloids, extract or tincture
(generic)
Oral: 0.27–0.33 mg/mL liquid
Clidinium (Quarzan)
Oral: 2.5, 5 mg capsules
Dicyclomine (generic, Bentyl, others)
Oral: 10, 20 mg capsules; 20 mg tablets; 10 mg/5 mL syrup
Parenteral: 10 mg/mL for injection
Flavoxate (Urispas)
Oral: 100 mg tablets
Glycopyrrolate (generic, Robinul)
Oral: 1, 2 mg tablets
Parenteral: 0.2 mg/mL for injection
Isopropamide (Darbid)
Oral: 5 mg tablets
l-Hyoscyamine (Anaspaz, Cystospaz-M, Levsinex)
Oral: 0.125, 0.15 mg tablets; 0.375 mg timed-release capsules; 0.125 mg/5 mL oral elixir and solution
Parenteral: 0.5 mg/mL for injection
Mepenzolate (Cantil)
Oral: 25 mg tablets
Methantheline (Banthine)
Oral: 50 mg tablets
Methscopolamine (Pamine)
Oral: 2.5 mg tablets
Oxybutynin (generic, Ditropan)
Oral: 5 mg tablets, 5 mg/5 mL syrup
Oxyphencyclimine (Daricon)
Oral: 10 mg tablets
Propantheline (generic, Pro-Banthine)
Oral: 7.5, 15 mg tablets
Scopolamine (generic)
Oral: 0.25 mg capsules
Parenteral: 0.3, 0.4, 0.65, 0.86, 1 mg/mL for injection
Tridihexethyl (Pathilon)
Oral: 25 mg tablets

Proton Pump Inhibitors
Omeprazole (Prilosec)
Oral: 10, 20 mg delayed-release capsules
Lansoprazole (Prevacid)
Oral: 15, 30 mg capsules

Mucosal Protective Agents
Misoprostol (Cytotec)
Oral: 100, 200 μg tablets
Sucralfate (Carafate)
Oral: 1 g tablets

Drugs for Motility Disorders & Selected Antiemetics
Cisapride (Propulsid)
Oral: 10, 20 mg tablets; 1 mg/mL suspension
Dronabinol (Marinol)
Oral: 2.5, 5, 10 mg tablets
Metoclopramide (generic, Reglan, others)

Oral: 5, 10 mg tablets; 5 mg/5 mL syrup
Parenteral: 5 mg/mL for injection
Ondansetron (Zofran)
Oral: 4, 8 mg tablets
Parenteral: 2 mg/mL for IV injection
Prochlorperazine (Compazine)
Oral: 5, 10, 25 mg tablets; 10, 15, 30 mg capsules; 1 mg/mL solution
Rectal: 2.5, 5, 25 mg suppositories
Parenteral: 5 mg/mL for injection

Selected Anti-inflammatory Drugs Used in Gastrointestinal Disease
Hydrocortisone (Cortenema, Cortifoam)
Rectal: 100 mg/60 mL unit retention enema; 90 mg/applicatorful intrarectal foam
Mesalamine (Asacol, Pentasa, Rowasa)
Oral: 400 mg tablets; 250 mg controlled-release capsules
Rectal: 4 g/60 mL suspension; 500 mg suppositories
Methylprednisolone (Medrol Enpack)
Rectal: 40 mg/bottle retention enema
Olsalazine (Dipentum)
Oral: 250 mg capsules
Sulfasalazine (generic, Azulfidine, others)
Oral: 500 mg tablets and enteric-coated tablets; 250 mg/5 mL suspension

Selected Antidiarrheal Drugs
Bismuth subsalicylate (Pepto-Bismol, others)
Oral: 262 mg chewable tablets; 262, 524 mg/15 mL suspension
Difenoxin (Motofen)
Oral: 1 mg (with 0.025 mg atropine sulfate) tablets
Diphenoxylate (generic, Lomotil, others)
Oral: 2.5 mg (with 0.025 mg atropine sulfate) tablets and liquid
Kaolin/pectin (generic, Kaopectate, others)
Oral (typical): 5.85 g kaolin and 260 mg pectin per 30 mL suspension
Loperamide (Imodium)
Oral: 2 mg tablets, capsules; 1 mg/5 mL liquid
Paregoric (generic)
Oral: 2 mg morphine (equivalent) per 5 mL liquid

Selected Laxative Drugs
Bisacodyl (generic, Dulcolax, others)
Oral: 5 mg enteric coated tablets
Rectal: 10 mg suppositories
Cascara sagrada (generic)
Oral: 325 mg tablets; 5 mL per dose fluid extract (approximately 18% alcohol)
Castor oil (generic, others)
Oral: liquid or liquid emulsion
Docusate (generic, Colace, others)
Oral: 50, 100, 240, 250 mg capsules; 100 mg

tablets; 50, 60, 150 mg/15 mL syrup; 50 mg/mL solution

Glycerin suppository (generic, Sani-Supp, Fleet Babylax)

Lactulose (Chronulac, Cephulac)
Oral: 10 g/15 mL syrup

Magnesium hydroxide [milk of magnesia, Epsom Salt] (generic)
Oral: 7–8.5% aqueous suspension

Methylcellulose
Oral: 450 mg/5 mL liquid

Mineral oil (generic, others)
Oral: liquid, jelly, or emulsion

Phenolphthalein (generic, Ex-Lax, others)
Oral: 60, 90, 97.2, 130 mg tablets; 65, 90, 97.2, 120 mg chewable tablets

Polycarbophil (Equalactin, Mitrolan, FiberCon, Fiber-Lax)
Oral: 500, 625 mg tablets; 500, 1250 mg chewable tablets

Polyethylene glycol electrolyte solution (CoLyte, GoLYTELY, others)

Oral: Powder for oral solution, makes one gallon (approx 4 L)

Psyllium (generic, Serutan, Metamucil, others)
Oral: 2.5, 3.4, 3.5, 4.94 g psyllium granules or powder per packet; 50%, 100% psyllium also available

Senna (Senokot, others)
Oral: 187, 217, 374, 600 mg tablets; 326 mg granules; 1.65 g senna (eq) per 1/2 tsp granules; 218 mg/5 mL syrup; 33.3 mg/mL liquid
Rectal: 652 mg suppositories

Drugs That Dissolve Gallstones

Chenodiol (Chenix)
Oral: 250 mg tablets

Monoctanoin (Moctanin)
Parenteral: 120 mL infusion bottle

Ursodiol (Actigall)
Oral: 300 mg capsules

REFERENCES

Pharmacokinetics

Lauritsen K, Laursen LS, Rask-Madsen J: Clinical pharmacokinetics of drugs used in the treatment of gastrointestinal diseases. (Two parts.) Clin Pharmacokinet 1990;19:11, 94.

Acid-Peptic Disease

Blum AL: Treatment of acid-related disorders with gastric acid inhibitors: The state of the art. Digestion 1990; 47(Suppl 1):3.

Burgess E, Muruve D: Aluminum absorption and excretion following sucralfate therapy in chronic renal insufficiency. Am J Med 1992;92:471.

Chamberlain CE, Peura DA: *Campylobacter (Helicobacter) pylori:* Is peptic disease a bacterial infection? Arch Intern Med 1990;150:951.

Farup PG et al: Low-dose antacids versus 400 mg cimetidine twice daily for reflux oesophagitis: A comparative, placebo-controlled, multicentre study. Scand J Gastroenterol 1990;25:315.

Galmiche JP et al: Double-blind comparison of cisapride and cimetidine in treatment of reflux esophagitis. Dig Dis Sci 1990;35:649.

Graham DY et al: Effect of treatment of *Helicobacter pylori* infection on the long-term recurrence of gastric or duodenal ulcer: A randomized, controlled study. Ann Intern Med 1992;116:705.

Gugler R, Allgayer H: Effects of antacids on the clinical pharmacokinetics of drugs: An update. Clin Pharmacokinet 1990;18:210.

Hetzel DJ: Controlled clinical trials of omeprazole in the long-term management of reflux disease. Digestion 1992;5(Suppl 1):35.

Lamberts SWJ et al: Octreotide. N Engl J Med 1996; 334:246.

Maton PN: Omeprazole. N Engl J Med 1991;324:965.

Maton PN et al: The effect of Zollinger-Ellison syndrome and omeprazole therapy on gastric oxyntic endocrine cells. Gastroenterology 1990;99:943.

McCarthy DM: Sucralfate. N Engl J Med 1991;325:1017.

Pope CE: Acid-reflux disorders. N Engl J Med 1994;331:656.

Ramirez B, Richter JE: Review article: promotility drugs in the treatment of gastro-esophageal reflux disease. Aliment Pharmacol Ther 1993;7:5.

Sachs G, Prinz C: Gastric enterochromaffin-like cells and the regulation of acid secretion. News Physiol Sci 1996;11:57.

Soll AH (moderator): Nonsteroidal anti-inflammatory drugs and peptic ulcer disease. Ann Intern Med 1991;114:307.

Soll AH et al: Medical treatment of peptic ulcer disease: Practice guidelines. JAMA 1996;275:622.

Sontag S et al: Cimetidine, cigarette smoking, and recurrence of duodenal ulcer. N Engl J Med 1984;311:689.

Walsh JH, Peterson WL: The treatment of *Helicobacter pylori* infection in the management of peptic ulcer disease. N Engl J Med 1995;333:984.

Walt RP: Misoprostol for the treatment of peptic ulcer and anti-inflammatory-drug-induced gastroduodenal ulceration. N Engl J Med 1992;327:1575.

Walt RP, Langman MJS: Antacids and ulcer healing. Drugs 1991;42:205.

Wilson DE: Prostaglandins in peptic ulcer disease: Their postulated role in the pathogenesis and treatment. Postgrad Med 1987;81:309.

Wolfe MM, Soll AH: The physiology of gastric acid secretion. N Engl J Med 1988;319:1707.

Motility Disorders

Binder HJ, Donowitz M: A new look at laxative action. Gastroenterology 1975;69:1001.

Drenth JPH, Engels LGJB: Diabetic gastroparesis: A critical appraisal of new treatment strategies. Drugs 1992; 44:537.

Drossman DA, Thompson WG: The irritable bowel syndrome: Review and a graduated multicomponent treatment approach. Ann Intern Med 1992;116:1009.

Fedorak RN, Field M, Chang EB: Treatment of diabetic diarrhea with clonidine. Ann Intern Med 1985;102:197.

Lynn RB, Friedman LS: Irritable bowel syndrome. N Engl J Med 1993;329:1940.

Tack J et al: Effect of erythromycin on gastric motility in controls and in diabetic gastroparesis. Gastroenterology 1992;103:72.

Gallstone Therapy

Hoffman AF: Nonsurgical treatment of gallstone disease. Annu Rev Med 1990;41:401.

Johnston DE, Kaplan MM: Pathogenesis and treatment of gallstones. N Engl J Med 1993;328:412.

Poupon RE et al: A multicenter, controlled trial of ursodiol for the treatment of primary biliary cirrhosis. N Engl J Med 1991;324:1548.

Inflammatory Bowel Disease

Hanaver SB: Inflammatory bowel disease. N Engl J Med 1996;334:841.

Klotz U et al: Therapeutic efficacy of sulfasalazine and its metabolites in patients with ulcerative colitis and Crohn's disease. N Engl J Med 1980;303:1499.

Kozarek RA: Review article: immunosuppressive therapy for inflammatory bowel disease. Aliment Pharmacol Ther 1993;7:117.

Lashner BA et al: Testing nicotine gum for ulcerative colitis patients. Dig Dis Sci 1990;35:827.

Schroeder KW, Tremaine WJ, Ilstrup DM: Coated oral 5-aminosalicylic acid therapy for mildly to moderately active ulcerative colitis: A randomized study. N Engl J Med 1987;317:1625.

Shanahan F, Targan S: Medical treatment of inflammatory bowel disease. Annu Rev Med 1992;43:125.

Watkinson G: Sulphasalazine: A review of 40 years' experience. Drugs 1986;32(Suppl 1):1.

Antiemetics

Aapro MS et al: Antiemetic efficacy of droperidol or metoclopramide combined with dexamethasone and diphenhydramine: Randomized open parallel study. Oncology 1991;48:116.

Beck TM et al: Efficacy of oral ondansetron in the prevention of emesis in outpatients receiving cyclophosphamide-based chemotherapy. Ann Intern Med 1993; 118:407.

Lane M et al: Dronabinol and prochlorperazine alone and in combination as antiemetic agents for cancer chemotherapy. Am J Clin Oncol 1990;13:480.

Marin J, Ibanez MC, Arribas S: Therapeutic management of nausea and vomiting. Gen Pharmacol 1990;21:1.

Mitchelson F: Pharmacological agents affecting emesis. A review. (Two parts) Drugs 1992;43:295, 443.

Stewart DJ: Cancer therapy, vomiting, and antiemetics. Can J Physiol Pharmacol 1990;68:304.

Tortorice PV, O'Connell MB: Management of chemotherapy-induced nausea and vomiting. Pharmacotherapy 1990;10:129.

Miscellaneous

Hendeles L et al: Treatment failure after substitution of generic pancrelipase capsules: Correlation with in vitro lipase activity. JAMA 1990;263:2459.

64

Therapeutic & Toxic Potential of Over-the-Counter Agents

Mary Anne Koda-Kimble, PharmD

In the USA, drugs are divided by law into two classes: those restricted to sale by prescription only and those for which directions for safe use by the public can be written. The latter category constitutes the nonprescription or over-the-counter (OTC) drugs. In 1995, the American public spent approximately $18 billion on well over 125,000 OTC products to medicate themselves for self-diagnosed ailments ranging from asthma to warts. These products represent about 700 active ingredients in various forms and combinations. It is thus apparent that many are no more than "me too" products advertised to the public in ways that suggest that there are significant differences between them. For example, there are over 100 different systemic analgesic products almost all of which contain aspirin, acetaminophen, salicylamide, phenacetin, nonsteroidal anti-inflammatory drugs (NSAIDs) such as ibuprofen, or a combination of these agents as primary ingredients. They are made different from one another by the addition of questionable ingredients such as caffeine or antihistamines; by brand names chosen to suggest a specific use or strength ("feminine pain," "arthritis," "maximum," "extra"); or by their special dosage form (enteric-coated tablets, liquids, sustained-release products, powders, seltzers). There is a price attached to all of these artificial features, and in most cases a less expensive generic product can be equally effective. It is probably safe to assume that the public is generally overwhelmed and confused by the wide array of products presented and will probably use those that are most heavily advertised.

Since 1972, the Food and Drug Administration has been engaged in a methodical review of OTC ingredients for both safety and efficacy. There have been two major outcomes of this review: (1) ingredients designated as ineffective or unsafe for their claimed therapeutic use are being eliminated from OTC product formulations (eg, antimuscarinic agents have been eliminated from OTC sleep aids); and (2) agents previously available by prescription only have been made available for OTC use because they were judged by the review panel to be generally safe and effective for consumer use without medical supervision (eg, topi-cal hydrocortisone 0.5% and 1%, diphenhydramine, several NSAIDs, clotrimazole, H_2 antagonists, topical minoxidil). Since the appointment of a new Nonprescription Drugs Advisory Committee in 1993, the rate of switches from prescription to OTC status has accelerated. Some OTC ingredients previously available in low doses only are now available in higher concentrations. Table 64–1 lists some prescription drugs that have been recommended for OTC use. Although few final regulations have been issued on these recommendations, the FDA's position has been to allow manufacturers to incorporate these ingredients into their OTC formulations upon publication of the review panel's preliminary report unless it (the FDA) finds compelling reason to dissent. Examples of other prescription drugs currently under consideration for OTC sales include sucralfate, nonsedating antihistamines, oral contraceptives, albuterol, and cromolyn.

There are three reasons why it is important for the clinician to be familiar with this class of products. First, many of the ingredients contained in these products are effective in treating common ailments, and it is important to be able to help the patient select a safe, effective product. As managed care practices direct clinicians to limit the cost of drugs they prescribe, many will begin to recommend effective OTC treatments to their patients, since these drugs are rarely paid for by the insurance plan. (See Table 64–2.) Second, many of the active ingredients contained in OTC drugs may worsen existing medical conditions or interact with prescription medications. (See Appendix II, Drug Interactions.) Finally, the misuse or abuse of OTC products may actually produce significant medical complications. Phenylpropanolamine, for example, a sympathomimetic included in many cold, allergy, and weight control products, has been abused by adolescents and is often sold as a cocaine or amphetamine substitute. In only two to three times the therapeutic dose, this drug can cause severe hypertension, seizures, and intracranial hemorrhage. A general awareness of these products and their formulation will enable clinicians to more fully appreciate the potential for OTC drug-related problems in their patients.

Table 64–1. Ingredients that have been recommended by the over-the-counter (OTC) review panel to be switched from prescription to OTC status.

Ingredient and Dosage	Indication	Single-Ingredient Product Examples or FDA Status
Systemic Acyclovir 200 mg	Antiviral	Advisory Committee voted "no" on January 12, 1996
Brompheniramine 4 mg every 4–6 hours	Antihistamine	Dimetane Extentabs
Chlophedianol hydrochloride 25 mg every 6–8 hours	Antitussive	None

Chlorpheniramine
  4 mg every 4–6 hours
  12 mg every 12 hours
	Antihistamine	Chlor-Trimeton, Teldrin
		Chlor-Trimeton Maximum Strength

Cholestyramine	Cholesterol-lowering agent	Advisory committee voted "no" on September 27, 1995
Cimetidine 200 mg twice weekly	Acid reducer	Tagamet HB
Clemastine fumarate 1.25 mg every 12 hours	Antihistamine	Tavist-1
Colestipol	Cholesterol-lowering agent	Not yet reviewed by Advisory Committee

Dexbrompheniramine maleate
  3 mg every 6–8 hours
  6 mg/12 hours (time-released)
	Antihistamine	Drixoral[2]

Diflunisal	Analgesic, antipyretic	Not yet reviewed by Advisory Committee
Diphenhydramine hydrochloride 25–50 mg every 4–6 hours	Antihistamine Antitussive Sleep aid	Benadryl Benylin Syrup Sominex 2, Sleep-Eze 3
Doxylamine succinate 25 mg single-dose only	Sleep aid	Unisom
Dyclonine hydrochloride 0.05–0.10%; 1–3 mg as lozenge	Oral local anesthetic, analgesic	Sucret's Maximum Strength Throat Spray; Lozenge
Famotidine 10 mg, up to 20 mg daily	Acid reducer	Pepcid AC

Fluoride (various salts)
  Sodium 0.05% rinse
  Stannous 0.1% rinse
  Acidulated phosphate 0.02% rinse
	Dental caries prophylaxis	Fluorigard
		Stan Care
		None

Ibuprofen
  200 mg every 4–6 hours
  7.5 mg/kg up to 4 times daily as
    a suspension
	Analgesic, antipyretic
	Pediatric dose
		Advil, Motrin, Nuprin
		Children's Motrin

Ketoprofen 12.5 mg every 4–6 hours	Analgesic, antipyretic	Actron, Orudis KT
Loperamide 4 mg, then 2 mg; 8 mg/d	Antidiarrheal	Imodium A-D
Methocarbimol	Muscle relaxant	Advisory Committee undecided as of March 28, 1996
Methoxyphenamine hydrochloride 100 mg every 4–6 hours	Antihistamine	None
Naproxen 200 mg every 4–6 hours	Analgesic, antipyretic	Aleve

Nicotine
  Various doses based on delivery
    system and instructions for use
	Smoking cessation	Patch: NicoDerm CQ
		Transdermal: Nicotrol
		Nasal spray: Nicotrol NS

Nicotine polacrilex 2 mg and 4 mg chewing pieces	Smoking cessation	Gum: Nicorette
Nizatidine	Heartburn prevention	Axid

(continued)

Table 64–1. Ingredients that have been recommended by the over-the-counter (OTC) review panel to be switched from prescription to OTC status (cont'd).

Ingredient and Dosage	Indication	Single-Ingredient Product Examples or FDA Status
Phenylpropanolamine hydrochloride 75 mg/12 hours (time-released)	Nasal decongestant	Allerest-12 Hour, Contac, Triaminic-12[3]
Pseudoephedrine hydrochloride and sulfate 60 mg every 4–6 hours; 240 mg maximum/24 hours 120 mg/12 hours (time-released)	Nasal decongestant	D-Feed, Sudafed Chlor-Trimeton Long-Acting Repetabs[3]
Pyrantel pamoate 11 mg/kg as single dose; 1 g maximum	Anthelmintic (pinworms)	Antiminth (Oral Suspension) Reese's Pinworm (Liquid)
Ranitidine 75 mg up to twice daily	Acid reducer	Zantac 75
Triprolidine hydrochloride 2.5 mg every 4–6 hours; 5 mg/12 hours (time-released)	Antihistamine	Actifed (various)[4]
Topical Butoconazole nitrate 2% cream; applicators for 3 days	Anticandidal	Femstat 3
Clotrimazole 1% lotion or cream 2 times daily	Antifungal	Lotrimin AF
Cromolyn Nasal solution 40 mg/mL	Allergic rhinitis	Nasalcrom
Ephedrine sulfate 0.1–1.25%	Hemorrhoidal vasoconstrictor	None
Epinephrine hydrochloride 0.005–0.01%	Hemorrhoidal vasoconstrictor	Pazo Ointment
Haloprogin 1%	Antifungal	None
Ketoconazole 1% shampoo	Dandruff	Approval recommended by Advisory Committee February 16, 1994; pending FDA approval
Miconazole nitrate 2%	Antifungal	Micatin cream, spray, powder, liquid
	Anticandidal	Monistat vaginal cream, suppositories
Miconazole nitrate 200 mg suppository	Vaginal yeast infection	Monistat 3
Minoxidil 2% solution, 1 mL twice daily	Hair grower	Rogaine
Nystatin 100,000 units/g	Anticandidal[1]	None
Oxymetazoline hydrochloride 0.05%	Nasal decongestant	Afrin, Dristan Long-Lasting, NeoSynephrine 12 Hour
0.025% solution or drops	Ocular vasoconstrictor	Ocu Clear
Permethrin 1% cream rinse	Pediculicide (head lice)	Nix
Phenylephrine hydrochloride 0.25%	Hemorrhoidal vasoconstrictor	None
Tioconazole 1%	Antifungal	None
Xylometazoline hydrochloride 0.01%	Nasal decongestant	Otrivin

[1]Despite review panel recommendation, the FDA has dissented from OTC use for this application at this time.
[2]No single-ingredient product available. Combined with pseudoephedrine 60 mg.
[3]No single-ingredient product available. Combined with chlorpheniramine 8–12 mg.
[4]No single-ingredient product available. Combined with pseudoephedrine 30–120 mg.

Table 64–2. Ingredients of known efficacy for selected over-the-counter (OTC) classes.

OTC Category	Ingredient and Dosage	Product Examples	Comments
Acid reducers (H$_2$ antagonists)	Cimetidine,[1] 200 mg twice daily	Tagamet HB (100 mg/tablet)	These products have been approved at lower than prescription doses for the relief of "heartburn, acid indigestion, and sour stomach." They should not be taken for longer than 2 weeks and are not approved for children.
	Famotidine,[1] 10 mg, up to 20 mg daily	Pepcid AC Acid Controller (10 mg/tablet)	
	Nizatidine,[1] 75 mg up to twice daily	Axid AR	
	Ranitidine,[1] 75 mg up to twice daily	Zantac 75 (75 mg per tablet)	
Acne preparations	Benzoyl peroxide, 2.5, 5, 10%	Generic, Benoxyl, Clearasil, Oxy-5, Oxy-10	One of the most effective acne preparations. Apply sparingly once or twice daily. Decrease dose if excessive skin irritation occurs.
Allergy and "cold" preparations	Chlorpheniramine, 4 mg every 4–6 hours; 12 mg every 12 hours	Generic, Chlor-Trimeton (4 mg/tab or 10 mL syrup), Long Acting Chlor-Trimetron[1] (8 mg/tab), Teldrin Time-Released Capsules[1] (8 mg and 12 mg/cap)	Antihistamines alone relieve most symptoms associated with allergic rhinitis or hay fever. Chlorpheniramine, brompheniramine, and clemastine cause less drowsiness than diphenhydramine, methapyriline, pyrilamine, doxylamine, and phentoloxamine. Occasionally, symptoms unrelieved by the antihistamine respond to the addition of a sympathomimetic.
	Brompheniramine, 4 mg every 4–6 hours; 12 mg every 12 hours	Symptom 3 (4 mg/10 mL), Dimetane Extentab[1] (12 mg)	
	Clemastine fumarate,[1] 1.34 mg every 12 hours	Tavist-1 (1.34 mg/tab)	
	Diphenhydramine,[1] 25–50 mg every 4–6 hours	Benadryl (25 mg/cap; 12.5 mg/5 mL elixir)	
	Chlorpheniramine (8–12 mg) with phenylpropanolamine	Contac, Triaminic-12	
	Clemastine fumarate (1.34 mg) with phenylpropanolamine (75 mg) every 12 hours	Tavist-D	
	Triprolidine HCl (2.5 mg) with pseudoephedrine (60 mg)	Actifed	
Analgesics and antipyretics	Aspirin, 300–600 mg every 4–6 hours	Generic, Bayer Aspirin (325 mg/tab)	There are numerous product modifications, including the addition of antacid, caffeine, and methapyriline; enteric-coated tablets and seltzers; long-acting or extra-strength formulations; and various mixtures of analgesics. None have any substantial advantage over a single-ingredient product. Acetaminophen lacks anti-inflammatory activity but is available as a liquid; this dosage form is used primarily for infants and children who cannot chew or swallow tablets. Aspirin should be used cautiously in certain individuals (see text). Avoid products that contain phenacetin, eg, A.S.A. compound, Bromo-Seltzer, A.P.C. Capsules. Extra-strength formulations contain 400–600 mg of active ingredient.
	Acetaminophen, 300–600 mg every 4–6 hours	Generic, Datril, Tylenol (325 mg/tab various strengths available)	
	Ibuprofen,[1] 200–400 mg every 4–6 hours	Generic, Advil, Nuprin, Mediprin (200 mg/tab)	
	Naproxen, 200 mg every 8–10 hours	Aleve (200 mg/tab)	
	Ketoprofen,[1] 12.5 mg every 4–6 hours	Actron (12.5 mg tablet) Orudis KT (12.5 mg tablet)	
Antacids	Magnesium hydroxide and aluminum hydroxide combinations	Gelusil, Gelusil II, Maalox No. 1, Maalox No. 2, Mylanta, Mylanta II, Wingel, others	Combinations of magnesium and aluminum hydroxide are less likely to cause constipation or diarrhea and offer high neutralizing capacity. The "II" formulations are approximately twice as potent on a meq/mL basis. The products listed are liquid products with a low sodium content.

(continued)

Table 64–2. Ingredients of known efficacy for selected over-the-counter (OTC) classes (cont'd).

OTC Category	Ingredient and Dosage	Product Examples	Comments
Anthelmintics (pinworms)	Pyrantel pamoate, 11 mg/kg (maximum: 1 g)	Antiminth (250 mg/5 mL), Reese's Pinworm (250 mg/5 mL)	Treat all members of the household. Consult physician for children under age 2 years or under 25 lb. Disinfection of linens and environment is required to prevent reinfection.
Antidiarrheal agents	Bismuth subsalicylate, 600 mg 4 times daily to prevent traveler's diarrhea	Pepto-Bismol (262 mg/tab or 524 mg/30 mL suspension)	Can turn tongue and stools black. Salicylates are absorbed and can cause tinnitus.
	Loperamide, 4 mg initially, then 2 mg after each loose stool, not to exceed 16 mg/d	Imodium (2 mg/cap or 1 mg/5 mL liquid)	A synthetic opioid that does not penetrate the CNS. Not considered a controlled substance. Avoid in febrile patients.
	Opium, powdered, 15–20 mg 1–4 times daily, not to exceed 2 days (> 1.5–2 mg morphine)	Diabismal suspension (0.47 mg/ mL), Donnagel-PG (0.8 mg/ mL), Infantol Pink (0.5 mg/mL)	A schedule V substance when combined with other antidiarrheal substances. Not available OTC in some states. Avoid use in febrile patients and those predisposed to toxic megacolon. CNS depression possible.
	Tincture of opium (paregoric), 4–5 mL 1–4 times daily, not to exceed 2 days. (1 mL paregoric contains 4 mg opium.)	Kaodene with Paregoric (0.125 mg/mL), Parepectolin (0.12 mg/ mL)	
Antifungal topical preparations	Clotrimazole, 1% cream or 100 mg vaginal inserts[1]	Fem-Care, Gyne-Lotrimin, Mycelex 7	Fungicidal. Effective for the treatment of tinea pedis, tinea cruris, and tinea corporis. Clotrimazole and miconazole also effective against *Candida albicans*. Insert one applicatorful or one insert at bedtime for 7 days.
	Tolnaftate, 1% solution, cream, or powder	Generic, Aftate, Dr. Scholl's Athlete Foot Products, Tinactin	
	Miconazole nitrate, 2% cream or 100 mg vaginal tablet[1]	Monistat-7	
Anti-inflammatory topical preparations	Hydrocortisone, 0.5%	Generic, Cortaid (cream, lotion, ointment), Dermolate, Lanacort	Used to temporarily relieve itching and inflammation associated with minor rashes due to contact or allergic dermatitides, insect bites, and hemorrhoids. Apply small amounts and thoroughly rub into skin 3 or 4 times daily.
	Hydrocortisone, 1% cream or spray.[1]	Generic, Caldecort, Cortizone 10, Lanacort 10, Maximum Strength Cortaid	
Antiseborrheal agents	Selenium sulfide, 1–2% Zinc pyrithione, 1–2%	Selsun Blue Many. Breck One, Head and Shoulders	Both are cytostatic agents that decrease epidermal turnover rates. Work into clean scalp for 5–10 minutes 2 or 3 times weekly. Selenium sulfide can be irritating to the eyes and skin.
Antitussives	Codeine, 10–20 mg every 4–6 hours (with guaifenesin)	Cheracol, Robitussin A-C (both contain 2 mg/mL)	In doses required for cough suppression, the addictive liability associated with codeine is low. Codeine is a schedule V narcotic, and its OTC sale is re-
	Dextromethorphan, 10–20 mg every 4 hours or 30 mg every 6 hours (with guaifenesin)	Cheracol D (2 mg/mL), 2/G-DM (3 mg/mL), Novahistine Cough Formula (5 mg/mL), Pertussin 8-Hour Cough Formula (1.5 mg/mL), Robitussin-DM (3 mg/mL)	stricted in some states. The efficacy of expectorants, which are included in almost all antitussives, is questionable. Guaifenesin has the least potential for toxicity. Watch for hidden ingredients in these products.
Decongestants	Topical Oxymetazoline Xylometazoline	Afrin Dristan Long Lasting Nasal Mist, Neo-Synephrine II, Sinex-L.A., Sinutab Nasal Spray	Topical sympathomimetics are effective in the acute management of rhinorrhea associated with common colds and allergies. Long-acting agents (oxymetazoline and xylometazoline) are generally preferred, though phenylephrine is equally effective. Oral decongestants have a prolonged duration of action but may cause more systemic

Table 64–2. Ingredients of known efficacy for selected over-the-counter (OTC) classes (cont'd).

OTC Category	Ingredient and Dosage	Product Examples	Comments
Deconges- tants (cont'd)	Phenylephrine	Allerest, Coricidin Nasal Spray, Neo-Synephrine, NTZ	effects. Pseudoephedrine has the least CNS stimulatory effect. Phenylpropanolamine is also effective. Phenylephrine is unpredictably absorbed.
	Oral Pseudoephedrine 60 mg every 4 hours or 120 mg every 12 hours	Novafed (30 mg/5 mL), Sudafed (30 mg/tab or 5 mL)	
	Phenylpropanol-amine 25 mg every 4 hours	Sudafed SA (120 mg/cap) No single-ingredient product available	
Expectorants	Guaifenesin (20 mg/mL): age >12, 200–400 mg every 4 hours; age 6–12, 100–200 mg every 4 hours; age 2–6, 50–100 mg every 4 hours	1/G, Nortussin, Robitussin Syrups	The only expectorant ingredient listed by FDA panel as having scientific evidence of safety and efficacy.
Laxatives	Bulk formers	Metamucil, Serutan	The safest laxatives for chronic use include the bulk formers and stool softeners. Saline laxatives and stimulants may be used acutely but not chronically (see text).
	Stool softeners: docusate sodium	Generic, Colace, Coloctyl, Doxinate	
	Saline laxatives	Phillips' Milk of Magnesia	
Pediculicides	Permethrin 1%[1]	NIX Cream Rinse	Apply to dry hair and scalp, wetting entire area. Leave on for 10 minutes. Lather with water and rinse. Avoid contact with eyes. Repeat once if reinfestation occurs. Comb out nits.
	Pyrethrums combined with piperonyl butoride	A-200 Pediculicide Shampoo and Gel; RID Lice Killing Shampoo	
Sleep aids	Diphenhydramine,[1] 25–50 mg at bedtime	Sominex 2, Sleep-Eze 3 (25 mg/tab or cap); Sleepinal (50 mg), Compoz (50 mg)	Diphenydramine, an antihistamine with well-documented CNS depressant effects, is now available over the counter for sedative use.
Smoking cessation aids	Nicotine	Nicoderm CQ (patch)	Quit rates associated with these products at 6 weeks exceed placebo (50% versus 27%). Quit rate after 1 year is about 25%. Review directions for use carefully, since self-titration and weaning are involved.
		Nicotrol (transdermal system)	
		Nicotrol NS (nasal spray)	
	Nicotine polacrilex	Nicorette Gum	

[1]Previously available by prescription only. Now available over the counter.

Table 64–2 lists examples of OTC products that may be used effectively to treat medical problems commonly encountered in ambulatory patients. The selection of one ingredient over another may be important in patients with certain medical problems or in patients taking certain prescription medications. These are discussed in detail in other chapters. The recommendations listed in Table 64–2 are based upon the efficacy of the ingredients and on the principles set forth in the following paragraphs:

(1) Select the product that is simplest in formulation with regard to ingredients and dosage form. In general, single-ingredient products are preferred. Although some combination products contain effective doses of all ingredients, others contain therapeutic doses of some ingredients and subtherapeutic doses of others. Furthermore, there may be differing durations of action among the ingredients, and there is always a possibility that the clinician or patient will be unaware of the presence of certain active ingredients in the product. Aspirin, for example, is present in many cough and cold preparations; a patient unaware of this may take separate doses of analgesic in addition to that contained in the cold preparation.

(2) Select a product that contains a therapeutically effective dose.

(3) Select a product that lists its ingredients and their amounts. The label of a product should always be read carefully, since ingredients may be changed without public notification or change of brand name.

(4) Recommend a generic product if one is available.

(5) Be wary of "gimmicks" or advertising claims of specific superiority over similar products.

(6) For children, the dose, dosage form, and palatability of the product will be prime considerations.

Certain ingredients in OTC products should be avoided or used with caution in selected patients because they may exacerbate existing medical problems or interact with prescription medications the patient is taking. Many of the more potent OTC ingredients are "hidden" in products where their presence would not ordinarily be expected (Table 64–3). This lack of awareness of the ingredients present in OTC products and the belief by many physicians that OTC products are "ineffective and harmless" may cause diagnostic confusion and perhaps interfere with therapy.

For example, innumerable OTC products, including cough and cold preparations, decongestants, and appetite control products, contain sympathomimetics. These agents should be avoided or used cautiously in insulin-dependent diabetics and patients with hypertension, angina, or hyperthyroidism. Aspirin should be avoided by individuals with active peptic ulcer disease, certain platelet disorders, or patients taking oral anticoagulants. Cimetidine, an H_2 receptor antagonist, is a well-known inhibitor of drug metabolism and can increase the toxicity of drugs such as phenytoin, theophylline, and warfarin.

Finally, overuse or misuse of OTC products may induce significant medical problems. A prime example is rebound congestion from the regular use of nasal sprays for more than 3 or 4 days. The improper and chronic use of some antacids (eg, aluminum hydroxide) may cause constipation and even impaction in elderly people as well as hypophosphatemia. Laxative abuse (chiefly by older people) can result in abdominal cramping and fluid and electrolyte disturbances. Insomnia, nervousness, and restlessness can result from the use of sympathomimetics or caffeine hidden in many OTC products (Table 64–3). The chronic systemic use of some analgesics containing large amounts of caffeine may produce rebound headaches, and long-term use of analgesics, especially those containing phenacetin, has been associated with interstitial nephritis. Acute ingestion of large amounts of aspirin or acetaminophen by adults or children causes serious toxicity. Antihistamines may cause sedation or drowsiness, especially when taken concurrently with sedative-hypnotics, tranquilizers, alcohol, or other central nervous system depressants. Finally, antihistamines, local anesthetics, antibiotics, antibacterial agents, counterirritants, p-aminobenzoic acid (PABA), preservatives, and deodorants contained in a myriad of OTC topical and vaginal products may induce allergic reactions.

There are two major drug information sources for OTC products. *Handbook of Nonprescription Drugs* is the most comprehensive resource for OTC medications; it evaluates ingredients contained in major OTC drug classes and lists the ingredients included in many OTC products. *Physicians' Desk Reference for Nonprescription Drugs,* a compendium of manufacturers' information regarding OTC products, is somewhat incomplete with regard to the number of products included and the consistency of information provided. Any clinician who seeks more specific information regarding OTC products should find these references useful.

Table 64–3. Hidden ingredients in over-the-counter (OTC) products.

Hidden Drug or Drug Class	OTC Class Containing Drug	Product Examples
Alcohol (percent ethanol)	Cough syrups, cold preparations	Comtrex (20%) Contac Nighttime Cold Medicine (25%) Cotussis (20%) Formula 44D (10%) Halls (22%) Novahistine DMX (10%) Nyquil Nighttime Cold/Flu Medicine (25%) Pertussin 8-Hour Cold Formula (9.5%) Prunicodeine (25%)
	Mouthwashes	Cepacol Mouthwash (14%) Listerine (27%) Scope (19%)
Antihistamines	Analgesics	Allerest Headache Strength Tablets Excedrin PM Sinarest Tablets
	Asthma products	Bronitin, Primatin M
	Cold/allergy products	(Many) Alka-Seltzer Plus Allerest Benylin Cough Syrup Chlor-Trimeton Contac Coricidin Co-Tylenol Dristan 4-Way Cold Tablets Novahistine NyQuil Sinarest Sine-Off Sinutab Super Anahist Triaminic Triaminicin
	Dermatologic products	Pyribenzamine Cream or Ointment
	Menstrual products	Midol Pamprin Sunril
	Motion sickness products, antiemetics	Bonine Dramamine Marezine
	Sleep aids	Compoz Nervine Nytol Sleep-Eze Sominex
	Topical decongestants	Dristan 4-Way Fast-Acting Menthol and Regular
Antimuscarinic agents	Antidiarrheals	Amogel Donnagel Donnagel-PG Quiagel
	Hemorrhoidal products	Wyanoids Hemorrhoidal Suppositories
Aspirin and other salicylates	Analgesics	(Many) Alka-Seltzer Anacin Aspergum Cope Ecotrin Excedrin Measurin Vanquish

(continued)

Table 64–3. Hidden ingredients in over-the-counter (OTC) products (cont'd).

Hidden Drug or Drug Class	OTC Class Containing Drug	Product Examples
	Antidiarrheals	Pepto-Bismol (bismuth subsalicylate)
	Cold/allergy preparations	Alka-Seltzer Plus Coricidin Sine-Off
	Menstrual products	Diurex (potassium salicylate)
	Sleep aids	Quiet World Tablets
Barbiturates	Asthma products	Asthmalixir Bronkotabs Primatene P Tedral
Caffeine	Analgesics	Anacin Cope Excedrin Vanquish
	Cold/allergy products	Dristan
	Menstrual/diuretic products	Aqua-Ban Tri-Aqua
	Stimulants	Caffedrine NoDoz Vivarin
	Weight control products	Anorexin Dexatrim
Estrogens	Hair creams	Le Kair
Local anesthetics (usually benzocaine)	Antitussives	Cepacol Troches Silexin Cough Tablets Spec T Sucrets Vicks Cough Silencers
	Dermatologic preparations	Americaine Bactine Dermoplast Nupercainal Cream or Ointment Medi-Quick Solarcaine Unguentine Spray Xylocaine Ointment
	Hemorrhoidal products	Americaine Lanacane Medicated Creme Nupercanainal Cream or Ointment Pontocaine
	Lozenges	Cepacol Troches Hold Spec-T Sore Throat Products Trokettes Vicks Throat Lozenges
	Toothache, cold sore, and teething products	Baby Orajel Benzodent Numzident Orabase B with Benzocaine
	Weight control products	Diet Ayds Diet Trim Tablets Dieutrim T.D.
Sodium (mg/tablet or mg/5 mL or as stated)	Analgesics	Alka-Seltzer Effervescent Pain Reliever and Antacid (567) Bromo-Seltzer (761) Fizrin Powder (673) Sodium salicylate (50 mg, 300 mg)

Table 64–3. Hidden ingredients in over-the-counter (OTC) products (cont'd).

Hidden Drug or Drug Class	OTC Class Containing Drug	Product Examples
	Antacids	Alka-Seltzer Effervescent Antacid (276) Bromo-Seltzer (761) BisoDol (157) Rolaids (53)
	Cough syrups	Coryban D (31) Cerose (38) Dristan (59) Pertussin 8-Hour Cough Formula (24) Formula 44 (68) Vicks Cough Syrup (54)
	Laxatives	Fleets Enema (500 mg, of which 250–300 mg is absorbed) Phospho-Soda (554)
Sympathomimetics	Analgesics	Allerest Headache Strength Tablets Sinarest Tablets Sine-Aid Sinus Headache Tablets
	Asthma products	Bronkaid Bronkotabs Primatene Tedral
	Cold/allergy preparations	(Many) Alka-Seltzer Plus Allerest Chlor-Trimeton Decongestant Contac Coricidin 'D' Decongestant Tablets Co-Tylenol Dristan 4-Way Cold Tablets Novafed Novahistine Sinus Tablets NyQuil Sinarest Sine-Aid Sine-Off Sinutab Sudafed Super Anahist Triaminicin
	Cough syrups	(Many) Cerose DM Formula 44D Robitussin-PE Triaminic Expectorant Triamincol
	Hemorrhoidal products	A-Caine Epinephricaine Rectal Ointment HTO Stainless Manzan Hemorrhoidal Tissue Ointment Pazo Hemorrhoid Ointment Wyanoids Ointment
	Lozenges	Spec-T Sore Throat/Decongestant Sucrets Cold Decongestant Formula
	Menstrual products	Femcaps
	Topical decongestants	(Many) Afrin Benzedrex Neo-Synephrine Hydrochloride NTZ Privin Sinex Vicks Inhaler
	Weight control products	Acutrim Appedrine Tablets Dexatrim Capsules Prolamine Capsules

REFERENCES

Estrogens in cosmetics: Med Lett Drugs Ther 1985;27:54.

Fredd SB: The OTC drug approval process. Am J Gastroenterol 1990;85:12.

Gossel TA: Implications of the reclassification of drugs from prescription-only to over-the-counter status. Clin Ther 1991;13:201.

Handbook of Nonprescription Drugs, 10th ed. American Pharmaceutical Association, 1993.

Hansten PD, Horn JR: Principles of H_2-antagonist drug interactions. In: *Drug Interactions and Update Quarterly.* Applied Therapeutics, 1993.

Kofoed LL: OTC drug overuse in the elderly: What to watch for. Geriatrics 1985;40:55.

Palmer HA: New OTCs: A selected review. Am Pharm 1992;NS32:26.

Pentel P: Toxicity of over-the-counter stimulants. JAMA 1984;252:1898.

Physicians' Desk Reference for Nonprescription Drugs, 15th ed. Medical Economics, 1995.

Smith MBH, Feldman W: Over-the-counter cold medications. A critical review of clinical trials between 1950 and 1991. JAMA 1993;269:2258.

Whelton A: Renal effects of over-the-counter analgesics. J Clin Pharmacol 1995;35:454.

Rational Prescribing & Prescription Writing

65

Paul W. Lofholm, PharmD, & Bertram G. Katzung, MD, PhD

A practitioner's decision to treat a patient assumes that the patient has been evaluated and diagnosed. The practitioner can then select from a variety of therapeutic approaches. Medication, surgery, psychiatric treatment, radiation, physical therapy, health education, counseling, further consultation, or no therapy are some of the options available. Of these options, drug therapy is by far the most commonly chosen. In most cases, this requires the writing of a prescription. A prescription is the prescriber's order to prepare or dispense a specific treatment—usually medication— for a specific patient. When a patient comes for an office visit, the physician or other authorized health professional will prescribe medications 67% of the time, and an average of one prescription per office visit is written because more than one prescription may be written at a single visit.

In this chapter, a plan for prescribing is presented. The physical form of the prescription, common prescribing errors, and legal requirements that govern various features of the prescribing process are then discussed. Finally, some of the social and economic factors involved in prescribing and drug use are described.

RATIONAL PRESCRIBING

Like any other process in medicine, writing a prescription should be based on a series of rational steps. These operations can be described as follows.

(1) Make a specific diagnosis: Prescriptions based merely on a desire to satisfy the patient's psychologic need for some type of therapy are often unsatisfactory and may result in adverse effects. A specific diagnosis, even if it is "presumptive," is required to move to the next step. In a 35-year-old woman with symmetric joint stiffness, pain, and inflammation that are worse in the morning and not associated with a history of infection, the diagnosis of rheumatoid arthritis would be considered. This diagnosis and the

reasoning underlying it should be shared with the patient.

(2) Consider the pathophysiology of the diagnosis selected: If the disorder is well understood, the prescriber is in a much better position to select effective therapy. For example, increasing knowledge about the mediators of inflammation makes possible more effective use of NSAIDs and other agents used in rheumatoid arthritis. The patient should be provided with the appropriate level and amount of information about the pathophysiology. Many disease-oriented public and private agencies (eg, American Heart Association, American Cancer Society, Arthritis Foundation) provide information sheets suitable for patients.

(3) Select a specific therapeutic objective: A therapeutic objective should be chosen for each of the pathophysiologic processes defined in the preceding step. In a patient with rheumatoid arthritis, relief of pain by reduction of the inflammatory process is one of the major therapeutic goals that defines the drug groups which will be considered. Arresting the course of the disease process in rheumatoid arthritis is a different therapeutic goal that might give rise to consideration of other drug groups and prescriptions.

(4) Select a drug of choice: One or more drug groups will be suggested by each of the therapeutic goals specified in the preceding step. Selection of a drug of choice from among these groups will follow from a consideration of the specific characteristics of the patient and the clinical presentation. For certain drugs, characteristics such as age, race, other diseases, and other drugs being taken are extremely important in determining the most suitable drug for management of the present complaint. In the example of the patient with probable rheumatoid arthritis, it would be important to know whether she has a history of aspirin intolerance or ulcer disease, whether the cost of medication is an especially important factor, and whether there is a need for once-daily dosing. Based on this information, a drug would probably be selected from the nonsteroidal anti-inflammatory group. If the patient is intolerant of aspirin and does not have ulcer disease but does have a need for low-cost treatment, ibuprofen would be a rational choice.

(5) Determine the appropriate dosing regimen: The dosing regimen is determined primarily by the pharmacokinetics of the drug in that patient. If the patient is known to have disease of the major organs required for elimination of the drug selected, adjustment of the "average" regimen will be needed. For a drug such as ibuprofen, which is eliminated mainly by the kidney, renal function should be assessed. If renal function is normal, the half-life of ibuprofen (about 2 hours) requires administration three or four times daily. The dosage suggested in drug handbooks and the manufacturer's literature is 400–800 mg four times daily.

(6) Devise a plan for monitoring the drug's action and determine an end point for the therapy: The prescriber should be able to describe to the patient the kinds of drug effects that will be monitored and in what way, including laboratory tests (if necessary) and signs and symptoms that the patient should report. For conditions that call for a limited course of therapy (eg, most infections), the duration of therapy should be made clear so that the patient will not stop taking the drug prematurely and will understand why the prescription probably need not be renewed. For the patient with rheumatoid arthritis, the need for prolonged—perhaps indefinite—therapy should be explained. The prescriber should also specify any changes in the patient's condition that would call for changes in therapy. For example, in the patient with rheumatoid arthritis, development of gastrointestinal bleeding would require an immediate change in drug therapy and a prompt workup of the bleeding. Major toxicities that require immediate attention should be explained clearly to the patient.

(7) Plan a program of patient education: The prescriber and other members of the health team should be prepared to repeat, extend, and reinforce the information transmitted to the patient as often as necessary. The more toxic the drug prescribed, the greater the importance of this educational program. The importance of informing and involving the patient in each of the above steps must be recognized, as shown by experience with teratogenic drugs (Shulman, 1989).

THE PRESCRIPTION

While a prescription can be written on any piece of paper (as long as all of the legal elements are present), it usually takes a specific form. A typical printed prescription form for outpatients is shown in Figure 65–1.

In the hospital setting, drugs are prescribed on a particular page of the patient's hospital chart called

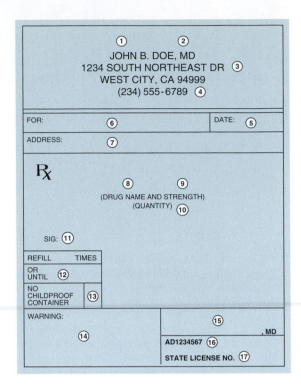

Figure 65–1. Common form of outpatient prescription. Circled numbers are explained in the text.

the physician's order sheet (POS) or a **chart order.** The contents of that prescription are specified in the medical staff rules by the hospital's Pharmacy and Therapeutics Committee. The patient's name is typed or written on the form; therefore, the orders consist of the name and strength of the medication, the dose, the route and frequency of administration, the date, other pertinent information, and the signature of the prescriber. The duration of therapy or the number of doses is often not specified; therefore, medications are continued until the prescriber discontinues the order or until it is terminated as a matter of policy routine, eg, a stop order policy.

A typical chart order might be as follows:

11/14/97
10:30 a.m.

> **(1) Ampicillin 500 mg IV q6h × 5 days**
> **(2) ASA 0.6 g per rectum q6h prn temp over 101**
>
> **[Signed] Janet B. Doe, MD**

Thus, the elements of the hospital chart order are equivalent to the central elements (8–11) of the outpatient prescription.

Whether in the hospital or in an office practice setting, the implications of each element of the prescription should be understood.

Elements of the Prescription

The first four elements (see circled numerals in Figure 65–1) of the outpatient prescription establish the identity of the prescriber: name, license classification (ie, professional degree), address, and office telephone number. Before dispensing a prescription, the pharmacist must establish the prescriber's bona fides and should be able to contact the prescriber by telephone if any questions arise. Element [5] is the date the prescription was written. It should be near the top of the prescription form or at the beginning (left margin) of the chart order. Since the order has legal significance and usually has some temporal relationship to the date of the patient-prescriber interview, a pharmacist should refuse to fill a prescription without verification by telephone if too much time has elapsed since its writing.

Elements [6] and [7] identify the patient by name and address. The patient's name and full address should be clearly spelled out.

The body of the prescription contains the elements [8] to [11] that specify the medication, the strength and quantity to be dispensed, the dosage, and complete directions for use. When writing the drug name (element [8]), either the brand name (proprietary name) or generic name (nonproprietary name) may be used. Reasons for using one or the other are discussed below. The strength of the medication (element [9]) should be written in metric units. However, the prescriber should be familiar with both systems now in use: apothecary and metric. For practical purposes, the following approximate conversions are useful:

1 grain (gr) = 0.065 grams (g), often rounded to 60 milligrams (mg)
15 gr = 1 g
1 ounce (oz) = 30 milliliters (mL)
1 teaspoonful (tsp) = 5 mL
1 tablespoonful (tbsp) = 15 mL
1 quart (qt) = 1000 mL
20 drops (gtt) = 1 mL
2.2 pounds (lb) = 1 kilogram (kg)
1 minim = 1 drop

The strength of a solution is usually expressed as the quantity of solute in sufficient solvent to make 100 mL; for instance, 20% potassium chloride solution is 20 grams of KCl per deciliter (g/dL). Both the concentration and the volume should be explicitly written out.

The quantity of medication prescribed should reflect the anticipated duration of therapy, the cost, the need for continued contact with the clinic or physician, the potential for abuse, and the potential for toxicity or overdose. Consideration should be given also to the standard sizes in which the product is available and whether this is the initial prescription of the drug or a repeat prescription or refill. If 10 days of therapy are required to effectively cure a streptococcal infec-

tion, an appropriate quantity for the full course should be prescribed. Birth control pills are often prescribed for 1 year or until the next examination is due; however, some patients may not be able to afford a year's supply at one time; therefore, a 3-month supply might be ordered, with refill instructions to renew three times or for 1 year (element [12]). Finally, when first prescribing medications that are to be used for the treatment of a chronic disease, the initial quantity should be small, with refills for larger quantities. The purpose of beginning treatment with a small quantity of drug is to reduce the cost if the patient cannot tolerate it. Once it is determined that intolerance is not a problem, a larger quantity purchased less frequently is sometimes less expensive.

The directions for use (element [11]) must be both drug-specific and patient-specific. The simpler the directions, the better; and the fewer the number of doses (and drugs) per day, the better. Patient noncompliance (failure to adhere to the drug regimen) is a major cause of treatment failure. To help patients remember to take their medications, prescribers often give an instruction that medications be taken at or around mealtimes and at bedtime. However, it is important to inquire about the patient's eating habits and other life-style patterns, since many patients do not eat three regularly spaced meals a day, especially if they are sick or dieting.

The instructions on how and when to take medications, the duration of therapy, and the purpose of the medication must be explained to each patient by the physician and by the pharmacist. (Neither should assume that the other will do it.) Furthermore, the drug name, the purpose for which it is given, and the duration of therapy should be written on each label so that the drug may be identified easily in case of overdose. An instruction to "take as directed" may save the time it takes to write the orders out but often leads to noncompliance, patient confusion, and medication error. The directions for use must be clear and concise to avoid toxicity and to obtain the greatest benefits from therapy.

Patient education has been of concern to the FDA and professional groups and has resulted in several programs. The United States Pharmacopeial Convention (USP) annually publishes a three-volume work entitled *USP DI* ("Drug Information"). The first volume contains information for the professional (prescriber) and the second consists of short informational notes prepared for patients' use in understanding the drugs they are given. Over 1000 medications are covered in the 1996 edition. Practitioners can also order patient information leaflets for the more commonly used drugs, in Spanish as well as English. Information about patient information sheets may be obtained from the USP Drug Information Division, 12601 Twinbrook Parkway, Rockville, MD 20852-1790. Large health maintenance organizations often have similar preprinted patient information sheets available for distribution.

Although directions for use are no longer written in Latin, many Latin apothecary abbreviations (and some others included below) are still in use. Knowledge of these abbreviations is essential for the dispensing pharmacist and often useful for the prescriber. Some of the abbreviations still used are listed in Table 65–1.

Elements [12] to [14] of the prescription include refill information, waiver of the requirement for child-proof containers, and additional labeling instructions (eg, name of drug on label, "may cause drowsiness," "do not drink alcohol"). Most pharmacists now put the name of the medication on the label unless directed otherwise by the prescriber, and some medications have the name of the drug stamped or imprinted on the tablet or capsule. Pharmacists should also place the expiration date for the drug on the label. If the patient or prescriber does not request waiver of child-proof containers, the pharmacist or dispenser must place the medication in such a container. Pharmacists may not refill a prescription medication without authorization from the prescriber. Prescribers may grant authorization to renew prescriptions at the time of writing the prescription or over the telephone. Finally, the prescriber may request that special warning notices be placed on the label by the pharmacist. Elements [15] to [17] are the prescriber's signature and other identification data.

PRESCRIBING ERRORS

All prescription orders should be legible, unambiguous, dated (and timed in the case of a chart order), and signed clearly for optimal communication between prescriber, pharmacist, and nurse. Furthermore,

Table 65–1. Abbreviations used in prescriptions and chart orders. *Note:* It is always safer to write out the direction without abbreviating.

ABBREVIATION	EXPLANATION	ABBREVIATION	EXPLANATION
ā	before	prn	when needed
ac	before meals	q	every
agit	shake, stir	qam, om	every morning
Aq	water	qd	every day
Aq dest	distilled water	qh, q1h	every hour
bid	twice a day	q2h, q3h, etc	every 2 hours, every 3 hours, etc
c̄	with		
cap	capsule	qhs	every night at bedtime
D5W, D$_5$W	dextrose 5% in water		
dil	dissolve, dilute	qid	four times a day
disp, dis	dispense	qod	every other day
elix	elixir	qs	sufficient quantity
ext	extract	rept, repet	may be repeated
g	gram	Rx	take
gr	grain	s̄	without
gtt	drops	SC, SQ	subcutaneous
h	hour	Sig, S	label
hs	at bedtime	sos	if needed
IA	intra-arterial	ss, s̄s̄	one-half
IM	intramuscular	stat	at once
IV	intravenous	sup, supp	suppository
IVPB	IV piggyback	susp	suspension
kg	kilogram	tab	tablet
mEq, meq	milliequivalent	tbsp, T	tablespoon (always write out "15 mL")
mg	milligram		
mcg, µg	microgram (always write out "microgram")	tid	three times a day
		tr, tinct	tincture
no	number	tsp	teaspoon (always write out "5 mL")
non rep	do not repeat		
OD	right eye	U (do not use this abbreviation)	units (always write out "units")
OS, OL	left eye		
OTC	over-the-counter	vag	vaginal
OU	both eyes	i, ii, iii, iv, etc	one, two, three, four, etc
p̄	after	ℨ	(in fluid measure, 3.7 mL)
pc	after meals	℥	
PO	by mouth		(in fluid measure, 29.6 mL)
PR	per rectum		

a good prescription or chart order should contain sufficient information to permit the pharmacist or nurse to discover possible errors before the drug is dispensed or administered.

Several types of prescribing errors are particularly common. These include errors involving omission of needed information; poor writing perhaps leading to errors of drug dose or timing; and prescription of drugs that are inappropriate for the specific situation.

Omission of Information

Errors of omission are common in hospital orders and may include instructions to "resume pre-op meds," which assumes that a full and accurate record of the "pre-op meds" is available; "continue present IV fluids," which fails to state exactly what fluids are to be given, in what volume, and over what time period; or "continue eye drops," which omits mention of which eye is to be treated as well as the drug, concentration, and frequency of administration. Chart orders may also fail to discontinue a prior medication when a new one is begun; may fail to state whether a regular or long-acting form is to be used; may fail to specify a strength or notation for long-acting forms; or may authorize "as-needed" (prn) use that fails to state what conditions will justify the need.

Poor Prescription Writing

Poor prescription writing is traditionally exemplified by illegible handwriting. However, other types of poor writing are common and often more dangerous. One of the most important is the misplaced or ambiguous decimal point. Thus ".1" is easily misread as "1," a tenfold overdose, if the decimal point is not unmistakably clear. This danger is easily avoided by always preceding the decimal point with a zero. On the other hand, appending an unnecessary zero after a decimal point increases the risk of a tenfold overdose, because "1.0 mg" is easily misread as "10 mg," whereas "1 mg" is not. The slash or virgule ("/") was traditionally used as a substitute for a decimal point. This should be abandoned because it is too easily misread as the numeral "1." Similarly, the abbreviation "U" for units should never be used because "10U" is easily misread as "100"; the word "units" should *always* be written out. Doses in micrograms should *always* have this unit written out because the abbreviated form ("μg") is very easily misread as "mg," a 1000-fold overdose! Orders for drugs specifying only the number of dosage units and not the total dose required should not be filled if more than one size dosage unit exists for that drug. For example, ordering "one ampule of furosemide" is unacceptable because furosemide is available in ampules that contain 20, 40, or 100 mg of the drug. Unclear handwriting can be lethal when drugs with similar names but very different effects are available, eg, acetazolamide and acetohexamide, methotrexate and metolazone (Huseby et al, 1991). In this situation, errors are best avoided by

noting the indication for the drug in the body of the prescription, eg, "acetazolamide, for glaucoma."

Inappropriate Drug Prescriptions

Prescribing an inappropriate drug for a particular patient results from failure to recognize contraindications imposed by other diseases the patient may have, failure to obtain information about other drugs the patient is taking (including over-the-counter drugs), or failure to recognize possible physicochemical incompatibilities between drugs that may react with each other. Contraindications to drugs in the presence of other diseases or pharmacokinetic characteristics are listed in the discussions of the drugs described in this book. The manufacturer's package insert usually contains similar information. Some of the important drug interactions are listed in Appendix II of this book as well as in package inserts.

Physicochemical incompatibilities are of particular concern when parenteral administration is planned. For example, when calcium and phosphate ion concentrations are excessively high in a total parenteral nutrition (TPN) solution, precipitation will occur. Similarly, the simultaneous administration of antacids or products high in metal content may compromise the absorption of many drugs in the intestine, eg, tetracyclines. The package insert and the *Handbook on Injectable Drugs* are good sources for this information.

COMPLIANCE

Compliance is the extent to which patients follow instructions. There are four types of noncompliance leading to medication errors.

(1) The patient fails to obtain the medication. Some studies suggest that one-third of patients never have their prescriptions filled. Some patients leave the hospital without obtaining their discharge medications, while others leave the hospital without having their prehospitalization medications resumed. Some patients cannot afford the medications prescribed.

(2) The patient fails to take the medication as prescribed. Examples include wrong dosage, wrong frequency of administration, improper timing or sequencing of administration, wrong route or technique of administration, or taking medication for the wrong purpose.

(3) The patient prematurely discontinues the medication. This can occur, for instance, if the patient incorrectly assumes that the medication is no longer needed because the bottle is empty or symptomatic improvement has occurred.

(4) The patient (or another person) takes medication inappropriately. For example, the patient may share a medication with others for any of several reasons.

Several factors encourage noncompliance. Some diseases cause no symptoms (eg, hypertension); patients with these diseases therefore have no symptoms to remind them to take their medications. Patients with very painful conditions, such as arthritis, may continually change medications in hope of finding a better one. Characteristics of the therapy itself can limit the degree of compliance; patients taking a drug once a day are much more likely to be compliant than those taking a drug four times a day. Various patient factors also play a role in compliance. Men living alone are much less likely to be compliant than married men of the same age. Packaging may also be a deterrent to compliance—elderly arthritic patients often have difficulty opening their medication containers. Lack of transportation as well as various social or personal beliefs about the use of medications are likewise barriers to compliance.

Strategies for improving compliance include enhanced communication between the patient and health care team members; assessment of personal, social, and economic conditions (often reflected in the patient's lifestyle); development of a routine for taking medications (eg, at mealtimes if the patient has regular meals); and provision of systems to assist taking medications (ie, devices that separate drug doses by day of the week, or medication alarm clocks that remind patients to take their medications); and mailing of refill reminders by the pharmacist to patients taking drugs chronically. The patient who is likely to discontinue a medication because of a perceived drug-related problem should receive instruction and education about how to monitor and understand the effects of the medication. Compliance can often be improved by enlisting the patient's active participation in the treatment.

LEGAL FACTORS (USA)

The United States government recognizes two classes of drugs: (1) over-the-counter (OTC) drugs and (2) those that require a prescription from a licensed prescriber (legend drugs). OTC drugs are those that can be safely self-administered by the layman for self-limiting conditions and for which appropriate labels can be written for lay comprehension. Half of all drug doses consumed by the American public are OTC drugs.

Physicians, dentists, podiatrists, and veterinarians—and, in some states, specialized pharmacists, nurses, physician's assistants, and optometrists—are granted authority to prescribe dangerous drugs (those bearing the federal legend statement, "Federal law prohibits dispensing without a prescription") on the basis of their training in diagnosis and treatment (see box: Who May Prescribe?). Pharmacists are authorized to dispense prescriptions pursuant to a prescriber's order provided that the medication order is appropriate and rational for the patient. Nurses are authorized to administer medications to patients subject to a prescriber's order.

WHO MAY PRESCRIBE?*

The right to prescribe drugs and much of the legal responsibility for any harm that derives from the prescription were largely limited to just two groups in the past: physicians and osteopaths. In recent years, this power has diffused and now includes—in a number of states and in varying degrees—pharmacists, nurse practitioners, physician's assistants, and optometrists (see Table 65–2). This development began with the growth of a sense of independence within different health professions and was actively promoted by their professional societies. The more recent development of large health maintenance organizations has greatly strengthened the movement because it offers these extremely powerful economic bodies a way to reduce their expenses.

For example, under a plan of pharmacist care, a patient diagnosed as asthmatic by a physician might be referred to a pharmacist for coordination and follow-up of therapy. The pharmacist would be responsible for generating a problem list, prescribing and dispensing the appropriate drugs after consultation with the physician, educating the patient with regard to his or her disease and medications, and then following the patient's responses to the medications by means of appropriate tests (peak airflow metering, etc).

The primary organizations controlling the privilege of prescribing in the USA are the state boards, under the powers delegated to them by the state legislatures. As indicated in Table 65–2, many state boards have attempted to reserve some measure of the primary responsibility for prescribing to physicians by requiring that the ancillary professional work with or under a physician according to a specific "protocol." In the state of California, this protocol must include a statement of the training, supervision, and documentation requirements of the arrangement and must specify referral requirements, limitations to the list of drugs that may be prescribed (ie, a formulary), and a method of evaluation by the supervising physician. The protocol must be in writing and must be periodically updated (An explanation of the scope of RN Practices, 1994).

---

*This section prepared with the assistance of Ronda Malone, BS.

Table 65–2. Prescribing authority of certain allied health professionals in selected states.

State	Pharmacists	Nurse Practitioners	Physician's Assistants	Optometrists
California	Yes, under protocol;[1] must be trained in clinical practice	Yes, see footnote 2	No	Yes, limited to certain drug classes
Florida	Yes, according to state formulary; protocol not required	Yes, see footnote 2	Yes, see footnote 2	Yes, limited to certain drug classes
Michigan	Yes, under protocol; must be specially qualified by education, training or experience	Yes, do not need physician supervision	Yes, see footnote 2	Yes, limited to certain drug classes
Mississippi	Yes, under protocol in an institutional setting	Yes, see footnote 2, under narrowly specified conditions	No	Yes, limited to certain drug classes
Nevada	Yes, under protocol, within a licensed medical facility	Yes, see footnote 2	Yes, see footnote 2	Yes, limited to certain drug classes
New Mexico	Yes, under protocol, must be "pharmacist clinician"	Yes, do not need physician supervision	Yes, see footnote 2	Yes, limited to certain drug classes
North Dakota	Yes, under protocol in an institutional setting	Yes, do not need physician supervision	Yes, see footnote 2	Yes, limited to certain drug classes
Oregon	Yes, under guidelines set by the state board	Yes, do not need physician supervision	Yes, see footnote 2	Yes, limited to certain drug classes
Texas	Yes, under protocol set for a particular patient in an institutional setting	Yes, do not need physician supervision	Yes, see footnote 2	Yes, limited to certain drug classes
Washington	Yes, under guidelines set by the state board	Yes, do not need physician supervision	Yes, see footnote 2	Yes, limited to certain drug classes

[1]Under protocol: see box: Who May Prescribe.
[2]In collaboration with or under the supervision of a physician.

Prescription drugs are controlled by the United States Food and Drug Administration as described in Chapter 5. The federal legend statement as well as the package insert are part of the packaging requirements for all prescription drugs. The package insert is the official brochure setting forth the indications, contraindications, warnings, and dosing for the drug.

The prescriber, by writing and signing a prescription order, controls who may obtain prescription drugs. The pharmacist may purchase these drugs, but they may be dispensed only on the order of a legally qualified prescriber. Thus, a "prescription" is actually three things: the physician's order in the patient's chart, the written order to which the pharmacist refers when dispensing, and the patient's medication vial with a label affixed.

While the federal government controls the drugs and their labeling and distribution, the state legislatures control who may prescribe drugs through their licensing boards, eg, the Board of Medical Examiners. Prescribers must pass examinations, pay fees, and—in the case of some states and some professions—meet other requirements for relicensure such as continuing education. If these requirements are met, the prescriber is licensed to order dispensing of drugs.

The federal government and the states further impose special restrictions on drugs according to their perceived potential for abuse (Table 65–3). Such drugs include opioids, hallucinogens, stimulants, and depressants (Chapter 32). Special requirements must be met when these drugs are to be prescribed. The Controlled Drug Act requires prescribers and dispensers to register with the Drug Enforcement Agency (DEA), pay a fee, receive a personal registration number, and keep records of all controlled drugs prescribed or dispensed. Every time a controlled drug is prescribed, a valid DEA number must appear on the prescription blank.

Prescriptions for substances with a high potential for abuse (class II) cannot be refilled. Prescriptions for class III, IV, and V drugs can be refilled, but there is a five-refill maximum, and in no case may the prescription be refilled after 6 months from the date of writing. Class II drug prescriptions may not be transmitted over the telephone, and some states require a

Table 65–3. Classification of controlled substances. (See inside front cover for examples.)

	Potential for Abuse	Other Comments
Class I	High	No accepted medical use; lack of accepted safety as drug.
Class II	High	Current accepted medical use. Abuse may lead to psychologic or physical dependence.
Class III	Less than I or II	Current accepted medical use. Moderate or low potential for physical dependence and high potential for psychologic dependence.
Class IV	Less than III	Current accepted medical use. Limited potential for dependence.
Class V	Less than IV	Current accepted medical use. Limited dependence possible.

special state-issued prescription blank. These restrictive prescribing laws are intended to limit the amount of drugs of abuse that are made available to the public. However, some states have recognized the underutilization of pain medications in the treatment of pain associated with chronic and terminal conditions. California, for example, has enacted an "intractable pain treatment" act that reduces the difficulty of renewing prescriptions for opioids. Under the provisions of this act, upon receipt of a copy of the order from the prescriber, eg, by fax, a pharmacist may write a "triplicate" prescription* for a Schedule II substance for a patient under hospice care or living in a skilled nursing facility.

Labeled & Unlabeled Uses of Drugs

In the USA, the FDA approves a drug only for the specific uses proposed and documented by the manufacturer in its New Drug Application (NDA; see Chapter 5). These approved (labeled) uses or indications are set forth in the package insert that accompanies the drug. For a variety of reasons, these labeled indications may not include all the conditions in which the drug might be useful. Therefore, a clinician may wish to prescribe the agent for some other, unapproved (unlabeled) clinical condition, often on the basis of adequate or even compelling scientific evidence. Federal laws governing FDA regulations and drug use place no restrictions on such unapproved use.† Even if the patient suffers injury from the drug, its use for an unlabeled purpose does not in itself constitute "malpractice." However, the courts may consider the package insert labeling as a complete listing of the indications for which the drug is considered

safe unless the clinician can show (from the literature, etc) that his or her use of the agent is considered reasonable by his or her peers.

SOCIOECONOMIC FACTORS

Generic Prescribing

Prescribing by generic name offers the pharmacist flexibility in selecting the particular drug product to fill the order and the patient a potential savings if there is price competition. The brand name of a popular sedative is, for example, Valium by Roche. The generic (public nonproprietary) name of the same chemical substance adopted by United States Adopted Names (USAN) and approved by the Food and Drug Administration (FDA) is diazepam. All diazepam drug products in the USA meet the pharmaceutical standards expressed in *United States Pharmacopeia (USP)*. However, there are several manufacturers, and prices vary greatly. For other drugs, the difference in cost between the trade-named product and generic products varies from less than twofold to more than 100-fold.

In some states and in many hospitals, pharmacists have the option of supplying a generically equivalent drug product even if a proprietary name has been specified in the order. If the physician wants a particular brand of drug product dispensed, handwritten instruction to "dispense as written" or words of similar meaning are required. Some government-subsidized health care programs and many third-party insurance payers require that pharmacists dispense the cheapest generically equivalent product in the inventory. However, the principles of drug product selection by private pharmacists do not permit substituting one therapeutic agent for another; ie, dispensing trichlormethiazide for hydrochlorothiazide would not be permitted without the prescriber's permission even though these two diuretics may be considered pharmacodynamically equivalent. Pharmacists within managed care organizations may follow different policies; see below.

It should not be assumed that every generic drug product is as satisfactory as the trade-named product,

---

*The "triplicate" is the special California prescription form required for Schedule II substances.

†"Once a product has been approved for marketing, a physician may prescribe it for uses or in treatment regimens or patient populations that are not included in the approved labeling. Such 'unapproved' or, more precisely, 'unlabeled' uses may be appropriate and rational in certain circumstances, and may, in fact, reflect approaches to drug therapy that have been extensively reported in medical literature."—FDA Drug Bull 1982;12:4.

though most generics are satisfactory. Bioavailability—the effective absorption of the drug product—varies between manufacturers and sometimes between different lots of a drug produced by the same manufacturer. In the case of a very small number of drugs, which usually have a low therapeutic index, poor solubility, or a high ratio of inert ingredients to active drug content, a specific manufacturer's product may give more consistent results. In the case of life-threatening diseases, the advantages of generic substitution are probably outweighed by the clinical urgency so that the prescription should be filled as written.

In an effort to codify bioequivalence information, the FDA publishes *Approved Drug Products With Therapeutic Equivalence Evaluations,* with monthly supplements, commonly called "the Orange Book." The book contains listings of multisource products in one of two categories: Products coded "A" are considered bioequivalent to all other versions of that product with a similar "A" coding. Products not considered bioequivalent are coded "B." Of the approximately 8000 products listed, 90% are coded "A." This information is also published in volume 3 of *USP DI.*

Mandatory drug product selection on the basis of price is rapidly becoming common practice in the USA as third-party payers (insurance companies, health maintenance organizations, etc) enforce money-saving regulations. If outside a managed care organization, the prescriber can sometimes override these controls by writing "dispense as written" on a prescription that calls for a brand-named product. However, in such cases, the patient may have to pay the difference between the dispensed product and the cheaper one.

Within most managed care organizations, formulary controls have been put in place that force the selection of less expensive medications whenever they are available. In a managed care environment, the prescriber often selects the drug group rather than a specific agent, and the pharmacy dispenses the formulary drug from that group. For example, if a prescriber in such an organization decides that a patient needs a thiazide diuretic, the pharmacy will automatically dispense the single thiazide diuretic carried in the organization's formulary.

Other Cost Factors

The private pharmacist bases his or her charges on the cost of the drug plus a fee for providing a professional service. Each time a prescription is dispensed, there is a fee. The prescriber controls the frequency of filling prescriptions by authorizing refills and specifying the quantity to be dispensed. Thus, the prescriber can save the patient money by prescribing standard sizes (so that drugs do not have to be repackaged) and, when chronic treatment is involved, by ordering the largest quantity consistent with safety and expense. Thus, optimal prescribing often involves consultation between the prescriber and the pharmacist.

REFERENCES

An explanation of the scope of RN practice including standardization procedures. Board of Registered Nursing, State of California, August 1994.

Bloom BS, Wierz DJ, Pauly MV: Cost and price of comparable branded and generic pharmaceuticals. JAMA 1986;256:2523.

California Business and Professions Code, Chapter 9, Division 2, Pharmacy Law. Department of Consumer Affairs, Sacramento, California, 1985.

Do we pay too much for prescriptions? Consumer Reports 1993;58:668.

Final Report: *Task Force on Prescription Drugs.* Department of Health, Education, and Welfare, 1969.

Frazier LM et al: Can physician education lower the cost of prescription drugs? Ann Intern Med 1991;115:116.

Friedman D et al: Physician attitudes toward and knowledge about generic drug substitution. N Y State J Med 1987;87:539.

Gennaro AR (editor): *Remington's Pharmaceutical Sciences,* 18th ed. Mack, 1990.

Huseby JS, Anderson P: Confusion about drug names. (Letter.) N Engl J Med 1991;325:588.

Jerome JB, Sagan P: The USAN nomenclature system. JAMA 1975;232:294.

King RE (editor): *Dispensing of Medication. A Practical Manual on the Formulation and Dispensing of Pharmaceutical Products,* 9th ed. Mack, 1984.

Krawelski JE, Pitt L, Dowd B: The effects of competition on prescription-drug product substitution. N Engl J Med 1983;309:213.

Kuehm SL, Doyle MJ: Medication errors: 1977 to 1988. Experience in medical malpractice claims. N J Med 1990;87:27.

Lindley CM et al: Inappropriate medication is a major cause of adverse drug reactions in elderly patients. Age Aging 1992;21:294.

Shulman SR: The broader message of Accutane. Am J Public Health 1989;79:1565.

Strom BL: Generic drug substitution revisited. N Engl J Med 1987;316:1456.

Trissel LA: *Handbook on Injectable Drugs,* 7th ed. American Society of Hospital Pharmacists, 1994. (With supplements.)

United States Pharmacopeial Convention: *1996 USP DI.* Vol 1: *Advice for the Health Care Professional;* Vol 2: *Advice for the Patient;* Vol 3: *Approved Drug Products and Legal Requirements,* 17th ed. United States Pharmacopeial Convention, 1997.

Use of approved drugs for unlabeled indications. FDA Drug Bull 1982;12:4.

Vagelos PR: Are prescription prices high? Science 1991; 252:1080.

WHO Drug Action Committee: *Model Guide to Good Prescribing.* WHO, 1994.

Wu AW et al: Do house officers learn from their mistakes? JAMA 1991;265:2089.

Appendix I: Vaccines, Immune Globulins, and Other Complex Biologic Products

I

Harry W. Lampiris MD, Daniel S. Maddix, PharmD, & Steven L. Barriere, PharmD

Vaccines and related biologic products constitute an important group of agents that bridge the disciplines of microbiology, infectious diseases, immunology and immunopharmacology. While a complete discussion of these agents is beyond the scope of this book, a listing of the most important preparations is provided here. The reader who requires more complete information is referred to the sources listed at the end of this appendix.

ACTIVE IMMUNIZATION

Active immunization consists of the administration of antigen to the host to induce formation of antibodies and cell-mediated immunity. Immunization is practiced to induce protection against many infectious agents and may utilize either inactivated (killed) materials or live attenuated agents (Table I–1). Desirable features of the ideal immunogen include complete prevention of disease, prevention of the carrier state, production of prolonged immunity with a minimum of immunizations, absence of toxicity, and suitability for mass immunization (eg, cheap and easy to administer). Active immunization is generally preferable to passive immunization—in most cases because higher antibody levels are sustained for longer periods of time, requiring less frequent immunization, and in some cases because of the development of concurrent cell-mediated immunity. However, active immunization requires time to develop and is therefore generally inactive at the time of a specific exposure (eg, for parenteral exposure to hepatitis B, concurrent hepatitis B IgG [passive antibodies] and active immunization are given to prevent illness).

Current recommendations for routine active immunization of children are given in Table I–2.

PASSIVE IMMUNIZATION

Passive immunization consists of transfer of immunity to a host using preformed immunologic products. From a practical standpoint, only immunoglobulins have been utilized for passive immunization, since passive administration of cellular components of the immune system has been technically difficult and associated with graft-versus-host reactions. Products of the cellular immune system (eg, interferons) have also been used in the therapy of a wide variety of hematologic and infectious diseases (Chapter 56).

Passive immunization with antibodies may be accomplished with either animal or human immunoglobulins in varying degrees of purity. These may contain relatively high titers of antibodies directed against a specific antigen or, as is true for pooled immune globulin, may simply contain antibodies found in most of the population. Passive immunization is useful for (1) individuals unable to form antibodies (eg, congenital agammaglobulinemia); (2) prevention of disease when time does not permit active immunization (eg, postexposure); (3) for treatment of certain diseases normally prevented by immunization (eg, tetanus); and (4) for treatment of conditions for which active immunization is unavailable or impractical (eg, snakebite).

Complications from administration of *human* immunoglobulins are rare. The injections may be moderately painful and rarely a sterile abscess at the injection site may occur. Transient hypotension and pruritus occasionally occur with the administration of IVIG products, but generally are mild. Individuals with certain immunoglobulin deficiency states (IgA deficiency, etc.) may occasionally develop hypersensitivity reactions to immune globulin that may limit therapy. Conventional immune globulin contains aggregates of IgG; it will cause severe reactions if given

Table I–1. Materials commonly used for active immunization in the United States.[1]

Vaccine	Type of Agent	Route of Administration	Primary Immunization	Booster[2]	Indications
Cholera	Inactivated bacteria	Subcutaneous, intramuscular, or intradermal	Two doses given at least 1 week apart, preferably 1 month apart	Every 6 months	Persons who work and live in highly endemic areas
Diphtheria-tetanus-pertussis (DTP)	Toxoids and inactivated whole bacteria	Intramuscular	See Table I–2		For all children
Diphtheria-tetanus-acellular pertussis (DTaP)	Toxoids and inactivated bacterial components	Intramuscular	See Table I–2		For use for the fourth or fifth dose (or both) of DTP in children ≥15 months of age
DTP-*Haemophilus influenzae* type b conjugate (DTP-Hib)	Toxoids, inactivated whole bacteria, and bacterial polysaccharide conjugated to protein	Intramuscular	See Table I–2		May be used in place of DTP and Hib when the 2 vaccines are administered at the same time
Haemophilus influenzae type b conjugate (Hib)	Bacterial polysaccharide conjugated to protein	Intramuscular	One dose (see Table I–2 for childhood schedule)	Not recommended	(1) For all children (2) Asplenia and other at-risk conditions
Hepatitis A	Inactivated virus	Intramuscular	One dose (administer at least 2–4 weeks before travel to endemic areas)	At 6–12 months for long-term immunity	(1) Travelers to hepatitis A endemic areas (2) Homosexual men (3) Illicit drug users (4) Chronic liver disease (5) Persons with occupational risk for infection
Hepatitis B	Inactive viral antigen	Intramuscular	Three doses at 0, 1, and 6 months (see Table I–2 for childhood schedule)	Not routinely recommended	(1) For all infants (2) Preadolescents, adolescents, young adults (3) Persons with occupational, lifestyle, or environmental risk (4) Hemophiliacs (5) Hemodialysis patients (6) Postexposure prophylaxis
Influenza	Inactivated virus or viral components	Intramuscular	One dose. (Children ≤12 years of age should receive split virus vaccine only; children < 9 who are receiving influenza vaccine for the first time should receive 2 doses administered at least 1 month apart.)	Yearly with current vaccine	(1) Adults ≥65 years of age (2) Persons with high risk-conditions (eg, asthma) (3) Medical care personnel

Table I–1. Materials commonly used for active immunization in the United States (cont'd).

Vaccine	Type of Agent	Route of Administration	Primary Immunization	Booster[2]	Indications
Measles	Live virus	Subcutaneous	Two doses at least 1 month apart	None	(1) Adults born after 1956 without a history of measles or live virus vaccination on or after their first birthday (2) Postexposure prophylaxis in unimmunized persons
Measles-mumps-rubella (MMR)	Live virus	Subcutaneous	See Table I–2	None	For all children
Meningococcal	Bacterial polysaccharides of serotypes A/C/Y/W-135	Subcutaneous	One dose	Unknown	(1) Travelers to areas with epidemic meningococcal disease (2) Asplenic individuals (3) Control of outbreaks in closed or semiclosed populations
Mumps	Live virus	Subcutaneous	One dose	None	Adults born after 1956 without a history of mumps or live virus vaccination on or after their first birthday
Pneumococcal	Bacterial polysaccharides of 23 serotypes	Intramuscular or subcutaneous	One dose	Repeat after 6 years in patients at high risk	(1) Adults ≥65 years of age (2) Persons at increased risk for pneumococcal disease or its complications
Poliovirus vaccine, inactivated (IPV)	Inactivated viruses of all 3 serotypes	Subcutaneous	Two doses 4–8 weeks apart, and a third dose 6–12 months after the second	One-time booster dose for travelers	Previously unvaccinated adults at increased risk for occupational or travel exposure to polioviruses
Poliovirus vaccine, oral (OPV)	Live viruses of all 3 serotypes	Oral	See Table I–2 for childhood schedule	One-time booster dose for travelers	(1) For all children (2) Alternative to IPV when there is < 4 weeks before travel
Rabies	Inactivated virus	Intramuscular or intradermal	**Preexposure:** 3 doses (IM or ID) at days 0, 7, and 21 or 28 **Postexposure:** 5 doses (IM only) at days 0, 3, 7, 14, and 28	Serologic testing every 6 months to 2 years in persons at high risk	(1) Preexposure prophylaxis in persons at risk for contact with rabies virus (2) Postexposure prophylaxis (administer with rabies immune globulin)
Rubella	Live virus	Subcutaneous	One dose	None	Adults without a history of rubella or live virus vaccination on or after their first birthday

Table I–1. Materials commonly used for active immunization in the United States (cont'd).

Vaccine	Type of Agent	Route of Administration	Primary Immunization	Booster[2]	Indications
Tetanus-diphtheria (Td or DT)[3]	Toxoids	Intramuscular	Two doses at least 4 weeks apart, and a third dose 6–12 months after the second	Every 10 years or at age 50	(1) All adults who have not been immunized as children (2) Postexposure prophylaxis if > 5 years has passed since last dose
Typhoid, Ty21a oral	Live bacteria	Oral	Four doses given 2 days apart	4 doses every 5 years	Risk of exposure to typhoid fever
Typhoid, Vi capsular polysaccharide	Bacterial polysaccharide	Intramuscular	One dose	Every 2 years	Risk of exposure to typhoid fever
Typhoid, heat-phenol-inactivated	Inactivated bacteria	Subcutaneous or intradermal	Two doses ≥4 weeks apart	Every 3 years	Risk of exposure to typhoid fever
Varicella	Live virus	Subcutaneous	Two doses 4–8 weeks apart in persons past their 13th birthday. (See Table I–2 for childhood schedule.)	Unknown	(1) For all children (2) Persons past their 13th birthday without a history of varicella infection or immunization
Yellow Fever	Live virus	Subcutaneous	One dose 10 days to 10 years before travel	Every 10 years	(1) Laboratory personnel who may be exposed to yellow fever virus (2) Travelers to areas where yellow fever occurs

[1]Dosages for the specific product, including variations for age, are best obtained from the manufacturer's package insert.
[2]One dose unless otherwise indicated
[3]Td = Tetanus and diphtheria toxoids for use in persons ≥7 years of age (contains less diphtheria toxoid than DPT and DT); DT = Tetanus and diphtheria toxoids for use in persons < 7 years of age (contains the same amount of diphtheria toxoid as DPT).

Table I–2. Recommended childhood immunization schedule.[1]

Age	Immunization	Comments
Birth to 2 months	Hepatitis B vaccine (HBV)	Administration should be at birth, with a second dose administered at 2 months of age for infants born to seronegative mothers. Infants born to seropositive mothers should receive the first dose at birth (with hepatitis B immune globulin), the second dose at 1 month of age, and the third dose at 6 months of age.
2 months	Diphtheria and tetanus toxoids and pertussis vaccine (DTP), Oral poliovirus vaccine (OPV), *Haemophilus influenzae* type b conjugate vaccine (Hib)[2]	
2–4 months	HBV	The second dose should be given at least 1 month after the first dose.
4 months	DTP, Hib, OPV	
6 months	DTP, Hib[2]	
6–18 months	HBV, OPV	Routine vaccination with OPV at 6 months of age is preferred. Vaccination at as late as 18 months of age is an acceptable alternative.
12–15 months	Measles-mumps-rubella vaccine (MMR), Hib	
12–18 months	DTP or diphtheria and tetanus toxoids and acellular pertussis vaccine (DTaP) at 15 months, Varicella vaccine	Varicella vaccine is recommended for all children from 18 months to the 13th birthday who have not been previously immunized and who lack a history of varicella infection.
4–6 years	DTP or DTaP, OPV	Administer at or before school entry.
4–6 years or 11–12 years	MMR	The second dose of MMR should be administered *either* at 4–6 years of age *or* at 11–12 years of age.
11–12 years	Diphtheria and tetanus toxoids (Td)	Vaccination at 14–16 years of age is an acceptable alternative.

[1]Data from MMWR Morbid Mortal Wkly Rep 1995;44(No. RR-5).
[2]Three Hib conjugate vaccines are available for use: (a) oligosaccharide conjugate Hib vaccine (HbOC), (b) polyribosylribitol phosphate-tetanus toxoid conjugate (PRP-T), and (c) *Haemophilus* b conjugate vaccine (meningococcal protein conjugate) (PRP-OMP). Children immunized with PRP-OMP at 2 and 4 months of age do not require a dose at 6 months of age.

intravenously. However, if the passively administered antibodies are derived from *animal* sera, hypersensitivity reactions ranging from anaphylaxis to serum sickness may occur. Highly purified immunoglobulins, especially from rodents or lagomorphs are the least likely to cause reactions. To avoid anaphylactic reactions, tests for hypersensitivity to the animal serum must be performed. If an alternative preparation is not available and administration of the specific antibody is deemed essential, desensitization can be carried out.

Antibodies derived from human serum not only avoid the risk of hypersensitivity reactions but also have a much longer half-life in humans (about 23 days for IgG antibodies) than those from animal sources (5–7 days or less). Consequently, much smaller doses of human antibody can be administered to provide therapeutic concentrations for several weeks. These advantages point to the desirability of

using human antibodies for passive protection whenever possible. Materials available for passive immunization are summarized in Table I–3.

LEGAL LIABILITY FOR UNTOWARD REACTIONS

It is the physician's responsibility to inform the patient of the risk of immunization and to employ vaccines and antisera in an appropriate manner. This may require skin testing to assess the risk of an untoward reaction. Some of the risks described above are, however, currently unavoidable; on the balance, the patient and society are clearly better off accepting the risks for routinely administered immunogens (eg, poliomyelitis and tetanus vaccines). For example, the in-

Table I–3. Materials available for passive immunization.[1]

Indication	Product	Dosage	Comments
Black widow spider bite	Antivenin (*Latrodectus mactans*), equine	1 vial (6000 units) IV or IM.	For persons with hypertensive cardiovascular disease or age < 16 or > 60 years.
Botulism	Botulism antitoxin (trivalent, types A, B, and E), equine	Consult the CDC.[2]	Treatment and prophylaxis of botulism. Available from the CDC.[1] Ten to 20 percent incidence of serum reactions.
Chronic lymphocytic leukemia (CLL)	Immune globulin (intravenous)[3]	Initial dose of 400 mg/kg IV every 3 weeks. Dosage should be adjusted upward if bacterial infections occur.	CLL patients with hypogammaglobulinemia and a history of at least one serious bacterial infection.
Cytomegalovirus	Cytomegalovirus immune globulin (intravenous)	**Bone marrow transplantation:** 1 g/kg weekly. **Kidney transplantation:** 150 mg/kg then 50 to 100 mg/kg every 2 weeks.	Treatment and prophylaxis of CMV infection in bone marrow and kidney transplantation.
Diphtheria	Diphtheria antitoxin, equine	20,000–120,000 units IV or IM depending on the severity and duration of illness.	Early treatment of respiratory diphtheria. Available from Connaught Laboratories (800-822-2463) or the CDC.[2] Anaphylactic reactions in ≥ 7% of adults and serum reactions in ≥ 5–10% of adults.
Hepatitis A	Immune globulin (intramuscular)	**Preexposure prophylaxis:** 0.02 ml/kg IM for anticipated risk of ≤ 3 months, 0.06 ml/kg for anticipated risk of > 3 months repeated every 4 to 6 months for continued exposure. **Postexposure:** 0.02 mL/kg IM as soon as possible after exposure up to 2 weeks	Preexposure and postexposure hepatitis A prophylaxis. The availability of hepatitis A vaccine may greatly reduce the need for preexposure prophylaxis.
Hepatitis B	Hepatitis B immune globulin (HBIG)	0.06 mL/kg IM as soon as possible after exposure up to 1 week for percutaneous exposure or 2 weeks for sexual exposure. 0.5 mL IM within 12 hours after birth for perinatal exposure.	Postexposure prophylaxis in nonimmune persons following percutaneous, mucosal, sexual, or perinatal exposure. Hepatitis B vaccine should also be administered.
Idiopathic thrombocytopenic purpura (ITP)	Immune globulin (intravenous)[3]	400 mg/kg IV daily for 2–5 consecutive days, depending on the platelet count and clinical response, or 1 g/kg once daily for 1 day or 2 consecutive days.	Response in children with ITP is greater than in adults. Corticosteroids are the treatment of choice in adults, except for severe pregnancy-associated ITP.
Kawasaki disease	Immune globulin (intravenous)[3]	400 mg/kg IV daily for 4 consecutive days within 4 days after the onset of illness. A single dose of 2 g/kg IV over 10 hours is also effective.	Effective in the prevention of coronary aneurysms. For use in patients who meet strict criteria for Kawasaki disease.
Measles	Immune globulin (intramuscular)	**Normal hosts:** 0.25 mL/kg IM. **Immunocompromised hosts:** 0.5 mL/kg IM (maximum dose of 15 mL for all patients).	Postexposure prophylaxis (within 6 days after exposure) in nonimmune contacts of acute cases.
Primary immunodeficiency disorders	Immune globulin (intravenous)[3]	Minimum effective dosage is 150 mg/kg every 3–4 weeks. Dosage should be adjusted to maintain the serum IgG concentration ≥ 400 mg/dL.	Primary immunodeficiency disorders include specific antibody deficiencies (eg, X-linked agammaglobulinemia) and combined deficiencies (eg, severe combined immunodeficiencies).
Rabies	Rabies immune globulin	20 IU/kg. If possible, up to one-half of the dose should be infiltrated around the wound and the remainder should be given IM in the gluteal area.	Postexposure rabies prophylaxis in persons not previously immunized with rabies vaccine. Must be combined with rabies vaccine.

Table I–3. Materials available for passive immunization (cont'd).

Indication	Product	Dosage	Comments
Rh isoimmuni- zation	Rh_o(D) immune globulin	The usual dose is 1 vial IM administered within 72 hours after delivery or termination of pregnancy.	To suppress the formation of anti-Rh_o(D) in Rh_o(D)-negative, D^u-negative women exposed to Rh-positive blood during delivery or pregnancy termination.
Rubella	Immune globulin (intramuscular)	0.55 mL/kg IM	Nonimmune pregnant women exposed to rubella who will not consider therapeutic abortion. Administration does not prevent rubella in the fetus of an exposed mother.
Snake bite (coral snake)	Antivenin (*Micrurus fulvius*), equine	At least 3–5 vials (30–50 mL) IV initially within 4 hours after the bite. Additional doses may be required.	Neutralizes the venom of the eastern coral snake and the Texas coral snake. Serum sickness occurs in almost all patients who receive > 7 vials.
Snake bite (pit vipers)	Antivenin (Crotalidae) polyvalent, equine	The entire dose should be given within 4 hours after the bite by the IV or IM route (1 vial = 10 mL): Minimal envenomation: 2–4 vials Moderate envenomation: 5–9 vials Severe envenomation: 10–15 vials Additional doses may be required.	Neutralizes the venom of rattlesnakes, copperheads, cottonmouths, water moccasins, and tropical and Asiatic crotalids. Serum sickness occurs in almost all patients who receive > 7 vials.
Tetanus	Tetanus immune globulin	**Postexposure prophylaxis:** 250 units IM. **Treatment:** 3000 to 6000 units IM.	Treatment of tetanus and postexposure prophylaxis of nonclean, nonminor wounds in inadequately immunized persons (< 2 doses of tetanus toxoid or < 3 doses if wound is > 24 hours old).
Vaccinia	Vaccinia immune globulin	Consult the CDC.[1,2]	Treatment of severe reactions to vaccinia vaccination, including eczema vaccinatum, vaccinia necrosum, and ocular vaccinia. Available from the CDC.[2]
Varicella	Varicella-zoster immune globulin	125 units/10 kg IM, up to 625 units. Higher doses may be required for immunocompromised hosts.	Postexposure prophylaxis in susceptible immunocompromised hosts, selected pregnant women, and perinatally exposed newborns.

[1]Passive immunotherapy or immunoprophylaxis should always be administered as soon as possible after exposure. Prior to the administration of animal sera, patients should be questioned and tested for hypersensitivity.
[2]Centers for Disease Control and Prevention, 404-639-3670.
[3]For an analysis of additional uses of intravenously administered immune globulin, see Ratko TA et al: Recommendations for off-label use of intravenously administered immunoglobulin preparations. JAMA 1995;273:1865.

cidence of paralytic poliomyelitis caused by the oral vaccine is currently estimated as ten cases per years in the USA. In the absence of vaccination, approximately 100,000 paralytic cases would be expected.

Manufacturers should be held legally accountable for failure to adhere to existing standards for production of biologicals. However, in the present litigious atmosphere of the US, the filing of large liability claims by the statistically inevitable victims of good public health practice has caused manufacturers to abandon efforts to develop and produce low-profit but medically valuable therapeutic agents such as vaccines. Since the use and sale of these products are subject to careful review and approval by government bodies such as the Surgeon General's Advisory Committee on Immunization Practices and the Food and Drug Administration, "strict product liability" (liabil-

ity without fault) may be an inappropriate legal standard to apply when rare reactions to biologicals, produced and administered according to government guidelines, are involved.

RECOMMENDED IMMUNIZATION OF ADULTS FOR TRAVEL

Every adult, whether traveling or not, must be immunized with tetanus toxoid and should also be fully immunized against poliomyelitis, measles (for those born after 1956), and diphtheria. In addition, every traveler must fulfill the immunization requirements of the health authorities of the countries to be visited.

These are listed in *Health Information for International Travel,* available from the Superintendent of Documents, US Government Printing Office, Washington, DC 20402. *The Medical Letter on Drugs and Therapeutics* also offers periodically updated recommendations for international travelers (see issue of March 1, 1996). Immunizations received in preparation for travel should be recorded on the International Certificate of Immunization. Note: Smallpox vaccination is not recommended or required for travel in any country.

REFERENCES

Academy of Pediatrics Committee on Infectious Diseases: Recommendations for the use of live attenuated varicella vaccine. Pediatrics 1995;9:791.

American College of Physicians Task Force on Adult Immunization and Infectious Disease Society of America: *Guide for Adult Immunization.* American College of Physicians, 1994.

American Hospital Formulary Service: *AHFS 95 Drug Information.* American Society of Health-System Pharmacists, 1995.

ASHP Commission on Therapeutics: ASHP therapeutic guidelines for intravenous immune globulin. Clin Pharm 1992;11:117.

Gardner P et al: Adult immunizations. Ann Intern Med 1996;12:35.

Gardner P, Schaffner W: Current concepts: Immunization of adults. N Engl J Med 1993;328:1252.

General recommendations on immunization: recommendations of the Immunization Practices Advisory Committee (ACIP). MMWR Morb Mortal Wkly Rep 1994;43:1.

Peter G: Current concepts: Childhood immunizations. N Engl J Med 1992;327:1794.

Prevention and control of influenza: recommendations of the Immunization Practices Advisory Committee (ACIP). MMWR Morb Mortal Wkly Rep 1995;44:1.

Recommendations for use of Haemophilus b conjugate vaccines and a combined diphtheria, tetanus, pertussis, and Haemophilus b vaccine: recommendations of the Immunization Practices Advisory Committee (ACIP). MMWR Morb Mortal Wkly Rep 1993;42:1.

Recommendations of the Advisory Committee on Immunization Practices (ACIP): use of vaccines and immune globulins in persons with altered immunocompetence. MMWR Morb Mortal Wkly Rep 1993;42:1.

Recommended childhood immunization schedule—United States, 1995. MMWR Morb Mortal Wkly Rep 1995;44:1.

Standards for pediatric immunization practices. MMWR Morb Mortal Wkly Rep 1993;42:1.

Typhoid immunization: recommendations of the Immunization Practices Advisory Committee (ACIP). MMWR Morb Mortal Wkly Rep 1994;43:1.

Update: Vaccine side effects, adverse reactions, contraindications, and precautions. MMWR Morb Mortal Wkly Rep 1996;45:1.

Appendix II: Important Drug Interactions & Their Mechanisms

II

Philip D. Hansten, PharmD

One of the factors that can alter the response to drugs is the concurrent administration of other drugs. There are several mechanisms by which drugs may interact, but most can be categorized as pharmacokinetic (absorption, distribution, metabolism, excretion), pharmacodynamic, or combined interactions. Knowledge of the mechanism by which a given drug interaction occurs is often clinically useful, since the mechanism may influence both the time course and the methods of circumventing the interaction. Some important drug interactions occur as a result of two or more mechanisms.

Pharmacokinetic Mechanisms

The gastrointestinal **absorption** of drugs may be affected by concurrent use of other agents that (1) have a large surface area upon which the drug can be adsorbed, (2) bind or chelate, (3) alter gastric pH, or (4) alter gastrointestinal motility. One must distinguish between effects on absorption rate and effects on extent of absorption. A reduction in only the absorption rate of a drug is seldom clinically important, whereas a reduction in the extent of absorption will be clinically important if it results in subtherapeutic serum levels.

The mechanisms by which drug interactions alter drug **distribution** include (1) competition for plasma protein binding and (2) displacement from tissue binding sites. Although competition for plasma protein binding can increase the free concentration (and thus the effect) of the displaced drug in plasma, the increase tends to be temporary owing to a compensatory increase in drug disposition. The clinical importance of protein binding displacement has probably been overemphasized; current evidence suggests that such interactions are unlikely to result in adverse effects. Displacement from tissue binding sites would tend to increase the blood concentration of the displaced drug. Such a mechanism may contribute to the elevation of serum digoxin concentration by concurrent quinidine therapy.

The **metabolism** of drugs can be stimulated or inhibited by concurrent therapy. Induction (stimulation) of hepatic microsomal drug-metabolizing enzymes can be produced by drugs such as barbiturates, carbamazepine, glutethimide, phenytoin, primidone, rifampin, and rifabutin. Enzyme induction does not take place quickly; maximal effects usually occur after 7–10 days and require an equal or longer time to dissipate after the enzyme inducer is stopped. Inhibition of metabolism generally takes place more quickly than enzyme induction and may begin as soon as sufficient hepatic concentration of the inhibitor is achieved. However, if the half-life of the affected drug is long, it may take a week or more to reach a new steady state serum level. Drugs that may inhibit hepatic microsomal metabolism of other drugs include allopurinol, amiodarone, androgens, chloramphenicol, cimetidine, ciprofloxacin, clarithromycin, diltiazem, disulfiram, enoxacin, erythromycin, fluconazole, fluoxetine, fluvoxamine, isoniazid, itraconazole, ketoconazole, metronidazole, miconazole, omeprazole, paroxetine, phenylbutazone, propoxyphene, quinidine, sulfonamides, and verapamil.

The renal **excretion** of active drug can also be affected by concurrent drug therapy. The renal excretion of certain drugs that are weak acids or weak bases may be influenced by other drugs that affect urinary pH. This is due to changes in ionization of the drug, thus altering its lipid solubility and therefore its ability to be absorbed back into the blood from the kidney tubule. For some drugs, active secretion into the renal tubules is an important elimination pathway. This process may be affected by concurrent drug therapy, thus altering serum drug levels and pharmacologic response.

Pharmacodynamic Mechanisms

When drugs with similar pharmacologic effects are administered concurrently, an additive or synergistic response is usually seen. The two drugs may or may not act on the same receptor to produce such effects.

Conversely, drugs with opposing pharmacologic effects may reduce the response to one or both drugs. Pharmacodynamic drug interactions are relatively common in clinical practice, but adverse effects can usually be minimized if the interactions are anticipated and appropriate countermeasures taken.

Combined Toxicity

The combined use of two or more drugs, each of which has toxic effects on the same organ, can greatly increase the likelihood of organ damage. For example, concurrent administration of two nephrotoxic drugs can produce kidney damage even though the dose of either drug alone may have been insufficient to produce toxicity. Furthermore, some drugs can enhance the organ toxicity of another drug even though the enhancing drug has no intrinsic toxic effect on that organ.

PREDICTABILITY OF DRUG INTERACTIONS

The designations listed in Table II-1 will be used here to *estimate* the predictability of the drug interactions. These estimates are intended to indicate simply whether or not the interaction will occur and do not always mean that the interaction is likely to produce an adverse effect. Whether the interaction occurs and produces an adverse effect or not depends upon (1) the presence or absence of factors that predispose to the adverse effects of the drug interaction (diseases, organ function, dose of drugs, etc) and (2) awareness on the part of the prescriber, so that appropriate monitoring can be ordered or preventive measures taken.

Table II–1. Important drug interactions.

HP = Highly predictable. Interaction occurs in almost all patients receiving the interacting combination.
P = Predictable. Interaction occurs in most patients receiving the combination.
NP = Not predictable. Interaction occurs only in some patients receiving the combination.
NE = Not established. Insufficient data available on which to base estimate of predictability.

Drug or Drug Group	Properties Promoting Drug Interaction	Clinically Documented Interactions

Alcohol	Chronic alcoholism results in enzyme induction. Acute alcoholic intoxication tends to inhibit drug metabolism (whether person is alcoholic or not). Severe alcohol-induced hepatic dysfunction may inhibit ability to metabolize drugs. Disulfiram-like reaction in the presence of certain drugs. Additive central nervous system depression with other central nervous system depressants.	**Acetaminophen:** [NE] Increased formation of hepatotoxic acetaminophen metabolites (in chronic alcoholics).
		 Anticoagulants, oral: [NE] Increased hypoprothrombinemic effect with acute alcohol intoxication.
		 Central nervous system depressants: [HP] Additive or synergistic central nervous system depression.
		 Insulin: [NE] Acute alcohol intake may increase hypoglycemic effect of insulin (especially in fasting patients).
		 Drugs that may produce a disulfiram-like reaction:
		     Cephalosporins: [NP] Disulfiram-like reactions noted with cefamandole, cefoperazone, cefotetan, and moxalactam.
		     Chloral hydrate: [NP] Mechanism not established.
		     Disulfiram: [HP] Inhibits aldehyde dehydrogenase.
		     Metronidazole: [NP] Mechanism not established.
		     Sulfonylureas: [NE] Chlorpropamide is most likely to produce a disulfiram-like reaction; acute alcohol intake may increase hypoglycemic effect (especially in fasting patients).

Allopurinol	Inhibits hepatic drug-metabolizing enzymes.	**Anticoagulants, oral:** [NP] Increased hypoprothrombinemic effect. **Azathioprine:** [P] Decreased azathioprine detoxification resulting in increased azathioprine toxicity. **Mercaptopurine:** [P] Decreased mercaptopurine metabolism resulting in increased mercaptopurine toxicity.
Antacids	Antacids may adsorb drugs in gastrointestinal tract, thus reducing absorption. Antacids tend to speed gastric emptying, thus delivering drugs to absorbing sites in the intestine more quickly. Some antacids (eg, magnesium hydroxide + aluminum hydroxide) alkalinize the urine somewhat, thus altering excretion of drugs sensitive to urinary pH.	**Digoxin:** [NP] Decreased gastrointestinal absorption of digoxin. **Iron:** [P] Decreased gastrointestinal absorption of iron with some antacids. **Itraconazole:** [P] Reduced gastrointestinal absorption of itraconazole due to increased pH (itraconazole requires acid for absorption). **Ketoconazole:** [P] Reduced gastrointestinal absorption of ketoconazole due to increased pH (ketoconazole requires acid for absorption). **Quinolones:** [HP] Decreased gastrointestinal absorption of ciprofloxacin, norfloxacin, enoxacin (and probably other quinolones). **Salicylates:** [P] Increased renal clearance of salicylates due to increased urine pH; occurs only with large doses of salicylates. **Sodium polystyrene sulfonate:** [NE] Binds antacid cation in gut, resulting in metabolic alkalosis. **Tetracyclines:** [HP] Decreased gastrointestinal absorption of tetracyclines.
Anticholinergics	*See* Antimuscarinics.	*See* Antimuscarinics.
Anticoagulants, oral	Metabolism inducible. Susceptible to inhibition of metabolism. Highly bound to plasma proteins. Anticoagulation response altered by drugs that affect clotting factor synthesis or catabolism.	*Drugs that may increase anticoagulant effect:* **Amiodarone:** [P] Inhibits anticoagulant metabolism. **Anabolic steroids:** [P] Alter clotting factor disposition? **Chloramphenicol:** [NE] Decreased dicumarol metabolism (possibly also warfarin). **Cimetidine:** [HP] Decreased anticoagulant metabolism. **Ciprofloxacin:** [NE] Probably inhibits anticoagulant metabolism. **Clofibrate:** [P] Mechanism not established. **Danazol:** [NE] Impaired synthesis of clotting factors? **Dextrothyroxine:** [P] Enhances clotting factor catabolism? **Disulfiram:** [P] Decreased anticoagulant metabolism. **Erythromycin:** [NE] Probably inhibits anticoagulant metabolism. **Fluconazole:** [P] Decreased warfarin metabolism. **Gemfibrozil:** [NE] Mechanism not established. **Lovastatin:** [NE] Probably decreased anticoagulant metabolism. **Metronidazole:** [P] Decreased anticoagulant metabolism. **Miconazole:** [NE] Decreased anticoagulant metabolism.

(continued)

Table II–1. Important drug interactions (cont'd).

HP = Highly predictable. Interaction occurs in almost all patients receiving the interacting combination.
P = Predictable. Interaction occurs in most patients receiving the combination.
NP = Not predictable. Interaction occurs only in some patients receiving the combination.
NE = Not established. Insufficient data available on which to base estimate of predictability.

Drug or Drug Group	Properties Promoting Drug Interaction	Clinically Documented Interactions
Anticoagulants, oral (cont'd)	(See preceding page.)	**Nonsteroidal anti-inflammatory drugs:** [P] Inhibition of platelet function, gastric erosions; some agents increase hypoprothrombinemic response (unlikely with ibuprofen or naproxen). **Phenylbutazone:** [HP] Inhibits anticoagulant metabolism. **Propafenone:** [NE] Probably decreased anticoagulant metabolism. **Quinidine:** [NP] Additive hypoprothrombinemia. **Salicylates:** [HP] Platelet inhibition with aspirin but not with other salicylates; [P] large doses have hypoprothrombinemic effect. **Sulfinpyrazone:** [NE] Mechanism not established. **Sulfonamides:** [NE] Inhibit anticoagulant metabolism; displace protein binding. **Thyroid hormones:** [P] Enhance clotting factor catabolism. **Trimethoprim-sulfamethoxazole:** [P] Inhibits anticoagulant metabolism; displaces from protein binding. *See also* Alcohol; Allopurinol. *Drugs that may decrease anticoagulant effect:* **Aminoglutethimide:** [P] Enzyme induction. **Barbiturates:** [P] Enzyme induction. **Carbamazepine:** [P] Enzyme induction. **Cholestyramine:** [P] Reduces absorption of anticoagulant. **Glutethimide:** [P] Enzyme induction. **Nafcillin:** [NE] Mechanism not established. **Phenytoin:** [NE] Enzyme induction; anticoagulant effect may increase transiently at start of phenytoin therapy due to protein-binding displacement. **Primidone:** [P] Enzyme induction. **Rifampin:** [P] Enzyme induction. *Effects of anticoagulants on other drugs:* **Hypoglycemics, oral:** [P] Dicumarol inhibits hepatic metabolism of tolbutamide and chlorpropamide. **Phenytoin:** [P] Dicumarol inhibits metabolism of phenytoin.
Antidepressants, tricyclic and heterocyclic	Inhibition of amine uptake into postganglionic adrenergic neuron. Antimuscarinic effects may be additive with other antimuscarinic drugs. Metabolism inducible.	**Barbiturates:** [P] Increased antidepressant metabolism. **Carbamazepine:** [NE] Enhanced metabolism of antidepressants. **Cimetidine:** [P] Decreased antidepressant metabolism. **Clonidine:** [P] Decreased clonidine antihypertensive effect. **Guanadrel:** [P] Decreased uptake of guanadrel into sites of action. **Guanethidine:** [P] Decreased uptake of guanethidine into sites of action. **Monoamine oxidase inhibitors:** [NP] Some cases of excitation, hyperpyrexia, mania, and convulsions, but many patients have received combination without ill effects. **Quinidine:** [NE] Inhibits antidepressant metabolism. **Selective Serotonin Reuptake Inhibitors (SSRIs):** [P] Fluoxetine and paroxetine inhibit CYP2D6 and decrease metabolism of antidepressants metabolized by this enzyme (eg, desipramine). Sertraline and fluvoxamine are only weak inhibitors of CYP2D6, but fluvoxamine inhibits CYP1A2 and CYP3A4 and thus can inhibit the metabolism of antidepressants metabolized by these enzymes. **Sympathomimetics:** [P] Increased pressor response to norepinephrine, epinephrine, and phenylephrine.
Antihistamines, nonsedating (terfenadine, astemizole)	Susceptible to inhibition of hepatic metabolism.	**Erythromycin:** [NP] Reduced antihistamine metabolism; possible cardiac arrhythmias. Clarithromycin may produce similar effects. **Itraconazole:** [NE] Decreased antihistamine metabolism, increased serum levels; possible ventricular arrhythmia. **Ketoconazole:** [P] Reduced antihistamine metabolism, increased serum levels, possible cardiac arrhythmia.

Table II–1. Important drug interactions (cont'd).

HP = Highly predictable. Interaction occurs in almost all patients receiving the interacting combination.
P = Predictable. Interaction occurs in most patients receiving the combination.
NP = Not predictable. Interaction occurs only in some patients receiving the combination.
NE = Not established. Insufficient data available on which to base estimate of predictability.

Drug or Drug Group	Properties Promoting Drug Interaction	Clinically Documented Interactions
Antihistamines (cont'd)	(See preceding page.)	**Nefazodone:** [NE] Possible decreased metabolism of antihistamine by CYP3A4; possible ventricular arrhythmia. **Selective serotonin reuptake inhibitors (SSRIs):** [NE] Fluoxetine and fluvoxamine inhibit CYP3A4 and probably decrease antihistamine metabolism; possible ventricular arrhythmia.
Antimuscarinics	Decreased gastrointestinal motility. This may increase bioavailability of poorly soluble drugs and reduce bioavailability of drugs degraded in gut. Combined use of more than one antimuscarinic or combination of an antimuscarinic with another drug with "hidden" antimuscarinic actions (especially OTC antihistamines) increases likelihood of antimuscarinic adverse effects.	**Combined antimuscarinics:** [P] Antimuscarinic adverse effects (eg, paralytic ileus, urinary retention, blurred vision). **Levodopa:** [P] Increased degradation of levodopa in gut; serum levodopa levels lowered.
Barbiturates	Induction of hepatic microsomal drug-metabolizing enzymes. Additive central nervous system depression with other central nervous system depressants.	**Beta-adrenoceptor blockers:** [P] Increased beta-blocker metabolism. **Calcium channel blockers:** [P] Increased calcium channel blocker metabolism. **Central nervous system depressants:** [HP] Additive central nervous system depression. **Corticosteroids:** [P] Increased corticosteroid metabolism. **Cyclosporine:** [NE] Increased cyclosporine metabolism. **Doxycycline:** [P] Increased doxycycline metabolism. **Estrogens:** [P] Increased estrogen metabolism. **Itraconazole:** [P] Increased itraconazole metabolism. **Ketoconazole:** [P] Increased ketoconazole metabolism. **Phenothiazines:** [P] Increased phenothiazine metabolism. **Quinidine:** [P] Increased quinidine metabolism. **Theophylline:** [NE] Increased theophylline metabolism; reduced theophylline effect. **Valproic acid:** [P] Decreased phenobarbital metabolism. *See also* Anticoagulants, oral; Antidepressants, tricyclic.
Beta-adrenoceptor blockers	Beta blockade (especially with nonselective agents such as propranolol) alters response to sympathomimetics with beta-agonist activity (eg, epinephrine). Beta-blockers that undergo extensive first-pass metabolism may be affected by drugs capable of altering this process. Beta-blockers may reduce hepatic blood flow.	*Drugs that may increase beta-blocker effect:* **Chlorpromazine:** [P] Decreased metabolism of propranolol. **Cimetidine:** [P] Decreased metabolism of beta-blockers that are cleared primarily by the liver, eg, propranolol. Less effect (if any) on those cleared by the kidneys, eg, atenolol, nadolol. **Furosemide:** [P] Decreased metabolism of propranolol. **Hydralazine:** [P] Decreased metabolism of propranolol. *Drugs that may decrease beta-blocker effect:* **Enzyme inducers:** [P] Barbiturates, phenytoin, and rifampin may enhance beta-blocker metabolism; other enzyme inducers may produce similar effects. **Nonsteroidal anti-inflammatory drugs:** [P] Indomethacin reduces antihypertensive response; other prostaglandin inhibitors probably also interact. *Effects of beta-blockers on other drugs:* **Clonidine:** [NE] Hypertensive reaction if clonidine is withdrawn while patient is taking propranolol. **Insulin:** [P] Inhibition of glucose recovery from hypoglycemia; inhibition of symptoms of hypoglycemia (except sweating); increased blood pressure during hypoglycemia. **Lidocaine:** [NE] Decreased clearance of intravenous lidocaine; increased plasma lidocaine levels.

(continued)

Table II–1. Important drug interactions (cont'd).

HP = Highly predictable. Interaction occurs in almost all patients receiving the interacting combination.
P = Predictable. Interaction occurs in most patients receiving the combination.
NP = Not predictable. Interaction occurs only in some patients receiving the combination.
NE = Not established. Insufficient data available on which to base estimate of predictability.

Drug or Drug Group	Properties Promoting Drug Interaction	Clinically Documented Interactions
Beta-adrenoceptor blockers (cont'd)	(See preceding page.)	**Prazosin:** [P] Increased hypotensive response to first dose of prazosin. **Sympathomimetics:** [P] Increased pressor response to epinephrine (and possibly other sympathomimetics); this is more likely to occur with nonspecific beta-blockers.
Bile acid-binding resins	Resins may bind with orally adminstered drugs in gastrointestinal tract. Resins may bind in gastrointestinal tract with drugs that undergo enterohepatic circulation, even if the latter are given parenterally.	**Acetaminophen:** [NE] Decreased gastrointestinal absorption of acetaminophen. **Digitalis glycosides:** [NE] Decreased gastrointestinal absorption of digitoxin (possibly also digoxin). **Methotrexate:** [NE] Reduced gastrointestinal absorption of methotrexate. **Thiazide diuretics:** [P] Reduced gastrointestinal absorption of thiazides. **Thyroid hormones:** [P] Reduced thyroid absorption. *See also* Anticoagulants, oral.
Calcium channel blockers	Verapamil, diltiazem, and possibly nicardipine (but not nifedipine) inhibit hepatic drug metabolizing enzymes. Metabolism of diltiazem, nifedipine, verapamil, and possibly other calcium channel blockers subject to induction and inhibition.	**Carbamazepine:** [P] Decreased carbamazepine metabolism with diltiazem and verapamil; possible increase in calcium channel blocker metabolism. **Cimetidine:** [NP] Decreased metabolism of calcium channel blockers. **Cyclosporine:** [P] Decreased cyclosporine metabolism with diltiazem, nicardipine, verapamil. **Phenytoin:** [NE] Increased metabolism of calcium channel blockers. **Rifampin:** [P] Increased metabolism of calcium channel blockers. *See also* Barbiturates, Theophylline.
Carbamazepine	Induction of hepatic microsomal drug-metabolizing enzymes. Susceptible to inhibition of metabolism.	**Cimetidine:** [P] Decreased carbamazepine metabolism. **Clarithromycin:** [P] Decreased carbamazepine metabolism. **Corticosteroids:** [P] Increased corticosteroid metabolism. **Cyclosporine:** [P] Increased cyclosporine metabolism. **Danazol:** [P] Decreased carbamazepine metabolism. **Diltiazem:** [P] Decreased carbamazepine metabolism. **Doxycycline:** [P] Increased doxycycline metabolism. **Erythromycin:** [NE] Decreased carbamazepine metabolism. **Estrogens:** [P] Increased estrogen metabolism. **Haloperidol:** [P] Increased haloperidol metabolism. **Isoniazid:** [P] Decreased carbamazepine metabolism. **Nefazodone:** Decreased carbamazepine metabolism. **Propoxyphene:** [HP] Decreased carbamazepine metabolism. **Selective serotonin reuptake inhibitors (SSRIs):** Fluoxetine and fluvoxamine decrease carbamazepine metabolism. **Theophylline:** [NE] Increased theophylline metabolism. **Troleandomycin:** [P] Decreased carbamazepine metabolism. **Verapamil:** [P] Decreased carbamazepine metabolism. *See also* Anticoagulants, oral; Antidepressants, tricyclic; Calcium channel blockers.
Chloramphenicol	Inhibits hepatic drug-metabolizing enzymes.	**Phenytoin:** [P] Decreased phenytoin metabolism. **Sulfonylurea hypoglycemics:** [P] Decreased sulfonylurea metabolism. *See also* Anticoagulants, oral.
Cimetidine	Inhibits hepatic microsomal drug-metabolizing enzymes. (Ranitidine and newer H$_2$ blockers do not appear to do so.) May inhibit the renal tubular secretion of weak bases. Purportedly reduces hepatic blood flow, thus reducing first-pass metabolism of highly extracted drugs. (However, the	**Benzodiazepines:** [P] Decreased metabolism of alprazolam, chlordiazepoxide, diazepam, halazepam, prazepam, and clorazepate but not oxazepam, lorazepam, or temazepam. **Carmustine:** [NE] Increased bone marrow suppression. **Ketoconazole:** [NE] Decreased gastrointestinal absorption of ketoconazole due to increased pH in gut; other H$_2$ blockers and proton pump inhibitors would be expected to have the same effect. **Itraconazole:** [NE] Decreased gastrointestinal absorption of itraconazole due to increased pH in gut; other H$_2$-receptor

Table II–1. Important drug interactions (cont'd).

HP = Highly predictable. Interaction occurs in almost all patients receiving the interacting combination.
P = Predictable. Interaction occurs in most patients receiving the combination.
NP = Not predictable. Interaction occurs only in some patients receiving the combination.
NE = Not established. Insufficient data available on which to base estimate of predictability.

Drug or Drug Group	Properties Promoting Drug Interaction	Clinically Documented Interactions
Cimetidine (cont'd)	ability of cimetidine to affect hepatic blood flow has been disputed.)	antagonists and proton pump inhibitors would be expected to have the same effect. **Lidocaine:** [P] Decreased metabolism of lidocaine; increased serum lidocaine. **Phenytoin:** [NE] Decreased phenytoin metabolism; increased serum phenytoin. **Procainamide:** [P] Decreased renal excretion of procainamide; increased serum procainamide levels. Similar effect with ranitidine but smaller. **Quinidine:** [P] Decreased metabolism of quinidine; increased serum quinidine levels. **Theophylline:** [P] Decreased theophylline metabolism; increased plasma theophylline. *See also* Anticoagulants, oral; Antidepressants, tricyclic; Beta-adrenoceptor blockers; Calcium channel blockers, Carbamazepine.
Cisapride	Susceptible to inhibition of metabolism by CYP3A4 inhibitors. High cisapride serum concentrations can result in ventricular arrhythmias.	**Clarithromycin:** [NP] Decreased metabolism of cisapride; possible ventricular arrhythmia. **Erythromycin:** [NP] Decreased metabolism of cisapride; possible ventricular arrhythmia. **Itraconazole:** [NP] Decreased metabolism of cisapride; possible ventricular arrhythmia. **Ketoconazole:** [NP] Decreased metabolism of cisapride; possible ventricular arrhythmia. **Nefazodone:** [NP] Possible decreased metabolism of cisapride by CYP3A4; possible ventricular arrhythmia. **Selective serotonin reuptake inhibitors (SSRIs):** [NP] Fluoxetine and fluvoxamine inhibit CYP3A4 and probably decrease cisapride metabolism; possible ventricular arrhythmia.
Cyclosporine	Metabolism inducible. Susceptible to inhibition of metabolism. (Tacrolimus appears to have similar interactions.)	**Aminoglycosides:** [NE] Possible additive nephrotoxicity. **Amphotericin B:** [NE] Possible additive nephrotoxicity. **Androgens:** [NE] Increased serum cyclosporine. **Barbiturates:** [P] Increased cyclosporine metabolism; reduced cyclosporine effect. **Carbamazepine:** [P] Increased cyclosporine metabolism; reduced cyclosporine effect. **Diltiazem:** [NE] Decreased cyclosporine metabolism; increased cyclosporine effect. **Erythromycin:** [NE] Decreased cyclosporine metabolism; increased cyclosporine effect. **Fluconazole:** [NE] Decreased cyclosporine metabolism; increased cyclosporine effect, especially with large fluconazole doses. **Ketoconazole:** [NE] Increased serum cyclosporine with nephrotoxicity; due to decreased cyclosporine metabolism. **Lovastatin:** [NE] Myopathy and rhabdomyolysis noted in patients taking both drugs. **Phenytoin:** [NE] Increased cyclosporine metabolism; reduced cyclosporine effect. **Rifampin:** [P] Increased cyclosporine metabolism; reduced cyclosporine effect. **Verapamil:** [NE] Decreased cyclosporine metabolism; increased cyclosporine effect. *See also* Barbiturates; Calcium channel blockers
Digitalis glycosides	Digoxin susceptible to inhibition of gastrointestinal absorption. Digitalis toxicity may be increased by drug-induced electrolyte imbalance (eg, hypokalemia). Digitoxin metabolism inducible. Renal excretion of digoxin susceptible	*Drugs that may increase digitalis effect:* **Amiodarone:** [P] Reduced renal digoxin excretion leads to increased plasma digoxin concentrations. **Diltiazem:** [P] Increased plasma digoxin (usually 20–30%) due to reduced renal and nonrenal clearance. **Erythromycin:** [NP] Increased gastrointestinal absorption of digoxin in certain patients; probably due to decreased inactivation of digoxin by intestinal flora.

(continued)

Table II–1. Important drug interactions (cont'd).

HP = Highly predictable. Interaction occurs in almost all patients receiving the interacting combination.
P = Predictable. Interaction occurs in most patients receiving the combination.
NP = Not predictable. Interaction occurs only in some patients receiving the combination.
NE = Not established. Insufficient data available on which to base estimate of predictability.

Drug or Drug Group	Properties Promoting Drug Interaction	Clinically Documented Interactions
Digitalis glycosides (cont'd)	to inhibition.	**Potassium-depleting drugs:** [P] Increased likelihood of digitalis toxicity. **Propafenone:** [P] Increased plasma digoxin levels. **Quinidine:** [HP] Reduced digoxin excretion; displacement of digoxin from tissue binding sites; digitoxin may also be affected. **Spironolactone:** [NE] Decreased renal digoxin excretion and interference with some serum digoxin assays. **Verapamil:** [P] Increased plasma digoxin levels. *Drugs that may decrease digitalis effect:* **Kaolin-pectin:** [P] Decreased gastrointestinal digoxin absorption. **Penicillamine:** [NE] Decreased plasma digoxin. **Rifampin:** [NE] Increased metabolism of digitoxin and possibly digoxin. **Sulfasalazine:** [NE] Decreased gastrointestinal digoxin absorption. *See also* Antacids; Bile acid-binding resins.
Disulfiram	Inhibits hepatic microsomal drug-metabolizing enzymes. Inhibits aldehyde dehydrogenase.	**Benzodiazepines:** [P] Decreased metabolism of chlordiazepoxide and diazepam but not lorazepam and oxazepam. **Metronidazole:** [NE] Confusion and psychoses reported in patients receiving this combination; mechanisms unknown. **Phenytoin:** [P] Decreased phenytoin metabolism. *See also* Alcohol; Anticoagulants, oral.
Estrogens	Metabolism inducible. Entero-hepatic circulation of estrogen may be interrupted by alteration in bowel flora (eg, due to antibiotics).	**Ampicillin:** [NP] Interruption of enterohepatic circulation of estrogen; possible reduction in oral contraceptive efficacy. Other oral antibiotics may have a similar effect. **Corticosteroids:** [P] Decreased metabolism of corticosteroids leading to increased corticosteroid effect. **Diazepam:** [NE] Decreased diazepam metabolism. **Griseofulvin:** [NE] Possible inhibition of oral contraceptive efficacy; mechanism unknown. **Phenytoin:** [NP] Increased estrogen metabolism; possible reduction in oral contraceptive efficacy. **Rifampin:** [NP] Increased estrogen metabolism; possible reduction in oral contraceptive efficacy. *See also* Barbiturates; Carbamazepine.
Iron	Binds with drugs in gastrointestinal tract, reducing absorption.	**Methyldopa:** [NE] Decreased methyldopa absorption. **Quinolones:** [P] Decreased absorption of ciprofloxacin. **Tetracyclines:** [P] Decreased absorption of tetracyclines; decreased efficacy of iron. **Thyroid hormones:** [P] Decreased thyroxine absorption. *See also* Antacids.
Levodopa	Levodopa degraded in gut prior to reaching sites of absorption. Agents that alter gastrointestinal motility may alter degree of intraluminal degradation. Antiparkinsonism effect of levodopa susceptible to inhibition by other drugs.	**Clonidine:** [NE] Inhibits antiparkinsonism effect. **Monoamine oxidase inhibitors:** [P] Hypertensive reaction (carbidopa prevents the interaction). **Papaverine:** [NE] Inhibits antiparkinsonism effect. **Phenothiazines:** [P] Inhibits antiparkinsonism effect. **Phenytoin:** [NE] Inhibits antiparkinsonism effect. **Pyridoxine:** [P] Inhibits antiparkinsonism effect (carbidopa prevents the interaction). *See also* Antimuscarinics.
Lithium	Renal lithium excretion sensitive to changes in sodium balance. (Sodium depletion tends to cause lithium retention.) Susceptible to drugs enhancing central nervous system lithium toxicity.	**ACE inhibitors:** [NE] Probable reduced renal clearance of lithium; increased lithium effect. **Diuretics (especially thiazides):** [P] Decreased excretion of lithium; furosemide may be less likely to produce this effect than thiazide diuretics. **Haloperidol:** [NP] Occasional cases of neurotoxicity in manic patients, especially with large doses of one or both drugs. **Methyldopa:** [NE] Increased likelihood of central nervous system lithium toxicity.

Table II–1. Important drug interactions (cont'd).

HP = Highly predictable. Interaction occurs in almost all patients receiving the interacting combination.
P = Predictable. Interaction occurs in most patients receiving the combination.
NP = Not predictable. Interaction occurs only in some patients receiving the combination.
NE = Not established. Insufficient data available on which to base estimate of predictability.

Drug or Drug Group	Properties Promoting Drug Interaction	Clinically Documented Interactions
Lithium (cont'd)		**Nonsteroidal anti-inflammatory drugs:** [NE] Reduced renal lithium excretion (except sulindac). **Theophylline:** [P] Increased renal excretion of lithium; reduced lithium effect.
Monoamine oxidase inhibitors (MAOIs)	Increased norepinephrine stored in adrenergic neuron. Displacement of these stores by other drugs may produce acute hypertensive response. MAOIs have intrinsic hypoglycemic activity.	**Antidiabetic agents:** [P] Additive hypoglycemic effect. **Dextromethorphan:** [NE] Severe reactions (hyperpyrexia, coma, death, probably "serotonin syndrome") have been reported. **Guanethidine:** [P] Reversal of the hypotensive action of guanethidine. **Narcotic analgesics:** [NP] Some patients develop hypertension, rigidity, excitation; meperidine may be more likely to interact than morphine. **Nefazodone:** [NE] Possible serotonin syndrome; avoid concurrent use. **Phenylephrine:** [P] Hypertensive episode, since phenylephrine is metabolized by monoamine oxidase. **Selective serotonin reuptake inhibitors (SSRIs):** [P] Fatalities have occurred due to serotonin syndrome; SSRIs are contraindicated in patients taking MAOIs. **Sympathomimetics (indirect-acting):** [HP] Hypertensive episode due to release of stored norepinephrine (amphetamines, ephedrine, isometheptene, phenylpropanolamine, pseudoephedrine). **Venlafaxine:** [NE] Possible serotonin syndrome; avoid concurrent use. *See also* Levodopa.
Nonsteroidal anti-inflammatory drugs (NSAIDs)	Prostaglandin inhibition may result in reduced renal sodium excretion, impaired resistance to hypertensive stimuli, and reduced renal lithium excretion. Most NSAIDs inhibit platelet function; may increase likelihood of bleeding due to other drugs that impair hemostasis. Most NSAIDs are highly bound to plasma proteins. Phenylbutazone may inhibit hepatic microsomal drug metabolism (also seems to act as enzyme inducer in some cases). Phenylbutazone may alter renal excretion of some drugs.	**ACE inhibitors:** [P] Decreased antihypertensive response. **Furosemide:** [P] Decreased diuretic, natriuretic, and antihypertensive response to furosemide. **Hydralazine:** [NE] Decreased antihypertensive response to hydralazine. **Methotrexate:** [NE] Possible increase in methotrexate toxicity (especially with anticancer doses of methotrexate). **Phenytoin:** [P] Decreased hepatic phenytoin metabolism. **Triamterene:** [NE] Decreased renal function noted with triamterene plus indomethacin in both healthy subjects and patients. *See also* Anticoagulants, oral; Beta-adrenoceptor blockers; Lithium.
Phenytoin	Induces hepatic microsomal drug metabolism. Susceptible to inhibition of metabolism.	*Drugs whose metabolism is stimulated by phenytoin:* **Corticosteroids:** [P] Decreased serum corticosteroid levels. **Doxycycline:** [P] Decreased serum doxycycline levels. **Methadone:** [P] Decreased serum methadone levels; withdrawal symptoms. **Mexiletine:** [NE] Decreased serum mexiletine levels. **Quinidine:** [P] Decreased serum quinidine levels. **Theophylline:** [NE] Decreased serum theophylline levels. **Verapamil:** [NE] Decreased serum verapamil levels. *See also* Cyclosporine, Estrogens.
		Drugs that inhibit phenytoin metabolism: **Amiodarone:** [P] Increased serum phenytoin; possible reduction in serum amiodarone. **Chloramphenicol:** [P] Increased serum phenytoin.

(continued)

Table II–1. Important drug interactions (cont'd).

HP = Highly predictable. Interaction occurs in almost all patients receiving the interacting combination.
P = Predictable. Interaction occurs in most patients receiving the combination.
NP = Not predictable. Interaction occurs only in some patients receiving the combination.
NE = Not established. Insufficient data available on which to base estimate of predictability.

Drug or Drug Group	Properties Promoting Drug Interaction	Clinically Documented Interactions
Phenytoin (cont'd)	(See preceding page.)	**Felbamate:** [P] Increased serum phenytoin. **Fluconazole:** [P] Increased serum phenytoin. **Fluoxetine:** [P] Increased serum phenytoin. **Isoniazid:** [NP] Increased serum phenytoin; problem primarily with slow acetylators of isoniazid. **Miconazole:** [P] Increased serum phenytoin. *See also* Cimetidine; Disulfiram; Phenylbutazone. *Drugs that enhance phenytoin metabolism:* **Rifampin:** [P] Decreased serum phenytoin levels.
Potassium-sparing diuretics (amiloride, spironolactone, triamterene)	Additive effects with other agents increasing serum potassium concentration. May alter renal excretion of substances other than potassium (eg, digoxin, hydrogen ions).	**ACE inhibitors:** [NE] Additive hyperkalemic effect. **Potassium supplements:** [P] Additive hyperkalemic effect; especially a problem in presence of renal impairment. *See also* Digitalis glycosides; Nonsteroidal anti-inflammatory drugs.
Probenecid	Interference with renal excretion of drugs that undergo active tubular secretion, especially weak acids. Inhibition of glucuronide conjugation of other drugs.	**Clofibrate:** [P] Reduced glucuronide conjugation of clofibric acid. **Methotrexate:** [P] Decreased renal methotrexate excretion; possible methotrexate toxicity. **Penicillin:** [P] Decreased renal penicillin excretion. **Salicylates:** [P] Decreased uricosuric effect of probenecid (interaction unlikely with less than 1.5 g of salicylate daily).
Quinidine	Metabolism inducible. Inhibits cytochrome P450 2D6. Renal excretion susceptible to changes in urine pH.	**Acetazolamide:** [P] Decreased renal quinidine excretion due to increased urinary pH; elevated serum quinidine. **Amiodarone:** [NE] Increased serum quinidine levels; mechanism not established. **Kaolin-pectin:** [NE] Decreased gastrointestinal absorption of quinidine. **Rifampin:** [P] Increased hepatic quinidine metabolism. *See also* Anticoagulants, oral; Antidepressants, tricyclic; Barbiturates; Cimetidine; Digitalis glycosides; Phenytoin.
Quinolone antibiotics	Susceptible to inhibition of gastrointestinal absorption. Some quinolones inhibit hepatic microsomal drug-metabolizing enzymes.	**Caffeine:** [P] Ciprofloxacin, enoxacin, pipedemic acid, and to a lesser extent, norfloxacin, inhibit caffeine metabolism. **Sucralfate:** [HP] Reduced gastrointestinal absorption of ciprofloxacin, norfloxacin, and probably other quinolones. **Theophylline:** [P] Ciprofloxacin, enoxacin, and to a lesser extent, norfloxacin inhibit theophylline metabolism; lomefloxacin and ofloxacin appear to have little effect. *See also* Antacids; Anticoagulants, oral.
Rifampin	Induction of hepatic microsomal drug-metabolizing enzymes.	**Corticosteroids:** [P] Increased corticosteroid hepatic metabolism; reduced corticosteroid effect. **Itraconazole:** [P] Increased itraconazole metabolism; reduced itraconazole effect. **Ketoconazole:** [NE] Increased ketoconazole metabolism; reduced ketoconazole effect. **Mexiletine:** [NE] Increased mexiletine metabolism; reduced mexiletine effect. **Sulfonylurea hypoglycemics:** [P] Increased hepatic metabolism of tolbutamide and probably other sulfonylureas metabolized by the liver (including chlorpropamide). **Theophylline:** [P] Increased theophylline metabolism; reduced theophylline effect. *See also* Anticoagulants, oral; Beta-adrenoceptor blockers; Calcium channel blockers; Cyclosporine; Digitalis glycosides; Estrogens.
Salicylates	Interference with renal excretion of drugs that undergo active tubular secretion. Salicylate renal excretion dependent on urinary pH when large doses of	**Carbonic anhydrase inhibitors:** [NE] Increased acetazolamide serum concentrations; increased salicylate toxicity due to decreased blood pH. **Corticosteroids:** [P] Increased salicylate elimination; possible additive toxic effect on gastric mucosa.

Table II–1. Important drug interactions (cont'd).

HP = Highly predictable. Interaction occurs in almost all patients receiving the interacting combination.
P = Predictable. Interaction occurs in most patients receiving the combination.
NP = Not predictable. Interaction occurs only in some patients receiving the combination.
NE = Not established. Insufficient data available on which to base estimate of predictability.

Drug or Drug Group	Properties Promoting Drug Interaction	Clinically Documented Interactions
Salicylates (cont'd)	salicylate used. Aspirin (but not other salicylates) interferes with platelet function. Large doses of salicylates have intrinsic hypoglycemic activity. Salicylates may displace drugs from plasma protein binding sites.	**Heparin:** [NE] Increased bleeding tendency with aspirin, but probably not with other salicylates. **Methotrexate:** [P] Decreased renal methotrexate clearance; increased methotrexate toxicity. **Sulfinpyrazone:** [HP] Decreased uricosuric effect of sulfinpyrazone (interaction unlikely with less than 1.5 g of salicylate daily). *See also* Antacids; Anticoagulants, oral; Probenecid.
Theophylline	Susceptible to inhibition of hepatic metabolism. Metabolism inducible.	**Benzodiazepines:** [NE] Inhibition of benzodiazepine sedation. **Diltiazem:** [P] Decreased theophylline metabolism; increased theophylline effect. **Clarithromycin:** [NE] Decreased theophylline metabolism; increased theophylline effect. **Erythromycin:** [P] Decreased theophylline metabolism; increased theophylline effect. **Fluvoxamine:** [P] Decreased theophylline metabolism; increased theophylline effect. **Smoking:** [HP] Increased theophylline metabolism; decreased theophylline effect. **Tacrine:** [P] Decreased theophylline metabolism; increased theophylline effect. **Ticlopidine:** [NE] Decreased theophylline metabolism; increased theophylline effect. **Troleandomycin:** [P] Decreased theophylline metabolism; increased theophylline effect. **Verapamil:** [P] Decreased theophylline metabolism; increased theophylline effect. *See also* Barbiturates; Carbamazepine, Cimetidine; Lithium, Phenytoin; Quinolones, Rifampin.

REFERENCES

Freedman MD, Olatidoye AG: Clinically significant drug interactions with the oral anticoagulants. Drug Saf 1994;10:381.

Hansten PD, Horn JR: *Drug Interactions, Analysis and Management.* Applied Therapeutics. [Quarterly.]

Jankel CA, Speedie SM: Detecting drug interactions: A review of the literature. Ann Pharmacother 1990;24:982.

Lam YWF, Shepherd AMM: Drug interactions in hypertensive patients: Pharmacokinetic, pharmacodynamic and genetic considerations. Clin Pharmacokinet 1990;18:295.

Quinn DI, Day RO: Drug interaction of clinical importance: An updated guide. Drug Saf 1995;12:393.

Riesenman C: Antidepressant drug interactions and the cytochrome P450 system: A critical appraisal. Pharmacotherapy 1995;15:84S.

Rizack MA (editor): *The Medical Letter Handbook of Adverse Interactions.* Medical Letter, 1997.

Tatro DS (editor): *Drug Interaction Facts.* Facts & Comparisons. [Quarterly.]

Index

NOTE: Page numbers in bold face type indicate a major discussion. A *t* following a page number indicates tabular material and an *i* following a page number indicates an illustration. Most drugs are listed under their generic names. Insofar as possible, when a drug trade name is listed, page references are for preparations available. For further detail refer to the generic name provided.

A cells (alpha cells), pancreatic, 685*t*
  glucagon secretion from, 685*t*, 701
A fibers, local anesthetics affecting, 429, 429*t*
Abbokinase, 561. *See also* Urokinase
Abciximab, 557
  preparations available, 561
Abdominal examination, in poisoned patient, 971
Abortion/abortifacients
  mifepristone for, 671–672
  prostaglandins for, 312–313
Abscess, amebic hepatic, treatment of, 851*t*, 852
Absence seizure, 404
  drugs for, **398–402, 404–405**
Absidia, empiric antimicrobial therapy and, 815*t*
Absorption, 4
  aging affecting, 989
  extent of, bioavailability and, 40–41
  in infants and children, 982, 984*t*
  interactions and, 1059
  rate of, bioavailability and, 41–42, 41*i*
  therapeutic drug monitoring and, 46
Abstinence syndrome, 503, 509. *See also* Withdrawal
Abuse, drugs of, **516–531**. *See also specific drug*
  cultural considerations and, 516–517
  neurobiology and, 517–518
ABVD regimen, in Hodgkin's disease, 907
Acarbose, 700–701
Acceptable daily intake (ADI), 945–946
Accolate, 340. *See also* Zafirlukast
Accommodative esotropia, cholinomimetics for, 100
Accumulation, 40
  time course of drug effect and, 43
Accumulation factor, 40
Accupril, 175, 213. *See also* Quinapril
Accutane, 1007. *See also* Isotretinoin
ACE (angiotensin converting enzyme), 295
  in renin-angiotensin system, 288–289, 288*i*

ACE inhibitors (angiotensin-converting enzyme inhibitors), **170–171**, 290, 291*i*, 293
  fetus affected by, 983*t*
  for heart failure, 197, 206–207, 210, 210*t*, 213, 291, 292*i*
  for hypertension, **170–171**
  preparations available, 175, 213
  time course of effect of, 42–43, 43*i*
Acebutolol, 138*t*, 143*i*, 145, **165**
  for hypertension, **165**
  preparations available, 150, 174, 240
  properties of, 144*t*
Aceon (perindopril), 175
Acephen, 600. *See also* Acetaminophen
Acetaldehyde metabolism, 373
Acetaminophen, **594–595**, 595*i*
  absorption of, in neonate, 984*t*
  half-life of
    aging affecting, 992*i*
    in neonate vs. adult, 985*t*
  ionization constant of, 6*t*
  metabolism of to hepatotoxic metabolites, 56, 57*i*
  in OTC preparations, efficacy of, 1033*t*
  pharmacokinetic/pharmacodynamic parameters of, 36*t*
  in neonate, 984*t*, 985*t*
  preparations available, 600
Acetazolamide, 246–249
  for glaucoma, 149*t*, 248, 248*t*
  ionization constant of, 6*t*
  preparations available, 259
  proximal tubule as site of action of, 242
  for seizures, **403**
  structure of, 247, 248*i*
Acetohexamide, 697*t*, **698**
Acetophenazine, preparations available, 480
Acetylation, 57*t*
  genetic polymorphisms affecting, 57–58, 58*t*
Acetylcholine (ACh), 77*t*, 85*t*, 349*t*, 351, 435*i*
  cardiovascular effects of, 94*t*, 95

in cholinergic transmission, 74, 75–77, 76*i*
in direct-acting cholinomimetic mechanism of action, 93
drugs blocking, 435. *See also* Antimuscarinic agents; Neuromuscular blocking drugs
  for parkinsonism, **457**, 457*t*
ligand-gated channels as receptors for, 20–21, 21*i*
molecular structure of, 92*i*
in neuromuscular transmission, 434–435, 435*i*
as neurotransmitter, 77*t*, 349*t*, 351
organ effects of, 94*t*
preparations available, 103
properties of, 93*t*
receptors for, 81–82, 81*t*, 434, 435*i*
  neuromuscular blocking drugs affecting, 439–442, 440*i*
second messenger for, 22*t*
structure of, 435*i*
Acetylcholinesterase
  in cholinergic transmission, 77
  mechanism of action of drugs inhibiting, 99
Acetylcysteine, as antidote, 977*t*
Acetylsalicylic acid, 580. *See also* Aspirin
  preparations available, 599
ACh (acetylcholine), 77*t*, 85*t*, 349*t*, 351, 435*i*
  cardiovascular effects of, 94*t*, 95
  in cholinergic transmission, 74, 75–77, 76*i*
  in direct-acting cholinomimetic mechanism of action, 93
  drugs blocking, 435. *See also* Antimuscarinic agents; Neuromuscular blocking drugs
  for parkinsonism, **457**, 457*t*
  ligand-gated channels as receptors for, 20–21, 21*i*
  molecular structure of, 92*i*
  in neuromuscular transmission, 434–435, 435*i*
  as neurotransmitter, 77*t*, 349*t*, 351

ACh (acetylcholine) *(cont.)*
  organ effects of, 94*t*
  preparations available, 103
  properties of, 93*t*
  receptors for, 81–82, 81*t*, 434, 435*i*
    neuromuscular blocking drugs affecting, 439–442, 440*i*
  second messenger for, 22*t*
  structure of, 435*i*
AChR (nicotinic receptors), 20–21, 21*i*, 81, 81*t*, 90, 91*t*, 434
  activation of, 94
  in central nervous system, 96
  drugs blocking, **114–115**
  in peripheral nervous system, 96
  toxicity of drugs affecting, 102
Achromycin V, 751. *See also* Tetracycline
α₁-Acid glycoprotein, drug concentration affected by, 47
Acid-peptic disease. *See also* Peptic ulcer disease
  drugs used in, **1017–1021**
Acidosis
  anion gap
    drug-induced, 973, 974*t*
    in ethylene glycol poisoning, 383
  metabolic
    hyperchloremic
      carbonic anhydrase inhibitors causing, 249
      potassium-sparing diuretics causing, 254
    in methanol poisoning, 382
Acids, weak
  definition of, 5
  ionization constants of, 6*t*
  ionization of, 5–7
Acne
  drugs for treatment of, **1006–1007**
    OTC preparations, efficacy of, 1033*t*
    topical antibiotics, **1001**
  oral contraceptives causing, 668
  rosacea, metronidazole for, 1001
Acneiform eruptions, lithium causing, 479
Aconitine, sodium channels affected by, 428
Acquired immunodeficiency syndrome
  drugs for, **795–799**, 795*t*, 796*i*. *See also specific type*
    importance of pharmacologic knowledge and, 799
    preparations available, 801
  M avium complex infections in, drugs for, 777
  tuberculosis risk in, isoniazid treatment and, 771–772
Acrivastine, 268*t*
Acromegaly, bromocriptine for, 614
ACTH (adrenocorticotropin/adrenocorticotropic hormone/corticotropin), 604*t*, **609–610**, 610*i*
  adrenocortical steroid treatment compared with, 645
  for inflammatory bowel disease, 1026

preparations available, 617
  receptors for, 604
  second messenger for, 22*t*
ACTH stimulation tests, 610
Acthar, 617. *See also* Corticotropin
Actidil, 284. *See also* Triprolidine
Actigall, 1028. *See also* Ursodiol
Actimmune, 940. *See also* Interferon-γ
Actinic keratoses, fluorouracil for, 1013
Actinomyces, empiric antimicrobial therapy and, 814*t*
Actinomycin D (dactinomycin), 894*t*, **896–897**
  immunosuppressive actions of, 929
Action potential
  antiepileptic drugs affecting, 387, 389, 389*i*, 392, 396, 397, 400
  cardiac, 216–220, 221*i*
    active cell membrane and, 219, 220*i*, 221*i*
    amiodarone affecting, 231, 235
    digitalis glycosides affecting, 203–204, 203*i*, 204*i*
    drugs prolonging, for arrhythmias, **235–236**, 240
    ionic basis of, 216–219
    resting potential affecting, 219–220, 220*i*
  increased threshold for, anesthetics causing, 415
Activase, 561. *See also* Alteplase
Activated charcoal, for poisoned patient, 975–976
Active immunization, **1051**, 1052–1054*t*, 1055*t*
Active metabolites, **55–56**, 57*i*. *See also* Reactive metabolites
Activin, 664–666
Acute exposure, to chemicals, 946
Acute leukemias, **905–906**
  adult, 905–906
  childhood, 905
  lymphoblastic, 905
  lymphocytic, 903*t*
  myelocytic, 903*t*
  myelogenous, 905–906
    as second malignancy, 913
  myelomonocytic, 903*t*
Acute respiratory distress syndrome, nitric oxide for, 322
Acyclovir, **788–791**, 790*i*, 792*t*
  in dermatologic therapy, **1004**
  mechanism of action of, 789, 791*i*
  OTC status of, 1031*t*
  pharmacokinetic/pharmacodynamic parameters of, 36*t*, 789–790
  preparations available, 801
  resistance to, 789
  topical, **1004**
Adalat, 175, 194. *See also* Nifedipine
Adapalene, for acne, 1007
Addiction, 516. *See also* Abuse
Addison's disease, 641
Adenine arabinoside (vidarabine), 792*t*, **794–795**

Adenocard, 240. *See also* Adenosine
Adenosine, 85*t*, 229*t*
  for arrhythmias, **237**
  clinical properties of, 229*t*
  membrane actions of, 228*t*
  preparations available, 240
Adenosine triphosphate (ATP), 77*t*, 85*t*
Adenylyl cyclase, in alpha₂ receptor activation, 121, 122*i*
ADH (antidiuretic hormone/vasopressin), **295–296**, **616–617**
  antagonists of, **255–256**, **285–286**
  dosage of, 616
  elevated levels of, 255
  factor VIII activity affected by, 560
  receptors for, **285–286**
  second messenger for, 22*t*
  structure of, 615*i*
  syndrome of inappropriate secretion of, 255
  water excretion affected by, 246, 246*i*, 255
ADI (acceptable daily intake), 945–946
Adipose tissue. *See also* Fat
  insulin affecting, 688–689, 688*t*
Adjuvants, 935
Administration, routes of
  bioavailability and characteristics and, 40*t*
  first-pass effect and, 42
Adrenal androgens, **647**
Adrenal cancer, 903*t*
Adrenal cortex, angiotensin II affecting, 289
Adrenal function, metyrapone in tests of, 648
Adrenal hyperplasia, congenital, 641–642
Adrenal suppression, corticosteroid treatment causing, 644–645
Adrenalin, 133–134, 340. *See also* Epinephrine
Adrenergic fibers, 75
Adrenergic neurons, 77–80, 78*i*
  antihypertensive agents blocking, 141, 146, **161–164**
Adrenergic transmission, 77–80, 78*i*
  cotransmitters in, 80–81
  β-Adrenoceptor kinase, 23, 25*i*
Adrenoceptor agonists, **118–134**. *See also* Alpha agonists; Beta agonists; Sympathomimetics
Adrenoceptor antagonists, **136–151**. *See also* Alpha-receptor blocking drugs; Beta-receptor blocking drugs
  H₁ receptor antagonists as, 268
  for hypertension, 141, 146, **164–166**
  preparations available, 150
  specificity of, 138*t*
Adrenoceptors (adrenergic receptors), 81, 81*t*, **118–120**, 119*t*. *See also* Alpha adrenoceptors; Beta adrenoceptors
  drugs activating, **118–134**. *See also* Alpha agonists; Beta agonists; Sympathomimetics

drugs blocking, **136–151**. *See also* Alpha-receptor blocking drugs; Beta-receptor blocking drugs
for hypertension, 141, 146, **164–166**
preparations available, 150
specificity of, 138*t*
ergot alkaloids affecting, 279*t*
in exocrine glands, 127
nomenclature for subtypes of, 120
regulation of, 122–123
selectivity of drugs for, 120, 129
Adrenocortical hyperfunction, 641–642
Adrenocortical insufficiency, 641
Adrenocorticosteroids, **635–652**. *See also* Corticosteroids; Glucocorticoids
ACTH treatment compared with, 645
antagonists of, **647–649**
preparations available, 650
antiandrogens affecting synthesis of, 677–678
for cancer chemotherapy, 899*t*
fetal lung maturation and, 643
inhibitors of synthesis of, **647–649**
preparations available, 650
for nonadrenal disorders, 643–644, 643*t*
synthetic, **640–646**
Adrenocorticotropin (ACTH/adrenocorticotropic hormone/corticotropin), 604*t*, **609–610**, 610*i*
adrenocortical steroid treatment compared with, 645
for inflammatory bowel disease, 1026
preparations available, 617
receptors for, 604
second messenger for, 22*t*
Adriamycin, 894*t*. *See also* Doxorubicin
Adrucil, 891*t*. *See also* Fluorouracil
Adverse reactions, 31–33
in elderly, **995–996**
new drug evaluation and, 70
Advil, 599. *See also* Ibuprofen
Aerobic bacterial infections, empiric antimicrobial therapy and, 814*t*
AeroBid, 340. *See also* Flunisolide
Aerosols, abuse of, 529
Aerosporin, 810. *See also* Polymyxin B
Afibrinogenemia, factor I for, 559*t*, 560
African trypanosomiasis. *See also* Trypanosoma (trypanosomiasis)
suramin for, 876
Afrin, 134. *See also* Oxymetazoline
Aftate (tolnaftate), 1002–1003
Afterdepolarizations, 222, 222*i*
Afterload, in cardiac function, 200
Agar, laxative effect of, 1023
Agar diffusion susceptibility testing, 817
Aging
adverse drug reactions and, **995–996**
androgen replacement therapy and, 676
anti-inflammatory drug use and, **995**
antimicrobial drug use and, **995**
cardiovascular drug use and, **994–995**
central nervous system drug use and, **993–994**

drug absorption affected by, 989
drug distribution affected by, 989, 990*t*
drug elimination affected by, 990–991, 991*t*, 992*i*
drug metabolism affected by, 59, 989–990, 990*t*
drug use and, **989–998**
practical aspects of, **996–997**
neuromuscular blockade affected by, 444–445
pharmacodynamic changes associated with, 991
pharmacokinetic changes associated with, 989–991, 992*i*
pharmacologic changes associated with, **989–991**, 992*i*
physiologic functions affected by, 989, 990*i*
Aging (organophosphate), 99
Agonists, 4, 9. *See also specific type*
binding molecule inhibition by, 4
partial, 4, 15–16, 16*i*, 17, 17*i*
receptor binding of, concentration-effect curves and, 11, 12*i*
Agranulocytosis, clozapine causing, 474
AHG (antihemophilic globulin/factor VIII), 549*t*
deficiency of, 559, 559*t*
preparations available, 561
recombinant, 560
therapeutic, 559*t*, **560**
AIDS
drugs for, **795–799**, 795*t*, 796*i*. *See also specific type*
importance of pharmacologic knowledge and, 799
preparations available, 801
M avium complex infections in, drugs for, 777
tuberculosis risk in, isoniazid treatment and, 771–772
Air pollutants, 945–946, **947–949**
threshold limit values for, 948*t*
Airway management, in poisoned patient, 970
Airways. *See also* Bronchial/bronchiolar smooth muscle
cytochrome P450-derived metabolites affecting, 310–311
hyperreactivity of, in asthma, 326–328, 327*i*, 329*i*
lipoxygenase metabolites affecting, 310–311
prostaglandins affecting, 309, 315
thromboxanes affecting, 309, 315
Akathisia, antipsychotic agents causing, 473
Akineton, 462. *See also* Biperiden
Albamycin, 768. *See also* Novobiocin
Albendazole, **862–865**, 862*i*
preparations available, 878
Albumin, drug concentration affected by levels of, 47
Albuterol (salbutamol), 334*i*
for asthma, 333

ionization constant of, 6*t*
preparations available, 340
Alcohol-barbiturate withdrawal, 520
Alcohol dehydrogenase, 373, 373*i*
in methanol poisoning, 382
Alcohol-drug interactions, 1061*t*
Alcohol withdrawal syndrome, management of, **379–380**
preparations available for, 383
Alcoholic cardiomyopathy, 376–377
Alcoholism, 372, 375–378, 519
management of acute withdrawal and, **379–380**
preparations available, 383
pharmacotherapy of, **380–382**
preparations available, 383
Alcohols, **372–385**
antimicrobial effects of, 805*t*, **806**
drug interactions and, 1061*t*
ethyl. *See also* Ethanol
antimicrobial effects of, 805*t*, 806
basic pharmacology of, **372–378**
clinical pharmacology of, **379–382**
ethylene glycol, 383
isopropyl
antimicrobial effects of, 805*t*, 806
osmolar gap caused by, 974*t*
methyl (methanol/wood alcohol), 382–383
in OTC preparations, hidden, 1037*t*
Aldactazide, 254*t*. *See also* Spironolactone
Aldactone, 254*t*, 259. *See also* Spironolactone
Aldehydes, antimicrobial effects of, 805*t*, **808**
Aldesleukin, 940. *See also* Interleukin-2
Aldicarb, 952*t*
Aldin, 950*t*
Aldomet, 175. *See also* Methyldopa
Aldose reductase inhibitors, **701**
Aldosterone, **646**
angiotensin II affecting biosynthesis of, 289
antagonists of, **253–254**, 253*i*, 254*t*
in blood pressure regulation, 154, 154*i*
oral contraceptives affecting, 667
progesterone affecting, 662
synthesis of, 636*i*
Aldosteronism, 642
Alendronate, 711, 711*i*
for osteoporosis, 711, 712, 718
for Paget's disease, 720
preparations available, 721
Aleve, 599. *See also* Naproxen
Alfaxolone, GABA-DBZ receptor chloride channel binding and, 361
Alfenta, 501*t*, 513. *See also* Alfentanil
Alfentanil, 511
pharmacokinetics of, 501*t*
preparations available, 513
Alferon N (interferon alfa-n3), 801
Alfuzosin, 139
ALG (antilymphocyte globulin), 929–930
Alkalinization of urine, carbonic anhydrase inhibitors for, 248

Alkalosis, metabolic
carbonic anhydrase inhibitors for, 248
hypokalemic
loop diuretics causing, 250
thiazides causing, 251
Alkeran, 890*t*. *See also* Melphalan
Alkylamines, 267*t*
structures of, 266*i*
Alkylating agents, **884–889**
dosage and toxicity of, 889, 890*t*
pharmacologic effects of, 885–888,
887*i*
resistance to, 885
structures of, 884, 886*i*
ALL (acute lymphoblastic leukemia),
905
All-*trans*-retinoic acid (etretinate)
in cancer chemotherapy, 901–902
fetus affected by, 983*t*
for psoriasis, **1007–1008**
Allegra, 267*t*, 283. *See also* Fexofenadine
Allergic reactions
cromolyn for, 330
drug, 30, **936–940**
to antipyschotics, 474
to cephalosporins, 735
clinical identification of, **939–940**
immediate (type I), 937, **937–939**,
937*i*, 938*i*
to insulin, 695
to isoniazid, 772
to local anesthetics, 432
to loop diuretics, 251
to penicillin, 731
to thiazides, 252
H$_1$ receptor antagonists for, 268–269
OTC preparations for
efficacy of, 1033*t*
hidden ingredients in, 1037*t*, 1038*t*,
1039*t*
Allopurinol, **598–599**, 598*i*, 892*i*
in cancer chemotherapy, 891*t*
drug metabolism inhibited by, 60*t*
for gout, 598
for idiopathic hypercalciuria, 719–720
interactions of, 1061*t*
ionization constant of, 6*t*
nucleoside phosphotransferases affected by, 829
preparations available, 600
Alloxanthine, 598*i*
Allylamines, topical, 786
Aloes, laxative effect of, 1023
Alpha adrenoceptors, 119, 119*t*
activation of, 120–121, 121*i*, 122*i*
in bladder, 126
distribution of, 124*t*
drugs blocking. *See also* Alpha-receptor blocking drugs
basic pharmacology of, **136–140**
clinical pharmacology of, **140–142**
for hypertension, 141, **165–166**,
175
ergot alkaloids affecting, 279*t*
eye controlled by, 148
selectivity of drugs for, 120, 120*t*, 129

Alpha$_1$ adrenoceptors, 81*t*, 119, 119*t*
activation of, 120–121, 121*i*
distribution of, 124*t*
selectivity of drugs for, 120, 120*t*
Alpha$_2$ adrenoceptors, 81*t*, 119, 119*t*
activation of, 121, 122*i*
distribution of, 124*t*
selectivity of drugs for, 120, 120*t*, 129
Alpha agonists
gastrointestinal smooth muscle affected by, 126
for glaucoma, 149*t*
local anesthetics combined with, 131,
427
mechanism of action of, 120–121,
121*i*, 122*i*
sedative effects of, 355
selectivity of, 120, 120*t*, 129
Alpha$_1$ agonists, mechanism of action of,
120–121, 121*i*
Alpha$_2$ agonists
gastrointestinal system affected by,
126
for glaucoma, 149*t*
mechanism of action of, 120–121,
122*i*
Alpha antagonists. *See* Alpha-receptor
blocking drugs
Alpha$_2$ antagonists, applications of, 142
Alpha-blockers. *See* Alpha-receptor
blocking drugs
Alpha carbon, sympathomimetic activity
and, 123–124
Alpha cells (A cells)
pancreatic, 685*t*
glucagon secretion from, 685*t*, 701
Alpha-difluoromethylornithine (DFMO),
ornithine decarboxylase affected
by, 831–833
Alpha-glucosidase inhibitors, **700–701**
preparations available, 703
Alpha interferon, 800, 926, 934*t*, 935
Alpha nerve fibers, local anesthetics affecting, 429*t*
Alpha-receptor blocking drugs
basic pharmacology of, **136–140**
clinical pharmacology of, **140–142**
for hypertension, 141, **165–166**, 175
mechanism of action of, 136
organ system effects of, 136–138
preparations available, 150, 175
reversible vs. irreversible, 136, 137*i*
selectivity of, 138*t*
Alphagan, 133. *See also* Brimonidine
Alprazolam, 356*i*, 365
biotransformation of, 357*i*
dosages of, 366*t*
pharmacokinetics of, 358*t*
preparations available, 369
for tremor, 459
Alprenolol, 138*t*
ionization constant of, 6*t*
Alprostadil (PGE$_1$), 306, 312*i*. *See also*
Prostaglandins
for impotence, 314
preparations available, 317
Altace, 175, 213. *See also* Ramipril

Alteplase, **555**. *See also* t-PA
for myocardial infarction, 555, 556
preparations available, 561
Alternagel, 1018*t*
Alternate-day dosing, for glucocorticoid
administration, 645
Altretamine (hexamethylmelamine), **888**,
890*t*
Aluminum hydroxide antacids, 1018*t*
in OTC preparations, efficacy of,
1033*t*
Alupent, 340. *See also* Metaproterenol
Alurate (aprobarbital), 369
Alzapam, 369, 423. *See also* Lorazepam
Alzheimer's disease
dihydroergotoxine for, 282
drugs used in, 994
Amanita muscaria mushroom poisoning,
102, 972*t*
treatment of, 113
Amantadine, **799–800**
for parkinsonism, **456–457**
preparations available, 462, 801
Amaryl, 697*t*, 703. *See also* Glimepiride
Ambenonium, 97
for myasthenia gravis, 101
preparations available, 103
Ambien, 366*t*, 369. *See also* Zolpidem
Amebiasis
chloroquine for, 842, 850, 851*t*, **852**
drugs for, **850–855**, 851–852*t*
Ameboma, treatment of, 852
Amenorrhea
bromocriptine for, 614
oral contraceptive use and, 668–669
Amethopterin, 891*t*. *See also* Methotrexate
Amicar, 561. *See also* Aminocaproic acid
Amidate, 423. *See also* Etomidate
Amide hydrolysis, 54*t*
Amifostine, **902**, 902*i*
Amikacin, 754*i*, **758**, 776
adverse effects of, 754, 758
pharmacokinetic/pharmacodynamic
parameters of, 36*t*
preparations available, 759
for tuberculosis, 771*t*, 776
Amikin, 759. *See also* Amikacin
Amiloride, 253, 253*i*, 254*t*
chemistry and pharmacokinetics of,
253, 253*i*
interactions of, 1068*t*
ionization constant of, 6*t*
preparations available, 259
Amine hypothesis, of depression, 483
Amine neurotransmitters, antidepressants
affecting, 487, 489*i*
Amine oxidases, 53*t*
Amino acids, 348–351
acidic, 351
excitatory, ligand-gated channels as
receptors for, 20–21
as neurotransmitters in CNS, 348–351
neutral, 350–351
Amino group substitution, beta receptor
activity affected by, 123

p-Aminobenzoic acid (PABA)
  sulfonamide structure and, 761, 762*i*
  as sunscreen, 1006
Aminocaproic acid, 548, 550*i*, 560–561
  preparations available, 561
Aminocarb, 952*t*
Aminoglutethimide, 647*i*, **648**
  in cancer chemotherapy, 899*t*, **900**
    for breast cancer, 909
  preparations available, 650
Aminoglycosides, **752–759**
  adverse effects of, 753–754
  mechanism of action of, 752
  once-daily dosing with, 757
  pharmacokinetics of, 753
  physical and chemical properties of,
    752, 753*i*, 754*i*
  resistance to, 752–753
Aminopenicillins, 731
Aminophylline, for asthma, preparations
  available, 340
Aminopterin, fetus affected by, 983*t*
Aminopyrine, half-life of, aging affecting, 992*i*
Aminosalicylic acid, 776, 776*i*
  for inflammatory bowel disease, 1025
  preparations available, 778
  for tuberculosis, 771*t*, 776
Amiodarone, **230–232**, 230*i*
  action potential duration affected by,
    231, 235
  for arrhythmias, **230–232**
  clinical properties of, 229*t*
  ionization constant of, 6*t*
  membrane actions of, 228*t*
  preparations available, 240
Amitriptyline, 484, 485*i*
  dosages of, 491*t*
  effects of, 489*t*
  half-life of, aging affecting, 992*i*
  for migraine headache, 282
  overdoses of, 972*t*
  pharmacokinetics of, 488*t*
  preparations available, 494
AML (acute myelogenous leukemia),
  905–906
  as second malignancy, 913
Amlodipine
  clinical properties of, 190*t*
  for hypertension, 169
  pharmacokinetics of, 189*t*
  preparations available, 175, 194
  vascular selectivity of, 190*t*
Δ-Amninobutyric acid, 77*t*, 349*t*,
  350–351
  antiepileptic drugs affecting, 387, 395,
    396–397, 397–398, 400
  baclofen affecting, 445–446, 446*i*
  barbiturates affecting, 360, 361*i*
  benzodiazepines affecting, 359–360
  ethanol affecting, 374
  in Huntington's disease, 460
  receptors for, 351
    ligand-gated channels as, 20–21
  in tardive dyskinesia, 461
  vigabatrin affecting, 395

Amobarbital
  half-life of, aging affecting, 992*i*
  preparations available, 369
Amodiaquine, for malaria, 839*i*
Amoxapine, 484, 485*i*
  adverse effects of, 493*t*
  dosages of, 491*t*
  effects of, 488, 489*t*
  overdoses of, 493
  pharmacokinetics of, 488*t*
  preparations available, 494
Amoxicillin, 726*i*, 731
  adverse reactions to, 732
  dosing guidelines for, 730*t*
  pharmacokinetic/pharmacodynamic
    parameters of, 36*t*, 726
  preparations available, 740
Amoxicillin/potassium clavulanate
  dosing guidelines for, 730*t*
  preparations available, 740
Amoxil, 740. *See also* Amoxicillin
AMPA receptors, antiepileptic drugs affecting, 387
  "Ampakines," for Alzheimer's disease,
    994
Amphenone B, 647*i*, **649**
Amphetamine, 124*i*, 128, 133, 521
  abuse of, 522
  chemistry and pharmacology of, 522,
    522*i*
  fetus affected by, 983*t*
  ionization constant of, 6*t*
  overdose of, 972*t*
  preparations available, 133
  structure of, 522*i*
Amphojel, 1018*t*
Amphotericin A, 780
Amphotericin B, **780–782**, 781*i*
  antiparasitic actions of, 836*t*
  for leishmaniasis, 855–856
  liposomal, 781
  pharmacokinetic/pharmacodynamic
    parameters of, 36*t*, 780–781
  preparations available, 786
  topical, **1003**
Ampicillin, 724, 726*i*, 731
  absorption of, in neonate, 984*t*
  adverse reactions to, 731–732
  in breast milk, 987*t*
  CSF penetration by, 820*t*
  half-life of, aging affecting, 992*i*
  ionization constant of, 6*t*
  pharmacokinetic/pharmacodynamic
    parameters of, 36*t*, 726
    in neonate, 984*t*
  preparations available, 740
Ampicillin-sulbactam, 737
  preparations available, 740
Amplification, in second messenger signalling, 27
Amprolium, thiamin transporter affected
  by, 834
Amrinone
  for heart failure, **205–206**
  preparations available, 213
Amsacrine, in cancer chemotherapy,
  900–901, 901*t*

Amyl nitrite
  abuse of, 184, 529
  for angina, 186*t*
  chemistry of, 181, 182*i*
  organ system effects of, 183
  pharmacology of, 182
  preparations available, 194
  structure of, 529*i*
Amylase, in pancreatic enzyme replacement products, 1023*t*
Amylin (islet amyloid
  polypeptide/IAPP), 684, 685*t*, **703**
Amytal, 369. *See also* Amobarbital
Anabolic steroids, **674–677**
  abuse of, 676
  preparations available, 680
  synthetic, 675, 675*t*
Anaerobic bacterial infections, empiric
  antimicrobial therapy and,
  814–815*t*
Anafranil, 494. *See also* Clomipramine
Analgesia. *See also* Pain
  as anesthesia stage, 410
  aspirin for, 581, 582
  in elderly, 993
  neural mechanisms of, 502–503, 504*i*
  opioid receptor distribution in,
    502–503, 504*i*
  opioids producing, 505, 507. *See also*
    Opioid analgesics
  OTC preparations for
    efficacy of, 1033*t*
    hidden ingredients in, 1037*t*, 1038*t*,
      1039*t*
Anaphylactic shock/anaphylaxis
  epinephrine for, 132
  penicillin causing, 731
Anaprox, 599. *See also* Naproxen
Anaspaz, 1027. *See also* Hyoscyamine
Anastrozole, **672**
  in cancer chemotherapy, 899*t*, **900**
    for breast cancer, 909
  preparations available, 680
Anazpax, 116. *See also* Hyoscyamine
Ancef, 741. *See also* Cefazolin
Ancobon, 786. *See also* Flucytosine
Ancylostoma duodenale (ancylostomiasis), drugs for infection with, 863*t*
  albendazole, 864
  pyrantel, 876
  tetrachloroethylene, 876
Androderm, 680. *See also* Testosterone
Androgen replacement therapy
  adverse effects of, 676–677
  for gynecologic disorders, 676
  in men, 675–676, 676*t*
Androgens, **674–677**
  abuse of, 676
  adrenal, **647**
  in cancer chemotherapy, 899*t*
  fetus affected by, 983*t*
  inhibition of synthesis of, 677–678
  for oral contraception in men, 679
  ovarian, 664
  preparations available, 680
  receptor inhibitors of, 678–679

Androgens *(cont.)*
suppression of, **677**, 678*i*
in cancer chemotherapy, 899*t*, 900
synthetic, 675, 675*t*
synthetic and degradation pathways
for, 663*i*
Androl-50, 680. *See also* Oxymetholone
Androstenedione, 674
Anectine, 448. *See also* Succinylcholine
Anemias
agents used in, **533–546**. *See also specific type*
androgens for, 676
aplastic, chloramphenicol causing,
744–745
autoimmune hemolytic, immunosuppressive agents for, 931*t*, 932
erythropoietin for, 544
folic acid deficiency causing, 537,
540, 542
iron deficiency, 534–536
lead toxicity causing, 378
megaloblastic, vitamin B_{12} and folic
acid deficiency causing, 537,
540–541
pernicious, 541–542
vitamin B_{12} deficiency causing, 537,
540, 541–542
Anesthesia, 409. *See also* Anesthetics
antimuscarinic drugs and, 111
dissociative, ketamine producing,
422
opioid analgesics in, 507–508
sedative-hypnotic drugs producing,
355*i*, 362
signs and stages of, **410–411**
surgical, 410
Anesthetics. *See also specific agent*
general, **409–424**
inhaled, 409, 410*i*, **412–419**, 413*t*
intravenous, 409–410, 411*i*,
419–423
neuromuscular blocking drug interaction and, 444
preparations available, 423
solubility of, 412, 413*i*, 414*i*
local, **425–433**
alpha agonists combined with, 131,
427
basic pharmacology of, **425–430**
clinical pharmacology of, **430–432**
H_1 receptor antagonists as, 268
neuromuscular blocking drug interaction and, 444
preparations available, 432–433
structure-activity characteristics of,
429
toxicity of, 430–432
vasoconstrictors combined with,
131, 427
"Angel dust" (phencyclidine)
abuse of, 525–526
overdose of, 526
psychosis produced by, as schizophrenia model, 470
structure of, 524*i*

Angina pectoris
angiospastic, 179, 186, 193
atherosclerotic, 179, 185–186,
192–193
beta-receptor blocking drugs for, 146,
147*i*, **191–192**, 192*i*, 193*t*
calcium channel blockers for, 179,
180, 180*i*, **186–191**, 193*t*
classic, 179, 185–186, 192–193
drugs for, **179–196**. *See also* Antianginal agents; Vasodilators
action of, 181
basic pharmacology of, **181–192**
clinical pharmacology of, **192–194**
of effort, 179, 185–186, 192–193
history of, 179–180
nitrates and nitrites for, **181–186**,
186*t*, 193*t*
pathophysiology of, **180–181**
unstable, 179, 186, 193–194
variant, 179, 186, 193
ergonovine in diagnosis of, 282
vasodilators for, **179–196**. *See also*
Vasodilators
vasospastic, 179, 186, 193
Angioedema, H_1 receptor antagonists for,
269
Angiospastic angina, 179. *See also*
Angina pectoris
management of, 193
nitrates for, 186
Angiostrongylus cantonensis (angiostrongyliasis), drugs for
infection with, 863*t*
albendazole, 865
Angiotensin, **287–291**, 288
biosynthesis of, **287–289**
oral contraceptives affecting, 667
second messenger for, 22*t*
Angiotensin I, 288, 288*i*
Angiotensin II, 85*t*, 288, 288*i*
actions of, **289**
inhibition of, **290–291**, 292*i*, 293
mechanisms of action of, **289–290**
receptors for, **289–290**
inhibition of, 175, 291, 292*i*, 293.
See also Angiotensin receptor-blocking drugs
Angiotensin antagonists, 290–291, 292*i*,
293
Angiotensin converting enzyme, 295
in renin-angiotensin system, 288–289,
288*i*
Angiotensin-converting enzyme inhibitors, **170–171**, 290, 291*i*, 293
fetus affected by, 983*t*
for heart failure, 197, 206–207, 210,
210*t*, 213, 291, 292*i*
for hypertension, **170–171**
preparations available, 175, 213
time course of effect of, 42–43, 43*i*
Angiotensin inhibitors, **169–172**
for hypertension, **169–172**
mechanisms and sites of action of,
170
preparations available, 175

Angiotensin receptor-blocking drugs,
291, 292*i*, 293
for hypertension, **171–172**
preparations available, 175
Angiotensin receptors, **289–290**
inhibition of, 175, 291, 292*i*, 293. *See
also* Angiotensin receptor-
blocking drugs
Angiotensinase, 289
Angiotensinogen, 288, 288*i*
Angle-closure glaucoma. *See also* Glaucoma
treatment of, 87
cholinomimetics for, 100
Anion gap acidosis
drug-induced, 973, 974*t*
in ethylene glycol poisoning, 383
Anion inhibitors, antithyroid action of,
627
Anion overdose, loop diuretics in management of, 250
Anisotropine
for gastrointestinal and genitourinary
conditions, 112*t*
preparations available, 115, 1026
Anisoylated plasminogen streptokinase
activator complex
(anistreplase/APSAC), 550*i*, 555
for myocardial infarction, 555, 556
preparations available, 561
Anistreplase, 550*i*, 555
for myocardial infarction, 555, 556
preparations available, 561
Annexins, 311
ANP/ANF (atrial natriuretic peptide/fac-
tor), 296–297, 296*i*
ligand-regulated transmembrane enzymes in signalling by, 19–20,
26
ANP_A receptor, 297
ANP_B receptor, 297
ANP_C receptor, 297
ANS (autonomic nervous system), **73–89**
anatomy of, **73–74**, 74*i*
antipsychotic agents affecting, 470*t*,
473
functional organization of, **82–85**
neurotransmitter chemistry of, **74–81**,
77*t*
nonadrenergic/noncholinergic neurons
in, **82**
organ system effects of, 82, 83*t*
pharmacologic modification of function of, **85–87**
renin secretion regulated by, 287–
288
Ansaid, 599. *See also* Flurbiprofen
Ansamycin, 778. *See also* Rifabutin
Anspor, 741. *See also* Cephradine
Antabuse, 383. *See also* Disulfiram
Antacids, **1017–1019**, 1018*t*
interactions of, 1061*t*
major constituents of, 1018*t*
OTC preparations
efficacy of, 1033*t*
hidden ingredients in, 1039*t*

Antagonism
  antimicrobial combination therapy
      and, 822
  competitive, oral anticoagulant inter-
      actions and, 554
  toxicity of chemical mixtures and, 946
Antagonist-precipitated withdrawal, 509
Antagonists, 4, 9
  chemical, 16
  competitive, 14–15, 14*i*
  irreversible, 14*i*, 15
  physiologic, 16–17
Anterior chamber of eye, 88*i*
Anthelmintic agents, **862–880**, 863–864*t*.
      See also specific type
  administration of, 862
  contraindications to, 862
  neurotoxic, 835
  OTC preparations, efficacy of, 1034*t*
  pediatric dosages of, 862
  preparations available, 878
Anthracyclines, **895–896**
Antiandrogens, **677–679**
  in cancer chemotherapy, 899*t*, 900
  preparations available, 680
  sites of action of, 678*i*
Antianginal agents, **179–196**
  action of, 181
  basic pharmacology of, **181–192**
  beta blockers, 146, 147*i*, **191–192**,
      192*i*, 193*t*
  calcium channel blockers, 179, 180,
      180*i*, **186–191**, 193*t*
  clinical pharmacology of, **192–194**
  nitrates and nitrites, **181–186**, 186*t*,
      193*t*
  principles of use of, 192
  vasodilators, **179–196**
Antiarrhythmic agents, **216–241**. *See
      also specific type*
  basic pharmacology of, **224–226**
  benefits and risks of use of, 238–239
  class I (sodium channel-blocking
      drugs), 226, **227–234**
  class II (beta adrenoceptor-blocking
      drugs), 146, 226, **234**
  class III (action potential prolonga-
      tion), 226, **235–236**
  class IV (calcium channel-blocking
      drugs), 226, **236**
  digitalis as, 208
  in elderly, 995
  mechanisms of action of, 224–226,
      226*i*
  membrane actions of, 228*t*
  neuromuscular blocking drug interac-
      tion and, 444
  preparations available, 240
  pretreatment evaluation and, 237–238
  principles in use of, **237–239**
  use- and state-dependent, 224
Antiasthma drugs. *See also specific agent
      and* Asthma
  approaches to development of, 308
  basic pharmacology of, **328–338**
  clinical pharmacology of, **338–339**

OTC preparations, hidden ingredients
      in, 1037*t*, 1038*t*, 1039*t*
  preparations available, 340
Antibacterial agents. *See* Antibiotics
Antibiotic-associated colitis, clindamycin
      and, 750
Antibiotics. *See also specific type and*
      Antimicrobial agents
  for acne, **1001**
  in cancer chemotherapy, **895–898**
  in dermatologic therapy, **1000–1001**
  empiric therapy with, 814–815*t*
  neuromuscular blocking drug interac-
      tion and, 444
  topical, **1000–1001**
Antibodies, 918*i*, 920*i*, 921. *See also* Im-
      munoglobulins
  as immunosuppressive agents,
      929–931
Anticancer drugs, **881–915**. *See also spe-
      cific agent and* Cancer chemother-
      apy
Anticholinergic drugs, **105–117**. *See also*
      Antimuscarinic agents; Antinico-
      tinic agents
  preparations available, 1026–1027
Anticholinoceptor effects, of H_1 receptor
      antagonists, 268
Anticoagulants
  basic pharmacology of, **548–555**
  clinical pharmacology of, **557–558**
  coumarin (oral), **551–555**. *See also*
      Warfarin
  interactions of, 1061–1062*t*
Anticonvulsants (antiepileptic drugs),
      386–408. *See also specific type*
  basic pharmacology of, **387–388**
  chemistry of, 387, 387*i*
  clinical pharmacology of, **403–404**
  for generalized seizures, **398–403**,
      404–405
  for infantile spasms, **405**
  mechanism of action of, 387
  overdose of, **406–407**
  for partial seizures and generalized
      tonic-clonic seizures, **388–398**,
      404
  preparations available, 407
  presents status of development of,
      386–387
  sedative-hypnotics as, 362, 402
  for status epilepticus, **405–406**
  teratogenicity of, **406**
  therapeutic strategy for use of, **404**
  toxicity of, **406–407**
  withdrawal from, **406**
Antidepressants, **483–495**. *See also spe-
      cific type*
  adverse effects of, 492, 493*t*
  basic pharmacology of, **484–490**
  chemistry of, 484, 485*i*, 486*i*, 487*i*
  clinical indications for, 490
  clinical pharmacology of, **490–493**
  dosages of, 491, 491*t*
      for acute episode, 491
      for maintenance treatment, 491–492
  drug selection and, 490–491

effects of, 488–490
  in elderly, 993
  fetus affected by, 983*t*
  interactions of, 392–393, 1062*t*
  overdoses of, 493, 972*t*
  patients unresponsive to, 492
  pharmacodynamics of, 487–490, 489*i*,
      489*i*
  pharmacokinetics of, 484–487, 488*t*
  plasma concentration monitoring and,
      492
  preparations available, 494
  second- and third-generation, 484,
      484*i*, 486*i*
  dosages of, 491*t*
  for acute episode, 491
      effects of, 488–489
      interactions of, 1062*t*
      overdoses of, 493
      pharmacokinetics of, 486, 488*t*
      preparations available, 494
  tricyclic, 484, 485*i*
      adverse effects of, 493*t*
      clinical indications for, 490
      dosages of, 491*t*
      effects of, 488
      fetus affected by, 983*t*
      interactions of, 1062*t*
      overdoses of, 493, 972*t*
      pharmacokinetics of, 484–486, 488*t*
      preparations available, 494
Antidiabetic drugs, **684–705**. *See also*
      Insulin; Oral hypoglycemic agents
Antidiarrheal drugs, **1024**
  antimuscarinic agents, 111–112
  opioid analgesics, 507
  OTC preparations
      efficacy of, 1034*t*
      hidden ingredients in, 1037*t*, 1038*t*
Antidiuretic hormone (ADH/vaso-
      pressin), **295–296**, **616–617**
  antagonists of, **255–256**, **285–286**
  dosage of, 616
  elevated levels of, 255
  factor VIII activity affected by, 560
  receptors for, **285–286**
  second messenger for, 22*t*
  structure of, 615*i*
  syndrome of inappropriate secretion
      of, 255
  water excretion affected by, 246, 246*i*,
      255
Antidotes, 976, 977*t*
Antiemetic actions, of H_1 receptor antag-
      onists, 268
Antiemetic drugs, **1022**
  OTC preparations, hidden ingredients
      in, 1037*t*
  preparations available, 1027
Antiepileptic drugs, **386–408**. *See also
      specific type*
  basic pharmacology of, **387–388**
  chemistry of, 387, 387*i*
  clinical pharmacology of, **403–404**
  for generalized seizures, **398–403**,
      404–405
  for infantile spasms, **405**

Antiepileptic drugs *(cont.)*
  mechanism of action of, 387
  overdose of, **406–407**
  for partial seizures and generalized
      tonic-clonic seizures, **388–398,
      404**
  preparations available, 407
  presents status of development of,
      386–387
  sedative-hypnotics as, 362, 402
  for status epilepticus, **405–406**
  teratogenicity of, **406**
  therapeutic strategy for use of, **404**
  toxicity of, **406–407**
  withdrawal from, **406**
Antiestrogens, **671–672**, 898–900, 899*t*.
    See also specific type
  in cancer chemotherapy, 898–900,
      899*t*
    for breast cancer, 909
  preparations available, 680
Antifolates, **761–765**. *See also specific
    type*
Antifols, sulfonamides or sulfones com-
    bined with, 846
Antifungal agents, **780–787**. *See also
    specific type*
  in dermatologic therapy, **1002–1004**
  preparations available, 786
  systemic, **1003–1004**
    for surface infections, **785–786**
    for systemic infections, **780–785**
  topical, 786, **1002–1003**
    OTC preparations, efficacy of,
        1034*t*
Antigen-antibody complexes, in hyper-
    sensitivity reactions, 921
  drug allergy and, 937, 939
Antigen-presenting cells, 917
Antihemophilic globulin (AHG/factor
    VIII), 549*t*
  deficiency of, 559, 559*t*
  preparations available, 561
  recombinant, 560
  therapeutic, 559*t*, **560**
Antiherpes agents, **788–795**. *See also
    specific agent*
Antihistamines, **265–270**. *See also* H$_1$ re-
    ceptor antagonists
  antiemetic actions of, 1022
  in dermatologic therapy, 1014*t*
  interactions of, 1062–1063*t*
  in OTC preparations, hidden, 1037*t*
  overdose of, 972*t*
  preparations available, 283–284
  sedative effects of, 355
Antihypertensive drugs, **153–178**. *See
    also specific type*
  alpha-receptor blockers, 141,
      165–166, 175
  angiotensin inhibition by, **169–172**.
      See also Angiotensin inhibitors
  basic pharmacology of, **155–172**
  beta-receptor blockers, 146, **164–165**,
      174–175
  clinical pharmacology of, **172–174**
  in elderly, 994

monotherapy versus polypharmacy
    with, 173
  outpatient therapy with, **172–173**
  preparations available, 174–175
  sites of action of, 155, 156*i*
  sodium balance altered by, **155–157**.
      See also Diuretics
  sympathetic nervous system function
      altered by, **157–166**. *See also*
      Sympathoplegics
  vasodilation caused by, **166–169**. *See
      also* Vasodilators
  water balance altered by, **155–157**.
      See also Diuretics
Anti-IgE monoclonal antibodies, for
    asthma, 338
Anti-inflammatory drugs
  for asthma, 339
  for dermatologic therapy, **1008–1009**,
      1010*i*, 1011*t*
  in elderly, **995**
  glucocorticoids as, 639
  topical, OTC preparations, efficacy of,
      1034*t*
Anti-inhibitor coagulant complex, prepa-
    rations available, 561
Anti-insulin antibodies, 695
Antilymphocyte globulin (ALG),
    929–930
Antimalarial agents, **838–850**. *See also
    specific agent*
  classification of, **838–840**
  in dermatologic therapy, 1014*t*
  in inflammation, **591**
  for malaria prophylaxis, **840–841**,
      840*t*
  for malaria treatment, **840–841**, 841*t*
  parasite life cycle and, **838**
  structures of, 839*i*
Antimetabolites (structural analogs),
    889–893
  in dermatologic therapy, 1014*t*
  mechanisms of action of, 889
Antimicrobial agents. *See also specific
    type*
  antagonism and, **822**
  bacteriostatic versus bactericidal, 818,
      818*t*
  beta-lactamase assay and, 817
  body fluid concentrations of, 819,
      820*t*
  choice of, 813, 814–815*t*, 816*t*
  clinical failure of, 817
  clinical use of, **812–826**
  combination therapy with, **821–822**
  CSF penetration by, 820*t*
  culture results and, **813–816**
  duration of, **817**
  in elderly, 995
  empirical therapy with, **812–813**
  for infections with known etiology,
      813–815
  monitoring response to, 817
  pharmacodynamics of, **817–819**
  pharmacokinetics of, **819–820**
  postantibiotic effect of, 818–819, 818*t*

for prophylaxis, **822–824**, 824*t*,
      824–825*t*
  in renal/hepatic impairment, 819, 819*t*
  route of administration of, 819
  serum concentrations of, 820
  susceptibility testing and, 816–817
  synergism and, 817, **821–822**
  toxicity of, management of, **820–821**
Antiminth, 878. *See also* Pyrantel
    pamoate
Antimonials, pentavalent and trivalent,
    antiparasitic actions of, 836*t*, **865**
Antimuscarinic agents, **105–110,
    110–114**
  for acid-peptic disease, 111, 1020
  for asthma, **335–336**, 339, 340
  basic pharmacology of, **105–110,
      335–336**
  clinical pharmacology of, **110–114,
      339**
  interactions of, 1063*t*
  for motion sickness, 110–111, 1022
  in OTC preparations, hidden, 1037*t*
  overdosage of, 972*t*
  physostigmine for, 101–102
  for parkinsonism, 106, 110, **457**, 457*t*
  preparations available, 115–116, 340
Antimycobacterial drugs, **770–779**. *See
    also specific type*
  for atypical mycobacterial infections,
      777, 777*t*
  for leprosy, **777–778**
  preparations available, 778–779
  for tuberculosis, **770–777**
Antineoplastic drugs, **881–915**. *See also
    specific agent and* Cancer
    chemotherapy
Antinicotinic drugs, **114–115**
Antiparasitic agents
  mechanisms of action of
    biochemical functions of parasite
        and host and, **834–836**
    enzymes found in parasites and,
        827–831
    enzymes indispensable to parasite
        and, **831–834**
    unknown, 836, 836*t*
  principles of therapy with, **827–837**
  targets of, 827, 828*t*
Antiparkinsonism effects, of H$_1$ receptor
    antagonists, 268
Antiplatelet drugs
  basic pharmacology of, **555–557**
  clinical pharmacology of, **557–558**
Antiprogestins, with prostaglandins, for
    abortion, 313
Antiprotozoal drugs, **838–861**. *See also
    specific type*
  for amebiasis, **850–855**
  for giardiasis, **857–858**
  for leishmaniasis, **855–856**
  for malaria, **838–850**
  for *Pneumocystis carinii* pneumonia,
      856–857
  preparations available, 858–859
  for trichomoniasis, **857–858**
  for trypanosomiasis, **856–857**

Antipruritic agents, **1013–1014**
Antipsychotic agents (neuroleptics), **464–475**
　advantages and disadvantages of, 471*t*, 475
　adverse effects of, 470*t*, 473–474
　basic pharmacology of, **464–470**
　chemical types of, 464–465, 466*i*, 467*i*
　clinical pharmacology of, **470–475**
　combinations of, 473
　differences among, 468–469
　dosage schedules for, 472–473
　dose relationships of, 472, 472*t*
　in elderly, 993
　interactions of, 474
　lithium combined with, 473, 477
　maintenance treatment and, 473
　overdoses of, 474
　plasma concentrations of, 472
　preparations available, 472, 480
　selection of, 471–472, 471*t*
　tardive dyskinesia caused by, 461
　teratogenic effects of, 474
　toxicity of, 474
Antipyretics
　aspirin as, 581, 582–583
　OTC preparations, efficacy of, 1033*t*
Antipyrine, half-life of, aging affecting, 992*i*
Antiretroviral agents, **795–799**, 795*t*, 796*i*. See also specific type
　importance of pharmacologic knowledge in use of, 799
　preparations available, 801
Antirheumatic drugs, slow-acting/disease modifying, 579, **590–593**
　preparations available, 599–600
Antischistosomal agents, 863*t*
Antiseborrhea agents, **1014**, 1014*t*
　OTC preparations, efficacy of, 1034*t*
Antisecretory drugs, **1019–1021**
　OTC preparations, efficacy of, 1033*t*
Antisepsis, 805*t*. See also Antiseptics
Antiseptics, **804–810**
　definition of, 805
　preparations available, 810
Antistaphylococcal penicillins, 724, 729–731
　dosing guidelines for, 730*t*
Antisteroid drugs, in cancer chemotherapy, **898–900**, 899*t*
Antithrombin III (AT III), 548–550, 559*t*
　preparations available, 561
　therapeutic, 559*t*
Antithrombotic drugs
　basic pharmacology of, **555–557**
　clinical pharmacology of, **557–558**
Antithymocyte globulin (ATG), 929–930
Antithyroid agents
　adjuncts to, 630–631
　basic pharmacology of, **626–628**
　clinical pharmacology of, **628–632**
　for Graves' disease, 630
　preparations available, 633
Antitussives
　opioid analgesics as, 505, 507, **512**
　preparations available, 514

OTC preparations
　efficacy of, 1034*t*
　hidden ingredients in, 1037*t*, 1038*t*, 1039*t*
Antivenin
　crotalid, for rattlesnake envenomation, 978, 1057
　Latrodectus mactans, for black widow spider bite, 1056*t*
Antivert, 284. See also Meclizine
Antiviral chemotherapy and prophylaxis, **788–802**. See also specific agent
　for dermatologic disorders, **1004**
　sites of action of, 788, 789*i*
Anturane, 600. See also Sulfinpyrazone
Anxiety
　beta-receptor blocking drugs for, 148
　management of, **363–364**, **364–365**
Aortic aneurysm, dissecting, beta-receptor blocking drugs for, 146
Apazone, 580*t*
APCs (antigen-presenting cells), 917
A.P.L., 617. See also Chorionic gonadotropin
Aplastic anemia, chloramphenicol causing, 744–745
Apnea, inhaled anesthetics affecting threshold for, 417
Apo B-48 (apolipoprotein B-48), 564
Apo B-100 (apolipoprotein B-100), 563, 564
Apocrine sweat glands
　autonomic activity/drugs affecting, 83*t*
　sympathomimetics affecting, 127
Apolipoprotein B, familial ligand-defective, 568
Apolipoprotein B-48 (Apo B-48), 564
Apolipoprotein B-100 (Apo B-100), 563, 564
Apparent volume of distribution, 34
Appendectomy, antimicrobial prophylaxis and, 824*t*
Appetite control. See also Weight control/weight reduction
　through serotonin, 276
Apraclonidine, 159
　for glaucoma, 132, 149*t*
　preparations available, 133
Apresoline, 175. See also Hydralazine
Aprobarbital, preparations available, 369
Aprotinin, 295, **561**
　preparations available, 561
APSAC (anisoylated plasminogen streptokinase activator complex/anistreplase), 550*i*, 555
　for myocardial infarction, 555, 556
　preparations available, 561
Aquachloral Supprettes, 369. See also Chloral hydrate
AquaMephyton, 561. See also Phytonadione
Aqueous diffusion, drug permeation by, 5
Ara-A (vidarabine), 792*t*, **794–795**
Ara-C (cytarabine), 891*t*, **892–893**, 893*i*
　mechanism of action of, 791*t*, 892–893

Arachidonic acid, **304–305**, 305*i*
　dietary manipulation of metabolism of, **316–317**
Aralen, 858. See also Chloroquine
Aramine, 134. See also Metaraminol
Arduan, 448. See also Pipecuronium
Area under the concentration-time curve, cumulative effects and, 43
Aredia, 721. See also Pamidronate
Arginine vasopressin (desmopressin acetate/DDAVP), 296, 615*i*, 616. See also Vasopressin
　dosage of, 616
　factor VIII activity affected by, 560, 616
Argyrol SS, 810. See also Silver
Arimidex, 680, 899*t*. See also Anastrozole
Aristocort, 650. See also Triamcinolone
Aristospan, 650. See also Triamcinolone
Armour Thyroid, 633. See also Thyroid desiccated
Aromatase inhibitors, in cancer chemotherapy, 899*t*, **900**
　for breast cancer, 672, 909
Aromatic diamidines, antiparasitic actions of, 836*t*
Aromatic hydrocarbons, **950**
Arousal, methylxanthines causing, 331
Arrhythmias
　action potential prolongation in management of, **235–236**
　alcohol consumption and, 377
　beta-receptor blocking drugs for, 146, **234**
　bromocriptine causing, 455
　calcium channel-blocking drugs for, **236**
　definition of, 216
　digitalis in management of, 208
　digitalis-induced, 204, 204*i*, 209
　drug-induced, 226, 238–239
　drugs for management of, **216–241**. See also Antiarrhythmic agents
　basic pharmacology of, **224–226**
　impulse formation disturbances causing, 222, 222*i*
　levodopa causing, 453
　mechanisms of, **222–224**
　after myocardial infarction, treatment of, 234
　neuromuscular blockers causing, 443–444
　nonpharmacologic therapy of, 238
　pretreatment evaluation of, 237–238
　resting potential–action potential relationship and, 219–220, 221*i*
　sodium channel blockers for, **227–234**
Arsenic poisoning, 960*t*, **963–964**
　dimercaprol for, 957, 964
Arsine gas poisoning, 964
Artane, 462. See also Trihexyphenidyl
Artemisinin (qinghaosu), for malaria treatment, 849–850
Arterial blood gases, in poisoning, 973
Arterial blood pressure. See Blood pressure

Arterial thrombosis, **558**

Arteries, direct-acting cholinomimetics affecting, 94*t*

Arteriovenous concentration gradient, anesthetic uptake and distribution affected by, 413–414

Arthritis
gouty
drugs for, **595–599**
preparations available, 600
nonsteroidal anti-inflammatory drugs for, 567
pathophysiology of, 595, 596*i*
rheumatoid
chronic inflammation in, 578, 579*t*
eicosanoids in, 316
gold compounds for, 591–592
penicillamine for, 593
septic, empiric antimicrobial therapy and, 816*t*

Arthropan (choline salicylate), 599

ASA, 580, 599, 1025. *See also* Aminosalicylic acid; Aspirin

Asacol, 1027. *See also* Mesalamine

Ascaris lumbricoides (ascariasis), drugs for infection with, 863*t*
albendazole, 864
ivermectin, 868
levamisole, 869
mebendazole, 869
piperazine, 873
pyrantel, 876

Ascites
cancer-related, **912**
diuretics for, 258

Asendin, 494. *See also* Amoxapine

Asparaginase, **901**, 901*t*

Aspartate, 349*t*, 351
ethanol affecting, 374

Aspergillus, empiric antimicrobial therapy and, 815*t*

Aspirin, **579–585**, 580*t*
adverse effects of, 583–584
analgesic effects of, 581, 582
anti-inflammatory action of, 316, 581, 582
antipyretic effects of, 581, 582–583
antithrombotic action of, **556–557**, 581–582, 583
in breast milk, 987*t*
dosage of, 583, 583*i*
efficacy of, 1033*t*
in elderly, 995
interactions of, 584–585
ionization constant of, 6*t*
mechanism of action of, 581, 582*i*
in OTC preparations, hidden, 1037–1038*t*
overdose toxicity of, 584
pharmacokinetic/pharmacodynamic parameters of, 36*t*, 580–582
preparations available, 599
prophylactic use of, 314–315
selection of, 583

Aspirols, 194. *See also* Amyl nitrite

Astemizole, 267*t*
active metabolites of, 266

cardiac toxicity of, 269
interactions of, 266, 269–270
preparations available, 283

Asthma, **325–342**
acute, management of, 339
antimuscarinic agents for, 109, 111
beta-receptor blocking drug toxicity and, 149
drugs for. *See also specific type*
approaches to development of, 308
basic pharmacology of, **328–338**
clinical pharmacology of, **338–339**
OTC preparations, hidden ingredients in, 1037*t*, 1038*t*, 1039*t*
preparations available, 340
methylxanthines for, **330–333**
pathogenesis of, **325–328**, 326*i*, 327*i*, 329*i*
sympathomimetics for, 132–133, 333

Astrocytoma, 912

AT$_1$ receptors, 289–290
losartan blocking, 289, 291, 293

AT$_2$ receptors, 289–290

AT III (antithrombin III), 548–550, 559*t*
preparations available, 561
therapeutic, 559*t*

Atabrine, 859. *See also* Quinacrine

Atarax, 267*t*, 283, 369. *See also* Hydroxyzine

Ataxia
carbamazepine causing, 393
phenytoin causing, 391

Atenolol, 138*t*, 143*i*, 145, **165**
for hypertension, **165**
pharmacokinetic/pharmacodynamic parameters of, 36*t*
preparations available, 150, 174, 194
properties of, 144*t*

ATG (atithymocyte globulin), 929–930

Atgam (lymphocyte immune globulin), 940

Atherogenesis, 563–564

Atheromas, calcium channel blockers affecting development of, 190

Atherosclerosis
hyperlipoproteinemia causing, 563
nitric oxide and, **322–323**

Atherosclerotic angina, 179
management of, 192–193
nitrates for, 185–186

Athetosis, 450, 460

Ativan, 366*t*, 369, 407, 423. *See also* Lorazepam

ATnativ, 561. *See also* Antithrombin III

Atolone, 650. *See also* Triamcinolone

Atonic seizures, 404
management of, 405

Atorvastatin, 573
preparations available, 576

Atovaquone, **857**
mitochondrial electron transporter affected by, 834

ATP (adenosine triphosphate), 77*t*, 85*t*

Atracurium, 436*i*, 438*t*
cardiovascular effects of, 443, 443*t*
effects of, 443*t*

pharmacokinetics of, 438–439, 438*t*
preparations available, 448

Atria (cardiac)
antimuscarinic agents affecting, 108–109
direct-acting cholinomimetics affecting, 94*t*, 95

Atrial arrhythmias, digitalis for, 208

Atrial natriuretic peptide (ANP), 296–297, 296*i*
ligand-regulated transmembrane enzymes in signalling by, 19–20, 26

Atrial tachycardia, paroxysmal, sympathomimetics for, 131

Atrioventricular block, 224, 225*i*

Atrioventricular node, direct-acting cholinomimetics affecting, 94*t*

Atropa belladonna, 105

Atropine, 105
adverse effects of, 113–114
as antidote, 977*t*
central nervous system affected by, 106
for cholinesterase inhibitor toxicity, 102, 977*t*
with diphenoxylate, 112, 511
distribution of, 106
for gastrointestinal and genitourinary conditions, 112*t*
ionization constant of, 6*t*
mechanism of action of, 106
metabolism and excretion of, 106
for muscarinic mushroom poisoning, 102
for myocardial infarction, 111
ophthalmologic uses of, 111*t*
overdosage of, 113–114, 972*t*
physostigmine for, 101–102, 113
pharmacokinetic/pharmacodynamic parameters of, 36*t*
preparations available, 115, 1026
source and chemistry of, 105
structure of, 105, 106*i*
for urinary disorders, 112, 112*t*

Atropine esterase, 106

Atrovent, 116, 340. *See also* Ipratropium

AUC (area under the concentration-time curve), cumulative effects and, 43

Auerbach's plexus (myenteric plexus), 74

Augmentin, 740. *See also* Amoxicillin/potassium clavulanate

Auranofin, 591, 592
for asthma, 339
preparations available, 599

Aurothioglucose, 591
preparations available, 599

Aurothiomalate (gold sodium thiomalate), 591, 592
preparations available, 599

Autoclaving, 809

Autocoids, 261. *See also* Histamine; Serotonin

Autoimmune disorders
chloroquine for, 842
drugs inducing, **939**

immunosuppressive agents for, 931*t*, 932–933
Autoimmune hemolytic anemia, immunosuppressive agents for, 931*t*, 932
Autoimmunity, 923
Autonomic drugs, ganglion-blocking drugs affecting response to, 115
Autonomic nerve endings, sympathetic and parasympathetic activity/drugs affecting, 83
Autonomic nervous system, **73–89**
 anatomy of, **73–74**, 74*i*
 antipsychotic agents affecting, 470*t*, 473
 functional organization of, **82–85**
 neurotransmitter chemistry of, **74–81**, 77*t*
 nonadrenergic/noncholinergic neurons in, **82**
 organ system effects of, 82, 83*t*
 pharmacologic modification of function of, **85–87**
 renin secretion regulated by, 287–288
Autonomic receptors, **81–82**, 81*t*
Autoplex, 560. *See also* Factor IX
Autoplex T (anti-inhibitor coagulant complex), 561
Autoreceptors, 84, 85*t*
Aventyl, 494. *See also* Nortriptyline
Avermectins, synaptic transmission affected by, 835
Avloclor, 858. *See also* Chloroquine
Axid, 284, 1026. *See also* Nizatidine
Axoaxonic synapses, 347, 348*i*, 351
Aygestin, 680. *See also* Norethindrone
Azacitidine, 891*t*, **893**, 893*i*
Azactam, 741. *See also* Aztreonam
Azapropazone, **588**
Azatadine, preparations available, 283
Azathioprine, 927–928, 928*i*
 immunosuppressive actions of, 927–928
 in inflammation, 591
 for inflammatory bowel disease, 1026
 preparations available, 940
Azelaic acid, **1007**
Azelex (azelaic acid), 1007
Azidothymidine, 795, 801. *See also* Zidovudine
Azimexon, 935–936
Azinphos-methyl, 951*t*
Azithromycin, **749**
 for MAC infections, 777
 preparations available, 751
Azlocillin, 731
Azmacort, 340. *See also* Triamcinolone
Azo reductions, 54*t*
Azoles, **783–785**, 784*i*
 oral, **1004**
  interactions of/contraindications to, 1004
 resistance to, 783
 topical, **786**, **1002**
AZT, 795, 801. *See also* Zidovudine

Aztreonam, 736
 CSF penetration by, 820*t*
 preparations available, 741
Azulfidine, 600, 768, 1027. *See also* Sulfasalazine

B₁ (bradykinin) receptors, 294
 antagonists of, 295
B₂ (bradykinin) receptors, 294
 antagonists of, 295
B cells (beta cells), pancreatic, 685*t*
 insulin secreted by, 685, 685*t*, 687*i*
 sulfonylureas affecting, 696
B fibers, local anesthetics affecting, 429, 429*t*
B lymphocytes, 921
Babesia, drugs for infection with, 855*t*
Babesiosis, quinine for, 848
Bacampicillin, preparations available, 740
Bacille Calmette-Guerin (BCG), 935
 preparations available, 940
Bacillus, empiric antimicrobial therapy and, 814*t*
Bacitracin, **739**
 in dermatologic therapy, **1000**
Baclofen, **446–447**, 446*i*
 preparations available, 448
 site of action of, 446*i*
Bacterial infections. *See also specific type*
 empiric antimicrobial therapy and, 814–815*t*
Bactericidal activity, 818, 818*t*
Bacteriostatic activity, 818, 818*t*
Bacteroides fragilis, empiric antimicrobial therapy and, 815*t*
Bactocill, 740. *See also* Oxacillin
Bactrim, 768, 859. *See also* Trimethoprim-sulfamethoxazole
BAL (dimercaprol/2,3-dimercaptopropanol), **957–958**, 957*i*
 preparations available, 966
Balantidium coli (balantidiasis), drugs for, 855*t*
 metronidazole, 858
Baldness, minoxidil for, 1014
Ballismus, 460
Balsalazide, for inflammatory bowel disease, 1025
Banthine, 116, 1027. *See also* Methantheline
Barbiturates, **355–363**
 abuse of, **519–521**
 for alcohol withdrawal syndrome, 380
 for anesthesia, 362, **420**
 biotransformation of, 358
 chemical classification of, 354–355, 357*i*
 dosages of, 366*t*
 drug metabolism induced by, 59*t*
 in elderly, 993
 fetus affected by, 983*t*
 interactions of, 368, 1063*t*
 oral anticoagulant interactions and, 554

organ level effects of, 360–362
 in OTC preparations, hidden, 1038*t*
 overdose of, 972*t*
 pharmacodynamics of, 359–362
 pharmacokinetics of, 355–359
 preparations available, 369
 sleep affected by, 362
 toxicity of, 367–368
 ultra-short-acting, **420**
Baroreflex, postural, in blood pressure regulation, 84*t*, 154, 155*i*
Bases, weak
 definition of, 5–6
 ionization constants of, 6*t*
 ionization of, 5–7
Basophils, histamine in, 261–262
Batrachotoxin, sodium channels affected by, 428
Bayer-205, 878. *See also* Suramin
BCG (Bacille Calmette-Guerin), 935
 preparations available, 935
BCNU (carmustine), 886*i*, **888**, 890*t*
BDZ receptors, 359
 heterogeneity of, 360
 ligand interactions and, 360
Beclomethasone, 336
 aerosol form of, 646
 preparations available, 340
Beclovent, 340. *See also* Beclomethasone
Beef insulin, 690*t*, 692
Beef tapeworm, drugs for infection with, 863*t*
 niclosamide, 871
Behavioral effects
 of antipsychotic agents, 473
 of bromocriptine, 455
 of levodopa, 454
Behavioral tolerance, 516
Belladonna, 108
 preparations available, 115, 1027
Benadryl, 267*t*, 283. *See also* Diphenhydramine
Benazepril
 for hypertension, 170
 preparations available, 175
Bendectin
 for nausea and vomiting of pregnancy, 269
 teratogenic effects of, 269
Bendroflumethiazide, 252*t*
 preparations available, 259
Benemid, 600. *See also* Probenecid
Benign essential tremor, 450
Benign prostatic hyperplasia, alpha-receptor blocking drugs for, 141
Bentyl, 115, 1027. *See also* Dicyclomine
Benylin DM, 514. *See also* Dextromethorphan
Benzalkonium
 preparations available, 810
 risks of use of, 808
Benzamycin (benzoyl peroxide with erythromycin), 1001
Benzathine penicillin, 729
 pharmacokinetics of, 727
 preparations available, 740

Benzene, 950, 950*t*
structure of, 529*i*
threshold limit values for, 948*t*
Benzene hexachlorides, 950–951, 950*t*
Benzene ring substitution, sympathomimetic activity and, 123
Benzestrol, 656
Benzisoxazole, 468*t*
Benzocaine
in OTC preparations, hidden, 1038*t*
preparations available, 432
properties of, 426*t*
structure of, 426*t*
Benzodiazepine agonists, 360
Benzodiazepine antagonists, 360, **363**
preparations available, 369
Benzodiazepine inverse agonists, 360
Benzodiazepines, **355–363**
abuse of, **519–521**
for alcohol withdrawal syndrome, 380
for anesthesia, 362, **420–421**
for anxiety, **364–365**
biotransformation of, 356–358, 357*i*
chemical classification of, 354, 356*i*
dosages of, 366*t*
in elderly, 993
interactions of, 368
organ level effects of, 360–362
overdose of, 972*t*
pharmacodynamics of, 359–362
pharmacokinetics of, 355–359, 358*t*,
402
preparations available, 369
receptors for, 359
heterogeneity of, 360
ligand interactions and, 360
for seizures, 362, **402**
sleep affected by, 362
toxicity of, 367–368
Benzoic acid, as preservative, 810
Benzomorphans, 498*i*, **512**
Benzo[*a*]pyrene, drug metabolism induced by, 59*t*
Benzothiadiazides, 251. *See also* Thiazides
Benzoyl peroxide, **1007**
with erythromycin, 1001
in OTC preparations, efficacy of,
1033*t*
Benzquinamide, 471
Benzthiazide, 252*t*
preparations available, 259
Benztropine, 107*i*
for parkinsonism, 457*t*
preparations available, 462
Benzyl benzoate, **1005**
o-Benzyl-*p*-chlorophenol, antimicrobial
effects of, 807–808
Bephenium, synaptic transmission affected by, 835
Bepridil, 188*i*, 190*t*, **236**
for arrhythmias, **236**
clinical properties of, 190*t*
pharmacokinetics of, 189*t*
preparations available, 194, 240
toxicity of, 191
vascular selectivity of, 190*t*

Beta-adrenoceptor kinase, 23, 25*i*,
122–123
Beta adrenoceptors, 118–119
activation of, 121–122
in bladder, 127
desensitization of, 23, 25*i*, 122–123
distribution of, 124*t*
drugs blocking. *See also* Beta-receptor
blocking drugs
basic pharmacology of, **142–146**
clinical pharmacology of, **146–149**
eye controlled by, 148
heart affected by, 125
selectivity of drugs for, 120, 120*t*,
129, 129*i*
in uterus, 126
vascular smooth muscle tone regulated
by, 124
Beta₁ adrenoceptors, 81*t*, 118, 119*t*
distribution of, 124*t*
heart affected by, 125
selectivity of drugs for, 120, 120*t*,
129, 129*i*
Beta₂ adrenoceptors, 81*t*, 118, 119*t*
in bladder, 127
in bronchial smooth muscle, 126
distribution of, 124*t*
heart affected by, 125
selectivity of drugs for, 120, 120*t*,
129, 129*i*
asthma treatment and, 333–334
vascular smooth muscle tone regulated
by, 124
Beta₃ adrenoceptors, 81*t*, 119, 119*t*
distribution of, 124*t*
Beta agonists
for asthma, 333–334
gastrointestinal smooth muscle affected by, 126
for heart failure, 197, **206**
mechanism of action of, 121–122
selectivity of, 120, 120*t*, 129, 129*i*
Beta-blockers. *See* Beta-receptor blocking drugs
Beta-carbolines, 360
Beta carbon, sympathomimetic activity
and, 124
Beta cells (B cells), pancreatic, 685*t*
insulin secreted by, 685, 685*t*, 687*i*
sulfonylureas affecting, 696
Beta interferon, 800, 926, 933, 934*t*, 935
preparations available, 940
Beta-lactam antibiotics, **724–737**. *See
also specific agent and* Penicillins
Beta-lactamase, penicillin resistance
caused by, 729–731
Beta-lactamase assay, 817
Beta-lactamase inhibitors, 731, **736–737**,
736*i*
Beta-lactamase resistant penicillins,
729–731
Beta nerve fibers, local anesthetics affecting, 429*t*
Beta-receptor blocking drugs
for angina, 179, **191–192**, 193*t*, 194
for anxiety, 365
for arrhythmias, 146, **234**, 240

basic pharmacology of, **142–146**
choice of, 148
clinical pharmacology of, **146–149**
discontinuation of use of, hazards of,
149
for glaucoma, 132, 143, 147, 148,
149*t*
for heart failure, 146, 207, 210
risks of use of, 149, 207
for hypertension, 146, **164–165**,
174–175
for hyperthyroidism, 147–148, **628**
interactions of, 1063–1064*t*
for myocardial infarction prevention,
557
organ system effects of, 142–145
overdose of, glucagon for, 703
preparations available, 150, 174–175,
194, 240
prophylactic use of, 557
renin secretion affected by, 290
sedative effects of, 355
selectivity of, 138*t*
structures of, 142, 143*i*
toxicity of, 148–149
Betadine, 810. *See also* Povidone-iodine
Betagan Liquifilm, 150. *See also* Levobunolol
Betamethasone, 640*t*
preparations available, 650
for stimulation of fetal lung maturation, 643
structure of, 641*i*
Betapace, 150, 240. *See also* Sotalol
Betaseron, 940. *See also* Interferon-β
Betaxolol, 138*t*, 145, **165**
for glaucoma, 147, 149*t*
for hypertension, **165**
preparations available, 150, 174
properties of, 144*t*
Betazole, 264
Bethanechol
gastrointestinal motility affected by,
1021
for gastrointestinal and urinary tract
disorders, 100
molecular structure of, 92*i*
preparations available, 103
properties of, 93*t*
Bethanidine, 161
Bezafibrate, 572
Bias, subject and observer, in new drug
evaluation, 67
Biaxin, 751. *See also* Clarithromycin
Bicalutamide, 679
preparations available, 680
Bicarbonate
in antacids, 1018*t*
as antidote, 977*t*
for methanol poisoning, 382
Bicillin, 740. *See also* Penicillin G benzathine
Bicuculline, GABA-DBZ receptor chloride channel binding and, 361
Bigeminy, digitalis-induced, 204, 204*i*
Biguanides, **699–700**, 700*t*
preparations available, 703

Bilarcil, 878. *See also* Metrifonate
Bile acid-binding resins, **572–573**
  combination therapy with, **575**
  interactions of, 1064*t*
Bilharziasis (*Schistosoma haematobium*),
    drugs for infection with, 863*t*
  antimony compounds, 865
  metrifonate, 870
  praziquantel, 874
Biliary tract
  antimicrobial prophylaxis for surgery
    of, 824*t*
  opioid analgesics affecting, 506
Bilivist, 633. *See also* Ipodate
Biltricide, 878. *See also* Praziquantel
Binding, plasma protein
  drug concentration affected by, 47, 48
  passage across placenta and, 979–980
  reduced, oral anticoagulant interac-
    tions and, 554
Binding molecules, agonist inhibition of,
    4
Binding sites. *See also* Drug receptors
  inert, 4
Bioaccumulation, environmental toxicity
    and, 947
Bioavailability, 40–42
  in infants and children, 982, 984*t*
Biomagnification, environmental toxicity
    and, 947
Biotransformation, **50–61**. *See also* Me-
    tabolism, drug
  clinical relevance of, **56–61**
  in drug disposition, **50–51**, 51*i*
  locations of, **51–52**
  microsomal mixed function oxidase
    system in, 51*i*, **52–55**, 52*i*, 56*t*
  need for, **50**
  phase I reactions in, 51, 51*i*, **52–55**,
    53–54*t*
  phase II reactions in, 51, 51*i*, **55**, 57*t*
  toxic products of, **55–56**, 57*i*. *See also*
    Reactive metabolites
Biperiden
  for parkinsonism, 457*t*
  preparations available, 462
Biphenyls, polychlorinated (PCBs/copla-
    nar biphenyls), 954
Bipolar affective disorder
  depression associated with, 483, 484*t*
  drugs for, **475–479**
  lithium for, 476–477
  nature of, 475
Bipyridines, for heart failure, **205–206**
Bipyridyl herbicides, **953–954**, 953*i*
Bisacodyl
  laxative effect of, 1023
  preparations available, 1027
Bismuth subsalicylate
  for acid-peptic disease, 1021
  in OTC preparations, efficacy of,
    1034*t*
  preparations available, 1027
Bisoprolol, **165**
  for hypertension, **165**
  preparations available, 150, 174
  properties of, 144*t*

Bisphosphonates, **710–711**, 711*i*
  bone mineral homeostasis affected by,
    710–711
  for hypercalcemia, 713
  for osteoporosis, 711, 712, 718*i*
  for Paget's disease, 720
Bithionol, **865–866**
  antiparasitic actions of, 836*t*, 865
  preparations available, 878
Bitin, 878. *See also* Bithionol
Bitolterol
  for asthma, 333
  preparations available, 340
Black widow spider bite, passive immu-
    nization for, 1056*t*
Blackwater fever, quinine in, 848
Bladder
  adrenoceptors in, 126–127
  antimuscarinic agents affecting, 110
  autonomic activity/drugs affecting, 83*t*
  direct-acting cholinomimetics affect-
    ing, 94*t*, 96
Blastocystis hominis, drugs for infection
    with, 855*t*
  metronidazole, 858
Blastomyces (blastomycosis)
  empiric antimicrobial therapy and,
    815*t*
  pentamidine for, 856
Bleach, antimicrobial effects of, 807
Bleeding
  breakthrough/withdrawal, oral contra-
    ceptive use and, 668
  factor IX concentrates for, 554
  heparin causing, 551
  oral anticoagulant interactions and,
    554
  postmenopausal, estrogen therapy
    causing, 660
Bleeding disorders, drugs for, **558–559**
Blenoxane, 894*t*. *See also* Bleomycin
Bleomycin, 894*t*, **897–898**
Blocadren, 150, 175. *See also* Timolol
Blood. *See also* Hematotoxicity
  chronic alcohol consumption affect-
    ing, 377–378
  drug distribution in, 39*t*
  eicosanoids affecting, 314
  lead toxicity and, 961
  local anesthetic toxicity and, 432
  oral contraceptives affecting, 667
Blood alcohol level
  clinical effects of alcohol consumption
    and, 374, 374*t*
  driving impairment and, 374
Blood cells
  cytochrome P450-derived metabolites
    affecting, 311
  lipoxygenase metabolites affecting,
    311
  prostaglandins affecting, 309,
    314–315
  thromboxanes affecting, 309, 314–315
Blood coagulation, 547–548
  drugs for disorders of, **547–562**. *See*
    also specific type
  estrogens affecting, 657

  mechanisms of, **547–548**
  oral contraceptives affecting, 667
  regulation of, 548, 550*i*
Blood disorders. *See also* Hematotoxicity
  carbamazepine causing, 393
  eicosanoids in, 314–315
  H_2 receptor antagonists causing, 272
  inhaled anesthetics causing, 419
  local anesthetics causing, 432
Blood flow
  coronary
    determinants of, 180
    nitroglycerin affecting, 183–184
  drug absorption affected by, in infants
    and children, 982
Blood:gas partition coefficient, for in-
    haled anesthetics, 412, 413*t*
Blood gases, in poisoning, 973
Blood loss, in iron-deficiency anemia,
    535
Blood pressure
  alpha-receptor antagonists affecting,
    136–138, 138*i*
  angiotensin converting enzyme in-
    hibitors affecting, 291, 292*i*
  angiotensin II affecting, 289
  autonomic control of, 83, 84*i*
  decreased, renal response to, 154
  elevated, 153–154. *See also* Hyperten-
    sion
  ganglion-blocking drugs affecting,
    115
  H_2 receptor antagonists affecting, 271
  histamine affecting, 263, 263*i*
  inhaled anesthetics affecting, 416–417
  kinins affecting, 294
  nitric oxide affecting, **322**
  regulation of, 84*t*, **153–155**
    normal, 154, 154*i*, 155*i*
    therapeutic implications of,
        154–155. *See also* Antihyper-
        tensive drugs
  sympathomimetic agents affecting,
    125–126, 125*t*, 126*i*
  vasopressin affecting, 295
Blood schizonticides, for malaria, 838
Blood schizonts, plasmodial, 838
Blood vessels. *See also under* Vascular
  autonomic activity/drugs affecting, 83*t*
  cholinesterase inhibitors affecting,
    99–100
  direct-acting cholinomimetics affect-
    ing, 94*t*
  ganglion-blocking drugs affecting,
    115
  sympathomimetic agents affecting,
    124–125, 125*t*
BNP (brain natriuretic peptide),
    296–297, 296*i*
Body fluids
  drug distribution in, 39*t*
  drug trapping in, 7*t*
Bone
  drug distribution in, 39*t*
  Paget's disease of, **720**
  parathyroid hormone affecting, 709*t*
  prostaglandins affecting, 310

Bone *(cont.)*
tetracyclines affecting, 747
vitamin D affecting, 709*t*
Bone loss, in osteoporosis, 717, 718*i*
Bone marrow disorders
amphotericin B causing, 783
anemia associated with, erythropoietin for, 544
chloramphenicol causing, 744–745
zidovudine causing, 796
Bone marrow growth factors (hematopoietic growth factors), **543–545**, 543*t*
in cancer chemotherapy, **902**
preparations available, 546
Bone marrow transplantation
in chronic myelogenous leukemia, 906
cyclosporine therapy and, 925, 932
immunosuppressive therapy and, 931*t*, 932
Bone mineral homeostasis, agents affecting, **706–722**
basic pharmacology of, **706–712**
clinical pharmacology of, **713–720**
hormonal
primary regulators, **706–709**
secondary regulators, **709–710**
nonhormonal, **710–712**
preparations available, 721
Bonine, 267*t. See also* Meclizine
Bopindolol, 145
Borrelia recurrentis, empiric antimicrobial therapy and, 815*t*
Botanical insecticides, **952**, 953*i*
Botox, 448. *See also* Botulinum toxin
Botulinum toxin
preparations available, 448
for spastic disorders, **448**
Botulism, passive immunization for, 1056*t*
Botulism antitoxin, 1056*t*
BPH (benign prostatic hyperplasia), alpha-receptor blocking drugs for, 141
BQ-123, 298, 300*i*
Bradycardia
neuromuscular blockers causing, 443–444
torsade de pointes and, 223
Bradycardia-tachycardia syndrome, lithium contraindicated in, 478
Bradykinin, 293, 294
antagonists of, 295
in inflammation, 579*t*
metabolism of, 295
receptors for, 294–295
Brain
cellular organization of, 347–348, 348*i*
inhaled anesthetics affecting, 417
Brain-derived neurotrophic factor, for parkinsonism, 458
Brain natriuretic peptide (BNP), 296–297, 296*i*
Brain tumors, **912**
Bran, laxative effect of, 1023

Branhamella catarrhalis, empiric antimicrobial therapy and, 814*t*
Breakthrough bleeding, oral contraceptive use and, 668
Breast, oral contraceptives affecting, 666
Breast cancer, 903*t*, **908–909**
aminoglutethimide for, 648
aromatase inhibitors for, 672
estrogen administration and, 660
oral contraceptive use and, 670
Breast-feeding. *See also* Breast milk; Lactation
drug use during, **986**, 987*t*
H_2 receptor antagonist use during, 272
oxytocin in milk ejection reflex and, 615
Breast milk. *See also* Breast-feeding; Lactation
drug trapping in, 7*t*
drugs detectable in, **986**, 987*t*
sedative-hypnotics in, 356
Breast tenderness, estrogen therapy causing, 660
Breathing, in poisoned patient, 970
Brequinar sodium, 927
Brethine, 340. *See also* Terbutaline
Bretylium, **235**, 235*i*
action potential duration affected by, 235
for arrhythmias, **235**
clinical properties of, 229*t*
membrane actions of, 228*t*
preparations available, 240
Bretylol, 240. *See also* Bretylium
Brevibloc, 150, 240. *See also* Esmolol
Brevicon, 665*t*
Brevital, 423. *See also* Methohexital
Bricanyl, 340. *See also* Terbutaline
Brimonidine
for glaucoma, 132, 149*t*
preparations available, 133
Bromide, for seizures, **403**
Bromocriptine, **455–456**, **614–615**
for hyperprolactinemia, 282, 614
for lactation suppression, 282, 614
for parkinsonism, **455–456**
preparations available, 462, 617
receptors affected by, 279*t*, 280
structure of, 279*t*
Bromphen, 283. *See also* Brompheniramine
Brompheniramine, 267*t*
in OTC preparations, efficacy of, 1033*t*
OTC status of, 1031*t*
preparations available, 283
Bronchial glands, direct-acting cholinomimetics affecting, 94*t*
Bronchial hyperreactivity, in asthma, 326–328, 327*i*, 328*i*
Bronchial/bronchiolar smooth muscle
antimuscarinic agents affecting, 109
autonomic activity/drugs affecting, 83*t*
beta-receptor blocking drugs affecting, 143
cytochrome P450-derived metabolites affecting, 310–311

direct-acting cholinomimetics affecting, 94*t*, 96
histamine affecting, 264
lipoxygenase metabolites affecting, 310–311
prostaglandins affecting, 309, 315
sympathomimetic agents affecting, 125, 333
thromboxanes affecting, 309, 315
Bronchoconstriction
in asthma, 325–328, 327*i*, 328*i*
eicosanoids in, 315
histamine-mediated, 264
Bronchodilation
antimuscarinic agents affecting, 109
drugs causing, **325–342**. *See also specific type*
basic pharmacology of, **328–338**
clinical pharmacology of, **338**
preparations available, 340
methylxanthines causing, 332
muscarinic antagonists causing, 335–336, 335*i*
nitric oxide for, 322
prostaglandins for, 315
sympathomimetics causing, 333–335
Bronchogenic carcinoma, **911**
Bronkephrine (ethylnorepinephrine), 340
Broth dilution susceptibility testing, 817
Brucella (brucellosis), empiric antimicrobial therapy and, 814*t*
streptomycin for, 755
Brugia
malayi, drugs for infection with, 863*t*
diethylcarbamazine, 866
adverse reactions and, 867
ivermectin, 868
timori, drugs for infection with, diethylcarbamazine, 866
Bucindolol, 145
for heart failure, 210
Bucladin (buclizine), 283
Buclizine, preparations available, 283
Budesonide, for asthma, 336
Bufadienolides, 201
Buformin, 699–700, 700*t*
Bulking laxatives, **1023–1024**
Bumetanide, 249, 249*i*
clinical indications/dosage of, 250*t*
contraindications to, 251
preparations available, 259
Bumex, 259. *See also* Bumetanide
Buparvaquinone, mitochondrial electron transporter affected by, 834
Bupivacaine
cardiotoxicity of, 432
ionization constant of, 6*t*
preparations available, 432
properties of, 426*t*
structure of, 426*t*
Buprenex, 501*t*, 513. *See also* Buprenorphine
Buprenorphine, 512
pharmacokinetics of, 501*t*
preparations available, 513
receptor subtype activity of, 502*t*

Bupropion, 484, 485*i*
  adverse effects of, 493*t*
  biogenic amine neurotransmitters affected by, 487
  dosages of, 491*t*
    for acute episode, 491
  effects of, 489*t*
  pharmacokinetics of, 488*t*
  preparations available, 494
Burimamide, 270
  history of development of, 63*t*
Burkholderia cepacia, empiric antimicrobial therapy and, 814*t*
Burns, neuromuscular blockade affected by, 444–445
BuSpar, 366*t*, 369. *See also* Buspirone
Buspirone, 276, 363–364
  for alcoholism, 381
  dosages of, 366*t*
  preparations available, 369
Busulfan, 886*i*, 890*t*
  fetus affected by, 983*t*
Butabarbital, preparations available, 369
Butamben picrate, preparations available, 432
Butesin Picrate (butamben picrate), 432
Butisol (butabarbital), 369
Butoconazole, OTC status of, 1032*t*
Butorphanol, 512
  pharmacokinetics of, 501*t*
  preparations available, 513
  structure of, 499*i*
Butoxamine, 138*t*, 146
Butyrophenones, 465, 466*i*, 468*t*
  advantages and disadvantages of, 471*t*
  for Huntington's disease, 460
Butyrylcholinesterase
  local anesthetics metabolized by, 427
  succinylcholine metabolized by, 439
BV-araU (sorivudine), **794**
BZ₁ receptor, 359, 360, 364
BZ₂ receptor, 359, 360

C6 (hexamethonium), 114, 114*i*
C fibers, local anesthetics affecting, 429, 429*t*
C-peptide (connecting peptide), 686, 686*i*
C-type natriuretic peptide (CNP), 296–297, 296*i*
Cabergoline, 615. *See also* Bromocriptine
Cafergot, 284. *See also* Ergotamine
Caffeine
  abuse of, 521
  for asthma, 330–333
  in breast milk, 987*t*
  chemistry and pharmacology of, 521, 522*i*
  with ergotamine, for migraine, 278
  in OTC preparations, hidden, 1038*t*
  structure of, 330*i*, 522*i*
Cal-Sup, 721. *See also* Calcium
Calan, 175, 194, 240. *See also* Verapamil
Calcifediol (25-hydroxyvitamin D), 707–709, 708*i*, 709*t*. *See also* Vitamin D

  in chronic renal failure, 717
  for intestinal osteodystrophy, 717
  preparations available, 721
Calciferol, 721. *See also* Ergocalciferol
Calcijex, 721. *See also* Calcitriol
Calcimar, 713, 721. *See also* Calcitonin
Calciparine, 561. *See also* Heparin
Calcipotriene, **1008**
Calcitonin, **710**
  in bone mineral homeostasis, 710
  for hypercalcemia, 713
  for osteoporosis, 718, 718*i*
  for Paget's disease, 720
  preparations available, 721
  salmon for hypercalcemia, 713
      preparations available, 721
Calcitonin gene-related peptide (CGRP), 77*t*, **300–301**
Calcitriol (1,25-dihydroxyvitamin D), 707–709, 708*i*, 709*t*. *See also* Vitamin D
  in chronic renal failure, 716–717
  for hypocalcemia, 715
  for intestinal osteodystrophy, 717
  for osteoporosis, 718
  preparations available, 721
Calcium
  abnormal serum levels of, **713–715**.
      See also Hypercalcemia;
      Hypocalcemia
  in acetylcholine release, 76–77
  bone mineral homeostasis and, 706, 707*i*
  in cardiac conduction, 216–219
  in cardiac contractility, 197–198, 198*i*
  as clotting factor, 549*t*
  digitalis interactions and, 205
  for hypocalcemia, 715
  intracellular
    local anesthetic action affected by, 428
    vascular tone affected by, 180, 181*i*
  preparations available, 721
  as second messenger, 24–26, 26*i*
Calcium carbonate, in antacids, 1018*t*
Calcium channel blockers
  for angina, 179, 180, 180*i*, **186–191**, 193*t*
  for arrhythmias, **236**, 240
  for asthma, 337–338
  chemistry of, 187, 188*i*
  clinical properties of, 190*t*
  clinical uses of, 191
  in heart failure, 210
  for hypertension, **169**
  interactions of, 1064*t*
  mechanism of action of, 187, 191
  organ system effects of, 187–190
  pharmacodynamics of, 187–190
  pharmacokinetics of, 187, 189*t*
  preparations available, 175, 194, 240
  toxicity of, 190–191, 190*t*
  vascular selectivity of, 190*t*
Calcium channels
  antiepileptic drugs affecting, 387
  cardiac, 219

  in CNS, 344
  properties of, 186, 187*t*
Calcium Sodium Versenate, 966. *See also* Edetate calcium disodium
Calderol, 721. *See also* Calcifediol
cAMP (cyclic AMP)
  in alpha₂ receptor activation, 121, 122*i*
  in muscarinic agonist binding, 94
  as second messenger, 23–24, 26*i*
    G proteins and, 21, 22
  vascular tone affected by, 181, 181*i*
Camphechlor (toxaphene), 950–951, 950*t*
Campothecins, **895**
Camptosar, 894*t*. *See also* Irinotecan
Campylobacter jejuni, empiric antimicrobial therapy and, 814*t*
Cancer. *See also specific type or organ or structure affected*
  as cellular disease, **881–882**
  chronic alcoholic consumption affecting risk of, 378
  drugs for, **881–915**. *See also specific agent and* Cancer chemotherapy
  estrogen therapy and, 660
  inhaled anesthetics causing, 418
  oral contraceptive use and, 670
  treatment modalities for, **882**
Cancer chemotherapy, **881–915**. *See also specific agent*
  adjuvant, 904–905
  basic pharmacology of, **884–902**
  cell cycle kinetics and, **883–884**, 884*i*, 884*t*
  clinical pharmacology of, **902–913**
  drug development and, **882**
  evaluation of tumor response to, **912–913**
  immunosuppressive therapy and, **924–925**
  investigational agents in, **902**
  myeloid growth factor treatment after, 545
  neoplastic cell burden and, **882–883**, 883*i*
  resistance to cytotoxic drugs and, 883–884, 885*i*
  second malignancies and, **913**
Cancer immunotherapy, **936**
Candida (candidiasis)
  empiric antimicrobial therapy and, 815*t*
  vulvovaginal, topical azoles for, 786, 1002
Cannabidiol (CBD), 526, 527*i*
Cannabinoids (cannabis), 526–528
  antiemetic actions of, 528, 1022
  structure of, 527*i*
Cannabinol (CBN), 527, 527*i*
Cantharidin, **1012–1013**
Cantil, 116, 1027. *See also* Mepenzolate
Capacity-limited elimination, 39
Capacity-limited protein binding, drug concentration affected by, 47
Capastat, 778. *See also* Capreomycin

Capillaria phillippinensis (intestinal capillariasis), drugs for infection with, 863*t*
  albendazole, 865
  mebendazole, 870
  thiabendazole, 877
Capoten, 175, 213. *See also* Captopril
Capreomycin, 775
  preparations available, 778
  for tuberculosis, 771*t*, 775
Captopril, 291*i*, 293
  for heart failure, 210, 210*t*
  for hypertension, 170, 171*i*
  pharmacokinetic/pharmacodynamic parameters of, 36*t*, 170
  preparations available, 175, 213
Carafate, 1027. *See also* Sucralfate
Carbachol
  for glaucoma, 149*t*
  molecular structure of, 92*i*
  preparations available, 103
  properties of, 93*t*
Carbamate insecticides, 952, 952*t*, 972*t*
Carbamates, 97, 97*i*
  absorption/distribution/metabolism of, 97–98
  mechanism of action of, 99
  toxicity of, 102
Carbamazepine, 391–393, 392*i*
  action potentials affected by, 387, 389*i*, 392
  effective/toxic plasma levels of, 405*t*
  fetus affected by, 983*t*
  interactions of, 1064*t*
  as mood-stabilizer, 475, 479
  pharmacokinetic/pharmacodynamic parameters of, 36*t*, 392–393
  preparations available, 407, 480
Carbamic acid, molecular structure of, 92*i*
Carbapenems, 737
  dosing guidelines for, 730*i*
  preparations available, 741
  structure of, 725*i*
Carbaryl (carbaril), 97, 97*i*, 952*t*
Carbenicillin, 731
  half-life of, aging affecting, 992*i*
  preparations available, 740
Carbenicillin indanyl sodium, 731
Carbenoxolone, for acid-peptic disease, 1021
Carbidopa, 451*i*
  with levodopa, 452*i*, 453
    preparations available, 462
  preparations available, 462
Carbimazole, 626, 626*i*
Carbinoxamine, 267*t*
  preparations available, 283
Carbocaine, 426*t*, 432. *See also* Mepivacaine
Carbofuran, 952*t*
Carbohydrate metabolism
  beta-receptor blocking drugs affecting, 143–145
  oral contraceptives affecting, 667
  progesterone affecting, 662

Carbohydrate tolerance, impaired, thiazides causing, 251–252
β-Carbolines, 360
Carbon monoxide, 947–948
  threshold limit values for, 948*t*
Carbon tetrachloride, threshold limit values for, 948*t*
Carbonic anhydrase inhibitors, 246–249
  urinary electrolyte patterns affected by, 257*t*
Carbonium ion, in alkylating drug mechanism of action, 885
Carbonyl reductions, 54*t*
Carboplatin, 890*t*
Carboprost, 312*i*
  for abortions, 313
  preparations available, 317
Carboxypenicillins, 731
Carcinoembryonic antigen, gastrointestinal cancer elaborating, 910
Carcinogenicity. *See also* Cancer
  of inhaled anesthetics, 418
  of metronidazole, 858
Carcinoid, 904*i*
Cardene, 175, 194. *See also* Nicardipine
Cardenolides, 200, 201. *See also* Cardiac glycosides
Cardiac arrest. *See also* Myocardial infarction
  sympathomimetics for, 131
Cardiac contractility
  autonomic activity/drugs affecting, 83*t*
  beta-receptor blocking drugs affecting, 149
  control of, 197–199, 197*i*
  digitalis glycosides affecting, 203, 203*i*
  ethanol affecting, 374
  histamine affecting, 264
  in low output failure, 200
Cardiac glycosides
  administration and dosage of, 208
  for arrhythmias, 208
  basic pharmacology of, 200–205
  chemistry of, 200–201, 201*i*
  clinical pharmacology of, 207–209
  endogenous, 202
  for heart failure, 207–209
  interactions of, 205, 208, 1065–1066*t*
  parasympathomimetic effects of, 204
  pharmacodynamics of, 202–205
  pharmacokinetics of, 201–202, 201*t*
  preparations available, 213
  toxicity of, 203–204, 204*i*, 208–209
    arrhythmias caused by, 204, 204*i*, 209
    effects of outside heart, 205
Cardiac muscle cells
  calcium channel blockers affecting, 188–189
  local anesthetics affecting, 430
Cardiac output, H_2 receptor antagonists affecting, 271
Cardiac performance, pathophysiology of, 199–200
Cardiac rhythm, normal, electrophysiology of, 216–220, 217*i*, 221*i*

Cardiac surgery, antimicrobial prophylaxis and, 824*t*
Cardiac toxicity
  of lithium, 478
  of thioridazine, 474
Cardiogenic shock
  after myocardial infarction, 211*t*, 212
  sympathomimetics for, 131
Cardiomyopathy, obstructive, beta-receptor blocking drugs for, 146
Cardioquin, 240. *See also* Quinidine
Cardiovascular disease. *See also* Heart disease
  antimuscarinic agents for, 111
  aspirin for prevention of, 557
  beta-receptor blocking drugs for, 146
  drug metabolism and, 60*t*
  eicosanoids in, 314
  estrogen replacement therapy affecting, 658
  sympathomimetics for, 130–131
Cardiovascular drugs, in elderly, 994–995
Cardiovascular system. *See also* Cardiovascular disease
  alpha-receptor antagonists affecting, 136–138, 138*i*
  antimuscarinic agents affecting, 108–109
  antipsychotic drugs affecting, 470
  autonomic control of, 82–84, 84*i*
  beta-receptor blocking drugs affecting, 142–143, 144*i*
  bromocriptine affecting, 455
  cholinesterase inhibitors affecting, 99–100
  direct-acting cholinomimetics affecting, 94–95, 94*t*
  drugs acting in, in elderly, 994–995
  eicosanoid metabolites affecting, 310
  ethanol affecting
    acute consumption, 374
    chronic consumption, 376–377
  ganglion-blocking drugs affecting, 115
  H_2 receptor antagonists affecting, 271
  histamine affecting, 263–264, 263*i*
  inhaled anesthetics affecting, 416–417
  kinins affecting, 294
  levodopa affecting, 453
  lipoxygenase metabolites affecting, 310
  local anesthetic toxicity and, 430–431
  methylxanthines affecting, 331
  neuromuscular blocking drugs affecting, 443–444, 443*t*
  opioid analgesics affecting, 505–506
  oral contraceptives affecting, 667
  in poisoning, 970
  prostaglandins affecting, 314–315
  sedative-hypnotics affecting, 362
  serotonin affecting, 274–275
  sympathomimetic agents affecting, 124–126, 125*t*
  thyroid hormones affecting, 625*t*

Cardizem, 175, 194, 240. *See also* Diltiazem
Cardura, 150, 175. *See also* Doxazosin
Carisoprodol
  for muscle spasm, 448
  preparations available, 448
Carmustine (BCNU), 886*i*, **888**, 890*t*
Carprofen, **588**
Carrier molecules, drug permeation by, 5
Carteolol, 138*t*, 145, **165**
  for glaucoma, 149*t*
  for hypertension, **165**
  preparations available, 150, 174
  properties of, 144*t*
Cartrol, 150, 174. *See also* Carteolol
Carvedilol, 138*t*, 145, **165**
  enantiomers of, dissociation constants of, 3, 3*t*
  for heart failure, 146, 210
  for hypertension, **165**
  preparations available, 150, 174
  properties of, 144*t*
Cascara
  laxative effect of, 1023
  preparations available, 1027
Casodex, 680. *See also* Bicalutamide
Castor oil, 1023
  preparations available, 1027
Catapres, 175. *See also* Clonidine
Catechol, 123*i*
Catecholamines, 127–128. *See also specific type and* Sympathomimetics
  biosynthesis of, 78–79, 79*i*
  as central neurotransmitters, 352
  metabolism of, 80*i*
  receptors for, 81–82, 81*i*
  second messenger for, 22*t*
Catechol-*O*-methyltransferase inhibitors, for parkinsonism, **456**
Cathartics
  for poisoned patient, 976, 976*t*
  saline, 1023–1024
Cathinone, 521
Caudal block, 431*i*
Caverject, 317. *See also* Alprostadil
CBD (cannabidiol), 526, 527*i*
CBG (corticosteroid-binding globulin), 635
CBN (cannabinol), 527, 527*i*
CCK (cholecystokinin), as neurotransmitter, 77*t*
CCNS (cell cycle-nonspecific agents), 883, 884*t*
CCNU (lomustine), 886*i*, **888**, 890*t*
CCS (cell cycle-specific agents), 883, 884*t*
CD2, 917
CD4 T cells, 917, 919*i*
CD8 T cells, 917, 919*i*
CEA (carcinoembryonic antigen), gastrointestinal cancer elaborating, 910
Ceclor, 741. *See also* Cefaclor
Cefaclor, 734
  preparations available, 741
Cefadroxil, 732–734
  dosing guidelines for, 730*t*
  preparations available, 740

Cefadyl, 741. *See also* Cephapirin
Cefamandole, 733*i*, 734
  half-life of, aging affecting, 992*i*
  preparations available, 741
Cefazolin, 732–734, 733*i*
  dosing guidelines for, 730*t*
  half-life of, aging affecting, 992*i*
  preparations available, 741
Cefepime, 735
  preparations available, 741
Cefibuten, 734–735
Cefixime, 734–735
  preparations available, 741
Cefizox, 741. *See also* Ceftizoxime
Cefmetazole, 734
  preparations available, 741
Cefobid, 741. *See also* Cefoperazone
Cefonicid, 734
  preparations available, 741
Cefoperazone, 733*i*, 734–735
  preparations available, 741
Ceforanide, 734
Cefotan, 741. *See also* Cefotetan
Cefotaxime, 733*i*, 734–735
  CSF penetration by, 820*t*
  dosing guidelines for, 730*t*
  preparations available, 741
Cefotetan, 734
  dosing guidelines for, 730*t*
  preparations available, 741
Cefoxitin, 733*i*, 734
  dosing guidelines for, 730*t*
  preparations available, 741
Cefpodoxime, 734–735
  preparations available, 741
Cefprozil, 734
  preparations available, 741
Ceftazidime, 734–735
  CSF penetration by, 820*t*
  dosing guidelines for, 730*t*
  preparations available, 741
Ceftin, 741. *See also* Cefuroxime
Ceftizoxime, 734–735
  preparations available, 741
Ceftriaxone, 733*i*, 734–735
  CSF penetration by, 820*t*
  dosing guidelines for, 730*t*
  preparations available, 741
Cefuroxime, 734
  axetil, 734
  dosing guidelines for, 730*t*
  CSF penetration by, 820*t*
  dosing guidelines for, 730*t*
  preparations available, 741
Cefzil, 741. *See also* Cefprozil
Cel-U-Jec, 650. *See also* Betamethasone
Celestone, 650. *See also* Betamethasone
Celiprolol, 138*t*, 145
  for heart failure, 210
  properties of, 144*t*
Cell cycle kinetics, in cancer chemotherapy, **883–884**, 884*i*, 884*t*
Cell cycle-nonspecific agents (CCNS), 883, 884*t*
Cell cycle-specific agents (CCS), 883, 884*t*
Cell growth, angiotensin II affecting, 289

Cell-mediated immunity, 917, 918–921, 919*i*
Cell wall synthesis, antibiotics interfering with, **724–742**, 727*i*, 728*i*, 729*i*
Cellular hypoxia, in poisoning, 970
Cellulitis, empiric antimicrobial therapy and, 816*t*
Celontin, 407. *See also* Methsuximide
Central integration, autonomic, 82
Central nervous system
  angiotensin II affecting, 289
  antimuscarinic drugs affecting, 106–107
  antipsychotic drugs affecting, 470*t*
  aspirin affecting, 584
  beta-receptor blocking drugs affecting, toxicity and, 148–149
  cholinesterase inhibitors affecting, 99
  depression of, in poisoning, 970
  digitalis toxicity affecting, 205
  direct-acting cholinomimetics affecting, 96
  drugs acting in, **343–353**. *See also specific type*
    cellular organization of brain and, **347–348**
    ion channels and, **344**
    methods for study of, 343–344
    neurotransmitters and, **346–347**, **348–353**, 349–350*t*
    sedative-hypnotics, **354–371**. *See also* Sedative-hypnotic drugs
    sites of action of, **345–346**
    stimulants
      abuse of, **521–524**
      OTC preparations, hidden ingredients in, 1038*t*
    synapse and synaptic potentials and, **344–345**
    use of in elderly, 993
  ergot alkaloids affecting, 278–280
  ethanol affecting
    acute consumption, 373–374
    chronic consumption, 375
  ganglion-blocking drugs affecting, 115
  glucocorticoids affecting, 639
  graded dose-dependent depression of, 354, 355*i*
  H_2 receptor antagonist side effects and, 272
  lead toxicity and, 961
  local anesthetic toxicity and, 430
  methylxanthines affecting, 331
  nitric oxide affecting, **323**
  opioid analgesics affecting, 504–505
  oral contraceptives affecting, 666–667
  in poisoned patient, 971–973
  prostaglandins affecting, 310
  sympathomimetic agents affecting, 127
  thyroid hormones affecting, 625*t*
Central nervous system disorders
  antimuscarinic agents for, 110–112
  sympathomimetics for, 133

Central nervous system drugs, **343–353**. *See also specific type*
cellular organization of brain and, **347–348**
ion channels and, **344**
methods for study of, 343–344
neurotransmitters and, **346–347**, **348–353**, 349–350*t*
sedative-hypnotics, **354–371**. *See also* Sedative-hypnotic drugs
sites of action of, **345–346**
stimulants
abuse of, **521–524**
OTC preparations, hidden ingredients in, 1038*t*
synapse and synaptic potentials and, **344–345**
use of in elderly, 993
Centrax, 366*t*, 369. *See also* Prazepam
Cephalexin, 732–734, 733*i*
dosing guidelines for, 730*t*
pharmacokinetic/pharmacodynamic parameters of, 36*t*
preparations available, 741
Cephalosporins, **732–736**
adverse effects of, 735–736
first-generation, **732–734**, 733*i*
dosing guidelines for, 730*i*
preparations available, 740–741
fourth-generation, **735**
preparations available, 741
preparations available, 740–741
second-generation, 733*i*, **734**
dosing guidelines for, 730*i*
preparations available, 741
structures of, 725*i*, 732, 733*i*
third-generation, 733*i*, **734–735**
dosing guidelines for, 730*i*
preparations available, 741
toxicity of, 736
Cephalothin, 732–734, 733*i*
pharmacokinetic/pharmacodynamic parameters of, 36*t*
preparations available, 741
Cephapirin, 732–734, 733*i*
preparations available, 741
Cephradine, 732–734, 733*i*
dosing guidelines for, 730*t*
half-life of, aging affecting, 992*i*
preparations available, 741
Cephulac, 1028. *See also* Lactulose
Cerebral infarct, after subarachnoid hemorrhage, nimodipine for, 189
Cerebral insufficiency, senile, dihydroergotoxine for, 282
Cerebral vasospasm, nimodipine for, 189
Cerebrospinal fluid, antimicrobial drug concentration in, 819, 820*t*
Cerebrovascular disease, oral contraceptive use and, 669
Cerebyx, 407. *See also* Fosphenytoin
Cerubidine, 894*t*. *See also* Daunorubicin
Cervical cancer, 903*t*
Cervidil, 317. *See also* Prostaglandin E$_2$
Cesarean section, antimicrobial prophylaxis and, 824*t*

Cestodes, drugs for infection with, 863–864*t*
Cetirizine, 267*t*, 268*t*
preparations available, 283
cGMP (cyclic GMP)
in muscarinic agonist binding, 93–94
vascular tone affected by, angina management and, 180, 181, 181*i*
CGP42112A, angiotensin receptor affinity for, 289
CGRP (calcitonin gene-related peptide) 77*t*, **300–301**
Charcoal, activated, for poisoned patient, 975–976
Chelators, **956–959**. *See also specific type*
preparations available, 966
Chemet, 966. *See also* Succimer
Chemical antagonists, 16. *See also* Antagonists
Chemical mixtures, exposure to, 946
Chemical synapses, 344–345
as sites of CNS drug action, 345–346, 345*i*
Chemical/hormonal contraception
in men, **679**
in women, 665*t*, **666–671**. *See also* Oral contraceptives
Chemoprophylaxis, **822–824**, 824*t*, 824–825*t*
Chemotherapy, cancer, **881–915**. *See also specific agent and* Cancer chemotherapy
Chenix, 1028. *See also* Chenodiol
Chenodiol, 1024–1025
preparations available, 1028
Children, drug therapy in, **982–985**
dosage amounts and, **987–988**
dosage forms and compliance and, **985–986**
Chirality (stereoisomerism), 3
Chlamydia
pneumoniae, empiric antimicrobial therapy and, 815*t*
psittaci, empiric antimicrobial therapy and, 815*t*
trachomatis, empiric antimicrobial therapy and, 815*t*
Chlophedianol, OTC status of, 1031*t*
Chlor-Trimeton, 267*t*, 283. *See also* Chlorpheniramine
Chloral hydrate, 357*i*, 364
in breast milk, 987*t*
dosages of, 366*t*
overdose of, 973*t*
preparations available, 369
Chlorambucil, 886*i*, 890*t*
for chronic lymphocytic leukemia, 906
fetus affected by, 983*t*
Chloramine T, antimicrobial effects of, 807
Chloramphenicol, **743–745**, 743*i*
in breast milk, 987*t*
drug metabolism inhibited by, 60*t*
interactions of, 745

pharmacokinetic/pharmacodynamic parameters of, 36*t*, 743
preparations available, 751
protein synthesis affected by, 743, 744, 744*i*
Chlorcyclizine, drug metabolism induced by, 59*t*
Chlordane, 950*t*
Chlordiazepoxide, 356*i*
for alcohol withdrawal syndrome, 380
biotransformation of, 357, 357*i*
distribution of, 355
dosages of, 366*t*
for drug withdrawal, 366
ionization constant of, 6*t*
pharmacokinetic/pharmacodynamic parameters of, 36*t*, 358*t*
preparations available, 369
Chlorfenvinphos, 951*t*
Chlorhexidine
antimicrobial effects of, 805*t*, **806**
preparations available, 810
Chloride channels
cromolyn and nedocromil affecting, 328
GABA-BDZ receptor, 359, 359*i*, 361
antiepileptic drugs affecting, 387
Chlorinated hydrocarbon insecticides, **950–951**, 950*t*
Chlorine, antimicrobial effects of, 805*t*, **807**
Chlorine dioxide, antimicrobial effects of, 807
p-Chloroamphetamine, serotonin affected by, 273, 277
Chloroform
abuse of, 529
threshold limit values for, 948*t*
toxicity of, 529
Chloroguanide (proguanil), 839*i*, **845–846**
for malaria chemoprophylaxis, 840*t*, 845
preparations available, 859
Chlorohist, 134. *See also* Xylometazoline
Chloromycetin, 751. *See also* Chloramphenicol
Chlorophenothane (DDT), 950–951, 950*t*, 953*i*
p-Chlorophenylalanine, serotonin affected by, 273, 277
Chloroprocaine, preparations available, 432
Chloroquine, 839*i*, **841–843**
for amebiasis, 842, 850, 851*t*, **852**
antiparasitic actions of, 836*t*, 842
for autoimmune disorders, 842
in inflammation, **591**
ionization constant of, 6*t*
for malaria chemoprophylaxis, 840*t*, 842
for malaria treatment, 841*t*, 842
pharmacokinetic/pharmacodynamic parameters of, 36*t*, 841–842
preparations available, 858

with primaquine, preparations available, 858
resistance to, 842
Chlorothiazide
in breast milk, 987*t*
dosages of, 252*t*
ionization constant of, 6*t*
preparations available, 259
structure of, 248*i*
Chlorotrianisene, 656, 656*i*, 657*t*
preparations available, 680
Chlorphenesin
for muscle spasm, 448
preparations available, 448
Chlorpheniramine, 267*t*
ionization constant of, 6*t*
in OTC preparations, efficacy of, 1033*t*
OTC status of, 1031*t*
preparations available, 283
structure of, 266*i*
Chlorphenoxy herbicides, **952–953**, 953*i*
Chlorpromazine, 466*i*, 468*t*
advantages and disadvantages of, 471*t*
in breast milk, 987*t*
dose relationships of, 472*t*
in elderly, 993
ionization constant of, 6*t*
ocular complications of therapy with, 474
pharmacologic effects of, 466–468
preparations available, 480
receptor binding by, 468, 469
seizures caused by, 473
Chlorpropamide, 697*t*, **698**
fetus affected by, 983*t*
ionization constant of, 6*t*
pharmacokinetic/pharmacodynamic parameters of, 36*t*
preparations available, 703
Chlorprothixene, preparations available, 480
Chlortetracycline, 745, 745*i*
pharmacokinetics of, 745–746
Chlorthalidone
dosages of, 252*t*
half-life of, aging affecting, 992*i*
pharmacokinetics of, 251
preparations available, 259
structure of, 252*i*
Chlorzoxazone
for muscle spasm, 448
preparations available, 448
Cholecalciferol (vitamin D₃), 707, 708*i*, 709*t*. See also Vitamin D
preparations available, 721
Cholecystokinin, as neurotransmitter, 77*t*
Choledyl (oxtriphylline), 340
Cholera
antimicrobial prophylaxis and, 824*t*
vaccine for, 1052*t*
Cholestasis, estrogen therapy and, 660
Cholesterol
amphotericin B binding and, 780
biosynthesis of, 565*i*
lipoproteins transporting, 563
Cholesteryl esters, 563

Cholestyramine, 572–573
OTC status of, 1031*t*
preparations available, 576
Choline esters, 92, 92*i*
properties of, 92, 93*t*
toxicity of, 102
Choline salicylate, preparations available, 599
Choline theophyllinate (oxtriphylline), 340
Cholinergic fibers, 74
Cholinergic neurons, in Huntington's disease, 450–451, 451*i*
Cholinergic poisoning, antimuscarinic agents for, 112
Cholinergic transmission, 75–77, 75*i*
cotransmitters in, 80–81
Cholinesterase inhibitors, 91, **96–100**. See also Indirect-acting cholinomimetics
neuromuscular blockade reversed by, 445
preparations available, 103
toxicity of, 102
antimuscarinic therapy for overdose and, 112
cholinesterase regenerator compounds for overdose and, 113
Cholinesterase regenerator compounds, 112–113
preparations available, 116
Cholinoceptors (cholinergic receptors), 77, 81, 81*t*, 90, 91*t*
drugs activating, **90–104**. See also Cholinomimetics
drugs blocking, **105–117**. See also Antimuscarinic agents; Antinicotinic agents
Cholinomimetics, **90–104**. See also specific agent
clinical pharmacology of, **100–102**
direct-acting, 91, 91*i*, **92–96**, 103
for glaucoma, 100, 149*t*
indirect-acting, 91–92, 91*i*, **96–100**, 103
mode of action of, **91–92**
overdoses of, 972*t*
preparations available, 103
spectrum of action of, **90–91**
toxicity of, 102, 972*t*
"CHOP" regimen, for non-Hodgkin's lymphoma, 908
Chorea, 450, 460. See also Huntington's disease
Choriocarcinoma, 903*t*, **909–910**
Chorionic gonadotropin, 612, **613–614**
preparations available, 617
second messenger for, 22*t*
Chorthalidone, oral anticoagulant interactions and, 554
Christmas disease, 559
factor IX for, 559*t*, 560
Christmas factor (factor IX/plasma thromboplastin component), 549*t*
deficiency of, 559, 559*t*, 560
therapeutic, 559*t*, 560
preparations available, 561

Chronic exposure, to chemicals, 946
Chronic leukemias, **906**
lymphocytic, 903*t*, **906**
passive immunization and, 1056*t*
myelogenous, 903*t*, **906**
Chronic obstructive pulmonary disease, antimuscarinic agents for, 109, 111
Chronic renal failure, bone mineral homeostasis and, **716–717**
Chronulac, 1028. See also Lactulose
Chylomicronemia, primary, 566–567, 567*t*
Chylomicrons, 565*t*
synthesis and catabolism of, 564
Ciamexon, 935–936
Ciclopirox olamine, **1002**
Cidofovir, 790*i*, 792*t*, **793**
Cigarette smoking
aids for cessation of, OTC preparations, efficacy of, 1035*t*
coronary disease and, 564
drug metabolism affected by, 59
fetus affected by, 983*t*
Ciglitazone, 701
Ciliary muscle
antimuscarinic agents affecting, 108, 111
autonomic activity/drugs affecting, 83*t*, 148
direct-acting cholinomimetics affecting, 94, 94*t*
ganglion-blocking drugs affecting, 115
Cimetidine, 270*t*, 1019–1020
clinical uses of, 272, 1020
drug metabolism inhibited by, 60*t*
history of development of, 63*t*
immunomodulating effect of, 936
interactions of, 273, 1064–1065*t*
organ system effects of, 271
in OTC preparations, efficacy of, 1033*t*
OTC status of, 1031*t*
pharmacokinetic/pharmacodynamic parameters of, 36*t*, 270*t*
preparations available, 284, 1026
toxicity of, 272
Cinchonism, 848
Cinobac, 768. See also Cinoxacin
Cinoxacin, 765, **767**
preparations available, 768
Cipro, 768. See also Ciprofloxacin
Ciprofloxacin, 765, 765*i*, 776
CSF penetration by, 820*t*
ionization constant of, 6*t*
for MAC infections, 777
pharmacokinetic/pharmacodynamic parameters of, 36*t*, 766, 766*t*
preparations available, 768
for tuberculosis, 771*t*, 776
Circular muscle, autonomic activity/drugs affecting, 83*t*
Circulation, in poisoned patient, 970
"Circus movement," 224
Cirrhosis, diuretics for, **258**

13-*Cis*-retinoic acid (isotretinoin)
   for acne, **1007**
   in cancer chemotherapy, 902
   fetus affected by, 983*t*
Cisapride, 276
   gastrointestinal motility affected by, 1021–1022
   interactions of, 1065*t*
   preparations available, 284, 1027
Cisatracurium, 438*t*
   effects of, 443*t*
   pharmacokinetics of, 438*t*, 439
   preparations available, 448
Cisplatin, **888–889**, 890*t*
Citanest, 426*t*, 433. *See also* Prilocaine
Citracal, 721. *See also* Calcium
Citrobacter, empiric antimicrobial therapy and, 814*t*
Citrovorum factor (leucovorin)
   with methotrexate, 891
   with pyrimethamine, 845–846
Cladribine, 891*t*, **892**
Claforan, 741. *See also* Cefotaxime
Clarithromycin, 747*i*, **749**
   for MAC infections, 777
   preparations available, 751
Claritin, 267*t*, 283. *See also* Loratadine
Claviceps purpurea, ergot alkaloids produced by, 277
Clavulanic acid, 731, **736–737**, 736*i*
Clearance, 34, 35–40
   aging affecting, 990, 991*t*
   diseases affecting, drug metabolism and, 60, 60*t*
   drug concentration and, 47
      initial predictions, 48
      revising predictions, 48–49
   in infants and children, 984–985
   poisoning and, 968–969
   therapeutic drug monitoring and, 46
Clemastine
   in OTC preparations, efficacy of, 1033*t*
   OTC status of, 1031*t*
   preparations available, 283
Cleocin, 751. *See also* Clindamycin
Clidinium
   for gastrointestinal and genitourinary conditions, 112*t*
   preparations available, 115, 1027
Clinafloxacin, 765
Clindamycin, **749–750**, 749*i*
   for malaria treatment, 841*t*
   preparations available, 751
   protein synthesis affected by, 744, 744*i*
   topical, for acne, 1001
Clinical trials, in new drug evaluation, 63*i*, **66–72**
   confounding factors in, 66–67
   evaluation of, 70–72
Clinoril, 599. *See also* Sulindac
Clioquinol, subacute myelo-optic neuropathy caused by, 854
Clistin, 267*t*, 283. *See also* Carbinoxamine
Clobazam, for seizures, 402

Clofazimine, 776–777
   for leprosy, **778**
   preparations available, 779
   for tuberculosis, 771*t*, 776–777
Clofibrate, 571*i*, 572
Clomid, 680. *See also* Clomiphene
Clomiphene, **671**, **673–674**
   preparations available, 680
Clomipramine, 485*i*
   dosages of, 491*t*
   effects of, 489*t*
   fetus affected by, 983*t*
   pharmacokinetics of, 488*t*
   preparations available, 494
Clonazepam
   as mood-stabilizer, 475
   preparations available, 369, 407
   for seizures, 362, 402, 407
Clonidine, 133, 158, 159, 159*i*, **160**
   for anxiety, 365
   for hypertension, 158, 159, 159*i*, **160**
   ionization constant of, 6*t*
   pharmacokinetic/pharmacodynamic parameters of, 36*t*
   preparations available, 175
   sedative effects of, 355
Clonogenic capability, of tumor stem cells, 881
Clonorchis sinensis (clonorchiasis/liver fluke), drugs for infection with, 863*t*
   albendazole for, 865
   praziquantel, 874
Clorazepate
   absorption of, 355
   for alcohol withdrawal syndrome, 380, 383
   biotransformation of, 355, 357, 357*i*
   dosages of, 366*t*
   pharmacokinetics, of, 358*t*
   preparations available, 369, 383, 407
   for seizures, 402, 407
Clorpactin (oxychlorosene), 810
Closed-angle glaucoma. *See also* Glaucoma
   treatment of, 87
      cholinomimetics for, 100
Closed-loop systems, for insulin administration, 693
Clostridium difficile
   antibiotic-associated colitis caused by, clindamycin and, 750
   empiric antimicrobial therapy and, 814*t*
   empiric antimicrobial therapy and, 814*t*
Clotrimazole, 784*i*
   in OTC preparations, efficacy of, 1034*t*
   OTC status of, 1032*t*
   preparations available, 786
   topical, 786, 1002
Clotrimazole-betamethasone dipropionate cream, 1002
Clotting, 547–548
   drugs for disorders of, **547–562**. *See also specific type*
   estrogens affecting, 657

   mechanisms of, **547–548**
   oral contraceptives affecting, 667
   regulation of, 548, 550*i*
Clotting factors (coagulation factors), 547, 549*t*. *See also specific type*
   deficiencies in, plasma fractions for, **559–560**, 559*t*
Cloxacillin, 729–731
   dosing guidelines for, 730*t*
   preparations available, 740
Clozapine, 467*i*, 468*t*, 472
   advantages and disadvantages of, 471*t*
   agranulocytosis caused by, 474
   dose relationships of, 472, 472*t*
   preparations available, 480
   receptor binding by, 468, 469
   seizures caused by, 473
Clozaril, 471*t*, 472*t*, 480. *See also* Clozapine
CMF regimen, for breast cancer, 908
CMV infections (cytomegalovirus infections)
   cidofovir for, 793
   foscarnet for, 794
   ganciclovir for, 793
   passive immunization for, 1056*t*
CNP (C-type natriuretic peptide), 296–297, 296*i*
CNS (central nervous system)
   angiotensin II affecting, 289
   antimuscarinic drugs affecting, 106–107
   antipsychotic drugs affecting, 470*t*
   aspirin affecting, 584
   beta-receptor blocking drugs affecting, toxicity and, 148–149
   cholinesterase inhibitors affecting, 99
   depression of, in poisoning, 970
   digitalis toxicity affecting, 205
   direct-acting cholinomimetics affecting, 96
   drugs acting in, **343–353**. *See also specific type*
      cellular organization of brain and, **347–348**
      ion channels and, **344**
      methods for study of, 343–344
      neurotransmitters and, **346–347**, **348–353**, 349–350*t*
      sedative-hypnotics, **354–371**. *See also* Sedative-hypnotic drugs
      sites of action of, **345–346**
      stimulants, abuse of, 521–524
      synapse and synaptic potentials and, **344–345**
   use of in elderly, 993
   ergot alkaloids affecting, 278–280
   ethanol affecting
      acute consumption, 373–374
      chronic consumption, 375
   ganglion-blocking drugs affecting, 115
   glucocorticoids affecting, 639
   graded dose-dependent depression of, 354, 355*i*

H$_2$ receptor antagonist side effects and, 272
lead toxicity and, 961
local anesthetic toxicity and, 430
methylxanthines affecting, 331
nitric oxide affecting, **323**
opioid analgesics affecting, 504–505
oral contraceptives affecting, 666–667
in poisoned patient, 971–973
prostaglandins affecting, 310
sympathomimetic agents affecting, 127
thyroid hormones affecting, 625*t*
CNS disorders (central nervous system disorders)
antimuscarinic agents for, 110–112
sympathomimetics for, 133
CNS drugs (central nervous system drugs), **343–353**. *See also specific type*
cellular organization of brain and, **347–348**
ion channels and, **344**
methods for study of, 343–344
neurotransmitters and, **346–347**, **348–353**, 349–350*t*
sedative-hypnotics, **354–371**. *See also* Sedative-hypnotic drugs
sites of action of, **345–346**
stimulants
abuse of, **521–524**
OTC preparations, hidden ingredients in, 1038*t*
synapse and synaptic potentials and, **344–345**
use of in elderly, 993
CO (carbon monoxide), **947–948**
threshold limit values for, 948*t*
Coagulation, 547–548
drugs for disorders of, **547–562**. *See also specific type*
estrogens affecting, 657
mechanisms of, **547–548**
oral contraceptives affecting, 667
regulation of, 548, 550*i*
Coagulation factors (clotting factors), 547, 549*t*. *See also specific type*
deficiencies in, plasma fractions for, **559–560**, 559*t*
Coal tar, for dermatologic therapy, **1009**
Cocaine, 521
abuse of, 522–523, 523*i*
cardiovascular effects of, 432
chemistry and pharmacology of, 521, 522*i*
fetus affected by, 983*t*
ionization constant of, 6*t*
as local anesthetic, 426*t*
overdose of, 972*t*
for pharmacologic hemostasis, 131
preparations available, 432
structure of, 426*t*, 522*i*
sympathomimetic actions of, 129
"Cocaine" babies, 523
Coccidioides immitis, empiric antimicrobial therapy and, 815*t*

Codeine, 511
with acetaminophen, preparations available, 514
with aspirin, preparations available, 514
in breast milk, 987*t*
as cough suppressant, 505, 512
ionization constant of, 6*t*
in opium, 496
in OTC preparations, efficacy of, 1034*t*
overdose of, 972*t*
pharmacokinetics of, 501*t*
preparations available, 513, 514
receptor subtype activity of, 502*t*
structure of, 498*i*
Cogentin, 462. *See also* Benztropine
Colace, 1027–1028. *See also* Docusate
Colchicine, **596–597**, 596*i*
preparations available, 600
"Cold" preparations, OTC
efficacy of, 1033*t*
hidden ingredients in, 1037*t*, 1038*t*, 1039*t*
Colestid, 576. *See also* Colestipol
Colestipol, 572–573
OTC status of, 1031*t*
preparations available, 576
Colitis, ulcerative, drugs used in management of, **1025–1026**
Collecting tubule, transport in/diuretic site of action and, **245–246**, 253, 256*i*
Colloidal bismuth compounds, for acid-peptic disease, 1021
Colon, cancer of, 903*t*, 910–911
Colony-stimulating factors, 543, 543*t*, 544–545, 933–935, 934*t*. *See also specific type*
Colorectal surgery, antimicrobial prophylaxis and, 824*t*
CoLyte
for gut decontamination, 976
preparations available, 1028
Coma
myxedema, 629
sedative-hypnotic drugs producing, 355*i*
Combantrin, 878. *See also* Pyrantel pamoate
Combination therapy
antimicrobial, **821–822**
cancer chemotherapy, in Hodgkin's disease, 907
diuretic, 254*t*, **256**
in hyperlipidemia, **575**
in tuberculosis, 772, 772*t*
Compactin, 573
Compazine, 480, 1027. *See also* Prochlorperazine
Competitive antagonism, 14–15, 14*i*
oral anticoagulant interactions and, 554
Complement, in innate immunity, 916–917, 917*i*
Complete heart block, sympathomimetics for, 131

Complex partial seizure, 403
Compliance/noncompliance, **1045–1046**
in elderly, 996
in pediatric pharmacology, 985–986
Compound 48/80, histamine release caused by, 262
Compound 50-235, as endothelin receptor antagonist, 298, 300*i*
Comprehensive Drug Abuse Prevention and Control Act, 68*t*
COMT (catechol-*O*-methyltransferase) inhibitors, for parkinsonism, **456**
Concentration
anesthetic uptake and distribution affected by, 413–414
in dermatologic pharmacology, 999
in infants and children, 984
interpretation of measurements of, **47–49**
target
dosage regimen design and, **43–45**
therapeutic monitoring and, 46
timing of samples taken for measurement of, 47
Concentration-effect curves, 11, 12*i*
Concentration-response relationships, **11–17**, 34, 35*i*. *See also* Dose-response relationships
Conduction, cardiac, digitalis glycosides affecting, 203–204, 203*i*, 204*i*, 204*t*
Condyloma acuminatum, podophyllum resin for, 1012
Congenital adrenal hyperplasia, 641–642
Congestive heart failure. *See* Heart failure
Conjugation, in biotransformation, 55, 57*t*
Connecting peptide (C-peptide), 686, 686*i*
Conscious sedation, 422
Constipation
laxatives for, **1023–1024**
in OTC preparations
efficacy of, 1035*t*
hidden ingredients and, 1039*t*
preparations available, 1027–1028
opioid analgesics causing, 506
Contraception
chemical/hormonal
in men, **679**
in women, 665*t*, **666–671**. *See also* Oral contraceptives
"morning after," 670, 671*t*
Contractile proteins, sensitivity of to calcium, 197
Contractility, cardiac/myocardial
autonomic activity/drugs affecting, 83*t*
beta-receptor blocking drugs affecting, 149
control of, 197–199, 197*i*
digitalis glycosides affecting, 203, 203*i*
ethanol affecting, 374
histamine affecting, 264
in low output failure, 200
Contrast media, iodinated, **627**

Convulsions. *See* Seizures
COPD (chronic obstructive pulmonary disease), antimuscarinic agents for, 109, 111
Coplanar biphenyls (polychlorinated biphenyls/PCBs), 954
Copper accumulation/poisoning, penicillamine for, 461, 958
Cordarone, 240. *See also* Amiodarone
Coreg, 150. *See also* Carvedilol
Corgard, 150, 174, 194. *See also* Nadolol
Coronary artery/coronary heart disease. *See also* Angina; Heart disease; Myocardial infarction
    alcohol consumption and, 377
    myxedema and, 628–629
    vitamin B$_{12}$ and folic acid in prevention of, 542–543
Coronary blood flow
    determinants of, 180
    nitroglycerin affecting, 183–184
Coronary steal phenomenon, 184
Cortef, 650. *See also* Hydrocortisone
Cortenema, 1027. *See also* Hydrocortisone
Corticosteroid-binding globulin (CBG), 635
Corticosteroids, **336–337, 925**. *See also* Adrenocorticosteroids; Glucocorticoids
    aerosol, preparations available, 340
    for asthma, 315, **336–337, 338–339**, 340
    in dermatologic therapy, 1014*t*
    for drug allergy, 938–939
    eicosanoid synthesis blocked by, 311, 315
    in elderly, 995
    immunosuppressive action of, **925**
    for inflammatory bowel disease, 1026
    receptors for, 18
    topical, **1008–1009**
        dermatologic disorders sensitive to, 1011*t*
        relative efficacy of, 1010*t*
Corticosterone, synthesis of, 636*i*
Corticotropin (ACTH/adrenocorticotropin/adrenocorticotropic hormone), 604*t*, **609–610**, 610*i*
    adrenocortical steroid treatment compared with, 645
    for inflammatory bowel disease, 1026
    preparations available, 617
    receptors for, 604
    second messenger for, 22*t*
Corticotropin-releasing hormone (CRH), 604*t*, **609**
    receptors for, 604
Cortifoam, 1027. *See also* Hydrocortisone
Cortisol (hydrocortisone), 640*t*. *See also* Glucocorticoids
    for acute adrenocortical insufficiency, 641
    for cancer chemotherapy, 899*t*
        for breast cancer, 909

for dermatologic therapy, 1008–1009
for inflammatory bowel disease, 1026, 1027
metabolic effects of, 644
for nonadrenal disorders, 643–644
in OTC preparations, efficacy of, 1034*t*
pharmacokinetics of, 635–636, 636*i*, 637*i*
preparations available, 650, 1027
structure of, 641*i*
synthesis of, 636*i*
Cortisone, 640*t*
    preparations available, 650
Cortone, 650. *See also* Cortisone
Cortrosyn, 617. *See also* Cosyntropin
Corvert, 240. *See also* Ibutilide
Cosmegen, 894*t*. *See also* Dactinomycin
Cosyntropin, 609, 610. *See also* Adrenocorticotropin
Cotazyme, 1023*t*
Cotransmitters, 75, 80–81
Co-trimoxazole (trimethoprim-sulfamethoxazole), **763–765**
    intravenous, 764, 768
    preparations available, 768, 859
Cough suppression
    opioid analgesics for, 505, 507, **512**
        preparations available, 514
    OTC preparations for
        efficacy of, 1034*t*
        hidden ingredients in, 1037*t*, 1038*t*, 1039*i*
Coumadin, 561. *See also* Warfarin
Coumarin anticoagulants, **551–555**. *See also* Warfarin
Coupling, receptor-effector, 11–14
Coupling molecules, 4
Covalent bonds, in drug-receptor interactions, 2
COX-I (PGH synthase-1), 305–306, 578, 585
    glucocorticoids affecting, 639
COX-II (PGH synthase-2), 305–306, 578, 585
    glucocorticoids affecting, 639
Cozaar, 175. *See also* Losartan
"Crack" cocaine, 522
Cramps, leg, quinine for, 848
Craniosacral (parasympathetic) division of autonomic nervous system, 73, 74*i*
    autonomic nerve activity/drugs affecting, 83*t*
    in central integration, 82
    digitalis effects and, 204
Craniotomy, antimicrobial prophylaxis and, 824*t*
Creeping eruption (cutaneous larva migrans), drugs for, 863*t*
    albendazole, 865
    ivermectin, 868
    thiabendazole, 877
Cresols, antimicrobial effects of, 805*t*
CRH (corticotropin-releasing hormone), 604*t*, **609**
    receptors for, 604

Crippling fluorosis, 712
Crixivan, 801. *See also* Indinavir
Crohn's disease, drugs used in management of, **1025–1026**
    metronidazole, 858
Cromakalim, 166
    for asthma, 338
Cromolyn, **328–330**, 328*i*, **339**
    for asthma, 315, **328–330, 339**
    for allergy, 939
    ionization constant of, 6*t*
    OTC status of, 1032*t*
    preparations available, 340
Crossover design, for clinical trials, 66–67, 67*t*
Cross-tolerance, with opioid analgesics, 509
Crotalid antivenin, for rattlesnake envenomation, 978, 1057
Crotamiton, **1005**
Cryoprecipitate, 560. *See also* Factor VIII
Cryptococcus, empiric antimicrobial therapy and, 815*t*
Cryptosporidium, drugs for infection with, 855*t*
Crystodigin, 213. *See also* Digitoxin
Cultures (microbial), interpretation of, **813–815**
Cuprimine, 462, 600, 966. *See also* Penicillamine
Curare, 434
Cushing's syndrome, 642
    iatrogenic, 644
    ketoconazole for, 648, 678
Cutaneous larva migrans (creeping eruption), drugs for, 863*t*
    albendazole, 865
    ivermectin, 868
    thiabendazole, 877
Cyanide poisoning
    hydroxocobalamin for, 543
    sodium nitrite for, 184–185
Cyanocobalamin, 537, 542, 546. *See also* Vitamin B$_{12}$
Cyclic AMP (cAMP)
    in alpha$_2$ receptor activation, 121, 122*i*
    as second messenger, 23–24, 26*i*
        G proteins and, 21, 22
    vascular tone affected by, 181, 181*i*
Cyclic GMP (cGMP)
    in muscarinic agonist binding, 93–94
    vascular tone affected by, angina management and, 180, 181, 181*i*
Cyclizine, 267*t*
    ionization constant of, 6*t*
    for motion sickness, 269
    preparations available, 283
    structure of, 266*i*
Cyclobenzaprine
    for muscle spasm, 448
    preparations available, 448
Cyclodienes, 950–951, 950*t*
Cyclogyl, 115. *See also* Cyclopentolate

Cyclooxygenases, 305–307. *See also* Prostaglandins; Thromboxanes
  effects of, 308–310
  glucocorticoids affecting, 639
Cyclopentolate
  ophthalmologic uses of, 111*t*
  preparations available, 115
Cyclophosphamide, 886*i*, 890*t*
  fetus affected by, 983*t*
  half-life of, aging affecting, 992*i*
  immunomodulating effect of, 936
  immunosuppressive actions of, 928
  metabolism of, 887*i*
  preparations available, 940
Cycloplegia, antimuscarinic agents causing, 108, 109*i*, 111, 111*t*
Cyclo-prostin, 317. *See also* Epoprostenol
Cycloserine, **739–740**, 775
  preparations available, 741, 778
  for tuberculosis, 771*t*, 775
Cyclospasm, 148
Cyclosporine, **925–926**, 932
  for inflammatory bowel disease, 1026
  interactions of, 1065*t*
  pharmacokinetic/pharmacodynamic parameters of, 36*t*, 925–926
  preparations available, 940
Cyklokapron, 561. *See also* Tranexamic acid
Cylert, 134. *See also* Pemoline
Cynapen, 740. *See also* Dicloxacillin
Cyproheptadine, 267*t*, 277
  preparations available, 283
Cyproterone, 678–679
  for chemical contraception in men, 679
CYPs, 55, 56*t*
  H₁ receptor antagonists metabolized by, 266, 269–270
  induction of, 54
  inhibition of, 55
  local anesthetics metabolized by, 427
Cysticercosis. *See also* Neurocysticercosis
  drugs for, 863*t*
Cystospaz-M, 116. *See also* Hyoscyamine
Cytadren, 650, 899*t*. *See also* Aminoglutethimide
Cytarabine, 891*t*, **892–893**, 893*i*
  fetus affected by, 983*t*
  immunosuppressive actions of, 928
  mechanism of action of, 791*i*, 892–893
Cytidine, 893*i*
Cytochrome P450 enzyme system, 52–55, 52*i*, 53–54*t*
  epoxygenase products and, 308
  effects of, 310–311
  H₂ receptor antagonists affecting, 271
  in human liver, 55, 56*t*
  induction of, 52–55
  inhibition of, 55
  local anesthetics metabolized by, 427

Cytokines, 933–935, 934*t*
  immunomodulatory action of, 933–935
  receptors for, 20, 21*i*
Cytomegalovirus infections
  cidofovir for, 793
  foscarnet for, 794
  ganciclovir for, 793
  passive immunization for, 1056*t*
Cytomegalovirus immune globulin intravenous, preparations available, 801
Cytomel, 633. *See also* Liothyronine
Cytoprotection, 315
Cytosar-U, 891*t*. *See also* Cytarabine
Cytosine arabinoside (cytarabine), 891*t*, **892–893**, 893*i*
  mechanism of action of, 791*i*, 892–893
Cytospaz-M, 1027. *See also* Hyoscyamine
Cytotec, 317, 1027. *See also* Misoprostol
Cytotoxic drugs. *See also* Cancer chemotherapy
  for immunosuppressive therapy, **927–929**
  for inflammatory bowel disease, 1026
  resistance to, 883–884, 885*i*
Cytotoxic T cells, 919–920, 919*i*
Cytovene, 801. *See also* Ganciclovir
Cytoxan, 890*t*, 940. *See also* Cyclophosphamide

D cells (delta cells), pancreatic, 685*t*
d4T (stavudine), 795*t*, 796*i*, **798**
  preparations available, 801
2,4-D (2,4-dichlorophenoxyacetic acid), 952–953, 953*i*
D₁ (DA₁) dopamine receptors, 81*t*, 119–120, 119*t*, 467
  activation of, 122
  distribution of, 124*t*
  levodopa affecting, 451
D₂ (DA₂) dopamine receptors, 81*t*, 119–120, 119*t*, 467, 468
  activation of, 122
  antipsychotic drugs affecting, 468
  distribution of, 124*t*
D₃ dopamine receptors, 81*t*, 120, 467
D₄ dopamine receptors, 81*t*, 119*t*, 120, 467
D₅ dopamine receptors, 81*t*, 119*t*, 120, 467
d-tubocurarine, 434. *See also* Tubocurarine
Dacarbazine, **888**, 890*t*
Dactinomycin (actinomycin D), 894*t*, **896–897**
  immunosuppressive actions of, 929
DADs (delayed afterdepolarizations), 222, 222*i*
DAG (diacylglycerol)
  in alpha receptor activation, 121, 121*i*
  in calcium/phosphoinositide second messenger system, 24, 26*i*

lithium affecting, 476, 476*i*
  in muscarinic agonist binding, 93
Dalfopristin, 750
Dalgan, 513. *See also* Dezocine
Dalmane, 366*t*, 369. *See also* Flurazepam
Dalteparin, 550
  preparations available, 561
Danaproid, 550
  preparations available, 561
Danazol, **672**
  factor VIII activity affected by, 560
  for oral contraception in men, 679
  preparations available, 680
Danocrine, 680. *See also* Danazol
Dantrium, 448. *See also* Dantrolene
Dantrolene, **447–448**, 447*i*
  preparations available, 448
Dapsone, **778**, 778*i*, 839*i*
  in dermatologic therapy, 1014*t*
  preparations available, 779
  with pyrimethamine, **847**
Daranide, 259. *See also* Dichlorphenamide
Daraprim, 859. *See also* Pyrimethamine
Darbid, 115–116, 1027. *See also* Isopropamide
Daricon, 116, 1027. *See also* Oxyphencyclimine
Darvon, 501*t*, 514. *See also* Propoxyphene
Darvon Compound-65, 514. *See also* Propoxyphene, with acetaminophen; Propoxyphene, with aspirin
Datura stramonium, 105
Daunorubicin (daunomycin), 894*t*, **895–896**, 895*i*
Daypro, 599. *See also* Oxaprozin
dDAVP (desmopressin acetate/arginine vasopressin), 296, 615*i*, 616. *See also* Vasopressin
  dosage of, 616
  factor VIII activity affected by, 560, 616
ddC (zalcitabine), 795*t*, 796*i*, **797**
  preparations available, 801
ddI (didanosine), 795*t*, **796–797**, 796*i*
  preparations available, 801
DDT (chlorophenothane), 950–951, 950*t*, 953*i*
Deadly nightshade, 105
Dealkylations, 53*t*
Deamination, 53*t*
9-Deazainosine, nucleoside phosphotransferases affected by, 829
Debrisoquin, 161
Debrisoquin-sparteine oxidation polymorphism, 58
Decadron, 650. *See also* Dexamethasone
Decadron Phosphate Respihaler, 340. *See also* Dexamethasone
Deca-Durabolin, 680. *See also* Nandrolone
Decapryn, 267*t*. *See also* Doxylamine
Decaris, 878. *See also* Levamisole
Dechlorination, 53*t*

Declomycin, 259, 751. *See also* Demeclocycline
Decongestants, OTC preparations
  efficacy of, 1034–1035*t*
  hidden ingredients in, 1037*t*, 1039*t*
Decontamination (microbial), 805*t*
Decontamination procedures, for poisoned patient, 974–976
Deep sedation, 422
Deep venous thrombosis, 558. *See also* Venous thrombosis
  fibrinolytic agents for, 555, 558
Deferoxamine, **959**, 977*t*
  preparations available, 546, 966
Defibrination syndrome, factor I for, 559*t*, 560
Degradability, environmental toxicity and, 947
Dehydration
  loop diuretics causing, 251
  osmotic diuretics causing, 255
Dehydroemetine, **852–853**, **867**
  for amebiasis, 850, **852–853**
  for ameboma, 852
  preparations available, 858
Dehydroepiandrosterone (DHEA), 647, 674
Dehydroepiandrosterone sulfate (DHEA sulfate), 647, 674
Dehydrogenations, 53*t*
Delalutin, 680. *See also* Hydroxyprogesterone
Delayed afterdepolarizations, 222, 222*i*
Delayed hypersensitivity, 921–923, 922*i*
  drug allergy and, 937
Delayed toxicity, 946
Delsym, 514. *See also* Dextromethorphan
Delta cells (D cells), pancreatic, 685*t*
Delta-Cortef, 650. *See also* Prednisolone
Delta-D, 721. *See also* Cholecalciferol
Delta nerve fibers, local anesthetics affecting, 429, 429*t*
Delta (δ) receptors, 501
  opioid activity at, 502*t*
Demadex, 259. *See also* Torsemide
Demecarium, preparations available, 103
Demeclocycline, 255–256, 745*i*
  oral dosage for, 746
  pharmacokinetics of, 745–746
  preparations available, 259, 751
Demerol, 501*t*, 513. *See also* Meperidine
Demser, 150. *See also* Metyrosine
Demulen, 665*t*
Dental caries, fluoride in prevention of, 712
15-Deoxyspergualin, 927
Depakene, 407, 480. *See also* Valproic acid
Depakote, 407, 480. *See also* Valproic acid
Depen, 462, 600, 966. *See also* Penicillamine
Dependence (drug). *See also specific agent or drug class*
  drug abuse and, 516
  therapeutic dose, 520

Depo-Estradiol, 680. *See also* Estradiol
Depo-Medrol, 650. *See also* Methylprednisolone
Depot medroxyprogesterone, for contraception, 670
Deprenyl, 451*i*, 456
  for Alzheimer's disease, 994
  preparations available, 462
Depression, 483
  drugs for management of, 490. *See also* Antidepressants
  in elderly, 993
  lithium for, 477
  oral contraceptive use and, 669
  pathogenesis of, 483
  types of, 484*t*
Dermatologic pharmacology, **999–1016**. *See also* Skin
  OTC preparations in, hidden ingredients in, 1037*t*, 1038*t*
Dermatophytes, imidazoles for infections caused by, 1002
Dermopathy, in hyperthyroidism, 632
DES (diethylstilbestrol), 656, 656*i*, 657*t*, 660
  in cancer chemotherapy, 899*t*
  fetus affected by, 983*t*
  preparations available, 680
Desacetylvinblastine, 893
Desensitization, 4, 23, 25*i*, 122–123
  to drugs, 939
Desferal, 546, 966, 977*t*. *See also* Deferoxamine
Desflurane, 410*i*, 419
  elimination of, 414, 415
  organ system effects of, 416–418
  preparations available, 423
  properties of, 413*t*
  solubility of, 412, 413*t*
Desiccated thyroid, 625–626. *See also* Thyroid hormones
  preparations available, 633
Desipramine, 485*i*
  dosages of, 491*t*
  effects of, 489*t*
  half-life of, aging affecting, 992*i*
  ionization constant of, 6*t*
  pharmacokinetics of, 488*t*
  preparations available, 494
Desmethyldiazepam, 356*i*, 357, 357*i*
Desmopressin acetate (DDAVP/arginine vasopressin), 296, 615*i*, 616. *See also* Vasopressin
  dosage of, 616
  factor VIII activity affected by, 560, 616
Desogen, 665*t*
Desogestrel, 661, 661*t*, 662*i*
Desoxycorticosterone (DOC), 640*t*, **646–647**
  electrical potential and potassium secretion affected by, 246, 247*i*
Desoxyn, 134. *See also* Methamphetamine
Desulfuration, 53*t*
Desyrel, 494. *See also* Trazodone

Detrusor muscle, direct-acting cholinomimetics affecting, 94*t*
Dexamethasone, 640*t*
  for asthma, preparations available, 340
  preparations available, 650
Dexamethasone suppression test, 642–643
Dexbrompheniramine, OTC status of, 1031*t*
Dexchlorpheniramine, preparations available, 283
Dexedrine, 133
Dexfenfluramine, 276
  preparations available, 284
Dexmedetomidine, 159
Dextroamphetamine, 521
  abuse of, 521
  preparations available, 133
Dextromethorphan, 512
  in OTC preparations, efficacy of, 1034*t*
  preparations available, 514
Dextrose challenge, in initial management of poisoned patient, 970
Dezocine, 512
  preparations available, 513
  receptor subtype activity of, 502*t*
DFMO (alpha-difluoromethylornithine), ornithine decarboxylase affected by, 831–833
DHAD (mitoxantrone), **901**, 901*t*
D.H.E.45, 284. *See also* Dihydroergotamine
DHEA (dehydroepiandrosterone), 647, 674
DHEA sulfate (dehydroepiandrosterone sulfate), 647, 674
DHET (dihydroxyeicosatrienoic acid), 308
DHPG, 793. *See also* Ganciclovir
DHT (dihydrotachysterol)
  in chronic renal failure, 716–717
  preparations available, 721
Diaβeta, 697*t*, 703. *See also* Glyburide
Diabetes insipidus
  desmopressin for, 616
  diuretics for, **259**
  nephrogenic, lithium causing, 255, 259, 478
  vasopressin for, 616
Diabetes mellitus, 684–685
  benefit of glycemic control in, 693–694, 694
  beta-receptor blocking drug use and, 149
  treatment of, **684–705**
  type I (insulin-dependent/IDDM), 684, 693
  type II (non-insulin-dependent/NIDDM), 684–685
    insulin treatment for, 693, 694
    oral hypoglycemics for, **696–701**
Diabinese, 697*t*, 703. *See also* Chlorpropamide
Diacylglycerol
  in alpha receptor activation, 121, 121*i*

in calcium/phosphoinositide second
messenger system, 24, 26*i*
lithium affecting, 476, 476*i*
in muscarinic agonist binding, 93
Dialysis. *See also* Hemodialysis
for poisoning, 975*t*, 976–977
with methanol, 382
Diamidines, aromatic, antiparasitic actions of, 836*t*
Diamox, 259. *See also* Acetazolamide
Diarrhea, drugs for, **1024**
antimuscarinic agents, 111–112
opioid analgesics, 507
OTC preparations
efficacy of, 1034*t*
hidden ingredients in, 1037*t*, 1038*t*
Diazepam, 356*i*
absorption of, 355
in neonate, 984*t*
for alcohol withdrawal syndrome, 380,
383
for anesthesia, 362, 420, 423
biotransformation of, 357, 357*i*
in breast milk, 987*t*
distribution of, 355
dosages of, 366*t*
for drug withdrawal, 366
fetus affected by, 983*t*
half-life of
aging affecting, 992*i*
in infants vs. adults, 985*t*
ionization constant of, 6*t*
as muscle relaxant, 366
overdose of, 973*t*
pharmacokinetic/pharmacodynamic
parameters of, 36*t*, 358*t*
in neonate, 984*t*, 985*t*
preparations available, 369, 383, 407,
423, 448
for seizures, 362, 402, 407
for spasticity, **445**, 446*i*, 448
for status epilepticus, 405
Diazinon, 951*t*
Diazoxide, **168–169**, 169*i*
preparations available, 175
Dibenzodiazepines, 468*t*
advantages and disadvantages of, 471*t*
Dibenzo-*p*-dioxins, polychlorinated
(PCDDs), 954
Dibenzofurans, polychlorinated
(PCDFs), 954
Dibenzoxazepine, advantages and disadvantages of, 471*t*
Dibenzyline, 150. *See also* Phenoxybenzamine
Dibucaine, preparations available, 432
Dibucaine number, 439
DIC (disseminated intravascular coagulation), 548
Dichloroacetamides, for amebiasis, 850
Dichlorodiphenyltrichloroethane (DDT),
950–951, 950*t*, 953*i*
Dichloroisoproterenol, 145
2,4-Dichlorophenoxyacetic acid (2,4-D),
952–953, 953*i*
Dichlorphenamide
for glaucoma, 248*t*

preparations available, 259
structure of, 248*i*
Dichlorvos, 951*t*
Diclofenac, 580*t*, 586*i*, **587**
preparations available, 599
Dicloxacillin, 729–731
dosing guidelines for, 730*t*
pharmacokinetics of, 726
preparations available, 740
Dicumarol, 554
in breast milk, 987*t*
drug metabolism inhibited by, 60*t*
structure of, 552*i*
Dicyclomine, 107*i*
for gastrointestinal and genitourinary
conditions, 112*t*
preparations available, 115, 1027
Didanosine, 795*t*, **796–797**, 796*i*
preparations available, 801
Dideoxycytidine (zalcitabine), 795*t*,
796*i*, **797**
preparations available, 801
Dideoxyinosine (didanosine), 795*t*,
796–797, 796*i*
preparations available, 801
Didronel, 721. *See also* Etidronate
Dieldrin, 950*t*
Dienestrol, 656
preparations available, 680
Dientamoeba fragilis, drugs for infection
with, 855*t*
Diet
drug metabolism affected by, 59
in hyperlipoproteinemia, **569–570**
inflammation affected by, 594
Diethylcarbamazine, **866–867**
adverse reactions to, 867
antiparasitic actions of, 836*t*, 866–867
preparations available, 878
Diethyldithiocarbamate (DTC), 936
Diethylpentenamide, drug metabolism
inhibited by, 60*t*
Diethylstilbestrol (DES), 656, 656*i*, 657*t*,
660
in cancer chemotherapy, 899*t*
fetus affected by, 983*t*
preparations available, 680
Difenoxin, 511, 1024
preparations available, 1027
Differin (adapalene), 1007
Diffuse neuronal systems, 347–348
Diffusion
aqueous, 5
Fick's law of, 5
lipid, 5
Diflucan, 786, 1004. *See also* Fluconazole
Diflunisal, 580*t*, **585**
OTC status of, 1031*t*
preparations available, 599
Digibind, 213, 977*t*. *See also* Digitalis
antibodies
Digitalis
administration and dosage of, 208
for arrhythmias, 208
basic pharmacology of, **200–205**
chemistry of, 200–201, 201*i*

clinical pharmacology of, **207–209**
for heart failure, **207–209**
interactions of, 205, 208, 1065–1066*t*
parasympathomimetic effects of, 204
pharmacodynamics of, 202–205
pharmacokinetics of, 201–202, 201*t*
preparations available, 213
Digitalis antibodies
for overdose/toxicity, 209, 977*t*
preparations available, 213
Digitalis toxicity, 203–204, 204*i*,
208–209
arrhythmias caused by, 204, 204*i*, 209
effects outside heart, 205
Digitoxin. *See also* Digitalis
clinical use of, 208*t*
pharmacokinetic/pharmacodynamic
parameters of, 36*t*, 201–202,
201*t*
preparations available, 213
Digoxin, 200, 201*i*. *See also* Digitalis
absorption of, in neonate, 984*t*
in breast milk, 987*t*
for chronic heart failure, 209, 210
clinical use of, 208*t*
in elderly, 994
half-life of
aging affecting, 992*i*
in infants vs. adults, 985*t*
pharmacokinetic/pharmacodynamic
parameters of, 36*t*, 201–202,
201*t*
in neonate, 984*t*, 985*t*
preparations available, 213
Digoxin immune fab, preparations available, 213
Dihydrocodeine, 511
ionization constant of, 6*t*
pharmacokinetics of, 501*t*
Dihydroergotamine
for migraine, 282
preparations available, 284
Dihydroergotoxine, for senile cerebral
insufficiency, 282
Dihydropteroate synthesis, enzymes for,
antiparasitic drugs affecting, 828
Dihydropyridines. *See also specific type*
clinical properties of, 190*t*
for hypertension, 169
pharmacokinetics of, 189*t*
vascular selectivity of, 190*t*
Dihydrostreptomycin, half-life of, aging
affecting, 992*i*
Dihydrotachysterol
in chronic renal failure, 716–717
preparations available, 721
Dihydrotestosterone, 675
Dihydroxyanthracenedione (DHAD/mitoxantrone), **901**, 901*t*
Dihydroxyeicosatrienoic acid (DHET),
308
Dihydroxyphenylalanine, 451*i*
1,25-Dihydroxyvitamin D (calcitriol),
707–709, 708*i*, 709*t*. *See also* Vitamin D
in chronic renal failure, 716–717
for hypocalcemia, 715

1,25-Dihydroxyvitamin D (calcitriol)
 (cont.)
  for intestinal osteodystrophy *(cont.)*
  for osteoporosis, 718
  preparations available, 721
24,25-Dihydroxyvitamin D (secalciferol), 707–709, 708*i*, 709*t*
Diiodohydroxyquin, 853, 859. *See also*
  Iodoquinol
Diiodotyrosine (DIT), 619
2,6-Diisopropylphenol (propofol), 411*i*,
  420*t*, **421–422**
  for deep sedation, 421, 422
  GABA-DBZ receptor chloride channel
   binding and, 361
  preparations available, 423
Dilacor, 194, 240. *See also* Diltiazem
Dilantin, 407. *See also* Phenytoin
Dilaudid, 501*t*, 513. *See also* Hydromorphone
Diloxanide, **853**
  for amebiasis, 850, 851*t*, **853**
  antiparasitic actions of, 836*t*, 853
  preparations available, 858
Diltiazem, 188*i*, 189*t*, 190*t*, 229*t*, **236**
  for angina, 193*i*
  for arrhythmias, **236**
  clinical properties of, 190*t*, 229*t*
  for hypertension, 169
  membrane actions of, 228*t*
  pharmacokinetic/pharmacodynamic
   parameters of, 36*t*, 187, 189*t*
  preparations available, 175, 194, 240
  for thyroid storm, 631
  vascular selectivity of, 190*t*
Dimenhydrinate, 267*t*
  preparations available, 283
  structure of, 266*i*
Dimercaprol (2,3-
  dimercaptopropanol/BAL),
  957–958, 957*i*
  preparations available, 966
Dimercaptosuccinic acid (DMSA), 956,
  957*i*, **958**
  preparations available, 966
Dimetan, 952*t*
Dimetane, 267*t*, 283. *See also*
  Brompheniramine
Dimethadione, 401–402
Dimethisterone, 661*t*, 662*i*
Dimethoate, 951*t*
2,5-Dimethoxy-4-methylamphetamine,
  521
Dimethylcysteine (penicillamine),
  592–593, 957*i*, **958–959**
  fetus affected by, 983*t*
  ionization constant of, 6*t*
  preparations available, 462, 600, 966
  for Wilson's disease, 461, 958
Dimethylphenylpiperazinium (DMPP),
  93, 93*i*
  central nervous system effects of, 96
Dimetilan, 952*t*
Dinoprostone (prostaglandin E₂), 306,
  312–313, 312*i*. *See also*
  Prostaglandins
  for abortion, 312–313

for labor facilitation, 313
  preparations available, 317
Dioctyl sodium sulfosuccinate (docusate)
  in OTC preparations, efficacy of,
   1035*t*
  preparations available, 1027–1028
  as stool softener, 1024
Diovan, 175. *See also* Valsartan
Dioxins, 953, 954
Dipentum, 1027. *See also* Olsalazine
Diphenhydramine, 267*t*
  antiemetic actions of, 1022
  for motion sickness, 269, 1022
  in OTC preparations, efficacy of,
   1033*t*, 1035*t*
  OTC status of, 1031*t*
  preparations available, 283
  structure of, 266*i*
Diphenoxylate, 511
  with atropine, 112, 511, 1024, 1027
  for diarrhea, 507, 511, 1024
  ionization constant of, 6*t*
  preparations available, 1027
  structure of, 499*i*
Diphtheria
  antimicrobial prophylaxis and, 824*t*
  passive immunization for, 1056*t*
Diphtheria-tetanus acellular pertussis
  vaccine, 1052*t*
Diphtheria-tetanus-pertussis vaccine,
  1052*t*
Diphyllobothrium latum (fish tapeworm),
  drugs for infection with, 863*t*
  niclosamide, 871
  praziquantel, 874
Dipivefrin
  for glaucoma, 132, 149*t*
  preparations available, 133
Diplopia
  carbamazepine causing, 393
  phenytoin causing, 391
Diprivan, 423. *See also* Propofol
Dipylidium caninum, drugs for infection
  with, 864*t*
Dipyridamole, preparations available,
  561
Direct-acting cholinomimetics, 91, 91*i*,
  92–96, 103
  preparations available, 103
  toxicity of, 102
Disalcid (salsalate), 599
Disease-modifying antirheumatic drugs
  (DMARDs), 579, **590–593**
  preparations available, 599–600
Disinfectants, **804–810**. *See also specific
  type*
  activities of, 805*t*
  preparations available, 810
Disinfection, 805*t*. *See also* Disinfectants
Disk diffusion susceptibility testing, 817
Disoprofol (propofol), 411*i*, 420*t*,
  421–422
  for deep sedation, 421, 422
  GABA-DBZ receptor chloride channel
   binding and, 361
  preparations available, 423

Disopyramide, **230**, 230*i*
  for arrhythmias, **230**
  clinical properties of, 229*t*
  membrane actions of, 228*t*
  pharmacokinetic/pharmacodynamic
   parameters of, 36*t*, 230
  preparations available, 240
Disseminated intravascular coagulation
  (DIC), 548
Dissociation constant, enantiomers and,
  3, 3*t*
Dissociative anesthesia, ketamine producing, 422
Distal convoluted tubule, transport in/di-
  uretic site of action and, **245**, 245*i*
Distribution, 4
  aging affecting, 989, 990*i*
  in infants and children, 982–984, 984*t*
  interactions and, 1059
  models of, 38*i*
  volume of, 34–35
   drug concentration and
    initial predictions, 47–48
    revising predictions, 48–49
   in infants and children, 982–984,
    984*t*
   poisoning and, 968
   therapeutic drug monitoring and, 46
Disulfamoylchloraniline, structure of,
  248*i*
Disulfiram, 380–381
  drug metabolism inhibited by, 60*t*
  interactions of, 1066*t*
  preparations available, 383
DIT (diiodotyrosine), 619
Ditropan, 116, 1027. *See also* Oxybutynin
Diucardin, 259. *See also* Hydroflumethiazide
Diuresis, forced, in poisoning, 978
Diuretics, **155–157**, **242–260**. *See also
  specific type and agent*
  basic pharmacology of, **246–256**
  carbonic anhydrase inhibitors,
   246–249
    urinary electrolyte patterns affected
     by, 257*t*
  clinical pharmacology of, **256–259**
  combination products, 254*t*, **256**
    urinary electrolyte patterns affected
     by, 257*t*
  dosing considerations for, 157
  for glaucoma, 149*t*
  for heart failure, 206, 209, **256–257**
    with "power failure," 212
    with pulmonary congestion,
     211–212
  for hypertension, **155–157**, **258**
  loop, 244–245, **249–251**
    development of, 248
    with potassium-sparing diuretics,
     256
    with thiazides, **256**
    urinary electrolyte patterns affected
     by, 257*t*
  mechanisms of action and hemodynamic effects of, 155–157

methylxanthines as, 332
modern, development of, 248
osmotic, **254–255**
OTC preparations, hidden ingredients in, 1038*t*
potassium-sparing, **253–254**, 253*i*, 254*t*
    interactions of, 1068*t*
    with loop agents or thiazides, **256**
    urinary electrolyte patterns affected by, 257*t*
preparations available, 259
renal tubule transport mechanisms and, **242–246**, 243*i*
selection of, 157
sites of action of, **242–246**, 243*i*
thiazide, **251–253**, 252*i*
    bone mineral homeostasis affected by, **711**
    development of, 248
    with loop agents, **256**
    with potassium-sparing diuretics, **256**
    urinary electrolyte patterns affected by, 257*t*
toxicity of, 157
Diuril, 259. *See also* Chlorothiazide
Divalproex, 407, 480. *See also* Valproic acid
DMARDs (disease-modifying antirheumatic drugs), 579, **590–593**
    preparations available, 599–600
DMPP (dimethylphenylpiperazinium), 93, 93*i*
    central nervous system effects of, 96
DMSA (succimer/dimercaptosuccinic acid), 956, 957*i*, **958**
    preparations available, 966
DNA gyrase inhibitors, **765–767**
DNA synthesis, vitamin B$_{12}$ and folic acid for, 537
Doan's Pills, 599. *See also* Magnesium salicylate
Dobutamine, 128, 129, 129*i*
    for heart failure, 206
    preparations available, 133, 213
Dobutrex, 133, 213. *See also* Dobutamine
DOC/DOCA (desoxycorticosterone), 640*t*, **646–647**
    electrical potential and potassium secretion affected by, 246, 247*i*
Docetaxel, 894*t*, **895**
Docosahexaenoic acids, in dietary manipulation of arachidonic acid metabolism, 317
Docusate (dioctyl sodium sulfosuccinate)
    in OTC preparations, efficacy of, 1035*t*
    preparations available, 1027–1028
    as stool softener, 1024
Dolobid, 599. *See also* Diflunisal
Dolophine, 501*t*, 513. *See also* Methadone
DOM, 521
Donepezil, for Alzheimer's disease, 994
Dopa (dihydroxyphenylalanine), 451*i*

Dopamine, 77*t*, 85*t*, 123*i*, 128, 349*t*, 352
    alcoholism and, 381
    antipsychotic agents affecting, 466–468
    biosynthesis of, 79*i*
    for cardiogenic shock, 212
    for heart failure, 206
    metabolism of, 80*i*
    as neurotransmitter, 77*t*, 349*t*, 352
    preparations available, 133, 213
    as prolactin inhibitor, 604, 604*t*, 614
    receptors for, 604
        levodopa affecting, 451
    in schizophrenia, 465
Dopamine agonists, **455**, **614–615**
    mechanism of action of, 122
    for parkinsonism, **455**
    selectivity of, 120, 120*t*
Dopamine antagonists, antipsychotic agents as, 466
Dopamine hypothesis, for schizophrenia, 465
Dopamine receptors, 81*t*, 119–120, 119*t*
    activation of, 122
    antipsychotic drugs affecting, 467–468, 468–469
    distribution of, 124*t*
    ergot alkaloids affecting, 279*t*, 280
    selectivity of drugs for, 120, 120*t*
Dopaminergic neurons
    antipsychotic drugs affecting, 466–467
    in parkinsonism, 450–451, 451*i*
Dopar, 462. *See also* Levodopa
Doral, 366*t*, 369. *See also* Quazepam
Doriden, 973*t*. *See also* Glutethimide
Dorsal root, local anesthetics affecting, 429*t*
Dorzolamide
    for glaucoma, 149*t*, 248
    preparations available, 259
Dosage regimen
    drug concentration measurements and, 47
    target concentration approach to, **43–45**
Dose
    loading, 45
    maintenance, 44
        calculation of, 45
    median effective (ED50), 28, 29
    median lethal (LD50), 29, 65–66
    median toxic (TD50), 29
    minimum lethal, 65
    "no effect," 65
    pediatric, **987–988**
Dose-effect curves, quantal, 29–30, 29*i*
    in poisoning, 969, 969*i*
Dose-response curve, shape of, 28–29, 28*i*
Dose-response relationships, **27–33**, 34, 35*i*. *See also* Concentration-response relationships
    beneficial versus toxic effects and, 31–33
    graded, 28, 28*i*
    poisoning and, 969, 969*i*

for inhaled anesthetics, 416
    in patients, 28–30
    poisoning and, 969, 969*i*
    for sedative-hypnotics, 354, 355*i*
    variations in, 30–31
Double-blind design, for clinical trials, 67
Doxacurium, 436*i*, 438*t*
    effects of, 443*t*
    preparations available, 448
Doxazosin, 138*t*, 139
    for hypertension, 165–166
    preparations available, 150, 175
Doxepin, 485*i*, **1013**
    in dermatologic therapy, **1013**
    dosages of, 491*t*
    effects of, 489*t*
    overdoses of, 972*t*
    pharmacokinetics of, 488*t*
    preparations available, 494
Doxorubicin, 894*t*, **895–896**, 895*i*
    for non-Hodgkin's lymphoma, 908
Doxycycline, 745*i*
    half-life of, aging affecting, 992*i*
    for malaria chemoprophylaxis, 840*t*, 849
    for malaria treatment, 841*t*, 849
    oral dosage for, 746
    parenteral dosage of, 746
    pharmacokinetics of, 745–746
    preparations available, 751, 858–859
    vestibular reactions to, 747
Doxylamine, 267*t*
    for nausea and vomiting of pregnancy, 269
    OTC status of, 1031*t*
    teratogenic effects of, 269
Dracontiasis
    mebendazole for, 870
    thiabendazole for, 877
Dracunculus medinesis (dracunculiasis), drugs for, 863*t*
    metronidazole, 858
Dramamine, 267*t*, 283. *See also* Dimenhydrinate
Drisdol, 721. *See also* Ergocalciferol
Drocode, 501*t*. *See also* Dihydrocodeine
Dromostanolone, 675*t*
Dronabinol, 528, 1022. *See also* Δ^9-Tetrahydrocannabinol
    preparations available, 1027
Droperidol, for anesthesia, 421, 471
Drospirenone, 649
Drug abuse, **516–531**. *See also specific drug*
    cultural considerations and, 516–517
    neurobiology and, 517–518
Drug allergy, **936–940**. *See also* Allergic reactions
Drug-body interactions, 3–4
Drug concentration
    interpretation of measurements of, **47–49**
    target
        dosage regimen design and, **43–45**
        therapeutic monitoring and, 46

Drug concentration (*cont.*)
    timing of samples taken for measurement of, 47
Drug-drug interactions, **1059–1060**, 1061–1069t
    combined toxicity and, **1060**
    metabolism and, 59–60, 59i, 60i, 1059
    pharmacodynamic mechanisms of, 1059–1060
    pharmacokinetic mechanisms of, 1059
    predictability of, **1060**
Drug-endogenous compound interactions, metabolism and, 60
Drug holidays, with levodopa therapy, 454
Drug monitoring, therapeutic, **45–47**
    of antidepressant levels, 492
    of lithium levels, 477–478
Drug permeation, 4, 5
Drug Price Competition and Patent Restoration Act, 68t
Drug-receptor bonds, 2–3
Drug-receptor interactions, 4. *See also* Drug receptors
Drug receptors, 2, **9–33**. *See also specific type*
    alterations in number or function of, drug responsiveness affected by, 30–31
    beneficial vs. toxic drug effects and, 31–33
    classes of, drug development and, **27**
    concentration-response relationship and, 9, **11–17**
        variations in drug responsiveness and, 30
    desensitization of, 23, 25i, 122–123
    discovery and description of, 10, 11i
    dose-response relationship and, 9, **27–33**
    effector coupling and, 11–14
    inert binding sites and, 4
    intracellular, for lipid-soluble agents, 18–19, 19i
    macromolecular nature of, **9–11**
    mediation of antagonists and, 9
    nomenclature for, 3
    selectivity of drug action and, 9, 120
    serpentine, 22–23, 24i
    signaling mechanisms and, **17–27**
    spare, 11–14
    structure-activity relationships and, 27
    variation in responsiveness and, 30–31
Drug resistance
    to activated protein C, 558
    to acyclovir, 789
    to alkylating agents, 885
    to aminoglycosides, 752–753
    to antimycobacterial drugs, 770
    to azoles, 783
    to chloroquine, 842
    to cytotoxic drugs, 883–884, 885i
    to erythromycin, 748
    to fluoroquinolones, 765–766, 767
    to gentamicin, 756
    to indinavir, 798
    to insulin, 695, 700

    to isoniazid, 771
    to kanamycin, 758
    to mefloquine, 843
    to mercaptopurine, 891
    to methotrexate, 890
    to penicillins, 725–726
    to primaquine, 844
    to proguanil, 845
    to pyrimethamine, 845
    to quinine, 847
    to streptomycin, 754
    to sulfonamides, 761
    to tetracyclines, 745
        overuse and, 747
    to thioguanine, 891
    to trimethoprim, 763
    to vancomycin, 727, 738
    to zidovudine, 795
Drug screening, in new drug evaluation, 64
Drug trapping, 6–7, 7i
Drugs. *See also specific agent and* Pharmacology
    absorption of, 4
        aging affecting, 989
        extent of, bioavailability and, 40–41
        in infants and children, 982, 984t
        interactions and, 1059
        rate of, bioavailability and, 41–42, 41i
        therapeutic drug monitoring and, 46
    accumulation of, 40
        time course of drug effect and, 43
    adverse reactions to
        in elderly, **995–996**
        new drug evaluation and, 70
    beneficial effects of, 31–33
    bioavailability of, 40–42
    biotransformation of, **50–61**
    classification of by group, 7
    clearance of, 34, 35–40
        concentration and, 47
            initial predictions, 48
            revising predictions, 48–49
        poisoning and, 968–969
        therapeutic drug monitoring and, 46
    cumulative effects of, 43
    delayed effects of, 43, 44i
    desensitization to, 939
    development of
        rational design and, 3
        receptor classes and, 27
    discovery of, **62–64**, 62i
    distribution of, 4, 34–35
        aging affecting, 989, 990i
        concentration and
            initial predictions, 47–48
            revising prediction, 48–49
        in infants and children, 982–984, 984t
        interactions and, 1059
        models of, 38i
        therapeutic drug monitoring and, 46
    duration of action of, 4
    elimination of, 5, 35–39
        aging affecting, 990–991, 991t
        capacity-limited, 39

    first-pass
        bioavailability and, 41, 41i, 42
        route of administration and, 42
    flow-dependent, 39
    in infants and children, 984–985
    models of, 38i
    evaluation of, preclinical, **62–72**
        in humans, **66–72**
    excretion of
        in infants and children, 984–985
        interactions and, 1059
    half-life of, 39–40
        therapeutic monitoring and, 46
    hypersensitivity (allergic) reaction to, 30
    idiosyncratic response to, 30
    immediate effect of, 42–43, 43i
    immunologic reactions to, **936–940**. *See also* Allergic reactions
        clinical identification of, **939–940**
    Internet information about, 8
    metabolism of. *See also* Biotransformation
        aging affecting, 59, 989–990, 990t
        clinical relevance of, **56–61**
        diet affecting, 59
        diseases affecting, 60–61, 60t
        drug-drug interactions and, 59–60, 59t, 60t
        drug-endogenous compound interactions affecting, 60
        environmental factors affecting, 59
        fetal, 980
        genetic factors affecting, 57–59, 58i, 58t
        individual differences in rate of, 57
        in infants and children, 984, 985t
        interactions and, 1059
        phase I, 51, 51i, **52–55**, 53–54t
        phase II, 51, 51i, **55**, 57t
        placental, 980
        sex (gender) affecting, 59
        to toxic products, **55–56**, 57i. *See also* Reactive metabolites
    misuse of, 516. *See also* Drug abuse
    molecular size of, 2
        passage across placenta and, 979
    monitoring, **45–47**
    nature of, 2–3
    orphan, 70
    physical nature of, 2
    prototype, 7
    reactivity of, receptor bonds and, 2–3
    shape of, 3
    side effects of, 31–33
    sources of information about, 7–8
    time course of effect of, **42–43**, 43i
    toxic effects of, 31–33
    variations in response to, 30–31
Drunkenness (acute alcohol intoxication), 374, 374t. *See also* Ethanol poisoning
    management of, **379**
DT vaccine, 1053t
DTaP vaccine, 1052t
DTC (diethyldithiocarbamate), 936

dTMP synthesis cycle, 540, 541*i*

DTP vaccine, 1052*t*

DTP-*Haemophilus influenzae* type b conjugate, 1052*t*

Ductus arteriosus, patent
indomethacin for, 589
prostaglandins for, 314

Dulcolax, 1027. *See also* Bisacodyl

Duodenal ulcers, peptic, H_2 receptor antagonists for, 271–272, 1019

Durabolin, 680. *See also* Nandrolone

Duragesic (Fentanyl Transdermal System), 513

Duranest, 426*t*, 432. *See also* Etidocaine

Durham-Humphrey Act, 68*t*

Duricef, 740. *See also* Cefadroxil

DV (dienestrol), 656
preparations available, 680

dVDAVP (arginine vasopressin/desmopressin acetate/DDAVP), 296, 615*i*, 616.
dosage of, 616
factor VIII activity affected by, 560, 616

Dwarf tapeworm, drugs for infection with, 863*t*
niclosamide, 871
praziquantel, 875

Dwarfism, 607

Dyazide, 254*t*. *See also* Triamterene

Dyclone, 432. *See also* Dyclonine

Dyclonine
OTC status of, 1031*t*
preparations available, 432

Dymelor, 697*t*, 703. *See also* Acetohexamide

DynaCirc, 175, 194. *See also* Isradipine

Dynorphins, 497
receptor subtype activity of, 502*t*

Dyphylline, for asthma, preparations available, 340

Dyrenium, 254*t*, 259. *See also* Triamterene

Dysbetalipoproteinemia, familial, 567*t*, 568

Dysentery, amebic, treatment of, 851*t*, 852

Dyskinesias
bromocriptine causing, 455
drug-induced, 460–461
levodopa causing, 453–454
tardive, 461, 473

Dysmenorrhea
nonsteroidal anti-inflammatory drugs for, 313–314
prostaglandins in, 313–314

Dysmorphogenesis, antipsychotic agents causing, 474

Dyspnea, after myocardial infarction, 211–212, 211*t*

Dysthymia, 383

Dystonia, 450, 460
antipsychotic agents causing, 473

E_{max} (maximum effect), therapeutic drug monitoring and, 47

E coli (*Escherichia coli*), empiric antimicrobial therapy and, 814*t*

E-Mycin, 751. *See also* Erythromycin

EACA (aminocaproic acid), 548, 550*i*, 560–561

Early afterdepolarizations (EADs), 222, 222*i*

Easprin, 599. *See also* Aspirin

EC50 (median effective concentration), 28

Echinococcus granulosus (hydatid disease), drugs for, 864*t* albendazole, 864 mebendazole, 869 praziquantel, 875 *multilocularis*, drugs for, 864*t* albendazole, 864

Echothiophate, 97, 98*i*
absorption/distribution/metabolism of, 98
for glaucoma, 149*t*
preparations available, 103

Econazole
preparations available, 786
topical, 1002

Ecotoxicology, 946, 947

"Ecstasy," 521

Ectoparasiticides, **1004–1005**

Ectopic pacemakers, autonomic activity/drugs affecting, 83*t*

ED50 (median effective dose), 28, 29

Edecrin, 259. *See also* Ethacrynic acid

Edema
diuretics for, **256–258**
histamine-induced, 263–264
idiopathic, diuretics for, **258**
lithium causing, 478

Edetate calcium disodium (EDTA), 956, 957*i*, **959**
preparations available, 966

EDRF (endothelium-derived relaxing factor). *See also* Nitric oxide
discovery of, 319, 320*i*
in kinin-mediated vasodilation, 294
muscarinic agonists releasing, 95

Edrophonium, 97, 97*i*
mechanism of action of, 99
in myasthenia gravis, 101
preparations available, 103

EDTA (edetate calcium disodium/ethylenediaminetetraacetate), 956, 957*i*, **959**
preparations available, 966

EEG (electroencephalogram), antipsychotic drugs affecting, 469

EET (epoxyeicosatrienoic acid), 308

Efedron, 133. *See also* Ephedrine

Effector molecules, 4

Effexor, 494. *See also* Venlafaxine

Efficacy (drug), maximal, 28, 28*i*

Effusions, malignant, **912**

EGF (epidermal growth factor), ligand-regulated transmembrane enzymes in signalling by, 19–20, 20*i*

Eicosanoids, **304–318**. *See also* specific type
basic pharmacology of, **308–311**
clinical pharmacology of, **311–317**
mechanisms of action of, **308–311**

organ system effects of, **308–311**
precursors of, **304–305**, 305*i*
preparations available, 317
synthesis of, **305–308**
inhibition of, **311**

Eicosapentanenoic acid, 556

Ejaculation, adrenoceptor function and, 127

Elavil, 494. *See also* Amitriptyline

Eldepryl, 462. *See also* Selegiline

Electrical activity of heart
digitalis glycosides affecting, 203–204, 203*i*, 204*i*, 204*t*
ionic basis of, 216–219
normal, **216–220**, 217*i*, 221*i*

Electrical potential, potassium and, 246, 247*i*

Electrocardiogram
digitalis glycosides affecting, 203–204, 203*i*, 204*i*, 204*t*
in poisoning, 075*i*, 974

Electroencephalogram (EEG), antipsychotic drugs affecting, 469

Electrolytes
lithium affecting, 476
in poisoning, 973

Electrostatic bonds, in drug-receptor interactions, 2

Elimination, 5, 35–39
aging affecting, 990–991, 991*t*
first-pass, 51
bioavailability and, 41, 41*i*, 42
route of administration and, 42
in infants and children, 984–985
models of, 38*i*

Elimite (permethrin), 1005

Elixirs, for infants and children, 985

Elixophyllin, 340. *See also* Theophylline

Elspar, 901*t*. *See also* Asparaginase

Embequin, 859. *See also* Iodoquinol

Emesis, in poisoned patient, 974–975

Emetine, **852–853**, **867**
for amebiasis, 850, **852–853**
for ameboma, 852
antiparasitic actions of, 836*t*
preparations available, 859

Eminase, 561. *See also* Anistreplase

Empirical antimicrobial therapy, **812–813**

Empirin Compound (codeine, with aspirin), 514

Emulsifying agents, 999

Enalapril, 291*i*, 293
for hypertension, 170
pharmacokinetic/pharmacodynamic parameters of, 36*t*, 171
preparations available, 175, 213

Enalaprilat
for hypertensive emergencies, 170
pharmacokinetics and dosage of, 171
preparations available, 175

Enalkiren, 291*i*, 293

Enantiomers, drug potency and, 3

Encainide, for arrhythmias, 234

Encephalitis, herpes simplex, acyclovir for, 790

Encephalopathy
  lead, 961
  portal-systemic, drugs for, **1026**
  Wernicke's, 376
Endocarditis
  antimicrobial prophylaxis and, 824t
  empiric antimicrobial therapy and,
    816t
  streptomycin for, 755
Endocrine dysfunction
  drug metabolism affected by, 61
  opioid analgesic use and, 510
Endocrine system
  antipsychotic drugs affecting,
    469–470, 470t, 473
  beta-receptor blocking drugs affecting,
    143–145
  chronic alcohol consumption affect-
    ing, 378
  disorders of, glucagon in testing for,
    702
  H₂ receptor antagonist side effects
    and, 272
  kinins affecting, 294
  oral contraceptives affecting, 667
  sympathomimetic agents affecting,
    127
Endocytosis, drug permeation by, 5
Endogenous depression, 483, 484t, 490.
    See also Depression
Endogenous opioid peptides, 497, 500i
Endometrial cancer, 903t
  estrogen administration and, 659,
    660
  oral contraceptive use and, 670
Endometriosis
  danazol for, 672
  gonadotropin-releasing hormones for,
    611
Endometrium, estrogens affecting, 657
β-Endorphin, 497
  receptor subtype activity of, 502t
Endothelins, **297–298**, 298i
  receptors for, 297–298
    antagonists of, 298, 300i
  signal transduction mechanisms of,
    298, 299i
Endothelium, autonomic activity/drugs
    affecting, 83t
Endothelium-derived relaxing factor. See
    also Nitric oxide
  discovery of, 319, 320i
  in kinin-mediated vasodilation, 294
  muscarinic agonists releasing, 95
Endozepines, 360
Enduron, 259. See also Methyclothiazide
Enflurane, 410i
  organ system effects of, 416–418
  preparations available, 423
  properties of, 413t
Englitazone, 701
Enkephalins, 77t, 85t
  receptor subtype activity of, 502t
Enovid, 665t
Enoxacin, 765i, 766t
  preparations available, 768

Enoxaparin, 550. See also Heparin
  preparations available, 561
  for venous thrombosis prevention, 558
ENS (enteric nervous system), 74, 75i
  nonadrenergic/noncholinergic neurons
    in, 82
  transmitter substances in, 77t
Enseals, 599. See also Aspirin
Entamoeba histolytica, amebiasis caused
    by, **850–855**
Enteric nervous system, 74, 75i
  nonadrenergic/noncholinergic neurons
    in, 82
  transmitter substances in, 77t
Enteric oxaluria, **720**
Enterobacter, empiric antimicrobial ther-
    apy and, 814t
Enterobius vermicularis (pinworm),
    drugs for, 863t
  albendazole, 864
  mebendazole, 869
  pyrantel, 876
Enterochromaffin cells, serotonin in, 273
Enterococcus, empiric antimicrobial ther-
    apy and, 814t
Enterocytozoon bieneusi, albendazole
    for, 865
Enteroglucagon, 701
Enterohepatic circulation, in digitoxin
    metabolism, 201–202
Enuresis, tricyclic antidepressants for,
    490
Envenomation, rattlesnake, **978**
Environmental factors, drug metabolism
    affected by, 59
Environmental persistence, toxicity and,
    947
Environmental pollutants, **954**
Environmental toxicology, 945–946
  insecticides and, 951, 952
Enzyme induction, in biotransformation,
    52–55
  drug-drug interactions and, 59, 59t
  oral anticoagulant interactions and,
    554
Enzyme inhibition, in biotransformation
  drug-drug interactions and, 59–60, 60t
  oral anticoagulant interactions and,
    554
Enzymes
  as drug receptors, 10
  endogenous, drug responsiveness af-
    fected by, 30
  iron content of, 534t
  ligand-regulated transmembrane,
    19–20, 20i
  in parasites, antiparasitic drugs affect-
    ing, **827–831**
Eosinophilia, tropical, drugs for, 863t
  diethylcarbamazine, 867
EP₁ receptor, 308
EP₂ receptor, 308
EP₃ receptor, 308
Ephedrine, 124i, 128
  for asthma, 333, 340
  ionization constant of, 6t

OTC status of, 1032t
  preparations available, 133, 340
Epidermal growth factor (EGF), ligand-
    regulated transmembrane enzymes
    in signalling by, 19–20, 20i
Epidural nerve block, 431i
Epilepsy. See also Seizures
  drugs for, **386–408**. See also
    Antiepileptic drugs
Epinephrine, 85t, 123i, 127
  for anaphylaxis, 132
  for asthma, 333, 340
  biosynthesis of, 79i
  cardiovascular system affected by,
    125t
  for glaucoma, 132, 149t
  ionization constant of, 6t
  local anesthetics combined with, 131,
    427
  metabolism of, 79–80, 80i
  OTC status of, 1032t
  for pharmacologic hemostasis, 131
  preparations available, 133–134, 340
Epivir, 801. See also Lamivudine
Epo (erythropoietin), 543, **543–544**, 543t
  preparations available, 546
Epoetin, 934t. See also Erythropoietin
Epoetin alfa, 544. See also Erythropoi-
    etin
  preparations available, 546
Epogen, 546. See also Epoetin alfa
Epoprostenol (prostacyclin/PGI₂), 306,
    312i, 547. See also Prostaglandins
  platelets affected by, 314–315
  preparations available, 317
  for pulmonary hypertension, 314
  second messenger for, 22t
  synthesis of, 306–307, 306i
Epoxidation, 53t
Epoxyeicosatrienoic acid (EET), 308
Epoxygenase products, 308
  effects of, 310–311
Epsom Salt (magnesium hydroxide),
    1018t
  in OTC preparations, efficacy of,
    1033t
  preparations available, 1028
EPSP (excitatory postsynaptic potential),
    344–345, 344i
Equalactin (polycarbophil), 1028
Equanil, 369. See also Meprobamate
ERE (estrogen response elements), 657
Erethism, 965
Ergocalciferol (vitamin D₂), 707, 709t.
    See also Vitamin D
  preparations available, 721
α-Ergocryptine, structure of, 279t
Ergoline, 278
Ergomar, 284. See also Ergotamine
Ergonovine (ergometrine)
  for migraine, 282
  for postpartum hemorrhage, 282
  preparations available, 284
  receptors affected by, 279t
  structure of, 279t
  toxicity of, 283
  uterine contractions caused by, 280

Ergostat, 284. *See also* Ergotamine
Ergosterol, amphotericin B binding and, 780
Ergot alkaloids, 139, **277–283**, 279*t*
  basic pharmacology of, **278–281**
  clinical pharmacology of, **281–283**
  mechanism of action of, 278–279, 279*t*
  organ system effects of, 278–281
  preparations available, 284
  receptors affected by, 278, 279, 279*t*
  structures of, 279*t*
  toxicity and contraindications of, 278, 283
Ergotamine
  ionization constant of, 6*t*
  for migraine, 282
  preparations available, 284
  receptors affected by, 279*t*
  structure of, 279*t*
  toxicity of, 278, 283
  vasospasm caused by, 278, 280, 280*i*, 281*i*
Ergotamine tartrate, 284. *See also* Ergotamine
Ergotism (ergot poisoning), 277, 278, 283
Ergotrate maleate, 284. *See also* Ergonovine
Ergotropic system, sympathetic system as, 82
Erosive esophagitis, H₂ receptor antagonists for, 272
Erythrocin, 751. *See also* Erythromycin
Erythrocytic stage, of *Plasmodium*, 838
Erythromycin, **747–748**, 747*i*
  gastrointestinal motility affected by, 1022
  interactions of, 748
  pharmacokinetic/pharmacodynamic parameters of, 36*t*, 748
  preparations available, 751
  resistance to, 748
  topical, for acne, 1001
Erythropoietin (Epo), 543, **543–544**, 543*t*, 934*t*
  preparations available, 546
Escherichia coli, empiric antimicrobial therapy and, 814*t*
Eserine (physostigmine), 97, 97*i*
  as antidote, 977*t*
  for antimuscarinic drug intoxication, 101–102
  for glaucoma, 149*t*
  ionization constant of, 6*t*
  mechanism of action of, 99
  preparations available, 103
Esidrix, 259. *See also* Hydrochlorothiazide
Eskalith, 480. *See also* Lithium
Esmolol, 138*t*, 146
  as antidote, 977*t*
  for arrhythmias, 234
  clinical properties of, 229*t*
  distribution and clearance of, 142, 144*t*
  membrane actions of, 228*t*

preparations available, 150, 240
  properties of, 144*t*
Esophagitis
  cholinomimetics for, sphincter tone and, 100
  erosive, H₂ receptor antagonists for, 272
Esotropia, accommodative, cholinomimetics for, 100
Essential hypertension, 153. *See also* Hypertension
Essential tremor, 459
Estazolam
  dosages of, 366*t*
  pharmacokinetics of, 358*t*
  preparations available, 369
Ester hydrolysis, 54*t*
  genetic polymorphisms affecting, 58, 58*t*
Estinyl, 680, 899*t*. *See also* Ethinyl estradiol
Estrace, 680. *See also* Estradiol
Estraderm, 680. *See also* Estradiol
Estradiol, 654, 655*i*, 656*i*, 657*t*. *See also* Estrogens
  ethinyl, 656*i*, 657*t*
    in cancer chemotherapy, 899*t*
    preparations available, 680
  pharmacokinetics of, 655*i*, 656
  preparations available, 680
  rate of production of, 655
Estriol, 654, 655*i*, 656*i*. *See also* Estrogens
  pharmacokinetics of, 656
Estrogen inhibitors/antagonists, **671–672**
  in cancer chemotherapy, **898–900**, 899*t*
  preparations available, 680
Estrogen receptor, in breast cancer, 898
Estrogen replacement therapy, 658–659, 659*i*
  for prevention and treatment of osteoporosis, 658, 717–718, 718*i*
Estrogen response elements (ERE), 657
Estrogens, **654–660**
  adverse effects of, 660
  in bone mineral homeostasis, **710**
  in cancer chemotherapy, 899*t*
  clinical uses for, 658–659
  conjugated, 657*t*
    preparations available, 680
  contraindications to, 660
  dosages of, 660
  effects of, 656–658
  for hypogonadism, 658
  inhibitors and antagonists of, **671–672**
    in cancer chemotherapy, **898–900**, 899*t*
    preparations available, 680
  interactions of, 1066*t*
  mechanism of action of, 656–657
  natural, 654–655
  for osteoporosis, 658, 717–718, 718*i*
  in OTC preparations, hidden, 1038*t*
  pharmacokinetics of, 655*i*, 656
  for postmenopausal hormonal therapy, 658–659, 659*i*

preparations available, 660, 680
  synthetic, 655–656, 656*i*, 657*t*
  synthetic and degradation pathways for, 663*i*
  topical preparations of, 659
Estrone, 654, 655*i*, 656*i*. *See also* Estrogens
  pharmacokinetics of, 656
  preparations available, 680
Estropipate, 657*t*
  preparations available, 680
Estrovis, 680. *See also* Quinestrol
ET_A receptors, 297–298
  antagonists of, 298, 300*i*
ET_B receptors, 297–298
  antagonists of, 298, 300*i*
ET-1, 297, 298*i*
  signal transduction mechanisms in action of, 298, 299*i*
ET-2, 297, 298*i*
ET-3, 297, 298*i*
Ethacrynic acid, 249
  chemistry of, 249, 249*i*
  clinical indications/dosage of, 250, 250*t*
  for glaucoma, 149*t*
  ionization constant of, 6*t*
  pharmacokinetic/pharmacodynamic parameters of, 250
  preparations available, 259
  toxicity of, 250–251
Ethambutol, 770, 771*t*, **773–774**, 774*i*
  in combination therapy, 772, 772*t*
  pharmacokinetic/pharmacodynamic parameters of, 36*t*, 774
  preparations available, 778
Ethanol
  abuse of, 519. *See also* Alcoholism
  acute consumption of, 373–375. *See also* Ethanol poisoning
    management of intoxication caused by, **379**
  as antidote, 977*t*
  antimicrobial effects of, 805*t*, 806
  basic pharmacology of, **372–378**
  in breast milk, 987*t*
  chronic consumption of, 375–378. *See also* Alcoholism
  clinical pharmacology of, **379–382**
  cross tolerance with sedative-hypnotics and, 363, 368
  dependence on, 375–376
  drug interactions and, 378–379
  drug metabolism inhibited by, 60*t*
  fetus affected by, 983*t*
  H₂ receptor antagonists affecting first-pass metabolism of, 271, 273
  metabolism of, 372–373, 373*i*
  for methanol poisoning, 382, 383, 977*t*
  mortality rates related to intake of, 377
  neurotoxic effects of, 376
  in OTC preparations, hidden, 1037*t*
  preparations available, 383
  teratogenic effects of, 378, 983*t*
  tolerance to, 375–376

Ethanol (cont.)
    withdrawal from, management of, **379–380**
    preparations available, 383
Ethanol poisoning, 972t, 974t
Ethanolamines, 267t
    structure of, 266i
Ethchlorvynol, 364
    drug metabolism induced by, 59t
    overdose of, 973t
    preparations available, 369
Ether, abuse of, 529
Ethinamate, preparations available, 369
Ethinyl estradiol, 656i, 657t
    in cancer chemotherapy, 899t
    preparations available, 680
Ethionamide, 775, 775i
    preparations available, 778
    for tuberculosis, 771t, 775
Ethmozine, 240. See also Moricizine
Ethnor, 878. See also Levamisole
Ethosuximide, **398–399**, 398i
    effective/toxic plasma levels of, 405t
    preparations available, 407
Ethotoin, **391**
    preparations available, 407
Ethrane, 423. See also Enflurane
Ethylene glycol, 383
Ethylene glycol poisoning, 974t
Ethylene oxide, for sterilization, 809
Ethylenediamines, 267t
    structure of, 266i
Ethylenediaminetetraacetate (EDTA), 956, 957i, **959**
    preparations available, 966
Ethyleneimonium ion, in alkylating drug mechanism of action, 885
Ethylestrenol, 675t
Ethylnorepinephrine, preparations available, 340
Ethynodiol, 661t
Ethyol (amifostine), **902**
Etidocaine
    preparations available, 432
    properties of, 426t
    structure of, 426t
Etidronate, 710–711, 711i
    for hypercalcemia, 713
    for osteoporosis, 711, 712, 718
    for Paget's disease, 720
    preparations available, 721
Etodolac, 580t, **588**
    preparations available, 599
Etomidate, 411i, 420t, **422**
    preparations available, 423
Etoposide, **894–895**, 894t
Etorphine, receptor subtype activity of, 502t
Etretinate. See also Retinoic acid
    in cancer chemotherapy, 901–902
    fetus affected by, 983t
    for psoriasis, **1007–1008**
Eulexin, 680, 899t. See also Flutamide
Euphoria, opioid analgesics causing, 505
Eurax, 1005. See also Crotamiton
Ewing's sarcoma, 911–912
Ex-Lax, 1028. See also Phenolphthalein

Excitatory amino acids, ligand-gated channels as receptors for, 20–21
Excitatory postsynaptic potential (EPSP), 344–345, 344i
Excitement, as anesthesia stage, 410
Excretion (drug)
    in infants and children, 984–985
    interactions and, 1059
    renal, Henderson-Hasselbalch equation and, 6, 7i
Exelderm, 786, 1002. See also Sulconazole
Exna, 259. See also Benzthiazide
Exocrine glands
    kinins affecting, 294
    sympathomimetics affecting, 127
Exocytosis, drug permeation by, 5
Exoerythrocytic stage, of Plasmodium, 838
Expectorants, OTC preparations, efficacy of, 1035t
Expedited Drug Approval Act, 68t
Exposure to chemicals
    duration of, 946
    mixtures and, 946
    routes of, 946
Extracellular water, drug distribution in, 39t
Extraction ratio, 41, 42
Extrapyramidal reactions, antipsychotic agents causing, 473
Extrinsic factor, 538. See also Vitamin B$_{12}$
Eye
    anterior chamber of, 88i
    antimuscarinic agents affecting, 107–108
    antipsychotic agents affecting, 474
    autonomic activity/drugs affecting, 83t, 148
    beta-receptor blocking drugs affecting, 143
    cholinesterase inhibitors affecting, 99
    direct-acting cholinomimetics affecting, 94, 94t
    disorders of
        antimuscarinic agents for, 111, 111t
        cholinomimetics for, 100
        sympathomimetics for, 132
    ganglion-blocking drugs affecting, 115
    pharmacology of, 148
    in poisoned patient, 971
    prostaglandins affecting, 310
    sympathomimetic agents affecting, 126
    thyroid hormones affecting, 625t

F cells (PP cells), pancreatic, 685t
FAC regimen, for breast cancer, 908
Factor I (fibrinogen), 547, 549t
    therapeutic, 559t, **560**
Factor II (prothrombin), 547, 549t
    therapeutic, 559t
Factor IIa (thrombin), 547
Factor III (tissue thromboplastin), 549t

Factor IV, 549t
Factor V (proaccelerin), 549t
    therapeutic, 559t
Factor VII (proconvertin), 547, 549i, 549t
    therapeutic, 559t
Factor VIII (antihemophilic globulin/AHG), 549t
    deficiency of, 559, 559t
    preparations available, 561
    recombinant, 560
    therapeutic, 559t, **560**
Factor IX (Christmas factor/plasma thromboplastin component), 549t
    deficiency of, 559, 559t, 560
    therapeutic, 559t, 560
    preparations available, 561
Factor IX concentrates, 559t, 560
    for oral anticoagulant-induced bleeding, 554
Factor X (Stuart-Prower factor), 549t
    activated, 547
    therapeutic, 559t
Factor XI (plasma thromboplastin antecedent/PTA), 549t
    therapeutic, 559t
Factor XII (Hageman factor), 549t
    therapeutic, 559t
Factor XIII (fibrin-stabilizing factor), 549t
    acquired antibodies to, immunosuppressive therapy for, 931t
    therapeutic, 559t
Factrel, 617. See also Gonadorelin
Fadrozole, 672
Famciclovir, 790i, **791–793**, 792t
    in dermatologic therapy, 1004
    preparations available, 801
Familial combined hyperlipoproteinemia, 567t, 568
Familial dysbetalipoproteinemia, 567t, 568
Familial hypercholesterolemia, 567t, 568, 569i
Familial hypertriglyceridemia, 567–568, 567t
Familial ligand-defective apolipoprotein B, 568
Familial tremor, 450, 459
Famotidine, 270t, 1019–1020
    clinical uses of, 272, 1020
    organ system effects of, 271
    in OTC preparations, efficacy of, 1033t
    OTC status of, 1031t
    preparations available, 284, 1026
    toxicity of, 272
Famvir, 801. See also Famciclovir
Fansidar (pyrimethamine-sulfadoxine), 764, **846–847**
    for malaria treatment, 841t, 845, 846
Fasciola hepatica (fascioliasis), drugs for infection with, 863t
    albendazole, 865
    bithionol, 865–866
    praziquantel, 875

Fasciolopsis buski, drugs for infection with, 863*t*
  niclosamide, 872
  praziquantal, 875
Fat
  autonomic activity/drugs affecting, 83*t*
  drug distribution in, 39*t*
  insulin affecting, 688–689, 688*t*
Fatty acids, omega-3, in dietary manipulation of arachidonic acid metabolism, 317
FDA (Food and Drug Administration), in new drug evaluation process, 67–68
Federal Food, Drug, and Cosmetic Act, 67, 68*t*
Feedback, negative
  in autonomic control of cardiovascular function, 84, 84*i*
  in presynaptic levels of autonomic function, 84
Feiba, 560. *See also* Factor IX
Feiba VH Immuno (anti-inhibitor coagulant complex), 561
Felbamate, **396**, 396*i*
Feldene, 599. *See also* Piroxicam
Felodipine
  clinical properties of, 190*t*
  for hypertension, 169
  pharmacokinetics of, 189*t*
  preparations available, 175, 194
  vascular selectivity of, 190*t*
Female infertility
  gonadotropin-releasing hormones for, 611–612
  human chorionic gonadotropin for, 612, 614
  human menopausal gonadotropins for, 612–613
  ovulation-inducing agents for, **672–673**
Female reproductive system. *See also* Reproductive organs
  antipsychotic drugs affecting, 469
  inhaled anesthetics affecting, 418–419
  maturation of, estrogens in, 657
  prostaglandins affecting, 310, 311–314
Fenbendazole, microtubules affected by, 835
Fenclonine (*p*-chlorophenylalanine), serotonin affected by, 273, 277
Fenfluramine, 276
Fenitrothion, 951*t*
Fenofibrate, 572
Fenoprofen, 580*t*, **586–587**
  preparations available, 599
Fenoterol, toxicity of, 335
Fentanyl, 420*t*, 421, 511
  pharmacokinetics of, 501*t*
  preparations available, 513
  receptor subtype activity of, 502*t*
  structure of, 499*i*
Fentanyl Oralet, preparations available, 513
Fentanyl Transdermal System, preparations available, 513

Fentanyl Transmucosal System, preparations available, 513
Ferritin, 534
  iron content of, 534*t*
Ferrous fumarate, 535*t*. *See also* Iron
Ferrous gluconate, 535*t*. *See also* Iron
Ferrous sulfate, 535*t*. *See also* Iron
Ferroxamine, 957*i*
Fetal alcohol syndrome, 378
Fetal drug metabolism, 980
Fetal hydantoin syndrome, 406
Fetal well-being, oxytocin challenge test in evaluation of, 615
Fetus
  adrenocorticosteroids for stimulation of lung maturation in, 643
  maternal drug use affecting, **979–982**. *See also* Pregnancy
  therapeutic drug actions in, 980
  toxic drug actions in, predictable, 980
Fever
  aspirin for, 581, 582–583
  prostaglandins affecting, 310
Fexofenadine, 267*t*, 268*t*, 270
  preparations available, 283
  structure of, 266*i*
FiberCon (polycarbophil), 1028
Fiber-Lax (polycarbophil), 1028
Fibrin inhibition, 548
Fibrin-stabilizing factor (factor XIII), 549*t*
  therapeutic, 559*t*
Fibrinogen (factor I), 547, 549*t*
  therapeutic, 559*t*, **560**
Fibrinolysis, 548, 550*i*
  inhibitors of, **560–561**. *See also* Aminocaproic acid
Fibrinolytic drugs
  basic pharmacology of, **555**
  for venous thrombosis, 558
Fick's law of diffusion, 5
50-235, as endothelin receptor antagonist, 298, 300*i*
Filariasis, drugs for, 863*t*
  diethylcarbamazine, 866
    adverse reactions and, 867
  ivermectin, 868
Filgrastim, 544. *See also* Granulocyte colony-stimulating factor
  in cancer chemotherapy, 902
  preparations available, 546
Finasteride, 678, 678*i*
  preparations available, 680
First-pass effect/elimination, 51
  of benzodiazepines, 356
  bioavailability and, 41, 41*i*, 42
  route of administration and, 42
Fish tapeworm, drugs for, 863*t*
  niclosamide, 871
FK 506 (tacrolimus), **926**
  preparations available, 940
Flagyl, 810, 859. *See also* Metronidazole
Flavin monooxygenase, 53*t*
Flavoxate, preparations available, 115, 1027
Flaxedil, 448. *See also* Gallamine

Flecainide, **233–234**
  for arrhythmias, **233–234**, 234
  clinical properties of, 229*t*
  membrane actions of, 228*t*
  preparations available, 240
Fleet Babylax, 1028. *See also* Glycerin suppositories
Fleet Phospho-Soda, 721. *See also* Phosphate
Fleroxacin, 766
Flexeril, 448. *See also* Cyclobenzaprine
Flexible regulation, in second messenger signaling, 27
Flolan, 317. *See also* Epoprostenol
Florinef, 650. *See also* Fludrocortisone
Floropryl, 103. *See also* Isoflurophate
Flovent, 340. *See also* Fluticasone
Flow-dependent elimination, 39
Floxin, 768. *See also* Ofloxacin
Fluconazole, 784*i*, 784*t*, **785**, 1004
  for dermatologic therapy, 1004
  preparations available, 786
Flucytosine, **782–783**, 782*i*
  preparations available, 786
Fludara, 891*t*. *See also* Fludarabine
Fludarabine, 891*t*, **892**
Fludrocortisone, 640*t*, **647**
  preparations available, 650
Fluid and electrolyte balance, chronic alcohol consumption affecting, 378
Fluidization, ethanol causing, 374
Flukes, drugs for, 863*t*
  niclosamide, 872
Flumadine, 801. *See also* Rimantadine
Flumazenil, 360, **363**, 367, 977*t*
  in initial management of poisoned patient, 971
  preparations available, 369
Flunarizine, for migraine headache, 282
Flunisolide, 336
  aerosol form of, 646
  preparations available, 340
Flunitrazepam, criminal use of, 521
Fluoride
  bone mineral homeostasis affected by, **712**
  for osteoporosis, 712, 718, 718*i*
  OTC status of, 1031*t*
  preparations available, 721
Fluorocarbons, inhalation of, 529
5-Fluorodeoxyuridine, nucleoside phosphotransferases affected by, 829
Fluorophenylindole, 468*t*
Fluoroquinolones, **765–767**
  adverse effects of, 766–767
  pharmacokinetics of, 766, 766*t*
  preparations available, 768
  sistance to, 765–766, 767
  structures of, 765*i*
Fluorosis, 712
Fluorouracil, 891*t*, **892**, 892*i*
  in dermatologic therapy, **1013**
Fluothane, 423. *See also* Halothane
Fluoxetine, 484
  adverse effects of, 493*t*
  for alcoholism, 381

Fluoxetine (cont.)
dosages of, 491t
for acute episode, 491
effects of, 489, 489t
interactions of, 492
for obsessive-compulsive disorder, 490
pharmacokinetic/pharmacodynamic
parameters of, 36t, 486–487,
488t
preparations available, 494
Fluoxymesterone, 675t, 676t
in cancer chemotherapy, 899t
preparations available, 680
Fluphenazine, 466i, 468t, 472
advantages and disadvantages of, 471t
dose relationships of, 472t
ionization constant of, 6t
preparations available, 480
Fluprednisolone, 640t
Flurazepam, 356i
biotransformation of, 357–358, 357i
dosages of, 366t
pharmacokinetics of, 358t
preparations available, 369
Flurbiprofen, 580t, 586i, **587**
preparations available, 599
Flutamide, 677, 679, 679i, 899t, 900
in cancer chemotherapy, 899t, 900
preparations available, 680
Fluticasone, for asthma, 336
preparations available, 340
Fluvastatin, 573, 574
preparations available, 576
Fluvoxamine
dosages of, 491t
interactions of, 492–493
pharmacokinetics of, 488t
preparations available, 494
Folacin, 546. See also Folic acid
Folic acid, **537–543**
chemistry of, 538, 538i, 539i
clinical pharmacology of, 540–543
clinical uses for, 542–543
for coronary artery disease prevention,
542–543
deficiency of, 542
anemias caused by, 537, 540, 542
for methanol poisoning, 383
pharmacodynamics of, 540, 541i
pharmacokinetics of, 539
preparations available, 546
structure of, 538i
Follicle-stimulating hormone (FSH),
604t, **612**, 653
in menotropins, 612–613
receptors for, 604
second messenger for, 22t
Folliculitis, lithium causing, 479
Food, Drug, and Cosmetic Act, 67, 68t
Food and Drug Administration (FDA), in
new drug evaluation process,
67–68
Forane, 423. See also Isoflurane
Formaldehyde, antimicrobial effects of,
805t, 808
Formalin, 808
Formoterol, for asthma, 334

Formycin B, nucleoside phosphotrans-
ferases affected by, 829
Fortaz, 741. See also Ceftazidime
48/80, histamine release caused by, 262
Fosamax, 721. See also Alendronate
Foscarnet, 790i, 792t, **793–794**
preparations available, 801
Foscavir, 801. See also Foscarnet
Fosfomycin, **739**
preparations available, 741
Fosinopril
for hypertension, 170
preparations available, 175, 213
Fosphenytoin, 388
preparations available, 407
Foxglove plant, digitalis derived from,
200
FR-139317, 298, 300i
Fragmin, 561. See also Dalteparin
Framycetin, 758
Frank-Starling law, in cardiac function,
200, 200i
Free radicals, in nitric oxide inactivation,
320–321
FSH (follicle-stimulating hormone),
604t, **612**, 653
in menotropins, 612–613
receptors for, 604
second messenger for, 22t
5-FU (fluorouracil), 891t, **892**, 892i
in dermatologic therapy, **1013**
Fulvin P/G, 786. See also Griseofulvin
Functional tolerance, 516
Fungal infections
dermatologic, drugs for, **1002–1004**
drugs for, **780–787**. See also specific
type
preparations available, 786
systemic, **1003–1004**
for surface infections, **785–786**
for systemic infections, **780–785**
topical, **786**, **1002–1003**
OTC preparations, efficacy of,
1034t
empiric antimicrobial therapy and,
815t
Fungizone, 786, 1003. See also Amphotericin B
Furacin (nitrofurazone), 810
Furadantin, 810. See also Nitrofurantoin
Furamide, 858. See also Diloxanide
Furosemide, 249
chemistry of, 249, 249i
clinical indications/dosage of, 250,
250t
contraindications to, 251
ionization constant of, 6t
pharmacokinetic/pharmacodynamic
parameters of, 36t, 250
preparations available, 259
toxicity of, 250–251
Fusobacterium, empiric antimicrobial
therapy and, 815t

G proteins, 21–23
alpha receptor activation and,
120–121, 121i, 122i

muscarinic receptor activation and, 90,
93–94
opioid receptor linkage and, 501–502,
502i, 503i
receptors and effectors for, 23t
in sympathomimetic mechanism of
action, 120–121
G-CSF (granulocyte colony-stimulating
factor), 543, 543t, 544–545, 934t,
935
in cancer chemotherapy, 902
preparations available, 546
recombinant human, 544
GABA (gamma-aminobutyric acid), 77t,
349t, 350–351
antiepileptic drugs affecting, 387, 395,
396–397, 397–398, 400
baclofen affecting, 445–446, 446i
barbiturates affecting, 360, 361i
benzodiazepines affecting, 359–360
ethanol affecting, 374
in Huntington's disease, 460
receptors for, 351
ligand-gated channels as, 20–21
in tardive dyskinesia, 461
vigabatrin affecting, 395
GABA_A receptors, 351
benzodiazepine and barbiturate binding to, 359, 359i
ethanol affecting, 374
GABA_B receptors, 351
baclofen affecting, 446
GABA-BDZ receptor chloride channel,
359, 359i, 361
antiepileptic drugs affecting, 387
Gabapentin, **396–397**
preparations available, 407
Galactorrhea, bromocriptine for, 614
Galanin, as neurotransmitter, 77t
Gallamine, 438t
effects of, 443t
preparations available, 448
Gallbladder disease, estrogen therapy
and, 660
Gallium nitrate
for hypercalcemia, 714
preparations available, 721
Gallstones, drugs for dissolution of,
1024–1025
preparations available, 1028
Gametocides, for malaria, 838
primaquine, 845
Gametocytes, plasmodial, 838
Gamimune N, 801. See also Immune
globulin intravenous
Gamma-aminobutyric acid, 77t, 349t,
350–351
antiepileptic drugs affecting, 387, 395,
396–397, 397–398, 400
baclofen affecting, 445–446, 446i
barbiturates affecting, 360, 361i
benzodiazepines affecting, 359–360
ethanol affecting, 374
in Huntington's disease, 460
receptors for, 351
ligand-gated channels as, 20–21

in tardive dyskinesia, 461
vigabatrin affecting, 395
Gamma interferon, 800, 926, 933, 934, 934*t*, 935
preparations available, 940
Gamma nerve fibers, local anesthetics affecting, 429*t*
Ganciclovir, 790*i*, 792*t*, **793**
mechanism of action of, 791*i*
preparations available, 801
Ganglion-blocking drugs, **114–115**, **160–161**
for hypertension, **160–161**
preparations available, 116, 175
procainamide as, 228
Ganite, 721. *See also* Gallium nitrate
Gantanol, 768. *See also* Sulfamethoxazole
Gantrisin, 768. *See also* Sulfisoxazole
Garamycin, 759. *See also* Gentamicin
Gastrectomy, vitamin B$_{12}$ deficiency after, 541–542
Gastric acid secretion. *See also* Gastrointestinal secretion
drugs affecting, **1019–1021**
OTC preparations, efficacy of, 1033*t*
H$_2$ receptor antagonists affecting, 270–271, 271*i*, 1019–1020
histamine affecting, 264, 1019*i*
histamine for testing, 265
prostaglandins affecting, 315
Gastric antisecretory drugs, **1019–1021**
OTC preparations, efficacy of, 1033*t*
Gastric cancer, 903*t*, 911
Gastric lavage, for poisoned patient, 975, 976*i*
Gastric ulcers, H$_2$ receptor antagonists for, 272
Gastrin-releasing peptide (GRP), 77*t*
Gastritis, aspirin causing, 583–584
Gastrocrom, 340. *See also* Cromolyn
Gastroduodenal surgery, antimicrobial prophylaxis and, 824*t*
Gastroesophageal reflux disorder, H$_2$ receptor antagonists for, 272
Gastrointestinal disorders. *See also* specific type
antimuscarinic agents for, 111–112, 112*t*
chloramphenicol causing, 744
cholinomimetics for, 100–101
drugs used in, **1017–1029**
eicosanoids in, 315
erythromycin causing, 748
prostaglandins for, 315
quinine causing, 848
tetracyclines causing, 746–747
Gastrointestinal motility
antimuscarinic agents affecting, 110
direct-acting cholinomimetics affecting, 94*t*, 96
drugs promoting, **1021–1022**
preparations available, 1027
H$_2$ receptor antagonists affecting, 270–271

Gastrointestinal secretion. *See also* Gastric acid secretion
antimuscarinic agents affecting, 110
autonomic activity/drugs affecting, 83*t*
direct-acting cholinomimetics affecting, 94*t*, 96
H$_2$ receptor antagonists affecting, 270–271, 271*i*
histamine affecting, 264
Gastrointestinal system
antimuscarinic agents affecting, 109–110, 110*i*
aspirin affecting, 583–584
autonomic activity/drugs affecting, 83*t*
bromocriptine affecting, 455
carcinoma of, **910–911**
cholinesterase inhibitors affecting, 99
chronic alcohol consumption affecting, 375
cytochrome P450-derived metabolites affecting, 310
decontamination of in poisoned patient, 974–976
digitalis toxicity affecting, 205
direct-acting cholinomimetics affecting, 94*t*, 96
drug absorption affected by function of, in infants and children, 982
enteric nervous system of, 74, 75*i*
ganglion-blocking drugs affecting, 115
histamine affecting, 264
lead toxicity and, 961–962
levodopa affecting, 453
lipoxygenase metabolites affecting, 310
methylxanthines affecting, 331–332
opioid analgesics affecting, 506
oral contraceptive use and, 669
parathyroid hormone affecting, 709*t*
prostaglandins affecting, 309
radiology of, glucagon for, 703
serotonin affecting, 275
sympathomimetics affecting, 126
thromboxanes affecting, 309
thyroid hormones affecting, 625*t*
vitamin D affecting, 709*t*
Gelusil, 1018*t*
Gemfibrozil, **571–572**, 571*i*
combination therapy with, 575
preparations available, 576
Gemonil (metharbital), 407
Gender, drug metabolism affected by, 59
Gene therapy, **936**
General anesthetics, **409–424**
inhaled, 409, 410*i*, **412–419**, 413*t*
intravenous, 409–410, 411*i*, **419–423**
neuromuscular blocking drug interaction and, 444
preparations available, 423
solubility of, 412, 413*i*, 414*i*
Generalized seizures, 387*t*, 403–404
drugs used in, **398–402**, **404–405**
secondarily, 403
Generalized tonic-clonic seizures, 403–404
drugs used in, **388–398**, **404**

Generic name, prescribing by, 1048–1049
Genetic polymorphism, in drug metabolism, 57–59, 58*i*, 58*t*
Genital herpes
acyclovir for, 790, 791
antimicrobial prophylaxis and, 824*t*
famciclovir for, 792
valacyclovir for, 791
Genitourinary disorders, sympathomimetics for, 132–133
Genitourinary system. *See also* Urinary tract
antimuscarinic agents affecting, 110, 110*i*
autonomic activity/drugs affecting, 83*t*
direct-acting cholinomimetics affecting, 96
ganglion-blocking drugs affecting, 115
opioid analgesics affecting, 506
sympathomimetic agents affecting, 126–127
Genora, 665*t*
Gentamicin, 754*i*, **755–756**
adverse effects of, 754, 756
in dermatologic therapy, **1000–1001**
half-life of, aging affecting, 992*i*
pharmacokinetic/pharmacodynamic parameters of, 36*t*
preparations available, 759
resistance to, 756
Geocillin, 740. *See also* Carbenicillin
Geref, 617. *See also* Sermorelin
Geriatric pharmacology, **989–998**. *See also* Aging
Gestodene, 661
GH (growth hormone/somatotropin), 604*t*, **606–608**
deficiency of, 607
receptors for, 604–605
GHRH (growth hormone-releasing hormone/sermorelin), 604*t*, **605**
receptors for, 604
GHRPs (growth hormone-releasing peptides), **605**
Giardia lamblia (giardiasis)
drugs for, 855*t*, 857–858
albendazole, 865
metronidazole, 858
purine metabolism in, 831, 832*i*
Gilles de la Tourette's syndrome, 450, 460
antipsychotic agents for, 470
Gingival hyperplasia, phenytoin causing, 391
Glaucoma
levodopa use and, 454
treatment of, 87, 149*t*
beta-receptor blocking drugs for, 132, 143, 147, 148, 149*t*
carbonic anhydrase inhibitors for, 248, 248*t*
cholinomimetics for, 100, 149*t*
diuretics for, 149*t*, 248, 248*t*
latanoprost for, 316
sympathomimetics for, 132, 149*t*

Glibenclamide, 697t. *See also* Glyburide
Glicentin, 701
Glimepiride, 697t, 698, 699
  preparations available, 703
Glioblastoma multiforme, 912
Glipizide, 697t, 698, 699
  preparations available, 703
Glomerulonephritis, acute, immunosup-
    pressive agents for, 931t
Glomerulopathy, minimal change,
    lithium causing, 478
GLP-1, 701
GLP-2, 701
Glucagon, 684, 685t, **701–703**, 702i
  A cell secretion of, 685t, 701
  as antidote, 977t
  for diagnostic testing, 702
  "gut," 701–702
  preparations available, 703
  second messenger for, 22t
  sulfonylureas affecting serum concen-
      trations of, 696
Glucocorticoid receptor elements (GRE),
    637, 638i
  progesterone receptor binding to, 662
Glucocorticoids, **593–594, 635–640,
    640–646**. *See also* Adrenocorticos-
    teroids; Corticosteroids
  for adrenal disorders, 641–643
  antagonists of, **647–649**
    preparations available, 650
  anti-inflammatory effects of, 639
  in bone mineral homeostasis, **710**
  catabolic effects of, 639
  contraindications to, 645
  for diagnosis, 642–643
  dosage schedules and forms for,
      645–646
  fetal lung maturation and, 643
  for hypercalcemia, 714
  immunosuppressive effects of, 639, **925**
  mechanism of action of, 18–19, 19i,
      637, 638i
  metabolic effects of, 638–639
  naturally occurring, **635–640**
  for nonadrenal disorders, 643–644,
      643t
  pharmacodynamics of, 640–641,
      647–640
  pharmacokinetics of, 635–636, 636i,
      637i, 640, 640t, 641i
  physiologic effects of, 638
  precautions in use of, 645
  preparations available, 650
  selection of, 645
  synthesis of, 635, 636i
  synthetic, **640–646**
  toxicity of, 644–645
  withdrawal from, 645
Glucophage, 703. *See also* Metformin
Glucose tolerance, impaired, thiazides
    causing, 251–252
Glucose transporters, insulin affecting,
    686–688, 688t
α-Glucosidase inhibitors, **700–701**
  preparations available, 703
Glucotrol, 697t, 703. *See also* Glipizide

Glururonidation, 57t
GLUT 1 to 5, 688, 688t
Glutamate, 349t, 351
  ethanol affecting, 374
Glutamic acid decarboxylase, in Hunt-
    ington's disease, 460
Glutaraldehyde, antimicrobial effects of,
    805t, 808
Glutathione, nitric oxide interaction and,
    321
Glutathione conjugation, 57t
Glutethimide, 357i, 364
  drug metabolism induced by, 59t
  overdose of, 973t
Glyburide, 697t, 698–699
  preparations available, 703
Glycerin suppositories
  preparations available, 1028
  as stool softener, 1024
Glycine
  as neurotransmitter in CNS, 349t,
      350–351
  spasmolytic actions of, 447
Glycine conjugation, 57t
Glycolipid synthesis, antiparasitic drugs
    affecting, 831
Glycolytic enzymes, antiparasitic drugs
    affecting, 833–834
Glycopeptides, dosing guidelines for,
    730i
Glycopyrrolate, 107i
  for gastrointestinal and genitourinary
      conditions, 112t
  preparations available, 115, 1027
Glydiazinamide, 697t. *See also* Glipizide
Glynase, 703. *See also* Glyburide
GM-CSF (granulocyte-macrophage
    colony-stimulating factor), 543,
    543t, 544–545, 934t, 935
  in cancer chemotherapy, 902
  in inflammation, 579t
  preparations available, 546
  recombinant human, 544–545
Gnathostomiasis, albendazole for, 865
GnRH (gonadotropin-releasing hor-
    mone), 604t, **611–612**, 653
  receptors for, 604
GnRH agonists (gonadotropin-releasing
    hormone agonists), in cancer
    chemotherapy, 899t, **900**
GnRH antagonists (gonadotropin-releas-
    ing hormone antagonists), 677
  for chemical contraception in men,
      679
Goiter
  nontoxic, **632**
  toxic, uninodular and multinodular,
      631
Goitrogens, nontoxic goiter caused by,
    632
Gold compounds, in inflammation,
    591–592
Gold sodium thiomalate (aurothioma-
    late), 591, 592
  preparations available, 599
Goldman-Hodgkin-Katz equation,
    218–219

GoLYTELY
  for gut decontamination, 976
  preparations available, 1028
Gonadal hormones and inhibitors,
    653–683. *See also specific hor-
    mone and* Ovary; Testis
Gonadorelin, **611–612**. *See also* Go-
    nadotropin-releasing hormone
  structure of, 611i
Gonadotropin-releasing hormone
    (GnRH), 604t, **611–612**, 653
  receptors for, 604
Gonadotropin-releasing hormone
    (GnRH) agonists, in cancer
    chemotherapy, 899t, **900**
Gonadotropin-releasing hormone
    (GnRH) antagonists, 677
  for chemical contraception in men,
      679
Gonadotropins, **612–613**
  oral contraceptives affecting pituitary
      secretion of, 667
Goserelin, 611, 677
  in cancer chemotherapy, 899t, **900**
  structure of, 611i
Gossypol, **679**, 679i
Gout
  drugs for, **595–599**
    preparations available, 600
  loop diuretics precipitating attacks of,
      250
  nonsteroidal anti-inflammatory drugs
      for, 567
  pathophysiology of, 595, 596i
GP IIB/IIIA receptors, drugs blocking,
    557
Graded dose-response relationships, 28,
    28i
  poisoning and, 969, 969i
Graft-versus-host syndrome, cy-
    closporine for, 925, 932
Grain, ergot alkaloid contamination of,
    277, 278
Gram-negative bacteria, empiric antimi-
    crobial therapy and, 814t
Gram-positive bacteria, empiric antimi-
    crobial therapy and, 814t
Gramicidin, in dermatologic therapy,
    1000
Grand mal seizures, 403–404
  drugs used in, **388–398**, 404
Granisetron, 277
  preparations available, 284
Granulocyte colony-stimulating factor
    (G-CSF), 543, 543t, 544–545,
    934t, 935
  in cancer chemotherapy, 902
  preparations available, 546
  recombinant human, 544
Granulocyte-macrophage colony-stimu-
    lating factor (GM-CSF), 543, 543t,
    544–545, 934t, 935
  in cancer chemotherapy, 902
  in inflammation, 579t
  preparations available, 546
  recombinant human, 544–545

Granulocytopenia, myeloid growth factor treatment for, 545

Grapefruit juice, terfenadine blood levels affected by, 268, 269–270

Graves' disease, **629–631**
neonatal, 632

Gray baby syndrome, 745

GRE (glucocorticoid receptor elements), 637, 638*i*
progesterone receptor binding to, 662

Grifulvin, 786. *See also* Griseofulvin

Grisactin, 786. *See also* Griseofulvin

Griseofulvin, 785, **1003**
in dermatologic therapy, **1003**
drug metabolism induced by, 59*t*
preparations available, 786

Growth factors, **543–545**, 543*t*
in cancer chemotherapy, **902**
preparations available, 546
myeloid, **544–545**
preparations available, 546

Growth fraction, cancer cells in, cell cycle-specific drugs and, 883

Growth hormone (GH/somatotropin), 604*t*, **606–608**
deficiency of, 607
receptors for, 604–605

Growth hormone-inhibiting hormone (somatotropin release-inhibiting hormone/SRIH/somatostatin), 604*t*, **605–606**, 606*i*
receptors for, 604

Growth hormone-releasing hormone (GHRH/sermorelin), 604*t*, **605**
receptors for, 604

Growth hormone-releasing peptides (GHRPs), **605**

Growth stimulators, androgens and anabolic steroids as, 676

GRP (gastrin-releasing peptide), 77*t*

Guaifenesin, in OTC preparations, efficacy of, 1035*t*

Guanabenz, 158
preparations available, 175

Guanadrel, 161
preparations available, 175

Guanethidine, **161–162**, 161*i*, 162*i*
for hyperthyroidism, 628
ionization constant of, 6*t*
preparations available, 175

Guanfacine, 158
preparations available, 175

Guanine, 892*i*

Guanosine, nucleoside phosphotransferases affected by, 829

N-Guanylhistamine, history of development of, 63*t*

Guedel's signs, 410

Guinea worm (dracunculiasis/*Dracunculus medinesis*), drugs for infection with, 863*t*
metronidazole, 858

"Gut dialysis," 976

"Gut glucagon," 701–702

Gynecologic disorders, androgen replacement therapy for, 676

Gynecomastia
digitalis toxicity causing, 205
potassium-sparing diuretics causing, 254

H_1 receptors, 262, 263*t*
bronchoconstriction mediated by, 264
cardiovascular effects of histamine and, 263–264, 263*i*

H_1 receptor antagonists, **265–270**
active metabolites of, 268
antiemetic actions of, 1022
basic pharmacology of, **265–268**
cardiovascular response to histamine and, 263–264, 263*i*
clinical pharmacology of, **268–270**
effects of, 267–268
interactions of, 269–270
for motion sickness, 268, 269, 1022
preparations available, 283–284
sedative effects of, 355
structure of, 266*i*
toxicity of, 269

H_2 receptors, 262, 263*t*
cardiac contractility affected by, 264
cardiovascular effects of histamine and, 263–264, 263*i*

H_2 receptor antagonists, **270–273**, 270*t*, **1019–1020**
for acid-peptic disease, **1019–1020**, 1026
basic pharmacology of, **270–271**
cardiovascular response to histamine and, 263–264, 263*i*
clinical pharmacology of, **271–273**
in combination therapy, 1020
development of, 62–64, 63*t*, 270
dosage of, 1020
immunomodulating effect of, 936
interactions of, 273
mechanisms of action of, 270
organ system effects of, 270–271
OTC preparations, 1020
efficacy of, 1033*t*
preparations available, 284, 1026
for refractory disease, 1020
toxicity of, 272, 1020

H_3 receptors, 262–263, 263*t*

H-BIG (hepatitis immune globulin), 801

Haemophilus influenzae, type B
antimicrobial prophylaxis and, 825*t*
vaccine for, 1052*t*

Hageman factor (factor XII), 549*t*
therapeutic, 559*t*

Hair creams, OTC preparations for, hidden ingredients in, 1038*t*

Hair loss, minoxidil for, 1014

Hairy cell leukemia, **907**

Halazepam
dosages of, 366*t*
preparations available, 369

Halcion, 366*t*, 369. *See also* Triazolam

Haldol, 471*t*, 472*t*, 480. *See also* Haloperidol

Haldol Decanoate, 480

Half-life ($t_{1/2}$), 39–40
aging affecting, 991, 992*i*
in neonates vs. adults, 985*t*
therapeutic drug monitoring and, 46

Hallucinogens
abuse of, **524–526**
ergot alkaloids as, 277, 278, 279

Halofantrine, for malaria treatment, 841*t*, 849

Halogenated aliphatic hydrocarbons, **949–950**

Halogenated hydroxyquinolines
for amebiasis, 850
antiparasitic actions of, 836*t*

Halogens, antimicrobial effects of, **806–807**

Haloperidol, 466*i*, 468*t*, 471–472
advantages and disadvantages of, 471*t*
dose relationships of, 472*t*
in elderly, 993
for Huntington's disease, 460
plasma concentrations of, 472
preparations available, 480
receptor binding by, 468, 469
for Tourette's syndrome, 460

Haloprogin, OTC status of, 1032*t*

Halotestin, 680, 899*t*. *See also* Fluoxymesterone

Halothane, 410*i*
elimination of, 414
hepatotoxicity of, 418
organ system effects of, 416–418
preparations available, 423
properties of, 413*t*
solubility of, 412, 413*i*, 413*t*

Handwashing, in infection prevention, 804–805

Harrison Narcotic Act, 68*t*

Hashimoto's thyroiditis, 628, 629*i*, 632

Hay fever
cromolyn for, 330
H_1 receptor antagonists for, 268–269

Hazard, toxicologic definition of, 946

HBIG (hepatitis immune globulin), 801, 1056*t*

hCG (human chorionic gonadotropin), 612, **613–614**
preparations available, 617

HDL (high-density lipoproteins), 563–564, 565*t*
deficiency of, **569**
synthesis and catabolism of, 566

Head injury, opioid analgesic use and, 510

Head and neck cancer, 903*t*

Head and neck surgery, antimicrobial prophylaxis and, 824*t*

Heart
antimuscarinic agents affecting, 108–109
autonomic activity/drugs affecting, 83*t*
beta-receptor blocking drugs affecting, 142–143, 144*i*
toxicity and, 149
cholinesterase inhibitors affecting, 99–100

Heart (cont.)
digitalis affecting, 202–204
direct-acting cholinomimetics affecting, 94–95, 94t
electrical activity of
digitalis glycosides affecting, 203–204, 203i, 204i, 204t
ionic basis of, 216–219
normal, **216–220**, 217i, 221i
enlargement of
angiotensin II affecting, 289
in heart failure, 199
ethanol affecting
acute consumption, 374
chronic consumption, 376–377
ganglion-blocking drugs affecting, 115
glucagon affecting, 702
H_2 receptor antagonists affecting, 271
lipoxygenases affecting, 310–311
methylxanthines affecting, 331
performance of, pathophysiology of, 199–200
sympathomimetic agents affecting, 125, 125i, 125t
transplantation of, immunosuppressive therapy and, 931t
Heart block, 224, 225i
complete, sympathomimetics for, 131
Heart disease. See also Cardiac/cardio-vascular disease
alcohol consumption and, 377
cholinesterase inhibitors for, 101
ischemic. See also Angina pectoris
beta-receptor blocking drugs for, 146, 147i, 192, 192i
vasodilators for, **179–196**
lithium causing, 478
sympathomimetics for, 131
thioridazine causing, 474
Heart failure, **197–215**
acute, **210–212**
angiotensin-converting enzyme inhibitors for, 197, 206–207, 210, 210t, 213, 291, 292i, 293
beta-receptor blocking drugs for, 146, 207
risks of use of, 149, 207
chronic, **209–210**, 209t, 210t
compensatory responses in, 199, 199i
diuretics for, 206, 209, **256–257**
with "power failure," 212
with pulmonary congestion, 211–212
drugs for, **197–215**. See also Cardiac glycosides
basic pharmacology of, **200–207**
clinical pharmacology of, **207–212**
preparations available, 213
pathophysiology of, **199–200**
positive inotropic drugs for, **205–206**, 207
in elderly, 994–995
sympathomimetics for, 131
vasodilators for, 207

Heart rate
cardiac function affected by, 200
histamine affecting, 263, 263i
Heat shock proteins (Hsp), 637, 657
Heavy metals
chelators for intoxication with, **956–959**
preparations available, 966
as disinfectants, **809**
toxicology of, **959–966**
Helicobacter pylori
in acid-peptic disease, 1017
empiric antimicrobial therapy and, 814t
Helminthic infections, drugs for, **862–880**, 863–864t. See also specific type
administration of, 862
contraindications to, 862
neurotoxicity of, 835
OTC preparations, efficacy of, 1034t
pediatric dosages of, 862
Helper T cells, 918, 919i
Hematopoiesis
chronic alcohol consumption affecting, 378
thyroid hormones affecting, 625t
Hematopoietic growth factors, **543–545**, 543t
in cancer chemotherapy, **902**
preparations available, 546
Hematotoxicity. See also Blood
of inhaled anesthetics, 419
of lead, 961
of quinine, 848
of sulfonamides, 763
Heme, 533
Hemocholiniums, 75–76
Hemochromatosis, 536
Hemodialysis, in poisoning, 975t, 976
with methanol, 382
Hemofil M, 561. See also Antihemophilic globulin
Hemoglobin, 533
iron content of, 534t
Hemolysis, quinine causing, 848
Hemolytic anemia
autoimmune, immunosuppressive agents for, 931t, 932
of newborn, Rh_o (D) immune globulin in prevention of, 930–931, 931t
Hemoperfusion, in poisoning, 975t, 977
Hemophilia
type A (classic), 559
desmopressin for, 616
factor VIII for, 559t, 560
type B, 559
factor IX for, 559t, 560
Hemorrhage, postpartum, ergot alkaloids for control of, 282
Hemorrhoidal OTC preparations, hidden ingredients in, 1037t, 1038t, 1039t
Hemosiderin, 534
iron content of, 534t
Hemosiderosis, 536

Hemostasis, 547
aspirin affecting, 556–557, 581–582, 583
pharmacologic, sympathomimetics for, 131
Henbane, 105
Henderson-Hasselbalch equation, 5–7
Henle, loop of, transport in/diuretic site of action and, **244–245**, 245i, 249, 250
Heparin, 548, **548–551**
preparations available, 561
structure of, 550, 550i
for venous thrombosis, 558
Hepatic abscess, amebic, treatment of, 851t, 852
Hepatic blood flow, inhaled anesthetics affecting, 418–419
Hepatic cirrhosis, diuretics for, **258**
Hepatic clearance
of benzodiazepines, 356–358
diseases affecting, drug metabolism and, 60, 60t
of ethanol, 372–373, 373i
Hepatic disease/impaired hepatic function. See also Hepatotoxicity
acetaminophen causing, 595
alcoholic, 375
antimicrobial use and, 819, 819t
diuretics for, **258**
drug metabolism affected by, 60, 60t
erythromycin causing, 748
H_2 receptor antagonists causing, 272
halothane causing, 418
isoniazid causing, 772
opioid analgesic use and, 510
tetracyclines causing, 747
Hepatitis
erythromycin causing, 748
isoniazid causing, 772
viral
active immunization for, 1052t
disinfection procedures and, 807
passive immunization for, 1056t
Hepatitis B immune globulin, 1056t
preparations available, 801
Hepatotoxicity. See also Hepatic disease/impaired hepatic function
halothane, 418
Heptachlor, 950t
Herbicides, **952–954**, 953i
bipyridyl, **953–954**, 953i
chlorophenoxy, **952–953**, 953i
HERG gene mutation, in long QT syndrome, 223
Heroin, 510
abuse of, 518
in breast milk, 987t
fetus affected by, 983t
methadone for detoxification and, 510–511, 519
overdose of, 972t
withdrawal from, 518
Herpes simplex virus
acyclovir for, 790, 791
antimicrobial prophylaxis for, 824t
foscarnet for, 794

idoxuridine for, 794
valacyclovir for, 791
vidarabine for, 795
Herpes zoster
famciclovir for, 792
sorivudine for, 794
valacyclovir for, 791
Herpesvirus infections, **788–795**. *See also specific agent*
Herplex, 801. *See also* Idoxuridine
HETE (hydroxyeicosatetraenoic acid), 307
effects of, 310–311
Heteroceptors, 84, 85*t*
Heterocyclic antidepressants (second- and third-generation antidepressants)
chemistry of, 484, 484*i*, 486*i*
dosages of, 491*t*
for acute episode, 491
effects of, 488–489
interactions of, 1062*t*
overdoses of, 493
pharmacokinetics of, 486, 488*t*
preparations available, 494
Heterophyes heterophyes (heterophyiasis), drugs for, 863*t*
niclosamide, 872
praziquantel, 875
Hetrazan, 878. *See also* Diethylcarbamazine
Hexachlorocyclohexane (lindane), 950*t*, **1004–1005**
Hexachlorophene
adverse effects of, 808
antimicrobial effects of, 805*t*
preparations available, 810
Hexamethonium, 114, 114*i*
Hexamethylmelamine (altretamine), **888**, 890*t*
Hexestrol, 656
5-HIAA (5-hydroxyindoleacetic acid), excretion of, serotonin synthesis measured by, 274
Hib vaccine, 1052*t*
Hibiclens, 810. *See also* Chlorhexidine
Hibistat, 810. *See also* Chlorhexidine
Hierarchical neuronal systems, 347, 348*i*
High-density lipoproteins (HDL), 563–564, 565*t*
deficiency of, **569**
synthesis and catabolism of, 566
Hiprex, 810. *See also* Methenamine hippurate
Hirsutism
oral contraceptives affecting, 668
phenytoin causing, 391
spironolactone for, 649
Hirudin, **551**
Hismanal, 267*t*, 283. *See also* Astemizole
Histamine, 85*t*, **261–265**, 350*t*
basic pharmacology of, **261–265**
chemical and mechanical release of, 262
clinical pharmacology of, **265**

contraindications for, 265
immunologic release of, 262
in inflammation, 262, 578, 579*t*
mechanism of action of, 262–263
as neurotransmitter in CNS, 350*t*
physiologic antagonists of, 265
provocative bronchial testing with, 264, 265
receptors for, 262–263, 263*t*
drugs blocking, **265–273**. *See also* H$_1$ receptor antagonists; H$_2$ receptor antagonists
release inhibitors and, 265
second messenger for, 22*t*
tissue and organ system effects of, 263–264
toxicity of, 265
Histamine agonists, 264–265
Histamine antagonists, **265–273**. *See also* H$_1$ receptor antagonists; H$_2$ receptor antagonists
Histoplasma capsulatum, empiric antimicrobial therapy and, 815*t*
Histrelin, 611
structure of, 611*i*
HIV infection
antimicrobial prophylaxis and, 825*t*
disinfection procedures and, 807
drugs for, **795–799**, 795*t*, 796*i*. *See also specific type*
importance of pharmacologic knowledge and, 799
preparations available, 801
tuberculosis risk in, isoniazid treatment and, 771–772
Hivid, 801. *See also* Zalcitabine
hMG (human menopausal gonadotropins), **612–613**
HMG-CoA reductase inhibitors, **573–575**, 573*i*
combination therapy with, **575**
HN2, 890*t*. *See also* Mechlorethamine
Hodgkin's disease, 903*t*, **907**
Homatropine
ophthalmologic uses of, 111*t*
preparations available, 115
Homeostatic response, autonomic, 83–84
Hookworm, drugs for, 863*t*
albendazole, 864
mebendazole, 869
pyrantel, 876
tetrachloroethylene, **876**
Hormonal contraception
in men, **679**
in women, 665*t*, **666–671**
Hormones
in cancer chemotherapy, **898–900**, 899*t*
for breast cancer, 909
local, 261. *See also* Histamine; Serotonin
Horner's syndrome, sympathomimetics for, 132
Household bleach, antimicrobial effects of, 807

HPETE (hydroperoxyeicosatetraenoic acid), 307, 307*i*
effects of, 310–311
HPMPC, 793. *See also* Cidofovir
Hsp (heat shock proteins), 637, 657
hsp90, 657
in glucocorticoid action, 18–19, 19*i*
HSV (herpes simplex virus)
acyclovir for, 790, 791
antimicrobial prophylaxis for, 824*t*
foscarnet for, 794
idoxuridine for, 794
valacyclovir for, 791
vidarabine for, 795
5-HT (5-hydroxytryptamine/serotonin), 77*t*, 85*t*, **273–277**, 349*t*, 352. *See also under* Serotonin
alcoholism and, 381
antidepressants affecting, 487. *See also* Serotonin reuptake inhibitors
appetite control and, 276
basic pharmacology of, **273–276**
clinical pharmacology of, **276–277**
in inflammation, 579*t*
LSD affecting, 525
mechanisms of action of, 274
as neurotransmitter, 77*t*, 349*t*, 352
receptors for, 274, 274*t*, 352
drugs blocking, **277**
ergot alkaloids affecting, 279, 279*t*
second messenger for, 22*t*
structure of, 273*i*
tissue and organ system effects of, 274–276
5-HT receptors, 274, 274*t*, 352
drugs blocking, **277**
ergot alkaloids affecting, 279, 279*t*
Human chorionic gonadotropin (hCG), 612, **613–614**
preparations available, 617
second messenger for, 22*t*
Human immunodeficiency virus infection
antimicrobial prophylaxis and, 825*t*
disinfection procedures and, 807
drugs for, **795–799**, 795*t*, 796*i*. *See also specific type*
importance of pharmacologic knowledge and, 799
preparations available, 801
tuberculosis risk in, isoniazid treatment and, 771–772
Human insulin, 690*t*, 691, 692
Human menopausal gonadotropins (hMG), **612–613**
Human proinsulin, 692
structure of, 686*i*
Humans, new drug evaluation in, 63*i*, **66–72**
Humatin, 759, 859. *See also* Paromomycin
Humatrope, 617. *See also* Somatotropin
Humegon. *See also* Menotropins
Humoral immunity, 917, 918*i*, 919*i*
Humorsol (demecarium), 103

Humulin, 690t, 691, 692. *See also* Insulin
Huntington's disease, 459–460
  neurons involved in, 450–451, 451i
Hycamtin, 894t. *See also* Topotecan
Hycanthone, antiparasitic actions of, 836t
Hydatid disease, drugs for, 864t
  albendazole, 864
  mebendazole, 869–870
  praziquantel, 875
Hydeltra-T.B.A., 650. *See also* Prednisolone
Hydralazine, **166–167**, 166i
  for heart failure, 197, 210t
  for hypertension, **166–167**
  ionization constant of, 6t
  pharmacokinetic/pharmacodynamic parameters of, 36t, 166–167
  preparations available, 175
  toxicity of, 167
Hydrea, 901t. *See also* Hydroxyurea
Hydrocarbons
  aromatic, **950**
  chlorinated insecticides, **950–951**, 950t
  halogenated aliphatic, **949–950**
Hydrochlorothiazide, 251
  in combination diuretics, 254t, **256**
  dosages of, 252t
  for idiopathic hypercalciuria, 719
  preparations available, 259
  structure of, 252i
Hydrocodone, 511
  with acetaminophen, preparations available, 514
  structure of, 498i
Hydrocortisone (cortisol), 640t. *See also* Glucocorticoids
  for acute adrenocortical insufficiency, 641
  for cancer chemotherapy, 899t
    for breast cancer, 909
  for dermatologic therapy, 1008–1009
  for inflammatory bowel disease, 1026, 1027
  metabolic effects of, 644
  for nonadrenal disorders, 643–644
  in OTC preparations, efficacy of, 1034t
  pharmacokinetics of, 635–636, 636i, 637i
  preparations available, 650, 1027
  structure of, 641i
  synthesis of, 636i
HydroDIURIL, 259. *See also* Hydrochlorothiazide
Hydroflumethiazide
  dosages of, 252t
  preparations available, 259
Hydrogen peroxide, antimicrobial effects of, 808–809
Hydrolyses, in biotransformation, 54t
Hydromorphone, 510
  pharmacokinetics of, 501t
  preparations available, 513
  structure of, 498i
Hydromox, 259. *See also* Quinethazone

Hydroperoxyeicosatetraenoic acid (HPETE), 307, 307i
  effects of, 310–311
Hydrophilic colloids, laxative effect of, 1023
Hydrophobic bonds, in drug-receptor interactions, 2
Hydroquinone, **1005**
Hydroxocobalamin, 537, 542, 546. *See also* Vitamin B_{12}
  for cyanide poisoning, 543
Hydroxychloroquine, 842. *See also* Chloroquine
  in inflammation, **591**
  preparations available, 599
Hydroxyeicosatetraenoic acid (HETE), 307
  effects of, 310–311
5-Hydroxyindoleacetic acid, excretion of, serotonin synthesis measured by, 274
Hydroxylations, 53t
Hydroxyprogesterone, 661t, 662i
  in cancer chemotherapy, 899t
  preparations available, 680
Hydroxyquinolines, halogenated
  for amebiasis, 850
  antiparasitic actions of, 836t
5-Hydroxytryptamine (5-HT/serotonin), 77t, 85t, **273–277**, 349t, 352. *See also under* Serotonin
  alcoholism and, 381
  antidepressants affecting, 487. *See also* Serotonin reuptake inhibitors
  appetite control and, 276
  basic pharmacology of, **273–276**
  clinical pharmacology of, **276–277**
  in inflammation, 579t
  LSD affecting, 525
  mechanisms of action of, 274
  as neurotransmitter, 77t, 349t, 352
  receptors for, 274, 274t, 352
    drugs blocking, **277**
    ergot alkaloids affecting, 279, 279t
  second messenger for, 22t
  structure of, 273i
  tissue and organ system effects of, 274–276
Hydroxyurea, **901**, 901t
25-Hydroxyvitamin D (calcifediol), 707–709, 708i, 709t. *See also* Vitamin D
  in chronic renal failure, 717
  for intestinal osteodystrophy, 717
  preparations available, 721
Hydroxyzine, 267t
  antiemetic actions of, 1022
  preparations available, 283, 369
Hygroton, 259. *See also* Chlorthalidone
Hylorel, 175. *See also* Guanadrel
Hymenolepis
  diminuta (rat tapeworm), drugs for, 864t
  nana (dwarf tapeworm), drugs for, 863t
    niclosamide, 871
    praziquantel, 875

Hyoscine, 105. *See also* Scopolamine
Hyoscyamine, 105. *See also* Atropine
  preparations available, 116, 1027
Hyoscyamus niger, 105
Hyperaldosteronism, 642
Hyperbaric oxygen, for carbon monoxide intoxication, 948
Hyperbilirubinemia, indinavir causing, 798
Hypercalcemia, **713–714**
  diuretics for, **258–259**
Hypercalciuria, idiopathic, **719–720**
Hyperchloremic metabolic acidosis
  carbonic anhydrase inhibitors causing, 249
  potassium-sparing diuretics causing, 254
Hypercholesterolemias, **568–569**
  familial, 567t, 568, 569i
  unclassified, 567t, 569
Hyperglycemia. *See also* Diabetes mellitus
  in obesity, biguanides for, 700
Hyperhidrosis, antimuscarinic agents for, 113
Hyperkalemia
  arrhythmias caused by, 218
  loop diuretics for, 250
  tassium-sparing diuretics causing, 254
  succinylcholine causing, 444
Hyperlipemia, 563
Hyperlipidemia, 563
  agents used in. *See also specific type*
    basic and clinical pharmacology of, **570–575**
    drug combinations and, **575**
    preparations available, 576
  thiazides causing, 252
Hyperlipoproteinemia, 563, 565t, **566–569**
  dietary management of, **569–570**
  familial combined, 567t, 568
  pathophysiology of, **564–566**
  secondary, **569**
  treatment guidelines for, 566t
Hypernatremia, osmotic diuretics causing, 255
Hyperparathyroidism, **715**
Hyperphosphatemia, **715**
Hyperpigmentation
  estrogen therapy causing, 660
  hydroquinone and monobenzone for, 1005
  oral contraceptives causing, 667–668, 668
Hyperprolactinemia, 282
  bromocriptine for, 282, 614
Hyperreactive drug response, 30
Hypersecretory conditions, gastric antisecretory drugs for, **1019–1021**
  H_2 receptor antagonists, 272
  OTC preparations, efficacy of, 1033t
Hypersensitivity reactions, 30, 921–923, 922i. *See also* Allergic reactions
Hyperstat IV, 175. *See also* Diazoxide
Hyperstimulation syndrome, 613

Hypertension, **153–155**
angiotensin-converting enzyme inhibitors for, **170–171**, 291, 292*i*, 293
chronic alcohol consumption and, 377
diagnosis of, 153
diuretics for, **155–157**, **258**
drugs for, 141, 146, **153–178**. *See also* Antihypertensive drugs
in elderly, 994
essential, 154
estrogen therapy and, 660
etiology of, 153–154
levodopa causing, 453
monotherapy versus polypharmacy for, 173
outpatient treatment of, **172–173**
during pregnancy, nitric oxide and, **322**
pulmonary
nitric oxide for, 322
prostacyclin for, 314
Hypertensive emergencies, 141, **173–174**
Hyperthermia
malignant, 418
dantrolene for, 447–448
in poisoning, 970
Hyperthyroidism (thyrotoxicosis), **629–632**
beta-receptor blocking drug use masking signs of, 149
beta-receptor blocking drugs for, 147–148, **628**
drug metabolism affected in, 61
excessive ingestion of thyroid hormone causing (thyrotoxicosis factitia), **631**
during pregnancy, 632
[131]I for treatment of, 627–628, 630
Hypertriglyceridemias, **566–568**
familial, 567–568, 567*t*
Hyperuricemia, loop diuretics causing, 250
Hypnosis, sedative-hypnotic drugs producing, 355*i*, 361–362
dosages for, 366*t*
Hypnotic, 354. *See also* Sedative-hypnotic drugs
Hypnozoites, plasmodial, 838
Hypocalcemia, **714–715**
Hypochlorite, antimicrobial effects of, 805*t*, 807
Hypoglycemia
glucagon for, 702
insulin causing, 694–695
quinine causing, 848
Hypoglycemic agents, **684–705**. *See also* Insulin; Oral hypoglycemic agents
Hypogonadism
androgen replacement therapy for, 675, 676*t*
estrogens for, 658
hypogonadotropic, hCG stimulation in evaluation of, 614

Hypokalemia
arrhythmias caused by, 218, 222, 223
diuretics causing, heart failure management and, 257
torsade de pointes caused by, 223
Hypokalemic metabolic alkalosis
loop diuretics causing, 250
thiazides causing, 251
Hypomagnesemia, loop diuretics causing, 250–251
Hyponatremia
loop diuretics causing, 251
thiazides causing, 252
Hypoparathyroidism, **716**
Hypophosphatemia, **715**
Hyporeactive drug response, 30
Hypotension, 455
neuromuscular blockers causing, 443
orthostatic/postural
antipsychotic drugs causing, 470
bromocriptine causing, 455
levodopa causing, 453
sympathomimetics for, 130
sympathomimetics for, 130
Hypothalamic hormones, **604–615**, 604*t*
Hypothyroidism, **628–629**, 629*t*
drug metabolism affected in, 61
Hypovolemia, after myocardial infarction, 211, 211*i*, 211*t*
Hypoxanthine, 598*i*, 892*i*
Hypoxia, cellular, in poisoning, 970
HypRho-D Mini-Dose, 940. *See also* Rh$_o$ (D) immune globulin micro-dose
Hysterectomy, antimicrobial prophylaxis and, 824*t*
Hytakerol, 721. *See also* Dihydrotachysterol
Hytrin, 150, 175. *See also* Terazosin

[131]I, 627–628
for Graves' disease, 630
preparations available, 633
IAPP (islet amyloid polypeptide/amylin), 684, 685*t*, **703**
Ibopamine, 128
Ibuprofen, 580*t*, **586**, 586*i*
ionization constant of, 6*t*
in OTC preparations, efficacy of, 1033*t*
OTC status of, 1031*t*
preparations available, 599
Ibutilide, **236**
action potential duration affected by, 235, 236
for arrhythmias, **236**
clinical properties of, 229*t*
membrane actions of, 228*t*
preparations available, 240
ICD (implantable cardioverter-defibrillator), 238
"Ice," 522
ICI-182780, 672
ICI-164384, 672
Idamycin, 894*t*. *See also* Idarubicin
Idarubicin, 894*t*, 896
Idiopathic hypercalciuria, **719–720**

Idiopathic thrombocytopenic purpura
immunosuppressive agents for, 931*t*, 932, 933
passive immunization for, 1056*t*
Idiosyncratic drug response, 30
IDL (intermediate-density lipoprotein), 563, 564, 565*t*
Idoxuridine, 792*t*, **794**
mechanism of action of, 791*i*
preparations available, 801
IDU/IUDR (idoxuridine), 792*t*, **794**
IFNs (interferons), **800**, **926**
immunosuppressive actions of, **926**
in inflammation, 579*t*
IgE
in asthma, 325–326
drugs targeting, 338
in histamine release, 262
in immediate hypersensitivity reaction, 921, 922*i*, 937*i*, 938*i*
drug allergy and, 937, **937–939**, 937*i*, 938*i*
IGFs (insulin-like growth factors), growth hormone effects and, 607
IgG anti-insulin antibodies, 695
IGIV (immune globulin intravenous), 930
preparations available, 801
IL-1 (interleukin-1), 934, 934*t*
in inflammation, 579*t*
IL-2 (interleukin-2), 933, 934*t*, 935
in inflammation, 579*t*
preparations available, 940
IL-3 (interleukin-3), 543, 543*t*, 545, 934, 934*t*
in inflammation, 579*t*
IL-4 (interleukin-4), 934, 934*t*
IL-5 (interleukin-5), 934*t*
IL-6 (interleukin-6), 543*t*, 934, 934*t*
IL-7 (interleukin-7), 934*t*
IL-8 (interleukin-8), 934*t*
IL-9 (interleukin-9), 543*t*, 934*t*
IL-10 (interleukin-10), 543*t*, 934*t*
IL-11 (interleukin-11), 543*t*, 934, 934*t*
IL-12 (interleukin-12), 934, 934*t*
IL-13 (interleukin-13), 934*t*
IL-14 (interleukin-14), 934*t*
IL-15 (interleukin-15), 934*t*
IL-16 (interleukin-16), 934*t*
IL-17 (interleukin-17), 934*t*
Ileum, contents of, drug trapping in, 7*t*
Ileus, postoperative, cholinomimetics for, 100
Ilosone, 751. *See also* Erythromycin
Ilotycin, 751. *See also* Erythromycin
Ilozyme, 1023*t*
Imexon, 935–936
Imidazoles, 783, 1002. *See also* specific type
Imidazoline receptor, 158, 159
Imidazopyridines, 360
GABA$_A$ receptor binding and, 359
Imipenem (imipenem/cilastin), 737
CSF penetration by, 820*t*
dosing guidelines for, 730*t*
preparations available, 741

Imipramine, 484, 485*i*
dosages of, 491*t*
effects of, 489*t*
half-life of, aging affecting, 992*i*
ionization constant of, 6*t*
for panic attacks, 490
pharmacokinetic/pharmacodynamic parameters of, 36*t*, 488*t*
preparations available, 494
for urinary disorders, 112
Imitrex, 284. *See also* Sumatriptan
Immediate hypersensitivity reactions, 921, 922*i*
to drugs, 937, **937–939**, 937*i*, 938*i*
Immune globulin intravenous (IGIV), 930, 1056–1057*t*
preparations available, 801
Immune insulin resistance, 695, 700
Immune system (immune response/immunity)
abnormal, **921–924**
adaptive, 917–921, 918*i*, 919*i*, 920*i*
in asthma, 325–326
chronic alcoholic consumption affecting, 378
drugs affecting, **916–944**. *See also* Immunopharmacology
preparations available, 940
eicosanoids affecting, 315–316, 316*i*
elements of, **916–936**
innate, 916–917, 917*i*
normal, **916–921**
tests of, **924**
Immunization, **1051–1058**. *See also* Vaccines
active, **1051**, 1052–1054*t*, 1055*t*
for adults, for travel, **1057–1058**
for children, recommended schedule for, 1055*t*
passive, **1051–1055**, 1056–1057*t*
Immunocompetence, tests of, **924**
Immunodeficiency diseases, 923–924. *See also* Acquired immunodeficiency syndrome
passive immunization and, 1056*t*
Immunoglobulins, 918*i*, 920*i*, 921. *See also specific type under Ig and* Antibodies
Immunomodulating agents, **933–936**
Immunopharmacology, **916–944**
immune system elements and, **916–946**
preparations available, 940
reactions to drugs and drug allergy and, **936–940**
Immunosuppressive agents, **925–933**
antibodies as, **929–931**
cancer chemotherapy agents and, **924–925**
clinical uses of, **931–933**, 931*t*
cytotoxic, **927–929**
glucocorticoids as, 639, **925**
in inflammation, **590–591**
for inflammatory bowel disease, 1026
interferons as, **926**
site of action of, 924*i*
Immunotherapy, cancer, **936**

Imodium, 1027. *See also* Loperamide
Implantable cardioverter-defibrillator, 238
Implantable contraceptive, 665*t*, 666, 670
Impotence
alpha-receptor antagonists for, 141–142
alprostadil for, 314
Impromidine, 264
Impulse conduction, arrhythmias caused by disturbances of, 224, 225*i*
Impulse formation, arrhythmias caused by disturbances of, 222, 222*i*
Imuran, 940. *See also* Azathioprine
Inactivated poliovirus vaccine, 1053*t*
Incertohypothalamic pathways, 467
Increased intraocular pressure. *See also* Glaucoma
management of, 87
beta-receptor blocking drugs for, 147, 148
cholinomimetics for, 100
osmotic diuretics for, 255
IND (Notice of Claimed Investigational Exemption for a New Drug), 63*i*, 68
Indapamide
dosages of, 252*t*
preparations available, 259
structure of, 252*i*
Inderal, 150, 174, 194, 240. *See also* Propranolol
Indinavir, 795*t*, **798**
preparations available, 801
Indirect-acting cholinomimetics, 91–92, 91*i*, **96–100**, 103
toxicity of, 102
Indocin, 599. *See also* Indomethacin
Indomethacin, 580*t*, 586*i*, **588–589**
half-life of, aging affecting, 992*i*
immunomodulating effect of, 936
pharmacokinetic/pharmacodynamic parameters of, 36*t*
preparations available, 599
Indoramin, 140
Industrial solvents, abuse of, 529
Infantile spasms, 404
management of, **405**
Infants, drug therapy in, **982–985**
dosage amounts and, **987–988**
dosage forms and compliance and, **985–986**
InFeD (iron dextran), 536, 546
Infertility
female
gonadotropin-releasing hormone for, 611–612
human chorionic gonadotropin for, 612, 614
human menopausal gonadotropins for, 612–613
ovulation-inducing agents for, **672–673**
male
gonadotropin-releasing hormone for, 612

human chorionic gonadotropin for, 614
human menopausal gonadotropins for, 613
Inflammation (inflammatory response), **578**
acute, 578
mediators of, 579*t*
aspirin affecting, 316, 581, 582
chloroquine in, **591**
chronic, 578
mediators of, 579*t*
dietary manipulation of, **594**
glucocorticoids affecting, 639
histamine in, 262, 578, 579*t*
kinins in, 294, 578, 579*t*
nitric oxide and, **324**
prostaglandins in, 316, 316*i*, 578, 579*t*
treatment of, **578–579**. *See also specific agent*
Inflammatory bowel disease, drugs used in management of, **1025–1026**
Influenza virus
amantadine and rimantadine for infection with, 799–800
antimicrobial prophylaxis and, 825*t*
vaccine for prevention of infection with, 1052*t*
INH (isoniazid), 770, **770–773**, 770*i*, 771*t*
in breast milk, 987*t*
in combination therapy, 772, 772*t*
drug metabolism inhibited by, 60*t*
preparations available, 778
resistance to, 771
Inhalants, abuse of, **529**
Inhalation route of administration
bioavailability and characteristics and, 40*t*
first-pass effect and, 42
Inhaled anesthetics, 409, 410*i*, **412–419**. *See also specific agent*
neuromuscular blocking drug interaction and, 444
newer compounds available, 419
Inhibin, 664–666
Inhibitory postsynaptic potential (IPSP), 345, 345*i*
Inocor, 213. *See also* Amrinone
Inocybe mushroom poisoning, 102
Inosiplex (isoprinosine), 935
Inositol phosphates, lithium affecting, 476, 476*i*
Inositol-1,4,5-trisphosphate (IP_3/$InsP_3$)
in alpha receptor activation, 120–121, 121*i*
in calcium/phosphoinositide second messenger system, 24
lithium affecting, 476, 476*i*
in muscarinic agonist binding, 93
Inotropic drugs, positive, for heart failure, **205–206**, 207
in elderly, 994–995
Inotropin, 133, 213. *See also* Dopamine
Insecticides, **950–952**
botanical, 952, 953*i*
carbamate, **952**, 952*t*

chlorinated hydrocarbon, **950–951**, 950*t*
organophosphorus (organophosphate/thiophosphate), 97, 98*i*, **951–952**, 951*t*
  absorption/distribution/metabolism of, 98–99
  toxicity of, 102
Insomnia
  management of, **363–364**
  sedative-hypnotic drugs for, 361–362, **365–366**
InsP$_3$ (inositol-1,4,5-trisphosphate/IP$_3$)
  in alpha receptor activation, 120–121, 121*i*
  in calcium/phosphoinositide second messenger system, 24
  lithium affecting, 476, 476*i*
  in muscarinic agonist binding, 93
Inspired air, anesthetic concentration in, 412
Insulin, 684, **685–695**, 685*t*
  chemistry of, 685, 686*i*
  complications of treatment with, 694–695
  concentration of, 690*t*, 692
  degradation of, 685
  delivery systems for, 693
  durations of action of, 689–691, 689*i*
  effects of, 686–689, 688*i*
  immunopathology of treatment with, 695
  ligand-regulated transmembrane enzymes in signalling by, 19–20
  measurement of blood levels of, 685
  mixtures of, 691–692
  in non-insulin-dependent diabetes, 693, 694
  preparations available, 689–693, 690*t*
  purity of, 692
  resistance to, 695, 700
  secretion of, 685, 687*i*
  species of, 690*t*, 692
  substances modifying release of, 696, 696*t*
  sulfonylurea therapy combined with, 699
  sulfonylureas affecting release of, 696
Insulin allergy, 695
Insulin analogs, 692–693
Insulin-like growth factors
  deficiency of, short stature and, 607
  growth hormone effects and, 607
Insulin lispro, 689–690, 690*t*
Insulin pumps, 693
Insulin receptor, 685–686, 687*i*
Insulin receptor substrate-1 (IRS-1), 686, 687*i*
Insulin resistance syndrome, 695
  biguanides for, 700
Insulinoma, 904*t*
Intal, 340. *See also* Cromolyn
Integrelin, 557
Integrin, platelet receptors for, drugs blocking, 557
Intention myoclonus, 405
Intention tremor, 450, 459

Interactions, drug-drug, **1059–1060**, 1061–1069*t*
  combined toxicity and, **1060**
  metabolism and, 59–60, 59*i*, 60*i*, 1059
  pharmacodynamic mechanisms of, 1059–1060
  pharmacokinetic mechanisms of, 1059
  predictability of, **1060**
Intercalated cells, 245, 246*i*
Interferon-α, 800, 926, 934*t*, 935
Interferon alfa-2a, preparations available, 801, 940
Interferon alfa-2b, preparations available, 801, 940
Interferon alfa-n3, preparations available, 801
Interferon-β, 800, 926, 933, 934*t*, 935
  preparations available, 940
Interferon-γ, 800, 926, 933, 934, 934*t*, 935
  preparations available, 940
Interferons, **800**, **926**, 933–935
  immunosuppressive actions of, **926**
  in inflammation, 579*t*
Interleukin-1, 934, 934*t*
  in inflammation, 579*t*
Interleukin-2, 933, 934*t*, 935
  in inflammation, 579*t*
  preparations available, 940
Interleukin-3, 543, 543*t*, 545, 934, 934*t*
  in inflammation, 579*t*
Interleukin-4, 934, 934*t*
Interleukin-5, 934*t*
Interleukin-6, 543*t*, 934, 934*t*
Interleukin-7, 934*t*
Interleukin-8, 934*t*
Interleukin-9, 543*t*, 934*t*
Interleukin-10, 934*t*
Interleukin-11, 543*t*, 934, 934*t*
Interleukin-12, 934, 934*t*
Interleukin-13, 934*t*
Interleukin-14, 934*t*
Interleukin-15, 934*t*
Interleukin-16, 934*t*
Interleukin-17, 934*t*
Interleukins, 934–935, 934*t*
Intermediate-acting insulin, 690–691, 690*t*
Intermediate-density lipoprotein (IDL), 563, 564, 565*t*
Internet, drug information on, 8
Intestinal capillariasis, drugs for, 863*t*
  albendazole, 865
  mebendazole, 870
  thiabendazole, 877
Intestinal flukes, drugs for, 863*t*
  niclosamide, 872
  praziquantel, 875
Intestinal osteodystrophy, **717**
Intoxication, alcohol, 374
  management of, **379**
Intracellular receptors, for lipid-soluble agents, 18–19, 19*i*
Intracranial pressure, reduction of, osmotic diuretics for, 255
Intragastric pressure, increased, succinylcholine causing, 444

Intramuscular route of administration, bioavailability and characteristics and, 40*t*
Intranasal route of administration, for opioid analgesics, 508
Intraocular pressure
  increased. *See also* Glaucoma
  management of, 87
    beta-receptor blocking drugs for, 147, 148
    cholinomimetics for, 100
    osmotic diuretics for, 255
  succinylcholine causing, 444
  prostaglandins affecting, 310
Intravenous anesthetics, 409–410, 411*i*, **419–423**, 420*t*
Intravenous route of administration, bioavailability and characteristics and, 40*t*
Intrinsic factor, in vitamin B$_{12}$ deficiency, 541–542
Intron (interferon alfa-2b), 801, 940
Inversine, 116, 175. *See also* Mecamylamine
Invirase, 801. *See also* Saquinavir
Inward rectifier channels, 217–218
Iodide metabolism, 619
Iodide organification, 619
Iodide trapping, 619
Iodides, **627**
  fetus affected by, 983*t*
  preparations available, 633
Iodinated contrast media, **627**
Iodine
  antimicrobial effects of, 805*t*, **806**
  deficiency of, goiter caused by, 632
  preparations available, 810
  radioactive, **627–628**
    in breast milk, 987*t*
    for Graves' disease, 630
Iodo-Niacin, 633. *See also* Potassium iodide solution
Iodophors, antimicrobial effects of, **806–807**
Iodoquinol, **853–854**, 853*i*
  for amebiasis, 851*t*, **853–854**
  preparations available, 859
Iodotope, 633. *See also* ^{131}I
Ion channels, **344**
  chemically activated/receptor-operated, 344
  ligand-gated, 20–21
  nicotinic receptor activation and, 90, 94
  voltage-gated, 344
Ion transport, lithium affecting, 476
Iopanoic acid, 627
  preparations available, 633
Iopidine, 133. *See also* Apraclonidine
IP$_3$ (inositol-1,4,5-trisphosphate/InsP$_3$)
  in alpha receptor activation, 120–121, 121*i*
  in calcium/phosphoinositide second messenger system, 24
  lithium affecting, 476, 476*i*
  in muscarinic agonist binding, 93

Ipecac syrup, for emesis induction in poisoned patient, 974–975
Ipodate, 627
  preparations available, 633
  for thyroid storm, 631
Ipratropium, 107*i*
  preparations available, 116, 340
  for respiratory disorders, 111
IPSP (inhibitory postsynaptic potential), 345, 345*i*
IPV (inactivated poliovirus vaccine), 1053*t*
Irinotecan, 894*t*, **895**
Iris
  autonomic activity/drugs affecting, 83*t*
  direct-acting cholinomimetics affecting, 94, 94*t*
IRL1038, 298, 300*i*
Iron, **533–536**
  distribution of, 533, 534*t*
  indications for supplemental use of, 534–535
  interactions of, 1066*t*
  oral therapy with, 535–536, 535*t*
  parenteral therapy with, 536
  preparations available, 546
  requirements for, 533–534
  toxicity of, 536
Iron deficiency anemia, 534–536
Iron dextran, 536, 546
Iron poisoning, deferoxamine for, 959
Irreversible antagonist, 14*i*, 15
Irritant laxatives, **1023**
IRS-1 (insulin receptor substrate-1), 686, 687*i*
Islet amyloid polypeptide (IAPP/amylin), 684, 685*t*, **703**
Islets of Langerhans, 684, 685*t*
Ismelin Sulfate, 175. *See also* Guanethidine
Ismo, 194. *See also* Isosorbide mononitrate
Iso-Bid, 194. *See also* Isosorbide dinitrate
Isobutyl nitrite, abuse of, 184
Isocaine, 426*t*. *See also* Mepivacaine
Isocarboxazid, 484
Isoetharine, 334*i*
  preparations available, 340
Isoflurane, 410*i*
  elimination of, 415
  preparations available, 423
  properties of, 413*t*
Isoflurophate, 97, 98*i*
  preparations available, 103
Isolan, 952*t*
Isoniazid (INH), 770, **770–773**, 770*i*, 771*t*
  in breast milk, 987*t*
  in combination therapy, 772, 772*t*
  drug metabolism inhibited by, 60*t*
  preparations available, 778
  resistance to, 771
Isophane insulin (NPH insulin), 690*t*, 691

Isoprenaline (isoproterenol), 123*i*, 128, 334*i*
  for asthma, 333, 340
  cardiovascular system affected by, 125*t*
  ionization constant of, 6*t*
  preparations available, 134, 340
Isoprinosine (inosiplex), 935
Isopropamide
  for gastrointestinal and genitourinary conditions, 112*t*
  preparations available, 115–116, 1027
Isopropanol
  antimicrobial effects of, 805*t*, 806
  osmolar gap caused by, 974*t*
Isoprostanes, 308
Isoproterenol, 123*i*, 128, 334*i*
  for asthma, 333, 340
  cardiovascular system affected by, 125*t*
  ionization constant of, 6*t*
  preparations available, 134, 340
Isoptin, 175, 194, 240. *See also* Verapamil
Isopto Carbachol, 103. *See also* Carbachol
Isopto Carpine, 103. *See also* Pilocarpine
Isopto Homatropine, 115. *See also* Homatropine
Isopto Hyoscine, 116. *See also* Scopolamine
Isordil, 194. *See also* Isosorbide dinitrate
Isosorbide dinitrate
  for angina, 186*t*
  chemistry of, 181, 182*i*
  pharmacology of, 182
  preparations available, 194
Isosorbide mononitrate
  for angina, 186*t*
  preparations available, 194
Isospora belli, drugs for infection with, 855*t*
Isotretinoin
  for acne, **1007**
  in cancer chemotherapy, 902
  fetus affected by, 983*t*
Isoxazolyl penicillins, 729–731
Isradipine
  clinical properties of, 190*t*
  for hypertension, 169
  pharmacokinetics of, 189*t*
  preparations available, 175, 194
  vascular selectivity of, 190*t*
Isuprel, 134, 340. *See also* Isoproterenol
Itraconazole, 784*i*, 784*t*, **785**, 1004
  for dermatologic therapy, 1004
  lovastatin interaction and, 574
  parasite sterol synthesis affected by, 831
  preparations available, 786
Ivermectin, **867–869**
  GABA-BDZ receptor chloride channel binding and, 361, 868
  preparations available, 878
  synaptic transmission affected by, 835, 868

JAK family (Janus-kinase family), 20, 21*i*
Jamestown weed (jimsonweed), toxicity of, 105, 972*t*
Janus-kinase family, 20, 21*i*
Jejunum, contents of, drug trapping in, 7*t*
Jenamicin, 759. *See also* Gentamicin
Jimsonweed (Jamestown weed), toxicity of, 105, 972*t*

K_d (dissociation constant), enantiomers and, 3, 3*t*
Kabikinase, 561. *See also* Streptokinase
Kala-azar, 855. *See also* Leishmania
Kallikrein-kinin system, 293–294, 293*i*
  drugs affecting, **295**
Kallikreins, 292
Kanamycin, 754*i*, **758–759**, 776
  adverse effects of, 754, 759
  in breast milk, 987*t*
  half-life of, aging affecting, 992*i*
  ionization constant of, 6*t*
  preparations available, 759
  for tuberculosis, 776
Kantrex, 759. *See also* Kanamycin
Kaolin, 1024
Kaolin/pectin, preparations available, 1027
Kaopectate (kaolin/pectin), 1027
Kaposi's sarcoma, AIDS-related, hCG for, 614
Kappa (κ) receptors, 501
  opioid activity at, 502*t*
Katayama syndrome, oxamniquine for, 872
Kawasaki disease, passive immunization for, 1056*t*
Kefauver-Harris Amendments, 67–68, 68*t*
Keflex, 741. *See also* Cephalexin
Keflin, 741. *See also* Cephalothin
Kefurox, 741. *See also* Cefuroxime
Kefzol, 741. *See also* Cefazolin
Kemadrin, 462. *See also* Procyclidine
Kenacort, 650. *See also* Triamcinolone
Kenalog, 650. *See also* Triamcinolone
Keratitis, herpes
  idoxuridine for, 794
  vidarabine for, 795
Keratoacanthoma, fluorouracil for, 1013
Keratoconjunctivitis, herpes, vidarabine for, 795
Keratolytic agents, **1011–1013**
Keratoses, fluorouracil for, 1013
Kerlone, 150, 174. *See also* Betaxolol
Ketalar, 423. *See also* Ketamine
Ketamine, 411*i*, 420*t*, **422–423**
  enantiomers of, potency and, 3
  hallucinogenic effects of, 525
  preparations available, 423
Ketanserin, 277
Ketoconazole, 647*i*, **648**, **784–785**, 784*i*, 784*t*, 1004
  for dermatologic therapy, 1004
  drug metabolism inhibited by, 60*t*, 783–784
  OTC status of, 1032*t*

parasite sterol synthesis affected by, 831
preparations available, 650, 786
steroid synthesis affected by, **648**, 678–679
topical, 1002
Ketoprofen, 580*t*, **587**
in OTC preparations, efficacy of, 1033*t*
OTC status of, 1031*t*
preparations available, 599
Ketorolac, 580*t*, **589**
preparations available, 599
Ketotifen, for drug allergy, 939
Ketrax, 878. *See also* Levamisole
Khat, 521
Kidney stones
carbonic anhydrase inhibitors causing, 249
potassium-sparing diuretics causing, 254
Kidneys
angiotensin II affecting, 289
autonomic activity/drugs affecting, 83*t*
in blood pressure regulation, 154, 154*i*
cytochrome P450-derived metabolites affecting, 311
disease of. *See also under Renal and Nephrotoxicity*
amphotericin B causing, 781
diuretics for, **257–258**
lithium causing, 478
drug excretion via, Henderson-Hasselbalch equation and, 6, 7*i*
glucocorticoids and, 639–640
inhaled anesthetics affecting, 417
lead toxicity and, 961
lipoxygenase metabolites affecting, 311
lithium affecting, 478
methylxanthines affecting, 332
opioid analgesics affecting, 506, 510
parathyroid hormone affecting, 709*t*
phenacetin affecting, 595
prostaglandins affecting, 309–310
renin synthesis and secretion by, 287–288
tetracyclines affecting, 747
thromboxanes affecting, 309–310
thyroid hormones affecting, 625*t*
transplantation of, immunosuppressive therapy and, 931*t*, 932
vitamin D affecting, 709*t*
Killer cells
lymphokine-activated, 921
natural, 921
Kininase I, 295
Kininase II, 295. *See also* Angiotensin-converting enzyme
in renin-angiotensin system, 288–289, 288*i*
Kininogens, 293
Kinins, **292–295**
actions of, **294**
biosynthesis of, **292–293**
formation of in plasma and tissues, **293–294**, 293*i*

mechanisms of action of, **294–295**
metabolism of, **295**
receptors for, **294–295**
antagonists of, 295
Kirby-Bauer susceptibility testing, 817
Klebsiella, empiric antimicrobial therapy and, 814*t*
Klonopin, 369, 407. *See also* Clonazepam
Koate-HP, 561. *See also* Antihemophilic globulin
Kogenate, 561. *See also* Antihemophilic globulin
Konakion, 561. *See also* Phytonadione
Koyne-80, 561. *See also* Factor IX (Christmas factor/plasma thromboplastin component), therapeutic
Kwell, 1005. *See also* Lindane
Kytril, 284. *See also* Granisetron

Labetalol, 136, 138*t*, 140, 143*i*, 145, **165**
for heart failure, 210
for hypertension, **165**
pharmacokinetic/pharmacodynamic parameters of, 36*t*
preparations available, 150, 174
properties of, 144*t*
Labial herpes, acyclovir for, 790, 791
Labor
oxytocin for induction of, 616
preterm, indomethacin in, 589
prostaglandins in facilitation of, 313
sedative-hypnotics before, 355–356
Lacrimal glands, direct-acting cholinomimetics affecting, 94*t*
Lacrimal secretion, antimuscarinic agents affecting, 108
Lactation. *See also* Breast-feeding; Breast milk
bromocriptine for suppression of, 282, 614
drug use during, **986**, 987*t*
H_2 receptor antagonist use during, 272
oxytocin in, 615
sedative-hypnotic use during, 356
Lactulose
laxative effect of, 1024
for portal-systemic encephalopathy, 1026
preparations available, 1028
Lamisil, 786. *See also* Terbinafine
Lamivudine, 795*t*, 796*i*, **797**
preparations available, 801
Lamotrigine, **396**, 396*i*
Lamprene, 779. *See also* Clofazimine
Langerhans, islets of, 684, 685*t*
Lanodoxin, 859. *See also* Iodoquinol
Lanoxicaps, 213. *See also* Digoxin
Lanoxin, 213. *See also* Digoxin
Lansoprazole
for acid-peptic disease, 1020
preparations available, 1027
Laplace relation, 185
Large intestinal fluke (*Fasciolopsis buski*), drugs for infection with, 863*t*
niclosamide, 872

Lariam, 859. *See also* Mefloquine
Larodopa, 462. *See also* Levodopa
Laron dwarfism, 607
Larva migrans
cutaneous (creeping eruption), drugs for, 863*t*
albendazole, 865
ivermectin, 868
thiabendazole, 877
visceral, drugs for, 863*t*
thiabendazole, 877
Lasix, 259. *See also* Furosemide
Lamisil, 1002. *See also* Terbinafine
Latanoprost, 306
for glaucoma, 316
preparations available, 317
Latrodectus mactans, antivenin for envenomation by, 1056*t*
Lavage, gastric, for poisoned patient, 976*i*
Laxatives, **1023–1024**
cathartic, for poisoned patient, 976, 976*t*
in OTC preparations
efficacy of, 1035*t*
hidden ingredients and, 1039*t*
preparations available, 1027–1028
LCD (liquor carbonis detergens), for dermatologic therapy, 1009
LD50 (median lethal dose), 29, 65
LDL (low-density lipoproteins), 563, 565*t*
estrogen replacement therapy affecting, 658, 659*i*
synthesis and catabolism of, 566
Lead compound, in new drug development, 63*i*, 64
Lead encephalopathy, 961
Lead poisoning, **959–963**, 960*t*
dimercaprol for, 957, 962
edetate calcium disodium for, 959, 962
succimer for, 958, 963
Leeches, medicinal, 551
Left ventricular function curve, 200, 200*i*
Leg cramps, quinine for, 848
Legionella, empiric antimicrobial therapy and, 814*t*
Leishmania (leishmaniasis), drugs for, **855–856**
braziliensis, 855*t*
donovani, 855*t*
mexicana, 855*t*
pentamidine, 856
stibogluconate, 855, 865
tropica, 855*t*
Lente insulin, 690–691, 690*t*
Lentinan, 935
Leprosy, drugs for, **777–778**
preparations available, 779
Leptophos, 951*t*
Leptospira, empiric antimicrobial therapy and, 815*t*
Lescol, 576. *See also* Fluvastatin
Letrozole, 672
Leu-enkephalin (leucine enkephalin), 497

Leucovorin
  with methotrexate, 891
  with pyrimethamine treatment,
    845–846
Leukemias, **905–907**
  acute, **905–906**
    adult, 905–906
    childhood, 905
    lymphoblastic, 905
    lymphocytic, 903*t*
    myelocytic, 903*t*
    myelogenous, 905–906
      as second malignancy, 913
    myelomonocytic, 903*t*
  chronic, **906**
    lymphocytic, 903*t*, **906**
      passive immunization and, 1056*t*
    elogenous, 903*t*, **906**
  hairy cell, **907**
Leukeran, 890*t. See also* Chlorambucil
Leukine, 546. *See also* Sargramostim
Leukocytes, glucocorticoids affecting,
    639
Leukocytosis, lithium causing, 479
Leukotriene A$_4$, 307
Leukotriene B$_4$, 307
Leukotriene C$_4$, 307–308
Leukotriene D$_4$, 308
Leukotriene pathway inhibitors, for
    asthma, **337**
  preparations available, 340
Leukotrienes, **304–318**. *See also*
    Eicosanoids
  biosynthesis of, 307–308, 307*i*
  bronchoconstriction caused by, 315
  effects of, 310–311
  in inflammation, 579*t*
Leuprolide, 611, 677
  in cancer chemotherapy, 899*t*, **900**
  structure of, 611*i*
Leustatin, 891*t. See also* Cladribine
Levallorphan, structure of, 499*i*
Levamisole, **869**, 935
  preparations available, 878, 940
  synaptic transmission affected by, 835
Levarterenol (norepinephrine), 77*t*, 85*t*,
    123*i*, 127–128, 350*t*, 352
  in adrenergic transmission, 78–80, 78*i*
  antidepressants affecting, 487
  biosynthesis of, 78–79, 79*i*
  ionization constant of, 6*t*
  metabolism of, 79–80, 80*i*
  as neurotransmitter, 77*t*, 350*t*, 352
  noradrenergic fiber release of, 74
  preparations available, 134
  receptors for, 81–82, 81*i*
  renin secretion affected by, 287–288
Levatol, 150, 174. *See also* Penbutolol
Levo-Dromoran, 501*t*, 513. *See also*
    Levorphanol
Levobunolol, 145
  for glaucoma, 149*t*
  preparations available, 150
Levocabastine, 268*t*
Levodopa, **451–455**
  with carbidopa, 452*i*, 453
    preparations available, 462

interactions of, 1066*t*
  ionization constant of, 6*t*
  monoamine oxidase inhibitor interac-
    tion and, 454, 456
  preparations available, 462
Levofloxacin, 765, 766*t*
Levomethadyl acetate, 511
  preparations available, 513
Levonantradol, 528
Levonorgestrel
  for male contraception, 679
  preparations available, 680
Levophed, 134. *See also* Norepinephrine
Levopropoxyphene, 512
Levorphanol, 511
  pharmacokinetics of, 501*t*
  preparations available, 513
  structure of, 499*i*
Levothroid, 633. *See also* Levothyroxine;
    Thyroxine
Levothyroxine, 625, 628. *See also* Thy-
    roxine
  with antithyroid drugs, for Graves'
    disease, 630
  preparations available, 633
Levoxyl, 633. *See also* Levothyroxine;
    Thyroxine
Levsinex, 116, 1027. *See also*
    Hyoscyamine
LFA-1, 917
LH (luteinizing hormone), 604*t*, **612**, 653
  in menotropins, 612–613
  receptors for, 604
  second messenger for, 22*t*
LHRH (luteinizing hormone-releasing
    hormone), **611–612**. *See also* Go-
    nadotropin-releasing hormone
Li$^+$ (lithium), **475–479**
  as ADH antagonist, 255–256
  adverse effects and complications of,
    478–479
  with antipsychotic agents, 473, 477
  in breast milk, 987*t*
  clinical indications and dosage for,
    255, 476–479
  dosage schedules for, 477
  in elderly, 993
  fetus affected by, 983*t*
  half-life of, aging affecting, 992*i*
  interactions of, 478, 1066–1067*t*
  maintenance treatment with, 478
  overdoses of, 479
  pharmacokinetic/pharmacodynamic
    parameters of, 36*t*, 255,
    475–476, 475*t*
  in pregnant patient, 478–479
  preparations available, 480
  serum monitoring of levels of,
    477–478
  toxicity of, 255–256
Librium, 366*t*, 369. *See also* Chlor-
    diazepoxide
Lice (pediculosis)
  benzyl benzoate for, 1005
  lindane for, 1005
  permethrin for, 1005
Lidanar, 472*t. See also* Mesoridazine

Lidocaine, **232–233**, 232*i*
  for arrhythmias, **232–233**
  clinical properties of, 229*t*
  half-life of, aging affecting, 992*i*
  ionization constant of, 6*t*
  as local anesthetic, 426*t*
  membrane actions of, 228*t*
  pharmacokinetic/pharmacodynamic
    parameters of, 36*t*, 233
  preparations available, 240, 432
  structure of, 426*t*
Lidone, 472*t. See also* Molindone
Ligand-defective apolipoprotein B, fa-
    milial, 568
Ligand-gated channels, 20–21
Ligand-regulated transmembrane en-
    zymes, 19–20, 20*i*
  endogenous, drug responsiveness af-
    fected by, 30
Lincomycin, 749
Lindane (hexachlorocyclohexane), 950*t*,
    1004–1005
Lioresal, 448. *See also* Baclofen
Liothyronine, 625. *See also* Triiodothyro-
    nine
  preparations available, 633
Liotrix, preparations available, 633
Lipase, in pancreatic enzyme replace-
    ment products, 1023*t*
Lipemia, 567–568
Lipid diffusion, drug permeation by, 5
Lipid-soluble agents
  intracellular receptors for, 18–19, 19*i*
  passage across placenta and, 979
Lipids
  estrogen replacement therapy affect-
    ing, 658, 659*i*
  oral contraceptives affecting metabo-
    lism of, 667
Lipitor, 576. *See also* Atorvastatin
Lipocortins, 311
Lipodystrophy, at insulin injection sites,
    695
Lipolysis, beta-receptor blocking drugs
    affecting, 143–145
Lipoproteins, 563–564, 565*t*
  disorders of, **566–569**, 567*t*
  estrogen replacement therapy affecting
    levels of, 658, 659*i*
  metabolism of, **564–566**, 565*i*
  structure of, 564
Liposomal amphotericin B, 781
Lipoxin A, 311
Lipoxin B, 311
Lipoxygenase, products of, 307–308,
    307*i*
  effects of, 310–311
  inhibition of synthesis of, 311
Liquor carbonis detergens (LCD), for
    dermatologic therapy, 1009
Lisinopril
  for heart failure, 210
  for hypertension, 170
  pharmacokinetics and dosage of, 171
  preparations available, 175, 213
Listeria, empiric antimicrobial therapy
    and, 814*t*

Lithium, **475–479**
  as ADH antagonist, 255–256
  adverse effects and complications of, 478–479
  with antipsychotic agents, 473, 477
  in breast milk, 987t
  clinical indications and dosage for, 255, 476–479
  dosage schedules for, 477
  in elderly, 993
  fetus affected by, 983t
  half-life of, aging affecting, 992i
  interactions of, 478, 1066–1067t
  maintenance treatment with, 478
  overdoses of, 479
  pharmacokinetic/pharmacodynamic parameters of, 36t, 255, 475–476, 475t
  in pregnant patient, 478–479
  preparations available, 480
  serum monitoring of levels of, 477–478
  toxicity of, 255–256
Livedo reticularis, amantadine causing, 457
Liver
  acetaminophen affecting, 595
  alcohol metabolized in, 372–373, 373i, 375
  autonomic activity/drugs affecting, 83t
  benzodiazepines metabolized in, 356–357
  chronic alcohol consumption affecting, 375
  disease/impaired function of. See also Hepatotoxicity
    acetaminophen causing, 595
    alcoholic, 375
    antimicrobial use and, 819, 819t
    diuretics for, **258**
    drug metabolism affected by, 60, 60t
    erythromycin causing, 748
    H_2 receptor antagonists causing, 272
    halothane causing, 418
    isoniazid causing, 772
    opioid analgesic use and, 510
    tetracyclines causing, 747
  first-pass elimination by, 51
    bioavailability and, 41, 41i, 42
    route of administration and, 42
  inhaled anesthetics affecting, 417–418
  insulin affecting, 688, 688t
  opioid analgesics metabolized by, 500–501
  oral contraceptives affecting, 667
  P450 enzymes in, 55, 56t
  transplantation of, immunosuppressive therapy and, 931t
Liver cancer, drug metabolism and, 60
Liver fluke, drugs for infection with, 863t
  albendazole, 865
  praziquantel, 874
Loa loa (loiasis), drugs for, 863t
  albendazole, 865

diethylcarbamazine, 866
  adverse reactions and, 867
  ivermectin, 868
Loading dose, 45
Lobeline, 92, 93, 93i
  central nervous system effects of, 96
Local anesthetics, **425–433**
  alpha agonists combined with, 131, 427
  basic pharmacology of, **425–430**
  clinical pharmacology of, **430–432**
  H_1 receptor antagonists as, 268
  neuromuscular blocking drug interaction and, 444
  in OTC preparations, hidden, 1038t
  preparations available, 432–433
  structure-activity characteristics of, 429
  toxicity of, 430–432
  vasoconstrictors combined with, 131, 427
Local hormones, 261. See also Histamine; Serotonin
Lodine, 599. See also Etodolac
Lodosyn, 462. See also Carbidopa
Loestrin, 665t
"Log-kill hypothesis," 883, 883i
Loiasis, drugs for, 863t
  albendazole, 865
  diethylcarbamazine, 866
    adverse reactions and, 867
  ivermectin, 868
Lomefloxacin, 765i, 766t
  preparations available, 768
Lomotil, 112, 1027. See also Diphenoxylate, with atropine
Lomustine (CCNU), 886i, **888**, 890t
Long-acting insulin, 690–691, 690t
Long QT syndrome, 223, 223i
Loniten, 175. See also Minoxidil
Loop diuretics, 244–245, **249–251**
  development of, 248
  with potassium-sparing diuretics, **256**
  with thiazides, **256**
    urinary electrolyte patterns affected by, 257t
  urinary electrolyte patterns affected by, 257t
Loop of Henle, transport in/diuretic site of action and, **244–245**, 245i, 249, 250
Lo/Ovral, 665t
Loperamide, 511, 1024
  in OTC preparations, efficacy of, 1034t
  OTC status of, 1031t
  preparations available, 1027
Lopid, 576. See also Gemfibrozil
Lopressor, 150, 174. See also Metoprolol
Loprox (ciclopirox olamine), 1002
Lorabid, 741. See also Loracarbef
Loracarbef, 734
  preparations available, 741
Loratadine, 267t
  preparations available, 283
Lorazepam, 356i
  absorption of, 355

for anesthesia, 420, 423
  biotransformation of, 357i
  distribution of, 355
  dosages of, 366t
  in elderly, 993
  pharmacokinetics of, 358t
  preparations available, 369, 407, 423
  for seizures, 362, 402, 407
  for status epilepticus, 405
Lortab (hydrocodone, with acetaminophen), 514
Losartan, 291, 292i, 293
  angiotensin receptor affinity for, 289, 291, 293
  for heart failure, 207
  for hypertension, 171–172
  preparations available, 175
Lotensin, 175. See also Benazepril
Lotrimin, 786, 1002. See also Clotrimazole
Lotrisone (clotrimazole-betamethasone dipropionate cream), 1002
Lovastatin, 573–574, 573i
  preparations available, 576
Lovenox, 561. See also Enoxaparin
Low-density lipoproteins (LDL), 563, 565t
  estrogen replacement therapy affecting, 658, 659i
  synthesis and catabolism of, 566
Low-level long-term exposure, to chemicals, 946
Low salt diet, for hypertension, 155, 172
Loxapine, 467i
  advantages and disadvantages of, 471t
  dose relationships of, 472t
  preparations available, 480
Loxitane, 471t, 472t, 480. See also Loxapine
Lozol, 259. See also Indapamide
Lp(a) hyperlipoproteinemia, 567t, 568–569
Lp(a) lipoprotein, 563, 565t
  synthesis and catabolism of, 566
LSD (lysergic acid diethylamide), 279
  abuse of, 524–526
  receptors affected by, 279, 279t
  structure of, 279t, 524i
LTA_4 (leukotriene A_4), 307
LTB_4 (leukotriene B_4), 307
LTC_4 (leukotriene C_4), 307–308
LTD_4 (leukotriene D_4), 308
Ludiomil, 494. See also Maprotiline
Lugol's solution, 633, 810. See also Iodine
Luminal, 369, 407. See also Phenobarbital
Luminal amebicides, 850
Lung. See also under Pulmonary and Respiratory
  direct-acting cholinomimetics affecting, 94i
Lung cancer, 903t, 911
Lung fluke (paragonimiasis), drugs for, 863t
  bithionol, 865–866
  praziquantel, 874

Lung maturation, fetal, adrenocorticosteroids for stimulation of, 643
Lupron, 611, 617, 899t. *See also* Leuprolide
Lupus erythematosus, procainamide causing syndrome like, 229
Luteinizing hormone (LH), 604t, **612**, 653
　in menotropins, 612–613
　receptors for, 604
　second messenger for, 22t
Luteinizing hormone-releasing hormone (LHRH), **611–612**. *See also* Gonadotropin-releasing hormone
Lutrepulse, 617. *See also* Gonadorelin
Luvox, 494. *See also* Fluvoxamine
Lymphocyte immune globulin, preparations available, 940
Lymphocytes, eicosanoids affecting, 315–316, 316i
Lymphokine-activated killer cells, 921
Lymphoma, **907–908**
　Hodgkin's, 903t, **907**
　non-Hodgkin's, 903t, **907–908**
　prednisone-sensitive, 898
Lynestrenol, 661t
Lyophilized factor VIII concentrates, 560. *See also* Factor VIII
Lysergic acid, structure of, 279t
Lysergic acid diethylamide (LSD), 279
　abuse of, 524–526
　receptors affected by, 279, 279t
　structure of, 279t
Lysodren, 650, 901t. *See also* Mitotane
Lysylbradykinin, 293, 294

M_1 muscarinic receptors, 81t, 91t, 108t
M_2 muscarinic receptors, 81t, 91t, 108t
M_3 muscarinic receptors, 81t, 91t, 108t
m_4 muscarinic receptors, 91t
m_5 muscarinic receptors, 91t
M-CSF (monocyte-macrophage colony-stimulating factor), 543, 543t, 545, 934t
Maalox, 1018t
MAC (minimum alveolar anesthetic concentration), 416
MAC (*Mycobacterium avium* complex), 777, 777t
Macrodantin, 810. *See also* Nitrofurantoin
Macroglobulinemia, 903t
Macrolides, **747–749**, 747i
　preparations available, 751
　protein synthesis affected by, 744, 744i
Macrophage colony-stimulating factor (M-CSF), 543, 543t, 545, 934t
Macrophages, glucocorticoids affecting functions of, 639
Macula densa, renin secretion controlled by, 287
Mafenide
　preparations available, 768
　topical, 763
Magan, 599. *See also* Magnesium salicylate

Magnesium
　for arrhythmias, **237**
　digitalis interactions and, 205
　preparations available, 240
Magnesium chloride, 240. *See also* Magnesium
Magnesium citrate, for poisoned patient, 976t
Magnesium hydroxide antacids (milk of magnesia), 1018t
　in OTC preparations, efficacy of, 1033t
　preparations available, 1028
Magnesium salicylate, 585
　preparations available, 599
Magnesium sulfate, for poisoned patient, 976, 976t
Maintenance dose, 44
　calculation of, 45
Major depressive episode (endogenous depression), 483, 484t, 490. *See also* Depression
Major histocompatibility complex proteins, 917, 920–921, 920i
Malaoxon, 98i
Malaria
　antimicrobial prophylaxis and, 825t, **840–841**, 840i
　drugs for, **591**, **838–850**. *See also* Antimalarial agents
Malathion, 97, 98i, 951t
　absorption/distribution/metabolism of, 98–99
Male infertility
　gonadotropin-releasing hormones for, 612
　human chorionic gonadotropin for, 613, 614
　human menopausal gonadotropins for, 613
Male reproductive system. *See also* Reproductive organs
　antipsychotic drugs affecting, 469
　prostaglandins affecting, 310, 314
Male sexual dysfunction
　alpha-receptor antagonists for, 141–142
　alprostadil for, 314
Malignant effusion, **912**
Malignant hyperthermia, 418
　dantrolene for, 447–448
Malignant melanoma, 904t, **911–912**
Maloprim, 847, 859. *See also* Pyrimethamine-dapsone
Mandelamine, 810. *See also* Methenamine mandelate
Mandol, 741. *See also* Cefamandole
Manic-depressive disorder (bipolar affective disorder)
　depression associated with, 483, 484t
　drugs for, **475–479**
　lithium for, 476–477
　nature of, 475
Manic episodes, drugs for, 470, **475–479**. *See also* Antipsychotic agents; Lithium

Mannitol, 254–255
　preparations available, 259
Mansil, 878. *See also* Oxamniquine
Mansonella, drugs for infection with
　diethylcarbamazine, 867
　ivermectin, 868
MAO (monoamine oxidase), in serotonin metabolism, 273–274
MAO inhibitors (monoamine oxidase inhibitors), **456**
　adverse effects of, 493t
　chemistry of, 484
　clinical indications for, 490
　dosages of, 491t
　　for acute episode, 491
　effects of, 489–490
　interactions of, 492, 1067t
　　with levodopa, 454, 456
　　with tyramine, 130
　overdoses of, 493
　for parkinsonism, **456**
　pharmacokinetics of, 487
　preparations available, 494
Maolate, 448. *See also* Chlorphenesin
Maprotiline, 484, 485i
　adverse effects of, 493t
　dosages of, 491t
　effects of, 488, 489t
　overdoses of, 972t
　pharmacokinetics of, 488t
　preparations available, 494
Marcaine, 426t, 432. *See also* Bupivacaine
Marezine, 267t, 283. *See also* Cyclizine
Marijuana, **526–528**
　antiemetic action of, 1022
Marinol, 528, 1027. *See also* Dronabinol
Mass therapy, of *W bancrofti* infections, diethylcarbamazine for, 867
Mast cells, histamine in, 261–262
Mastectomy, for breast cancer, 908
Maternal drug actions, 980
Matulane, 890t. *See also* Procarbazine
Maxair (pirbuterol), 340
Maxaquin, 768. *See also* Lomefloxacin
Maximal efficacy, 28, 28i
Maximum effect, therapeutic drug monitoring and, 47
Maxipime, 741. *See also* Cefepime
Maxzide, 254t. *See also* Triamterene
Mazotti reaction, 868
MBC (minimum bactericidal concentration), 816
MDA (methylenedioxyamphetamine), 521
MDMA (methylenedioxymethamphetamine), 521
　structure of, 524i
Measles
　active immunization for, 1052t
　passive immunization for, 1056t
Measles-mumps-rubella vaccine, 1053t
Mebadin, 858. *See also* Dehydroemetine
Mebaral (mephobarbital), 369, 407
Mebendazole, **869–870**, 869i
　microtubules affected by, 834–835, 869
　preparations available, 878

Mecamylamine, 114, 114*i*
  preparations available, 116, 175
Mechlorethamine, 886*i*, 890*t*
Meclan, 1001. *See also* Meclocycline
Meclizine, 267*t*
  for motion sickness, 269
  preparations available, 284
Meclocycline, 1001
Meclofenamate, 580*t*, **588**
  preparations available, 599
Meclomen, 599. *See also* Meclofenamate
Mectizan, 878. *See also* Ivermectin
Median effective concentration (EC50), 28
Median effective dose (ED50), 28, 29
Median lethal dose (LD50), 29, 65–66
Median toxic dose (TD50), 29
Medical pharmacology, definition of, 1.
  See also Pharmacology
Medrol, 650. *See also* Methylpred-
  nisolone
Medrol Enpack, 1027. *See also* Methyl-
  prednisolone
Medroxalol, 145
Medroxyprogesterone, 661*t*, 662*i*, 664
  in cancer chemotherapy, 899*t*
  depot, for contraception, 670
  preparations available, 680
Medullary depression, as anesthesia
  stage, 410–411
Medullary-periventricular pathway,
  467
Mefenamic acid, 586*i*, **588**
  preparations available, 599
Mefloquine, 839*i*, **843–844**
  for malaria chemoprophylaxis, 840*t*,
    843
  for malaria treatment, 841*t*, 843
  preparations available, 859
  resistance to, 843
  teratogenicity of, 844
Mefoxin, 741. *See also* Cefoxitin
Megace, 680, 899*t*. *See also* Megestrol
Megacolon, cholinomimetics for, 100
Megaloblastic anemia, vitamin defi-
  ciency causing, 537, 540–541
Megestrol acetate, 661*t*
  in cancer chemotherapy, 899*t*
  preparations available, 680
Meissner's plexus (submucosal plexus),
  74
MEL₁ receptor, 275
Melanocyte-stimulating hormone, second
  messenger for, 22*t*
Melanoma, 904*t*, **911–912**
Melarsen, antiparasitic actions of, 836*t*
Melatonin, 275
  receptors for, 275
Mellaril, 471*t*, 472*t*, 480. *See also* Thior-
  idazine
Melphalan, 886*i*, 890*t*
Membrane-stabilizing action, of beta-
  receptor blocking drugs, 145
Menaquinone (vitamin K₂), 558–559
Meniere's syndrome, H₁ receptor antago-
  nists for, 269

Meningitis
  empiric antimicrobial therapy and,
    816*t*
  intrathecal gentamicin for, 756
Meningococcal infections
  antimicrobial prophylaxis and, 825*t*
  empiric antimicrobial therapy and,
    814*t*
  vaccine for, 1053*t*
Menopause, 653, 654
Menotropins, 612, **612–613**
Menstrual cycle, 653–654, 654*i*
Menstrual products, OTC preparations,
    hidden ingredients in, 1038*t*, 1039*t*
Menstruation, iron-deficiency anemia
    and, 535
Mental disturbances
  bromocriptine causing, 455
  levodopa causing, 454
MEOS (microsomal ethanol oxidizing
    system)/mixed function oxidase
    system), 373, 373*i*
  in drug biotransformation, 51*i*, **52–55**,
    52*i*, 56*t*
Mepacrine, 859. *See also* Quinacrine
Mepenzolate
  for gastrointestinal and genitourinary
    conditions, 112*t*
  preparations available, 116, 1027
Meperidine, 511
  abuse of, 518
  overdose of, 972*t*
  pharmacokinetic/pharmacodynamic
    parameters of, 37*t*, 501*t*
  preparations available, 513
  receptor subtype activity of, 502*t*
  structure of, 499*i*
Mephentermine, preparations available,
    134
Mephenytoin, **391**
  genetic polymorphisms affecting me-
    tabolism of, 58
  preparations available, 407
Mephobarbital, preparations available,
    369, 407
Mephyton, 561. *See also* Phytonadione
Mepivacaine
  preparations available, 432
  properties of, 426*t*
  structure of, 426*t*
Meprednisone, 640*t*
Meprobamate, 357*i*, 364
  for anxiety, 365
  distribution of, 355
  as muscle relaxant, 366
  preparations available, 369
Meprolone, 650. *See also* Methylprednisolone
Merbromin, preparations available, 810
Mercaptopurine, **891–892**, 891*t*, 892*i*
  immunosuppressive actions of,
    927–928
  for inflammatory bowel disease, 1026
Mercurochrome (merbromin), 810
Mercury
  as disinfectant, **809**
  intoxication with, 960*t*, **964–966**

dimercaprol for, 957, 965–966
penicillamine for, 958–959, 965
Meropenem, 737
Merozoites, plasmodial, 838
Mersol, 810. *See also* Thimerosal
Merthiolate, 810. *See also* Thimerosal
Mesalamine. *See also* Aminosalicylic
    acid
  for inflammatory bowel disease, 1025
  preparations available, 1027
Mesantoin, 407. *See also* Mephenytoin
Mescaline
  abuse of, 524–526
  structure of, 524*i*
Mesolimbic-mesocortical pathway, 467
Mesoridazine
  dose relationships of, 472*t*
  preparations available, 480
Mestinon, 103. *See also* Pyridostigmine
Mestranol, 656*i*
Mesylate, 966. *See also* Deferoxamine
Met-enkephalin (methionine enkephalin),
    497
Metabolic acidosis
  hyperchloremic
    carbonic anhydrase inhibitors caus-
      ing, 249
    potassium-sparing diuretics causing,
      254
  in methanol poisoning, 382
Metabolic alkalosis
  carbonic anhydrase inhibitors for,
    248
  diuretics causing, heart failure man-
    agement and, 257
  hypokalemic
    loop diuretics causing, 250
    thiazides causing, 251
Metabolism
  antipsychotic agents affecting, 473
  autonomic activity/drugs affecting,
    83*t*
  beta-receptor blocking drugs affecting,
    143–145
  drug. *See also* Biotransformation
    aging affecting, 59, 989–990, 990*t*
    clinical relevance of, **56–61**
    diet affecting, 59
    diseases affecting, 60–61, 60*t*
    drug-drug interactions and, 59–60,
      59*t*, 60*t*
    drug-endogenous compound inter-
      actions and, 60
    environmental factors affecting, 59
    fetal, 980
    genetic factors affecting, 57–59,
      58*i*, 58*t*
    individual differences in rate of, 57
    in infants and children, 984, 985*t*
    interactions and, 1059
    phase I, 51, 51*i*, **52–55**, 53–54*t*
    phase II, 51, 51*i*, **55**, 57*t*
    placental, 980
    sex (gender) affecting, 59
    to toxic products, **55–56**, 57*i*. *See
      also* Reactive metabolites
  estrogens affecting, 657

Metabolism *(cont.)*
  sympathomimetic agents affecting, 127
  thyroid hormones affecting, 625*t*
Metabolites, toxic, **55–56**, 57*i. See also* Reactive metabolites
Metagonimus yokogawai (metagonimiasis), drugs for, 863*t*
  niclosamide, 872
  praziquantel, 875
Metamucil, 1028. *See also* Psyllium
Metanephrines, 80, 80*i*
Metaprel, 340. *See also* Metaproterenol
Metaproterenol, 333, 334*i*
  preparations available, 340
Metaraminol
  ionization constant of, 6*t*
  preparations available, 134
Metastasis, 881
Metaxalone
  for muscle spasm, 448
  preparations available, 448
Metformin, 699–700, 700*t*
  preparations available, 703
Methacholine
  enantiomers of, potency and, 3
  molecular structure of, 92*i*
  properties of, 93*t*
Methacycline, 745*i*
  pharmacokinetics of, 745–746
  preparations available, 751
Methadone, 510–511
  in breast milk, 987*t*
  fetus affected by, 983*t*
  for heroin detoxification, 510–511, 519
  ionization constant of, 6*t*
  overdose of, 972*t*
  pharmacokinetics of, 501*t*
  preparations available, 513
  receptor subtype activity of, 502*t*
Methallenestril, 656, 656*i*, 657*t*
Methamphetamine, 128, 521
  abuse of, 522
  ionization constant of, 6*t*
  preparations available, 134
Methandrostenolone (methandienone), 675*t*
Methanol (wood alcohol) poisoning, 382–383, 974*t*
Methantheline
  for gastrointestinal and genitourinary conditions, 112*t*
  preparations available, 116, 1027
Metharbital, preparations available, 407
Methdilazine, preparations available, 284
Methedrine, 521. *See also* Methamphetamine
Methemoglobin, nitrites in formation of, 184
Methenamine hippurate, **804**
  preparations available, 810
Methenamine mandelate, **804**
  preparations available, 810
Methergine (methylergonovine), 284
Methestrol, 656

Methicillin, 729–731
  adverse reactions to, 731
  preparations available, 740
Methimazole, 626–627, 626*i*
  for Graves' disease, 630
  preparations available, 633
  for thyroid storm, 631
Methionine-enkephalin (met-enkephalin), 497
Methionyllysylbradykinin, 284, 293
Methocarbamol
  for muscle spasm, 448
  OTC status of, 1031*t*
  preparations available, 448
Methohexital, 362, 420
  preparations available, 423
Methomyl, 952*t*
Methotrexate, **590–591**, **889–891**, 890*i*
  for asthma, 339
  dosage and toxicity of, 890–891, 891*t*
  fetus affected by, 983*t*
  half-life of, aging affecting, 992*i*
  immunosuppressive actions of, 928–929
  in inflammation, **590–591**
  ionization constant of, 6*t*
  pharmacokinetic/pharmacodynamic parameters of, 37*t*
  preparations available, 600
  resistance to, 890
Methotrimeprazine, half-life of, aging affecting, 992*i*
Methoxamine, 124*i*, 128
  preparations available, 134
Methoxsalen, **1006**
Methoxychlor, 950*t*
Methoxyflurane, 410*i*
  preparations available, 423
  properties of, 413*t*
  solubility of, 412, 413*t*
Methoxyphenamine, OTC status of, 1031*t*
Methscopolamine
  for gastrointestinal and genitourinary conditions, 112*t*
  preparations available, 116, 1027
Methsuximide, **399**
  preparations available, 407
Methyclothiazide
  dosages of, 252*t*
  preparations available, 259
Methycycline, oral dosage for, 746
N-Methyl-CD-aspartate, 351
  ethanol affecting, 374
  ketamine affecting, 422
Methylation, 57*t*
Methylbenzene (toluene), 950
  structure of, 529*i*
  threshold limit values for, 948*t*
Methyl-CCNU (semustine), 886*i*, **888**, 890*t*
Methylcellulose
  laxative effect of, 1023
  preparations available, 1028
Methyldopa, 158, **158–160**, 158*i*
  ionization constant of, 6*t*
  preparations available, 175
  renin secretion affected by, 290

Methylenedioxyamphetamine, 521
Methylenedioxymethamphetamine, 521
  structure of, 524*i*
6-Methylergoline, structure of, 279*t*
Methylergonovine, preparations available, 284
Methylethylketone, structure of, 529*i*
Methylhistamine, 264–265
Methylmercury intoxication, 965
Methylphenidate, 128–129, 521
  preparations available, 134
1-Methyl-4-phenyl-1,2,5,6-tetrahydropyridine, in parkinsonism, 458, 459
Methylprednisolone, 640*t*
  dosing schedules for, 645
  preparations available, 650, 940, 1027
Methyl *tert*-butyl ether, 1025
Methyltestosterone, 675*t*, 676*t*
  preparations available, 680
Methylthiouracil, fetus affected by, 983*t*
Methylxanthines, for asthma, **330–333**
  preparations available, 340
Methyprylon, 364
Methysergide
  ionization constant of, 6*t*
  for migraine, 282
  preparations available, 284
  receptors affected by, 279*t*
  structure of, 279*t*
  toxicity of, 283
Metiamide, 270
  history of development of, 63*t*
Meticorten, 650. *See also* Prednisone
Metipranolol
  for glaucoma, 149*t*
  preparations available, 150
Metoclopramide
  antiemetic action of, 1022
  gastrointestinal motility affected by, 1021–1022
  preparations available, 1027
Metocurine, 438*t*
  cardiovascular effects of, 443, 443*t*
  effects of, 443*t*
  preparations available, 448
Metolazone, 256
  dosages of, 252*t*
  preparations available, 259
  structure of, 252*i*
Metoprolol, 138*t*, 143*i*, 145, **165**, 194
  distribution and clearance of, 142, 144*i*
  half-life of, aging affecting, 992*i*
  for hypertension, **165**
  ionization constant of, 6*t*
  pharmacokinetic/pharmacodynamic parameters of, 37*t*
  preparations available, 150, 174, 194
  properties of, 144*t*
  for tremor, 459
Metrifonate, **870–871**
  antiparasitic actions of, 836*t*, 870
  preparations available, 878
Metrodin, 617. *See also* Urofollitropin
Metronidazole, **803**, **857–858**, 857*i*
  for amebiasis, 850, 851*t*, **854**
  for ameboma, 852

fetus affected by, 983*t*

pharmacokinetic/pharmacodynamic parameters of, 37*t*, 857

preparations available, 810, 859

pyruvate:ferredoxin oxidoreductase affected by, 829

topical, for acne rosacea, 1001

Metubine, 448. *See also* Metocurine

Metyrapone, **647–648**, 647*i*

Metyrosine

for pheochromocytoma, 141

preparations available, 150

Mevacor, 576. *See also* Lovastatin

Mevalonate, 573*i*

Mexiletine, **233**, 233*i*

for arrhythmias, **233**

clinical properties of, 229*t*

membrane actions of, 228*t*

preparations available, 240

Mexitil, 240. *See also* Mexiletine

Mezlocillin, 731

preparations available, 740

MHC proteins, 917, 920–921, 920*i*

Miacalcin, 721. *See also* Calcitonin

MIC (minimal inhibitory concentration), 816

Micatin, 786, 1002. *See also* Miconazole

"Mickey Finn," 520–521

Miconazole, 784*i*

in OTC preparations, efficacy of, 1034*t*

OTC status of, 1032*t*

parasite sterol synthesis affected by, 831

preparations available, 786

topical, 786, 1002

MICRhoGAM, 940. *See also* Rh₀ (D) immune globulin micro-dose

Micrometastases, adjuvant chemotherapy for, 904–905

Micronase, 697*t*, 703. *See also* Glyburide

Micronor, 665*t*, 680. *See also* Norethindrone

Microsomal mixed function oxidase system (microsomal ethanol oxidizing system), 373, 373*i*

in drug biotransformation, 51*i*, **52–55**, 52*i*, 56*t*

Microsomes, 52

Microtubules, antiparasitic agents affecting, 834–835

Micturition, antimuscarinic agents affecting, 110

Midamor, 254*t*, 259. *See also* Amiloride

Midazolam, 411*i*, 420*t*

for anesthesia, 362, 420, 420*t*, 421, 423

pharmacokinetic/pharmacodynamic parameters of, 37*t*

preparations available, 369, 423

Midodrine, 128

preparations available, 134

Mifepristone (RU 486), **648**, **671–672**

with prostaglandins, for abortion, 313

Migraine headache

amitriptyline for, 282

ergot alkaloids for, 281–282

toxicity and, 278, 283

estrogen therapy and, 660

flunarizine for, 282

propranolol for, 148, 282

sumatriptan for, 282

Milbemycins, synaptic transmission affected by, 835

Milk ejection reflex, oxytocin affecting, 615

Milk of magnesia (magnesium hydroxide), 1018*t*

in OTC preparations, efficacy of, 1033*t*

preparations available, 1028

Milontin, 407. *See also* Phensuximide

Milophene, 680. *See also* Clomiphene

Milrinone

for heart failure, **205–206**

preparations available, 213

Miltown, 369. *See also* Meprobamate

Mimicry, synaptic, 346–347

Mineral oil

preparations available, 1028

as stool softener, 1024

Mineralocorticoids, 640*t*, **646–647**

antagonists of, **649**

preparations available, 650

receptors for, 18

Mini-Gamulin Rh, 940. *See also* Rh₀ (D) immune globulin micro-dose

Minimal change glomerulopathy, lithium causing, 478

Minimal inhibitory concentration (MIC), 816

Minimum alveolar anesthetic concentration, (MAC), 416

Minimum bactericidal concentration (MBC), 816

Minimum lethal dose, 65

Minipress, 150, 175. *See also* Prazosin

Minitran, 194. *See also* Nitroglycerin

Minocin, 751. *See also* Minocycline

Minocycline, 745*i*

clinical uses of, 746

oral dosage for, 746

pharmacokinetics of, 745–746

preparations available, 751

vestibular reactions to, 747

Minoxidil, **167–168**, 167*i*

in dermatologic therapy, **1014**

OTC status of, 1032*t*

for heart failure, 210*t*

for hypertension, **167–168**

preparations available, 175

potassium channels and, 181

Mintezol, 878. *See also* Thiabendazole

Miochol, 103. *See also* Acetylcholine

Miosis, 148

opioid analgesics causing, 505

Miostat, 103. *See also* Carbachol

Mirtazapine, 484, 486*i*

biogenic amine neurotransmitters affected by, 487

dosages of, 491*t*

effects of, 489*t*

pharmacokinetics of, 488*t*

preparations available, 494

Misoprostol, 306, 312*i*

for acid-peptic disease, 1021

with antiprogestins, for abortion, 313

preparations available, 317, 1027

MIT (monoiodotyrosine), 619

Mithracin, 721, 894*t*. *See also* Mithramycin

Mithramycin (plicamycin)

bone mineral homeostasis affected by, **711**

for cancer chemotherapy, 894*t*, **897**

for hypercalcemia, 714

for Paget's disease, 720

preparations available, 721

Mitochondrial electron transporter, antiparasitic agents affecting, 834

Mitomycin, 894*t*, **897**, 897*i*

Mitotane, 647*i*, **648–649**, **901**

in cancer chemotherapy, 901*t*

preparations available, 650

Mitoxantrone, **901**, 901*t*

Mitral regurgitation, myocardial infarction and, 211*t*, 212

Mitrolan (polycarbophil), 1028

Mivacron, 448. *See also* Mivacurium

Mivacurium, 436*i*, 438*t*

cardiovascular effects of, 443, 443*t*

effects of, 443*t*

neostigmine interaction and, 445

pharmacokinetics of, 438*t*, 439

preparations available, 448

Mixed alpha and beta agonists, selectivity of, 120, 120*t*

Mixed alpha and beta antagonists, selectivity of, 138*t*

Mixed function oxidase system (microsomal ethanol oxidizing system), 373, 373*i*

in drug biotransformation, 51*i*, **52–55**, 52*i*, 56*t*

Mizoribine, 927

MLCK (myosin light chain kinase), 24

MMR vaccine, 1053*t*

Moban, 472*t*, 480. *See also* Molindone

Mobidin, 599. *See also* Magnesium salicylate

Mobility, environmental toxicity and, 947

Moclobemide, 484, 487*i*

Moctanin, 1028. *See also* Monoctanoin

Modicon, 665*t*

Moduretic, 254*t*. *See also* Amiloride

Moebequin, 853. *See also* Iodoquinol

Moexipril

for hypertension, 170

preparations available, 175

Molecular size of drug, 2

passage across placenta and, 979

Molindone, 467*i*

dose relationships of, 472*t*

preparations available, 480

Monistat, 786, 1002. *See also* Miconazole

Monoamine oxidase, in serotonin metabolism, 273–274

Monoamine oxidase inhibitors (MAO inhibitors), **456**
  adverse effects of, 493*t*
  chemistry of, 484
  clinical indications for, 490
  dosages of, 491*t*
    for acute episode, 491
  effects of, 489–490
  interactions of, 492, 1067*t*
    with levodopa, 454, 456
    with tyramine, 130
  overdoses of, 493
  for parkinsonism, **456**
  pharmacokinetics of, 487
  preparations available, 494
Monoamines. *See also specific type*
  as central neurotransmitters, 352
Monobactams, **736**
  preparations available, 741
  structure of, 725*i*
Monobenzone, **1005**
Monocid, 741. *See also* Cefonicid
Monoclate, 561. *See also* Antihemophilic globulin
Monoctanoin, 1025
  preparations available, 1028
Monocyte-macrophage colony-stimulating factor (M-CSF), 543, 543*t*, 545
Monoiodotyrosine (MIT), 619
Monopril, 175, 213. *See also* Fosinopril
Monurol, 741. *See also* Fosfomycin
Mood-stabilizing drugs, **475–479**. *See also specific type and* Lithium
  preparations available, 480
MOPP regimen, in Hodgkin's disease, 907
Moraxella catarrhalis, empiric antimicrobial therapy and, 814*t*
Moricizine, **234**
  for arrhythmias, **234**
  clinical properties of, 229*t*
  membrane actions of, 228*t*
  preparations available, 240
"Morning after" contraception, 670, 671*t*
Morning sickness, H$_1$ receptor antagonists for, 269
Morphinans
  mixed agonist-antagonists/partial agonists, **512**
  strong agonists, **511**
  structures of, 498*i*
Morphine, 510
  abuse of, 518
  for anesthesia, 421
  ionization constant of, 6*t*
  in opium, 496
  organ system effects of, 504–506
  overdose of, 972*t*
  pharmacokinetic/pharmacodynamic parameters of, 37*t*, 501*t*
  preparations available, 513
  for pulmonary edema, 212
  receptor subtype activity of, 502*t*
  structure of, 498*i*
Motility, gastrointestinal
  antimuscarinic agents affecting, 110

direct-acting cholinomimetics affecting, 94*t*, 96
drugs promoting, **1021–1022**
H$_2$ receptor antagonists affecting, 270–271
preparations available, 1027
Motion sickness
  antimuscarinic agents for, 110–111, 1022
  H$_1$ receptor antagonists for, 268, 269, 1022
  OTC preparations for, hidden ingredients in, 1037*t*
  scopolamine for, 107, 110–111, 269, 1022
Motofen, 1027. *See also* Difenoxin
Motrin, 599. *See also* Ibuprofen
Mountain sickness, carbonic anhydrase inhibitors for, 248–249
Mouth, in poisoned patient, 971
Mouthwashes, hidden ingredients in, 1037
Movement disorders, **450–463**. *See also* Parkinsonism
  preparations of drugs for, 462
Moxalactam, 734–735
6-MP (mercaptopurine), **891–892**, 891*t*, 892*i*
  immunosuppressive actions of, 927–928
  for inflammatory bowel disease, 1026
MPTP (1-methyl-4-phenyl-1,2,5,6-tetrahydropyridine), in parkinsonism, 458, 459
MTX (methotrexate), **590–591, 889–891**, 890*i*
  for asthma, 339
  dosage and toxicity of, 890–891, 891*t*
  fetus affected by, 983*t*
  half-life of, aging affecting, 992*i*
  immunosuppressive actions of, 928–929
  in inflammation, **590–591**
  ionization constant of, 6*t*
  pharmacokinetic/pharmacodynamic parameters of, 37*t*
  preparations available, 600
  resistance to, 890
Mu (μ) receptors, 501
  opioid activity at, 502*t*
Mucociliary function, inhaled anesthetics affecting, 417
Mucomyst (acetylcysteine), 977*t*
Mucoraceae, empiric antimicrobial therapy and, 815*t*
Mucosal protective agents
  for acid-peptic disease, **1021**
  preparations available, 1027
Multiple myeloma, 903*t*, **908**
Mumps vaccine, 1053*t*
Mupirocin, **803**
  in dermatologic therapy, **1000**
Muromonab-CD3 (OKT3), 930
  preparations available, 940
Muscarine, 90, 92, 93*i*. *See also* Muscarinic receptors
  toxicity of, 102

Muscarinic receptor-blocking drugs, **105–110, 110–114**
  for asthma, **335–336, 339**, 340
  basic pharmacology of, **105–110, 335–336**
  clinical pharmacology of, **110–114, 339**
  overdosage of, physostigmine for, 101–102
  preparations available, 115–116, 340
Muscarinic receptors, 81, 81*t*, 90, 91*t*, 108*t*
  activation of, 93–94
  atropine selectivity for, 106
  in central nervous system, 96
  toxicity of drugs affecting, 102
Muscimol, for tardive dyskinesia, 461
Muscle-derived differentiation factor, for parkinsonism, 458
Muscle pain, succinylcholine causing, 444
Muscle spasm
  acute, drugs for management of, **448**
  drugs for management of, **445–448**.
    See also specific agent
  preparations available, 448
Muscle/musculoskeletal system. *See also* Skeletal muscle; Smooth muscle
  insulin affecting, 688*t*
  relaxation of
    drugs causing, **434–449**. *See also* Neuromuscular blocking drugs; Spasmolytic drugs
    sedative-hypnotics producing, 362, 366
  thyroid hormones affecting, 625*t*
Mushroom poisoning, 102
  treatment of, 113
Mustargen, 890*t*. *See also* Mechlorethamine
Mutagenicity
  of inhaled anesthetics, 418
  of metronidazole, 858
  of quinine, 848
Mutamycin, 894*t*. *See also* Mitomycin
Myambutol, 778. *See also* Ethambutol
Myasthenia gravis, cholinesterase inhibitors for, 101
Mycelex, 786, 1002. *See also* Clotrimazole
Mycifradin, 759. *See also* Neomycin
Mycobacterium (mycobacterial infections)
  atypical, **777**, 777*t*
  avium complex, 777, 777*t*
    antimicrobial prophylaxis and, 825*t*
  chelonae, 777*t*
  drugs for, **770–779**
    preparations available, 778–779
    streptomycin, 754–755
  empiric antimicrobial therapy and, 815*t*
  fortuitum, 777*t*
  kansasii, 777, 777*t*
  leprae, **777–778**
    empiric antimicrobial therapy and, 815*t*
  marinum, 777*t*

scrofulaceum, 777*t*
tuberculosis, **770–777**. *See also* Tuberculosis
   empiric antimicrobial therapy and, 815*t*
ulcerans, 777*t*
Mycobutin, 778. *See also* Rifabutin
Mycophenolate mofetil (RS-61443), 927
Mycoplasma pneumoniae, empiric antimicrobial therapy and, 815*t*
Mycostatin, 786. *See also* Nystatin
Mydriacyl, 116. *See also* Tropicamide
Mydriasis
   antimuscarinic agents causing, 108, 109*i*, 111, 111*t*
   levodopa causing, 454
Myeloid growth factors, **544–545**
   preparations available, 546
Myeloma, 903*t*, **908**
Myelosuppression, zidovudine causing, 796
Myenteric plexus (plexus of Auerbach), 74
Myidil, 284. *See also* Triprolidine
Mykrox, 259. *See also* Metolazone
Mylanta, 1018*t*
Myleran, 890*t*. *See also* Busulfan
Myocardial contractility
   autonomic activity/drugs affecting, 83*t*
   beta-receptor blocking drugs affecting, 149
   control of, 197–199, 197*i*
   digitalis glycosides affecting, 203, 203*i*
   ethanol affecting, 374
   histamine affecting, 264
   in low output failure, 200
Myocardial hypertrophy
   angiotensin II affecting, 289
   in heart failure, 199
Myocardial infarction
   acute heart failure after, **210–212**
      subsets in, 211–212, 211*t*
   antimuscarinic agents for pain of, 111
   arrhythmias after, treatment of, 234
   aspirin for prevention of, 557
   beta-receptor blocking drugs affecting outcome of, 146, 147*i*, 192, 192*i*
      risks of use of, 149
   oral contraceptive use and, 669
   thrombolytic agents for, 555, 556
Myocardial oxygen demand, determinants of, 180, 180*t*
Myocardial oxygen supply, determinants of, 180
Myocardial remodeling
   angiotensin-converting enzyme inhibitors affecting, 289
   in heart failure, 199
Myochrysine, 599. *See also* Gold sodium thiomalate
Myoclonic jerking, 404
   drugs used for, 405
Myoglobin, iron content of, 534*t*
Myopathy, alcoholic, 376–377
Myoproic Acid, 407. *See also* Valproic acid

Myosin light chain kinase, 24
Mysoline, 407. *See also* Primidone
Mytelase, 103. *See also* Ambenonium
Myxedema, 628–629
   pretibial, 632
Myxedema coma, 629

N_M nicotinic receptors, 81*t*, 91*t*
N_N nicotinic receptors, 81*t*, 91*t*
Na^+-K^+ ATPase
   in cardiac conduction, 216–217
   in cardiac contractility, 198–199
   cardiac glycoside inhibition of, 202
Na^+-K^+-$2Cl^-$ cotransporter
   in distal convoluted tubule, 245
   in loop of Henle, 244, 245*i*, 250
Nabumetone, 580*t*, 586*i*, **588**
   preparations available, 599
N-acetylpepstatin, renin inhibited by, 290
Nadolol, 143*i*, 145, **165**
   distribution and clearance of, 142, 144*t*
   for hypertension, **165**
   preparations available, 150, 174, 194
   properties of, 144*t*
Nafarelin, 611
   structure of, 611*i*
Nafcil, 740. *See also* Nafcillin
Nafcillin, 724, 725, 726*i*, 729–731
   adverse reactions to, 731
   CSF penetration by, 820*t*
   dosing guidelines for, 730*t*
   preparations available, 740
Naftifine
   preparations available, 786
   topical, 786, **1002**
Naftin, 786, 1002. *See also* Naftifine
Nalbuphine, 511–512
   pharmacokinetics of, 501*t*
   preparations available, 513
   receptor subtype activity of, 502*t*
Nalfon, 599. *See also* Fenoprofen
Nalidixic acid, 765, **767**
   preparations available, 768
Nallpen, 740. *See also* Nafcillin
Nalmefene, 512–513
   preparations available, 514
Nalorphine, structure of, 498*i*
Naloxone, 512–513, 977*t*
   in initial management of poisoned patient, 971
   preparations available, 514
   receptor subtype activity of, 502*t*
   structure of, 498*i*
Naltrexone, 512–513
   for alcoholism, 381–382, 383
   preparations available, 383, 514
   structure of, 498*i*
   for treatment of opioid abuse, 519
Nandrolone, 675*t*
   preparations available, 680
Naphazoline, preparations available, 134
Naprosyn, 599. *See also* Naproxen
Naproxen, 580*t*, **586–587**
   in OTC preparations, efficacy of, 1033*t*

OTC status of, 1031*t*
   preparations available, 599
Naqua, 259. *See also* Trichlormethiazide
Narcan, 514, 977*t*. *See also* Naloxone
Narcotic, 496. *See also* Opioid analgesics
Narcotic antagonists (opioid antagonists), 498–499*i*, **512–513**
   preparations available, 514
   for treatment of opioid abuse, 519
Nardil, 494. *See also* Phenelzine
Naropin, 426*t*, 433. *See also* Ropivacaine
Nasal insulin delivery, 693
Nasalcrom, 340. *See also* Cromolyn
Nasopharyngeal glands, direct-acting cholinomimetics affecting, 94*t*
Natriuretic peptides, **296–298**, 296*i*
Natural killer cells, 921
Naturetin, 259. *See also* Bendroflumethiazide
Nausea. *See also* Motion sickness; Vomiting
   drugs for control of, **1022**
   estrogen therapy causing, 660
   H_1 receptor antagonists preventing, 268
   opioid analgesics causing, 505
   in pregnancy, H_1 receptor antagonists for, 269
Navane, 471*t*, 472*t*, 480. *See also* Thiothixene
Navelbine (vinorelbine), 894*t*
NDA (New Drug Application), 63*i*, 69
Nebcin, 759. *See also* Tobramycin
Nebirolol, for heart failure, 210
Necator americanus (necatoriasis), drugs for, 863*t*
   albendazole, 864
   pyrantel, 876
   tetrachloroethylene, 876
Nedocromil
   for asthma, **328–330**, 328*i*, **339**
   preparations available, 340
Nefazodone, 484, 486*i*
   adverse effects of, 493*t*
   biogenic amine neurotransmitters affected by, 487
   dosages of, 491*t*
      for acute episode, 491
   interactions of, 492–493
   pharmacokinetics of, 488*t*
   preparations available, 494
Negative feedback control
   in autonomic control of cardiovascular function, 84, 84*i*
   in presynaptic levels of autonomic function, 84
NegGram, 768. *See also* Nalidixic acid
Neisseria
   gonorrhoeae, empiric antimicrobial therapy and, 814*t*
   meningitidis
      antimicrobial prophylaxis and, 825*t*
      empiric antimicrobial therapy and, 814*t*
Nelfinavir, 799
   preparations available, 801
Nelova, 665*t*

Nematodes, drugs for, 863*t*
Nembutal, 369, 407. *See also* Pentobarbital
Neo-Antergan, 267*t*. *See also* Pyrilamine
Neo-Calglucon, 721. *See also* Calcium
Neoendorphins, 497
Neomycin, **758–759**
  adverse effects of, 754, 759
  in dermatologic therapy, **1000–1001**
  for portal-systemic encephalopathy, 1026
    preparations available, 759
Neonate
  chloramphenicol toxicity in, 745
  cocaine addiction in, 523
  drug therapy in, **982–985**
  Graves' disease in, 632
  hemolytic anemia in, Rh$_o$ (D) immune globulin in prevention of, 930–931, 931*t*
  meningitis in, empiric antimicrobial therapy and, 816*t*
  opioid analgesic withdrawal in, 510
  pneumonia in, empiric antimicrobial therapy and, 816*t*
  respiratory disorders in, nitric oxide for, 322
Neosar, 940. *See also* Cyclophosphamide
Neostigmine, 97, 97*i*
  for gastrointestinal and urinary tract disorders, 100–101
  mechanism of action of, 99
  mivacurium interaction and, 445
  for myasthenia gravis, 101
  neuromuscular blockade reversed by, 445
  preparations available, 103
Neo-Synephrine, 134. *See also* Phenylephrine
Neo-Synephrine 12 Hour, 134. *See also* Oxymetazoline
Neo-Synephrine Long-Acting, 134. *See also* Xylometazoline
Nephritis, chronic interstitial, lithium causing, 478
Nephrogenic diabetes insipidus, lithium causing, 255, 259, 478
Nephrolithiasis
  diuretics for, **258**
  indinavir causing, 798
Nephrotic syndrome, bone mineral homeostasis and, **719**
Nephrotoxicity. *See also* Renal disease
  of amikacin, 758
  of aminoglycosides, 753–754
  of cidofovir, 793
  of gentamicin, 756
  of inhaled anesthetics, 418
  of tobramycin, 758
Nernst equation, 218
Nerve endings
  histamine affecting, 264
  kinins affecting, 294
  serotonin affecting, 275
Nerve fibers, local anesthetics affecting, 429, 429*t*

Nervous system. *See also* Central nervous system; Neurologic disease
  antipsychotic agents affecting, 473
  autonomic, **73–89**. *See also* Autonomic nervous system
  enteric, 74, 75*i*
    transmitter substances in, 77*t*
  lithium affecting, 478
  peripheral
    chronic alcohol consumption affecting, 376
    direct-acting cholinomimetics affecting, 96
    local anesthetic toxicity and, 430
    nitric oxide affecting, **323–324**
    prostaglandins affecting, 310
  in poisoned patient, 971–973
  serotonin affecting, 275–276
Nesacaine (chloroprocaine), 432
Netilmicin, 754*i*, **758**
  preparations available, 759
Netromycin, 759. *See also* Netilmicin
Neupogen, 546. *See also* Filgrastim
Neural tube defects, fetal, folic acid in prevention of, 543
Neuritis, retrobulbar, ethambutol causing, 774
Neurobiology, in drug abuse, 517–518
Neuroblastoma, 903*t*
Neurocysticercosis
  albendazole for, 864–865
  praziquantel for, 874–875
Neuroendocrine system
  opioid analgesics affecting, 506
  prostaglandins affecting, 310
Neuroleptanesthesia, 421
Neuroleptic malignant syndrome, 474
Neuroleptics (antipsychotic agents), **464–475**
  advantages and disadvantages of, 471*t*, 475
  adverse effects of, 470*t*, 473–474
  basic pharmacology of, **464–470**
  chemical types of, 464–465, 466*i*, 467*i*
  clinical pharmacology of, **470–475**
  combinations of, 473
  differences among, 468–469
  dosage schedules for, 472–473
  dose relationships of, 472, 472*t*
  in elderly, 993
  interactions of, 474
  lithium combined with, 473, 477
  maintenance treatment and, 473
  overdoses of, 474
  plasma concentrations of, 472
  preparations available, 472, 480
  selection of, 471–472, 471*t*
  tardive dyskinesia caused by, 461
  teratogenic effects of, 474
  toxicity of, 474
Neurologic disease
  beta-receptor blocking drugs for, 148
  chronic alcohol consumption causing, 376
Neuromuscular blocking drugs, **434–445**
  age affecting response to, 444–445

basic pharmacology of, **435–442**
  chemistry of, 435, 435*i*, 436*i*, 437*i*
  clinical pharmacology of, **442–445**
  depolarizing, 435
    effects of, 444
    mechanism of action of, 439–442, 440*i*, 440*t*, 441*i*
    pharmacokinetics of, 439
    skeletal muscle paralysis caused by, 442–443, 443*i*
  disease affecting response to, 444–445
  interactions of, 444
  nondepolarizing, 435
    mechanism of action of, 439, 440*i*, 440*t*, 441*i*
    pharmacokinetics of, 435–439
    reversal of, 445
    skeletal muscle paralysis caused by, 442, 442*i*
  preparations available, 448
  properties of, 438*t*
  for seizures, 445
  structures of, 435, 435*i*, 436*i*, 437*i*
  for ventilation control, 445
Neuromuscular junction
  cholinesterase inhibitors affecting, 100
  direct-acting cholinomimetics affecting, 96
  disorders of, cholinesterase inhibitors for, 101
  normal function of, 434–435, 435*i*
Neurontin, 407. *See also* Gabapentin
Neuropathy, peripheral
  isoniazid causing, 773
  lead toxicity causing, 961
Neuropathy target esterase, organophosphorus insecticides affecting, 951–952
Neuropeptide Y, 77*t*, 85*t*, **301**
Neurosurgery, antimicrobial prophylaxis and, 824*t*
Neurotensin, **300**
Neurotoxicant anthelmintics, 835
Neurotoxicity, of local anesthetics, 430
Neurotransmitters, **74–81**, 77*t*, **348–353**, 349–350*t*. *See also specific type*
  for alcoholism, 381
  antidepressants affecting, 487, 489*i*
  drugs acting on, 345–346
  identification of, **346–347**
  lithium affecting, 476
  localization of, 346
  in parkinsonism, 458
  prostaglandins affecting, 310
  release of, 346
  synaptic mimicry and, 346–347
Neurotrophic factors, for parkinsonism, 458
Neutra-Phos, 721. *See also* Phosphate
Neutral protamine Hagedorn insulin (NPH insulin), 690*t*, 691
New Drug Application (NDA), 63*i*, 69
Newborn
  chloramphenicol toxicity in, 745
  cocaine addiction in, 523
  drug therapy in, **982–985**
  Graves' disease in, 632

hemolytic anemia of, Rh$_o$ (D) immune globulin in prevention of, 930–931, 931*t*
    meningitis in, empiric antimicrobial therapy and, 816*t*
    opioid analgesic withdrawal in, 510
    pneumonia in, empiric antimicrobial therapy and, 816*t*
    respiratory disorders in, nitric oxide for, 322
NHL (non-Hodgkin's lymphoma), 903*t*, **907–908**
Niacin (nicotinic acid)
    for hyperlipidemia, **570–571**
        combination therapy with, **575**
    preparations available, 576
Nicardipine
    clinical properties of, 190*t*
    for hypertension, 169
    pharmacokinetics of, 189*t*
    preparations available, 175, 194
    vascular selectivity of, 190*t*
Niclocide, 878. *See also* Niclosamide
Niclosamide, **871–872**, 871*i*
    antiparasitic actions of, 836*t*, 871
    preparations available, 878
Nicorandil, for angina, mechanism of action of, 183
Nicotine, 90, 92, 93*i*, 521. *See also* Muscarinic receptors
    central nervous system effects of, 96
    as insecticide, 952
    ionization constant of, 6*t*
    in OTC preparations, efficacy of, 1035*t*
    OTC status of, 1031*t*
    peripheral nervous system effects of, 96
    toxicity of, 102
Nicotine dependence, 521, 524
Nicotine polacrilex
    in OTC preparations, efficacy of, 1035*t*
    OTC status of, 1031*t*
Nicotinic acid (niacin)
    for hyperlipidemia, **570–571**
        combination therapy with, **575**
    preparations available, 576
Nicotinic receptors, 20–21, 21*i*, 81, 81*t*, 90, 91*t*, 434
    activation of, 94
    in central nervous system, 96
    drugs blocking, **114–115**
    in peripheral nervous system, 96
    toxicity of drugs affecting, 102
Nifedipine
    chemistry of, 187, 188*i*
    clinical properties of, 190*t*
    for hypertension, 169
    pharmacokinetic/pharmacodynamic parameters of, 37*t*, 189*t*
    preparations available, 175, 194
    toxicity of, 190–191
    vascular selectivity of, 190*t*
Nifurtimox, trypanothione reductase affected by, 829
Nigrostriatal pathway, 467

Nimbex, 448. *See also* Cisatracurium
Nimodipine
    cerebral blood vessels affected by, 189
    clinical properties of, 190*t*
    pharmacokinetics of, 189*t*
    preparations available, 194
    vascular selectivity of, 190*t*
Nimotop, 194. *See also* Nimodipine
Nipride, 175. *See also* Nitroprusside
Niridazole, antiparasitic actions of, 836*t*
Nisoldipine
    clinical properties of, 190*t*
    for hypertension, 169
    pharmacokinetics of, 189*t*
    preparations available, 175, 194
    vascular selectivity of, 190*t*
Nitrates
    for angina, **181–186**, 186*t*, 193*t*
        beneficial and deleterious effects of, 185–186, 185*t*
        cGMP affected by, 180
    chemistry of, 181, 182*i*
    clinical use of, 186
    for heart failure, 210*t*
        with "power failure," 212
    mechanism of action/clinical effects of, 181*i*, 182–183, 185–186, 185*t*
    organ system effects of, 183–185
    pharmacodynamics of, 182–185
    pharmacology of, 182
    preparations available, 194
    tolerance to, 185
    toxicity of, 185
Nitrazepam, 356*i*
    for seizures, 362, 402
Nitrendipine
    clinical properties of, 190*t*
    pharmacokinetics of, 189*t*
    vascular selectivity of, 190*t*
Nitric oxide, **319–324**, 353. *See also* Endothelium-derived relaxing factor
    in asthma, 338
    cGMP affected by, angina management and, 180, 181, 181*i*, 182–183
    effects of, **322–324**
    endogenous, discovery of, **319**, 320*i*
    inactivation of, **320–321**
    in kinin-mediated vasodilation, 294
    as neurotransmitter, 77*t*, 353
    platelets affected by, 184
    synthesis of, **319–320**, 320*t*, 321*i*, 321*t*
    in transmembrane signalling, 18, 26
Nitric oxide synthase, 319, 320*t*, 353
Nitrites
    abuse of, 184
    chemistry of, 181, 182*i*
    for cyanide poisoning, 184–185
    mechanism of action of, 181*i*
    organ system effects of, 183–184
    pharmacodynamics of, 182–185
    pharmacology of, 182
    preparations available, 194
    tolerance to, 185
    toxicity of, 185

Nitro-Bid, 194. *See also* Nitroglycerin
Nitro-Dur, 194. *See also* Nitroglycerin
Nitro reductions, 54*t*
Nitrofurantoin, **804**
    preparations available, 810
Nitrofurazone, preparations available, 810
Nitrogard, 194. *See also* Nitroglycerin
Nitrogen dioxide, 949
    threshold limit values for, 948*t*
Nitrogen mustard, 890*t*. *See also* Mechlorethamine
Nitrogen oxides, **949**
Nitroglycerin
    for angina, 179, 181–186, 186*t*
    chemistry of, 181, 182*i*
    clinical use of, 186
    for heart failure, 197
    organ system effects of, 183–185
    pharmacodynamics of, 182–185
    pharmacology of, 182
    preparations available, 194
Nitroimidazoles. *See also specific type*
    for amebiasis, 850, **854**
Nitrol, 194. *See also* Nitroglycerin
Nitrong, 194. *See also* Nitroglycerin
Nitroprusside, **168**, 168*i*
    for cardiogenic shock, 212
    for heart failure, 197
        with "power failure," 212
    preparations available, 175
Nitrosamines, carcinogenicity of, 185
Nitrosoglutathione, 321
Nitrosureas, 886*i*, **888**
Nitrous oxide, 410*i*
    abuse of, 529
    elimination of, 414
    preparations available, 423
    properties of, 413*t*
    solubility of, 412, 413*i*, 413*t*
Nivaquine, 843, 858. *See also* Chloroquine
Nix (permethrin), 1005
Nizatidine, 270*t*, 1019–1020
    clinical uses of, 272, 1020
    organ system effects of, 271
    in OTC preparations, efficacy of, 1033*t*
    OTC status of, 1031*t*
    preparations available, 284, 1026
    toxicity of, 272
Nizoral, 650, 786, 1002, 1004. *See also* Ketoconazole
NMDA receptors, 351
    antiepileptic drugs affecting, 387
    ethanol affecting, 374
    ketamine affecting, 422
    nitric oxide affecting, 323
N-methyl-CD-aspartate, 351
    ethanol affecting, 374
    ketamine affecting, 422
NO (nitric oxide), **319–324**, 353. *See also* Endothelium-derived relaxing factor
    in asthma, 338
    cGMP affected by, angina management and, 180, 181, 181*i*, 182–183

NO (nitric oxide) *(cont.)*
  effects of, **322–324**
  endogenous, discovery of, **319**, 320*i*
  inactivation of, **320–321**
  in kinin-mediated vasodilation, 294
  as neurotransmitter, 77*t*, 353
  platelets affected by, 184
  synthesis of, **319–320**, 320*t*, 321*i*,
    321*t*
  in transmembrane signalling, 18, 26
NO synthase (nitric oxide synthase), 319,
    320*t*, 353
"No effect" dose, 65
Nocardia, empiric antimicrobial therapy
    and, 814*t*
Nolahist (phenindamine), 284
Nolvadex, 680, 899*t*. *See also* Tamoxifen
Nonadrenergic/noncholinergic neurons,
    82
  nitric oxide affecting, 323–324
  transmitter substances in, 77*t*
Noncompliance/compliance, **1045–1046**
  in elderly, 996
  in pediatric pharmacology, 996
Non-Hodgkin's lymphoma, 903*t*,
    907–908
Non-NMDA channels, 351
Nonspecific neuronal systems, 347–348
Nonsteroidal anti-inflammatory drugs
    (NSAIDs), **579–590**. *See also spe-*
    cific agent
  chemistry of, 585
  clinical pharmacology of, **589–590**
  COX-I and COX-II and, 305, 585
  for dysmenorrhea, 313–314
  in elderly, 995
  interactions of, 1067*t*
  pharmacodynamics of, 585
  pharmacokinetics of, 585–586
  preparations available, 599
  prostaglandin formation blocked by,
    311
  special indications for, **588–589**
  thromboxane formation blocked by,
    311
Nontoxic goiter, **632**
Noradrenaline (norepinephrine), 77*t*, 85*t*,
    123*i*, 127–128, 350*t*, 352
  in adrenergic transmission, 78–80, 78*i*
  antidepressants affecting, 487
  biosynthesis of, 78–79, 79*i*
  ionization constant of, 6*t*
  metabolism of, 79–80, 80*i*
  as neurotransmitter, 77*t*, 350*t*, 352
  noradrenergic fiber release of, 74
  preparations available, 134
  receptors for, 81–82, 81*i*
  renin secretion affected by, 287–288
Noradrenergic fibers, 75
Noradrenergic neurons, 77–80, 78*i*
Noradrenergic receptors, 81. *See also*
    Adrenoceptors
Noradrenergic transmission, 77–80, 78*i*
  cotransmitters in, 80–81
Norcet (hydrocodone, with aceta-
    minophen), 514
Norcuron, 448. *See also* Vecuronium

Nordette, 665*t*
Nordiazepam, clorazepate conversion to,
    355
Norepinephrine, 77*t*, 85*t*, 123*i*, 127–128,
    350*t*, 352
  in adrenergic transmission, 78–80, 78*i*
  antidepressants affecting, 487
  biosynthesis of, 78–79, 79*i*
  ionization constant of, 6*t*
  metabolism of, 79–80, 80*i*
  as neurotransmitter, 77*t*, 350*t*, 352
  noradrenergic fiber release of, 74
  preparations available, 134
  receptors for, 81–82, 81*i*
  renin secretion affected by, 287–288
Norethindrone, 661*t*, 662*i*
  preparations available, 680
Norethynodrel, 661*t*
Norflex, 448. *See also* Orphenadrine
Norfloxacin, 765, 765*i*, 766, 766*t*
Norgestimate, 661
L-Norgestrel, 661*t*, 666, 670 preparations
    available, 680
Norinyl, 665*t*
Norlutin, 680. *See also* Norethindrone
Normal flora, tetracyclines affecting, 747
Normodyne, 150, 174. *See also* Labetalol
Noroxin, 768. *See also* Norfloxacin
Norpace, 240. *See also* Disopyramide
Norplant, 665*t*, 680. *See also* Lev-
    onorgestrel
Norpramin, 494. *See also* Desipramine
Nor-QD, 665*t*, 680. *See also* Norethin-
    drone
Nortriptyline, 485*i*
  dosages of, 491*t*
  drug metabolism inhibited by, 60*t*
  effects of, 489*t*
  pharmacokinetic/pharmacodynamic
    parameters of, 37*t*, 488*t*
  preparations available, 494
Norulate, 680. *See also* Norethindrone
Norvasc, 175, 194. *See also* Amlodipine
Norvir, 801. *See also* Ritonavir
NOS (nitric oxide synthase), 319, 320*t*,
    353
Noscapine, 512
Notec, 369. *See also* Chloral hydrate
Notice of Claimed Investigational Ex-
    emption for a New Drug (IND),
    63*i*, 68
Novantrone, 901*t*. *See also* Mitoxantrone
Novobiocin, **767**
  preparations available, 768
Novocain, 426*t*, 433. *See also* Procaine
Novolin, 690*t*, 692. *See also* Insulin
NPH insulin, 690*t*, 691
NPY (neuropeptide Y), 77*t*, 85*t*, **301**
NSAIDS (nonsteroidal anti-inflammatory
    drugs), **579–590**. *See also specific*
    agent
  chemistry of, 585
  clinical pharmacology of, **589–590**
  COX-I and COX-II and, 305, 585
  for dysmenorrhea, 313–314
  in elderly, 995
  interactions of, 1067*t*

pharmacodynamics of, 585
pharmacokinetics of, 585–586
preparations available, 599
prostaglandin formation blocked by,
    311
special indications for, **588–589**
thromboxane formation blocked by,
    311
Nubain, 501*t*, 513. *See also* Nalbuphine
Nucleoside phosphotransferases, antipar-
    asitic agents affecting, 829, 830*i*
Numorphan, 501*t*, 514. *See also* Oxy-
    morphone
Nupercainal (dibucaine), 432
Nuprin, 599. *See also* Ibuprofen
Nuromax, 448. *See also* Doxacurium
Nursing (breast-feeding). *See also* Breast
    milk; Lactation
  drug use during, **986**, 987*t*
  H$_2$ receptor antagonist use during, 272
  oxytocin in milk ejection reflex and,
    615
Nutrition, chronic alcohol consumption
    and, 375
Nutropin, 617. *See also* Somatotropin
Nystagmus, phenytoin causing, 391
Nystatin, **786**
  OTC status of, 1032*t*
  preparations available, 786
  topical, **1003**

O$_3$ (ozone), **949**
  threshold limit values for, 948*t*
Obesity, hyperglycemia in, biguanides
    for, 700
Observer bias, in new drug evaluation,
    67
Obsessive-compulsive disorder, antide-
    pressants for, 490
Occlusion/occlusive dressings, in derma-
    tologic pharmacology, 999
Occupational toxicology, 945
Octreotide, 606, 606*i*
  for acid-peptic disease, 1020–1021
  in cancer chemotherapy, 899*t*
Ocufen, 599. *See also* Flurbiprofen
Ocular disorders, antipsychotic agents
    causing, 474
Ocusert, 103. *See also* Pilocarpine
Ocusert Pilo-40, 103. *See also* Pilo-
    carpine
Ofloxacin, 765, 765*i*, 766*t*, 776
  preparations available, 768
  for tuberculosis, 771*t*, 776
Ogen, 680. *See also* Estropipate
Ohm's law, 217
OK432 (picibanil), 935
OKT3 (muromonab-CD3), 930
  preparations available, 940
Olanzapine, 467*i*, 468*t*, 471
  advantages and disadvantages of, 471*t*
  dose relationships of, 472*t*
  preparations available, 480
  receptor binding by, 468
Olsalazine
  for inflammatory bowel disease, 1025
  preparations available, 1027

Omega-3 fatty acids, in dietary manipulation of arachidonic acid metabolism, 317
Omeprazole
   for acid-peptic disease, 272, 1020
   preparations available, 1027
Omnipen, 740. *See also* Ampicillin
On-off phenomenon, with levodopa, 454
Onchocerca volvulus (onchocerciasis), drugs for, 863*t*
   diethylcarbamazine, 866–867
      adverse reactions and, 867
   ivermectin, 868
   suramin, 876
Oncogenes, 881
Oncovin, 894*t*. *See also* Vincristine
Ondansetron, 277
   antiemetic action of, 1022
   preparations available, 284, 1027
Open-angle glaucoma. *See also* Glaucoma
   treatment of, 87, 149*t*
      cholinomimetics for, 100
Open-loop systems, for insulin administration, 693
Ophthalmologic disorders. *See also* Eye
   antimuscarinic agents for, 111, 111*t*
   cholinomimetics for, 100
   sympathomimetics for, 132
Ophthalmopathy, in hyperthyroidism, 631–632
Ophthalmoscopic examination, antimuscarinic agents for, 111, 111*t*
OPIDP (organophosphorus ester-induced delayed polyneuropathy), 951–952
Opioid analgesics, **496–512**. *See also specific agent*
   abuse of, **518–519**
   for anesthesia, **421**
   as antitussive, 512
   basic pharmacology of, **496–506**
   classification and chemistry of, 496–497, 498–499*i*
   clinical pharmacology of, **506–510**
   contraindications/cautions in therapy with, 510
   dependence on, 503–504, 508, 509, 518
   effects of, 504–506
   in elderly, 993
   endogenous, 497, 498*i*
   full/strong agonists, 496, 498–499*i*, **510–511**
      mixed agonist-antagonists used with, 510
   history of use of, 496
   interactions of, 506–507, 507*t*, 510
   mechanism of action of, 501–504
   mild to moderate agonists, 498–499*i*, **511**
   mixed agonist-antagonists, 497, 498–499*i*, 502*t*, **511–512** effects of, 506 pure agonists used with, 510
   overdose of, 509–510, 972*t*
   partial agonists, 497, **511–512**
   pharmacodynamics of, 501–506

pharmacokinetics of, 497–501, 501*t*
preparations available, 513–514
receptor subtype activity of, 501, 502*t*
routes of administration of, 508
source of, 496
spinal action of, 502, 502*i*, 504*i*
supraspinal action of, 502, 504*i*
tolerance to, 503–504, 505*t*, 508–509, 518
toxic/undesired effects of, 506, 507*t*, 508–510
uses of, 507–508
withdrawal from, 503, 509, 518
   in newborn of addicted mother, 510
Opioid antagonists, 498–499*i*, **512–513**
   preparations available, 514
   for treatment of opioid abuse, 519
Opioid peptides, 350*t*
   endogenous, 497, 498*i*
   as neurotransmitters, 77*t*, 350*t*
   receptor subtype activity of, 502*t*
Opioid receptors, 501–503, 502*t*, 503*i*
Opisthorchis (opisthorchiasis), drugs for, 863*t*
   albendazole, 865
   praziquantel, 874
Opium. *See also* Opioid analgesics
   in OTC preparations, efficacy of, 1034*t*
   source of, 496
Opium Exclusion Act, 68*t*
Optimine (azatadine), 283
Optipranolol, 150. *See also* Metipranolol
OPV (oral poliovirus vaccine), 1053*t*
Oragraffin, 633. *See also* Ipodate
Oral anticoagulants, **551–555**. *See also* Warfarin
Oral contraceptives, 665*t*, **666–671**
   adverse effects of, 668–670
   beneficial effects of, 671
   in breast milk, 987*t*
   clinical uses of, 668
   contraindications and cautions with use of, 670
   drug metabolism inhibited by, 60*t*, 667
   effects of, 666–668
   mechanism of action of, 666
   for men, **679**
   postcoital, 670, 671*t*
   with progestins alone, 670
Oral gold
   for asthma, 339
   for inflammation, 591–592
Oral hypoglycemic agents, **696–701**. *See also specific type*
Oral poliovirus vaccine, 1053*t*
Oral route of administration, bioavailability and characteristics and, 40*t*
Orap, 480. *See also* Pimozide
Organ transplantation
   immunosuppressive therapy and, 931–932, 931*t*
   nitric oxide and, **323**
   rejection of
      cell–mediated, prostaglandins affecting, 315–316
      nitric oxide and, 323

Organic nitrites, abuse of, 529
Organolead poisoning, 962, 963
Organophosphates, 97, 98*i*
   absorption/distribution/metabolism of, 98–99
   as insecticides, 97, 98*i*, **951–952**, 951*t*
      absorption/distribution/metabolism of, 98–99
      toxicity of, 102
   mechanism of action of, 99
   toxicity of, 102, 972*t*
Organophosphorus ester-induced delayed polyneuropathy (OPIDP), 951–952
Orgaran, 561. *See also* Danaproid
Orinase, 697*t*, 703. *See also* Tolbutamide
Orlaam, 513. *See also* Levomethadyl acetate
Ornidazole, for amebiasis, 850
Ornithine decarboxylase, antiparasitic drugs affecting, 831–833
Orphan Drug Act, 68*t*, 70
Orphan drugs, 70
"Orphan receptors," 637
Orphenadrine
   for muscle spasm, 448
   for parkinsonism, 457*t*
   preparations available, 448, 462
Orthoclone, 930. *See also* OKT3
Ortho Dienestrol, 680. *See also* Dienestrol
Ortho-Novum, 665*t*
Orthopedic surgery, antimicrobial prophylaxis and, 824*t*
Orthostatic hypotension (postural hypotension)
   antipsychotic agents causing, 470
   bromocriptine causing, 455
   levodopa causing, 453
   sympathomimetics for, 130
Ortho-Tri-Cyclen, 665*t*
Orudis, 599. *See also* Ketoprofen
Os-Cal, 721. *See also* Calcium
Osmitrol, 259. *See also* Mannitol
Osmolality, serum, in poisoning, 973–974
"Osmolar gap," in poisoning, 074*t*, 973–974
Osmotic diuretics, **254–255**
Osteodystrophy
   intestinal, **717**
   renal, vitamin D for, 717
Osteogenic sarcoma, 904*t*, 911–912
Osteomalacia, phenytoin causing, 391
Osteoporosis, **717–719**
   androgens for, 676
   bisphosphonates for, 711, 712, 718, 718*i*
   calcitonin for, 718, 718*i*
   estrogen replacement therapy in prevention and treatment of, 658, 717–718, 718*i*
   fluoride for, 712, 718, 718*i*
   vitamin D for, 718
OTC agents (over-the-counter agents), **1030–1040**, 1031–1035*t*
   hidden ingredients in, 1037–1039*i*

Otitis media
    antimicrobial prophylaxis and, 825t
    empiric antimicrobial therapy and, 816t
Ototoxicity
    of amikacin, 758
    of aminoglycosides, 753–754
    of gentamicin, 756
    of loop diuretics, 250
    of tobramycin, 758
Otrivin, 134. *See also* Xylometazoline
Ouabain, pharmacokinetics of, 201, 201t, 202
Ovarian cancer, 903t, **910**
    oral contraceptive use and, 670
Ovary, **653–674**
    disturbances in function of, 654
    hormonal contraception and, 665t, **666–671**
    hormones produced by, **664–666**
        antagonists of, **671–672**
        in cancer chemotherapy, 898–900, 899t
        preparations available, 680
    estrogens, **654–660**
    progestins, **661–664**, 661t
    oral contraceptives affecting, 666
    ovulation-inducing agents and, **672–673**
Ovcon, 665t
Over-the-counter agents (OTC agents), **1030–1040**, 1031–1035t
    hidden ingredients in, 1037–1039i
Overdoses. *See also specific agent and* Poisoning
    deliberate, sedative-hypnotics used for, 367
    pharmacokinetic process affected by, 969
Ovral, 665t
Ovrette, 665t, 680. *See also* Norgestrel
Ovulation, agents inducing, **672–673**
Oxacillin, 726i, 729–731
    adverse reactions to, 731
    dosing guidelines for, 730t
    preparations available, 740
Oxaluria, enteric, **720**
Oxamniquine, **872–873**
    antiparasitic actions of, 836t, 872
    preparations available, 878
Oxandrin, 680. *See also* Oxandrolone
Oxandrolone, 675t
    preparations available, 680
Oxantel pamoate, **873**
    preparations available, 878
    synaptic transmission affected by, 835
Oxantel/pyrantel pamoate, **873**
    preparations available, 878
Oxaprozin, 580t, **587**
    preparations available, 599
Oxazepam, 356i
    absorption of, 355
    biotransformation of, 357, 357i
    dosages of, 366t
    in elderly, 993
    pharmacokinetics of, 358t
    preparations available, 369, 383

Oxazolidinediones, **401–402**
Oxcarbazepine, 392i, **393**
Oxiconazole
    preparations available, 786
    topical, 1002
Oxidations
    cytochrome P450-dependent, 52–55, 52i, 53–54t
    cytochrome P450-independent, 54t
    genetic polymorphisms affecting, 58, 58t
Oxidative dealkylations, 53t
Oxidizing agents, antimicrobial effects of, 805t
Oxidizing air pollutants, 947
Oxime agents, for cholinergic poisoning, 112–113
Oxistat, 786, 1002. *See also* Oxiconazole
Oxolinic acid, 765
Oxotremorine, 92–93, 93i
Oxprenolol, 145
Oxtriphylline, for asthma, preparations available, 340
Oxybutynin, 112
    for gastrointestinal and genitourinary conditions, 112, 112t
    preparations available, 116, 1027
Oxychlorosene, preparations available, 810
Oxycodone, 511
    abuse of, 518
    with acetaminophen, 511
    with aspirin, 511
    pharmacokinetics of, 501t
    preparations available, 514
    structure of, 498i
Oxygen, for carbon monoxide intoxication, 948, 977t
Oxygen demand, myocardial, determinants of, 18, 180t
Oxygen supply, myocardial, determinants of, 180
Oxymetazoline, 128
    in OTC preparations, efficacy of, 1034–1035t
    OTC status of, 1032t
    preparations available, 134
Oxymetholone, 675t
    preparations available, 680
Oxymorphone, 510
    pharmacokinetics of, 501t
    preparations available, 514
    structure of, 498i
Oxyphencyclimine
    for gastrointestinal and genitourinary conditions, 112t
    preparations available, 116, 1027
Oxyphenonium, for gastrointestinal and genitourinary conditions, 112t
Oxytetracycline, 745, 745i
    pharmacokinetics of, 745–746
    preparations available, 751
Oxytocin, **615–616**, 615i
Oxytocin challenge test, fetal well-being evaluated with, 615
Ozone, **949**
    threshold limit values for, 948t

P170 glycoprotein, verapamil affecting, 190
P450 enzyme system, 52–55, 52i, 53–54t
    epoxygenase products and, 308
    effects of, 310–311
    H_2 receptor antagonists affecting, 271
    in human liver, 55, 56t
    induction of, 52–55
    inhibition of, 55
    local anesthetics metabolized by, 427
P450-2D6 inhibitors, interactions of, 492
P450-3A4 inhibitors, interactions of, 492–493
PABA (*p*-aminobenzoic acid)
    sulfonamide structure and, 761, 762i
    as sunscreen, 1006
Pacemaker activity, sympathomimetics affecting, 125
Pacemaker potential, 219
Pacemaker rate
    determinants of, 222, 222i
    quinidine affecting, 227
Pachymaran, 935
Paclitaxel, 894t, **895**
PAE (postantibiotic effect), 818–819, 818t
Paget's disease of bone, **720**
Pain. *See also* Analgesia
    aspirin for, 581, 582
    chronic, tricyclic antidepressants for, 490
    opioid analgesics for, 506–508. *See also* Opioid analgesics
    sensation of
        histamine and, 264
        kinins and, 294
        local anesthetics blocking, 429
        serotonin and, 275
PALE (postantibiotic leukocyte enhancement), 818–819
Paludrine, 859. *See also* Proguanil
PAM (pralidoxime)
    for cholinergic poisoning, 112–113, 977t
    preparations available, 116
Pamelor, 494. *See also* Nortriptyline
Pamidronate, 711, 711i
    for hypercalcemia, 713
    preparations available, 721
Pamine, 116, 1027. *See also* Methscopolamine
Panadol, 600. *See also* Acetaminophen
Pancreas
    cancer of, 903t, 911
    endocrine, **684–685**, 685t
Pancrease, 1023t
Pancreatic enzyme replacement products, **1023**, 1023t
Pancreatic hormones, **684–705**, 685t. *See also specific type*
Pancreatic polypeptide (PP), 684, 685t
Pancreatin, 1023
Pancreatitis
    didanosine causing, 797
    hyperlipoproteinemia causing, 563
Pancrelipase, 1023

Pancuronium, 435*i*, 437*i*, 438*t*
  effects of, 443*t*
  preparations available, 448
Panic disorder, antidepressants for, 490
Panic reactions, hallucinogenics causing,
    526
Papaverine, for male sexual dysfunction,
    141
Para-aminobenzoic acid
  sulfonamide structure and, 761, 762*i*
  as sunscreen, 1006
Parabens, as preservative, 810
Paradione, 407. *See also* Paramethadione
Paraflex, 448. *See also* Chlorzoxazone
Paragonimus westermani (paragonimia-
    sis), drugs for, 863*t*
  bithionol, 865–866
  praziquantel, 874
Paraldehyde, preparations available, 369
Paralysis agitans, 450–459. *See also*
    Parkinsonism
Paramethadione, 401–402
  preparations available, 407
Paramethasone, 640*t*
Paraoxon, 98*i*
Paraplatin, 890*t*. *See also* Carboplatin
Paraquat, 953–954, 953*i*
Parasites
  biochemical functions in, **834–836**
  drugs for infections caused by,
      827–837. *See also* Antiparasitic
      agents
  enzymes found in, **827–831**
  enzymes indispensable in, **831–834**
Parasympathetic (craniosacral) division of
    autonomic nervous system, 73, 74*i*
  autonomic nerve activity/drugs affect-
      ing, 83*t*
  in central integration, 82
  digitalis effects and, 204
Parasympathomimetics, 90
Parathion, 97, 98*i*, 951*t*
  absorption/distribution/metabolism of,
      98–99
Parathion-methyl, 951*t*
Parathyroid hormone (PTH), **706–707**
  abnormal serum levels of, 715–716
  in bone mineral homeostasis, 706–707
  second messenger for, 22*t*
  vitamin D interaction and, **709**, 709*t*
Paravertebral nerve block, 431*i*
Paregoric, 1027
Pargyline, **163–164**
Parkinsonism (paralysis agitans/Parkin-
    son's disease), **450–459**
  antimuscarinic agents for, 106, 110,
      457, 457*t*
  bromocriptine for, **455–456**
  drug-induced, **458**, 459, 473
  experimental approaches to manage-
      ment of, **457–458**
  H_1 receptor antagonists affecting, 268
  neurons involved in, 450–451, 451*i*
  pharmacologic management of,
      451–457, **458**. *See also specific*
      agent
    preparations available and, 462

surgical procedures in management of,
    457
Parlodel, 462, 615. *See also* Bromocriptine
Parnate, 494. *See also* Tranylcypromine
Paromomycin, 758
  for amebiasis, 851*t*, **854**
  antiparasitic actions of, 836*t*, 854
  preparations available, 759, 859
Paroxetine
  dosages of, 491*t*
  effects of, 489, 489*t*
  interactions of, 492
  pharmacokinetics of, 488*t*
  preparations available, 494
Paroxysmal atrial tachycardia, sympath-
    omimetics for, 131
Partial agonists, 4, 15–16, 16*i*, 17, 17*i*
Partial pressure, of anesthetic gas, 412
Partial seizures, 387*t*, 403
  drugs used in, **388–398**, **404**
Partial thromboplastin time (PTT), for
    heparin monitoring, 551
Parvaquinone, mitochondrial electron
    transporter affected by, 834
PAS, 778. *See also* Aminosalicylic acid
Passive immunization, **1051–1055**,
    1056–1057*t*
Pasteurization, 805*t*
Patent ductus arteriosus
  indomethacin for, 589
  prostaglandins for, 314
Pathilon, 116, 1027. *See also* Tridihex-
    ethyl
Patient-controlled analgesia (PCA), 508
Pavulon, 448. *See also* Pancuronium
Paxil, 494. *See also* Paroxetine
Paxipam, 366*t*, 369. *See also* Halazepam
PBPs (penicillin-binding proteins), 725
PBZ, 267*t*, 284. *See also* Tripelennamine
PCA (patient-controlled analgesia), 508
PCBs (polychlorinated biphenyls/copla-
    nar biphenyls), 954
PCDDs (polychlorinated dibenzo-*p*-diox-
    ins), 954
PCDFs (polychlorinated dibenzofurans),
    954
PCP (phencyclidine)
  abuse of, 525–526
  fetus affected by, 983*t*
  overdose of, 526, 972*t*
  psychosis produced by, as schizophre-
      nia model, 470
  structure of, 524*i*
PCPA (*p*-chlorophenylalanine), serotonin
    affected by, 273, 277
PD123177, 291, 292*i*
  angiotensin receptor affinity for, 289
PDGF (platelet-derived growth factor)
  in inflammation, 579*t*
  ligand-regulated transmembrane en-
      zymes in signalling by, 19–20
  second messenger for, 22*t*
Pectin, 1024
Pediatric pharmacology, **982–985**
  dosage forms and compliance and,
      985–986
  drug dosage amounts and, **987–988**

Pediculicides. *See also* Pediculosis
  OTC preparations, efficacy of, 1035*t*
Pediculosis
  benzyl benzoate for, 1005
  lindane for, 1005
  permethrin for, 1005
Peganone, 407. *See also* Ethotoin
Pelamine, 284. *See also* Tripelennamine
PEMA (phenylethylmalonamide), 394*i*,
    395
Pemoline, 128–129
  preparations available, 134
Pen injectors, for insulin administration,
    693
Pen-Vee K, 740. *See also* Penicillin V
Penbutolol, 138*t*, 145, **165**
  distribution and clearance of, 142,
      144*t*
  for hypertension, **165**
  preparations available, 150, 174
  properties of, 144*t*
Penetrex, 768. *See also* Enoxacin
Penicillamine (dimethylcysteine),
    592–593, 957*i*, **958–959**
  fetus affected by, 983*t*
  ionization constant of, 6*t*
  preparations available, 462, 600, 966
  for Wilson's disease, 461, 958
Penicillin-binding proteins, 725
Penicillin G, 724, 726*i*, 728
  absorption of, in neonate, 984*t*
  CSF penetration by, 820*t*
  dosing guidelines for, 730*t*
  half-life of, aging affecting, 992*i*
  preparations available, 740
  units and formulations of, 724–725
Penicillin G benzathine, 729
  pharmacokinetics of, 727
  preparations available, 740
Penicillin G procaine, 729
  half-life of, aging affecting, 992*i*
  pharmacokinetics of, 727
  preparations available, 740
Penicillin V, 728–729
  dosing guidelines for, 730*t*
  preparations available, 740
Penicillins, **724–732**
  adverse reactions to, 731–732
  antipseudomonal, 724
  antistaphylococcal, 724, 729–731
    dosing guidelines for, 730*t*
  beta-lactamase resistant, 729–731
  in breast milk, 987*t*
  clinical uses of, 728–731
  dosing guidelines for, 730*t*
  excretion of in infants and children,
      985
  extended-spectrum, 724, 731
    dosing guidelines for, 730*i*
  isoxazolyl, 729–731
  mechanism of action of, 725, 727*i*,
      728*i*, 729*i*
  pharmacokinetics of, 726–728
  preparations available, 740
  resistance to, 725–726
  side chains of, 724, 726*i*
  structure of, 724, 725*i*

Penicillins *(cont.)*
  use/misuse of, problems associated
    with, 732
Penis, autonomic activity/drugs affecting,
    83*t*
Pentam, 859. *See also* Pentamidine
Pentamidine, **856–857**
  preparations available, 859
Pentasa, 1027. *See also* Mesalamine
Pentavalent antimonials, antiparasitic ac-
    tions of, 836*t*, **865**
Pentazocine, 512
  effects of, 506
  ionization constant of, 6*t*
  pharmacokinetics of, 501*t*
  preparations available, 514
  receptor subtype activity of, 502*t*
  structure of, 499*i*
Penthrane, 423. *See also* Methoxyflurane
Pentids, 740. *See also* Penicillin G
Pentobarbital, 357*i*
  dosages of, 366*t*
  ionization constant of, 6*t*
  overdose of, 973*t*
  preparations available, 369, 407
Pentostam, 859. *See also* Stibogluconate
Pentothal, 423. *See also* Thiopental
Pentoxifylline, for asthma, preparations
    available, 340
Pepcid, 284, 1026. *See also* Famotidine
Pepstatin, renin inhibited by, 290
Peptic ulcer disease
  antimuscarinic agents for, 111, 1020
  aspirin/NSAID use and, 584
  drugs used in, **1017–1021**
  glucocorticoids and, 639, 644
  H_2 receptor antagonists for, 271–272,
    1019–1020
  levodopa use and, 454
Peptide hormone inhibitors, in cancer
    chemotherapy, 899*t*
Peptides
  as central neurotransmitters, 352
  vasoactive, **287–303**. *See also specific*
    type
Peptidyl dipeptidase (PDP/converting en-
    zyme), 295. *See also* Angiotensin-
    converting enzyme
  in renin-angiotensin system, 288–289,
    288*i*
Pepto-Bismol (bismuth subsalicylate),
    1021, 1027
Peptococcus, empiric antimicrobial ther-
    apy and, 814*t*
Peptostreptococcus, empiric antimicro-
    bial therapy and, 814*t*
Peracetic acid, antimicrobial effects of,
    808–809
Percocet, 514. *See also* Oxycodone, with
    acetaminophen
Percodan, 501*t*, 514. *See also* Oxycodone
Perfloxacin, 765*i*, 766, 766*t*
Performance anxiety (stage fright), beta-
    receptor blocking drugs for, 148
Pergolide, **456**, 614
  dopamine receptors affected by, 280,
    456
  preparations available, 462

Pergonal, 617. *See also* Menotropins
Periactin, 267*t*, 283. *See also* Cyprohep-
    tadine
Peridex, 810. *See also* Chlorhexidine
Peridural nerve block, 431*i*
Perinatal pharmacology, **979–988**
Perindopril, preparations available, 175
Peripheral nervous system
  chronic alcohol consumption affect-
    ing, 376
  direct-acting cholinomimetics affect-
    ing, 96
  local anesthetic toxicity and, 430
  nitric oxide affecting, **323–324**
  prostaglandins affecting, 310
Peripheral neuropathy
  isoniazid causing, 773
  lead toxicity causing, 961
Peripheral vascular disease
  alpha-receptor blocking drugs for,
    141
  prostaglandin E and prostacyclin for,
    314
Peripheral vasodilation, after myocardial
    infarction, 211*t*, 212
Peristalsis, direct-acting cholinomimetics
    affecting, 94*t*, 96
Peritoneal dialysis, in poisoning, 976
Peritonitis, empiric antimicrobial therapy
    and, 816*t*
Permapen, 740. *See also* Penicillin G
    benzathine
Permax, 462, 617. *See also* Pergolide
Permeation, drug, 4, 5
Permethrin, **1005**
  in OTC preparations, efficacy of,
    1035*t*
  OTC status of, 1032*t*
Permitil, 471*t*, 472*t*, 480. *See also*
    Fluphenazine
Pernicious anemia, 541–542
Peroxygen compounds, antimicrobial ef-
    fects of, **808–809**
Perphenazine, 466*i*
  dose relationships of, 472*t*
  preparations available, 480
  receptor binding by, 468
Persantine (dipyridamole), 561
Persistent chemicals, environmental toxi-
    cology and, 951
Pertofrane, 494. *See also* Desipramine
Pertussis, antimicrobial prophylaxis and,
    825*t*
Pesticides (insecticides), **950–952**
  botanical, **952**, 953*i*
  carbamate, **952**, 952*t*
  chlorinated hydrocarbon, **950–951**,
    950*t*
  organophosphorus
    (organophosphate/thiophos-
    phate), 97, 98*i*, **951–952**, 951*t*
  absorption/distribution/metabolism
    of, 98–99
  toxicity of, 102
Petit mal seizure, 404
  drugs for, **398–402**, **404–405**
Pfizerpen, 740. *See also* Penicillin G

PGE$_1$ (prostaglandin E$_1$/alprostadil), 306,
    312*i*. *See also* Prostaglandins
  for impotence, 314
  preparations available, 317
PGE$_2$ (dinoprostone), 306, 312–313,
    312*i*. *See also* Prostaglandins
  for abortion, 312–313
  for labor facilitation, 313
  preparations available, 317
PGF$_{2\alpha}$, 306, 312*i*. *See also*
    Prostaglandins
  for abortion, 312, 313
  for labor facilitation, 313
PGH synthase-1 (COX-I), 305–306, 578,
    585
  glucocorticoids affecting, 639
PGH synthase-2 (COX-II), 305–306,
    578, 585
  glucocorticoids affecting, 639
PGI$_2$ (prostacyclin/epoprostenol), 306,
    312*i*, 547. *See also* Prostaglandins
  for hypertension, 314
  platelets affected by, 314–315
  preparations available, 317
  second messenger for, 22*t*
  synthesis of, 306–307, 306*i*
pH, urinary, manipulation of in poisoned
    patient, 978
Pharmacodynamics
  aging affecting, 991
  definition of, 4
  drug therapy in pregnancy and,
    980–982
  in neonate, 985
  pharmacokinetics and, **34–49**. *See*
    also Concentration-response re-
    lationships; Dose-response re-
    lationships
  in poisoning, **969**
  principles of, 4
  therapeutic drug monitoring and, 47
Pharmacokinetics, **34–42**
  aging affecting, 989–991, 992*i*
  definition of, 4
  drug concentration measurements and,
    47–49
  drug therapy in pregnancy and,
    979–980
  in infants and children, 982–985
  pharmacodynamics and, **34–49**. *See*
    also Concentration-response re-
    lationships; Dose-response re-
    lationships
  in poisoning, **968–969**
  principles of, 4–7
  target concentration approach to
    dosage regimen and, **43–45**
  therapeutic drug monitoring and, 46
Pharmacologic potency, 28, 28*i*
Pharmacologic profile, development of,
    64, 65*t*
Pharmacology. *See also* Drugs
  definition of, 1
  dermatologic, **999–1016**. *See also*
    Skin
  geriatric, **989–998**. *See also* Aging

history of, 1–2
pediatric, **982–985** dosage forms and compliance and, **985–986** drug dosage amounts and, **987–988**
perinatal, **979–988**
Phase 1 clinical testing, in new drug evaluation, 63*i*, 68–69 Phase I reactions, in drug biodisposition, 51, 51*i*, **52–55**, 53–54*t*
benzodiazepines undergoing, 356
Phase 2 clinical testing, in new drug evaluation, 63*i*, 69
Phase II reactions, in drug biodisposition, 51, 51*i*, **55**, 57*t*
benzodiazepines undergoing, 356–357
Phase 3 clinical testing, in new drug evaluation, 63*i*, 69
Phase 4 clinical testing, in new drug evaluation, 63*i*, 69
Phenacemide, **391**
preparations available, 407
Phenacetin, **595**, 595*i*
Phenanthrenes
mild to moderate, **511**
mixed agonist-antagonists/partial agonist, **511–512**
strong, **510**
structures of, 498*i*
Phencyclidine (PCP)
abuse of, 525–526
fetus affected by, 983*t*
overdose of, 526, 972*t*
psychosis produced by, as schizophrenia model, 470
structure of, 524*i*
Phendimetrazine, preparations available, 134
Phenelzine, 484, 487*i*
dosages of, 491*t*
for acute episode, 491
pharmacokinetics of, 487
preparations available, 494
Phenergan, 267*t*, 284. *See also* Promethazine
Phenformin, 699–700, 700*t*
Phenindamine, preparations available, 284
Phenindione, structure of, 552*i*
Phenmetrazine, 128, 521
abuse of, 521
structure of, 522*i*
Phenobarbital, 357*i*, **393–394**, 394*i*
absorption of, in neonate, 984*t*
for anxiety, 365
in breast milk, 987*t*
dosages of, 366*t*
drug metabolism induced by, 59*t*
for drug withdrawal, 366
effective/toxic plasma levels of, 405*t*
half-life of
aging affecting, 992*i*
in infants vs. adults, 985*t*
overdose of, 973*t*
pharmacokinetic/pharmacodynamic parameters of, 37*t*
in neonate, 984*t*, 985*t*
preparations available, 369, 407

for seizures, **393–394**, 407
for status epilepticus, 406
Phenolphthalein
laxative effect of, 1023
preparations available, 1028
Phenols/phenolics, antimicrobial effects of, 805*t*, **807–808**
Phenothiazines, 267*t*, 464–465, 466*i*, 468*t*, 471
advantages and disadvantages of, 471*t*
antiemetic action of, 1022
dyskinesias caused by, 460
in elderly, 993
for Huntington's disease, 460
pharmacologic effects of, 466–468
structure of, 266*i*
Phenoxybenzamine, 137*i*, 138*t*, 139, 166
for pheochromocytoma, 140–141, 140*i*
preparations available, 150
Phenprocoumon, 554–555
Phensuximide, **399**
preparations available, 407
Phentolamine, 136, 137*i*, 138–139, 138*t*, 166
cardiovascular effects of, 138, 138*i*
for male sexual dysfunction, 141
for pheochromocytoma, 140–141
preparations available, 150
for vasoconstrictor excess, 141
Phenurone, 407. *See also* Phenacemide
Phenylbutazone, 586*i*, **589**
drug metabolism induced by, 59*t*
drug metabolism inhibited by, 60*t*
half-life of, aging affecting, 992*i*
oral anticoagulant interactions and, 554
Phenylephrine, 124*i*, 128
cardiovascular system affected by, 125*t*
ionization constant of, 6*t*
ophthalmic applications of, 132
in OTC preparations, efficacy of, 1035*t*
OTC status of, 1032*t*
preparations available, 134
Phenylethylamine, 123, 123*i*
Phenylethylmalonamide (PEMA), 394*i*, 395
Phenylheptylamines
mild to moderate agonists, **511**
strong agonists, **510–511**
structures of, 498*i*
o-Phenylphenol, antimicrobial effects of, 807–808
Phenylpiperidines
mild to moderate agonists, **511**
strong agonists, **511**
structures of, 498*i*
Phenylpropanolamine, 129
in OTC preparations, efficacy of, 1035*t*
OTC status of, 1032*t*
preparations available, 134
Phenytoin, **388–391**, 388*i*
absorption of, in neonate, 984*t*

action potentials affected by, 387, 389, 389*i*
for alcohol withdrawal syndrome, 380
in breast milk, 987*t*
drug metabolism induced by, 59*t*
effective/toxic plasma levels of, 405*t*
fetus affected by, 983*t*
half-life of, 985*t*
interactions of, 1067–1068*t*
ionization constant of, 6*t*
pharmacokinetic/pharmacodynamic parameters of, 37*t*, 389–391
in neonate, 984*t*, 985*t*
preparations available, 407
for seizures, **388–391**
for status epilepticus, 406
teratogenicity of, 406, 983*t*
Pheochromocytoma, 140–141, 140*i*
histamine in diagnosis of, 265
pHisoHex, 810. *See also* Hexachlorophene
Phocomelia, thalidomide causing, drug testing methods affected by, 67
Phos-Ex, 721. *See also* Calcium
PhosLo, 721. *See also* Calcium
Phosphate
abnormal serum levels of, **715**
bone mineral homeostasis and, 706, 707*i*
for hypercalcemia, 714
preparations available, 721
Phosphatidylinositol, thromboxane binding affecting metabolism of, 308
Phosphatidylinositol-4,5-bisphosphate (PIP$_2$), in calcium/phosphoinositide second messenger system, 24, 26*i*
Phosphodiesterase inhibitors, for heart failure, 197, 205–206
Phosphoinositides, as second messenger, 24–26, 26*i*
Phospholine, 103. *See also* Echothiophate
Phospholipase A$_2$, in arachidonic acid release, 304, 305*i*
Phospholipase C, in calcium/phosphoinositide second messenger system, 24, 26*i*
Phosphonomycin, 739
Phosphorylation, in second messenger signalling, 26–27
Phosphotransferases, nucleoside, antiparasitic agents affecting, 829
Photochemical air pollutants, 947
Photosensitization, tetracyclines causing, 747
Phthalylsulfathiazole (sulfathalidine), 762*i*
Physiologic antagonism, 16–17
Physiologic dependence. *See also* specific agent or drug class
drug abuse and, 516
Physostigmine (eserine), 97, 97*i*
as antidote, 977*t*
for antimuscarinic drug intoxication, 101–102
for glaucoma, 149*t*

Physostigmine (eserine) *(cont.)*
ionization constant of, 6*t*
mechanism of action of, 99
preparations available, 103
Phytonadione (vitamin K₁), 558–559
for oral anticoagulant-induced bleeding, 554
preparations available, 561
structure of, 552*i*
Picibanil (OK432), 935
Picrotoxin, GABA-DBZ receptor chloride channel binding and, 361
Pigmentation (skin). *See also* Hyperpigmentation
agents affecting, **1005–1006**
Pilo-20, 103. *See also* Pilocarpine
Pilocarpine, 92, 93*i*
cardiovascular effects of, 95
for glaucoma, 149*t*
ionization constant of, 6*t*
preparations available, 103
toxicity of, 102
Pilomotor smooth muscle, autonomic activity/drugs affecting, 83*t*
Pima, 633. *See also* Potassium iodide solution
Pimozide, 467*i*
preparations available, 480
receptor binding by, 468
for Tourette's syndrome, 460
Pinacidil, 166
Pindolol, 138*t*, 143*i*, 145, **165**
for hypertension, **165**
ionization constant of, 6*t*
preparations available, 174
properties of, 144*t*
Pinworm (*Enterobius vermicularis*),
drugs for, 863*t*
albendazole, 864
mebendazole, 869
pyrantel, 876
Pioglitazone, 701
PIP₂ (phosphatidylinositol-4,5-bisphosphate), in calcium/phosphoinositide second messenger system, 24, 26*i*
Pipecuronium, 437*i*, 438*t*
effects of, 443*t*
preparations available, 448
Piperacetazine, dose relationships of, 472*t*
Piperacillin, 731
dosing guidelines for, 730*t*
preparations available, 740
with tazobactam, preparations available, 740
Piperazine (anthelmintic), **873**
preparations available, 878
synaptic transmission affected by, 835, 873
Piperazines, 267*t*
advantages and disadvantages of, 471*t*
for motion sickness, 269
structure of, 266*i*
Piperidines, 267*t*
structure of, 266*i*
Pipracil, 740. *See also* Piperacillin
Pirbuterol, preparations available, 340

Pirenzepine, 107*i*
for acid-peptic disease, 1020
gastric acid secretion affected by, 110, 1020
Piroxicam, 580*t*, 586*i*, **588**
preparations available, 599
Pitocin, 617. *See also* Oxytocin
Pitressin Synthetic, 617. *See also* Vasopressin
Pituitary gland, thyroid relationships and, 620, 623*i*
Pituitary hormones, 604*t*
anterior, **604–615**
posterior, **615–617**
Pityrosporum orbiculare, imidazoles for infection caused by, 1002
Placebo response, new drug evaluation and, 67
Placental barrier. *See also* Pregnancy
sedative-hypnotics crossing, 355–356
Placental drug metabolism, 980
Placidyl, 369, 973*t*. *See also* Ethchlorvynol
Plague
antimicrobial prophylaxis and, 825*t*
streptomycin for, 755
Plant systemics, organophosphorus insecticide, 951
Plaquenil, 599. *See also* Hydroxychloroquine
Plasma, drug distribution in, 39*t*
Plasma cholinesterase (pseudocholinesterase)
local anesthetics metabolized by, 427
succinylcholine metabolized by, 439
Plasma concentration monitoring, therapeutic, **45–47**
of antidepressant levels, 492
of lithium levels, 477–478
Plasma fractions, for bleeding disorders, **559–560**
Plasma protein binding
drug concentration affected by, 47, 48
passage across placenta and, 979–980
reduced, oral anticoagulant interactions and, 554
Plasma thromboplastin antecedent (PTA/factor XI), 549*t*
therapeutic, 559*t*
Plasma thromboplastin component (Christmas factor/factor IX), 549*t*
deficiency of, 559, 559*t*
therapeutic, 559*t*, 560
preparations available, 561
Plasmin, 548, 550*i*, 555
Plasminogen, 549*t*, 550*i*, 555
Plasmodium
falciparum, 838–840
resistance to, 840, 840*t*
life cycle of, **838**
malariae, 838–840
ovale, 838–840
vivax, 838–840
Platelet adhesion, 547
Platelet aggregation, 547
aspirin affecting, 314

calcium channel blockers affecting, 190
heparin-induced, thromboembolism and, 551
prostaglandins affecting, 308, 309, 314–315
Platelet-derived growth factor (PDGF)
in inflammation, 579*t*
ligand-regulated transmembrane enzymes in signalling by, 19–20
second messenger for, 22*t*
Platelets, 547
aspirin affecting, **556–557**, 581–582, 583
drugs affecting, 555–557
in hemostasis, 547
nitrates/nitrites affecting, 184
nitric oxide affecting, **323**
prostaglandins affecting, 308, 309, 314–315
receptors for, drugs blocking, 557
regulation of function of, 555
Platinol, 890*t*. *See also* Cisplatin
PLC (phospholipase C), in calcium/phosphoinositide second messenger system, 24, 26*i*
Plendil, 175, 194. *See also* Felodipine
Plexus of Auerbach (myenteric plexus), 74
Plexus of Meissner (submucosal plexus), 74
Plicamycin (mithramycin)
bone mineral homeostasis affected by, **711**
for cancer chemotherapy, 894*t*, **897**
for hypercalcemia, 714
for Paget's disease, 720
preparations available, 721
Pneumococcal infections, vaccine for, 1053*t*
Pneumococcemia, antimicrobial prophylaxis and, 825*t*
Pneumocystis carinii pneumonia
antimicrobial prophylaxis and, 825*t*
atovaquone for, **857**
drugs for, 855*t*, **856–857**
pentamidine for, **856–857**
primaquine for, 845
Pneumocystosis. *See also Pneumocystis carinii* pneumonia
pentamidine for, 856
Pneumonia, empiric antimicrobial therapy and, 816*t*
Podofilox. *See also* Podophyllotoxin
in dermatologic therapy, **1012**
Podophyllotoxin, **894–895**, **1012**
Podophyllum resin, in dermatologic therapy, **1012**
Poisoning, **968–978**. *See also specific agent causing*
antidotes in, 976, 977*t*
approach to patient and, **970**
decontamination procedures for, 974–976
history and physical examination in, 971–973
initial management in, **970–978**

laboratory and X-ray procedures in evaluation of, 973–974
screening tests for, 974
toxicodynamics and, **969**
toxicokinetics and, **968–969**
toxin elimination in, 976–977
Polamine (dexchlorpheniramine), 283
Poliovirus vaccine
inactivated, 1053*t*
oral, 1053*t*
Pollutants, 945
air, 945–946, **947–949**
environmental, **954**
Polycarbophil, preparations available, 1028
Polychlorinated biphenyls (PCBs/coplanar biphenyls), 954
Polychlorinated dibenzo-*p*-dioxins (PCDDs), 954
Polychlorinated dibenzofurans (PCDFs), 954
Polycillin, 740. *See also* Ampicillin
Polycythemia vera, 903*t*
Polydipsia, lithium causing, 478
Polyethylene glycol electrolyte solution (CoLyte/GoLYTELY)
for gut decontamination, 976
preparations available, 1028
Polymorphism, genetic, in drug metabolism, 57–59, 58*i*, 58*t*
Polymyxin B
in dermatologic therapy, **1000**
preparations available, 810
Polymyxins, **803–804**
Polyneuropathy, organophosphorus ester-induced delayed, 951–952
Polythiazide
dosages of, 252*t*
preparations available, 259
Polyuria, lithium causing, 478
Polyvinyl pyrrolidone (PVP/povidone-iodine)
antimicrobial effects of, 805*t*, **806–807**
preparations available, 810
POMC (prepro-opiomelanocortin), 497, 500*i*
Ponstel, 599. *See also* Mefenamic acid
Pontocaine, 426*t*, 433. *See also* Tetracaine
"Poppers," 529
Pork insulin, 690*t*, 692
Pork tapeworm, drugs for infection with, 863*t*
niclosamide, 871
Porphyromonas, empiric antimicrobial therapy and, 815*t*
Portal-systemic encephalopathy, drugs for, **1026**
Positive inotropic drugs, for heart failure, **205–206**, 207
in elderly, 994–995
Postantibiotic effect (PAE), 818–819, 818*t*
Postantibiotic leukocyte enhancement (PALE), 818–819
Postcoital contraceptives, 670, 671*t*

Postmenopausal bleeding, estrogen therapy causing, 660
Postmenopausal hormonal therapy, 658–659, 659*i*
Postoperative pain control, PCA for, 508
Postpartum hemorrhage, ergot alkaloids for control of, 282
Postreceptor effects, of antidepressants, 487–488
Postsynaptic regulation, autonomic, 85, 87*i*
Postural baroreflex, in blood pressure regulation, 154, 155*i*
Postural hypotension (orthostatic hypotension)
antipsychotic agents causing, 470
bromocriptine causing, 455
levodopa causing, 453
sympathomimetics for, 130
Postural tremor, 450
Posture, 721. *See also* Calcium
Potassium
for arrhythmias, **237**
in cardiac conduction, 216–219
digitalis interactions and, 205
effects of, 218
electrical potential affected by, 246, 247*i*
Potassium channel openers
for angina, 181
for asthma, 338
Potassium channels
cardiac, 217–218
in CNS, 344
Potassium equilibrium potential, 218
Potassium iodide solution
preparations available, 633
for thyroid storm, 631
Potassium-sparing diuretics, **253–254**, 253*i*, 254*t*
interactions of, 1068*t*
with loop agents or thiazides, **256**
urinary electrolyte patterns affected by, 257*t*
Potassium wasting, carbonic anhydrase inhibitors causing, 249
Potency (pharmacologic), 28, 28*i*
Potentiation, toxicity of chemical mixtures and, 946
Povidone, antimicrobial effects of, 805*t*
Povidone-iodine (PVP/polyvinyl pyrrolidone)
antimicrobial effects of, 805*t*, **806–807**
preparations available, 810
"Power failure," after myocardial infarction, 211*t*, 212
PP (pancreatic polypeptide), 684, 685*t*
PP cells (F cells), pancreatic, 685*t*
Practolol, half-life of, aging affecting, 992*i*
Pralidoxime
for cholinergic poisoning, 112–113, 977*t*
preparations available, 116
Pramipexole, for parkinsonism, 456

Pramoxine, **1014**
preparations available, 433
Pravachol, 576. *See also* Pravastatin
Pravastatin, 573, 574
preparations available, 576
Prax, 433. *See also* Pramoxine
Prazepam
biotransformation of, 357, 357*i*
dosages of, 366*t*
pharmacokinetics of, 358*t*
preparations available, 369
Praziquantel, **873–875**
antiparasitic actions of, 836*t*, 874
preparations available, 878
Prazolam, biotransformation of, 358
Prazosin, 136, 137*i*, 138*t*, 139, **165–166**
for hypertension, **165–166**
mechanisms and sites of action of, 165
pharmacokinetic/pharmacodynamic parameters of, 37*t*, 166
preparations available, 150, 175
Precocious puberty, medroxyprogesterone for, 664
Precose, 703. *See also* Acarbose
Prednisolone, 640*t*
preparations available, 650
structure of, 641*i*
Prednisone, 640*t*
in breast milk, 987*t*
for cancer chemotherapy, 899*t*
dosing schedules for, 645
for drug allergy, 938
for inflammatory bowel disease, 1026
preparations available, 650, 940
Prednisone-sensitive lymphomas, 898
Preeclampsia, nitric oxide and, 322
Pregnancy
alcohol use during, 378
anesthesia during, 418–419
antiepileptic drug use during, 401, **406**
antipsychotic drug use during, 474
autonomic activity/drugs affecting uterus and, 83*i*
cocaine abuse during, 523
drug therapy in, **979–982**
folic acid deficiency during, 542
folic acid supplementation during, 543
glucocorticoid use during, 640
H_2 receptor antagonist use during, 272
hypertension during, nitric oxide and, **322**
hyperthyroidism during, 632
hypothyroidism and, 629
lithium use during, 478–479
nausea and vomiting of, H_1 receptor antagonists for, 269
opioid analgesic use and, 510
valproic acid and sodium valproate use during, 401
warfarin use during, 552, 558
Pregnyl, 617. *See also* Chorionic gonadotropin
Prekallikreins, 292, 294
Preload, cardiac performance affected by, 199–200, 200*i*
Prelone, 650. *See also* Prednisolone

Preludin, 521. *See also* Phenmetrazine
Premarin, 680. *See also* Estrogens
Premature labor, beta agonist therapy for, 132
Premature ventricular contractions, after myocardial infarction, treatment of, 234
Prenalterol, 129, 129*i*
Prepidil, 317. *See also* Prostaglandin E₂
Preprodynorphin, 497, 500*i*
Preproenkephalin, 497, 500*i*
Prepro-opiomelanocortin (POMC), 497, 500*i*
Prescription Drug User Fee Act, 68*t*
Prescription writing/prescription, **1041–1050**
  abbreviations used in, 1044*t*
  authority for, 1046–1047, 1047*t*
  classification of controlled substances and, 1043*t*
  compliance and, **1045–1046**
  cost factors and, 1048–1049
  elements of, 1042*i*, 1043–1044
  errors associated with, **1044–1045**
  generic, 1048–1049
  labeled and unlabeled uses of drugs and, 1048
  legal aspects of, **1046–1048**, 1047*t*
  rational approach to, **1041–1042**
  socioeconomic factors and, **1048–1049**
Preservatives, disinfectants used as, **809–810**
PresTab, 703. *See also* Glyburide
Presynaptic regulation, autonomic, 84–85, 85*t*
Preterm labor, indomethacin in, 589
Pretibial myxedema, 632
Prevacid, 1027. *See also* Lansoprazole
Prevotella, empiric antimicrobial therapy and, 815*t*
Prilocaine
  blood disorders caused by, 432
  preparations available, 433
  properties of, 426*t*
  structure of, 426*t*
Prilosec, 1027. *See also* Omeprazole
Primacor, 213. *See also* Milrinone
Primaquine, 839*i*, **844–845**
  antiparasitic actions of, 836*t*, 844
  for malaria chemoprophylaxis, 840*t*, 844
  for malaria treatment, 841*t*, 844
  preparations available, 859
  resistance to, 844
Primaxin, 741. *See also* Imipenem
Primidone, **394–395**, 394*i*
  effective/toxic plasma levels of, 405*t*
  preparations available, 407
  for tremor, 459
Principal cells, 245
Prinivil, 175, 213. *See also* Lisinopril
Priscoline, 150. *See also* Tolazoline
Privine (naphazoline), 134
PRL (prolactin), 604*t*, **614**
  adenomas secreting, bromocriptine for, 614

bromocriptine affecting secretion of, 282
  receptors for, 604–605
Proaccelerin (factor V), 549*t*
  therapeutic, 559*t*
Proadifen, cytochrome P450 inhibition by, 55
ProAmatine, 134. *See also* Midodrine
Probalan, 600. *See also* Probenecid
Pro-Banthine, 116, 1027. *See also* Propantheline
Probenecid, 596*i*, 597
  interactions of, 1068*t*
  preparations available, 600
Procainamide, **228–230**, 228*i*
  for arrhythmias, **228–230**
  clinical properties of, 229*t*
  ionization constant of, 6*t*
  membrane actions of, 228*t*
  pharmacokinetic/pharmacodynamic parameters of, 37*t*, 228–230
  preparations available, 240
Procaine
  ionization constant of, 6*t*
  preparations available, 433
  properties of, 426*t*
  with propoxycaine, preparations available, 433
  structure of, 426*t*
Procaine penicillin, 729
  half-life of, aging affecting, 992*i*
  pharmacokinetics of, 727
  preparations available, 740
Procan, 240. *See also* Procainamide
Procarbazine, **888**, 890*t*
Procardia, 175, 194. *See also* Nifedipine
Prochlorperazine, 471
  antiemetic action of, 1022
  preparations available, 480, 1027
Proconvertin (factor VII), 547, 549*i*, 549*t*
  therapeutic, 559*t*
Procrit, 546. *See also* Epoetin alfa
Proctitis, HSV, acyclovir for, 790
Procyclidine
  for parkinsonism, 457*t*
  preparations available, 462
Profasi, 617. *See also* Chorionic gonadotropin
Profilnine Heat-Treated, 561. *See also* Factor IX
Progabide, spasmolytic actions of, 447
Progesterone, 661, 661*t*, 662*i*
  effects of, 662–663
  inhibitors and antagonists of, **671–672**
  mechanism of action of, 662
  pharmacokinetics of, 661*t*, 662–662, 663*i*
  preparations available, 680
  synthetic and degradation pathways for, 663*i*
Progesterone receptor, in breast cancer, 898
Progestins, **661–664**, 661*t*
  in cancer chemotherapy, 899*t*
  clinical uses of, 664
  contraception with, 670

contraindications/cautions/adverse effects of, 664
  effects of, 662–664
  mechanism of action of, 662
  natural (progesterone), 661, 662–664
  pharmacokinetics of, 661–662, 661*t*, 663*i*
  preparations available, 680
  synthetic, 661, 661*t*, 662*i*, 664
Proglucagon, 702*i*
Proglycem, 175. *See also* Diazoxide
Prograf, 940. *See also* Tacrolimus
Proguanil (chloroguanide), 839*i*, **845–846**
  for malaria chemoprophylaxis, 840*t*, 845
  preparations available, 859
Proinsulin, 692
  structure of, 686*i*
Prokine, 546. *See also* Sargramostim
Prolactin (PRL), 604*t*, **614**
  bromocriptine affecting secretion of, 282
  receptors for, 604–605
Prolactin-secreting adenomas, bromocriptine for, 614
Proleukin, 940. *See also* Interleukin-2
Prolixin, 471*t*, 472*t*, 480. *See also* Fluphenazine
Prolixin Decanoate, 480
Prolixin Enanthate, 480
Proloprim, 768. *See also* Trimethoprim
Promazine
  ionization constant of, 6*t*
  preparations available, 480
Promethazine, 267*t*, 471
  antiemetic action of, 1022
  ionization constant of, 6*t*
  for motion sickness, 6*t*, 1022
  preparations available, 284
  structure of, 266*i*
Pronestyl, 240. *See also* Procainamide
Propafenone, **234**
  clinical properties of, 229*t*
  membrane actions of, 228*t*
  preparations available, 240
Propantheline, 107*i*
  for gastrointestinal and genitourinary conditions, 112*t*
  preparations available, 116, 1027
Propicillin, half-life of, aging affecting, 992*i*
Propine, 133. *See also* Dipivefrin
Propiverine, 112
Proplex, 561. *See also* Factor IX (Christmas factor/plasma thromboplastin component), therapeutic
Propofol, 411*i*, 420*t*, **421–422**
  for deep sedation, 421, 422
  GABA-DBZ receptor chloride channel binding and, 361
  preparations available, 423
Propoxur, 952*i*
Propoxycaine, with procaine, preparations available, 433
Propoxyphene, 511
  with acetaminophen, 511

with aspirin, 511
pharmacokinetics of, 501*t*
preparations available, 514
structure of, 498*i*
Propranolol, 138*t*, 143*i*, 145
for arrhythmias, 234
bioavailability of, 142, 144*t*
in breast milk, 987*t*
clinical properties of, 229*t*
distribution and clearance of, 142, 144*t*
dosing of, 164
for essential tremor, 459
half-life of, aging affecting, 992*i*
for hypertension, **164**
for hyperthyroidism, 148, 628
ionization constant of, 6*t*
mechanisms and sites of action of, 164
membrane actions of, 228*t*
for migraine headache, 148, 282
pharmacokinetic/pharmacodynamic parameters of, 37*t*, 164
preparations available, 150, 174, 194, 240
properties of, 144*t*
renin secretion affected by, 290
for schizophrenia, 475
as standard for beta-blocker selection, 148
for thyroid storm, 631
toxicity of, 148–149, 164
Propulsid, 284, 1027. *See also* Cisapride
Propylene glycol, as keratolytic agent, **1011–1012**
Propylthiouracil (PTU), 626–627, 626*i*
in breast milk, 987*t*
fetus affected by, 983*t*
for Graves' disease, 630
ionization constant of, 6*t*
preparations available, 633
Proscar, 680. *See also* Finasteride
ProSom, 366*t*, 369. *See also* Estazolam
Prostacyclin (PGI₂/epoprostenol), 306, 547. *See also* Prostaglandins
platelets affected by, 314–315
preparations available, 317
for pulmonary hypertension, 314
second messenger for, 22*t*
synthesis of, 306–307, 306*i*
Prostaglandin E, 85*t*. *See also* Prostaglandins
second messenger for, 22*t*
Prostaglandin E₁ (alprostadil), 306, 312*i*. *See also* Prostaglandins
for impotence, 314
preparations available, 317
Prostaglandin E₂ (dinoprostone), 306, 312–313, 312*i*. *See also* Prostaglandins
for abortion, 312–313
for labor facilitation, 313
preparations available, 317
Prostaglandin endoperoxide synthases, products of, 305–307. *See also* Prostaglandins

Prostaglandin F₂α, 306, 312*i*. *See also* Prostaglandins
for abortion, 312–313
for labor facilitation, 313
Prostaglandins, **304–318**. *See also* Eicosanoids
for abortion, 312–313
for acid-peptic disease, 1021
blood affected by, 314–315
bronchoconstriction caused by, 315
bronchodilation caused by, 315
in cardiovascular disorders, 314
for dysmenorrhea, 313–314
effects of, 308–310
female reproductive system affected by, 310, 311–314
in inflammation, 316, 316*i*, 578, 579*t*
in kinin-mediated vasodilation, 294
for labor facilitation, 313
male reproductive system affected by, 310, 314
receptors for, 308
structures of, 312*i*
synthesis of, 306–307, 306*i*
Prostaphlin, 740. *See also* Oxacillin
Prostate cancer, 903*t*, **910**
androgen suppression for, 677
gonadotropin-releasing hormones for, 611
Prostatic hyperplasia, benign, alpha-receptor blocking drugs for, 141
Prostatic secretions, drug trapping in, 7*t*
Prostigmin, 103. *See also* Neostigmine
Prostin, 317. *See also* Alprostadil
Prostin E2, 317. *See also* Prostaglandin E₂
Protamine
for heparin-induced bleeding, 551
preparations available, 561
Protease inhibitors, **798–799**
Protein anabolic agents, androgens and anabolic steroids as, 676
Protein binding
capacity-limited, 47
drug concentration affected by, 47, 48
passage across placenta and, 979–980
reduced, oral anticoagulant interactions and, 554
Protein C, 548, 549*t*
activated, resistance to, 558
deficiency of, 558
Protein kinase C, in calcium/phosphoinositide second messenger system, 25, 26*i*
Protein S, 548, 549*t*
deficiency of, 558
Protein synthesis, antibiotics interfering with, **743–751, 752–760**
mechanism of action and selectivity of, 744
Proteins, as drug receptors
regulatory, 9–10
structural, 10
transport, 10
Proteus, empiric antimicrobial therapy and, 814*t*

Prothrombin (factor II), 547, 549*t*
therapeutic, 559*t*
Protirelin (thyrotropin-releasing hormone/TRH), 604*t*, **608**, 620, 623*i*
receptors for, 604
second messenger for, 22*t*
Proton pump inhibitors
for acid-peptic disease, 1020
preparations available, 1027
Protopam, 116. *See also* Pralidoxime
Prototype drugs, 7
Protriptyline, 485*i*
dosages of, 491*t*
effects of, 489*t*
half-life of, aging affecting, 992*i*
pharmacokinetics of, 488*t*
preparations available, 494
Protropin, 617. *See also* Somatrem
Proventil, 340. *See also* Albuterol
Provera, 680, 899*t*. *See also* Medroxyprogesterone
Proximal tubule, transport in/diuretic site of action and, **242–244**, 244*i*, 254, 255
Prozac, 494. *See also* Fluoxetine
Pseudocholinesterase
local anesthetics metabolized by, 427
succinylcholine metabolized by, 439
Pseudodepression, antipsychotic agents causing, 473
Pseudoephedrine
ionization constant of, 6*t*
in OTC preparations, efficacy of, 1035*t*
OTC status of, 1032*t*
preparations available, 134
Pseudomonas
aeruginosa, empiric antimicrobial therapy and, 814*t*
cepacia, empiric antimicrobial therapy and, 814*t*
Pseudomonic acid A (mupirocin), in dermatologic therapy, **1000**
Psilocybin
abuse of, 524–526
structure of, 524*i*
Psoralens, for repigmentation, 1006
Psoriasis, drugs in management of, **1007–1008**
Psychiatric disorders
benzodiazepines for, 366–367
lithium toxicity and, 478
Psychologic dependence. *See also* specific agent or drug class
drug abuse and, 516
Psychosis, 464
drugs for treatment of, **464–475**. *See also* Antipsychotic agents
glucocorticoids and, 644
levodopa contraindicated in, 454
Psyllium
laxative effect of, 1023
preparations available, 1028
PTA (plasma thromboplastin antecedent/factor XI), 549*t*
therapeutic, 559*t*

PTC (plasma thromboplastin component/Christmas factor/factor IX), 549*t*
deficiency of, 559, 559*t*
therapeutic, 559*t*, 560
preparations available, 561
Pteroylglutamic acid, 538, 546. *See also* Folic acid
PTH (parathyroid hormone), **706–707**
abnormal serum levels of, 715–716
in bone mineral homeostasis, 706–707
second messenger for, 22*t*
vitamin D interaction and, **709**, 709*t*
PTT (partial thromboplastin time), for heparin monitoring, 551
PTU (propylthiouracil), 626–627, 626*i*
in breast milk, 987*t*
fetus affected by, 983*t*
for Graves' disease, 630
ionization constant of, 6*t*
preparations available, 633
Puberty
constitutional delay in onset of, hCG stimulation in evaluation of, 614
precocious, medroxyprogesterone for, 664
Pulmonary blood flow, anesthetic gas uptake and distribution affected by, 412–414
Pulmonary congestion, after myocardial infarction, 211–212, 211*t*
Pulmonary disease. *See also under Respiratory*
antimuscarinic agents for, 111
eicosanoids in, 315
nitric oxide for, **322**
sympathomimetics for, 131–132
Pulmonary edema, acute, opioid analgesics for pain management in, 507
Pulmonary embolism
fibrinolytic agents for, 555
management of, 558
Pulmonary function, impaired, opioid analgesic use and, 510
Pulmonary function testing, histamine in, 264, 265
Pulmonary hypertension
nitric oxide for, 322
prostacyclin for, 314
Pulmonary ventilation, anesthetic gas tension and, 412, 414*i*
Pupillary constrictors, antimuscarinic agents affecting, 107–108
Pupillary dilators, sympathomimetic agents affecting, 125
Pure Food and Drug Act, 67, 68*t*
Purine antagonists, **891–892**
Purine phosphoribosyl transferases, antiparasitic drugs affecting, 831, 832*i*
Purinethol, 891*t*. *See also* Mercaptopurine
Purpura, idiopathic thrombocytopenic immunosuppressive agents for, 931*t*, 932, 933
passive immunization for, 1056*t*

PVCs (premature ventricular contractions), after myocardial infarction, treatment of, 234
PVP (polyvinyl pyrrolidone/povidone-iodine)
antimicrobial effects of, 805*t*, **806–807**
preparations available, 810
Pygmies, 607
Pyramat, 952*t*
Pyrantel pamoate, **876**
in OTC preparations, efficacy of, 1034*t*
OTC status of, 1032*t*
preparations available, 878
synaptic transmission affected by, 835, 876
Pyrazinamide, 770, 771*t*, **774**, 774*i*
in combination therapy, 772, 772*t*
preparations available, 778
Pyrethrin, 953*i*
Pyrethrum, 952
in OTC preparations, efficacy of, 1035*t*
Pyridostigmine
for myasthenia gravis, 101
neuromuscular blockade reversed by, 445
pharmacokinetic/pharmacodynamic parameters of, 37*t*
preparations available, 103
Pyridoxine (vitamin B$_6$), 770*i*
levodopa interactions and, 454
Pyrilamine, 267*t*
preparations available, 284
Pyrimethamine, 839*i*, **845–846**
ionization constant of, 6*t*
for malaria treatment, 841*t*, 845
preparations available, 859
resistance to, 845
with sulfonamide, 764. *See also* Pyrimethamine-sulfadoxine
for toxoplasmosis, 845–846
Pyrimethamine-dapsone, **847**
preparations available, 859
Pyrimethamine-sulfadoxine (Fansidar), 764, **846–847**
for malaria treatment, 841*t*, 845, 846
Pyrimidine antagonists, **892–893**
Pyrimidines, 762*t*
Pyrolan, 952*t*
Pyrophosphoric acid, 711, 711*i*
Pyruvate:ferredoxin oxidoreductase, antiparasitic agents affecting, 828–829
Pyruvate phosphate dikinase, antiparasitic agents affecting, 829
PZA (pyrazinamide), 770, 771*t*, **774**, 774*i*
in combination therapy, 772, 772*t*
preparations available, 778

Qinghaosu (artermisinin), for malaria treatment, 849–850
Quantal dose-effect curves, 29–30, 29*i*
in poisoning, 969, 969*i*
Quantrel, 878. *See also* Oxantel pamoate

Quarzan, 115, 1027. *See also* Clidinium
Quaternary ammonium compounds, antimicrobial effects of, 805*t*, **808**
Quazepam
dosages of, 366*t*
pharmacokinetics of, 358*t*
preparations available, 369
Questran, 576. *See also* Cholestyramine
Quetiapine, 467*i*
dose relationships of, 472*t*
effects of, 469
preparations available, 480
Quide, 472*t*. *See also* Piperacetazine
Quinacrine, 839*i*, **850**, **876**
antiparasitic actions of, 836*t*
preparations available, 859
Quinagolide, 615. *See also* Bromocriptine
Quinapril
for heart failure, 210
for hypertension, 170
preparations available, 175, 213
Quinestrol, 656*i*, 657*t*
preparations available, 680
Quinethazone
dosages of, 252*t*
preparations available, 259
structure of, 252*i*
Quinidex Extentabs, 240. *See also* Quinidine
Quinidine, **227–228**, 227*i*, **848**
action potential duration affected by, 235
for arrhythmias, **227–228**
clinical properties of, 229*t*
interactions of, 1068*t*
ionization constant of, 6*t*
for malaria treatment, 841*t*, **848**
membrane actions of, 228*t*
pharmacokinetic/pharmacodynamic parameters of, 37*t*, 227–228
preparations available, 240, 859
Quinidine gluconate, 140, 859. *See also* Quinidine
Quinidine polygalacturonate, 140. *See also* Quinidine
Quinidine sulfate, 240. *See also* Quinidine
Quinidine syncope, 227
Quinine, **847–848**
antiparasitic actions of, 836*t*, 847
interactions and, 848
for malaria chemoprophylaxis, 848
for malaria treatment, 841*t*, 847–848
preparations available, 859
resistance to, 847
Quinolones. *See also* Fluoroquinolones
interactions of, 1068*t*
preparations available, 768
Quinupristin, 750

Rabies
active immunization and, 1053*t*
passive immunization and, 1056*t*
Rabies immune globulin, 1056*t*
Radial muscle, autonomic activity/drugs affecting, 83*t*

Radioactive iodine, **627–628**
  in breast milk, 987*t*
  for Graves' disease, 630
Rafoxanide, antiparasitic actions of, 836*t*
Ramipril
  for heart failure, 210
  for hypertension, 170
  preparations available, 175, 213
Ranitidine, 270*t*, 1019–1020
  clinical uses of, 272, 1020
  interactions of, 273
  organ system effects of, 271, 271*i*
  in OTC preparations, efficacy of, 1033*t*
  OTC status of, 1032*t*
  pharmacokinetic/pharmacodynamic parameters of, 37*t*, 270*t*
  preparations available, 284, 1026
  toxicity of, 272
Rapamycin (sirolimus), 927
Rattlesnake envenomation, **978**
Rauwolscine, 138*t*
Ravocaine, with Novocain (propoxycaine and procaine), 433
Reactive depression, 483, 484*t*. *See also* Depression
Reactive metabolites, 55–56, 57*i*
  antihistamines and, 268
  benzodiazepines forming, 357*i*, 358
  phenoxybenzamine forming, 136, 137*i*
Receptive substance, 9. *See also* Drug receptors
Receptor-effector coupling, 11–14
Receptor-operated channels, 344
Receptors, 9. *See also* Drug receptors
  agonist binding by, concentration-effect curves and, 11, 12*i*
  antidepressants affecting activity of, 487–488
Recombinant human erythropoietin, 544. *See also* Erythropoietin
Recombinant human G-CSF, 544. *See also* Granulocyte colony-stimulating factor
Recombinant human GM-CSF, 544–545. *See also* Granulocyte-macrophage colony-stimulating factor
Recombinant tissue plasminogen activator (rt-PA), discovery and development of, 71
Recombinate, 561. *See also* Antihemophilic globulin
Rectal route of administration
  bioavailability and characteristics and, 40*t*
  first-pass effect and, 42
  for opioid analgesics, 508
Red thrombus, 547
Reducing air pollutants, 947
Reductase inhibitors, **573–575**, 573*i*
  combination therapy with, **575**
Reductions, in biotransformation, 54*t*
Redux, 276, 284. *See also* Dexfenfluramine
Reed-Sternberg cells, 907
Reentry, 224, 225*i*
  nonpharmacologic therapy of, 238

Reflux, gastroesophageal, H_2 receptor antagonists for, 272
Regitine, 150. *See also* Phentolamine
Reglan, 1027. *See also* Metoclopramide
Regular insulin, 690, 690*t*
Regulatory proteins, as drug receptors, 9–10
Rejection, transplant
  cell-mediated, prostaglandins affecting, 315–316
  nitric oxide and, 323
Relafen, 599. *See also* Nabumetone
Relaxin, 666
Relefact, 617. *See also* Protirelin
Remeron, 494. *See also* Mirtazapine
Remifentanil, 511
  preparations available, 514
Remikiren, 291*i*, 293
Remodeling, myocardial
  angiotensin-converting enzyme inhibitors affecting, 289
  in heart failure, 199
Renal disease/impaired renal function. *See also* Nephrotoxicity
  amphotericin B causing, 781
  antimicrobial use and, 819, 819*t*
  diuretics for, **257–258**
  lithium causing, 478
  opioid analgesic use and, 510
Renal failure
  acute
    loop diuretics in management of, 250
    potassium-sparing diuretics causing, 254
  ADH antagonists causing, 256
  anemia in, erythropoietin for, 544
  bone mineral homeostasis and, **716–717**
  phenacetin and, 595
Renal function tests, in poisoning, 973
Renal osteodystrophy, vitamin D for, 717
Renal stones
  carbonic anhydrase inhibitors causing, 249
  potassium-sparing diuretics causing, 254
Renal transplantation, immunosuppressive therapy and, 931*t*, 932
Renal tubular acidosis, tetracyclines causing, 747
Renal tubules, transport mechanisms in/diuretic site of action and, **242–246**, 243*i*
Renal vascular receptor, renin secretion controlled by, 287
Renese, 259. *See also* Polythiazide
Renin, 287–288
  in blood pressure regulation, 154, 154*i*
  inhibitors of action of, 290, 291*i*, 293
  inhibitors of secretion of, 290, 293
  pharmacologic alteration of release of, 288
Renin-angiotensin system, 287
  chemistry of, 288*i*
  inhibition of, **290–291**, 292*i*, 293
Renoquid, 768. *See also* Sulfacytine

ReoPro, 561. *See also* Abciximab
Reproductive organs
  lead toxicity and, 961
  lipoxygenase metabolites affecting, 311
  prostaglandins affecting, 310, 311–314
  thyroid hormones affecting, 625*t*
Reserpine, **162–163**, 163*i*
  for Huntington's disease, 460
  preparations available, 175
  serotonin affected by, 273, 277
Resistance
  to activated protein C, 558
  to acyclovir, 789
  to alkylating agents, 885
  to aminoglycosides, 752–753
  to antimycobacterial drugs, 770
  to azoles, 783
  to chloroquine, 842
  to cytotoxic drugs, 883–884, 885*i*
  to erythromycin, 748
  to fluoroquinolones, 765–766, 767
  to gentamicin, 756
  to indinavir, 798
  to insulin, 695, 700
  to isoniazid, 771
  to kanamycin, 758
  to mefloquine, 843
  to mercaptopurine, 891
  to methotrexate, 890
  to penicillins, 725–726
  to primaquine, 844
  to proguanil, 845
  to pyrimethamine, 845
  to quinine, 847
  to streptomycin, 754
  to sulfonamides, 761
  to tetracyclines, 745
    overuse and, 747
  to thioguanine, 891
  to trimethoprim, 763
  to vancomycin, 727, 738
  to zidovudine, 795
Resistance (vascular), alpha-receptor antagonists affecting, 136
Resochin, 858. *See also* Chloroquine
Respiration, sedative-hypnotics affecting, 362
Respiratory depression, opioid analgesics causing, 505
Respiratory disorders
  antimuscarinic agents for, 111
  eicosanoids in, 315
  nitric oxide for, **322**
  sympathomimetics for, 131–132
Respiratory rate, inhaled anesthetics affecting, 417
Respiratory syncytial virus infection, ribavirin for, 800
Respiratory system. *See also* Bronchial/bronchiolar smooth muscle
  antimuscarinic agents affecting, 109
  beta-receptor blocking drugs affecting, 143
  cholinesterase inhibitors affecting, 99

Respiratory system (cont.)
  direct-acting cholinomimetics affect-
    ing, 94t, 96
  inhaled anesthetics affecting, 417
  progesterone affecting, 662
  prostaglandins affecting, 309, 315
  serotonin affecting, 275
  sympathomimetic agents affecting, 125
  thromboxanes affecting, 309, 315
  thyroid hormones affecting, 625t
Response axis, 28, 28i
Response elements, 18
Rest tremor, 459
Resting potential, cardiac action potential
    affected by, 219–220, 220i
Restoril, 366t, 369. See also Temazepam
Retavase, 561. See also Reteplase
Reteplase, **555**
  for myocardial infarction, 555, 556
  preparations available, 561
Retin-A, 1006–1007. See also Retinoic
    acid
Retinitis, CMV
  cidofovir for, 793
  foscarnet for, 794
  ganciclovir for, 793
Retinoic acid/retinoic acid derivatives,
    1006i
  for acne, **1006–1007**
  in cancer chemotherapy, **901–902**
  topical, 1006–1007
Retrobulbar neuritis, ethambutol causing,
    774
Retrocollis, antipsychotic agents causing,
    473
Retrovir, 801. See also Zidovudine
Reverse potential, 218
Reverse transcriptase inhibitors,
    795–798. See also specific type
Reverse triiodothyronine (rT₃), 621i
Revex, 514. See also Nalmefene
ReVia, 383, 514. See also Naltrexone
Rezulin, 703. See also Troglitazone
Rh isoimmunization, passive immuniza-
    tion for, 930–931, 931t, 1057t
Rhₒ (D) immune globulin micro-dose,
    930–931, 931t, 1057t
  preparations available, 940
Rheumatic fever, antimicrobial prophy-
    laxis and, 825t
Rheumatoid arthritis
  chronic inflammation in, 578, 579t
  eicosanoids in, 316
  gold compounds for, 591–592
  penicillamine for, 593
Rheumatrex, 600. See also Methotrexate
Rhinitis, allergic
  cromolyn for, 330
  H₁ receptor antagonists for, 268–269
Rhizopus, empiric antimicrobial therapy
    and, 815t
rHuEpo (recombinant human erythropoi-
    etin), 544. See also Erythropoietin
rHuG-CSF (recombinant human granulo-
    cyte colony-stimulating factor),
    544. See also Granulocyte colony-
    stimulating factor

rHuGM-CSF (recombinant human gran-
    ulocyte-macrophage colony-stimu-
    lating factor), 544–545. See also
    Granulocyte-macrophage colony-
    stimulating factor
Ribavirin, **800**
  preparations available, 801
Rickets
  nutritional, **716**
  vitamin D-dependent, **719**
  vitamin D-resistant, **719**
Ridaura, 599. See also Auranofin
Rifabutin, 776
  for MAC infections, 777
  preparations available, 778
  for tuberculosis, 771t, 776
Rifadin, 778. See also Rifampin
Rifampin, 770, 771t, **773**
  in combination therapy, 772, 772t
  drug metabolism induced by, 59t, 773
  interactions of, 1068t
  for leprosy, **778**
  oral anticoagulant interactions and,
    554, 773
  pharmacokinetic/pharmacodynamic
    parameters of, 37t, 773
  preparations available, 778
Right ventricular infarction, 211t, 212
Rigidity, truncal, opioid analgesics caus-
    ing, 505
Rimactane, 778. See also Rifampin
Rimantadine, **799–800**
  preparations available, 801
Risk, toxicologic definition of, 946
Risperdal, 472t, 480. See also Risperi-
    done
Risperidone, 467i, 468t, 472
  advantages and disadvantages of, 471t
  dose relationships of, 472t
  preparations available, 480
  receptor binding by, 468
Ritalin, 134, 521. See also
    Methylphenidate
Ritanserin, 277
  for alcoholism, 381
Ritodrine, 129, 129i
  for premature labor, 132
Ritonavir, 795t, **798–799**
  preparations available, 801
Robaxin, 448. See also Methocarbamol
Robinul, 115, 1027. See also Glycopy-
    rrolate
Rocaltrol, 721. See also Calcitriol
Rocephin, 741. See also Ceftriaxone
Rocuronium, 437i, 438t
  effects of, 443t
  pharmacokinetics of, 438, 438t
  preparations available, 448
Roferon (interferon alfa-2a), 801, 940
Rogaine, 175, 1014. See also Minoxidil
Rohypnol, criminal use of, 521
Romazicon, 369, 977t. See also
    Flumazenil
Rondomycin, 751. See also Methacycline
"Roofies," criminal use of, 521
Ropinirole, for parkinsonism, 456

Ropivacaine
  cardiotoxicity of, 432
  CYPs in metabolism of, 427
  preparations available, 433
  properties of, 426t
  structure of, 426t
Roquinimex, 935
Rotenone, 952, 953i
Roundworms, drugs for, 863t
Routes of administration
  bioavailability and characteristics and,
    40t
  first-pass effect and, 42
Rowasa, 1027. See also Mesalamine
RP59500, 750
RS-61443 (mycophenolate mofetil (RS-
    61443)), 927
rT₃ (reverse triiodothyronine), 621i
rt-PA (recombinant tissue plasminogen
    activator), discovery and develop-
    ment of, 71
RU 486 (mifepristone), **648**, **671–672**
  with prostaglandins, for abortion, 313
Rubella
  active immunization for, 1053t
  passive immunization for, 1057t
Rufen, 599. See also Ibuprofen
"Run," in amphetamine abuse, 522
Ryanodine, 447
Rythmol, 240. See also Propafenone
RZRβ, 275

SAARDs (slow-acting antirheumatic
    drugs/disease-modifying an-
    tirheumatic drugs), 579, **590–593**
  preparations available, 599–600
Safety testing, in new drug development,
    63i, **64–66**, 66t
  in phase 4 clinical trials, 69, 69t
St. Anthony's fire, 277
Salbutamol (albuterol), 334i
  for asthma, 333
  ionization constant of, 6t
  preparations available, 340
Salicylates, **579–585**, 580t, 581i. See
    also Aspirin
  half-life of, 985t
  for inflammatory bowel disease,
    1025–1026
  interactions of, 1068–1069t
  nonacetylated, **585**
  in OTC preparations, hidden,
    1037–1038t
  overdose of, 972t
  preparations available, 599
Salicylhydroxamic acid (SHAM), glycol-
    ysis affected by, 834
Salicylic acid, 1011i
  ionization constant of, 6t
  pharmacokinetic/pharmacodynamic
    parameters of, 37t
  topical, **1011**
Salicylism, 584
  following topical application, 1011
Salicylsalicylate (salicylsalicylic acid),
    585
  preparations available, 599

Saline cathartics, 1023–1024
Saline diuresis, for hypercalcemia, 713
Saline laxatives, in OTC preparations, efficacy of, 1035t
Salivary glands
  antimuscarinic agents affecting, 110, 110i
  direct-acting cholinomimetics affecting, 94t, 96
  sympathomimetics affecting, 127
Salmeterol, 334, 334i
  preparations available, 340
Salmon calcitonin. *See also* Calcitonin
  for hypercalcemia, 713
  preparations available, 721
Salmonella, empiric antimicrobial therapy and, 814t
Salmonine, 721. *See also* Calcitonin
Salsalate, preparations available, 599
Saluron, 259. *See also* Hydroflumethiazide
Sandimmune, 940. *See also* Cyclosporine
Sandostatin, 617, 899t. *See also* Octreotide
Sani-Supp, 1028. *See also* Glycerin suppositories
Sanitization, 805t
Sansert, 284. *See also* Methysergide
Saquinavir, 795t, **799**
  preparations available, 801
Saralasin, 290–291
  angiotensin receptor affinity for, 289
  for hypertension, 171i, 172
Sarcoma, 904t, **911–912**
  Ewing's, 911–912
  osteogenic, 904t, 911–912
Sarcoplasmic reticulum
  calcium released from, cardiac contractility and, 197–198
  calcium stored in, cardiac contractility and, 198
Sargramostim, 544–545. *See also* Granulocyte-macrophage colony-stimulating factor
  in cancer chemotherapy, 902
  preparations available, 546
Savorquin, 859. *See also* Iodoquinol
Saxitoxin, sodium channels affected by, 428
Scabies
  benzyl benzoate for, 1005
  crotamiton for, 1005
  ivermectin for, 868
  permethrin for, 1005
  sulfur for, 1005
  thiabendazole for, 877
SCF (stem cell factor), 543, 543t, 545
Schilling test, 540–541
  in pernicious anemia, 541
Schistosoma (schistosomiasis)
  haematobium (bilharziasis), drugs for infection with, 863t
  antimony compounds, 865
  metrifonate, 870
  praziquantel, 874

japonicum, drugs for infection with, 863t
mansoni, drugs for infection with, 863t
  oxamniquine, 872
  praziquantel for, 874
praziquantel for, 874
Schizoaffective disorders, drugs for, 470. *See also* Antipsychotic agents
  lithium, 477
Schizophrenia, 464
  dopamine hypothesis for, 465
  drugs for treatment of, **464–475**. *See also* Antipsychotic agents
Scopolamine, 105
  deliriant effects of, 525–526
  distribution of, 106
  eye affected by, 109i
  for gastrointestinal and genitourinary conditions, 112t
  ionization constant of, 6t
  for motion sickness, 107, 110–111, 269, 1022
  ophthalmologic uses of, 111t
  overdose of, 972t
  preparations available, 116, 1027
  transdermal absorption of, 105–106, 110–111
Scorpion venom, sodium channels affected by, 428
Scratch test, for drug allergy, 938
Screening tests, in poisoning, 974
Seasickness. *See also* Motion sickness
  scopolamine for, 107, 110–111
Sebaquin, 859. *See also* Iodoquinol
Seborrhea, drugs for, **1014**, 1014t
  OTC preparations, efficacy of, 1034t
Secalciferol (24,25-dihydroxyvitamin D), 707–709, 708i, 709t
Secobarbital, 357i
  dosages of, 366t
  drug metabolism inhibited by, 60t
  preparations available, 369
Seconal, 369. *See also* Secobarbital
Second messengers
  G proteins and, 21–23
  lithium affecting, 476, 476i
Secondarily generalized seizure, 403
Secretory tissue, histamine affecting, 264
Sectral, 150, 174, 240. *See also* Acebutolol
Sedation
  conscious, 422
  deep, 422
  H_1 receptor antagonists causing, 267–268
  opioid analgesics causing, 505
  sedative-hypnotic drugs producing, 355i, 360–361
  dosages for, 366t
Sedative, 354. *See also* Sedative-hypnotic drugs
Sedative-autonomic drugs, 355
Sedative-hypnotic drugs, **354–371**. *See also specific agent and* Barbiturates; Benzodiazepines
  abuse of, **519–521**

for alcohol withdrawal syndrome, 365, 368, 379–380
for anxiety, **364–365**
basic pharmacology of, **354–364**
chemical classification of, **354–355**, 356i, 357i
clinical pharmacology of, **364–368**
clinical uses of, 365t, **366–367**
criminal use of, 520–521
dependence on, 362–363, 368, 519–520
dosages of, 366t
dose-response curves for, 354, 355i
in elderly, 993
interactions of, 368
newer agents, **363–364**
older agents, 354, 357i, **364**
overdose of, 972t, 973t
preparations available, 369
for sleep problems, **365–366**
tolerance to, 362–363, 368, 519–520
toxicity of, **367–368**
withdrawal from, 363, 368, 520
Seizures
  antipsychotic agents causing, 473
  classification of, 387t, **403–404**
  drugs for, **386–408**. *See also* Antiepileptic drugs
  neuromuscular blocking drugs, 445
  sedative-hypnotics, 362, 402
  in poisoning, 970, 971, 973
Seldane, 267t, 284. *See also* Terfenadine
Selective serotonin reuptake inhibitors
  adverse effects of, 493t
  for alcoholism, 381
  chemistry of, 484, 486i
  clinical indications for, 490
  dosages of, 491t
    for acute episode, 491
  effects of, 489
  interactions of, 492–493
  overdoses of, 493
  pharmacokinetics of, 486–487, 488t
  preparations available, 494
Selegiline, 451i, 456
  for Alzheimer's disease, 994
  preparations available, 462
Selenium, in OTC preparations, efficacy of, 1034t
Semen, prostaglandins affecting, 310
Seminal vesicles, autonomic activity/drugs affecting, 83t
Semustine (methyl-CCNU), 886i, **888**, 890t
Senile cerebral insufficiency, dihydroergotoxine for, 282
Senna
  laxative effect of, 1023
  preparations available, 1028
Senokot, 1028. *See also* Senna
Sensitivity, target organ, therapeutic drug monitoring and, 47
Sensorcaine, 432. *See also* Bupivacaine
Sensory nerves. *See also* Nerve endings
  kinins affecting, 294
Septata intestinalis, albendazole for infection with, 865

Septic arthritis, empiric antimicrobial therapy and, 816*t*
Septic shock, nitric oxide and, **322**
Septicemia, empiric antimicrobial therapy and, 816*t*
Septisol, 810. *See also* Hexachlorophene
Septra, 768, 859. *See also* Trimethoprim-sulfamethoxazole
Serax, 366*t*, 369, 383. *See also* Oxazepam
Serentil, 472*t*, 480. *See also* Mesoridazine
Serevent, 340. *See also* Salmeterol
Serine protease inhibitors, **561**
Serlect, 472*t*, 480. *See also* Sertindole
Sermorelin (growth hormone-releasing hormone/GHRH), 604*t*, **605**
 receptors for, 604
Seromycin, 741, 778. *See also* Cycloserine
Serophene, 680. *See also* Clomiphene
Seroquel, 472*t*. *See also* Quetiapine
Serotonergic neurons, 273
Serotonin, 77*t*, 85*t*, **273–277**, 349*t*, 352
 alcoholism and, 381
 antidepressants affecting, 487. *See also* Serotonin reuptake inhibitors
 appetite control and, 276
 basic pharmacology of, **273–276**
 clinical pharmacology of, **276–277**
 in inflammation, 579*t*
 LSD affecting, 525
 mechanisms of action of, 274
 as neurotransmitter, 77*t*, 349*t*, 352
 receptors for, 274, 274*t*
  drugs blocking, **277**
  ergot alkaloids affecting, 279, 279*t*
  second messenger for, 22*t*
 structure of, 273*i*
 tissue and organ system effects of, 274–276
Serotonin agonists, **276–277**
 preparations available, 284
Serotonin antagonists, **277**
 H$_1$ receptor antagonists as, 268
 preparations available, 284
Serotonin receptor antagonists, **277**
Serotonin reuptake inhibitors
 adverse effects of, 493*t*
 for alcoholism, 381
 chemistry of, 484, 486*i*
 clinical indications for, 490
 dosages of, 491*t*
  for acute episode, 491
 effects of, 489
 interactions of, 492–493
 overdoses of, 493
 pharmacokinetics of, 486–487, 488*t*
 preparations available, 494
Serotonin syndrome, 273
Serpasil, 175. *See also* Reserpine
Serpentine receptors, 22–23, 24*i*
Serratia, empiric antimicrobial therapy and, 814*t*
Sertindole, 467*i*, 468*t*
 dose relationships of, 472*t*

preparations available, 480
 receptor binding by, 468–469
Sertoli cells, 674
Sertraline, 489
 dosages of, 491*t*
 effects of, 489*t*
 pharmacokinetics of, 488*t*
 preparations available, 494
Serum osmolality, in poisoning, 973–974
Serum sickness, drugs causing, **939**
 penicillin, 731
Serutan, 1028. *See also* Psyllium
Serzone, 494. *See also* Nefazodone
Sevoflurane, 410*i*, 419
 elimination of, 414
 organ system effects of, 416–418
 preparations available, 423
 properties of, 413*t*
Sex (gender), drug metabolism affected by, 59
Sex hormone-binding globulin (SHBG), 674
Sex steroids
 in cancer chemotherapy, **898–900**, 899*t*
 receptors for, 18
 cancer and, 898
Sexual dysfunction, male, alpha-receptor antagonists for, 141–142
SHAM (salicylhydroxamic acid), glycolysis affected by, 834
SHBG (sex hormone-binding globulin), 674
Sheep liver fluke (fascioliasis), drugs for, 863*t*
 albendazole, 865
 bithionol, 865–866
Shigella, empiric antimicrobial therapy and, 814*t*
Shock
 cardiogenic, after myocardial infarction, 211*t*, 212
 septic, nitric oxide and, **322**
 sympathomimetics for, 130–131
Short-acting insulins, 690, 690*t*
Short stature, 607
SIADH (syndrome of inappropriate ADH secretion), 255
Sick sinus syndrome
 lithium contraindicated in, 478
 quinidine in patients with, 227
Signalling mechanisms, **17–27**, 18*i*
 calcium as second messenger and, 24–26, 26*i*
 cAMP as second messenger and, 23–24, 26*i*
 cGMP as second messenger and, 26
 cytokine receptors and, 20
 G proteins and, 21–23, 23*t*
 interplay among, 26
 intracellular receptors for lipid-soluble agents and, 18–19
 ligand-gated channels and, 20–21
 ligand-regulated transmembrane enzymes and, 19–20, 20*i*
 phosphoinositide as second messenger and, 24–26, 26*i*

phosphorylation and, 26–27
 receptor desensitization and, 23
 second messengers and, 21–23, 23–26, 26*i*
 tyrosine kinases and, 19–20, 20*i*
Silo-filler's disease, 949
Silvadene, 768. *See also* Silver sulfadiazine
Silver
 as disinfectant, **809**
 preparations available, 810
Silver nitrate, antimicrobial effects of, 809
Silver sulfadiazine
 for burns, 763, 809
 preparations available, 768
Simple partial seizure, 403
Simvastatin, 573, 574
 preparations available, 576
Sinemet, 453, 462. *See also* Carbidopa, with levodopa
Sinequan, 494. *See also* Doxepin
Single-blind design, for clinical trials, 67
Sinoatrial node, 216, 217*i*
 autonomic activity/drugs affecting, 83*t*
 direct-acting cholinomimetics affecting, 94*t*
Sinusitis, empiric antimicrobial therapy and, 816*t*
Sirolimus (rapamycin), 927
Sisomicin, 755
Skelaxin, 448. *See also* Metaxalone
Skeletal muscle
 autonomic activity/drugs affecting, 83*t*
 calcium channel blockers and, 189
 methylxanthines affecting, 332
 neuromuscular blocking drugs causing paralysis of, 442–443, 442*i*, 443*i*
Skeletal muscle relaxants, **434–449**. *See also* Neuromuscular blocking drugs; Spasmolytic drugs
Skin
 autonomic activity/drugs affecting, 83*t*
 decontamination of in poisoned patient, 974
 drugs for disorders of, **999–1016**. *See also specific type*
  acne preparations, **1006–1007**
  antibacterial agents, **1000–1001**
  antifungal agents, **1001–1004**
  anti-inflammatory agents, **1008–1009**, 1010*t*, 1011*t*
  antipruritic agents, **1013–1014**
  antiseborrhea agents, **1014**
  antiviral agents, **1004**
  concentration gradient and, 999
  dosing schedule and, 999
  ectoparasiticides, **1004–1005**
  keratolytic agents, **1011–1013**
  occlusion affecting efficacy of, 999
  OTC preparations, hidden ingredients in, 1037*t*, 1038*t*
  penetration variables and, 999
  pigmentation and, **1005–1006**
  psoriasis agents, **1007–1008**

regional variation in penetration and, 999
trichogenic agents, **1014**
vehicles for, 999, **999–1000**
oral contraceptives affecting, 667–668
in poisoned patient, 971
sunscreens for protection of, **1006**
thyroid hormones affecting, 625*t*
Sleep
drugs for induction of (sleep aids)
OTC preparations
efficacy of, 1035*t*
hidden ingredients in, 1037*t*, 1038*t*
sedative-hypnotics, 361–362, **365–366**
prostaglandins affecting, 310
Sleep disorders
management of, **363–364**
sedative-hypnotic drugs for, 361–362, **365–366**
Slo-Phyllin, 340. *See also* Theophylline
Slow acetylators, 58
Slow-acting antirheumatic drugs (SAARDs/disease-modifying antirheumatic drugs), 579, **590–593**
preparations available, 599–600
Slow-reacting substance of anaphylaxis, 308
Small intestinal flukes (*Heterophyes heterophyes/Metagonimus yokogawai*), drugs for infection with, 863*t*
niclosamide, 872
Smoking
aids for cessation of, OTC preparations, efficacy of, 1035*t*
coronary disease and, 564
drug metabolism affected by, 59
fetus affected by, 983*t*
Smooth muscle. *See also specific organ*
autonomic activity/drugs affecting, 83*t*
calcium channel blockers affecting, 187–188
cytochrome P450-derived metabolites affecting, 310–311
ergot alkaloids affecting, 281
ethanol affecting, 374–375
glucagon affecting, 702
histamine affecting, 264
lipoxygenase metabolites affecting, 310
methylxanthines affecting, 332
nitrates/nitrites affecting, 184
prostaglandins affecting, 309
thromboxanes affecting, 309
SMS 201-995 (octreotide), 606, 606*i*
Snake bites (rattlesnake envenomation), **978**
passive immunization for, 1057*t*
SO₂ (sulfur dioxide), **948**
threshold limit values for, 948*t*
Sodium
in cardiac conduction, 216–219
dietary restriction of, for hypertension, 155, 172

intracellular concentration of, in cardiac contractility, 198–199
in OTC preparations, hidden, 1038–1039*t*
Sodium antimony gluconate, 859. *See also* Stibogluconate
Sodium balance, antihypertensive drugs affecting, **155–157**. *See also* Diuretics
Sodium bicarbonate
in antacids, 1018*t*
as antidote, 977*t*
for methanol poisoning, 382
Sodium-calcium exchanger, in cardiac contractility, 198
Sodium channel-blocking drugs, 226, **227–234**. *See also specific type*
for arrhythmias, 226, **227–234**
local anesthetics as, 428, 428*i*
preparations available, 240
Sodium channels, 217
amiodarone affecting, 231
antiepileptic drugs affecting, 387, 389, 389*i*, 392, 396, 397, 400
in CNS, 344
lidocaine affecting, 232, 232*i*
local anesthetics affecting, 428, 428*i*
resting potential–action potential relationship and, 219–220, 221*i*
Sodium fluoride (fluoride)
bone mineral homeostasis affected by, **712**
for osteoporosis, 712, 718, 718*i*
OTC status of, 1031*t*
preparations available, 721
Sodium hypochlorite, antimicrobial effects of, 805*t*, 807
Sodium Iodide I 131 Therapeutic, 633. *See also* ¹³¹I
Sodium nitroprusside, **168**, 168*i*
preparations available, 175
Sodium-potassium pump (Na⁺-K⁺ AT-Pase)
in cardiac conduction, 216–217
in cardiac contractility, 198–199
cardiac glycoside inhibition of, 202
Sodium salicylate, 585
preparations available, 599
Sodium sulfate, for poisoned patient, 976*t*
Sodium thiosalicylate, preparations available, 599
Sodium valproate, 389*i*, **399–401**. *See also* Valproic acid
effective/toxic plasma levels of, 405*t*
as mood-stabilizer, 475, **479**
preparations available, 407
Solaskil, 878. *See also* Levamisole
Solfanal, 599. *See also* Aurothioglucose
Solu-Cortef, 650. *See also* Hydrocortisone
Solu-Medrol, 650, 940. *See also* Methylprednisolone
Solvents, **949–950**
industrial, abuse of, 529
threshold limit values for, 948*t*
Soma, 448. *See also* Carisoprodol

Soman, 97, 98*i*
Somatostatin (somatotropin release-inhibiting hormone/SRIH/growth hormone-inhibiting hormone), 604*t*, **605–606**, 606*i*, 684, 685*t*
receptors for, 604
Somatostatin analog (octreotide), 606, 606*i*
Somatotropin (growth hormone/GH), 604*t*, **606–608**
deficiency of, 607
receptors for, 604–605
Somatotropin release-inhibiting hormone (SRIH/somatostatin/growth hormone-inhibiting hormone), 604*t*, **605–606**, 606*i*, 684, 685*t*
receptors for, 604
Somatrem, 607. *See also* Growth hormone
Sorbitol
laxative effect of, 1024
for poisoned patient, 976, 976*t*
Sorbitrate, 194. *See also* Isosorbide dinitrate
Sorivudine, 790*i*, 792*t*, **794**
Sotalol, 144*t*, 229*t*, **235**, 235*i*
action potential duration affected by, 235
for arrhythmias, 146, 234, **235**
membrane actions of, 228*t*
preparations available, 150, 240
properties of, 144*t*, 229*t*
Spare receptors, 11–14
Sparfloxacin, 765, 766, 766*t*
Sparine, 480. *See also* Promazine
Spasmolytic drugs, **445–448**. *See also specific agent*
preparations available, 448
Spectazole, 786, 1002. *See also* Econazole
Spectinomycin, **759**, 759*i*
preparations available, 759
Spectrobid (bacampicillin), 740
"Speed," 521. *See also* Methamphetamine
"Speedball," 523
Sphincters
bladder
autonomic activity/drugs affecting, 83*t*
direct-acting cholinomimetics affecting, 94*t*
gastrointestinal, direct-acting cholinomimetics affecting, 94*t*
Spinal nerve block, 431*i*
Spirochetal infections, empiric antimicrobial therapy and, 815*t*
Spironolactone, 253, 253*i*, 254*t*, 649, 649*i*, 679
antiandrogen effects of, 679
in breast milk, 987*t*
chemistry and pharmacokinetics of, 253, 253*i*
half-life of, aging affecting, 992*i*
interactions of, 1068*t*
with oral anticoagulants, 554
pharmacodynamics of, 253
preparations available, 259

Splanchnic vessels, autonomic activity/drugs affecting, 83*t*

Sporanox, 786, 1004. *See also* Itraconazole

Sporonticidal agents, for malaria, 838

Sporothrix schenkii, empiric antimicrobial therapy and, 815*t*

SRIH (somatotropin release-inhibiting hormone/somatostatin/growth hormone-inhibiting hormone), 604*t*, **605–606**, 606*i*, 684, 685*t*
    receptors for, 604

SRS-A (slow-reacting substance of anaphylaxis), 308

SSKI, 633. *See also* Potassium iodide solution

SSRIs (selective serotonin reuptake inhibitors)
    adverse effects of, 493*t*
    for alcoholism, 381
    chemistry of, 484, 486*i*
    clinical indications for, 490
    dosages of, 491*t*
        for acute episode, 491
    effects of, 489
    interactions of, 492–493
    overdoses of, 493
    pharmacokinetics of, 486–487, 488*t*
    preparations available, 494

Stadol, 501*t*, 513. *See also* Butorphanol

Stage fright (performance anxiety), beta-receptor blocking drugs for, 148

Stanozolol, 675*t*
    preparations available, 680

Staphcillin, 740. *See also* Mezlocillin

Staphylococcal beta-lactamase, penicillin resistance caused by, 729–731

Staphylococcal infections
    empiric antimicrobial therapy of, 814*t*
    penicillins for, 729–731

Staphylococcus aureus, empiric antimicrobial therapy and, 814*t*

STATs, 20, 21*i*

Status epilepticus, management of, **405–406**

Stavudine, 795*t*, 796*i*, **798**
    preparations available, 801

Steatorrhea, pancreatic enzyme replacement products for, 1023

Stelazine, 472*t*, 480. *See also* Trifluoperazine

Stem cell factor (SCF), 543, 543*t*, 545

Stem cells, tumor, 881

Stenotrophomonas maltophilia, empiric antimicrobial therapy and, 814*t*

Stereoisomers (chirality), 3

Sterilants, **809**
    definition of, 805
    preparations available, 810

Sterilization, 805*t*. *See also* Sterilants

Steroids. *See also* Adrenocorticosteroids; Corticosteroids; Glucocorticoids
    anabolic, **674–677**
        abuse of, 676
        preparations available, 680
        synthetic, 675, 675*t*

in cancer chemotherapy, **898–900**, 899*t*

Sterol synthesis, parasite, antiparasitic agents affecting, 829–831

Stibogluconate
    for leishmaniasis, 855, 865
    preparations available, 859

Stilphostrol, 680. *See also* Diethylstilbestrol

Stimate, 617. *See also* Desmopressin

Stimulant laxatives, **1023**

Stimulants
    abuse of, **521–524**
    OTC preparations, hidden ingredients in, 1038*t*
    overdose of, 972*t*

Stimulus-secretion coupling, calcium channel blockers affecting, 189–190

Stomach
    cancer of, 811, 903*t*
    contents of, drug trapping in, 7*t*

Stool softeners, **1024**
    OTC preparations, efficacy of, 1035*t*

"STP," 521

Streptase, 561. *See also* Streptokinase

Streptococcus
    agalactiae, empiric antimicrobial therapy and, 814*t*
    empiric antimicrobial therapy and, 814*t*
    group B
        antimicrobial prophylaxis for exposure to, 824–825*t*
        empiric antimicrobial therapy and, 814*t*
    pneumoniae, empiric antimicrobial therapy and, 814*t*
    pyogenes, empiric antimicrobial therapy and, 814*t*
    viridans, empiric antimicrobial therapy and, 814*t*

Streptogramins, **750**
    protein synthesis affected by, 744, 744*i*

Streptokinase, 548, 550*i*, **555**
    for myocardial infarction, 555, 556
    preparations available, 561

Streptomycin, 753*i*, **754–755**, **774–775**
    adverse effects of, 754, 755, 775
    fetus affected by, 983*t*
    mechanism of action of, 752
    preparations available, 759, 779
    for tuberculosis, 754–755, 770, 771*t*, 775

Stretch reflex arc, 445, 446*i*

Stroke
    aspirin affecting risk of, 314
    oral contraceptive use and, 669

Strongyloides sterocoralis (strongyloidiasis), drugs for, 863*t*
    albendazole, 864
    ivermectin, 868
    mebendazole, 870
    thiabendazole, 877

Structural analogs (antimetabolites), **889–893**

in dermatologic therapy, 1014*t*
    mechanisms of action of, 889

Structural proteins, as drug receptors, 10

Structure-activity relationships, 27
    of local anesthetics, 429

Strychnine, ionization constant of, 6*t*

Stuart-Prower factor (factor X), 549*t*
    activated, 547
    therapeutic, 559*t*

Subacute myelo-optic neuropathy (SMON), 854

Subacute thyroiditis, **631**

Subarachnoid hemorrhage, nimodipine for prevention of sequelae of, 189

Subcutaneous route of administration, bioavailability and characteristics and, 40*t*

Subject bias, in new drug evaluation, 67

Sublimaze, 501*t*, 513. *See also* Fentanyl

Sublingual route of administration, first-pass effect and, 42

Submucosal plexus (plexus of Meissner), 74

Substance P, 77*t*, **299–300**, 352

Succimer (DMSA), 956, 957*i*, **958**
    preparations available, 966

Succinylcholine, 434, 438*t*
    cardiovascular effects of, 443–444, 443*t*
    effects of, 443*t*, 444
    mechanism of action of, 439–442, 440*i*, 440*t*, 441*i*
    pharmacokinetics of, 438*t*, 439
    preparations available, 448
    skeletal muscle paralysis caused by, 442–443, 443*i*
    structure of, 435, 435*i*

Sucralfate
    for acid-peptic disease, 272, 1021
    preparations available, 1027

Sudafed, 134. *See also* Pseudoephedrine

Sufenta, 501*t*, 514. *See also* Sufentanil

Sufentanil, 511
    pharmacokinetics of, 501*t*
    preparations available, 514

Sular, 175, 194. *See also* Nisoldipine

Sulbactam, 731, **736–737**, 736*i*

Sulbenicillin, half-life of, aging affecting, 992*i*

Sulconazole
    preparations available, 786
    topical, 1002

Sulfacetamide
    preparations available, 768
    topical, 763

Sulfacytine, 762*t*
    preparations available, 768

Sulfadiazine, 762–763, 762*i*, 762*t*, 839*i*
    ionization constant of, 6*t*
    for malaria, 839*i*, 841*t*
    preparations available, 768
    with pyrimethamine, 764

Sulfadoxine, 762*t*, 763
    with pyrimethamine (Fansidar), 764, **846–847**
        for malaria treatment, 841*t*, 845, 846

Sulfaguanidine, dihydropteroate synthesis affected by, 828
Sulfamethizole, 762*t*
  half-life of, aging affecting, 992*i*
  preparations available, 768
Sulfamethoxazole, 762, 762*i*, 762*t*
  CSF penetration by, 820*t*
  pharmacokinetic/pharmacodynamic parameters of, 37*t*
  preparations available, 768
Sulfamylon, 768. *See also* Mafenide
Sulfanilamide, 762*i*
  development of modern diuretics and, 248
  dihydropteroate synthesis affected by, 828
  structure of, 248*i*
Sulfapyridine, 762*t*
  ionization constant of, 6*t*
Sulfasalazine, **593**, 763
  for inflammatory bowel disease, 1025
  preparations available, 600, 768, 1027
Sulfate conjugation, 57*t*
Sulfathalidine (phthalylsulfathiazole), 762*i*
Sulfathiazole, dihydropteroate synthesis affected by, 828
Sulfinpyrazone, 596*i*, 597
  oral anticoagulant interactions and, 554
  preparations available, 600
Sulfisoxazole, 762, 762*i*, 762*t*
  preparations available, 768
Sulfonamides, **761–763**
  absorption of, in neonate, 984*t*
  actions of, 761, 762*i*
  adverse reactions to, 763
  dihydropteroate synthesis affected by, 828
  for malaria, **846–847**
  pharmacokinetics of, 761, 762*t*
    in neonate, 984*t*
  preparations available, 768
  resistance to, 761
Sulfones
  dihydropteroate synthesis affected by, 828
  for leprosy, **778**
  for malaria, **846–847**
Sulfonylureas, **696–699**, 697*t*. *See also* specific type
  efficacy and safety of, 698
  insulin therapy combined with, 699
  mechanism of action of, 696–697
  preparations available, 703
  second-generation, **698–699**
  secondary failure and, 699
  tachyphylaxis to, 699
Sulfur, for scabies, **1005**
Sulfur dioxide, **948–949**
  threshold limit values for, 948*t*
Sulindac, 580*t*, **587**
  preparations available, 599
Sumatriptan, 276
  for migraine headache, 282
  preparations available, 284
Sunscreens, **1006**

Sunshades, 1006
Superinfection, with cephalosporins, 736
Superoxide dismutase, nitric oxide affected by, 321
Suppositories, rectal
  bioavailability and characteristics and, 40*t*
  first-pass effect and, 42
Supprelin, 617. *See also* Histrelin
Suprane, 423. *See also* Desflurane
Suprax, 741. *See also* Cefixime
Suramin, **876**
  preparations available, 878
Surface area, pediatric dosage calculation from, 988, 988*t*
Surgical prophylaxis, 822–823, 824*t*
Surital, 423. *See also* Thiamylal
Surmontil, 494. *See also* Trimipramine
Susceptibility testing, 816–817
Suspensions, for infants and children, 985
Sweat glands
  antimuscarinic agents affecting, 110
  autonomic activity/drugs affecting, 83*t*
  direct-acting cholinomimetics affecting, 94*t*
  sympathomimetic agents affecting, 127
Symmetrel, 462, 801. *See also* Amantadine
Sympathetic nerve fibers, local anesthetics affecting, 429*t*
Sympathetic (thoracolumbar) division of autonomic nervous system, 73, 74*i*
  autonomic nerve activity/drugs affecting, 83*t*
  in central integration, 82
  renin secretion regulated by, 287–288
Sympathomimetics, **118–134**. *See also* specific agent
  alpha carbon substitutions and, 123–124
  amino group substitution and, 123
  for asthma, **333–335**, 340
  basic pharmacology of, **118–130**
  benzene ring substitutions and, 123
  beta carbon substitutions and, 124
  clinical pharmacology of, **130–133**
  for glaucoma, 132, 149*t*
  for heart failure, 206, 213
  mode and spectrum of action of, 118
  molecular mechanisms of action of, **120–123**
  organ system effects of, **124–127**
  in OTC preparations, hidden, 1039
  preparations available, 133–134, 213, 340
  receptor-selective, 129, 129*i*
  toxicity of, **133**, 334–335
Sympathoplegics, for hypertension, **157–166**
  centrally acting, **158–160**
  preparations available, 175
Synapses, **344–345**
Synaptic mimicry, 346–347
Synaptic potentials, **344–345**, 344*i*, 345*i*

Synaptic transmission, antiparasitic agents affecting, 835
Synaptotagmin, 77
Synarel, 617. *See also* Nafarelin
Syncope, quinidine, 227
Syndrome of inappropriate ADH secretion, 255
Synechia, antimuscarinic agents for prevention of, 111
Synergism
  antimicrobial combination therapy and, 821–822
  oral anticoagulant interactions and, 554
  toxicity of chemical mixtures and, 946
Synergy studies, 817
Synthroid, 633. *See also* Levothyroxine; Thyroxine
Syntocinon, 617. *See also* Oxytocin
Syprine, 462, 966. *See also* Trientine

$t_{1/2}$ (half-life), 39–40
  aging affecting, 991, 992*i*
  in neonates vs. adults, 985*t*
  therapeutic drug monitoring and, 46
T$_3$ (triiodothyronine)
  basic pharmacology of, **621–626**
  biosynthesis of, 619, 620*i*
  chemistry of, 621, 621*i*
  effects of, 623–625, 625*t*
  interactions of, 621–622, 624*t*
  mechanism of action of, 623, 624*i*
  pharmacokinetics of, 621–623, 622*t*
  reverse (rT$_3$), 621*i*
  structure of, 621*i*
T$_4$ (thyroxine)
  basic pharmacology of, **621–626**
  biosynthesis of, 619, 620*i*
  in breast milk, 987*t*
  chemistry of, 621, 621*i*
  dosages of, 628
  effects of, 625*t*
  interactions of, 621–622, 624*t*
  mechanism of action of, 623, 624*i*
  peripheral metabolism of, 620, 620*i*, 621*i*
  pharmacokinetics of, 621–623, 622*t*
  structure of, 621*i*
  toxicity of, 628
2,4,5-T (2,4,5-trichlorophenoxyacetic acid), 952–953, 953*i*
T cell receptor (TCR), 917
T foetus, purine phosphoribosyl transferases as targets in, 831
T helper lymphocytes, 918, 919*i*
T lymphocytes, in immunity, 917–918
t-PA (tissue plasminogen activator), 548, 550*i*, **555**
  for myocardial infarction, 555, 556
  recombinant (rt-PA), discovery and development of, 71
Tacaryl (methdilazine), 284
TACE, 680. *See also* Chlorotrianisene
Tachycardia, paroxysmal atrial, sympathomimetics for, 131
Tachykinins, 350*t*
  as neurotransmitters in CNS, 350*t*

Tachyphylaxis, 30
Tacrine, 100, 994
Tacrolimus (FK 506), **926**
  preparations available, 940
Taenia (taeniasis)
  albendazole for, 865
  mebendazole for, 870
  praziquantel for, 874
  saginata (beef tapeworm), drugs for, 863*t*
    niclosamide, 871
  solium (pork tapeworm), drugs for, 863*t*
    niclosamide, 871
Tagamet, 284, 1026. *See also* Cimetidine
Talwin, 501*t*, 514. *See also* Pentazocine
Tambocor, 240. *See also* Flecainide
Tamoxifen, 660, **671**, **898–900**, 899*i*, 899*t*
  for breast cancer, 909
  fetus affected by, 983*t*
  preparations available, 680
Tamsulosin, 139
Tapazole, 633. *See also* Methimazole
Tapeworms, drugs for, 863–864*t*
  niclosamide, 871
Tar compounds, for dermatologic therapy, **1009**
Taractan (chlorprothixene), 480
Tardive dyskinesia, 461, 473
Target concentration
  dosage regimen design and, **43–45**
  therapeutic monitoring and, 46
Target organs, sensitivity of, therapeutic drug monitoring and, 47
Tavist, 283. *See also* Clemastine
Taxanes, **895**
Taxol, 894*t*. *See also* Paclitaxel
Taxotere, 894*t*. *See also* Docetaxel
Tazidime, 741. *See also* Ceftazidime
Tazobactam, 731, **736–737**, 736*i*
3TC (lamivudine), 795*t*, 796*i*, **797**
  preparations available, 801
TCAs (tricyclic antidepressants)
  adverse effects of, 493*t*
  chemistry of, 484, 485*i*
  clinical indications for, 490
  dosages of, 491*t*
    for acute episode, 491
  effects of, 488
  fetus affected by, 983*t*
  interactions of, 1062*t*
  overdoses of, 493, 972*t*
  pharmacokinetics of, 484–486, 488*t*
  preparations available, 494
TCDD (2,3,7,8-tetrachlorodibenzo-*p*-dioxin), 953, 953*i*, 954
TCR (T cell receptor), 917
TD50 (median toxic dose), 29
Td vaccine, 1053*t*
TDE (tetrachlorodiphenylethane), 950*t*
TEA (tetraethylammonium), 114, 114*i*
Teeth, tetracyclines affecting, 747
Tegison, 1007. *See also* Etretinate
Tegopen, 740. *See also* Cloxacillin
Tegretol, 407, 480. *See also* Carbamazepine

Teicoplanin, **739**
Teldrin, 283. *See also* Chlorpheniramine
Telenzepine, gastric acid secretion affected by, 110
Telepaque, 633. *See also* Iopanoic acid
Telopar, 878. *See also* Oxantel/pyrantel pamoate
Temaril (trimeprazine), 284
Temazepam
  absorption of, 355
  biotransformation of, 357
  dosages of, 366*t*
  pharmacokinetics of, 358*t*
  preparations available, 369
Tempra, 600. *See also* Acetaminophen
Tenex, 175. *See also* Guanfacine
Teniposide, **894–895**
Tenizolamide, for brain tumors, 912
Tenormin, 150, 174, 194. *See also* Atenolol
Tensilon, 103. *See also* Edrophonium
Tension, of anesthetic gas, 412
Teratogen, definition of, 982
Teratogenesis
  counseling and, 982
  drugs causing, 980–982, 981*i*
    antiepileptic drugs, **406**
    antipsychotic agents, 474
    bendectin, 269
    doxylamine, 269
    ethanol, 378
    mechanisms of, 980–982
    mefloquine, 844
    phenytoin, 406
    quinine, 848
    warfarin, 552, 558
Terazosin, 138*t*, 139
  for hypertension, 165–166
  preparations available, 150, 175
Terbinafine, **785–786**
  preparations available, 786
  topical, 786, **1002**
Terbutaline, 129*i*, 334*i*
  for asthma, 333, 340
  ionization constant of, 6*t*
  pharmacokinetic/pharmacodynamic parameters of, 37*t*
  for premature labor, 132
  preparations available, 340
Terfenadine, 267*t*
  active metabolites of, 266, 268
  cardiac toxicity of, 269
  interactions of, 266, 269–270
  preparations available, 284
  structure of, 266*i*
Terramycin, 751. *See also* Oxytetracycline
p-Tertiary amylphenol, antimicrobial effects of, 807–808
Teslac (testolactone), 680
Testex, 680. *See also* Testosterone
Testicular cancer, 903*t*, **910**
Testicular descent, hCG testing in evaluation of, 613–614
Testis, **673–679**
  cancer of, 903*t*, **910**
  chemical contraception and, **679**

hormones produced by, **674–677**
  suppressors of, **677–679**
    in cancer chemotherapy, 899*t*, 900
    preparations available, 680
Testoderm, 680. *See also* Testosterone
Testolactone, preparations available, 680
Testosterone, 674, 675, 675*t*
  adverse effects of, 676
  for androgen replacement therapy, 675–676, 676*t*
  in cancer chemotherapy, 899*t*
  for oral contraception in men, 679
  ovarian, 664
  preparations available, 680
Tetanus, passive immunization for, 1057*t*
Tetanus-diphtheria vaccine, 1053*t*
Tetanus immune globulin, 1057*t*
Tetrabenazine, for Huntington's disease, 460
Tetracaine
  preparations available, 433
  properties of, 426*t*
  structure of, 426*t*
2,3,7,8-Tetrachlorodibenzo-*p*-dioxin (TCDD), 953, 953*i*, 954
Tetrachlorodiphenylethane (TDE), 950*t*
Tetrachloroethylene, **876**
  threshold limit values for, 948*t*
Tetracycline, 745, 745*i*
  in breast milk, 987*t*
  fetus affected by, 983*t*
  half-life of, aging affecting, 992*i*
  for malaria treatment, 841*t*
  oral dosage for, 746
  pharmacokinetic/pharmacodynamic parameters of, 37*t*, 745–746
  preparations available, 751
  topical, for acne, 1001
Tetracyclines, **745–747**
  adverse reactions to, 746–747
  for amebiasis, 850, 854–855
  antimicrobial activity of, 745
  chemistry of, 745
  clinical uses of, 746
  overuse of, medical and social implications of, 747
  pharmacokinetics of, 745–746
  preparations available, 751
  protein synthesis affected by, 744, 744*i*, 745
  resistance to, 745
    overuse and, 747
  structures of, 745*i*
Tetraethylammonium, 114, 114*i*
Tetrahydroaminoacridine (tacrine/THA), 100, 994
Δ^9Tetrahydrocannabinol (THC), 526–527, 527*i*
  antiemetic action of, 528, 1022
  clinical effects of, 528
  mechanism of action of, 527–528
  therapeutic uses of, 528, 1022
Tetrahydrozoline, preparations available, 134
Tetrodotoxin, sodium channels affected by, 428
TF (tissue factor), 547, 549*i*

TFPI (tissue factor pathway inhibitor), 547–548

6-TG (thioguanine), **891–892**, 891*t*, 892*i*

TGFβ (transforming growth factor-beta), ligand-regulated transmembrane enzymes in signalling by, 19–20

T$_H$1, 918

T$_H$2, 918

THA (tacrine/tetrahydroaminoacridine), 100, 994

Thalidomide
  drug testing methods affected by experience with, 67
  fetus affected by, 983*t*
  immunosuppressive actions of, 927

THC (Δ^{9}tetrahydrocannabinol), 526–527, 527*i*
  antiemetic action of, 528, 1022
  clinical effects of, 528
  mechanism of action of, 527–528
  therapeutic uses of, 528, 1022

Theelin, 680. *See also* Estrone

Theo-24, 340. *See also* Theophylline

Theo-Dur, 340. *See also* Theophylline

Theobromine, 330*i*
  for asthma, 330–333

Theophylline, 330–333, 330*i*
  for asthma, 332–333
  in breast milk, 987*t*
  half-life of, 985*t*
  interactions of, 1069*t*
  ionization constant of, 6*t*
  pharmacokinetic/pharmacodynamic parameters of, 37*t*, 331–332
    in neonates, 985*t*
  preparations available, 340

Therapeutic dose dependence, 520

Therapeutic drug monitoring, **45–47**
  of antidepressant levels, 492
  of lithium levels, 477–478

Therapeutic index, 29

Thermoregulation
  antimuscarinic agents affecting, 110
  autonomic activity/drugs affecting, 83*t*
  ganglion-blocking drugs affecting, 115

Thiabendazole, **877–878**
  preparations available, 878

Thiamine
  deficiency of, in Wernicke-Korsakoff syndrome, 376
  in initial management of poisoned patient, 970–971
  preparations available, 383

Thiamine transporter, antiparasitic agents affecting, 834

Thiamylal, 420
  preparations available, 423

Thiazides, **251–253**, 252*i*
  bone mineral homeostasis affected by, **711**
  development of, 248
  for diabetes insipidus, 259
  for hypertension, 258
  for idiopathic hypercalciuria, 719
  with loop agents, **256**
    urinary electrolyte patterns affected by, 257*t*

with potassium-sparing diuretics, **256**
  urinary electrolyte patterns affected by, 257*t*

Thiazolidinedione derivatives, **701**
  preparations available, 703

Thienobenzodiazepine, 468*t*

Thimerosal
  antimicrobial effects of, 809
  preparations available, 810

Thioamides, **626–627**, 626*i*

Thiobarbiturates, distribution of, 355

Thiocyl (sodium thiosalicylate), 599

Thioguanine, **891–892**, 891*t*, 892*i*

Thiopental, 362, 411*i*, 420, 420*t*
  distribution of, 355, 420, 421*i*
  preparations available, 423

Thiophosphate insecticides, 97, 98*i*
  absorption/distribution/metabolism of, 98–99

6-Thiopurines, **891–892**

Thiopurinol, nucleoside phosphotransferases affected by, 829

Thioridazine, 466*i*
  advantages and disadvantages of, 471*t*
  cardiac toxicity of, 474
  dose relationships of, 472*t*
  in elderly, 993
  half-life of, aging affecting, 992*i*
  ionization constant of, 6*t*
  preparations available, 480
  receptor binding by, 468

Thiosalicylate, preparations available, 599

Thiosulfil, 768. *See also* Sulfamethizole

Thiotepa, 886*i*, 890*t*

Thiothixene, 466*i*, 468*t*, 471–472
  advantages and disadvantages of, 471*t*
  dose relationships of, 472*t*
  preparations available, 480

Thioxanthenes, 465, 466*i*, 468*t*
  advantages and disadvantages of, 471*t*

Thoracic surgery, antimicrobial prophylaxis and, 824*t*

Thoracolumbar (sympathetic) division of autonomic nervous system, 73, 74*i*
  in central integration, 82
  renin secretion regulated by, 287–288

Thoracys, 935. *See also* Bacille Calmette-Guerin

Thorazine, 471*t*, 472*t*, 480. *See also* Chlorpromazine

Thorn apple, 105

Threadworm (*Strongyloides stercoralis* /strongyloidiasis), drugs for, 863*t*
  albendazole, 864
  ivermectin, 868
  mebendazole, 870
  thiabendazole, 877

Threshold limit values (TLV), 945, 948*t*

Thrombin (factor IIa), 547

Thrombocytopenic purpura, idiopathic immunosuppressive agents for, 931*t*, 932, 933
  passive immunization for, 1056*t*

Thromboembolism
  drugs for, **557–558**
  fibrinolytic agents for, 555, 558

oral contraceptive use and, 667, 669
  paradoxical, heparin-induced platelet aggregation and, 551
  tetracyclines causing, 747

Thrombogenesis, 547–548, 548*i*
  drugs for management of disorders associated with, **547–562**. *See also specific type*

Thromboplastin
  plasma component (Christmas factor/factor IX), 549*t*
    deficiency of, 559, 559*t*
    preparations available, 561
  tissue (factor III), 549*t*

Thromboplastin time, partial (PTT), for heparin monitoring, 551

Thromboxane A$_2$ (TXA$_2$), 547, 556
  aspirin affecting, 556

Thromboxanes, **304–318**, 305. *See also* Eicosanoids
  blood affected by, 314–315
  bronchoconstriction caused by, 315
  effects of, 308–310
  receptors for, 308
  synthesis of, 306–307, 306*i*

Thrombus
  formation of, 547–548, 548*i*
  red, 547
  white, 547

Thymic humoral factor, 933

Thymopentin, 933

Thymopoietin, 934*t*

Thymosin, 933

Thymosin α-1, 933

Thypinone, 617. *See also* Protirelin

Thyrar, 633. *See also* Thyroid desiccated

Thyroglobulin, 619

Thyroid desiccated, 625–626. *See also* Thyroid hormones
  preparations available, 633

Thyroid dysfunction
  amiodarone causing, 231
  drug metabolism affected in, 61

Thyroid function tests, normal values for, 622*t*

Thyroid gland
  abnormal stimulators of, 620
  autoregulation of, 620
  cancer of, 903*t*, **910**
  control of function of, 620, 622*t*, 623*i*
  enlargement of
    in nontoxic goiter, 632
    toxic goiter, 631
  lithium affecting, 478
  neoplasms of, **632**
  physiology of, **619–620**, 620*i*, 621*i*
  pituitary relationships and, 620, 623*i*

Thyroid hormones
  basic pharmacology of, **621–626**
  biosynthesis of, 619, 620*i*
  chemistry of, 621, 621*i*
  clinical pharmacology of, **628–632**
  effects of, 625*t*
  excessive ingestion of (thyrotoxicosis factitia), **631**
  interactions of, 621–622, 624*t*
  mechanism of action of, 623, 624*i*

Thyroid hormones *(cont.)*
  peripheral metabolism of, 620, 620*i*, 621*i*
  pharmacokinetics of, 621–623, 622*t*
  preparations available, 625–626, 633
  receptors for, 18
  structures of, 621*i*
  transport of, 619
Thyroid-stimulating hormone (TSH/thyrotropin), 604*t*, **608–609**, 620
  receptors for, 604
  second messenger for, 22*t*
Thyroid-stimulating immunoglobulin (TSI/TSH receptor-stimulating antibody), 620
  in Graves' disease, 630
  neonatal Graves' disease caused by, 632
Thyroid storm, 631
Thyroid Strong, 633. *See also* Thyroid desiccated
Thyroidectomy, for Graves' disease, 630
Thyroiditis
  Hashimoto's, 628, 629*t*, 632
  subacute, **631**
Thyrolar (liotrix), 633
Thyrotoxic crisis, 631
Thyrotoxicosis (hyperthyroidism), **629–632**
  beta-receptor blocking drug use masking signs of, 149
  beta-receptor blocking drugs for, 147–148, **628**
  drug metabolism affected in, 61
  factitia, **631**
  [131]I for treatment of, 627–628, 630
Thyrotropin-releasing hormone (TRH/protirelin), 604*t*, **608**, 620, 623*i*
  receptors for, 604
  second messenger for, 22*t*
Thyroxine-binding globulin, oral contraceptives affecting, 667
Thyroxine (T₄)
  basic pharmacology of, **621–626**
  biosynthesis of, 619, 620*i*
  in breast milk, 987*t*
  chemistry of, 621, 621*i*
  dosages of, 628
  effects of, 625*t*
  interactions of, 621–622, 624*t*
  mechanism of action of, 623, 624*i*
  peripheral metabolism of, 620, 620*i*, 621*i*
  pharmacokinetics of, 621–623, 622*t*
  structure of, 621*i*
  toxicity of, 628
Thytropar, 617. *See also* Thyrotropin
Tiagabine, **397–398**, 398*i*
Ticar, 740. *See also* Ticarcillin
Ticarcillin, 726*i*, 731
  with clavulanate potassium, preparations available, 740
  dosing guidelines for, 730*t*
  preparations available, 740
Tice, 935. *See also* Bacille Calmette-Guerin (BCG)

Ticlid, 561. *See also* Ticlopidine
Ticlopidine, **557**
  preparations available, 561
Tics, 450, 460
Tidal volume, inhaled anesthetics affecting, 417
Tilade, 340. *See also* Nedocromil
Time course of drug effect, **42–43**, 43*i*
Timentin, 740. *See also* Ticarcillin
Timolol, 138*t*, 143*i*, 145
  for glaucoma, 147, 149*t*
  for myocardial infarction prevention, 557
  preparations available, 150, 175
  properties of, 144*t*
Timoptic, 150. *See also* Timolol
Tinactin (tolnaftate), 1002–1003
Tincture of iodine, preparations available, 810
Tincture of opium, in OTC preparations, efficacy of, 1034*t*
Tindal (acetophenazine), 480
Tinea nigra palmaris, thiabendazole for, 877
Tinea versicolor, imidazoles for, 1002
Tinidazole, for amebiasis, 850
Tioconazole, OTC status of, 1032*t*
Tiotropium, for COPD, 111
Tissue amebicides, 850
Tissue factor, 547, 549*i*
Tissue factor pathway inhibitor, 547–548
Tissue plasminogen activator (t-PA), 548, 550*i*, **555**
  for myocardial infarction, 555, 556
  recombinant (rt-PA), discovery and development of, 71
Tissue schizonticides, for malaria, 838
Tissue thromboplastin (factor III), 549*t*
Tixocortol pivalate, for inflammatory bowel disease, 1026
Tizanidine, 159, **447**
  preparations available, 448
TLV (threshold limit values), 945, 948*t*
TMP-SMZ (trimethoprim-sulfamethoxazole), **763–765**
  intravenous, 764, 768
  preparations available, 768, 859
TNFα (tumor necrosis factor-α), 934–935, 934*t*
  in inflammation, 579*t*
TNFβ (tumor necrosis factor-β), 934*t*
Tobramycin, 754*i*, **756–758**
  adverse effects of, 754, 758
  pharmacokinetic/pharmacodynamic parameters of, 37*t*, 756
  preparations available, 759
Tocainide, **233**, 233*i*
  for arrhythmias, **233**
  clinical properties of, 229*t*
  membrane actions of, 228*t*
  pharmacokinetic/pharmacodynamic parameters of, 37*t*
  preparations available, 240
Tocolytic, indomethacin as, 589
TOCP (triorthocresyl phosphate), toxicity of, 951–952
Tofranil, 494. *See also* Imipramine

Tolazamide, 697*t*, **698**
  preparations available, 703
Tolazoline, 136, 137*i*, 138*t*, 139
  ionization constant of, 6*t*
  preparations available, 150
Tolbutamide, 697*t*, **698**
  in breast milk, 987*t*
  ionization constant of, 6*t*
  pharmacokinetic/pharmacodynamic parameters of, 37*t*
  preparations available, 703
Tolectin, 599. *See also* Tolmetin
Tolerance, 30, 516. *See also specific agent or drug class*
Tolinase, 697*t*, 703. *See also* Tolazamide
Tolmetin, 580*t*, 586*i*, **588**
  preparations available, 599
Tolnaftate, **1002–1003**
  in OTC preparations, efficacy of, 1034*t*
Tolrestat, 701
Tolterodine, 112
Toluene, 950
  structure of, 529*i*
  threshold limit values for, 948*t*
Tonic-clonic seizures, generalized, 403–404
  drugs used in, **388–398**, 404
Tonocard, 240. *See also* Tocainide
Tooth (teeth), tetracyclines affecting, 747
Topamax, 407. *See also* Topiramate
Topical (transdermal) route of administration
  bioavailability and characteristics and, 40*t*
  for dermatologic medications, 999–1000
  first-pass effect and, 42
  for opioid analgesics, 508
Topicycline, 1001. *See also* Tetracycline
Topiramate, **397**, 397*i*
  preparations available, 407
Topoisomerase II, fluoroquinolone blockade of, 765
Topoisomerse IV, fluoroquinolone blockade of, 765
Topotecan, 894*t*, **895**
Toprol, 150. *See also* Metoprolol
Toradol, 599. *See also* Ketorolac
Tornalate, 340. *See also* Bitolterol
Torsade de pointes, 223, 223*i*
  bepridil causing, 191
  H₁ receptor antagonists causing, development of active metabolites and, 268
  quinidine causing, 227, 239
Torsemide
  clinical indications/dosage of, 250*t*
  contraindications to, 251
  pharmacokinetics of, 250
  preparations available, 259
Torticollis, antipsychotic agents causing, 473
Torulopsis, empiric antimicrobial therapy and, 815*t*
Total body water, drug distribution in, 39*t*

Tourette's syndrome, 450, 460
   antipsychotic agents for, 470
Toxaphenes, 950–951, 950*t*
Toxic goiter, uninodular and multinodu-
      lar, **631**
Toxic metabolites, **55–56**, 57*i. See also*
      Reactive metabolites
Toxicity. *See also specific substance*
   definition of, 946
   delayed, 946
   drug-drug interactions and, 1060
Toxicity testing, in new drug develop-
      ment, 63*i*, **64–66**, 66*t*
Toxicodynamics, **969**
Toxicokinetics, **968–969**
Toxicology, **945–955**. *See also specific
      substance*
   definition of, 1
   environmental, 945–946
      insecticides and, 951, 952
   environmental considerations in,
      946–947
   occupational, 945
   terms/definitions used in, **946**
Toxicology screen, 974
Toxocariasis
   albendazole for, 865
   diethylcarbamazine for, 867
Toxoplasma (toxoplasmosis)
   antimicrobial prophylaxis and, 825*t*
   gondii, drugs for, 855*t*
   pyrimethamine for, 845–846
t-PA (tissue plasminogen activator), 548,
      550*i*, **555**
   for myocardial infarction, 555, 556
   recombinant (rt-PA), discovery and
      development of, 71
TPO (thymopoietin), 934*t*
Tracrium, 448. *See also* Atracurium
Tramadol, 512
   preparations available, 514
Trandate, 150, 174. *See also* Labetalol
Tranexamic acid, 560
   preparations available, 561
Transderm-Nitro, 194. *See also* Nitro-
      glycerin
Transdermal (topical) route of adminis-
      tration
   bioavailability and characteristics and,
      40*t*
   for dermatologic medications,
      999–1000
   first-pass effect and, 42
   for opioid analgesics, 508
Transferrin, iron content of, 534*t*
Transforming growth factor-beta, ligand-
      regulated transmembrane enzymes
      in signalling by, 19–20
Transmembrane enzymes, ligand-regu-
      lated, 19–20, 20*i*
   endogenous, drug responsiveness af-
      fected by, 30
Transmembrane signalling, **17–27**, 18*i.
      See also* Signalling mechanisms
Transplant rejection
   cell-mediated, prostaglandins affect-
      ing, 315–316
   nitric oxide and, 323

Transplantation
   immunosuppressive therapy and,
      931–932, 931*t*
   nitric oxide and, **323**
Transport proteins, as drug receptors, 10
Tranxene, 366*t*, 369, 383, 407. *See also*
      Clorazepate
Tranylcypromine, 484, 487*i*
   dosages of, 491*t*
   pharmacokinetics of, 487
   preparations available, 494
Trasylol, 561. *See also* Aprotinin
Travel, recommended immunizations
      and, **1057–1008**
Traveler's diarrhea, antimuscarinic
      agents for, 111–112
Trazodone, 484, 485*i*
   adverse effects of, 493*t*
   dosages of, 491*t*
   effects of, 488–489, 489*t*
   pharmacokinetics of, 486, 488*t*
   preparations available, 494
Trecator-SC, 778. *See also* Ethionamide
Tremor, 450, 459
   beta-receptor blocking drugs for, 148
   lithium causing, 478
Trental (pentoxifylline), 340
Treponema, empiric antimicrobial ther-
      apy and, 815*t*
Tretinoin. *See also* Retinoic acid for
      acne, 1006–1007
TRH (thyrotropin-releasing
      hormone/protirelin), 604*t*, **608**,
      620, 623*i*
   receptors for, 604
   second messenger for, 22*t*
Triamcinolone, 640*t*
   aerosol form of, 646
   for asthma, 336, 646
      preparations available, 340
   preparations available, 650
   structure of, 641*i*
Triamterene, 253, 253*i*, 254*t*
   chemistry and pharmacokinetics of,
      253, 253*i*
   interactions of, 1068*t*
   preparations available, 259
Triazolam, 356*i*
   absorption of, 355
   biotransformation of, 357*i*, 358
   distribution of, 355
   dosages of, 366*t*
   pharmacokinetics of, 358*t*
   preparations available, 369
   toxicity of, 367
Triazoles, 783, 783*i. See also specific
      type*
Trichinella spiralis (trichinosis), drugs
      for, 863*t*
   mebendazole, 870
Trichlorfon, 951*t*
Trichlormethiazide
   dosages of, 252*t*
   preparations available, 259
1,1,1-Trichloroethane, threshold limit
      values for, 948*t*
Trichloroethanol, 357*i*, 364

Trichloroethylene
   structure of, 529*i*
   threshold limit values for, 948*t*
2,4,5-Trichlorophenoxyacetic acid (2,4,5-
      T), 952–953, 953*i*
Trichogenic agents, **1014**
Trichomonas vaginalis (trichomoniasis)
   metronidazole for, 857–858
   pyrimidine metabolism in, 829, 830*i*
   treatment of, **857–858**
Trichostrongylus
   drugs for, 863*t*
      levamisole, 869
      mebendazole, 869
   orientalis, pyrantel for, 876
Trichuris trichiura (trichuriasis), drugs
      for, 863*t*
   albendazole, 864
   mebendazole, 869
Tricyclic antidepressants
   adverse effects of, 493*t*
   chemistry of, 484, 485*i*
   clinical indications for, 490
   dosages of, 491*t*
      for acute episode, 491
   effects of, 488
   fetus affected by, 983*t*
   interactions of, 1062*t*
   overdoses of, 493, 972*t*
   pharmacokinetics of, 484–486, 488*t*
   preparations available, 494
Tridihexethyl
   for gastrointestinal and genitourinary
      conditions, 112*t*
   preparations available, 116, 1027
Tridil, 194. *See also* Nitroglycerin
Tridione, 407. *See also* Trimethadione
Trientine (triethylenetramine), **959**
   preparations available, 462
   for Wilson's disease, 461, 959
Triethylenemelamine, 886*i*
Triethylenethiophosphoramide, 890*t. See
      also* Thiotepa
Triethylenetramine (trientine), **959**
   preparations available, 462
   for Wilson's disease, 461, 959
Trifluoperazine, 466*i*
   dose relationships of, 472*t*
   preparations available, 480
Triflupromazine, preparations available,
      480
Trifluridine (trifluorothymidine), 792*t*,
      794
   preparations available, 801
"Trigger" calcium, in cardiac contractil-
      ity, 198, 198*i*
Trigone (bladder), direct-acting choli-
      nomimetics affecting, 94*t*
Trihexyphenidyl
   for parkinsonism, 457*t*
   preparations available, 462
Triiodothyronine (T$_3$)
   basic pharmacology of, **621–626**
   biosynthesis of, 619, 620*i*
   chemistry of, 621, 621*i*
   effects of, 623–625, 625*t*
   interactions of, 621–622, 624*t*

Triiodothyronine (T₃) (cont.)
mechanism of action of, 623, 624*i*
pharmacokinetics of, 621–623, 622*t*
reverse (rT₃), 621*i*
structure of, 621*i*
Trilafon, 472*t*, 480. *See also* Perphenazine
Tri-Levlen, 665*t*
Trilostane, **649**
Trimeprazine, preparations available, 284
Trimethadione, 401–402, 401*i*
fetus affected by, 983*t*
preparations available, 407
Trimethaphan, 114, **161**
Trimethoprim, **763–765**, 839*i*
actions of, 762*i*
adverse effects of, 764–765
CSF penetration by, 820*t*
pharmacokinetic/pharmacodynamic parameters of, 37*t*, 762*t*
preparations available, 768
resistance to, 763
Trimethoprim-sulfamethoxazole, **763–765**
intravenous, 764, 768
preparations available, 768, 859
Trimipramine, 485*i*
dosages of, 491*t*
preparations available, 494
Trimpex, 768. *See also* Trimethoprim
Tri-Norinyl, 665*t*
Triorthocresyl phosphate (TOCP), toxicity of, 102, 951–952
Triostat, 633. *See also* Liothyronine
Trioxsalen, **1006**
Tripelennamine, 267*t*
preparations available, 284
structure of, 266*i*
Triphasil, 665*t*
"Triple response," histamine causing, 264
Tripotassium dicitrato bismuthate, for acid-peptic disease, 1021
Triprolidine
in OTC preparations, efficacy of, 1033*t*
OTC status of, 1032*t*
preparations available, 284
Trisulfapyrimidines. *See also* Sulfonamides
preparations available, 768
Trivalent antimonials, antiparasitic actions of, 836*t*, **865**
Trobicin, 759. *See also* Spectinomycin
Troglitazone, 701
preparations available, 703
Troleandomycin, drug metabolism inhibited by, 60*t*
Tronothane, 432. *See also* Pramoxine
Trophoblastic neoplasms, 903*t*
Trophotropic system, parasympathetic system as, 82
Tropical eosinophilia, drugs for, 863*t*
diethylcarbamazine, 867
Tropicamide, 107*i*
ophthalmologic uses of, 111*t*
preparations available, 116

Trovafloxacin, 765
Truncal rigidity, opioid analgesics causing, 505
Trusopt, 259. *See also* Dorzolamide
Trypanosoma (trypanosomiasis)
brucei brucei, glycolytic pathway in, 833, 833*i*
brucei gambiense, drugs for, 855*t*
suramin, 876
brucei rhodesiense, drugs for, 855*t*
suramin, 876
cruzi, drugs for, 855*t*
drugs for, **856–857**
pentamidine, 856
Trypanothione reductase, antiparasitic agents affecting, 829
Trypsin, in pancreatic enzyme replacement products, 1023*t*
TSH (thyroid-stimulating hormone/thyrotropin), 604*t*, **608–609**, 620
receptors for, 604
second messenger for, 22*t*
TSH receptor-stimulating antibody (TSH-R Ab[stim]/thyroid-stimulating immunoglobulin/TSI), 620
in Graves' disease, 630
neonatal Graves' disease caused by, 632
TSI (thyroid-stimulating immunoglobulin/TSH receptor-stimulating antibody), 620
in Graves' disease, 630
neonatal Graves' disease caused by, 632
Tuberculosis
antimicrobial prophylaxis and, 825*t*
drugs for, 771*t*
combination therapy, 772, 772*t*
first-line, 770–775, 771*t*
preparations available, 778–779
resistance to, 770
second-line, 771*t*, **775–777**
streptomycin for, 754–755
Tuberoinfundibular system, 467
Tubocurarine, 434, 435, 436*i*, 438*t*
cardiovascular effects of, 443, 443*t*
effects of, 443*t*
mechanism of action of, 439, 440*i*, 440*t*
pharmacokinetic/pharmacodynamic parameters of, 37*t*, 438*t*
preparations available, 448
skeletal muscle paralysis caused by, 442, 442*i*
Tubulins, antiparasitic agents affecting, 834–835
Tularemia, streptomycin for, 755
Tumor necrosis factor-α, 934, 934*t*, 935
in inflammation, 579*t*
Tumor necrosis factor-β, 934*t*
Tumor stem cells, 881
Tumor suppressor genes, 881
Tums, 721. *See also* Calcium
Tusal (sodium thiosalicylate), 599
TXA₂ (thromboxane A₂), 547, 556
aspirin affecting, 556

Tylenol, 600. *See also* Acetaminophen
with codeine, 514
Tylox (oxycodone, with acetaminophen), 514
Typhoid vaccine, 1054*t*
Tyramine, 129–130, 130*t*
Tyrosine kinases, receptor, 19–20, 20*i*
Tyzine (tetrahydrozoline), 134

Ulcerative colitis, drugs used in management of, **1025–1026**
Ultane, 423. *See also* Sevoflurane
Ultiva, 514. *See also* Remifentanil
Ultram, 514. *See also* Tramadol
Ultra-short-acting insulin (insulin lispro), 689–690, 690*t*
Ultraviolet light, with psoralens, for repigmentation, 1006
Unasyn, 740. *See also* Ampicillin-sulbactam
Unipen, 740. *See also* Nafcillin
Uniphyl, 340. *See also* Theophylline
United States Pharmacopeial Convention, 1043
Univase, 175. *See also* Moexipril
Unstable angina, 179
management of, 193–194
nitrates for, 186
Upper motor neuron disease, neuromuscular blockade affected by, 444–445
Uracel, 599. *See also* Sodium salicylate
Uracil, 892*i*
Urapidil, 140, 166
Urea, in dermatologic therapy, **1012**
Urecholine, 103. *See also* Bethanechol
Ureidopenicillins, 731
Ureters, antimuscarinic agents affecting, 110
Urex, 810. *See also* Methenamine hippurate
Uric acid, 598*i*
Uricosuric agents, **597**
Urinary alkalinization, carbonic anhydrase inhibitors for, 248
Urinary antiseptics, **804**
Urinary obstruction, alpha-receptor blocking drugs for, 141
Urinary pH manipulation, in poisoning, 978
Urinary tract. *See also* Genitourinary system
cholinesterase inhibitors affecting, 99
Urinary tract disorders
antimuscarinic agents for, 112, 112*t*
cholinomimetics for, 100–101
sulfonamides causing, 763
Urinary tract infections
antimicrobial prophylaxis and, 825*t*
fluoroquinolones for, 766
Urination (micturition), antimuscarinic agents affecting, 110
Urine, drug trapping in, 7*t*
Urine volume, increasing, osmotic diuretics for, 255
Urispas (flavoxate), 115, 1027
Urofollitropin, 612, **612–613**

Urogenital trichomoniasis, metronidazole for, 857–858
Urokinase, 548, 550*i*, **555**
  for myocardial infarction, 555
  preparations available, 561
Ursodiol, 1024–1025
  preparations available, 1028
Urticaria, H₁ receptor antagonists for, 268–269
USP DI, 1043
Uterus
  adrenoceptors in, 126
  choriocarcinoma of, **909–910**
  ergot alkaloids affecting, 279*t*, 280
  ethanol affecting, 375
  inhaled anesthetics affecting, 418
  opioid analgesics affecting, 506
  oral contraceptives affecting, 666
  during pregnancy, autonomic activity/drugs affecting, 83*t*
  prostaglandins affecting, 310

V_d (volume of distribution), 34–35. *See also* Distribution
  drug concentration and
    initial predictions, 47–48
    revising predictions, 48–49
  poisoning and, 968
  therapeutic drug monitoring and, 46
V_1 receptors, 295–296, 616
V_2 receptors, 295, 616
V-Cillin, 740. *See also* Penicillin V
Vaccines, **1051–1058**
  active immunization and, **1051**, 1052–1054*t*, 1055*t*
  for adults, for travel, **1057–1058**
  cytokines as adjuncts to, 934
  legal liability for untoward reactions and, **1055–1057**
  passive immunization and, **1051–1055**, 1056–1057*t*
Vaccinia, passive immunization for, 1057*t*
Vaccinia immune globulin, 1057*t*
Vagina, cancer of, estrogen therapy and, 660
Vaginal secretions, drug trapping in, 7*t*
Valacyclovir, **791**, 792*t*
  in dermatologic therapy, 1004
  preparations available, 801
Valium, 366*t*, 369, 383, 407, 423, 448, 973*t*. *See also* Diazepam
Valmid (ethinamate), 369
Valpin, 115, 1026. *See also* Anisotropine
Valproate, 389*i*, **399–401**. *See also* Valproic acid
  effective/toxic plasma levels of, 405*t*
  as mood-stabilizer, 475, **479**
  preparations available, 407
Valproic acid, **399–401**, 400*i*. *See also* Valproate
  fetus affected by, 983*t*
  as mood-stabilizer, 475, **479**
  pharmacokinetic/pharmacodynamic parameters of, 37*t*, 400
  preparations available, 407, 480

Valsartan, 291
  for hypertension, 171–172
  preparations available, 175
Valtrex, 801. *See also* Valacyclovir
Vanceril, 340. *See also* Beclomethasone
Vancocin, 741. *See also* Vancomycin
Vancoled, 741. *See also* Vancomycin
Vancomycin, **737–739**
  CSF penetration by, 820*t*
  dosing guidelines for, 730*t*
  pharmacokinetic/pharmacodynamic parameters of, 37*t*, 738
  preparations available, 741
  resistance to, 727, 738
Vansil, 878. *See also* Oxamniquine
Vantin, 741. *See also* Cefpodoxime
Vaporole, 194. *See also* Amyl nitrite
Variant angina, 179. *See also* Angina pectoris
  ergonovine in diagnosis of, 282
  management of, 193
    nitrates for, 186
Varicella
  active immunization for, 1054*t*
  passive immunization for, 1057*t*
  sorivudine for, 794
Varicella-zoster immune globulin, 1057*t*
  preparations available, 801
Varicella zoster virus, acyclovir for, 790–791
Vascor, 194, 240. *See also* Bepridil
Vascular disease
  oral contraceptive use and, 669
  peripheral
    alpha-receptor blocking drugs for, 141
    prostaglandin E and prostacyclin for, 314
Vascular resistance, alpha-receptor antagonists affecting, 136
Vascular smooth muscle. *See also* Vasoconstriction; Vasodilation
  calcium channel blockers affecting, 187–188
  depolarization of, angina management and, 180–181, 182–183
  ergot alkaloids affecting, 278, 280, 280*i*, 281*i*
  nitrates/nitrites affecting, 183–184, 183*i*
  nitric oxide affecting, **322**
  prostaglandins affecting, 309
  sympathomimetic agents affecting, 124
  thromboxanes affecting, 309
Vascular surgery, antimicrobial prophylaxis and, 824*t*
Vascular tone, determinants of, 180–181
Vasculitis, immune, drugs causing, 939
Vasoactive intestinal peptide, 77*t*, **298–299**
Vasoactive peptides, **287–303**. *See also* specific type
Vasoconstriction. *See also* Vascular smooth muscle
  alpha agonist infiltration causing, phentolamine for relief of, 141

endothelins causing, 297–298
  signal transduction mechanisms in, 298, 299*i*
  ergot alkaloids causing, 278, 280, 280*i*, 281*i*, 283
  thromboxanes causing, 309
  vasopressin causing, 295–296
Vasodilation. *See also* Vascular smooth muscle
  kinins causing, 294
  neurotensin causing, 300
  nitric oxide causing, 322
  peripheral, after myocardial infarction, 211*t*, 212
  prostaglandins causing, 309
  substance P causing, 299
  vasoactive intestinal peptide causing, 298–299
Vasodilators
  for angina, **179–196**
    basic pharmacology of, **181–192**
    clinical pharmacology of, **192–194**
  compensatory responses to, 166, 167*i*
  for heart failure, 207, 209–210, 210*t*
  for hypertension, **166–169**
  mechanisms and sites of action of, 166
  preparations available, 175
Vasopressin (antidiuretic hormone/ADH), **295–296**, **616–617**
  antagonists of, **255–256**, **285–286**
  dosage of, 616
  elevated levels of, 255
  factor VIII activity affected by, 560, 616
  receptors for, **285–286**
  second messenger for, 22*t*
  structure of, 615*i*
  syndrome of inappropriate secretion of, 255
  water excretion affected by, 246, 246*i*, 255
Vasospasm, 547
  ergotamine and ergonovine causing, 278, 281*i*, 283
Vasospastic angina, 179. *See also* Angina pectoris
  management of, 193
    nitrates for, 186
Vasotec, 175, 213. *See also* Enalapril
Vasotocin, 295–296
Vasoxyl, 134. *See also* Methoxamine
Vatronol, 133. *See also* Ephedrine
V-Cillin, 740. *See also* Penicillin V
Vecuronium, 437*i*, 438*t*
  effects of, 443*t*
  pharmacokinetics of, 438, 438*t*
  preparations available, 448
Veins, direct-acting cholinomimetics affecting, 94*t*
Velban, 894*t*. *See also* Vinblastine
Velnacrine, for Alzheimer's disease, 994
Velosef, 741. *See also* Cephradine
Velosulin, 690*t*, 692. *See also* Insulin
Venlafaxine, 484, 486*i*
  adverse effects of, 493*t*

Venlafaxine *(cont.)*
  dosages of, 491*t*
    for acute episode, 491
  effects of, 489*t*
  pharmacokinetics of, 486, 488*t*
  preparations available, 494
Venous thrombosis, **558**
  fibrinolytic agents for, 555, 558
  oral contraceptive use and, 669
  tetracyclines causing, 747
Ventilation
  neuromuscular blocking drugs in control of, 445
  pulmonary, anesthetic gas tension and, 412, 414*i*
Ventolin, 340. *See also* Albuterol
Ventricles (cardiac), direct-acting cholinomimetics affecting, 94*t*, 95
Ventricular arrhythmias, beta-receptor blocking drugs for, 147
Ventricular infarction. *See also* Myocardial infarction
  right, 211*t*, 212
Ventricular septal defect, myocardial infarction and, 211*t*, 212
VePesid, 894*t*. *See also* Etoposide
Verapamil, 189*t*, 190*t*, 229*t*, **236**
  for arrhythmias, **236**
  chemistry of, 187, 188*i*
  clinical properties of, 190*t*, 229*t*
  for hypertension, 169
  membrane actions of, 228*t*
  P170 glycoprotein affected by, 190
  pharmacokinetic/pharmacodynamic parameters of, 37*t*, 187, 189*t*, 236
  preparations available, 175, 194, 240
  vascular selectivity of, 190*t*
Veratridine, sodium channels affected by, 428
Veratrum alkaloids, antihypertensive effect of, 157
Verelan, 175. *See also* Verapamil
Vermizine, 878. *See also* Piperazine
Vermox, 878. *See also* Mebendazole
Verruca vulgaris. *See also* Warts
  cantharidin for, 1012–1013
Versed, 369, 423. *See also* Midazolam
Very low density lipoproteins (VLDL), 563, 565*t*
  synthesis and catabolism of, 564–566
Vesamicol, 76
Vesnarinone, for heart failure, 205, 206
Vesprin (triflupromazine), 480
Vestibular disturbances
  aminoglycosides causing, 753–754
  H$_1$ receptor antagonists for, 269
  scopolamine for, 107, 269
  streptomycin causing, 755
  tetracyclines causing, 747
Vibramycin, 751, 858–859. *See also* Doxycycline
Vibrio, empiric antimicrobial therapy and, 814*t*
Vicodin (hydrocodone, with acetaminophen), 514

Vidarabine, 792*t*, **794–795**
  mechanism of action of, 791*i*
  preparations available, 801
Videx, 801. *See also* Didanosine
Vigabatrin, **395**, 395*i*
Vinblastine, **893**, 893*i*, 894*t*
Vincristine, 893*i*, **894**, 894*t*
  immunosuppressive actions of, 928
Vindesine, 893
Vinorelbine, 894*t*
Vinzolidine, 893
Viokase, 1023*t*
VIP (vasoactive intestinal peptide), 77*t*, **298–299**
Vira-A, 801. *See also* Vidarabine
Viracept, 801. *See also* Nelfinavir
Viral infections
  dermatologic, **1004**
  drugs for, **788–802**. *See also specific agent*
    sites of action of, 788, 789*i*
Virazole, 801. *See also* Ribavirin
Viridans streptococci, empiric antimicrobial therapy and, 814*t*
Viroptic, 801. *See also* Trifluridine
Visceral larva migrans, drugs for, 863*t*
  thiabendazole, 877
Visken, 150, 174. *See also* Pindolol
Vistaril, 283, 369. *See also* Hydroxyzine
Vital signs, in poisoned patient, 971
Vitamin B$_6$ (pyridoxine), 770*i*
  levodopa interactions and, 454
Vitamin B$_{12}$, **537–543**
  chemistry of, 537–538, 537*i*
  clinical pharmacology of, 540–543
  clinical uses for, 542–543
  for coronary artery disease prevention, 542–543
  deficiency of, 541–542
    anemias caused by, 537, 540, 541–542
  pharmacodynamics of, 539–540, 540*i*
  pharmacokinetics of, 538–539
  preparations available, 546
  structure of, 537*i*
Vitamin D, **707–709**
  in bone mineral homeostasis, 707–709
  in chronic renal failure, 716–717
  deficiency of, 716
  for hypocalcemia, 715
  for intestinal osteodystrophy, 717
  metabolites of, 707–709, 708*i*, 709*t*
    loss of in nephrotic syndrome, 719
    preparations available, 721
  for osteoporosis, 718
  parathyroid hormone (PTH) interaction and, **709**, 709*t*
  phenytoin affecting metabolism of, 391
  preparations available, 721
  receptors for, 18
Vitamin D$_2$ (ergocalciferol), 707, 709*t*. *See also* Vitamin D
  preparations available, 721
Vitamin D$_3$ (cholecalciferol), 707, 708*i*, 709*t*. *See also* Vitamin D
  preparations available, 721

Vitamin D-dependent rickets, **719**
Vitamin D-resistant rickets, **719**
Vitamin E, for parkinsonism, 457
Vitamin K, **558–559**
  altered physiologic control loop for, 554
  oral anticoagulant interactions and, 554
Vitamin K$_1$, 558–559
  for oral anticoagulant-induced bleeding, 554
  preparations available, 561
  structure of, 552*i*
Vitamin K$_2$, 558–559
Vitamin K cycle, 552, 553*i*
Vivactil, 494. *See also* Protriptyline
VLDL (very low density lipoproteins), 563, 565*t*
  synthesis and catabolism of, 564–566
VM-26 (teniposide), **894–895**
Voiding, antimuscarinic agents affecting, 110
Voltage-gated ion channels, 344
Voltaren, 599. *See also* Diclofenac
Volume of distribution, 34–35. *See also* Distribution
  drug concentration and
    initial predictions, 47–48
    revising predictions, 48–49
  poisoning and, 968
  therapeutic drug monitoring and, 46
Volume expansion, extracellular, osmotic diuretics causing, 255
Vomiting. *See also* Nausea
  drugs for control of, **1022**
  opioid analgesics causing, 505
  in pregnancy, H$_1$ receptor antagonists for, 269
  serotonin receptors in, 276
von Willebrand's disease
  desmopressin for, 616
  factor VIII for, 559*t*
VP-16 (etoposide), **894–895**, 894*t*
Vulvovaginal candidiasis, topical azoles for, 786, 1002
VZV (varicella zoster virus), acyclovir for, 790–791

Warfarin, **551–555**
  administration and dosage of, 553–554
  in breast milk, 987*t*
  fetus affected by, 983*t*
  interactions of, 554, 554*t*
  ionization constant of, 6*t*
  pharmacokinetic/pharmacodynamic parameters of, 37*t*, 551–552, 553*i*
  preparations available, 561
  structure of, 552*i*
  teratogenic effects of, 552, 558, 983*t*
  toxicity of, 552–553
  for venous thrombosis treatment, 558
Warts
  cantharidin for, 1012–1013
  podofilox for, 1012
  podophyllum resin for, 1012

Water balance, antihypertensive drugs affecting, **155–157**. *See also* Diuretics
Water conjugation, 57*t*
Water excretion
    antidiuretic hormone affecting, 246, 246*i*
    diuretics enhancing, **254–256**
Weak acids
    definition of, 5
    ionization constants of, 6*t*
    ionization of, 5–7
Weak bases
    definition of, 5–6
    ionization constants of, 6*t*
    ionization of, 5–7
Weight control/weight reduction
    in hypertension management, 172
    OTC preparations for, hidden ingredients in, 1038*t*, 1039*t*
    serotonin in, 276
Weight gain
    with antipsychotic drug treatment, 473
    oral contraceptives causing, 668
Wellbutrin, 494. *See also* Bupropion
Wernicke-Korsakoff syndrome, 376
Wernicke's encephalopathy, 376
WH-2721 (amifostine), **902**
Wheal-and-flare response, histamine causing, 264
Whipworm, drugs for infection with, 863*t*
White thrombus, 547
Wilms' tumor, 903*t*
Wilson's disease, 461
    penicillamine for, 461, 958
    trientine for, 461, 959
WIN 64338, kallikrein-kinin system affected by, 295
Winstrol, 680. *See also* Stanozolol
Withdrawal
    from alcohol, management of, **379–380**
        preparations available for, 383
    from antiepileptic drugs, **406**
    from glucocorticoids, 645
    from opioid analgesics, 503, 509, 518
        antagonist-precipitated, 509
        in newborn of addicted mother, 510
    from sedative-hypnotics, 363, 368, 520

sedative-hypnotics for management of, 365, 368, 379–380
Withdrawal bleeding, oral contraceptive use and, 668
Wolff-Parkinson-White syndrome, 224
Wood alcohol (methanol), 382–383
World Wide Web, drug information on, 8
Wound infections, surgical, antimicrobial prophylaxis and, 822–823, 824*t*
Wucheria bancrofti, drugs for infection with, 863*t*
    diethylcarbamazine, 866
        adverse reactions and, 867
    ivermectin, 868
Wyamine (mephentermine), 134
Wytensin, 175. *See also* Guanabenz

Xalatan, 317. *See also* Latanoprost
Xanax, 366*t*, 369. *See also* Alprazolam
Xanthine, 598*i*
    structure of, 330*i*
Xanthomonas maltophilia, empiric antimicrobial therapy and, 814*t*
Xenobiotics, 50
Xomen H-65, 930
Xylocaine, 240, 426*t*, 432. *See also* Lidocaine
Xylometazoline, 128
    in OTC preparations, efficacy of, 1034–1035*t*
    OTC status of, 1032*t*
    preparations available, 134

Yellow fever vaccine, 1054*t*
Yew tree, taxanes derived from, 895
Yodoxin, 853. *See also* Iodoquinol
Yohimbine, 138*t*, 140

Z track injection technique, for iron administration, 536
Zafirlukast, 337*i*
    for asthma, 337
        preparations available, 340
Zalcitabine, 795*t*, 796*i*, **797**
    preparations available, 801
Zanaflex, 448. *See also* Tizanidine
Zantac, 284, 1026. *See also* Ranitidine
Zarontin, 407. *See also* Ethosuximide
Zaroxolyn, 259. *See also* Metolazone

Zebeta, 150. *See also* Bisoprolol
Zectran, 952*t*
Zefazone, 741. *See also* Cefmetazole
Zelate, 174. *See also* Bisoprolol
Zemuron, 448. *See also* Rocuronium
Zental, 878. *See also* Albendazole
Zephiran, 810. *See also* Benzalkonium
Zerit, 801. *See also* Stavudine
Zestril, 175, 213. *See also* Lisinopril
Zidovudine, **795–796**, 795*t*, 796*i*
    anemia caused by, erythropoietin for, 544
    mechanism action of, 791*i*
    pharmacokinetic/pharmacodynamic parameters of, 37*t*, 795
    preparations available, 801
    resistance to, 795
Ziegler's enzyme, 53*t*
Zileuton, 315, 337*i*
    for asthma, 337
    preparations available, 340
Zinacef, 741. *See also* Cefuroxime
Zinc acetate, for Wilson's disease, 461
Zinc pyrithione, in OTC preparations, efficacy of, 1034*t*
Zinc sulfate, for Wilson's disease, 461
Zithromax, 751. *See also* Azithromycin
ZK 98734, 672
Zocor, 576. *See also* Simvastatin
Zofran, 284, 1027. *See also* Ondansetron
Zoladex, 617, 899*t*. *See also* Goserelin
Zollinger-Ellison syndrome, H_2 receptor antagonists for, 272
Zoloft, 494. *See also* Sertraline
Zolpidem, 355, 360, 364
    dosages of, 366*t*
    preparations available, 369
Zonalon, 1013. *See also* Doxepin
Zonisamide, **398**, 398*i*
Zoster (herpes zoster)
    famciclovir for, 792
    sorivudine for, 794
    valacyclovir for, 791
Zosyn (piperacillin, with tazobactam), 740
Zovirax, 801, 1004. *See also* Acyclovir
Zyflo, 340. *See also* Zileuton
Zyloprim, 600, 891*t*. *See also* Allopurinol
Zyprexa, 472*t*, 480. *See also* Olanzapine
Zyrtec, 267*t*, 283. *See also* Cetirizine